FOURTH EDITION

DRUGS

Use, Misuse, and Abuse

Richard G. Schlaadt
University of Oregon

Peter T. Shannon
Emerald Center for Behavior Change

Prentice Hall, Englewood Cliffs, NJ 07632

Library of Congress Cataloging-in-Publication Data

Schlaadt, Richard G.
    Drugs : use, misuse, and abuse / Richard G. Schlaadt, Peter T.
Shannon. — 4th ed.
        p.   cm.
    Includes bibliographical references and index.
    ISBN 0-13-220450-9
    1. Drugs.   2. Psychotropic drugs.   3. Drug utilization — United
States.   4. Substance abuse — United States.   I. Shannon, Peter T.
II. Title.
RM301.S43   1994   93-39822
362.29 — dc20   CIP

TO MY WIFE JAN AND FOUR CHILDREN:
MIKE, PHIL, KATHY, AND STEVE.
THANKS FOR YOUR CONTINUED SUPPORT.
LOVE, DICK

Acquisitions editor: Ted Bolen
Editorial/production supervision: Patricia V. Amoroso
Interior design: Christine Wolf
Cover design: Design Lab
Project coordinators: Herb Klein and Kelly Behr

©1994,1990,1986,1982 by Prentice-Hall, Inc.
A Paramount Communications Company
Englewood Cliffs, New Jersey 07632

Printed in the United States of America
10 9 8 7 6 5 4 3 2 1

0-13-220450-9

Prentice-Hall International (UK) Limited, *London*
Prentice-Hall of Australia Pty. Limited, *Sydney*
Prentice-Hall Canada Inc., *Toronto*
Prentice-Hall Hispanoamericana, S.A., *Mexico*
Prentice-Hall of India Private Limited, *New Delhi*
Prentice-Hall Japan, Inc., *Tokyo*
Simon & Schuster Asia Pte. Ltd., *Singapore*
Editora Prentice-Hall do Brasil, Ltda., *Rio de Janeiro*

CONTENTS

PREFACE   xvii

CHAPTER 1   INTRODUCTION   1

The Gray Area   1

Individual Differences   2
Quality Control   2
Set   3
Setting   4
Legality   4

Perspective on Drugs   4

Trends in Drug Abuse   5
Illegal Drug Tab Dropping   6
Caffeine   7
Alcohol   7
Nicotine   7
Stimulants and Sedatives   8
Marijuana   9
Hallucinogens   9
Opiates   10
Volatile Substances   10

Drug Technology   10

Over-the-Counter Drugs   12
Commercial Drugs   13
Recreational Drugs   13
Herbal Preparations   14
Illegal Drugs   14

Summary   14

CHAPTER 2   THEORIES OF DRUG USE   16

Introduction   16

Psychological Factors   17

Recreation and Social Facilitation   17
Sensation Seeking and Risk Taking   18
Religious and Spiritual Factors   20
Altered States   20
Rebellion and Alienation   21
Personality Traits   21
Personal Habits   22

Sociological Factors, Peer Pressure, Family
and Group Entry   23

Advertising   25
National Trends   25

Dependency States   26

Dependency   26
Psychological Perspectives   26
Sociological Perspectives   27
Biological Perspectives   28
Dependency Pain   28
Genetic Factors and Dependency   32

Summary   33

CHAPTER 3   THE DRUG SCENE   36

Introduction   36

The Youth Drug Scene   38

Background   38
Drugs on Campus   42
Drugs in the Military   44
Drugs and Athletics   46

The Adult Drug Scene   52

Alcohol   53
Tranquilizers and Sedative-Hypnotics   53
Nicotine   54
Caffeine   54
Aspirin   54
Amphetamines   55
Marijuana   55
Opiates   55
The Workplace   55
Drug Testing   57

The Older American Drug Scene 60

    Types of Drug Use 61

Summary 63

CHAPTER 4

PHARMACOLOGY: BASIC CONCEPTS OF DRUG ACTIVITY 68

Pharmacological Theories and Discoveries 68

    Fountain of Youth 69
    Endorphins 69

Consumer Safety 70

    The Chemical (Drug) Being Considered 70
    The Receptor Mechanisms Affected 71
    The Dosage and the Method of Administration 71
    The Kinds of Drug Interactions That Will Likely
        Take Place 74
    The Potential for Allergic Reactions 74
    The Potential for Tolerance and the Potential
        for Physical Dependence 75

Anatomy and Physiology 75

    The Nervous System as an Electrical System 75
    The Central Nervous System 77
    The Peripheral Nervous System 81

Summary 87

CHAPTER 5

STIMULANTS 89

Amphetamines 89

    Introduction 89
    Dextroamphetamine 92
    Methamphetamines (Crank, Speed, and Meth) 93
    Methamphetamine: Ice 95

Methylphenidate (Ritalin) 97

    Physical and Psychological Effects 97
    Hyperkinesis or Attention-Deficit Hyperactive
        Disorder 98
    Educating the Hyperkinetic Child 99

Cocaine 101

    Introduction 101
    History 102
    Physiological and Pharmacological Effects 103
    Psychological-Physiological Dependency 107
    Dopamine 108

Cocaine and Suicide 108
Cocaine as an Aphrodisiac 108
Crack 108
Problems with Cocaine and Crack 111
Hospitals and Drug Addicts 115
Crack and Heroin 115
Cocaine Anonymous 115

Caffeine (Xanthines) 116

Introduction 116
History 120
*The Controversy over Research Findings
   on Caffeine* 120
Physical Effects 122
Caffeinism 125
Decaffeinated Coffee 126
Suggestions for Decreasing Use of Caffeine 127

Look-Alikes 127

Summary 127

CHAPTER 6   TOBACCO: AMERICA'S NUMBER ONE PREVENTABLE HAZARD   135

Introduction 135

History 136

Chemistry 136

The 1979 Surgeon General's Report 138

Physiological Effects 138

Gases 139

Chronic Disease 140

Cardiovascular Disease 140
Strokes 141
Respiratory Diseases 141
Lung and Other Cancers 142

Side Effects 143

Metabolism 143
Appetite Reduction 143
Pregnancy and Fetal Nutrition 144
Exercise and Physical Performance 145
Sexual Activity 145
Other Health Factors 146
Combining Alcohol and Tobacco 147
Nicotine and Coffee Intake 147
Vitamins 147

Psychological Effects 147

    The Smoking Habit 147
    Reasons for Smoking and Not Smoking 147
    Advertising 148
    Types of Smokers 149
    Women 149
    Minorities 150
    Adolescents 151

Alternatives to Smoking and Consequent
   Problems 151

Kicking the Habit 152

    Smoking Cessation 152
    The Quitting Process 153
    Government Support 154
    Methods 154
    Benefits of Quitting 154
    Changing to Other Forms of Tobacco
      Consumption 156

Tobacco and the Nonsmoker 161

    Effects of Tobacco Smoke on Nonsmokers 161
    Nonsmokers' Rights 163
    Selling Tobacco to Children 164
    Exporting Tobacco 165

Diversification 167

Summary 167

CHAPTER 7   DEPRESSANTS 174

Sedative-Hypnotics 175

    Classification 175
    Physical Effects 175
    Barbiturates 175

Minor Tranquilizers 177

    Classification 177
    History 178
    Physical Effects 178
    Valium (Diazepam) 179
    Librium (Chlordiazepoxide) 183

Major Tranquilizers (Antipsychotics) 183

    Classification 183
    Current Use 184
    Physical Effects 184

Deliriants (Volatile Substances)   185

    Classification   185
    History   185
    Physical Effects   186
    Psychological Effects   186

Designer Drugs   187

    MDMA   187
    Fentanyl   188
    Meperidine   188
    Testing Problems   188

Summary   188

CHAPTER 8   ALCOHOL: AMERICA'S NUMBER ONE DRUG PROBLEM   192

Introduction   192

Consumption in the United States   194

    Youth   194
    Adults   195
    The Elderly   196

History   197

Why Do People Drink?   197

    Advertising   198
    Peer Acceptance, Search for Adulthood, and Rebellion   199
    Recreation and Enjoyment   199
    Changing Sex Roles   199
    Sex   199
    Family Influence   200

Physiological Effects   200

    Circulatory System and Blood   200
    Nervous System   203
    Liver   205
    Digestive System   206
    Kidneys   207
    Body Temperature   207
    Fetal Alcohol Syndrome and Fetal Alcohol Effect   207
    Cancer   208
    Testosterone Level   208
    Women   209
    Combining Alcohol with Other Drugs   209

Effects of Drinking on the Individual
   and Society   210

   Economic Costs   210
   Adolescent Drinking   212
   Effects of Alcohol by Ethnic Group and Race   212
   Crime   213
   The Homeless   213
   Violence   213
   Suicide   214
   Warning Labels   214

Alcoholism   214

   What Is Alcoholism?   214
   Causes   221
   B-Endorphins   223
   Blood Enzymes   223
   Biological Marker   224
   Brain   224
   Types of Alcoholics   224
   Alcoholism Among Women   225
   Treatment and Rehabilitation Services   226
   Treatment Approaches   227
   Alcoholism and the Family   231

The Movement Against Drunk Driving   234

   Mothers Against Drunk Drivers   234
   Students Against Driving Drunk   234

Responsible Drinking   234

Summary   235

CHAPTER 9   OPIATES   242

Nonsynthetic Opiates   242

   Morphine   243
   Heroin   245
   Codeine   250

Synthetic Opiates   250

   Methadone   250
   Propoxyphene Hydrochloride (Darvon)   252

Drug Abuse-Related Legislation   253

   The National Addiction Rehabilitation
      Administration   253
   Earlier Legislation   254

Detoxification   255

    General Effects   256

Therapeutic Approaches   257

    Small-Group Support   257
    Therapeutic Communities   258
    Personal Responsibility and Commitment   258
    The Young User   259

Methadone Maintenance   259

    Introduction   259
    Interim Methadone Clinic   260
    Possible Hazards and Side Effects   261
    The Process   262
    Rate of Success   263
    Social Implications of Methadone-
      Maintenance Programs   265

Does Any Treatment Work?   265

    Maturing Out   265

Summary   265

CHAPTER 10   HALLUCINOGENS   270

Background   270

Site of Action   271

LSD   271

    Introduction   271
    Psychophysiological Effects   272
    LSD and Society   273
    Use in Mind-Control Research   275
    Use in Medical Research   275

Mescaline (Peyote)   276

    Introduction   276
    Psychophysiological Effects   277

Psilocybin   278

    Introduction   278
    Psychophysiological Effects   278

PCP   279

    Introduction   279
    PCP and Society   280
    Psychophysiological Effects   281

Summary   283

CHAPTER 11 MARIJUANA: CONTINUING CONTROVERSY   285

Introduction   285

Marijuana Use in the World   285
Marijuana Use in the United States   286
Decreasing Popularity   287

Pharmacological Classification   288

Physiological Effects   288

Extent of Effects on Body Functions   289
Pulmonary Effects   290
Cardiovascular Complications   292
Effects on the Immune System   293
Effects on Endocrine Functioning   293
Psychomotor Impairment   294
Genetic Damage   295
Effects on the Brain   296
Memory   297
Tolerance   298

Psychological Effects   298

Adolescents' Perceptions   300
Peer Influences   300
Effects on School Performance   300
Aggression   301
Social Conversation   301
Family Cohesiveness   301
Psychopathology   301
Amotivational Syndrome   302
Flashbacks   302

Therapeutic and Medical Uses of Marijuana   302

Glaucoma   303
Cancer   303
Medical Applications   303

Economics   304

Workplace   304
Marijuana Crops   304

Legalization   305

Proponents of Legalization   306
Opponents of Legalization   306

Summary   306

CHAPTER 12   OVER-THE-COUNTER DRUGS: WHAT YOU CAN GET
              WITHOUT A PRESCRIPTION   311

              Introduction   311

                  Self-Monitoring and Self-Care   312
                  Development of OTCs in the United States   314
                  Reform   315
                  What Sets Prescription and Nonprescription
                      Apart?   315

              Nostrums   317

              Salicylates (Aspirin)   317

                  History   317
                  Physical Effects   317
                  Side Effects   318
                  Therapeutic Effectiveness   319
                  Toxicology   321
                  Aspirin: The Miracle Drug   322
                  Acetaminophen   323
                  Ibuprofen   323

              Laxatives   324

                  Introduction   324
                  Laxative Use   325

              Cough Relievers (Antitussives)   325

                  The Cough   325
                  Reducing the Severity   325

              Antihistamines   326

              Vitamins and Minerals   327

                  Introduction   327
                  Specific Use   330
                  Specific Vitamins   330
                  Megavitamin Madness   333

              The Elderly and OTC Drugs   333

              Diet Pills   334

              Food Labels   334

              Summary   335

CHAPTER 13   PRESCRIPTION AND OTHER DRUGS OF INTEREST   340

              New Drug Applications   341

                  New Medicines and Delivery   342

Placebos   343

   Introduction   343
   Individual Differences   344
   Social Environment and Situational Variables 344
   Administration, Frequency, and Cost 344
   The Power of Suggestion   345

Antibiotics   345

   Classification   345
   History   346
   Effects   346
   Resistance to Antibiotics   346
   Misuse   347

Drugs for the Mentally Ill   348

   Antidepressants   348
   Prozac   349
   Clozapine (Brand Name Clozaril) 350

Accutane   350

Lithium   351

   Classification   351
   Pharmacology   351
   Medical Use   351

Contraceptives   352

   History   352
   Composition and Use   352
   Mechanism   352
   Possible Side Effects   353
   A Pill for Males   355
   Depro Provera   355
   Norplant   356
   RU 486   357

Fertility Pills   358

   Introduction   358
   Method of Treatment   358
   Possible Side Effects   359
   Multiple Births   359

Menopause and Estrogen Replacement
   Therapy   359

Acquired Immunodeficiency Syndrome   360

   Azidothymidine   360
   Dextran Sulfate   360
   Drug 566   361

Streptokinase 361

Cholesterol-Lowering Agents 361

Peptide T 362

Food Additives 362

Introduction 362
History 363
Preservatives 364
Nitrites and Nitrates 365
Adverse Effects 365
Sucrose (Sugar) 365
Nutrasweet 366

Summary 367

CHAPTER 14   THE CONSUMER AND DRUG LEGISLATION 372

Introduction 372

The Physician's Role 372

Physicians' Versus Pharmacists' Dispensing 374

The Patient's Role 375

Consumers 375

The Drug Industry 376

Profit and Production 377
Marketing and Advertising 377
Research and Development 378
The High Cost of Prescription Drugs 378
Brand-Name Versus Generic Drugs 379
The Orphan Drug Act 381

Drug Use and the Law 382

Victimless Crimes 383
Should We Legalize Drugs? 383
Intervention Programs 384
A War on Drugs with Real Troops 385
Drug Vigilantes 386

A History of Major Drug-Related Legislation 386

Regulation of Opiates: 1865–1905 386
The Pure Food and Drug Act, 1906 387
The Shanghai Conference, 1909 387
The Harrison Narcotic Act, 1914 387
Prohibition, 1920 388
Importation of Heroin Banned, 1924 388
Linder *v.* United States, *1925* 389

Porter Narcotic Farms Bill, 1929   389
Federal Bureau of Narcotics, 1930   389
The Marijuana Tax Act, 1937   389
The Food, Drug, and Cosmetic Act, 1938   390
The Boggs Amendment, 1951   390
The Narcotic Drug Control Act, 1956   390
The Kefauver–Harris Amendments, 1962   390
Robinson v. California, 1962   391
The Community Mental Health Centers Act,
  1963   391
The Drug Abuse Control Amendments, 1965   391
The Narcotic Addict Rehabilitation Act, 1966   392
The Comprehensive Drug Abuse Prevention
  and Control Act (The Controlled
  Substances Act), 1970   392
The Anti-Drug Bill, 1988   396
Consumer Legislation   400

Decriminalization   401

Marijuana   401
Opiates   402

Summary   405

Milestones in Attempted Drug Regulation   406

CHAPTER 15

PREVENTION: EDUCATION AND ALTERNATIVES   411

Introduction   411
A New Philosophical Perspective   412

Drug-Education Programs   412

The Role of the School   412
Teachers   414
Educational Approaches   414
Counselors   417

The Role of Parents   418

The Influence of Peers   421

Natural Helpers   421
Drug Abuse Response Team   421
Student Athletic Summer Institute   422

School and Community Cooperation   422

Project Impact   422
Hampton Intervention and Prevention
  Project (Hampton, Virginia)   423
Seattle School Development Project   423

Soulbeat I 423
Community Together 424

Mass Media 424

The Harvard Alcohol Project 424

Alternatives 425

Exercise 426
Wilderness Experiences 428
Work 429
Social and Political Activism 429
Religion 430
Biofeedback 431
Meditation 433

Summary 435

CHAPTER 16   TREATMENT OF DRUG ABUSE 439

Introduction 439

Addiction and Dependency 440
Infant Addiction 441
Intervention 441

Treatment Approaches 441

Adolescent Treatment 442
Adult-Treatment Programs 445
Employers 446
Key Components 446
Examples of Adult-Treatment Programs 449

Fighting Drugs with Drugs 454

Alcohol Treatment 454
Heroin Treatment 455
Cocaine Treatment 456

Relapse 458

Summary 459

GLOSSARY 463

INDEX 469

PREFACE

The fourth edition of *Drugs: Use, Misuse, and Abuse* greatly expands the former editions with sweeping updates and incorporates new research findings; a new glossary; inclusion of charts, pictures, graphs, and boxes; a revised chapter on prevention, which adds sound educational approaches as well as alternatives to drugs; and finally, a new chapter on treatment of drug abuse. This edition is longer in length and considerably more comprehensive in scope than the previous editions.

Chapter 1 offers an overview of drugs, describes the "gray area" of drug use, and incorporates several new research findings on drug use by various populations and age groups in the United States. Chapter 2 describes the delicate balance among the psychological, sociological, and biological reasons why people use drugs. New studies on family, peers, suicide, and pain have been added to show how easily this balance can be disrupted. Chapter 3 deals with the ever-changing drug scene, describing how there are as many different drug scenes as there are people. This chapter focuses on the youth, adult, and older American drug scenes. The National Household and National Senior High School study results show an overall decline in drug use in the United States. Also, employers are becoming more involved with the drug problem and it is estimated that over two-thirds of the Fortune 500 companies, along with the Department of Transportation, have installed drug-testing programs. A closer look at older Americans and their drug problems is also addressed. Chapter 4 provides an overview of pharmacology and physiology. New concepts are emerging on, "Do humans need to get high?", and new drug discoveries about hGH (Somatropin) to stay youthful and new findings on the effects of endorphins are discussed.

Chapter 5 focuses on stimulants or "uppers," such as amphetamines, methamphetamines (including ICE), cocaine, ritalin, and caffeine. There is an enlarged section on the overall crack problem, new findings on attention-deficit hyperactive disorder, and some discussion of the controversy over what problems caffeine does or does not cause. Chapter 6 presents dramatic new findings on smoking and smokeless tobacco. Approximately one in four adults currently smoke. More Americans appear to be quitting smoking but more are dying—

nearly 450,000 a year—from smoking-related illnesses as habits from the 1950s and 1960s take an increasing toll. Nicotine gum and nicotine patches appear to be helping individuals quit their smoking habit. Government and businesses are starting to place restrictions on the hiring of employees who smoke.

Chapters 7 through 9 focus on "downers." In Chapter 7, "Depressants," the section on Valium has been enlarged. Also, the designer drug section has been expanded (although not all designer drugs are depressants). Chapter 8 presents new findings on alcoholism. Fetal Alcohol Syndrome (FAS) and Fetal Alcohol Effect (FAE) are discussed as growing problems among drinking women. It should be stressed that FAS and FAE are 100 percent preventable. Also, children of alcoholics (and adult children of alcoholics) are given special attention. The increase in the number of children and adolescents who are becoming alcoholics is discussed as a growing problem. Also included is the role of alcohol dehydrogenase in contributing to the inability of women to metabolize alcohol as rapidly as men. Finally, greater discussion is given to how alcohol is related to such issues as violence and the homeless. Chapter 9 takes a new look at heroin in medicine, opiate dependency, combining crack with heroin (called "chasing the dragon"), and research on the effectiveness of methadone and other drugs to curb the craving for heroin.

Chapter 10 presents some of the latest research findings on LSD, mescaline (especially peyote being used as part of tribal ceremonies by Native Americans), psilocybin, and phencyclidine (PCP). Chapter 11 discusses the controversy surrounding higher-potency marijuana and some of the potential health hazards for regular users. Chapter 12 offers an expanded look at the potential for harm from over-the-counter drugs if consumer safety rules are not closely followed. Chapter 13 presents several new discoveries and technological advances that are changing the types of prescription drugs and the methods of using them. Some of the newer discoveries can be extremely beneficial in helping individuals with a variety of ailments. New steps have also been taken to speed up the drug approval process.

The final three chapters deal with drug control, prevention of abuse, and treatment. Chapter 14 discusses the importance of physicians, pharmacists, and patients cooperating in the treatment of patients, and some new attempts to reduce the cost of prescription drugs. The use of generic drugs, orphan drugs, new regulations, and drug laws will be included. Chapter 15 stresses prevention through a comprehensive approach (using a variety of educational approaches for grades K–12) involving schools, teachers, parents, peers, counselors, law enforcement officials, and community groups all working together to reduce the drug problem. Alternatives to drugs are also discussed in this chapter. Chapter 16 is new and stresses a variety of drug treatment programs for different age groups as well as a series of new drugs being used to assist in treatment. Relapse is discussed as a part of treatment. The overall prognosis for treatment has greatly improved with more approaches and more agencies available to help those with drug dependencies.

C H A P T E R
1

INTRODUCTION

THE GRAY AREA

The United States is a drug-oriented nation. Media messages concerning the benefits—or dangers—of drug use continually bombard us. According to physician Andrew Weil,

> the use of drugs to alter consciousness is nothing new. It has been a feature of all human life in all places on the earth and in all ages of history . . . the ubiquity of drug use is so striking that it must represent a basic human appetite. Yet many Americans seem to feel that the contemporary drug scene is something new, something qualitatively different from what has gone before. This attitude is peculiar because all that is really happening is a change in drug preference.[1]

Though the messages are frequent, they are often "gray"—a combination of fact and fiction that the listener must sort through. Research reports are often conflicting or contradictory. For example, one report suggests that taking an aspirin every other day may help prevent heart attacks, while another states that aspirin may increase the chances of a stroke. Another report finds that one alcoholic drink a day may help prevent a heart attack, but it also suggests that this same amount may contribute to breast cancer in women. Still another research report finds that caffeine may contribute to high blood pressure, anxiety, insomnia, and fibrocystic breast disease; other reports state that the evidence in these areas is inconclusive. Half truths and sensationalism distort drug-related discussions and make accurate assessment of the drug scene difficult. Wide variation in drug use and its effects on the individual further obscures attempts to clarify the issues surrounding drug use.

Five aspects of the "**gray area**" of drug use need to be probed: (1) individual differences in reactions to drugs, (2) quality control—or lack of it, (3) effect of drug use on a drug user's expectations, (4) the influence of setting, and (5) the relation of a drug's legality to its effectiveness and to the treatment of those who use it.

INDIVIDUAL DIFFERENCES

Individuals are unique in their reactions to drugs. Too often we issue blanket statements about how people will react to a drug. Such generalizations must be carefully examined, since most are based on "normal reaction" to a drug. Health status, size, age, sex, time of day, personal expectations, dosage, previous experience, and surroundings all influence the effect of a given drug on a given individual. For example, penicillin is valuable in combating certain diseases, but people who are allergic to it experience unpleasant and adverse reactions following its use. Physicians and pharmacists anticipate that 3 to 5 percent of any given population may be allergic to a given drug. In short, not all individuals react the same way to a drug.

QUALITY CONTROL

Federal Food and Drug Administration (FDA) procedures and regulations make it extremely difficult to introduce a new drug on the market. Before a new drug can be approved, pharmaceutical companies must expend considerable time and money putting it through a series of rigorous tests to determine its safety and effectiveness. (The effects of the drug thalidomide have demonstrated the importance of such testing.) In spite of this extensive research, a few individuals will suffer complications from using the drug. Medical drug use needs to be regulated and monitored if its possible benefits are to be maximized.

Further down the line of quality control, the pharmacist must fill each prescription to the exact chemical amount specified. A lesser amount might be totally ineffective and a greater amount might cause adverse reactions. The final responsibility for quality control rests with the individual. Self-medication or irresponsible use of drugs is likely to result in adverse reactions.

However, in addition to regularly prescribed and over-the-counter drugs, which have been approved for use, there are also "street drugs"—prescription drugs as well as other drugs that "street manufacturers" cut and dilute for

Gray Area

A combination of fact and fiction the listener must sort through in the drug field. Research reports are often conflicting or contrary. Half truths and sensationalism distort drug-related discussions and make accurate assessments of the drug scene difficult. Wide variation in drug use and its effects on the individual further obscures attempts to clarify the issues surrounding drug use.

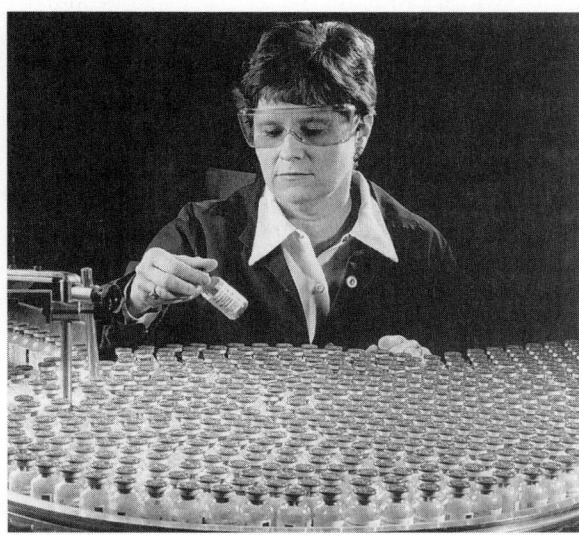

Quality Control of Prescription
Drugs
Source: John Coletti/Stock Boston

sale. A prescription drug such as amphetamine, for example, can make its way onto the street through various illicit channels and be sold as a stimulant, perhaps cut with cocaine. Because there is no quality control on the street, one drug may be substituted for another. Caffeine-pill look-alikes can be substituted for amphetamine pills, for example, resulting in a nice profit for the "manufacturer."

Street-produced drugs are suspect for a number of reasons. First, they are often impure and adulterated. Second, some of the preferred chemical constituents may be unavailable and less desirable components may be substituted for them. Third, the qualifications of the street "pharmacist" are sometimes as suspect as the equipment being used. As a result, drug potency and purity often vary from batch to batch. Finally, street manufacturers are often on the move to avoid police detection, and this leaves them little time to follow proper procedures: distillation and filtration processes that might normally occur in legal environments often do not exist on the street.

SET

Set means people's expectations of a drug—what they think it will do for them. Set, in other words, deals specifically with one's *internal* environment and personality characteristics. The set will not always guarantee a particular experience, but it can have a great effect. For example, expectations of a pleasurable experience can often bring one about, as in the case of students who thought they were taking marijuana feeling high when in actuality they had been smoking Sir Walter Raleigh tobacco.[2] At the other end of the spectrum, people who are very depressed or frustrated prior to drug use are likely to feel more so afterward.

SETTING

The setting consists of the people and the environment in which a drug is taken. Setting can greatly influence the drug's effect. It primarily involves the *external* social and physical environment. Being among friends at a festive, pleasurable New Year's Eve party may enhance a drug experience. But a tense setting, as in situations where there is anger, fighting, depression, or the fear of being arrested, can produce anxiety. Research by John Reed on controlled drinking in a simulated bar confirms this belief in the setting's influence. Reed studied three groups: group I members were given alcohol; group II members were told they were drinking alcohol but were not given any; and group III members were told they had not been given alcoholic beverages but actually had been. Group I responded in an intoxicated manner, as would be expected, but group II responded the same way, even though they had not been given alcohol. Group III exhibited traits of sobriety even though they were drinking alcoholic beverages.[3]

LEGALITY

If a drug can be used legally, anxiety may not be associated with its use. Illegal drug use, on the other hand, can often bring feelings of danger and fear. Such risk taking may enhance or decrease the effectiveness of any drug.

The heavy drug user (the alcoholic, heroin dependent, and others) is gradually being viewed as ill rather than criminal. Efforts are under way to decriminalize the use of some drugs and make sentencing for drug possession uniform. Many individuals feel that present laws actually create criminals rather than help those with problems. More emphasis is being placed on prevention and treatment, as we will see.

PERSPECTIVE ON DRUGS

In the following pages we present an overview on drugs that will set the stage for the more specific coverage in the chapters to come. This perspective portrays the total drug scene in relation to society without implying that any one drug is of greater or lesser importance to the individual. The use of drugs is not limited to any socioeconomic group. Today drugs are used in affluent suburbs and middle-class neighborhoods as well as the ghetto.

The FDA distinguishes drug use, misuse, and abuse as follows. *Drug use* is the taking of a drug for its intended purpose and in an appropriate amount, frequency, strength, and manner. *Drug misuse* is the taking of a substance for a purpose, but not in the appropriate amount, frequency, strength, or manner. *Drug abuse* is the deliberate use of a substance for other than its intended purpose, in a manner that can damage health or ability to function.

The American drug-use pattern began to shift from the primary use of alcohol and tobacco toward hallucinogens, marijuana, amphetamines, and barbiturates in the early 1960s—the beginning of the period (which extended through the 1980s) commonly referred to as the Age of Anxiety. The numerous reasons for this shift are discussed throughout the book. But one general reason is stress. As mental and emotional pressures increased, millions of Americans began taking doses of stimulants, depressants, and hallucinogenic drugs each day. Today, the majority of adults rarely go through a week without consuming alcohol in some form. Large numbers also regularly use sedatives to help them sleep and stimulants to keep them awake for prolonged periods.

TRENDS IN DRUG ABUSE

According to the 1990 National Household Survey on Drug Abuse, there is an increasing downward trend in drug abuse.[4]

- Current prevalence rates for use of any illicit drug among persons 12 years of age and older continued to decrease from 23 million drug users (12.1 percent) in 1985, to 14.5 million users (7.3 percent) in 1988 to 13 million users (6.4 percent) in 1990.

- The number of current cocaine users decreased significantly from 2.9 million (1.5 percent) in 1988 to 1.6 million (0.8 percent) in 1990, continuing a previous decline. This represents a 72 percent decrease in the number of current cocaine users since 1985, when there were an estimated 5.8 million (2.9 percent) current cocaine users.

- Current cigarette use dropped from 32 percent in 1985 to 29 percent in 1988, and presently stands at 27 percent (probably lower), representing a significant decrease from 1988. This represents a 3.5 million decrease in the number of cigarette smokers in the last two years. The previous three year period, 1985–1988, experienced a 3.2 million decrease, for a total decrease of 6.7 million persons since 1985.

- There were 102.9 million current drinkers of alcoholic beverages in 1990 compared with 105.8 million in 1988, and 113.1 million in 1985. The alcohol-use rates in 1985, 1988, and 1990, for those 12 and over, are 59 percent, 53 percent, and 51 percent, respectively.

Overall drug use decreased by 11 percent from 1988 to 1990.[5] Former Health and Human Services Secretary Louis W. Sullivan stated, "This news is encouraging and will most certainly provide reinforcement to the millions of people who have been working so diligently to eliminate the drug abuse problems that have affected so many of us."[6] Sullivan further reported, "Despite this impressive good news about our progress in reversing our nation's drug using habits, however, many pockets of serious drug problems remain." While overall drug abuse declined to 6.4 percent in any current illicit use, demographic subgroups with higher rates included young adults age 18–25 years (14.9 percent), blacks (8.6 percent), individuals in large metropolitan areas (7.3 percent), those living in the West (7.3 percent), and the unemployed population (14.0 percent).

Sullivan also reported some encouraging news about high school students. "For the first time in the 16 years the annual survey [National High School Senior Drug Abuse Survey] has been conducted, less than half of the students surveyed have tried any illicit drug. This is truly a sign of progress

**FIGURE 1–1 CURRENT OVER-
ALL DRUG USE (IN THOUSANDS
OF USERS)**
Source: Household Survey

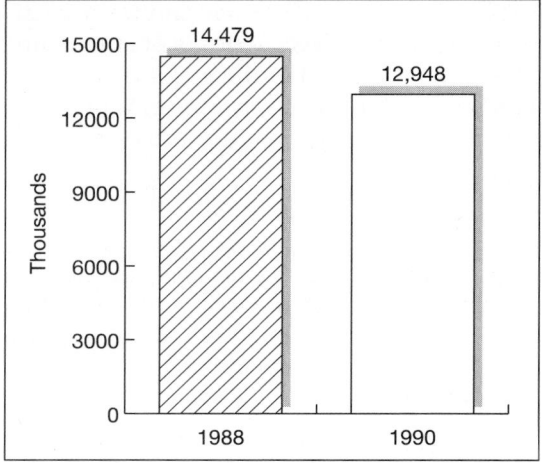

toward the goal of achieving a drug-free society."[7] Sullivan expressed his concern, however, about the continued high rates of cigarette smoking by high school seniors noted in the survey. The survey found no decrease from 1989 to 1990 in daily cigarette smoking, which has remained at virtually the same rate over the past seven surveys.

ILLEGAL DRUG TAB DROPPING

The downward trend in drug abuse appears to be accompanied by a downward trend in sales of illegal drugs. The Office of National Drug Control Policy issued a report stating that in 1990 Americans shelled out more than $40 billion for illegal drugs.[8] That reflects a decline from an estimated $49.8 billion in 1989 and $51.6 billion the year before. The 1990 total included $17.5 billion for cocaine, $12.3 billion for heroin, $8.8 billion for marijuana, and $1.8 billion for other drugs.[9] For comparison, the report said Americans spend $44 billion a year on alcoholic beverages and $37 billion a year on

**FIGURE 1–2   ILLICIT DRUGS: HOW
MUCH AMERICA'S USERS SPEND**
Source: Office of National Drug Policy For comparison, the report said Americans spend $44 billion a year on alcoholic beverages and $37 billion a year on tobacco products. The Pharmaceutical Manufacturers Association says Americans spent $38.6 billion on prescription drugs in 1990.

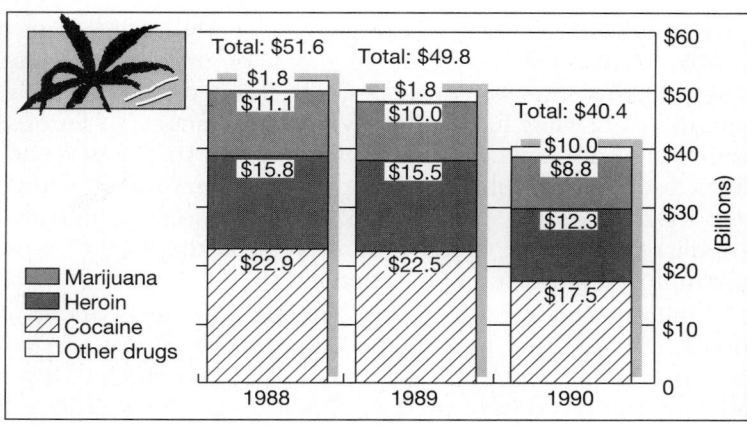

tobacco products. The Pharmaceutical Manufacturers Association says Americans spent $38.6 billion on prescription drugs in 1990.

CAFFEINE

Caffeine is a stimulant found in tea, coffee, cola drinks, chocolate, and aspirin. Although the use of other stimulants, such as amphetamines, is seriously discouraged, the use of beverages containing caffeine is commonly accepted. The coffee break, in fact, has become a regular part of many Americans' lives. Recently, however, greater attention has been focused on the adverse effects caffeine may have—high blood pressure, anxiety, and insomnia.

ALCOHOL

Alcohol remains king of the drug scene: It is the most commonly abused drug in the United States today, often used to relieve anxiety and tension. Of the estimated 100 million people who use alcohol, approximately 10 million are classified as alcoholics.[10] Drinking problems cost society approximately $43 billion a year in lost production, medical costs, and other expenses.[11] In fact, according to some sources, the economic cost of alcohol abuse and alcoholism may be as high as $120 billion annually.[12] Roughly $20 billion is spent each year on alcohol; it is a substantial element of the economy.[13]

NICOTINE

"Warning: The Surgeon General Has Determined That Cigarette Smoking Is Dangerous to Your Health." This well-known warning appears on the label of every pack of cigarettes sold in the United States, yet despite it, approximately 47 million Americans smoke an estimated 590 billion cigarettes yearly. The number of adults using tobacco products *has* declined in recent years, but alarming use trends continue among the young. The use of chewing tobacco has recently increased.

Tobacco is the second leading drug problem in the United States, and the surgeon general has cited it as the primary cause of preventable disease. New

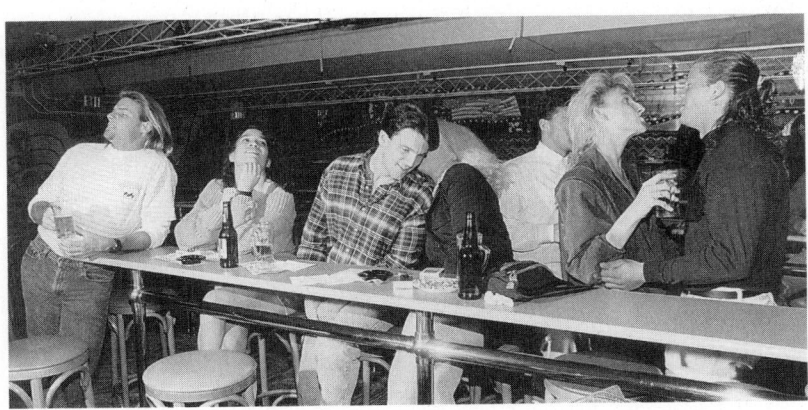

College Students Socializing at a Local Tavern
Source: Spencer Grant/Photo Researchers

strategies are currently being employed to reduce cigarette consumption: utilizing alternative ingredients, lengthening filters, and reducing tar and nicotine are meeting with limited success. Stressing alternatives to smoking and providing detoxification clinics and educational programs may prove somewhat successful as well.

Strong political debate is taking place over the rights of nonsmokers, and many states have passed laws requiring public business meetings to restrict the use of cigarettes to protect nonsmokers. The marketing and use of tobacco products are also surrounded by controversy, the tobacco industry and smokers promoting "smokers' rights" and scientists, environmental groups, health groups, and nonsmokers promoting "nonsmokers' rights." There also appears to be growing concern that society and specifically the government should *not* use tax dollars to pay medical costs incurred from smoking cigarettes. In short, people who smoke should pay their own medical bills, it is argued.

STIMULANTS AND SEDATIVES

The use of stimulants and sedatives, both legal and illegal, is widespread in American society.

Crack

Cocaine mixed with baking soda and water over a hot flame. The substance is then dried. The soapy-looking substance that results can be broken up into rocks and smoked. These rocks are approximately five times as strong as cocaine. Crack is normally smoked, and because it is such a pure drug, it takes much less time to achieve the desired high. One puff of a pebble-sized rock produces an intense high that lasts 20 minutes.

Stimulants   Many individuals use stimulants such as amphetamines and caffeine to remain alert, increase work capacity, alleviate fatigue, and induce a sense of euphoria. Prescription stimulants are available in a limited supply for dieting, hyperactivity, and the sleeping disorder narcolepsy. Over-the-counter stimulants containing caffeine are available from drugstores and supermarkets, and the sale of illicit stimulants to students, those working graveyard or swing shifts, and long-haul truck drivers is common. Since 1972 the federal government has attempted to restrict by law the production and dispensing of prescription stimulants by pharmaceutical houses because of the illicit routes along which the products are often diverted.

Many stimulants can be harmful. Repeated use may lead to tolerance, and increased dosages may then be required to produce the original stimulation. Intravenous use of methamphetamines, the most potent amphetamine, by "speed freaks" in San Francisco during the late 1960s often resulted in psychotic episodes brought on by the sleep deprivation experienced during the "speed run." The use of cocaine, among the most powerful of the available stimulants and in great demand as a recreational drug, may result in psychological dependence. "Crack" cocaine has become an extremely popular and heavily used stimulant, and "ice," a form of methamphetamine, is starting to emerge as a popular newer street drug.

Sedatives   Physicians frequently prescribe sedatives to relieve a number of ills. Sedatives have sleep-inducing properties; they are also prescribed at lower dosage for daytime relaxation and for the relief of anxiety. Valium and Librium have replaced many of the barbiturate-based sedatives. Currently, middle-aged women rely on sedatives for relief of anxiety and insomnia more than their male counterparts do. In November 1983 the Lemmon Company, the only remaining manufacturer of methaqualone, announced that it would no longer produce the drug and would destroy its remaining stockpiles of it. The company cited as reasons the widespread illicit use of the substance and government pressures to ban its preparation.[14]

Designer drugs, both stimulant and depressant, such as **Ecstasy, Fentanyl,** and **Meperdine** are also being found more frequently on the drug scene.

MARIJUANA

The use of marijuana has become commonplace in recent years because of its availability and relative inexpensiveness, and because results of medical studies indicate some of its dangers have been exaggerated. The early 1970s saw a growing movement toward the decriminalization of marijuana, and possession of small amounts of marijuana was downgraded from a criminal act to a misdemeanor in several states. Since Oregon established a law in 1973 making possession of less than an ounce of marijuana a misdemeanor resulting in a maximum fine of $100, 11 other states, including New York, California, Ohio, and Michigan, have passed similar legislation.[15] However, in 1991 Oregon changed its law and imposed stiffer penalties. Possession of small amounts of marijuana (less than an ounce) is a Class C misdemeanor punishable by a maximum 30-day jail term and a $500 fine. Alaska and other states are also reevaluating their marijuana laws.

Marijuana depresses the central nervous system, producing a sense of relaxation in most individuals. Although occasional disorientation and confusion may result, marijuana usually calms people and is often used recreationally as a mild sedative. Its minimal side effects and its capacity to alleviate stress and reduce tension, to produce a sense of euphoria and a feeling of lightness, and to alter and intensify perceptions have made it a popular drug.

HALLUCINOGENS

Hallucinogenic, or psychedelic, drugs such as LSD were widely used in the United States among middle-class youth in the 1960s and early 1970s. Though the use of LSD continues, its popularity seems to have declined in favor of less powerful drugs having organic (natural) sources (psilocybin and mescaline from mushrooms, and peyote).

Hallucinogenic drugs alter and frequently enhance the processing of sensory and emotional information in brain centers, and for this reason their use appears to coincide with a person's search for individuality and an understanding of life. Depending on the dosage, the expectations of the drug experience, and the physical and emotional settings of the individual, LSD can chemically facilitate a person's sense of well-being and awareness of body functions. If the dosage is too great and/or the setting is unsupportive or inappropriate, LSD may trigger distortions of the environment, causing anxiety or, in more severe forms, psychological crisis and trauma.

Ecstasy

An amphetaminelike drug that is an analog of MDA. Street names include MDMA, MDA, Adam, Ecstasy, XTC. It produces LSD effects (minus hallucinations) such as increased self-awareness, removes communication barriers, and seems to remove the fear response.

Fentanyl

An intravenous analgesic-anesthetic that is a flavored preanesthetic medication, anesthetic, and postsurgical analgesic. Fentanyl analogs are now being used as designer drugs like China White and synthetic heroin. They are extremely potent and make overdose a serious risk.

OPIATES

Heroin is the most widely used of the opiate drugs, but accurate figures on the extent of its use are difficult to obtain. Some studies estimate that 10 percent of heroin users are dependent on the drug and mainline (inject) it; the remaining 90 percent are weekend "chippers," who inhale or snort it as a recreational activity or inject it just beneath the skin. Heroin-dependent individuals are found in all professions, socioeconomic strata, and communities. Most are under 35.

Methadone maintenance programs have been implemented to treat opiate-dependent people. Though still controversial, methadone, a synthetic opiate that blocks the euphoria given by heroin (but is nonetheless dependency-producing itself), coupled with strong psychological support and counseling, can often be a viable alternative to heroin dependence.

VOLATILE SUBSTANCES

The use of volatile inhalants, such as gasoline, glue, and typewriter correction fluid, is usually limited to elementary and junior high students. Regardless of the user's age, the misuse of such substances can be fatal. When death occurs, however, it is difficult to determine if it has been caused by inhalation of the fumes or suffocation from placing an inhaling aid, such as a plastic bag, over the nostrils and mouth.

DRUG TECHNOLOGY

Drug technology and the production of new drugs have grown astonishingly in recent decades. Forty-five years ago, physicians had at their disposal only 12 to 20 chemotherapeutic agents. Today more than 22,000 prescription "name" products are available to physicians.[16] (This figure is misleading, since

"Shooting Up Heroin"
Source: Arlene Collins/Monkmeyer Press

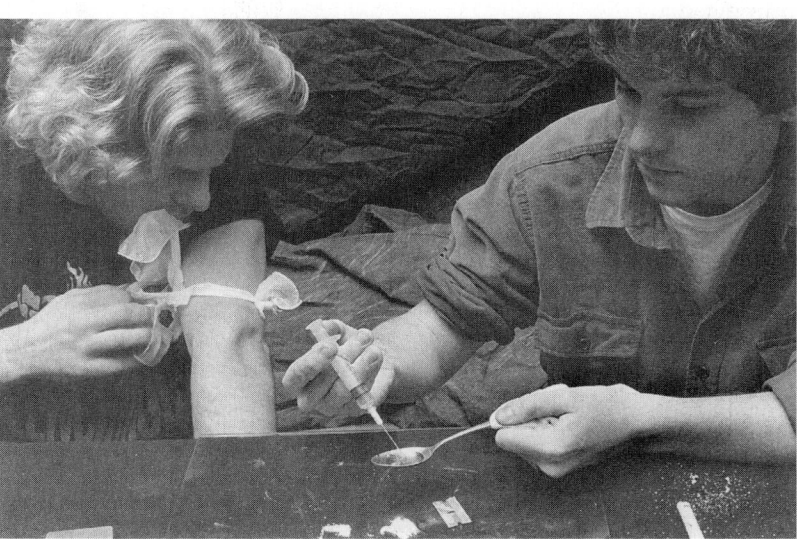

the same drug may be listed in the *Physician's Desk Reference* 20 or more times under different names.)

The combination of this rapid increase in prescription drugs and a growing trend among the general population to visit a physician regularly has had several notable effects. Average life expectancy has increased dramatically. New hygienic procedures, passed on from physician to patient, are reducing the incidence and severity of disease. Refinements in certain drugs have alleviated pain and suffering. Millions of people now benefit from the wise and judicious dispensation of prescription drugs by physicians.

Despite the positive changes drug use has brought about, available data suggest that adverse drug reactions afflict large portions of the population, causing hundreds of thousands of unnecessary hospitalizations and thousands of needless deaths. There are far more iatrogenic (medically induced) illnesses or deaths than is commonly realized by the general public. Evidence from the limited studies done to date indicates that between $3 and $4 billion in direct and indirect drug-induced damage is done each year. Current estimates of deaths caused by adverse drug reactions vary from 6,000 per year to as many as 140,000.[17]

Some of the responsibility for these figures rests with physicians, who "are lamentably ill-instructed in clinical pharmacology, a hardly recognized specialty for which no formal training is usually given,"[18] but who must select the correct prescription from the thousands of chemotherapeutic agents at their disposal. Some studies have gone so far as to say that "even where fully tested and established drugs are concerned, most of the adverse reactions are the direct result of the indiscriminate and overindulgent prescribing habits of physicians who often rely solely on advertisers' copy for their guidance."[19]

Current trends in prescriptive practices also invite possible adverse drug reactions or drug abuse. A substantial number of the psychoactive agents prescribed, many of them stimulants or sedatives, can be unknowingly abused. The phenomenon of **polypharmacy**—many sources supplying one person with medications that may be harmful when taken concurrently—is another cause of drug abuse.

Although doctors realize the negative effects of polypharmacy and although they are inadequately trained in giving prescriptions,

> prescribe they do, often with alacrity and apparent casualness and often without knowing that the patient may already be dosing himself with all kinds of heavily advertised medicines bought over-the-counter, which may greatly affect his reaction to the prescribed drug . . . . Certain hospital surveys have identified patients who are taking up to 30 different preparations a day. Small wonder new diseases develop, and who is to say whether the symptoms are caused by the original complaint or by the drug combination given to treat it?[20]

One study found that 40 percent of patients receive drugs prescribed by two or more physicians and are therefore more liable to dangerous drug interactions.[21]

Patients themselves may also be contributing markedly to the high rates of adverse drug reactions and drug-induced death. Noncompliance with a

Polypharmacy
A term applied to the use of several drugs at the same time. A person may be taking several prescriptions from several doctors.

physician's instructions can bring about serious consequences ranging from the failure of the drug to affect the disease to intensification of the disease and even death. Studies have indicated that noncompliance in the case of prescription drugs runs as high as 85 percent, with the highest incidence seen in nonhospitalized patients. On the other hand, many patients pressure their physician to overprescribe, particularly in the case of tranquilizers, currently one of the most frequently dispensed medications. Many drug experts, both within and outside the FDA, insist that drug abuse and adverse reactions must be combated by (1) improving physicians' training and sources of clinical-drug information; (2) developing informed consent procedures that provide detailed descriptions of drug effects, proper utilization of preparations, and patient prescription monitoring; and (3) informing the public about the effects and responsible use of drugs.

A recent trend concerning prescription drugs could have substantial adverse effects on street-drug users: Drug enforcement officials are suggesting that almost half the drugs now seen on the street market are diverted pharmaceutical drugs. It is estimated that approximately 13,000 physicians and pharmacists (2 percent of the registered population) are involved in this diversion.[22]

OVER-THE-COUNTER DRUGS

The number of over-the-counter (OTC) drugs has also expanded dramatically. Forty-five years ago only 50 to 60 products were available without prescription; currently, more than 300,000 medications are available at the local drugstore.[23] Many of these preparations are geared to minor ailments, including aspirin for headaches, laxatives for gastrointestinal upset, sleeping aids for insomnia, and antihistamines for hay fever. The public is willing to pay to obtain relief from these ailments, and consequently OTC drugs continue to be big business.

Television advertising is a key factor in OTC sales: One in every eight commercials advertises a drug.[24] But drug experts point out that advertising creates false expectations for relief by stressing drug benefits without discussing side effects or contraindications (inadvisable uses of the drug). And though the public expects consistent alleviation of ailments through chemical use, physicians know all too well that a drug's benefit may be reduced by negative side effects.

Because of consumer concern about the safety and effectiveness of OTC products, the FDA engaged in an extensive review of OTC medications from 1972 to early 1984. Several FDA panels reviewed more than 700 ingredients, many of them several times because of their use in different products. The panels found that only about one third of the ingredients were effective and safe; the rest required additional proof from manufacturers if the products containing them were to remain available for sale. This does not mean that two thirds of all OTC drug products are unsafe. Most products have safe and effective ingredients even if they contain other ingredients that are ineffective.[25]

Over-the-counter drugs represent the largest drug market openly available to consumers. Yet most people who obtain OTC products rarely have the pharmacological training to ensure proper drug usage. Since noncompliance with physicians' instructions occurs frequently, one must assume it occurs with OTC product instructions at an equal or greater rate.

COMMERCIAL DRUGS

Commercial drugs include food additives, industrial chemicals and inorganic wastes introduced into the atmosphere and water supply, household chemicals (cleaners, detergents, polishes, and the like), and cosmetics. Most of the commercial drugs utilized today were not available 15 years ago.

In previous years, consumer interest focused on the danger of children being poisoned by household chemicals or factory workers being exposed to industrial chemicals. Today so many new substances have such far-reaching effects that the recognition of any risks associated with them has lagged far behind appreciation of their benefits. The general public usually becomes aware of possible dangers only when some tragic event becomes news.[26]

Exposure to chemicals in the environment has been increasingly recognized as a major cause of cancer in humans. The National Cancer Institute has reported that more than 80 percent of the cancer in humans can be prevented by the reduction of exposure to certain natural or synthetic chemicals in foods, household products, and industrial by-products found in the air and water.[27] In passing the Delaney Amendment in 1958, Congress sought to prohibit the use of substances capable of producing cancer in humans. Consumers must be warned in supermarkets and workers at work sites by special notices of hazardous and carcinogenic materials. The Environmental Protection Agency also oversees efforts under the Toxic Substances Act to ensure that exposure to carcinogens is reduced. However, scientists still warn that Americans may have to make major changes in their diet (which for many is too high in fat) and use of tobacco products, and that rigid standards of air and water quality must be maintained, to ensure reduced cancer rates.

RECREATIONAL DRUGS

Recreational drugs are chemical agents that adults may legally consume, including alcohol (in beer, wine, distillates), nicotine (in cigarettes, snuff, cigars, pipe tobacco), and caffeine (in coffee, tea, soft drinks, chocolate). Large segments of the population take such substances for relaxation, stimulation, and, in some cases, social acceptance.

Advertising in the print and electronic media promotes extensive use and availability of recreational drugs. Yet, despite this exposure, little effort is made to ensure that individuals are taught judicious and responsible use. Irresponsible drug consumption can result in psychological and physiological dependence, medical complications, traffic accidents, violent crimes, high treatment costs, imprisonment, court costs, loss of work productivity, broken homes, scarred interpersonal relationships, and death.

To help people make better-informed and more realistic decisions about their drug-consuming behaviors, and to help them learn what drugs can provide in terms of self-growth and recreational activity, significant educational efforts must be made, starting at the elementary school level. Adults, too, must be educated to understand appropriate alcohol levels for driving, potential interactions between alcohol and other drugs, appropriate consumption of caffeine, and methods of reducing nicotine use.

HERBAL PREPARATIONS

Herbal chemicals, those occurring naturally in plants, have been used since the earliest times. Today, more than half of all available prescription and OTC products are derived from plant chemicals.[28]

An individual who obtains a preparation from a plant is obtaining all the chemicals the plant uses for its metabolism. In a pharmaceutical (synthetic) preparation, the single desired chemical has been isolated from the others and provided in the correct dosage, which is somewhat difficult to estimate when using bulk quantities of a plant. Whether a drug is organic or synthetic, it will be metabolized in the body by the same processes. The renewed public interest in herbal preparations, however, has been fostered by the public belief that organic drugs are inherently better than synthetic chemicals.

ILLEGAL DRUGS

Illegal drugs are those chemicals that government authorities have determined to be subject to abuse or that are capable of causing severe harm. Among them are marijuana, amphetamines, cocaine, opiates, sedatives, and tranquilizers. Laws have been passed to prevent the public from obtaining or distributing these drugs, and to deter and punish people who attempt to use them without a physician's prescription.

SUMMARY

To gain a solid understanding of drugs and their use, one must consider several factors. The topic is highly emotionally charged; it is heavily laden with individual biases; it is inundated with myths and inaccurate information; it is subject to rapid change in valid data. Often these factors conflict with one another, and as a result the drug scene is a "gray area" of unanswered questions and vague issues. Individual differences, quality control, set, setting, and legal implications must all be considered. And it must be understood that it is often difficult to put drugs in a realistic perspective. For example, alcohol and tobacco, both legal drugs for those of age, probably lead to more health and economic problems than do illicit drugs. A full range of drug education is therefore necessary.

Because of the increasing number of drugs available for prescription, OTC, and recreational use, an awareness of drug technology is highly important. With physicians unable to remain informed on all the drugs currently available for treatment, with billions of dollars paid each year for licit and illicit drugs, with over-the-counter drugs filling drugstores and supermarkets, and with drug advertising and promotion the big business it is, today's consumer must be informed and responsible if he or she is to use drugs rationally.

INTRODUCTION
N O T E S

1. From *The Natural Mind,* by Andrew Weil. Copyright 1972 by Andrew Weil. Reprinted by permission of the publisher, Houghton Mifflin Company.

2. A graduate student report presented to a Drugs in Society class at the University of Oregon, March 1985, Eugene, Oregon.

3. Lecture by Peter Shannon to a Drugs in Society class at the University of Oregon, January 1978.

4. National Institute on Drug Abuse, "Summary of Findings from the 1990 National Household Survey on Drug Abuse," NIDA Capsules, CAP 20 (Rockville, Md.: U.S. Department of Health and Human Services, Public Health Service, Alcohol, Drug Abuse, and Mental Health Administration, 1990).

5. Ibid.

6. U.S. Department of Health and Human Services, *HHS News,* RPO 729, (December 19, 1990).

7. National Institute on Drug Abuse, "Summary of Findings from the 1990 National Household Survey on Drug Abuse."

8. "Illicit Drugs: How Much Americans Spend," *Register-Guard* (Eugene, Oregon), June 20, 1991, p. 5A.

9. Ibid.

10. "The Sobering Cost of Alcoholism," *Science News* 114, no. 18 (October 28, 1978):293.

11. Ibid.

12. Office of Technological Assessment, *The Effectiveness and Costs of Alcoholism Treatment* (Washington, D.C.: U.S. Government Printing Office, 1983), p. 3.

13. Bryan R. Luce, "Smoking and Alcohol Abuse: A Comparison of Their Economic Consequences," *New England Journal of Medicine* 298, no. 10 (March 9, 1978):569.

14. "Quaaludes 'Dead,' Agents Claim," *Register-Guard* (Eugene, Oregon), August 19, 1984, p. 17D.

15. *Focus on Alcohol and Drug Issues* 3, no. 1 (January/February 1980):2.

16. Lecture by Mark Miller to a Drugs in Society class at the University of Oregon, April 1980.

17. N. S. Irey, "Deaths Due to Adverse Drug Reactions," *Journal of the American Medical Association* 231, no. 1 (January 6, 1975):22–23; J. Kock-Weser, "Fatal Reactions to Adverse Drug Reactions," *New England Journal of Medicine* 291, no. 6 (August 8, 1974):302–3.

18. Special Commission on Internal Pollution, "Toward Assessing the Chemical Age," *Journal of the American Medical Association* 234, no. 5 (November 3, 1975):509.

19. Ibid.

20. Ibid.

21. George J. Caranasos, Ronald B. Stewart, and Leighton E. Cluff, "Drug Induced Illness Leading to Hospitalization," *Journal of the American Medical Association* 228, no. 6 (May 6, 1974):716–17.

22. *Pharmaceutical Manufacturers Association Newsletter* 25, no. 24 (July 4, 1983):2.

23. Lecture by Mark Miller.

24. "Television Advertising and Drug Use: Health Care Sociology," *Drug Intelligence and Clinical Pharmacy* 11, no. 8 (August 1977), p. 2.

25. "Panels' Review Completed," *FDA Consumer,* February 1984:32–33.

26. Special Commission on Internal Pollution, "Toward Assessing the Chemical Age."

27. American Cancer Society, *1981 Cancer Facts and Figures* (New York, 1981).

28. Lecture by Mark Miller.

THEORIES
OF DRUG USE

INTRODUCTION

Different individuals use different drugs for different reasons. Whereas one will use alcohol to facilitate interaction at a cocktail party, another may smoke marijuana as a political statement. The reasons individuals use psychoactive substances vary as much as the individuals themselves: to find sexual fulfillment, to seek spiritual enlightenment, to have fun, to produce mood fluctuations, to enhance athletic performance, to reduce inhibitions in bar settings, to fight boredom, to satisfy curiosity, to be "in" as opposed to "left out."

The many reasons for psychoactive substance use are similar to those for drug dependence, but they can be broken down into two major groups: psychological (interpersonal) and sociological (environmental). The two are not mutually exclusive, since personal and societal factors work in consort to determine behavior. Theories on the nature of dependency states fall into three camps—psychological, sociological, and biological—which again are not mutually exclusive. A composite of the three areas offers an explanation of drug dependency.

PSYCHOLOGICAL FACTORS

RECREATION AND SOCIAL FACILITATION

The American cocktail party is a setting in which drug use and the reasons for use are plentiful. Alcohol is in demand at such occasions because it facilitates interpersonal and group dynamics through its capacity to depress the central nervous system. Alcohol and other recreational drugs may foster a sense of camaraderie and co-adventure, and may fulfill the need or desire to feel good. Therefore, individuals who feel poorly and want to feel better may use these drugs; so may individuals who already feel fine.

People use drugs recreationally simply to enhance social facilitation and to feel good—at cocktail parties, at football games, on Friday at the local watering hole, in restaurants, on picnics, and during lazy afternoons. Social drug use brings people together. It helps to create an atmosphere in which openness becomes appropriate and people share more of themselves than they normally would. The character armoring, as Reich would say, may become less rigid. Alexander Shilgin, who synthesized the hallucinogen STP, comments:

> In drinking, there is this marvelous level, somewhere during the second martini; you can't say what's happening, but suddenly everything is a little bit brighter, conversation a little bit more relaxed, the music is suddenly proper, you are fitting into the environment. That's the goal of alcohol drinking. I find it a fabulous moment.[1]

Finding that level is a goal shared by a significant segment of the drinking population. Again, as an amplification of the cocktail party, social drug use promotes communication by allowing the possibility of a shared feeling or experience. In short, people use drugs to communicate and because it is ritualistic fun.

A recent study found a linkage to illicit substance in adolescent males and their levels of shyness and sociability.[2] The main findings include higher use of illicit substances in the shy male subjects than the unshy males. When com-

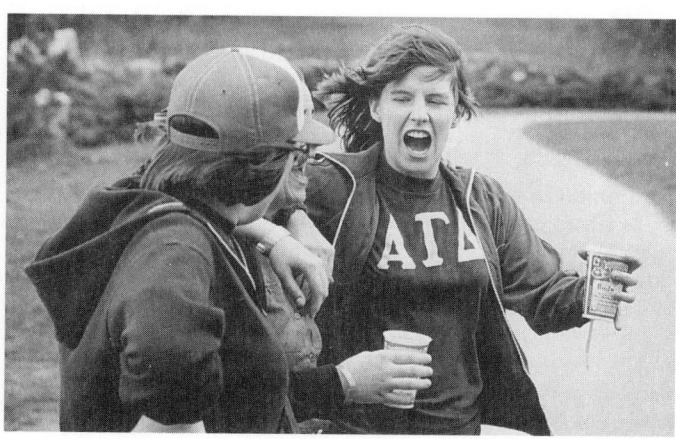

Fraternity–Sorority "Party Time"
Source: James L. Shaffer/Photoedit

bined with high-level sociability factors, high shyness levels seem to moderately indicate higher usage levels of cocaine and marijuana (with the exception of hallucinogenic substances). Adolescents, it is hypothesized, turn to illicit substances in order to overcome their shyness in social situations. They seem to lack the tools and confidence to be able to interact in a social setting without the crutch of the substance. Although this may not be the only factor in the whole arena, it surely is one of the bigger reasons for substance abuse.

SENSATION SEEKING AND RISK TAKING

The present emphasis on sports, the preponderance of sex and violence in films and television, videogames, and computers, and the level of drug dependency already displayed by millions of people give credence to the current need for stimulating experiences—the pursuit of sensation. But heightened and exciting experiences become increasingly difficult to achieve as people build up tolerance to sensation and need new regions to explore. It may be that

> football and hockey spectacles are a pallid substitute for the corny productions of the Roman Coliseum. In past centuries, war, conquest, and exploration, along with saturnalias, tournaments, public executions, and orgiastic feasts, fed the hunger for unusual and arousing experience . . . . In 19th century America, the more adventurous struck out for the frontier when life on the eastern seaboard became tame and predictable. Ever since our ancestors settled in permanent locations, boredom has been a problem that varies with the need for survival.[3]

Sensory bombardment through high technology has led to sensory numbing.

Individuals vary in their susceptibility and reaction to boredom. Security in a well-defined and repetitious lifestyle is not a goal, but a plague. Psychologist Marvin Zuckerman explains: " 'Boredom' is the term we use to describe the negative feeling produced by lack of change in the environment . . . . Boredom drives us to seek relief in the form of risky adventures, artistic creation, sex, alcohol, drugs, and even aggression. It is a demand for stimulation and varied experience."[4]

Pioneering sensory-deprivation research by John Lilly proved that in an environment where stimuli are constant, uniform, and never changing, the "bored" mind will initiate auditory and visual hallucinations to keep cognitively awake and stimulated. Describing his work with the National Institute of Mental Health (NIMH) in Bethesda, Maryland, Lilly wrote:

> In the absence of all stimulation it was found that one quickly makes up for this by an extremely heightened awareness and increasing sensory experience in the absence of known means of external stimulation . . . . I went through dreamlike states, trancelike states, mystical states. In all of these states, I was totally intact, centered, and there . . . . I went through experiences in which other people apparently joined me in this dark silent environment. I could actually see them, feel them and hear them. At other times I apparently tuned in on networks of communication that are normally below our levels of awareness, networks of civilizations way beyond ours. I

did hours of work on my own hinderances to understanding myself, or my life situation.[5]

The need for periodic variation in sensory stimuli may be a biological function, according to Zuckerman. The basic survival needs for food, drink, and warmth must be satisfied, but following such satisfaction we do not usually sit and hibernate, waiting for the next upswing in the internal-need cycle. Human beings, like other mammals, have the urge to explore their environment. We spend a great deal of our time playing in our physical and social surroundings.

Sensation seeking may be a general trait—not restricted to any one sensory modality—experienced by all human beings to some degree. Its particular expression may depend on the range of environmental options available, and psychoactive drug use may be one of those options.[6]

Ralph Keyes, author of *Chancing It: Why We Take Risks,* defines "risk" as "something that causes fear and has the possibility of failure."[7] Gayle Maleskey states that the problem with risk is that every individual has a very subjective view about fear and failure, which may vary with time and circumstance.[8] Not only that, the risk taker is in the position to determine what is genuinely risky. As a result, switching jobs may be a high risk for one individual while jumping out of an airplane is a low risk for another individual.

Why take risks? According to Frank Farley, "it's important to take risks to grow and experience life . . . . If you don't expose yourself to new experiences and new ideas, you remain the same. And change is a very important part of personal growth. Satisfying your curiosity about the world around you, about people and yourself requires a certain amount of risk taking."[9] One reason **high-risk** sports are popular is because they are a ground for success: success in the fact that you are faced with fear repeatedly and learn to overcome it. The reward is that "you discover how exciting, even ecstatic, confronting fear can be." Some people turn to drugs for the excitement of an unknown experience.

NIMH brought together a group of psychologists, brain scientists, and others at a conference on "Self-Regulation and Risk-Taking Behavior."[10] After probing into many risky activities, the participants at the conference came to the conclusion that "the U.S. culture as a whole is in the midst of an epidemic of violent and self-destructive risk-taking behavior." Debilitation and premature death are more often the result of behavioral and environmental conditions than disease: This includes drinking and drug and eating disorders.

Those scientists attending the 1987 conference fear an "epidemic" of risk-taking behavior in the United States. According to Leonard Zegan, a psychiatrist, the culture extols heroes—will overlook maladaptive behavior (such as extreme risk taking) as long as you succeed, while at the same time has high expectations for safety. Although risk taking has positive elements such as courage, creativity, curiosity, and growth, many individuals lack the decision-making skills necessary for making healthy, intelligent choices.

High-Risk Factors
An individual who has high potential for substance abuse may have the following high-risk factors: unconventionality (a need or tendency to rebel), uncontrolled emotions (expressed as impulsiveness), intrapsychic functioning (depression), interpersonal relations (when expressed in terms of aggression), and nonachievement (described not as a lack of ability but as a lack of motivation).

RELIGIOUS AND SPIRITUAL FACTORS

Some people use drugs to gain spiritual enlightenment and to enhance religious ceremonies. Medical studies have determined that psychoactive substances can produce profound perception changes that can enhance and/or facilitate spiritual experiences. The Native American church of the American Southwest and the Tarahumara and Huichol Indians of Mexico utilize the peyote cactus, whose plant buttons contain mescaline.[11] Hindu religious rites call for the use of ganja (bhang), a rich, potent tea made from cannabis.

> To the Hindu, the hemp plant is holy. A guardian lives in "bhang" . . . bhang is the joy giver, the sky flier, the heavenly guide, the poor man's heaven, the soother of grief . . . . No god of man is as good as the religious drinking of bhang. The students of the scriptures of Benares are given bhang before they sit to study. At Benares, Vjjain and other holy places, yogis take deep draughts of bhang, that they may center their thoughts on the eternal.[12]

When used in a religious setting—be it a temple or the desert—alcohol, cannabis, and psychedelic drugs can elevate the emotional intensity of a person's perceptions.

ALTERED STATES

From a strictly pharmacological standpoint, psychoactive substances increase the intensity of mood. By causing changes in the neurotransmitter levels of serotonin, dopamine, and norepinephrine, the reticular activating system (the human sensory-screening mechanism) becomes less able to filter out indigenous environmental stimuli. Individuals use drugs in this way to alter their thinking patterns, enhance sensation, and experience new sensations.

From a metaphysical viewpoint, drugs are often used to enhance reflection and to find new ways of looking at oneself and the world. Ken Kesey, author of *One Flew over the Cuckoo's Nest* and *Sometimes a Great Notion,* calls this "looking at the books." In Buddhism, everything one does is

Preparation for a Peyote Ritual
Source: Ira Block/The Image Bank

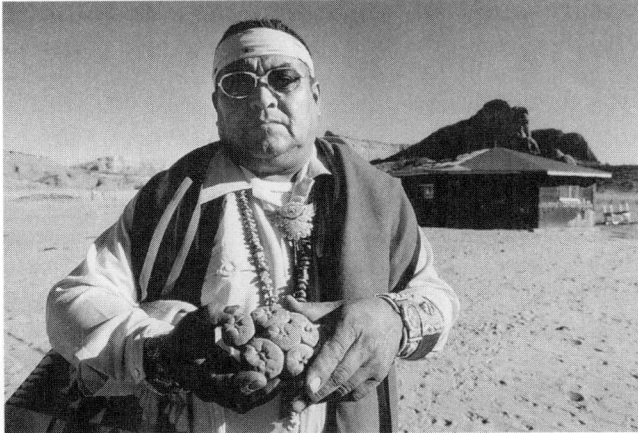

recorded in time and stored up as karma (the impact a person has during his or her existence). The books are the track record of one's life. More than a few have taken psychoactive substances to look at the books. Though some have unlocked important clues to their inner selves, others have been shattered by the experience.

REBELLION AND ALIENATION

On college campuses in the early 1960s, students were told to "turn on, tune in, and drop out." Then Harvard professor Timothy Leary, along with fellow academician Richard Alpert (later to become Ram Dass) extolled the virtues of thinking along alternative pathways: War was wrong; conspicuous material consumption was an illusion; people should strive for harmony with nature. Young people were asked to seek new perspectives, to redefine priorities, and they were told that hallucinogens could facilitate this process. Such motives for drug use became tantamount to a cultural revolution.

Many students accepted Leary's message. They began to find fault with many of the standards and values of the time. To express their rejection of these middle-class values, they grew their hair long, dressed in nontraditional clothes, listened to antiestablishment music. They expressed their discontent conspicuously, and drug use was a part of that expression.

Drug use became a way people could reveal something of themselves. It was also used to make political and social statements. In the late 1960s, marijuana was smoked openly as a counterculture flag-flying gesture; it was flaunted before those who deemed it illegal. The dissident users were telling mainstream America that they were not accepting traditional American values, that a change in attitudes and laws was needed. Some changes were eventually undertaken, but many people ended up behind bars for their antiestablishment acts.

Some individuals use drugs to cope with alienation (Who am I? Where am I going?); others use drugs to combat depression and dysphoria (feeling unwell, impatient, restless), to experience euphoria, and to remove themselves from the boredom of their existence. They may be living at a rat-race pace, competing to the point of emotional if not physical death, unable to make any sense of or to accept their existence. Therefore, they bring in the "fog"—the chemical haze that envelops their consciousness and muffles their perceptions. The fog can be delivered by alcohol, marijuana, Valium, Seconal, methaqualone, the phenothiazines, Prolixin, Dalmane, Sinequan, glue, PCP, or any number of other substances. The fog may not last long initially, but with repeated doses it will stay as long as one desires.

PERSONALITY TRAITS

According to a longitudinal study by Judith Brook and her colleagues, certain personality traits that are allowed to be carried into adolescence indicate a high potential for substance abuse.[13] The study identifies five observable characteristics as "high-risk factors": unconventionality (a need or tendency to rebel), uncontrolled emotions (expressed as impulsiveness), intrapsychic functioning (depression), interpersonal relations (when expressed in terms of aggression), and nonachievement (described not as a lack of ability but as a lack of motivation). Brook and her associates state that successful intervention and the prevention of these characteristics from being carried from childhood to adolescence may significantly decrease the likelihood of substance abuse.

Similar findings were reported in a study by Erich Labouvre and Connell McGee.[14] Adolescents who used drugs heavily scored lower on achievement, cognitive-structuring, and harm-avoidance tests and higher on tests measuring impulsiveness, exhibitionism, autonomy, and affiliation and play.

Although suicide may not be a reason for taking drugs, the use of drugs may be attributed as a reason why many young people attempt or commit suicide. Studies during the past two decades suggest a significant association between suicidal behavior and the use of psychoactive substances among adolescent populations. Over the past two decades there has been a measurable increase in adolescent use of psychoactive substances. Likewise, from 1950 through 1990, there was a 305.4 percent increase in the suicide rate for 15- to 19-year-old white males. Likewise, white female adolescents had an increase of 66.7 percent during the same time period.[15] Frank Crumley found evidence for an association between (1) substance abuse and adolescent suicide and attempted suicide, (2) substance abuse and the frequency of medical seriousness of suicide attempts, (3) substance abuse and depression, and (4) alcohol abuse and firearm suicide by adolescents. It would be pure speculation to state the extent to which the use of psychoactive substances is associated with adolescent suicidal behavior. However, it appears that the use of these substances should be added to the roster of risk factors for adolescent suicidal behavior.

PERSONAL HABITS

In a 1984 survey given to 379 boys and 464 girls in grades 9–12 in California, students were asked 70 questions about their personal life and the problems they saw in their parents. Among the respondents, "43 girls and 34 boys were identified who indicated never using alcohol, other drugs, or nicotine products."[16] The nonuser group was then compared with the user group. "The overall picture of the invulnerable subjects was one of generally better physical and mental health and academic achievement."[17] Users, on the other hand, were more likely to describe themselves as tense and hyper, bored and stingy. But the most interesting difference between the two groups was the parallel between user problems and parent problems. Twenty-five percent of the users reported that one or both parents had problems with drugs. Users were also more likely to report having had an unhappy childhood.

In a study of cocaine users and nonusers, the users generally reported a much higher consumption of nicotine, coffee, and alcoholic beverages.[18] They also did less daily planning and organizing, engaged in fewer relaxing activities, and ate fewer balanced meals. The hypothesized lower levels of exercise in the cocaine users were not found, however; perhaps the self-report nature of the study prompted the users to exaggerate the levels of exercise they reported. The researchers concluded that cocaine users indulge in a more unhealthy lifestyle than nonusers, confirming their initial hypothesis.

SOCIOLOGICAL FACTORS: PEER PRESSURE, FAMILY, AND GROUP ENTRY

Peer-group pressure influences our activity phenomenally. We copy the activities and behavior of our **peers** as a way of learning social behavior and gaining acceptance. Behavior acquired through environmental influence is visible in the young of many species as they learn survival techniques. In humans, drug consumption is often a group-entrance requirement.

In gaining entrance to a group, we prove ourselves to the group and to ourselves. When drugs are involved, there is a challenge of strength, if not survival: "It is not unlike the game of chicken, but instead of testing oneself against the fear of a high speed head-on collision with another automobile, the 'contest' is an internal one which tests one's ability to come as close as possible to a psychotic 'crash' or even go over the line and then return unscathed."[19]

So-called primitive societies still have initiation rites. Young men go out into the woods to spend a specified amount of time on their own. If they survive to return to the group, they have passed the test of "manhood." This trial becomes more difficult if a particular task is required, such as slaying an animal or returning with an object that requires hazardous efforts to obtain.

Modern society does not often provide this overt testing for group entrance. Ritualized ceremonies, where they are still practiced, now serve this purpose. Jewish bar mitzvahs, fraternity and sorority initiations, licensing tests for the professions, fraternal-club initiations, and chugging contests provide avenues for testing.

Once individuals have been accepted into the group, socialization continues. It determines their behavior, dress, skill acquisition, interests, speech, and so on. In short, the group can help establish and maintain an individual's self-concept and orientation and how he or she views and reacts to the world.[20] Such direction can include use of psychoactive substances.

The family also affects attitudes toward drug use, although its effect, more pronounced in a child's earlier years, diminishes as peer influence increases. Parent figures are powerful models, and young children model their behavior in much the same fashion individuals seeking group entrance do. For example, children born into alcoholic families are more likely to become alcohol-abusive or -dependent than those growing up in families in which alcohol use is nonexistent to moderate.

A study was done to determine if cohesiveness and adaptability within a family would play a role in an adolescent's use of illicit substances.[21] Cohesion was defined as a family where family members have emotional bonding toward one another. Adaptability referred to family power, negotiation styles, role relationships, and relationship rules. Researchers hypothesized

Peer Group Pressure
We copy the activities and behavior of our peers as a way of learning social behavior and gaining acceptance. In gaining entrance to a group, we prove ourselves to the group and to ourselves. Once individuals have been accepted to the group, socialization continues. It determines an individual's behavior, dress, skill acquisition, interests, speech, and so on.

Peers
Student-to-student support.

that students coming from families that were both very high and very low, or were either high and low, in cohesion, adaptability categories would be more inclined to use illicit substances. The findings indicate that students who came from highly structured and rigid families tended to report greater use and experimentation of illicit substances than students from families that were too loose; they all proved to have greater problems than the balanced families. The support from the balanced families seemed to give the students enough self-confidence to reject the temptations of drug use.

A problem some parents have is that they tell their children not to drink or take drugs, but then they themselves drink martinis and beer and use "adult culture" drugs, such as sleeping pills and tranquilizers. This gives children mixed messages. The "do as I say, not as I do" approach does not work well. Rather, parents should practice what they preach. For example, The Seventh-Day Adventists and the Mormons preach and *live* abstinence from drugs. Six ways to "drug-proof" children are[22]

1. Set a good example of abstinence.
2. Educate your children about the danger of drugs as early as age five or six.
3. Give short-term rewards for not using drugs.
4. Identify problems early and know signs of drug use.
5. Get help in a treatment program when you recognize a problem.
6. Be supportive of follow-up treatment and forgive your children.

Overall, "experts estimate that 2.3 to 3 million persons are homeless annually and that families are approximately 30 percent of the homeless population."[23] A recent study of the homeless in Baltimore, Maryland, came up with very high, alarming statistics: Eighty-five percent of homeless men and 67 percent of homeless women suffered from a substance-abuse problem. These statistics may be a significant factor contributing to the high number of people living on the streets, as drug abuse inhibits one's physical and emotional well-being while keeping one from performing the necessary steps to meet life's basic needs.

Children who are victims of an alcoholic, dysfunctional family are more likely to drink than those not from a dysfunctional family. It has been shown that the average age at which people start to drink is 12.5 years and that more than 3 million of the 10 million alcoholics in the United States are teenagers.[24] There are approximately 17 million young people in our country today, and 3.3 million of them are problem drinkers.[25] Children of alcoholics experience more problems, though, because they have traits of the alcoholic personality and they try to get drunk more often. And many of them become social outcasts, which causes them to drink even more.

Group structure may have an effect on drug use. Gary Selnow and William Crano have found that adolescents in ad hoc groups are more likely to use drugs and alcohol than those in more formal groups, which have more traditional norms and values and some form of adult supervision.[26]

One study that directly addressed the issue of peer pressure found that students who reported a positive relationship with their parents drank less and had more confidence in their ability to accomplish school-related tasks.[27] The study concluded that adolescent drinking patterns were influenced more by the esteem gained from positive parental relationships and academic success than by esteem received from peers.

Peer clusters are essentially a person's friends and the overall network of acquaintances whom he or she grows up with or spends time with.[28] Peer clusters serve as an important social influence on youth. Psychosocial theories contend that, for youth, the social effects of taking drugs are more important than the physiological effects.[29] Peer pressure, whether subtle or overt, is a very real aspect of a youth's life. Drug abuse is often the result of direct influence of peer drug associations. Not all peer clusters consist of youth who use drugs. Many factors combine to create a drug problem. Socioeconomic status, family strength, environment, and deviant role models are only a few of the factors that contribute to drug-using peer cultures. However, drug users show a much higher rate of interaction with deviant peers, whereas nondrug users seem to interact with mostly nondeviant peers.[30]

ADVERTISING

Advertising is a huge business in today's society, and many advertisers are clever at what they do; they want to get the consumer to buy their product and have some brand loyalty at the same time. How do they go about doing that? Some of the beer and wine companies, for example, target the younger population, those 21 years of age and under, and get them hooked on their products before they are even old enough to buy them legally.[31] Also, many large companies use sports superstars or movie stars to influence the young to buy the products they represent.

NATIONAL TRENDS

Cycles of drug abuse tend to sweep across the country in waves and appear to stimulate use of a particular drug or drugs. The late Norman E. Zinberg, a former psychiatrist at Harvard, believed shifting patterns in drug abuse are a sign of the times. Cocaine became the drug of the 1980s because it is a stimulant and people were looking for action, whereas the psychedelics were selected in the early 1960s because people were looking inward and reflecting on the direction of society. The nation has gone through four major waves of drug use, beginning with LSD in the 1960s, marijuana in the mid- to late 1960s, heroin from 1969 to 1971, and cocaine and crack in the late 1970s and 1980s.[32] The wave of the 1990s appears to be a fast-acting form of the stimulant methamphetamine (popularly known as "ice").

Although there have been several societal waves of drug use, drug researchers have found that (1) drug use varies tremendously from region to region, even city to city; (2) drugs of choice move with some predictability through the social-class structure; and (3) rather than a simple succession of drugs in use, one drug will piggyback on another, complicating efforts at prevention.[33]

DEPENDENCY STATES

DEPENDENCY

What causes addiction or dependency? Robert Millman, director of the Alcohol and Drug Abuse Service at New York Hospital–Cornell Medical Center, sees two basic models for addiction.[34] "The first attribute is the compulsive behavior to psychological difficulties, such as the need to mask pain. The second blames it all on chemical dependency." Percentages of people fall into each category. Edward Khantziank, the principal psychiatrist for Substance Abuse at Cambridge Hospital, is a proponent of the theory that drug use is a subtle form of self-medication—meaning the person uses it to cope with emotional conflicts and shortcomings.[35] However, according to John Grabowski, a researcher at the University of Texas Health Center in Houston, "the notion of an addictive personality is conceptionally just not very useful. It presumes all sorts of things about preaddiction I don't think we are capable of doing."[36] He concluded that it would be more realistic to construct a profile entailing all the characteristics, both internal and external. There are several different factors that contribute to the making of an addict, one being a healthy, functioning nervous system, as well as the interaction of personality, environment, biology, and social acceptability. It appears that some people turn to drugs for psychological reasons, while others become physically "hooked" after their first use of the particular substance.

PSYCHOLOGICAL PERSPECTIVES

Personality, Psychoanalytic, and Existential Views   There are many ways of looking at drug dependency. Some suggest that certain individuals have an "addictive personality," a constitution disposed to the use of narcotics or other drugs. These people argue that ending drug dependency requires a restructuring of the user's personality. Freudians, on the other hand, argue that drug use is a case of unresolved childhood conflicts—that narcotics use is an immature response of acting out, rather than dealing with, these conflicts. And existentialists argue that life's unresolved conflicts constantly bombard people with insurmountable pressures but offer no viable means of relief. Thus, for some, drug use may be viewed as self-treatment for internal distress.[37] But as Manuel M. Pearson and Ralph B. Little note, self-treatment may lead to addiction:

> The addict . . . has a special psychological relationship with his addicting drug—a pathological dependency upon the agent which he needs and without which he cannot deal with the stressful factors in his life situation.
>
> Later on, such a dependency produces the pathological craving, a central feature of all addiction that is reflected in the subsequent reorientation of his existence. Obtaining and taking this drug becomes his way of life.[38]

The necessary state for addiction is *preaddiction* or a *predilection* for addiction. Before using a drug, people experience certain feelings or drives that prepare them for becoming drug-dependent. Potential users may be unaware of their vulnerability to dependency.

People inclined toward drug use usually suffer from psychological tensions that, left unabated, become painful and may produce a state of helplessness. Such a state may bring on self-deprecation and depression, exacerbating the problem and contributing to further tension and loss of self-esteem. This cycle of negativism may result in the use of psychoactive substances and, depending on the intensity of the predependent state, drug dependence.[39] The gratifying use of narcotics relieves the tension and may be tantamount to a return to the womb, where frustrations are nonexistent and the painful realities of existence have little impact.

Generally speaking, the personality traits of a drug abuser may include (1) difficulty handling frustration, anxiety, and depression; (2) an urge for immediate gratification of desires; (3) difficulty relating with others; (4) low self-esteem; (5) impulsiveness, risk taking, and little regard for health; and (6) resistance to authority.

The Adlerian Theory of Ego Compensation   The Adlerian interpretation of drug dependency focuses on the perceived inferiority complex of the user. The theory states that neurotic symptoms develop to safeguard an individual's self-esteem. The "perceived inferiority causes withdrawal from social participation and leads to compensatory maneuvers. Drug abuse would be such a maneuver."[40]

The person who is drug-dependent would like to succeed, but all too often can't. Drug taking becomes an excuse to relinquish responsibility for failure. It takes on the role of scapegoat: "If I only didn't have this drinking problem, I could succeed."[41] Drug dependency becomes a self-fulfilling prophecy.

Basic to the Adlerian view of addiction is the theme of weak-ego compensation by a source other than the individual. The drug is supposedly taken to strengthen the normal defense mechanisms that have failed the user in coping with stress: The user actually believes that the drug will help him or her to overcome the obstacles to gratification and unleash restricted potentials and powers.[42]

SOCIOLOGICAL PERSPECTIVES

Sociological perspectives hold that humanity is responsible for drug dependency. The origin of this theory can be found in the urban ghetto, where men and women have to "fight like hell" in order to stay alive, let alone enjoy themselves. Ghetto conditions are a constant reminder that the occupants are living in the dirtiest, most run-down part of the city—and not by choice, but by necessity. What's happening in the classrooms is often not what's happening in the real world. Consequently, even if there were job possibilities related to their education, ghetto children cannot avail themselves of those possibilities because they've quit school by the time they're of working age. The area is impoverished, legitimate employment is simply not a reality, and learning takes place in the streets. The ghetto can be a living nightmare. There is a sense of hopelessness and defeat among dwellers in our city slums, the sense, among young people today, to belong to a group and their consequent drift into groups of heroin users . . . . An addict relapses, according to some sociological theories, because he returns to the same neighborhood where he became addicted and associates with addicts once more.[43]

Can it be any wonder that people in these environments are continually on edge, angry, depressed, and frustrated? That interpersonal relationships are at best taut and frayed, and at worst brutally violent? The familiar names include Detroit, Harlem, and, the most infamous, Watts. No money, no jobs, rats, deteriorating buildings, tremendous noise and overcrowding, garbage, and littered streets—the chain of frustration can easily lead ghetto dwellers to seek escape—in drug use. The "no hope but dope" scenario is finally enacted.

But we also have the other extreme: Individuals who have too much become bored and unhappy.

BIOLOGICAL PERSPECTIVES

In comparison with psychological and sociological theories, biological explanations of dependency are relatively new. Such explanations emphasize that psychological and sociological causes of drug dependency are only part of the picture, and that biochemistry is also a factor, involving cellular dependency on the molecules of certain chemicals. This viewpoint states what may occur to the chemistry of the body with repeated exposure to psychoactive substances. It also tells us that an individual may remain, or become, drug-dependent in spite of a harmonious mental state and environment.

Explaining human behavior, maladaptive or otherwise, in terms of biological abnormalities is enticing. It has already been seen to be easier to define and correct mental disorders by biological means than by psychological and sociological ones, and test-tube solutions may be easier to secure, and less costly, than sweeping social and interpersonal change. Of course, biochemical theorists gloss over or deny the idea that the world is incorrect, preferring to say that the individual is simply "out of synch," thus eliminating the need to confront and change the social order.

There is some validity to the biological argument. Even so, far too often treatment of people with problems consists of making them fit into society, rather than acknowledging that their problems stem from living in an often crazy world. Helping individuals adapt to the existing social order with pills, potions, and surgery can be a quick and inexpensive "cure." But any objective thinker will see that the biochemical perspective must address the important psychological and sociological aspects of dependency as well as its physiological aspects. The combination of the three will give a complete explanation of dependency states.

DEPENDENCY PAIN

Many studies have concluded that there is a strong relationship between drug use and experienced pain. Drug use is proportional to experienced pain. It is the intensity of the pain the user experiences that primarily determines whether he or she will choose the immediate relief the next dose promises in spite of mounting costs, which can be deferred. The problem arises, however, because the addict often cannot identify the pain or cause of drug use. Therapy, then, begins with pinpointing the source of pain that is so great that it causes persons to choose immediate relief and ruin all aspects of their lives, which essentially increases the pain.

The two sources of pain are external and internal. External are environmental sources that are unstimulating, impoverished, and depriving of a person. After constant exposure, avoidance can begin through a pattern of seeking temporary relief with substance use. Internal sources are much more vague, since subjective distress is usually a little more than a sense that life could be better but the means for attaining the better state are elusive or unreachable. Three important considerations regarding pain are the following: (1) addictive or dependent use of drugs is initiated by acute pain and then catalyzed by conditioning and neurochemical changes; (2) pain can arise from internal and external sources; and (3) when internal psychological, the source of pain is commonly profound disregard for self.[44]

Biochemical Theory   Current trends in research may mean that some day dependency conditions for all psychoactive substances will be explained in biochemical terms. Opiate dependency is presently explained in this manner—as a response to repeated administrations of the opiate molecule in its natural or synthesized form (opium, morphine, heroin, demerol, dilaudid, percodan). The time required for an individual to become drug-dependent may vary from months to years, depending on the frequency of drug use and the dosage.

Simply stated, the body gradually adapts to the presence of the opiate molecule with repeated exposure to it. At some point the body becomes so adapted that the molecule becomes a necessity for proper physiological functioning. Further research may lead to the application of this theory to other psychoactive substances as well.

The foundation for a biochemical theory of opiate dependency was being set by the mid-1970s.[45] For some time it was suggested that certain areas of the brain, and the central nervous system in general, were particularly sensitive to opiates, that certain receptor mechanisms or binding sites specifically received opiate molecules administered into the body. Recent research indicates that opiate-receptor mechanisms are actually binding sites for an internally produced chemical. What, then, becomes of this chemical in the presence of the opiate molecule? What is its own function? Furthermore, will it bind with the opiate-receptor mechanisms following discontinuation of opiate use? Researchers are still investigating these questions.

Enkephalins and Endorphins   The existence of the opiate-receptor mechanism was first established in a 1977 article in *Neurosciences Research Program Bulletin.* The stumbling block in identifying the receptor mechanism was that opiates, like most other compounds, bind to virtually any bio-

Enkephalins and Endorphins

Enkephalins are neurotransmitters of specific neuronal systems in the brain that mediate the integration of sensory information having to do with pain and emotional behavior. The body's own natural morphinelike pain killer, endorphin, centers in the numerous pleasurable sensations associated with the body's natural secretion of this "magical" hormone. Endorphins, or their receptors, are responsible not only for their widely known anesthetic effect but also for the intensity of other emotional states, such as happiness, depression, compulsiveness, masochism, excitation, sexual satisfaction, and hunger.

logical or nonbiological membrane. Research studies by Avram Goldstein at the Stanford University School of Medicine and Solomon H. Snyder and Candice B. Pert at the Johns Hopkins School of Medicine eventually broke the ice. Using membrane fragments from homogenized brain cells and radioactively labeled Naloxone (an opiate antagonist), they conducted tests that established the phenomenon of specific binding to receptor mechanisms.[46]

After the receptor mechanisms had been identified, research could be directed to how they function. Many neurotransmitter systems (systems in which chemicals released by nerve endings modulate the firing of other nerve cells, thereby transmitting messages) and brain functions were known to be distributed throughout the brain. If opiate-receptor distribution were to mirror some specific brain property, then opiate action might be implicated as a necessary component of the property. Because opiates are pain killers, the brain structures involved in pain were natural suspects. Of the two known pathways implicated in the perception of pain, the pathway for duller, more chronic, and less localized pain is relieved quite effectively by opiates. The other pathway, which transmits sharp, localized pain, is poorly relieved by opiates.[47] The paleospinothalmic (opiate-affected) pain pathway consists of many interconnected nerve cells, most of which lack a fatty myelin insulation and therefore conduct impulses rather slowly.

Distribution measurements indicated striking parallels between the opiate-affected pain pathways and opiate-receptor mechanisms. Opiate-receptor binding occurs at high density in the limbic system, which mediates emotion in humans.[48] Furthermore, this binding appears to affect memory and spatial orientation (the awareness of where one is in relation to the environment). Says Snyder:

> Clearly man was not made with morphine inside him. The existence in all vertebrates of specific opiate receptor sites strongly indicated the presence of a natural morphine like substance in the brain, possibly a neurotransmitter, that acts at these sites.
>
> Opiates, like most other drugs that affect the mind, are thought to act primarily at synapses in the brain, the specialized regions where the terminal of a nerve fiber makes a junction with the outer membrane of another nerve cell and chemically modulates its activity . . . . It appears that the opiate receptor is associated with synaptic regions of the brain.
>
> Since neurotransmitters act as synapses, the opiate receptor appeared to function very much like a receptor site for a natural neurotransmitter substance in the brain.[49]

This reasoning eventually led to the discovery of the endogenous (internally produced) neurotransmitter.[50] Experiments conducted by researchers John Hughes and Hans W. Kasterlitz of the University of Aberdeen provided the evidence of a morphinelike neurotransmitter. Subsequent studies by Lars Terenius of the University of Uppsala and by Pasternak and Snyder independently identified the same substance. Hughes and Kasterlitz isolated the factor from the brain of pigs and named it *enkephalin,* from the Greek word meaning "in the head." A similar peptide (an intermediate between the amino acids and peptones in the synthesis of protein) is beta endorphine, which is also found in the pituitary gland. "Enkephalins are neurotransmitters of specific neuronal systems in the brain that mediate the integration of sensory information having to do with pain and emotional behavior, and that subserve unidentified functions as well."[51] With the discovery of enkephalin came a new theory of opiate dependence.

Years of research have thus provided a fairly clear model of the biochemistry of opiate dependence. Opiate-receptor mechanisms in the body facilitate the amelioration of certain types of pain throughout the central nervous system and the gastrointestinal tract and bind with the body's own morphinelike substances, enkephalin and beta endorphine, found in the pituitary gland. In the presence of administered opiates, enkephalin release is reduced, though its production continues. But continual opiate administration results in a complete stoppage of enkephalin release. If opiate use is discontinued, the receptor mechanisms are left without any chemical counterpart, and a series of intracellular events occur that lead to withdrawal symptoms. Eventually, enkephalin, in the absence of opiates, is gradually reintroduced into the system and begins to neutralize the elevated nucleotide levels. This return to normal chemical levels signifies the termination of the withdrawal symptoms.[52]

Sometimes, however, the desire to use opiates returns after total withdrawal. The cause for this is unclear, though it may be that enkephalin levels or the level of their release never quite returns to the predependent level. As a result, the feeling remains that there should always be just a little more, and therefore the need for just a little more.

What application this model of opiate dependency has to other dependency-producing psychoactive substances is not clear at this time, but it is possible that similar situations result from the use of other mind-altering drugs. As Snyder states,

> in a formal sense the processes of tolerance and physical dependence are the same for most classes of drugs. Hence, if one could understand the biochemical mechanisms involved for one class, such as the opiates, one would know something about what was happening with drugs in other classes.[53]

The current research on the body's own natural morphinelike pain killer, endorphin, centers in the numerous pleasurable sensations associated with the body's natural secretion of this "magical" hormone. Endorphins, or their receptors, are responsible not only for their widely known anesthetic effect but also for the intensity of other emotional states, such as happiness, depression, compulsiveness, masochism, excitation, sexual satisfaction, and hunger.

Studies show there is a direct link between autistic children who inflict self-injuries and the masochist.[54] This is due, in fact, to the "pleasure" felt by the sudden release of endorphins upon the pain centers in our brain after self-inflicted injury. The result is very similar to what happens after a major injury, such as a burn: Endorphins enter our bloodstream and delay signals of pain to the brain for several hours. The "runner's high"—the pleasant feeling experi-

A "Runner's High"
Source: Topham/The Image Works

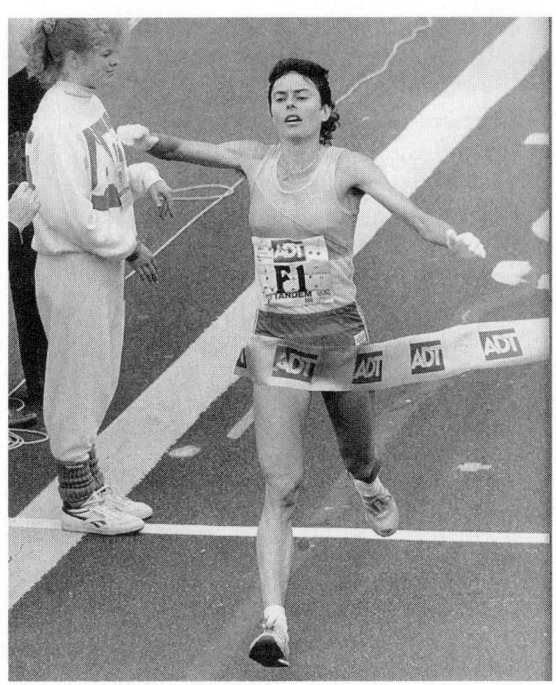

enced during and after structured, regulated exercise—is also similar. Like-wise, the pleasant sensations accompanying the eating of certain foods con-taining fats and sugars is now thought to result from endorphin release throughout the body directly after eating.[55] Currently, much research is being done on the role endorphins play in the eating disorders of anorexia and bulimia. It is known that food deprivation stimulates the release of opiates in the brain, and this "reward" may explain the complexity and low success of treatment of victims of these disorders. Endorphin research is still in its early stages, but the findings are encouraging.

GENETIC FACTORS AND DEPENDENCY

Researchers are accumulating a great deal of information associating genetic factors with addiction. Studies show how the brain is affected by both cocaine and alcohol.[56] They recognized a certain portion of the brain as the "reward system." Cocaine and alcohol differ in many ways, but the notion that they somehow stimulate a common brain reward system is a concept that is being revived from the 1950s. The theory basically is that a drug such as cocaine stimulates the reward system directly, producing such intense pleasure that one wants to repeat the experience. These researchers also rec-ognized the fact that the neurotransmitters in the body are altered a great deal when a drug is administered, and that this also may be the "biological" reason for addiction.

RANKING OF MOST ADDICTING DRUGS

A ranking of drugs according to their addictive potential is as follows: (1) central nervous system stimulants (especially cocaine), (2) opiates, (3) alcohol, (4) sedative-hypnotics, (5) nicotine, (6) anxiolytics, (7) marijuana, (8) inhalants, and (9) PCP.[57]

SUMMARY

The reasons for the use of psychoactive drugs are as varied as the individuals who use them, but most can be categorized as either psychological (interpersonal) or sociological (environmental). These factors, which work in consort to affect human behavior, include peer pressure, parental-behavior modeling, cohesiveness and adaptability within a family, homelessness, the need for mood alterations, interpersonal and social communication, stress reduction and relaxation, risk-taking behaviors, religious and spiritual enlightenment, sexual enhancement, personal awareness, sensation seeking, political expression, coping with alienation, and advertising.

THEORIES OF DRUG USE
N O T E S

1. Quoted in David Rorvik, "Mood Drugs," *Penthouse* 10, no. 4 (December 1978), p. 15.

2. Randy M. Page, "Shyness and Sociability: A Dangerous Combination for Illicit Substance Use in Adolescent Males?" *Adolescence* 25, no. 100 (Winter 1990):803–6.

3. Marvin Zuckerman, "The Search for High Sensation," *Psychology Today* 11, no. 9 (February 1978):38. Reprinted with permission from *Psychology Today Magazine*. Copyright © 1978 American Psychological Association (APA).

4. Ibid.

5. Reprinted from *The Center of the Cyclone* by John C. Lilly. Copyright ©1972 by John C. Lilly. Reprinted with permission of The Julian Press, Inc. The quotation appears on pages 42–43 of the Crown Publishers edition (New York, 1972).

6. Zuckerman, "The Search for High Sensation," p. 40.

7. Gale Maleskey, "How Gutsy Are You? (Risk Taking)," *Prevention* 40, (January 1988):66–73.

8. Ibid.

9. Ibid.

10. Rick Weiss, "Risk Taking: Do We Dare?" *Current Health* 299 (January 1988):26–29.

11. Louise A. Richards, "Role of Society," in *Drug Abuse: Clinical and Basic Aspects,* ed. Sachindra N. Pradham and Samarendra N. Dutta (St. Louis: C. V. Mosby, 1977), p. 511.

12. Quoted in Solomon H. Snyder, "What We Have Forgotten about Pot: A Pharmacologist's History," *New York Times Magazine,* December 13, 1970, p. 125.

13. Judith S. Brook, Martin Whitman, Ann Scovell Gordon, and Patricia Cohen, "Dynamics of Childhood and Adolescent Personality Traits and Adolescent Drug Use," *Developmental Psychology* 22 (1986):403–14.

14. Erich W. Labouvre and Connell R. McGee, "Relation of Personality to Alcohol and Drug Use in Adolescence," *Journal of Consulting and Clinical Psychology* 54 (1986):289–93.

15. Frank E. Crumley, "Substance Abuse and Adolescent Suicidal Behavior," *Journal of the American Medical Association* 263 (June 13, 1990):3051–56.

16. Albert Martson, "Adolescents Who Apparently Are Vulnerable to Drug, Alcohol, and Nicotine Use," *Adolescence* 23, no. 91 (Fall 1988):93–95.

17. Ibid., 93–95.

18. Felipe G. Castro, Michael D. Newcomb, and Karen Cadish, "Lifestyle Differences between Young Adult Cocaine Users and Their Nonuser Peers," *Drug Education* 17, no. 2 (1987):89–109.

19. Lester Grinspoon, *Marijuana Reconsidered* (New York: Bantam, 1971), p. 202.

20. Richards, "Role of Society," p. 506.

21. Laura S. Smart, Thomas R. Chibucos, and Larry A. Didler, "Adolescent Substance Use and Perceived Family Functioning," *Journal of Family Issues* 11, no. 2 (June 1990):208–25.

22. Stephen Arterbur and Mary Thomsen, "Drug-Proof Your Kids," *Vibrant Life* 6, no. 7 (November/December 1990):28–29.

23. Linda Weinreb and Ellen L. Bussuk, "Substance Abuse: A Growing Problem among Homeless Families," *Family Community Health* 13, no. 1 (May 1990):55–63.

24. Donna J. Hymes, "Alcoholism: Yes, It Can Happen to You," *Current Health* 2 (February 1987):19.

25. Ibid.

26. Gary Selnow and William D. Crano, "Formal vs. Informal Group Affiliations: Implications for Alcohol and Drug Use among Adolescents," *Journal of Studies of Alcohol* 47 (1986):48–52.

27. D. L. Yanish and J. Battle, "Relationship between Self-Esteem, Depression and Alcohol Consumption among Adolescents," *Psychology Reports* 57 (1985):331–34.

28. E. R. Oetting and Fred Beauvais, "Common Elements in Youth Drug Abuse: Peer Clusters and Other Psychosocial Factors," *Journal of Drug Issues* 2 (Spring 1987):133–47.

29. Ibid.

30. José Manuel Otgero Lopez; Lourdes Redondo; Martin Miron; and Luengo Angeles, "Influence of Family and Peer Group on the Use of Drugs by Adolescents," *The International Journal of Addictions* 24, no. 11 (1989):1065–82.

31. "The Ad Made Me Do It," *Current Health,* November 1990, pp. 16–18.

32. Dan Hurley, "The Cycles of Craving," *Psychology Today,* July/August, 1989, p. 56.

33. Ibid.

34. David Gelman, et al., "Roots of Addiction," *Newsweek,* February 20, 1989, pp. 52–57.

35. Ibid.

36. Ibid.

37. Jerome Jaffe, "Drug Addiction and Drug Abuse," in *The Pharmacological Basis of Therapeutics,* 6th ed., ed. Alfred Goodman Gilman, Louis S. Goodman, and Alfred Gilman (New York: Macmillan, 1980), p. 543.

38. Manuel M. Pearson and Ralph B. Little, "The Addictive Process in Unusual Addictions: A Further Elaboration of Etiology," *The American Journal of Psychiatry* vol. 125:9, pp. 1166–71, March 1969. Copyright © 1969, The American Psychiatric Association. The quotation appears on page 1166. Used with permission.

39. Ibid.

40. Ronald A. Steffenhagen, "Drug Abuse and Related Phenomena: An Adlerian Approach," *Journal of Individual Psychology* 30, no. 2 (November 1974):240–41.

41. Ibid.

42. Pearson and Little, "The Addictive Process in Unusual Addictions," p. 1669.

43. Jaffe, "Drug Addiction and Drug Abuse," p. 543.

44. Robert Gugliemo and Arthur P. Sullivan, "Chronic Imperceptible Pain as a Cause of Addiction," *Journal of Drug Education* 15, (1985):381–87.

45. See, for example, Solomon Snyder and Steven Matthysse, eds., "Opiate Receptor Mechanisms," *Neurosciences Research Program Bulletin* 13, no. 1 (1977):48–53.

46. Solomon H. Snyder, "Opiate Receptors and Internal Opiates," *Scientific American* 236, no. 3 (March 1977):53.

47. Ibid., p. 48.

48. Ibid.

49. Ibid., p. 49.

50. Snyder and Matthysse, "Opiate Receptor Mechanisms."

51. Snyder, "Opiate Receptors and Internal Opiates," pp. 48–53.

52. Ibid.

53. Ibid.

54. Janet L. Hopson, "A Pleasurable Chemistry," *Psychology Today* 22 (July/August 1988):29–33.

55. Ibid., p. 33.

56. Deborah M. Barnes, "The Biological Tangle of Drug Addiction," *Science* 241 (July 22, 1988):415–17.

57. Carlton K. Erikson, Martin A. Javaors, and William W. Morgan, "Drug Dependence: Defining the Issues," *Advances in Alcohol and Substance Abuse* 9, no. 1–2 (1990):1–7.

CHAPTER
3

THE DRUG
SCENE

INTRODUCTION

As mentioned in Chapter 1, drug use appears to be on the decline in the United States. Table 3–1 offers an excellent overview of drug-use trends by various populations. Despite the fact that use is on a downward trend, the United States remains the biggest market for illegal drug trade. There are 40 million illegal drug users throughout the world, and half of these users are in the United States.[1] The use of drugs has become such a large problem that it has become one of our country's top priorities.

Giving law enforcement responsibility for solving society's drug problems is unfair. For any product, demand generates supply. The demand for drugs has contributed to the rise in the number of suppliers from producing countries.[2] Demand has also resulted in the increasing number of drug producers, followed by a rise in output with subsequent drop in price. Law enforcement is working very hard to reduce the supply of drugs, but society must also work to reduce demand.

In addition to being a major law enforcement problem, drug abuse in the United States is implicated in one third to half of lung cancers and coronary

TABLE 3-1 OVERVIEW OF THE 1990 NATIONAL HOUSEHOLD SURVEY ON DRUG ABUSE
Annual Drug Use, 1972 to 1990

Youth Age 12–17								
	1972	1974	1976	1977	1979	1982	1985	1988	1990
Marijuana	—	18.5%	18.4%	22.3%	24.1%	20.6%	19.7%	12.6%	11.3%
Hallucinogens	3.6	4.3	2.8	3.1	4.7	3.6	2.7	2.8	2.4
Cocaine	1.5	2.7	2.3	2.6	4.2	4.1	4.0	2.9	2.2
Heroin	*	*	*	0.6	*	*	*	0.4	0.6
Nonmedical Use of									
Stimulants	—	3.0	2.2	3.7	2.9	5.6	4.3	2.8	3.0
Sedatives	—	2.0	1.2	2.0	2.2	3.7	2.9	1.7	2.2
Tranquilizers	—	2.0	1.8	2.9	2.7	3.3	3.4	1.6	1.5
Analgesics	—	—	—	—	2.2	3.7	3.8	3.0	4.8
Alcohol	—	51.0	49.3	47.5	53.6	52.4	51.7	44.6	41.0
Cigarettes	—	—	—	—	13.3**	24.8	25.8	22.8	22.2
Any Illicit Use	—	—	—	—	26.0	22.0	23.7	16.8	15.9

Young Adults Age 18–25								
	1972	1974	1976	1977	1979	1982	1985	1988	1990
Marijuana	—	34.2%	35.0%	38.7%	46.9%	40.4%	36.9%	27.9%	24.6%
Hallucinogens	—	6.1	6.0	6.4	9.9	6.9	4.0	5.6	3.9
Cocaine	—	8.1	7.0	10.2	19.6	18.8	16.3	12.1	7.5
Heroin	—	0.8	0.6	1.2	0.8	*	0.6	0.3	0.5
Nonmedical Use of									
Stimulants	—	8.0	8.8	10.4	10.1	10.8	9.9	6.4	3.4
Sedatives	—	4.2	5.7	8.2	7.3	8.7	5.0	3.3	2.0
Tranquilizers	—	4.6	6.2	7.8	7.1	5.9	6.4	4.6	2.4
Analgesics	—	—	—	—	5.2	4.4	6.6	5.5	4.1
Alcohol	—	77.1	77.9	79.8	86.6	87.1	87.2	81.7	80.2
Cigarettes	—	—	—	—	46.7**	47.2	44.3	44.7	39.7
Any Illicit Use	—	—	—	—	49.4	43.4	42.6	32.0	28.7

Older Adults Age 26+								
	1972	1974	1976	1977	1979	1982	1985	1988	1990
Marijuana	—	3.8%	5.4%	6.4%	9.0%	10.6%	9.5%	6.9%	7.3%
Hallucinogens	—	*	*	*	0.5	0.8	1.0	0.6	0.4
Cocaine	—	*	0.6	0.9	2.0	3.8	4.2	2.7	2.4
Heroin	—	*	*	*	*	*	*	0.3	0.1
Nonmedical Use of									
Stimulants	—	*	0.8	0.8	1.3	1.7	2.6	1.7	1.0
Sedatives	—	*	0.6	*	0.8	1.4	2.0	1.2	0.8
Tranquilizers	—	*	1.2	1.1	0.9	1.1	2.8	1.8	1.0
Analgesics	—	—	—	—	0.5	1.0	2.9	2.1	1.9
Alcohol	—	62.7	64.2	65.8	72.4	72.0	73.6	68.6	66.6
Cigarettes	—	—	—	—	39.7**	38.2	36.0	33.7	31.9
Any Illicit Use	—	—	—	—	10.0	11.8	13.3	10.2	10.0

Source: National Institute on Drug Abuse, Division of Epidemiology and Prevention Research, NIDA Capsules, "National Household Survey on Drug Abuse," CAP 21 (Rockville, Md.: U.S. Department of Health and Human Services, Public Health Service, Alcohol and Mental Health Administration, 1990).

− Estimate not available

* Low precision—no estimate shown

** Includes only persons who ever smoked at least five packs.

heart disease in adults and in the majority of violent deaths (homicides, suicides, and accidents in youths).[3]

This chapter focuses on three groups involved in the drug scene—youths, adults, and older adults. We realize that there are many subgroups as well. However, these three categories will give us a start in clarifying some of the general differences among the various inhabitants of the drug scene. This chapter offers an overview of the drug scene; greater detail will be provided in later chapters.

Our culture accepts some types of drug consumption while penalizing those using other types of drugs. For example, alcohol, caffeine, and nicotine are legal and often thought of as innocuous drugs, but marijuana and cocaine are classified as illegal and dangerous substances. Whatever the drug, the problem of misuse has grown to astounding proportions. Patterns of intense drug taking have reached virtually all classes of society. The consumer can pick from many thousands of drugs now available. Furthermore, each generation seems to vary in its motivation for drug use. Youths, possessing the exuberance of young life and feeling pressures to succeed, often use drugs to satisfy the need for sensation or confidence. Adults, burdened with the pressures of family, advancing age, and the world of work, may use drugs to rest and relax. Older Americans are motivated toward drug use to ease physical pain as well as the pain of lost family and friends, fixed incomes, and sleepless nights. Drug use is a part of most people's lives.

THE YOUTH DRUG SCENE

BACKGROUND

The contemporary youth drug scene encompasses a vast number of people, from all socioeconomic classes, in their teens and early twenties. These people are confronted with rapid change, too many choices, and computerized technology that often leads to depersonalization. They face difficult and confusing decisions about education, religion, work, and the directions they will choose for their lives. Because of the tensions such decisions can bring, many youths look to drugs to temporarily escape or to look inward for solutions.

A recent study has found that drug users are increasingly younger, that use begins as early as elementary school. It has also been found that there is a growing propensity toward polydrug use (the use of several drugs), with younger students imitating the drug-taking behavior of classmates and friends.[4] Group acceptance plays a key role in this increasing drug taking. Many youths do not have the strength or the desire to resist peer pressure and often find themselves with drug-related problems. Consistent with these facts are the yearly increases in the number of liquor- and marijuana-related arrests of those under 18.

Our society is based on drugs. Nearly everyone relies upon them to cure aches and pains as well as for recreational purposes. Drug use begins very early. Chemical substances are given to infants and toddlers. Children are frequently treated with prescription drugs, over-the-counter remedies, or home remedies. In addition, youngsters are often given chemicals such as vitamins. As kids enter school they continue to use prescription and over-the-counter drugs. However, there is usually a dramatic increase in the use of caffeine in the form of chocolate, cocoa, or cola drinks.

During grades 4, 5, and 6, recreational illicit drug use and abuse begin to appear. The types of drugs used to get high are often aerosols and inhalants. These substances give a quick high and are everyday items—for example, glue—that are easily obtained. As children continue to use these substances, they often begin to experience irritation. However, they are not willing to give up the high, so they turn to other drugs. Grade schoolers may begin using tobacco, marijuana, alcohol, or amphetamines. It is alarmingly easy for children as young as 11 or 12 to obtain drugs.[5]

Children often have their first experience with alcohol in grades 5 and 6. Many of these children have older siblings who are drinkers, or alcoholic parents. At the junior high, alcohol and marijuana use increases; it is often associated with school dances or other evening functions. The ease of buying drugs such as marijuana and speed contributes to their increased use at the junior high level. At the high school there is much greater use of a wider variety of drugs. Serious problems, such as dependency and drug-related accidents and fatalities, are more frequent.

Alcohol and tobacco cigarettes continue to be widely used by high school–age and younger students, but the use of the latter appears to be leveling off or declining. Cigarettes are frequently smoked in emulation of adults or as a status symbol. Girls from 12 to 18 seem to be the fastest-growing group of tobacco smokers, but this increase has leveled off recently to the point where about the same percentage of boys and girls smoke.

Abuse of alcoholic beverages by youth is tolerated by some parents because they fear their child's use of other drugs and believe alcohol is not as habit forming or dangerous. In addition, the use of alcohol does not carry a social stigma for them, and the legal consequences for its use are not as severe as those for other drugs. In effect, most parents are more familiar with alcohol than with other drugs and can identify with its effects. Alcohol is still generally thought to be the drug used in the greatest *quantity* by youth.

Four surveys in Northeast Ohio questioned students on frequency of drug use, reasons for taking drugs, and smokeless tobacco use.[6] These surveys were supposed to inform us of the drug trends these students go through in school, including pressures from society. The ten categories of drugs most used by students were reported to be as follows:

1. coffee
2. aspirin
3. cigarettes
4. alcohol
5. marijuana
6. inhalants
7. cocaine

8. amphetamines

9. barbiturates

10. narcotics

Inhalants, alcohol, cigarettes, amphetamines, coffee, and narcotics all showed the highest percentage reported in ten years for both males and females.

One of the most important findings of this survey was a steady increase in the perceived harm associated with the use of all drugs except coffee and aspirin. A second major finding was that females perceived a higher health risk than males in using all categories of drugs.

Two substances used by young people require special attention—alcohol and crack. Nearly all adolescents have experimented with alcohol. This does not mean that they all use it regularly. Even so, alcohol use among teenagers is common at parties and tied very closely with socializing. Many teenagers view drinking as being cool and grown up. What is not cool are alcohol's physical and mental effects on the body, particularly a body that is still growing, and the number of injuries and deaths caused by drinking and driving. Drinking is thought to be common among teenagers because alcohol is easy to obtain and fairly inexpensive. Many teenagers feel that it is fine to drink as long as they do not use other drugs because alcohol is not as bad as marijuana, cocaine, speed, or downers—or so they think. And, as we have seen, parents often accept drinking by their kids in exchange for their not taking "harder" drugs. What most parents and kids do not realize is that alcohol use is often a precursor to the use of other drugs, not to mention its other hazardous effects.

Crack has received much publicity recently because of its sudden emergence as a powerful and lethal substance. True crack provides an intense high almost instantly, leaving plenty of opportunity for accidental overdose and death. Because it is fairly easy to obtain and inexpensive compared with other drugs, crack is fast becoming a popular drug among young people.

Aside from dangerous behavior, there are the physical and mental consequences of taking a chemical. Drugs block, retard, or distort the most crucial human capacities, and this loss of function is rewarded by surpassingly pleasurable sensations. According to educator Richard Hawley:

> American children are most likely to make their initial decision to try intoxicating drugs between the ages of 12 and 16: during the peak years of adolescent growth. During these years, every cell and tissue of the body is either altered or replaced altogether. Sexual potency, nearly all of one's adult skeletal stature, and the capacity for higher-order mental functions are produced during this developmental surge.[7]

Hawley continues by saying, "Chemically anesthetizing oneself with drugs serves only to delay maturation—or in some cases to replace it altogether—often with lifelong consequences."[8]

The use of steroids in high schools has become a problem, and the drugs are gaining a following among nonathletes. Instead of taking steroids to make themselves bigger and stronger for athletic competition, high school boys are taking the drugs to "bulk up for the girls."[9] There is pressure on high school students to look good physically, and many boys perceive steroids to be a shortcut to an attractive, muscular body.

A study done by two psychology professors from the University of California, Los Angeles, gives some frightening results but also offers some consoling ones.[10] The study watched 700 teenagers from the area over an eight-year period. This is a reliable longitudinal study, one of the first of its kind to determine the effects that teenage drug and alcohol use can have on later life. The study positively says large doses of drugs throughout the teenage years leads to problems in adulthood. Those who used drugs and alcohol in their teens tend to divorce more rapidly, have problems keeping jobs, commit more crimes, and are generally not as happy with their lives as their counterparts as adults. One consolation this study has for parents is that teens who just try drugs once a month or so are left unaffected.

The results of the 1990 High School Senior Survey on Drug Abuse, an annual survey sponsored by the National Institute on Drug Abuse and conducted by the University of Michigan, indicate a continuing drop in the percentage of high school seniors and young adults who are using illicit drugs.[11] For the first time in the 16 years this annual survey has been conducted, less than half the students surveyed have tried an illicit drug. This is part of a continuing decline since the 1980s, when up to 66 percent of seniors had tried an illicit drug at least once. Some of the significant findings of this survey include the following:

- Crack use by high school seniors decreased significantly between 1989 and 1990. In 1990, 0.7 percent of seniors had used crack within the past month, which is half the 1989 rate of 1.4 percent. Annual use of crack also decreased significantly by about two-fifths, from 3.1 percent in 1989 to 1.9 percent in 1990.

- All measures of marijuana use decreased significantly between 1989 and 1990. Lifetime prevalence of marijuana use decreased significantly from 43.7 percent in 1989 to 40.7 percent in 1990. Annual prevalence decreased from 29.6 percent in 1989 to 27.0 percent, and current use decreased from 16.7 percent to 14.0 percent between 1989 and 1990. Marijuana remains the most widely used illicit drug among high school seniors.

- Annual use of PCP decreased from 2.4 percent in 1989 to 1.2 percent in 1990, continuing an almost 60 percent decline from 1985. The percentage of seniors using PCP in the past month decreased from 1.43 percent in 1989 to 0.4 percent in 1990.

- Rates of cigarette smoking by high school seniors continued to be high. There was no decrease from 1989 to 1990 in daily cigarette smoking, which has remained virtually the same rate over the past seven surveys. The proportion of seniors who smoked at least one cigarette daily has remained around 19 percent since 1984, and the percentage of seniors who smoked a half pack a day has remained around 11 percent since 1986.

- Current use of alcohol decreased, from 60.0 percent in 1989 to 57.1 percent in 1990. The percentage of seniors reporting daily alcohol use remained around 4 percent in 1989 and 1990. The percentage of seniors who had five or more drinks in a row within the past two weeks also remained about the same, 33.0 percent in 1989 and 32.2 percent in 1990.
- The percentage of seniors saying they see "great risk" in trying cocaine in the crack or powder form increased significantly. Since 1987, the first year data on crack were collected, the proportion seeing great harm in using crack regularly has increased from 84.6 percent to 91.6 percent.
- Follow-up data on the young adults who are in college show that lifetime, annual, and current cocaine use decreased significantly between 1989 and 1990. Lifetime use decreased from 14.6 percent in 1989 to 11.4 percent in 1990; annual use from 8.2 percent to 5.6 percent; and current use from 2.8 percent to 1.2 percent.

DRUGS ON CAMPUS

The social values that swept the nation's campuses in the 1960s are now shared by many students and deeply influence the whole of society. According to Daniel Yankelovich, "These new values are not simply a matter of adopting a freer, more casual life style. They symbolize a profound value transformation affecting every phase of life."[12]

These values can be divided into three domains: (1) moral norms, consisting of more liberal sexual attitudes, changes in one's relation to authority institutions, different attitudes toward churches and organized religion as a behavior guide, and a change in traditional concepts of patriotism and national allegiance; (2) new values pertaining to the Protestant work ethic, marriage, family, and success defined in terms of money; and (3) a vague but intense concern with self-fulfillment, a feeling that there must be more to life than just working to make ends meet.[13] Drug use is associated with each of the three areas: It is often considered an expression of political consciousness; it may cause a person to relinquish obligations to friends and country; and it may initiate dissatisfaction with work and work-related problems.

In college, marijuana, alcohol, cocaine, and amphetamines are the drugs of choice. (See Table 3–2).

College students who are involved with drugs appear to differ vastly from students who don't use drugs. Drug users are usually nonconformists in terms of academic performance, political activity, religious conviction, and involvement with the law.[14] According to Armand Nicholi, the more frequently students use marijuana, the more nonconforming and rebellious they are. Students who use harder drugs are even more deviant than the marijuana users. Users in general are more involved in stealing, brawling, vandalism, and truancy.

Users and nonusers also differ in religious faith. Nicholi cites statistics showing that 45 percent of nonusers report that their faith is very important to them, compared with 21 percent of marijuana and hard drug users.[15]

The number of college students who have experimented with cocaine, or are choosing to use cocaine instead of marijuana, has increased substan-

TABLE 3.2   COLLEGE STUDENTS SURVEY ON DRUG USE, 1980–1989

The following tables are part of the nationwide survey of drug use among high school seniors, conducted annually for the National Institute on Drug Abuse by the University of Michigan Institute for Social Research. Each year since 1977, some participants from all previously graduated high school classes have been followed through the use of mailed questionnaires. These follow-up surveys include a sample of about 1,200 full time American college students one to four years past high school.

Trends in Annual Prevalence of Fourteen Types of Drugs Among College Students 1–4 Years beyond High School

Percent who used in the last twelve months

	1980	1981	1982	1983	1984	1985	1986	1987	1988	1989
Approx. Wtd. N-	(1040)	(1130)	(1150)	(1170)	(1110)	(1080)	(1190)	(1220)	(1310)	(1300)
Marijuana	51.2	51.3	44.7	45.2	40.7	41.7	40.9	37.0	34.6	33.6
Inhalants [b]	3.0	2.5	2.5	2.8	2.4	3.1	3.9	3.7	4.1	3.7
Hallucinogens	8.5	7.0	8.7	6.5	6.2	5.0	6.0	5.9	5.3	5.1
LSD	6.0	4.6	6.3	4.3	3.7	2.2	3.9	4.0	3.6	3.4
Cocaine	16.8	16.0	17.2	17.3	16.3	17.3	17.1	13.7	10.0	8.2
Crack [c]	NA	NA	NA	NA	NA	NA	1.3	2.0	1.4	1.5
Heroin	0.4	0.2	0.1	0.0	0.1	0.2	0.1	0.2	0.2	0.1
Other Opiates [a]	5.1	4.3	3.8	3.8	3.8	2.4	4.0	3.1	3.1	3.2
Stimulants [a]	22.4	22.2	NA	NA	NA	NA	NA	NA	NA	NA
Stimulants, Adjusted [a,d]	NA	NA	21.1	17.3	15.7	11.9	10.3	7.2	6.2	4.6
Sedatives [a]	8.3	8.0	8.0	4.5	3.5	2.5	2.6	1.7	1.5	1.0
Barbiturates [a]	2.9	2.8	3.2	2.2	1.9	1.3	2.0	1.2	1.1	1.0
Methaqualone [a]	7.2	6.5	6.6	3.1	2.5	1.4	1.2	0.8	0.5	0.2
Tranquilizers [a]	6.9	4.8	4.7	4.6	3.5	3.6	4.4	3.8	3.1	2.6
Alcohol	90.5	92.5	92.2	91.6	90.0	92.0	91.5	90.9	89.6	89.6
Cigarettes	36.2	37.6	34.3	36.1	33.2	35.0	35.3	38.0	36.6	34.2

Source: National Institute on Drug Abuse, NIDA Capsules, "College Students Survey on Drug Use 1980–1989," CAP 16 (Rockville; Md.: U.S. Department of Health and Human Services, Public Health Service, Alcohol and Drug Abuse and Mental Health Administration, 1990).

Notes: NA indicates data not available.

[a] Only drug use which was not under a doctor's orders is included here

[b] This drug was asked about in four of the five questionnaire forms. M is four fifths of N indicated

[c] This drug was asked about in one of the five questionnaire forms in 1986 (M is one fifth of N indicated), and in two of the five questionnaire forms thereafter (N is two fifths of N indicated)

[d] Based on the data from the revised question, which attempts to exclude the inappropriate reporting of non-prescription stimulants

tially. The University of Michigan's Institution for Social Research (ISR) released a follow-up study of drug users revealing that an estimated 30 percent of all students have used cocaine by the end of their fourth year in college.[16] This use continues past college: An estimated 40 percent of all people age 26 or 27 who have completed high school and college have tried cocaine.

Studies indicate that few students associate any risk with experimenting with cocaine, even though its addictive potential and other medical dangers are known publicly. However, these studies were published before the highly publicized deaths of star athletes Len Bias and Don Rogers. Bias collapsed and died from the effects of cocaine ingestion two days before he was to sign with the Boston Celtics. A few days later Rogers, of the Cleveland Browns, died a similar death the night before he was to be married. It remains to be seen whether these deaths have influenced college students' perceptions of the medical risks associated with cocaine use.

DRUGS IN THE MILITARY

In 1988, both licit and illicit drug use was shown to be higher among men in the military services than among civilians of the same age. In the early 1970s, however, drug use in the military was more than simply high—it reached epidemic proportions in Vietnam.

Drug Use by Servicemen in Vietnam   The unusual setting and circumstances of the Vietnam War provide a unique perspective on the drug scene. In Southeast Asia, all varieties of drugs except hallucinogens were plentiful, inexpensive, and easy to obtain.[17] Initially, marijuana was the most popular drug among American servicemen there, so much so that the rate of use grew to alarming proportions, even in the field of combat. Eventually, this extensive use became of great concern to the military and to a number of

Vietnam Soldier Smoking
Marijuana
Source: AP/Wide World Photos

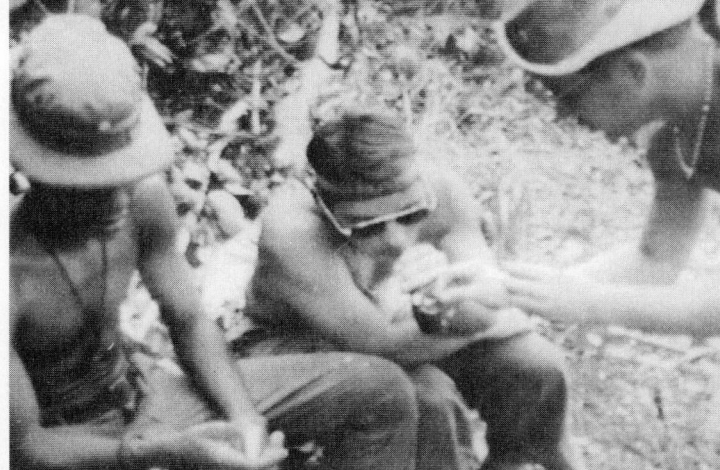

stateside politicians, resulting in rigid controls and sanctions regarding marijuana use. At that point servicemen were forced to seek alternatives, and they
turned to opiates, which were also readily available and inexpensive. In time
purified heroin became the most commonly used opiate by American GIs.
Injection, the stateside method of heroin administration, was rare. Vietnam
heroin, because of its high purity, was usually smoked or inhaled. Thus the
geographical setting, in which heroin was easily accessible, played an important role in the Vietnam drug scene.

By the early 1970s, drug use by servicemen in Vietnam was epidemic.
Chemical tests as well as various military surveys showed that by 1972
approximately 7 percent of Army enlisted men were using heroin. In 1974,
counselors in the Army drug program estimated that well over half of the
lower-ranking enlisted men were using hashish or marijuana.[18]

Reasons for Drug Use in Vietnam   One of the most common reasons for drug use in Vietnam was a desire to escape mental and physical pain
and fear. The social setting was also a factor, since military morale was generally very low, few regarded their duty as useful, and off-duty time was often
boring and frustrating. Since many soldiers felt that Vietnam was not part of
the "real world," behavior was permitted there that would not normally have
been condoned stateside.[19] There was also the cultural shock associated with
combat in a foreign country. Finally, peer pressure played a significant role in
soldiers' drug involvement.

Treatment for Returning Vietnam Veterans   In December 1970,
the United States Army took responsibility for treatment and prevention of
drug abuse. The program the Army developed consisted of diagnosis, drug-
education classes, rehabilitation through group therapy and medication,
cooperation with civilian authorities in reducing drug traffic, and amnesty for
those who voluntarily sought treatment. The Free Radical Assay Technique
(FRAT) was used to detect heroin in the urine; other tests measured barbiturate, amphetamine, opiate, and methadone involvement. Treatment centers
were set up in barracks, hospitals, and prisonlike settings. Diagnosis was
made by a physician, and treatment ranged from four days to two weeks.

Many soldiers, however, lacked trust in the military justice system. They
considered amnesty a hoax and felt they would be harassed if they joined the
program.[20] Servicemen participated in the program primarily out of fear of not
returning home on time, or fear of punishment or prosecution. The Army's
goal of total elimination of the drug problem may have been unrealistic.

Conclusion   What lessons may be learned from the Vietnam experience? First, as shown by the Army's attempt to stop marijuana use, high-pressure
drug control is usually ineffective and may instead promote a switch to other
drugs. Second, the belief that a drug problem can be eliminated by cutting off
the drug's availability is incorrect. Third, people usually seek periodic escape as
a way of coping with stressful situations; one of the means of escape can be drug
use or abuse. Fourth, a high rate of drug use may be a response to a specific set-

ting, as demonstrated by returning servicemen who reverted to preservice patterns of drug use, which included high marijuana use and amphetamine, barbiturate, and narcotics use, in descending order of frequency.

The U.S. military services have long condoned and at times encouraged the use of alcohol. In ancient times, the victors of a war would celebrate with an elaborate feast that included large quantities of alcohol. More recently the military has made available liquor rations to soldiers and sailors. For example, in World War II, Air Force pilots were given a 2-ounce shot of liquor after returning from a combat mission "to relieve stress."[21] Alcohol has not only been used in wartime settings; it has been used extensively in peacetime social activities as well—"hail and farewells," "dining-ins," military balls, and so on.

To cut down on the use of alcohol, the U.S. military will not promote any official or unofficial function that "glamorizes" abuse of alcohol through drinking contests, games, or initiations. In addition, nonalcoholic beverages are to be made available at any function. Violation of these rules will subject the violator to failure-to-obey-an-order regulations.[22] Furthermore, unit commanders are to publicize that the abuse of alcohol and other drugs will not be condoned within their unit and that commissioned and noncommissioned officers who drink will set examples of responsible drinking. A study done in fall 1985 showed that the number of heavy drinkers among the 2.1 million men and women in the armed forces decreased from 14 percent in 1982 to 11.9 percent in 1985. However, the number of moderate drinkers increased from 29.5 percent to 31.1 percent, suggesting that alcohol problems are still present in the military.[23]

As a result, the Army has developed an alcohol-abuse program that provides general policies for preventing and controlling alcohol abuse. The program also recommends treatment and rehabilitation techniques. The program focuses on four key areas: prevention, identification, detoxification, and rehabilitation. In addition to these extensive programs, bartenders in officers' and NCO clubs can now be held responsible for serving those who are intoxicated. This has led to a "designated driver" program that allows one person in a group to receive free soft drinks so that he or she remains sober to drive.[24] There are other incentives as well. At Warren Air Force Base in Wyoming, everyone in a squadron that has no drunk driving offenses within the previous six months gets an extra day off. This type of peer pressure seems to be working.[25]

DRUGS AND ATHLETICS

Introduction   Drug use has been reported throughout the sports world, from amateur athletics to professional sports. Most of the drugs used come under two headings: restorative and ergogenic (additive). Restorative drugs are used with the intent of returning the athlete to a previous level of proficiency following illness, injury, or performance anxiety. These drugs may include antiinflammatory agents, pain killers, and tranquilizers used as muscle relaxants. Ergogenic drugs are used with the intent of enhancing an athlete's normal ability. These drugs may include anabolic steroids and amphetamines.

The use of ergogenic aids is a growing problem in today's athletic community and has led to rigid drug testing. An ergogenic aid is defined as any substance that will improve not only athletic performance but work level as well. Therefore, it may be inferred that industrial workers share the same interest in ergogenic aids that discus throwers might have. Athletes have used a variety of supposedly ergogenic substances to improve performance. Alcohol, amphetamines, anabolic steroids, caffeine, hormones, and protein supplements are examples.

Drug Use in College and Amateur Athletics   The reports on college athletic drug use are somewhat ambiguous. Numerous claims have been made about the pregame use of novocaine and other analgesics, amphetamines, and tranquilizers for muscle relaxation, but it is difficult to estimate the amount of drugs being used. College coach Tom Ecker, however, says, "It's a great rarity today for someone to achieve athletic success who doesn't take drugs."[26]

Steroids   Along with amphetamines, anabolic steroids are probably the most prevalent drugs used today by athletes in international competition. "Introduced in the late 1950's, anabolic steroids are synthetic derivatives of the male hormone testosterone. They stimulate a building up, or anabolic, process in the body through synthesis of protein for muscle growth and tissue repair."[27] Athletes use steroids for a variety of reasons. "First of all, competitors have discovered that anabolic steroids allow them to recover more quickly from workout sessions, which in turn makes more intense training possible."[28] They also use them to increase aggressiveness and build strength. Overall, athletes use steroids to gain a competitive edge.

Steroids

Anabolic steroids are synthetic derivatives of the male hormone testosterone. They stimulate a building up, or anabolic, process in the body through synthesis of protein for muscle growth and tissue repair. Athletes have discovered that anabolic steroids allow them to recover more quickly from workout sessions, which in turn makes more intense training possible.

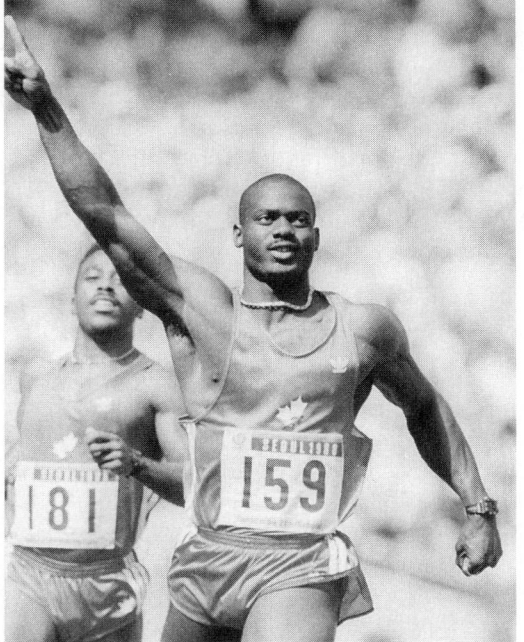

Positive Steroid Test Takes Away Gold Medal
Source: AP/Wide World Photos

ANABOLIC STEROIDS[29]

Examples:

Dianabol, synthetic testosterone, all steroids banned by the International Olympic Committee.

Common Users:

Athletes requiring muscularity and strength; some athletes in almost every sport are using steroids today, including football and the Olympic sports of weightlifting, wrestling, track and field, rowing, boxing, and cycling.

Athletic Benefits:

Increased lean muscle mass and secondary strength when used in conjunction with training; no medical support exists to indicate that steroids alone increase muscularity or strength; the notion held by some athletes that steroids help injuries to mend more quickly is medically unfounded.

When the Body Gets Too Much:

Anabolic steroids are synthetic versions of the naturally occurring male hormone testosterone. The two substances have pharmacological action and side effects that are very similar. In mature males, 2.5–10 milligrams of testosterone are secreted by the body each day to promote various body processes. Steroid use often introduces up to an additional 100 milligrams of testosterone into the system daily. When testosterone levels get too high, the hypothalamus in the brain starts to shut down the body processes involving the hormone. These processes include, in men, stimulation and maintenance of the sex organs, including the penis, prostate gland, and semen sacs. In women, little testosterone is naturally produced, so an impact on the body is felt quickly, leading to the development of masculine body characteristics. Other processes influenced by testosterone and at risk to shut down are development of bones and muscles, skin maintenance, hair growth, and emotional response.

Male Reproductive System:

Too much testosterone or related substances, that is, steroids, prompts the pituitary gland to stop producing the hormone gonadotropin. This in turn stops the testicles from producing testosterone, which leads to a distortion of male characteristics, such as testicular atrophy, lowered sperm count, sterility (reversible), priapism (painful, prolonged erection), prostate enlargement, and frequent or continuing erections. When steroids are stopped, the testosterone-producing function may remain shut down, leading to an imbalance of male and female hormones.

Cardiovascular:

Steroids can cause fluid retention, which in turn can lead to high blood pressure. Steroids also lower high-density lipoproteins (HDLs) in the blood. These HDLs help rid the body of cholesterol. In some cases, production of low-density lipoproteins (LDLs), which promote the production of cholesterol, increases. Too much cholesterol leads to a buildup of plaque on the walls of arteries. Clogged arteries can result in stroke or heart attack.

Liver:

Steroid users risk peliosis hepatitis, a disease in which the liver and sometimes the splenic tissue is replaced with blood-filled cysts. These cysts sometimes have little impact on liver functions but at other times have been associated with liver failure. The cysts are often not detected until life-threatening liver failure or intra-abdominal bleeding develops. Withdrawal from steroids usually results in the complete disappearance of the disease. Liver cell tumors are also a possible side effect. The tumors are most often benign, but some fatal malignant tumors have been reported. Withdrawal from steroids often results in the recession of the tumors or stops their progression. Like the cysts in peliosis hepatitis, these tumors are often not detected until life-threatening circumstances develop.

Female Reproductive System:

These side effects are the result of masculinization due to increased testosterone and include enlargement of the clitoris, uterine atrophy, irregularity or cessation of menstrual cycle, increased body hair, deepening of the voice, shrinkage of breast size, and masculinization of female fetuses in pregnant women.

Adolescents:

Bone growth is among the body processes that can shut down with steroid use. Adolescents on steroids may find their muscle bulking up, but bone growth stops with premature fusion of the epiphysis—growth center—of long bones. Permanently stunted growth results. There is a risk until bones stop growing, generally at age 18 in boys and 16 in girls. Other side effects experienced by adolescents include penis enlargement and increased frequency of erections in boys and masculinization in girls.

Psychological:

Psychological side effects of steroids are just beginning to be recognized and studied. Of greatest concern is aggressive behavior or "roid" rage, characterized by displays of violence or prolonged temper tantrums. Other effects can be mood swings, increased libido, and depression and other withdrawal symptoms when steroids are stopped.

SIDE EFFECTS OF STEROID ABUSE[30]

Altered liver function, sometimes causing hepatitis and possibly causing liver cancer

Altered blood metabolism, potentially leading to a buildup of plaque in blood vessels, a major cause of strokes and heart attacks

High blood pressure

Nosebleeds

Atrophy of testicles, sometimes to the point of sterility

Clitoral enlargement and cessation of menstruation in women

Early onset of male-pattern baldness

Growth of body hair and dark facial hair in women; sometimes male-pattern baldness in women

Increased aggressiveness

Development of breast tissue and tender nipples in men, sometimes requiring breast-reduction surgery

Deeper voice

Acne

Stunted growth of long bones in adolescents

Athletes take anabolic steroids in a cyclic manner, with "drug holidays" between periods of use. They usually start with a low dose, progressively increase the amount until the maximum dose is reached, then taper the dosage until the drug is completely withdrawn. This pyramiding achieves an optimal anabolic effect while minimizing the chance of detection during competition.[31] Other athletes "stack the pyramid," using numerous drugs and varying the dosage throughout the cycle. No scientific evidence supports the idea that "stacking" or "pyramiding" the drugs is more effective than other methods of using them, or that it minimizes the harmful side effects of steroid use.

The dosages used by athletes vary widely, but they may be as high as 40 times the therapeutic amounts. Most anabolic steroid regimens include a combination of injectable and oral preparations. The majority of athletes obtain their drugs illegally; 20 percent of the respondents to one survey claimed to have received them by prescription.[32] An average midcycle dosage is about 200 milligrams daily. At the very top of the stack, however, a person could be taking as much as 600 milligrams a day.

Not all research findings on steroids are negative. Steroids still fulfill their original purpose of increasing the intake of protein to build muscles in patients suffering from chronic diseases and to protect blood cells from destruction by radiation and chemotherapy.[33] In addition, steroids are used in the treatment of burns, hormonal imbalances, certain bone diseases, such as osteoporosis, and some cases of effeminacy. Last, they can help control muscle-wasting diseases and certain kinds of anemia and speed healing after surgery or long illness.

Male high school students reported that the main reason for taking anabolic steroids was to boost athletic performance. But there were a surprising number who took the drug just to improve their appearance at school.[34] The more and more that appearance plays a role in popularity, especially in high school, the more you will see males trying to increase their size just to get attention. A study was done to determine the extent of steroid use and knowledge about the drug.[35] When asked about the side effects of steroid use, they found only 30 percent of users were able to identify stunted growth, 38 percent liver disease, 35 percent cancer of the liver, and 18 percent acne. Of the users, 22 percent were not aware of any complications associated with steroid use.

Professional Sports   Some professional athletes take amphetamines to "get up" and barbiturates or depressants to "come down." In general, professional football players appear to use amphetamines in three ways.[36] The first is ingestion of high doses (30 to 150 milligrams or more) only on game days for pain relief and the induction of rage. (A linebacker recalled a game in which he took a little extra amphetamine: "I was bouncing all over the field. . . . I was running and jumping along the sidelines hollering, I'm a superplayer, they can't block me. No one can block me, it was really funny, I knew what I was saying but I just didn't care."[37] The second involves taking lower doses (5 to 30 milligrams) on game days to increase speed and combat pain. The third, also used for weight control by other professional athletes, such as jockeys, boxers, and wrestlers (approximately 15 milligrams per day), is usually confined to the first several weeks of summer camp and the preseason, when overweight players must lose weight quickly.

The results of abuse of these drugs are often dramatic and carry over from the playing field to the players' family life as well.[38] Pathological jealousy, wife abuse, drinking binges, fighting, and various physiologic ailments can be caused by such abuse, and other drugs, such as sleeping pills, may be needed to bring the players down. Bob Lundy, Miami Dolphins trainer, comments: "I've seen players in a daze as late as Tuesday after Sunday's game. . . . Some need a week to come down after a game. It's a continuous cycle; pepped up, drunk (or tranquilized), hung over, and pepped up.[39]

The impact of cocaine on the professional sports arena has been incredible. A number of lives and teams have been devastated by this white powder. The acknowledgment of cocaine in the sporting world has been fairly recent.

But the presence of this very powerful psychoactive substance in professional sports has been increasingly documented since the mid-1970s. More and more professional athletes have been linked to its use.

In 1985 the National Basketball Association enacted the toughest drug regulations in professional sports history. Detection of cocaine use could result in a lifetime ban from the sport. These measures were drafted in response to drug-related incidents involving a number of name players, including David Thompson of Denver, John Drew of Atlanta, Michael Ray Richardson of the New York Knicks, and John Lucas of Houston.

What all of this points out, among other things, is that professional athletes have been favored targets of drug traffickers. This is nothing new, really. The main difference is in the drugs being trafficked. Professional athletes cannot escape drug traffickers, who hang out at every arena, restaurant, and hotel making themselves available for purchases. The public is led to believe by the media that the life of professional athletes is exciting, glamorous, and full of "the jazz." In reality, quite often, nothing could be further from the truth. Athletes are human and fall to the same temptations as others in our society. The endless repetition of one-night stands, hotel rooms, and restaurant food makes the travel life of the professional athlete tiring and, worse yet, boring. Cocaine use is in many instances tantamount to an antiboredom remedy.

The mandate is clear. Each professional league must enforce strict measures concerning drug use and abuse. The drug-related media notoriety showered on athletes in the 1980s can be reversed. It is obvious that without the external motivation of enforcement the status of professional athlete will continue to decline, further lessening the attractiveness of professional sports in general.

THE ADULT DRUG SCENE

Four major drug groups are used by adults: (1) alcohol, (2) barbiturates, tranquilizers, and sedatives, (3) nicotine, and (4) caffeine. Drugs used with less frequency include aspirin, amphetamines, marijuana, and opiates.

The following update on adult use comes from the 1990 National Household Survey on Drug Abuse (Table 3–1):[40]

- Overall in 1990, 74.4 million Americans age 12 or older (37 percent of the population) had tried marijuana, cocaine, or other illicit drugs at least once in their lifetime.

- Almost 27 million Americans (13.3 percent) used marijuana, cocaine, or other illicit drugs at least once in the past year.

- Among young adults (18 to 25 years old) 28.7 percent used an illicit drug in the past year and 14.9 percent used an illicit drug at least once during the past month; among adults (26 years old and over), 10.0 percent used an illicit drug in the past year and 4.6 percent used an illicit drug at least once during the past month.

- The overall current (past-month) prevalence rate for any illicit drug use (12 years old and over) was 6.4 percent. Rates for males and females are

7.9 percent and 5.1 percent, respectively. In addition to males, other demographic subgroups with rates in excess of the overall rate are those for blacks (8.6 percent), large metro areas (7.3 percent), those living in the West (7.3 percent), and the unemployed population (14.0 percent).

- Over 4.8 million, or 8 percent, of the 60.1 million women 15–44 years of age (the height of childbearing years) have used an illicit drug in the past month. Slightly over 0.5 million, or 0.9 percent, used cocaine and 3.9 million (6.5 percent) used marijuana in the past month.

- Among 18–34-year-old full-time employed Americans, 24.4 percent used an illicit drug in the past year, and 10.5 percent used an illicit drug in the past month. Of these full-time workers, 9.2 percent used marijuana, and 2.1 percent used cocaine in the past month.

ALCOHOL

Alcohol use is widespread among adults: Approximately 70 to 75 percent use it. Though most adults are moderate drinkers, some become alcohol-dependent. The majority of these are males, though more and more women are now drinking.

The problem drinker and the alcoholic encounter many problems. They may expect a 10- to 12-year decrease in life expectancy. They may experience personal problems, including love-relationship difficulties. A tremendous economic loss may result from their drinking, affecting them and their families as well as the nation. In addition, approximately half of all fatal motor-vehicle accidents and one third of all suicides are alcohol-related.[41]

Alcohol is also responsible for half of adult deaths by fire and plays a significant role in drowning. The overall economic costs of alcoholism are difficult to estimate. In terms of lost production, health expenses, violent crimes, and traffic accidents, alcoholism and alcohol misuse have been estimated to cost from $43 billion to $120 billion a year.[42]

TRANQUILIZERS AND SEDATIVE-HYPNOTICS

According to the National Clearinghouse for Drug Abuse Information, studies of the late 1960s and early 1970s showed widespread adult use of both tranquilizers and sedative-hypnotics (barbiturates and nonbarbiturates), with the former more popular.[43] Seventy percent of all adults in a 1974 California study frequently used sedative-hypnotics, and 10 percent used minor tranquilizers. Almost twice as many women as men are frequent tranquilizer users, and Caucasians, people between 30 and 60 from middle-socioeconomic classes, and people with higher education levels are most likely to be regular users.[44]

What complications arise from heavy depressant use? The short-term psychological and behavioral effects of barbiturates are similar to those of another depressant, alcohol.[45] Depending on conditions, a low dose can either relax or excite a person. Heavy use, however, may cause apathy, reduced drive, and reduced ambition. It may also cause death (often in combination with alcohol), from accidental overdose or suicide.[46] Such abuse occurs more frequently among women (80 percent) than among men (20 percent). If barbiturates are used in high enough doses to cause tolerance and dependence, withdrawal may lead to convulsions severe enough to be life-threatening.

NICOTINE

Generally speaking, cigarette smoking is more common among males than females, in cities than in small towns, among people from 20 to 44, and among alcoholics than nonalcoholics. It is least common among people 65 and older. As the hazards of smoking have become better known, more and more people have succeeded in quitting the habit. Doctors have been leaders—less than 21 percent now smoke. Still, many Americans die each year of cigarette-induced heart attacks, lung cancer, chronic bronchitis, and emphysema. The amount of cigarette-induced illness and loss of work, money, and enjoyment of life is proportionately heavy.

CAFFEINE

Although caffeine is found in chocolate and cola drinks, most adults in the United States ingest it through coffee. The National Center for Health Statistics reports that adult Americans currently average about three cups of coffee per day, or about 12 pounds per year.[47] Alfred Gilman and Louis Goodman report that

> over indulgence in xanthine* beverages may lead to a condition that might be considered one of chronic poisoning. Central nervous stimulation results in restlessness and disturbed sleep; myocardial stimulation is reflected in cardio-irregularities; essential oils of coffee may cause some gastro intestinal irritation; and diarrhea is a common symptom.[48]

Quite frequently a dependent caffeine user experiences prolonged headaches during periods of abstinence from caffeine, only to find relief several minutes after drinking one cup of coffee.

The morning cup of coffee and coffee breaks are definitely part of the American lifestyle. And because so many people drink coffee, it has somehow become legitimate to consume the stimulant it contains. The consumption of coffee, with its relatively low cost and easy availability, has become an accepted ritual of socialization.

ASPIRIN

According to Oakley Ray, "There are over 300 aspirin-containing products on the American market. Each day Americans gobble down about 44 million aspirin tablets. Twenty-one tons of aspirin (acetylsalicylic acid) a day."[49] If we consider the tremendous availability and use of aspirin, the high incidence of toxic reactions (salicylate poisoning) that may result in death (the number one cause of poisoning in children under five) and the incidence of aspirin-related gastrointestinal disorders should come as no surprise. The toxicity of the salicylates in aspirin is underestimated, and they should not be viewed as a harmless household remedy. Aspirin would have great difficulty being approved by the FDA as an over-the-counter drug on the basis of today's knowledge and standards.

AMPHETAMINES

At one time, overweight adults used amphetamines to control their appetite. Others used them to overcome fatigue and to keep alert while driving. Now, however, amphetamine use is not nearly as widespread among American adults. Production and prescription rates dropped dramatically in the mid-1970s. Still, adults with long working hours or taxing schedules may find the temporary relief offered by amphetamines extremely desirable. In 1972 federal regulatory agencies began to limit the production of amphetamines by pharmaceutical companies. In 1978 the FDA removed amphetamines as an approved medication for obesity, and the legitimate medical use of amphetamines (for such conditions as narcolepsy) is much lower today.[50]

MARIJUANA

The use of marijuana as a psychoactive substance has become more and more popular with adults. Many of those who began as youthful marijuana users have continued their use into their adult years. Lessening fear of physical harm from marijuana and the lessening legal penalties for possession of it have made the drug more acceptable.

OPIATES

For most adults, narcotic abuse begins in response to pain. Adults also take opiates to relieve anxiety and to enjoy the strong euphoric effect the drugs offer. Once tolerance develops, though, it becomes necessary to increase the amount taken to achieve the desired effect: Continued use and increased amounts may lead to dependence. According to the National Clearinghouse for Drug Information:

> Figures show that more than half [of narcotic dependents] are under 30 years of age. . . . All narcotic addiction in the United States is not limited to heroin users. Some middle-aged and older people who take narcotic drugs regularly to relieve pain can also become addicted. So do some people who can obtain opiates easily, such as doctors and nurses. They take injections to keep going under pressure and eventually find themselves locked into narcotic addiction.[51]

THE WORKPLACE

Daily use of illegal drugs, not to mention legal ones, is common in the U.S. workplace today. No longer can it be said that drug use on the job amounts to a few isolated incidents. Drugs have invaded industry, from factory workers to white-collar middle management on up to chief executive officers. "Substance abuse . . . is costing the business community $160 billion a year and is responsible for eroding productivity, industrial accidents, absenteeism and tardiness, and inflating health care costs."[52] General Motors estimates it lost $1 billion alone due to substance abuse. This raised the cost of a GM car by over $400. Pinkerton Security estimated that 80 percent of corporate theft and pilferage it investigates is substance-abuse related. GM also reported that the average substance abuser was at work only 140 out of 240 working days before treatment. The United States has the worst drug problem of any of the industrialized Western nations.[53] Sixty percent of all drugs produced in the world are consumed in the United States.

Business and industry are concerned not only about the increased use of drugs on the job but about the wider acceptance of drug use, the greater availability of drugs, and the increased variety of drugs taken. Alcohol is still the most abused drug on the job, followed by marijuana and cocaine. Here is one illustration of the wider acceptance of drugs in the workplace:

> "I've been on jobs where the foreman actually passes out stuff to make sure the work gets done," says John E. Neece, a building union leader in California. "Sometimes 90 percent of the crew have been doing uppers."[54]

Cocaine use is extensive, accepted, and steadily growing in financial centers from coast to coast. "One reason for the increase in use and acceptance is that the generation of people who used drugs other than alcohol in the 1960s and 1970s are growing older and taking their drug habits to the workplace."[55]

Industry is finally realizing that it has a very real and costly problem on its hands. Though some companies choose to ignore the problem, others, with an extremely limited understanding of drugs, are nevertheless attempting to confront it. It is a difficult situation for industry, since very few companies have established drug policies and many supervisors lack training in dealing with drug users. It is also difficult for a supervisor who has a two-martini lunch to discipline an employee for smoking a joint during lunch. Even so, companies are starting to spell out drug policies stating what will happen to those caught using drugs.

A Firestone Tire and Rubber Company study completed in mid-1983 found that drug users were 36 times as likely to be involved in a plant accident and 2.5 times more likely to require absences lasting more than a week than employees who didn't use drugs.[56] The increased concern over industrial accidents directly caused by employees using drugs has spread to the public. For example, in September 1982 in Livingston, Louisiana, a freight train derailed and two tank cars carrying chemicals exploded and burned. About 3,000 people who lived within five miles of the accident site had to be evacuated for up to two weeks, and environmental damage was extensive. The National Transportation Safety Board found that impairment of the engineer's faculties by alcohol had contributed to the accident.[57]

American companies are attempting to fight the "war on drugs."[58] Many are making jobs conditional on whether or not a potential employee is found drug-free. Citicorp is declining to hire anyone who tests positive for amphetamines, barbiturates, cocaine, or heroin. Adolf Coors brewing company is refusing to back down from its use of undercover investigators trying to detect workers who are using and selling drugs. Georgia Power is using trained dogs to sniff out drugs in employees' lunchboxes and cars.

Corporations such as Whirlpool and General Motors utilize undercover detective agencies because they cannot afford not to.[59] The U.S. Chamber of Commerce found that recreational drug users are one-third more likely to come to work late and twice as likely to leave work early. Drug-using employees are two and a half times more likely to miss eight or more days of work and four times more likely to be involved in injuries while working. The Drug-Free Workplace Act of 1988 also pushes this issue, as it requires companies with federal contracts to "clean house" or lose their contracts. A specific example of how much even one drug-using employee can cost a company is a 1987 train wreck caused by a train engineer who smoked a joint while at his post. This wreck killed 16 people, injured 175, and cost Conrail and Amtrak $106 million.[60]

Employee-assistance programs (EAPs) seem to be a growing trend among companies. A number of companies immediately fire anyone who fails a test of drug use. However, employees who admit to a drug problem before taking the test are granted leave to seek treatment, which is kept confidential. EAPs are being expanded to include therapy for all types of drug use. Many companies are funding EAPs to save money in the long run, and they find that the employees so served are extremely productive. "When you're able to help an employee save his life," says Frank Price, head of the Owens-Illinois EAP in Atlanta, "there's dedication that dollars and cents can't buy."[61] Business and industry are starting to deal with their growing drug problem through a variety of approaches. With more experience, it is hoped, they will be able to improve these approaches.

DRUG TESTING

Drug testing has become a major concern for many people in our society. Some feel it is an infringement of one's rights, but others support it to ensure that performance, mental or physical, is not impaired. Drug testing has also been introduced to reduce illicit drug use.

Drug testing versus the right to privacy is a very important issue among the workforce today. There are four general categories of testing: (1) testing prospective employees, (2) testing for cause (after "observing a significant degradation" in an employee's performance), (3) periodic testing (announced, tests everyone, considered fairer than random), and (4) random testing (most controversial, provides the greatest deterrence).[62]

The biggest problems most employers face with drugs is inconsistency when enforcing the policy and a failure to educate employees on what their policy is. Legally, companies face the issue of a person's right to privacy (Fourth Amendment). Many people agree that drug testing is necessary for those employed in "safety-sensitive" jobs, but then the problem of who determines what is a "safety-sensitive" job and what isn't arises. Generally a good drug-testing policy would "limit the testing to safety-sensitive" or "national-security-related jobs," limit testing to instances where drug abuse is already suspected, notify employees of the general program in advance, and follow proper procedure (confidentiality, prohibiting frontal observation).[63]

Employee Assistance Program (EAP)
A formal broad-based approach to helping maintain a healthy workplace. It has been established to assist with employees' personal problems that affect the work situation. Drug problems and drug testing are a major focus of most employee assistance programs.

Drug Testing
It has been introduced to reduce illicit drug use. A urine test is required to determine whether or not drugs are present in the employee. Some say it is an infringement of one's rights, but others support it to ensure that performance, mental or physical, is not impaired. The test is used to keep employees off drugs so a safe work environment can be maintained.

Lining Up for a Drug Test
Source: UPI/Bettmann

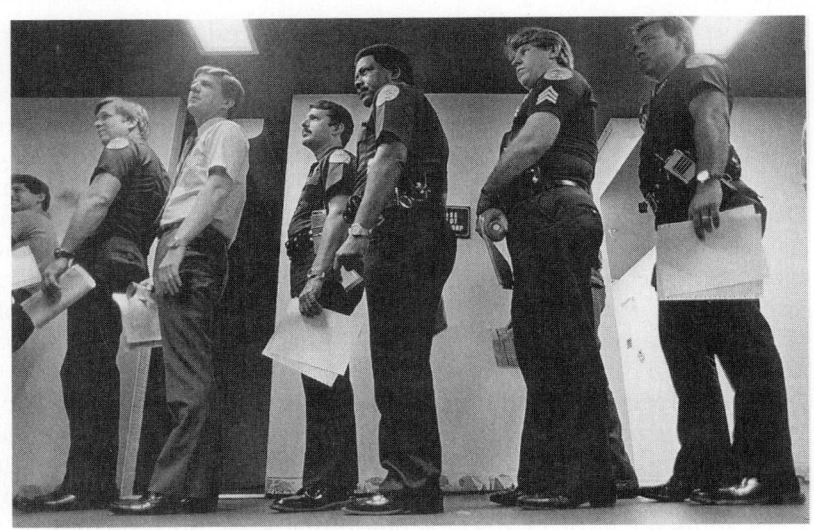

It is estimated that over half of the *Fortune* 500 companies along with the U.S. Department of Transportation have drug-testing programs in effect. Their main purpose for maintaining these programs is to deter drug abuse. Corporations are also sensitive to the public's concern for wanting those who hold "responsible" positions, such as pilots, police officers, bus drivers, or fire fighters, to be drug-free. They are also looking for ways of maintaining a safe workplace and keeping insurance costs down.[64] Experts estimate that between 10 percent and 23 percent of all U.S. workers use dangerous drugs on the job.[65] How reliable are urinalysis methods? Drug testing guidelines for federal agencies specify use of immunoassays for initial screenings and gas chromatography/mass spectometry for the confirmation test. Gas chromatography coupled with mass spectometry (GC/MS) had evolved as the preferred method for confirmation of a positive urine screening test.[66]

The value of drug testing is severalfold. It is preventive, rehabilitative, and reinforcing. Companies that have initiated drug testing along with education and training programs have experienced a decrease in accidents, a drop in absenteeism, and a significant containment in medical-benefit cost.

Privacy in the workplace is going to be a controversial issue in the 1990s. Also, people on drugs can endanger other workers and cost an employer millions of dollars in liability claims. However, some people do not want to be tested for drugs because they feel that their privacy is being invaded. Solving this dilemma boils down to finding a proper balance between the common good and personal freedom. The issue of confidentiality and release of information is always a great concern. The records of alcohol- and drug-abuse clients in an EAP may be protected by federal statutes.

But is testing legal? Yes, where there is just cause to test; where the test is used to help the employee or ensure safety; and where the employee's confidentiality is protected.[67] In addition, employers have the right to protect the company's reputation and to keep the public trust in the company's mainte-

EMPLOYEE DRUG USE[68]

Evidence That May Suggest Drug Use at the Workplace

- Absenteeism
- Theft
- Arrests of employees outside work
- Referrals to the EAP
- Anecdotal evidence (i.e., observed drug use)
- Quality control problems
- Unsafe work practices

Typical Drug-Abusing Worker

- Late three times more than nonabusing employees
- Requested early dismissal or time off during work 2.2 times more often than nonabusing co-workers
- Had 2.5 times as many absences of eight days or more
- Was five times more likely to file a workmen's compensation claim
- Was involved in accidents 3.6 times more often than other employees

nance of certain behavior standards on the part of its employees. Law enforcement personnel, professional sports teams, some government workers, medical personnel, and pharmaceutical company employees are examples of groups who must maintain certain behavioral standards.

In March of 1989, the Supreme Court upheld the drug-testing issue by a 7–2 vote.[69] They also upheld by a 5–4 vote that the U.S. Customs Service employees seeking a drug-enforcement post be subject to urine tests as well. Attorney General Dick Thournburg said, "The court recognized the government should take all necessary and reasonable steps to prevent drug use by employees in sensitive positions." The private sector is now following federal guidelines in initiating their policies; however, the results of many lawsuits against private drug testing are still pending.

Tests are legally valid and can be used in a court of law. The amount of weight this evidence has in a given case, though, depends on the court and/or arbitrator.[70] A refusal to be tested can be considered evidence that the person was under the influence.[71] Where safety may not be at stake but company policy has been broken, the company has the right to request a test. Employee refusal is grounds for discharge. With adequate safeguards such as

fair notice to employees and confidentiality protection, testing will become
an accepted part of the approach to employee-assistance programs.

THE OLDER AMERICAN DRUG SCENE

As recently as the turn of the century, the average life span in the United
States was approximately 49 years; by 1980 it had risen to 73 years. Furthermore, it is estimated that by the year 2000 there will be 31 million Americans
over 65, representing almost 13 percent of the population. Drug technology
has contributed to this increase in longevity by eliminating and/or helping
control many infectious and chronic diseases.[72]

In the next 25 years the U.S. population is expected to grow by 16 percent for those 65 to 74 years of age, 60 percent for those 75 to 84, and nearly
100 percent for those over 85.[73] Presently, those over 65 represent 12 percent of the population but account for 30 percent of the American drug
industry's $17.3 billion in sales in 1984.[74] One may infer from these projec-
tions and statistics that the demand for drugs by those 65 and older will
increase dramatically. This demand will tax the creative skills of the medical
community, which is already failing to deal with the drug problems of the
elderly. Although the aged have much to gain through proper and necessary
drug use, they are at an increased risk of drug problems because of their
decreased sensory abilities, other physiological changes, polypharmacy, a
greater potential for adverse drug reactions, voluntary misuse, and, for some,
the overuse of psychotropic medications in nursing homes (a setting where
the aged have little or no control over drug intake).

The elderly are in a unique situation regarding drugs. Their physical systems are degenerating, and they often have one or more chronic diseases. To
complicate things, they make extensive use of multiple medications. The
average older person takes from three to seven medications at the same
time.[75] Polypharmacy is one aspect of drug use that is central to the problems
among older people. "Polypharmacy can be the result of multiple chronic
conditions, multiple physicians, lack of coordination of care, illusive symptomatology, and drugs given to counteract the side effects of other drugs."[76]
Thirty-five percent of office visits by older persons result in polypharmacy
and establish a risk for adverse drug reactions.[77] Over-the-counter drugs complicate the use of clinical drugs, since the elderly are some of the greatest
users of the former. According to a University of Michigan study, elderly
women living alone on a $3,000-to-$8,000 annual income are most likely to
develop drug problems. Statistically, this group takes seven prescription
drugs and five over-the-counter medications.[78]

In the past, elderly drug-dependents were not considered drug abusers
by professionals because long-term drug-dependents generally die before age
60 and those who survive have given up drugs.[79] But senior citizens show a
dramatic lack of drug knowledge, considering it of little benefit to them, and
this often causes drug abuse. In a study of the level of drug knowledge and
misconceptions among senior citizens, half of the subjects thought there
were risks involved in taking prescribed medicine; 60 percent believed some

medications should not be mixed with certain foods; and the majority believed that drugs could be habit forming. In addition, over 70 percent were unaware of the side effects of aspirin and 60 percent used laxatives to stimulate a bowel movement.[80]

Although numerous medications are prescribed to many older Americans, the medications are rarely designed in terms of dosage and method of administration for the aged person. Because the bodies of the aged weigh less, have less fluid, and metabolize things less quickly than those of younger individuals, the dosage for one may not be the dosage for another and this misdosage can lead to some deleterious effects. These effects include overdosage, synergism with other medications, and more severe complications.[81]

TYPES OF DRUG USE

To better understand the older American drug scene, we will consider four ways in which seniors use drugs: (1) proper use of drugs, (2) misuse of drugs, (3) accidental abuse of drugs, and (4) purposeful use of dependency-causing drugs.

Proper Use   Proper drug use involves refraining from taking several drugs that may have been prescribed by different physicians for different conditions. A doctor will often write a prescription without knowing that other physicians are treating the same patient. The elderly often dwell upon the increasing debilitation of their bodies, and many ingest multitudes of drugs to help themselves feel young again. Illness and the approach of death often cause extreme depression, and seniors also take drugs to alleviate this condition, as well as loss of appetite and weight, sleep disturbances, and constipation.

Misuse of Drugs   Senior patients may become drug-dependent without their physician's or their own knowledge. They may visit several physicians at a time, each for a different condition, and be prescribed a different drug by each. They may also "repeatedly self-administer drugs and . . . eventually come to feel that they cannot carry on normal everyday activities unless they take drugs."[82] As tolerance to the drugs develops, some increase the dosage at will.

Adverse drug reactions (ADRs) are unwanted or unexpected results of drug use. They can become very serious in the elderly because they are often ignored. Symptoms of such reactions are often dismissed by physicians and patients alike.

Noncompliance is another dimension of the misuse of drugs by the elderly. A recent study showed that "only 22 percent of prescriptions were being taken properly—and 31 percent were being misused in a manner which posed a serious threat to the patient's health."[83] Many of the elderly fail to understand that many medications are prescribed to prevent problems from developing, and they will often stop taking them when symptoms do not appear or when they are alleviated or become less observable. "Various studies of older patients [have] indicated that 50 to 60 percent of them make medication errors or simply don't take their medicine at all."[84]

Many nursing homes are resorting to powerful sedatives and antipsychotic drugs to keep their elderly residents manageable. However, these drugs are being overused, and there are a growing number of lawsuits that attribute the deaths of nursing-home residents to inappropriate medication.[85]

Though nursing-home staffs may overmedicate their patients to keep them quiet or happy, sometimes producing undesirable mental conditions as well as adverse physical problems, there is no indication that all or even most physicians are unconcerned about their elderly patients. Most of those physicians who do incorrectly prescribe do so out of frustration and/or lack of knowledge about the aged patient and the drugs themselves. They may prescribe medications without realizing the undesirable side effects they can produce. This may lead to a vicious cycle of drug-induced diseases, including fainting spells, slurred speech, rashes, constipation, and an increased tendency to bruise easily.

Accidental Abuse of Drugs   Many cases of accidental abuse of drugs are caused by improper self-administration. The elderly may not have enough information to take a certain drug wisely. They may not be able to read the label or remember to take the medication at the proper time. Or there may be so many drugs in the medicine cabinet that selecting the appropriate one is difficult.

As many as 25 percent of patients 80 or over experience adverse drug reactions, compared with 9.9 percent for younger adults.[86] Another study found that adverse drug reactions occurred in 3 to 8 percent of hospitalized patients under 59, but in 11 to 21 percent of those over 60.[87]

Only through comprehensive client teaching, dissemination of information on drugs to the elderly, utilization of "significant others" (family, friends, and other close social supports) as a support system, and education of health-care workers in the effects of polypharmacy can the problem of accidental drug misuse in the elderly be reduced.

Purposeful Use of Dependency-Causing Drugs   Until recently, it was assumed that drug dependency was almost nonexistent among the elderly. However, several reports and studies now reveal that drug dependency is not so rare in that segment of the population.

As with other age groups, alcohol is commonly used by the elderly. Alcohol-related problems, such as health or marital problems, affect about 10 percent of the elderly. Male Caucasians are more likely to drink, and drink heavily, than members of other racial groups. Late onset of alcoholism seems to correspond to losses of loved ones, social deprivation, loss of status, and boredom. The man who is 75 or older and has lost his wife seems to be the most vulnerable to alcohol dependency. Elderly alcoholics usually began drinking heavily in their forties or fifties, but they receive voluntary treatment more often than younger alcoholics and consequently respond to and complete therapy programs much more frequently. Perhaps this is because they experience more alcohol-induced health problems.

Alcoholism among the elderly may increase, inasmuch as people are living longer and drinking more on average, and because alcohol-treatment services for the elderly are greatly lacking. But since geriatric alcoholics often drink primarily to cope with physical, social, and emotional problems, they

> respond readily to a therapeutic regime combining antidepressant medication with resocialization. They just stop drinking, and they do it without the assistance of Alcoholics Anonymous or Antabuse [a substance used in the treatment of alcoholism].
>
> The geriatric alcoholic's problems are clearly reactive. He responds readily when he finds a sympathetic ear for his problem, when he feels that someone is concerned about him. Once his depression lifts, he discovers that he doesn't need alcohol to adapt gracefully and effectively to the stress of aging.[88]

SUMMARY

We are a drug-oriented society, with many types of drugs and reasons for drug use. In fact, the United States still remains the biggest market for drug use in the world. However, there is some good news. Overall, drug use appears to be on a downward trend in the United States. For the first time in 16 years the 1990 High School Senior Survey on drug abuse reported that less than half the students surveyed had tried illicit drugs. Young people favor alcohol and nicotine, and continue to use various hallucinogens, volatile substances, and amphetamines. Initiation to cocaine (crack) and heroin usually begins in youth and may continue into the early adult years as well. Youths take drugs to get high or relax while going to school, during social activities, in the military, and in athletics. Drug abuse in athletics has reached such a high level that greater restrictions and punitive action are being applied. Many high school males are taking steroids to improve their appearances.

Adult drug use focuses on tranquilizers, alcohol, nicotine, and caffeine. Though males still constitute most of the alcohol-dependent population, there has been a large increase in female alcoholics since 1980, and the number appears to be growing rapidly. Adults also smoke marijuana, a behavior they have carried over from their youth. Amphetamine use has dropped in recent years, but cocaine has become prevalent among a growing number of adults. Heroin continues to be the most notorious illicit drug. Business and industry now find it necessary to monitor many of their employees and executives because of great financial losses associated with drug abuse on the job. Substance abuse is costing the business community $160 billion per year by eroding productivity, industrial accidents, absenteeism, and inflating health-care costs. Employee Assistance Programs are becoming more involved in drug testing to protect workers.

Among older Americans we find a disproportionate amount of prescription drugs being used. Older Americans also have more problems with misuse and accidental use of medicines than do other groups. Another area of growing concern is nursing homes and convalescent centers, where drugs are frequently overprescribed to quiet patients or to make them happy.

THE DRUG SCENE
N O T E S

1. Mary Ellen Sullivan, "Drugs: The World Picture," *Current Health,* February 1990, pp. 4–10.

2. Jerome Skolnkk, "Searching for an Answer," *USA Today,* July 1990, pp. 16–18.

3. Mary Ann Pentz, et al., "A Multicommunity Trial for Primary Prevention of Adolescent Drug Abuse," *Journal of the American Medical Association* 2671 (June 9, 1989) :3259–66.

4. Lawrence Ziomkowski, Rodney Mulder, and Donald Williams, "Drug Use between Delinquent and Non-Delinquent Youth," *Intellect* 104, no. 2367 (July/August 1975):36.

5. See, for example, "1983 Drug Use Questionnaire," issued by Youth Help, Inc., Hoquiam, Wash.

6. Peitro J. Pascale, "Trend Analysis of 4 Large-Scale Surveys of High School Drug Use, 1977–1986," *Journal of Drug Education* 18, no. 3 (1988):221–32.

7. Hawley, "School Children and Drugs," pp. K1–K8.

8. Ibid.

9. Patrick Murphy, "Steroids: Not Just for Athletes Anymore," *Physician and Sportsmedicine* 14, no. 6 (June 1986):48.

10. "What Drugs Do and Don't Do to Teens," *U.S. News & World Report,* August 1, 1988, p. 8.

11. "The High School Senior Survey," Sponsored by National Institute of Drug Abuse (NIDA) and conducted by the University of Michigan, Institute for Social Research. HHS News, U.S. Department of Health and Human Services, News Release, January 24, 1991.

12. Daniel Yankelovich, "Drug Users vs. Drug Abusers: How Students Control Their Drug Crisis," *Psychology Today* 9, no. 5 (October 1975):39. Reprinted from *Psychology Today Magazine.* Copyright © 1975 Ziff-Davis Publishing Company.

13. Ibid., p. 41.

14. Armand M. Nicholi, Jr., "College Students Who Use Psychoactive Drugs for Nonmedical Reasons," *Journal of American College Health* 33, no. 2–6 (April 1985):189.

15. Ibid., p. 190.

16. "Ranks of Cocaine Users Continue to Grow for a Decade after High School," *Drugs and Drug Abuse Education Newsletter* 17, no. 7 (July 1986):61–65.

17. "Vietnam Heroin Abuse Drops, but Problem Still Severe," *Journal of the American Medical Association* 219, no. 10 (March 6, 1972):1280.

18. Cited in ibid.

19. Ibid.

20. See John F. Greden and Donald W. Morgan, "Amnesty's Impact upon Drug Use: A Pre/Post Study," *American Journal of Psychiatry* 129, no. 4 (October 1972):123–25.

21. U.S. Department of the Army, *A Commander's, Supervisor's and Physician's Guide to Alcohol Abuse,* Pamphlet 600-17 (Washington, D.C., 1973).

22. U.S. Department of the Army, *Alcohol and Drug Abuse Prevention and Control Program,* Pamphlet 600-85 (Washington, D.C., 1986), pp. 600–685.

23. Cited in Richard Hallovan, "On Alert at an MX Missile Base," *New York Times,* January 28, 1987, p. A20.

24. Ibid.

25. Ibid.

26. Quoted in Jack Scott, "It's Not How You Play the Game but the Pill You Take," *New York Times Magazine,* October 1971, p. 12.

27. Jack C. Horn, "A Dangerous Edge," *Psychology Today* 17 (November 1983):68.

28. "The Doping of Amateur Sports," *Macleans* 95 (June 21, 1982):41.

29. "Anabolic Steroids and Their Side Effects," *Anchorage Daily News,* September 15, 1988, p. D.

30. Compiled by the *Register-Guard* (Eugene, Oregon), November 6, 1988, section c, p. 3, from various publications.

31. Gary Perlmutter and David T. Lowenthal, "The Use of Anabolic Steroids by Athletes," *American Family Physician* 32, no. 4 (October 1985):208.

32. Ibid.

33. "The Doping of Amateur Sports," p. 41.

34. Kathy A. Facklemann, "Male Teenagers at Risk of Steroid Abuse," *Science News* 134, no. 25 (December 17, 1988):391.

35. Ibid.

36. Arnold J. Mandell, "The Sunday Syndrome," *Journal of Psychedelic Drugs* 10, no. 4 (October/December 1978):379–84.

37. Quoted in Bil Gilbert, "Drugs in Sports," *Sports Illustrated* 30, no. 25 (June 23, 1969):27.

38. Mandell, "The Sunday Syndrome."

39. Quoted in Bil Gilbert, "Problems in a Turned on World," *Sports Illustrated* 30, no. 26 (June 30, 1969):30.

40. National Institute on Drug Abuse, "National Household Survey on Drug Abuse."

41. Secretary of Health, Education and Welfare, *Alcohol and Health Report* (New York: Scribner's, 1970), pp. 417–19.

42. Office of Technological Assessment, *The Effectiveness and Costs of Alcoholism Treatment* (Washington, D.C.: U.S. Government Printing Office, 1983), p. 3.

43. Department of Health, Education and Welfare, *CNS Depressants* (Washington D.C.: National Clearinghouse for Drug Abuse Information, 1974), pp. 7–8.

44. Cited in ibid.

45. *Commission of Inquiry into the Non-Medical Use of Drugs: Final Report* (Ottawa: Crown, 1973), pp. 417–19.

46. American Cancer Society, *1980 Facts and Figures* (New York, 1980), p. 144.

47. Jill Andresky, "The Caffeine Controversy," *Consumer Digest* 20, no. 6 (1981):31–34.

48. Alfred Gilman and Louis S. Goodman, eds., *The Pharmacological Basis of Therapeutics,* 4th ed. (London and Toronto: Macmillan, 1971), pp. 367–68.

49. Oakley S. Ray, *Drugs, Society and Human Behavior,* 2nd ed. (St. Louis: C. V. Mosby, 1978), p. 208.

50. Michael Dolan, "Clamping Down on 'Uppers,' " *American Pharmacy* 18 (new series), no. 4 (April 1978):18.

51. Department of Health, Education and Welfare, *Fact Sheet 6,* no. 1 (Washington, D.C.: National Clearinghouse for Drug Abuse Information, 1974), p. 2.

52. Robert M. Strutman, "Can We Stop Drug Abuse in the Workplace?" *USA Today,* July 1990, pp. 18–20.

53. Ibid.

54. Quoted in Jo Brecher et al., "Taking Drugs on the Job," *Newsweek,* August 22, 1983, p. 52.

55. Quoted in Stephen J. Sanswee, Thomas Petzinger, Jr., and Gary Putka, "High Fliers:

Use of Cocaine Grows among Top Trades in Financial Centers," *Wall Street Journal,* September 12, 1983. Reprinted by permission of *Wall Street Journal,* © Dow Jones & Company, Inc., 1983. All Rights Reserved.

56. Sidney Cohen, *Drug Abuse and Alcoholism Newsletter* 12, no. 6 (1983):1.

57. Bill Paul, "Danger Signal: Alcohol and Drug Use by Railroad Crewman Poses Threat to Safety," *Wall Street Journal,* August 16, 1983, p. 1.

58. "Mission Just Possible," *The Economist,* September 30, 1989, p. 72.

59. John Schwartz, "Using Spies to Win a War," *Newsweek,* November 6, 1989, pp. 56–57.

60. Ibid.

61. Brecher et al., "Taking Drugs on the Job."

62. Joyce Frieden, "Corporate America's Response to Substance Abuse," *Business and Health* 8, no. 7 (July 1990):32–42.

63. Frieden, "Corporate America's Response to Substance Abuse."

64. Marvin D. Felt, "Drug Testing: A Research Strategy," *Compensation and Benefits Management* 6, no. 3 (Spring 1990):219–24.

65. National Institute on Drug Abuse, "Drug Abuse Curriculum."

66. Ibid.

67. David G. Evans, "Is It Legal, Is It Fair? Alcohol and Drug Testing in Industry," *U.S. Journal* 9, no. 2 (February 1985).

68. National Institute on Drug Abuse, Office of Workplace Initiatives, "Drug Abuse Curriculum for Employees Assistance Programs Professionals," DHHS Publication No. (Adm) 89-1587 (Rockville, Md.: U.S. Department of Health and Human Services. Alcohol, Drug Abuse and Mental Health Administration).

69. Alan Sanders, "A Boost for Drug Testing," *Time,* April 13, 1989, p. 62.

70. Evans, "Is It Legal, Is It Fair?"

71. Ibid.

72. "Drugs and the Elderly," *OPEN: Oregon Prevention and Education Newsletter* 2, no. 1 (January/February 1980):50.

73. Peter P. Lamy, "Hazards of Drug Use in the Elderly," *Postgraduate Medicine,* July 1984, p. 50.

74. Francesca Lunzer, "Bitter Pills," *Forbes,* June 3, 1985, pp. 203–4.

75. Rein Tideiksaar, "Drug Noncompliance in the Elderly," *Hospital Physician,* March 1984, pp. 92–101.

76. Pearl S. German and Lynda C. Burton, "Clinicians, The Elderly and Drugs," *Journal of Drug Issues* 19, no. 2 (1989):221–22.

77. Ibid.

78. "Aged Women at High Risk for Drug-Related Problems," *Geriatrics,* March 1985, pp. 26–27.

79. Emil Pascarelli, "Old Drug Addicts Do Not Die, Nor Do They Just Fade Away," *Geriatric Focus* 11, no. 5 (1972):1.

80. Emil Pascarelli et al., "Drug-Related Behavior, Knowledge and Misconceptions among a Selected Group of Senior Citizens," *Journal of Drug Education* 8, no. 2 (1978):85–92.

81. William Ira Bennet, "Monitoring Drugs for the Aged," *New York Times Magazine,* December 13, 1987, pp. 73–74.

82. Walter L. Way, *The Drug Scene: Help or Hang Up?* (Englewood Cliffs, N.J.: Prentice-Hall, 1970), p. 17.

83. William Nolen, "Doctor's Orders: Why Patients Should Never Ignore Them," *Fifty Plus,* April 1984, p. 52.

84. Hecht, "Medicine and the Elderly," p. 2.

85. Steven Findlay, "Is Grandma Drowsy, or Is She Drugged?" *U.S. News & World Report,* June 12, 1989, p. 68.

86. Beverly G. Clark and Robert E. Vestal, "Adverse Drug Reactions in the Elderly: Case Studies," *Geriatrics* 39, no. 12 (December 1984):53.

87. William G. Berlinger and Ronald Spector, "Adverse Drug Reactions in the Elderly," *Geriatrics* 39, no. 5 (May 1984):40.

88. Sheldon Zimberg, "The Geriatric Alcoholic on a Psychiatric Couch," *Geriatric Focus* 2, no. 5 (1972):1.

*Xanthines are alkaloids (chemicals capable of neutralizing acids) found in a variety of plants throughout the world. The chemical family Xanthines includes caffeine, theophylline, and theobromine.

C H A P T E R
4

PHARMACOLOGY

Basic Concepts
of Drug Activity

Without knowledge of the pharmacological properties of drugs, it is hard for people who have taken drugs to understand why the mind and body change during the drug experience. Scientists are constantly presenting new discoveries to the public. For example, in 1975 neuroscientists discovered enkephalin and endorphin.[1] These hormones are thought to be the body's own source of relief from pain and disabling emotions, binding with receptors in the brain and inhibiting pain signals there.[2] They may also improve memory. Furthermore, they may offer an explanation for acupuncture analgesia.[3] In addition to reducing pain, enkephalin and endorphin may effectively treat depression and schizophrenia.[4]

PHARMACOLOGICAL THEORIES AND DISCOVERIES

Do humans need to get high? Ronald Siegel, a research pharmacologist at the UCLA School of Medicine, argues that the human desire to seek out pleasure through the use of caffeine, nicotine, alcohol, opium, marijuana, or cocaine is a "universal and inescapable fact of life."[5] Siegel is not alone in his view that "the desire to alter one's state of consciousness is a drive as essential as hunger, thirst, and sex." Siegel says that society would be better off accepting the fact that we seek pleasure through drugs and invent a nonaddictive and less harmful alternative. Siegel's drug would be nontoxic and nonaddictive and would provide pleasure or stimulation within limits. The drug would not allow the user to lose control or overdose. Although this is an interesting concept, other experts in the field disagree with Siegel on his views about building a better drug. Andrew Weil, of the University of Arizona College of Medicine, says, "There is a real danger in thinking there is a perfect drug that won't interfere with psychological and spiritual growth and without the potential for dependence and damage."[6]

FOUNTAIN OF YOUTH

Pharmacology is always looking for ways to improve the quality and quantity of life. Somatropin, also known as human growth hormone, hGH, is naturally produced in our bodies by the pituitary gland. This hormone seems to be what keeps us young, as the amount produced in our bodies decreases as we get older. In the mid-1980s two companies solved the problems with hGH. Genetech Incorporated and Eli Lilly & Company developed a synthetic hGH hormone.[7] This breakthrough is helping scientists study hGH, since before supplies were limited and expensive.

Daniel Rudman, a doctor at the Medical College of Wisconsin in Milwaukee, tested hGH on 12 older men ages 61–81 and found amazing results.[8] In the first six months the men lost body fat by an average of 14.4 percent, got more muscular, had a 7.1 percent increase in skin thickness, and had their natural hGH levels increased back to a youthful amount.

This drug not only reverses aging but has also been proven to help people who have pituitary gland problems. The FDA has approved its use in the treatment of abnormally short children who have pituitary deficiencies. The reduction of fat may reduce the risk of heart disease. The only side effect caused by injecting this drug is a small increase in blood pressure.

ENDORPHINS

The current research on the body's own natural morphinelike pain killer, endorphin, centered on the numerous pleasurable sensations associated with the body's natural secretion and release of this "magical" hormone. Endorphins or their receptors are not only responsible for their widely known anesthetic effect but also for the induced intensity of other emotional states, such as happiness, depression, compulsiveness, masochism, excitation, sexual satisfaction, and hunger.[9]

Studies show there is a direct link between autistic children who inflict self-injuries or pain and the masochist.[10] This is due, in fact, to the "pleasure" felt by a sudden release of endorphins upon the pain centers in our brain after self-inflicted injury. The result is very similar to a circumstance after a major injury, such as experienced by a burn victim, when the body's natural endorphin hormones enter the bloodstream and delay signals of pain to the brain area for several hours after the injury. A "runner's high," or the natural high experienced in structured, regular exercise, may lead to feelings of well-being or actual highs after exercise. Pleasure sensations from eating certain foods (i.e., fats and sugars) is now thought to be from endorphin released throughout the body directly after eating.

Currently, much research is being done on the effects of endorphins upon the eating disorders of anorexia and bulemia; food deprivation enhances the release of opiates in the brain, and this "reward" may explain the complexity and low success of treating victims of these disorders. Endorphin research is still in its early stages, and the findings are encouraging.

CONSUMER SAFETY

Responsible consumer safety requires one to consider seven basic points in deciding whether or not to take a drug.[11]

1. the chemical being considered
2. the receptor mechanisms affected
3. the dosage and the method of administration
4. the kinds of drug interactions that will likely take place
5. the potential for allergic reactions
6. the potential for tolerance
7. the potential for physical dependence

THE CHEMICAL (DRUG) BEING CONSIDERED

A drug is a compound that affects the chemical functioning of the organism that ingests it. It may cause changes in bodily processes or behaviors. The

Nader Expresses Concern About Consumer Safety and Drugs
Source: AP/Wide World Photos

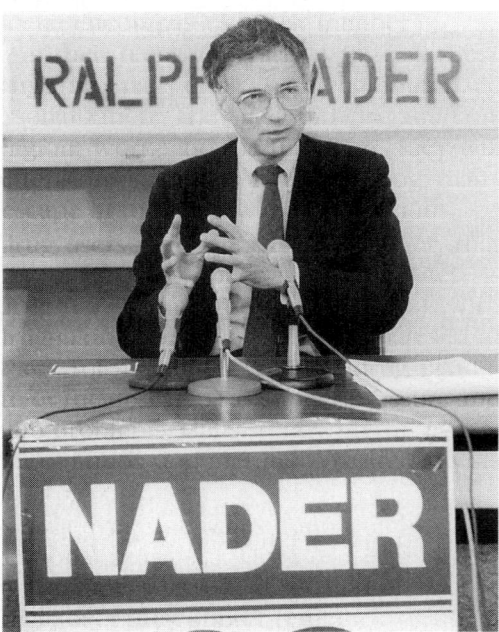

water we drink, the air we breathe, and the food we eat are all chemicals producing various effects in our bodies.

To maintain life, an organism must produce, or otherwise obtain, various chemicals. When a chemical must be obtained from substances taken into the body, it must be determined how the chemical will affect the system.

THE RECEPTOR MECHANISMS AFFECTED

The chief determinant of the effects of a drug is its site of action within the body. Current theories on drug action suggest that chemical receptors within the body provide chemical sites coded to receive specific chemical substances. When a drug finds its chemical-receptor mechanism (binding site), which is part of a large chemometabolic pathway, the interaction of the drug with that mechanism will eventually alter the function of the pathway. Chemicals that bind to one or more of these binding sites will either fulfill normal biochemical functions or alter them and thus our bodily activities as well.

A drug, binding at these scattered receptors, can have a wide variety of actions and effects. When these are beneficial, they define a drug's therapeutic or medical use. An *adverse reaction* occurs when a drug produces unexpected or undesirable effects. The desired effect is usually considered the main effect; the unwanted responses are labeled the *side effects.* More serious side effects include toxic reactions and elevated or lowered blood pressure.[12]

THE DOSAGE AND THE METHOD OF ADMINISTRATION

The amount of a drug present at a binding site determines the intensity or depth of the body's response to the drug's characteristic actions. Therapeutic effects are obtained only when specific concentrations of the drug are present at the appropriate receptors. Incorrect concentrations can result in a lack of action, toxic reactions, or other alterations in the expected effects.

How much of a chemical must be taken for it to be effective? Each drug has its own optimum dose that will achieve maximum benefits with minimal side effects. Surprisingly, the best effects of many drugs are achieved at low

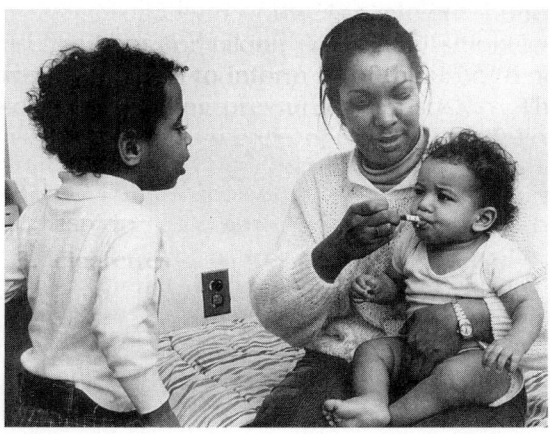

A Mother Administering the Proper Medicine Dosage to Her Baby
Source: Alice Kandell/Photo Researchers

dosages. To determine how effective a drug will be, a person should know how the action of the drug is affected by body mass (weight). (Convert pounds to kilograms [2.2 pounds equal 1 kilogram] and multiply by the amount of the drug that has been determined through research to produce the maximum beneficial effects and minimum side effects. Then compare the resultant figure with the specified dosage.)

Absorption is an important pharmacological factor in drug activity. Drugs must be lipid-soluble (soluble in fat but insoluble in water) in order to cross cell membranes, which contain substantial amounts of lipid fats. Non-lipid-soluble chemicals may not penetrate cell membranes in sufficient quantities to affect the cells. As a drug enters the system, it will usually move from a region of higher concentration of molecular volume per specific surface area to a region of lower concentration; when it is unable to do this, special transport mechanisms (such as the binding of a drug to a protein molecule, which can enter a cell) go into effect. The body continually releases energy-stored nutrients and uses them to maintain a chemical equilibrium. Depending on the drug and the transport mechanism it is using, more or less energy will be required to absorb the drug before sufficient concentrations have been reached to produce the desired effect.

Distribution of a drug is dependent on absorption. The blood vessels of the brain, however, are surrounded by a fatty sheath that limits the entry of many drugs. This decreased permeability of the capillaries of the brain to certain substances is frequently called the *blood-brain barrier.* This term is widely used for distinguishing drugs that can penetrate the brain from those that cannot.[13]

Many areas of the body store drugs rather than distribute them. Some of these storage depots are fat reservoirs (for drugs with high lipid solubility), bones (for heavy metals and tetracyclines), and plasma proteins (for drugs with an affinity for albumin).

Some drugs become active only after the liver transforms them biologically; others are initially active and become inactive after biotransformation. Still others may be active at one site in the body, go through biotransformation to become inactive at that site, then transfer to another site where they become active again. These transformation factors add to some of the unpredictable effects a drug can have, but after transformation the drug's metabolites (a substance produced by metabolism) are usually filtered out and excreted by the liver and kidneys.

The *dose-response curve,* a fundamental concept in pharmacology, illustrates how different levels of a drug in the body can produce different behavioral effects.[14] This S-shaped curve (see Figure 4–1) shows that up to a certain level (the bottom of the curve), the concentration of a drug does not produce suitable effects to warrant continued administration at that level. The dose-time curve (Figure 4–2), which is usually bell-shaped, shows that increasing the dose beyond a certain level may prolong the effects, but the effects themselves will not increase. What may increase are the side effects.

Body weight and sex are also important factors in drug activity. A specific dosage, given both to a large person and to a small person, will affect the

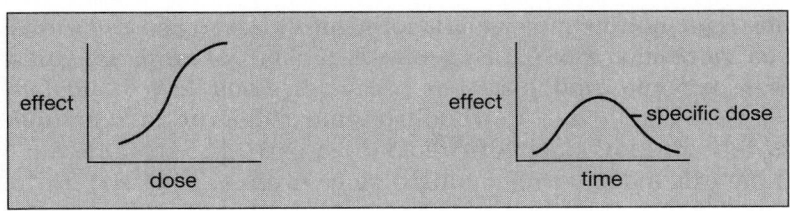

FIGURE 4–1 DOSE-RESPONSE CURVE

FIGURE 4–2 DOSE-TIME CURVE

smaller person more strongly (other factors being equal), since he or she has less tissue and blood to absorb it. Also, a woman will respond differently to a drug than will a man of the same size because her body contains a higher ratio of fat. Drugs that have an affinity for stored fat may thus have prolonged effects in women. Individual metabolism affects the concentration of a drug at its receptor and the rate at which that concentration is reached. Thus, it also helps determine a drug's effects.

The way a drug is administered affects the onset of its effects, the duration of its action, and its potency. In general, substances injected into the bloodstream act quickly, last a short time, and produce a great effect. Inhalation, ingestion, or inunction (rubbing into the skin to achieve a systemic effect) may be used when an immediate high dosage is not required.

Ingestion   Drugs that are ingested are normally taken in pill or liquid form. Once swallowed, the drug goes mainly to the stomach, where some of the chemical will be broken down, then to the small intestine, bloodstream, liver, and so on. It can take 20 to 40 minutes for a drug to enter the bloodstream and finally reach the receptor site; the original dosage may be diluted and changed somewhat by the time it finally arrives. Certain drugs may not have the proper chemical charge and shape to enter the bloodstream when ingested and will be eliminated as waste. Those drugs must therefore be taken through oral inhalation or intravenously.

Inhalation   Inhalation is a drawing in through the nasal passage; oral inhalation, a drawing in through the mouth. Though almost any nonliquid form of a chemical can be inhaled, only a few psychoactive substances are generally taken in this fashion. The most common of these are cocaine and, to a lesser extent, amphetamines, heroin, and volatile substances such as glue; marijuana and cigarettes, and, again, some volatile substances are orally inhaled. Drugs that are inhaled are lipid-soluble and can pass quickly into the bloodstream. However, since there is only a small amount of blood in the lungs, drugs need to be inhaled often to obtain the desired effects.

Injection

INTRAVENOUS (IV).   Drugs administered intravenously are placed directly into the bloodstream. Because of their immediate absorption and rapid distribution throughout the circulatory system, their full potency is felt very quickly. It is sometimes difficult to treat a person who has intravenously injected a lethal dose of a drug such as heroin, since the person receives full dosage in a very short time.

INTRAMUSCULAR (IM).   Here the drug is injected directly into the muscle tissue and then gradually filters out into the bloodstream. This form of injection usually takes more time than an intravenous injection to reach the binding sites, since absorption is slower. This prevents an inundation of the receptors by the drug.

SUBCUTANEOUS.   These injections go into the dermal layers of the skin. Since such shots have a slower absorption rate than intramuscular injections, they can further slow the onset of effects, depending on the solubility of the drug.

Inunction   A drug administered by inunction is rubbed into the skin, and from there it works its way into the bloodstream.

THE KINDS OF DRUG INTERACTIONS THAT WILL LIKELY TAKE PLACE

A drug interaction occurs when two or more drugs are administered concomitantly; the responses are unexpected, unusual, or amplified. Such responses are the results of one drug altering the actions of another. One chemical may, for instance, affect another's absorption into the bloodstream, its distribution to receptor sites, or its rate of elimination from the body. The actions of any administered drug, as well as normal bodily processes, may be changed in these ways. Any chemical taken into the body, moreover, may compete with those already present.

Women need to be educated about drug use during pregnancy. Drug interactions are therefore inevitable in a great number of pregnant women. In addition, pregnant women must be extremely careful to avoid teratogens, "substances that cause abnormalities in the unborn child. . . . Teratogens can inflict their damage in two ways. Some act indirectly by interfering with the blood flow through the placenta."[15] The effects of drugs on an unborn child can be influenced by several factors: (1) the susceptibility of the unborn child to the effects of a chemical circulating from the mother's bloodstream into the uterus, (2) the dose or amount of the teratogen, and (3) the time of exposure during pregnancy.

THE POTENTIAL FOR ALLERGIC REACTIONS

Hypersensitivity
Drugs interact with bodily chemicals to produce allergic reactions. The initial sign of hypersensitivity may be a skin rash or development of an asthmatic condition.

Because every person has a unique biochemical makeup, each administration of a drug is much like an experiment. Occasionally, drugs interact with bodily chemicals to produce allergic reactions. These **hypersensitivity** reactions may not present themselves initially, or even every time the drug is used.

Hypersensitivity is difficult to predict. By taking a lower dose of a drug upon first use, a person has a greater chance of avoiding a possible allergic reaction. The initial sign of hypersensitivity may be a skin rash or development of an asthmatic condition. A severe reaction may result in anaphalactic shock, respiratory depression, convulsions, or death.

Though some 3 to 5 percent of our population are hypersensitive, reacting very quickly to very small amounts of a drug, some individuals are *hyposensitive:* They require extra amounts of a drug to gain the desired effects. Other people may experience a **synergistic** response. In this case a combination of two drugs, such as alcohol and barbiturates, may have geometric rather than arithmetic effects.

Synergistic
When a combination of two or more drugs are taken and may have geometric rather than arithmetic effects.

THE POTENTIAL FOR TOLERANCE
AND THE POTENTIAL FOR PHYSICAL DEPENDENCE

The continued presence of a drug can cause its receptor site to lose sensitivity. In addition, when drugs are put into the body, the liver responds with enzymes to break them down. Increasing amounts are then required to exceed the liver's efficiency and produce the desired effects. *Tolerance* is the body's ability to adapt to existing drug dosage, thereby reducing or eliminating the desired effects; dose increases are then needed to produce these effects. *Physical dependence* occurs when certain drugs, in higher concentrations made necessary by tolerance, cause various biochemical transformations that in turn cause the system to become dependent on the presence of these drugs. Under these circumstances, if the drug is not taken or does not reach its receptor site in sufficient concentration, a syndrome of physical responses (withdrawal) will occur.

Cocaine is an example of a drug that was once considered psychologically but not physiologically addictive. In the last few years, however, doctors have discovered otherwise.[16] Cocaine has a variety of pharmacological effects on the central nervous system and on nerve conduction. It is thought to act like dopamine, a neurotransmitter, in the brain. The short-term effect of cocaine is a euphoria produced by excess dopamine. But the long-term effect is depression because the excess dopamine is metabolized and washed out of the body. This depression creates a craving for more cocaine.[17] Although dopamine in the brain is thought to mediate reinforcement, and although it is often assumed that cocaine's inhibition of dopamine uptake underlies this reinforcement, there are no data on receptor binding that support this notion.[18]

ANATOMY AND PHYSIOLOGY

THE NERVOUS SYSTEM AS AN ELECTRICAL SYSTEM

To better understand how drugs can affect the body, we need to first understand how the nervous system works (see Figure 4–3). The nervous system consists of billions of *neurons* (nerve cells). A neuron usually consists of dendrites, a cell body (soma), and an axon with its terminals. The dendrites receive signals from other neurons, summarize the information, and transfer it to the soma for production of a nerve impulse. After the impulse is generated, it travels down the axon to the terminals, which contact the dendrites

FIGURE 4–3   THE NERVOUS SYSTEM

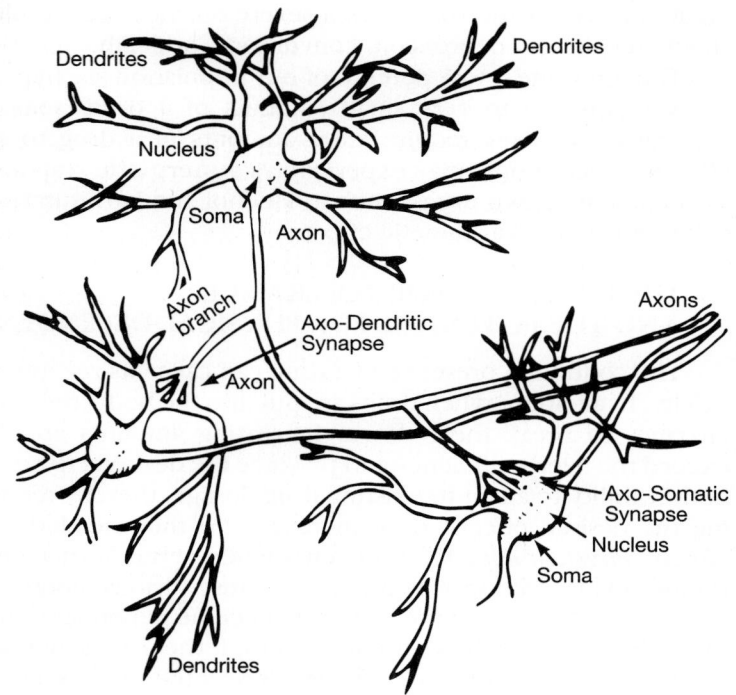

of other neurons or other terminals. The gap between a terminal and another neuron is called a synapse, and when a signal has jumped this gap it migrates to a receptor site. A neuron will not fire, however, unless sufficient excitatory receptor sites in the dendrites bring the cell to an electrochemical threshold, where it will start an impulse of its own.

In an unstimulated state, a nerve's membrane (the layer surrounding the neuron) normally has many more potassium ions inside it than outside, and many more sodium and chloride ions outside than inside. Ions are atoms with a positive or negative charge, and when they move they form a current, which is simply a flow of charges. When allowed to move freely, ions travel from a region where they are of higher concentration to a region where they are less concentrated; if the difference in concentration between the two areas is large, more ions flow (producing a greater electrical current) than if the difference is small. As ions travel along a neuron, the membrane becomes selectively permeable, opening certain "channels" or "gates" to allow some of the ions to pass through; it is this flow of ions that constitutes the electrical signal we call an impulse, or *action potential.* Drugs that affect the sodium and potassium levels in and around a neuron might alter the quality of the impulse by making the cell capable of firing faster or slower. Coding of information in the nervous system usually is affected by frequency of firing rather than on the amplitude of the impulse.

Consequently, each receptor site (which is either excitatory, bringing the cell closer to threshold, or inhibitory, sending it farther away) will have only a partial influence on the readiness of the neuron to fire. In this sense, the excitatory and inhibitory signals from other cells are summarized, and this information is transformed into the all-or-nothing impulse.

The neuron membrane is semipermeable, allowing only certain molecules and atoms to move through it (notably, potassium, sodium, and chloride ions). Physicians closely monitor a patient's sodium and potassium levels in surgery to prevent shock. As an impulse travels along, the membrane changes its permeability so as to admit sodium ions and then potassium ions, each flowing in a different direction, and it is these local ion flows, or currents, that constitute the impulse. The way a drug alters the body's pH level (its acid-alkaline balance) is very important. Drugs can thus affect currents by changing the sodium or potassium levels, and hence the degree to which they pass through neuron membranes, or by altering the permeability of the membrane itself.

Most drugs, however, do not affect nerve currents through the membrane. The great majority of psychoactive drugs alter the signal at the synapse. When an impulse comes along, vesicles in the terminal release neurotransmitters into the gap, which migrate to receptor sites in a few thousandths of a second. The transmitters activate the receptor, which then releases the transmitters back into the gap, where they are either taken into the terminal again for reuse or deactivated by a special chemical (monoamine oxidase) residing in the synapse.

When a drug is taken, it can change an impulse by altering the release, activation, reuptake, or deactivation of transmitters. Since a drug can affect impulses throughout the nervous system, which includes the brain and the spinal cord, it can affect all life functions, memory, and personality.

There may be as many as 30 different neurotransmitters; we will deal only with the most prevalent. *Acetylcholine* (ACH) is an excitatory transmitter in skeletal muscles and an inhibitory one in heart muscle. Appropriately, neurons that use ACH are called *cholinergic. Serotonin* acts as a transmitter in many parts of the central nervous system; neurons using it are termed *serotonergic. Adrenergic* neurons use *dopamine* or *norepinephrine* (NE) as transmitters.

THE CENTRAL NERVOUS SYSTEM

There are two major divisions of the nervous system: the central nervous system and the peripheral nervous system. The central nervous system (Figure 4–4), or CNS, includes the brain and the spinal cord. There are several substructures in the brain that are significant in the actions of certain drugs.

Hypothalamus and Pituitary Gland   The hypothalamus is like the central processing unit of a computer. It is the foundation of the mammalian brain, which originated some 30,000 years ago. Also known as the *prehistoric brain,* the hypothalamus is the seat of many major life-support functions. In a sense, because of its neurological design, we can also think of it as a switchboard. Communication between the brain and the pituitary gland, which secretes hormones, occurs through the hypothalamus. Because of this, what affects the brain can affect the pituitary.

**FIGURE 4–4   THE CENTRAL
NERVOUS SYSTEM**

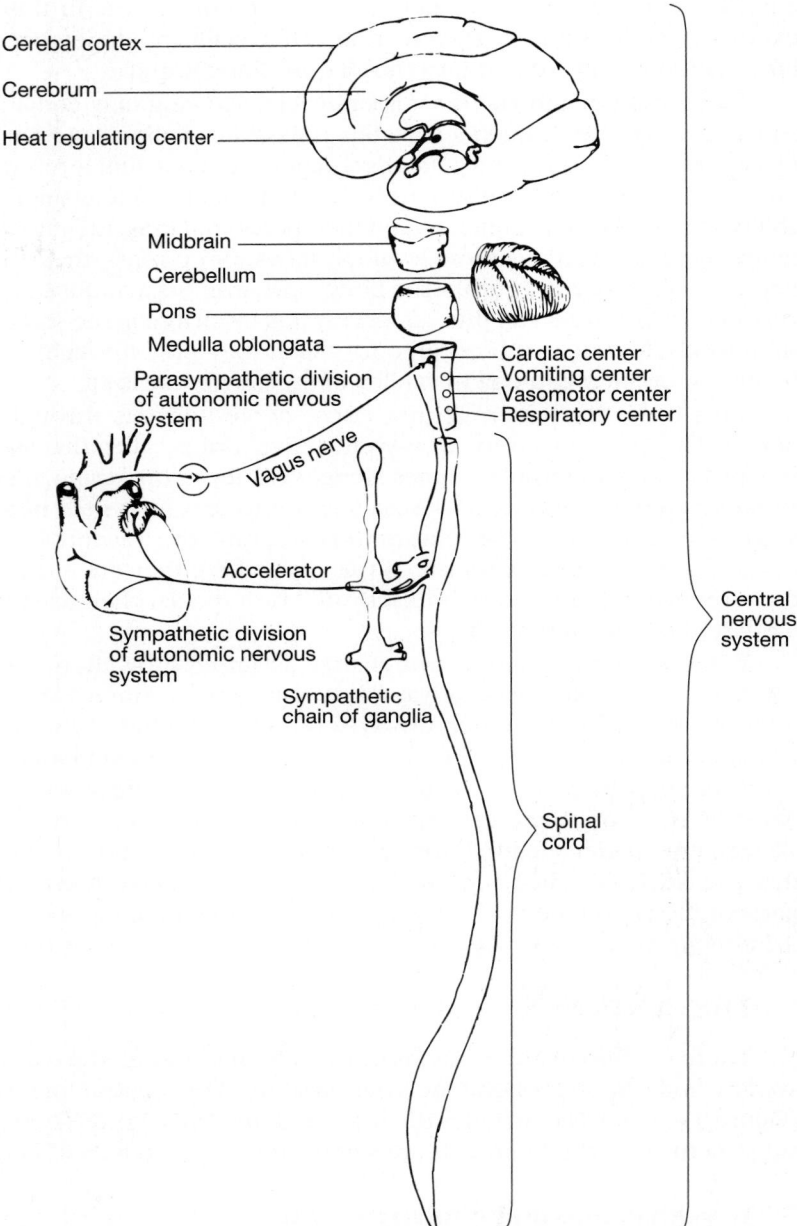

Cerebal cortex

Cerebrum

Heat regulating center

Midbrain

Cerebellum

Pons

Medulla oblongata

Parasympathetic division
of autonomic nervous
system

Vagus nerve

Accelerator

Sympathetic division
of autonomic nervous
system

Sympathetic
chain of ganglia

Cardiac center
Vomiting center
Vasomotor center
Respiratory center

Central
nervous
system

Spinal
cord

The hypothalamus regulates many of the functions of *homeostasis*—the
body's need to keep its biological systems in balance. The sleep-waking cycle
is housed here, as are hunger, thirst, sexual behavior, blood pressure, and
body temperature. This tiny cerebral component also coordinates and selects
which major pathways will be affected by analgesics, and it appears to be a

factor in many behavioral and chemical dependencies, such as alcoholism and other drug abuse, compulsive gambling, sexual offenses, and obesity. Many of these dependencies are influenced by the relationship between the hypothalamus and the rest of the limbic and endocrinal system (the system that regulates hormone levels, which in turn affect emotions). The general adaptation syndrome or stress response is likewise housed in the hypothalamus.

Medial Forebrain Bundle   A tract of nerve fibers runs through both sides of the hypothalamus. When electrodes implanted in this area are stimulated, humans report pleasurable sensations and will do work, such as pressing a lever, to receive them. This area of the brain is sometimes referred to as the pleasure center.

Periventricular System   The major part of the periventricular system consists of the periventricular nuclei, located above and to either side of the hypothalamus. The system is mainly cholinergic—that is, it transmits acetylcholine. Electrical stimulation of the area produces sensations of displeasure in humans, leading to the view that the system is a punishment center.

Reticular Formation (Ascending Reticular Activating System)
This structure is located in the brain stem (see Figure 4–5), just behind the hypothalamus. It receives all types of internal and external stimuli and in turn

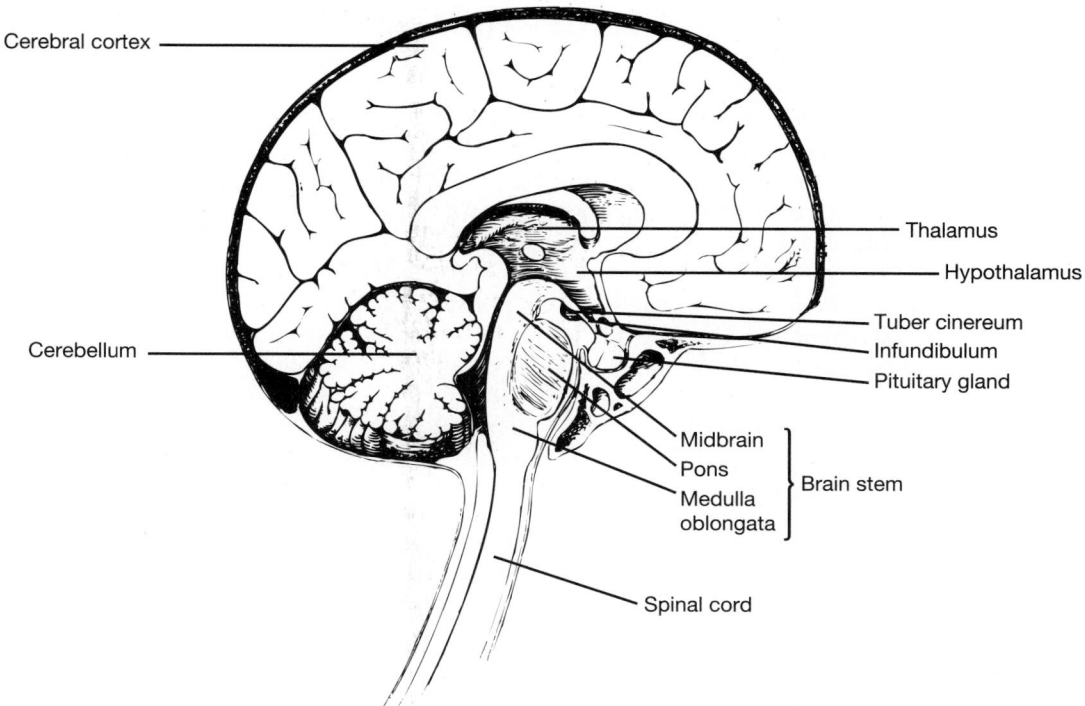

Cerebral cortex

Thalamus

Hypothalamus

Tuber cinereum

Infundibulum

Pituitary gland

Cerebellum

Midbrain
Pons
Medulla oblongata
} Brain stem

Spinal cord

FIGURE 4–5   THE BRAIN

projects messages to many parts of the cerebral cortex. The reticular formation acts as a switchboard, helping to sort impulses and direct them to the appropriate area of the brain. Many of the neurons in the reticular formation have collaterals (branches) from their axons. Each neuron can then send its signals to more than one area of the brain. One primary function of the formation is to regulate the *arousal level* of the cortex, which varies from alertness to sleep, by performing what might be called an evaluation of incoming stimuli.

Medulla   The medulla oblongata is located in the lower part of the brain stem (which comprises all parts of the brain except the cerebellum and the cerebral hemispheres). The medulla has intimate connections with the reticular formation and is hence involved to some extent with the regulation of arousal. The medulla also receives inputs from the vestibular apparatus for balance and initiates reflex responses of the head. When an individual hears a noise, the information is sent simultaneously to both the reticular formation and the medulla.

The medulla works with the hypothalamus to regulate many autonomic (automatic) functions of the body—breathing, heart rate, blood pressure, and pupil dilation. When an individual dies from an overdose of a depressant drug, the cause is usually depression of the medulla. The speed at which food moves through the digestive system and the vomiting reflex are also mediated by the medulla. The medulla is influenced by both the cortex and the internal status of the body. In short, it is involved in motor responses and homeostasis.

Raphae Nuclei   The raphae nuclei are clusters of cell bodies lying above the medulla and just behind the hypothalamus. Like the cells in the reticular formation, these cells act on the ability of the cortex to receive sensory input, but they use serotonin as a transmitter substance instead of norepinephrine. According to one theory, the raphae nuclei inhibit the arousal of the reticular formation and the cortex, producing a state of light sleep.[19] Since most serotonergic neurons in the CNS are located in the raphae, drugs that affect serotonin levels (LSD, for example) will alter the functioning of these nuclei and perhaps cause new behaviors.

Cerebral Cortex   The cerebral cortex is one of the newest structures in the original mammalian brain, and its existence distinguishes mammals from other vertebrates. However, no enormous differences separate humans from other mammals. Humans may have more *nuclei* (nerve cell centers) than the rat, but both brains are organized similarly. The cerebral cortex covers all other structures in a series of convolutions, or folds, to conserve space. Fully half the cells of the nervous system reside in the cortex.[20]

Language, abstract thought, personality, and the more subtle influences on how we interpret emotion seem to reside in the cerebral cortex. Learning and memory, on the other hand, are situated throughout the brain.

Several bands of accumulated nerve tracts, the corpus callosum, lie along the midline of the brain. The cerebral hemispheres communicate with each other by sending impulses along the fibers running through the corpus callosum. When these bands are cut, the individual suddenly has two completely separate brains, each capable of independent thought and independent response. Testing of epileptic patients who have had this operation reveals a functional diversity. In most people, the left hemisphere is found to be very good at language and linear thought but very bad at interpreting spatial images. Just the opposite occurs in the right hemisphere. These findings have led to the speculation that one side of the brain functions linearly while the other is adept at perceiving things in their entirety.[21]

Specific cerebral functions are indigenous to specific cerebral components. On the other hand, there are systemwide memory and personality influences, which are not restricted to the left or the right hemisphere. Thus, we can view a single thought as involving billions of neurons firing in immensely complicated circuits, or we can view a thought as the firing of a single cell. Research on the vision of monkeys brought on the discovery that some neurons fire only when they "see" a line in their visual field. Other neurons are most excited when a series of lines appears in a certain pattern.

THE PERIPHERAL NERVOUS SYSTEM

Many of the nerves in the peripheral nervous system constitute the autonomic nervous system, which mediates the automatic functions of the body, such as heart rate and digestion. Two further divisions of the autonomic nervous system are the *sympathetic* and the *parasympathetic* systems.

Most body organs have nerves structured for innervation (arousal), according to Walter Cannon's "fight-or-flight" hypothesis. When the sympathetic division dominates, heart rate, blood pressure, respiration, and perspiration increase; pupils dilate to allow wider peripheral vision; blood is diverted from the digestive system to the skeletal muscles; and adrenaline is released. In peripheral-skeletal-muscle blood vessels and in sweat glands, the sympathetic transmitter is ACH. All other nerve innervation utilizes norepinephrine.

TABLE 4-1   EFFECTS OF THE SYMPATHETIC AND PARASYMPATHETIC NERVOUS SYSTEMS ON SELECTED BODY STRUCTURES

Structure	Sympathetic Effect	Parasympathetic Effect
Heart rate	increase	decrease
Blood pressure	increase	decrease
Respiration	increase	decrease
Digestive system	inhibition	activation
Pupils	dilation	constriction
Salivary glands	decrease in secretion	secretion
Skin blood vessels	constriction	dilation
Sweat glands	secretion (ACH)	(no effect)

Source: Oakley S. Ray, Drugs, *Society, and Human Behavior*, 3rd ed. (St. Louis: C.V. Mosby, 1983).

TABLE 4–2 SUMMARY OF DRUG INFORMATION

	Effects	Side Effects	Adverse Effects	Potential for Addiction	Withdrawal Symptoms
STIMULANTS (Benzedrine, Dexedrine, methamphetamines, methadrine, Ritalin, etc.)	increased wakefulness, reversal of fatigue, depressed appetite, reduction of narcolepsy	dry mouth, increased perspiration, enlarged pupils, talkativeness, nervousness, involuntary trembling, restlessness, excitability, tension, anxiety, nausea, hot flashes, and bruxism; cramps, increased heart rate, and stimulation of force of heart contractions and breathing	headaches, palpitations, delirium, circulatory collapse, vomiting, malnutrition, and paranoia; depletion of the body's energy stores; GI disorders, liver and stomach disorders, and nerve damage	slowly increasing tolerance; high potential for psychological addiction; possible mild physical dependence	renewed desire to take more of the drug; overwhelming fatigue; severe depression; occasional suicidal tendencies
COCAINE	numbness—used as a local anesthetic in surgery; dilated pupils; strong stimulation of the CNS; increased motor activity	increased heart rate and blood pressure; increased respiration rate and depth of respiration *From free-basing:* chest pain, sore throat, hoarse voice, shortness of breath	*Large dosage:* tremors, convulsive movements, respiratory and cardiac failure *Excessive dosage:* hallucinations, paranoid delusions, cocaine "bugs," insomnia, weight loss, financial extinction, and accidental OD	very rapidly increasing tolerance; very high potential for psychological addiction	irritability, discomfort, strong desire to repeat use; physical exhaustion; severe depression possibly leading to suicide

TABLE 4-2 (CONTINUED)

	Effects	Side Effects	Adverse Effects	Potential for Addiction	Withdrawal Symptoms
SEDATIVE-HYPNOTICS (Barbiturates: Seconal Tuinal, Nembutal, etc.)	relaxation and sleep	range from subtle changes in mood and sedation to sleep and coma; typical effects are a reduction in attention span, less awareness of external stimuli, and a decreased ability to perform intellectual tasks	nausea, dizziness, confusion, impaired mental state, and allergic reactions such as swelling of the face; dermatitis, skin lesions, fever, delirium, convulsions, and degenerative changes in the liver	rapidly increasing tolerance; high physical and psychological potential for addiction	sweating, insomnia, vomiting, tremors, paranoia, and a short temper; excessive dreaming, nightmares, and in extreme cases hallucinations and seizures
QUAALUDES	relief of nervous tension, promotion of sleep	dreamy moods, lowered inhibitions	headache, hangover, menstrual disturbance, tongue changes, dry mouth, rashing at the angles of the mouth, nosebleeds, depersonalization, dizziness, skin eruption, pain in the extremities, diarrhea, anorexia, anxiety, nausea, and restlessness	increasing tolerance; high physical and psychological potential for addiction; high potential for accidental OD	irritability, vomiting, headaches, seizures, cramps, tremors, sleeplessness, mania, convulsions, and death

TABLE 4–2 (CONTINUED)

	Effects	Side Effects	Adverse Effects	Potential for Addiction	Withdrawal Symptoms
MINOR TRANQUILIZERS (Valium, Librium, Miltown, Serax, etc.)	reduction in neuromuscular activity and thereby a reduction in environmental awareness; easier relaxation	motor impairment, speech disturbance, shortened attention span, and reduced sex drive; reduced feelings of aggression, increased sociability, and drowsiness progessing towards sleep	apathy, illogical fears, low blood pressure, fainting, chills, rashes, upset stomach, disorientation, blurred vision; bladder, menstrual, and ovulary irregularities; sleep disturbance; if taken with alcohol, a toxic or fatal reaction can occur	rapidly increasing tolerance with high potential for crosstolerance; high physical and psychological potential for addiction	anxiety, muscle twitches, insomnia, headache, fever, nausea, vomiting, abdominal cramps, sweating, and convulsions; death is possible
ALCOHOL	relaxation, euphoria, and lessened inhibitions	slight increase in heart rate, sweating, dilation of blood vessels, moderately lower blood pressure, appetite stimulation, increased gastric secretion, and increased urine production; levels of fat and protein affected	inability to perform simple motor activities, blackout, facilitation of hypothermia, irritation and inflammation of the linings of the oral cavity, esophagus, and stomach, violent behavior, fetal alcohol syndrome, cirrhosis of the liver, permanent kidney damage, brain damage, congestive heart failure, unconsciousness, and death	tolerance increases depending on amount consumed and period of time of consumption; very high potential for physiological and psychological addiction	irritability, sleeplessness, tremors, sweating, hallucinations, seizures, delirium, tachycardia, and low-grade fever

TABLE 4–2 (CONTINUED)

	Effects	Side Effects	Adverse Effects	Potential for Addiction	Withdrawal Symptoms
OPIATES (heroin, codeine, morphine, Darvon, Dilaudid, Percodan, Talwin, methadone, Demerol)	relief of pain and promotion of sleep	constricted pupils, reduced respiration and pulse, drowsiness, loss of appetite, sweating, elevated blood-sugar level, constipation, and impotence	hepatitis, blood poisoning, inflammation of the membranes lining the heart, dizziness, headache, and possible coma or death	extremely rapidly increasing tolerance; very high physical and psychological potential for addiction	*12–24 hours:* restlessness *24–48 hours:* dilated pupils, anorexia, gooseflesh, restlessness, irritability, and tremors *48–72 hours:* increasing irritability, insomnia, marked anorexia, violent yawning, severe sneezing, lacrimation, weakness, vomiting, intestinal spasm, and diarrhea; elevated blood pressure, marked chilliness alternated with flushing
HALLUCINOGENS (LSD, mescaline, psilocybin)	altered sensory perception; stimulation of the sympathetic nervous system leading to heightened sensitivity to stimuli; synesthesia (blending of senses)	dilated pupils, rise in body temperature and blood pressure; increased heartbeat, possible moderate rise in blood sugar, nausea, headache, loss of appetite, dizziness, and mild tremors; visual distortions, distorted depth perception	hallucinations, severe paranoia, "bad trips," accidental or deliberate death	rise in tolerance not likely unless taken on a continued basis over a long period—increased dosage then needed to achieve desired effects; psychological addiction very possible	

TABLE 4–2 (CONTINUED)

	Effects	Side Effects	Adverse Effects	Potential for Addiction	Withdrawal Symptoms
PCP	anesthesia	*Moderate dose:* numbness, blurred vision, muscular dysfunction, dizziness, profuse sweating, flushing, increased blood pressure, and rapid heartbeat; spaciness, problems with perception and coordination, bloodshot eyes, impaired speech	anxiety, depression, sporadic outbreaks of violent behavior, and accidental death	definite possibility of psychological addiction	none known
MARIJUANA	intoxication, euphoria, enhanced congeniality, relaxed passivity	mild dilation of the blood vessels in the extremities, slight increase in blood flow to the arms and legs, reduction of body temperature; slightly elevated blood pressure, dry mouth, appetite stimulation	irritation of the throat and lungs; cardiovascular complications; possible damage to the immune system; alteration of endocrine function; psychomotor impairment	possible tolerance; potential for addiction depending on frequency of use and amount used	short-term anxiety, panic, impairment of short-term memory, disturbance in thought patterns, lapses in attention, depersonalization, mental confusion, flashbacks, paranoid thoughts

Source: Martin Chess, drug counselor, Serenity Lane, Inc., Alcohol Treatment Center, Eugene, OR 97401. Reprinted with permission.

The parasympathetic system is very specific in its innervation: It seems to work toward maintenance and repair of the body. When the parasympathetic supersedes the sympathetic, heart rate, blood pressure, and respiration become slow and regular; blood is diverted from the skeletal muscles to the digestive glands (where motility, or movement, is increased); and pupils constrict. Sweat glands are not affected because they are innervated only by the sympathetic system. The neurotransmitter involved in parasympathetic reactions is always ACH. A special condition exists in the heart: It makes rhythmic contractions without outside intervention because of a spontaneous release of potassium. Here ACH has an inhibitory effect. (The excitatory or inhibitory effect of a transmitter depends on the nature of the receptor site.) If the majority of receptor sites are excitatory or ACH, then ACH may be described as an excitatory transmitter; but not all receptors are excited—some may be inhibited by the transmitter. Some of the effects of the sympathetic and parasympathetic nervous systems are listed in Table 4–1.

Table 4–2 describes the effects, side effects, adverse effects, potential for addiction, and withdrawal symptoms for several drugs that are commonly abused.

SUMMARY

How drugs affect the human body is a fascinating process. Neuron cells and synapses relay drug messages, but the human body is able to alter the effects of drugs on the various parts of the nervous system. It can also manufacture its own drugs, such as enkephalin and endorphin, to meet its specific needs.

We must consider several basic factors if we are to be safe consumers of drugs, whether prescription, over-the-counter, or recreational. These factors include the chemical being considered; the receptor mechanisms to be affected; the dosage; the kinds of drug interactions that will likely take place; and the potential for allergic reactions, tolerance, and physical dependence. Additional pharmacological knowledge and more understanding of the physiological effects of drugs will give us more insight into what happens when we take various drugs.

Pharmacology
N   O   T   E   S

1. David N. Leff, "Brain Chemistry May Influence Feeling, Behavior," *Smithsonian* 9, no. 3 (June 1978):64.
2. David N. Leff, "The Pain Killers," *Time,* December 4, 1978, p. 96.
3. Elizabeth Frost, "Acupuncture and Hypnosis," *New York State Journal of Medicine* 78, no. 1 (September 1978).
4. Elizabeth Frost, "Endorphin for Emotions: A Good Beta," *Science News* 114, no. 20 (November 11, 1978):326.
5. Jonathan Beaty, "Do Humans Need to Get High?" *Time,* August 21, 1989, p. 58.

6. Ibid.

7. Bill Lawren, "The Hormone That Makes Your Body 20 Years Younger," *Longevity,* October 1990, pp. 31–36.

8. Ibid.

9. Janet L. Hopson, "A Pleasurable Chemistry," *Psychology Today* 22 (July/August, 1988):29–33.

10. Ibid.

11. Elizabeth Frost, "Consumer Safety Rules," in *Drug Information Center (DIC) Handout* (Eugene: University of Oregon, 1979).

12. Robert M. Julien, *A Primer of Drug Action,* 3rd ed. (San Francisco: W. H. Freeman & Company, 1981), pp. 75–76.

13. Ibid., p. 76.

14. See A. Goth, *Medical Pharmacology* (St. Louis: C. V. Mosby, 1972), p. 8.

15. Guttman, "Drugs and Pregnancy: A Risky Mix."

16. Peggy Mann, "Breakthrough against Cocaine," *Reader's Digest* 130 (April 1, 1987):185–94.

17. Ibid., p. 187.

18. Mary C. Ritz et al., "Cocaine Receptors on Dopamine Transporters Are Related to Self Administration of Cocaine," *Science* 237 (September 1987):1219–23.

19. M. Jouvet, "The States of Sleep," *Scientific American* 216, no. 2 (February 1967):14.

20. D. Kimble, *Psychology as a Biological Science* (Pacific Palisades, Calif.: Goodyear, 1973).

21. M. Gazzaniga, "The Split Brain in Man," *Scientific American* 211, no. 2 (August 1967):24–29.

CHAPTER
5

STIMULANTS

AMPHETAMINES

INTRODUCTION

The most common amphetamine derivatives currently available are amphetamine (Benzedrine), dextroamphetamine (Dexedrine), and methamphetamine (Methedrine or Desoxyn). The following information pertains to all these derivatives, unless otherwise noted.

Description and History Amphetamines are powerful CNS stimulants, particularly effective on the reticular formation and the cerebral cortex. They are synthetic substances belonging to a class of drugs known as sympathomimetics—drugs that mimic actions of the sympathetic nervous system, the division of the autonomic nervous system that increases the rate of body functions.

Amphetamines and all other sympathomimetics have the following actions:

An Assortment of Amphetamines
Source: Gatewood/The Image Works

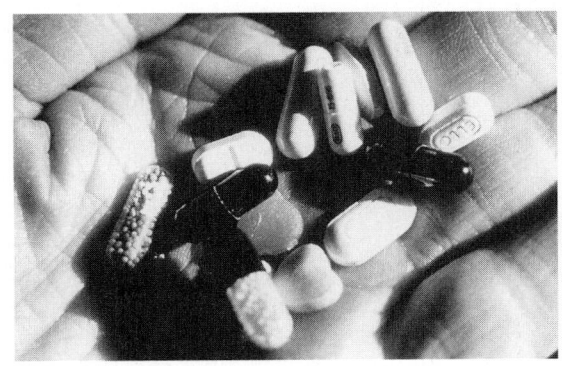

1. excitatory action on smooth muscles, such as those in blood vessels supplying the skin and mucous membranes, and on secretions from the salivary glands

2. inhibitory action on other smooth muscles, such as those in the intestinal wall, the bronchial tubes, and blood vessels supplying skeletal muscles

3. excitation of heart action, resulting in increased heart rate and force of contraction

4. metabolic actions, such as an increase in the conversion of glycogen into sugar in the liver and muscles, and the liberation of free fatty acids from fatty tissues

5. excitatory action on the central nervous system resulting in respiratory stimulation, increased wakefulness, and prevention as well as reversal of fatigue

6. reduction in appetite[1]

Amphetamines may also cause dryness of the mouth, loss of appetite, increased perspiration, enlarged pupils, talkativeness, nervousness, involuntary trembling, restlessness, excitability, aggressive behavior, tension, anxiety, insomnia, nausea, hot flashes, and **bruxism** (grinding of the teeth).

Bruxism

A grinding of the teeth that often occurs in heavy methamphetamine users.

Though amphetamines were synthesized as long ago as 1887, the first significant investigation into their pharmacology and therapeutic application was begun in 1927. Ten years later, amphetamines became available as prescription drugs. They were used to treat narcolepsy, a disease producing an uncontrollable urge to sleep, and, paradoxically, to alleviate hyperactivity in children. With continued clinical use, amphetamines were eventually found to produce other major effects, including appetite suppression and stimulation.

In the early 1930s the pharmaceutical company of Smith, Kline and French used Benzedrine in decongestant inhalers that were sold to the public.[2] The stimulating effect of the drug was first recognized when some people began chewing the wicks of the inhalers for kicks. Laws were soon passed prohibiting over-the-counter sale of Benzedrine, but in 1937 the drug was approved by the American Medical Association as a prescription medication.[3] The most popular illicit use of amphetamines is in the form of ingestion of Dexedrine tablets. Intravenous methamphetamine use, though more notorious, is much less frequent now than it was in the late 1950s and the 1960s, when it spread throughout the United States. Injectable amphetamine was an alternative to opiate dependency, and unethical distribution of the drug by a few physicians made amphetamines easy to obta

Although closer legal controls were aced on amphetamine prescriptions, a black market 1971 amphetamines and methamphetami ral controls.[4] Continued feder 1971 and 1972 that focus tion amphetamines, and illi

Phy lating effects of ampheta cts may last from 4 to 14 h imilated into the bloodstre changed in the urine up t

Amphe control center in the hypot .[6] Though initially helpful s rapid tolerance develop as increased the dose or ch

Amphetam as providing temporary mood elevation is not the *source* of such stimulation: As amphet ally interact with the central nervous system, they release stored energy from the body's mitochondria cellular reserves. Continued use of amphetamines leads to depletion of these energy stores.

If amphetamines or other stimulants are used regularly at high dosages, tolerance will occur. Tolerance builds slowly but steadily as an adaptation at the cellular level in the CNS makes the user less sensitive to the drug's effects. Serious gastrointestinal, liver, and stomach disorders can occur, since the mechanism in the liver that metabolizes amphetamines is impaired with continued use. Another mechanism of tolerance may be that high doses of amphetamines inhibit appetite markedly, causing the urine to be strongly acid. Since excretion of amphetamines is much faster when the urine is acidic, a heavy user must keep increasing his or her dose to obtain the desired effects.[7]

Prolonged use of large doses of amphetamines can lead to severe anxiety reactions, overaggressiveness, and paranoia.[8] Recent medical evidence suggests that over time it may also cause severe arterial degeneration.[9]

The average patient with amphetamine psychosis began with pills, usually Benzedrine (Bennies) or Dexedrine. As tolerance rapidly increased, the user increased the potency of the doses and decreased intervals between doses to maintain the same level of effectiveness. Soon the user switched from pills to injections.

Abrupt cessation of high doses of amphetamines creates no classic *physiological* withdrawal syndrome. It does produce marked *psychological* changes, however, including renewed desire for the drug, overwhelming fatigue, and severe depression (occasionally provoking suicide).[10] If amphetamines have been self-prescribed to combat depression, the "crash" that follows abrupt cessation of use will generally result in an even deeper depression.

Medical Use   Until recently, amphetamines were often prescribed to help overweight people reduce. However, many physicians are currently limiting such usage because of the drug's side effects. Additionally, as tolerance develops, increased dosage is necessary. Following discontinuation of amphetamines, previous eating habits often return and lost weight is gained back. Furthermore, amphetamines have little effect in suppressing the appetite of individuals whose major substance of misuse is food.

As we have noted, amphetamines have also been used in the treatment of narcolepsy. By increasing alertness they reduce the need to sleep that this disorder creates. On the other hand, they have been used in the treatment of certain hyperkinetic disorders in children. Hyperactivity and/or minimal brain dysfunction in children are primarily treated with amphetamine and its analog methylphenidate (the generic name for Ritalin), but there is dispute over such use of these drugs. Though the drugs are calming in some instances, it remains unclear why amphetamines produce this effect.[11]

Amphetamines are also useful in treating brain damage or "senility" in geriatric patients. In patients with cellular damage, the drug stimulates and improves the function of the remaining cells. It also increases the amount of *epinephrine* (an adrenalin transmitter) in those whose natural level of adrenalin has diminished with age.

Narcolepsy
A condition or disease causing an individual to keep falling asleep.

Misuse and Abuse   Many people still take amphetamines for the wrong reasons: quick pep-me-ups, extended wakefulness, weight control, and recreation.[12] The FDA is attempting to prevent such use by recommending that prescriptions of amphetamines be limited to those who have minimal brain dysfunction or **narcolepsy**. In general, the FDA feels that misuse of amphetamines will decrease if fewer amphetamines are produced.

DEXTROAMPHETAMINE

Dextroamphetamine (Dexedrine) stimulates the cerebral cortex. It does not act on the peripheral or autonomic nervous system, but it does increase blood pressure.[13] The drug depresses the sense of smell and the ability to taste sweet food. It suppresses appetite and can produce euphoria. Used to treat Parkinson's disease, it helps increase epinephrine availability in geriatrics, perception skill, and judgment capabilities and performance, and decreases the need for sleep. Often obtained illicitly, the pills are sometimes known as Dexies or cross-tops, because of the cross that divides each pill into four sections.

METHAMPHETAMINES (CRANK, SPEED, AND METH)

Speed, or methamphetamine hydrochloride (Methedrine), is a powerful stimulant to the nervous system that has been used for a generation. Similar to Benzedrine, methamphetamine is more potent. Speed or crank can be snorted, injected, or taken in a beverage and offers an intense euphoria. Of course, a concern with intravenous use is the risk of hepatitis, infection, or AIDS from exchanging needles. Methamphetamine is made in a growing number of clandestine laboratories, and the drug "speed" is surging across the West and could soon rival crack.[14] Speed keeps users awake and under the influence for several days.

The drug depresses the appetite, is used in treating narcolepsy, relieves symptoms of Parkinson's disease, and has been used in the treatment of obesity.[15] Methamphetamine produces greater cortical stimulation than other amphetamines, has a more rapid and prolonged onset, and has less intense effects on the peripheral system and the heart. When abused, however, it can cause progressive inflammation of the medium and small arteries throughout the body, resulting in permanent damage to the kidneys, intestines, liver, and pancreas.

The Speed-Taking Ritual   Most users of methamphetamine begin by taking the drug orally. Initial doses range from 10 milligrams to 20 milligrams, but a compulsive user may eventually increase to 250 to 1,000 milligrams per day, since tolerance develops rapidly. Once doses get this high, intravenous injections may begin. The powder used in this illicit preparation of speed is often termed *crystal*. In the early stages of intravenous use, the user finds that three or four doses (20 to 30 milligrams each) are enough. In time, this dose may elevate to 200 milligrams or more. (Most pills on the legal market contain 5 to 10 milligrams of an active amphetamine.)

Even before an intravenous user withdraws the needle, she or he feels an intense and buzzing euphoria. Elation and hyperactivity last for several hours, and there is no desire for food or sleep. The user has a sense of markedly enhanced physical strength and increased mental capacity. A *speed freak* may "shoot up" every three to four hours for five or six days before crashing from exhaustion and lack of sleep. Sleep can last anywhere from 12 hours to four days, depending on the intensity of the trip. Extreme hunger usually follows sleep. Once this hunger is satisfied, however, a profound depression can occur.[16]

Increased doses and frequent use of methamphetamines lead to toxicity and potential amphetamine psychosis. Various signs of these conditions are bruxism[17] and touching and picking at the extremities and especially the face.[18] A first sign of **amphetamine psychosis** is fear or suspicion: The user feels uneasy but is not quite sure why. The fear soon becomes intense, causing paranoia and a specific delusion. This amphetamine-induced paranoia causes a high rate of violence among speed freaks. Users feel they are the target of some sort of surveillance, that they are being watched by the police or by friends. They feel that their friends are no longer trustworthy and are "out

Speed Freak
A heavy amphetamine user who may "shoot up" every three or four hours for five or six days before crashing from exhaustion or lack of sleep.

Amphetamine Psychosis
A condition where a user of amphetamines starts having fear and suspicion and an uneasy feeling. The fear soon becomes intense, causing paranoia and a specific delusion. This amphetamine-induced paranoia causes a high rate of violence among amphetamine (speed) users.

to get them." Consequently users often arm themselves "for their own protection" and try to assault those who are "threatening" them. In this sense, the expression "speed kills" is most appropriate.

Another unique personality trait of amphetamine users is compulsive, repetitious behavior. Users can repeat the same action hour after hour without fatigue or boredom. Patients who suffer from full-blown amphetamine psychosis are preoccupied with taking apart complex mechanical structures. They are usually so confused, however, that they cannot reassemble them.[19]

A fully developed toxic syndrome is characterized by vivid visual, auditory, and sometimes tactile hallucinations. In amphetamine psychosis, imaginary snakes or insects crawling on or under the skin are envisioned,[20] and one's sense of reality is greatly changed. Because of such symptoms, it is extremely difficult to distinguish amphetamine psychosis from true schizophrenia. However, rapid recovery usually occurs with the discontinuation of amphetamine use if the toxic and psychotic state has not lasted too long.

The relapse rate of amphetamine users after withdrawal seems to be high. A small percentage of amphetamine users seem to be able to function socially and professionally by restricting their intake, but others show progressive impairment punctuated by hospitalization.

Adverse Effects   A number of adverse effects can result from methamphetamine use. Needle contamination from intravenous use can lead to serious complications, including serum hepatitis, endocarditis, thrombophlebitis, and other forms of infection.[21] Users have a false sense of unlimited energy, which may result in improper self-care or create or reinforce medical and psychiatric problems.[22] There are also a number of side effects that the excessive user may experience—headaches, irritability, palpitations, delirium, circulatory collapses, nausea, vomiting, diarrhea, and abdominal cramps.[23] Nonhealing ulcers, brittle fingernails, bruxism, liver disease, and hypersensitivity have been associated with massive doses of the drug.[24] Malnutrition and weight loss are other major concerns, since speed decreases the desire for food and increases energy output.

Treatment   Treatment for the methamphetamine user, particularly one experiencing psychosis, should include hospitalization. Psychiatric hospitalization at the point of crashing may help to avert a further cycle of amphetamine highs and withdrawal crashes. Chlorpromazine, a tranquilizer, is often used in the treatment of psychosis and may be used to block the central and peripheral effects of amphetamines.

Crank Laboratories   Many crank dealers have moved their operation into the country to elude the law. This is because of the strong, unpleasant odor from the manufacturing process that makes laboratories detectable in crowded cities.[25] A crack dealer needs only $10,000 for chemicals and $2,000 for a laboratory to make $200,000 worth of crank.

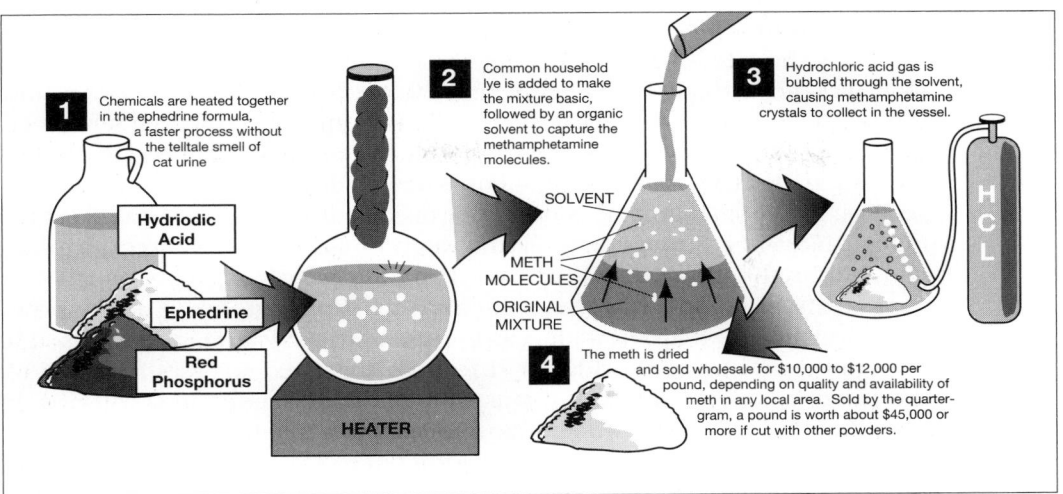

FIGURE 5–1   HOW METH IS MADE

Source: (Bill Bishop, "New Recipe Finding Favor with Meth Makers," *Register-Guard* (Eugene, Oregon), July 28, 1991, p. 4C.)

Price and Availability   Speed at about $30 per gram is one of the most affordable drugs, along with being fairly easy to obtain. Once sold in pill form, speed is now sold as a loose powder in vials or small envelopes and is usually white.[26]

Dumping Meth Lab Wastes   The production of meth often results in property being destroyed. The problem arises when the meth is already made and a toxic waste is left behind. These toxic wastes can be hydrogen chloride gas and lead acetate or even explosive wastes such as ether and red phosphorus.[27] Law enforcement officers dread "taking down" a meth lab because of the risk of these toxic wastes and highly explosive materials. Specially trained teams usually make these arrests. Unfortunately, the smell tends to permeate the trailer, apartment, or house that has been used as a lab, and it is almost impossible to get rid of the odor. In some cases the buildings must be torn down and rebuilt. This creates another problem because most builders don't want to tear down a building that has been exposed to toxic wastes.[28] Sometimes a special team, wearing protective equipment, will have to be called to tear down the structure.

Since the cookers of meth are not able to call up a professional disposal service, they dump the waste wherever it is handy, such as in backyard pits, creeks, and roads and down bathtub drains. This further contaminates dwellings and pollutes the soil and water.

METHAMPHETAMINE: ICE

"**Ice**" in America, "shabu" in Japan, and "hipproppon" in Korea—all these words describe the most potent and addicting form of a methamphetamine to date.[29] Ice is a free-base form of methamphetamine that can

Ice

A stronger form of amphetamine. It is a pure form of methamphetamine hydrochloride, more dangerous than cocaine because of its purity and because the effects last for hours compared to minutes with cocaine use.

be smoked in a pipe at a temperature around 100°F. The base itself does not carry the effects that ice produces, so it is thought that the meth crystal is washed with another chemical.[30] The chemical is not yet known, and it is suspected that Asian chemists may be the only ones to know what it is. Its intense highs last from 8 to 24 hours and result in an immediate euphoria and increased alertness. Its euphoria is described as "amping" by addicts. Ice is smoked and is odorless, making it easy to conceal. According to Mike Sager, rather than getting high or some sort of buzz from ice, you feel bright, awake, and happy.[31] The drug simply makes you feel fantastic without making you feel as if you were on a drug. Ice is a very powerful drug, but it is not new. It was invented by the Japanese, who used it in liquid form during World War II to revitalize tired soldiers. This led to thousands of addictions, and it was consequently banned in the 1950s. It was then relocated in Korea. Japan is the drug's biggest market, but approximately 130,000 Koreans are addicted to ice.[32] Korean drug organizations and gangs (Korean Power, or K. P.) are now trying to spread ice throughout the United States. Korean chemists in Taiwan supply ice to a trafficking network. Ice is threatening to become the next major drug wave to hit the United States and has the potential to turn into an even more serious problem than crack, according to unpublished U.S. intelligence analysis.[33] Hawaii has been hit hard with ice, which has bypassed cocaine and marijuana as Hawaii's biggest drug problem. Intelligence analysts believe methamphetamine labs in the United States will begin to manufacture the drug very soon because of the large profit potential. One estimate is that $700 worth of chemicals could net about $1.6 million. A ranking intelligence official stated that if ice gains even a minor foothold in the United States, it could overrun the country "in a matter of weeks, months, tops."[34]

There are some dangers associated with the drug. A most common side effect is the voices people hear inside their heads.[35] Many people also experience hallucinations—of bugs crawling all over their bodies, for example. Other side effects include paranoia, fatal kidney failure, lung disorders, and long-term psychological damage. The smoking method allows the stimulant to go directly to the brain instead of being filtered through the blood, liver, and kidneys. After a time the brain becomes so flooded with the drug that there results an imbalance that is similar to paranoid schizophrenia.[36] Hawaiian hospitals are now having to take care of ice babies, who seem to be even more damaged and go through more severe withdrawals than crack babies.[37] According to staff, ice babies are even more difficult to handle than cocaine babies. Unfortunately, the drug is expected to be popular among women, who generally favor a drug that is smoked.[38]

Compared to crack cocaine, ice is more expensive ($50 for *less* than a gram compared to crack, which costs $3 to $20 for *less* than a gram), but the high from ice lasts up to 20 hours (see comparison Table 5–1). Since the term of the high is much longer, those on binges find ice a cheaper drug than the others.

TABLE 5–1 COMPARISON CHART

	Crack	Methamphetamine (Speed)	Ice
FORM	White/brown rock chips	Powder, liquid, tablets	Clear, quartzlike chips
ROUTE OF ADMINISTRATION	Smoking	Injection, oral, snorting, smoking	Smoking
PHYSICAL PROPERTIES	Botanical	Pharmaceutical	Pharmaceutical
PLACE OF ORIGIN	South America	U.S., Europe, Far East	U.S., Taiwan, Korea, Philipines
COST PER GRAM	$75–$100	$50–$125	$200–$400
LENGTH OF HIGH	20 minutes	4–5 hours	8–24 Hours
TYPICAL USER	Inner-city youth	White, working-class male/female	White/Asian working-class male/female
EFFECTS	Short, intense euphoria followed by a sharp crash; violent impulses, highly addictive	Intense, much longer euphoria; tremendous energy and heightened sexual potency; violent and paranoid impulses	Euphoria; tremendous energy, confusion, paranoia, nausea, vomiting, coma, possibly death

METHYLPHENIDATE (RITALIN)

Ritalin increases blood pressure, stimulates the central nervous system, and has been used in treating epileptic seizures. It has also been used for a wide variety of clinical conditions, such as obesity, depression, hyperactivity, behavioral disorders in children, and excessive sleepiness. Ritalin is less potent than amphetamines but more potent than caffeine. Its effectiveness has still not been fully evaluated and remains controversial.

PHYSICAL AND PSYCHOLOGICAL EFFECTS

Side Effects The side effects of Ritalin are similar to, though less severe than, the adverse reactions caused by amphetamines. They may consist of nausea, dry mouth, nervousness, restlessness, dizziness, headache, and palpitations. More common reactions are loss of appetite, abdominal pain, weight loss during long-term Ritalin therapy, insomnia, and **tachycardia** (accelerated heartbeat).[39] The long-term use of Ritalin to control hyperactivity is under debate, since continual medication suppresses growth and causes weight loss.

Tachycardia

A fast heartbeat. This is a common condition in amphetamine users and increases the concern for heart damage.

Tolerance Because of the length of time Ritalin stays in the body, a hyperactive child being treated with the drug must receive the dosage around noon if he or she is to sleep at night. It takes the liver approximately 24 hours to break down Ritalin, which is somewhat shorter than the time other drugs take to be eliminated. Thus tolerance can develop more readily with Ritalin than with other drugs.

Dependence   Most available evidence indicates that the use of Ritalin in the treatment of hyperactive children does not cause psychological dependence. Of particular concern following the cessation of hyperactivity and Ritalin use, however, is whether the child will want to use other drugs to cope with the stresses of adolescence.[40]

HYPERKINESIS OR ATTENTION-DEFICIT HYPERACTIVE DISORDER

Attention-Deficit Hyperactive Disorder (ADHD)

A recent term used to describe hyperactivity.

The prescription of Ritalin has increased tenfold over the last 20 years and more than 1 million children with hyperactivity or "attention-deficit disorder" are taking the drug.[41] Although Ritalin is classified as an amphetamine, it has a calming effect on **"attention-deficit hyperactive disorder" (ADHD)** children and helps them increase their attention span. Some say that academic performance is increased, but others may disagree. Safer and Krager studied the effectiveness of stimulant medication in the elementary and middle schools.[42] The study found that stimulant medication was effective in the reduction of hyperactivity and inattentiveness. The effect was more pronounced in the elementary school students than in older kids. However, according to psychiatrist Peter S. Jensen of the Eisenhower Army Medical Center, stimulant drugs such as Ritalin cause unintended psychological effects on hyperactive children and their families.[43] When medication becomes the only treatment offered to the hyperactive children, youngsters often perceive themselves as "bad," causing them to suffer from loss of self-esteem.

Jensen further explains that when assessing both the parents' and the children's feelings toward administering stimulants, both the parents and the children say the medication is a "magic bullet." For if a youngster's behavior doesn't improve, parents respond by increasing the dosage given. Children, on the other hand, begin to disclaim responsibility for their behavior and, instead, claim they need the "good pill" to control themselves. Some of the side effects from Ritalin include headaches, insomnia, stunted growth, and a variety of nervous tics.

Several methods are used to assess children who exhibit characteristics of ADHD: interviews with parents; interviews with and observation of the child; behavior-rating scales completed by parents, teachers, and significant others in the child's life; physical examination; neurological examination; and allergy evaluation.[44] Parent and child interviews and behavior-rating scales are most often used. Psychological testing is valuable for determining the specific nature of the child's deficits and strengths. Approximately 5 percent of elementary school children have been diagnosed as hyperactive, the problem occurring more frequently in boys.[45]

Hyperactivity is the most common complaint of parents who bring their children to mental-health facilities; some say it accounts for 40 percent of all cases.[46] Robert Smith and John Netsworth believe this condition is based on some inborn error of metabolism, but organic brain damage is usually not detectable.[47]

Childhood hyperactivity is characterized by a combination of behaviors: short attention span and distractibility, restlessness, poor impulse control, excessive motor activity, learning difficulties, and emotional liability. The child may be easily frustrated, aggressive, destructive, and apparently antisocial. Behavioral problems may come about from poor verbal skills and problems with conception, perception, memory, attention, impulse control, and motor functions (jumping, running, or otherwise moving about somewhat out of control). Although the mechanism of treatment is not understood, hyperactive children do respond to stimulant medication.

There are two points to consider when treating a hyperactive child: The child is difficult to cope with and has difficulty coping.[48] One must be sure which of these problems to deal with and which approach is appropriate. Giving a child Ritalin to help him or her cope may be justifiable, but doing so to help others cope with the child is an infringement of his or her rights.

EDUCATING THE HYPERKINETIC CHILD

Behaviors associated with hyperactivity are usually not noticed or are not much of a problem until the child begins school. In the classroom, however, such behaviors can create a classroom management problem, and learning difficulties may occur. As parents, teacher, and physician work with the hyperkinetic child, they should examine their roles, since their feelings and attitudes are altered by the behaviors they are judging.

Children who use Ritalin will frequently be identified by their teachers because of the learning deficiencies they exhibit. When instructors recognize these symptoms, they should be prepared to alter their teaching materials to meet the children's needs. Expressing negative attitudes about the children or the use of Ritalin may seriously impair the medical treatment and reduce the drug's usefulness in the school environment.

Alternative Treatments for Hyperactivity   There are other ways, besides using Ritalin, to treat hyperactivity: (1) behavior modification, (2) caffeine, (3) reduction of food additives, and (4) electromyographic biofeedback. Behavior modification is an attractive alternative because it is nonchemical. A study of hyperactive elementary school children was done in 1977 to find out if stimulant drugs could be withdrawn immediately, or at least reduced gradually, and be replaced with behavioral therapy; parent and teacher feedback was used in evaluating the progress of the children. The study showed that behavioral treatment improved the condition of unmedicated children by over 33 percent. Social behavior significantly improved and was related to the amount of the parents' commitment to the treatment group.[49] Another study, conducted in Atlanta and Chicago, found behavior modification of definite value in reducing symptoms of minimal brain dysfunction and hyperkinesis. This study focused on rewarding positive school performance in math and reading activities. Results indicated that school-work as well as behavior skills improved with behavior modification.[50]

The use of caffeine to treat hyperactivity is grounded in research: "A pilot study substituting caffeine in the form of two cups of regular coffee a day suggests that caffeine may be an alternative to a Schedule II [Ritalin-based] drug."[51] (Schedule II drugs include opium, codeine, morphine, methadone, cocaine, and amphetamines.) Caffeine has a calming effect on some hyperkinetic children, and treatment with it is free. The theory behind caffeine use in hyperactivity came to light when Robert Schnacker noted an unusually high rate of coffee drinking in young hyperkinetic children. When asked why they drank so much coffee, the children replied, "It calms me down" or "I can do better in school."

Benjamin Feingold found that food additives in hyperkinetic children's diets affected their behavior. When the children ate only food containing no additives, their hyperactivity would markedly decrease or disappear entirely. Dr. Feingold designed a diet that eliminated artificial colors and flavors and certain preservatives, including those in breakfast cereals, desserts, meats, soft drinks, flavored yogurt, colored cheeses, butter, margarine, gum, vitamins, toothpastes, cough drops, and candy.[52] Fruits such as apples, apricots, berries, cherries, currants, grapes, raisins, nectarines, oranges, and peaches, once thought to contain naturally occurring salicylates, were also banned from the diet; but recent analysis has found little or no salicylate in some of these fruits. Salicylate-containing foods are now permitted in some Feingold diets. Despite the diets' successes, however, results of several recent studies have led researchers to question the idea that diet control is the ultimate panacea for hyperactivity.[53]

The fourth alternative is electromyographic biofeedback training for the reduction of muscle tension. Such training

> involves the use of electronic equipment to monitor a subject's physiological processes (which are normally not attended to and not under "voluntary" control) and then [makes] these processes known to the subject by means of some external stimulus such as a light or tone. This "externalization" of information about internal functioning ultimately allows the subject to gain voluntary control over his internal physiological systems.[54]

This alternative is relatively new, and further research is needed before it can be employed extensively in the schools.

Physicians are concerned that adverse publicity and public opinion may affect the medical use of Ritalin for people with attention-deficit hyperactivity. Such publicity includes questions about the drug's possible harmful side effects and the perceived eagerness with which doctors prescribe it. The medical community maintains that because Ritalin has been the same for many years with some addition of behavior therapy, cognitive training, and dietary manipulation, that the proper use of stimulant drugs is still good treatment.

One of the major public concerns is that Ritalin is being overused: Sales of the drug have surged since 1985. Another public concern is that the desire of teachers and other adults to control children's behavior, coupled with the overly broad definition of hyperactivity and the excessive use of Ritalin, may result in hyperactive children becoming drug addicts. In the final analysis, before prescribing anything for attention-deficit hyperactivity disorder, there should be a comprehensive diagnosis and evaluation, proper baseline assessment, and family involvement."[55]

There appears to be a new problem associated with the use of Ritalin: Ritalin is gaining in popularity as a drug of abuse among adults.[56] Prescriptions of Ritalin account for one half of the cases of abuse. Ironically, this drug when purchased at a pharmacy costs 35¢ for a 10-milligram tablet; the price on the street increases to $5 per tablet.

A large dose of Ritalin provides the effects of amphetamines—with the possible benefit of relatively high safeguards involving quality control. Abusers often combine narcotics, which generally provides a sedative effect, with Ritalin to produce the "speedball" effect, with the Ritalin counteracting the narcotic's depressive attribute. Ritalin causes tolerance to develop rather fast, and often a user, an adult family member of a hyperactive child, will get multiple prescriptions from several doctors.

COCAINE

INTRODUCTION

Cocaine is a potent and rapid-acting stimulant, an alkaloid derived from the leaves of the *Erythroxylon* coca plant. Coca paste is extracted from the leaves of the plant where it grows high in the Andes mountains and is then smuggled to northern Chile, Argentina, or southern Colombia, where it is processed. A typical processing compound employs 1,000 people, may have as many as 19 separate laboratories, and is capable of producing 300 tons of cocaine a year. Pure cocaine is fine, opalescent, white, fluffy, odorless, and bitter-tasting.

Cocaine was the most popular illegal stimulant of the 1980s. A recent medical journal report estimated that over 25 million Americans had tried the drug and that every day another 5,000 take their first dose.[57] Until the early 1980s cocaine was used mainly by the wealthy. Now it is also used by students, by heroin addicts who want an extra lift, and by lower-income groups.

The nationwide epidemic of cocaine addiction not only appears to have swept all socioeconomic levels but is an increasing problem for women. More women are turning up at drug-treatment centers and joining self-help groups.

According to Ronald Dougherty, director of the chemical-abuse recovery service at Benjamin Rush Hospital, a psychiatric institution in Syracuse, New York, 53 percent of the women referred for treatment for cocaine abuse are younger than 30, compared with 25 percent of the men. Women tend to use cocaine in greater quantity, between $500 and $1,000 worth a week, compared with $300 for men. The price of cocaine has generally been dropping and now ranges from approximately $60 to $150 per gram. "Women start earlier and are into larger amounts," said Dougherty. "With increased use, and increasing problems, women are getting into trouble with the law, with their employers and with their families."[58]

HISTORY

It is thought that a pre-Inca tribe began to cultivate the coca plant because the wild leaves were unfit for chewing. By the end of the fourteenth century, use of the plant by the peasantry was widespread as a means of relieving hunger while increasing strength and endurance.[59] To this day, Indians in the mountainous areas of Peru and Bolivia use cocaine to help themselves tolerate the cold and suppress their hunger.

In 1884 young Sigmund Freud became interested in cocaine. He had read of the substance's beneficial effects, and he purchased a quantity of it to use in treating those of his patients who suffered from heart disease and nervous exhaustion. Eventually Freud was to experiment with it himself, since he suffered from depression, chronic fatigue, and various neurotic symptoms. After using the drug, he found that a mood of disfavor turned to one of cheer.

Freud experimented with cocaine for three years, then discontinued the drug's use and no longer prescribed it for his patients. He and a number of his colleagues had become concerned about prolonged and excessive use of the drug.

The same year Freud became interested in cocaine, an ophthalmologist friend of his, Karl Koller, did intensive experimental studies on its numbing effect. The drug became popular immediately and was used in eye surgery and dentistry. William Halsted, the father of modern American surgery and one of the founders of the Johns Hopkins Medical School, was the first to use cocaine extensively as a local anesthetic in surgery. The drug caught on with writers. In one of his stories Sir Arthur Conan Doyle had Sherlock Holmes injecting cocaine three times a day, and speculation has it that Robert Louis Stevenson wrote *The Strange Case of Dr. Jekyll and Mr. Hyde* with the help of the drug.[60]

In 1888 Asa G. Chandler took a momentous step in the history of popular beverages when he bought the rights to an almost completely unknown proprietary elixir called Coca-Cola. Initially very few knew that cocaine was an additive in the drink (giving a new meaning to "the pause that refreshes"), but when the slang term for Coca-Cola became *dope,* Chandler's company became worried about its corporate image. Passage of the Pure Food and Drug Act in 1906 forced elimination of cocaine from Coke, and in 1914 the Harrison Narcotic Act made cocaine use illegal except for limited medical purposes.

In the late 1960s illicit use of "coke" began to spread, especially among rock and movie performers. The Grateful Dead went so far as to popularize cocaine use in their song "Casey Jones." Today cocaine is one of the most popular drugs for those able to afford it. Heroin is the only street drug more expensive.

In the early 1980s cocaine was promoted as a relatively safe, nonaddicting, and euphorian agent. Because people thought it was safe, they tried it. By

1986, the National Institute on Drug Abuse said 3 million Americans abused cocaine; that's about five times the number for heroin.[61]

Some of the following cocaine highlights were reported in the 1990 National Household Survey on Drug Abuse:[62]

- Among the 6.2 million people who used cocaine in the past year, 662,000 (10.6 percent) used the drug once a week or more and 336,000 (5.4 percent) used the drug daily or almost daily throughout the year. Although the number of past-year and past-month cocaine users has decreased significantly since the peak year 1985, frequent or more intense use has not decreased. Of the 12.2 million past-year cocaine users in 1985, an estimated 647,000 used the drug weekly and 246,000 used it daily or almost daily.

- Rates for use of cocaine in the past year declined for youth (12–17 years old) from 4.0 percent in 1985 to 2.9 percent in 1988 to 2.2 percent in 1990. For young adults (aged 18–25), the rates for 1985, 1988, and 1990 are 16.3 percent, 12.1 percent, and 7.5 percent, respectively. These decreases between 1985 and 1990 were statistically significant for both age groups.

- Approximately 1.4 percent of the population 12 years old and over have used crack at some time in their lives, and one half of 1 percent used crack during the past year. These rates changed very little from those in 1988. This translates to about 1 million past-year users for each year, 1988 and 1990. Past-year use in 1990 is highest among males (0.8 percent), blacks (1.7 percent), and the unemployed (1.3 percent). By age group, the highest rate is for young adults 18–25 years old (1.4 percent).

However, policy makers have sometimes misconstrued the full picture of cocaine abuse in the United States by relying on one-dimensional data from government-sponsored surveys of drug use in American households and among high school seniors.[63] The problem is that the numbers cited invariably reflect an undercount of the very populations most likely to regularly use cocaine—the homeless, heroin addicts, school dropouts, and prisoners.

PHYSIOLOGICAL AND PHARMACOLOGICAL EFFECTS

Cocaine is a very powerful drug that has a variety of effects on the central nervous system, such as increased heart rate and increased nerve stimulation, and it causes strong feelings of well-being and euphoria. The euphoria lasts 15 to 40 minutes, which makes it desirable to use cocaine more often than other stimulants such as amphetamines. Cocaine dependence usually occurs in 2 to 4 years, with cocaine "binges" an increasing occurrence as time goes by. Abusers may average two or three binges every week. It lowers anxiety and social inhibitions while increasing alertness, energy, self-esteem, and sexuality. The drug offers an intense high. A more clinical description of cocaine's effect on the user follows:

Cocaine alters the synaptic transmission in the central nervous system and produces an excess of norepinephrine and dopamine at the postsynaptic receptor sites by blocking their presynaptic uptake. This results in an adren-ergic response, manifested by hypertension, tachycardia, mydriasis, hyper-glycemia, hyperthermia ("cocaine fever"), and most important with respect to morbidity, a predisposition to seizure and arrhythemias.[64]

In other words, cocaine attacks and blocks the reuptake of dopamine into the cell that releases it, thus making an excess amount of dopamine available to be taken up by other neurons. Cocaine acts as a shield, causing neurotrans-mitters to keep producing the chemical. Cocaine has severe effects on the brain. It can produce headaches, seizures, or strokes.[65] These effects can take place several hours or even days after the drug is taken. As the dose is increased, so are the depth of respiration and the heart rate. Large doses may cause tremors and convulsive movements, medullary depression, and respi-ratory and cardiac failure.

Cocaine numbs the sensory- and motor-nerve endings and causes blood vessels to contract, resulting in decreased stimulation. Euphoria is felt, accompanied by an increase in mental alertness, dilated pupils, heightened muscular strength, a decrease in hunger, and an increase in talkativeness and sexual stimulation. Cocaine works on the peripheral nervous system, which releases the neurotransmitter norepinephrine. With excessive dosages, cocaine can produce hallucinations and paranoid delusions, including itch-ing; cocaine bugs (the sensation of insects moving under or on the skin, clin-ically known as formication); the sensation of people brushing against the body; smoke, gasoline, fecal, and other foul odors; and voices calling and whispering.

Cocaine can cause sudden death by triggering the "chaotic heart rhythm called ventricular fibrillation. Cocaine can overwork the heart, forcing it to beat too fast and powerfully.[66] As the heart tires, it becomes susceptible to irregularities in its normal rhythm, which can cause it to stop. Cocaine can also cause coronary-artery spasm, a sudden narrowing of the arteries leading to the heart. Such spasms can cause blood to clot, even in otherwise normal arteries. These spasms restrict the flow to the heart and cause heart attacks or dangerous heartbeat irregularities.

Basically, the drug's effects are unpredictable. Cocaine can kill a person even if the heart is in perfect shape. The size of the dose is unimportant. After a single dose, superbly conditioned athletes like Len Bias and Don Rogers have succumbed to the potent and variable effects of cocaine.

A study done in Brookhaven National Laboratory in Upton, New York, involved researchers injecting healthy volunteers with radioactivity-labeled cocaine at doses far too small to induce addiction or a high.[67] They found that the drug binds strongly to heart cells, especially those in the left ventricle. From this it was suggested that cocaine overdose may pose a triple threat to the heart. It was already known that cocaine abuse can cause heart failure through its indirect effects of constricting blood vessels and manipulating the brain to disrupt normal heart rhythm. The new finding of cocaine binding directly to cardiac tissue suggests that cocaine may slow the passage of sodium ions into the heart cells and stimulate the release of the neurotransmitter norepinepherine, which may lead to irregular heartbeat, or arrhythemia. It was also found that large concentrations of the drug bind to the aorta and may account for some of the blood-vessel damage associated with cocaine overdoses.

There are several ways to take cocaine. It may be swallowed, but this is not as effective as other methods because of poor absorption in the gastrointestinal tract. The most common method is to snort the drug (sniff it through the nose). The powder is first chopped fine with a razor blade and arranged into lines or columns on a piece of glass. The user may then inhale the cocaine through a rolled-up dollar bill, an empty pen cartridge, a straw, or a "coke spoon." In some cases, a tightly rolled hundred-dollar bill (chic!), a diamond-studded straw, or a gold tooter becomes part of the ritual.

When the powder is sniffed, the blood vessels in the nose are constricted and their blood supply is reduced. Chronic rhinitis (inflammation of the sinus membrane) and, in general, greater vulnerability to upper respiratory infection are adverse effects of snorting.[68] Furthermore, less experienced and less meticulous sniffers will incur damage to the nasal pathways from their less thoroughly chopped cocaine. (Some of the materials added to cocaine, such as sugars—especially mannitol—cause clumping, and the synthetic lidocaine, with which cocaine is cut or mixed, makes the crystals harder to chop.) Recreational use of cocaine has also been linked to coronary-artery spasms and myocardial infarction.[69] In addition, cellulose granulomas have been found in the lungs of the recreational sniffer.

Injecting cocaine produces an intense and exhilarating rush, but one that is short-lived because of the drug's rapid metabolization by the liver. The active ingredients in cocaine that is injected may have been cut with inert ingredients. Such nondrug cuts are usually insoluble in the blood and veins and become emboli that lodge in the arterioles and capillary beds of the vein. Intravenous administration provides the highest plasma concentration (the drug gets directly into the bloodstream and in a higher concentration) in the shortest period, but this carries the added risk of contaminated needles. Oral, muscular, and other forms of administration take longer, and the drug becomes diluted before entering the blood. Moreover, deaths from acquired immune deficiency syndrome (AIDS) have been reported among intravenous cocaine shooters from San Francisco to New York City.[70]

Binge use is common, with users sharing a needle for injection many times in a short period, unlike that of the heroin addict, who falls asleep after injection.

A relatively new and more intense form of cocaine known as free-base is being used in affluent circles of the United States. It is unique in its dramatic effects, cost, and possible health hazards. Free-base cocaine is popular because it produces a stronger high and because the process by which it is made eliminates some of the cutting agents. Cocaine hydrochloride (street-market cocaine) is dissolved in water, and a solvent (usually petroleum ether or ammonia) is added to release the cocaine alkaloid from the salt and other adulterants. A stronger base is then added to neutralize the acid content. The solvent rises to the top, where it can be filtered or drawn off. As the solvent evaporates, the cocaine salt oxidizes and what is left is cocaine base. The volatile nature of this process sometimes has explosive consequences.

This method gets rid of most, but not all, possible cuts in cocaine. Sugars such as mannitol and lactose are eliminated. However, cocainelike salts remain. Since most cocaine sold on the streets is far from pure, what is left after the free-base process is often less than half the original amount.

Free-base cocaine is water-soluble and can be smoked or injected. The high is rapid, powerful, and short-lived, much like the high from injection. The euphoria and feelings of energy last only a few minutes, but the effects on the autonomic nervous system include prolonged pupil dilation, increased blood pressure, and increased heart and respiratory rates. The euphoria is quickly followed by irritability and discomfort. This extreme shift creates a strong desire to continue free-basing. Some people have turned to heroin or other depressants to relieve the aftereffects. Side effects from chronic free-basing include chest pains, sore throat, hoarse voice, shortness of breath, swollen mouth glands, and an aching, flulike feeling. The increased heart rate and blood pressure caused by cocaine could cause problems for people with high blood pressure. Some users have been hospitalized for ammonia poisoning when they haven't taken the time to rinse the ammonia-soaked powder in water during the final extraction stage. A few instances of bronchitis have occurred, but exactly what constant use of free-base will do to the lungs remains to be seen.

The greatest danger is the possibility of overdose, since in smoking free-base, as in injecting, a high blood level of the drug is assimilated quickly. Although individual tolerance levels vary, any more than 20 milligrams of cocaine per kilogram of body weight will severely impair the respiratory control center in the brain and the user may die of cardiorespiratory arrest.[71]

As we have noted, users often feel compelled to continue free-basing in order to keep the euphoria and avoid the postuse depression; they eventually find themselves physically and financially exhausted. Heavy users experience insomnia, weight loss, and paranoia.

One of the common problems surrounding cocaine is how quickly one starts to abuse the drug. The half-life of cocaine in plasma is 1.5 hours, but because the effect felt by the user is for only 45 minutes, the user may overdose more easily. Because the user has this shortened euphoria he or she may go on binges lasting as long as a week and averaging 12 hours.[72] Further, although stimulants magnify the pleasure, "they do not distort it." Because of this, and because users are reinforced by others for their energy and skill while using drugs, they tend to repeat the usage.[73]

This leads to the user's lack of attention to other personal issues, including family, health, and work. Cocaine's adverse effects—disinhibition, hypersexuality, impaired judgment, grandiosity, heart damage, hypervigilance, compulsively repeated actions, and extreme psychomotor activation—are usually, but not always, associated with the high dose. These adverse effects can lead to accidents, criminal behavior, and atypical sexual behavior; and adverse effects occur in about 80 percent of regular cocaine users.[74]

PSYCHOLOGICAL-PHYSIOLOGICAL DEPENDENCY

As mentioned earlier, many users binge on cocaine. Afterward they crash, and this is generally characterized by extreme exhaustion. Symptoms of withdrawal include anergia (low energy), apathy, and low ability to experience pleasure. It usually takes 6 to 18 weeks to break the habit, although cravings can occur for weeks, months, or even years afterward.

The neurophysiological properties of cocaine are such that the drug locks people into continuous use.[75] Cocaine was once considered a safe recreational drug. However, research indicates that cocaine has negative psychological and physiological effects. Daily and binge users may experience confusion, anxiety,

HOW COCAINE ASSAULTS THE BODY

Cocaine's chief effects are on the nervous system and blood vessels. Researchers have found these direct and indirect actions from ingesting cocaine either in its powder form or in crack pellets:

Blood vessels	Constriction of blood vessels.
	Quick rises in blood pressure.
	Angina
Heart	Reduced flow of oxygenated blood to heart.
	Cellular damage.
	Irregularity or increased rate of heartbeat.
	Heart attacks.
Brain, nervous system	Arterial constriction or breaking of weakened artery, leading to stroke.
	Seizures, tremors, delirium, and psychosis.
Abdomen	Constriction of blood supply to intestines.
Liver	Destruction of cells.
Lungs	Accumulation of fluid.
Nasal passages	Damage to cells in lining of nose.
	Loss of sense of smell.
Reproductive system	With long-term use, difficulty in maintaining erection and ejaculating for males and difficulty in reaching orgasm for females.

Lawrence K. Altman, "Cocaine's Many Dangers: The Evidence Mounts," *New York Times*, January 26, 1988, p. C3.

depression, short tempers, and paranoia and they may neglect responsibilities. In acute cases cocaine psychosis may be sustained. A cocaine psychotic becomes paranoid and experiences auditory and visual hallucinations and/or "coke bugs," which give the user the feeling that bugs are crawling beneath the skin. The effects upon the body may be as minor as a runny nose or as severe as death. The drug may induce epilepsy and cause angina and irregular heartbeat. Cocaine has caused death by creating respiratory paralysis, convulsions, and allergic reactions. Cocaine's strength as a reinforcer may explain its addicting nature. The physiological effects seen primarily as reinforcers may also be strengthened by secondary effects.

DOPAMINE

Researchers at the National Institute on Drug Abuse Addiction Research Center found a regular site for dopamine possibly responsible for cocaine's strong addiction. With the presence of cocaine in the system, the chemical process that removes the neurotransmitter dopamine from the synaptic cleft is severely inhibited.[76] The result is that neurons are not able to relax their messages; cocaine thus prolongs the effect of dopamine.

COCAINE AND SUICIDE

Analysis done by the National Institute of Drug Abuse and Johns Hopkins University School of Medicine determined that using cocaine dramatically increases the likelihood that a suicide attempt will occur, sometimes increasing the risk by as much as 62 percent.[77] Cocaine use provides for a greater chance of attempted suicide than either clinical depression or alcohol abuse.

COCAINE AS AN APHRODISIAC

A study of 228 coke users and ex-users who weren't associated with treatment programs was conducted to determine if cocaine is an aphrodisiac.[78] The study found that men have a greater level of cocaine-induced sexual enhancement than women do. In males, orgasm can be prolonged and premature ejaculation prevented, but this is by no means automatic. In fact, more often than not, cocaine use among males leads to some kind of sexual impairment, ranging from lack of arousal to an inability to perform. Freebasers and snorters generally have the same level of sexual dysfunction, but injectors suffer the most problems with sex.

Whether cocaine acts as an aphrodisiac depends heavily on individual differences such as gender, dosage, set, and setting. It was found, however, that the longer one uses large doses of cocaine, the more likely he or she is to have sexual trouble.

CRACK

Crack is cocaine mixed with baking soda and water over a hot flame. The substance (which is 90 percent pure cocaine) is then dried. The "soapy-looking substance" that results can be broken up into rocks and smoked.[79] These rocks are approximately five times as strong as cocaine.[80] Crack gets its name from the popping noises it makes when it is smoked.

Because crack is such a pure drug, it takes much less time to achieve the desired high. One puff of a pebble-sized rock produces an intense high that lasts about 20 minutes. The user can usually get three or four "hits" off the rock before it is used up. Crack is generally purchased in small plastic vials containing two or three rocks. The price for a vial is usually $10 to $20.

In May 1987 police discovered a new form of crack. Instead of a rocklike substance, it resembled the common aspirin. This new style of crack is being sold under names such as "easy access" or "press." The name *press* is derived from the way the "pills" are made. The dealer simply takes the crack and presses it into a mold.[81] The aspirin-sized pellets of the drug are being sold for $8 each. The user must smoke it; just ingesting the pill would not be as efficient in producing the desired high.

As compared to snorting cocaine powder, smoking free-base produces a more intense, more rapid high (euphoria), a greater concentration of the drug in the bloodstream and the brain, and a more powerful compulsion in the user to repeat the experience. Within 7 to 15 seconds, the cocaine is flooding the brain cells, but absorption is blocked so the chemicals just flood the spaces between the cells and continuously excite the nerves. The user's pulse rate increases and he or she seems to feel an incredible sense of euphoric energy and becomes alert, confident, and very talkative. The high from each dose lasts about 20 minutes and is followed immediately by feelings of irritability, agitation, and intense cravings for more cocaine.[82]

"Crack is often used in binges lasting one to three days at a time. During the course of a binge, the drug is smoked continuously until money and drug supplies are depleted or the user collapses from physical exhaustion. As much as 10 to 15 grams of cocaine, or even several ounces of the drug, may be consumed during a binge."[83]

Unlike cocaine addiction, which takes three to four years to develop, a crack user may become addicted in six to ten weeks.[84] Addiction is accelerated by the speed in which crack is absorbed through the lungs (it hits the brain within seconds after use) and by the intensity of the high.

Crack can be mixed with different substances to alter its effects as well as its looks. The following are just a few of the more popular mixtures and their intended effects:[85]

MIXER	EFFECTS
yeast	expands the amount
vitamin B12	Adds color and flavor to crack
speed	helps sustain the amphetamine rush
Valium	user "stays cool" during the rush
PCP	a wild, more sustained high ("space-basing")
heroin	minimizes the intense crash ("speedballing")

Physiological and Psychological Effects   A person can become physiologically, psychologically, and socially addicted to crack. When the person smokes crack, the brain's neurotransmitters (dopamine, serotonin, and norepinephrine) are triggered and released, which causes the euphoric feeling. However, the cocaine blocks the return of these neurotransmitters to the nerve cells for reuse. So, with repeated use, the individual's brain is squeezed of its neurotransmitters. The absence of the drug and the loss of the neurotransmitters force the body into a state of withdrawal.[86] The body craves stimulation but is not getting it from the drug or, to a lesser degree, the body.

Although it takes several weeks to become physically addicted to crack, people can become psychologically addicted after smoking it just a few times. Because of the immediate, extreme high, even very limited use is enough to make them feel they have to have the drug again.

Crack gradually destroys the body. Seconds after use, the blood vessels constrict, the heart rate rapidly increases, the brain is intensely stimulated, blood pressure quickly rises, body temperature rises, and the pupils of the eyes dilate. With continued use, the effects get worse. The user experiences sore throat or hoarseness, shortness of breath, weight loss, high blood pressure, and increasing confusion. The long-term effects can be devastating—emphysema, yellowish skin, loss of teeth, sores (due to scratching for "crack bugs"), psychological damage, malnutrition, and heart problems.[87]

People who smoke crack, whether for the first time or the fiftieth time, are risking their lives and maybe those of others as well. The intense crack high can be too much for the body, causing respiratory arrest, heart attack, or convulsions. Crack addicts feel such a need for the drug and may be experiencing such horrible depression while crashing that their chances of committing a crime are enormously increased. It is this despair that has led to the numerous violent crimes committed by "crack heads." For example, in New York City a young man threw his eight-year-old niece off an apartment balcony because the child's mother refused to give him crack.[88] In another case a 24-year-old man killed his girlfriend with a 9-inch butcher knife after smoking six pellets of crack.[89] Such horror stories are numerous.

"What makes crack so addicting is that it produces such a high," says Dr. Kleber. "When you snort cocaine, the high lasts for awhile, but it is not very strong. You can walk away from it. But when you smoke crack, the high is so intense that you go out after more."[90]

Animal Experiments   Researchers recently found interesting results with rats that were hooked up to an intravenous source of cocaine.[91] If they pushed the lever, they would get the drug. The rats did virtually nothing but push the lever. Within a month, they had lost 40 percent of their body weight and were dead. Another group of rats were hooked up to an intravenous source of heroin. They, too, pushed the lever to get the drug, but they also managed to eat and sleep. All were alive and apparently healthy a month later.

Researchers find that cocaine works in the brain by absorbing essential chemicals, most notably dopamine, that normally one nerve requires to excite another, but only briefly. After doing their work, these chemicals are quickly absorbed by the nerves and the excitement ends. But with cocaine, dopamine is not absorbed and continues to excite nerve cells. The result is that nerve stimulation rises to a crescendo with no relief, causing the feeling of euphoria.

Medical Consequences   The medical consequences of smoking crack can include brain seizures, lung damage, heart attack, stroke, neurological impairment, chronic cough, chest congestion, black phlegm, wheezing, burning of the lips, throat, and tongue, and weight loss.[92] The fatal overdose reaction to cocaine is much greater with crack because of the large drug doses delivered to the brain. Inhaling purified cocaine gets the substance into the bloodstream faster (within 20 seconds) than snorting at higher concentrations.

PROBLEMS WITH COCAINE AND CRACK

Crime on the Streets   America once thought of drug-related crime in terms of heroin, with stable organized-crime groups managing the distribution, with junkies stealing for the price of a fix and then nodding off. In contrast, the crack high reinforces aggression and feelings of power. Crack is distributed by younger, wilder, more heavily armed gangs. They arrogantly intimidate whole communities and make war on each other to control the lucrative business.

Kids Who Sell Crack   Crack has brought with it an assortment of problems. There are now three levels of drug-related jobs for kids on the streets.[93] The first is the lookout. Lookouts are young kids who warn dealers whenever police are in the area. These kids receive $100 a day. The next level is runner. Runners are older kids who transport drugs to various dealers in an area. These kids make $300 a day. The final level is dealer. Dealers actually peddle the drugs throughout the community. Because these kids are on the front lines, they earn up to $3,000 a day. Drug lords prefer to use children to sell drugs because they are not at risk to serve a jail sentence.

Crack Gangs   In the 1970s, gangs were proud of their area. They defended what was theirs, the neighborhood in which they were raised. However, with crack the priorities have changed focus to drugs and money.[94] It appears the use of crack has become more important than the gang itself. Gangs are not protectors of the land anymore but, instead, drug and money dealers involved in endless numbers of crimes and murders. Gang members are of deep concern to the communities, especially when innocent people die because they are in the wrong place at the wrong time during a shootout. In cities throughout the United States the outbreak of crack has resulted in more gang killings than ever before. In 1987, for example, there were 387 reported gang killings in Los Angeles County, and in 1988 the number climbed to about 450. The most saddening and maddening thing about gang killings is that the majority of victims are innocent bystanders caught in a crossfire.

In Los Angeles, the black street gangs, the Bloods and the Crips, have the corner on the crack market.[95] Gangs fight to get a monopoly on the drug market, and they care little about life, not expecting to live over the age of 25 themselves.

Increasing Number of Homicides   In 1987, 20,096 people were murdered in the United States.[96] It is estimated that the number of homicides will continue to increase as long as crack is popular. Dealers degrade the bodies of their victims by riddling a body with several bullets or decapitating it.[97] In other words, crack dealers appear to have total disregard of the value of human beings.

One reason for the homicides is that dealers have sophisticated weapons. They begin by buying or stealing bulletproof vests, silencers, military assault guns, and automatic pistols. Indeed, in many cases the drug gangs have more gun power than the police. Kids, especially poor ones, are enticed into the drug business because of the large amounts of money they can make. They are attracted by the dealers' expensive material items, their stereos, cars, jewelry, and automatic weapons.[98]

In 1989, Washington, D.C., became the city with the highest crime rate in America.[99] Other cities, such as Philadelphia, New York, and Kansas City, offer the same scenario. The drug problem is highly visible, with everyday deals taking place on many street corners, youths toting guns and flaunting more money than their parents have ever seen, and very young children running around and watching for police.[100] These children know no other way of life. Either they have seen their parents work hard and get nowhere (because of a lack of education) or they have witnessed their parents using drugs and thus believe it is acceptable. Another problem arises when parents know their children are stealing and making money; because they are getting part of it, the parents accept the situation or are even happy with it. Youngsters in these communities often lack the self-discipline needed to grow up in a neighborhood where they are constantly exposed to drugs.[101] During the past three years crack use has also grown to epidemic proportions in New York City. Despite the more than $500 million spent by the city in the last fiscal year on drug-related enforcement alone—more than twice the amount spent in 1986—the presence of crack is more pervasive, more violent, and more insidious in its effect on New Yorkers, particularly the poor.[102]

Crack Houses   The crack house, whose ancestor is the opium den of the 1960s, is a convenient place to use the drug.[103] Crack houses are usually old warehouses or boarded-up buildings; they are normally so heavily guarded that police would rather ignore their presence than risk their lives busting them. Inside, the user can buy crack along with an assortment of other drugs that supposedly make the crack high better or the crash less intense. Within these fortresses you can find representatives of every stratum of the community, from the common junkie to a businessman on his lunch break.[104]

There is a very complicated system of supply and distribution in these houses, many of which are run by the same organization. These organizations tend to be street gangs who are expanding their business from pushing marijuana on the streets to shuttling a crack operation among a series of rundown houses to avoid detection by the police. Crack houses all have one thing in common: no shortage of customers.[105]

However, many people in the neighborhood, especially in the bigger cities, are getting tired of crack houses and the crimes associated with them.[106] The residents in nearby apartments are tired and scared: They are tired simply because the police are having a difficult time busting people. Residents are fighting back in many ways: by developing a sophisticated arsenal of weapons; by organizing street patrols, to break up the rhythm of the crack dealers; by performing block watches and giving information to beat police; by serving civil court evictioning; and even sometimes, by hiring private security forces to patrol the neighborhood.[107] The police in New York City feel they are being helped tremendously when residents take steps to clean up their own neighborhoods.

Women on Crack   People agree that the crack epidemic poses what may be called the greatest threat to this country's future. What is seldom said is that crack is taking a disproportionate toll on women, whether or not they are addicted.[108] Many women take crack not only to experience the euphoria but to ease the pressures of modern life. A poll taken by the 1-800-COCAINE hotline found that the average female caller was 25 years of age.[109] Of those who admitted to having a problem, 50 percent stated they were involved in some kind of violent activity because of their cocaine use. The reasons women found themselves with a cocaine habit varied; however, all of these women were low in self-esteem. Many said that cocaine "fills the emptiness," an emptiness that seems able to be filled only with this wonder drug that gives them energy and the feeling they can conquer the world. Some women describe the great thrill they receive when introduced to a new drug, and it is also a thrill for many of these women to keep their habit hidden.

Crack and Pregnancy   There are approximately 375,000 babies born on crack, and that may be a very low estimate.[110] Cocaine or crack babies, as they are called, are more likely to be born prematurely or die before birth. When a pregnant woman takes cocaine, it triggers spasms in the baby's blood vessels, which can severely restrict the flow of oxygen and nutrients for long periods.

FETAL HAZARDS.   The first detailed studies of babies exposed to cocaine before birth suggest that the widely used drug is causing an epidemic of damaged infants, some of whom may be impaired for life because their mothers used cocaine even briefly during pregnancy.[111] The new research has found a wide spectrum of ill effects that can result from fetal exposure to cocaine. These include retarded growth in the womb and subtle neurological abnor-

Caring for Abandoned Crack
Babies
Source: AP/Wide World Photos

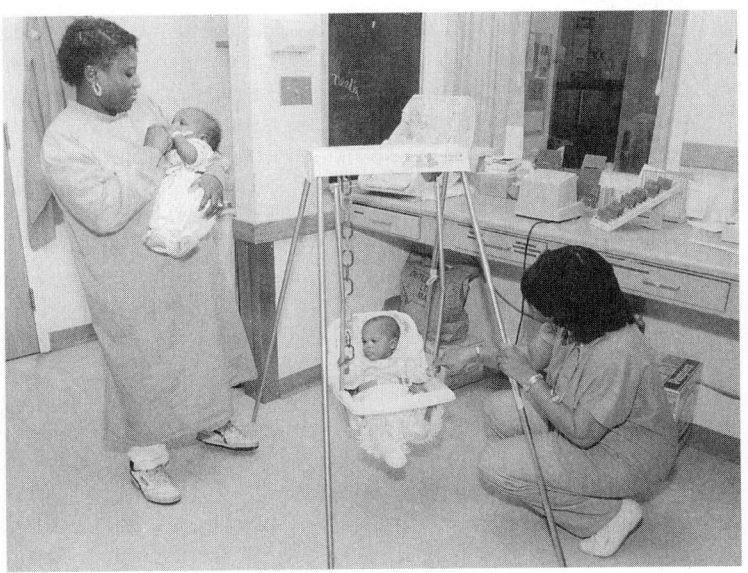

malities, which may afflict a majority of exposed newborns. In more extreme cases, cocaine can cause loss of the small intestine and brain-damaging strokes.[112] Even if a women stops the drug once pregnancy is diagnosed or uses it only intermittently, her baby can suffer physical and behavioral problems. The research suggests that a single cocaine "hit" during pregnancy can cause fetal damage.[113]

CRACK BABIES.   Babies born to untreated addicts show signs of withdrawal within a few hours of birth. Cocaine babies are usually wide-eyed and very irritable. They cry or scream often, sleep little, and may have trouble gaining weight because of excessive activity. Addicts' babies are also much more likely to be premature, to be undersized, and to have difficulties in sucking, swallowing, and breathing. They tremble constantly unless wrapped securely in blankets and maintained on a high dose of a sedative such as phenobarbital, from which they are later gradually withdrawn.[114]

CRACK BABIES' ENVIRONMENT.   Once crack babies survive pregnancy and birth, they are still often confronted with a poor environment. "People who start using got to find money. Children aren't fed. Mothers sell their food stamps. Young women sell their bodies, and that's often done in front of the children. Even when heroin was at its worse, it wasn't like this—it wasn't openly done."[115] More and more infants, neglected or abandoned by their parents, are left in hospital units until they go into foster care.

GRANDMOTHERS BEAR BURDEN.   To an extent that even hardened child-welfare mothers find shocking, grandmothers have become the parents of last resort, forced into a second round of child rearing because their own children are lost to crack cocaine.[116] Grandmothers have always played a powerful role in poor, inner-city families, offering respite and inspiration, but never before have so many assumed full responsibility for their children's children.

Crack Children   Babies born from crack-addicted mothers are difficult to care for almost from the moment of birth. They are either extremely irritable or very lethargic, and they have poor sucking abilities and irregular sleeping patterns. Recently, as the first generation of crack babies has grown older, it has been observed that these children are hyperactive, are slow in learning, and have trouble relating to other people.[117] Teachers describe their behavior as operating on instinctual levels. Oftentimes these children are withdrawn and have trouble playing or even talking with other kids. Early intervention and individual attention seem to be crucial in helping these crack-born children.

There is no specific treatment for cocaine babies. Therapists must therefore work with the mothers. They teach women what to do with babies who have long crying jags and are unresponsive. The mothers need to be treated before they conceive, but it is often difficult to get them into treatment. Many of them come to the hospital in the last stages of delivery and are so high that treatment is probably the last thing on their minds.

HOSPITALS AND DRUG ADDICTS

At its simplest level, doctors say, the rise of crack has hurt hospitals by greatly increasing the numbers of patients, including growing casualties of battles for drug turf. On a deeper level, it has lengthened hospital stays by complicating illnesses and spawning fear of theft or assault among doctors, nurses, and other patients.[118] Health officials are concluding that crack is playing a major role in encouraging the unsafe sex and intravenous-drug abuse by which AIDS is spread.

Doctors say that crack's starkest impact has been the rise of violence involving teenage drug-dealing gunners, whose turf wars and vendettas send a steady flow of patients into a hopelessly overworked emergency room.

CRACK AND HEROIN

A highly addictive mixture of crack and smokable heroin is emerging as the new drug of choice among some of New York City's chronic drug abusers, city and state drug-treatment officials say.[119] The mixture is deadly because it combines the physical addiction of heroin with the intense high of crack. The new mixture of crack and heroin lengthens the crack high and reduces the intensity of the depression that follows it. (This mixture is called "chasing the dragon.")

The drug combination is sometimes sold premixed and generally costs about $10 a dose, roughly twice as much as a dose of crack. Although it has not been found outside New York City, it is likely to appear in other large cities where crack is already available.

COCAINE ANONYMOUS

In 1984 a fellow named Jack helped found a new organization called Cocaine Anonymous (CA), which applied the principles of Alcoholics Anonymous to cocaine use. Today there are over 1,600 CA meetings held in over 46 states and Canada. These programs serve over 60,000 members.

MEDICAL USE

Cocaine has been used by doctors as a topical (local) anesthetic since 1884, when Freud began experimenting with the drug. But by the 1890s the medical community had begun to feel that its use was often more harmful than therapeutic. In the early 1900s a number of cocaine derivatives were synthesized to improve the drug's medical usefulness. These cocaine synthetics—Novocain (procaine) and Xylocaine—did not stimulate the nervous system as cocaine did and were extensively used as local anesthetics. Despite its drawbacks, cocaine is still used by many ophthalmologists and ear, nose, and throat specialists. It is used to dilate the pupil in certain inflammatory diseases of the eye and is sometimes used following cataract surgery to prevent perforations in the vitreous body. During a tear-duct operation, gauze is often saturated in cocaine crystals and then applied as a local anesthetic and to control bleeding.

The effects and potential use of cocaine for treatment of depressed patients were studied by Robert Post and Frederick Goodwin at the National Institute of Mental Health in Bethesda, Maryland.[120] They concluded that although cocaine can elicit positive changes, such as elation, it also elicits ambivalence and deep depression, leading them to dismiss its use as an antidepressant.

CAFFEINE (XANTHINES)

INTRODUCTION

If we had to identify the drug that has had the greatest impact on civilization, caffeine would be a top contender. Xanthines, the family of chemicals that includes caffeine, are the oldest stimulants known. Today caffeine is perhaps the most widely used drug, constituting a regular portion of the American diet. The drug can be found in many substances, the most common of which are listed in Tables 5-2, 5-3, and 5-4.

Caffeine is one of the most widely used stimulant drugs in the United States. Americans consume approximately 45 million pounds of caffeine every year in such substances as coffee, tea, soft drinks, cocoa products, chocolate, and various over-the-counter and prescription drugs.[121]

Caffeine is a socially acceptable drug. Each day over 80 percent of Americans consume beverages containing the equivalent of two to three cups of caffeinated coffee.[122] Most people know that coffee, tea, and soft drinks contain caffeine, and they drink these beverages for their stimulating effects. These effects include an increase in alertness, motor performance, and the capacity for work and a decrease in fatigue. Users of caffeine may find that it helps in performing a repetitive task, and it may improve muscular endurance in a physically demanding job. The increase for work capacity may be due in part to caffeine's ability to increase the level of fatty acids in the blood, which are used for energy. Otherwise, the increases in work capacity, alertness, and motor performance are the result of caffeine's influence on the central nervous system. These benefits are generally acceptable in America's culture; caffeine use is found in the workplace, in places of recreation, and in the home.

TABLE 5–2   CAFFEINE CONTENT OF BEVERAGES AND FOODS

Item	Average Milligrams Caffeine	Range
Coffee (5-oz. cup)		
Brewed, drip method	115	60–180
Brewed, percolator	80	40–170
Instant	65	30–120
Decaffeinated, brewed	3	2–5
Decaffeinated, instant	2	1–5
Tea		
Brewed, major U.S. brands (5-oz. cup)	40	20–90
Brewed, imported brands (5-oz. cup)	60	25–110
Instant (5-oz. cup)	30	25–50
Iced (12-oz. cup)	70	67–76
Cocoa (5-oz. glass)	4	2–20
Chocolate milk (8 oz.)	5	2–7
Milk chocolate (1 oz.)	6	1–15
Dark chocolate, semisweet (1 oz.)	20	5–35
Baker's chocolate (1 oz.)	26	26
Chocolate-flavored syrup (1 oz.)	4	4

Source: *FDA Consumer* (Washington, D.C.: Department of Health and Human Services, 1983), p. 3.

TABLE 5–3   CAFFEINE CONTENT OF SOFT DRINKS

Brand	Milligrams Caffeine (12-oz. serving)
Sugar-Free Mr. PIBB	58.8
Mountain Dew	54.0
Mellow Yello	52.8
TAB	46.8
Coca-Cola	45.6
Diet Coke	45.6
Shasta Cola	44.4
Shasta Cherry Cola	44.4
Shasta Diet Cola	44.4
Mr. PIBB	40.8
Dr. Pepper	39.6
Sugar-Free Dr. Pepper	39.6
Big Red	38.4
Sugar-Free Big Red	38.4
Pepsi-Cola	38.4
Aspen	36.0
Diet Pepsi	36.0
Pepsi Light	36.0
RC Cola	36.0
Diet Rite	36.0
Kick	31.2
Canada Dry Jamicia Cola	30.0
Canada Dry Diet Cola	1.2

Source: Institute of Food Technologists (IFT), 1983, based on data from the National Soft Drink Association, Washington, D.C. The IFT also reports that there are at least 68 varieties of soft drinks produced by 12 leading bottlers that have no caffeine. *FDA Consumer* (Washington, D.C.: Department of Health and Human Services, 1983), p. 4.

TABLE 5–4   CAFFEINE CONTENT OF PRESCRIPTION AND OVER-THE-COUNTER DRUGS

Prescription Drugs	Milligrams Caffeine (pill or liquid)
Cafergot (for migraine headache)	100
Fiorinal (for tension headache)	40
Soma Compound (pain relief, muscle relaxant)	32
Darvon Compound (pain relief)	32.4

Nonprescription Drugs	
Weight-Control Aids	
Codexin	
Dex-A-Diet II	200
Dexatrim, Dexatrim Extra Strength	200
Dietac capsules	200
Maximum Strength Appedrine	100
Polamine	140
Alertness Tablets	
Nodoz	100
Vivarin	200
Analgesic/Pain Relief	
Anacin, Maximum Strength Anacin	32
Excedrin	65
Midol	32.4
Vanquish	33
Diuretics	
Aqua-Ban	100
Maximum Strength Aqua-Ban Plus	200
Permathene H2 Off	200
Cold/Allergy Remedies	
Coryban-D capsules	30
Triaminicin tablets	30
Dristan Decongestant tablets and	
Dristan A–F Decongestant tablets	16.2
Duradyne-Forte	30

Source: FDA's National Center for Drugs and Biologics. *FDA Consumer* (Washington, D.C.: Department of Health and Human Services, 1983), p. 4.

Coffee is the consumer's second choice of beverage, after soft drinks.[123] But coffee consumption in the United States has been declining: In 1986 it was 26.3 gallons per person, compared with 37.8 gallons in 1965. Health concerns regarding caffeine have been cited as the major reason for this decline. (Shortly we will examine the controversy over some of these concerns.)

However, caffeine does not have long-term ill effects on health, except for people with diabetes. But to avoid any side effects, one should consume caffeine in moderation—no more than 500 milligrams per day.[124]

The medical community is concerned with caffeine for various reasons. Caffeine can change the effectiveness of other drugs, it can cause or compli-

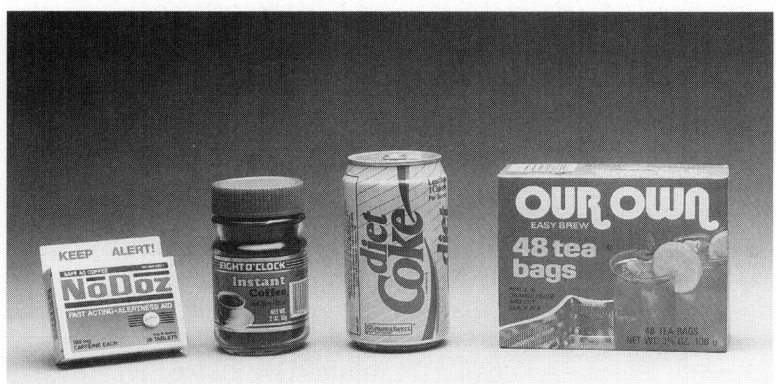

All These Products Contain Caffeine
Source: Steve Goldberg/Monkmeyer Press

cate health problems, it can help in the treatment of some diseases, and it is believed to be associated with some chronic illnesses.[125]

Three quarters of the caffeine in our diets is found in coffee. However, coffee is just one source of caffeine. The caffeine taken out of coffee (in the process of making decaffeinated coffee) is bought by the soft-drink industry. Cola drinks contain some caffeine naturally, but more is added during manufacturing. Non-cola drinks may also contain large quantities of caffeine—a fact not always realized when these are given to children. Caffeine can also be found in prescription drugs (APC, Darvon, and others) and over-the-counter analgesics (Empirin, Anacin, and other pain relievers). It has been estimated that an American's daily intake of caffeine from all sources is 210 milligrams per day.

As a member of the methylate xanthines, caffeine has stimulating effects that are often pleasant:

> After taking caffeine, one is capable of greater sustained intellectual effort and a more perfect association of ideas. There is also a keener appreciation of sensory stimuli, and reaction time to them is appreciably diminished. This accounts for the hyperesthesia, sometimes unpleasant, which some people experience after drinking too much coffee. In addition, motor activity is increased; typists, for example, work faster and with fewer errors. However, recently acquired motor skill in a task involving delicate muscular coordination and accurate timing may . . . be adversely affected. These effects may be brought on by the administration of 150 to 250 milligrams of caffeine, the amount contained in one or two cups of coffee or tea.[126]

Americans may have more of a physiological and/or psychological dependence on caffeine than on all other drugs combined. Some individuals experience a jittery feeling, a slight loss of motor coordination, and insomnia after consuming it. Even small amounts increase anxiety, irritate the stomach lining, and may be undesirable for certain cardiac patients. However, the morning cup of coffee is so much a part of America that we seldom look upon its consumption as a drug habit.

As you can see in Table 5–3, caffeine is also found in many common medications. It is added to cold, headache, allergy, stay-awake, and other remedies, both prescription and nonprescription. The Food and Drug Administration's National Center for Drugs and Biologics reports that more than 1,000 OTC drugs list caffeine as an ingredient.[127]

HISTORY

Caffeine has a long history, dating back thousands of years, as the world's most commonly used psychotropic drug. There are many reports of Stone Age people making beverages from caffeine-containing plants.

The history of caffeine use, like that of many other drugs, is surrounded by myth and supposition. Legend has it that coffee was discovered by a friar in an Arabian convent after he witnessed the stimulating effect the berries of a coffee plant had on goats.[128] Actually, coffee was first introduced as a medicine in England and Europe but became popular as a nonalcoholic drink. The "medicine" became so popular that about the middle of the seventeenth century coffeehouses (known as "penny universities") were established where people could listen to learned figures as well as politicians for a cup of coffee bought for a penny. Despite its popularity, coffee drinking was outlawed at various times in both Arabia and England because it was considered an intoxicating beverage that often led to discussions of rebellion and slander of those in power.

Tea was first known of in China, where it was used primarily as a medicine, as early as 4700 B.C. Later it was introduced as a beverage, and around 1600 it was shipped by the Dutch and British from their colonies in the East to Europe. By the 1700s, tea was being shipped to America, where it eventually became involved in the infamous battle over taxation. Participants in the Boston Tea Party deposited many cases of the herb into the waters of Boston Harbor in a statement that eventually resulted in war.

Coca, obtained from the seeds of the theobroma tree, also contains caffeine. Coca drinking spread during the sixteenth century in Spain and Mexico. Today the major coca supplier is Africa. Chocolate, first manufactured by the Dutch in the early 1800s, also contains caffeine, although the active ingredient is theobromine, a methylated xanthine.

THE CONTROVERSY OVER RESEARCH FINDINGS ON CAFFEINE

There is a lot of controversy over whether caffeine is related to chronic diseases. Studies have associated coffee drinking with more than 100 diseases and disorders, including pancreatic cancer and heart disease. But they have failed to confirm a cause-and-effect relationship between high coffee intake and health, except to prove that such intake aggravates certain gastrointestinal problems and causes jitteriness.[129] Researchers may never be able to establish a direct link between the popular beverage and a number of suspected health hazards.

There have been numerous studies on the effects of caffeine on cardiovascular disease, hypertension, pancreatic cancer, and fibrocystic breast disease. The results of these studies frequently conflict. Some studies note other variables may be contributing to their results.[130] Tobacco use, alcohol use, high fat intake, and high sodium consumption are examples of such variables. A few of these conflicting studies will be presented—then you decide which are the most conclusive.

Cardiovascular Disease   Let us first examine some studies on caffeine and cardiovascular disease. A study conducted in collaboration with the Boston Drug Surveillance Program was carried out in 24 Boston-area hospitals on the incidence of myocardial infarction and coffee consumption. In the study,

> a positive association between coffee consumption and acute myocardial infarction was confirmed by analysis of data from a multipurpose survey of 12,759 hospitalized patients, including 440 with a diagnosis of acute myocardial infarction. As compared with those who drink no coffee, the risk of infarction among those drinking one to five or six or more cups of coffee per day is estimated to be increased by 60 to 120 percent, respectively. This association could not be attributed to compounding by age, sex, past coronary heart disease, hypertension, congestive heart failure, obesity, diabetes, smoking or occupation, nor could it be explained by the use of sugar with coffee.[131]

Control studies support an elevated risk of myocardial infarction among men and women with high coffee intakes.[132] The definition that was used for high coffee intake was over five cups per day, which results in a 2.5-fold risk of coronary heart disease in drinkers as compared to nondrinkers. However, some concern arose over these findings, because many of the men and women studied died of unrelated causes instead of coffee. "Our data support the conclusion that caffeinated coffee as it is currently consumed by men and women in the United States causes no substantial increase in the risk of coronary heart disease or stroke."[133]

Constant stimulation of the nervous and cardiac systems by caffeine may be a factor in cardiac problems. Caffeine ingestion also causes a significant rise in serum-free fatty acids (or triglyceride level) in the blood, causing further heart problems.

Caffeine and Cholesterol   A 1985 study at Stanford University showed that men who drank three or more cups of coffee a day had higher cholesterol associated with heart disease than those who drank two cups or less.[134] Another study reports that "heavy coffee consumption appears to be an independent risk factor of coronary heart disease."[135] These studies show that caffeine affects the cardiovascular disease. But other research, such as the Framingham Heart Study, did not show such a correlation.[136]

Currently scientists are doing many studies on the incidences of heart disease as related to coffee drinkers. Research has shown that there is a relationship between coffee drinking and body blood-cholesterol level.[137] The greater the coffee intake, the higher the cholesterol level and the more likely that heart disease will occur. The studies also show that the level of cholesterol can be reduced by decreasing the amount of caffeine consumption. Researchers from Norway found that those who drank boiled coffee had higher cholesterol levels than those who drank brewed coffee.[138]

Recently Robert Superko of Stanford University and his colleagues were awarded a $450,000 grant from the National Institutes of Health to take a more rigorous look at the effects of caffeine.[139] They studied 180 healthy non-smoking men whose blood-cholesterol levels were below 200 milligrams (the point where increased risk of heart disease is thought to begin). For four months all 180 drank three to six cups of regular coffee, another third stopped drinking coffee, and the rest drank decaffeinated coffee. Two months later all characteristics were the same except that the low-density lipoproteins (LDL, a harmful kind of cholesterol) in the blood of the decaffeinated drinkers was up 9 percent. That indicates enough to boost their long-term risk of heart attack or other health-related problems by 12 to 14 percent.

Superko suspects that the chemicals left from the coffee bean after the decaffeination process could be responsible for the LDLs. He feels more studies should be conducted to see if similar findings occur.

Conditions such as cardiovascular disease and hypertension have not been fully substantiated at this time. While research reports in these areas have not been fully substantiated, they remain as possible risks for one to consider when consuming caffeine.

Studies of pancreatic cancer and fibrocystic breast disease also show conflicting results. For example, a Harvard study that associated pancreatic cancer with caffeine use was challenged by a later study.[140] Fibrocystic breast disease, which affects about half of all women in their reproductive years, has been associated by some studies with caffeine use. But the American Cancer Institute has found no association between the two. Another study of caffeine consumption and fibrocystic breast disease determined "that caffeine avoidance need not be recommended routinely for women who have fibrocystic disease but are otherwise healthy."[141]

An interesting study comparing the effect of caffeine in coffee with that of asthma medication found that caffeine widens the air passages in the lungs, allowing asthmatics to breathe easier and more deeply.[142] Since coffee is only 40 percent as potent as the asthma drug, one would have to drink excessive amounts of it to get the same results. Therefore coffee should not replace asthma medication, but it could be used as an alternative in emergencies.

Caffeine consumption and several symptoms of premenstrual syndrome were studied among 295 college sophomores aged 18 to 21.[143] The symptoms included depression, tiredness, irritability, anxiety, headaches, breast swelling and tenderness, craving for salty foods, constipation, and acne. It was found that as the level of caffeine consumption increased so did the severity of the symptoms.

PHYSICAL EFFECTS

When a person drinks two cups of coffee (150 to 300 milligrams of caffeine), the effects begin in 15 to 30 minutes. Metabolism, body temperature, and blood pressure increase. Other effects include increased urine production, higher blood-sugar levels, hand tremors, a loss of coordination, decreased appetite, and delayed sleep. Extremely high doses may cause nausea, diarrhea, sleeplessness, trembling, headache, and nervousness. Poisonous doses of caffeine occur occasionally and may result in convulsions, breathing failure, and death.[144]

Effects on the Central Nervous System   In general, caffeine acts on certain neurotransmitters that stimulate the central nervous system. A large dose of caffeine stimulates the central nervous system at all levels. The drug's effect on the cortex allows the user a clearer, more productive, and more rapid flow of thought, increased cerebral efficiency, and no drowsiness or fatigue. As a result of cortical stimulation, the individual is more alert, has a better memory, forms judgments more quickly, learns faster (temporarily), and has a decreased reaction time. The sense of touch may be more discriminating and the sense of pain more keen.[145] However, insomnia, restlessness, and excitement may occur, sometimes progressing to sensory disturbances such as ringing in the ears and flashing lights. Tachycardia and respiratory quickening can also occur,[146] although death is quite unlikely, since the toxic dose in humans is over 10 grams, or 70 to 100 cups of coffee.

Caffeine acts as a substitute for adenosine, a naturally occurring chemical found in the brain that acts like a neurotransmitter. Adenosine suppresses brain cells that increase alertness and elevate mood. Caffeine attaches to adenosine's receptor sites, blocking adenosine action on cells. It therefore allows brain cells that increase alertness to become available.[147]

Alertness and Wakefulness   The general conclusions from research on alertness indicate that caffeine users (not abstainers) require caffeine in the morning to achieve a sufficient state of alertness and readiness to face the day's tasks. Also, in the absence of caffeine, users may experience symptoms of mild withdrawal, which are relieved dramatically by caffeine intake.[148] Symptoms may appear approximately 12 to 16 hours after the last dose of caffeine.

The results of a study of the wakefulness effects of caffeine on 230 medical students contained the following information: (1) Caffeine prolonged the time required to fall asleep and disturbed the soundness of sleep when administered in a dose of 150 to 200 milligrams in coffee before bedtime; (2) caffeine caused distinctly less wakefulness in subjects who habitually drank a great deal of coffee; and (3) some subjects, among those who drank the most coffee, experienced morning headache after about 18 hours without caffeine (but if a single dose of 150 milligrams was given the previous evening, the headache was prevented).[149] A study of 1,500 undergraduate college students found that the group consuming the most caffeine had a higher frequency of psychophysiological disorders and lower academic performance.[150]

Pregnant Women and Birth Defects   Medical consultants advise pregnant women to give up coffee drinking in order to prevent birth defects. Some may recommend that women substitute decaffeinated coffee for caffeinated coffee. However, the FDA research prompting physicians to advise pregnant women to abstain from drinking coffee was done on rats that were given astronomically large amounts of caffeine at one time; furthermore, there have been no direct links of birth defects and caffeine in humans.[151] What this research did show was that caffeine stops adenosine receptor sites in cells (depressant in body), which explains a person's alertness after having caffeine.

Weight Loss   Caffeine also markedly affects the body's sugar metabolism: Excesses of the drug have been linked to hypoglycemia (deficient glucose levels). This low sugar level can result in weakness, marked perspiration, fatigue, and fainting.

The metabolic half-life of caffeine averages from several hours to several days, depending upon age, sex, hormonal status, medications being taken, and smoking habits. Infants and children do not metabolize and eliminate caffeine as rapidly as adults, so the effects of the substance last longer in them—as much as three to four days in newborns.[152]

Some new evidence shows that drinking one cup of coffee a day can result in loss of weight. Researchers have found that one cup of coffee can boost metabolic rate, which means that more calories are being burned. It was also found that if overweight people drink caffeinated products during their meals, more calories will be burned after finishing.[153]

Research has shown that caffeine may be able to increase metabolism by about 3 to 4 percent, thereby keeping off a few unwanted extra pounds.[154] Scientists measured metabolism with caffeine and without. They found that an average of 75 to 110 more calories a day were used by the people ingesting caffeine.[155] Even more calories were burned if caffeine was taken after a meal. Metabolism increased by about 25 to 30 percent.

Researchers believe that one of the reasons caffeine may help burn calories is that it enables more fat to move out of the body stores and into the bloodstream. Studies at the University of Bologna in Italy showed that three cups of coffee a day mobilize more than 38 percent more fat.[156] Five cups a day mobilize even more at 58 percent more fat than using no coffee at all.

Ergogenic Aid   Many experiments on caffeine as an ergogenic aid have had conflicting research results, which may be due to several different factors including who is being tested, amount of training, and nutritional state. The conclusions of current tests show that even though caffeine increases plasma free fatty acid concentrations, it doesn't have a metabolic or neuromuscular effect, and therefore it would not serve as an ergogenic aid in habitual caffeine consumers (200 milligrams a day).[157]

Infertility   For women trying to become pregnant, the latest news is to cut down, if not eliminate, the use of caffeine in the diet. A recent study by the National Institute of Health found that moderate consumption of caffeine by 104 women caused 50 percent less chance of conception in all of them.[158] The researchers found that the women who drank more than one cup of coffee or two or more pops a day were "consistently less likely to become pregnant" than their counterparts who consumed less. Although this is the conclusion, the study was small and should not therefore lead one to conclude that fertility is greatly affected by caffeine in a detrimental way.[159]

A new, retrospective study by the Centers for Disease Control (CDCs) reports that there is no correlation between caffeine consumption and infertility.[160] On the average, fertile women who drank more than two cups of coffee per day took about the same time to conceive as did women who drank less than one cup per month. The study conducted by the centers involved 2,817 pregnant women, and 1,818 infertile women (defined as not conceiving after one year of unprotected intercourse). In short, researchers found no link between caffeine and inability to conceive.[161]

However, fertility experts claim that caffeine significantly affects fertility.[162] Benjamine Younger of the American Fertility Society points out that if a patient has medically unexplained infertility, cutting down on caffeine consumption is a reasonable thing to do at the very least. Coffee and cola consumers should consider the possibility of a caffeine-fertility connection if they are having difficulty becoming pregnant.

CAFFEINISM

Caffeine may not fit technical definitions of substances to which people may become addicted, but "withdrawal headache" from a decrease in caffeine consumption is well documented.[163] There is also a measurable, temporary depression that occurs with caffeine abstinence. Although the literature is divided on the potential of caffeine to produce tolerance and dependence, it is evident that the substance has a hold over a large number of people. A high dose of caffeine (over 600 milligrams, less for some), perhaps in the form of five cups of coffee or more, can cause anxiety, nervousness, and insomnia, and these have been recognized as symptoms of **caffeinism.**[164] Some feel tolerance may develop with use of over 500 to 600 milligrams of caffeine per day. A regular user of caffeine develops a tolerance and may crave the drug in order to "get going." A person going through withdrawal may be accident-prone and irritable.

Caffeinism
A condition characterized by a "withdrawal headache" from a decrease in caffeine consumption and by a temporary depression.

Caffeine does act as an addictive drug in that it induces cravings, causes physical dependence, and leaves the consumer with withdrawal symptoms. It is possible to get hooked on as little as 100 milligrams of caffeine a day. The American Psychiatric Association has added caffeinism to its *Diagnostic and Statistical Manual of Mental Disorders.* Caffeinism includes automatic signs, diureses, gastrointestinal disturbances, insomnia, and symptoms mimicking anxiety disorders.[165]

Liver and Pancreas   The body normally releases glucose reserves in the liver as energy for physiological functioning. This release of glucose leads to increased availability of insulin from the pancreas, which reduces elevated blood-sugar levels.[166] When blood sugar is lowered, fatigue often results. Thus results the desire for the time-honored coffee break. Several cups of coffee and a donut will raise the glucose level again. Then insulin will be released to bring the blood-sugar level back down. This process is continuous in the body's attempt to establish a balance among its chemical constituents. But with excessive fluctuations in daily functions, the liver's reserve, the pancreas, the nervous system, and the cardiac system will be subject to strain.

Diuretic Action   Caffeine is a diuretic: It causes an increased production of urine.

Gastric Upset   Persons with a predisposition toward ulcers may exhibit an abnormal response to caffeine ingestion and suffer some gastric upset.

Use with Children   Twelve ounces of a cola drink can produce significant reactions in children. Walter Silver, of the Maimonides Medical Center in New York, found tachycardia and insomnia in otherwise healthy preadolescent cola drinkers. Both of these complaints disappeared when the beverage was withdrawn. Silver claims that "children are more susceptible than adults to excitation by xanthines, [and that] we should . . . withdraw these beverages from our children's diet."[167]

Skeletal Muscles   The xanthines, particularly caffeine, make skeletal muscles less susceptible to fatigue by increasing their capacity for muscular activity.

Fibrocystic Breast Disease

Lumps, nodules, and thickenings in the breast tissue of women. Caffeine and related substances are suspected of increasing the supply of Camp, a growth-promoting compound in breast tissue. Women with fibrocystic breasts have an increased risk of developing breast cancer.

Fibrocystic Breast Disease   **Fibrocystic breast disease** is a common and worrisome complaint of many women. The characteristic lumps, nodules, and thickenings in the breast tissue are benign yet hard to distinguish from cancerous tissue, and they may impede the diagnosis of cancer. Furthermore, women with fibrocystic breast disease have an increased risk of developing breast cancer.

For women who have fibrocystic breast disease, caffeine was thought to be the culprit. However, recent studies indicate that eliminating caffeine causes a decrease in fibrocystic lumps, but caffeine isn't exactly a direct cause of them.[168] As of now, there is no definite connection between cancer and caffeine intake.

DECAFFEINATED COFFEE

Since recent research has suggested that caffeine may cause birth defects, many women have switched to decaffeinated coffee. But is decaffeinated coffee safe? Decaffeination is a process using water, heat, and a solvent. A hot-water solution removes the caffeine from the beans and an organic solvent removes the caffeine from the water, which is then reused. From the standpoint of taste, the process has advantages. From the standpoint of safety, however, the use of a solvent is questionable.

Many people are concerned about their caffeine intake, so they now drink decaffeinated coffee, which accounts for more than 20 percent of the coffee drinkers today.[169] Decaffeinated coffees made in the United States are usually treated with caffeine solvent, methylene chloride. Unfortunately, this chemical is suspected of being a carcinogen (cancer-causing substance).[170] However, most blends contain only about two parts per million. The Food and Drug Administration permits up to ten parts per million. The decaffeination process itself strips the beans of most of the body and flavor. The chemical solvent methylene chloride was thought to be dangerous, but it evaporates at 100° to 120°F and beans are usually roasted at 350° to 425°F.[171] More expensive steam-decaffeinated coffee can be obtained at many specialty shops.

SUGGESTIONS FOR DECREASING USE OF CAFFEINE

Caffeine has had a long history of safe use by humans everywhere. However, if you feel you need to cut back, here are some suggestions: (1) Select decaffeinated coffee, tea, or soft drinks; (2) mix caffeinated and decaffeinated coffee grounds together before making coffee; (3) limit your consumption of caffeinated beverages to a prescribed number and then gradually switch to decaffeinated beverages; and (4) limit the amount of chocolate that you eat.[172]

LOOK-ALIKES

After restrictions were placed on production and distribution of amphetamines in the early 1970s, there was an initial disruption of the flow of these drugs to the illicit street market. In the late 1970s, however, new, nontraditional companies started manufacturing and distributing what have since been called look-alike stimulants. These companies usually use three over-the-counter cold preparations: caffeine, ephedrine, and phenylpropanolamine. When these three ingredients are combined into a single preparation, they produce stimulatory side effects that are somewhat similar to the arousal and alertness caused by amphetamines. The drugs obtained the title *look-alikes* because their manufacturers packaged them in a variety of pills and capsules whose letters and markings gave them the appearance of prescription medications.

Large numbers of these preparations are now consumed each year in the United States, and they are frequently advertised in drug-oriented magazines and other publications. Side effects can include high blood pressure, which could make sensitive individuals more prone to strokes. More routine side effects consist of mild to severe headache and possibly mild to moderate stomach irritation. With prolonged frequent use, tolerance can develop such that large amounts taken over time are required to obtain the desired effects of the drug.[173]

SUMMARY

A number of stimulants are currently used in the United States. Amphetamines, for example, may help people to overcome fatigue, improve performance, prevent narcolepsy, or lose weight. For some, methamphetamine ("speed") is used to experience exhilaration. However, intravenous injection of these drugs can lead to serious health hazards and have deleterious social consequences. In addition, the process of manufacturing and dumping "meth" waste is becoming very hazardous and poisonous to the environment. Another current form of methamphetamine, called *ice,* is extremely potent and is used primarily in Korea, Japan, and Hawaii.

Methylphenidate (Ritalin) is sometimes used to calm children who suffer from attention-deficit hyperactive disorder (ADHD). This particular use has led to considerable controversy, with some claiming that behavioral modification, use of caffeine, reduction of food additives, or electromyographic biofeedback could accomplish the same goal without the possibility of the child becoming dependent on drugs as a coping mechanism.

Cocaine has seen limited medical application as an anesthetic for surgery. Because of its euphoria-producing properties, however, it has gained great street popularity. However, recent research has indicated that cocaine may not be a safe drug because of the increasing number of heart attacks it causes in otherwise healthy users. Crack, a newer form of cocaine, is smoked and takes much less time for a user to achieve a high. This form of cocaine has led to crack addicts, gangs who sell crack, and pregnant women using crack who produce physically and mentally damaged babies.

A drug that millions of Americans use regularly is caffeine, found in beverages such as coffee, tea, cocoa, and soft drinks. Caffeine can also be found in prescription and over-the-counter analgesics.

STIMULANTS
N O T E S

1. Stanley Einstein, *Beyond Drugs* (New York: Pergamon Press, 1975), p. 52.

2. "Amphetamine: Alcohol and Drug Fact Sheet," *Drug Information Center (DIC)* (Eugene: University of Oregon, 1979), p. 1.

3. Ibid.

4. Ibid.

5. Ibid.

6. Ibid.

7. Peter Ognibere, "Amphetamines and Barbiturates," *New Republic* 168, no. 5 (February 3, 1973):130.

8. Department of Health, Education and Welfare, *Amphetamine,* Report Series 28, no. 1 (Washington, D.C.: National Clearinghouse for Drug Abuse Information, 1974), p. 3.

9. "Amphetamine," p. 1.

10. Thomas Weisman, *Drug Abuse and Drug Counseling* (Cleveland: Press of Case Western Reserve University, 1972), p. 90.

11. "Clinical Aspects of Amphetamine Abuse," *Journal of the American Medical Association* 240, no. 21 (November 17, 1978):2317–19.

12. Michael Dolan, "Clamping Down on Uppers," *American Pharmacy* 18, no. 4 (April 1978):18–23.

13. "Amphetamine," p. 1.

14. Jane Gross, " 'Speed's' Gain in Use Could Rival Crack, Drug Experts Warn," *New York Times,* November 27, 1988, p. A1.

15. Ibid.

16. Louis S. Goodman and Alfred Gilman, eds., *The Pharmacological Basis of Therapeutics,* 4th ed. (New York: Macmillan, 1970), p. 294.

17. *Dorland's Illustrated Medical Dictionary,* 24th ed. (Philadelphia: Saunders, 1965), p. 245.

18. Goodman and Gilman, *The Pharmacological Basis of Therapeutics.* p. 294.

19. Ibid., p. 295.

20. Edward Brecher et al., *Licit and Illicit Drugs* (Boston: Little, Brown, 1972), p. 285.

21. "Amphetamine," p. 1.

22. Einstein, *Beyond Drugs,* p. 54.

23. Ibid.

24. *The Nonmedical Use of Drugs: An Interim Report of the Canadian Government Commission on Inquiry* (Ottawa: Penguin, 1970), p. 85.

25. James N. Baker, "The Newest Drug War," *Newsweek,* April 3, 1989, pp. 20–22.

26. Erika Reider Mark, "Dangerous New Drugs on the Teen Market," *Good Housekeeping,* April 1989, pp. 235–36.

27. Gordon Witkin, "The Midnight Dumpers," *U.S. News & World Report,* January 9, 1989, p. 57.

28. Ibid.

29. Michael A. Lerner, "The Fire of 'Ice,' " *Newsweek,* November 27, 1989, pp. 37ff.

30. Dean Kuipers, "ICE," *Spin,* November 1989, pp. 37–39.

31. Mike Sager, "Death in Venice," *Rolling Stone,* September 22, 1988, p. 64.

32. Lerner, "The Fire of 'Ice.' "

33. "Wishing for `The Good Old Crack Days'?" *Drugs and Drug Abuse Education Newsletter* (April 1990): 1, 45, 47.

34. Ibid.

35. Sager, "Death in Venice."

36. Ibid.

37. Lerner, "The Fire of 'Ice.' "

38. Constance Holden, " 'Ice Age' in Hawaii," *Science* 246, no. 4932 (November 17, 1989):1648.

39. "Amphetamine," p. 1.

40. A. F. Charles, "Case of Ritalin: Drugs for Hyperactive Children," *New Republic* 165, no. 17 (October 23, 1971):17–19.

41. Richard E. Vatz and Lee S. Weinberg, "The Hyperactivity Myth and Drugs in the Classroom," *USA Today,* September 1988, pp. 89–90.

42. "Stimulant Medication in Hyperactive Children," *American Family Physicians* 40, no. 5 (November 1989):279.

43. B. Bower, "Kids Talk about the "Good Pill," *Science News* 135 (May 27, 1989):332.

44. Harriette C. Johnson, "Drugs, Dialogue, or Diet: Diagnosing and Treating the Hyperactive Child," *National Association of Social Workers* 4, no. 8 (March 1988):349–53.

45. Alexander Lucas and Morris Weiss, "Methylphenidate Hallucinesis," *Journal of the American Medical Association* 217, no. 8 (August 23, 1971):377.

46. Robert L. Sprague, Kenneth R. Barnes, and John Werry, "Methylphenidate and Thorazine: Learning, Reaction Time, Activity and Classroom Behavior in Disturbed Children," *American Journal of Orthopsychiatry* 40, no. 4 (July 1970):615.

47. Robert M. Smith and John Netsworth, *The Exceptional Child: A Functional Approach* (New York: McGraw-Hill, 1975).

48. C. J. Weithorn and R. Ross, "Stimulant Drugs for Hyperactivity: Some Disturbing Questions," *American Journal of Orthopsychiatry* 46, no. 1 (January 1976):171.

49. Susan G. O'Leary and William E. Pelham, "Behavior Therapy and Withdrawal of Stimulant Medication in Hyperactive Children," *Pediatrics* 61, no. 2 (February 1978):211–17.

50. Garnun Gray, "Order in the Classroom: Drugging for Deportment," *Nation* 221, no. 14 (November 1, 1975):424.

51. Robert C. Schnacker, "Caffeine as a Substitute for Schedule II Stimulants in Hyperkinetic Children," *American Journal of Psychiatry* 130, no. 7 (July 1973):297.

52. "The Feingold Diet for Hyperactive Children," *Medical Letter* 20, no. 12 (June 16, 1978):56.

53. J. Preston Harley and Charles G. Mathews, "The Hyperactive Child and the Feingold Controversy," *American Pharmacy* 18, no. 6 (June 1978):44–46; C. K. Connors and C. H. Goyette, "The Effects of Certified Food Dyes on Behavior: A Challenge Test," *Clinical Drug Evaluation Unit Program* 7 (1977):18–19; Jeffrey Mattes and Rachel Gittleman-Klein, "A Cross-Over Study of Artificial Food Colorings in a Hyperkinetic Child," *American Journal of Psychiatry* 135, no. 8 (August 1978):987–88.

54. Reprinted from *Journal of Learning Disabilities,* "Use of Electromyographic Biofeedback in Control of Hyperactivity," by Brand Lendell and Mimi Lupin, Volume 8, Number 7, September 1975. The Professional Press, Inc., 101 E. Ontario Street, Chicago, IL 60611.

55. Virginia S. Cowart, "The Ritalin Controversy: What's Made This Drug's Opponents Hyperactive?" *Journal of the American Medical Association* 259, no. 17 (May 6, 1988):2522.

56. Ann Ivey Fulton and William R. Yates, "Family Abuse of Methamphetamines," *American Family Physician* 38, no. 2 (August 1988):143–45.

57. A. Washton and N. Stone, "The Human Cost of Cocaine Use," *Medical Aspects of Human Sexuality* 18, no. 11 (November 1984):122.

58. Quoted in "Cocaine Addiction: A Growing Problem for Women," *Register-Guard* (Eugene, Oregon), February 18, 1985, p. B5.

59. "Cocaine: Alcohol and Drug Fact Sheet," *Drug Information Center (DIC)* (Eugene: University of Oregon, 1979).

60. "Dr. Jekyll and Mr. Cocaine," *Science News* 99, no. 16 (April 17, 1971):264.

61. Frank H. Gawin and Everett H. Ellingwood, Jr., "Cocaine and Other Stimulants in Action, Abuse and Treatment," *New England Journal of Medicine* 318, no. 18 (May 5, 1988):1173–82.

62. National Institute on Drug Abuse, Division of Epidemiology and Prevention Research, "National Household Survey on Drug Abuse," NIDA Capsules. CAP 21, (Rockville, Md.: U. S. Department of Health and Human Services, Public Health Service, Alcohol, Drug Abuse, Mental Health Administration, 1990).

63. David Whitman, "The Streets Are Filled with Coke," *U.S. News & World Report,* March 5, 1990, pp. 24–25.

64. Gawin and Ellingwood, "Cocaine and Other Stimulants."

65. Steven S. Hull, Jr, "Cocaine's Harmful Side Effects," *Science* 248 (April 13, 1990):166.

66. "Cocaine and Sudden Death," *Mayo Clinic Health Letter* 7, no. 5 (May 1989):6–7.

67. R. Cowen, "Probing Cocaine in the Heart and Brain," *Science News* 137 (June 30, 1990):406–7.

68. G. Gay, "You've Come a Long Way, Baby! Coke Time for the New American Lady of the Eighties," *Journal of Psychoactive Drugs* 13, no. 4 (October/December 1981):297–316.

69. J. Schachne et al., "Coronary-Artery Spasm and Myocardial Infarction Associated with Cocaine Use," *New England Journal of Medicine* 13, no. 4 (June 1983):297–316.

70. *Pharmaceutical Chemical Newsletter* 12, no. 5 (September/October 1983):p. 1.

71. "Cocaine: Alcohol and Drug Fact Sheet," p. 78.

72. Gawin and Ellingsworth, "Cocaine and Other Stimulants."

73. Ibid.

74. Ibid.

75. "Cocaine: The Consequences of Use," *Consumer Research* 71, no. 1 (January 1988):18–21.

76. "Stimulants," *Journal of the American Medical Association* 258 (December 10, 1987):3362.

77. Frederick K. Goodwin, "Cocaine and Suicide Attempts," *Journal of the American Medical Association* 259 (June 10, 1988):3314–15.

78. Patrick T. MacDonald et al., "Heavy Cocaine Use and Sexual Behavior," *Journal of Drug Issues* 18, no. 3 (Summer 1988):437–55.

79. Dody Tsiabtar, " 'Crack' Making Its Violent Presence Felt in New York," *Washington Post,* June 13, 1987, p. A3.

80. Jill Nelson, "Cracking Up," *Essence,* January 1987, p. 66.

81. Howard French, "Police Discover Crack in Tablet Form," *New York Times,* May 23, 1987, p. A50.

82. Rene Noorbergen, "Cocaine—America's Newest Epidemic," *Vibrant Life,* March/April 1987, p. 11.

83. Ibid.

84. Peter Kerr, "Battle against Crack," *New York Times,* June 27, 1986, p. A14.

85. Nelson, "Cracking Up," p. 65.

86. Jacob Lamar, "Crack: A Cheap and Deadly Cocaine Is a Spreading Menace," *Time,* June 2, 1986, p. 17.

87. Ibid., p. 18.

88. Ibid., p. 17.

89. Ibid.

90. Gina Kolata, "Drug Researchers Try to Treat a Nearly Unbreakable Habit," *New York Times,* June 25, 1988, p. A1.

91. Ibid.

92. Noorbergen, "Cocaine—America's Newest Epidemic."

93. Jacob V. Lamar, "Kids Who Sell Crack," *Time,* May 9, 1988, pp. 20–33.

94. Sager, "Death in Venice."

95. Morgan Tanner, "CRACK IN AMERICA: L.A. Drug Gangs Create a Depraved New World," *Soldiers of Fortune,* June 1989, p. 40.

96. Larry Marty, "A Tide of Drug Killing," *Newsweek,* January 16, 1989, pp. 44–45.

97. Ibid.

98. Ibid.

99. Tom Morganthau, "Murder in Capital," *Newsweek,* March 13, 1989, pp. 16–19.

100. Tom Morganthau, "Children of the Underclass," *Newsweek,* September 11, 1989, pp. 16–24.

101. Ibid.

102. Michael Marriott, "After 3 Years, Crack Plague in New York Only Gets Worse," *New York Times,* February 20, 1989, p. A1.

103. Nelson, "Cracking Up," p. 66.

104. Ibid.

105. Malcom W. Klein and Cheryl Maxson, "Rock Sales in South Los Angeles," *Sociology and Social Research* 69 (July 4, 1985):561–65.

106. Eric Podey, "Fighting Back against Crime," *New York Times,* January 23, 1989, p. 31.

107. Ibid.

108. Elizabeth Wynhausen, "Cracked Out," *Ms.,* September 1988, pp. 67–75.

109. Aimee Lee Ball, "White Lies Cocaine: The Dirty Little Secret in the Age of Clean," *Newsweek,* April 3, 1989, pp. 20–22.

110. Ellen Hopkins, "Childhood's End," *Rolling Stone,* October 18, 1990, pp. 66–72, 108–9.

111. Jane E. Brody, "Cocaine Litany of Fetal Risk Grows," *New York Times,* September 6, 1988, p. C1.

112. Ibid.

113. Ibid.

114. Sandra J. Weber, "Mothers on Drugs, Addicts at Birth," *New York Times,* January 29, 1989, p. 1.

115. Wynhausen, "Cracked Out."

116. Jane Gross, "Grandmothers Bear a Burden Sired by Drugs," *New York Times,* April 9, 1989, p. A1.

117. Barbara Kantrowity, "The Crack Children," *Newsweek,* February 12, 1990, pp. 62–63.

118. Howard French, "Crime and Fear Follow Crack into Hospitals," *New York Times,* May 19, 1989, p. A1.

119. Michael Marriott, "Potent Crack Blend in the Streets Lures a New Generation to Heroin," *New York Times,* July 13, 1989, p. A1.

120. Robert M. Post, Joel Kotin, and Frederick K. Goodman, "The Effects of Cocaine on Depressed Patients," *American Journal of Psychiatry* 1 (March 1978):411.

121. Les Stanwood, "C Is for Coffee, Chocolate, Cola, and Caffeine," *Current Health* 17, no. 4 (December 1990):11–13.

122. Arthur Heller, "Caffeine and Your Health," *Shape* (September 1987):58.

123. Paterson, Bruce. "Caffeine: Villain or Victim?" *Consumer Research* 71, no. 3 (March 1988):16–19.

124. Ibid., p. 79.

125. D. Edwards, "Drug Side Effects or Java Jitters," *Science News* (October 17, 1987):255.

126. Louis Goodman and Alfred Gilman, "Xanthines," in *The Pharmacological Basis of Therapeutics,* 4th ed., ed. Goodman and Gilman, pp. 358–70.

127. Chris Lecos, "The Latest Caffeine Scorecard," *FDA Consumer,* OHHS Publication No. (FDA) 84-2184 (Washington, D.C.: Department of Health and Human Services, 1984).

128. Goodman and Gilman, "Xanthines," p. 199.

129. Steve Eisenberg, "Looking for the Perfect Brew," *Science News* 133, no. 16 (April 1988):252–53.

130. Heller, "Caffeine and Your Health," p. 201.

131. Hershel Jick et al., "Coffee and Myocardial Infarction," *New England Journal of Medicine* 289, no. 2 (July 12, 1973):63–67.

132. Diedrick Gobbee et al., "Coffee, Caffeine and Cardiovascular Disease in Men," *New England Journal of Medicine* 323, no. 15 (October 1990):1026.

133. Ibid.

134. A. LaCroix et al., "Coffee Consumption and the Incidence of Coronary Heart Disease," *New England Journal of Medicine* (October 1986):277.

135. Heller, "Caffeine and Your Health," p. 60.

136. Paula Dranov, "Caffeine Redeemed?" *Health* 19, no. 11 (November 1987):70.

137. Editors, "Is Coffee Safe?" *Consumer Reports,* September 1987, p. 529.

138. Liz Applegate "Nutrition on Caffeine," *Runner's World* 24 (November 1989): 22–24.

139. "Yuppi Health Shock," *The Economist,* November 25, 1990, no. 313:98.

140. S. Wicklund, "Caffeine Consumption and Fibrocystic Breast Disease: No Relationship?" *American Journal of Nursing* 86 (December 1986):1387–89.

141. Ibid.

142. S. L. Schiwall, "Asthma Relief That's Brewed by the Cup," *Prevention* 38 (November 1986):127.

143. A. M. Rossingnol, "Caffeine-Containing Beverages and Premenstrual Syndrome in Young Women," *American Journal of Public Health* 75 (November 1985):1335–37.

144. National Institute on Drug Abuse, *Stimulants and Cocaine,* DHHS Publication No. (ADM) 83-1304 (Washington, D.C.: U.S. Government Printing Office, 1983).

145. Betty Bergerson and Elsie E. Krug, *Pharmacology in Nursing,* 14th ed. (St. Louis: C. V. Mosby, 1979), p. 360.

146. Ibid.

147. Melvin Konner, "Caffeine High," *New York Times,* January 17, 1988, pp. 47–48.

148. Brecher et al., *Licit and Illicit Drugs,* p. 202.

149. A. Goldstein, "Wakefulness Caused by Caffeine," *Naunyn-Schmiedebergs Arch in Pathopharmacology* 248 (1964):269–78.

150. K. Gilliland and D. Andress, "Ad Lib Caffeine Consumption, Symptoms of Caffeinism, and Academic Performance," *American Journal of Psychiatry* 138, no. 4 (April 1981):180.

151. Editors, "Is Coffee Safe?"

152. "Caffeine," *Contemporary Nutrition Newsletter* 9, no. 5 (May 1984).

153. Liz Applegate, "Nutrition on Caffeine," *Runner's World* 24 (November 1989):22–24.

154. Kimberly Hamilton, "The Weight Loss Perk," *Health* 5, no. 21 (November 1989):32.

155. Ibid.

156. Ibid.

157. Mark Tarnopolsky, "Physiological Responses to Caffeine during Endurance Running in Habitual Caffeine Users," *Medicine and Science in Sports and Exercise* (February 1989):419–23.

158. Mary Hager, "Latest Infertility Suspect: Caffeine," *Newsweek,* January 23, 1989, p. 60.

159. Ibid.

160. Sarah Williams, "Caffeine, Conception: No Correlation," *Science News,* February 10, 1990, no. 137:93–95.

161. Ibid.

162. "Latest Infertility Suspect: Caffeine," *Newsweek,* January 23, 1989.

163. D. Sawyer, H. Julia, and A. Turin, "Caffeine and Human Behavior: Arousal, Anxiety, and Performance Effects," *Journal of Behavioral Medicine* 5, no. 4 (1982):415–39.

164. F. W. Furlong, "Possible Psychiatric Significance of Excessive Coffee Consumption," *Canadian Psychiatric Association Journal* 20 (1975).

165. J. P. Bradley and A. Petree, "Caffeine Consumption and Expectancies of Caffeine-Enhanced Performance, and Caffeinism Symptoms among University Students," *Journal of Drug Education* 20, no. 4 (1990):319–27.

166. J. Lin Boniface and Reginald E. Haist, "Effects of Some Modifiers of Insulin on Insulin Biosynthesis," *Endocrinology* 92, no. 3 (March 1973):735–42.

167. Walter Silver, "Insomnia, Tachycardia, and Cola Drinkers," *Pediatrics* 47, no. 3 (March 1971):35.

168. Carol L. Otis and Roger Goldingay, "To Brew or Not to Brew," *Women's Sports and Fitness* 12, no. 3 (April 1990):12.

169. Corby Krummer, "Is Coffee Harmful?" *The Atlantic,* July 1990, pp. 92–96.

170. James P. Sweeney and Clifford J. Sherry. "How Safe Is Caffeine?" *Vibrant Life,* May/June 1986, p. 28.

171. Krummer, "Is Coffee Harmful?"

172. Paterson, "Caffeine: Villain or Victim?"

173. See "Look-Alike Drugs: Information Fact Sheet," *Drug Information Center (DIC)* (Eugene: University of Oregon, 1981).

TOBACCO

America's Number One Preventable Hazard

INTRODUCTION

More Americans are quitting smoking but more are dying from smoking-related illnesses—nearly 450,000 a year—as habits of the 1950s and 1960s take an increasing toll.[1] The national Centers for Disease Control (CDC) reported that 434,175 Americans died from smoking in 1988, up 11 percent from the 390,000 deaths attributed to smoking in 1985.

According to William Roper, director of the Atlanta-based Centers for Disease Control, "The problem is, we are now paying for what happened 20, 30 years ago, when large numbers of people smoked in large amounts.[2] The burden includes more than 100,000 annual deaths from lung cancer; 30,851 other cancer deaths (such as mouth cancers and pancreatic cancer); 202,802 deaths from a range of cardiovascular diseases such as heart disease and arterial disease; 82,857 deaths from respiratory diseases such as bronchitis and emphysema. In addition, there were 2,552 deaths of infants attributed to mother's smoking and 1,303 burn deaths in fires caused by smoking.

Former health secretary Louis Sullivan stated that smoking costs the country more than $52 billion annually in health-care costs and lost productivity.[3] Sullivan stated that the economic consequences of smoking cost each American $221 a year largely in health-care and insurance costs.

The 1990 National Household Survey on Drug Abuse reports the following on tobacco:[4]

- Nearly three quarters of the American population (73.2 percent) have tried cigarettes, and slightly over a quarter (26.7 percent) are past-month (current) smokers—a decrease from 28.8 percent in 1988. Current use of cigarettes among youth is almost 12 percent; 32 percent among young adults; and 28 percent among adults 26 and over.
- Four percent of youth and 6 percent of young adults used smokeless tobacco during the past month. These data indicate little change from 1988.

C. Everett Koop, the past surgeon general, names cigarette smoking "the chief preventable cause of death" and calls for a smoke-free environment by the year 2000. Earlier in 1988 Koop declared nicotine in cigarettes as addictive as cocaine and heroin.[5]

HISTORY

In the almost 500 years since European explorers first saw Native Americans smoking tobacco, a great segment of the world population has become dependent on the extremely harmful products made from this plant. Ironically, tobacco first became popular in Europe for its supposed curative powers and was looked upon by some as a panacea for health problems. The smoking of tobacco spread rapidly across Europe and eventually the entire world.

Early on, tobacco was smoked through a pipe. But in the mid-nineteenth century, this form of tobacco use decreased in Europe and the United States and was replaced by chewing tobacco. Spittoons became an accepted part of the era, and near the end of the nineteenth century half of all the tobacco consumed in the United States was chewed. Later, cigars and cigarettes were introduced. Their consumption increased steadily, and in 1885 over 1 billion cigarettes were sold.

Researchers have also discovered that the risk to women smokers in the United States is increasing.[6] Studies have shown that middle-aged women who smoke are having more heart attacks. In fact, women smokers of all ages are subject to coronary artery disease. Smoking, regardless of age and regardless of the amount, is not safe. According to a Harvard study, men and women now have the same risk of developing coronary disease; before, the risk was high for men alone. Among women who smoke 25 cigarettes a day, 81 percent of deaths are from coronary artery disease, attributed to smoking.[7]

CHEMISTRY

Cigarette smoke from burning tobacco consists of a mixture of approximately 3,000 chemical substances that are dangerous to living tissue.[8] These substances include (1) droplets of tars and other compounds, which form 40 percent of the smoke; (2) nicotine, a drug that is poisonous in higher concentrations; and (3) a dozen gases, including carbon monoxide, hydrogen cyanide, and nitrous oxides. The toxicity of these gases and compounds, coupled with nicotine, is responsible for many of the cigarette-related premature deaths that occur each year in the United States.

Tar and nicotine in cigarettes are usually present in the ratio of 10 to 1.[9] Research has shown tobacco tars to be carcinogenic (cancer-producing) when applied to the skin or bronchial tubes of mice and other laboratory animals. Other chemicals in tobacco tar are co-carcinogens (substances that do not themselves cause cancer but stimulate the growth of certain cancers when combined with other chemicals). For example, the phenols present in tar are not inherently carcinogenic but may combine with benzopyrene, another substance in tar, to produce cancer.

A combination of hydrogen cyanide, tars, and the drying effect of cigarette smoke paralyzes or destroys the action of the cilia, the mucus-covered hairlike structures that keep the lungs free from mucus, germs, and dirt. Eventually, the bronchial tubes become saturated with a brown, sticky coating of hydrogen cyanide, tars, and other foreign matter. In attempting to dislodge this matter many smokers develop a "smoker's cough" or "hack."[10]

Cigarettes contain significantly large amounts of nicotine alkaloid. Pharmacologically, nicotine, which is liberated from tobacco by the heat produced by combustion, is classified as a stimulant. Clinical findings indicate that its major effects on the body are respiratory stimulation and gastrointestinal hyperactivity, since nicotine is readily absorbed from oral and gastrointestinal mucosa, the respiratory tract, and the skin.[11] Because deeper inhaling takes place in cigarette smoking, the smoker inhales more tars, nicotine, and **carbon monoxide** from cigarettes than from cigars or pipes. Nicotine in snuff and chewing tobacco is absorbed through buccal (cheek and mouth) membranes, rather than from inhalation.

Cigarettes contain from 0.7 to 3.0 percent nicotine, or 0.5 to 2.0 milligrams per cigarette,[12] depending on the type of tobacco. The amount absorbed into the bloodstream varies with the moisture content of the tobacco, the amount of filter added, the length of the cigarette, heat, the rapidity of smoking, and the depth of inhalation, but conservative estimates place it at approximately 90 percent (0.45 to 1.8 milligrams). Though 60 milligrams is considered a lethal dose, as little as 4 milligrams in novice or infrequent users may occasionally produce alarming symptoms—giddiness, nausea, vomiting, abdominal cramping, a cold sweat, and vasomotor collapse.[13]

Smoke is readily absorbed by the body, and some of its nicotine goes directly to the brain. Eighty to ninety percent of the nicotine absorbed is metabolized by the liver before it is excreted by the kidneys.[14] The amount excreted depends on the pH of the urine; four times as much is excreted when the urine is acid. Absorbed nicotine can be transferred to infants during breast feeding by mothers who smoke.

Carbon Monoxide
An odorless, colorless, and poisonous gas possessing an affinity for hemoglobin 250 times that of oxygen. It is one of the gases given off in cigarette smoke, and it literally drives oxygen out of body cells.

THE 1979 SURGEON GENERAL'S REPORT

In 1979, the surgeon general reported "overwhelming" evidence that smoking contributes directly to disease and death.[15] Surgeon General Julius Richmond noted that this conclusion was based on a 1,200-page report of a "review and reappraisal" of research accumulated over the previous 15 years. According to former secretary of health, education and welfare Joseph Califano, the document revealed smoking to be more dangerous than supposed in a 1964 surgeon general's report. Califano contended that the report "demolished" claims by cigarette manufacturers that there is no proven link between smoking and cancer and chronic diseases. Additional surgeon general reports have further validated these extremely conclusive findings on the harmful effects of smoking, especially in regard to cardiovascular diseases, cancer, and chronic obstructive lung disease.

Among the findings the 1979 surgeon general's report reemphasized are these:

1. Smokers, male and female, die from a variety of ailments at a rate two-thirds higher than nonsmokers.
2. The risk goes up as the amount smoked goes up. For example, two-pack-a-day smokers have a death rate twice as high as nonsmokers.
3. Women are dying from lung cancer at a rate three times as high as in 1964.
4. Coronary heart disease from smoking causes more premature deaths than lung cancer and other lung diseases.
5. Pipe and cigar smokers "experience overall mortality rates that are slightly higher than those of nonsmokers, but at rates substantially lower than those of the cigarette smokers."
6. Smokers of low-tar and nicotine cigarettes run lower risks of lung cancer and coronary heart disease but "may in fact increase their hazard if they begin smoking more cigarettes or inhaling more deeply."
7. Children or adolescents who smoke may suffer immediate harm in the form of lung damage and respiratory problems.
8. Ninety percent of the people who smoke "have either tried to quit smoking or would probably quit, if only they could find an effective way to do so."[16]

PHYSIOLOGICAL EFFECTS

Nicotine affects the brain and the spinal cord as well as the peripheral nervous system. It can cause increased blood pressure, increased heart rate, reduced skin temperature, release of epinephrine (adrenalin), and increased gastrointestinal activity. The substance also exerts an antidiuretic action for two to three hours (reducing urine formation), increases tone and motor activity of the bowel (occasionally causing diarrhea), stimulates then depresses production of saliva and bronchial secretions, vasoconstricts the blood vessels of the skin, increases the amounts of free fatty acids in the bloodstream, increases platelet adhesiveness (a blood-clotting factor), and decreases DNA synthesis of lymphocytes, consequently altering the body and its steady-state mechanisms. Consistent with the effects of other stimulants, nicotine-caused excitation of the brain is followed by a period of postuse depression. Skeletal muscle activity, including the work of the diaphragm, which affects breathing, is reduced because of neuronal-function depression. Nerve fibers coming from the muscles are also affected, leading to a marked reduction in muscle tone that may be involved in the relaxation that accompanies smoking.

Nicotine in tobacco smoke stimulates brain cells and speeds up the heart rate, creating a state of alertness. This is why most people like this particular substance. At the same time, though, it relaxes the muscles in your body. If you take a higher dose, you could become extremely depressed rather than alert. People can become addicted to this drug very easily. The more you use nicotine, the more your system needs to get the same result. Discontinuation of the drug may result in withdrawal symptoms including restlessness and anxiety, irritability, depression, and dizziness. Though withdrawal is not fatal, it can be extremely uncomfortable, difficult, and prolonged.

GASES

Carbon monoxide (CO), hydrogen cyanide, and nitrous oxides are gases in cigarette smoke that affect the homeostatic condition of the circulatory and respiratory systems. Carbon monoxide is an odorless, colorless, and poisonous gas possessing an affinity for hemoglobin 250 times that of oxygen.[17] It impairs oxygen transportation to body tissues in at least two ways: by competing with oxygen for hemoglobin-binding sites and by increasing the affinity of the remaining hemoglobin for oxygen, thereby strengthening the oxyhemoglobin bond and making it difficult for the tissues to draw oxygen away from the hemoglobin. Body tissues receive oxygen, but not as much as they would under normal circumstances. Carbon monoxide literally drives the oxygen out of the body's red blood cells. As a result, the oxygen-carrying capacity of the blood is impaired and the body lacks sufficient quantities of this necessary element.

Hydrogen cyanide, a powerful, rapidly acting blood and nerve poison, is the element in cigarette smoke that is most responsible for the impairment of cilia function in the lungs. Removal of this poisonous gas from the smoke allows the cilia to continue to work until overcome by other harmful elements in the smoke.

Nitrous oxides have a deleterious effect on macrophages—the large, vacuum-cleaner-like white cells that live in the fluid that lines the inner surfaces of the lungs and that serve as cleaning mechanisms along with the cilia. Macrophages attack invading particles that are inhaled by digesting them or transporting them to the bronchioles, where they are transferred to the lymphatic system and removed from the lungs. Studies conducted at the University of Pittsburgh showed that when rabbit macrophages were exposed to high concentrations of nitrous dioxide (NO_2), the number of microbes eaten by the macrophages were reduced and the microbe-killing capacity of the defending cells was also lowered.[18]

CHRONIC DISEASE

Cigarette smoking is the cause of one in every six deaths in the United States and is responsible for cardiovascular disease, emphysema, cancer, and low birth weight.[19] Unfortunately, this cost is paid for by all of us—smokers and nonsmokers alike. Nonsmokers pay through state-supported public welfare programs that provide benefits to those disabled by smoke-related diseases and to their survivors. They also pay in the form of increased insurance premiums and increased prices for consumer goods as a result of smokers' high rates of absenteeism from work.

The cost of smoking in terms of lost health and depleted economic resources has become astronomical. For example, a middle-aged man who smokes two packs of cigarettes per day will incur an average of more than $56,000 in costs of illness in his lifetime as a direct cause of smoking.[20]

Under a Federal Trade Commission plan that went into effect in October 1985, four new warnings are rotated on all cigarette packs. These warnings are listed in Figure 6–1.

CARDIOVASCULAR DISEASE

The amount of smoking-induced damage to the cardiovascular system is directly proportional to the number of cigarettes smoked, the age smoking began, and the number of years the user has been smoking. Since nicotine increases both heart rate and blood pressure, smokers respond with sustained increases in blood pressure, which increase the work load of the heart. The chronic hyperactivity of the sympathetic nervous system, caused by nicotine absorption, is also a predisposing factor in heart disease and myocardial infarction.[21]

An increase in coronary-artery blood flow after smoking parallels the rise in systemic blood pressure and ventricular output. In a study of nine patients

FIGURE 6-1 Read the Tobacco Warning Labels
Source: Ogust/The Image Works

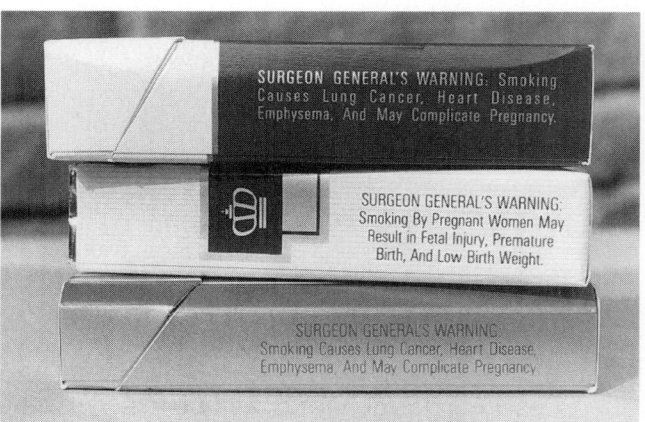

who smoked regularly and always inhaled freely, a significant rise in arterial pressure five minutes after smoking a cigarette was reported.[22]

Carbon monoxide interferes with circulation by increasing material membrane permeability, creating edema (abnormal accumulation of fluid), and inviting cholesterol deposits. These deposits may eventually lead to arteriosclerosis, considered to be the first stage of many dangerous circulatory conditions. Approximately 90 percent of all patients with symptoms of arteriosclerosis are smokers; very few are nonsmokers.

Another circulatory disease associated with nicotine is Buerger's disease. Patients with this problem have decreased blood flow to the extremities, which in extreme cases requires amputation.

In the 1983 surgeon general's report, *Health Consequences of Smoking: Cardiovascular Disease,* the key finding was that *cigarette smoking* should be considered the most important known modifiable risk factor for heart disease in the United States. The report stated that up to 30 percent of all coronary deaths are related to smoking.[23] This appears to reaffirm the statistics from the Framington Heart Study, which links cigarette smoking to sudden death due to heart disease. Furthermore, "cigarette smoking is the most significant risk factor for sudden death in men."[24] It is thought that smoking might cause sudden death by increasing the adrenalin and carbon-monoxide levels, making platelets stickier, irritating the myocardium, or raising the blood pressure.

Another significant relationship is that between smoking and coronary bypass operations. For years, physicians have known that smoking causes changes in blood chemistry that facilitate plaque buildup in arteries, which in turn leads to heart attacks and strokes. But it is only in the past few years that we have seen just how important smoking is as a cause of blockage of coronary arteries. One team of physicians found that 92 percent of their coronary bypass patients under the age of 40 were smokers.

STROKES

Smoking is now blamed for 26,500 stroke deaths per year.[25] Smokers are more likely than nonsmokers to die from cerebrovascular disease, a condition in which hardening of blood vessels in the brain may lead to a stroke. Both the carbon monoxide and the nicotine in tobacco affect the adhesiveness of platelets—the main clotting factor in blood—in the brain, speeding the formation of clots.[26] Nicotine also causes blood vessels to constrict, reducing the passageways by which blood reaches the brain. If these arteries become too constricted, the blood supply is greatly diminished or cut off and the smoker suffers a stroke.

RESPIRATORY DISEASES

Cigarette cough is so common—it afflicts millions of Americans—that it is accepted as normal rather than as the warning of damage to the lungs that it actually is. Shortness of breath and the nagging smoker's cough are the cumulative effect of toxic chemicals found in tobacco smoke. Tars, nicotine,

Chronic Bronchitis
An inflammation of the bronchial tubes often caused by smoking tobacco cigarettes.

Emphysema
A lung disease in which the lungs lose their normal elasticity and retain abnormal amounts of air. Smoking destroys the tiny air sacs in the lungs, where oxygen is absorbed into the body, resulting in a loss of oxygen absorption and subsequent loss of breath.

hydrogen cyanide, and nitrous oxides are associated with the lung diseases of **chronic bronchitis** and **emphysema,** known together as chronic obstructive pulmonary disease (COPD).[27]

In the case of smoking-induced bronchitis, cigarette smoke irritates and inflames the air passages (bronchi) leading from the windpipe to the lungs. After prolonged smoking, the cilia become useless and tars build up. This buildup causes a reduction in normal respiration, resulting in regular coughing and regurgitation of phlegm—the body's way of attempting to expel the foreign particles the cilia can no longer eliminate. The only "cure" for this vicious cycle is to quit smoking and give the lungs a chance to resume normal functioning.

Emphysema is a lung disease in which the lungs lose their normal elasticity and retain abnormal amounts of air. Smoking destroys the tiny air sacs in the lungs, where oxygen is absorbed into the body, resulting in a loss of oxygen absorption and a subsequent loss of breath. Breathing becomes extremely difficult, and people with advanced emphysema may use 80 percent of their strength just in breathing. The condition is extremely agonizing and usually ends in heart failure. Since damaged lung tissue can never be replaced, there is no real cure, but quitting smoking will stop the disease from progressing. Nonsmokers can also develop emphysema, but such cases are considerably less common.

The overall conclusion of the 1984 surgeon general's report on smoking is that

> cigarette smoking is the major cause of chronic obstructive lung disease in the United States for both men and women. The contribution of cigarette smoking to chronic obstructive lung disease morbidity and mortality far outweighs all other factors.[28]

LUNG AND OTHER CANCERS

Since the surgeon general's *1964 Smoking and Health Report,* over 43 million Americans have voluntarily quit smoking. According to recent studies, voluntary quitting has saved over 200,000 premature deaths. The number of smokers in this country has fallen from about 70 million at the time of the *1964 Smoking and Health Report* to 47 million today. A smaller percentage of American adults smoke today than at any other time since the Great Depression.

In 1989 we celebrated the twenty-fifth anniversary of that 1964 report by looking at the new U.S. surgeon general's report on tobacco. Although there has been a favorable change in smoking behaviors and attitudes, many people continue to die from the effects of smoking. One in six deaths in the United States is caused by smoking, and the 1989 report shows tobacco is more detrimental than people originally suspected.[29] Two thirds of those fatalities are from cardiovascular disease, lung cancer, and respiratory ailments like emphysema.[30] Lung cancer rates leveled off for men, but the average male smoker is still 22 times more likely to die from lung cancer than a nonsmoker. Lung cancer for women has reached an all-time high and is now the number one killer for women, surpassing breast cancer.

The Centers for Disease Control also said 3,825 Americans died from lung cancer caused by others' smoking, or "passive smoke."[31] However, the CDC's statistical formulas do not yet include passive smoking deaths from heart diseases, which a recent study estimated at 37,000 a year.[32]

SIDE EFFECTS

METABOLISM

Smoking tends to stimulate the adrenalin-releasing effect of nicotine; the cessation of smoking depresses energy consumption and favors fat- and carbohydrate-deposit formations. Since carbohydrates tend to aggravate the process of weight gain through the action of insulin, a low-carbohydrate, low-fat diet such as the Mayo Clinic diet may be useful after quitting.[33]

There is conflicting evidence concerning the release of fatty acids as an effect of nicotine. One research team examined the effects of cigarette smoking on blood-lipid values in ten healthy volunteers between the ages of 20 and 40. The results showed that cigarette smoking caused a prompt rise in free fatty acids and a delayed rise in serum triglycerides.[34] Some data indicate increased serum-cholesterol levels in heavy smokers, whereas other data reveal no correlation.[35]

APPETITE REDUCTION

Contrary to common knowledge, studies have shown that nonsmokers do not generally eat more than smokers, nor do they exercise less. In fact, when researchers performed tests on smokers at rest, the results indicated that nicotine itself caused an increase in basal metabolic rate, showing that smokers burn more calories than nonsmokers during periods of inactivity.[36] Surveys have shown, however, that most smokers smoke not while completely at rest, but while performing light activities such as desk work or housework. This light activity not only increases the metabolic rate on its own, but when combined with nicotine, can raise one's metabolic rate by two or three times. Research has shown that an increase in nicotine consumption results in a proportional increase in metabolic rate, indicating that the two events are dependent on each other.[37] These results have proven that the metabolic effect of nicotine may play a much greater part in accounting for body-weight differences between smokers and nonsmokers than was previously believed.

Research has found that smokers weigh 5 to 10 pounds less than nonsmokers of comparable age and height. However, smokers' body fat accumulates primarily around the waist and increases the risk for developing cardiovascular disease, as well as for developing diabetes.[38] The researchers found that although total weight and body mass were lower among smokers compared to nonsmokers, the waist circumference and the waist-hip ratio in smokers were greater than in the nonsmokers (this variance increased in proportion with the actual number of cigarettes smoked daily).

Tobacco smoke has been implicated in gastrointestinal disturbances. The volume and acidity of continuous gastric secretions are decreased in normal subjects who smoke, and the acidity of the basal gastric secretion often decreases in patients with peptic ulcers who smoke. Smoking tends to increase the motor activity of the colon. Also, smokers have a high propensity for losing lower-esophageal sphincter pressure, resulting in heartburn from gastric reflex.

Cigarette smoking apparently interferes with the body's normal immunological defenses. A two-year study found that 50 percent more heavy smokers were hospitalized for one reason or another than nonsmokers. Even light smoking may have an effect on cellular immunity.[39] Harkey, who performed some of the earliest studies on the antigenicity of nicotine (its ability to elicit a specific immunologic response), could not exclude the possibility that nicotine may act as a hapten (a compound that is not antigenic itself but reacts with an antibody and conveys antigenic specificity when combined with another compound). Silvette and colleagues reviewed several papers dealing with the immunology of nicotine and concluded that nicotine was antigenic.[40]

PREGNANCY AND FETAL NUTRITION

Women who smoke during pregnancy tend to give birth to smaller babies, probably because of the increased carboxyhemoglobin level in their bloodstream.[41] This condition reduces their oxygen level, resulting in less oxygen being available to the fetus. A second probable cause of smaller babies is that nicotine decreases hunger, causing the mother to eat less and thereby reducing the nutrients available to the developing fetus.

Spontaneous Abortions   Although several investigators have found a significantly higher dose-related incidence of spontaneous abortion among cigarette smokers than among nonsmokers, the lack of control of significant variables does not permit conclusions to be drawn. Ingestion of nicotine, however, has been proved to cause spontaneous abortions in animals.[42]

As part of a prenatal program in the United States, 50,000 pregnant women and children were studied. It was determined that the risk of miscarriage and infant death increases for women who smoke cigarettes prior to pregnancy (depending on the quantity of cigarettes smoked and the duration of smoking).[43] Other findings from the study indicate that smoking before pregnancy may damage the small arteries in the uterus, depriving the fetus of necessary oxygen and nutrients. This damage may be permanent and affect future pregnancies. Furthermore, the risk of sudden infant death syndrome (SIDS) is increased by approximately 50 percent when the mother smokes during pregnancy.

Stillbirth and Neonatal Deaths   In 1964, the Public Health Service (PHS) reported 46,000 stillbirths associated with pregnant women who smoked. The PHS also noted a decrease in deaths if smoking was given up by the fourth month of pregnancy. Butler, in 1969, found a highly significant association between maternal smoking after the fourth month and both late-fetal and neonatal deaths. Pregnant women who smoked had a higher late-fetal mortality rate than pregnant women who did not smoke.[44] Passive smoke or environmental tobacco smoke (ETS) was also shown to be harmful.[45]

Nicotine in Mothers' Milk   The surgeon general's 1972 and 1973 reports cited findings concerning nicotine in the milk of nursing mothers.[46] For example, Rerlman found nicotine in the milk of all mothers he had tested who smoked. There was a direct relationship between the concentration of nicotine in the milk and the number of cigarettes smoked.[47]

Anomalies   Some research indicates a higher incidence of congenital malformation, such as cleft lip and cleft palate, in infants born to smokers. In a study of 100 mothers (37 smokers and 63 nonsmokers),[48] two fetuses of smokers had Klinefelter's syndrome*. Erickson, Kallen, and Westerholm identified a relationship between smoking and the rate of infant birth malformations.[49] In their study of hospital records concerning such malformations, they found a significant increase in cleft lip or palate in infants born to women who smoked.

EXERCISE AND PHYSICAL PERFORMANCE

A reduction in the oxygen-carrying capacity of the red blood cells—which occurs from smoking—means a reduction in physical capacity. Smoking also causes swelling of the mucous membranes in the trachea and the bronchial tubes, leading to increased airway resistance; extra effort is needed to get air in and out of the lungs. The alveoli (air sacs) in the lungs may also receive a reduced amount of oxygen. During exercise, when the demand on the respiratory system is elevated, the increased respiratory resistance caused by smoking may be noticeable.

During heavy exercise, the oxygen cost of exhaling for chronic smokers is on the average twice as great as that for nonsmokers. This is true even if only a few cigarettes are smoked within one hour prior to exercise. In heavy smokers (people who smoke 20 to 30 cigarettes per day for at least 27 years), the cost is nearly four times that of nonsmokers. If no cigarettes are smoked within 24 hours prior to exercise, the oxygen cost is still about 60 percent higher than that for nonsmokers.[50]

SEXUAL ACTIVITY

Smoking impairs sexual performance in two primary ways: (1) The CO intake reduces the blood's oxygen level and impairs the production of the male sex hormone testosterone, and (2) the nicotine intake constricts the blood vessels, which need to swell to cause sexual excitement and erection in males. A study by Carl Schirren also found severe disturbance of sperm motility in a group of men who smoked. Their sperm counts were low, and the sperm that were present were sluggish, displaying low motility. Schirren reported that stopping smoking resulted in a considerable improvement in sperm motility within six to ten weeks.[51]

*A condition in which the sex-chromosome constitution is abnormal, in that a Y chromosome is associated with more than one X chromosome. A Klinefelter male may appear normal, or be very tall, sterile, or mentally retarded.

The reduced lung capacity in smokers also affects sexual activity by lowering stamina, and thus it affects the ability to prolong the sexual experience. In addition, nicotine discolors the teeth and causes bad breath, reducing the smoker's sexual attractiveness. It is no mere coincidence that patients of sex counselors and doctors report that after they quit smoking, their sex lives improve.[52]

OTHER HEALTH FACTORS

Nicotine and Oral Contraceptives   The Walnut Creek study of the long-term effects of the use of oral contraceptives on health,[53] started in 1969, has provided a good deal of nicotine-related information. The study, involving 17,929 suburban, predominately white women, found that smoking may increase the likelihood of subarachnoid hemorrhage (bleeding between portions of the brain). The risk to cigarette smokers was 5.7 times that to nonsmokers, and the risk to smokers who used oral contraceptives was 22 times that to women who neither smoked nor used oral contraceptives.

A study of the interactions of oral contraceptives and nicotine showed increased urinary levels of epinephrine and norepinephrine.[54] (Norepinephrine is a hormone that stimulates the sympathetic nervous system, which mediates functional activity. Therapeutically it is useful for maintaining blood pressure in acute hypotensive states, central vasomotor depression, and hemorrhage.) In addition, continual circulatory fluctuations resulting from smoking and oral-contraceptive use are known to increase the risk of myocardial infarction.[55]

Periodontal Disease   Tobacco smokers have much higher rates of periodontal disease, which can cause excessive damage to the gums. Trench mouth and loss of teeth from gum damage may also be caused by cigarette smoking.

Effectiveness of Medication   The 1979 surgeon general's report on smoking and health reveals that smoking alters the effectiveness of some medications.[56] For example, theophylline, used for treating acute and chronic asthma and bronchitis, and pentazocine, a prescription narcotic antagonist and pain killer, must be taken in larger doses by smokers than nonsmokers; overdoses are therefore possible if smoking habits vary. It has also been suggested that vaccines are less effective in smokers than in nonsmokers, and responses to diagnostic tests may be affected by smoking. The level of white blood cells, the size of red blood cells, and the time required for blood clotting are also adversely affected by smoking.[57] Smoking diminishes the effects of many medications because it accelerates the metabolism of many drugs and also reduces the blood flow to skin, thereby reducing insulin absorption in smokers.[58] Therefore, it not only is bad for the heart, lungs, circulation, and respiration but can nullify the effects of medications taken to cure or heal other ailments or needs.

COMBINING ALCOHOL AND TOBACCO

It was discovered that over 90 percent of the people (male and female) who went in for alcohol treatment were also smokers.[59] It seems that the combination of alcohol and nicotine has a "multiplicative" effect when oral and pharyngeal cancer are concerned. Just smoking or just drinking increases one's risk for this type of cancer, but when combined the risk is tremendously increased.

NICOTINE AND COFFEE INTAKE

From a psychological standpoint, smoking may fill a behavioral need for oral stimulation. Studies indicate that smokers may further fulfill this need with additional oral habits, such as greater alcohol and coffee intake. From a physiological standpoint, caffeine and nicotine work together to affect homeostasis. Hickey and colleagues suggest that tobacco smoking and coffee may be self-selected behavioral regulators of the homeostatic process.[60]

VITAMINS

Smoking causes changes in plasma and leukocyte concentrations of vitamin C and impairs biochemical functions of this vitamin. Vitamin B-12 is metabolized in the body's detoxification of the cyanide released from tobacco in smoking. Some heavy smokers develop amblyopia (an eye disease), which is reversed by either vitamin B-12 supplements or termination of smoking. There is evidence that smoking may also alter the metabolism of lipids, carbohydrates, proteins, and other vitamins, such as B-6.[61]

PSYCHOLOGICAL EFFECTS

THE SMOKING HABIT

Smoking involves more than just a physiological addiction to nicotine. Various psychological and social factors work together to cause an individual to start smoking. Unfortunately, the habit is usually initiated with naive intentions, but social forces reinforce the smoking behaviors until the individual develops physical dependence on the drug and then cannot quit without experiencing some type of withdrawal.

As with other forms of nonmedical drug use, the initial experimentation and regular use of tobacco begin in youth. Initiation of the behavior depends on three factors:

1. an opportunity to engage in the behavior
2. a high degree of curiosity about the effects
3. the discovery that smoking is a way to express conformity with the behaviors of others or to rebel

REASONS FOR SMOKING AND NOT SMOKING

People begin smoking for many reasons: curiosity, boredom, peer pressure and social acceptance, expression of independence and maturity, parental example, imitation of supposed glamorous social figures, low (or high) academic achievement, response to stress, relief of tension (Figure 6–2). Smoking often induces feelings of stimulation or tranquility in addition to an increased sense of well-being and improved working efficiency. The habit is relaxing and pleasurable to many and is seen as a means of facilitating communication, a way to role-play, and a way to fill time.

Cigarette smoking received a boost in popularity during World War I, when troops were given free cigarettes by the tobacco companies. In the midst of worry, homesickness, and the nerve-racking experience of warfare, cigarettes acted as a peacemaker to the central nervous system. They numbed the nerve endings and reduced the perception of both pleasurable and unpleasant sensations. Their threat to health was of limited importance, since the men could die in battle the next day.

The results of surveys of sex-role convergence and aging effects, smoking initiation, and current smoking and smoking behavior of men and women professionals indicate that men smokers still exceeded women smokers as of 1975 but that presently more women than men are smoking. Women smokers may have taken up the habit to identify with males and achieve liberation from the traditional female stereotype, a supposition supported by the fact that women employed outside the home are more likely to smoke than housewives.

ADVERTISING

Targeting specific demographic groups seems to be a fact of economic life for tobacco manufacturers. Since young women, less-educated blue-collar workers, and blacks apparently cling to the smoking habit more than other groups, cigarette advertising will surely continue to focus on them.[62]

In February 1990 protests from civil-rights groups and Secretary of Health and Human Services Louis Sullivan forced R. J. Reynolds to scrap plans for a cigarette called Uptown, aimed at blacks. However, in March a marketing proposal leaked anonymously to an antismoking group that revealed Reynolds seemed to have another target in its sights: young (age 18 to 24), white, working-class women. Dubbed "virile females" in a campaign recommended by a marketing agency, these women, R. J. Reynolds seems to

FIGURE 6–2 THE MAIN PSYCHOSOCIAL FACTORS DETERMINING THE ONSET OF SMOKING.
On the Right are the positive reinforcers or incentives to smoke. On the Left are the factors that discourage smoking.
Source: M.A.H. Russel, "Tobacco Dependence: Is Nicotine Rewarding or Aversive?" *Practitioner* 212 (1974):791–800 (London: Morgan Crampion, Ltd.). Used with permission.

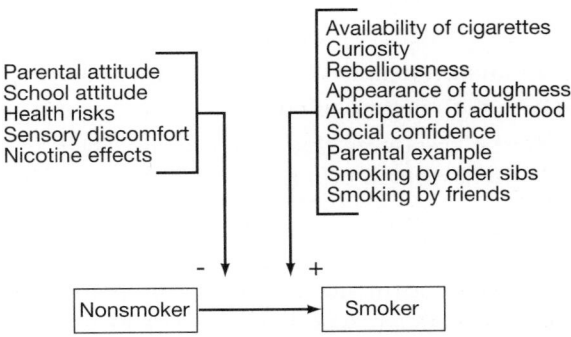

believe, are among society's most vulnerable women—and most apt to fall for the new cigarettes, to be called Dakota. They state that these women, who have little education, work in entry-level service or factory jobs and enjoy going to hot-rod and "monster truck" events with their boyfriends. Oriented firmly in the present, they're unlikely to have absorbed information about smoking's long-term health risks to themselves and, if pregnant, to their unborn.[63]

TYPES OF SMOKERS

Habitual Smokers   In this pattern, smokers are hardly aware that they have a cigarette in their mouth. For these people, smoking may once have been an important sign of status, but now it is simply automatic. The act of smoking enhances the habitual smoker's mood and feelings of competency.

Positive-Effect Smokers   Here smoking serves as a stimulant, producing pleasure, relaxation, or heightened enjoyment, as at the end of a meal. Smokers in this pattern may most enjoy the handling of a cigarette or the sense and sight of the smoke curling out of their mouths. Beginning smokers may fall into this pattern to demonstrate their defiance of their parents.

Negative-Effect Smokers   This is sedative smoking, using the habit to reduce distress, fear, shame, or disgust, or any combination of these feelings. People in this pattern may not smoke at all under normal circumstances, but they may reach for a cigarette when things go badly.

Addicted Smokers   These smokers are always aware they are smoking. They are also aware of not smoking, since the lack of nicotine builds a need and desire for it, and discomfort sets in. The increasing need leads to a growing expectation that a cigarette will reduce the discomfort—and it does give relief, but just for a moment. For dependent smokers, the pleasure of smoking is real, just as the buildup of discomfort when not smoking is real, and sometimes rapid and intolerable.

WOMEN

Smoking today is becoming just as attractive and popular to women as it has been to men over the years. Women who were almost free from cardiovascular diseases and lung diseases are not free anymore. The U.S. surgeon general has estimated that smoking is responsible for "around 40 percent of heart disease deaths, 55 percent of lethal strokes and among women of all ages 80 percent of lung cancer and 30 percent of all cancer deaths."[64] Smoking is also affecting women's health in ways that are specific to women.[65] Cervical cancer is higher in women who smoke than in nonsmokers. Smoking also affects women's reproductive health: There is an increase in low birth weight, miscarriages, and earlier menopause. Low birth weight becomes an increasing concern for women of underdeveloped countries that already have a high mortality rate as well as malnutrition and poverty.

Smoking kills over half a million women each year in the industrialized world. Throughout the world, tobacco has been named the cause of 2.7 million deaths per year. By the year 2025 this death toll may increase to 8 million deaths per year.[66]

Women who kick the habit of smoking have a declined risk of first heart attack. The risk reduction in women should provide a new incentive for women to quit their smoking habit. Studies show that smoking has steadily declined in the United States in the past decades, but the trend among females is less robust than among males. Women are known to have lower success rates when it comes to kicking the habit than men. Instead of quitting, it has been noted that women switch to low-tar brands. Data drawn from 3,000 women show that the risk of heart attack three years after a woman quits is "virtually indistinguishable" from that of a woman who has never smoked before.[67]

In general, men smoke more than women, but smoking among men seems to be decreasing. The problem is that the smoking trend for women is starting to parallel that of men.[68] And not only is women's use of cigarettes increasing, but it is harder to get women to quit once they've started.

MINORITIES

Antismoking campaigns have lowered the prevalence of cigarette smoking in adults but have not been equally successful in all ethnic and socioeconomic groups. Blacks are more likely to smoke than white adults, who in turn are more likely to smoke than Hispanics.[69] One interesting finding among Hispanics was that acculturation plays a role in smoking behavior. The less acculturated were more likely to smoke. This study points out that *it now appears to be educational differences rather than ethnic differences that determine smoking behavior.*

Although the onset of smoking begins later for black youth than for white youth, blacks have a higher percentage of cigarette smokers than whites.[70] Specifically, 45 percent of black men and 30 percent of black women smoke compared to 37 percent of white men and 30 percent of white women who smoke.

According to the Centers for Disease Control, smoking-related diseases kill proportionately more blacks than whites. Yet the tobacco lobby turns to blacks for support. This is because the tobacco industry gives generous contributions to the National Association for the Advancement of Colored People, the Congress of Racial Equality, the National Urban League, and other minority organizations.[71] The tobacco lobby still clings to an economic argument: Smoking restrictions place an unfair economic burden on businesses such as restaurants. But now the industry is trying a constitutional argument: Smoking restrictions discriminate against minorities and violate civil liberties. "In 1987, when the New York City Council was preparing to impose tough smoking bans, Hazel Dukes, president of the state NAACP, argued that the proposal was unfair to blacks because it would permit white executives to smoke in their private offices while the rank and file, many of them black, could not smoke in common areas."[72]

ADOLESCENTS

The percentage of adults who smoke has decreased since recent evidence has been available discussing the harms of tobacco. Research and educational efforts have made a significant impact on motivating individuals to quit and to prevent the onset of smoking. However, according to the 1991–1992 school year survey conducted by Parents Resource Institute for Drug Education (PRIDE), smoking and drug use were on the rise again among young people, especially junior high students and blacks.[73] The students, in questionnaires distributed by teachers, were asked about their usage of drugs in ten categories: cigarettes, beer, wine coolers, liquor, marijuana, cocaine, uppers, downers, hallucinogens, and inhalants. This study's results reverse the previous trend in which the survey found that drug use among students dropped or stayed the same.

Early intervention has had the most lasting effects. "Cigarette promotion and advertising expenditures have grown from $261 million in 1964 to $2 billion in 1984."[74] Education needs to be promoted widely to overpower these advertising campaigns. To look at what we need to do in the next 25 years, researchers need to examine carefully marketing campaigns aimed at enticing adolescents into tobacco use.[75]

ALTERNATIVES TO SMOKING AND CONSEQUENT PROBLEMS

Since the early 1960s, because of the publicizing of the deleterious effects of tars and nicotine, cigarette companies have reduced the amount of these substances in their cigarettes and have begun large-scale manufacturing of filtered cigarettes. Unfortunately, even though the dependency-producing agent (nicotine) has been reduced, the poisonous gases have remained constant, and in a few cases even increased.[76] It is also unfortunate that the fraction of nicotine removed from the mainstream smoke by a filter is very small. To avoid nicotine's vascular effects, one would have to use a filter that passes no smoke at all.

Since nicotine is the element in cigarettes that produces the desired effects, smokers draw more deeply and inhale more often when they smoke low-nicotine brands. Consequently, they increase their tar and gas intake. The Snell Laboratories programmed smoking machines to behave like smokers who take faster puffs and inhale deeply. They tested six low-tar, low-nicotine brands and found that in almost every instance the quantity of gas increased, sometimes dramatically. Hence, smoking filtered, low-nicotine brands may produce more of the three poisonous gases than nonfilter brands.[77]

Nicotine gum has been discussed in several studies as a less harmful substitute for smoking. The idea may sound like a vast improvement over smoke inhalation, but most studies list many drawbacks. The main problem is that the gum is absorbed through the throat and lungs. Chewing it may also release three times as much nicotine as a cigarette, but the effect takes longer to achieve. This slower effect produced by buccal absorption may, however, produce less dependency in the tobacco chewer. On January 13, 1984, the Food and Drug Administration finally approved the use of nicotine chewing gum as a prescription drug for use in quitting smoking. Merrel Dow Pharmaceuticals was authorized to begin marketing Nicorette (Nicotine Resin Complex) in the United States.[78] Nicorette has been called "a nicotine-laced chewing gum prescribed by doctors as a chemical crutch for reforming smokers."[79] The problem is that it is also addicting. A large portion of the 100,000 new Nicorette users each month are nicotine abusers. Nicorette chewing gum can be a very useful way to quit smoking as long as it is used correctly. "An estimated 1 million smokers in the United States have succeeded in quitting with its help."[80] The problems lie with those who abuse it.

Another new approach being experimented with is nicotine skin patches. The patches, which are like large Band-Aids infused with nicotine, are stuck to any spot on the upper torso. The nicotine is gradually leached through the skin and into the bloodstream, much like the way hand cream is absorbed. The patches initially release 21 milligrams of nicotine every 24 hours, the equivalent of smoking about a pack of cigarettes a day. After 6 weeks, the smoker uses a 14 milligram patch for 2 weeks, then a 7 milligram patch for 2 weeks. The patches cost about $115 a month. It will take time to determine the effectiveness of nicotine skin patches.

Other efforts are being made to develop methods of delivering a maximum of nicotine to the bloodstream of tobacco dependents with a minimum of smoke to their lungs. This would reduce or eliminate the hazards of lung cancer, although the effects of nicotine on the body would continue. Efforts presently under way include development of a short cigarette with a high nicotine content; a cigarette with noninhalable smoke; smoke-free ways to deliver nicotine to the lungs, as in nicotine inhalers; and methods of ingesting nicotine through the mouth, perhaps in pill form.[81] Obviously, these alternatives are not as desirable as discontinuing the nicotine-consuming act itself or selecting nonchemical alternatives to smoking.

Future research should also concentrate on producing a nicotine substitute that has no adverse effects on the heart or other organs but satisfies the craving for nicotine. Development of this alternative is possible because of the numerous molecules closely related chemically to nicotine, many of which are known to have no effects on heart action.

KICKING THE HABIT

SMOKING CESSATION

Experts claim that smokers who have problems quitting may be biologically inclined to become addicted to nicotine. However, quitting is easier now than in the past due to various strategies. Interestingly, by combining methods, a person can be even more successful. However, by combining too many strategies, smokers can be unsuccessful, possibly due to losing their self-reliance.

Three essential elements for success include (1) preparation for quitting, (2) awareness of physiological and social sides of addiction, and (3) follow-up support.[82] Approximately 90 percent give up cigarettes on their own without treatment. The more times a person quits, the more chance for success. A person who fails should seek out health-maintenance organizations, hospitals, health clubs or associations, or company programs. Success claims by commercial programs should be considered with skepticism. People who want to stop smoking should refrain from using over-the-counter pills, special filters, and nonprescription chewing gum because there is no evidence they will work.

A heart attack seems to be the most successful way to quit smoking.[83] Doctors seem to have the most influence with cardiac patients, with a 43 percent success rate. Besides nicotine chewing gum, transdermal patches, support groups, and techniques like rapid smoking, where the smoker takes a puff every seven seconds, have shown success. Acupuncture and hypnosis work for some but haven't been scientifically tested.

THE QUITTING PROCESS

Many people have quit on their own, so not all people need a structured program to stop smoking. Both smoking leaders and the clients need to recognize when the smoker is ready to give up smoking. Smoking has many reinforcements other than just the addictive effects.

One of the most fearful concerns of a smoker trying to kick the habit is the weight gain associated with quitting. Weight gain is widespread. However, it has been estimated that a person would have to gain up to 125 pounds to experience the same health risks as smoking one pack of cigarettes a day.[84] So weight gain concern is more about cosmetics than health. Smoking does help to keep weight gain down by increasing metabolism and reducing appetite, and food may remain in a smoker's stomach longer than it does in a nonsmoker's stomach, giving the feeling of more satiety.

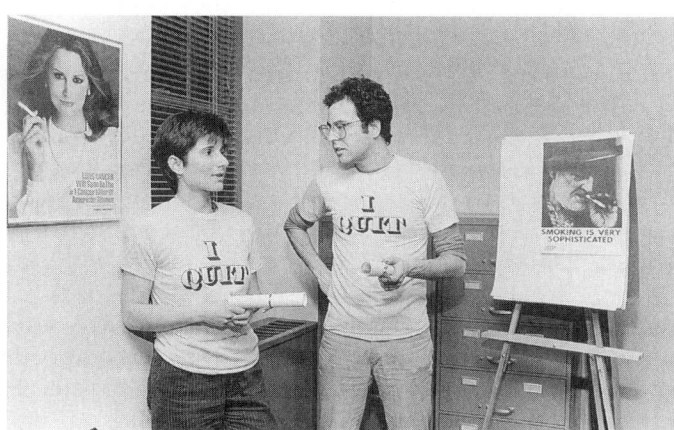

Giving Up the Habit
Source: Hazel Hankin/Stock Boston

GOVERNMENT SUPPORT

Some of the first major steps to prevent smoking were initiated in April 1989. Bills to Congress included a 32¢ tax on each pack of cigarettes, a smoking ban on all domestic airplane flights, and prohibition of tobacco advertisements and cigarette sales in vending machines.[85] Congress hasn't willfully supported these bills against the tobacco companies. After all, it is the tobacco companies who share their billion-dollar industry, for the tobacco industry is one of the largest contributors to congressional campaigns. In 1988 tobacco industries gave $1 million to incumbents.[86] As a result, Congress isn't in any hurry to attack the tobacco industry. In fact, in many cases politicians protect their interests by trading votes with other politicians. The tobacco industry's strategy is to put smoking in a libertarian context, the argument being that it's an individual's right to choose.

METHODS

Behavioral Programs   The American Lung Association (ALA), American Cancer Society (ACS), and American Heart Association (AHA) have united in a goal of a smoke-free society by the year 2000. All have initiated programs to maintain the new nonsmoking lifestyle. The ALA has Freedom from Smoking, the ACS offers an I Quit Kit and FRESHSTART, and the AHA has Save a SweetHEART. These programs also attempt to counter the billions of dollars spent on cigarette advertising each year by the tobacco industry.

Company Programs   Companies are now beginning to realize that they can save money in the long run by investing in quit-smoking programs for their employees. Health-insurance premiums for employees are a growing concern for America's major corporations, for they are being dramatically influenced by the growing number of cigarette-induced diseases. The latest studies indicate that all told, it costs our country about $3 for every pack of cigarettes sold. However, if a single smoking employee were to kick the habit, total savings for the employer would exceed $34,000.[87] Employers now have the information they need to determine the savings they could expect from implementing a smoking-cessation program for employees or their family members. For example, Campbell Soup, American Telephone and Telegraph, Johns-Manville, and Boeing Aircraft employ consultants who help workers quit smoking. It is now clear that *smoking control among employees and their dependents is the single most cost-effective way of containing health-care costs for employers.*

BENEFITS OF QUITTING

Regardless of the number of years a person has been smoking, chances for longer life and good health are greatly improved once he or she has stopped. Digestive and eating patterns change, absorption of food is greater, appetite is improved, and both the taste of food and the sense of smell are better.

SEVEN-DAY PLAN TO STOP SMOKING[88]

Day 1

Make a list of reasons why you want to stop and post it where you can see it. Then throw out all your cigarettes and buy just one pack at a time. Buy a brand you do not really like and make it lower in tar and nicotine content than your usual brand. Place a record-keeping chart on your cigarettes, numbering each cigarette and describing your feelings. Finally, do not empty the ashtrays.

Day 2

Stock up on celery and carrot sticks to chew on instead of smoking a cigarette. After dinner take a walk so you feel healthy and good about what you are doing.

Day 3

Always ask yourself, "Do I really need this cigarette?" Instead of a cigarette relax and do a deep breathing exercise. Set a definite period of time to go without smoking. Change cigarettes again and choose an even lower nicotine and tar level.

Day 4

Throw away all lighters and matches. Find a situation you usually smoke in and decide not to smoke then.

Day 5

Do not buy any more cigarettes. Announce to friends and family you are quitting. Take all butts and put them in a big jar—if you are tempted to smoke open the jar and sniff.

Day 6

Do not smoke for 24 hours. Go places that you are not allowed to smoke. Do not drink alcohol.

Day 7

Do not smoke for 24 hours. Open a bank account for all the money you will save and buy something special after a set amount of time. Remember if you backslide and have a cigarette, just try again and have determination.

Circulation improves as the blood vessels begin to expand to normal size, returning blood pressure to normal, slowing pulse rate, and increasing heart efficiency; even facial complexion improves. The ex-smoker is less tired, and often rises earlier in the morning and is more alert during the day.

Precancerous cells in the respiratory tract are gradually replaced by new ones. The breathing rate decreases, and there is an increase in maximal breathing capacity. A better exchange of oxygen between the lungs and the circulatory system also results. Conditions such as bronchitis improve and coughing disappears. Emphysema patients breathe more easily and many asthma conditions improve considerably.

There are monetary benefits to quitting as well. A heavy smoker can save up to $20,000 in a lifetime by putting cigarettes aside. Insurance premiums can be lowered, since insurance companies offer lower rates to nonsmokers, realizing that smoking endangers health and shortens life expectancy and that cigarette smokers are more accident-prone. These various benefits, along with the risks of smoking, are summarized in Table 6–1.

In a September 1990 report, the U.S. surgeon general, Antonia Novello, offered scientific proof that elderly people can benefit from kicking the smoking habit.[89] If America's seniors quit, they will increase their life expectancy and reduce their risk of illnesses such as heart, lung, and vascular disease. Also, more than 13 million smokers are over age 50, and most of them are men. "Approximately 34 percent of men aged 50 to 59 and 20 percent of men 60 and older smoke."[90]

CHANGING TO OTHER FORMS OF TOBACCO CONSUMPTION

Though some people kick the smoking habit through any of a number of treatment programs, including behavior modification, role playing, aversion therapy, and self-monitoring, others simply turn to other forms of tobacco consumption. Pipe and cigar smoking, chewing tobacco, and snuff are increasing in popularity as the hazards of cigarette smoking are brought into the foreground.

Pipe and Cigar Smoking   People who smoke pipes and cigars instead of cigarettes reduce some hazards to their health but increase others. Since most pipe and cigar smoke isn't inhaled, the harmful particles and poisonous gases it contains don't reach lung tissue or pass into the bloodstream. As a result, pipe and cigar smokers' chances of developing coronary heart disease or severe lung diseases are less than those of cigarette smokers. However, when people who smoke pipes and cigars do inhale, as they do with certain brands and sometimes because of the cigarette-inhaling habit, their chances of developing serious heart and lung diseases are even higher than those of cigarette smokers. These chances increase in direct proportion to how deeply they inhale and how often.[91]

Tobacco smoke that is not inhaled still affects the site it touches. Hot smoke lingers inside the mouth and can travel into the throat and windpipe,

TABLE 6-1   RISKS OF SMOKING AND BENEFITS OF QUITTING

Risks of Smoking	Benefits of Quitting	Relative Risks: Filter–Tipped, Low T/N Brands
Risk: Shortened life expectancy. 25-year-old 2-pack-a-day smokers have life expectancy 8.3 years shorter than nonsmoking contemporaries. Other smoking levels: proportional risk.	*Benefit:* Reduces risk of premature death cumulatively. After 10–15 years, ex-smokers' risk approaches that of those who've never smoked.	Reduced risk of death from certain diseases (see below) implies increased life expectancy.
Risk: Lung cancer. Smoking cigarettes "major cause in both men and women."	*Benefit:* Gradual decrease in risk. After 10–15 years, risk approaches that of those who never smoked.	Filter tips reduce risk, but it is still 5 times that of nonsmokers. Low-T/N brands reduce male risk by 20 percent, female risk by 40 percent.
Risk: Larynx cancer. In all smokers (including pipe and cigar) it's 2.9 to 17.7 times that of nonsmokers.	*Benefit:* Gradual reduction of risk after smoking cessation. Reaches normal after 10 years.	Filter tips reduce risk 24 to 49 percent.
Risk: Mouth cancer. Cigarette smokers have 3 to 10 times as many oral cancers as nonsmokers. Pipes, cigars, chewing tobacco also major risk factors. Alcohol seems synergistic carcinogen with smoking.	*Benefit:* Reducing or eliminating smoking/drinking reduces risk in first few years; risk drops to level of nonsmokers in 1–15 years.	(no identified benefit)
Risk: Cancer of esophagus. Cigarettes, pipes and cigars increase risk of dying of esophageal cancer about 2 to 9 times. Synergistic relationship between smoking and alcohol.	*Benefit:* Since risks are dose related, reducing or eliminating smoking/drinking should have risk-reducing effect.	(no identified benefit)
Risk: Cancer of bladder. Cigarette smokers have 7 to 10 times risk of bladder cancer as nonsmokers. Also synergistic with certain exposed occupations: dyestuffs, etc.	*Benefit:* Risk decreases gradually to that of nonsmokers over 7 years.	(no identified benefit)
Risk: Cancer of pancreas. Cigarette smokers have 2 to 5 times risk of dying of pancreatic cancer as nonsmokers.	*Benefit:* Since there is evidence of dose-related risk, reducing or eliminating smoking should have risk-reducing effect.	(no identified benefit)

TABLE 6–1   (CONTINUED)

Risks of Smoking	Benefits of Quitting	Relative Risks: Filter-Tipped, Low T/N Brands
Risk: Coronary heart disease. Cigarette smoking is major factor; responsible for 120,000 excess U.S. deaths from coronary heart disease (CHD) each year.	*Benefit:* Sharply decreases risk after one year. After 10 years ex-smokers' risk is same as that of those who never smoked.	Low-T/N male smokers had 12 percent lower CHD rate, female low-T/N smokers 19 percent lower than high-T/N smokers.
Risks: Chronic bronchitis and pulmonary emphysema. Cigarette smokers have 4–25 times risk of death from these diseases as nonsmokers. Damage seen in lungs of even young smokers.	*Benefit:* Cough and sputum disappear during first few weeks. Lung function may improve and rate of deterioration slows down.	(no identified benefit)
Risks: Stillbirth and low birthweight. Smoking mothers have more stillbirths and babies of low birthweight—more vulnerable to disease and death.	*Benefit:* Women who stop smoking before fourth month of pregnancy eliminate risk of stillbirth and low birthweight caused by smoking.	(no identified benefit)
Risks: Children of smoking mothers smaller, underdeveloped physically and socially, years after birth.	*Benefit:* Since children of nonsmoking mothers are bigger and more advanced socially, inference is that not smoking during pregnancy might avoid such underdeveloped children.	(no identified benefit)
Risk: Peptic ulcer. Cigarette smokers get more peptic ulcers and die more often of them; cure is more difficult in smokers.	*Benefit:* Ex-smokers get ulcers but these are more likely to heal rapidly and completely than those of smokers.	(no idenfitifed benefit)
Risk: Allergy and impairment of immune system.	*Benefit:* Since these are direct, immediate effects of smoking, they are obviously avoidable by not smoking.	(no identified benefit)
Risks: Alters pharmacologic effects of many medicines, diagnostic tests, and greatly increases risk of thrombosis with oral contraceptives.	*Benefit:* Majority of blood components elevated by smoking return to normal after cessation. Nonsmokers on Pill have much lower risks of thrombosis.	(no identified benefit)

Source: American Cancer Society, *Dangers of Smoking...Benefits of Quitting and Relative Risks of Reduced Exposure* (New York, 1980).

even into the upper breathing passages. Smoke can be dissolved in saliva and absorbed in the mucous membranes of the mouth, and it can be swallowed and enter the digestive tract. The incidence of cancer of the mouth, throat, larynx, and stomach is high—even higher than for cigarette smokers, according to some studies—and pipe smoking, either alone or in combination with other forms of smoking, seems to be a direct cause of cancer of the lip. Also, malignant skin tumors grow more rapidly and in larger numbers in animals whose skin has been painted with cigar tars rather than cigarette tars.[92]

In general, smokers who limit themselves to pipes and cigars live longer than cigarette smokers, yet they do not live as long as nonsmokers.[93] There is some evidence, too, that cigarette smokers who cut down on cigarettes and substitute cigars and pipes somewhat decrease their chance of premature death.

Smokeless Tobacco   Since the 1970s there has been a resurgence in the use of all forms of smokeless tobacco in the United States.[94] Today's users are more sophisticated than those of yesterday, and apparently more considerate than those old-timers who were not overly concerned about where they spat. Smokeless tobacco is being heavily promoted through the mass media by well-known sports personalities and entertainers.

DIPPING AND CHEWING.   **Snuff dipping** consists of placing a pinch of powder tobacco (which is sold in cans) between the cheek and gum, whereas chewing tobacco consists of placing a leaf tobacco (which comes in a pouch) or plug (in the form of a brick) in the area near the inner cheek.[95] A "chaw" is a golf-ball-size quid of leaf or plug tobacco. "Chewing clubs," complete with charters, membership cards, and even T-shirts emblazoned with mottos such as "Don't Spit On Me," have been spawned in high schools and colleges by this new tobacco craze.

The tobacco industry's advertising campaign is designed to appeal to impressionable young males, especially elementary through college-age students and athletes. And in fact most smokeless tobacco is used by adolescent males. It is no accident that macho sports idols provide the basis for the appeal. The use of smokeless tobacco and the resultant nicotine dependency are enhanced by the habits and traditions that are closely associated with our societal sports. Users were once characterized as rural or "backwoodsy." The tough mountain man or cowboy always had a chew during his survival trips. This image faded with the advent of widely televised sports figures who use tobacco. Those athletes and cowboy celebrities who currently tout smokeless tobacco help legitimize the image of the user as a manly, athletic type. "In sports such as baseball, football and softball, smokeless tobacco is as firmly ingrained as are H_2O buckets, strapping tape, and pine tar."[96]

Use of smokeless tobacco by athletes merely mirrors its use in our society as a whole: An estimated 12 million individuals age 12 and older use smokeless tobacco in the United States today.[97] Young adolescents are the most apt to convert because they want to express new identities, often symbolically, by such gestures as smoking. In middle adolescence youths experiment with

Snuff Dipping
Snuff dipping consists of placing a pinch of powder tobacco (which is sold in cans) between the cheek and gum.

substances for the same reason, but also for psychoactive effects. The use of smokeless tobacco fulfills both purposes. The status and tradition of the athlete compel young athletes to start using smokeless tobacco, and the nicotine dependency ensures continuance of its use and the tradition. It's a vicious circle, one in which male adolescents can be trapped and, what with smokeless tobacco and cancer awareness, confused.

Dental caries, receding gums, and greater wear and tear on the enamel are associated with smokeless tobacco use. Chemical analysis of various smokeless tobacco products has shown large variations in sugar concentrations in different tobacco products and different brands, including some sold in the United States. Pouch and plug tobacco had a higher sugar content than snuff, pipes, or cigars, ranging from 13.6 percent to 65.7 percent.[98] Shannon and Trodahl analyzed the percentage of sucrose and glucose in pouch, plug, and powdered tobacco.[99] They found a smaller range among pouch and plug brands—1.0 percent to 16.0 percent sucrose and 2.2 percent to 13.1 percent glucose. This level of glucose is high enough to adversely affect diabetics' blood-glucose levels if they swallowed the tobacco. Besides the sweeteners, researchers have found different flavorings, additives, and median fluoride content in smokeless tobacco. Plug tobacco has been found to contain 1.35 parts per million (ppm) of fluoride; pouch, 56 ppm; and snuff, 18 ppm. The various smokeless tobacco products therefore appear to vary widely in fluoride and sugar content, and "plug and pouch forms tend to have higher concentrations of both sugar and fluoride when compared to snuff."[100]

On the average a smoker is 16 times more at risk to exposure to nitrosamines as nonsmokers. The smokeless tobacco user gets 165 times the combined amount of nitrosamines found in beer, cosmetics, and bacon in the United States.[101] Along with nitrosamines, other carcinogens, including polynuclear aromatic hydrocarbons and radiation-emitting polonium-210 are found in smokeless tobacco.[102] Each of these compounds adds its influence to the initiation and promotion of various cancers.

Smokeless tobacco doesn't cause cancer the first time it is placed in the mouth. But the risk of cancer progresses through frequency, duration, and placement. "Smokeless tobacco can lead to . . . non-cancerous oral conditions, particularly oral leukoplakia (white patches or plaques of oral mucosa [the mouth lining]) and gingival recession."[103] The severity of oral leukoplakia reflects varying degrees of 3,000 chemical substances and may persist or progress with continued smokeless tobacco use. There are three degrees of severity. The first is reddening and irritation. Second, the gums become wrinkled, forming valleys, and the lesions are more pronounced. Last comes the development of leukoplakia, which leads to cancer. Leukoplakia (a white plaque on the gums, cheek, or roof of the mouth) may appear after even a year of use.[104] This is a precancerous sign that can eventually lead to permanent removal of the teeth, salivary glands, tongue, portions of the jaw, or sections of the neck and cheek.

There have been smokeless tobacco users who have lost part of their jaw to cancer. Continued use gives prospect for salivary gland damage, which in turn further supports the association between leukoplakia and cancer. Limited evidence shows that "loss of salivary gland function can result in the decreased production of saliva and the ultimate loss of a protective buffer for the oral epithelium and the teeth against exogenous factors such as infectious agents including dental caries."[105] In short, smokeless tobacco is not a safe alternative to smoking tobacco.

Clove Cigarettes   In various parts of the country there has been an increase in the use of clove cigarettes. Quite often these are passed off as safe substitutes for tobacco cigarettes. However, anyone contemplating smoking these cigarettes should first consider the following facts:

1. Clove cigarettes contain 60 percent tobacco and 40 percent ground cloves, clove oil, and other ingredients.
2. On the average, clove cigarettes contain higher levels of tar, nicotine, carbon monoxide, and carbon dioxide than regular commercial cigarettes.
3. Clove oil (eugenol) is on the FDA's list of chemicals that are "generally recognized as safe," but only when it is consumed orally in its unburnt form.
4. Clove oil stimulates the central nervous system and can result in delirium, hallucinations, and seizures.
5. Clove oil affects the cardiovascular system by lowering blood pressure. This causes sweating, weakness, dizziness, and ringing in the ears.
6. Clove oil is an irritant that can burn the body's mucous membranes, resulting in coughing, hoarseness, and difficulty in breathing. It is also an anesthetic, which is why the burning sensation is not apparent.
7. Commercial cigarettes dipped in clove oil are more dangerous than imported clove cigarettes because of the quality of the clove oil.[106]

TOBACCO AND THE NONSMOKER

EFFECTS OF TOBACCO SMOKE ON NONSMOKERS

The chemicals in tobacco smoke are derived from two sources: **mainstream smoke** and **sidestream smoke.** *Mainstream* smoke is inhaled from the burning tobacco by the user, and *sidestream* smoke rises from the cigarette, cigar, or pipe as it burns. Since each individual has a particular technique of smoking, different concentrations of substances are found in exhaled mainstream smoke, depending on the tobacco product, the composition of the tobacco, and the degree of inhalation by the smoker. These concentrations, together with the harmful sidestream smoke, put the nonsmoker in a dangerous position when exposed to another person's smoke. Regardless of the controversy surrounding this issue, "passive smoking" or "involuntary smoking" can harm the nonsmoker's health.

Anyone who breathes the smoke from another person's cigarette, cigar, or pipe is a passive smoker. A passive smoker is usually in more danger of respiratory problems than the smoker, because the smoker will just puff at a cig-

Mainstream Smoke
Smoke that is inhaled from the burning tobacco by the user.

Sidestream Smoke
Smoke that rises from the cigarette, cigar, or pipe as it burns. Because each individual has a particular technique of smoking, different concentrations are found in exhaled mainstream smoke, depending on the tobacco product, the composition of the tobacco, and the degree of inhalation by the smoker. These concentrations, together with the harmful sidestream smoke, put the nonsmoker in a dangerous position when exposed to another person's smoke.

Second-Hand Smoking
and Nonsmoker's Rights
Source: Steve Goldberg/Monk-
meyer Press

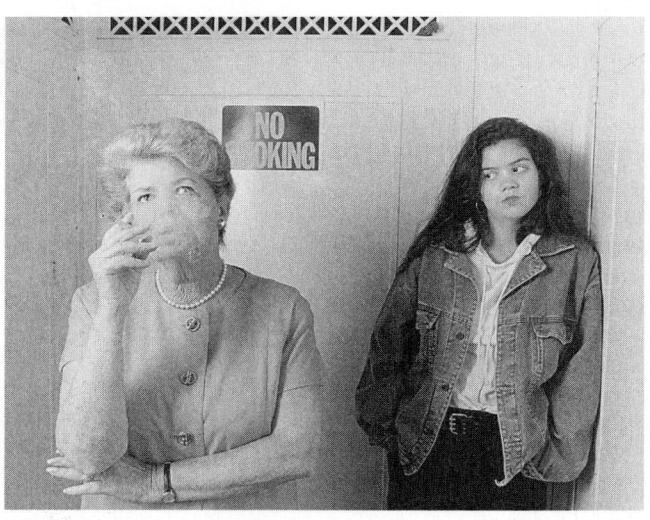

arette to get the nicotine while the people surrounding the smoker will
deeply inhale the smoke. Tobacco smoke can harm passive smokers in the
following ways: (1) Young children are more likely to have respiratory problems and require medical attention if raised by smoking than nonsmoking parents; (2) adults who have never smoked are significantly more likely to get
lung cancer if married to smokers than if not; and (3) many people suffer eye
and nose irritation when exposed to tobacco smoke.[107] Also, the children of
smokers have a 20 to 80 percent greater risk of respiratory problems than
other children. They are more likely to have respiratory infections, bronchitis, and pneumonia during their first year of life, due in part to their exposure
to cigarette smoke.

The amount of carbon monoxide smoking puts into the environment is
also of major concern to the nonsmoker. The level of this gas varies with (1)
the size of the space in which the smoking occurs (dilution of CO), (2) the
number and type of tobacco products smoked (CO production), and (3) the
amount and effectiveness of ventilation (CO removal). Fifty CO ppm is considered safe, according to the American Conference of Government Industrial Hygienists. Researchers have found that only under conditions of
unusually heavy smoking and poor ventilation did CO levels exceed this maximum safe limit. However, even with adequate ventilation, the measured CO
levels did exceed the maximum ambient level of 9 ppm.[108]

To determine the amount of carbon monoxide absorbed by the passive
smoker, a team of researchers measured changes in the carboxyhemoglobin
levels in nonsmokers exposed to cigarette-smoke-filled environments. In a
well-ventilated room with a CO level of 4.5 ppm, no change in COHb levels of
nonsmokers was found. Without ventilation, the CO level rose to 30 ppm and
the COHb level increased from 0.9 to 2.1 percent in two hours. In another
experiment, where the CO level was measured at 38 ppm and ventilation was
poor, the COHb level increased from 1.6 to 2.6 percent in nonsmokers.[109]

These increases in COHb levels may not significantly affect a healthy adult, but they can produce deleterious effects in people with angina pectoris or coronary heart disease. In angina pectoris, the volume of blood able to be pumped through the heart muscle decreases under exercise stress. If oxygen-carrying capacity is reduced by the presence of CO in the blood, a person's ability to perform physical activity is shortened. COHb levels necessary to bring on this discomfort are within the levels produced by passive smoking. At these same CO levels, CO has been shown to decrease cardiac contractility in persons with coronary heart disease. Also, the heart's functional reserve is reduced.[110]

Cigarette-smoke-filled environments have also been found to cause slight deterioration in some psychomotor performance, especially in attentiveness and cognitive function. Resultant CO levels, however, do not impair one's ability to operate a motor vehicle.[111]

There are very few instances when the concentration and quantity of cigarette smoke are great enough to cause permanent damage or chronic disease. Exposure to cigarette smoke can result, however, in conjunctival (eye) irritation, dry throat, and the breathing of unpleasant odors. Passive inhalation of sidestream smoke from cigars and pipes can also cause the heart to beat faster, the blood pressure to rise, and the CO level in the blood to rise.

NONSMOKERS' RIGHTS

Antismokers are campaigning for their rights, and their voices are increasingly affecting public regulations on smoking. Some 33 states have passed laws prohibiting smoking in public places, except in designated smoking areas, and are issuing citations for disobedience of the specified laws. Smoking and nonsmoking sections in airplanes, restaurants, and trains are now commonplace. But change will take time.

With only one in four Americans smoking, nonsmokers are the clear majority in the United States. This majority has long been silent, but now nonsmokers are beginning to speak out because they are seeing how second-hand (sidestream) smoke affects them. It has been shown that even when a smoker inhales, two thirds of the smoke goes into the environment. Sidestream smoke has a higher concentration of noxious compounds than mainstream smoke: Some studies show that it has twice as much tar and nicotine and three times as much benzopyrene and carbon monoxide.[112]

Greater attention is being called to the presence of sidestream smoke in the workplace. Nonsmokers who work in a smoking environment have been shown to have a dysfunction in the small airways of the lungs. A recent study showed that 50 percent of nonsmoking employees have reported difficulty in working near a smoker.[113] Another 36 percent have been forced to move to a different desk due to second-hand smoke

The number of state and federal laws restricting smoking at the workplace has been increasing. For example, a Massachusetts law forbids new police officers and firefighters from smoking on or off the job.[114] All of the current 21,300 state and municipal police officers and 600 new firefighters will be expected to abide by the law. This law is supposed to help lower health-care and pension costs for these public employees, who have been shown to receive higher accidental-disability pensions than other public employees, whether for on-the-job stress, heart ailments, or (in firefighters) lung cancer and emphysema.

The National Interagency Council on Smoking and Health has highlighted three additional ways in which nonsmokers'-rights groups appear to be gaining support.

Churches Question the Morality of the Tobacco Industry   The North Carolina Council of Churches has issued a report questioning the morality of the billion-dollar tobacco industry.[115] Although tobacco employs more than 150,000 North Carolinians, although the state manufactures more than half of all American cigarettes, and although North Carolina farms raise almost 40 percent of the tobacco grown in America, the report questions the morality of making money from a product that poses such great health risks. The report was prepared to stimulate discussion of this issue from North Carolina's pulpits.

San Francisco   In a victory for nonsmokers, voters in San Francisco narrowly approved an ordinance believed to establish a precedent likely to be followed by other major municipalities. The ordinance prohibits smoking in the private-sector workplace as well as in public areas.[116] It was passed in spite of massive opposition by the tobacco industry, which invested a reported $12.58 per vote (a total of about $1.3 million) to kill the measure. Violators of the new law (employers) may be fined up to $500 a day for noncompliance.

Smokers Support Nonsmokers   A recent national survey has revealed that for the first time a majority of Americans—including both smokers and nonsmokers—now believe "smokers should refrain from smoking in the presence of nonsmokers."[117] According to the survey, released by the ALA, an overwhelming 82 percent of nonsmokers and a surprising 55 percent of current smokers agree that smokers should not light up among nonsmokers. A majority of the smokers prefer designated smoking areas in the workplace, in restaurants, and on airplanes, trains, and buses. It appears that the nonsmokers' movement is gaining momentum.

SELLING TOBACCO TO CHILDREN

A very important measure in reducing the number of smokers is to delay the onset period of smoking. Recently, there has been growing concern about the easy availability of cigarettes and smokeless tobacco for those under the age of 18. The sale of tobacco to anyone under 18 years of age is illegal in 43 states and the District of Columbia. Even so, these laws are ignored by the tobacco industry, retailors, and law officers. More than 3 million children under 18 in America smoke. These kids buy 947 million packages of cigarettes a year and 26 million cans of smokeless tobacco.[118]

Both the tobacco industry and the government profit from these illegal sales to children. About 3 percent of all tobacco-sales profits come from the sale to children. That 3 percent is around $1.23 billion from cigarettes and another $32.5 million a year from smokeless tobacco.

At the city level, laws need to be reinforced more. Some communities have started fighting the sale of tobacco to children. What they have set up works in five steps: (1) Make the sale a civil rather than a criminal offense; (2) make provisions for law enforcement to get tough without a lot of extra expenses; (3) license tobacco vendors locally; (4) impose penalties of fines and loss of license; (5) restrict vending machines and free samples.[119]

Despite the law forbidding the sale of cigarettes to anyone under 18 years of age, 87 percent of merchants are selling anyway. One billion packs of cigarettes go to teens every year. These facts startled Officer Bruce Tabot of Woodridge, Illinois, and started him on a journey to cut the easy access of cigarettes for kids.[120] First he conducted his own survey in his hometown, which revealed 83 percent of the town's merchants were selling to minors. Then in March 1989 he drafted a new city ordinance licensing the sale of tobacco products. Signs were posted next to displays telling minors that the sale of cigarettes to minors was prohibited by law: Merchants now risked not a $50 fine but a $500 fine, and a limit minimum-age of 18 was put into effect for the purchase of tobacco. The ordinance also limited free distribution to stores. This type of activity is being duplicated throughout the United States to stop the sale of tobacco to adolescents.

The state of Minnesota recently banned cigarette vending machines in 20 communities.[121] Many cities in various states have now banned cigarette vending machines.[122] The United States Senate is also proposing legislation to ban cigarette vending machines from areas accessible to children.[123]

EXPORTING TOBACCO

Tobacco sales continue to decrease, and it appears they will continue to do so even more. Only about 25 percent of Americans smoke, with a great number trying to quit.[124] The tobacco industry is now looking for new places to sell its cigarettes. These places seem to be other countries. This has stirred an angry debate between the U.S. medical community and the U.S. government. The federal government is allowing exporting of cigarettes to other countries even though cigarettes are the number one cause of preventable disease. The cigarettes being exported are even worse than the ones being sold in the United States. They have more tar in them and have no warning labels, and yet the U.S. international trade representative has said once again "that cigarettes are a harmless commodity."[125] It appears that tobacco brings in too much money to the government for anyone to stop exporting.

The United States has pressured Third World countries to accept importation of cigarettes under threat of economic or defense sanctions.[126] Section 301 of the 1974 Trade Act permits the U.S. government to take punitive action against other countries if it is determined that the U.S. exporters are experiencing "unfair" or "discriminatory" trade restrictions. President Ronald Reagan directed that Section 301 be used to influence cigarette trade with Japan, South Korea, and Taiwan. Reagan aides successfully lobbied on behalf of the tobacco companies.[127]

Tobacco companies are advertising and selling overseas. Exports of tobacco rose 20 percent in 1991 alone.[128] Although it is now illegal to show tobacco of any form in advertisements on television in the United States, it is perfectly legal to show advertisements in Tokyo, Manila, and Seoul.

Cigarette exports since 1986 have reached 2.6 million, mainly because Japan, South Korea, and Taiwan—under U.S. government pressure—opened their markets to our imports.[129] Thailand does not want the United States to import goods because it will cut into their monopoly of tobacco products. The U.S. competition, however, believes this is unfair, since they have already been hurt by the ban on television advertising. In 1989 the tobacco companies were focusing on Thailand and urging sanctions under Section 301. Thailand had been engaging in a successful antismoking campaign for 20 years and in 1987 approved a proposal for a total ban on cigarette consumption. On September 19, 1989, the U.S. trade representative held hearings on the matter.[130] One witness was Surgeon General C. Everett Koop (whose testimony, it is speculated, would not have been cleared by the White House had he submitted it for approval), who called efforts to force Thailand to accept importation of cigarettes "unconscionable" and "deplorable." He called it "hypocrisy for the United States to export tobacco" in light of the U.S. war on drugs and efforts to stop cocaine from entering this country, when "last year [1988] in the United States, 2,000 people died from cocaine and in that same year, cigarettes killed 390,000 people."[131] The United States is forcing advertisement rights in Thailand, where the country's own laws outlaw cigarette advertising, and threatening to stop all importing from Thailand.[132] The Thai government claims that the United States is not watching out for the health of the Thai people but, rather, exploiting them.

Apparently, in the slow economy of China, cigarettes are an excellent way for the Chinese government to make money.[133] The Chinese government sells the cigarettes on commission, so it gives cigarette manufacturers lots of warehouse and dock space to keep their stock; under this arrangement, the government takes free profit from the cigarette companies, risk-free. Also, smoking in many foreign countries is now a symbol of social status. "For every inch lost in the States, a foot is gained abroad."[134]

Recently legislation has been written to protect these developing countries. The Tobacco Reform Act would require warnings on cigarettes sold in other countries, restrict advertising as it is in the United States, and prevent the executive branch from "encouraging the imposition of import duties and quotas as a way to push tobacco overseas."[135]

In many of the developing countries, smoking is now more common among teenage girls than boys. It is estimated that 50 percent of the men and only 5 percent of women in developing countries smoke.[136] In the past 20 years death rates of women from lung cancer have more than doubled in

Japan, Norway, Poland, Sweden, and the United Kingdom.[137] These rates have increased over 200 percent in Australia, Denmark, and New Zealand, and increased 300 percent in Canada and the United States.

DIVERSIFICATION

When the 1964 surgeon general's report was released, the American tobacco industry was dominated by six large cigarette manufacturers. These corporations had few nontobacco interests. By 1984 the situation was markedly different. The big six had emerged as multinational conglomerates with financial interests reaching from pet food to insurance underwriting, from breweries to security services. Table 6–2 illustrates an example of these dramatic changes away from tobacco production by the tobacco companies. There appears to be growing concern about the future of U.S. tobacco sales, and companies are beginning to diversify, in case sales drop rapidly. The antismoking movement is growing in the United States.

SUMMARY

The use of tobacco in the United States goes back to the Native Americans, who introduced tobacco to Columbus. It was commonly accepted thereafter, until it became associated with various diseases. The 1979 surgeon general's

TABLE 6–2   DIVERSIFICATION IN THE TOBACCO INDUSTRY, 1984

Tobacco Manufacturer (conglomerate owner or affiliate)	Tobacco Brands	Other Representative Products
R.J. Reynolds Tobacco Company (R.J. Reynolds Industries)	Camel, Winston, Salem, Sterling, Bright, Doral, More, Century, Now, Vantage, Winchester, Work Horse Chew, Prince Albert, Carter Hall, Madeira Gold	Kentucky Fried Chicken, Canada Dry, Del Monte, Chun King oriental foods, Hawaiian Punch, Morton Frozen Foods, Patio Mexican foods, Snap-E-Tom, Milk Mate, A-1 Steak Sauce, Escoffier Sauces, Grey Poupon, Ortega Mexican foods, My-T-Fine, Brer Rabbit Molasses, College Inn, Vermont Maid, Heublein, Inc. (Arrow Cordials, Black Velvet, Cuervo, Don Q Rum, Irish Mist, Jose Cuervo, Popov, Simirnoff, The Club Cocktails, Yukon Jack, Inglenook Wines, Napa Valley Wines, Harveys Bristol Creme, Lancer's Vin Rose)

Source: Annual company reports (1982 or 1983) and news releases, complied by William J. Bailey, "Opportunity or Threat: Tobacco Industry," *Smoking and Health Reporter* 1, no.4 (July 1984):10–11. National Interagency Council on Smoking and Health. Used with permission.

report stated that the smoking of tobacco cigarettes is directly related to an increase in heart problems, lung and other cancers, and respiratory diseases such as emphysema. It also interferes with metabolism, increases the number of stillborn and neonatal deaths, appears in the milk of nursing mothers, reduces availability of oxygen during exercise, and contributes to many other health problems. More Americans are quitting smoking but more are dying from smoking-related illnesses as habits of the 1950s and 1960s take an increasing toll. Smoking costs the country more than $52 billion annually in health care costs and lost productivity.

Smokers derive pleasure from the effects of smoking, but once a person is dependent on tobacco, it is difficult to stop smoking. Clinics have been organized to help smokers kick the habit, and smoking has been made somewhat safer by the addition of filters and the reduction of nicotine in tobacco products. Alternative uses of tobacco, such as chewing, pipe and cigar smoking, and snuff, may help some to give up cigarette smoking, but these forms of tobacco also harm one's health.

Nonsmokers have mobilized to protect themselves from the health dangers of passive breathing of tobacco smoke. Their efforts have led to smoking and nonsmoking sections in restaurants and airplanes and to the prohibition of smoking in some public places.

Because of the harmful effects of smoking, there is an increasing movement away from smoking. Even the tobacco industry senses this movement, as evidenced in its increasing diversification away from tobacco products. Tobacco companies are spending enormous sums of money in advertising to reach specific demographic groups such as women and less-educated blue-collar workers. In addition, tobacco companies are looking for new markets in foreign countries.

Tobacco

N O T E S

1. "Smoking Costs Nation More Than $52 Billion a Year," *Register-Guard* (Eugene, Oregon), February 21, 1990, p. 6A.

2. Ibid.

3. Ibid.

4. National Institute on Drug Abuse, Division of Epidemiology and Prevention Research, "National Household Survey on Drug Abuse," NIDA Capsules, CAP 21 (Rockville, Md.: U.S. Department of Health and Human Services, Public Health Service, Alcohol, Drug Abuse and Mental Health Administration, 1990).

5. Ethel Gofen, "Report on Smoking: 1988," *Current Health* 2 (November 1988):3–9.

6. J. Eisenberg, "Smoking Raises Female Heart Attack Risk," *Science,* November 28, 1988, p. 341.

7. Ibid.

8. "Risks in Low Tar Smokers," *The Journal Canadien* 6, no. 7 (July 1, 1977).

9. Oakley S. Ray, *Drugs, Society and Human Behavior*, 3rd ed. (St. Louis: C. V. Mosby, 1983). Reproduced with permission.

10. American Cancer Society, *Dangers of Smoking . . . Benefits of Quitting and Relative Risks of Reduced Exposure* (New York, 1980), pp. 413–29.

11. Louis S. Goodman and Alfred Gilman, *The Pharmacological Basis of Therapeutics*, 4th ed. (New York: Macmillan, 1970), p. 115.

12. Ray, *Drugs, Society and Human Behavior*, pp. 100–106.

13. J. W. Hurst et al., *The Heart, Arteries and Veins* (New York: McGraw-Hill, 1974), pp. 1563–66.

14. Goodman and Gilman, *The Pharmacological Basis of Therapeutics*, 4th ed.

15. Department of Health, Education and Welfare, *1979 Surgeon General's Report* (Washington, D.C., 1979), p. 29.

16. Ibid.

17. Center for Disease Control, *The Health Consequences of Smoking* (Washington, D.C.: Department of Health, Education and Welfare, 1975).

18. See Walter S. Ross, "Poison Gases in Your Cigarettes: Hydrogen Cyanide and Nitrous Oxides," *Reader's Digest* 109, no. 656 (December 1976):92–98.

19. Anne Elixhauser, "The Costs of Smoking and the Cost Effectiveness of Smoking-Cessation Programs," *Journal of Public Health Policy*, Summer 1990, pp. 218–37.

20. National Interagency Council on Smoking and Health, "New Study Reveals: Smoking Costs an Extra $56,000 in Health Related Expenses over Lifetime," *Smoking and Health Reporter* 1, no. 4 (July 1984):7. Copyright © 1984 National Interagency Council on Smoking and Health. Used with permission.

21. American Cancer Society, *Dangers of Smoking*.

22. G. A. Cellini et al., "Direct Arterial Pressure, Heart Rate, and Electro-Cardiography during Cigarette Smoking of Unrestricted Patients," *American Heart Journal* 89, no. 1 (January 1975):18–25.

23. *Health Consequences of Smoking: Cardiovascular Disease*, 1983 Surgeon General's Report (Rockville, Md.: U.S. Department of Health and Human Services, Public Health Service, Office on Smoking, 1983), p. 384.

24. "Medical News: Can You Alter Your Heart Disease Risk?" *Journal of the American Heart Association* 245, no. 19 (May 15, 1981):1904, 1907.

25. "A Stroke Alert Sounds for Smokers," *U.S. News & World Reports*, January 23, 1989, p. 9.

26. Hurst et al., *The Heart, Arteries and Veins*, pp. 1563–66.

27. Center for Disease Control, *The Health Consequences of Smoking*.

28. *Health Consequences of Smoking: Chronic Obstructive Disease*, 1984 Surgeon General's Report (Rockville, Md.: U.S. Department of Health and Human Services, Public Health Service, Office on Smoking, 1984), p. 312.

29. Anastasiam Toufexis, "A Not-So-Happy Anniversary," *Time*, January 23, 1989, p. 54.

30. Ibid.

31. "Toll Blamed on Smoking Still Goes Up," *Register-Guard*, February 1, 1991, p. 3A.

32. Ibid. p. 3A.

33. Public Health Service, *The Health Consequences of Smoking* (Washington, D.C.: Department of Health, Education and Welfare, 1967).

34. Cited in H. Van Vunakis et al., "Nicotine and Cotenine in the Amniotic Fluid of Smokers in the Second Trimester of Pregnancy," *American Journal of Obstetrics and Gynecology* 120, no. 1 (September 1, 1974):62–64.

35. Hurst et al., *The Heart, Arteries and Veins*.

36. R. Weiss, "Nicotine Boosts a Busy Body's Metabolism," *Science News*, April 8, 1989, p. 214.

37. Ibid.

38. "Effects of Smoking on Fat Distribution," *American Family Physician* 41, no. 5 (May 1990):1620.

39. G. H. Neher, "Nicotine-Induced Depression of Lymphocyte Growth," *Toxicology and Applied Pharmacology* 27, no. 2 (February 1974):253–58.

40. Cited in Luther Terry, "Pushing the Anti-Smoking Crusade in New Directions," *Today's Health* 51, no. 1 (June 1973).

41. American Cancer Society, *Dangers of Smoking*, p. 413.

42. Ibid.

43. "Smoking and Pregnancy," *Family Health* 2, no. 5 (May 1979):32.

44. Cited in American Cancer Society, *Dangers of Smoking*, p. 414.

45. Lois A. Fingerhut, "Smoking before, during, and after Pregnancy," *American Journal of Public Health* 80, no. 5 (May 1990):541–44.

46. Cited in American Cancer Society, *Dangers of Smoking*, p. 414.

47. Cited in ibid.

48. Cited in ibid.

49. A. Erickson, B. Kallen, and P. Westerholm, "Cigarette Smoking as an Etiologic Factor in Cleft Lip and Palate," *American Journal of Obstetrics and Gynecology* 135, no. 3 (October 1, 1979):348–51.

50. Donald K. Mathews and Edward L. Fox, *The Physiological Basis of P. E. and Athletics* (Philadelphia: Saunders, 1971), pp. 178–79.

51. Cited in Genell J. Subak-Sharpe, "Is Your Sex Life Going Up in Smoke?" *Today's Health* 52, no. 8 (August 1974):65.

52. Cited in ibid.

53. Diana Petitt and John Wingerd, "Use of Oral Contraceptives, Cigarette Smoking and the Risk of Subarachnoid Hemorrhage," *Lancet* 2, no. 8083 (July 29, 1978):234–35.

54. F. P. Zuspan and N. Davis, "The Effect of Smoking and Oral Contraceptives on the Urinary Excretion of Epinephrine and Norepinephrine," *American Journal of Obstetrics and Gynecology* 135, no. 8 (December 15, 1979):1012.

55. Ibid.

56. Department of Health, Education and Welfare, *1979 Surgeon General's Report*, p. 85.

57. "Drug Effects Can Go Up in Smoke," *FDA Consumer* 13, no. 2 (March 1979):18.

58. William S. Bond, "Smoking's Effects on Medications," *American Druggist*, July 1989, pp. 24–26.

59. Janet K. Bobo, "Nicotine Dependence and Alcoholism Epidemiolgy and Treatment," *Journal of Psychoactive Drugs* 21, no. 3 (July/September 1989):323–28.

60. R. Hickey et al., "Coffee Drinking, Smoking, Pollution, and Cardio-Vascular Disease: A Problem of Self Selection," *Lancet* 1, no. 7810 (May 5, 1973):1003.

61. Department of Health, Education and Welfare, *1979 Surgeon General's Report*, p. 68.

62. Tom Morganthau, "Cigarettes in Search of a Target," *Newsweek*, March 5, 1990, pp. 18–20.

63. Ibid.

64. Amanda Amos and Claire Chollat-Traquet, "Women and Tobacco," *World Health*, April-May 1990, pp. 7–8.

65. Ibid.

66. Ibid.

67. R. Weiss, "Heart Risks Drop in Women Ex-Smokers," *Science News* 137, no. 4 (January 27, 1990):55.

68. J. Pierce et al., "National Age and Sex Differences in Quitting Smoking," *Journal of Psychoactive Drugs* 21, no. 3 (July/September 1989):293–98.

69. David Keopke, Brian R. Flay, and C. Anderson Johnson, "Health Behaviors in Minority Families: The Case of Cigarette Smoking," *Family and Community Health,* 13, January 1990, pp. 35–43.

70. Gilbert J. Botvin et al., "A Psychological Approach to Smoking Prevention for Urban Black Youth," *Public Health Reports* 104, no. 6 (November/December 1989):573–82.

71. M. Miller, "A New Tobacco Alliance," *Newsweek,* February 13, 1989, p. 20.

72. Ibid.

73. "Study: Teen Drug Use on Rise," *The Register-Guard,* Eugene, Oregon, Monday, October 19, 1992, 3A.

74. Ellen Bonaguro and John Bonaguro, "Tobacco Use among Adolescents: Directions for Research," *American Journal of Health Promotion* 4, no. 1 (September/October 1989).

75. Ibid.

76. See Ross, "Poison Gases in Your Cigarettes," pp. 92–98.

77. Cited in ibid., pp. 92–95.

78. National Interagency Council on Smoking and Health, "Model Program Launched: Dow Chemical Begins Massive Smoking Cessation Project in Texas," *Smoking and Health Reporter* 1, no. 4 (July 1984):6. Copyright © 1984 National Interagency Council on Smoking and Health. Used with permission.

79. Jennifer Foote, "Out of Cigarettes and into Chewing Gum," *Newsweek* August 22, 1988, p. 64.

80. Ibid.

81. Edward M. Brecher et al., *Licit and Illicit Drugs* (Boston: Little, Brown, 1972), pp. 241–44.

82. Erica E. Good, "How to Stop Smoking and Stick with It," *U.S. News & World Report,* August 1, 1988, pp. 59–60.

83. Ibid.

84. Jennifer Klein et al., "Understanding the Issues in Smoking Cessation," *Health Values* 13, no. 4 (July 1989):44–49.

85. Andy Plattner, "Big Tobacco's Toughest Road," *U.S. News & World Report,* April 17, 1989, p. 26.

86. Ibid.

87. John R. Seffrin, "Freedom of Choice?" *Smoking and Health Reporter* 1, no. 4 (July 1984):3. Copyright © 1984 National Interagency Council on Smoking and Health. Used with permission.

88. American Cancer Society, *Quitter's Guide: 7 Day Plan to Help You Stop Smoking Cigarettes* (New York, 1987).

89. "Older Smokers Who Kick the Habit . . ." *Aging Research and Training News* 13, no. 18 (October 1990):138.

90. Ibid.

91. Department of Health, Education and Welfare, *1979 Surgeon General's Report,* p. 65.

92. Oregon Lung Association, *Pipe and Cigarette Smoking* (Eugene, 1977).

93. National Institute on Education, *Teen-age Smoking Survey* (Washington, D.C.: Department of Health, Education and Welfare, 1978), p. 65.

94. A. G. Christen and E. D. Glover, "The Case against Smokeless Tobacco: Five Facts for the Health Professional to Consider," *Journal of the American Dental Association* 101, no. 3 (1980):464–69. Copyright by the American Dental Association. Reprinted by permission.

95. Ibid.

96. Steven W. Edwards, Elbert D. Glover, and Katheline L. Schroeder, "Effects of Smokeless Tobacco on Heart Rate and Neuromuscular Reactivity in Athletes and Nonathletes," *Physician Sportsmedicine* 15, no. 7 (July 1987):142.

97. Ibid.

98. Brian A. Burt and Jane A. Weintraub, "Peridontal Effects and Dental Caries Associated with Smokeless Tobacco Use," *Public Health Reports* 102, no. 1 (January/February 1987):30.

99. Cited in ibid.

100. Cited in ibid.

101. Mervyn G. Harding and William Andress, "Fire without Smoke," *Vibrant Life,* March/April 1990, pp. 19–20.

102. Ibid.

103. Blolet et al., "Health Consequences of Using Smokeless Tobacco."

104. Judy Folkenberg, "Oral Cancer on Rise," *FDA Consumer* (December 1989/January 1990):24–25.

105. Ibid.

106. Oregon Lung Association, *The Lung and Short of It* (Eugene, 1985).

107. E. Marshall, "Involuntary Smokers Face Health Risk," *Science* 234 (November 28, 1986):1066.

108. Center for Disease Control, *The Health Consequences of Smoking,* p. 65.

109. Ibid.

110. Ibid.

111. Ibid.

112. American Lung Association, *Second Hand Smoke* (1986).

113. Cited in ibid.

114. Alan Cooperman, "Massachusetts Smoking Ban Fires Up Police," *Oregonian* (Portland), October 17, 1988.

115. National Interagency Council on Smoking and Health, "Churches Question `Morality' of North Carolina Tobacco Industry," *Smoking and Health Reporter* 1, no. 4 (July 1984):7. Copyright © 1984 National Interagency Council on Smoking and Health. Used with permission.

116. Michael Lespaire, "San Franciscans Vote to Require Non-Smoking Work Areas," *Smoking and Health Reporter* 1, no. 2 (January 1984):5. Copyright © 1984 National Interagency Council on Smoking and Health. Used with permission.

117. National Interagency Council on Smoking and Health, "Even Smokers Agree That They Shouldn't Smoke in the Presence of Non-Smokers," *Smoking and Health Reporter* 1, no. 4 (July 1984):10–11. Copyright © 1984 National Interagency Council on Smoking and Health. Used with permission.

118. Joseph R. DiFranza and Joe B. Tye, "Who Profits from Tobacco Sales to Children?" *Journal of the American Medical Association* 263 (May 23–30, 1990):2784–87.

119. Ibid.

120. "Would You Sell Cigarettes to Children?" *Saturday Evening Post,* September 1990, pp. 50–72.

121. "Cigarette Machines Curbed," *New York Times,* April 1990.

122. David Altman, "Reducing the Illegal Sale of Cigarettes to Minors," *Journal of the American Medical Association* 261, no. 1 (January 6, 1989):80–84.

123. Ibid.

124. Marsha F. Goldsmith, "Fight against Tobacco Addiction Moving into International Arena," *Journal of the American Medical Association* 263 (June 13, 1990):2989–90.

125. Ibid.

126. Alexander Cockburn, "Beat the Devil," *The Nation,* October 30, 1989, pp. 482–83.

127. Ibid.

128. Goldsmith, "Fight against Tobacco Addiction."

129. Barbara Rudolph, "Fuming over a Hazardous Export," *Time,* October 2, 1989, p. 82.
130. Cockburn, "Beat the Devil."
131. Ibid.
132. Goldsmith, "Fight against Tobacco Addiction."
133. "When Will We Stop Foreign Cigarettes?" *Beijing Review,* October 10–16, 1988, p. 40.
134. Plattner, "Big Tobacco's Toughest Road."
135. Cockburn, "Beat the Devil."
136. Amos and Chollat-Traquet, "Women and Tobacco."
137. Ibid.

CHAPTER
7

DEPRESSANTS

Hypnotics

Drugs used to induce sleep.

Depressants, or "downers," are drugs that decrease awareness and response of incoming stimuli by depressing the central nervous system. Major depressants include alcohol, sedative-**hypnotics,** tranquilizers, deliriants, and opiates. The use and effects of downers can cause problems. All slow down the body and mind, particularly the senses. They are dangerous and are most frequently involved in the overdose cases treated in emergency rooms.[1] They also are most frequently responsible for drug-related deaths. All have the potential for addiction, increased tolerance, and a very dangerous withdrawal sickness. A dangerous effect of downers is that they all potentiate each other. This means that the depressant effect multiplies when two types are taken with another drug, for example, alcohol. It takes very little to overdose on a combination of downers. Three major depressants—sedative-hypnotics, minor and major tranquilizers, and deliriants (volatile substances)—are probed in this chapter.

SEDATIVE-HYPNOTICS

CLASSIFICATION

Drugs classified as sedative-hypnotics may differ chemically, but they produce similar effects.[2] Their action is chiefly one of CNS depression, though the precise mechanism of this effect is not known. Both barbiturates and nonbarbiturate drugs are included in this class, as well as a wide variety of organic and synthetic compounds.

PHYSICAL EFFECTS

Hypnotics are used to bring on sleep; sedatives are usually used to induce a milder degree of CNS depression, such as anxiety relief. In most instances, the same substances can be used for both sedation and hypnosis, depending on the dose. Large doses depress the cerebral cortex, the respiratory system, and the cardiovascular system.

Sedative-hypnotics impair judgment and motor coordination. Side effects can include nausea, vomiting, headache, drowsiness, gastric upset, rashes, and hangover. Excitement, blurred vision, facial numbness, an aftertaste, and fever can also occur. And if an individual is hypersensitive to a drug in this class, more serious reactions are possible. A further hazard is that the difference between therapeutic and lethal dose levels is often minimal.

Sedative-hypnotics can produce both psychological and physiological dependence. Symptoms of withdrawal from long-term use are far more severe than they are for alcohol and require close medical supervision. In therapeutic use, the dangers of dependence and sudden withdrawal are greater than those from direct toxic side effects.[3]

BARBITURATES

The basic ingredient of the barbiturate family of drugs is barbituric acid. Various members of the family include phenobarbital, pentobarbital, amobarbital, and secobarbital.

Classification   Barbiturates are classified by duration of action: They are either ultrashort (30 minutes to 3 hours), short (3 to 6 hours), intermediate (6 to 12 hours), or long-acting (12 to 24 hours). Ultrashort barbiturates produce anesthesia within one minute of intravenous administration. The most commonly used of these drugs is thiopental.

Among the short-acting barbiturates are pentobarbital, secobarbital, and amobarbital. It takes from 15 minutes to 40 minutes for these drugs to go into effect.

Butabarbital is the most commonly used intermediate barbiturate. Its onset time is generally 30 to 45 minutes.

Long-acting barbiturates have onset times of up to one hour. This category of barbiturates includes barbital and phenobarbital.

History   Barbiturates were among the first drugs of the twentieth century designed to produce relaxation and sleep. Discovery of their hazardous effects, including physiological dependence, brought about a search for substitutes. Numerous compounds were developed, but many of them, including Valium and Librium, were also found to have hazardous effects, such as severe physiological dependence. Barbiturates are now rarely used for medical purposes.

Physical Effects   Barbiturates affect the user in many ways, ranging from subtle changes in mood and sedation to sleep and coma. Typical effects are a reduction in attention span, less awareness of external stimuli, and a decrease in the ability to perform intellectual tasks. Barbiturates also decrease the amount of sleep spent in dreaming (rapid-eye-movement, or REM, sleep). Children and elderly users, however, may experience excitement rather than sedation.

These drugs are sold in capsules, tablets, and sometimes liquid form or suppositories. The effects of barbiturates, in many ways, are similar to alcohol. Small amounts produce calmness and relax muscles. Somewhat larger doses can cause slurred speech, staggering gait, poor judgment, and slow, uncertain reflexes. These effects make it dangerous to drive a car or operate machinery. Large doses can cause unconsciousness and death.

Continued barbiturate use often results in tolerance and may eventually result in physical dependence. Pregnant women who ingest large doses of barbiturates throughout pregnancy (or during the last three months) run the risk of congenital dependency in their infants.[4] During chronic barbiturate intoxication, nausea, dizziness, confusion, and an impaired mental state occur. Allergic reactions, though rare, are also possible, resulting in swelling of the face, dermatitis, skin lesions, fever, delirium, convulsions, and degenerative changes in the liver.[5] When administered to expectant mothers, barbiturates may cause fetal oxygen deficiency, which may result in birth defects, brain damage, or death. When taken with alcohol, barbiturates exert a powerful synergistic effect, which may lead to accidental overdose or become an avenue to suicide.

Withdrawal from barbiturates is far more severe than withdrawal from alcohol or heroin and can be life-threatening without medical supervision. Initial withdrawal symptoms include sweating, insomnia, vomiting, tremors, paranoia, and a short temper. Excessive dreaming and nightmares can occur, and hallucinations and seizures have been reported in extreme cases.

Medical Use   Barbiturates account for 25 percent of the mood-altering prescriptions written for anxiety, insomnia, and epilepsy. The withdrawal from barbiturate addiction or dependency is considered to be the most dangerous of any drug, including heroin. Nearly 5,000 deaths occur each year involving barbiturates, and approximately 25,000 trips are made to the emergency room for overdose as a result of barbiturate abuse.[6]

Because of the large number of nonbarbiturate sedatives and tranquilizers currently available, the medical uses of barbiturates are limited today to the treatment of insomnia, certain convulsive disorders, and, to a lesser extent, anxiety. There is some evidence that thiopental, a barbiturate-analgesic, may prevent brain damage when given immediately following the loss of oxygen.[7] Harvey Shapiro, an anesthesiologist at the University of California, also found

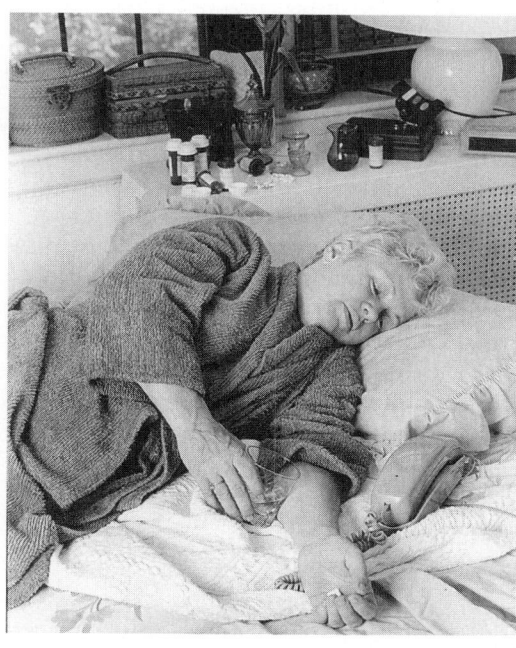

Overdose on Alcohol and Prescription Drugs
Source: Shirley Zeiberg

that thiopental reduced brain swelling during operations, as well as lessening cerebral pressure and improving blood circulation.[8]

Abuse   There are several nonmedical uses of barbiturates that can be classified as barbiturate abuse. The first is for maintenance of an anxiety-free state of chronic intoxication.

The second is for stimulation, to amplify altered moods. Such episodic intoxication is found most commonly in young adults or teenagers, often at parties.

Barbiturates are also taken to counteract the effects of amphetamines, or to ease withdrawal from heroin.[9] The heroin dependent may also supplement his or her heroin doses with barbiturates when the supply is low, or unknowingly administer heroin cut with barbiturates. Although this pattern of use characterizes a relatively small number of individuals, it is by far the most hazardous because tolerance can develop and because lethal doses may accidentally be taken.

Barbiturates are sometimes taken in combination with alcohol. Recently, however, people have become aware of the hazards (coma and death) of this, and mixing of these drugs seems to be declining.

MINOR TRANQUILIZERS

CLASSIFICATION

The word *tranquilizer* describes a number of drugs with differing chemical structures. The three major chemical families of **minor tranquilizers** are meprobamate and its analogues (Soma, Miltown, Equanil); benzodiazepines (Librium, Valium); and dephenylmethanes (Suavitil, Softran).

Minor Tranquilizers
Drugs used to help relieve anxiety or tension.

HISTORY

Introduced in 1955 as the first minor tranquilizer, meprobamate (Miltown) was originally prescribed for the treatment of mild to moderate anxiety and mild psychoneurotic or psychosomatic complaints. The drug previously used to treat these problems, barbituric acid, was being used less often because of its adverse effects, including physical dependence. The new minor tranquilizer allowed for a wider variation of dose to achieve the desired results. In a world seeking immediate relief from tension and anxiety, this drug and the others in its class found rapid acceptance.

Acceptance soon turned to widespread use—related, some feel, to overprescribing by physicians. Some researchers estimate that as much as 50 percent of minor-tranquilizer prescriptions are unnecessary.[10]

Though all segments and professions in society now use tranquilizers as a coping device (Valium is sometimes referred to as the "executive Excedrin"), tranquilizers simply postpone finding solutions to the problems they are taken to cure. It is hoped that this knowledge, along with knowledge of the drugs' negative effects, will bring about a decline in their use.

PHYSICAL EFFECTS

Tranquilizers are taken as antianxiety drugs that relax neuromuscular activity. Drug therapy has become common in stress management by relaxing people with a lot of anxiety. The class of drugs most commonly prescribed for this purpose are benzodiazepines, which are referred to as minor tranquilizer or antianxiety agents.[11]

Valium and Librium are two commonly prescribed tranquilizers and are effective and safe if used properly, but they may produce physical and psychological dependence if abused. In the United States as many as 2.5 million adults—over 75 percent of them women—have been taking these drugs on a regular basis for more than a year.[12] Although there are some medical conditions, such as panic attacks and certain phobias, that do require extended use of tranquilizers, most prescriptions of minor tranquilizers are for temporary use to fight anxiety and insomnia.

Tranquilizers reduce neuromuscular activity, thereby reducing environmental awareness and facilitating relaxation. Motor coordination, speech patterns, attention span, and libido (sex drive) are all affected. Feelings of aggression are reduced and feelings of sociability occasionally increase. With increasing dosages, drowsiness progresses toward sleep.

Minor tranquilizers have a number of known side effects. These include apathy; illogical fears; low blood pressure; fainting; chills; rashes; upset stomach; disorientation; blurred vision; bladder, menstrual, and ovulary irregularities; and sleep disturbances. If taken with alcohol, toxic and sometimes fatal reactions can occur. The euphoria the drugs produce also promotes psychological dependence. With repeated use, tolerance, as well as cross-tolerance (tolerance for one drug extending to tolerance for another), develops. However, the lethal dose level does not rise. Dose escalation brings one closer to death more quickly than with other drugs. Withdrawal symptoms following

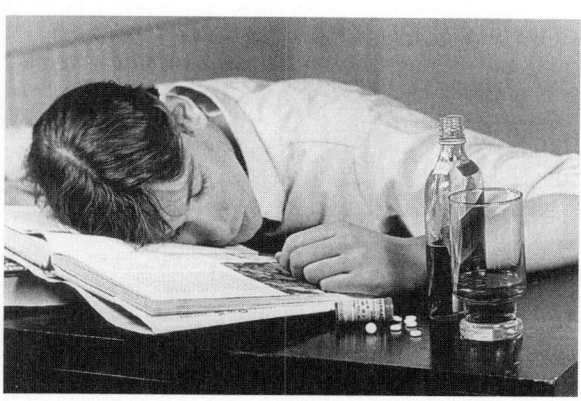

Student Passes Out After Combining
Alcohol with Other Drugs
Source: Laima Druskis

chronic administration of large doses are similar to the symptoms of withdrawal from alcohol and barbiturates: anxiety, muscle twitches, insomnia, headache, fever, nausea, vomiting, abdominal cramps, sweating, and convulsions; death is possible.

The more recently developed minor tranquilizers—benzodiazepine derivatives—are considered safer than older forms. Their dose-response curves are flat (except for diazepam), which means that increased dosage does not always produce increased effect. Hence, benzodiazepine derivatives used in therapeutic doses rarely act strongly on respiration and normally do not result in psychological depression that could lead to suicide.

VALIUM (DIAZEPAM)

Derived from the Latin word meaning "to be strong and well," **Valium** is an antianxiety agent and a muscle relaxant and produces antiepileptic effects without sedation. It is used to treat anxiety and muscle spasms, as a preanesthetic for heart patients, in the early stages of labor, and to control cerebral palsy, convulsive attacks, and low-back pain. Unfortunately, very little is known about how Valium works.[13]

Diazepam (Valium)
An antianxiety agent and muscle relaxant that produces antiepileptic effects without sedation.

History   Developed in 1961 by Leo Sternbach, a chemist for Roche Laboratories, Valium became the most prescribed drug in the world. In 1978, over 45 million prescriptions were written for it; in 1980, it was estimated that 10 to 15 percent of all Americans took Valium sometime during the previous year. According to the Drug Abuse Warning Network (DAWN), Valium is the most abused medicine in this country.[14] Approximately 30 percent of Valium prescriptions are for anxiety and insomnia, 15 to 18 percent for muscle spasms, 2 to 3 percent for epilepsy and cerebral palsy, and 45 percent for anxiety-related psychosomatic or organic illness (such as ulcers).

Many tranquilizer users are upper- or upper-middle-class and/or white-collar workers, retired persons, or unemployed.[15] The National Institute of Mental Health and the National Institute on Drug Abuse estimate that women users outnumber men by 2.5 to 1.[16] Changing social roles, more leisure time, employment pressures, poor self-image and insecurity, problems in child rearing, and the so-called empty-nest syndrome are among the oft-cited reasons why women become dependent on tranquilizers.[17] Furthermore, there is speculation that women use tranquilizers more than men because they see their physicians more often than men. And because women are generally more able to discuss their frustrations and their physical and emotional pain, their physician's treatment often includes the prescription of tranquilizers to ease the discomfort.

Valium is a popular street drug as well as a prescription drug. The Philadelphia Veterans Administration Drug Dependence Treatment and Research Center has noted an increase in the use, misuse, and abuse of Valium among opiate dependents. Valium is also used by heroin dependents, particularly those undergoing methadone treatment, as it supplements the CNS-depressing effects of methadone while adding its own antianxiety properties.

Doctors often overprescribe these drugs possibly because they don't take the time to examine thoroughly the actual condition of their patients and end up giving them far more than they need for short-time use and thus trigger the potential for addiction. "Obviously, there are some physicians who ignore the data on these drugs and overprescribe," says Bonnie B. Wilford, director of the American Medical Association's (AMA) department of substance abuse.[18] "But we have come a long way in educating physicians about the potential for addiction, and overall most doctors are more cautious than they were even 10 years ago about prescribing them for long periods."

Physical Effects   Valium may cause the user to become drowsy and less alert. The drug also causes respiratory depression, a decrease in memory and motor functions, and occasional decreases in arterial pressure. Valium should be used cautiously by those with liver and kidney impairments and should not be used by women who are pregnant or nursing. In July 1970, the FDA ordered manufacturers of tranquilizers to issue warnings to physicians that these drugs should be avoided by women during the first trimester of pregnancy. Subsequent studies associated Valium and the incidence of cleft palate and lips in babies.[19] Children of mothers who used Valium in the first trimester had four times greater incidence of this congenital defect. Furthermore, babies born to Valium users tend to be hypoactive, exhibiting abnormally low muscle tension for the first 24 hours following delivery.[20]

A number of side effects are also associated with Valium use. These include lethargy, skin rashes, menstrual and ovulatory irregularities, blood abnormalities, conjunctivitis (pink eye), drowsiness, insomnia, fatigue, changes in emotional reactions, irritability, overexcitement, hostility and confusion, headaches, double vision, constipation, hypertension, stammering, changes in libido, nausea, slurred speech, perspiration, and thirst.[21]

VISUAL-MOTOR REACTION TIME.   The frequency of diazepam use has caused many to wonder whether this compound adversely affects visual-motor reaction time. If so, the user's ability to drive a car or perform other daily functions could be affected. To answer this question, two researchers conducted an experiment.[22]

Subjects were tested for impaired reaction time before diazepam was administered. They were tested again after an oral dose of 0.2 milligrams per kilogram of body weight. Another group of subjects were given a placebo instead of diazepam. Both groups were tested two and four hours after taking the drug or placebo. Results showed little retardation of reaction time, even though the dose given in the experiment was higher than the dose suggested for many disorders. The researchers concluded that when diazepam is taken as directed, there is little risk of impaired reaction time, but that doses greater than 0.2 milligrams per kilogram would most likely adversely affect reaction time.

COGNITIVE PROCESSES.   A team of researchers tested normal subjects (no organic brain impairment) by orally administering 10 milligrams of diazepam.[23] They then tested the memory and auditory abilities of the subjects, seeking a negative effect on both memory and auditory vigilance. The most important impairment was found to occur in attention and immediate recognition.

LONG-TERM MEMORY LOSS.   The research on Valium (diazepam) by Steven Mewaldt of Marshall University has found that Valium not only induces sleepiness and relaxes muscles but also has the effect of interfering with long-term memory.[24] Further experiments have supported his theory. These experiments provide the evidence that Valium interferes with the function of GABA, a neurotransmitter that is involved in memory function. This blockage of memory does depend upon how often one takes the drug, how much is taken, and at what time of the day it is taken. Mewaldt states, "If people are taking diazepam as a sleeping aid, it will probably be gone by the time they wake up. But if taken during the day that presents a concern."[25]

Synergism   Valium alone thus has significant bodily effects, and in combination with other drugs it can be even more dangerous. It has been found, for example, that when Valium is combined with ethanol (alcohol), the plasma levels of Valium increased, probably because Valium is more soluble in ethanol than in water, thus increasing the permeability of Valium in

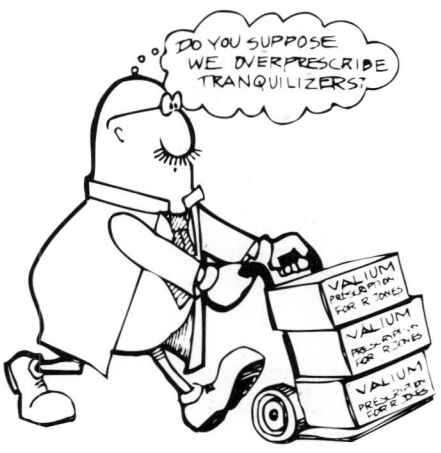

the blood.[26] It has also been noted that "acceleration by ethanol of the absorption of diazepam (Valium[R]) is important and provides a more complete explanation of the marked sedation that can follow this combination of drugs. . . . Overdose with diazepam alone is remarkably safe, but combined with alcohol can produce central nervous system depression and death."[27]

Dependence and Withdrawal   Withdrawal from benzodiazepines produces a hyperexcitable state that is opposite to the normal sedative and inhibitory effects of the drug. These signs and symptoms include anxiety, hyperactivity, agitation, insomnia, and depression. Visual hallucinations and paranoia may also occur. The onset of withdrawal differs depending on the duration of action of the specific benzodiazepines. It can take days or weeks to develop but a detoxification program is essential to control the problem.

Because of the way the benzodiazepines affect the brain, rebounding from these drugs can be very difficult.[28] Benzodiazepines help control the level of anxiety that we feel because of the way they affect cells in the brain. After these cells become dependent on these drugs, they react much more negatively to anxiety when they must do without. If someone has taken these drugs for a long time, he or she should *not* stop taking this medication suddenly. Sudden withdrawal from this group of drugs could cause serious mental distress or even psychotic reactions. Reducing intake gradually is the best way to withdraw; however, in order to do this reasonably and effectively, hospitalization may be required.

Today emotional disturbances are given as the most common reason for medical prescription of Valium. The drug is used to help patients cope with anxiety or depression. Valium is prescribed by 97 percent of all general practitioners and internists. The average daily use of Valium is 15 milligrams. It has been noted that because Valium creates a feeling of relaxation, euphoria, well-being, and uninhibitedness, users gradually increase their dosage above the prescribed amount.[29] When this happens, users form a psychological dependence on the drug.

Valium occupies the spotlight of controversy because researchers failed to recognize its apparent addiction capabilities when it was first being used years ago. Valium has a high rate of abuse because it is so easy to increase the dosage and become dependent and because it rarely proves fatal.

Nursing Homes   It is quite difficult to put a relative into a nursing home and now there is more concern: Many nursing homes are resorting to powerful sedatives to keep residents docile.[30] The drugs are being widely overused, and there is a growing number of lawsuits attributed to deaths of nursing home residents. Experts say the reasons behind the resurgence of the practice include an aging population in nursing homes, with more residents in their eighties and nineties who suffer from mental confusion.[31] "In some cases drugs are justified," but in many they are not. A proportion of demented patients scream and bite, kick and punch those around them.

Drugged Drivers   At the Southern California Research Institute and at UCLA, psychologist Herbert Moskowitz and study engineer Alison Smiley gave subjects 15 milligrams of diazepam (a commonly prescribed dose) daily

NURSING HOMES

Hal Willard, a writer for *Newsweek,* wrote a story about his 90-year-old mother, who was a patient in a nursing home and was experiencing blackouts and falling.[32] After moving her to another nursing home, it was discovered that his mother had been given a powerful antipsychotic tranquilizer called Mellaril, which drugged her into a helpless stupor. Once the drug stopped being administered, his mother made a remarkable recovery. With an estimated 1.5 million Americans living in nursing homes, there is growing concern that they not be sedated by abusing prescribed tranquilizers.

for eight days and had them drive a simulator.[33] After one day, driving skills were impaired; after eight days, subjects had trouble controlling their speed on curves, following the car ahead, and dividing their attention to monitor pedestrians, traffic signals, and signs.

Suicide Attempts   Benzodiazepines are often used in suicide. However, they are generally considered to be safe with low suicide potential, despite strong evidence that suggests benzodiazepines foster suicidal thoughts and actions. They are a depressant just like alcohol and can cause depression, anxiety, and suicide ideation.[34]

LIBRIUM (CHLORDIAZEPOXIDE)

The only major chemical difference between Librium and Valium is that Valium is not as soluble in water. Librium is a brand name, chlorodiazepoxide the chemical name. Librium is used as much as Valium—as an antianxiety agent, for muscle relaxation, and in various drug-withdrawal treatments. It has been used in the treatment of geriatric patients to reduce the chances of overexertion and in emotional crises. It has also been used to treat emotionally disturbed children.

Physical Effects   Librium has longer-lasting physiological effects than Valium, and a greater potential for dependence when used in excess. The drug produces mild drowsiness, fatigue, and a reduced ability to coordinate voluntary muscle movement. In some instances, it may cause skin rash, nausea, mild headache, and either an increased or decreased sex drive. Librium may depress blood pressure as well as pulse rate, lower body metabolism, and increase appetite. In large doses, it can produce a partial or complete suspension of respiration.

Librium's euphoric effects may lead some patients to psychological dependence, and tolerance can occur in only a few weeks of use. Physical dependence may ultimately occur, producing hyperexcitability, insomnia, vomiting, tremors, muscle twitching, anxiety, and depression. As with Valium, withdrawal from Librium should be medically supervised.

MAJOR TRANQUILIZERS (ANTIPSYCHOTICS)

CLASSIFICATION

Major Tranquilizers

Antipsychotics grouped on the basis of their widespread medical use: treatment and management of certain acute psychological disorders, notably schizophrenia and other severe conditions.

Antipsychotics, or "**major tranquilizers,**" are grouped on the basis of their most widespread medical use: treatment and management of certain acute psychological disorders, notably schizophrenia and other severe conditions.[35] There are four recognized groups of antipsychotics: the Rauwolfia alkaloids, the phenothiazines, the thioxanthines, and the butyrophenones. Although these groups are chemically dissimilar and their modes of action different, they all act on the central nervous system to block, inhibit, or retard signals along nerve pathways.

The physiological theory of schizophrenia, for which phenothiazine use is indicated, holds that auditory and visual hallucinations are caused by inadequate sorting of relevant and irrelevant stimuli within the brain. Confusing the relevant (pertinent) and irrelevant (or possibly unreal) stimuli might lead to a highly disoriented state. The structures involved in brain arousal and the evaluation and filtering of relevant stimuli include the reticular formation and its ascending reticular activating system (ARAS).

Situated along the brain stem (the part of the spinal cord that leads to the cerebellum and cerebral cortex), the ARAS samples all sensory impulses coming into the brain, and then alerts the cerebrum to receive information. Barbiturates and other sedative-hypnotics directly suppress ARAS neuronal activity. However, phenothiazines appear to depress the *input* reaching the ARAS, thus limiting the amount of information transmitted to it and in turn to the cerebrum. Although the patient is awake, there is decreased sensory input into the ARAS.

CURRENT USE

The growing use of antipsychotic preparations in the behavior management of chronic forms of psychosis, senility, and violent behavior has led some experts to credit these drugs with reducing the number of patients requiring hospitalization or institutionalization. Major tranquilizers make certain uncontrollable individuals less harmful to themselves and others.

PHYSICAL EFFECTS

Though the CNS-depressant action of the antipsychotics varies with the particular drug, the dose, the duration of application, and individual metabolic factors, mild doses generally produce a marked decrease in the intensity of neural activity in the brain. Thus, the impact of emotions is reduced, and awareness of internal and external events is minimized. Antipsychotics will bring on sedation accompanied by significantly reduced motor activity and muscle tone, and they will lower blood pressure, pulse rate, and body temperature as well.

Antipsychotics, like all drugs, produce contraindications (adverse reactions) in a certain percentage of individuals. These reactions can involve any of the bodily systems, producing anemia; weight gain; dry mouth; altered liver, kidney, or bladder functions; swollen tongue; and emotional dependence. Hypersensitivity reactions may include diarrhea, nausea, vomiting, and fever. Major tranquilizers are also able to cross the placental barrier and reportedly produce prolonged side effects and birth defects in the newborn.

Long-term therapy with antipsychotics may lead to a condition called tardive dyskinesia. This drug-induced nervous disorder is manifested in involuntary movements of the jaws, lips, and tongue. The condition is more common in the middle-aged or elderly, and once developed, the pattern of uncontrollable chewing, puckering of lips, and repetitive tongue protrusions may become irreversible.[36]

The lethal levels of antipsychotics depend on the specific preparation, on individual metabolic factors, and on whether the user exhibits tolerance, chemical hypersensitivity, or multidrug use. When antipsychotics interact with alcohol, antihistamines, or opiates, the combined depressant effects are greater than the sum of the effects of the substances taken singly.

DELIRIANTS (VOLATILE SUBSTANCES)

Volatile substances are breathable chemicals that produce psychoactive (mind-altering) vapors. People do not usually think of volatile substances (inhalants) as drugs because most of them were never intended to be used that way. The usual pattern of use is for children to start experimenting with inhalants around age 12 and stop by at least age 22. The effects produced by inhalants are similar to that of alcohol intoxication and are rapid but subside within minutes. Inhalants are found at home in glue, paints, nail-varnish remover, dry-cleaning fluids, and degreasing compounds.[37] Others are propellant gases in aerosols and fire extinguishers, or fuels (petrol or cigarette-lighter gas). Sometimes to heighten the effect a plastic bag is placed over the face or head. Of course, this places the user at the additional risk of suffocation by the bag sealing over the mouth and nose if the user should pass out.

Inhalant solvent vapors are absorbed through the lungs and rapidly reach the brain. Breathing and heart rates are depressed, and repeated or deep inhalation can result in an overdose, causing disorientation, loss of control, and unconsciousness. Generally the sniffer recovers quickly but may experience a mild hangover in the form of a headache and poor concentration for about a day.[38]

CLASSIFICATION

Volatile substances inhaled as psychoactive drugs may be broken into three classes: the volatile hydrocarbon solvents, aerosols, and anesthetics. The volatile hydrocarbon solvents are used primarily as commercial solvents.

Their power as solvents plus their tendency to evaporate quickly make them desirable for use in materials where quick drying is required or convenient,[39] such as in plastic-model cement and typewriting correction fluid. Some of the more highly refined petroleum products, such as gasoline and lighter fluid, are also included in this group.[40]

The anesthetics are considered more exotic than the solvents and aerosols, since they are generally less easy for the general public to obtain. One of the anesthetics often inhaled is chloroform. Although only limited research has been performed on these compounds, they seem to closely resemble various CNS depressants in their effects.

HISTORY

Before their medical applications were known, anesthetics such as nitrous oxide (laughing gas) and ether were frequently used for recreational purposes. Some deliriants have also been used during historical periods of stress (war, scarcity, depression) as a substitute for drugs that were more socially acceptable but unavailable. Presently deliriants are used in cleaning compounds, spray cans, model-airplane glue, and many industrial products.

One of the most striking features of volatile substances is their availability. For example, one survey found it was possible to purchase 38 different products containing volatile solvents from a single service station–hardware store.[41] Also, there are at least 300 products currently offered in aerosol form.[42] The lack of regulations on the sale of these products has contributed to their abuse among adolescents since the early 1960s. This abuse has led to the limiting of model-cement sales in some states to certain age categories and to the addition of certain chemical agents with unpleasant side effects to volatile substances. It is hoped that these side effects will be severe enough to discourage inhalation of the substances.

Studies indicate that the regular inhalant user is likely to be a sixth or seventh grader.[43] This stereotypical user is usually male, performs poorly in school, and comes from a low socioeconomic background. Adolescents are most likely to abuse inhalants (especially glue) during periods of distress or discomfort.

PHYSICAL EFFECTS

Volatile substances are rapidly transported across the blood-brain barrier. In low doses, they produce arousal and euphoria typical of CNS depressants. Several inhalations produce intoxication characterized by alterations in judgment, hyperactivity, and some lack of behavioral control. With increased doses, activity is further reduced and sedation becomes pronounced. High doses can produce hilarity, dizziness, a floating sensation, and hallucinations.

Solvents have caused temporary changes in kidney, liver, and bone-marrow functions and have affected responses to certain psychological tests.[44] Other deliriant compounds are caustic enough to produce mouth ulcers and severe stomach distress. Appetite reduction may also be caused, leading to nutritional disorders. Inert-gas propellants in aerosols can cause asphyxiation or freeze the vocal cords when inhaled.

Some users of volatile substances report side effects that include confusion, headache, lack of coordination, and watery eyes. Large doses often cause nausea, vomiting, or runny nose. Heavy sedation caused by these drugs can be characterized by stupor, respiratory depression, and unconsciousness, and it may lead to death.

PSYCHOLOGICAL EFFECTS

For many, the psychological effects of inhaling volatile substances are very pronounced. These effects include impaired judgment, confusion, hyperactivity, lack of behavioral control, fright, and tenseness. Acute, though temporary, psychosis has also been observed.[45]

DESIGNER DRUGS

These drugs got their name from the increasing sophistication of chemists in illicit laboratories, who are now producing drugs designed to fit the tastes of individual clients.[46] However, in an attempt to reduce some of the confusion caused by the term's varied applications, Donald R. Wasson has defined designer drugs as "substances wherein the psychoactive properties of a scheduled drug have been retained, but the molecular structure has been altered in order to avoid prosecution under the Controlled Substances Act."[47] Three main types of designer drugs are MDMA (3,4 methylenedioxymethamphetamine), fentanyl analogues, and meperidine analogues. Some designer drugs have had 1,000 to 6,000 times the potency of heroin and have produced accelerated aging, acute paranoia, irreversible brain damage, and premature death among users.[48]

In 1986 the Analogs Act allowed the DEA to ban drugs that are chemically similar to drugs already banned.[49] This act bans not only drugs similar to chemically made up drugs but also drugs that have similar effects on the body as previously banned drugs. Although the law may have passed, designer drugs remain very popular. Designer drugs can be either stimulants or depressants, depending on the chemicals being altered. The names of designer drugs are often abbreviations of their chemical formulas.

The tragic fact of this is that these drugs are 20 to 2,000 times more powerful than scheduled drugs, making them lethal to novice or low-grade users.[50] Designer drugs are addictive and can produce severe side effects such as memory loss, headaches, and paranoia by selectively killing brain cells. In some cases, they leave users so brain damaged they resemble people with advanced Parkinson's disease, paralyzed for life. Because they are often sold as the real drug, such as heroin, users have no way of knowing the potency.

Analogues are easily made in small labs by amateur scientists. A $500 investment in good lab equipment can yield $2 million worth of drugs.[51] Millions of dollars' worth of these drugs can be cooked up and shipped in just a matter of days.

MDMA

This amphetamine-like drug is an analogue of MDA. Street names include MDMA, MDA, Adam, **Ecstasy,** and XTC. It produces LSD effects (minus the hallucinations) such as increased self-awareness, removes communication barriers, and seems to remove the fear response. Thousands of young professionals and students are buying MDMA. One reason might be that MDMA's forerunner, MDA, was known as an aphrodisiac. However, MDMA is preferred because it produces a less troublesome high than MDA. MDMA produces such side effects as increased heart rate and blood pressure, irregular heartbeat, panic attacks, anxiety, sleep disorders, drug craving, and rebound depression.[52]

Synthesized about 70 years ago for use as an appetite suppressant, Ecstasy is now sold in tablets and capsules for a cost of about $20 a dose. The effects last for about six hours. Unfortunately, the long-term effect of the drug on a person's brain is unknown. However, Ecstasy may have long-term damaging effects on the brain, according to Stanford researcher Stephen Peroutka.[53] He has found that the drug damages brain cells in animals, suggesting that it may do the same thing in humans. Conclusive studies in humans have not been performed.

FENTANYL

This drug was introduced as an intravenous analgesic-anesthetic in 1968 and is now a favored preanesthetic medication, anesthetic, and postsurgical analgesic. **Fentanyl** is probably used in over 70 percent of all surgeries in the United States and is a respected drug.[54] It is very potent and short-acting (thirty minutes in duration).

A heroin substitute, Fentanyl is the most popular drug in the doctor scene.[55] It is also a "fast-acting" narcotic that is injected to get a stimulated high. Some believe that the Fentanyl analog is more addictive than crack.

Fentanyl analogues are excellent substitutes for heroin because they work just like it in terms of duration, euphoric effect, and ability to block pain. Sold by such names as China White, Synthetic Heroin, and Fentanyl, these analogues are coming into demand among heroin addicts, some of whom feel they contain less adulterants than heroin. Other fentanyl analogues, such as alpha-methyl fantanyl and 3-methyl fentanyl, are several times more powerful and could shut down respiration and kill a novice user who has not built up tolerance. Their potency makes overdose a very serious risk.

MEPERIDINE

Meperidine analogues (MPPP and MPTP) are, like fentanyl analogues, sold as Synthetic Heroin and China White, and are also offered as Zoom or even cocaine. Initial exposure to these drugs leads to disorientation, hallucinations, blurred vision, nodding off, difficulties in speech and swallowing, intermittent jerking of limbs, slow movement, and tremor. This slow movement may be abruptly followed by a "freezing up"—rigidity of the extremities and inability to move.

TESTING PROBLEMS

A major clinical problem is that the presence of these drugs cannot be detected by normal tests for opiates. Most laboratories can test at parts per million in body fluids, but fentanyl testing involves parts per billion.[56] Presently, there is only one laboratory in the country, aside from the Drug Enforcement Agency's, that can measure MPPP in forensic tests. Obviously, this is a tremendous problem in terms of medical diagnosis and reduces the possibility of effective treatment.

SUMMARY

Despite the number of medical problems that are effectively met by proper and judicious use of barbiturates, abuse of these substances remains one of America's hidden drug problems. To combat this problem, physicians have begun diagnosing and treating underlying disorders before relying on barbiturate use.

Tranquilizers are the number one prescription drug in the United States, with minor tranquilizers, including Valium and Librium, the most frequently prescribed. Minor tranquilizers reduce stress, anxiety, and tension as well as aiding in muscle relaxation and working as mild analgesics. However, many physicians are presently reassessing their prescribing of tranquilizers, and it is hoped that people will learn to cope rather than rely on these drugs. The side effects of minor tranquilizers, the potential hazard when they are combined with alcohol or other depressants, and the genuine possibility of psychological and physical dependence make these drugs dangerous.

Major tranquilizers have been effective in the treatment of severe and chronic psychological disorders in that they reduce potential self-harm and allow clinicians to make therapeutic contact. Despite their tremendous medical potential, however, they can cause harmful side effects.

Volatile substances are also CNS depressants and are found in three forms: volatile hydrocarbon substances, aerosols, and anesthetics. Abuse of volatile hydrocarbon substances includes glue sniffing and inhaling typing correction fluid and gasoline fumes; aerosol abuse includes inhaling propellants that have been used in deodorants and hair sprays; and anesthetic abuse includes inhaling more exotic solvents such as chloroform. Deliriants' psychophysiological effects include euphoria, confusion, and increased hilarity, and lead to sleep or coma. Research indicates that regular use leads to changes in kidney and liver functions and a reduction of appetite. The effect on the brain is still not known with certainty.

Designer drugs, such as MDMA, fentanyl analogues, and meperidine analogues, are appearing on the drug scene with greater frequency. Unfortunately, these drugs have potentially extreme health hazards. Their extremely high potency could lead to heart damage, irreversible brain damage, or premature death.

Depressants
N O T E S

1. John Reinhold, "Thumbs Down on Downers," *Current Health,* April 1988, pp. 16–17.

2. "Sedatives and Hypnotics: Alcohol and Drug Fact Sheet," *Drug Information Center (DIC)* (Eugene: University of Oregon, 1979).

3. Ibid.

4. Pauline Postotnick, "Pregnancy and Drugs," *FDA Consumer* 12, no. 8 (October 1978):7–10.

5. "Barbiturates: Alcohol and Drug Fact Sheet," *Drug Information Center (DIC)* (Eugene: University of Oregon, 1979).

6. Reinhold, "Thumbs Down on Downers," p. 17.

7. Owen Davis, "Saving the Brain When Accident or Stroke Halts Oxygen," *Science Digest* 84, no. 3 (September 1978):39–42.

8. Cited in M. Clark and B. Castel, "Saving Coma Victims," *Newsweek,* May 22, 1978, pp. 20–22.

9. "Barbiturates."

10. John Pekkanen, "The Impact of Promotion on Physicians' Prescribing Patterns," *Journal of Drug Issues* 6, no. 1 (Winter 1976):14.

11. Cheryl Gutman, "Treating Stress with Drugs," *Current Health* 15, no. 2 (October 1988):19–21.

12. Joseph Alper, "Tranquilizers: A User's Guide," *Health* 29, no. 11 (November 1988):35–39, 86.

13. Susan Edmiston, "The Medicine Everybody Loves," *Family Health* 10, no. 1 (January 1978):25–28.

14. Ibid., 52.

15. Annabel Hecht, "Tranquilizers: Use, Abuse, and Dependency: FDA Requirements," *FDA Consumer* 12, no. 8 (October 1978):20–33.

16. Penelope McMillan, "Women and Tranquilizers: A Special Report," *Ladies Home Journal* 93, no. 1 (November 1976):167.

17. Hecht, "Tranquilizers: Use, Abuse, and Dependency."

18. Alper, "Tranquilizers," p. 39.

19. Mark Safra and Godfrey P. Oakley, Jr., "Association between Cleft Lip with or without Cleft Palate and Prenatal Exposure to Diazepam," *Lancet* 2 (September 13, 1975); Betty Smith, "Tranquilizer Hazards," *Drug Survival News* 7, no. 2 (October 1978):5.

20. R. E. Kron et al., "Neonatal Narcotic Abstinence: Effects of Pharmacotherapeutic Agents and Maternal Drug Usage on Nutritive Sucking Behavior," *Journal of Pediatrics* 88, no. 4 (April 1976).

21. Elmar G. Lutz, "Allergic Conjunctivitis Due to Diazepam," *American Journal of Psychiatry* 132, no. 5 (May 1975):548.

22. James Barbee and Iryna L. Black, "Effects of Diazepam on Visuomotor Reaction Time," *Perceptual and Motor Skill* 60 (1985):106–11.

23. Peter P. Roy-Byrne, Thomas W. Uhde et al. "Effects of Diazepam on Cognitive Processes in Normal Subjects," *Psychopharmacology* 91, no. 1 (January 1987):30–33.

24. Susan Chollar, "Diazepam," *Psychology Today,* January 1988, p. 12.

25. Ibid.

26. S. L. Hayes et al., "Ethanol and Oral Diazepam Absorption," *Drugs* 14, no. 1 (July 1977):68.

27. Ibid., p. 69.

28. Alper, "Tranquilizers."

29. Robert M. Julien, *A Primer of Drug Action* (San Francisco: W. H. Freeman & Company, 1981), pp. 53–54, 122–23.

30. Steven Findlay, "Is Grandma Drowsy, or Is She Drugged?" *U.S. News & World Report,* June 12, 1989, p. 68.

31. Ibid.

32. Hal Willard, "At 90, the Zombie Shuffle," *Newsweek,* February 20, 1989, p. 10.

33. Rebecca Coffey, "Drugged Driving: Behind the Wheel, Valium May Kill," *Science Digest* 94 (September 1988):15.

34. Miller and Gold, "Identification and Treatment of Benzodiazepine Abuse."

35. "Antipsychotics: Alcohol and Drug Fact Sheet," *Drug Information Center (DIC)* (Eugene: University of Oregon, 1979).

36. M. D. Long, *The Essential Guide to Prescription Drugs,* 4th ed. (New York: Harper & Row, 1985), p. 923.

37. Social Issues Resource Series, "Glue Sniffing," *Richmond Times-Dispatch,* March 16, 1987, p. 24.

38. Ibid.

39. *The Non-Medical Use of Drugs: Final Report of the Canadian Government Commission of Inquiry* (Ottawa: Crown, 1973), p. 439.

40. James Gamage and E. Lief Zerkin, "The Deliberate Inhalation of Volatile Substances," *National Clearinghouse for Drug Abuse Information* 30, no. 1 (1974):4.

41. *The Non-Medical Use of Drugs,* p. 4.

42. Gamage and Zerkin, "The Deliberate Inhalation of Volatile Substances," p. 4.

43. Wayne R. Mitic, "Adolescent Inhalant Use and Perceived Stress," *Journal of Drug Education* 17, no. 2 (1987):113.

44. "Volatile Substances: Alcohol and Drug Fact Sheet," *Drug Information Center (DIC)* (Eugene: University of Oregon, 1980).

45. *The Non-Medical Use of Drugs,* p. 443.

46. Robert J. Roberton, "Designer Drugs: Analogy Game, Excerpts from Congressional Testimony," *Grassroots* (1986):27, 32.

47. David Smith and Richard B. Seymour, "Classification of Designer Drugs," *The Journal* 12, no. 15 (November 1985):1.

48. "Designer Drugs: Murder by Molecule," *U.S. News & World Report,* August 5, 1985, p. 14.

49. Bruce Eisner, "Your Head Is under Arrest," *Omni* 10, no. 9 (June 1988):35.

50. Hal Straus, "From Crack to Ecstasy," *American Health,* June 1988, pp. 50–54.

51. Gary Merritt, "The Danger of Designer Drugs," *Mademoiselle,* July 1989, pp. 160–61, 212.

52. L. Dunn, "Designer Meperidine and MPTP Contamination," *Pharm Alert* 16, no. 2 (1986).

53. "Ecstasy Drug Tied to Brain Damage," *New York Times,* January 17, 1989, p. C11.

54. Smith and Seymour, "Classification of Designer Drugs," p. 1.

55. John Pekkanen, "Confessions of Doctors on Drugs," *Hippocrates,* November 1988, p. 92.

56. Roberton, "Designer Drugs," pp. 27, 32.

CHAPTER
8

ALCOHOL

America's Number One
Drug Problem

INTRODUCTION

You have asked me how I feel about whiskey. Well, here's how I stand on the question. If, when you say whiskey, you mean that devil's brew, the poison spirit, the bloody monster that defiles innocence, dethrones reason, destroys the home and creates misery, poverty, yes, literally takes the bread from the mouths of little children, if you mean the evil drink that topples the Christian man from the pinnacle of righteous, gracious living and causes him to descend to the pit of degradation, despair, shame, and helplessness, then I am certainly against it with all my heart.

But, if when you say whiskey, you mean the oil of conversation, the philosophic wine, the ale consumed when good fellows get together, that puts a song in their hearts and laughter on their lips, the warm glow of contentment in their eyes; if you mean Christmas cheer, if you mean the stimulating drink that puts the spring in an old man's footsteps on a frosty morning, if you mean the drink whose sale puts untold millions of dollars into our treasury which are used to provide tender care for our little crippled children, our blind, our deaf, our dumb, our pitiful aged and infirm, to build highways and hospitals and schools, then certainly I am in favor of it. This is my stand and I will not compromise.[1]

In view of such feelings toward alcohol, it is not surprising that the drug is one of the most widely used and abused by people of all ages and backgrounds in our society. There are approximately 90 to 100 million regular users of alcohol, and 9 to 12 million classified as alcoholics. Alcohol leads to more problems for individuals, families, and society as a whole than any other drug in the United States.

Alcohol is classified as a CNS depressant that produces analgesia. Several alcohols (ethyl, n-butyl, and amyl) are produced by the fermentation process, in which certain yeasts convert the carbon, hydrogen, and oxygen of sugar and water into ethyl alcohol and carbon dioxide. Most natural fermentation will lead to about 14 percent alcohol. Distillation, a process in which alcohol is added to an already fermented beverage, produces a higher alcoholic content, often more than 50 percent by volume. Ethyl alcohol (100 percent ethanol) is also known as absolute alcohol. *Proof* refers to the percentage of pure alcohol in a beverage. The percentage of alcohol is always half the proof (100 percent alcohol would be 200 proof). The term *proof alcohol* dates back to early America, when alcohol was used to help ignite gunpowder. Unless the alcohol concentration in the powder was at least 50 percent, the gunpowder would not ignite. Table 8–1 indicates the approximate percentage of alcohol in various beverages.

Consumption of alcohol worldwide is increasing as more and more countries become industrialized. The alcohol industry is becoming more concentrated as distilleries and breweries fast become multinational companies. This trend is leading to the production of all kinds of alcohol. What this means is not that beer-drinking countries are giving up their beer and wine-drinking countries their wine, but that all are adding beverages over and above these preferred drinks.[2]

TABLE 8–1 APPROXIMATE PERCENTAGE OF ALCOHOL IN VARIOUS ALCOHOLIC BEVERAGES

Alcoholic Beverage	Percentage of Alcohol by Volume
Table wines (still, white, sparkling, red, and rosé)	10–22
Aperitifs, dessert wines, flavored wines	17–20
Beer	3–6
Ale	6–8
Hard cider	5–10
Whiskey	42–52
Brandy	40–50
Rum	34–46
Gin	37–50
Vodka	37
Liqueurs	30–65

CONSUMPTION IN THE UNITED STATES

It is clear that Americans are drinking more beer than wine or distilled spirits. Per capita consumption for Americans 14 and older is nearly 30 gallons of beer each year. This is equivalent to 320 12-ounce cans of beer. Americans consume nearly as much ethanol from beer (49 percent) as from wine (12 percent) and distilled spirits (39 percent) combined.[3]

YOUTH

The 1990 National High School Senior Drug Abuse Survey reported that the drop from the peak year (1980) to 1990 for every senior student having used alcohol is only about 4 percent: "This is the first year ever that fewer than 9 out of 10 students report alcohol use, even trying it once."[4] More specifically the survey stated:

- Nearly all high school seniors (89.5 percent) have used alcohol. Two thirds (57.1 percent) have used in the past month and 32.2 percent have had five or more drinks in a row on at least one occasion in the past two weeks, indicating a slight decline since 1989.

The following was true for those 12–17 years of age:

- Almost half (48.0 percent) of young people ages 12 to 17 have tried alcohol at least once in their lifetime. Of the 8.2 million who used alcohol within the past year, 4.9 million used at least once in the past month, and 1 million used alcohol once a week or more.[5]

Early onset of alcohol and other drug use is one of the strongest predictors of later dependency problems. A recent study found that the likelihood of developing a drug disorder depends on the age that the drug use starts. The best predictor is when the onset of use is prior to age of 15.[6] This study showed that 34 percent started drinking in middle school and 14 percent started in elementary. The age at which children begin to drink has been getting younger and younger. The study also shows that students who started drinking in elementary school and middle school had significantly higher problems with alcohol abuse than those who started in high school or college. There appears to be a linear relationship present: The earlier a student begins drinking, the more he or she tends to consume and the more alcohol-related problems there are in college.[7]

A study found that fifth-grade students with positive self-esteem are less likely to be influenced to drink alcohol through peer pressure.[8] It is important that parents and schools work on activities to build positive self-esteem in children.

Recent literature suggests that the variables associated with teenage drug use are many and conflicting. A study conducted in Georgia and South Carolina found associations between student drinking, behavior, and several variables such as liberal attitudes toward drinking, an older age of the child, and having a drink at an earlier age.[9] The most significant predictor of student drinking is whether or not the student's best friend drinks, as well as the student's own attitudes about drinking.

In influencing students' alcohol attitude and providing a knowledge of risk factors through education programs, a concerted effort must be taken by parents and the community. Also, as peers have a significant influence on adolescent alcohol use, future research should focus on early peer-group interactions to determine how peer influences may start alcohol use in our youth.

It is estimated that presently 200,000 children and adolescents are admitted in public and private drug- and alcohol-treatment centers, but this represents only 10 percent of the total number of children and adolescents needing to be treated.[10] Barriers include lack of coordination, shortage of facilities, gaps in insurance, communities that oppose treatment centers, and money—which is the main barrier.

According to the Department of Health and Human Services (1987), there is substantial evidence that legislation raising the drinking age in most states to 21 years of age has reduced the number of alcohol-related traffic accidents significantly.[11] The Insurance Institute of Highway Safety did a study of 26 states that raised the legal drinking age to 21 between 1975 and 1984. The study showed a 13 percent drop in the number of fatal crashes caused by alcohol by 18- and 19-year-old drivers.

Alcohol consumption, however, has been on the decrease in college-age students since 1981, following a similar trend of decrease in the total population.[12] Another possible reason for decreased use is the increased attention these problems are receiving from the media, and from education and community groups.

Alcoholism is one of the biggest problems all colleges have. Many clubs, especially sororities and fraternities, have used liquor as part of their initiation and/or functions. In 1988 two Princeton University students were fined $500 and sentenced to 30 days in jail for serving liquor to minors.[13] Also, 39 pledges were hospitalized after being blindfolded and having the other club members pour liquor down their throats. One person remained in a coma for 24 hours. Though Princeton University president Harold Shapiro disapproved of the drinking incident, he disagreed with the sentences, saying they were "excessive."[14]

College students drink to relieve tensions, meet new people, or belong to a fraternity or sorority; they also drink because of a low level of campus activity and low academic performance (suggested as cause and effect).[15] In addition, women are less satisfied with alcohol than men, freshmen are more dissatisfied with consumption than upperclassmen, and people who are involved with campus activities are less likely to consume large amounts of alcohol.

ADULTS

According to the 1990 National Household Survey on Drug Abuse:[16]

- There were 102.9 million current drinkers of alcoholic beverages in 1990 compared with 105.8 million in 1988 and 113.1 million in 1985. The alcohol-use rates in 1985, 1988, and 1990, for those aged 12 and over, are 59 percent, 53 percent, and 51 percent, respectively.

- The decline in the rates of lifetime alcohol use seen between 1985 and 1988 (from 56 percent to 50 percent) for youth continued in 1990 to 48 percent. Past-year use was 41 percent in 1990 and has experienced a steady decline since 1979. In 1990 less than 25 percent of youth have had at least one drink during the past month. This is similar to 1988 survey results.

- For young adults, the prevalence of alcoholic beverage use is substantially higher than for youth: 88 percent have tried alcohol, 80 percent have used alcohol in the past year, and 63 percent have used alcohol during the preceding month. Although this represents little change from 1988, drinking alcohol has steadily declined since 1985. The 1990 rates for drinking among young adults in the past year and past month are significantly lower than those reported in 1985 (87 percent and 71 percent, respectively in 1985).

- Of the 133 million people age 12 and older (66 percent of the population) who drank alcohol in the past year, nearly one third, or 42 million, drank at least once a week.

It is estimated that "twenty percent of the population drinks eighty percent of the alcohol consumed each year. This minority drinks nearly five billion fifths of eighty-proof liquor per year."[17] Far-reaching medical effects from such drinking include fetal alcohol syndrome, mental retardation, and physical abnormalities.

THE ELDERLY

Of the estimated 25 million people in the United States over the age of 65, 10 to 15 percent are believed to suffer from alcohol- or drug-related problems.[18] Much of the drug-related abuse stems from prescription or over-the-counter medications rather than street drugs. The National Institute of Alcohol and Alcoholism estimates that 12 percent of older men and women are heavy to problem drinkers with about two thirds of these being long-time users and the other third having started later in life. Those who begin later in life often have an emotional crisis or social upheaval, such as the loss of a spouse or retirement, which has an effect on their use of alcohol. People over the age of 65, who make up 12 percent of the population, use one fourth of all medications.[19]

There is much talk over the issue of polydrug use among the elderly.[20] They use one or maybe many drugs to relax their bodies. Alcohol appears to be their drug of choice; however, its use in combination with other drugs can be very dangerous.

Cynthia Robbins reports some interesting information about the elderly after a survey of 8,038 subjects that also included some interviews.[21] The following four factors can be noted relating to the demographic increases in alcohol use and abuse in the elderly: (1) The general trend since World War II has been an increase in alcohol consumption populationwide. This, combined with the increased numbers of elderly, needs to be considered. (2)

There has been a general increase in alcohol use by women, partly related to increased acceptability. (3) The elderly population tends to live longer than previously. And (4) the amount of prescription drugs used by the elderly has increased dramatically. The major implication here is the synergistic effects of alcohol with other drugs.

Two additional considerations are important also: the effect of alcohol on the older body, and the psychological changes associated in role changing.[22] In older adults, alcohol takes longer to filter through the body. Due to decreased body-water levels, a small amount of alcohol can have a large effect. Role changes, caused by life transitions such as retirement or spousal death, may have a profound effect on the use of alcohol. Employment and marital status are other important considerations. The study made clear that young people abuse alcohol far more than do older adults, but 10 percent of the elderly population do have some sort of drinking problem.[23]

Physicians are becoming more aware of older drinkers and how alcohol can affect their health and functioning. Of the estimated 10 million alcoholics in the United States, 3 million of them are over 60.

HISTORY

According to paleontologists, the ingredients necessary to synthesize alcohol (sugar, water, yeast, and heat) were present on earth at least 200 million years ago. Evidence of the drug's use dates back to 6400 B.C.; both intoxicating beverages (wines and stronger drinks) as well as their effects were well known to the Egyptians, ancient Hebrews, Greeks, and Romans.[24]

The date of the discovery of distillation remains a mystery. The Arabians were apparently distilling alcohol by A.D. 900, however, and in the mid-1600s a Dutch physician distilled alcohol by using juniper berries in an effort to produce a diuretic. The diuretic, known as *jenever,* was later called gin.[25]

Alcohol in colonial America consisted mainly of beer, wine, hard cider, and rum. Political problems concerning alcohol led to the "Whiskey Rebellion" in Pennsylvania in 1794, and social problems led to the temperance movement, which culminated in 1920 with the passage of the Eighteenth Amendment and its prohibition of the manufacture and sale of any alcoholic beverage. Prohibition endured for thirteen years but did not eliminate the problems associated with alcohol.

WHY DO PEOPLE DRINK?

There are many reasons people drink. Reasons often offered by junior high students include

1. acceptance by peers
2. the smart thing to do
3. a way to forget troubles
4. habit
5. advertising

6. movies
7. examples set by older people
8. taste
9. rebellion against authority

These reasons can apply to people of every age who drink. The findings of a recent study on the reasons for drinking included the following: excitement seeking, escape, and social pressure.[26] Females seemed to be most affected by the escape aspect of drinking. Males tended to drink for excitement and felt social pressure more than females.

ADVERTISING

When alcohol is advertised to consumers, it is often depicted as a way to gain greater health, sexier lives, rugged individualism, and social sophistication. Its sphere of influence is shown to encompass recreation, work, and business; it's promoted as a casual yet indispensable part of social life. Through advertising, alcohol, like hundreds of thousands of other products, has become a part of our national buying pattern.

The alcohol industry is a major advertiser that heavily promotes its product. A progressively more concentrated group of giant conglomerates are promoting alcohol products through mass advertising, which is a tax-deductible business expense. The alcohol industry's budget for its advertising is many times greater than all the funds spent publicly and privately each year on alcohol-prevention campaigns. One annual tabulation showed that the distilled-spirits industry spent $160 million on advertising, the beer industry more than $100 million, and the wine makers more than $50 million.[27]

Advertising Makes Alcohol Attractive
Source: David Striekler/Monkmeyer Press

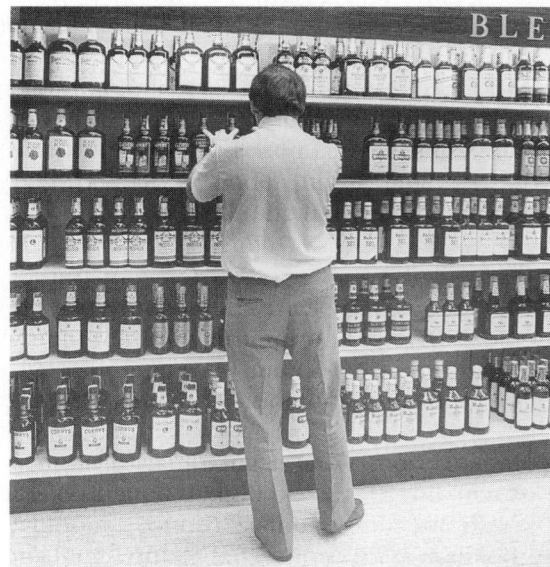

PEER ACCEPTANCE, SEARCH FOR ADULTHOOD, AND REBELLION

It seems extremely important for young people to feel accepted by their peers. It is also important to them to be thought of as adults in control of their own lives. These two points, in combination, are reasons for teenage drinking. Many teenagers drink to take on the role of adults, and many others drink to be accepted by that group. Young people seem to regard drinking as a badge of adulthood, of virility. They also see it as a way to rebel against adults or society in general when they feel thwarted by them.

RECREATION AND ENJOYMENT

Studies show that most adults drink for recreation and enjoyment. Alcohol makes one feel good. Small amounts of alcohol cause a euphoric, relaxed feeling. After a couple of drinks everything looks better and problems seem less devastating. Drinking helps people to feel more comfortable and less inhibited during social gatherings, thus making it easier to get to know others and enjoy themselves.

Moderate drinking is thought to aid in socialization and the reducing of tension. Small amounts of alcohol can truly enhance many situations. It's when alcohol gets to be *the* situation that the problems begin. Alcoholics and potential alcoholics increase their dependence on alcohol to constantly make situations easier and more enjoyable. Instead of having a few drinks at the party, they will have a few drinks just to feel like going to the party.

CHANGING SEX ROLES

Changing sex roles have affected the numbers of women with alcohol problems. Women who have left the home and entered the traditionally male working world are encouraged by advertising to consume greater quantities of alcohol. Their involvement in more extensive social and business situations exposes them to heavy drinking, and the increased stress they undergo in new roles may also lead to alcoholism. Women now make up about 50 percent of all alcoholics.

SEX

Alcohol consumption before sex is very popular because it can reduce inhibitions and often induces a sense of increased arousal. What alcohol does is make sex more fun to think about, but that's the extent of it.[28] As Shakespeare recognized, "Drink . . . provokes desire, but it takes away the performance." Recent research has supported this statement: Tests have revealed that more alcohol causes less physical arousal, regardless of what the person thinks. Another study showed that alcohol caused testosterone levels in males to drop to as much as five times less than normal.

A recent study of the effects of alcohol on women's sexual behavior determined that drinking seemed to enhance feelings of womanliness.[29] The study noted, however, that alcohol hindered their subjects' ability to gain satisfying interactions with men. The study also found that heavy-drinking women were generally more sexually active than nondrinkers or light drinkers. These women were also found to have had sex more frequently at an early age and were currently more sexually active than their lighter- or nondrinking counterparts. Citing their inability to develop satisfying relationships, the study indicated that heavy-drinking women were unable to receive sexual fulfillment much of the time and tended to have a lower regard for feminine ideals.

FAMILY INFLUENCE

A recent study compared alcohol use and consumption of parents to their offspring after 17 years.[30] Results indicate that a father's drinking habits were significantly associated with drinking of the adult sons. The strength of the associations varied according to what category of drinking (abstainer, low volume, medium volume, or high volume) that the father fell into. A majority of the abstainers' sons were drinkers, but in low volume, and they were less likely than drinkers' sons to be high-volume drinkers. Sons of medium-volume drinkers were more likely to be in the medium category than any other category. High-volume drinkers' sons were more likely to be either low- or high-volume drinkers. Daughters had about a 38 percent likelihood of being in the same drinking category as their fathers. Daughters of abstaining mothers were much more likely to abstain than those of drinkers. Mothers in the high-volume drinking category had 50 percent of their daughters who were also high-volume drinkers. Having both parents as abstainers increased the likelihood that offspring would be abstainers. When both parents were abstainers, 95 percent of the females were also abstainers or very low volume drinkers and 0 percent were high-volume drinkers. When both parents were drinkers, the likelihood of a son being a high-volume drinker was twice as high as when neither parent drank. The study clearly shows the influence and positive association of parental drinking on offspring, especially on female offspring.[31] Other studies also support this finding.[32]

PHYSIOLOGICAL EFFECTS

"Alcohol is a depressant that acts as an anesthetic on the CNS. It is absorbed unchanged in the stomach and small intestine and is disseminated by the blood to all parts of the body, including the brain."[33] Though people may feel stimulated and less inhibited after drinking an alcoholic beverage, their central nervous system is actually being depressed. Problem drinkers and alcoholics should be greatly concerned about these effects, since the mortality rate for alcoholics is about 2.5 times that for the normal population.[34]

CIRCULATORY SYSTEM AND BLOOD

Pulse rate and total blood flow are increased by the consumption of alcohol. "In moderate quantities, alcoholic beverages slightly increase the heart rate, slightly dilate blood vessels in arms, legs, and skin, moderately lower blood pressure, stimulate appetite, increase production of gastric secretion, and markedly stimulate urine output."[35] Levels of lipoproteins (substances in the blood consisting of various fats and proteins) are also affected: High-density lipoproteins (HDL) increase and low-density lipoproteins (LDL) decrease. Reports indicate that this may be why daily consumption of small to moderate amounts of alcohol can prevent heart disease.[36] Studies by the National Heart, Lung, and Blood Institute reveal that moderate drinking (one to two drinks a day) and exercise are linked to higher levels of blood protein, which in turn appears to help protect against coronary heart disease.[37] Research findings suggest that high-density lipoproteins clear away cholesterol deposits from the walls of coronary arteries. Previous research indicated that low-density lipoproteins carry cholesterol, which leads to fatty deposits in blood vessels and increased coronary risk. By contrast, HDL appears to remove cholesterol from the body. Recent studies, including the Framingham Heart Study, have shown that persons with high levels of HDL were less likely to suffer heart attacks.

Recently there has been a reaffirmation of beliefs that occasional drinking (two drinks a day) lowers the mortality rate due to a decrease in heart attacks.[38] Simply stated, drinkers are found to have higher levels of HDL cholesterol. Alcohol raises HDL levels and protects coronary arteries from arteriosclerosis, and with less arteriosclerosis moderate drinkers live longer. However, not all agree. Some say alcohol increases HDL_3; however, it is HDL_2 that protects against heart disease.[39] Exercise appears to elevate HDL_2, and some feel an evening jog may be more beneficial than an evening drink. Still another theory is that in alcoholics, the effect may primarily be on the HDL_2 subfraction, while in the general population it may primarily raise the HDL_3.[40] Leslie Klevay, who is a nutritionist at the Department of Agriculture, believes lack of copper in people's diets can cause clogged arteries.[41] Klevay has found that rats given alcohol as opposed to water lived six times longer. The rats that consumed beer also had lower blood cholesterol and fewer enlarged hearts. Through separate studies on the rats it was found that pure alcohol did not have the same profound effects on rats that beer did, so maybe, Kelvay suggests, beer contains some other ingredient that works with the alcohol to help rats absorb more copper from food. The controversy continues; however, it is hoped that researchers will finally clarify the mystery of alcohol and its effects on reducing heart attacks.

But caution should be used in increasing alcohol consumption. Chronic excessive use of alcohol causes lesions in the muscular tissue of the heart and can lead to congestive heart failure. Also, it has long been known that in healthy humans alcohol doses equivalent to two to five ordinary drinks (30 to 75 milliliters) slightly increase heart rate, blood pressure (systolic more than diastolic), and cardiac output.[42] In other words, regular consumption of large amounts of alcohol, regardless of race or sex, is associated with a substantially higher prevalence of high blood pressure. Furthermore, W. P. Castell, director of the Framingham Heart Study, has stated that some "people are born with a biological makeup that can enhance the addictive qualities of alcohol."[43] He pointed out that "it could be very dangerous to tell some people that two drinks a day will be good for them when their makeup will not allow them to stop at two. Thus, what starts out as prudent advice may turn into advice that could lead to cardiac death from alcohol myopathy (toxic disorder of the heart muscle), rather than to an extension of life by lower coronary atherosclerosis (fatty deposits)."[44]

It has been found that abstinence significantly reduces blood pressure and strokes. Chronic alcoholism is associated with dysfunction of the heart and injury to skeletal muscle. Because addicted individuals frequently delay medical assistance, complications become more extensive, although abstinence plays an important role in treating and correcting heart conditions. A Swedish study linked alcohol abuse and smoking with coronary death and found that for smoking alcoholics this increased fourfold compared to nonalcoholic nonsmokers and threefold for nonsmoking alcoholics; both smoking and alcohol abuse were independently associated with coronary death.[45]

Alcohol abuse primarily affects the heart and cardiovascular system in the following ways.[46] The first is that alcohol abuse is associated with hypertension; it is related to elevated levels of systemic arterial pressure. This hypertension usually disappears with hospitalization, but only if alcohol is withdrawn. A second effect of alcohol on the cardiovascular system is both atrial and ventricular dysrhythmias, or "holiday heart syndrome," which is flutter and fibrillation of the atrial. This is usually present several days after a drinking binge. It is like a withdrawal syndrome. The third effect of alcohol on the heart muscle is the production of a cardiomyopathic ventricle. This occurs after prolonged periods of exposure. In 30 percent of patients it may be reversible if abstention from alcohol is achieved. However, a line of studies indicate that alcohol use on a moderate daily basis may suppress heart-muscle disease.

As we have seen, when people begin drinking they become relaxed and euphoric; they may say and do things they would not do under normal circumstances. When their blood-alcohol content (BAC) reaches .05 to .10 percent, however, a depressant action begins to interfere with ability to function. Most states hold .10 blood-alcohol content to be the point of legal intoxication—the point at which people can no longer safely operate an automobile.

At .10 to .20, additional CNS depression makes it more obvious that a person is intoxicated. The individual may not be able to walk a straight line, close his or her eyes, touch fingers together, or perform other simple motor activities. At .20 to .30, a drinker is highly intoxicated. At this point, control is lost and the drinker may change from being the life of the party to being strongly sedated. When blood alcohol reaches .40 to .50, the drinker becomes unconscious. At .50 to .60, death may occur.

Blackout may occur with almost any level of alcohol in the body, though usually it is experienced at higher levels of intoxication and after chronic alcohol intake. Blackout is a temporary form of amnesia. While the individual is drinking, he or she is conscious, ambulatory, and appears in control. On the following day, however, much of the time spent drinking is completely forgotten. Blackouts are thought to be an early warning signal in the progression toward alcoholism.

The percentage of alcohol in the blood can be estimated by the number of drinks consumed in relation to body weight. Table 8–2 shows the number of drinks a person needs to reach a blood-alcohol level, or concentration, of .08 in one hour. Pacing alcohol consumption over a longer period will help to prevent intoxication, as will having food in the stomach, since food helps slow absorption.

Prolonged use of substantial amounts of alcohol has been found in a large proportion of patients with unexplained cardiomyopathy, who make up 2 to 3 percent of those hospitalized for heart disease. But abstinence from alcohol produces a good recovery rate in early stages of the disease and can lead to marked recovery even in advanced stages.

NERVOUS SYSTEM

Chronic alcoholism has been shown to cause brain damage in a number of individuals. In fact, many studies have suggested that at least 50 percent of people who have been drinking heavily for years will develop some sort of brain disorder by the time they are 40.[47] Such alcohol-related brain damage may at least partially reverse itself once a person stops using alcohol. One study reported that parts of destroyed brain cells actually begin to grow back after alcohol use has been discontinued.

Alcohol's first CNS-depressing action is exerted on the cerebrum, the part of the brain responsible for inhibitions, judgments, and reasoning. When this area is sedated, thought processes become jumbled and disorganized. The finer grades of discrimination, memory, concentration, and insight are also dulled and finally submerged. When the cerebrum is affected, the cerebral cortex is also restricted. Motor processes become disrupted; outbursts and quick changes in mood can occur.

The cerebellum, the part of the brain that controls the senses, is affected next. Vision dims, the field of vision eventually narrows; sound becomes distorted and hearing levels are lowered. Gradually the remaining senses—smell, taste, and touch—are also impaired.

The last part of the brain to be affected is the medulla, the vital brain center that monitors respiration. When alcohol sedates the medulla, respiration may be impaired and breathing may eventually cease.

TABLE 8–2   NUMBER OF DRINKS IN ONE HOUR NEEDED TO REACH A BAC OF APPROXIMATELY .08 PERCENT

Weight Kg.	Lbs.	Number of drinks						
45	100	1	2					Legal
54	120	1	2	3				Oregon
63	140	1	2	3				BAC Limit for
72	160	1	2	3	4			Driving
81	180	1	2	3	4			.08%
90	200	1	2	3	4	5		
99	220	1	2	3	4	5	6	
108	240	1	2	3	4	5	6	

One drink = 1.05 oz. of 80-proof liquor = 5oz. of 12% wine = 12oz. of 5% beer.

The potentially damaging effects of alcoholism on the brain are of increasing concern. Light and moderate social drinkers appear to experience a loss of some intellectual abilities, even when sober, as a result of drinking. The degree of impairment appears directly related to the amount the social drinker usually consumes each time he or she drinks; frequency of drinking does not appear important. According to Elizabeth Loftus, the evidence suggests that years of partygoing take no inevitable toll. However, it seems that as far as memory is concerned, it would be better to have one drink every day than to save up until Saturday and splurge with seven drinks.[48] Even though the same amount of alcohol is ingested in both cases, the effects on the brain are apparently different. *The amount of alcohol consumed in one setting is critical.* As research continues, additional insight should be gained into the effects of moderate drinking on the brain.

Brain atrophy has been reported in anywhere from 50 percent to 100 percent of alcoholics.[49] New evidence suggests that heavy social drinking may also result in brain atrophy. The notion that brain damage from chronic alcohol abuse is irreversible is being reexamined. Several studies have shown partial reversal of brain atrophy and neuropsychological impairment in the abstinent alcoholic. One team of researchers has suggested that the brain damage often accompanying chronic alcohol abuse is caused only in part by malnutrition. That is, those areas of the brain that are particularly vulnerable to ethanol damage—the hippocampus (part of the cerebral cortex) and the cerebellum—are affected by some as yet unclear aspect of chronic alcohol abuse distinct from malnutrition. Although the precise destructive action of alcoholism remains a mystery, members of the research team have formu-

The Amount of Alcohol Consumed in
One Sitting Is Critical
Source: Akos Szilvas/Stock Boston

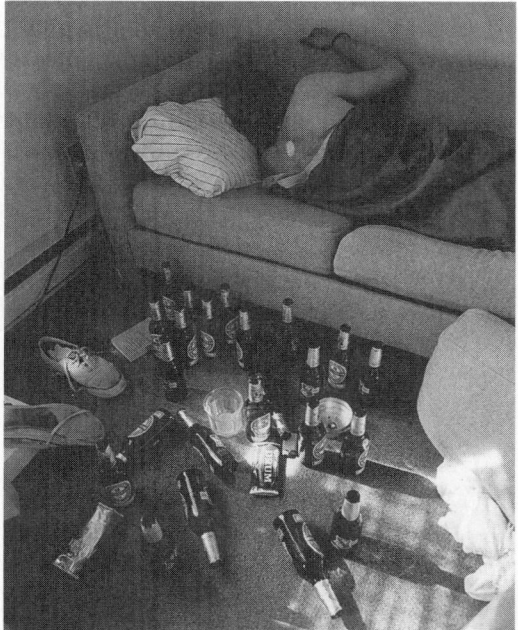

lated several hypotheses. They suggest that ethanol—or its metabolite, acetaldehyde—could be indirectly toxic by inhibiting protein synthesis in the brain. Or it could be that alcohol serves to obstruct the flow of blood to areas of the brain that mediate functioning.

Memory   Researchers at the National Institute on Alcohol Abuse and Alcoholism have shown that alcohol alters the function of the brain's N-Methyl-D-asparate (NMDA) receptor system.[50] The NMDA receptor, along with a calcium channel it controls, plays an important part in memory. Two research groups have shown that alcohol inhibits functioning of the NMDA receptor in cultured neuronal cells at concentration levels of 40 to 50 milligrams daily, a level expected in the brain areas that are thought to process memory, including the hippocampus and the cerebellum. Although it has been known that heavy drinking leads to a certain amount of brain-cell damage, this research points out that even responsible amounts of alcohol can alter the function of the brain.

Alcoholic Blackout   Alcoholic blackout refers to a state of antero-grade amnesia.[51] This is loss of memory for recent events with retention of remote ones. While the patient is intoxicated, he or she is not unconscious or even stuporous. The memory deficit often goes unnoticed until later and then is mistakenly viewed as retrograde amnesia. Retrograde amnesia is a loss of memory for events occurring before the onset of the current disease. In this state, the abuser is unable to form new memories or remember what was said even a few minutes before. Memory loss is related to isolated episodes of binge drinking, such as at fraternity initiation parties or a twenty-first-birthday celebration. Although blackouts are not necessarily a sign of alcoholism and are not always a sign of advanced disease, there is correlation between the number of blackouts an individual has in a year and the number of times the person becomes intoxicated each month.

Hangover   Anne B. Simons describes the hangover as nature's way of punishment. Symptoms include a throbbing headache, nausea, vomiting, thirst, and generally feeling like death warmed over.[52] Medically, a hangover is a mild version of alcohol withdrawal syndrome. The headache is caused by alcohol's relaxation of the blood vessels. Once stretched they impinge on the neighboring nerves and trigger pain. The nausea and vomiting are caused by alcohol's stomach irritation and its effects on the central nervous system. Thirst is caused by alcohol's diuretic action (it causes dehydration).

LIVER

Cirrhosis of the liver is one of the more serious physiological problems related to alcohol. Statistical evidence linking cirrhosis and alcohol consumption includes the following:

1. Cirrhosis is seven times as common in heavy drinkers as in nondrinkers.

Cirrhosis

After the ingestion of relatively small amounts of alcohol, the accumulation of fat in the liver can be detected. Alcohol is thought to be toxic to the liver and interferes with acetaldehyde, the intermediate by-product of alcohol metabolism. In heavy drinkers the continued use of alcohol leads to cirrhosis of the liver, which can be fatal.

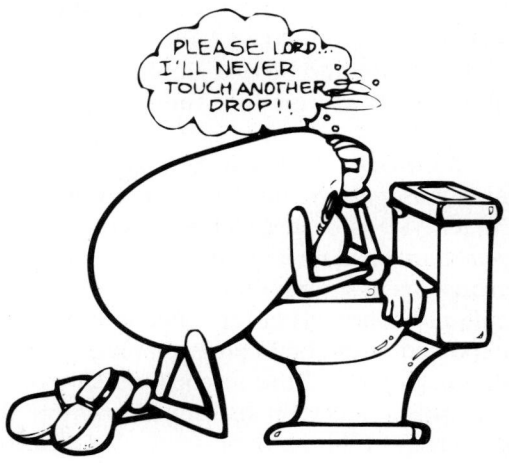

2. There is a high association of the extremes of high intake (1.5 gallons per capita) and low intake (0.5 gallons per capita).
3. There is a positive relationship between increases in intake, amount, and duration on the one hand, and cirrhosis on the other.[53]

Some scientists think that proper nutrition will provide effective protection against cirrhosis. Others have indicated that alcohol itself appears to be toxic to the liver, and that physicians should caution alcoholic patients not to rely on a nutritious diet as a safeguard and continue alcohol abuse.[54] After the ingestion of relatively small amounts of alcohol, the accumulation of fat in the liver can be detected. Cirrhosis is the sixth leading cause of death of adults in the United States, and it is estimated that alcohol is directly toxic to the liver when nutritional factors are controlled.[55]

Acetaldehyde, the intermediate by-product of alcohol metabolism, appears to be one of the major villains in the onset of alcoholic drinking, and the trouble probably begins in the liver. Researchers have found that the same amount of alcohol given to alcoholics and nonalcoholics produced much higher blood acetaldehyde levels in alcoholics. It is thought that this is due in part to a malfunctioning of the liver's enzymes. Also, the rate of breakdown of acetaldehyde into acetate is performed at about half the normal rate, apparently because of the accumulation of acetaldehyde.

DIGESTIVE SYSTEM

Moderate alcohol use may help the digestive system since it causes an increased flow of saliva and gastric juices. It may also alleviate distressing moods that interfere with digestion. Alcohol may harm digestion, however, by irritating the linings of the oral cavity, esophagus, and stomach. The pyloric sphincter, a muscle valve that separates the stomach from the small intestine, will contract and cause vomiting when sufficiently irritated by alcohol.

Because alcohol takes priority in being digested, heavy drinking that accompanies a meal may interfere with the digestion of the food.[56] The alcohol ties up the liver's transport system and uses enzymes and oxidation pathways needed for digesting food. As a result, some of the food is not converted into forms the body can use or store and necessary vitamins and minerals are lost.

While heavy drinkers consume alcohol, replacing other nutritious foods in their diet, over half the total calorie intake comes from alcohol. Similarly, drinking a lot of alcohol reduces hunger. The diets of heavy drinkers are high in fat and sodium and can result in chronic malnutrition. The liver is most susceptible.

True vitamin and mineral deficiencies occur in people who drink too much alcohol and don't eat enough food.[57] The body can become deficient in folic acid, which is important for making proteins and cell development. Another deficient mineral is zinc, which can lead to the inability to grow and heal. Hair loss, skin changes, and decreased sense of taste are also effects of zinc deficiency. Thiamin deficiency would cause the body to go through mental changes, anorexia, and muscle weakness.

A study on the effect of alcohol on body weight revealed surprising results for women: Alcohol users tended to lose weight. In contrast, there was little if any change in the body weight of men who drank.[58] It is believed that the different types of alcohol consumed may play a large part in these findings. Males drink more beer, which is more fattening; females tend to drink more wine and hard liquor.

KIDNEYS

When alcohol is consumed, blood vessels in the kidneys dilate, causing increased urine production.[59] Increased urine production is also caused when alcohol affects the brain centers responsible for maintaining body water. Excessive use of alcohol can cause permanent kidney damage.

BODY TEMPERATURE

Ingestion of alcohol induces a false feeling of warmth because it increases blood flow to the skin and stomach. Actually, the increased blood flow may cause increased sweating, resulting in rapid heat loss and the lowering of the body temperature. Large amounts of alcohol will depress the hypothalamus, the mechanism that controls body temperature, also resulting in a decrease in body temperature. Thus, drinking alcoholic beverages to keep warm in cold environments not only doesn't work but may actually facilitate hypothermia (subnormal body temperature).

FETAL ALCOHOL SYNDROME
AND FETAL ALCOHOL EFFECT

In 1973 the term *fetal alcohol syndrome* (**FAS**) was coined to designate the pattern of growth retardation, physical defects, and mental retardation found in infants born to women who drank heavily and extensively during

Fetal Alcohol Syndrome (FAS)
A pattern of growth retardation, physical defects, and mental retardation found in infants born to women who drink heavily and extensively during pregnancy. The severe cases are called FAS, while the milder cases are referred to as Fetal Alcohol Effect (FAE).

pregnancy.[60] Fetal alcohol syndrome and its more subtle variant, fetal alcohol effect (FAE), are umbrella terms used to describe the condition affecting the scarred offspring of drinking mothers.[61] There has been a lot of information recently on FAS, which happens when a pregnant woman drinks too much alcohol, causing children who have special problems such as underdevelopment, mental retardation, curvature of the spine, and facial abnormalities. What many people have not heard about, though, is the less severe form of FAS called fetal alcohol effect, which can be brought on by moderate drinking while pregnant. Effects on the child can include emotional problems, insomnia, and inability to deal with stress in school and on the job. People need to realize that any alcohol the expectant mother consumes will pass on to the bloodstream of the unborn fetus, basically causing a state of intoxication.

The Centers for Disease Control estimates that more than 8,000 alcohol-damaged babies are born each year with FAS, or 2.7 babies for every 1,000 live births, and some 65,000 with FAE.[62] Others feel that these figures are low. On some Native American reservations, 25 percent of all children are reportedly afflicted.

The University of Washington in Seattle conducted a longitudinal study on a sample of 421 mothers who reported drinking during pregnancy, and their children.[63] The researchers found a significant relationship between alcohol consumption during pregnancy and a lower IQ in the offspring.

The tragedy of FAS is that it is entirely preventable. If a woman, even an alcoholic one, stops drinking before she becomes pregnant, her fetus will not develop FAS or any alcohol-related birth defects. In other words, FAS and FAE are 100 percent preventable.

CANCER

Heavy alcohol consumption has been related to increased risk of cancer at various sites, especially the mouth, pharynx, larynx, and esophagus. Cancer risk is further increased for heavy drinkers who use tobacco.[64]

Alcohol may be a carcinogen, according to molecular biologists Heinz Fraenkel-Conrat and Bea Singer.[65] These researchers say that alcohol and acetaldehyde combine in test-tube experiments to chemically change DNA. The altered DNA is similar to that produced by other carcinogens. According to the researchers, the DNA changes occurred at concentrations of alcohol and acetaldehyde that would be found in one or two drinks. They believe that moderate alcohol consumption could cause cancer.[66]

A link between moderate alcohol consumption and breast cancer has been discovered. Women who drink more than three times a week have a 40 to 50 percent higher risk of developing breast cancer.

TESTOSTERONE LEVEL

It is now felt that alcohol can affect offspring by altering the sperm.[67] A test was conducted on male rats where they were kept continually intoxicated for 39 days, weaned from alcohol, and mated two weeks later with females who didn't drink. The results showed that in appearance the rats were the same as the control group, but when tested in a maze with food as the reward, it took them 50 percent longer to complete it. Learning and hormonal differences were found between the control and test groups. The finding correlated with findings dealing with sons of alcoholic humans.[68]

Research is currently going on to determine alcohol's effect on sperm and a connection with FAS.[69] Numerous studies have shown that acute or chronic ingestion of alcohol results in lowered testosterone in the serum of males of all species. This reduction may cause impotency, loss of libido, breast enlargement, loss of facial hair, and testicular atrophy in male alcoholics.[70]

WOMEN

Men and women respond in different ways when using alcohol. For example, compared to men of similar size who drink the same amount of alcohol as women, the women wind up with more alcohol in their bloodstream. Women are also much quicker to develop alcohol-related ailments, such as liver disease.

People used to believe that men could hold their liquor better than women because of their body size and weight. Another explanation was that women carry more fat and less water than men, and as a result, liquor in women is less diluted. Recently a team of Italian and American researchers have found a better explanation: "Women have far smaller quantities of the protective enzyme alcohol dehydrogenase that breaks down alcohol in the stomach."[71]

Researchers have made another interesting discovery concerning alcoholic men. They have found that these men have about half as much alcohol dehydrogenase as men who are not alcoholics.[72] Also, women alcoholics showed almost no alcohol dehydrogenase in their stomachs at all.

It is usually recommended that people drink moderately, but findings suggest clinicians need to redefine moderate alcohol consumption because "what is moderate for a man is not for a woman" or for patients taking certain prescription drugs.[73]

A major concern is the number of women with alcohol-abuse problems, including teenagers and women in their twenties, whose numbers have risen dramatically over the past 40 years.[74] More than 60 percent of American women now drink alcoholic beverages, the highest percentage ever. It is estimated that 12 to 16 percent are heavy drinkers (three to five drinks a day).

Women afflicted with alcoholism tend to be less visible than men. Many drink at home and alone. Therefore, alcohol abuse among women has been called a "hidden" or "invisible" problem.[75] Although women drink less than men, their alcohol-related health hazards may be greater. Many medical complications result from abuse of alcohol.

COMBINING ALCOHOL WITH OTHER DRUGS

When alcohol is mixed with other drugs, it may decrease, increase, or multiply the effects of the original drug.[76] There is a decrease in the effectiveness of the secondary substance when alcohol is combined with prescription drugs as well as when taking vitamins. Alcohol increases the effects of another drug by adding its own properties to those of the drug, as seen frequently with the use of marijuana. This particular combination has been a frequent cause of death from traffic accidents among teenagers.

The alcohol-and-other-drug combinations can also be harmful in the way they affect certain organs of the body. Chronic alcohol use can damage the liver. Alcohol also damages the heart and when combined with crack cocaine can be fatal. Even combining alcohol and aspirin may cause ulcers and internal bleeding. There is also the synergistic effect, which multiplies the drug actions. With such drugs as sedative-hypnotics and antianxiety agents, alcohol may cut the lethal dose in half.[77]

EFFECTS OF DRINKING ON THE INDIVIDUAL AND SOCIETY

At least one national survey has emphasized the *social* rather than the physical effects of drinking.[78] Adverse social effects include economic costs, interpersonal problems (a spouse, friend, or relative either threatened to break off the relationship or actually did so), problems with the police (being questioned, warned, or arrested for drinking or drunkenness), and automobile or other accidents involving personal injury or property damage.

ECONOMIC COSTS

The economic costs of alcoholism and alcohol abuse are estimated at nearly $117 billion a year, including $18 billion for premature deaths, $66 billion in reduced work effort, and $13 billion for treatment.[79]

Job-Related Problems   Alcohol consumption even in minimal amounts tends to increase the rate of accidents at work. It is estimated that about 10 to 30 percent of occupational accidents are preceded by alcohol intake. Even in modest amounts, alcohol affects the reflexes and judgment of people whose jobs involve a risk of accidents (driving or operating machines, working at heights, and so on) and people who have executive responsibility.[80]

There is evidence, especially from developed countries, that persons engaged in certain occupations are at particularly high risk of developing alcohol problems. Unfavorable psychological conditions of work (such as isolation, monotony, low pay, pressure to increase output, and lack of career opportunities) may contribute to poor morale, stressful situations, and psychological disturbance. These in turn may encourage alcohol use and lead to a new set of problems.

Motor-Vehicle Accidents   The third largest economic cost of drinking, after lost productivity and health and medical costs, is that of alcohol-related motor-vehicle accidents. The drinking driver is a menace to everyone on the road. Alcohol impairs vision, coordination, judgment, sensation of speed, and depth perception, making the driver careless or uninhibited. Of the 50,000 people killed in traffic accidents each year, half are killed by drinking drivers; millions more are injured. The risk of motor-vehicle accidents tends to increase in proportion to the blood-alcohol concentration of the driver.

Fifteen states impound the cars or license plates of people convicted of drunk driving. Massachusetts authorities may lift the license of any tavern found to have served five or more people convicted of drunk driving. Other states have developed ways to single out the drunk driver. Ohio, for example, puts orange plates on the car of a person convicted of drunk driving.

In the mid-1980s, "with oil prices and interest rates low, more and more Americans [bought] boats—and as traffic on the waterways increase[d], so [did] the toll of drinking and driving afloat."[81] Boating accidents have become the second leading cause of transportation injuries. The U.S. Coast Guard estimates that at least half of these accidents are alcohol-related. "And a National Transportation Safety Board study concludes that drinking may be a factor in 80% of the 1,000 or so boating fatalities that occur each year."[82]

According to studies, there is now substantial evidence that the legislation changing the drinking age to 21, instead of 18 or 19, has produced marked reductions in those traffic accidents that are alcohol-related.[83] Some evidence comes from the state of Michigan, which raised its drinking age to 21. There was a 16 percent reduction in single-vehicle nighttime crashes and a 19 percent reduction in police-reported, alcohol-involved injury. The insurance industry's Institute of Highway Safety conducted a study in 1985 and examined automobile fatalities of 26 states that raised the drinking age some time between 1975 and 1984. The finding shows a 13 percent reduction in fatal car crashes.

During recent years, many states have passed harsher laws for driving under the influence of alcohol. By using large fines, sentencing people to jail, and taking away licenses, states are trying to lower the percentage of drunk drivers. Along with raising the drinking age to 21, many states are passing laws stating that an individual driving with a blood-alcohol concentration of .08 instead of .10 is legally intoxicated.

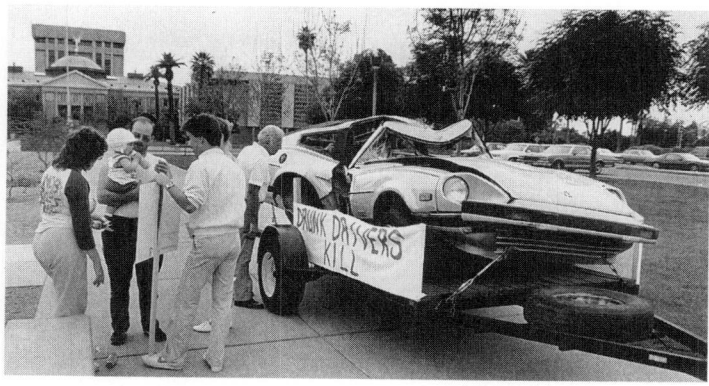

Drinking and Driving Do Not Mix
Source: Spencer Grant/Stock Boston

Nonvehicle Accidents   Research has shown that alcohol is involved in about half of nonvehicle accidents. It is implicated, for example, in up to 50 percent of adult deaths from fires, and in 50 to 68 percent of drownings.[84]

ADOLESCENT DRINKING

Although many adults chuckle over their first experiments with alcohol, youthful drinking is no joke. Alcohol is the most commonly used drug among adolescents.[85] Nearly half of all teens who commit suicide are intoxicated at the time. In 1986 more than 3,500 teens died in alcohol-related car crashes. Perhaps in part because of this, the drinking age has been changed to 21 in all states, with Wyoming being the last to convert, in the summer of 1987.[86] The earlier a person begins drinking, the greater his or her risk of becoming an alcoholic.[87]

ADOLESCENTS AND ALCOHOL

- One out of ten people who drink becomes alcoholic. This amounts to about 17 million Americans, 4.5 million of whom are teenagers.
- One out of 20 high school seniors drinks daily.
- The average age people start drinking is now 12.9 years.
- Of the 25,000 people who die each year in drunk-driving accidents, 5,000 are 15-to-19-year-olds. Fourteen teenagers die each day in drunk-driver accidents.
- Adolescents are the only age group in which the mortality rate has increased in the past 20 years. This is largely due to drunk-driving accidents.

Source: Roberts, Fitzmahan, and Associates, *Teen and Alcohol* (Portland: Oregon Drug and Alcohol Information Center, 1987).

EFFECTS OF ALCOHOL
BY ETHNIC GROUP AND RACE

Alcohol has existed for thousands of years. Some ethnic groups—the Jews and Italians, for example—have used alcohol for 7,000 years or more. These groups experience relatively low rates of alcoholism.[88] At the other end of the spectrum, Native Americans and Eskimos have been exposed to alcohol for only 200 to 300 years. Their rates of alcoholism are quite high, perhaps 80 to 90 percent in some areas.

Lower rates of alcoholism are also found among East Asians.[89] Studies indicate that roughly half of all Japanese men exhibit the flushing response to alcohol. Men with this response have been found to be significantly less likely than men without the response to drink daily, to drink during the day, and to stop at bars. These men, according to research, metabolize all the alcohol they consume, and thus none is left over to be converted to acetaldehyde. Apparently these men appear to be missing a gene present in some alcoholics.[90] Comparing the habits of Caucasians with homeland Asians as well as American Asians reveals that many Asians lack the enzyme ADLH-I, which is produced by the liver and is used in metabolizing alcohol.[91]

CRIME

Alcohol is closely associated with certain forms of crime. Individuals under the influence resort more frequently to physical assaults, domestic violence, disorderly conduct, and rape. In the case of homicide, a blood-alcohol level above .10 has been found in 67 percent of offenders nationwide determined to be drinking at the time of the crime. For aggravated assault, the figure is an estimated 80 percent.[92] The combined cost of violent crimes and the social responses to alcohol problems is estimated at over $10 billion per year.

THE HOMELESS

Chronic alcoholics and drug abusers are now the fastest-growing group among those living in the streets and shelters, so much so that substance abuse is slightly *more* prevalent among the new homeless than among their predecessors of the 1950s and 1960s, when the skid-row image of the homeless was predominant.[93] Almost 40 percent of the homeless are substance abusers and chronic alcoholics. Three main reasons for this emergence of out-of-control homeless people include the reduction of available shelters or "skid rows" in lieu of urban-renewal projects, the decriminalization of vagrancy and public drunkeness, and the emergence of highly addictive crack.[94]

VIOLENCE

About 100,000 deaths occur and approximately 500,000 people are injured each year because of alcohol.[95] Generally speaking, when people drink they become more aggressive and less afraid. As a result, alcohol plays an important role in violent crimes. A study conducted at the University of New Mexico reported that 35 percent of rapists were alcoholics and half were drinking at the time of rape.[96] Another college study found that 55 percent of the men who acknowledged committing a sexual assault were under the influence of alcohol, and 53 percent of the women who were victims were under the influence.[97] Also, each year 30,000 suicides have alcohol in their blood at the time of their death.

Alcohol is also a cause of many accidents on and off the road. Over half the drowning victims have been drinking. A French study found 69 percent of abuse and neglect cases were related to alcohol abuse.[98]

SUICIDE

More men than women commit suicide, but suicide attempts are more frequent by women. Suicide is one of the more frequent causes of death among alcoholics.[99] This relationship between alcoholism and suicide has been related to depression and other psychiatric disorders, to erosion of social networks, and to disrupted interpersonal relationships.

The risk of suicide among alcoholics is about 30 times greater than it is in the general population. Among Native Americans, five of the top ten causes of death are alcohol-related: accidents, cirrhosis, alcoholism, suicide, and homicide. Among ethnic groups, Native Americans appear to have the highest prevalence of drinking problems. According to figures released by the Indian Health Service, suicide rates among Indians below age 35 are 2.4 to 3.3 times as great as they are among all U.S. citizens in the same age groups.[100] According to Calvin Frederic, chief of the Disaster Assistance and Mental Health Section of the National Institute of Mental Health, many Native Americans

> don't feel they have anywhere to go. They're caught between a desire to move out of their own sphere into a more modern society and a desire to maintain the traditions of their old lives. Yet the realities of today make it impossible to continue their old way of life. They wind up frustrated. They drink heavily, become depressed, and become self destructive.[101]

The self-destruction takes the form of accidents, murders, and suicides.

WARNING LABELS

The surgeon general is attempting to get the word out on the potential danger of alcohol by affixing warning labels.[102] The labels would warn that alcohol may be addictive, that there are risks of hypertension, cancer, and liver disease; in addition they would warn against drunk driving and fetal alcohol syndrome. But will true problem drinkers or alcoholics take notice?

ALCOHOLISM

WHAT IS ALCOHOLISM?

There are some who believe alcoholism is a disease, and some who do not. According to one definition, alcoholism is "a chronic disease, or disorder of behavior, characterized by the repeated drinking of alcoholic beverages to an extent that exceeds customary dietary use or ordinary compliance with the social drinking customs of the community, and which interferes with the drinker's health, interpersonal relations or economic functioning."[103] The American Medical Association had earlier come to a similar conclusion, and in 1956 it formally acknowledged that alcoholism was to be included in the treatment realm of medical science. Furthermore, both the American Medical Association and the American Bar Association have declared that alcoholics are entitled to the same rights and privileges under the law and the same medical treatment granted to persons with other diseases. The National Institute on Alcohol Abuse and Alcoholism views alcoholism as a treatable dysfunction from which as many as two thirds of those affected can recover (though they cannot return to drinking). Many states now allow chronic alcoholism to be a defense against drunkenness charges and refer chronic drunk drivers to appropriate treatment resources rather than sending them to jail.

By the most conservative estimates, 10 percent of the people in this country suffer from alcoholism. The average alcoholic affects four or more people—family and friends—in a serious way. That means that 50 percent of the population of the United States live in close contact with alcoholism, a disease that affects people physically, mentally, emotionally, and spiritually.[104]

When discussing alcoholism, chemical dependency, and/or physiological addiction to alcohol, we need to keep in mind the three phenomena of tolerance, withdrawal, and compulsive use. Alcohol use is a response to the relationship between *tolerance* and *withdrawal.* Withdrawal leads to irritability and sickness. *Compulsive use* is a result of high tolerance and the desire to avoid withdrawal. It is the absolute need to keep the system medicated with the quantity of alcohol needed to prevent withdrawal symptoms.

Alcoholism is a chronic disease. In many cases it is present years prior to diagnosis. It is a progressive disorder: Left untreated, it intensifies. It is a disease, interestingly enough, that seems to continue despite sobriety; alcoholics who decide to resume drinking do not start at the beginning but continue where they would have been had they not stopped drinking. Even in the absence of alcohol use, characteristics of the disease seem to continue developing.

The biochemistry of the disease can be explained in fairly simple terms. The ethanol molecule, when ingested, is quickly metabolized in the blood system, primarily by the liver. The initial stages of metabolism by hepatic protein enzymes result in alcohol being transformed into acetaldehyde, which is closely related to the famous pickling agent formaldehyde. Because of its poisonous nature it is quickly transformed into acidic acid (vinegar) and then into carbon dioxide and water, which are eliminated through breathing and urination. This process occurs when normal drinkers consume alcohol. However, the metabolism of an alcoholic is dramatically different in one sense. Though most of the alcohol is transformed and eliminated in the fashion just described, approximately 1 percent of it is diverted to an alternative fate. It is this fate that results in biochemical dependency. This very small percentage of residual alcohol combines with the neurotransmitter dopamine to form an addictive alkaloid called **tetrahydraisoquardrelone (THIQ)**. This substance is closely related to the opium family, especially morphine. Furthermore, THIQ combines with other neurotransmitters in the central nervous system to form other similarly addictive alcoholoids. It is now thought that for the most part these substances are not truly metabolized and eliminated from the central nervous system; they remain within the system to act, it appears, much in the same fashion as heroin. Hence, "once an alcoholic, always an alcoholic," for reasons similar to those causing opiate dependency. This explains why after 20 years of sobriety one may return to the use of alcohol.

Tetrahydraisoquardrelone (THIQ)

Most of alcohol is transformed and eliminated by the body; however, approximately 1 percent of it is diverted to an alternative fate. It is this fate that results in biochemical dependency. This very small percentage of residual alcohol combines with the neurotransmitter dopamine to form an addictive alkaloid called tetrahydraisoquardrelone (THIQ). This substance is closely related to the opium family, especially morphine. THIQ combines with other neurotransmitters in the central nervous system to form other similarly addictive alcoholoids.

Though the jury is still out on this theory, it appears that several supplemental factors are occurring simultaneously in a number of alcoholics. One of these is that the livers of many alcoholics have an insufficiency of ADH (alcoholdehydrogenase). This insufficiency lowers their ability to metabolize alcohol at a sufficient rate. Hence, the active ingredient remains in the system longer in an alcoholic than in normal drinkers. One can hypothesize that this prolonged presence in the system allows more diversion of the alcohol to the "dopamine connection."

Furthermore, it appears that a person can not only contract a carrier-type and pass it on through birth but can also become a transmitter, even if there is no prior history of alcoholism in the family. People from nonalcoholic families who eventually drink to the point of developing the disorder can transfer the carrier-type to their children. Research on these theories is still being evaluated, but it appears they will eventually be proved true.

There is also a psychological component to this biochemical model that further predisposes one to alcoholism. The behavioral theory of learning has two major aspects: instrumental or operant conditioning and classical conditioning. The first includes the stimulus-response-reward relationship, in which a precipitating factor causes the individual to respond by consuming alcohol; the reward consists of the desired effects. One of the best examples is the five o'clock happy hour on Friday afternoon following a hard day (or week) of work. People meet at their favorite watering hole to respond to that hard period of work by consuming alcohol for the desired effect of conviviality, good cheer, and relaxation. Most people drink in partial response to this behavioral principle. The stimuli may be varied, the response is to drink, and the rewards may also vary. The classical-conditioning aspect consists of anticipation of the reward prior to the consumption of alcohol. The anticipated feeling of relaxation furthers the reinforcement offered by that upcoming drinking episode.

Heredity may be an important factor in predisposition to certain reactions to alcohol.[105] In human studies, twins raised in different family settings tended toward the same alcohol-related behaviors. The implication that genetic makeup can have an effect is gaining support. However, one should note that fewer than half of all children of an alcoholic parent develop alcohol problems, and only a portion of those become dependent.

The central nervous system is where the physical differences would be manifested if genetics are an important factor in predisposition. Some studies suggest that brain electrical activity in alcoholics and nonalcoholics differ in fundamental ways.[106] Further, they suggest that these changes are in place largely before dependence, and this becomes an argument for the genetic model. Other studies have examined electrical makeup possibly related to dependence.

Some recent findings tend to confirm long-suspected genetic links in alcoholism.[107] Children of alcoholic parents were four times more at risk of becoming alcoholics themselves, even if they were raised by nonalcoholic adoptive parents.

Recently, medical researchers unveiled what looks like a partial answer. Their suspect: a gene that affects the brain's handling of dopamine, one of the chemicals involved in the body's response to alcohol. Kenneth Blum of the University of Texas, San Antonio, and Ernest Noble of UCLA reported that an aberrant form of the so-called dopamine D_2 receptor gene was strongly associated with alcoholism in the small group of people they studied.[108] The finding could lead to radical new strategies for preventing and treating drinking problems, but it won't yield a complete explanation of why people become alcoholics. Even if larger studies confirm the role of the D_2 receptor gene, it will remain but one piece of a large and complex puzzle.[109]

At adulthood, those with alcoholic parents were four times more likely to be alcoholics. Also, the costs of alcoholism to the person, family, and country are staggering. "One of four hospital beds are filled by someone with an alcohol-related problem. Twenty percent of the nation's total health-care costs of 427 billion dollars are attributable to alcohol use. And finally, thirty-eight percent of all families listed alcohol-related problems."[110]

Appetite needs are normally met by a dampening mechanism that comes from satisfactory interpersonal relations. But when a boy or a girl cannot relate effectively to the parent of the same sex, the normal mechanism for dampening a particular need is unavailable. Because of this, alcohol offers a medicinal effect when consumed. Individuals in an alcohol-using society discover sooner or later that alcohol either allows them to relate to others or relieves them of the sense of need to do so. Either way, alcohol use is perceived by the alcoholic to be a solution. It is not an accident that Alcoholics Anonymous is as successful as it is because of the emotional bonding occurring within its group structure. There are a number of stages in alcoholism:

1. *The well individual.* The use of alcohol has not yet damaged the individual's physical, social, or economic capacities. There is no reason for concern regarding his or her use of alcohol.

2. *The episodic excessive drinker.* The frequency of drinking has begun to increase to the point where the individual is visibly intoxicated up to 12 times per year. Initial signs of health impairment do not necessarily include evidence of addiction. However, there may be secondary damage related to alcohol—trauma (a shocklike effect on the system) or accident—and also primary damage (reversible). Other symptoms may include transient nutritional deficiencies that reverse with the cessation of drinking and proper nutritional treatment.

3. *The habitual excessive drinker.* Intoxication episodes equal or surpass 13 per year. Damage to health continues as in stage 2. Interpersonal and social relationships begin to show signs of deterioration as the individual loses long-time friends, is separated or divorced, and so on. Social relationships now *necessarily* involve alcohol use and other heavy users. Economic costs progress to the loss of employment because of alcohol abuse. The individual may be temporarily employed in a setting in which the employer has a specific interest in treating alcoholism and is inclined to tie job security to a treatment plan promoting recovery.

4. *Alcohol addiction; physiological changes.* The frequency of drinking has progressed to the point of inability to abstain even one day. Health continues to deteriorate: There is additional documentation of withdrawal symptomatology, including delirium tremens, hallucinations, shakes, sweats, whips-and-jangles seizures, and so on. Interpersonal and social relationships continue to deteriorate, as does the individual's capacity for financial self-support.

5. *Alcohol addiction; irreversible damage.* The frequency of drinking continues as in stage 4, with further evidence of permanent physiological deterioration. There are a variety of areas in which the body can be dramatically harmed, including the hepatic, gastrointestinal, cardiovascular, and central and peripheral nervous systems. A variety of psychiatric concerns can develop, such as Korsicoff's syndrome and Wernicky's disorder. In this late stage of deterioration one can lose control of the bladder and bowels as well. These are only a few examples of the excessive medical deterioration that develops in the late stages of alcoholism.

6. *Death.*

These stages include a variety of specific cognitive-behavioral indicators by which the disease can be diagnosed. Many of these indicators appear among virtually all alcoholics. Some of the indicators are as follows:

1. *Symptomatic drinking.* The drinker begins to use alcohol to satisfy conditions of his or her inner environment, for personal rather than social reasons. The social setting becomes an excuse, rather than the reason, for drinking.

2. *Increased tolerance.* The individual can drink more with less apparent effects. The psychophysiological systems adapt to the presence of the ethanol molecule so effectively that larger quantities of alcohol are tolerated.

3. *Blackouts (alcoholic amnesia).* The individual has no recall of events during these periods, which can last from several minutes to several hours or days. During the blackouts the individual may not appear to be intoxicated and may carry on conversations or perform a variety of other behavioral functions, such as driving a car with apparent control. However, at a later date the individual cannot remember any of the events taking place.

4. *Sneaking drinks.* Because of his rising tolerance to alcohol and dependence on its anxiety-relieving properties, the individual needs to drink more in order to gain satisfaction from the experience. A need arises to find ways to consume more alcohol than his companions without revealing himself. The individual may drink before going to a party or bring along a concealed supply to be consumed away from companions. This is often quite confusing to his social-drinking friends, who may see him becoming intoxicated while apparently consuming the same quantity as other guests. This is the

same individual who is embarrassed when observed drinking in a secluded area.

5. *Preoccupation with drinking.* Drinking has now become an increasingly important role in the individual's life and seems to dominate her thinking.

6. *Gulping drinks.* The individual is becoming more and more concerned with the biochemical effects of alcohol and is less concerned with the social setting and conviviality.

7. *Avoidance of references to drinking.* Sensing the change in his drinking behavior and probably experiencing some related guilt, the individual tends to avoid discussions of his drinking behavior. When such discussions are unavoidable, he understates the amount and frequency of his drinking. This is a hallmark characteristic of alcoholism.

8. *Increased frequency of blackouts.* The fear and discomfort created by the frequency of blackouts is overshadowed by the individual's need to secure the medicinal effects of alcohol.

9. *Loss of control.* Gradually, and often imperceptibly to the individual, she exercises less and less control of the amount consumed, intending 1 or 2 but having 10 or 15. This loss of control often identifies itself in the form of a series of "benders." The individual may be able to abstain for relatively long periods, but with the first ingestment of a small quantity of alcohol a demand is set that ceases only when advanced intoxication makes further intake impossible—in other words, drinking to the point of passing out. Once drinking has begun, only situational or circumstantial factors stop it, such as running out of alcohol or money or becoming physically unable to continue drinking. Interventions on the part of concerned others will also stop drinking in this instance. The individual may seek to sustain a certain amount of alcohol in her system 24 hours a day.

10. *Creation of an alibi system.* With loss of control the patient begins to develop a system of excuses. The individual believes these rationalizations and feels that his drinking is a result rather than a cause of the problems.

11. *Reproof by family.* If the alcoholic is married, drinking will affect the family, materially and emotionally, and family members will react with pleading, cajoling, threats, and other forms of emotional bribery in an effort to stop the alcoholic's drinking. Eventually the family rejects the alcoholic.

12. *Extravagance.* The alcoholic will often become extravagant, "buying the house a drink," placing long-distance phone calls, or making unnecessary or costly purchases. Quite often this is done while she is intoxicated.

13. *Aggression.* As the illness progresses the individual may reveal deep-seated but repressed hostility through aggressive behavior. He will often strike out at those closest to him—family members and close friends. The individual may also unconsciously use this aggressive behavior as a

means of seeking rejection to confirm his own feelings of inadequacy and to once again give himself an excuse for continued drinking.

14. *Persistent remorse.* Following periods of heavy drinking the alcoholic is plagued by persistent deep guilt and remorse, and on some level she is aware of the effect of her drinking on her own life as well as those of family members. This characteristic often involves sincere promises to herself and others to modify her drinking behavior. These attempts are usually unsuccessful.

15. *Water wagon.* The individual resolves to take control of himself in a very drastic fashion by stopping drinking altogether. Usually, however, he relapses and resumes his drinking patterns.

16. *Changes in drinking pattern.* After unsuccessful attempts to go on the wagon, the alcoholic will try other forms of controlling her drinking—switching types of beverages, drinking only at certain times or only in certain places, and so on.

17. *Loss of friends.* By now the use of alcohol has become so problematic that the individual begins to lose even his best friends. At this point, because of the rejection of people he has known over a long period, the individual is forced to drink with people he may at one point have considered his inferiors. However, these are people with whom he shares a common denominator—alcohol dependency.

18. *Vocational difficulties.* The person's alcoholism interferes with her ability to secure and maintain gainful employment. Typically, she drinks on the job, is absent because of hangovers, is late for work, and is less productive and more hazardous in her behavior. Frequent job changes and firings occur.

19. *Changing family habits.* The individual's family pattern changes in response to his unpredictable behavior. The family begins to withdraw from social and community activities; the children's performance in school may drastically deteriorate, and children may isolate themselves from their peers. Hostility, guilt, and aggression strain the family to the breaking point.

20. *Medical complications.* Many alcoholics experience physical difficulties due in part to their generally poor nutrition and the presence of extremely high amounts of alcohol and acetaldehyde in their system. A variety of medical disorders can occur.

21. *Resentment.* The individual becomes increasingly resentful of her growing isolation from the community, her family, and her friendship group. A certain amount of paranoia and suspiciousness culminates in feelings of persecution.

22. *The geographic cure.* With his world falling around him and having failed to abstain or modify his drinking behavior, the alcoholic may attempt to control his drinking by seeking a completely new environment. This means packing the bags and moving; it may or may not include the family.

23. *Protecting the supply.* The illness has reached such a point that alcohol is the only salvation. It is the only means of escaping from or dealing with a world that is increasingly frustrating and painful. The thought of being caught without the ability to drink becomes frightening. At this point the individual will foresake almost everything else to safeguard the means of supplying alcohol.

24. *Morning drinking.* The medicinal value of alcohol now requires the individual to start drinking from the moment she gets up. This drinking continues throughout the day and into the evening, when the individual literally drinks herself to sleep. Morning drinking is often done in response to severe hangovers as well.

25. *The moment of truth.* At this point the alcoholic has reached rock bottom. Death faces him squarely. He is at the crossroads in his life, forced to make a decision between life and death. The sad reality is that 35 of 36 alcoholics not in treatment (not choosing prolonged sobriety) die!

CAUSES

Although research indicates a significant relationship between hereditary (genetic) factors and alcoholism, results from such research remain inconclusive. Since alcoholism occurs in the children of total abstainers, social environment may also be a factor. Finally, physiological factors, such as nutritional deficiencies and/or lowered blood-chloride levels, may contribute to alcoholism. Acetaldehyde synthesis and metabolism may be the keys to explaining biochemical alcohol dependency. Further research in all these areas is crucial.

Several studies focusing on alcoholism in twins indicate a genetic factor in drinking behavior. However, the evidence for a genetic *determinant* remains inconsistent. Studies done with adoptees separated at an early age from their biological parents indicate that sons and daughters of alcoholics are four times as likely to become alcoholics as are sons and daughters of nonalcoholics, whether raised by alcoholic parents or nonalcoholic parents.[111] In a study of familial incidence of alcoholism, "rates of alcoholism [were found to be] substantially higher in relatives of alcoholics than in relatives of nonalcoholics."[112] Among the conclusions from that study are these:

> Almost one-third of any sample of alcoholics will have at least one parent who was an alcoholic; if one member of a family is an alcoholic, 82 percent of the time there is at least one other alcoholic in the family; while data support the widely held view that alcoholism can be a familial disease, it is important to realize that [this] is not sufficient to allow the finding of a hereditary or environmental etiology of alcoholism.[113]

The usefulness of studies seeking genetic factors in alcoholic families is limited by the environmental influences of an alcoholic household. Even so, the risk for alcoholism in identical and fraternal twins has been compared in research. Twins share a very similar environment, so theoretically they should develop equal rates of the disorder. Identical twins share 100 percent of their genes, fraternal twins 50 percent. If genetic influences exist, then identical twins should have a higher incidence of alcoholism. Most recent studies have born this out, finding twice the incidence of the disorder among identical twins. Adopted-away children of alcoholics—those who are raised by someone other than biological relatives—have offered the strongest evidence of genetic influences in alcoholism. The data have consistently shown a three- to fourfold increase in risk for sons of alcoholics who were adopted away, even if they were raised in an nonalcoholic environment.[114] These data reinforce the findings of the research by Rutstein and colleagues cited earlier.

Theodore Reich suggests that six factors are inherited in families susceptible to alcoholism:[115]

1. Personality traits.
2. The addictive process.
3. Protective factors: These are shown with respect to alcohol-dehydrogenase deficiency. This can also lead to protection within the *environment.*
4. Psychiatric disorders: Community as well as hospital samples show comorbidity of alcoholism and psychiatric disorders in families. This condition is, unfortunately, not rare in children.
5. Medical complications: Neurological damage may be passed on and may lead to alcoholism (and related problems).
6. Effects on chromosomes and/or female reproduction. These exemplify problems other than genetic.

Recent research indicates that a disorder called antisocial personality (ASP) may be genetically linked to alcoholism. ASP shows up in childhood and is characterized by "impulsivity, egocentricity, short attention span, sensation-seeking, aggressiveness, and poor socialization."[116] Twenty-five percent of the alcoholic population has this disorder, compared with about 3 percent of the general population. Psychiatrist Ralph Tarter contends that these characteristics in children may be "a behavioral manifestation of a genetic vulnerability to both alcoholism and ASP."[117]

That ASP appears to have a genetic component is significant. Certain childhood disorders precede the development of ASP, alcoholism, or both. One such disorder is attention deficit, which can result in short attention span, impulsivity, and hyperactivity. Tarter, after several extensive studies, has concluded that there is a severe form of alcoholism, linked with behavioral tendencies, that may be associated with brain defect. This defect occurs in the areas of the brain that control temperament and behavior.[118]

There are also some who feel that an "alcoholic personality" is a cause of alcoholism. According to this theory, individuals who find tension relief through alcohol may in time become behaviorally conditioned by the positive reinforcement. Unfortunately, research in this area is often contradictory and nonspecific. Researchers have found significant relationships, however, between a person's self-concept and alcoholism.[119] Alcoholics often have dependent personalities and lack a good self-image.

B-ENDORPHINS

Endorphins are substances released from the limbic system in the brain that have been tied to learning, memory, sex drive, temperature regulation, hormone regulation during puberty, reproduction, and mental illnesses such as depression and schizophrenia. These opioid peptide compounds react with receptors on certain brain cells located in known pain pathways and centers; they also interact with B-endorphins. B-endorphins are found in large concentrations in the limbic system and cerebral spinal fluid. They inhibit the firing of certain neurons and also produce a sense of euphoria. Immediately after exercise many athletes experience a "runner's high" caused by B-endorphin release in the limbic system. B-endorphins, therefore, contribute to a sense of well-being and pain reduction. When ethanol is ingested, it results in postsynaptic membrane transport changes that increase opiate-receptor stimulation. Alcohol has been shown to increase exogenous B-endorphin levels, while decreasing endogenous production.[120] Research by Genazzani and colleagues suggests that although similar conditions exist for other narcotic substances, those substances do not alter the natural levels of B-endorphins and enkephalins as much as ethanol does.[121]

In 1983 Blum developed a "psychogenetic theory of drug-seeking behavior," hypothesizing that individuals who are prone to drug abuse have a genetic deficiency in their peptidyl opiate systems.[122] Blum also contends that continued exposure to ethanol may be caused by the fact that long-term use depresses endogenous peptidyl opiate production. In a nutshell, the more one drinks, the fewer natural opiates one produces endogenously, and the more one needs to drink to feel good.[123]

Genazzani and colleagues studied 29 alcoholics and discovered that their ACTH (adrenocorticotrophic hormone) levels were four times normal levels.[124] ACTH is released by the pituitary gland in response to stress. It can inhibit the activity of endorphins, resulting in greater overall stress. These researchers also found that the B-endorphin levels of their population were less than one-third that of normal.[125]

BLOOD ENZYMES

Although alcohol abuse is not difficult to identify, the line between alcoholism and heavy drinking is often indistinguishable. However, molecular pharmacologist Boris Tabakoff states that blood-enzyme testing shows a great deal of promise in testing for alcoholism.[126] Tabakoff and his team examined the blood of 128 males— 95 alcoholics and 33 nonalcoholics. By examining the activity of two enzymes, monoamine oxidase and adeylate cyclase, they were able to identify three quarters of the alcoholics and nonalcoholics. Tabakoff found a decrease in monoamine oxidase activity when the samples were saturated with alcohol. Adeylate cyclase activity also decreased when exposed to cesium fluoride. This outcome occurred in all blood samples taken from the alcoholics. Tabakoff and many other scientists believe that the accuracy of such tests will be dramatically improved as they are repeated and refined, resulting in what may become a foolproof test for alcoholism.

BIOLOGICAL MARKER

Researchers at the University of Wisconsin–Madison may have discovered a biological marker associated with alcoholism.[127] Phosphatidylethanol is an alcohol derivative. A simple blood test could determine susceptibility to alcoholism. These researchers discovered phosphatidylethanol while studying ways to regulate growth of cancer cells. When an alcohol solvent was used in these experiments, phosphatidylethanol was produced. Tests were conducted on 24 alcoholic men from 18 years of age to 52 years of age and 24 nonalcoholic men with no family history of alcoholism. "Men were tested because they have a greater risk of inheriting a predisposition to alcoholism." Results indicated that "almost half the alcoholics registered phosphatidylethanol levels about twice those observed in the nonalcoholic group and in the remaining alcoholics."[128] Far more information about the effects of phosphatidylethanol on alcoholism are now being conducted.

BRAIN

Alcohol abuse is linked with serotonin levels and "turnover" in the brain. Alcohol appears to play an important part in speeding up the turnover, and probably the depletion as well, of serotonin in the brain.[129]

Studies suggest that low serotonin turnover in the brain might be a factor in violent suicide attempts by depressed people. Researchers have found that impulsive arsonists and impulsive violent offenders with antisocial or intermittent-explosive personality disorders have a low concentration of the major metabolite of serotonin in the cerebrospinal fluid and show a tendency toward low blood sugar after an oral sugar load.[130]

Most of these people turn to alcohol for self-medication, which proves to be counterproductive. Alcohol does cause an immediate increase in the release of serotonin from presynaptic neurons, but chronic alcohol use may actually cause a deficiency in serotonergic neurotransmission.

Abnormal brain patterns, particularly in sons of alcoholics, seem to be the key to the elusive "biological marker" for alcoholism that many researchers are looking for. Begleiter and colleagues discovered that both alcoholic fathers and their sons had significantly low P3 voltage readings compared with the nonalcoholic population. They concluded that reduced P3 amplitude may indicate a predisposition to alcoholism.[131]

TYPES OF ALCOHOLICS

Blum has suggested that alcoholics can be divided into three categories according to existing biochemical differences.[132] He theorizes that type 1 alcoholics have a genetic deficiency of endogenous opiates; type 2 individuals have high stress levels that correspond with elevated amounts of ACTH, and a low level of endogenous opiates; and type 3 alcoholics begin drinking for unknown reasons, but as they consume more and more alcohol, endogenous B-endorphin production decreases and receptor sites are altered. Because type 3 alcoholics experience a decline in the effectiveness of

B-endorphin systems, they find themselves drinking more and more to achieve an everyday sense of well-being.

ALCOHOLISM AMONG WOMEN

In recent years there has been a marked increase in the number of reported female alcoholics, and some researchers estimate that nearly half of the country's 10 million alcoholics are female.[133] Although there is no typical alcoholic woman, there appear to be social and emotional problems that distinguish women alcoholics from men. In addition, female alcoholics seem to share certain physical characteristics and notable behavior patterns. For example, women alcoholics who have been the subjects of studies have said they felt warm, loving, considerate, and expressive when drinking.

For years there has been a double standard of acceptable behavior for women, one that does not include drinking. For example, the heavy-drinking man is often accepted but a heavy-drinking woman is often criticized.[134] In some social settings, drinking by women may be associated with sophistication and maturity. But in general, it has been stigmatized as immoral, a betrayal of a woman's "proper role" of wife and mother. It is becoming increasingly difficult for the modern woman to conform to society's expectations, to achieve the "superwoman" goal of playing the roles of career woman, wife, mother, lover, and so on, while maintaining a sense of family.[135]

There are some indications that women's new lifestyle is changing their drinking habits and placing them in different drinking situations. A study of suburban and urban populations of women alcoholics showed that the suburban housewife is the most secretive in her drinking and the professional woman the least secretive.[136] The National Institute on Alcohol Abuse and Alcoholism reports that eight of ten working women between the ages of 21 and 34 drink, and that the average age of working women who drink dropped during the 1970s from 40 to 30. In fact, almost two of three women now being treated for alcoholism are under 35.[137] Also, there is a higher rate of alcoholism among employed women than among homemakers; married working women are especially prone.[138]

Women's roles and responsibilities have changed dramatically since the early 1970s. Paralleling their rise in status, opportunity, and pay, however, has been an increase in stress, aggression, stress-related diseases, and alcoholism.[139]

The now widespread phenomenon of alcoholism in women can be attributed to an increase in their actual number, an increase in the number of women alcoholics "coming out of the closet," or both.[140] Even in adolescents, the drinking patterns of boys and girls are converging to the point that many girls are as likely to drink as much as boys.

The guilt expressed by female alcoholics in treatment predominates most counseling sessions.[141] Their drinking is often covered and protected by spouse and family, which often delays them from seeking treatment. The husband is often embarrassed by his wife's drinking and feels it may reflect poorly on his masculinity, so he tries to hide the problem. Interestingly, a husband is more likely to leave a wife with alcohol problems than a wife is to leave an alcohol-abusing husband.[142]

TREATMENT AND REHABILITATION SERVICES

Although there are many places that an alcoholic can go for help, no recovery program will succeed until the alcoholic recognizes that his or her alcoholism is a problem and, most important, accepts the need for help. The alcoholic must be determined to recover and ready to seek a solution. Since each person is different, the individual's recovery program depends on the length of addiction and the attitudes of family and friends. A good environment is a key to success for the recovering alcoholic. When an alcoholic who is committed to recovery reverts to drinking, this does not mean that the treatment has failed. Rather, it could be viewed as confirmation to the alcoholic that abstinence is the only alternative.

Though myths, stigmas, and misunderstandings make it difficult for the alcohol-dependent person to obtain the help he or she needs, a wide variety of facilities, programs, and agencies do exist to treat alcoholism. The philosophies and methods of these programs differ, but the ultimate goal of each is to either stop or control the intake of alcohol. Generally available services include alcoholism-information programs, general hospitals, mental-health facilities, and rehabilitation clinics. Halfway houses, outpatient clinics, community human-service organizations, and volunteer-run organizations such as Alcoholics Anonymous (AA) are also located in many areas.

Volunteer-Run Organizations   Alcoholics Anonymous is probably the best-known alcoholism-treatment organization run by volunteers. Unlike other organizations, AA does not participate in political or public policy action related to either the causes of or the problems associated with alcoholism. Its activities are devoted only to maintaining and encouraging abstinence by alcoholics.

General Hospitals   Until recently, general hospitals offered little or no treatment for alcohol dependents. The American Hospital Association now has a national plan, however, to promote alcoholism programs in all general hospitals and to extend such programs into community treatment systems for alcoholics.[143] Hospital admission policies have also been changed in order to admit alcoholics with the diagnosis of alcoholism into general wards. Specialized wards in certain hospitals have been made available to the nonprofessional community to provide and conduct alcoholism programs.

Intermediate Care (Halfway Houses)   After failing many times to move the alcoholic from the therapeutic milieu back into community life, alcoholic rehabilitation workers saw the need for some form of intermediate care. The result of this need was the halfway house, where information about alcoholism could be disseminated, shelter and security provided, and residents eased back into a life of sobriety and community living. Halfway houses are sometimes given governmental support but are usually run by nonprofit community groups interested in alcoholism treatment and recovery. Professionals may be available for medical or psychological treatment.

TREATMENT APPROACHES

Drug Treatment   For many years, various drugs have been used to treat alcoholic patients. Recently, however, clinical examinations and controlled double-blind studies have shown that these drugs are not as effective as they were once thought to be.[144] The early success of most of the drugs appears to have been due to the patient's eagerness to be cured, rather than to the drugs' ability to cure. Some of these drugs, including disulfiram (Antabuse), tranquilizers, antidepressants, and lithium, are still utilized in treating alcohol dependency, but they are only one component of a total treatment program.

DISULFIRAM (ANTABUSE).   As we have seen, alcohol ingestion causes an increased acetaldehyde concentration in the blood. Antabuse appears to inhibit liver enzymes that are needed to oxidize acetaldehyde, producing symptoms that serve as a deterrent to further alcohol drinking.[145]

Antabuse has a slow absorption rate and may take from 3 hours to 12 hours to become effective. Tolerance and dependency do not develop, but the interaction of the drug with alcohol may produce numerous adverse effects, such as a rise in blood pressure, deep flushing, a sensation of warmth, decreased respiratory efficiency and oxygen debt, accelerated heart rate, severe dizziness, nausea, and vomiting. A rapid fall in blood pressure, unconsciousness, and death are extreme possibilities. Antabuse should therefore be administered only after a complete physical examination and under close medical supervision.

Despite widespread use of Antabuse, some clients can have serious adverse reactions to the drug, including strong psychotic reactions. In fact, the widespread practice of court-mandated Antabuse therapy for repeat alcohol offenders may not be producing the intended effects, since the best treatment rates with Antabuse are seen when clients voluntarily admit themselves to an Antabuse program.[146]

TRANQUILIZERS AND ANTIDEPRESSANTS.   Tranquilizers and antidepressants are an inexpensive way to treat large numbers of patients. The goal of such treatment is to reduce patient anxiety and concomitantly the need for alcohol.[147] Efforts to determine these drugs' effectiveness have been relatively few. However, the results of a double-blind study of ten different psychopharmacologic agents indicated that none of the drugs was superior to a placebo in producing *significant* abstinence.

LITHIUM.   Lithium, a soft metal belonging to the alkali group, is a more recent addition to the drug treatment of alcoholism. Researchers at Memorial University in Newfoundland report that 36 percent of patients undergoing lithium treatment were still abstaining from alcohol after six months of treatment.[148]

The value of Lithium as an effective treatment for alcoholics has been challenged recently, however.[149] Some feel it is not effective, although it may help a subgroup of alcoholics—those who may be depressed.

Detoxification

A medical program designed to assist the dependent with withdrawal symptoms and help restore his or her general health with good nutrition and hygiene instructions. Proper detoxification allows the patient to start a treatment program in improved health. It is difficult for treatment to be successful when the patient is still ill.

Detoxification   **Detoxification,** the process by which a substance foreign to the body is changed to a compound or compounds more easily excretable, is the necessary first step in the successful rehabilitation of an alcohol dependent. Most detoxification programs do not require expensive or elaborate medical facilities, but many alcoholics entering such programs need specific medical attention.

Self-Help Programs   There are several groups whose supportive interaction helps members remain sober. As we have noted, the most well-known of these groups is Alcoholics Anonymous, founded in 1935 by two alcoholics who were searching for a self-help approach to alcoholism.

AA membership does not require dues, only the admission of being an alcoholic and the desire to stay sober while helping other alcoholics do the same. AA depends primarily on a spiritual approach and unselfish devotion to other recovering alcoholic members.[150] Rehabilitation includes discussion of day-to-day problems.

Throughout the years this group has become very strong and helped thousands of recovering alcoholics to become sober. It has also changed considerably, allowing for people of all races, religious backgrounds, ethnic backgrounds, and sexual preferences to live with this disease. In 1990 there were 1.5 million AA groups around the world. Having this many groups has become a necessity because there are now over 29 million alcoholics. This is about 12 percent of the population. After the American Medical Association declared alcoholism a disease in 1956, AA was accepted by society and more people were willing to admit they had a disease.

Alcoholics Anonymous has a high rate of recovery for those who stay with it. The program has qualities similar to those of group therapies, yet it also has some qualities that are rather unique. The following is a list of some of the "curative" or "healing" qualities of AA, and a description of each:[151] The box on page 229 lists the 12-step approach to recovery.

There are three other groups related to AA: Al-Anon, Al-a-teen, and Al-a-tot. Al-Anon was founded around 1940 when wives of AA members found that they too had problems—coping with alcoholic husbands (early AA groups were invariably *all men*) and finding ways in which they could help their husbands fight alcoholism.[152] Supportive discussion is the key to Al-Anon's effort, and with the increasing number of female alcoholics the group now has male members as well.

Al-a-teen came into being in 1957 because many children of alcoholics felt uneasy trying to relate to older people in Al-Anon groups. These children were often embarrassed and distrustful, and they were more willing to seek and accept advice from their contemporaries. Al-a-tot was founded for similar reasons to help preteenage children of alcoholics. Both groups are supported and sponsored by Al-Anon.

The question often arises, "Can alcoholics become social drinkers?" In the majority of cases the answer is no. According to AA philosophy, a return to normal or social drinking is impossible because of the alcoholic's biophysiological makeup. AA remains steadfast in its belief that alcoholism is a progressively irreversible disease characterized by the inevitable loss of control over alcohol use.

12 STEPS TO A NEW LIFE

Many rehab units urge patients to join Alcoholics Anonymous, whose 12 steps have been used to battle everything from drug abuse to compulsive overeating.

1. We admitted we were powerless over alcohol—that our lives had become unmanageable.

2. Came to believe that a Power greater than ourselves could restore us to sanity.

3. Made a decision to turn our will and our lives over to the care of God, as we understood Him.

4. Made a searching and fearless moral inventory of ourselves.

5. Admitted to God, to ourselves, and to another human being the exact nature of our wrongs.

6. Were entirely ready to have God remove all these defects of character.

7. Humbly asked Him to remove our shortcomings.

8. Made a list of all persons we had harmed, and became willing to make amends to them all.

9. Made direct amends to such people wherever possible, except when to do so would injure them or others.

10. Continued to take personal inventory and when we were wrong promptly admitted it.

11. Sought through prayer and meditation to improve our conscious contact with God, as we understood Him, praying only for knowledge of His will for us and the power to carry that out.

12. Having had a spiritual awakening as the result of these steps, we tried to carry this message to alcoholics and to practice these principles in all our affairs.

Sharon Begley et al., "12 Steps to a New Life," *Newsweek*, May 11, 1987, p. 66.

Rational Recovery   Rational Recovery (RR) groups lean more on willpower than on any higher power. "Where AA calls drinking a disease and urges members to acknowledge their own helplessness against it, the alternative groups emphasize taking personal responsibility for kicking the habit."[153] Rational Recovery shuns the religious element. It tries to help members recognize the sort of "crooked" thinking that sets up impulsive behavior.

RR rejects AA's notion of powerlessness and insists that you do have a choice. That choice, Rational Recovery insists, is the essence of the drinking problem. AA holds that alcoholics are never cured and must attend meetings the rest of their lives. Their critics contend that AA simply substitutes one kind of dependency for another. Rational Recovery seems to be gaining a large following, and the "taking charge of your own destiny" approach is gaining popularity. Ironically, some individuals subscribe to both AA and RR at the same time.

Crisis Intervention   Treating alcoholism is a long process that involves not only the alcoholic but also his family. There are many methods of treatment, but the first step in any process of detoxification is for the alcoholic to admit he has a problem and make a commitment to do something about it. Often this comes about because of a crisis in the alcoholic's life that is a direct result of alcohol abuse. For example, he might have received a drunk-driving ticket, had an automobile accident when he was drunk, lost his spouse when she couldn't deal with the problem any longer, or hurt himself or someone else while under the influence. Once the person admits to having a problem, *then* he can be treated.

Sometimes this takes "tough love" on the part of family members or friends. This means that the alcoholic is not protected or sheltered but instead is confronted with the facts. Specific written documentation of what has happened when the alcoholic drinks must be presented to the alcoholic in a non-emotional, nonthreatening manner. Such an approach will help lead to early **intervention.** In a nutshell, this is the approach called crisis intervention.

The family must first decide that it is not just a personal problem but a family problem and that they must all learn to identify with and talk about the addiction. They gather, at first without the dysfunctional member, to identify the problem. They make lists of several significant instances when the behavior has been a direct disruption to normal family functioning. They must decide to confront the alcoholic before he or she hits rock bottom. By moving "the bottom up" the family does not have to wait until the alcoholic does something detrimental to himself or others.[154]

The family must then decide what treatment options are probably most plausible, given the environment in which the abuser lives. All this is prior to the confrontation. Participants take heart in the statistic that states that 90 percent of all people confronted in this way begin treatment of some kind.

Finally, they rehearse what it is that each family member is going to say to the alcoholic and how it will be said. They decide when would be a good time for the intervention. Early morning before work or on a Saturday might be desirable. That way, the family will have a chance to intervene before the person starts drinking for the day and disappears.

The actual intervention might lead to admitting the alcoholic into a treatment center; however, the family should also decide what they will do if the individual refuses to go for help. An intervention that doesn't lead to immediate treatment should not be viewed as a failure. It will at least bring the problem out in the open and require the alcoholic to start thinking about his or her future. Some families ask the alcoholic to move out if he or she won't go for treatment.

Sometimes, though, the family and friends of the alcoholic are referred to as ***co-dependents,*** because without realizing it they help the alcoholic to continue living her life with the problem. For example, they might constantly bail her out of jail, make excuses for her, or even give her the money to buy her

Intervention

A process where an attempt is made by family, friends, and an alcohol-and drug-treatment counselor to stop substance abuse before a person bottoms out with the illness. It is a carefully executed process wherein friends, in a loving and caring manner, express their concern about the dependent's problem and cite specific examples of behaviors they have observed while the dependent was under the influence of alcohol or other drugs. It is the goal of the intervention to get the dependent into a treatment center for help.

Co-Dependent

Family and friends of the alcoholic are often referred to as co-dependents because without realizing it they help the alcoholic to continue living his or her life with the problem. They offer excuses for the alcoholic's behavior and may even provide money to bail the alcoholic out of jail.

alcohol. They need help just as the alcoholic does. Intervention, if carefully worked out early, can do a great deal to stop alcoholism in its early stages.

Intervention is often thought of as a positive group effort. However, it may have a negative "side effect" on the family.[155] In some cases it has been shown that intervention has resulted in significant damage to the family unit or one of its members. Counselors should be aware that intervention can be difficult for the family and should be handled with care. It is vital to recognize that the final step in intervention is the recovery of the family and not just the alcoholic.

Group Therapy   Regardless of the medical treatment needed, the alcohol dependent will usually participate in a counseling or psychotherapy program to help deal with immediate problems and to recognize factors underlying drinking patterns. Such treatment seems to be most effective when employed by a group of men and women similarly affected.

Psychodrama, a method of learning through role playing, is a treatment method often used in group therapy. Its primary goals are to improve the individual's failing self-image[156] and to improve behavioral patterns. Psychodrama has proved effective because of its ability to deal with the variety of problems, personalities, and situations confronting the alcoholic.

Abstinence   Since midcentury abstinence-oriented ideology has dominated the strategies and procedures used to treat alcoholism. This ideology holds that the alcoholic is unable to regulate his or her rate of alcohol intake, that this loss of control is inevitable and irreversible, and that any return to normal or socially accepted levels of consumption is impossible.[157]

Clearly, alcohol and drug treatment has become big business. On any given day approximately 600,000 people are undergoing treatment, with 100,000 in hospitals or residential treatment centers and the rest in outpatient programs.[158] In addition, over 38,000 AA groups meet regularly, and 4,500 clinics, hospitals, halfway houses, and other institutions specialize in treating chemical abuse.

A typical inpatient treatment program will run for about 28 to 32 days. It will include detoxification, education, counseling (individual, group, and family), nutritional analysis, education, and possibly some exercise, and it will expect the patients to attend AA, NA, or CA meetings. Most will follow the 12 steps of Alcoholics Anonymous. Aftercare is critical in keeping patients from relapsing. These aftercare programs may consist of weekly meetings for a year or longer.

It should be noted that more information about treatment will be presented in the chapter on treatment.

ALCOHOLISM AND THE FAMILY

Most people will now admit that the alcoholic is a sick person, but only recently have people begun to realize that it is the whole family that suffers from the disease. Since the family is the main socializing agent in this country, it is important to study the impact of alcoholism on the family and the family's influence on the onset of alcoholism. Do certain kinds of families raise alcoholics? Can the actions of family members actually enable and encourage another member to drink? Some theorists believe that the family has a strong influence on the alcoholic's drinking behavior and that the study of the alcoholic family can lead to more effective treatment methods.

Alcoholism destroys the relationships at the core of the family. The roles of each member become twisted and turned as he or she tries to deal with the alcoholic. The woman who used to be a lover, friend, and wife to her husband is changed into mother, protector, and nursemaid. Even the children's roles change. These roles have been described numerous times in the literature and are usually stated as follows:

1. *Enabler:* This person is usually the spouse of the dependent or the one with the closest involvement. This persons tends to take over for the alcoholic and make choices for him or her. The enabler will usually take the blame for many things that go wrong and take care of the alcoholic when he or she is sick. The enabler is constantly running interference and making excuses for the alcoholic.

2. *Hero* or *achiever:* Usually the oldest child has excessive achievements, becomes a family caretaker, and tries to please people.

3. *Problem child* or *scapegoat:* Often the middle child becomes rebellious and defies authority. The problem child provides distraction from the alcoholic. He or she may also have learning problems as well as problems in school.

4. *Lost child* or *quiet child:* The role of this child is to offer relief to the family system. He or she is uninvolved and spends a lot of time on his or her own activities.

5. *Mascot:* Frequently the youngest child becomes a comedian and tries to provide fun and humor to make a happy family.

Children of Alcoholics

Children who are victims of an alcoholic, dysfunctional family. They are more likely to become drinkers than children who are not from a dysfunctional family. They experience more problems because they have traits of the alcoholic personality and many of them become social outcasts, which causes them to drink even more.

Children of Alcoholics

Dealing with the far-reaching effects of alcoholism strains the entire family of an alcoholic.[159] When one family member is an alcoholic, the whole family suffers. An estimated 28 million Americans are trying to cope with the often delayed, but always severe, effects of living with an alcoholic parent.[160] Twenty-one million are 18 or older, and many have carried the emotional scars of their childhood into their adult years. The remaining 7 million, who are 18 or younger, live in an atmosphere of anxiety, tension, confusion, and denial.[161] Many have no idea of what a normal family life is like.

Nearly every child who grows up in an alcoholic home suffers in significant and long-term ways.[162] The unpredictability of the alcoholic, plus embarrassment, often keeps the children from bringing friends home, or in some cases from having any friends at all.[163] Psychosomatic ailments such as headaches, upset stomachs, and insomnia are common, and many children suffer from depression and loneliness.

The central facts of an alcoholic family are secrecy and denial. Perhaps the most significant pressure of all in an alcoholic home is keeping the parent's drinking a secret—not letting the neighbors find out, not even talking openly inside the family. The children become co-conspirators in this pact of silence.

Bennett and colleagues extensively compared children having at least one alcoholic parent and children with nonalcoholic parents. The variables studied included intelligence, cognitive achievement, psychological and physical disorders, impulsivity-hyperactivity, social competence, learning problems, behavioral problems, and self-esteem. In 9 out of the 17 tests, the children of alcoholics scored lower, although both populations fell within the normal ranges. The most startling results of this study were that the children of alcoholic parents scored significantly lower on four tests of intelligence and cognitive performance and on two tests of self-concept.[164]

The psychological damage to children of alcoholic parents is astounding. Both physical abuse and incest are more likely to occur in alcoholic families.[165] Children of alcoholic families are sent to foster homes at three times the rate of children raised in nonalcoholic families, are more likely to commit suicide, and are more likely to become delinquents.

Adult Children of Alcoholics　　Adult children of alcoholics (ACoA) must cope with problems such as the inability to get close to someone in a relationship, the need for constant control over everything, and guilt and other emotions. According to alcohol counselor Jeanette Murray, ACoA need to focus on a vision of a healthier future.[166] To accomplish this they must go through the steps of (1) growing up, (2) growing out, and (3) coming home. *Growing up* consists of reconstructing the past in a realistic way. This may involve group support and counseling. ACoA must learn more about the makeup of an alcoholic's family, the various roles members assume, and the denial, and they must realize that the alcoholic family is not a "normal" family. ACoA can no longer feel responsible for their parents. *Growing out* means no longer having to accept responsibility for the alcoholic parent. This step allows the ACoA to continue to care for his or her family but to assume responsibility for his or her own life. *Coming home* deals with developing new relationships and eliminating defenses, denial, and compulsive behaviors. Here, ACoA accept the positive and negative experiences of living in an alcoholic family. They learn to grieve the loss of the childhood they never had because they were too busy being responsible for their alcoholic parent(s). They learn to be responsible for themselves and give up the need to look after and control others.

As ACoA grow older, they find many resources to help them. They may seek professional therapy. The support group that seems most successful is the Adult Children of Alcoholics, which is based on the same principles as Alcoholics Anonymous. In ACoA the person learns that he or she can no longer blame the past for his or her maladaptive behaviors of today. In ACoA they find a solution: to become loving parents themselves.

THE MOVEMENT AGAINST DRUNK DRIVING

MOTHERS AGAINST DRUNK DRIVERS

Mothers Against Drunk Drivers (MADD) is a grass-roots movement whose members are concerned citizens, men and women, victims and nonvictims. Its goals are first to keep the issue of drunk driving alive by making people aware of the problem and second to mobilize the public to help individuals modify their drinking habits. To these ends, they have chosen to make drunkenness and drunk driving socially unacceptable. In the words of the MADD Mission Statement, "Mothers against Drunk Driving mobilizes victims and their allies to establish the public conviction that impaired driving is unacceptable and criminal, in order to promote corresponding public policies, programs, and accountability.[167]

MADD was started by Candy Lightner, whose daughter Cari was struck and killed by a drunk driver near her home in Fair Oaks, California. The driver who hit Lightner's daughter had a prior arrest for hit-and-run driving and drunk driving and had been released from custody on bail only two days before killing Cari. The driver was sentenced to two years in prison but was made to serve only 16 months in a work camp. Angry and frustrated, Candy Lightner protested a judicial system that allowed someone with a history of drunk driving to continue to drive. She finally decided to develop a powerful nationwide group to do something about it.

In addition to the goals just mentioned, MADD educates citizens on how they can be individually responsible, organizing community efforts to fight drunk driving, reforming laws relating to drunk driving, and conducting programs for victims of drunk drivers. MADD has been very successful in reducing the legal blood-alcohol content in various states and has initiated several effective programs to limit drinking and driving.

STUDENTS AGAINST DRIVING DRUNK

Students Against Driving Drunk (SADD) was started in September 1981 as part of a mandatory health-education program for sophomores at Wayland High School near Boston. The program was developed under the leadership of Robert Anastas, who has made curriculum materials for others desiring to start a SADD program. The students organized for the following reasons: to help save their own lives and the lives of others; to educate students on the problem of drinking and driving; to develop peer counseling among students about alcohol use; and to increase public awareness and prevention of alcohol abuse everywhere.

RESPONSIBLE DRINKING

It should be stressed that the vast majority of social drinkers imbibe for pleasure and other beneficial effects. Some feel the time has come to inform those who choose to drink to do so in a responsible manner—in moderation. We have seen that there are an estimated 100 million or more regular alcohol users in the United States and approximately 10 million or more alcoholics. A considerable amount of energy has gone into encouraging abstinence, and enormous sums of money have been spent on the problem of alcoholism. However, what is being done for the over 90 million social drinkers to keep them from losing control?

It appears that the social drinker will receive greater attention in the future. A few suggestions are being offered. One is to limit alcohol consumption to one drink per hour. One drink is defined as 12 ounces of beer *or* 4 ounces of wine *or* 1.5 ounces of 80-proof distilled liquor. Going beyond this amount can lead to problems. Another suggestion is not to mix alcohol with other drugs because of possible synergistic effects.

The following guidelines can help you prevent drunkenness if you are hosting a social gathering:

Don't serve alcohol only. Many people will behave responsibly when other beverages are available.

Serve food first. The more food in the stomach, the slower the rate of alcohol absorption. However, avoid serving salty snacks: They just make people more thirsty.

Don't serve alcohol to someone who already appears intoxicated.

Don't allow an intoxicated person to drive.

When necessary, advise guests that they should drink responsibly at your social functions.[168]

SUMMARY

Alcohol-related problems far exceed problems related to any other psychoactive drug found in the United States. However, national surveys indicate a gradual downward trend in the use of alcohol. The psychological effects of drinking extend to almost every sector of society; the physiological effects range from loss of coordination to death. Alcohol may be a major contributing factor in violence and suicide. Prolonged drinking may lead to cirrhosis of the liver, brain impairment, heart problems, and fetal alcohol syndrome.

There has been national recognition of the problems associated with irresponsible drinking. Mothers Against Drunk Driving (MADD) has been able to create a national awareness about not drinking and driving. States are lowering the limits for legal intoxication and many drivers are volunteering to remain sober while their passengers drink.

Individuals are more aware of drinking in a responsible manner. Also, through increased education and television programs, the general public is better informed about what to do if a person's drinking is getting out of control. It is no longer necessary to hit rock bottom before getting help for alcoholism. Many individuals are treated through crisis intervention before they can develop serious drinking problems.

Though debate continues over whether alcoholism is a disease, hospitals, intermediate-care facilities (halfway houses), and drug-treatment and detoxification programs all work to help the alcoholic. In addition, self-help groups, group therapy, and family counseling provide support systems for medical care.

In addition to various treatment options available for the alcoholic, families, including children of alcoholics and adult children of alcoholics, are receiving more help.

Alcohol
N O T E S

1. Quoted in Wayne Polen, Garen Len, and Gail Vive, *Alcoholism: A Treatment Manual* (New York: Gardner Press, 1979), p. 14.
2. "Worldwide Consumption Continues to Climb," *U.S. Journal of Drug and Alcohol Dependence* 5, no. 2 (March 1981):19.
3. *Alcohol and Health,* Fourth Special Report to the U.S. Congress from the Secretary of Health and Human Services (Rockville, Md.: National Institute on Alcohol Abuse and Alcoholism, 1981).
4. "The High School Senior Drug Abuse Survey," Sponsored by National Institute of Drug Addiction (NIDA) and conducted by the University of Michigan, Institute for Social Research. HHS News, U.S. Department of Health and Human Services, News Release, January 24, 1991.
5. National Institute on Drug Abuse, "Facts about Teenagers and Drug Abuse," NIDA Capsules, CAP 17 (Rockville, Md.: U.S. Department of Health and Human Services, Public Health Service, Alcohol, Drug Abuse, and Mental Health Administration, 1991).
6. Gerardo Gonzalez, "Early Onset of Drinking as a Predictor of Alcohol Consumption and Alcohol-Related Problems in College," *Journal of Drug Education* 19, no. 3 (1989):225–30.
7. Ibid.
8. Romania Miller, "Positive Self-Esteem and Alcohol and Drug Related Attitudes among School Children," *Journal of Alcohol and Drug Education* 33, no. 3 (Spring 1988):26–30.
9. Mary Ann Forney, Paul D. Forney, and William K. Ripley, "Predictor Variables of Adolescent Drinking," *Advances in Alcohol and Substance Abuse* 8, no. 2 (1989):97–113.
10. "Treatment Now Available to Only 10% of Addicted Teens: Funding Lack Seen as Chief Barrier," *Drugs and Drug Abuse Education* 20, no. 5 (May 1989):1, 52–54.
11. Gerardo M. Gonzalez, "Effects of Drinking Age on Reduced Consumption of Alcohol Reported by College Students, 1981–1986," *Journal of Drug Issues* 20, no. 1 (Winter 1990):67–73.
12. Ibid.
13. "Campus Dryout (Crackdown on Alcohol Abuse in Colleges)," *Time,* June 6, 1988, pp. 70–73.
14. Ibid.
15. Leonard Goodwin, "Social Psychological Bases for College Alcohol Consumption," *Journal of Alcohol and Drug Education* 36, no. 1 (Fall 1990):83–95.
16. National Institute on Drug Abuse, Division of Epidemiology and Prevention, "National Household Survey on Drug Abuse," NIDA Capsules, CAP 21, (Rockville,

Md.: U.S. Department of Health and Human Services, Public Health Service, Alcohol, Drug Abuse, and Mental Health Administration, 1990).

17. Jean Kinney, "America's Silent Epidemic," *American Legion Magazine,* January 1989, pp. 26–27.

18. Gail Rosenblum, "A Sobering Story: *New Choices for the Best Years,*" 29, no. 5, May 1989, 62–69.

19. Ibid.

20. John Minnis, "Toward an Understanding of Alcohol Abuse among the Elderly," *Journal of Alcohol and Drug Education* 33, no. 3 (Spring 1988):32–39.

21. Cynthia Robbins, "Social Roles and Alcohol Abuse among Older Men and Women," *Family and Community Health* 13, no. 4 (January 1991):37–47.

22. Ibid.

23. Ibid.

24. Richard H. Blum et al., *Society and Drugs* (San Francisco: Jossey-Bass, 1970).

25. Ibid.

26. Grace M. Barnes and Michael Windle, "Similarities and Differences in Correlates of Alcohol Consumption and Problem Behaviors among Male and Female Adolescents," *International Journal of Addictions* 23, no. 7 (1988):707–28.

27. Meyer Kalzper, Ralph Ryback, and Marc Hertzman, "Alcohol Beverage Advertisement and Consumption," *Journal of Drug Issues* 8, no. 4 (Fall 1978):339–53.

28. "Drugs and Alcohol: The Aphrodisiacs That Aren't," *Executive Fitness Newsletter* 2, no. 17 (August 23, 1980):1–2.

29. Richard A. Zucker, Victor A. Battistach, and Ginette B. Langer, "Sexual Behavior, Sex-Role Adaptation to Drinking in Young Women," *Journal of Studies on Alcohol* 42, no. 5 (May 1981):457–65.

30. Daniel W. Webster et al., "Familial Transmission of Alcohol Use: Parent and Adult Offspring Alcohol Use over 17 years—Tecumseh, Michigan," *Journal of Studies on Alcohol* 50 (1989):557–66.

31. Ibid.

32. Rona Preli and Howard Protinsky, "Aspects of Family Structures in Alcoholic, Recovered, and Nonalcoholic Families," *Journal of Marital and Family Therapy,* July 1988, no. 14:311–13.

33. David A. Works, *New Hope, New Responsibilities* (Washington, D.C.: Department of Transportation, 1974), p. 7.

34. *NIAAA Information and Feature Service* No. 84 (June 1, 1981):6.

35. National Institute of Mental Health, *Alcohol and Alcoholism* (Chevy Chase, Md., 1970), p. 22.

36. See, for example, Charles H. Hennekens et al., "Effects of Beer, Wine, and Liquor in Coronary Deaths," *Journal of the American Medical Association* 242, no. 18 (November 2, 1979):1973.

37. Cited in *Alcohol and Health,* Fourth Special Report, p. 30.

38. Staff, "Alcohol, Heart Disease, and Mortality," *Harvard Medical School Health Letter* 14, no. 7 (May 1989):1–2.

39. Nancy Clark, "Social Drinking and Athletics," *The Physician and Sports Medicine* 17, no. 10 (October 1989):95–100.

40. J. Cauley and L. Kuller, "Studies on the Association between Alcohol and High Density Lipoprotein Cholesterol: Possible Benefits and Risks," *Advances in Alcohol and Substance Abuse* (1987):53–64.

41. Denise Grady, "Give That Rat a Bud," *Discover* 11, no. 9 (September 1990):16.

42. W. P. Castell, "Editorial," *Journal of the American Heart Association* 242, no. 18 (1985):2000.

43. Ibid.

44. Ibid., p. 4.

45. Timothy J. Regan, "Alcohol and the Cardiovascular System," *Journal of the American Medical Association* 264, no. 3 (July 18, 1990):337–381.

46. Louis G. Lange and Paula Kinnunen, "Cardiovascular Effects of Alcohol," *Advances in Alcohol and Substance Abuse* 6, no. 3 (1987):47–50.

47. "Alcohol and Brain Damage: Circle the Wagons," *Science News* 116 (October 20, 1979):262.

48. Elizabeth F. Loftus, "Did I Really Say That Last Night? Alcohol, Marijuana, and Memory," *Psychology Today* 13, no. 10 (1980):48. Reprinted with permission from *Psychology Today*. Copyright © 1980 American Psychological Association (APA).

49. "Alcohol-Related Brain Damage Subject of Research," *NIAA Information and Feature Service,* no. 81 (April 1, 1981):4.

50. F. K. Goodwin, "Only Two Drinks May Affect Memory," *Journal of the American Medical Association* 261 (May 12, 1989):2604.

51. D. C. Vinson, "Acute Transient Memory Loss," *Journal of American Family Physicians* 39 (May 1989):249–54.

52. Anne B. Simons, "Hangover: The Morning After," *Medical Self Care,* January/February 1988, no. 44:24–25.

53. N. Spritz, "Review of Literature Linking Alcohol Consumption with Liver Disease and Atherosclerotic Disease," *American Journal of Clinical Nutrition* 32, no. 12 (December 1979):2654.

54. "Liquor Hurts Livers, Regardless of Diet," *Journal of the American Medical Association* 228, no. 4 (April 22, 1974):449.

55. *Alcohol and Health,* Fifth Special Report to the U.S. Congress from the Secretary of Health and Human Services (Washington, D.C., 1984), p. 8.

56. Harvey Grachow and Kathleen Sobocinske, "Lite Drinking," *Health,* February 6, 1986, p. 6.

57. Terri Mendoza and Carolyn Gloeckner, "Alcohol and Nutrition," *Current Health* 17, no. 2 (October 1990):20–25.

58. David F. Williamson, Michelle R. Foreman, and Nancy J. Binkin, "Alcohol and Body Weight in United States Adults," *American Journal of Public Health* 77 (October 1987):1324.

59. N. Kessel and H. Walton, *Alcoholism* (London: MacGibbon & Kee, 1965), p. 25.

60. See K. L. Jones et al., "Pattern of Malformation in Offspring of Chronic Alcoholic Mothers," *Lancet* 1, no. 7815 (June 9, 1973):1267–71.

61. Charles Leerhsen, "Pregnancy + Alcohol = Problems," *Newsweek,* July 31, 1989, p. 57.

62. Dorris Michael, "A Desperate Crack Legacy," *Newsweek,* June 25, 1990, p. 6.

63. Bruce Bower, "Drinking While Pregnant Risks Child's IQ," *Science News* 135 (February 4, 1989):68.

64. *NIAAA Information and Feature Service,* April, 1981, no. 32:4.

65. "Researchers Say Alcohol May Have a Link to Cancer," *Los Angeles Times,* June 4, 1988.

66. Ibid.

67. John Horgan, "When Dad Drinks," *Scientific American* 262, no. 2 (February 1990):23.

68. Andrea Dorfman, "Alcohol's Youngest Victim," *Time,* August 28, 1989, p. 60.

69. Ibid.

70. Jones et al., "Pattern of Malformation," p. 1267.

71. Anastasia Toufexis, "Why Men Can Outdrink Women," *Time,* January 22, 1990, p. 61.

72. Ibid.

73. J. Raloff, "Women and Alcohol: A Gastric Disadvantage," *Science News,* January 21, 1990, pp. 39–40.

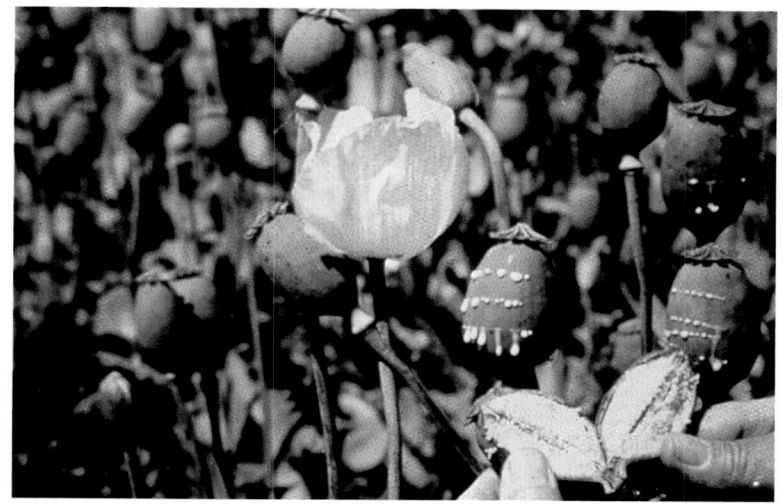

POPPY CAPSULE
The milky substance from the opium plant is incised out and air-dried to form a brownish gummy substance. The raw opium gum is changed to smoking opium by a simple heating process, and may then be eaten or smoked. (DEA)

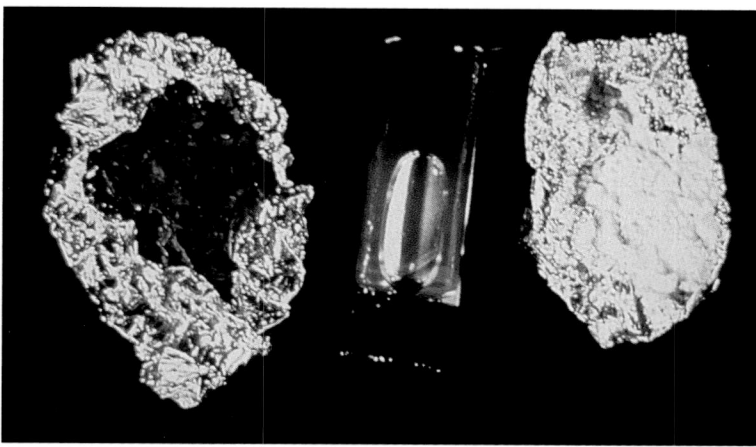

PHENCYCLIDINE (PCP)
First synthesized in the late 1950s, PCP was intended for use as an animal tranquilizer. On April 1, 1979, all legal manufacturing of the drug in the United States was banned. Despite this restriction, PCP is relatively easily obtained because it is simple to produce. It can be injected, taken orally, or smoked. (DEA)

MEXICAN HEROIN
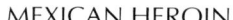
It is usually brown, instead of white, because of the method used to process the opium. Mexican heroin is not brown as a result of impurities. (DEA)

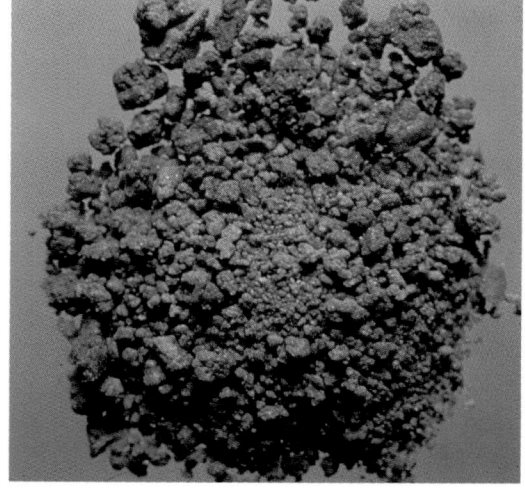

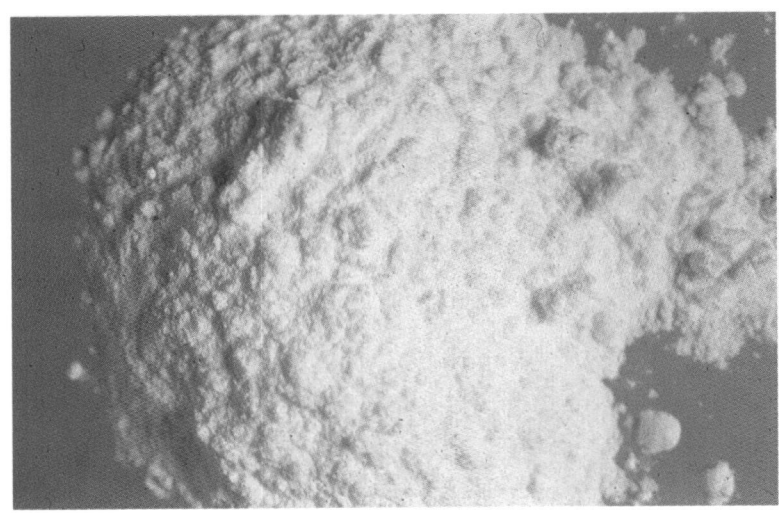

S. W. ASIAN HEROIN
This is heroin that comes from the "Golden Crescent" (Iran, Afghanistan, and Pakistan). Although the Pakistani government outlawed all poppy growing in 1979, many farmers still grow the crop because poppy cultivation brings them almost ten times as much money as the next most profitable crop. (DEA)

MORPHINE PREPARATION
In 1805 the major active constituent of opium, an alkaloid, was isolated and named morphine after the Greek god of dreams, Morpheus. Morphine is about ten times more potent than opium. (DEA)

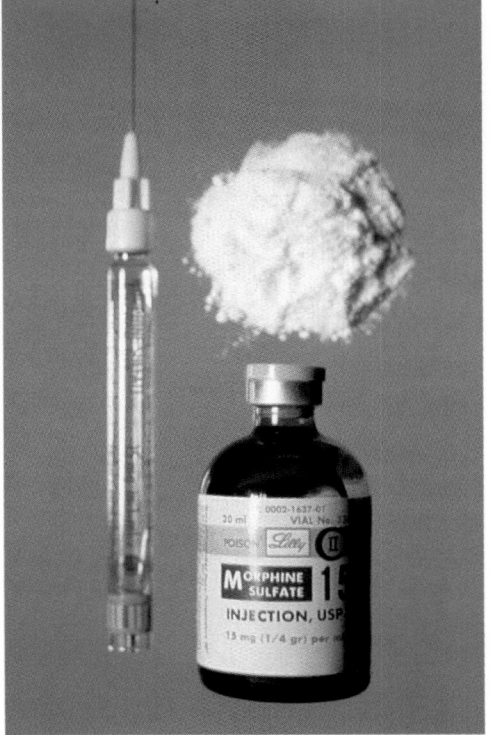

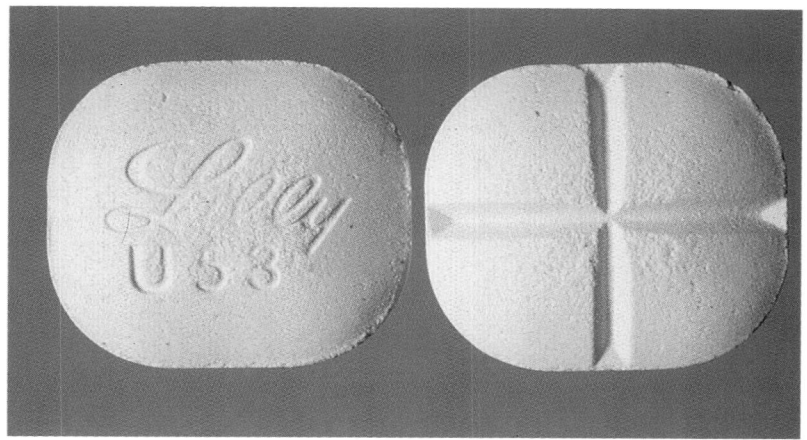

METHADONE HCl DISKETS
While many drug treatment programs still use the liquid form of
methadone with orange juice, taken orally, some are now switching
to methadone HCl Diskets because they are easier to administer to
patients. (DEA)

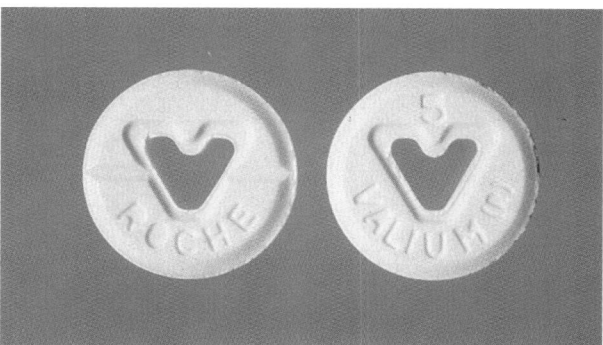

VALIUM
Valium, or diazepam, is an antianxiety agent and a
muscle relaxant that produces antiepileptic effects
without sedation. It is used to treat anxiety and
muscle spasms, as a preanesthetic for heart patients,
in the early stages of labor, and to control cerebral
palsy, convulsive attacks, and low-back pain.

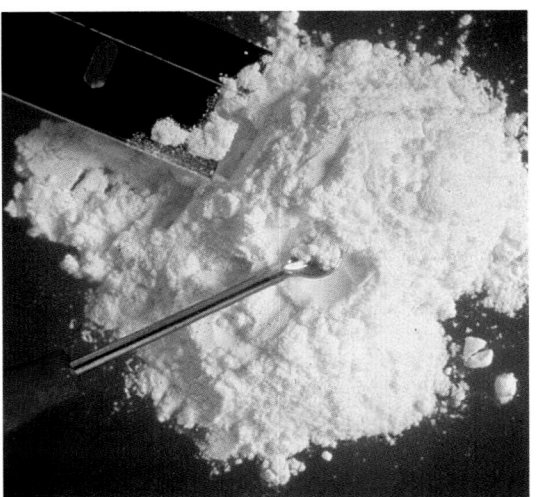

COCAINE HYDROCHLORIDE
A stable compound of cocaine, this is a fine powder that can be snorted through the nasal passage. It cannot be smoked. (DEA)

HASHISH OIL
This substance is made by boiling hashish (resin from the flowering tops of the marijuana plant) in a solvent and filtering out the solids. The final product is between 15 and 60 percent THC (delta-9 tetrahydrocannabinol), the active substance in marijuana. (DEA)

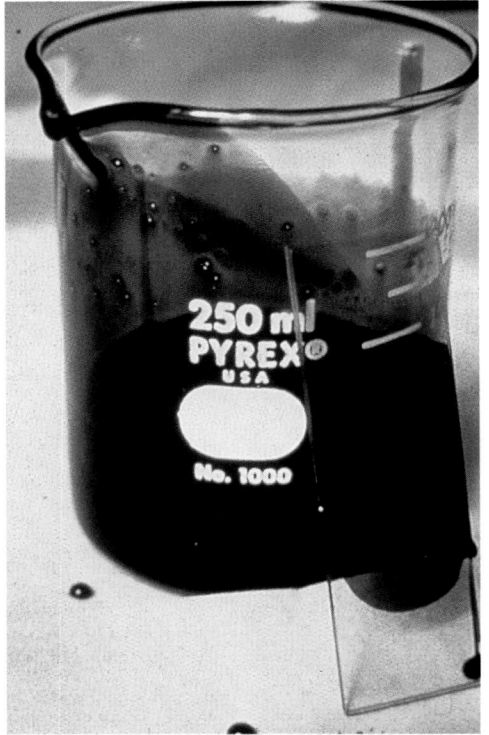

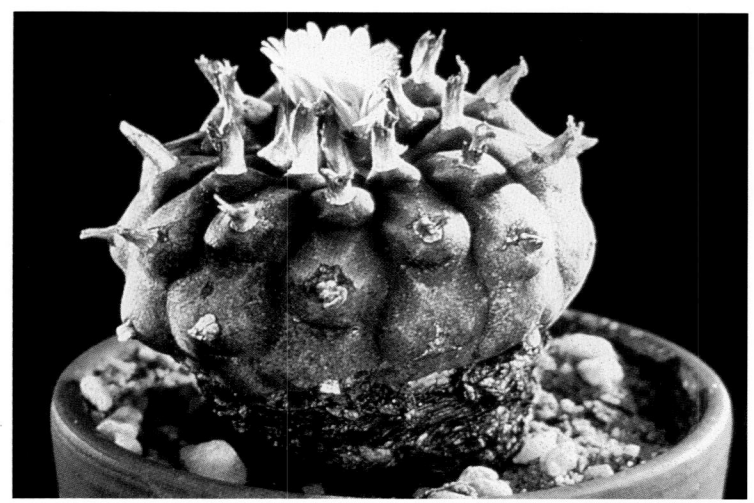

PEYOTE CACTUS
Mescaline is derived from peyote "buttons," the dried tops of several species of cactus. Once dried, peyote buttons can be ingested in raw form, but they are usually extremely bitter and can cause nausea or vomiting. Native Americans regard the cactus as God's special gift to them and equate its effects with the workings of the divine spirit. (DEA)

PSILOCYBE MUSHROOM
Psilocybin is a chemical derivative of the Psilocybe Mexica mushroom. The mushroom has been used by Aztec Indians in the belief that it would help establish communication with the spiritual world. Currently the drug has no medical use. It is usually taken orally, as dried mushrooms or in tablet form, or it may dried, ground, and added to food. (DEA)

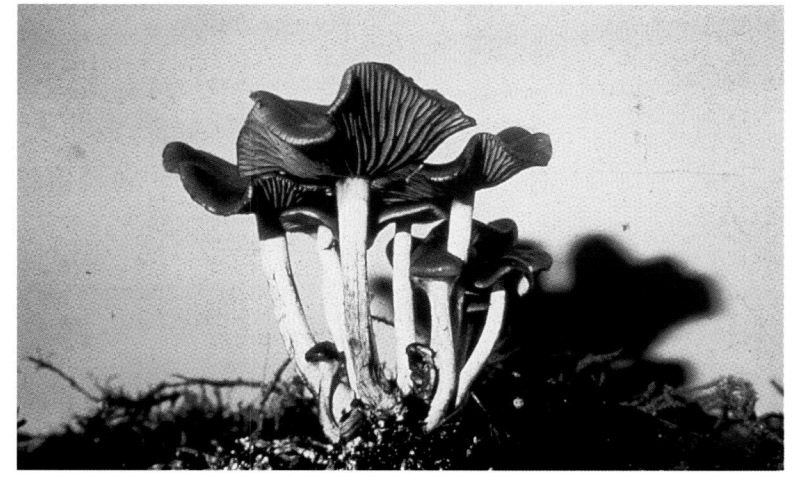

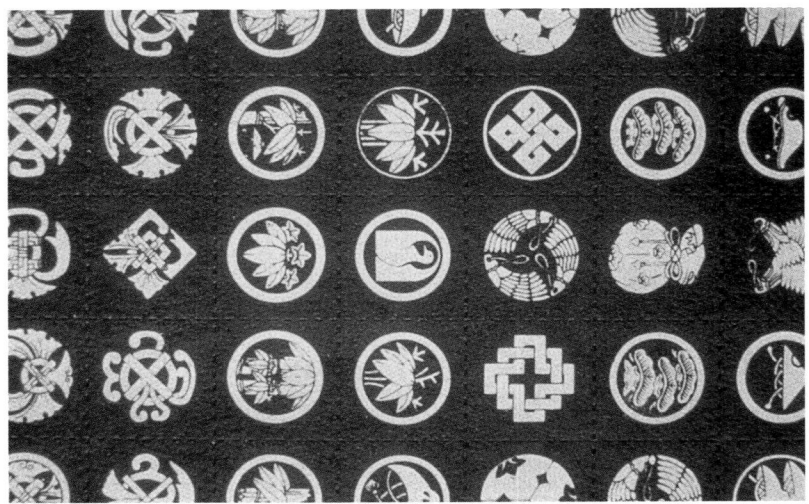

LSD BLOTTER PAPER
Diluted drops of LSD are placed on blotter paper. Usually the paper has been printed with some sort of art work, such as dragons or popular comic-strip characters. It is then cut up into tiny pieces, usually one-quarter to one-half the size of a small postage stamp. (DEA)

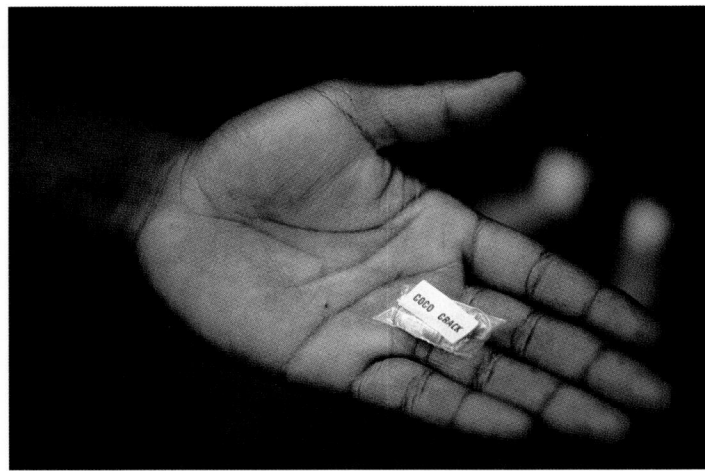

CRACK VIALS
Crack is generally purchased in small plastic vials containing two or three rocks. One puff of a pebble-sized rock produces an intense high that lasts about 20 minutes. The price for a vial is usually $10 to $20. (Wesley Bocxe/Photo Researchers)

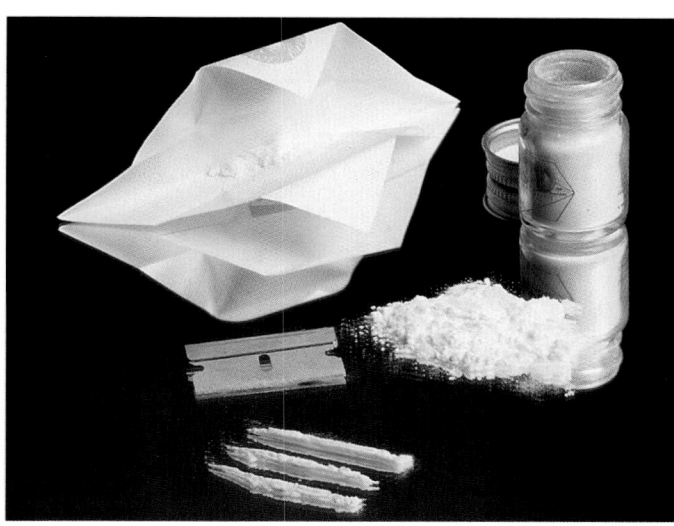

COCAINE WITH A CUTTING AGENT, MANNITOL
Sometimes cutting agents are used to dilute the substance and allow more profit to be made by the dealer. In addition, some of the cutting agents are laxative in nature and help reduce the constipation that is caused by a slowing of peristalsis that frequently occurs in users. (Bobbie Kingsley/Photo Researchers)

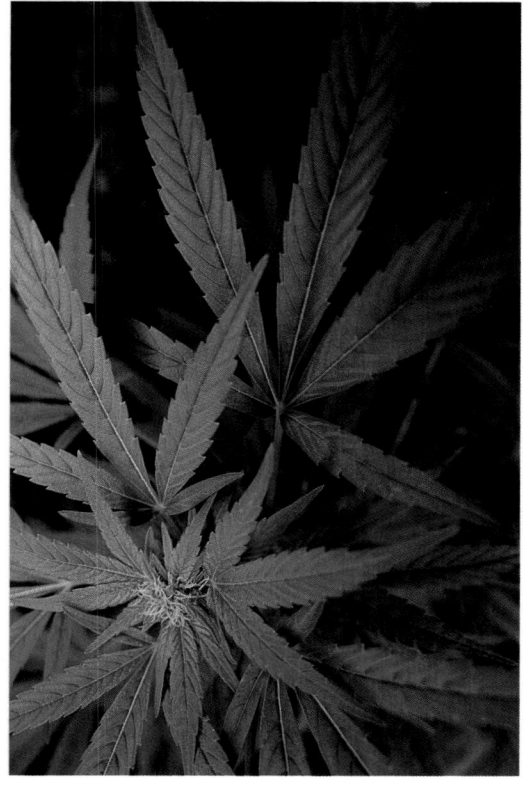

MARIJUANA PLANT
Marijuana (grass, pot, weed, dope) is the common name for a drug made from the plant Cannabis sativa. The psychoactive ingredient is delta-9-tetrahydrocannabinol (THC), although there are more than 420 chemicals in the cannibas plant. The type of plant, the weather, the soil, the time of harvest, selective cultivation, and other factors determine this amount of potency. Most of the THC found in marijuana comes from the leaves and flowering tops, as well as from the resin taken from the leaves. Some of the stem and stocks of the plant have been used to make hemp rope. (Don King /The Image Bank)

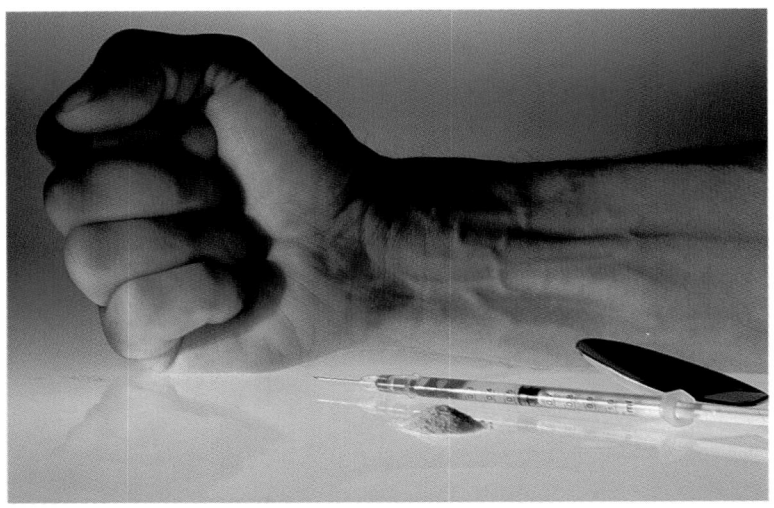

HEROIN INJECTION EQUIPMENT
Usually included in this equipment are a spoon, syringe, ligature (to tie off a blood vessel), and matches to heat the material. One of the dangers of heroin use is the sharing of needles with others and coming in contact with blood that may be infected with AIDS. (Oscar Burriel/Latin Stock/Science Photo Library/Photo Researchers)

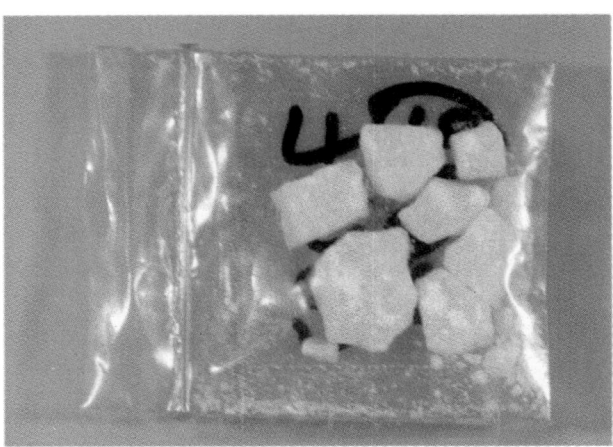

ICE
Ice is a freebase form of methamphetamine that can be smoked in a pipe at a temperature of around 100 degrees. The base itself does not carry the effects that ice produces, so it is thought that the meth crystal is washed with another chemical. The chemical is not yet known and it is suspected that Asian chemists may be the only ones to know what it is. Its intense highs last from 8 to 24 hours and result in an immediate euphoria and increased alertness. (Kermani/Liaison)

74. Ibid.

75. Ibid.

76. Les Stanwood, "The Double Whammy of Alcohol and Drugs," *Current Health 2* 17, (October 1990):26–27.

77. Ibid.

78. *Alcohol and Health,* Fifth Special Report, p. 25.

79. J. Lewis Lord, "Coming to Grips with Alcoholism," *U.S. News & World Report* 103, no. 6 (1987):56.

80. *NIAAA Information and Feature Service,* April 1, 1981, no. 82:4–5.

81. "A Few Too Many on the Water," *Newsweek,* August 3, 1987, p. 22.

82. Ibid.

83. Gonzalez, "Effects of Drinking Age on Reduced Consumption."

84. *NIAAA Information and Feature Service* No. 82 (April 1, 1981):5.

85. Mary Conroy, "Is Your Child an Alcoholic?" *Better Homes and Gardens* no. 3 (May 1988):72–76.

86. Bob Cohn, "The Menace on the Roads," *Newsweek* 110, no. 25 (December 21, 1987):42–43.

87. Roberts, Fitzmahan and Associates, 66, *Teens and Alcohol* (Portland: Oregon Drug and Alcohol Information Center, 1987).

88. James Milan, *Under the Influence* (New York: Bantam, 1981), pp. 45–46.

89. Ibid., p. 45.

90. Michael J. Stoil, "The Case of the Missing Gene," *Alcohol Health and Research World,* Winter 1987/88, no. 6:130.

91. Johnson, C. Renold et al., "Asians, Asian-Americans and Alcohol," *Journal of Psychoactive Drugs* 22, no. 1 (January/March 1990):45–51.

92. "Counting the Cost," *Bottom Line* 3, August 1980, no. 4:10–14.

93. David Whitman, "The Return of Skid Row," *U.S. News & World Report,* January 15, 1990, pp. 27–29.

94. Ibid.

95. Goodman, Susan, "Agony Without Ecstasy—Alcohol and Violence," *Current Health 2,* 17 (October 1990):28–29.

96. Ibid.

97. Antonia Abbey, "Acquaintance Rape and Alcohol Consumption on College Campuses: How Are They Linked?" *Journal of American College Health* 39, no. 4 (January 1991):165–169.

98. Op. cit.

99. Edith S. Liasansky Gomberg, "Suicide Risks among Women with Alcohol Problems," *American Journal of Public Health* 79 (1989):1363–65.

100. Cited in *NIAA Information and Feature Service,* no. 82, p. 4.

101. Quoted in ibid., p. 3.

102. Beryl L. Benderly, "Saving the Children," *Health* 21, no. 12 (December 1989):74–75.

103. Department of Health, Education and Welfare, *Alcohol and Alcoholism* (Rockville, Md., 1981), p. 89.

104. O'Connell-Cahill, "Whiskey River Please Run Dry: Alcoholism in the Christian Family," *U.S. Catholic,* February 1986, p. 51.

105. Sean O'Conner, Victor Hesselbrock, and Lance Bauer, "The Nervous System and the Predisposition to Alcohol," *Alcohol and Health and Research World* 14, no. 2 (1990):90–97.

106. Ibid.

107. "Roots of Addiction," *Newsweek,* February 20, 1989, pp. 52–57.

108. Editorials, "Finding the Gene(s) for Alcoholism," *Journal of the American Medical Association* 263, no. 15 (April 18, 1990):2094–5.

109. Geofrey Crowley, "The Gene and the Bottle," *Newsweek,* April 30, 1990, p. 59.

110. Jean Kinney, "America's Silent Epidemic," *American Legion Magazine* 126, no. 1, January 1989, pp. 26–27.

111. David Rutstein, Richard Veech, and D. Phil, "Genetic Factors and Alcoholism," *New England Journal of Medicine* 298, no. 20 (May 18, 1978):1140–41.

112. Nancy Cotton, "The Familial Incidence of Alcoholism," *Journal of Studies on Alcohol* 40, no. 1 (January 1979):89–112.

113. Ibid., p. 89.

114. Marc A. Schuckit, "Genetic Aspects of Alcoholism," *Annals of Emergency Medicine* 15, no. 9 (September 1986):993.

115. Theodore Reich, "Beyond the Gene," *American Health and Research World* 12, no. 2 (Winter 1987/88).

116. Constance Holden, "Genes, Personality and Alcoholism," *Psychology Today* 19, no. 1 (January 1985):38–44.

117. Quoted in ibid.

118. Ibid.

119. Albert J. Yakichuk, "A Study of the Self-Concept Evaluations of Alcoholics and Non-alcoholics," *Journal of Drug Education* 8, no. 1 (1978):41–47.

120. Susan Speece, "B-endorphins and THIQ and Their Relationship to Alcoholism," *American Biology Teacher* 49, no. 1 (1987):37–39.

121. G. Genazzani et al., "Central Deficiency of B-endorphin in Alcohol Addicts," *Clinical Endocrinology and Metabolism* 55, no. 3 (1982):583–86.

122. K. Blum, "Alcohol and Central Nervous System Peptides," *Substance and Alcohol Actions/Misuse* 4 (1983):73–87.

123. Ibid., p. 583.

124. Genazzani et al., "Central Deficiency of B-endorphin in Alcohol Addicts," p. 584.

125. Ibid.

126. Boris Tabakoff et al., "Differences in Platelet Enzyme Activity between Alcoholics and Nonalcoholics," *New England Journal of Medicine* 318 (1988):134–39.

127. Gerald Mueller, "Blood Test Linked to Alcohol Risk," *Science News* 135, no. 1 January 7, 1989, p. 13.

128. Ibid.

129. "Serotonin May Be Key Link between Alcohol, Drugs, Violence," *Drugs and Drug Abuse Newsletter* 107 (January 1986):1–5.

130. Ibid.

131. H. Begleiter et al., "Event-related Brain Potentials in Boys at Risk for Alcoholism," *Science* 225 (1984):1493–96.

132. Blum, "Alcohol and Central Nervous System Peptides," pp. 73–87.

133. "The New Alcoholics," *Glamour,* March 1983.

134. J. Langone, *Women Who Drink* (Reading, Mass.: Addison-Wesley, 1980), p. 2.

135. Ibid.

136. E. N. Corrigan, *Alcoholic Women in Treatment* (New York: Oxford University Press, 1980).

137. "A Special Redbook Report," *Redbook,* June 1982, p. 77.

138. "The New Alcoholics," p. 18.

139. "Effects of Women's New Roles," *USA Today,* February 1985, p. 14.

140. Ibid.

141. "Female Alcoholics: Are They Different?" *Focus on Family,* November/December 1984, p. 16.

142. Ibid.

143. *Alcohol and Health,* Special Report to the U.S. Congress by the Secretary of Health, Education and Welfare (Rockville, Md.: Department of Health, Education and Welfare, 1974).

144. Ibid.

145. John Guarnaschelli, Edward Zapanto, and Frederick Pitts, "Intercranial Hemorrhage Associated with the Disulfiram-Alcohol Reaction," *Bulletin of the Los Angeles Neurological Societies* 37 (January 1972):19–23.

146. "Antabuse: A Special Report," *Amethyst: Multnomah County Alcohol and Drug Scene* 3, no. 7 (September 1979).

147. E. J. Larkin, *The Treatment of Alcoholism: Theory, Practice and Evaluation* (Toronto: Addiction Research Foundation of Ontario, 1974), p. 19.

148. "Lithium Treatment for Alcoholics," *Science News* 114, no. 16 (October 14, 1978).

149. B. Bower, "Lithium Dissolves as Alcoholism Treatment," *Science News,* May 20, 1989, p. 309.

150. National Institute on Alcohol Abuse and Alcoholism, *Treating Alcoholism* (Washington, D.C.: Department of Health, Education and Welfare, 1974), p. 10.

151. David F. Machell, "Alcoholics Anonymous: A Wonderful Medication with Some Possible Side Effects," *Journal of Alcohol and Drug Education* 34, no. 3 (Spring 1989):80–84.

152. Morris E. Chafetz and Harold W. Demono, *Alcoholism and Society* (New York: Oxford University Press, 1962), p. 167.

153. David Gelman, Elizabeth Ann Leonard, and Binnie Fisher, "Clean and Sober—And Agnostic," *Newsweek,* July 8, 1991, pp. 62–63.

154. Mary Lance, "Either Get Treatment for Your Drinking, or Leave This Family," *Medical Self Care,* January/February 1990, pp. 28, 33, 72.

155. D. F. Machelle, "Alcoholism and Alcohol Education," *Alcohol Drug Education,* Spring 1987, pp. 47–48.

156. Ruth Fox, *Alcoholism: Behavioral Research, Therapeutic Approaches* (New York: Springer, 1967), p. 218.

157. E. M. Jellineck, *The Disease Concept of Alcoholism* (Chicago: Hillhouse Press, 1960), p. 1.

158. William Prochnau, "The Last Resort," *Vogue,* February 1989, pp. 347–49.

159. Molly Malone, "Dependent on Disorder: Children of Alcoholics Are Finding Each Other—and Paths to a Better Life," *Ms.* 15, no. 8 (February 1987):50.

160. Jan Marks, "The Children of Alcoholics," *Parents* 61, no. 3 (March 1986), p. 105.

161. Elizabeth Stark, "Forgotten Victims: Children of Alcoholics," *Psychology Today* 21, no. 1 (January 1987):59.

162. Marks, "The Children of Alcoholics," p. 105.

163. Stark, "Forgotten Victims."

164. L. Bennet et al., "Cognitive and Emotional Problems of Alcoholics," *American Journal of Psychiatry* 45, no. 2 (February 1988):351.

165. D. W. Behling, "Alcohol Abuse as Encountered in 51 Instances of Reported Child Abuse," *Clinical Pediatrician* 18 (1979):87–88, 90–91.

166. Jeanette Murray, lecture to a class on chemical dependency at the University of Oregon, February 2, 1988.

167. Suzan Brook, "Victims and MADD's Mission," *MADDVocate,* 1, no. 2 (Fall 1988):2.

168. "Using Alcohol Responsibly," *Drug Information Center (DIC)* (Eugene: University of Oregon, 1983).

CHAPTER
9

OPIATES

Opiates

Drugs, sometimes called narcotics, which are derived from opium (the thickened juice of the opium poppy), that are used to induce sleep and remove pain.

NONSYNTHETIC OPIATES

Opiates, sometimes called narcotics, are drugs derived from opium (the thickened juice of the opium poppy) that are used to induce sleep and relieve pain. Opium has been in existence since at least 4000 B.C., when it was known as "the plant of joy."[1] Raw opium was highly regarded by the early physicians Hippocrates in Greece and Galen in Rome, and it spread into Europe and China during the first century A.D.

In 1805, the major active constituent of opium, an alkaloid, was isolated and named morphine after the Greek god of dreams, Morpheus. Codeine, another alkaloid, was isolated approximately 30 years later. Heroin, a semi-synthetic drug produced by synthesizing acetic anhydride (a common industrial acid) and morphine, was produced in 1874. With the use of these drugs and the invention of the hypodermic needle, opiates were employed freely and approved for general use. As late as 1906, the American Medical Association even believed heroin to be nonaddictive.

Many reasons are given for the widespread use of opium, but according to

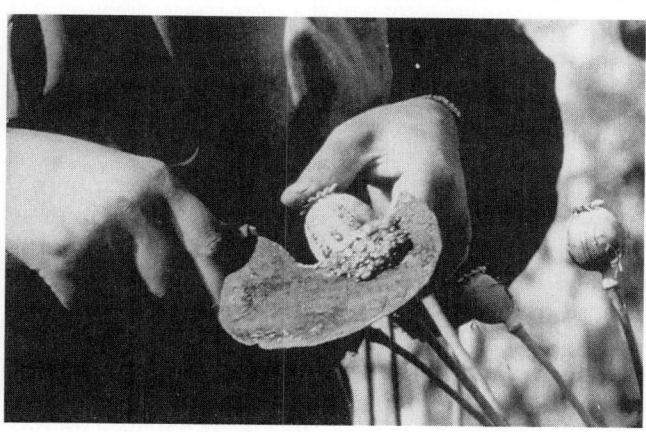

Scraping the Plant for
Raw Opium
Source: Drug Enforcement
Administration

Norman Taylor, a noted botanist, the main reasons are that it is cheap to produce, readily available, and the greatest chemical flight from reality known.[2] Opium's unlicensed cultivation is forbidden in most countries, but it is grown nonetheless in Turkey, Asia Minor, Macedonia, the former Yugoslavia, Bulgaria, Iran, China, and India and transported for distribution. Raw opium can be prepared for smoking by dissolving, boiling, roasting, or fermenting. Americans seldom use opium in its raw state, preferring its derivatives morphine and heroin.

Pakistan, Afghanistan, and Iran are the largest producers of illicit opium in the world.[3] A problem for these countries is that many of their citizens are very poor because of war and food shortages; growing and selling opium is a cash crop for them. After the crops are harvested they are sent out through North Africa and then Europe. Finally they make their way over to the United States. These markets pose large problems for countries like the United States and for the North Atlantic Treaty Organization (NATO).

However, it should also be noted that according to the Drug Enforcement Administration, world production of opium doubled in the late 1980s.[4] The new poppy fields are widespread in Mexico and Guatemala. Local police in those areas say the drug is "flooding the markets." The purity of heroin has soared from 10 percent or less to anywhere from 30 percent to 50 percent. The higher purity and stable prices make it economical for users to smoke rather than inject the drug. This could cause an entire new generation to use heroin without the risk of AIDS from needle use.

Smoking or eating opium produces dullness or stupor, and in larger doses it may produce sleep, coma, or even death. Tolerance and physical dependence will result with repeated use, as will psychological dependence. Once dependence has set in, opium users often continue to take the drug not to seek a high but rather to remain free from withdrawal symptoms.

MORPHINE

Morphine is about ten times stronger than opium and takes effect much more rapidly. It can be pure white, off-white, or light brown and can be purchased as a cube, capsule, tablet, or powder, or in solution. Intravenous injection gets the medication into the bloodstream for immediate transportation. But use of hypodermic syringes must be carefully regulated so that drugs are injected in the proper dosage and so that dirty needles, which lead to such conditions as AIDS, hepatitis, blood poisoning, and endocarditis (inflammation of the membranes lining the heart), are avoided.

Morphine acts as a primary and continuous depressant on respiratory action in the brain stem.[5] It decreases the amount of oxygen and carbon dioxide that is exchanged, depresses the coughing center, and stimulates the vomiting center.[6] Some researchers also believe that free morphine leaves the blood and concentrates in the tissues such as the kidneys, liver, and lungs.[7]

Individuals intoxicated by morphine have pinpoint pupils that do not react to light. If they inject the drug frequently, vein membrane walls break down, eventually forming scar tissue referred to as *tracks*. Although the blue discoloration caused by the needle may disappear, the tracks will remain permanently.

Morphine is one of the most useful drugs available for acute and chronic pain. Physicians have been using it for this purpose since the middle of the nineteenth century. The World Drug Organization has designated it an "essential drug" that should be available everywhere for medical use."[8] However, governments around the world are so concerned about the abuse of narcotics that they have developed strict laws banning the manufacturing and importing of such drugs. Many governments do not distinguish between legitimate drug use and drug abuse, thus preventing those in severe pain from receiving relief from morphine. Even in the United States many state governments, fearing abuse, limit the amount of morphine that is distributed, causing many to suffer needlessly. Narcotics are still underused in this country for the treatment of cancer pain.[9]

Many people are suffering with pain that cannot effectively be alleviated with existing treatments. Physicians are reluctant to prescribe morphine, which is the safest, most effective pain killer known for constant, severe pain.[10] Unfortunately, it can also be addictive for some. Because of this fear, physicians are afraid of turning patients into addicts and end up giving doses that are too small or not given often enough to suppress pain. However, when used for pain, addiction is rare. Addiction appears to be the result only in some users who take it for its psychological effects. Those who take morphine for pain may have some initial tolerance with their required dose, raising gradually and then stabilizing.[11]

According to research conducted by Richard J. Weber of the National Institute of Diabetes and Digestive and Kidney Diseases and of the National Institute of Mental Health (NIMH), in addition to killing pain, morphine may prove helpful in suppressing natural killer-cell activity to destroy viral infected cells and destroy cancer cells.[12] They injected six groups of male rats with enough morphine to make them drowsy. A seventh group was used as a control. Three hours after the injection the researchers took cells from the rats' spleens, mixed them with cancer cells, and measured killer cells' ability to destroy their tumor targets. The results were a "dramatic" drop in killer-cell performance.

HEROIN

When first synthesized in 1874, heroin was thought to be a cure for morphine addiction. It was soon discovered, however, that heroin is twice as likely to produce dependency as morphine and is ten times stronger. It is usually found as a white, odorless, crystalline powder that dissolves in water.

Since heroin is a CNS depressant, drowsiness follows injection, the pupils constrict, respiration and pulse are slowed, and, after large doses, coma or death may occur. The danger of dependency seems to be greater than for other opiate agents because tolerance develops more rapidly (about twice as fast as with morphine).

The government estimates that there are about 750,000 heroin users in the United States.[13] DAWN, the government's Drug Abuse Warning Network, did a study and found that in 27 cities, heroin and cocaine use had caused deaths to triple to 627 between 1985 and 1989. According to DAWN, the number could go even higher. Heroin is currently being sold for $10 for a .05 gram bag. It is thus within the reach of the young and poor.

Chronic use of heroin by pregnant women may result in a variety of obstetrical complications.[14] Heroin dependency may cause poor nutrition and inadequate hygiene, and it may involve other drugs that can contribute their own complications. Babies born to chronic users also run the risk of congenital heroin dependence and may need special care for several weeks following delivery, though withdrawal symptoms may not show. Many of these infants have low birth weights, but this has not been attributed to heroin use alone.

Since the beginning of the 1980s, researchers have tried to find more about what heroin does to pregnant women and the developing fetus. "There are an estimated 100,000 [heroin-dependent] women of childbearing age in the United States and they give birth to almost 10,000 babies each year."[15] Some of the effects of addiction can be passed on to a fetus, leading to retardation, behavioral abnormalities, and delayed development of the muscular and nervous systems. Even methadone and other heroin substitutes can cause these problems. Symptoms will occur in about 75 percent of newborns of heroin-dependent mothers. Methadone-dependent mothers may have infants that go through withdrawal symptoms. Another major reason for problems with newborns is that heroin-dependent mothers rarely have proper prenatal care.[16]

Withdrawal Symptoms   Symptoms of withdrawal from heroin can be violent and long-lasting:

About 12 or 24 hours after the last dose, the addict may fall into a tossing, restless sleep known as the "yen," which may last several hours but from which he awakens more restless and more miserable than before. As the syndrome progresses . . . dilated pupils, anorexia (loss of appetite), gooseflesh, restlessness, irritability, and tremor [set in]. . . . at 48 to 72 hours . . . the patient exhibits increasing irritability, insomnia, marked anorexia, violent yawning, severe sneezing, lacrimation, and coryza (inflammation of nasal mucous membrane with profuse nasal mucous discharge). Weakness and vomiting are common, as are intestinal spasm and diarrhea. Heart and blood pressure are elevated. Marked chilliness, alternating with flushing (skin reddening) and excessive sweating, is characteristic. Pilomotor activity (contraction of skin's smooth muscle causing hairs to stand erect) resulting in waves of gooseflesh (*curtis anserina*) is prominent, and skin resembles that of a plucked turkey. This feature is the basis of the expression "cold turkey" to signify abrupt withdrawal without treatment. Abdominal cramps and pains in the bones and muscles of the back and extremities are also characteristic, as are the muscle spasms and kicking movements that may be the basis for the expression "kicking the habit." . . .

The failure to take food and fluids, combined with vomiting, sweating and diarrhea, results in marked weight loss, dehydration, . . . and disturbance in acid-base balance. Occasionally there is cardiovascular collapse. . . .

. . . In addition, there seem to be subtle behavioral manifestations of protracted abstinence that include the incapacity to tolerate stress, a poor self-image, and overconcern about discomfort.[17]

Nonphysical Dependence   According to Stewart, de Witt, and Eikelboom, recent behavioral and neuropharmacological findings suggest that opiates (and stimulants) act on common neurochemical systems of the brain to generate appetitive states that maintain drug behavior.[18] It has become clear, they say, through comparative study of drug self-administration by humans and by laboratory mammals, that the part of the brain that regulates appetite has a particular affinity for depressant drugs such as heroin and morphine. Their study of the reactions of animals to these drugs not only is directly relevant to our understanding of drug abuse but may provide us with important information about the control of appetitive behavior and about the neural substrate of the motivational systems of the brain.[19]

It has been demonstrated that physical dependence is not necessary for opiates to be sought and taken. Yet the prevailing view has been that continued self-administration of opiates is a function of the need to reduce or avoid withdrawal. Stewart and colleagues quote other studies that show that the initial acquisition of opiates that are self-administered can occur rapidly in an animal having no previous drug experience, and that opiate use can be maintained over long periods at doses too low to bring on withdrawal or deprivation.

Likewise, the conditions surrounding relapse to drug taking by individuals who have been drug-free for long periods suggest that avoidance of withdrawal or desire to reduce need does not provide an adequate account of drug-taking behavior. Reexposure to the environment previously associated with drug taking leads to relapse in a large percentage of experienced but drug-free individuals, even after prolonged abstinence.

Maddox and Desmond studied the effect of opioid use on 248 addicts in San Antonio for three years. They found that moving away from the environment of regular use led to abstinence, but upon return to San Antonio, 81 percent of the addicts relapsed within one month.[20] Three reasons they suggest for abstinence through relocation are reduced availability, separation from conditioned stimuli, and separation from models. In short, physical dependence may not be the only reason people crave drugs.

Heroin-Related Deaths   For opiate dependents who do not kick the habit, opiate poisoning (**overdose**) can occur. Numerous deaths have been attributed to overdoses, though some researchers in the field suggest that many of these deaths were *not* a result of too much heroin.

When an individual dies in the absence of a physician who can determine the cause of death, it becomes the duty of the local coroner or medical examiner to determine it. Following the autopsy, no coroner wants to be faced with inquiries from the press, police, and anxious family members without knowing the cause of death. Milton Halpern, a physician, states that

> in some fatal acute cases, the rapidity and type of reaction do not suggest overdose alone but rather an overwhelming shocklike process due to sensitivity to the injected material. The toxicologic examination of the tissues in such fatalities, where the reaction was so rapid that the syringe and needle were still in the vein of the victim when the body was found, demonstrated only the presence of alkaloid, not overdosage. In other acute deaths, in which the circumstances and autopsy findings were positive, the toxicologist could not even find any evidence of alkaloid in the tissues or body fluids. Thus, there does not appear to be any quantitative correlation between the acute fulminating lethal effect and the amount of heroin taken.[21]

Others interested in drug abuse have identified the sugar and quinine adulterants often added to heroin as the true culprits of overdose-attributed deaths. Michael M. Baden, one-time deputy chief medical examiner of New York City, states that

> the majority of [heroin] deaths are due to an acute reaction to the intravenous injection of the heroin-quinine-sugar mixture. This type of death is often referred to as an "overdose" which is a misnomer. Death is not due to a pharmacological overdose in the vast majority of cases.[22]

Further speculation about heroin-related deaths centers in the area of synergism. On many occasions, heroin is used with other CNS depressants, such as alcohol and barbiturates, and combining such drugs may amplify their chemical effects, causing death. Administering an opiate to an already depressed central nervous system may simply be too severe.

Three of the most publicized overdose deaths of the 1970s were those of rock performers Jimi Hendrix, Janis Joplin, and Jim Morrison. In particular, Janis Joplin "drank like an F. Scott Fitzgerald legend."[23] On October 19, 1970, shortly after her death, *Time* reported:

> The quart bottle of Southern Comfort that she held aloft onstage was at once a symbol of her load and a way of lightening it. . . . Last week, . . . returning to her Hollywood room after a late-night recording session and some hard drinking with friends at a nearby bar, she apparently filled a hypodermic needle with heroin and shot it into her left arm. The injection killed her.[24]

. . . Not to mention the Southern Comfort. However, her death was attributed strictly to overdose.

Heroin is back on the streets and is more potent and more plentiful than ever.[25] But what alarms drug experts most is the increasing popularity of smoking heroin as opposed to injecting it. Smoking opens up the specter of

Overdose

Taking an excessive amount of a drug, such as heroin, or a combination of several drugs and adulterants that may lead to death.

heroin addiction to a whole new population. Authorities report that growing numbers of crack addicts are smoking heroin with crack, which is called "chasing the dragon." Addicts are doing this because it prolongs the high while slowing down the racing feeling of crack and reducing anxiety, depression, and paranoia that would otherwise occur when crack wears off.[26]

Heroin Dependents' Lifestyles   A researcher examined the life histories of 30 hard-core heroin addicts, paying close attention to their criminal record and the types of crimes they committed.[27] He proposed that the addicts learned specific skills that enabled them to support their habits. They gravitated toward certain crimes more often than not because of these skills and their years on the street. The criminal addicts saw themselves as entrepreneurs of a sort: They saw a challenge in getting the drug, akin to that of business people who set goals for themselves in the business world.[28] Most of the addicts relied on one or two types of crime to support their habit, but they could perpetuate other crimes as well if they had to. However, they were more often caught and jailed while trying to commit crimes other than the ones they usually committed. The women tended to participate in more crimes traditionally committed by women: prostitution, shoplifting, forgery, and drug dealing. Most of the addicts prepared meticulously for their crimes, spending days or weeks learning the patterns of their victims—all in order to meet the expense of their addiction.

Does crime cause drug use, or does addiction to drugs lead to crime? Several large-scale studies in the United States have suggested that a general increase in criminality commonly occurs in conjunction with heroin use. For example, one team of researchers examined two hypotheses: Heroin addict criminality is a consequence of addiction, and the principal explanation of the association between drug use and crime is likely to be found in subcultural attachment.[29] In studying 32 hard-core addicts, they discovered (1) childhood and early-adolescent experiences that may be predisposing factors for eventual drug involvement, (2) initial encounters with various drugs, (3) the evolution of the addict's drug and criminal careers, (4) patterns of activity during peak periods, and (5) preferences for types of crimes and drugs. All the respondents in this study felt that their drug and criminal careers happened independently. The researchers concluded that two general factors shape and influence the drug and crime careers of addicts: availability of the drug and the addict's lifestyle. Most addicts maintain normal, predictable daily routines. Many work conventional jobs.

Stages of Dependency   After interviewing many former and current heroin addicts, Charles Faupel concluded that addicts have a code of ethics, and that adherence to that code is determined by which of the following stages the addict is in.[30]

OCCASIONAL USER.   Two factors limit drug availability in this stage—income and inexperience in the drug subculture, which in turn limits access to dealers. Those in this stage have very structured lives in terms of school, sports, or jobs.

STABILIZED JUNKIE.   This stage is characterized by increasing familiarity with the subculture. Users learn how to locate dealers, prepare drugs, and inject themselves. They become familiar with the art of hustling, since the cost of their habit can no longer be supported by a job or allowance. Still, users maintain a very structured life.

FREEWHEELING JUNKIE.   This stage is characterized by a disruption of the addict's structured life. This disruption is often caused by a "big score" or "sting," which enables the addict to go for a number of days without hustling. Availability goes up with the increasing income, as does use.

STREET JUNKIE.   This stage is characterized by low drug availability and minimal life structure. At this point the addict lives from fix to fix, almost unable to maintain the simplest routines. Hygiene and nutrition suffer, and the addict takes on the appearance of the stereotypical "junkie." All subculture ethics are gone as the addict struggles to maintain his or her habit. He will steal from his own family, perhaps even kill in order to get what he feels he needs to survive.

Heroin and AIDS   In recent years the problems of heroin addiction took a back seat in the media to the resurgence of cocaine and the problems related to its use. Now, with the spread of **AIDS,** heroin is back in the spotlight. It has been estimated that as many as 60 percent of the 200,000 heroin addicts in New York City may carry the virus.[31] In New York City a pilot program has been launched in which free syringes are distributed to addicts along with information about the spread of the AIDS virus through sexual avenues and the sharing of needles. Law enforcement officials and clergy oppose the program, saying it will only promote crime. Health officials claim it is necessary to stop the spread of AIDS in the addict population and into the heterosexual population.[32]

AIDS
Acquired Immunodeficiency Syndrome. This life-threatening disease is often spread by sharing syringes while injecting various drugs.

Medical Uses   A five-year study was conducted by the Sloan-Kettering Cancer Center in New York City on the efficacy of various analgesics. Heroin was included in this study, since there has been growing support for making heroin available to terminally ill cancer patients experiencing intractable pain (pain so intense that patients are aware of nothing else). The medication presently provided to such patients is either given in dosages too small to help or must be continually increased because tolerance is reached. Available studies suggest that heroin would aid terminal patients with intractable pain, but legislators and others are afraid legalization will increase street use.

Proponents of heroin use for terminally ill patients with intractable pain feel that such use is safe and invaluable. Surprisingly, the use of heroin in this way alone does not lead to addiction even when it is administered regularly.[33] In the United States, various groups have actively sought to reintroduce heroin into the medical community. The following two acts, among others, show that their voices are being heard:

1. The Compassionate Pain Relief Act (H.R. 5290) would give physicians the freedom and responsibility to provide heroin to patients who need it. H.R.

5290 also states specifically that heroin would be available only to cancer patients whose pain is not relieved by conventional analgesics.

2. The Waxman Bill (as amended and approved in March 1984 by the Committee on Energy and Commerce) would allow distribution of heroin according to prescriptions written by physicians registered under section 302 of the Controlled Substances Act, and then only through hospitals, pharmacies, or hospices.[34]

A growing number of people, especially in Great Britain, where heroin is legal, feel that the lawful availability of heroin poses no greater security threat than similar drugs do. The Heroin Movement created in 1974 by the National Committee for the Treatment of Intractable Pain has helped foster initial efforts in the United States in pain research, terminal care, and studies on the comfort of patients.[35] Pain control is discussed openly on rounds: Nurses and doctors are beginning to be concerned now not about addiction but about giving enough of the right narcotic to the suffering patient. American medicine appears to be giving serious consideration to placing heroin on the prescribed drug list.

Great Britain has been administering heroin and morphine to terminally ill patients with intractable pain for a number of years. Both drugs are prescribed in English hospices and treatment centers. Hospices, in fact, often prefer heroin to morphine because it has fewer side effects (less nausea and vomiting, reduced **constipation** potential, reduced anorexia) and is highly soluble in water, making it a substantially stronger analgesic. A specialist at St. Thomas's Hospital in London stated, "But when prescribed for pain the pain eats up the addictive qualities of heroin."[36]

CODEINE

Codeine, derived from morphine, is less effective than morphine in inducing sleep and alleviating pain. It is widely used in cough medicines, through which it appears to exert analgesic and antitussive (cough-reduction) effects on the central nervous system. It is also found in pills for treating various types of mild to moderately severe pain. Little is known, however, about the location and nature of codeine's effects.

In therapeutic doses, the side effects of codeine are seldom serious, but may include such gastrointestinal reactions as nausea, vomiting, constipation, and dizziness. The drug possesses a certain potential for dependence, but the incidence of abuse does not remotely approach that of morphine or heroin. The lethal dose of codeine is not known with certainty.[37]

SYNTHETIC OPIATES

METHADONE

Methadone is a synthetic narcotic classified as a CNS depressant. Its effects are similar to those of morphine, though they develop more slowly and persist longer.[38] First synthesized during World War II, the drug is cur-

---

Constipation

A condition in which the feces become hard and dry because fluid is not absorbed quickly enough to produce softer stools.

Methadone

A synthetic narcotic classified as a CNS depressant. Its effects are similar to those of morphine, though they develop more slowly and persist longer. Methadone blocks the high given by heroin and has been used in treatment of heroin dependency. The user substitutes methadone for heroin until he or she can be gradually withdrawn from heroin. This removes the heroin high and the withdrawal symptoms caused when heroin is no longer used.

rently approved for uses in reduction of severe pain and detoxification and maintenance treatment for opiate dependents. Methadone is a white crystalline powder that is soluble in alcohol and water and may be injected or drunk.

Methadone is a synthetic, addictive opiate used as a substitute for heroin. In 1963 it was discovered that dependence on heroin can be transferred to methadone. Given a daily oral dose of methadone, an addict can be stabilized, or "maintained," in a condition where his or her physical yearning for heroin is eliminated.[39] Although still addicted to a drug, the user is free from the necessity of continued "hustling" to meet the need for heroin.

The controversial development of methadone maintenance and the problems of the individual suggest the complex issues involved in the use of technology as a quick solution to profound social problems. The problem of heroin addiction has been variously described in moral, social, psychological, legal, and medical terms. The use of methadone involves a decision to define it as a medical problem and to focus on the most manageable and most easily understood of the problems of the addict—his physiological need.

Because methadone maintenance and detoxification programs have become widespread since the early 1980s, more methadone has been available on the illicit market, and "drug-program abuse" is frequent. Diversion of medication, missed medication, lost medication, medicine supplementation, multiple registrations of patients, and other forms of program abuse exist throughout the country.

Methadone has been used to rid addicts of the crippling financial and physical burden of heroin addiction. Now, the National Institute on Drug Abuse (NIDA), a federal research agency, is trying to develop drugs that can supplement or replace methadone as treatment for addiction. A drug called buprenorphine has been approved by the U.S. Food and Drug Administration as an analgesic for acute, chronic pain.[40] It is an opioid and comes in two forms, injectable liquid and tablet. This will be discussed more fully in the chapter on treatment.

Physical Effects   Methadone produces a loss of appetite, constriction of pupils, sweating, reduced respiration, elevated blood-sugar levels, constipation, the release of antidiuretic hormones, drowsiness, and impo-

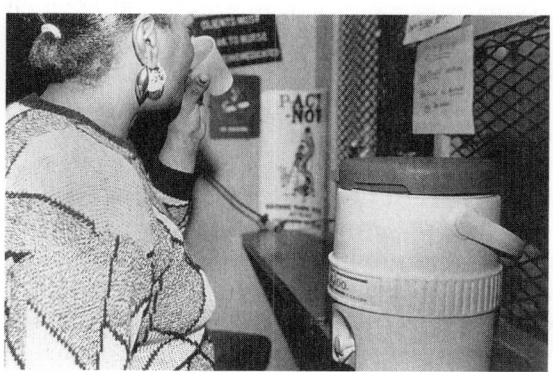

Former Heroin Addict Receives Methadone with Orange Juice
Source: Griffin/The Image Bank

tence. It has less hypnotic action than morphine but is very dependency-producing. Methadone is absorbed rapidly after administration—within 10 minutes it can be found in significant concentrations in plasma. Like other opiate analgesics, it quickly leaves the blood and localizes in the lungs, liver, kidneys, and spleen. Concentration levels in the brain reach their peak one or two hours following administration. The drug readily crosses the placental barrier and enters into a fetal circulation, and it may produce a methadone-dependent infant.

Withdrawal in Infants   Studies have been made of infants born to mothers taking methadone; these cases have been compared with those of infants born to mothers who used heroin during pregnancy.[41] Withdrawal symptoms exhibited by the methadone group were approximately the same as, though a bit less pronounced than, those exhibited by heroin-dependent infants. Other studies concur in finding milder withdrawal symptoms in methadone-dependent babies, but one study found that longer treatment was needed for those infants.[42]

Overdose   Acute methadone poisoning may result from clinical, accidental, or deliberate overdose (suicide attempts). By the time the patient reaches medical assistance, he or she may be asleep or stuporous; a large overdose may result in a deep coma from which there is no arousal.

PROPOXYPHENE HYDROCHLORIDE (DARVON)

Propoxyphene hydrochloride (best known under its trade name of Darvon), a white crystalline powder that is water-soluble and usually combined with aspirin or acetaminophen, was first synthesized in 1953. It was considered a medical breakthrough because it had the potency of codeine but not its side effects or potential for abuse or dependency. Unfortunately, this initial optimism was short-lived, since research later proved that Darvon was structurally related to methadone.[43] Darvon is generally taken to relieve mild pain.

Propoxyphene Hydrochloride (Darvon)

A white crystalline powder that is water-soluble and usually combined with aspirin or acetaminophen to relieve mild pain. It was considered a medical breakthrough because it had the potency of codeine but not the side effects or potential for dependency. Unfortunately, this initial optimism was short-lived, since research later proved that Darvon was structurally related to methadone and could cause psychological dependency.

Physical Effects   Many of the people who become dependent on Darvon were first introduced to the drug when it was prescribed by their physician for specific pain relief. Users then went on to use the drug for every physical discomfort they encountered, without further consulting their doctor. Many found the Darvon-produced euphoria a pleasant relief from the problems of day-to-day life. The drug can eventually lead to psychological dependence.

For most individuals, recommended doses do not cause clinically significant changes of respiration, blood pressure, or pulse rate. Research indicates, however, that Darvon may impair cognition and motor-skill coordination. Adverse reactions can include dizziness, headache, sedation, insomnia, skin rashes, and gastrointestinal disturbances (including nausea, vomiting, abdominal pain, and constipation).

Continual ingestion of large doses of Darvon will produce physical dependence. As tolerance develops, the dosage must be increased approximately every six weeks to obtain the desired effects. The drug can be easily abused, since it is not thought of as one of the strongest synthetic opiates. The claim is now being made that Darvon is one of the deadliest prescription drugs in the United States.

Accidental or intentional overdose of Darvon has symptomatology similar to that of opiate overdose and includes convulsions, coma, respiratory depression, and severe cardiovascular depression. In 1978, over 600 deaths were attributed to Darvon.[44]

DRUG ABUSE–RELATED LEGISLATION

THE NATIONAL ADDICTION REHABILITATION ADMINISTRATION

Established by Congress in 1966, the National Addiction Rehabilitation Administration (NARA) marked a major shift in this country's policy on opiate dependence. For the first time since the Harrison Act became effective in 1914, the problem of opiate dependence was looked at from a medical rather than a legal-criminal point of view.[45] That is, the advent of the NARA marked a national acceptance of such dependence as an illness rather than an act punishable by imprisonment.

Pilot Programs   The major effect of the NARA legislation was the establishment, under the auspices of the National Institute of Mental Health and the Department of Justice, of medical treatment programs in Lexington, Kentucky, and Fort Worth, Texas. Opiate dependents convicted of drug-related offenses could be sent there instead of to prison, under the following terms:

> (1) The user could be committed for treatment rather than criminal prosecution of a drug-related crime. If the offense was non-violent in nature, the Surgeon General of the Public Health Service took responsibility for examination, treatment, and rehabilitation. (2) If the user was already convicted of a crime, [he] could be committed to the Attorney General for treatment at one of the centers. The treatment period was not to exceed 10 years or the maximum sentence period for [the] crime. (3) The user could voluntarily submit himself to the Attorney General for treatment at one of the centers. This form of civil commitment could be implemented even if criminal charges for an offense didn't exist.[46]

The Lexington facility comprised two treatment centers. One was operated in conjunction with the Department of Psychiatry at the University of Kentucky Medical Center. This program consisted of an outpatient center within the university hospital and provided crisis intervention, individual psychotherapy, referral, education and family counseling, vocational training, job placement, and legal intervention.

The other center, the NIMH's Clinical Research Center (CRC), is a comprehensive residential in-patient facility. Services include detoxification, therapeutic community setting, group and individual therapy, encounter groups, sensitivity and self-awareness groups, vocational training, supervised work assignments, social services referral, job placement, legal intervention, medical-health care, and recreational therapy.[47]

The treatment program at the latter was not unlike one at an average large inpatient psychiatric facility. The admitting procedure included a complete history of drug use, a family history, education and vocational history, psychological testing, and physical examination. A physician then made a diagnosis and instituted specific treatment based on the patient's data. If the patient was physically dependent on opiates at the time of admission, he or she was placed in a detoxification ward. The treatment procedure included the administration of 60 to 100 milligrams per day of methadone, followed by incremental reductions of approximately 10 milligrams per day.

Follow-up studies tracking 1,912 Lexington "graduates" one to four years after their release showed that only 6.6 percent of them had abstained from further drug use through this period. A second study involving 453 former patients spot-checked at six months, two years, and five years following release found a total of only 12 who had abstained through the five-year period.[48] "Almost all [became] readdicted and reimprisoned early in the [next] decade and for most the process [has been] repeated over and over again."[49]

EARLIER LEGISLATION

As laws dealing with narcotics failed, new legislation repeatedly increased the severity of the penalty for drug-related offenses. In 1909, three federal laws specified only a two-year imprisonment for narcotics use. In 1917, the Harrison Act increased this period to five years. Ten years became the typical penalty in 1922, and some states provided for sentences of 20, 40, and up to 99 years. During the 1950s, the death penalty and life imprisonment were added to federal statutes as well as to some state codes.

This mandatory sentencing, however, failed to close down illicit drug trafficking. Subsequent federal and state legislation was then enacted depriving convicted narcotics users of the right to parole or time off for good behavior. But these actions too were ineffective, and drug dealing continued to grow. What the laws did bring about was the imprisonment of noncriminal addicts as well as addicts engaged in drug-related crime.

Many deplored what they felt was the injustice of laws stipulating mandatory sentencing for drug addiction. In 1969 Stanley Yolles, director of the National Institute of Mental Health, testified to that effect before the House Select Committee on Crime:

This type of law has no place in a system devised to control an illness. It has no place being used for individuals who are addicted to drugs. This type of law angers us as doctors, because it should not be applied to people who are sick. It destroys hope on the part of the person sentenced—hope of help, hope of starting a fresh life. It's totally contradictory to the whole concept of medicine. A prison experience is often psychologically shattering. The young person is exposed to severe assaults. He may for the first time learn criminal ways. Such mandatory sentences destroy the prospects of rehabilitation.[50]

The Supreme Court eventually ruled that punishment for simply being drug-dependent was cruel and unusual. But the federal government and several states were still able to incarcerate opiate dependents by sending them to "rehabilitation centers" under an imprisonment procedure called civil commitment. One of the largest civil-commitment programs was launched by the state of California. Many convicted drug users in California were sent to the California Rehabilitation Center. There they were detained up to seven years, spending part of their time confined within the center and the remaining time as outpatients after being paroled.[51] Vocational rehabilitation and educational advancement through high school were offered. But five times a month, for at least the first six months, users had to submit to both planned and spontaneous drug tests. Following parole, a halfway house helped ex-residents to readjust to community life. A resident became eligible for final discharge after three drug-free years as an outpatient, but of the 5,300 persons admitted between 1961 and 1965, only 27 were finally discharged.[52]

DETOXIFICATION

If you go for medical detoxification, you will probably be given methadone, today's "preferred" substitute drug.[53] Still, even with methadone, you are going to feel some physical pain, although not much, and the roughest part of withdrawal will be mental, dealing with depression that is often a part of the abstinence syndrome.

Detoxification for former heroin users who have been maintained on high doses of methadone is difficult.[54] In the past, the patient's daily maintenance dose (as high as 70 to 100 milligrams) was reduced by 3 to 5 milligrams a day. But withdrawal symptoms often appeared when the dose fell below 20 milligrams, and many patients continued to feel uncomfortable, irritable, and tired; they also experienced pain, diarrhea, and premature ejaculations for months after detoxification ended. Today, many medical researchers believe methadone detoxification should be extended for as long as four to six months.[55]

A clue to what may complicate detoxification of methadone-maintenance patients was recently uncovered by two studies of former patients that found lower endorphin levels persisting for 6 to 12 months after methadone had ended. If little of the body's own pain- and discomfort-relieving chemicals is reaching their receptors, it's understandable that former methadone users might feel lousy much of the time.[56]

There is great interest now in a nonnarcotic drug for detoxification of narcotic addicts. Not only might such a drug help detoxification of methadone patients, but it would meet the needs of narcotic users who are reluctant to take methadone to detoxify (some addicts fear that because of methadone's potency, they will wind up with heavier habits than they started with). In addition, a nonnarcotic would make it possible to start antagonist therapy immediately after detoxification (eliminating the present need to wait until the patient is free from all residual methadone effects). Clonidine, a drug now used to treat hypertension, has shown some ability to relieve symptoms of narcotic withdrawal and is being studied as a substitute for methadone (see chapter 16).

Many opiate addicts genuinely want to become opiate-free, but traditional withdrawal techniques result in high rates of dropout and early relapse. Acute methadone detoxification was induced by intravenous administration of naloxone hydrochloride during simultaneous intravenous sedation with midazolam hydrochloride, a fully reversible short-acting benzodiazepine, in seven patients addicted to opiates.[57] Within hours the patients tolerated full doses of naltrexone. This technique enables patients to transfer easily, quickly, and safely from methadone to naltrexone maintenance.

This rapid and safe approach permits opiate detoxification to be greatly accelerated without any damage; it's also economical in terms of treatment costs and time away from work. In the future, very long-acting opiate antagonists should be used after rapid detoxification to block opiate receptor sites for a longer time so as to interrupt the vicious circle of addiction.

A study reported that combined clonidine and naltrexone treatment allowed 38 of 40 patients addicted to methadone to withdraw completely in four to five days.[58] Clonidine reduced the intensity of naltrexone-induced withdrawal symptoms. Clonidine significantly decreased blood pressure without producing syncope and caused sedation, but no other clinical problems. The withdrawal symptoms of anxiety, anorexia, insomnia, restlessness, and muscular aching were more resistant but were mild or nonexistent at discharge. Clonidine-naltrexone treatment should succeed with patients receiving methadone doses up to 50 milligrams per day, facilitate naltrexone maintenance, and apply to many clinical settings. In other words, the clonidine and naltrexone treatment proved to be highly effective and well tolerated.

Methadone is the widely used opiate detoxicant because it is easily absorbed and is able to "block" heroin's euphoria. As we have seen, when opiate use ends, the withdrawal symptoms of yawning, perspiration, lacrimation, rhinorrhea, and "yen" sleep begin and pupil dilation, gooseflesh, tremors, hot and cold flashes, aching bones and muscles, and anorexia set in. At this point, methadone treatment begins. (Doctors must also be sure that patients do not fake symptoms to secure a prescriptive dose.) Doses of methadone are administered in 10-to-40-milligram amounts for two to three days and then reduced by 20 percent a day. This schedule may be extended for those unable to tolerate it (though it should not exceed 21 days), but an even shorter detoxification program should be encouraged.[59]

GENERAL EFFECTS

Detoxification and withdrawal are not enjoyable experiences. Their severity, however, is often overstated, and with proper medical treatment they *can* be relatively painless. On the street, drug dependents already suf-

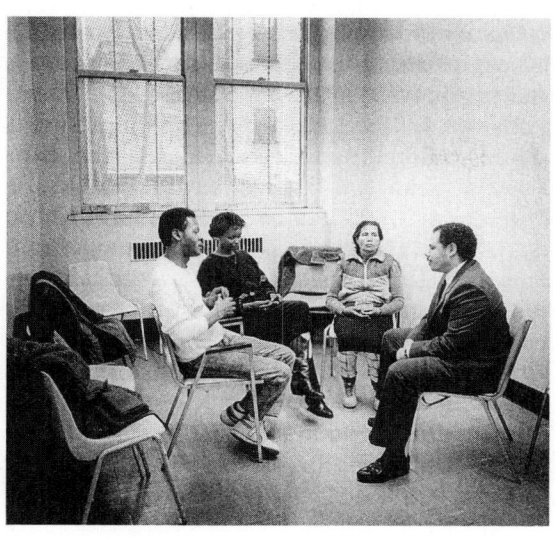

Small Group Counseling Session
Source: Griffin/The Image Works

fering from malnutrition and an array of drug-related illnesses may go through withdrawal with hallucinations, convulsions, weight loss, nausea, vomiting, diarrhea, temperature flashes, muscle cramps, and pain. Because they expect the worst, the worst may happen. Under clinical care, however, discomfort can be controlled, drug-related medical problems can be treated, and medical personnel can help to reduce anxiety by conveying a sense of ease and optimism. When detoxification has been carried out, good nutrition and hygiene instruction can be provided and plans can be made for continued treatment and follow-up.

THERAPEUTIC APPROACHES

Whereas some opiate dependents try to break their habit with chemicals such as methadone, others prefer to try a chemical-free approach. Most of the latter programs involve groups of individuals in noninstitutional treatment centers; the goal of the programs is positive psychological change, resulting from group pressure and reinforcement.

SMALL-GROUP SUPPORT

A number of groups whose aim is to help drug dependents work on their problems have sprung up across the country. Members of these groups feel that shared goals, values, and beliefs, plus a sense of personal responsibility and the chance to participate in one's own treatment, will help to bring about an end to drug addiction. Jerome Frank, professor of psychiatry at Johns Hopkins Medical School, agrees that group pressures, kept in proper perspective, *can* be very beneficial to the individual:

> An important over-all beneficial effect of group methods with inpatients, as well as outpatients, is to restore to patients a sense of individuality and of some control over their destinies. The expectation that they are capable of

self-control and of assuming some degree of responsibility for themselves and others, which is implicit in all forms of group therapy, bolsters their self-respect, stimulates their hopes and in general, helps to restore their morale.[60]

Group pressures and influences are frequently utilized in small-group encounter sessions. In these meetings, between 8 and 12 persons meet for a predesignated amount of time to handle individual and interpersonal difficulties. Through these meetings, participants hope to begin seeing themselves as responsible for their own actions. Meetings often become quite intense, with participants pouring out emotions, frustrations, and tears. But physical violence is not tolerated, and although no topic is immune from discussion, the emphasis is on present and personal behavior.[61]

THERAPEUTIC COMMUNITIES

Synanon

A drug-free therapeutic community where a dependent individual lives and attempts to gain control over bits of her actions and become responsible. No drugs are allowed in this community

The idea of group pressure as a drug-free way to achieve opiate independence is carried a step further in the therapeutic community. Here, in such communities as Daytop, Odyssey House, Phoenix House, Liberty Park Village, and **Synanon,** members (who join voluntarily) must submit to organization rules, relinquish all personal assets, and be responsible for assigned tasks. Members reinforce each other as they attempt to gain control over their actions and become responsible.

The success of these programs as a way of treating opiate dependency has not been substantial. By the mid-1960s, leaders of the Synanon community were ready to admit that they were not achieving the results they had hoped for. With few exceptions, Synanon "graduated" no drug-abstinent individuals. Members thought to be cured promptly relapsed when they left the security of the community.

A major reason for the failure of therapeutic communities seems to be that they are too self-contained and isolated, too unlike the "real" world. Day and night, members are reinforced and supported; their own egos become subservient to the group, and drug-using desires are completely repressed. When members choose to leave, they are faced with pressures and temptations their community had selectively eliminated. Returning to a "normal" environment can cause a relapse into narcotic-seeking behavior.

The future of therapeutic communities remains unclear. Some may become ongoing treatment facilities where recovered users would permanently live and work. Others may offer postdependence-syndrome assistance, since techniques they have developed seem effective. Therapeutic communities are an alternative to the institutional approach. But although they do offer good treatment, by no means are they a cure.[62]

PERSONAL RESPONSIBILITY AND COMMITMENT

Traditional drug treatment in the United States has been oriented toward heroin and similar narcotics.[63] However, alcohol and cocaine programs are increasing in number and in their new approaches to treatment. It's important to find appropriate help based on personal resources (family, friends, work, internal motivation) and deep involvement, regardless of the drugs being used. Therapy groups, education, and individualized recovery plans and follow-up care are important elements in success.[64] But treatment alone does not get a person off drugs. Personal responsibility and commitment do. Treatment can only help. A change in behavior is a three-step process: (1) motivation to act, (2) maximization of success, and (3) maintenance of new behavior.

THE YOUNG USER

A young, novice user, whose physiological adaptation to heroin may be minimal or nonexistent, may feel little or no postwithdrawal craving following detoxification. Early stages of novice use result predominantly from curiosity to experience the rush or high. As a result of his or her age and lack of experience, the young user hasn't seen and felt the severity of the street lifestyle of the opiate user. Therapy is less than desirable to such users because of the fascination of running and hustling in the streets. Attempts at treatment often present themselves as threatening coercion.

The task of therapy must transcend basic detoxification techniques because physiological dependence rarely constitutes the sole problem. The major problem is not dependence on the drug but infatuation with the heroin lifestyle.

METHADONE MAINTENANCE

INTRODUCTION

When first presented as a form of opiate-dependency treatment, methadone maintenance was predicted to produce positive results. Since then, however, a number of problems have dimmed that optimism, including the discovery that methadone is even more capable of causing dependence than heroin. Despite the method's shortcomings, methadone maintenance remains the technique most used for the treatment of opiate dependency.

Marie Nyswander and Vincent P. Dole proposed the idea of methadone maintenance in 1964. While studying the metabolic processes of drug dependents undergoing methadone detoxification, Nyswander and Dole noticed a definite attitude change in patients when methadone was administered past the usual ten-day detoxification period. Said Dole, "The interesting thing about methadone maintenance is that it permits people to become whatever they potentially are, whereas dependents, under the pressure of drug abuse and drug seeking, look very much the same. When [drug dependents are] freed from this dependency, they differentiate and become part of the spectrum of humanity."[65]

Nyswander and Dole found that therapeutic dose levels of methadone were able to assuage opiate desire without producing euphoria or disabling sedation. Because of cross-tolerance, methadone is also able to block an opiate's euphoric affects. Methadone can produce its own euphoria, however, when taken by a nonstabilized patient in high doses, and large doses of heroin can also break methadone's euphoria block. Treatment should include only gradual methadone dose increases. Dose levels can be stabilized over time. The rationale behind the method's use makes it a plausible treatment:

> In absence of a cure . . . it is traditional medical practice to attempt to ameliorate the symptoms or effects of the disease, and to rehabilitate the patient as far as possible to a plausible way of life. . . . Methadone maintenance therapy offers an effective means of managing the illness of heroin addiction—not to cure it, but to counter its effects.[66]

Methadone maintenance designed exclusively for narcotic addicts involves the daily oral administration of methadone, an addictive synthetic narcotic, in order to suppress opioid-drug craving and stave off withdrawal symptoms. Maintenance should be augmented by counseling, including educational and vocational counseling. Family counseling may be offered as well.

Methadone maintenance is one alternative that offers many addicts a reasonable chance of achieving sobriety. It is widely available in hospital outpatient programs and both public and private clinics. Admission to methadone programs is limited by federal regulations to users who are over 16 and have been *addicted* for at least one year.

There is some disagreement about the optimum dosage for maintenance.[67] "High-doses" advocates believe in gradually increasing the amount of the drug until the patient receives enough to prevent even substantial amounts of another narcotic having an effect. "Low-dose" advocates aren't concerned with "narcotic blockade" (block the high provided by the drug) and use a relatively small amount of methadone, just enough to control the craving for heroin and avoid symptoms of withdrawal. Experts in the field argue that methadone dose determination should always be a matter of good clinical judgment on the part of an experienced physician, not a matter to be decided by regulatory agencies or philosophy. The majority of patients ultimately fall into a range of effective doses, with 50 mg. generally accepted as the lowest effective dose. Optimum dose for most patients is 80 mg., plus or minus 20 mg.[68] At properly prescribed maintenance levels, methadone does not produce euphoria. Side effects may include drowsiness, sweating, constipation, and some loss of sexual interest and capacity to achieve orgasm.[69]

How well does methadone maintenance work for patients who do not attempt to withdraw? Effectiveness of methadone programs is generally measured by how long patients continue to participate, by their employment or other productive activity, and by the degree of criminal involvement. Studies of patients by John Ball and others consistently show that the longer a patient remains in treatment, the better the treatment outcome. That is, criminal behavior and elicit drug use decrease, while productive behavior, including employment, increase.[70]

INTERIM METHADONE CLINIC

A study by Yancovitz and others entitled "A Randomized Trial of an Interim Methadone Maintenance Clinic" is an addition to the list of controlled clinical trials on the effectiveness of methadone.[71] It shows that the medically supervised administration of a daily dose of methadone to heroin addicts on the waiting list for conventional treatment reduces heroin consumption even in the absence of the usual supportive services (intensive counseling, social assistance, supplementary care). By reducing intravenous drug use this minimal treatment, when combined with providing free condoms and counseling on risk behavior, also reduces the risk of acquiring or transmitting AIDS.

The importance of this finding is more practical than theoretical because the phenomenon of pharmacological blockade with methadone, and the attendant reduction of craving for opiates, has been documented by many studies during the past 25 years.[72] Not surprisingly, the purely pharmacological effects of methadone are invariant over a wide range of cultural and economic conditions. However, the full value of pharmacological support with minimal social services needs to be tested by additional controlled studies under field conditions.

POSSIBLE HAZARDS AND SIDE EFFECTS

The main hazards of methadone are overdosing by stabilized patients and use by nonstabilized children and adults. Making the drug available only in tablet form (to be taken orally) can cut down on the danger of overdosing, since it is very difficult for a user to overdose on orally ingested methadone, even in high doses. Labeling and putting the methadone in hard-to-reach locations in the refrigerator when used by the patient at home should protect unknowing adults and children. Making the substance available only in powder form also cuts down on illicit intravenous injection, since the powder is potent only in oral form.

Various side effects have been reported with initial methadone intake, especially during the first one to six weeks, when the body adapts to the continuing presence of the drug. Uncomfortable side effects usually occur in the evening, at least eight hours after methadone ingestion, and can include constipation, delayed ejaculation, more frequent urination, numbness in the hands and feet, hallucinations, insomnia, nausea, vomiting, muscle pains, anorexia, and excessive perspiration. Weight gain and the need to drink more fluids can also occur, as can the feeling of oversedation and confusion. Side effects are usually minimal, however, and very seldom warrant the discontinuance of treatment. If side effects do become too unpleasant, a dose reduction of 10 milligrams followed by a buildup to the desired therapeutic dose level will usually solve the problem, since side effects occur in response to specific dose levels.[73]

Though some side effects may appear, premethadone symptoms (caused by street heroin use) show improvement once the user begins to stabilize on methadone. Headaches, joint pains, hiccups, diarrhea, loss of sexual desire, nervousness, runny nose, urination difficulty, and a general feeling of unhappiness either lessen or disappear. The patient's expectations once treatment has begun also play an important role in the reduction of symptoms and in his or her general feeling of well-being.

How methadone use affects pregnancy is still uncertain. Carl Zelson, professor of pediatrics at New York Medical College, has reported that babies born to methadone users are likely to experience more severe consequences than those born to heroin users. Zelson lists the findings of a study of 91 infants born to heroin- and methadone-dependent mothers at New York's Metropolitan Hospital Center:

1. More methadone babies (42) than heroin [babies] developed withdrawal signs, and symptoms of the former were more severe. . . .
2. Five methadone babies suffered convulsive seizures compared to two of the heroin babies.
3. Twelve of the methadone babies and five of the heroin babies had jaundice. In the methadone group, five of these were serious as opposed to only two in the heroin group.
4. Almost one-half of both groups had sub-average birth weights and abnormal sleep patterns.[74]

In another study, however, M. E. Strauss of Johns Hopkins University's department of psychology found that in a compared-subject controlled study of 72 nondependent pregnant women and 72 methadone-dependent pregnant women (all receiving prenatal care), the rates of pregnancy illness, pregnancy complications, and labor and delivery characteristics of the two groups did not differ.[75]

Withdrawal from congenital drug dependence usually occurs within 48 hours of birth. Since newborns are not as heavily dependent on the drug as their mothers, brief medication to relieve the withdrawal and detoxification stress usually returns the infants to a normal state. Increasing tolerance or psychological dependence is not evident.

THE PROCESS

Methadone maintenance may be viewed as a process. During phase 1 low doses—30 to 40 milligrams—are given. Physiological responses are monitored to determine the patient's tolerance level. For three to six weeks, dosage is increased until a level of stabilization is reached—a point where the patient is comfortable, has no craving for opiates, and experiences no euphoria following an opium injection. When stabilization is reached, the dosage level is usually 60 to 100 milligrams a day.

In phase 2, the patient comes to the clinic daily to receive his or her methadone. The patient may leave a urine sample that will be tested for methadone level and the presence of other drugs, such as alcohol, other opiates, amphetamines, or barbiturates (an admission urine and eight random urine specimens are required by federal law during the first year of treatment). During this time, the patient may obtain continual medical care and social rehabilitation along with job consultation, vocational training, educational guidance, and counseling.

Phase 3 begins after behavior stabilizes. At this point, the patient is considered partially rehabilitated and may begin taking one or more days' worth of methadone home for self-administration. After three months, federal law permits a reduction in clinic attendance to three times per week, if approved by the physician, although the patient may receive no more than a two-day supply of medication. After two years of substantial progress, the physician may approve a reduction to two clinic visits per week with a three-day take-home supply of medication. After three consecutive years of rehabilitation, with no major behavior problems, the patient may be approved for one weekly clinic visit and a six-day supply of medication. A urine specimen must be given and tested once per month for use of illicit drugs. It should be noted that this schedule is permitted by federal regulation; states may implement more stringent requirements. It should also be noted that illicit drug use, criminal activity, or other behavioral problems result in increased required clinical visits and a reduced take-home supply of medication.

Discontinuance of methadone may lead to post-withdrawal syndrome and a resurfacing of the desire for heroin. Clinical evidence indicates that such a desire can return even to patients who have been stable more than five years.

RATE OF SUCCESS

Just how successful is methadone maintenance? There are several reasons why the program should meet with success: Because the drug can be obtained legally, it lessens the patient's guilt about desiring and taking narcotics, and reduces the need for self-punishment; it is relatively inexpensive compared with street heroin, and this often eliminates the need to steal to pay for it; since it is fully effective when taken orally, it eliminates the possibility of needle infections and blood-vessel damage; it breaks up the ritual of injecting, which is often the high point of heroin use; and because it is long-acting, it will not subject the user to the psychological "bouncing" reported by many heroin users.

Early findings by an independent evaluation team from the Columbia University School of Public Health, charged with evaluating the success of methadone programs, were very favorable. A later five-year follow-up study on the Santa Clara County Methadone Program indicated that fully one third of those who participated in the program (drinking at least one methadone dose) were still abstaining from heroin five years later. Furthermore, the overwhelming majority of these people were no longer using methadone.[76]

But there are a number of criteria on which to base program evaluations. The first, of course, is the percentage of reduced opiate use. Others are the amount of substitution of alcohol, barbiturates, or amphetamines for heroin, patient return to employment or to a job-training program, improvement in physical and psychological health, and degree of continuing criminal activity. In other words, one should consider not only reduced drug use but also the patient's overall quality of life.

Many feel the relationship between methadone maintenance and reduction in criminal activities is an important indicator of progress for both patient and program. A *Consumers Union Report* states that in one treatment program

91% of the patients had been in jail [prior to treatment], and all of them had been more or less continually involved in criminal activities. . . . Since entering the treatment program, 88% of the patients show arrest-free records. The remainder have had difficulties with the law . . . the only possible conclusion is that the great majority of addicts placed on methadone, despite pre-existing handicaps such as poverty, poor health, little education, prison records, and years of addiction, became self-supporting as well as law-abiding while on methadone.[77]

Others, however, feel that crime reduction is not a true indicator of methadone-maintenance effectiveness. These critics feel that many dependents are criminals and that, drug use or not, it is reasonable to assume they will remain criminal. "Various studies of known addicts have shown that between one-half [and] three-fourths were known to be delinquent before turning to drugs."[78]

Admissions criteria for early methadone-maintenance programs may have led to the initial success statistics. Participants were carefully selected, with psychotics, adolescents, and multiple-drug users specifically excluded. Patients needed to be particularly enthusiastic about joining the program. In some clinics, patients had a good employment record and a stable family record prior to dependency. By choosing only those users with the highest potential for success, the programs denied help to the people most in need of treatment. Success rates may have been high because harder-to-treat individuals did not participate.

Perhaps illustrative of the current fate of many methadone-maintenance programs is one implemented in the early 1980s by Alameda County, California, for heroin addicts residing there. The methadone and follow-up counseling would be paid for by the county for two years after entry into the program. The methadone was distributed daily, and tests were administered to detect continuing heroin abuse. Three years after the program started, the county contracted for a study on its overall effectiveness. County officials wanted to decide whether the program was worthwhile and whether it should be continued in its existing form.

The study consisted of interviews with 110 people who had participated in the treatment program for the prescribed two years of county payment.[79] The interview sought to find whether the majority of the patients were still addicted to heroin or if they were drug-free. The results were not encouraging. Over 90 percent of the patients were either still addicted to heroin at the end of two years or were still using methadone, either paying for it themselves or receiving it in another government-funded program. The overall relapse rate was deemed too high to continue the program in its existing form, and other alternatives were sought by the county.

It is easy to see that methadone maintenance is not a panacea for opiate dependency. It is, however, widely used and *can* help rehabilitate a dependent. With a large and dedicated staff, adequate facilities, sufficient funding, various diversified therapy programs (group and individual), educational-improvement opportunities, vocational-training and job-placement services, and health care (medical and nutritional), methadone maintenance can be effective.

SOCIAL IMPLICATIONS OF METHADONE-MAINTENANCE PROGRAMS

Critics charge that methadone-maintenance programs gloss over the social and economic conditions that drive people to opiate use and work only at controlling and pacifying addicts. Some feel that the programs are a potential form of group repression and covert social control, and reported accounts of methadone-linked sexual impotence arouse fears of population control and seemingly indefinite periods of chemotherapy.

DOES ANY TREATMENT WORK?

Despite the success of many opiate-dependency treatment programs, some individuals in the field feel that no rehabilitation program can really help a user with a long-term habit, someone whose lifestyle is totally identified with a drug-using subculture. A review of clinical treatment at the U.S. Public Health Service hospitals in Lexington, Kentucky, and Ft. Worth, Texas, shows that users treated at these facilities were antisocial prior to dependence and that behavior change was difficult to achieve.[80] Various other studies attempting to assess psychopathology in opiate users point to numerous cases of inappropriate anger, distrust, disbelief in "real" relationships, immaturity, passivity, dependency, low pain threshold, inability to perceive delayed gratification, and a strong ability to manipulate others.[81] Such ingrained tendencies and characteristics make rehabilitation difficult, but not impossible.

MATURING OUT

On the other end of the spectrum, the absence of treatment can sometimes result in a cure. For reasons that remain vague and unsubstantiated, a large percentage of individuals who need clinical services but don't seek or receive them seem to recover on their own. For opiate users, time may be the answer. By the time users reach their mid-thirties they often become spontaneously abstinent. The onset of middle age may make their previous lifestyle unwarranted. "Addiction [that] begins in late adolescence when the person is faced with multiple inner drives and major decisions [may burn] out when his life becomes more stabilized through 'some process of emotional homeostasis.' "[82] This may be true for as many as one third of known users.[83]

SUMMARY

Opium has existed for centuries. The class of opium drugs known as opiates has tremendous pain-relieving properties as well as the ability to produce one of the most powerful euphoric states known. Opiates often lead to psychophysiological dependence, and their legal use in the United States is therefore restricted to prescribed medical situations.

Morphine was the first pain killer to be derived from opium. Heroin soon followed, but both drugs were found to produce dependence with regular use. However, because of heroin's effectiveness, there is increasing legislative support for legalizing heroin for terminally ill cancer patients. In recent years, methadone, a synthetic opiate, has been used to treat heroin dependency. Methadone blocks the euphoria of and desire for heroin, but unfortunately also may lead to dependence. Under proper medical supervision and with proper counseling, however, methadone can be an effective treatment for heroin dependence.

Until recently, Darvon, a dependence-producing synthetic drug very similar to methadone, was easy to obtain and was routinely prescribed by most physicians for virtually every pain or physical discomfort. Recently, however, various government agencies and the medical community have become aware of its abuse and its propensity for contributing to overdose. Prescription of the drug is now greatly curtailed.

On the legal side of drug use, the National Addiction Rehabilitation Administration represented the first attempt to address drug abuse in medical rather than judicial terms. For the first time in recent history, drug-dependents were thought of as needing medical treatment, not punishment. The establishment of the NARA marked the beginning of a more positive attitude toward the problem of drug dependency.

A number of treatment options are available to drug-dependents. These include psychotherapy, peer pressure, chemotherapy, detoxification, job training, narcotic antagonists, and self-control, monitoring, and aversive stimuli. These approaches meet with varying success, depending on the sincerity of the individual in treatment, the training and attitudes of the staff, and the factors precipitating use and dependency.

Opiates
N O T E S

1. John B. Williams, *Narcotics and Hallucinogens* (Encino, Calif.: Glencoe Press, 1967), p. 129.
2. Norman Taylor, *Narcotics* (New York: Dell Pub. Co., 1966), p. 38.
3. "Southwest Asian Heroin: Pakistan, Afghanistan, and Iran," *Drug Enforcement* (Summer 1981):2–11.
4. "Hello Heroin," *The Economist* (September 8, 1990):33.
5. Louis S. Goodman and Alfred Gilman, eds., *The Pharmacological Basis of Therapeutics,* 4th ed. (New York: Macmillan, 1970), p. 243.
6. Williams, *Narcotics and Hallucinogens,* p. 134.
7. Goodman and Gilman, *The Pharmacological Basis of Therapeutics,* p. 248.
8. Robert Angarola, "World Narcotics Consumption," *American Journal of Nursing* 88 (July 1988):1021–25.
9. Ibid., p. 1022.
10. Ronald Melzack, "The Tragedy of Needless Pain," *Scientific American* 262, no. 2 (February 1990):27–33.
11. Ibid.

12. K. A. Fackelmann, "Brain and Immunity: Mapping the Link," *Science News* 136 (July 15, 1989):36.

13. Dan Goodgame, "Heroin Comes Back," *Time,* February 19, 1990, p. 63.

14. *The Non-Medical Use of Drugs: Final Report of the Canadian Government Commission of Inquiry* (Ottawa: Crown, 1973), p. 318.

15. "U.S. Heroin Addicts Bear 10,000 Babies a Year," *Canadian Journal* 10, no. 1 (1981).

16. Ibid.

17. Jerome H. Jaffe, "Drug Addiction and Drug Abuse," in *The Pharmacological Basis of Therapeutics,* 5th ed., ed. Louis S. Goodman and Alfred Gilman (New York: Macmillan, 1975), p. 296.

18. J. Stewart, H. de Witt, and R. Eikelboom, "Role of Unconditioned and Conditioned Drug Effects in the Self-Administration of Opiates and Stimulants," *Psychological Review* 91 (1984):251–68.

19. Ibid. p. 251.

20. J. F. Maddox and D. P. Desmond, "Residence Relocation Inhibits Opiate Dependence," *Archives of General Psychiatry* 39 (1982):1313–17. Copyright © 1982 American Medical Association. Used with permission.

21. Edward M. Brecher et al., *Licit and Illicit Drugs* (Boston: Little, Brown, 1972), pp. 104–5.

22. Quoted in ibid., p. 108.

23. Quoted in ibid., p. 113.

24. Quoted in ibid.

25. Gordon Witkin, "The Return of a Deadly Drug Named Horse," *U.S. News & World Report,* August 14, 1989, p. 31–32.

26. Ibid.

27. Charles E. Faupel, "Heroin Use, Street Crime and the 'Main Hustle': Implications for the Validity of Official Crime Data," *Deviant Behavior* 7, no. 1 (1987):31–45.

28. Ibid., p. 31.

29. C. E. Faupel and C. B. Klockars, "Drugs-Crime Connections and Elaborations from the Life Histories of Hard Core Addicts," *Social Problems* 34 (February 1987):54–68.

30. Charles E. Faupel, "Drug Availability, Life Structure, and Situational Ethics of Heroin Addicts," *Urban Life* 15 (January 1987):395–419.

31. C. Gorman, "The Lesser of Two Evils," *Time,* February 15, 1986.

32. Ibid.

33. John Strang and Les Kay, "How the Media Abuse Heroin," *New Scientist,* October 18, 1984, p. 62.

34. See Allen M. Mondzac, "In Defense of the Reintroduction of Heroin into American Medical Practice and H.R. 5290: The Compassionate Pain Relief Act," *New England Journal of Medicine* 311 (August 23, 1984):532–35. Copyright © 1984 Massachusetts Medical Society. Reprinted with permission of the *New England Journal of Medicine.*

35. Ibid.

36. Ken Walker, "How a Medical Journalist Helped to Legalize Heroin in Canada," *Journal of Drug Issues* 21, no. 1 (Winter 1991):141–47.

37. *Codeine* (New York: Marc K and Co., 1969), p. 4.

38. Williams, *Narcotics and Hallucinogens,* p. 25.

39. Dorthy Nelkin, *Methadone Maintenance: A Technological Fix* (New York: George Braziller, 1973), p. 4.

40. John Harold, "Lukewarm Turkey," *Scientific American* 260, no. 2 (March 1989):32–36.

41. Saul Blatman, "Neonatal and Follow-Up," in *Proceedings of the Third National Conference on Methadone* (1970), p. 82.

42. Leonard Class and Hugh E. Evans, "Narcotic Withdrawal in the Newborn," *American Family Physician* 6, no. 1 (July 1972):76.

43. Deborah Sternlicht, "The Prescribing of Darvon," *Street Pharmacologist* 2, no. 3 (June/July 1979):4–8.

44. "Stir over Darvon," *Time,* December 4, 1978, p. 96.

45. National Institute of Mental Health, *The Narcotic Addict Rehabilitation Act of 1966* (Washington, D.C.: Public Health Service, 1969), p. 2.

46. National Institute of Mental Health, *Narcotics: Some Questions and Answers* (Washington, D.C.: Public Health Service, 1970), p. 3.

47. Deena D. Watson, *National Directory of Drug Abuse Treatment Programs* (Washington, D.C.: National Institute of Mental Health, 1972), pp. 146–47.

48. Brecher et al., *Licit and Illicit Drugs,* p. 69.

49. Ibid., p. 13.

50. Quoted in ibid., p. 57.

51. Brecher et al., *Licit and Illicit Drugs,* p. 71.

52. *The Challenge of Crime in a Free Society: A Report by the President's Commission on Law Enforcement and Administration of Justice* (New York: Avon Books, 1968), pp. 518–19.

53. *How to Get Off Drugs,* "A Rolling Stone Press Book," (New York: Simon & Schuster, First Fireside Edition, 1986), pp. 46–47, 96–99, 112–17.

54. Ibid.

55. Ibid.

56. Ibid.

57. Norbert Loimer et al., "Technique for Greatly Shortening the Transition from Methadone to Naltrexone Maintenance to Patients Addicted to Opiates," *American Journal of Psychiatry* 148 (1991):933–35.

58. Dennis S. Charney, George R. Heninger, and Herbert D. Kleber, "The Combined Use of Clonidine and Naltrexone as a Rapid, Safe, and Effective Treatment of Abrupt Withdrawal from Methadone," *American Journal of Psychiatry* 143 (1986):831–37.

59. George M. Henry, "Treatment and Rehabilitation of Narcotic Addiction," in *Research Advances in Alcohol and Drug Problems,* vol. 1, ed. Robert J. Gibbins et al. (New York: John Wiley, 1980), pp. 267–68.

60. Jerome D. Frank, *Persuasion and Healing,* 2nd rev. ed. (Baltimore: Johns Hopkins, 1973).

61. M. D. Rosenthal, S. Mitchell, and Bias D. Vincent, "Phoenix House: Therapeutic Communities for Drug Addicts," *Hospital and Community Psychiatry* 20, no. 1 (January 1969):29.

62. Brecher et al., *Licit and Illicit Drugs,* p. 82.

63. James Q. Wilson, "Heroin Solution: The Fix," *New Republic,* October 25, 1982, p. 24.

64. Ira Mothner and Alan Weitz, "Get Off Coke," *Rolling Stone,* June 7, 1984, p. 29.

65. Marie E. Nyswander, "Methadone Therapy for Heroin Addiction: Where Are We? Where Are We Going?" *Drug Therapy* 1, no. 1 (January 1971):23.

66. Quoted in Brecher et al., *Licit and Illicit Drugs,* p. 139.

67. *How to Get Off Drugs.*

68. J. Thomas Payte and Elizabeth T. Khuri, "Principles of Methadone Dose Determination," in *State Methadone Maintenance Treatment Guidelines,* Mark W. Parrino, Consensus Panel Chair. Published by the U.S. Center for Substance Abuse Treatment (1992).

69. *How to Get Off Drugs.*

70. J. C. Ball et al., *The Effectiveness of Methadone Maintenance Treatment.* New York: Springer-Verlag, 1991.

71. S. R. Yancovitz et al., "A Randomized Trial of an Interim Methadone Maintenance Clinic," *American Journal of Public Health* 81 (1991):1185–1202.

72. Vincent P. Dole, "Interim Methadone Clinics: An Undervalued Approach," *American Journal of Public Health* 81 (September 1991):1111–12.

73. Ibid., p. 24; Brecher et al., *Licit and Illicit Drugs,* pp. 153–54.

74. Carl Zelson, "Methadone and Heroin," *Archives of Internal Medicine* 132 (July 1973):9.

75. M. E. Strauss et al., "Methadone Maintenance during Pregnancy: Pregnancy, Birth and Neonate Characteristics," *American Journal of Obstetrics and Gynecology* 120, no. 7 (December 1, 1974):895–99.

76. Avram Goldstein, "Heroin Maintenance: A Medical View," *Journal of Drug Issues* 9, no. 3 (Summer 1979):344.

77. Quoted in Brecher et al., *Licit and Illicit Drugs,* pp. 142–43, 148.

78. James Q. Wilson, Mark H. Moore, and I. David Wheat, Jr., "What Public Policy toward Heroin?" *Current Health* 147 (January 1973):16, 19.

79. Marsha Rosenbaum and Jerome Beck, "Money for Methadone: Preliminary Finds from a Study of Alameda County's New Maintenance Policy," *Psychopharmacology* 91, no. 1 (1987):30–33.

80. Henry, "Treatment and Rehabilitation of Narcotic Addiction," p. 283.

81. Ibid., p. 284.

82. Ibid., p. 291.

83. Ibid.

HALLUCINOGENS

BACKGROUND

Hallucinogenic drugs have been in use for a very long time. American Indians have historically used a hallucinogen, peyote, for religious ceremonies. The more recent use of hallucinogenic drugs for "recreational" purposes began in the 1950s.

People take hallucinogens for their unique psychophysiological effects. Each of these drugs has a slightly different effect, but for the most part they elicit a common set of responses: (1) sensory-perceptual (distorted time sense; altered sensations of colors, sounds, and shapes, ultimately developing into complex hallucinations and synesthesia, or mixing of the senses); (2) psychic (dreamlike feelings, depersonalization, rapid and often profound alterations of affect, such as depression or elation); and (3) somatic (dizziness, tingling skin, weakness, tremor, nausea, and increased reflexes).[1]

The use of hallucinogenic drugs greatly increased from 1965 on. Because of numerous reports of "bad experiences," the drugs were considered dangerous. The Federal Bureau of Narcotics and Dangerous Drugs has placed them in Schedule 1, the most restrictive class. In addition, many people are prejudiced against hallucinogens because of their association with the countercultural movement of the 1960s.

Since about 1979 there has been a gradual return of interest in psychedelic drugs.[2] This is indicated by a decrease in the hysteria surrounding the issue of their use and by the emergence of new information. Psychedelic-drug takers often adopt ethics similar to those in societies where such drugs are accepted, ethics that constructively integrate the drug "high" with ongoing life. But it is difficult to determine whether these drugs will ever be fully accepted again in the United States.

Hallucinogens, or psychedelics, are drugs that affect a person's perceptions, sensations, thinking, self-awareness, and emotions. They include such drugs as LSD, mescaline, and psilocybin. Some hallucinogens come from natural sources, such as mescaline from peyote cactus. Others, such as LSD, are synthetic or manufactured. The effects of psychedelics are undetectable. It depends on the amount taken, the user's personality, mood, and expectations, and the surroundings in which the drug is used. Usually, the user feels the first effects of the drug 30 to 90 minutes after taking it. The physical effects include dilated pupils, higher body temperature, increased heart rate and blood pressure, sweating, loss of appetite, sleeplessness, dry mouth, and tremors. Sensations and feelings change, since the hallucinogens alter a person's sense of time and self. The user may feel several different emotions at once or swing repeatedly from one emotion to another. Sensations may seem to "cross over," creating **synesthesia** (a blending of senses) by giving the user the feeling of "hearing" colors and "seeing" sounds, for example.[3] All these changes can be frightening and cause panic.

When looking back on the 1960s one's recollection is always marked by the "Summer of Love" and the heyday of America's counterculture.[4] It was a bewildering time made even more so by LSD, mescaline, and psilocybin.

SITE OF ACTION

Much of the research on hallucinogenic drugs has focused on a neurotransmitter in the brain called serotonin. It was discovered early on that many of the major hallucinogens had a molecular structure similar to that of serotonin.[5] Studies of brain neurochemistry in animals following administration of hallucinogens have reported changes in serotonin. Although it may seem naive to say that the complex variety of the hallucinatory experience is mediated by a single neurotransmitter system, this is exactly what happens. Once the drug acts upon the brain, the serotonin triggers a multitude of changes involving much of the enormous complexity of the brain.

LSD

INTRODUCTION

LSD (lysergic acid diethylamide-25) is the most potent psychoactive drug available. Originally synthesized by Swiss chemist Albert Hoffman in the mid-1940s, LSD was to be used as a headache remedy. From the time Hoffman

Synesthesia
The ingestion of hallucinogenic drugs may lead to a blending of the senses where one perceives one is smelling noises or tasting sounds. Administration of hallucinogens changes the serotonin in the brain, and serotonin further triggers a multitude of changes involving the complexity of the brain.

discovered the drug, it quickly became a psychological-research tool. Its hallucinogenic properties weren't discovered for several years, until Hoffman accidentally inhaled the substance and began to experience peculiar psychological changes.[6] Further tests revealed other potentially dangerous effects, such as chromosome damage, fetal abnormalities, and psychotic reactions. In 1965, after widespread experimental use by young people, purchase and use of LSD were made illegal.

PSYCHOPHYSIOLOGICAL EFFECTS

Whereas most drugs are taken in milligrams (thousandths of grams), LSD is taken in micrograms (millionths of grams), usually 50 to 300 micrograms. Depending on the dose, effects may last from 6 to 12 hours. If LSD were taken continuously over a long period, increased dosages would be required to achieve desired effects. However, because LSD is so powerful, most users do not take it frequently.

Researchers theorize that LSD works by stimulating the raphae nuclei. This section of the brain uses serotonin, which LSD chemically resembles, and is responsible for regulating incoming sensory information and outgoing muscular impulses. Researchers hypothesize that LSD increases the sensitivity of this brain region and allows more information to flow to higher brain regions, including those responsible for vision and emotion. Users may therefore experience heightened sensitivity to environmental stimuli, which can lead to distortions in perception (depth, touch/texture, color, sound, and balance). As we have seen, synesthesia may also occur.

A secondary action of LSD is to increase activity in the sympathetic nervous system, resulting in pupil dilation and a rise in body temperature, blood pressure, and heart rate. In addition to a slight rise in blood-sugar levels, users have also reported on occasion nausea, headaches, loss of appetite, dizziness, and mild tremors.

The effects of LSD vary with the dose, purity, setting, expectations, and motivations of the user. Smaller doses (25 to 75 micrograms) may cause slight perceptual alterations; large doses (300 to 600 micrograms) may result in mystical experiences or severe paranoia. Pleasant expectations and planned use help to increase the chances of a pleasant experience, but unexpected or unwanted use can have serious consequences. Many people never fully recover from bad trips. Many bad trips, which may be induced by sensory overload or unresolved emotional problems, can be resolved if a person acting in a nonthreatening manner "talks down" the individual in a supportive environment. Occasionally, severe anxiety reactions may require mild tranquilization or psychiatric follow-up after the drug effects have ended.

Research has shown changes in the mental functions of heavy use of LSD, but they are not present in all cases. Heavy users sometimes develop signs of organic brain damage, such as impaired memory and attention span, mental confusion, and difficulty with abstract thinking.[7] These signs may be strong or they may be subtle. It is not known whether such mental changes are permanent or if they disappear when LSD is stopped. Whether LSD does or does not increase creativity remains an unanswered question. All that can be definitely said about the effect of hallucinogenic drugs on the creative process is that a strong feeling of creativeness accompanies many of the experiences.[8]

Another possible adverse reaction to LSD is the **flashback,** a spontaneous reoccurrence of feelings that may have been experienced during an LSD trip weeks, months, or even years earlier. It has been estimated that flashbacks occur in approximately 5 percent of LSD users, although severe flashbacks or psychotic reactions are considerably rarer. Flashbacks, most of which are short, are not always a negative: Some users report them to be an unexpected bonus of the LSD experience. Many of the flashbacks that have been studied clinically center in unresolved problems, repressed fears, or frightening experiences while under the influence of the drug.

Researchers today are finding that the hallucinogenic effects of LSD are affecting former users as much as 20 years after they quit taking the drug.[9] Research is finding that the flashbacks (Post Hallucinogenic Sensory Disorder) experienced by former LSD users can often be induced by sounds, images, flashing lights, or something that triggers the memory of a former trip. It is thought that drugs like LSD "probably exert their influence at specific neuron receptor sites for the transmitter serotonin."[10] Flashback suffers seem to be unable to shut out certain visual stimuli, possibly due to a change in certain receptor sites, leaving them overly sensitized and thus allowing them to receive signals that are usually suppressed. The flashbacks many former LSD users experience are very similar to those experienced by posttrauma victims. It is quite possible that those who suffer from flashbacks are simply experiencing a very vivid memory or that they may have at one time damaged their temporal lobes, but the common link between many patients is former LSD use. Currently there is no *cure* for flashback; however, benzodiazepines (Valium) are the drugs commonly used in treatment.

Flashback

A spontaneous reoccurrence of feelings that may have been experienced during an LSD trip (and with some other drugs also) weeks, months, or even years earlier. It has been estimated that flashbacks occur in approximately 5 percent of LSD users.

LSD AND SOCIETY

It was Timothy Leary who raised LSD to national prominence with talk of mystical visions, egoless states, and trips within the mind. The drug was quite popular in the early 1960s, and articles depicting its evils—chromosome breakage, birth defects, insanity, and death and physical harm caused by users on bad trips—did little to discourage the acid's use. Growing concern over the drug's use, however, led to passage of the Drug Abuse Control Amendments in 1965. LSD, along with depressants, stimulants, and other hallucinogenic drugs, were placed under the heading *dangerous drugs,* and their manufacture, processing, and distribution or sale became a federal offense.

This legislation sparked the beginning of a decrease in LSD use. From 1970 to 1980 dramatic reductions were noted, and current government surveys show that no more than 1 percent of the teenage/young-adult population uses LSD.

AN LSD CASE STUDY

About five years ago five friends drove from Seattle, Washington, to Eugene, Oregon, to attend a rock concert at Autzen Stadium. During the concert the group used blotter acid. One of the members decided to leave the concert. He got into a car and drove approximately twenty miles south on the freeway and turned off at a town named Cottage Grove. He got out of the car at the freeway exit and left the vehicle there. An older couple approached him and asked if he was okay. He asked them for a gun and they promptly left and contacted the state police. He entered the community and went from house to house requesting a gun. One of the houses where he stopped belonged to an off-duty state policeman, whose wife answered the door and told the man she did not have a gun. When the man left she told her husband, who was in another part of the house. He picked up his gun and went after the man, who had picked up a claw hammer from the policeman's garage. When the police officer caught up with the young man he noticed he had captured a small child and was swinging the hammer downward toward the child's head. The policeman reacted quickly and shot the young man through the heart, killing him. An autopsy indicated the young man had swallowed blotter acid and also had some back at his unattended vehicle. The policeman was cleared of any wrongdoing, and the child survived the ordeal.[11]

LSD seems to be making a name for itself again. The revival has been especially prevalent in California and in large urban centers in the East and Midwest. Involvement seems to center in some of the old organizations and old-timers getting back into the business.[12] Some drug-abuse experts believe the slight increase is due to the unusual amount of new publicity about LSD in the media, along with a fascinating variety of brands of the drug now available. More people are taking notice of a subject that has not been newsworthy in recent years.

LSD use in the 1980s was very different from the "vintage" LSD use of the 1960s and 1970s. In the early days, sugar cubes and animal crackers were among the favored ways of delivering doses of the drug, but these fell from favor because of their bulk. From the mid-1960s to the mid-1970s, LSD in the form of tablets dominated the street acid market. Eventually these gave way to increasingly smaller formats, particularly small gelatin chips known as *windowpanes,* tiny pellets known as *microdots,* and the dominant format—*blotter.*[13] In the last-named format, diluted drops of the drug are placed on blotter paper. Usually the paper has been printed with some sort of artwork, such as dragons or popular comic-strip characters. It is then cut up into tiny pieces, usually one-quarter to one-half the size of a small postage stamp. Some blotters have slotlike perforations for easy separation.[14]

Blotter

Diluted drops of LSD are placed on blotter paper and this is referred to as blotter acid. Small sections or squares are torn off and consumed by a user.

The idea behind smaller forms of the drug is to make it as undetectable as possible. The smaller-is-better ethic in LSD marketing is due to the minuteness of effective psychoactive doses of LSD. As we have seen, as little as 25 micrograms can produce noticeable perceptual and cognitive changes. One key difference between today's LSD and that of the past is potency. Most acid today is not as strong as it was in previous years. The average LSD dose now ranges from 40 to 60 micrograms. This compares with an average dose of 150 to 200 micrograms a decade ago. Some feel the lower dosage produces a more manageable reaction and may account for the increasing use of LSD.

USE IN MIND-CONTROL RESEARCH

Research into possible LSD uses has been carried out in several areas. In 1949, the U.S. Central Intelligence Agency (CIA) and various military agencies began exploring the use of drugs and other exotic methods for mind control. On April 3, 1953, Richard Helms proposed to CIA director Allen Dulles that a program for covert use of biological and chemical materials to this end be set up.[15] It was approved and called MKULTRA.

In the early days of this program, six Technical Services Staff professionals investigated LSD. A small amount, the CIA and the military felt, could turn strong-willed individuals away from their most basic perceptions and make them susceptible to manipulation. In November 1953, they "tested" a group of scientists from the Army Chemical Corps Special Operations Division at Fort Detrich in Maryland. One of the scientists, Frank Olson, became psychotic and jumped from a hotel window to his death. Because of this type of problem and the extensive cover-up it entailed, the CIA decided to experiment with underworld prostitutes and drug dependents, who would be less likely to draw attention to the experiment.[16] Safe houses were set up in New York and San Francisco where drugs were disguised in food, drink, and cigarettes. Despite the extensive testing, however, the agencies came up with no positive results. LSD-initiated mind control was impossible because of the many differences among the people tested. After all these years the Frank Olson case, among others, is being brought to public attention.

USE IN MEDICAL RESEARCH

Investigators have researched LSD use in a number of other situations. Some success has been noted in the use of LSD to help terminally ill patients cope with death, and one researcher has hopes for the drug's use in other areas of life stress, such as major decision making, psychosomatic illness, and dealing with reality.[17] LSD has been used in the treatment of neurosis and as an aid to therapy and self-concept in the treatment of sexual deviancy, mental illness, pain in cancer patients, and frigidity. Thus far, however, LSD does not appear to be a highly desirable therapeutic agent.

LSD's relation to birth defects has also been studied. In cooperation with a pediatrician, three researchers studied 120 infants born to a sample of LSD users. They concluded that "there is no evidence of a relation between parental LSD exposure and major congenital defects in their offspring."[18] *However, no chemical known to science has been proved to be entirely harmless for all pregnant women and their babies during all stages of pregnancy.*[19]

Psychotherapists have used LSD in experiments on increasing the receptivity of patients to undergoing therapy or dealing with personal problems. Most of their research, however, has failed to document significant therapeutic benefits other than an increase in patient morale. The drug has *not* proved to be the long-sought chemical key to schizophrenia. LSD has been shown to be of some value in treating autistic children, but the improvement rapidly reverses when the use of the drug is stopped. Similarly, attempts at treating chronic alcoholics with LSD have not met with long-term success, and in what limited successes there were, it was not thought that LSD was the decisive factor. Some successes have been obtained in treating cancer patients and amputees.

According to Los Angeles psychiatrist and University of California Medical School professor Oscar Janigar, LSD can assist artistic development. Janigar has released the results of a study he did before the 1962 ban on LSD drug testing. In the study, Janigar had several artists paint a Hopi kachina doll, then ingest 2 micrograms of LSD per kilogram of body weight and paint the doll again. The artists wrote about their experience and filled out a questionnaire, and were interviewed a month later and a year later. The contrasts between the "before" and "after" paintings were remarkable. The "before" paintings were realistic, predictable, and drawn to scale. However, the LSD-inspired paintings were abstract, symbolic, brighter, and more emotional and tended to use more canvas.

Janigar explains that perhaps the brain has "schools of art" and that LSD is a means of opening some of these schools or connecting them so as to expose the mind to its capabilities. Upon meeting 25 years later for the revealing of Janigar's findings, all of the artists said the experience had taught them an impressionistic approach. Some even said the experience was the most beneficial they had ever had. According to Janigar, LSD will not make a good painter a great painter, but it is "an additional tool to use to explore the greater depth of what [the artist] is looking for."[20] He advocates more controlled studies of the drug.

MESCALINE (PEYOTE)

INTRODUCTION

Mescaline is derived from peyote "buttons," the dried tops of several species of cactus. Long used in American Indian religious ceremonies, peyote is said to have first become known through a revelation in a woman's dream. The substance is similar to strychnine and morphine, but is not physiologically active in humans aside from psychoactive effects.

Once dried, peyote buttons can be ingested in raw form, but they are usually extremely bitter and can cause nausea and vomiting. Synthetically produced mescaline has a better taste and less intense side effects, and it can be liquefied, encapsulated, or made into tablets.

Peyote was first studied in the United States by Lewis Lewin, who extracted mescaline and adrenaline alkaloids from the plant. Lewin categorized mescaline as a "phantasticant" substance "capable of exercising [its] chemical power on all senses, but . . . particularly the visual and auditory spheres as well as the general sensibility."[21] Study of the plant, Lewin felt, would aid in the understanding of psychotic mental states.

Though LSD was at the heart of the psychedelic-drug movement, mescaline use became popular too, since its "trip" was not as intense and was therefore more manageable. Use has been curtailed, however, since mescaline is now classified as a dangerous drug under state and national drug laws. It may still be used in religious practices of the Native American church, and medically it is used as a tincture for angina pectoris, as a respiratory stimulant for pneumonia patients, and as a cardiac tonic.

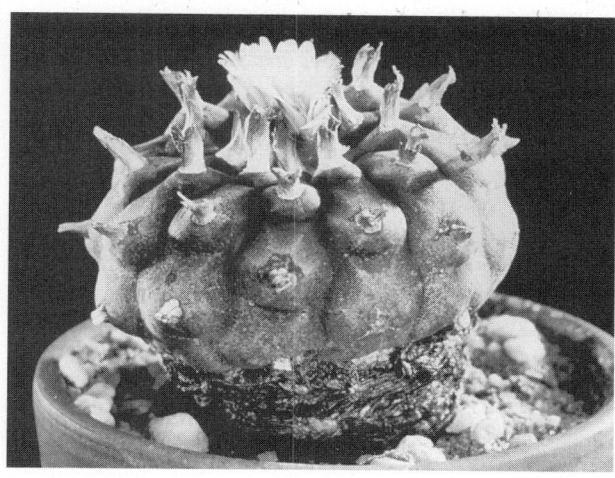

The Peyote Cactus
Source: Drug Enforcement
Administration

Some of the Native American church rites were influenced by early Christianity, but slices of peyote have replaced the sacramental bread and wine. Native Americans regard the cactus as God's special gift to the Indians and equate its effects with the workings of the divine spirit. Their use of mescaline is limited to healing religious services only; the drug is not to be used for recreational purposes.

Perhaps the safest place to take peyote is within the church.[22] The church knows the safest ways and requirements necessary before ingestion. Worshipers who take peyote see visions and participate in experiences that draw all together and facilitate adherence toward the church's teaching. It is written in the Bible that "anyone who eats the loaf or drinks the cup of the Lord carelessly will have to answer for a sin against the body and blood of the Lord."[23] This rule could also apply to peyote. It is to be used for its intended religious purpose only.

The purpose of peyote in the congregation is to minimize external stimuli and to allow the spiritually clarifying effect of the psychedelic sacrament to come through to the individual uncontaminated. Drug laws may be wrong if they violate freedom of religion as guaranteed in the Bill of Rights.[24] The church guides the taker of peyote in how to use it safely. First, the taker must be free of all pain, since the drug can greatly exaggerate the pain. Second, no alcohol can be in the system. Third, the drug is best taken on an empty stomach. The church believes peyote can promote general welfare, both social and religious, of the community. The peyote is also taken to encourage enlightenment, which is the realization that life is a dream and the externality of relations an illusion.

PSYCHOPHYSIOLOGICAL EFFECTS

Mescaline's primary effects are similar to those of LSD, focusing on sensory perception, particularly the audiovisual realm. With eyes closed, numerous colors and images may be visualized. With eyes open, mescaline users may be attracted to one particular object and may focus on it for a long

Peyote Ritual

Native Americans regard the peyote cactus as God's special gift to them and equate its effects with the workings of the divine spirit. Slices of peyote have replaced the sacramental bread used in other services, and the use is limited to religious healing services only; the drug is not to be used for recreational purposes. Several states have made it legal for Native Americans to use peyote.

> ## PEYOTE MEETING
>
> As part of the Native American church, rites were influenced to a degree by early Christianity, but slices of peyote replaced the sacramental bread and wine. Native Americans regard the cactus as God's special gift to the Indians and equate its effects with the workings of the divine spirit.
>
> The religious services are called meetings and they usually last from sundown to sunup.[25] Before entering into the tepee (usually where the meetings are held), a person must be clean inside and out. He must be free of drugs, including alcohol, and will usually take a sweat bath in a sweat-house and then go through a purification ceremony in which sage, juniper, or sweet grass is smoked. A woman who is in time of her moon (menstruation) is not allowed to enter the tepee, but she can sit outside if she wishes. These are very strict rules taken very seriously by the members of the Native American church. Peyote is not considered a drug but, rather, a medicine. It is a living gift from the Creator, not a picture or statue they pray to.

period. Synesthesia may occur, and the sense of time may diminish or vanish. Thoughts that are ordinarily suppressed may come to the surface, and users are sometimes quite sensitive to new ideas. Mood swings usually occur soon after ingestion.

Mescaline users may experience visual distortion as well as acuity. Spatial relationships and objects may seem to grow or shrink, and depth perception can become distorted.

PSILOCYBIN

INTRODUCTION

Psilocybin is a chemical derivative of the *Psilocybe Mexicana* mushroom. Fifteen species of this mushroom can be found growing wild in the United States or Canada, usually in moist areas such as wet meadows, pastures, and forests.

The psilocybin mushroom was worshiped in Guatemala as long ago as 1000 B.C.,[26] and it appears that Aztec Indians consumed it in the belief that it would help to establish communication with the spirit world. Currently the drug has no medical use, but it is being researched as a possible aid in experimental psychiatry and therapy. Psilocybin is usually taken orally, as dried mushrooms or in tablet form, or it may be dried, ground, and added to food.

PSYCHOPHYSIOLOGICAL EFFECTS

Once ingested, psilocybin is converted by an enzyme in the stomach into psilocin.[27] The effects of the drug, which are similar to those of LSD, usually begin 25 to 40 minutes later and generally last from three to eight hours. The

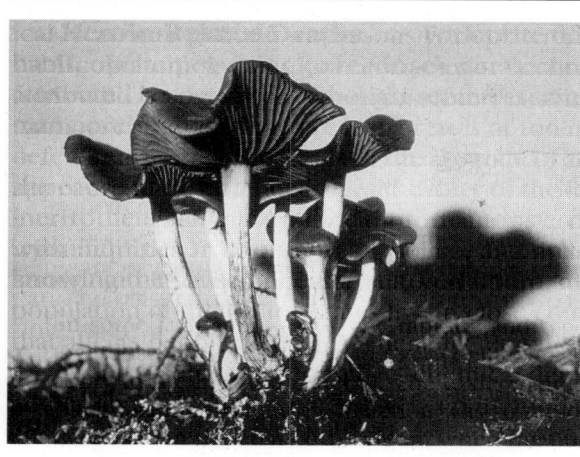

Psilocybe Mushrooms
Source: Drug Enforcement Administration

central nervous system is affected, and changes in time and space perception, wakefulness, attentiveness, suggestibility, and distractability occur.

The physiological effects of psilocybin include dilation of the pupils, an increase in deep-tendon reflex, and an increase in pulse rate, blood pressure, and body temperature.[28] The user may experience tingling on the skin surface and weak to strong involuntary limb movements. Intoxication from psilocybin, much like intoxication from mescaline, may result in muscular relaxation and emotional dysfunctions such as extreme hilarity and loss of concentration. The user may smell pleasant but unfamiliar odors, and have illusions and hallucinations.

The use of psilocybin may also result in swings of emotion, from marked euphoria to marked depression or anxiety. Hazards of the drug include acute paranoia and accidental or deliberate death, though no deaths have been directly related to overdose.

Due to the increasing popularity of psilocybin, the number of people collecting the mushroom for use and sale has increased dramatically in recent years. The increase in availability of the drug is a legitimate cause for concern. Property owners are becoming angry with trespassers. Increasing numbers of "**shroomers**" are being prosecuted for trespassing in the Pacific Northwest and the southeastern United States, where the mushrooms grow abundantly. Another danger is the high potential for mistaking a poisonous mushroom for psilocybin. It is estimated that toxic species outnumber psilocybin species by at least 10 to 1. Many mushroom pickers are not aware of this and so are especially vulnerable to mushroom poisoning.[29]

Shroomers
People who collect mushrooms for use and sale. Selection of the right kind of mushroom is very important because many mushrooms are poisonous and ingestion could lead to death.

PCP

INTRODUCTION

PCP (phencyclidine) is a difficult drug to classify. Many think of it as a hallucinogen, though it also produces depressant, stimulant, analgesic, and anesthetic effects.[30]

First synthesized in the late 1950s, PCP was intended for use as an animal tranquilizer and as an anesthetic in surgery on humans.[31] It produced such unwanted and unpleasant side effects, however, that experimental studies with humans were soon discontinued. In 1969, PCP became available "for veterinary use only," but on April 1, 1979, all legal manufacturing of the drug in the United States was banned.[32] Despite this restriction, PCP is relatively easily obtained because it is easy to produce. The drug can be injected, taken orally, or smoked.

Eighty percent of first-time PCP users describe a pleasurable experience.[33] The experiences associated with PCP are often described as sensory isolation, sedation, disequilibrium, and altered perceptions. Auditory hallucinations and image distortions may occur, producing a feeling of doom, paranoia, and violence. Common physical effects are a blank stare and rapid and involuntary eye movements. Effects include increased heart rate and blood pressure, flushing, sweating, dizziness, and numbness. When large doses are taken, effects include drowsiness, convulsions, coma, and death. The high, or euphoric state, lasts an average of three to four hours. It's the most unpredictable drug on the street, known to increase a person's strength five times. Recovery may take 12 hours or more.

PCP is considered a unique drug because it does different things to different people. Some categorize PCP as a designer or psychedelic drug. It's a hallucinogen, but it can also be a stimulant or a depressant.

PCP is available in a number of different forms. It can be a pure white crystalline powder, or a tablet or capsule. An average dose is 5 to 10 milligrams. The effects go away in 12 hours, and it can take as long as four days before the drug is eliminated from the body. PCP can be swallowed, smoked, sniffed, or injected. The results of the Substance Abuse and Sexual Concerns Project, a cooperative effort between Haight-Ashbury Free Medical Clinic and the Institute for the Advanced Study of Human Sexuality, indicated that PCP is smoked about 70 percent of the time, ingested in pill form 20 percent of the time, inhaled intranasally approximately 5 percent of the time, and injected intravenously 5 percent of the time.[34] PCP is sometimes sprinkled with marijuana or parsley and smoked. Those marijuana cigarettes laced with PCP cost between $10 and $15, and a week's supply is about $30.

PCP AND SOCIETY

PCP, commonly known as "angel dust" or "rocket fuel," first came into popular street use in San Francisco in 1967. Many early PCP experimenters soon rejected it as undesirable. In spite of its reputation, however, PCP was increasingly seen on the street because of its cheapness, availability, and ability to masquerade as other popular street drugs, such as THC (tetrahydrocannabinol), mescaline, or cocaine. It is still cheap and available, and despite its dangers it continues to be a drug of choice. Many take the drug simply to prove that they can handle it, and its use is spreading, some feel to epidemic proportions.

According to current data, PCP abuse is an increasingly regional problem, with Maryland, California, and the District of Columbia having the largest problem.[35] On the other hand, 32 states reported fewer than 300 PCP treatment admissions. When looking at the number of drug-treatment admissions in state-supported facilities, PCP abusers have a very low number of admissions. The reason for the decline in PCP use may be its availability. PCP is less available and more expensive than other illicit drugs like crack cocaine. It appears dealers are switching from selling PCP to selling crack cocaine.[36] Thus crack cocaine is more available and less expensive than PCP, explaining the decline.

PSYCHOPHYSIOLOGICAL EFFECTS

PCP is a powerful drug even in small quantities. It affects the entire body, particularly the cerebral cortex, and tolerance can develop quickly. In large doses the drug acts as a tranquilizing depressant, often inducing coma or comatose-like behavior. All too often, PCP results in psychotic episodes, seizures, violent behavior, and death.

PCP is most often smoked, but taking the drug in tablet or capsule form or snorting pure powder affords a larger dose. Injecting or snorting the drug produces almost immediate effects; effects from smoking may take 15 minutes to appear.[37] The experience can vary: Users report that PCP makes them feel as if they're in another world—a fantasy world that is sometimes pleasant, sometimes not. When the high wears off, users often feel mildly depressed, irritable, and alienated from their surroundings.

Generalized numbness, blurred vision, muscular dysfunction, and dizziness may occur, and profuse sweating, flushing, increased blood pressure, and rapid heartbeat are typical. A mild dose of 3 to 8 milligrams produces "spaciness," problems with perception and coordination, numbness, increased blood pressure, bloodshot eyes, and impaired speech. A dose of 10 to 20 milligrams produces indifference to pain, sweating and flushing, drooling, distorted vision, bulging eyeballs, muscle rigidity, verbal inhibition, mental and physical retardation (a general slowing down), and a total inability to comprehend time and space.[38] Larger amounts of the drug may cause users to appear drunk and may lead to confused speech and distorted vision. Thinking, remembering, and making decisions can be very difficult.

PCP changes how users see their own bodies and things around them. Speech, muscle coordination, and vision are affected, senses of touch and pain are dulled, and body movements are slowed. Time seems to "space out." A temporary mental disturbance, or a disturbance of the user's thought processes (a PCP psychosis), may last for days or weeks. Long-term PCP users report memory and speech difficulties, as well as hearing voices or sounds that do not exist. The biggest and most obvious danger of PCP is the drug's unpredictability.[39] Everytime a user lights up a PCP-laced joint, it's a spin of the big psychotic roulette wheel. There is a thin line between a numb, depersonalized high and a full-blown raging psychosis.

A few hypotheses have been formulated on how PCP works in the body. One claims that PCP attaches itself to one particular site along the nerve terminals, blocking a potassium channel.[40] These postassium channels directly affect the nerve cell by either reducing or increasing the release of neuro-transmitters, which communicate nerve impulses from one cell to another. Once this channel is blocked, the chemical imbalance is changed and more neurotransmitters are released. If this "overactivity" in the brain is caused by PCP, then it could explain the violent behavior that appears to coincide with this drug.

Another theory is that PCP interrupts signals that normally flow along neurons in the brain bearing a receptor called NMDA receptor.[41] The receptors bind to the amino acids, then they release and cross a small synapse. This opens a channel that lets calcium ions into the inside of the nerve, triggering an impulse and thus relaying the electrical signal from the tail of one nerve to the next. PCP stops calcium from getting into sites.[42] The users show symptoms of schizophrenia. Sometimes dulling of the neurons may be useful, however. The flow of oxygen to the brain is impaired during such unpleasant events as strokes, heart attacks, and shortness of breath. For these victims of oxygen starvation, electrical activity may reduce the risk of brain damage prior to resuscitation.

Another hypothesis is that PCP blocks a major chemical messenger in the brain called glutamic acid, or glutamate.[43] If there is too much glutamate in the brain, it will cause the neurons to work hard and they will die. For example, if someone has a heart attack, blood and oxygen stop going to the brain." Animal research and tissue culture is showing that PCP-related compounds block an excess of glutamate. By doing this, they prevent brain damage. Not only is it stated that treatment for schizophrenia is possible, but epilepsy as well.

Scientists think PCP may prove useful for study of brain functions or lead to treatment for epilepsy or schizophrenia.[44] The unique properties of the drug include binding to specific brain receptors. These receptors are in the limbic region of the brain, which regulates a person's emotions.

Long-Term Effects   Many users who take PCP regularly experience disturbances in memory, judgment, concentration, and perception long after they stop taking the drug.[45] Long-term users are also subject to recurring bouts of anxiety and depression and sporadic outbreaks of violent behavior.

Hazards   Though a PCP overdose may be lethal, more PCP users die from accidents caused by drug-induced behavior than from the drug itself. People on PCP have drowned in shallow water because they weren't able to tell which way was up. Others have had auto accidents, fallen off roofs, and fallen out of windows because of the drug's intoxicating effects.[46] PCP use has also been linked to suicides, drowning from sedation, and self-inflicted wounds.

PCP is one of the most powerful and abused drugs today. PCP-intoxicated individuals are prone to paranoia, unpredictable behavior, and psychotic reactions. They are capable of terrifying, almost superhuman acts of violence.

SUMMARY

LSD, mescaline, and psilocybin are hallucinogenic drugs that were particularly popular in the 1960s and early 1970s. They affect sensory perception and can lead to a variety of adverse psychological conditions. LSD causes the most severe effects and its action lasts the longest. All the drugs are illegal to purchase, except mescaline when used by the Native American church in religious services.

Another hallucinogenic drug, phencyclidine (PCP), was originally used by veterinarians as an animal tranquilizer. It is still popular today with young people, though it was deemed illegal in 1979. Use of PCP can lead to confusion, convulsions, psychosis, and even death.

Hallucinogenic drugs seem to gain periodic popularity, and then their usage decreases. They are now used with a somewhat clearer idea of what to expect than in the past.

Hallucinogens

N O T E S

1. Barry Jacobs, "How Hallucinogenic Drugs Work," *American Scientist* 75, no. 4 (August 1987):386.

2. Elvin D. Smith, "Evolving Ethics in Psychedelic Drug Taking," *Journal of Drug Issues* 18, no. 2 (Spring 1988):201–14.

3. National Institute on Drug Abuse, *Hallucinogenic and PCP,* DHHS Publication No. (ADM) 83-1306, (Washington, D.C.: Department of Health and Human Services, Public Health Service, Alcohol, Drug Abuse and Mental Health Administration, 1983).

4. Walter Clemons, "America' Long, Strange Trip," *Newsweek,* August 24, 1987, pp. 63–64.

5. Jacobs, "How Hallucinogenic Drugs Work," p. 201.

6. Bernard Aaronson and Humphrey Osmond, *Psychedelics* (New York: Doubleday, 1970).

7. National Institute on Drug Abuse, *Hallucinogenics and PCP.*

8. Oscar Janiger and Marion Dobkin De Rios, "The Effects of LSD on Creativity," *Journal of Psychoactive Drugs* 21, no. 1 (January/March 1989):129–34.

9. Steve Nadis, "After Lights," *Omni* 12, no. 5 (February 1990):24, 96.

10. Ibid.

11. Presented to a drug class at the University of Oregon by Terry Beckkedahl, an Oregon State Police criminologist.

12. *Drug Survival News,* November/December 1981, pp. 12–13. Reprinted with permission of Do It Now Foundation, Phoenix, AZ.

13. Ibid., p. 13.

14. Ibid.

15. John Marks, "Sex, Drugs, and the CIA: The Shocking Search for an Ultimate Weapon," *Saturday Review* 6, no. 3 (February 3, 1979). Copyright © 1979 by *Saturday Review.* All rights reserved. Reprinted with permission.

16. Ibid.

17. Ralph Metzger, "Reflection on LSD Ten Years Later," *Journal of Psychedelic Drugs* 10, no. 2 (April/June 1978):137–40.

18. William H. McGlothlin, Robert S. Sparkes, and David O. Arnold, "Effect of LSD on Human Pregnancy," *Journal of the American Medical Association* 212 (June 1, 1970):1483.

19. Edward M. Brecher et al., *Licit and Illicit Drugs* (Boston: Little, Brown, 1972), p. 390.

20. Cited in Robert B. Tucker, "Acid Test," *Omni,* November 16, 1987, p. 16.

21. Quoted in A. Hoffer and H. Osmond, *The Hallucinogens* (New York: Academic Press, 1967), p. 2.

22. Thomas Lyttle, "Drug Based Religious and Contemporary Drug Taking," *Journal of Drug Issues* 18 (1988):271–284.

23. Ibid.

24. Ibid.

25. A May 1988 interview with Bonnie Teeman, who is the wife of a Choctaw Indian chief.

26. Jeremy Sandford, *In Search of the Magic Mushroom.*

27. R. Schultes and Albert Hofmann, *The Botany and Chemistry of Hallucinogens* (Springfield, Ill.: Chas. C. Thomas, 1973), pp. 22–23.

28. L. E. Hollister, *Chemical Psychoses: LSD and Related Drugs* (Springfield, Ill.: Chas. C. Thomas, 1968), p. 52.

29. Richard H. Schwartz, "Hallucinogenic Mushroom," *Clinical Pediatrics* 27, no. 2 (February 1988):70–74.

30. Sidney Cohen, "PCP (Angel Dust): New Trends in Treatment," *Drug Abuse and Alcoholism Newsletter* 7, no. 6 (July 1978):1–3.

31. National Institute on Drug Abuse, *PCP* (Washington, D.C.: Department of Health, Education and Welfare, 1977) pp. 1–2.

32. Richard Geary, "PCP (Phencyclidine): An Update," *Journal of Psychedelic Drugs* 2, no. 4 (October/December 1979):265.

33. Joseph A. Barone, "Phencyclidine and Related Drugs," *Journal of Drug Education* (1989):201–4.

34. D. E. Smith, et al., "PCP and Sexual Dysfunction," *Journal of Psychedelic Drugs* 12, no. 3–4 (July/December 1980):269–73.

35. Dennis L. Thombs, "A Review of PCP Abuse, Trends, and Perceptions," *Public Health Reports* 104, no. 4 (July/August 1989):325–28.

36. Ibid.

37. "Phencyclidine: PCP," *National Clearinghouse for Drug Abuse Information* 14, no. 2 (March 1978):1–11.

38. Mark L. Richards et al., "Phencyclidine Psychosis," *Drug Intelligence and Clinical Pharmacy* 13, no. 6 (June 1979):336–39.

39. Tom McNicol, "PCP: The Cheap Thrill with a High Price," *Rolling Stone,* March 24, 1988, pp. 82–84.

40. Joshua Fischman, "The Angel Dust Connection," *Psychology Today,* July 1986, pp. 68–69.

41. "Designer Drugs: A Silver Lining," *The Economist* 310 (January 21, 1989):24.

42. Ibid.

43. Joyce Price, "From Lab to the Street and Back," *Insight,* August 10, 1987, p. 82.

44. Ibid.

45. National Institute on Drug Abuse, *PCP,* p. 2.

46. Ibid., pp. 3–4.

CHAPTER 11

MARIJUANA

Continuing Controversy

INTRODUCTION

Marijuana is a drug made from the chopped leaves, stems, and seeds of the cannabis plant. It has been used as an intoxicant and an herbal medication in various parts of the world for centuries, and it is still used by many people today. Its variable effects and uncertain hazards, however, make it a most controversial drug.

MARIJUANA USE IN THE WORLD

The first detailed description of cannabis appeared in a medical book prepared by the legendary Chinese emperor Shen-Nung in 2700 B.C.,[1] but archaeological data suggest that cannabis's use goes back at least 6,000 years.[2] Early uses of cannabis included smoking it as part of purification rituals and using it to relieve pain during surgery. Hashish, the resin of the marijuana plant, was eaten and drunk in Arabian countries during the Middle Ages.

Cannabis use did not spread to western Europe until the late 1700s; its therapeutic uses were studied intently by a British physician named

O'Shaughnessy in 1843.[3] Quasi-medical and medical use of a variety of cannabis preparations, including elixers and medicines, occurred in North America later in that century, but nonmedical consumption of cannabis in North America did not appear until the twentieth century. Presently, marijuana appears to be the fourth most popular psychoactive substance in the world,[4] preceded only by caffeine, nicotine, and alcohol.

MARIJUANA USE IN THE UNITED STATES

Marijuana actually became a popular recreational drug in the United States during the 1920s and immediately after alcohol prohibition. Because alcohol was becoming scarce, people began turning to pot. People began to see "tea pads" being established. Tea pads were much like the opium dens (early smoking in closed rooms or "dens" that occurred in China) we have heard about. They were a place where people could go to get high and forget about their problems for awhile. By 1930 New York City had about 500 tea pads, and it was rumored that marijuana could be easily obtained.[5] However, when prohibition ended, alcohol returned as the recreational drug of choice.

During the early 1900s, marijuana was *incorrectly* classified as a narcotic in the popular and legal literature. No comprehensive scientific study of the drug had been done in this country, but it was *assumed* to be a narcotic and its use was linked to violent crimes and insanity by the media and federal narcotics officers. In 1932 the National Conference on Uniform State Laws included marijuana provisions in the Uniform Narcotic Drug Act. In late 1937 Congress adopted the Marijuana Tax Act, which prohibited the use of marijuana.[6]

Though marijuana was used earlier in this century, it gained great popularity in the 1960s. It is now the fourth most widely used drug in the United States. Many young people are introduced to marijuana by their peers, usually acquaintances, friends, sisters, or brothers. People often try drugs such as marijuana because they feel pressured by peers to be part of the group. Students have reported some of the following reasons for using marijuana: to have a good time with friends; to get high; to relieve boredom; to enhance the effects of other drugs; and to cope with stress. It is interesting to examine some of the reasons former daily users have discontinued their habit: loss of interest in getting high; concern about harmful psychological effects; and concern about their loss of energy and ambition.

Today's marijuana is up to 20 times stronger than the drug used in the 1960s; hashish is up to 100 times stronger.[7] Researchers already know that marijuana affects personality and intellectual development, emotional growth, learning, memory, and psychomotor functions.[8] They are now looking at the drug's physical effects. It is now known that THC—the psychoactive element in marijuana—stays in the body for weeks. Higher doses increase health risks, and it seems there is no safe level for use.[9]

With the escalation of opiate-use violations in the 1950s, corresponding marijuana penalties were increased at the request of federal drug officials. Eventually, first-offense possession of marijuana was made a felony punishable by lengthy imprisonment. Marijuana was also reclassified as a Schedule 1 drug under the[10] Comprehensive Drug Abuse Prevention and Control Act of 1970, and as such it cannot be marketed but it can be used for research. Currently the Department of Health and Human Services is considering a proposal to reclassify marijuana as a Schedule 2 drug so that it might become a prescribed medicine for glaucoma and chemotherapy.[11] Several states have already passed laws allowing marijuana to be used in the treatment of certain patients.

DECREASING POPULARITY

Despite this law and the former social stigma attached to the drug, marijuana use thrived in the 1970s in all segments of society. With this increased use came increased interest in safety while using marijuana. It has been reported that after alcohol, more people use or have used marijuana than any other mind-altering substance. It is estimated that in the United States, 25 percent of the population have used marijuana at least once.

Pot smoking peaked in 1978 and has declined since, especially among teenagers.[12] The 1980s marked the beginning of a steady decline, and by 1986 the rates had dropped to 1975 levels.[13] Two different interpretations have been offered to explain the recent decline in marijuana use.[14] The first is that young people in recent years have become more conservative and less trouble-prone in general. The second is that there have been relatively specific changes in views about marijuana and the risks associated with its use. These two interpretations are not mutually exclusive, but they have important and distinctly different implications, especially with respect to drug-abuse prevention efforts. The number of high school seniors who smoke marijuana daily fell by over half from 1978 to 1986. The 1990 National Household Study provides the following information on the status of marijuana:[15]

- Marijuana remains the most commonly used illicit drug in the United States. Approximately 66.5 million Americans (33.1 percent) have tried marijuana at least once in their lives. Nearly 3 million youths, over 15 million young adults, and in excess of 48 million adults aged 26 and older have tried marijuana.

- In 1990 the lifetime rate of marijuana use for youths was 14.8 percent while the rate of young adults was 52.2 percent. These rates have been steadily decreasing since 1979, when they were 31 percent and 68 percent respectively.

- Rates of past-month use of marijuana did not change significantly between 1988 and 1990, decreasing slightly from 5.9 percent to 5.1 percent. Rates were highest for males (6.4 percent), blacks (6.7 percent), and the unemployed (12.3 percent).

- Of the 20.5 million people who used marijuana (at least once) in the past year in 1990, over one quarter, or 5.5 million, used the drug once a week or more.

PHARMACOLOGICAL CLASSIFICATION

The pharmacological classification of cannabis has been the subject of much public misunderstanding. Such controversy is most likely caused by the fact that under various conditions and doses, the drug may have stimulant, sedative, analgesic, and hallucinogenic effects. Scientists contributing to the First Report of the National Commission on Marijuana and Drug Abuse felt that marijuana should be listed in a category by itself. The authors of the report stated that "pharmacologically speaking, cannabis is unique and distinct from psychomimetics [drugs that mimic a psychotic disorder], opiates, barbiturates and amphetamines."[16]

Cannabis Sativa

The scientific name for marijuana (pot, weed, dope).

Marijuana (grass, pot, weed, dope, etc.) is the common name for a drug made from the plant **Cannabis sativa.** The psychoactive ingredient is **delta-9-tetrahydrocannabinol (THC)**, although "there are more than 420 chemicals [in the] sixty-one cannabis plants."[17] The amount of THC in marijuana determines its potency. The type of plant, the weather, the soil, the time of harvest, selective cultivation, and other factors determine this amount. **Hashish,** or hash, is made by taking resin from the leaves and flowers of the marijuana plant and pressing them into cakes or slabs.

Delta-9-Tetrahydracannabinol (THC)

The psychoactive ingredient in the marijuana plant that determines its potency.

Marijuana contains 1 to 3 percent THC, hashish 3 to 6 percent, and hash oil 30 to 50 percent.[18] Pure THC is almost never available, except for research.

PHYSIOLOGICAL EFFECTS

Hashish

Hash is the resin from the leaves and flowers of the marijuana plant. This resin (hashish) is pressed into cakes or slabs.

THC is highly **fat-soluble,** which means it is attracted to fat molecules anywhere in the body. It is slowly metabolized by the liver, and 80 percent of it is excreted by the intestines through feces and the remaining 20 by the kidneys.[19] When smoked it passes through the alveoli of the lungs and into the bloodstream, where it binds to lipoproteins and finds its way into parts of the body where fat is present. It accumulates and stays in fat in the brain, liver, lungs, and spleen. Twenty percent of the THC from a joint, inhaled, will be absorbed by the body. Its half-life is up to one week. It takes one to three months and sometimes longer for the THC to be completely eliminated by the body.[20]

Fat-Soluble

Drugs that are stored in fatty tissue. THC is fat-soluble and some of it is stored in fatty tissue, where it may stay for a month or more.

Homegrown Marijuana Plant
Source: Jery Howard/Stock Boston

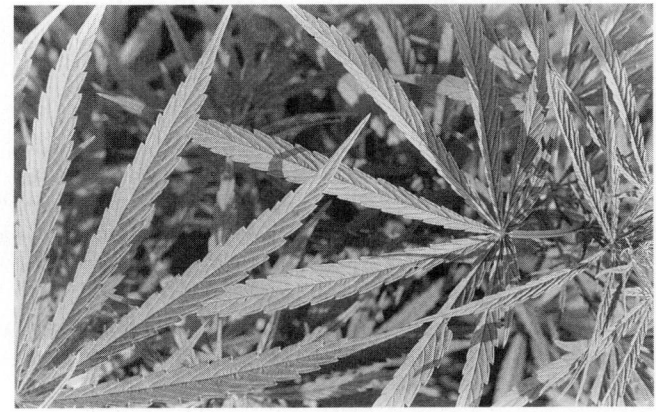

The physiological effects of marijuana smoking are worse than those of tobacco cigarette smoking. Marijuana leads to some of the same problems but is potentially more harmful. UCLA researchers have found that there is nearly five times more carbon monoxide and three times as much tar inhaled into the lungs when one smokes a marijuana cigarette.[21] Carbon monoxide has been linked to coronary heart disease and tar has been associated with cancer. A user may get a false sense of security from smoking only a few marijuana cigarettes a day. But it has been found that smoking one marijuana cigarette is equal to smoking five tobacco cigarettes and is equally damaging.[22] These differences are due in part to the chemical makeup of the two substances and to the different ways they are smoked. Each puff of a marijuana cigarette is on average 70 percent greater in volume and is inhaled 60 percent longer than the average puff of a tobacco cigarette.[23] Cigarette users take more puffs, but marijuana smokers inhale more deeply. Another study showed that smokers of three to four marijuana cigarettes a day suffered bronchitis and damage to the breathing passage equal to that of people who smoked one pack of tobacco cigarettes a day.[24] Because of poor combustion, marijuana smoke produces 50 percent more hydrocarbons than tobacco smoke; hydrocarbons are the chemicals associated with lung cancer.

Marijuana may be smoked in various ways or ingested in the form of baked goods or tea. When eaten, the effect on the lungs is much less. When it is smoked, its effects usually last from two to four hours; if the drug is ingested, effects may last 5 to 12 hours. Physiological responses include mild dilation of the blood vessels in the extremities, a slight increase in blood flow to the arms and legs, and a slight reduction of body temperature through heat loss. Blood pressure is slightly elevated, and reddened eyes and a dry mouth can be expected. Although appetite is usually stimulated, blood-sugar levels remain largely unaffected.

The hazards of marijuana use are related both to the drug itself and to the method of administration. Acute effects, such as psychological dependence, can occur with high doses or chronic use. On occasion anxiety reactions have been reported, and there are rare cases of hallucination-caused physical harm with very large doses, usually when the drug was eaten.

EXTENT OF EFFECTS ON BODY FUNCTIONS

Marijuana is absorbed into the bloodstream through the lungs or intestines, depending on the route administered, and then distributed to different parts of the body. As we have seen, THC is fat-soluble and some of it is stored in fatty tissue, where it may stay for a month or more. The metabolites are then slowly excreted from the body in urine and feces. THC and other cannabinols accumulate in the fatty linings of the cells and are released back into the bloodstream over many days. Studies of experienced users show that the half-life of THC metabolites is 50 hours.[25]

Though it is known that marijuana is an active intoxicant that affects body functions, the extent of its effects, both positive and negative, is difficult to determine. J. Thomas Underleider, Shaffer Commission member, has stated that "no intoxicant or, for that matter, no drug is totally safe or harmless. However, it is my opinion that marijuana involves only minimal harm to the user."[26] Backing up that theory are the findings of a careful review of the literature and of the testimony of health officials, which revealed that not a single human in the United States has ever died solely from marijuana use.[27]

Edward Senay, director of the Drug Abuse Center at the University of Chicago says, "Pot produces an addiction of a severity not known years ago."[28] Regular pot smokers build up a tolerance to the drug and need larger doses to achieve the same high. There are noticeable changes in brain waves during withdrawal from marijuana, and small amounts of THC remain in the blood and body fat for weeks after use has stopped. Although no conclusive evidence has been found on the development of cannabis dependence, the development of a pronounced tolerance has been found.[29] It is rare that such a tolerance develops without a physical dependence as well. The severity of withdrawal symptoms is usually a function of the degree of tolerance developed, but this again seems to be false for marijuana. A few cases of withdrawal syndrome have been observed with symptoms such as anxiety, hyperirritability, aggressiveness, tremors, insomnia, and hallucinations, but none of these symptoms was severe.

C. Everett Koop, former surgeon general of the U.S. Public Health Service stated the known or suspected chronic effects of marijuana use are the following:[30]

- impaired short-term memory and slow learning
- impaired lung function similar to that found in cigarette smokers (with more serious effects following extended use)
- decreased sperm count and sperm motility
- interference with ovulation and prenatal development
- impaired immune response
- possible adverse effects on heart function
- by-products of marijuana remaining in the body fat for several weeks with unknown consequences

PULMONARY EFFECTS

Marijuana smoking can have harmful pulmonary effects. Lung tissue continually exposed to marijuana smoke exhibits changes as serious as, or possibly more serious than, those found in tissues of heavy cigarette smokers. Chronic marijuana use has been seen to impair lung function in otherwise healthy subjects.[31] Heavy marijuana and/or hashish use can also cause chronic bronchitis, emphysema, and fibrosis.[32] Residuals of smoked marijuana have been shown to be carcinogenic to animal skin.

One possible reason for the apparently greater damage done by marijuana is that a joint is usually smoked differently than a tobacco cigarette. A joint is smoked until the very end, which is where most of the tar, cannabinol, and resins accumulate. Moreover, it is inhaled more deeply, so the chem-

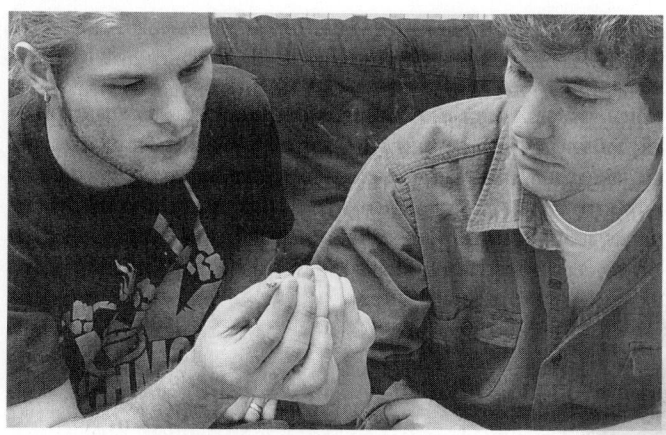

Sharing a Marijuana "Joint"
Source: Arlene Collins/Monkmeyer Press

icals have longer contact with lung tissue. Additionally, there is evidence that if marijuana is readily available, the number of marijuana cigarettes consumed (up to ten joints daily) may approach that of tobacco cigarettes.[33]

The research done so far on the effects of marijuana on the lungs shows it to be at least an irritant. The evidence suggests that marijuana with its many chemicals leads to damage similar to that from tobacco. However, more research is still needed to determine long-term effects in relation to dose and frequency.

It seems logical that the high amount of tobacco smoke that enters the average cigarette smoker's air passageways should put him or her at a higher risk than a marijuana smoker. However, according to Sidney Cohen, two factors equalize the risk:

1. Typical cigarette smokers do not inhale smoke deep into the bronchial passages, or if they do, it's for a short time. Marijuana is inhaled as deeply as possible.

2. In recent years, there has been an increase in the amount of marijuana smoked per individual.[34]

An interesting study was recently conducted by the University of California at Los Angeles that measured the carbon monoxide in the blood and inhaled tar in the lungs of men who smoked tobacco or marijuana cigarettes.[35] The researchers found that a single marijuana cigarette may be as unhealthy as smoking five cigarettes made of tobacco. The same scientists had concluded that habitual smoking of three or four marijuana cigarettes a day caused the same amount of bronchitis symptoms and lung-cell damage as smoking more than 20 tobacco cigarettes daily. Marijuana smoking resulted in three times the amount of tar inhaled and one-third more tar retained in the lungs and respiratory tract.

A study conducted at the University of Arizona, in 990 subjects between the ages of 15 and 40, found that those who smoked marijuana were almost twice as likely as a complete nonsmoker to report phlegm and wheezing.[36] On some tests of lung function, marijuana smokers had worse results than those who were only tobacco smokers. Significant abnormalities were found in a test for airway obstruction of pot smokers, more so in men than women, probably because men tended to smoke more often.[37]

Both marijuana and tobacco smoke contain about the same amount of tar. It takes only a few months for marijuana smokers' lungs to be as damaged as tobacco smokers' lungs get in many years.[38] There may be two reasons for this. One is that the chemical found in marijuana, THC (delta-9-tetrahydrocannabinol) alone can destroy cells. Another reason is that marijuana smokers inhale deeper and hold smoke in their lungs longer.

These findings are consistent with those in a study conducted at the University of California Los Angeles School of Medicine. The California study showed that marijuana cigarettes contain more harmful materials than those found in tobacco cigarettes.[39] Approximately five times the amount of carbon monoxide (which has been associated with coronary diseases) and three times the amount of tar is inhaled from a marijuana cigarette versus a tobacco cigarette and is deposited in the airway of the individual. There is increased exposure to these substances with marijuana because inhaling is generally deeper and breath-holding longer.

The lungs of anyone who smokes daily are bound to be damaged. However, tobacco smokers tend to smoke more *daily* than marijuana smokers, so the level of damage may not differ that much between the two.

A large number of people view marijuana smoking as harmless, relaxing, and possibly beneficial. Decades ago, a strikingly similar belief prevailed about cigarette smoking. After the 1964 surgeon general's report came out, the latter changed dramatically. "In terms of knowledge about the effects of marijuana, I suspect we are now where we were 20 years ago in cigarette smoking," says Donald T. Frederickson, assistant dean at New York University's Post Graduate School of Medicine.[40] Of growing concern is the potentially harmful effects of today's marijuana, which is so much stronger than that of the 1960s.

CARDIOVASCULAR COMPLICATIONS

Cardiovascular problems resulting from marijuana use may be relevant only to the elderly or to persons with preexisting cardiac disorders.[41] American Medical Association reports emphasize that the use of marijuana by patients with impaired heart function may precipitate chest pain more rapidly, following less effort, than the smoking of tobacco cigarettes.[42] "Marijuana accelerates the rate at which the heart contracts and may temporarily weaken the strength of contractions, making it potentially dangerous for people with certain cardiac conditions."[43] Though this and similar evidence is limited, warnings against marijuana use for heart patients and others who may have impaired cardiac function seem justified.[44]

There is good evidence that the smoking of marijuana typically causes acute changes in the heart and circulation. However, there is controversy surrounding the issue of how it affects the "normal," healthy individual. According to a study by the Committee of the Institute on Medicine, there is no evidence of a permanently deleterious effect on the cardiovascular system.[45] However, evidence shows that marijuana increases the work of the heart, usually by raising the heart rate—as much as 50 percent, or from approximately 70 beats per minute to as many as 150 beats per minute, depending on the amount of THC in the cigarette—and in some persons by raising the blood pressure. This effect is only temporary and lasts up to a few hours. When the heart rate goes up, the heart itself needs more oxygen to work harder. Smoking marijuana or tobacco cigarettes decreases the supply of available oxygen to the body. This work load poses a threat to persons with hypertension, cerebrovascular disease, and coronary atherosclerosis. It is thought that those with preclinical coronary heart disease may experience symptoms such as angina when smoking marijuana.

Coronary heart disease has been directly related to tobacco smoking. As mentioned before, marijuana and tobacco share similar ingredients. Marijuana too may some day be linked to coronary heart disease. As of now, the research is limited and inconclusive on this issue.

At least one research paper indicates that it may be very dangerous for cardiac patients to combine marijuana with alcohol.[46] Intense nausea, vomiting, and a drop in heart rate from 150 to 36 beats per minute have occurred in subjects using both of these drugs.

EFFECTS ON THE IMMUNE SYSTEM

Marijuana may act as an immunosuppressant, a substance that inhibits the body's response to disease. The data from hospital studies thus far are contradictory.

Some have demonstrated mild immunosuppressant effects, but others, using the same or similar methods, have found no differences in the immune system between normals and chronic marijuana smokers. No animal or human studies have yet determined if marijuana smokers are more prone to infections or other diseases.[47] Researchers are concerned that further research may not yield definitive findings, and because of the widespread use of marijuana, even weak immunosuppressive effects are alarming.

The immune system is important in protecting the body from bacteria, viruses, and cancerous cells. Studies on cell cultures show that THC affects the development of immune-system cells that would ordinarily develop into monocytes, a type of white blood cell; the cells are induced to mature partially, but they never develop the functions necessary for a proper immune response.[48] The possible consequences of a suppressed system caused by marijuana could lead to a number of health problems.

EFFECTS ON ENDOCRINE FUNCTIONING

The issue of marijuana's possible effect on endocrine functioning was first raised in 1972. In 1974, the first experimental evidence that marijuana causes a reduction in serum testosterone, the principal male sex hormone, was published. Low sperm counts in heavy marijuana users have also been indicated,[49] though the significance of this finding is yet to be evaluated. Studies of chronic hashish users in Greece also indicate a diminution of sperm count and alterations in the cellular characteristics of the spermatozoa in otherwise normal young males.[50]

Wylie Hembree did an interesting study on 16 young men.[51] He hospitalized them for three months, which increased the control of the study. The first month they were not allowed to smoke any marijuana. The second month they could smoke as much as they wanted; they averaged 12 joints per day, with 2 percent THC concentration. The third month they also did not smoke. It was found that during the second month, sperm count decreased by an average of 40 percent; sperm motility decreased by an average of 20 percent. Also, a slight increase in the number of abnormal sperm was seen. This last observation suggests a possible link that has not been determined. When marijuana is smoked its effects are immediate, and when its use is stopped the counts go back to normal. The question is: What happens over long periods—can these effects be permanent?

A Boston City Hospital study showed that women who smoked pot during pregnancy were five times more likely than non–pot-smoking pregnant women to deliver infants with features considered compatible with fetal alcohol syndrome.[52] This suggests a synergistic effect of marijuana and alcohol on the newborn.

It has been proven that marijuana changes the hormone levels in both men and women. Marijuana temporarily lowers the level of sex hormone in men and decreases the number, quality, and motility of sperm, but the impact on fertility is unknown.[53]

Women who smoke marijuana heavily may experience menstrual irregularities, including failure to ovulate. Doctors urge pregnant women and nursing women to treat pot with the same caution they give to alcohol and tobacco.

Many clinical studies have been done that show smoking marijuana during pregnancy has detrimental effects on the fetus.[54] Marijuana use has been associated with many difficulties such as prematurity, low birth weight, decreased maternal weight gain, complications of pregnancy, and difficult labor, among others.

Inconsistent findings on the effects of marijuana on fetal growth may be due to difficulties in accurately identifying marijuana users. Research indicates that women are more likely to underreport the use of marijuana, an illegal substance, than the use of cigarettes or alcohol, legal substances.[55]

PSYCHOMOTOR IMPAIRMENT

The Department of Health, Education and Welfare's 1979 report *Marijuana and Health* states that there is clear-cut evidence that marijuana impairs reaction time, motor coordination, and visual perception, making it dangerous for people to drive, fly, or operate machinery while intoxicated by the drug.[56] At the Fifth World Congress of Psychiatry in 1978, Danish investigators offered proof that cannabis reduces driving skills.[57] Braking time was shown to slow down after cannabis use, as was time of response to sound.

Illusions were reported to occur and sudden flights of ideas caused confusion and anxiety in new situations. Responses involving eye-hand coordination were impaired, and the more complex the situation became, the slower the response.

Research also indicates that with a severity directly related to dose, marijuana impairs motor coordination and affects tracking and the sensory and perceptual functions important for safe driving and the operation of other machines; impairs short-term memory; and slows learning. The drug appears to alter the sense of time, reduce one's ability to do things that require concentration, and affect the swift reactions that are so essential in driving a car or operating machinery.

Driving experiments show that marijuana use affects a wide range of skills needed for safe driving. Thinking and reflexes are slowed, making it hard for the driver to respond to sudden, unexpected events.[58] Also, the driver's ability to track (stay in lane) through curves, to brake quickly, and to maintain speed and the proper distance between cars is affected. Research shows that these skills are impaired for at least four to six hours after smoking a single marijuana cigarette, long after the high is gone. If a person drinks alcohol while using marijuana, the risk of an accident is greatly increased. Errors can be made in reading the speedometer while driving. The effects of marijuana are greatest immediately after smoking (unlike alcohol) and decline slowly over a period of hours.[59] In one study 60 percent of subjects failed a police field-sobriety test two and a half hours after smoking ad lib doses of marijuana, even though the THC plasma content of some had declined to negligible levels. In another study, researchers found evidence of adverse effects persisting for four to seven hours after smoking. In sum, the studies have shown that detectable blood levels of THC are present in 11 to 20 percent of drivers in fatal accidents, or as many as 37 percent of young California males.[60] Studies also have shown that 81 to 87 percent of THC-related fatalities involved alcohol, with 59 to 68 percent at levels of legal intoxication.

Despite such evidence that marijuana impairs driving ability, it is likely that more marijuana users than ever before now drive while high. In limited surveys, 60 to 80 percent of those questioned indicated that they sometimes drive while high.

GENETIC DAMAGE

Early reports of increased chromosomal breakage and human cell–culture abnormalities resulting from marijuana use have *not* been corroborated by recent research. Reports do indicate, however, that marijuana may increase the number of lung cells containing abnormal levels of chromosomes and may also increase the number of white blood cells showing abnormally low levels of chromosomes.

Early research has also indicated that cannabis, or one or more of its chemical components, may inhibit DNA metabolism in abnormal (carcinogenic) animal cells while leaving normal cells unaffected. If such preferential inhibition also occurs in humans, marijuana may turn out to be of chemotherapeutic value as an anticancer agent.[61] Further study may also substantiate current indications that cannabis, its synthesized components, or chemically related drugs might prove useful in preventing organ rejection in human organ-transplant surgery.[62]

EFFECTS ON THE BRAIN

According to some reports, marijuana has acute effects on the brain, including chemical and electrophysiological changes.[63] Its most clearly established acute effects are on mental functions and behavior. However, other studies have found no persuasive evidence that marijuana causes overt changes in the brain.[64] Computerized studies of users of marijuana reveal no gross changes in brain structure.

We also know that THC is stored in fat and that the brain is one-third fat.[65] All nerve-cell axons are covered in a fat sheath. Like opiates and some other drugs, THC has no specific reception site in the brain, but it interacts with several neurotransmitters.

THC has been found to affect the medulla oblongata, located in the brain stem. This is where the nausea center is located, and THC has been found to inhibit nausea and vomiting. This could have positive effects for cancer patients receiving chemotherapy.[66] But it also creates a danger for youngsters who are drinking while smoking pot: because they don't get sick they tend to drink more than normal—possibly to the point of death.[67]

Research on Brain Damage   When two samples of young men with histories of heavy cannabis smoking were studied in Missouri and Massachusetts, brain scans showed no evidence of cerebral atrophy. However, researchers Harold Kolansky and William Moore suggest that biochemical and even structural cerebral changes occur with chronic long-term cannabis use.[68] Symptoms of these changes include apathy, disturbed self-awareness, confusion, and unrealistic understanding, but such symptoms disappear 3 to 24 months after marijuana use has ended. Marijuana-caused intoxication also produces minimal and transient changes in brain waves, but as we have noted, results of brain-wave studies are still unclear and inconsistent.

Many studies have been done on marijuana's adverse effects on memory, attention, and perception. However, these effects were rarely significant four hours after use. The increase of marijuana consumption and recent airplane accidents involving pilots testing positive for THC prompted a study of marijuana's effects on the performance of pilots up to 24 hours after use.[69]

Ten certified pilots were tested in a flight simulator before smoking the drug. They were to perform a standard maneuver involving a takeoff, climb, two turns, and a landing and requiring changes in latitude, longitude, altitude, angle of bank, angle of climb, rate of climb, and velocity. All the pilots were observed and recorded by computer. Distance off center on landing was also recorded.

One hour after smoking a marijuana cigarette containing 19 milligrams of THC—the equivalent of a strong social dose—the pilots were instructed to perform the same task. They did so again 4 and 24 hours after ingestion.

Even after 24 hours, all the variables differed significantly when compared with the results of the test taken before the drug was smoked. The number and magnitude of the changes in lateral movement, vertical movement, and throttle were of specific concern. The difficulty pilots had in aligning and landing precisely in the center of the runway was alarming. Twenty-four hours after ingestion, landings were 50 percent off the base mark. One pilot even missed the runway. Such errors in actual flight, combined with wind and turbulence, could easily cause a major accident. Perhaps most disquieting of all, the pilots were unaware of their impaired performance!

Miles Herkenham and his colleagues at the National Institute of Mental Health recently mapped out the location of THC receptors in the brain.[70] They discovered that most of the receptors are in the hippocampus, where scientists believe memory consolidation occurs. This is also where the external may get translated into a spatial and cognitive map. They also found receptors throughout the cortex, which is the site for higher cognition. This distribution helps explain marijuana's detrimental effects on memory, mental activity, and spatial orientation. There were very few receptors in the brainstem, where critical life-support controls are based. This might explain why it is hard to die from even high doses of the drug. Also, some of the receptors in the spinal cord might explain pot's analgesic effects.

The researchers at the National Institute of Mental Health were aided by luck when they stumbled upon a cannabinoid receptor. They originally were searching for receptor genes when they stumbled upon the cannabinoid. Lisa Matsuday and her researchers compared the maps of Herkenham and his colleagues and have cloned a gene that gives rise to the receptor molecules that cannabinoids bind to the brain.[71] This discovery could lead to new pharmaceuticals based on marijuana. The potential importance of cannabinoids is that they may be useful as analgesics for treating asthma, glaucoma, and nausea and vomiting often caused by cancer chemotherapy.

MEMORY

The marijuana high is caused by chemicals called cannabinoids, especially THC, which interferes with the signals between the nerve cells, causing jumbled thought and distortions of perception.[72] The user may become illogical, forgetful, and clumsy. Short-term memory and learning ability are curtailed for students after smoking.[73] This could be a serious problem for students, especially frequent smokers. High doses cause irritability, anxiety, and hallucinations. The higher the dosage, the greater the memory loss.

A study was conducted by Richard Schwartz of Georgetown School of Medicine in Washington, D.C. Schwartz had noted that teenagers who abuse marijuana can suffer from problems with their short-term memory up to six weeks after they stop smoking the drug. Schwartz and his colleagues noticed that marijuana-abusing teenagers in drug-treatment programs often had trouble remembering rules and their following conversations. It has been found that marijuana is attracted to brain cells, and that marijuana impairs motor coordination and slows learning as well as affects short-term memory. There is the possibility that brain damage may occur in some people who use the drug.[74]

Some studies done previously demonstrated the effects of long-term marijuana use on memory impairment.[75] These studies were done a long time ago, and since then the potency of the active ingredient in marijuana, tetrahydrocannabinol, has increased as much as 250 percent in some cases. The results showed that the long-term marijuana users had significantly lower memory scores than the other two groups. After about six weeks of supervised abstinence in an inpatient program, the adolescents in the cannabis-using group showed improvement on several of the memory tests. The results of the test are thought to show that adolescents who use marijuana excessively have selective short-term memory deficits that continue for at least six weeks after discontinuing the drug.[76]

TOLERANCE

Tolerance to marijuana has been demonstrated in both humans and animals. Although tolerance can develop rapidly after only a few small doses, it disappears at an equally rapid rate for many who are affected. Large doses administered to animals result in tolerance lasting for longer periods. Tolerance to marijuana does not necessarily have health implications unless it should lead to stronger and more frequent doses with adverse consequences, such as stronger respiratory effects.

PSYCHOLOGICAL EFFECTS

These psychoactive effects are remarkably varied. Perceptions of color, sounds, patterns, textures, and tastes may be altered. Mood varies considerably: a sense of increased well-being is frequently experienced, but anxiety and depression may be enhanced as well. Drowsiness or hyperactivity and hilarity may occur. Passivity and apathy are often noted. Ideas may appear to be disconnected, rapidly flowing, and altered in emphasis and importance. Individuals may become more talkative or more withdrawn. Time seems to pass slowly, with little activity needed and no sense of boredom. Users describe long periods of listening to music or reading. Problems may appear to be less pressing or more urgent. Smokers describe the ability to observe their own intoxication, including anxiety and paranoid ideation. Occasional users often attempt to facilitate concentration at a concert or a movie or enhance sensual experiences.[77]

Marijuana use, in some individuals, tends to interfere with psychological functioning, personality development, and emotional growth. Long-term users of marijuana may become psychologically dependent. They may have a hard time limiting their use, they may need more of the drug to get the same effect, and they may develop problems with their jobs and personal relationships. They risk the danger of the drug becoming the most important aspect of their lives.

How marijuana affects the user depends not only on the dose taken but also on how experienced the smoker is. Small doses of cannabis generally

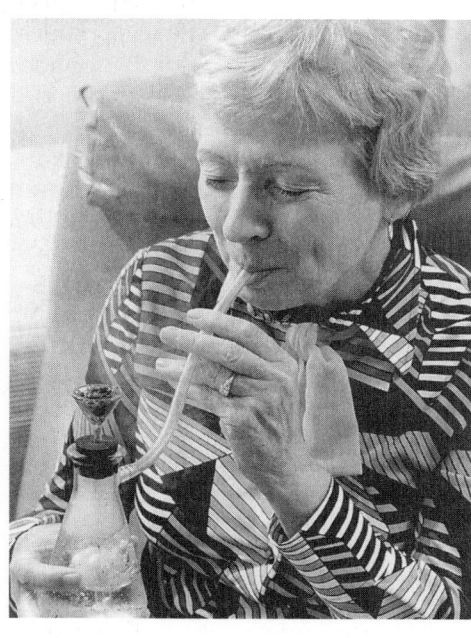

Research on Marijuana
Source: Ira Block/The Image Bank

elicit euphoria, enhance congeniality, and effects moods of passivity. At moderate doses, the effects are intensified and may be accompanied by some impairment of short-term memory, disturbances in thought patterns, lapses in attention, subjective feeling of unfamiliarity, depersonalization, and sensory distraction. Large doses bring on a further loosening of emotional and social restraints, a deeper feeling of relaxation or euphoria, and stronger distortions of time and space. In other words, marijuana responses are unpredictable. The drug may causes drowsiness or hyperactivity. One smoker may become chatty, another withdrawn, or the same user may experience both effects but on different occasions. The most common unpleasant side effects are paranoia and anxiety.

During a marijuana high, which lasts for two to four hours, users often experience relaxation and altered perception of signals, sounds, tastes, and cravings for snacks, especially sugary ones, and they consume more calories.[78]

This role of experience is reflected in Richard Schwartz's description of three phases of marijuana use in adolescence.[79] The first is the initial phase. Here the user is influenced by peer pressure, set, setting, and personality. The first experience usually includes anxiety, nausea, headache, palpitations, dizziness, and weakness. The user may experience an intense fear of losing control and dying. With an increase in use the person becomes high and has a feeling of well-being, serenity, omnipotence, and distortion of time perception.

The second phase is characterized by good feeling. The user knows how to get high. Time and energy go into getting high that would normally be spent developing other interests and lifestyles. Feelings of guilt, fear, and deception increase with frequency of use.

The third phase is dependence. Adolescents who frequently use pot have a difficult time coping with life's normal stresses and frustrations. Problems are usually blamed on outside sources. The initial euphoria subsides, and malaise, irritability, apathy, inertia, and depression set in.

When the use of marijuana is stopped, these symptoms usually go away. There is some evidence to support the notion of dependence, but it is not conclusive. Abrupt discontinuation has caused nausea, vomiting, sweating, tremors, and sleep disturbance. It has also been found to result in restlessness and irritability, depending upon the amount ingested.[80]

ADOLESCENTS' PERCEPTIONS

A recent study supports the idea that the junior high school age group tends to perceive behaviors, such as the use of marijuana, as more prevalent than they actually are.[81] They also found that those who engage in an activity are more likely to overestimate its prevalence. The "False Consensus Effect" is defined as users' perceptions that "their behavior is similar to other people's behavior. . . . Subjects usually believed others would do as they do in hypothetical and real situations."[82] This "False Consensus Effect" seems to be widespread when the behavior under consideration is drug use, and this concept is implicitly used by many researchers to explain why some people might initiate drug use.

PEER INFLUENCES

Many young people are introduced to marijuana by their peers, usually acquaintances, friends, sisters, and brothers. People try such drugs because they feel pressured by peers to be part of a group, to have a good time with friends, to get high, to relieve boredom, to enhance the effects of other drugs, and to cope with stress. Surprisingly enough, the reasons given by daily users for discontinuing their habit are loss of interest in getting high, concern about harmful physical and psychological effects, and concern about their loss of energy and ambition. While marijuana use seems to be on the decrease, it is too early to tell whether the decrease will continue or is merely a pause in the rise.

EFFECTS ON SCHOOL PERFORMANCE

Marijuana has been interfering with the education of a lot of youngsters today.[83] It is relatively cheap and easy to get hold of. It makes youngsters "feel good." The biggest explanation for early marijuana uses by youths is that they were bored, so the got "stoned" before, between, and after class. They actually believe that marijuana is helping them in the long run to stay alert, but "even though a marijuana smoker may believe he or she is very alert and has heightened senses, in reality the spaced-out student is missing a good deal of lecture."

When a stoned student does manage to pay attention to what a teacher is saying, the material is more difficult to understand than if the student were straight. Also, the information may only make it to the short-term memory. Later this information will not be there.

THC has been shown to lower alertness and retard learning and memory.[84] The higher the dosage, the greater the loss of memory. If a student could pay attention in class to a lecture, the problem will be storing that information into long-term memory. When exam time comes, student recall is difficult. Students have also reported that in their experience, marijuana impaired motivation, or the desire to learn, as well as learning itself.

AGGRESSION

Does marijuana cause an increase in human physical aggression? The results show "the subjects in the low dose condition tended to respond in more of an aggressive manner than subjects in moderate and high dose conditions."[85] Also, "The subjects in the high dose condition behaved in a relatively non-aggressive manner throughout the experimental session." The results of the study confirmed the belief that marijuana does not significantly "increase, instigate, precipitate, or enhance aggressive behavior."

SOCIAL CONVERSATION

The effects of smoked marijuana on social conversation have also been researched.[86] Speech was monitored in seven one-hour sessions following smoking by the subjects. The marijuana produced significant decreases in speech quantity by the users in comparison with the nonusers in the study. The subjects' self-reports showed further that marijuana does not increase communication, in opposition to the general rule that drugs increase social interaction. The active ingredients of marijuana produced significant decreases in speech quantity of the users versus the nonusers in the study. Heart rate was increased and the self-reports showed that the users said they felt high and sedated. Finally, it was stated that marijuana does not increase communication, in opposition to the general rule that drugs increase social interaction.

FAMILY COHESIVENESS

It has generally been found that a loving parent-child relationship is linked to reduced likelihood of the child's use of drugs.[87] The cohesiveness of the family unit appears to influence drug use by children. Adolescent involvement in family decisions is also associated with less drug use.

PSYCHOPATHOLOGY

The most common adverse psychological reaction to marijuana among American users is acute anxiety.[88] This reaction is an intense response to the perspective and distortion of reality marijuana generally produces. The reaction appears to be more common in relatively inexperienced users, although unexpectedly high doses of cannabis can cause panic in the more experienced user as well. Symptoms of acute anxiety generally respond to sensitive assurance and diminish soon after the effects of the marijuana recede.[89]

Transient mild paranoia is another adverse reaction common to marijuana users. Those who are characterized by more paranoid defense mechanisms are less likely to experience other acute adverse reactions. If users are concerned about their drug experience and/or the circumstances of use, anxiety and mild paranoid reactions to the drug are likely to occur. In a study of college student users, Naditch and colleagues found that those who were hypochondriacs, who felt less in control of their lives, and who were more at the mercy of external events were more likely to have adverse reactions to marijuana and other psychoactive drugs.[90]

AMOTIVATIONAL SYNDROME

There is still uncertainty over whether chronic marijuana use causes or results from apathy, listlessness, and associated personality difficulties. A much-disputed alleged effect of cannabis, however, the "amotivational syndrome," purports that individuals who smoke the drug become apathetic, lose interest in work, and suffer from a general lack of motivation.

Schwartz has also described an "amotivational syndrome" that occurs in long-term users.[91] This syndrome is characterized by decreased goals and ambitions, abnormal amounts of apathy, mood swings, and irritability. The user may show impaired short-term memory, confused thinking, and inability to master new problems. Amotivational users have been described as passive, slothful, sluggish, and lacking in ambition. This syndrome has been presented as the reason for poor school performance and personality deterioration, especially in adolescents.

FLASHBACKS

Marijuana flashbacks—spontaneous recurrences of feelings and perceptions similar to those produced by use of the drug—have been reported by some users.[92] Such experiences may range from the quite vivid re-creation of a drug-related experience to a much milder form of remembrance. A survey of U.S. Army personnel who used marijuana found that flashbacks occurred in both frequent and infrequent users and were not necessarily related to LSD use. It has since been reliably reported, however, that although flashbacks under the influence of marijuana are rare, individuals who have used LSD previously may be slightly more likely to have LSD-like flashbacks when they use marijuana.[93] The cause of flashbacks is still uncertain, but those who have experienced them usually require little or no treatment.[94]

THERAPEUTIC AND MEDICAL USES OF MARIJUANA

Though cannabis presently has limited medical application, studies indicate that the drug may have a bright future as a chemotherapeutic agent. Glaucoma and cancer are two diseases now undergoing experimental treatment with cannabis.

GLAUCOMA

Glaucoma is a disease in which the retina, the part of the eyeball that receives the image from the lens, degenerates. It is caused by intraocular pressure, which eventually reduces available intraocular fluids and secretions. Because marijuana enables blood vessel membranes to relax and expand in an elastic fashion, it creates more space for the blood to flow and thus reduces pressure. When marijuana is used to reduce intraocular pressure, it allows intraocular fluids to remain at sufficient levels.

Though there has been a good deal of controversy over marijuana's use in glaucoma treatment, the *Randall vs. FDA* lawsuit in the District of Columbia has upheld the legality of that use. The suit determined that physicians could be licensed to prescribe cannabis for glaucoma treatment,[95] and at least four states (New Mexico, Florida, Illinois, and Louisiana) have passed laws legalizing marijuana for research and treatment purposes.[96]

According to the federal government's National Eye Institute, however, no definitive clinical studies have been completed on marijuana. Some doctors therefore feel that the assumption that marijuana is safe and effective for glaucoma treatment is misleading and could result in serious ocular damage and other side effects. For example, Frank Newell, chairman of the Department of Ophthalmology at the University of Chicago, states that "in order to reduce the pressure on the eye, one would have to smoke a joint every two hours day and night!"[97]

But THC can now be made into eyedrops for the treatment of glaucoma. Synthetically produced THC has no impurities, unlike natural THC, and is safer to use.

CANCER

Studies at UCLA and other research centers have evaluated THC's capacity to alleviate various symptoms of cancer as well as side effects of chemotherapy.[98] The drug compares very favorably with Compazine, the standard but pharmacologically inconsistent drug of choice for these side effects. Researchers at the Sydney Farber Cancer Institute have also substantiated THC's effectiveness as a therapeutic adjunct in the treatment of cancer.[99] Because it often induces relaxation, the drug may additionally find application as an antianxiety agent in cancer treatment. This use may be of great value because of the recognized link between emotional distress and cancer propagation. A large-scale study in California has found marijuana to be a safe and effective way of reducing the side effects of radial chemotherapy given to cancer patients in that state.[100] Nine hundred patients who had failed to respond to normal antinausea treatments were given marijuana, to eat in capsules or to smoke in cigarettes. Almost 60 percent reported that the drug relieved the vomiting and nausea associated with chemotherapy.

MEDICAL APPLICATIONS

Sidney Cohen of the Neuropsychiatric Institute of UCLA was considered the most knowledgeable scientist in the United States on the medical use of marijuana. He felt that other drugs will eventually take the place of marijuana, but until these are developed, marijuana should remain available to patients if it helps them. Marijuana has been used to combat many of the following ailments.[101]

1. *Anorexia Nervosa:* Although there are more effective drugs to treat this disease, many users say that their appetite is increased by pot.

2. *Withdrawal from alcohol and opiates:* Marijuana can be taken with Antabuse (a medicine that causes a severe reaction when taken with alcohol) but has not been shown to help with withdrawal.

3. *Epilepsy:* Some patients have reported seizures despite the use of marijuana; others say marijuana helps a lot. One of the nonpsychoactive cannabinoid plants has helped in grand mal epilepsy.

4. *Asthma:* Although marijuana smoking does cause initial relief from bronchial constriction, continued smoking worsens the condition.

5. *Bacterial infections:* Marijuana may be used as an antibiotic with certain types of bacteria when applied to the skin.

6. *Muscle cramps:* Marijuana has been shown to help relax muscles, but it does no better than another drug, Baclofen.

7. *Tumors:* Studies of animals have shown THC to have tumor-suppressing effects. However, it does not compare with chemotherapy. On the other hand, another cannabinoid has been shown to increase tumor growth.

In spite of these uses, according to Cohen, marijuana will never become an accepted drug, because (1) it will be found to contain over 1,000 chemicals, and we now know of only 400; (2) it is an unstable substance; (3) it has a poor shelf life; and (4) it contains a lot of things, such as a fungus, that we don't want in our systems.

ECONOMICS

WORKPLACE

Research compiled by Kiam Associates determined that marijuana users represent a greater threat to workplace safety than cocaine users.[102] According to the results of this research, 8 percent of all full-time employees in the United States use illegal drugs; among workers between the ages of 18 and 25 years, the number is 19 percent. Among those who use illegal substances at least once a month, 87.5 percent use marijuana, whereas the number of employees who use cocaine at least once a month is statistically insignificant. The research also revealed that the level of job-performance impairment after using marijuana can last as long as 24 hours after ingestion, whereas job-performance impairment from using cocaine dissipates after only a few hours.

MARIJUANA CROPS

Since marijuana is a leading agricultural crop, possibly number one in the United States, it is imperative that we learn as much as possible about this most widely used illicit drug. In 1984 the House Select Committee on

Narcotics and Abuse said the annual U.S. pot crop could be worth $10 to $50 billion.[103]

Another concern has been mentioned by the U.S. Forest Service. Marijuana growers first started moving into the national forests in the late 1970s. The growers were attracted to the areas because of their remoteness and because it is difficult to prove ownership of a marijuana patch on public property. In 1988 law enforcement officers raided 3,034 marijuana plantations hidden in 156 national forests in 44 states, and they estimate they detected only 40 percent of the sites.[104]

The growers have a number of effects in our national forests. The areas are dangerous to campers and hikers because of armed guards and booby traps used to protect their products. (There were 75 cases of assaults against citizens in 1987). Their fertilizers pollute streams. Poisons are spread to kill animals that might graze on their plants, and fires have been set in retaliation for raids. The U.S. Forest Service lists 835,000 acres of national forests as off-limits because they cannot guarantee people's safety or manage them for resources, wildlife, and recreation. Now methamphetamine labs are moving into the areas. In 1987 there were 83 cases that involved meth labs.

In 1988 the Forest Service was finally given the authority to arrest drug producers on federal lands and Congress appropriated the funds to enforce the laws. Every state is working to develop a program to fight against marijuana planting, tightening state laws governing drug convictions, and encouraging citizens to help by reporting concealed gardens. The Forest Service is on the attack burning plants, closing labs, arresting producers, and getting growers jailed. It should be stressed that this concentrated attack on growers is forcing many of them inside, where they use grow lights in buildings to grow their crops.

Police say that due to the series of busts on the West Coast, farmers have been driven indoors. Because of this the price of marijuana has gone up. The back pages of pro-marijuana magazines are currently filled with ads for greenhouse supplies. Indoor gardening is sweeping the country, and an average basement with the latest equipment can yield $30,000 to $50,000 a year.[105]

Marijuana growth patterns have changed from large patches to smaller clumps and indoor gardens, which are more difficult for law enforcement officers to detect. The "traditional" drug grower is no longer the most common type of drug grower. We are seeing an increase in nontraditional growers like teachers, engineers, carpenters, and rural farmers.[106]

LEGALIZATION

On November 6, 1990, Alaska moved from one of the most lenient states on marijuana possession to one of the toughest states concerning the possession of pot.[107] In 1975 pot was legalized in Alaska. At that time an individual could have in his home up to 4 ounces of pot. If someone had excessive amounts of marijuana, the fine was only $100.

Today Alaska has changed. It is no longer isolated. The eyes of the nation can focus on Alaska with lightening speed through television cameras. The oil pipe has brought big business to Alaska. The people have grown more conservative. The citizens of Alaska now recognize marijuana as a health risk. Alaska passed legislation in 1990 to forbid any amounts of marijuana and to fine anyone in possession of pot $1000.[108]

PROPONENTS OF LEGALIZATION

Proponents feel a way to solve the drug problem is legalization of marijuana.[109] This would be accomplished by much stricter laws and consequences regarding hard drugs (e.g., heroin and cocaine). With legalization of marijuana, liquor stores would become the point of sale. The age restriction would be the same as for alcohol. The government could tax pot, with the revenue used to finance hard-drug treatment programs. If pot were taxed, it would generate an estimated $11 billion per year. Currently about $1.2 billion in state and federal money is spent annually on drug treatment.

The theory is that if marijuana were legalized, its distribution could be controlled. Also, users would have a safe place to get it, and this would put the pushers out of business. The legalization of this drug would free up the police force to allow them to put more money into cracking down on the illegal drug pushers.

OPPONENTS OF LEGALIZATION

Opponents feel that by legalizing marijuana we may be increasing the number of dependents considerably.[110] Legalization addresses only one aspect of drug use—preventing criminality—without raising the question of how people can be persuaded not to use drugs in the first place. Proponents of this view believe that more time needs to be spent looking at the underlying problems of drug users, spending much more time educating the public, and stopping drugs in source countries.

Also, with the newer and more potent form of marijuana, there are many physical effects that may result from heavy drug use. Usage affects short-term memory, the lungs, and coordination, and it impairs perception. The heart works harder, increasing blood pressure, and, it may have an overall negative effect on the body.

In the final analysis, how will marijuana affect one's health? Will it cause as many problems as tobacco? What will the long-term-use effects be on an individual? If legalized, would use escalate? What would be the effect of driving "under the influence"? In other words, an important health issue must also be considered when proposing legalization.

SUMMARY

Marijuana use has permeated American society. Marijuana smoking peaked in the United States in 1978 and has declined since. The newer high potency marijuana is causing increasing health problems. Pulmonary diseases, cardiovascular problems, psychomotor conditions, short-term memory loss, and psychological problems appear to be related to the use of marijuana. New research findings are starting to clarify the potential problems this drug might cause. On the other hand, research may also find new medical uses for the drug.

Marijuana

N O T E S

1. Norman Taylor, *Narcotics: Nature's Dangerous Gifts* (New York: Dodd, Mead, 1966), p. 20.
2. *Cannabis: A Report of the Canadian Government Commission of Inquiry into the Non-Medical Use of Drugs* (Ottawa: Crown, 1972).
3. "Marijuana: Alcohol and Drug Fact Sheet," *Drug Information Center (DIC)* (Eugene: University of Oregon, 1979).
4. John Kaplan, *Marijuana: The New Prohibition* (New York: World Publishing, 1972), p. 23.
5. Taylor, *Narcotics.*
6. National Commission on Marijuana and Drug Abuse, *Marijuana: A Signal of Misunderstanding* (New York: New American Library, Signet, 1972), p. 21.
7. Donna J. Hymes, "Marijuana Update: New Reasons to `Keep Off the Grass,'" *Current Health 2* (March 1987):18.
8. Ibid., p. 19.
9. Ibid.
10. "News Release: State of Oregon Marijuana Survey," *Grassroots,* April 1978, pp. 19–21.
11. Stuart Nightingale and Seymour Perry, "Marijuana and Heroin by Prescription: Recent Developments at the State and Federal Level," *Journal of the American Medical Association* 24, no. 4 (January 26, 1979):373–75.
12. Winifred Gallagher, "Marijuana: Is There New Reason to Why?" *American Health,* March 1988, pp. 92–101.
13. Jerald G. Backman, et al., "Explaining the Decline in Marijuana Use," *Journal of Health and Social Behavior* 29 (March 1988):92–112.
14. Ibid.
15. National Institute on Drug Abuse, Division of Epidemiology and Prevention, "National Household Survey on Drug Abuse," NIDA Capsules, CAP 21 (Rockville, Md.: U.S. Department of Health and Human Services, Public Health Service, Alcohol, Drug Abuse, and Mental Health Administration, 1990).
16. *Marijuana and Health,* First Report to the U.S. Congress by the Secretary of Health, Education and Welfare (Washington, D.C.: U.S. Government Printing Office, 1979), p. 56.
17. Milan Korocock, "News Report Underlines Health Hazards," *Focus on Alcohol and Drug Issues: Marijuana Update,* September/October 1982, p. 4. See also National Commission on Marijuana and Drug Abuse, *Marijuana.*
18. Gabriel G. Nahas, "Cannabis: Toxicological Properties and Epidemiological Aspects," *Medical Journal of Australia* 145 (July 21, 1986):82.
19. Quoted in Peggy Mann, *Marijuana Alert: The Health Hazards* (New York: McGraw-Hill, 1985), p. 97.
20. Ibid.
21. Cited in Janny Scott, "Pot Takes a Hit on Health Damage," *Los Angeles Times,* February 11, 1988, p. 14.

22. Ibid.

23. Ibid.

24. Ibid.

25. Horocock, "News Report Underlines Health Hazards," p. 4.

26. Quoted in Norman E. Zinberg, "The War over Marijuana," *Psychology Today* 10, no. 7 (December 1976):102. Reprinted from *Psychology Today Magazine.* Copyright © 1976 American Psychological Association (APA).

27. Zinberg, "The War over Marijuana," p. 102.

28. Hymes, "Marijuana Update," pp. 18–21.

29. David R. Compton, William L. Dewey, and Billy R. Martin, "Cannabis Dependence and Tolerance Production," *Advances in Alcohol and Substance Abuse* 9, No. 1–2, (1990):129–45.

30. *Marijuana and Health,* Ninth Report to the U.S. Congress by the Secretary of Health and Human Services (Rockville, Md.: National Institute on Drug Abuse, 1982).

31. Ibid., p. 20.

32. R. L. Henderson, F. S. Tennant, and R. Guerny, "Respiratory Manifestations of Hashish Smoking," *Archives of Otolaryngology* 95 (March 1972):248; Sidney Cohen, "Marijuana: A New Ball Game?" *Drug Abuse and Alcoholism Newsletter* 8, no. 4 (May 1979).

33. S. Cohen et al., "A 94-Day Cannabis Study," in *Pharmacology of Marijuana,* ed. M. C. Braude and S. Szara (New York: Raven Press, 1976), p. 621.

34. Sidney Cohen, "Marijuana: Pulmonary Issues," *Drug Abuse Newsletter* 9, (January 1980).

35. Peter Bridge, "Lungs Hit Harder by Pot Than by Cigarettes," *Science News* 136 (November 18, 1989):332.

36. "Marijuana: Rough Stuff," *Harvard Medical School Health Letter* 14 (November 1988):4–5.

37. Ibid.

38. William Steele, "The Downside of Smoking Tobacco and Marijuana," *Current Health* 2 16, no. 6 (November 1989):24–26.

39. Editors, "Lungs Hit Harder by Pot Than by Cigarettes," *Science News* 133, no. 8 (February 20, 1988):120.

40. Quoted in Doyle, "Marijuana and the Lungs," p. 4.

41. Zinberg, "The War over Marijuana"; Cohen et al., "A 94-Day Cannabis Study."

42. Cited in R. Prakash et al., "Effects of Marijuana and Placebo Marijuana on Hemodynamics in Coronary Disease," *Clinical Pharmacology of Therapeutics* 18, no. 1 (July 1975):94.

43. "The Medical View," *Time* 113, no. 5 (January 29, 1979):27. Reprinted by permission from *Time, The Weekly Newsmagazine;* copyright Time Inc. 1979.

44. Ibid.

45. Institute on Medicine, *Marijuana and Health* (Washington, D.C.: National Academic Press, 1982), pp. 50–52.

46. A Sulkowski and L. Vachon, "Side Effects of Simultaneous Alcohol and Marijuana Use," *American Journal of Psychiatry* 134, no. 6 (June 1977):691.

47. Institute on Medicine, *Marijuana and Health,* pp. 50–52.

48. Lori Olivenstein, "The Perils of Pot," *Discover,* June 1988, p. 18.

49. *Marijuana and Health,* Ninth Report, p. 18.

50. W. C. Hembree et al., "Marijuana Effect upon the Human Testis," *Clinical Research* 24, no. 3 (1976); C. N. Stefanis and M. R. Issidorides, "Cellular Effects of Chronic Cannabis Use in Man," in *Marijuana: Chemistry, Biochemistry and Cellular Effects,* ed. G. G. Nahas (New York: Springer-Verlag, 1976).

51. Cited in Nahas, "Cannabis," pp. 158–59.

52. Cited in ibid.

53. Gallagher, "Marijuana," pp. 93–104.

54. Barry M. Lester and Melanie Dreher, "Effects of Marijuana Use during Pregnancy on Newborn Cry," *Child Development* 60 (1989):765–70.

55. B. Zuckerman, "Effects of Maternal Marijuana and Cocaine Use on Fetal Growth," *New England Journal of Medicine* 320 (March 23, 1989):762–68.

56. *Marijuana and Health,* First Report, p. 18.

57. "Cannabis and Driving Skills," *Canadian Medical Association Journal* 107 (August 19, 1978):269–70.

58. National Institute of Mental Health, *Marijuana* (Washington, D.C.: U.S. Government Printing Office, 1983).

59. Dale H. Gieringer, "Marijuana, Driving, and Accident Safety," *Journal of Psychoactive Drugs* 20 (January/March 1988).

60. Ibid.

61. *Marijuana and Health,* Ninth Report, p. 23.

62. Ibid.

63. Ibid., p. 2.

64. Institute on Medicine, *Marijuana and Health,* p. 3.

65. Nahas, "Cannabis," p. 82.

66. Mann, *Marijuana Alert,* pp. 184–85.

67. Ibid., p. 184.

68. Harold Kolansky and William T. Moore, "Toxic Effects of Chronic Marijuana Use," *Journal of the American Medical Association* 222, no. 1 (October 2, 1972):35–41.

69. Jerome A. Yesavage and Leirer Von Otto, "Carry-Over Effects of Marijuana Intoxication on Aircraft Pilot Performance: A Preliminary Report," *American Journal of Psychiatry* 142 (November 1985):1325–29.

70. R. Weiss, "Marijuana's Brain Receptors Mapped," *Science News,* November 26, 1988, p. 350.

71. Jean Marx, "Marijuana Receptor Gene Cloned," *Science* 249, no. 4969 (August 10, 1990):624–26.

72. William Steele, "The Downside of Smoking Tobacco and Marijuana," *Current Health* 16, no. 3, (November 1989):24–24.

73. Gallagher, "Marijuana."

74. Richard H. Schwartz, "Marijuana Mangles Memory," *Science News* 136, no. 22 (November 18, 1989):332.

75. "Marijuana Use and Memory Loss," *American Family Physician* 41, no. 3 (March 1990):930–31.

76. Ibid.

77. R. B. Miilman and R. Sbrislio, "Patterns of Use and Psychopathology in Chronic Marijuana Users," *Psychiatric Clinic North America* 3 (September 9, 1986):536.

78. Gallagher, "Marijuana."

79. Richard H. Schwartz, "Marijuana Mangles Memory," p. 332.

80. Ibid., p. 201.

81. M. Sheppard and A. Margaret, "Adolescents' Perceptions of Cannabis Use by Their Peers: Does It Have Anything to Do with Behavior?" *Journal of Drug Education* 19, no. 2 (1989):147–64.

82. Ibid.

83. Kay Porterfield, "Grass Gets an F," *Current Health* 15, no. 5 (January 1989):20–23.

84. Ibid.

85. R. Myerscough and S. Taylor, "The Effects of Marijuana on Human Physical Aggression," *Journal of Personality and Social Psychology,* 49 (December 1985):1541–46.

86. Stephen T. Higgins and Maxine L. Stitzer, "Acute Effects of Marijuana on Social Conversation," *Psychopharmacology* 89, no. 2 (January 1986): 234–38.

87. John D. Hundleby and William G. Mercer, "Family and Friends as Social Environments and Their Relationship to Young Adolescents' Use of Alcohol, Tobacco, and Marijuana," *Journal of Marriage and the Family* 49 (February 1987):151–64.

88. J. A. Hilikas, "Marijuana Use and Psychiatric Illness," in *Marijuana,* ed. Miller; R. E. Meyer, "Psychiatric Consequences of Marijuana Use: The State of the Evidence," *Marijuana and Health Hazards: Methodologic Issues in Current Research,* ed. J. R. Tinklenberg (New York: Academic Press, 1975).

89. *Marijuana and Health,* Ninth Report, p. 27.

90. M. P. Naditch, P. C. Alker, and P. Joffe, "Individual Differences and Setting as Determinants of Acute Adverse Reactions to Psychoactive Drugs," *Journal of Nervous and Mental Disease* 284 (1971):792.

91. Schwartz, "Frequent Marijuana Use in Adolescence," p. 201.

92. *Marijuana and Health,* Ninth Report, p. 29.

93. Institute on Medicine, *Marijuana and Health,* p. 126.

94. M. D. Stanton, J. Mintz, and R. M. Franklin, "Drug Flashbacks, II: Some Additional Findings," *International Journal of the Addictions* 11, no. 1 (1976).

95. Norman E. Zinberg, "On Cannabis and Health," *Journal of Psychedelic Drugs* 11, no. 1–2 (January/June 1979):135.

96. Perry Bethesday, "Marijuana and Heroin by Prescription?" *Journal of the American Medical Association* 241, no. 4 (January 26, 1979):373–75.

97. Mann, *Marijuana Alert.*

98. Sidney Cohen, "Marijuana as Medicine," *Psychology Today* 11, no. 11 (April 1978):60.

99. Donald Sweet, "Marijuana for Drug-Induced Nausea and Vomiting," *Journal of the American Medical Association* 243, no. 12 (March 28, 1980):1265.

100. "Cancer Patients Turned On," *New Scientist* 96 (December 16, 1982):709.

101. Cited in Janny Scott "Researchers Suggest New Marijuana Hazard," *Oregonian* (Portland), February 1, 1988.

102. Mark A. Hofmann, "Marijuana Bigger Threat Than Cocaine," *Business Insurance,* September 30, 1990, pp. 71–72.

103. "Increasing U.S. Pot Crop," *Register-Guard* (Eugene, Oregon), January 8, 1985.

104. Richard Wolkomir and Joyce Wolkomir, "Drug Outlaws in Our National Forests," *Reader's Digest* 133, no. 798 (October 1988):193–200.

105. Ed Rosenthal, "A Bumper Crop of Hothouse Marijuana," *Newsweek,* August 15, 1988, p. 26.

106. Work Clemens et al., "The Greening of America: 80's Style," *U.S. News & World Report,* May 29, 1989.

107. Charles P. Wohlforth, "Off the Pot," *New Republic,* December 3, 1990, pp. 9–10.

108. Ibid.

109. Andrew Kupfer, "What to Do About Drugs," *Fortune,* June 20, 1988, p. 39.

110. Ibid.

OVER-THE-COUNTER DRUGS

What You Can Get Without a Prescription

INTRODUCTION

One of the traditions we have inherited from our ancestors is self-medication. The advertising industry has taken advantage of this tradition by promoting hundreds of thousands of drugs that can be purchased without prescription "over the counter." Cold and cough medications, vitamins, laxatives, analgesics, and an assortment of potions, ointments, and balms are big over-the-counter sellers, as are antihistamines, which are the most commonly used sedative-hypnotics.[1] Over-the-counter (OTC) drugs are readily obtained and are believed by consumers to be safe as well as helpful in the treatment of a disease or in the alleviation of some of its symptoms.

As many as 300,000 medicines have been estimated to be available for over-the-counter purchase. Reliable information on the efficiency and effectiveness of these drugs is crucial to the consumer. Most people fail to realize that many things they consume daily contain drugs. Due to the wide availability of OTC medicines many people forget that they are in fact drugs. We need to be cautious about what we are putting into our bodies and realize

A Wide Range of Over-The-
Counter Drugs
Source: Irene Springer

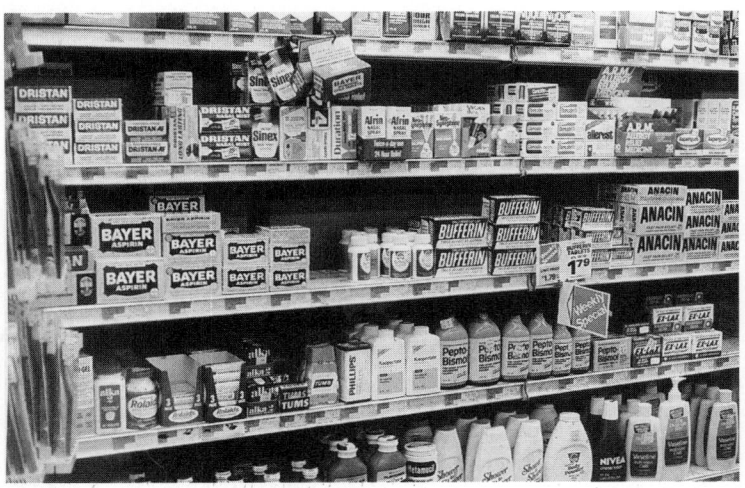

that adverse reactions might take place. Interactions may occur not only between two drugs but between a drug and something in our diet or the environment.[2]

The OTC drug business is a multibillion dollar industry that depends mainly on advertising for its income. In fact, it spends 20 to 40 percent of its income on advertising.[3] Because of the way these advertisements are presented, most people do not realize that OTC "medicines" can have adverse effects and even become addictive. In fact, it has been found that two thirds of OTC drugs are ineffective and can be unsafe.[4]

In the United States today, OTC drugs represent the largest drug market openly available to the consumer. What society does not understand is that we support the use of drugs through the sale of OTC remedies. Of course, most of the remedies do not contain enough of a drug to harm most individuals. Rather, the major problem is in the misuse and abuse of these drugs, either accidentally or purposefully. Since it has been found that noncompliance with prescriptions and with instructions from physicians is common, it is assumed that noncompliance with directions for OTC drugs also occurs.

Nonprescription drugs can be just as lethal as those our physician prescribes. They can aggravate existing conditions or even mask the symptoms of an underlying disease so that prompt corrective procedures by a physician are postponed. OTC drugs are capable of a variety of actions in our systems. "Within the last 30 years, many OTC drugs have assumed greater importance because of their ability to interact unfavorably with some widely used prescription drugs.[5]

SELF-MONITORING AND SELF-CARE

Part of an individual's responsibility in health care is appropriate self-medication. Surveys indicate that as many as 40 million Americans self-medicate with OTC drugs.[6] This can be a valuable alternative for individuals, for they can make their own decisions about their own symptoms and learn to take care of themselves. The options for health care, if the symptoms are not obviously serious, include the use of OTC drugs. Although self-medication is an important step in taking care of oneself, the role of the physician should not be excluded, especially in more serious illness. If misused, every type of OTC drug can become a potential problem. Some of the problems a person might encounter when using OTC drugs include improper choice of medication to treat illness, taking too large a dose, and in some cases, addiction.

Every year Americans spend about $15 billion on nonprescription drugs and $26 billion on prescription drugs.[7] It also appears that the public may not be well informed about taking drugs. People resort to **self-care** for minor ailments because it is an easy, convenient, relatively inexpensive alternative to medical consultation. They should realize, however, that medicine often doesn't take away symptoms but only covers them up. Self-care consumers seem to be at risk no matter which direction they turn.

Self-Care
Taking care of oneself in lieu of going to a physician.

Despite their popularity, OTC drugs can be hazardous if directions for their use are not followed and if improper self-diagnoses are made. In fact, it appears that many consumers are getting hooked on OTC drugs. Consumers need to be warned against relying too heavily on nasal sprays, laxatives, eye drops, stay-awake pills, sleeping pills, and codeine cough syrup.[8] The FDA enforces laws to protect consumers from danger, but consumers can best protect themselves by taking only the drugs they need, not overbuying or keeping drugs for long periods, not combining drugs carelessly, not continuing to use a drug if symptoms of illness persist, reading and following directions for use, and seeking professional advice before combining drugs.[9] To help consumers use products properly, manufacturers should list the common or generic names and the quantities of active ingredients, instructions for using the drug, and simple, direct warnings of possible side effects as well as limitations of the drug's effectiveness (many drugs are not effective except as placebos).

Because OTC drugs are sold in a competitive market, much depends on how they are advertised, as well as on how effectively they relieve symptoms. Advertisers appeal to consumers in every possible way—through emotions, faddism, bias, fear, envy, greed, even lust. Researcher Lois Debakey lists the following classic techniques that are used to promote over-the-counter drugs:

1. Bandwagon—Every mother I know buys brand X children's aspirin, so why don't you?

2. Testimonial—I drank antacid and I feel great; next time you need an antacid try the one I use.

3. The Down Home Approach—Standing by his barn Grandpa tells you about the analgesic he uses for his arthritis; if it's good enough for him, it's good enough for you.

4. The Authority Figure—A man in a white coat who looks like a doctor says he knows what is best and if you're smart you'll use what he suggests.[10]

Self-indulgence is another emotional appeal; it is coupled with the implication of instant relief and the idea that people should feel perfect every day. Announcement of a new scientific breakthrough is still another way advertisers try to win consumers.

DEVELOPMENT OF OTCs IN THE UNITED STATES

Patent medicines popular in England were imported to the American colonies soon after British migration to this country. The first American-patented medicine was Samuel Lee's "Bilious Pills," registered in 1796. Other medicines soon followed, many of which contained opiates. Alcohol, too, was a major constituent of patent drugs, often constituting 25 to 50 percent of the product.[11] Other ingredients found in these patent medicines included morphine, cocaine, caffeine, and belladonna.[12] Claims of the drugs' effectiveness were grossly overstated, and many advertisements stated that the medicines were cure-alls available from doctors, pharmacies, general grocery stores, and traveling shows and by mail.[13]

As pioneers moved westward, where doctors and pharmacists were in short supply, self-medication became a widespread method of health care. Early settlers had to rely on European folklore, Indian remedies using domestic plants, and the word of traveling entertainers. Patent medicines were an $80-million-a-year business by 1900.[14]

By the 1980s, the number of nonprescription preparations and the popularity of self-medication had increased greatly, but so had the incidence of adverse reactions. Though these drugs are more sophisticated than early patent medicines, they are still potentially dangerous, for several reasons:

1. Most have unclear label instructions.
2. Most contain several ingredients.
3. Many can be used for multiple symptoms.
4. The public considers them safe.
5. The public believes the government would never allow the sale of a dangerous product.[15]

FDA

The Federal Drug Administration, a government agency that oversees the production of over-the-counter drugs and prescription drugs to determine their safety and effectiveness.

There is a great deal of literature that reveals that many people may not attempt to read or follow the instructions on the bottles. The reason for this misuse of OTC products is that some may lack basic knowledge or reading skills to self-medicate safely.[16] Last year, more than 10,000 people died from using drugs such as pain relievers, cold pills, and diet pills that were purchased over-the-counter. These deaths occurred from misuse. The reason OTCs are available without prescriptions is that the **FDA** has determined them to be safe and effective—when used as directed. Recent studies have shown that many OTCs are simply not used as directed—and that their use can cause potentially dangerous results.[17]

REFORM

At the turn of the century, health hazards from patent medicines became a political issue. Outrage at the effects of adulterated foods eventually resulted in the passage of the 1906 Food and Drug Act, which affected OTC drugs by lowering their alcohol content to 17 percent and limiting opiates to prescription medicines. The act also divided drugs into proprietary (over-the-counter) drugs and ethical (prescription) drugs. It was intended to stop misleading advertising and consumer ignorance, but these problems remain a major concern today.

Since 1972 the FDA has had panels of nongovernmental experts reviewing more than 17 major classes of over-the-counter preparations. In 1984, after reviewing the 300,000 or so drug products marketed under various names, the advisory panels reported that only about one third of the ingredients were effective as well as safe for their intended use.[18] The remaining ingredients required additional proof if manufacturers were to be allowed to continue to market them. The report did not imply that only one third of all over-the-counter drug products contain ingredients that are safe and effective. Instead it meant that although many products contain ingredients that are safe, they may also have other ingredients whose safety has not yet been determined.

The panel recommendations are currently being incorporated into regulatory action, but already this review has allowed some new products to be sold over the counter to consumers (cortisone, fluoride rinses, new antihistamine and cold ingredients, and new nighttime sleeping aids). It has also quickly removed other ingredients that were deemed obvious hazards (Methapyrilene in sleep aids, hexachlorophene in soaps).

Earlier panel recommendations included placement of an ingredient into one of three categories. Category I contains ingredients considered safe and effective. Category II includes ingredients definitely shown to be unsafe or ineffective (panels have the power to recommend removal of any ingredient from the market that they consider dangerous). Category III is for ingredients that seem to need further testing. The pharmaceutical industry has supported such categorization and review, and on its own initiative has removed several proposed Category II ingredients from the market.

Procter and Gamble (P&G), one of the largest marketers of OTC drugs, is becoming bigger and more powerful than ever before.[19] In 1988 the company led domestic sales with $542 million and spent $652 million companywide to research and develop new products. Three well-known P&G products are NyQuil, Pepto-Bismol, and Metamucil. The interest of drug makers and consumer companies in such ventures reflects an increasing sense that the OTC side of the drug business will grow faster than prescription sales.[20]

WHAT SETS PRESCRIPTION AND NONPRESCRIPTION APART?

What sets prescription and nonprescription drugs apart, besides laws and availability, are the labels. Prescription drugs usually have serial numbers, name of dispenser, date, and patient's name. More information is available from the physician, but that is it.[21]

316

OVER-THE-COUNTER-DRUGS

Read the Labels on Over-The-Counter Drugs
Source: Steve Goldberg/Monkmeyer Press

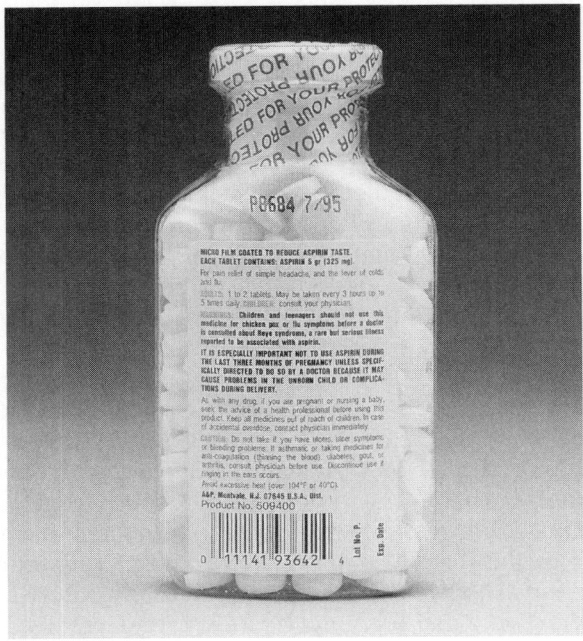

On the other hand, over-the-counter drug labels contain much more information. The FDA has restrictions requiring more information on OTC labels, due mainly to lack of contact between the pharmacist and the doctor. The following is a list of what should appear on an OTC product label.[22]

- Name and address of manufacturer and lot number.
- Name of product and type of drug.
- A statement of active ingredients.
- Declaration of dye Yellow No. 5. Many other inactive ingredients are voluntarily listed.
- Amount of product in container.
- Indications for use and symptoms.
- Directions for use and symptoms.
- Warnings or cautions. Some products may not be good for children, may cause drowsiness, and so on. Medicine taken internally must warn pregnant women to check with their doctors first. Another common warning is "Keep out of the reach of children"—even though adults are the only ones able to open the container.
- Drug interactions precautions—another abstract in this set focuses on interactions of drugs and food.
- Expiration date—not all will have one.

NOSTRUMS

A **nostrum** is a drug that is developed by an individual to help cure a disease or condition. In most cases the drug has not been tested and the claims are very suspect. Nostrums often proclaim they can prevent aging, for example. Americans spend about $2 billion a year on these nostrums.[23] Government regulators have lost track of all these new products, and they don't have the budget or the staff to investigate the claims. Federal laws also prohibit the government from policing the food-supplement industry. They can investigate only when the marketers make "specific health boasts."

Nostrum
A consumer product that is promoted by its maker. It may, or may not, be of any value.

SALICYLATES (ASPIRIN)

HISTORY

The modern history of salicylates began in 1852, when salicylic acid was first synthesized and found to have many useful properties. In 1874, Kalbe and Lauteman developed a procedure to produce the acid.[24] Its antiseptic properties enabled it to be used as a preservative to prevent milk and meat spoilage. During surgery it was used as an antiseptic and to treat infectious diseases.

Acetylsalicylic acid, commonly known as aspirin, was produced by the reaction of acetylchloride and sodium salicylate. For years it was an obscure chemical with no known therapeutic applications. Such therapeutic use was finally discovered in Germany when a man suffering from chronic rheumatoid arthritis approached his son, who was working with Bayer, to help find relief. Several different salicylate compounds were concocted, and finally acetylsalicylic acid proved successful. Salicylates were then used to treat a wide variety of diseases during the late nineteenth century.

It was not long, however, before the strong analgesic action of aspirin was recognized. Its greatest use soon became that of pain relief, particularly muscular pain and headache. Today it is the most popular of all drugs, both prescription and over-the-counter. Americans consume 16,000 tons of aspirin tablets a year, which equals 80 million pills, and spend about $2 billion a year for nonprescription pain killers, many of which contain aspirin drugs.[25]

PHYSICAL EFFECTS

Most scientists today will tell you that aspirin works by slowing down the production of chemicals called prostaglandins.[26] The 20 or so members of this chemical family are found in every tissue and regulate some of the body's most vital functions. When prostaglandins are produced in the wrong place, at the wrong time, or in too high amounts, however, the result can be fever, menstrual cramps—even a heart attack. Fortunately, aspirin seems to block the negative effects of prostaglandins without completely eliminating their positive effects. "Aspirin can subdue the part we can do without—pain, swelling, redness, and fever—without completely shutting down the body's defenses," says Saul Bloomfield, professor of internal medicine and pharmacology at the University of Cincinnati.[27]

When you cut your finger or skin your knee, prostaglandins help stop the bleeding by signaling tiny blood particles called platelets to clump together, plugging up the open blood vessel. But this same reaction can wreak havoc if clots form in the wrong places: In people with diseased blood vessels, that may lead to a heart attack or stroke (which involves the brain). By keeping the platelets from clumping in the first place, aspirin can prevent these disasters.[28] This theory has been borne out by several studies showing that people who have had a heart attack or a temporary loss of blood flow to the brain called TIA (transient ischemic attack) can cut their risk of having another by taking a daily dose of aspirin.

Salicylates are absorbed from the stomach and intestinal tract, then selectively distributed to the nervous system.[29] When they affect the hypothalamus, they reduce fever. When they affect certain sites in the upper spinal cord, they bring pain relief. Salicylates also block production of pain-producing plasma particles, causing further pain relief. As the chemicals move through the system, they dilate blood vessels, causing mild heat loss and sweating as well as a reduction in blood pressure.

Respiration is not normally affected by therapeutic doses (300 milligrams to one gram). Larger doses, however, are capable of stimulating brain respiratory-control centers, resulting in hyperventilating and excessive levels of oxygen and carbon dioxide in the body. If high dosages are continued over prolonged periods, severe potassium depletion may result, leading to general fatigue and dizziness.[30]

Long-term salicylate use can also produce serious gastric disturbances. Irritation of the protective mucosal stomach lining and mild to severe abdominal bleeding are often associated with prolonged salicylate therapy.[31] Since aspirin can also decrease blood coagulability, its use can also aggravate existing abdominal bleeding.

Intoxication from salicylates may be mild or severe, depending on the dosage. Mild intoxication, termed salicylism, is characterized by tinnitus (ringing in the ears), dizziness, headache, and disorientation. Severe intoxication produces marked mental confusion and gastric irritation, and internal tissue bleeding may be noted. Toxic doses—approximately 20 grams—produce changes in the body's acid-base balance, shifting the pH of body fluids. Death from overdose is possible, especially for children five and younger. Approximately 15 percent of all childhood poisoning deaths are aspirin-related.

Some individuals experience adverse responses to even small doses of salicylates. Some users fall victim to severe allergic shock reactions to the drugs, as well as severe asthma attacks if they are particularly hypersensitive. For these individuals, aspirin substitutes such as acetaminophen are advised.

SIDE EFFECTS

Extensive use of aspirin can cause numerous side effects. These may include gastrointestinal bleeding, nausea, vomiting, activation of peptic ulcer, bone-marrow depression, hepatitis with jaundice, and eventually kidney damage. When aspirin interacts with other drugs, such as alcohol, Vitamin C, some diuretics, antidiabetic drugs, insulin, or penicillin, it can increase or decrease their effectiveness, and in combination with some of them it can cause toxicity and increased stomach sensitivity.

It should be stressed that thousands of Americans are hospitalized for adverse drug reactions every year and many die. One of the most dangerous drugs is the OTC drug aspirin.[32] Aspirin and ibuprofen take away pain and inflammation by blocking the action of prostaglandins, which help maintain a protective mucous lining in the stomach. Therefore, twenty percent of users of these drugs develop severe gastric ulcers, and an estimated 10,000 die from hemorrhages each year.[33] The same drugs can harm or kill people who are dehydrated from vomiting or diarrhea, or whose blood flow is diminished by age or by other medications. The FDA is requiring that labeling of all oral and rectal OTC aspirin-containing products carry a warning that the product should not be used by women in the last trimester of pregnancy unless directed by a physician. To bring the consumer's attention to the new warning, it must be in bold print as follows:[34]

IT IS ESPECIALLY IMPORTANT NOT TO USE [ASPIRIN OR CABASPIRIN CALCIUM, AS APPROPRIATE] DURING THE LAST 3 MONTHS OF PREGNANCY UNLESS SPECIFICALLY DIRECTED TO DO SO BY A DOCTOR BECAUSE IT MAY CAUSE PROBLEMS IN THE UNBORN CHILD OR COMPLICATIONS DURING DELIVERY.

The new warning is in addition to an already required general pregnancy-nursing warning that states, "As with any drug, if you are pregnant or nursing a baby, seek the advice of a health professional before using this product."

THERAPEUTIC EFFECTIVENESS

Aspirin is recommended for four therapeutic uses: (1) as an analgesic, to relieve mild to moderate nonspecific pain; (2) as an antipyretic, to reduce fevers of over 101°F (though this may mask the need for more elaborate treatment); (3) as an antiinflammatory agent, to reduce inflammation in arthritis and other inflammatory conditions; and (4) to decrease platelet aggregation—that is, to keep platelets from adhering and clotting. Aspirin's effectiveness in these four areas has been applied to many diseases, but the drug is particularly useful in relieving the effects of rheumatoid arthritis. It may also prove to be critical in preventing heart attacks.

Rheumatoid Arthritis   Most doctors agree that the salicylates, particularly aspirin, are effective in relieving arthritis. A member of the American Rheumatic Association states that "either in the form of aspirin or sodium salicylate, the salicylates are the most useful drugs in the treatment of rheumatoid arthritis, and in a considerable proportion of patients, aspirin is the only drug needed.[35] The most effective dose is approximately 7 to 10 grams per day, unless side effects necessitate a dose reduction. Aspirin's antiinflammatory action is the main reason aspirin is used to treat arthritis, a disease in which joints become inflamed. Aspirin also successfully treats other effects of arthritis, however, relieving pain, reducing morning stiffness, and lessening swelling and immobility.

Heart Attacks and Strokes   Though the value of using aspirin to prevent heart attacks has not been completely determined, aspirin is known to hinder blood clotting.[36] In 1974 a British study found that out of 600 heart-attack patients who ingested one aspirin daily, 25 percent had fewer subsequent heart attacks than those who took placebos.[37] A study by the Boston Collaborative Drug Surveillance program found that heart attack was half as common to regular aspirin takers as it was to individuals who seldom took aspirin. It also concluded that first as well as recurrent nonfatal heart attacks were less likely among regular aspirin takers. The study warned, however, that evidence "fell short of establishing that ASA [aspirin] prevents heart attacks.[38]

By 1978 aspirin was known to be effective in preventing strokes. This knowledge prompted its use in the treatment of atherosclerosis, a narrowing of the blood vessels that can lead to myocardial infarctions. The exact dose needed to prevent heart attacks is still uncertain, but an extensive myocardial-infarction study nonetheless recommended routine aspirin use for the prevention of myocardial infarctions.

What concerns physicians most, however, is the remote possibility that aspirin's anticlotting action can cause internal bleeding. In fact, the Public Health Service showed a slight increase in the number of brain hemorrhages (a kind of stroke) among aspirin takers.[39] Ironically, an aspirin may be helpful to those who have had a stroke. A study done in March 1988 showed that stroke patients who took aspirin recovered lost mental capabilities by 17 percent to 21 percent a year, while those untreated got progressively worse.[40] This occurs because aspirin interferes with the process in which blood platelets form together to cause a clot. A recent study showed that aspirin can prevent strokes in people who have never had a stroke before.[41] While taking an aspirin a day or a clot-retarding drug called warfarin for a little more than a year, 716 stroke-prone men and women had 81 percent fewer strokes than the 528 who had previously tried taking a placebo. More research is needed to learn if aspirin's anticoagulant (agent that stops clots) may actually reduce further strokes in individuals who have had strokes or have atherosclerosis.

Other recent studies have also indicated that aspirin is of value in the treatment of coronary disease. The Public Health Service investigated the effect of aspirin on cardiovascular disease in 22,000 male U.S. physicians ages 40 to 84.[42] The physicians were randomly assigned to receive one of four treatments: (1) buffered aspirin and beta carotene, a vitamin A precursor (50 milligrams); (2) buffered aspirin and beta carotene placebo; (3) aspirin placebo and beta carotene, and (4) aspirin placebo and beta carotene placebo. The participants were given their allotted treatment in the form of one pill every other day. After about 4.8 years of follow-up, it was found that the incidence of myocardial infarction among those physicians taking the active aspirin was reduced by nearly half. Interestingly, strokes were slightly more numerous among aspirin takers. The effects of beta carotene on cardiovascular disease have not yet been determined.

Should aspirin be used therapeutically to prevent myocardial infarction? The answer is not always. Because participation in the study was confined to physicians who had no history of myocardial infarction, stroke, local anemia, or local diminution in the blood supply, the study was limited. Furthermore, those men with liver or renal disease, gout, or peptic ulcer were excluded along with those who could not tolerate aspirin. Therefore, prescribing aspirin to the general population as a method of reducing the risk of cardiovascular disease is still premature.

TOXICOLOGY

Though aspirin appears to rank as one of the safest drugs used today, it can cause gastric hemorrhage, bronchial asthma, and mild bleeding. These adverse reactions can be serious and even fatal, and some consumers feel that all medications that contain aspirin should be available only by prescription. Efforts have been made to have warning labels placed on containers of aspirin medications. The childproof top is another attempt to prevent adverse reactions.

Reye's Syndrome   The Food and Drug Administration warns that children who have chicken pox, flu, or late-winter flulike symptoms should not be given aspirin. A high percentage of children who suffer or die from a rare liver disorder known as **Reye's syndrome** turn out to have been treated with aspirin for chicken pox or flu symptoms.[43] Whether or how aspirin enhances this risk is not currently known, but acetaminophen does not have this risk.

Reye's Syndrome
A rare liver disease associated with taking aspirin while having chicken pox or flu. It is most common in children.

Gastrointestinal Bleeding   Aspirin seems to have an affinity for the stomach. It accumulates there after oral dosages and increases gastric salicylate levels following intravenous infusion.[44] As we have noted, aspirin is believed to have an effect on the protective mucous lining of the stomach,[45] and "ingestion of aspirin, in doses of 1 to 3 g. day [3 to 12 tablets], will induce acute gastrointestinal bleeding in about 70 percent of normal individuals."[46] Such bleeding can result in iron-deficiency anemia and, more seriously, massive gastric hemorrhage. Hemorrhage is especially possible in aspirin takers suffering from peptic ulcers.

Bleeding Tendency   In relatively high doses—3 grams (about 12 tablets) or more per day for a week—aspirin prevents clotting.[47] Even the ingestion of a single dose of 0.3 to 1.2 grams prolongs clotting time by several minutes in normal persons and to a much greater degree in people with bleeding disorders. The tendency to bleed may last for four to seven days, and though this would normally be of little significance, during surgery it could produce serious complications. Aspirin should therefore be avoided prior to surgery, especially by people with bleeding disorders.

Hypersensitivity Reactions   Hypersensitivity (allergic) reactions to salicylates are commonly manifested as skin eruptions, edema, and asthma. The symptoms are generally characterized either by sudden weakness, sweating, fainting, and collapse, as in an asthmatic attack, or by an acute rash. One study estimated that approximately 1 in 500 people is sensitive to aspirin, and that only a small percentage of these experience severe reactions.[48] Fatalities have occurred, however, after the ingestion of only a small dose of aspirin.

Asthma is the allergic reaction to aspirin that has received the most attention. "In a review of drug sensitivity [it was] found that 19 drugs or groups of drugs may precipitate asthma. Of these, aspirin is the only one to do so.[49] Despite these findings, it appears that aspirin is rarely the sole cause of asthmatic attack.

Migraine Headaches   Research indicates that one aspirin tablet taken every other day cuts the risk of migraine headaches.[50] Aspirin, which reduces clumping of key bloodclotting components called platelets, might help block the debilitating and poorly understood series of events that produce migraine symptoms. About 18 million people in the United States suffer these painful attacks, which may begin with a period of tiredness followed by nausea, visual hallucinations, and gripping pain that can last for hours. Although migraine symptoms are well known, their cause remains a mystery. Researchers believe that migraines start when platelets clump together and release a neurotransmitter called serotonin. The serotonin causes arteries in the brain to constrict and dilate, initiating a sequence that seems to produce migraine symptoms.[51]

ASPIRIN: THE MIRACLE DRUG

Recent research shows that aspirin can do a lot more than just kill pain. Many health professionals and scientists say they think aspirin could help combat AIDS and cancer because of its effect on the immune system.[52] Aspirin boosts the body's production of interferon and interleukin-2, both of which are important parts of the body's immune system. The National Institutes of Health is sponsoring 35 studies of aspirin's therapeutic role in conditions ranging from hearing loss to allergies.[53] In 1987, researchers at Rush Presbyterian St. Luke's Medical Center in Chicago tested a chemical cousin of aspirin on patients with Kaposi's sarcoma.

Aspirin might be effective in treating eye disease. In 1986 researchers in England found that aspirin and other analgesics could halve the risk of cataracts.[54] The National Institutes of Health is studying whether aspirin can treat retinopathy, a condition where blood-vessel walls thicken to restrict the blood supply to the retina.

Studies have also shown that aspirin can reduce eclampsia (high blood pressure late in pregnancy). Eclampsia can lead to miscarriage or birth defects.[55]

ACETAMINOPHEN

For people who cannot take aspirin, acetaminophen is an acceptable substitute. The drug is marketed in the United States under approximately 50 brand names—Tylenol, Datril, Liquiprin, and others. Acetaminophen is effective in reducing fever and decreasing pain, and it does not produce gastric irritation or intestinal bleeding or appear to have any effect on platelet formation.[56] Despite this benign appearance, the drug can still cause serious liver damage and even death if an overdose is taken.[57] Symptoms of an overdose may include nausea, vomiting, diarrhea, abdominal pain, and drowsiness.

Is acetaminophen better than acetylsalicylic acid? Despite the claims made by advertising agencies, both drugs are very good pain relievers. Aspirin is less expensive,[58] but for patients with gout, patients taking anticoagulants, pregnant women, and persons with allergies to aspirin or asthma, acetaminophen is the better choice. For those who need an antiinflammatory medicine, however, aspirin is the better choice, since it is much more effective in reducing inflammation.

Acetaminophen accounts for about 37 percent of the nation's $2.5-billion annual over-the-counter sales of pain pills. Aspirin represents 43 percent and ibuprofen 29 percent.[59] Aspirin, acetaminophen, and ibuprofen are the only important ingredients in over-the-counter pain relievers. Aspirin and ibuprofen interfere with prostaglandins, which stimulate pain nerves and cause inflammation.[60] But prostaglandins also help rebuild torn tissues. So these drugs are good for pain and some muscles but may slow the healing process. Acetaminophen also interferes with pain-causing chemicals but has no effect on inflammation. It is good for dental pain or menstrual cramps. All three reduce fever.

IBUPROFEN

Some people who are allergic to aspirin are also allergic to **ibuprofen** (Advil, Nuprin, Motrin) though they may not know it. Ibuprofen can cause fluid retention and swelling, gastrointestinal bleeding, and kidney disorders. Its use can also be harmful to those with high blood pressure.[61] Unlike aspirin, however, an overdose is rarely fatal. Clinical studies show that ulcers and possibly perforation occur in 1 percent of patients who take a prescription dosage (1600 milligrams) of ibuprofen daily for three to six months and in 2 to 4 percent of these treated for one year.[62]

Opthalmologists have reported that some of their female patients have reported visual disturbances after taking ibuprofen for migraine headaches.[63] The vision improved after the patients stopped using ibuprofen. Overall, visual disturbances associated with ibuprofen are considered rare.

Available without a prescription since 1985, ibuprofen has captured about 20 percent of the $2.5-billion nonprescription–pain-reliever market. As the prescription drug Motrin, it has annual sales of $46 million.[64]

Ibuprofen
An OTC medication that acts similarly to aspirin in that it blocks prostaglandin effects; however, it does not cause stomach upset or gastric ulcers.

LAXATIVES*

INTRODUCTION

There is a durable attitude, spanning many centuries and many cultures, that associates excrement with evil and its elimination with the expiation of guilt. The practical result is that most people of our society still regard even transitory constipation as something to be directly and promptly treated with a laxative.[65]

Today, advertisements constantly state that for good health and well-being we should be "regular" in our bowel movements. Irregularity (constipation), aftermeal discomfort, and headaches will disappear if we just take a laxative. To help us on our way, over 700 proprietary drugs that promote defecation are manufactured and made available each year. Over $200 million are spent on these nonprescription laxatives and other elimination aids, and between 15 and 30 percent of people over 60 take more than one laxative dose per week.[66]

Millions of people are "laxative junkies" with the most habit-forming laxatives containing phenophale.[67] The laxatives work by irritating the lining of the intestines, which in turn irritates the nerves that cause the muscle to contract. People who use laxatives for a prolonged period of time develop a sluggish colon. Eventually paralysis can occur in the intestine, which, ironically, leads to further constipation problems. A common addiction, especially with older patients, is laxatives.[68] The muscle tone in their gastrointestinal tract decreases with age, so unless they add bulk to their diet, they are prone to constipation.

Constipation

A condition in which the feces become hard and dry because fluid is not absorbed quickly enough to produce softer stools.

It is usually recommended that people experiencing **constipation** try exercising, drinking water, eating a diet with roughage, eating breakfast, and responding as quickly as possible when they have a natural urge to defecate. Reduction of stress also is helpful for some individuals.

Despite its popularity, taking a laxative is rarely appropriate for children and only occasionally appropriate for adults. It is not true that daily defecation is necessary for good health. Many people in perfect health have bowel movements every two to three days or longer without ill effect.[69] Supposed constipation may simply be slow movement of feces through the large intestine—slow but perfectly adequate for the system. A panel of scientists who reviewed OTC laxative products for the FDA stated that "there is widespread overuse of self-prescribed laxatives. . . . The Panel is concerned because many people are using laxatives that don't need them."[70]

This overuse can be dangerous. Continued unnecessary doses can lead to dependence on laxatives for normal bowel movements, a need for strong medication, or a malfunctioning of the gastrointestinal tract. If a laxative is

---

*Though drugs that cause evacuations of the intestine (bowel movements) are generally referred to as laxatives, cathartics and purgatives are often incorrectly included in this category. A laxative causes increased peristalsis (wavelike contractions of the intestine) by increasing or decreasing the water content of fecal matter, producing a soft, well-formed stool. A cathartic, on the other hand, causes a more drastic fluid evacuation and is almost always associated with increased motor activity in the intestines. A purgative is a more energetic agent than a cathartic or a laxative.[71] Despite these differences, and for purposes of simplicity and consistency, only the term *laxative* will be used in this text.

taken to relieve abdominal pain, cramps, nausea, or vomiting, the intestinal activity the laxative produces can cause further irritation. Laxatives can also rupture an inflamed appendix, greatly increasing the risk of serious illness.[72]

LAXATIVE USE

Constipation will generally alleviate itself if it isn't perpetuated with continual laxative use. Before resorting to chemical relief for constipation, people should be aware of the range of normal bowel function; respond to the need to defecate when it is first felt; add fiber to their diet; resist hurrying breakfast; exercise; and have patience. If a laxative is truly needed, a doctor or pharmacist should be consulted, because evidence suggests that individuals purchasing proprietary laxatives do not receive proper counsel concerning the merits and toxicity of these products. "There is no class of nonprescription drugs in which professional guidance is needed more than with the use of laxatives."[73]

COUGH RELIEVERS (ANTITUSSIVES)

Almost half of all Americans say they bought nonprescription drugs to relieve their aches, pains, or sniffles in the last six months.[74] In 1988 there were expenditures of $1.6 billion on cold medications, cough drops and syrups, nasal decongestants, and sore-throat remedies. With no cure yet for the common cold, people see little sense in spending time and money on a doctor's visit when promised relief is as close as the nearest supermarket. Most cold sufferers merely seek something they hope will help get them through the day or let them sleep through the night. The pharmaceutical industry has filled store shelves with as many as 250 cough and cold remedies.[75] About 36 major brands of cough and cold medications are on the market already, with as many as six varieties per brand, and drug firms constantly plan new offerings for winter, when sales peak.

THE COUGH

A cough can be defined as a sudden expulsion of air from the lungs. In the clinical sense it is a form of protection because it is an automatic attempt to release foreign matter from the esophagus. Coughs can result from a number of causes, ranging from irritation to pulmonary fibrosis.

REDUCING THE SEVERITY

Effective antitussives reduce the severity of a cough several ways. First, they depress the medullary center. Second, they tend to block impulse transmission in the nervous system. Third, they interfere with the impulses of the cough reflex. Fourth, they remove irritants by facilitating bronchial drainage.

Cough syrups contain either an expectorant or an antitussive; however, the FDA has found most expectorants are ineffective.[76] So researchers recommend using only a single-ingredient antitussive. The only antitussives classified as both safe and effective by the FDA are destromethorphan and codeine.[77] Experts suggest using antihistamines that contain either chlorophreniramine or brompheiramine, as these cause less sedation. Antihistamines are not effective for colds, and those with asthma should not use OTC antihistamines. Experts are continually saying that the first rule of the use of any drug is that more is not necessarily better. In fact, more can be dangerous. People with pulmonary obstructive problems, such as asthma, are recommended to stay away from these OTCs.

Codeine is the most effective opiate for reducing the severity of a cough. It can lead to tolerance and physical dependency, but in small doses it is rated high as an antitussive because it is rapidly absorbed following administration. Effects are generally felt 15 to 30 minutes after use, and relief is maintained for between four and six hours. Codeine combined with aspirin appears to be the most effective antitussant, but choosing the best product from the 50,000 nonprescription items now marketed for coughs, colds, allergies, and bronchial conditions can be complicated.

For those who don't wish to use codeine, a number of nonopiate substitutes are available. The most commonly used is most likely dextromethorphan, because it is as potent as codeine but does not produce dependency. Such nonnarcotic antitussives also do not lead to significant abuse problems, which codeine preparations can.

ANTIHISTAMINES

In 1910 a naturally occurring hormone named histamine was discovered. The hormone was found to release valuable antibodies that attack various bacteria, viruses, chemicals, and antigens (foreign bodies). Though this pharmacological action was both remarkable and necessary for protecting the body from disease, it was often found to result in vasodilation and blood vessel permeability; increased secretions that cause sneezing, runny nose and eyes, congestion, and itching; nausea; and changes in various smooth muscles, glands, and connective tissue.[78] To combat these side effects, **antihistamines** were developed; they offered relief by temporarily reducing histamine release.*

Antihistamines are most commonly found in "cold," "allergy," or "hay fever" preparations, since pollen, dust, bee stings, and enzymes are notable promoters of histamine release. They are also employed in tranquilizers, decongestants, antitussives, anticonvulsants, local anesthetics, and antinausea and motion-sickness medicines,[79] because their action can relieve sinus congestion, itching, nausea, insomnia, and restlessness and can reduce skin eruptions.

Not all antihistamine effects are beneficial, however. Side effects include drowsiness; a sense of weakness; dryness of the nose, mouth, and throat; and constipation. Rare, adverse reactions, which indicate the drug is not working properly and for which a physician should be quickly consulted, include allergic reactions (hives, itching), headaches, dizziness, inability to concen-

Antihistamines

Combat the effects of the naturally occurring hormone named histamine, which helps protect the body by increasing secretions that cause sneezing, running nose and eyes, congestion, itching, and nausea. Antihistamines offer relief by temporarily reducing histamine release.

*In 1947 a pregnant woman attending the Johns Hopkins allergy clinic was given a new drug to control her hives. It so happened that she suffered from car sickness as well. When reporting to the clinic the following week, she mentioned that not only had the new medicine taken care of her hives, it had also prevented her usual sickness when she traveled in the streetcar. Stimulated by this observation, Leslie N. Gay, chief of the clinic's allergy department, and Paul E. Carliner sought other victims of motion sickness to test the new drug. Later, when the drug proved itself, it was given the name Dramamine.

trate, nervousness, blurred or double vision, and difficulty urinating. A physician should also be consulted if a person develops signs of nausea or vomiting; severe behavioral disturbances such as confusion, excitement, or delirium; or any unusual bleeding or bruising.

Although antihistamines alone can be obtained only with a prescription, when combined in low dosages with other drugs they are available over the counter. Because they often cause drowsiness, all products containing them must have a warning label to that effect.[80] Antihistamines should not be taken by individuals who need to be alert; are hypertensive; have severely dry mucous membranes; are taking certain other drugs, particularly depressants; or are pregnant.[81]

VITAMINS AND MINERALS

INTRODUCTION

Vitamins are organic compounds necessary in small amounts for normal growth and maintenance of life. They transform foods into energy, but do not provide energy or build or maintain body parts. There are 13 or more of them, occurring naturally in foods and synthetically in vitamin preparations.

The vitamins and minerals sold over-the-counter in the United States are a billion-dollar business.[82] Though a well-balanced diet will usually meet all the body's vitamin needs (see Table 12–1), anyone who feels the need for vitamins or minerals can get them in drugstores, supermarkets, and health-food stores; from door-to-door salespeople; or through the mail. Despite their popularity, some vitamins and minerals may be dangerous if taken by the wrong people or in excessive dosages.

Vitamin and mineral products are sold in the United States with one of two labels: dietary supplement (intended to increase total dietary intake of one or more essential vitamins or minerals) and nonprescription drug (sold to prevent or treat a specific vitamin or mineral deficiency, such as one resulting from pregnancy, nursing, alcoholism, or intestinal disease).

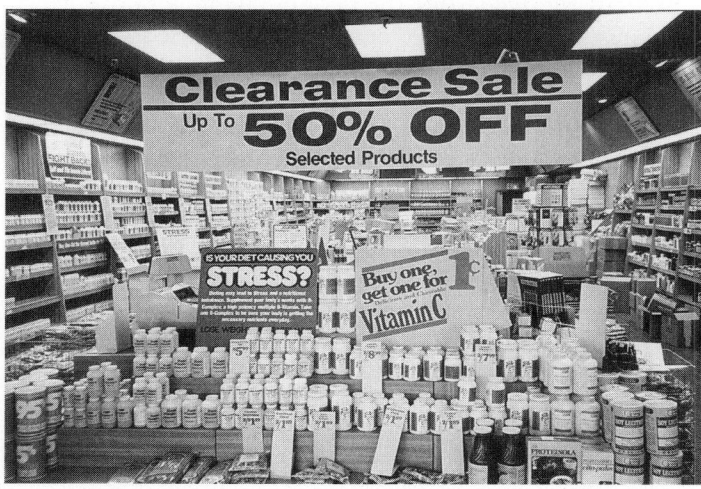

Is There Too Much Emphasis on Taking Vitamins?
Source: Mike Mazzachi/ Stock Boston

TABLE 12-1   U.S. RECOMMENDED DAILY ALLOWANCES OF VITAMINS

	Unit	Infants (0–12 months)	Children under 4 Years	Adults and Children 4 or more Years	Pregnant or Lactating Women
*Vitamin A	IU	1,500	2,500	5,000	8,000
*Vitamin D	IU	400	400	400	400
*Vitamin E	IU	5	10	30	30
Vitamin C	mg	35	40	60	60
Folacin (folic acid)	mg	0.1	0.2	0.4	0.8
Thiamine (B$_1$)	mg	0.5	0.7	1.5	1.7
Riboflavin (B$_2$)	mg	0.6	0.8	1.7	2.0
Niacin	mg	8	9	20	20
Vitamin B$_6$	mg	0.4	0.7	2	2.5
Vitamin B$_{12}$	mcg	2	3	6	8
Biotin	mg	0.05	0.15	0.3	0.3
Pantothenic acid	mg	3	5	10	10

IU = international unit
mg = milligram
mcg = microgram

*Fat-soluble vitamins.
Source: FDA Consumer (Washington, D.C.: U.S.Government Printing Office, April 1979).

A nongovernmental panel created by the FDA has evaluated the safety and effectiveness of all over-the-counter vitamin and mineral products sold as drugs. According to the panel, only nine vitamins and three minerals are safe and effective as over-the-counter drugs. The nine vitamins are C, B$_{12}$, folic acid, niacin, B$_6$, riboflavin, thiamine, A, and D. The panel determined that biotin, choline, vitamin E, and pantothenic acid should not be sold as single-ingredient, nonprescription drugs because deficiencies of these vitamins are virtually nonexistent. The panel also felt that vitamin K should be available by prescription only, since it is particularly dangerous for people taking anticoagulants.

More than a hundred miscellaneous ingredients, including apricots, brewer's yeast, buckwheat, comfrey root, hesperidin, kelp, lecithin, malt extract, molasses, rose-hips powder, and wheat germ, some of which are natural sources of vitamins and minerals, were considered inappropriate by the panel for inclusion in vitamin-mineral preparations. Such ingredients were excluded because they do *not* contribute to the product's effectiveness to treat or cure deficiencies. Combination products were deemed appropriate, however, because conditions that cause deficiencies usually involve more than one nutrient. Combinations that include any of the approved vitamins or any of the approved vitamins plus approved minerals were classified safe and effective as over-the-counter drugs. Pantothenic acid and vitamin E, which should not be sold as single ingredients, can be included in vitamin-mineral combinations that do not contain any other fat-soluble vitamins.

As for minerals, the panel said that calcium, iron, and zinc are safe and effective for single-ingredient use. Copper, fluoride, iodine, magnesium, manganese, phosphorus, and potassium were deemed inappropriate for over-the-counter sales because deficiencies are rare and because some of these minerals can be dangerous in high doses. The panel also pointed out that there is no need for multimineral preparations. This recommendation was made because multiple-mineral deficiencies rarely occur as a result of one condition.

It is common knowledge that trace elements of vitamins and minerals can improve overall health as well as improve conditions like schizophrenia, Down's syndrome, and impotence. However, other evidence suggests that increasing vitamin requirements may do more than help sometimes.

Requirements for the Recommended Daily Allowance (RDA) were "based on data on elimination of diseases and avoidance of toxicity in large numbers of healthy people."[83] If taking vitamins on a daily basis, one should not surpass the maximum RDA for the particular vitamin or mineral.

Table 12–2 outlines some of the adverse effects of excessive vitamin and mineral intake.

TABLE 12–2   ADVERSE EFFECTS OF EXCESSIVE VITAMIN AND MINERAL INTAKE

Vitamins	Adverse Effects
Vitamin A	Teratogen (affect formation or bring forth of a condition), encephalopathy, pseudotumor (false tumor) cerebi, hyperkeratosis (hypertrophy of bone tissue), bone pain, hyperkeratosis
Vitamin B_1	Tachycardia (fast heartbeat), fatty liver
Riboflavin	Itching, uriticarea, paresthesias
Niacin	Flushing, hepatotoxicity (substance or poison in the liver), increased uric acid, cardiac arrhythmia
Vitamin B_6	Polyneuropathy (simultaneous involvement of several nerves) paresis
Folate	Masks Vitamin B_{12} deficiency
Vitamin C	Modifies drug and vitamin metabolism, diarrhea, renal stones
Vitamin D	Teratogen, hypercacemia, renal failure, metastic calcification in the brain
Vitamin E	Fatigue, headache, delayed wound healing, increased bleeding, muscle weakeness
Minerals	
Chromium	Respiratory disease (rare)
Cobalt	Bone marrow toxicity (rare), hyperplasia
Copper	Gastrointestinal and CNS toxicity
Fluoride	Fluorosis (absorbing toxic doses of fluoride, tooth and bone abnormalities)
Iodine	Hyperthyroidism, thyroid abnormalities
Iron	Acute: gastrointestinal bleeding, CNS toxicity; chronic: hemosiderois (iron-containing substance found in liver)
Manganese	CNS toxicity
Molybdenum	Gout
Selenium	CNS and renal toxicity, hair loss
Zinc	Cholesterol abnormalities, teratogen
Lithium	Interactions with minerals, teratogen

Source: American Family Physician 35 (March 1987): 282.

SPECIFIC USE

The nongovernmental panel found that many manufacturers listed unverifiable claims and did not post adequate warnings on their products. They felt labels should be reworded to state that preparations should be used only "when the need for such therapy has been determined by a physician." They also recommended that labels include specific doses to be taken, and that listings be required of all ingredients in these preparations.

The panel felt there are a number of claims that labels should not be allowed to make:

1. claims of special effectiveness, such as "high" or "super" potency

2. claims that a product is "natural," because there is no evidence that natural forms of vitamins and minerals are better than synthetic ones

3. claims that vitamin C is useful for treating such conditions as the common cold, atherosclerosis, allergy, mental illness, corneal ulcers, thrombosis, anemia, or pressure sores

4. claims that vitamin A is of value in treating warts on the bottom of the feet, acne or other skin diseases, dry and wrinkled skin, stress ulcers, respiratory infections, or eye disorders

5. claims that vitamin D is effective in lowering blood cholesterol levels or in preventing or curing osteoporosis in the elderly

6. claims that any preparation is especially effective in geriatric use

7. claims that folic-acid preparations can prevent folic-acid deficiency in women taking oral contraceptives

8. claims that vitamin B_6 is useful for preventing kidney stones or controlling vomiting in pregnant women

9. claims that vitamin B_1 (thiamine) helps stimulate mental response or is useful in treating skin disease, multiple sclerosis, infections, cancer, or impotence

Recommendations by the vitamin-mineral panel were received by the FDA as part of the agency's effort to review all nonprescription drugs. The recommendations and a proposed monograph or "recipe book" for vitamin-mineral preparations were published in the March 16, 1979, *Federal Register*. A final monograph was expected in 1986, and six months after its publication manufacturers who sell vitamin and mineral preparations as drugs must reformulate and relabel their products to comply with the monograph. If compliance is not achieved, products must be removed from the market.[84]

SPECIFIC VITAMINS

Vitamin A (Retinol)   Vitamin A is an oil-soluble vitamin that is stored in the liver. It is necessary for new cell growth and healthy tissues and is essential for seeing in dim light. Besides night blindness and other eye maladies, a vitamin A deficiency can cause dry, rough skin that may become more susceptible to infection.

Vitamin A is found in foods in two forms: as carotene, a yellow pigment in green and yellow vegetables and yellow fruits that the human body converts to vitamin A, and as vitamin A itself, found in animals who have formed it from carotene and store it in body tissues. Good sources of vitamin A are liver, eggs, and milk.

Large doses of vitamin A can cause increased pressure inside the skull. This pressure so mimics symptoms of a brain tumor that tumors have been suspected in several patients whom hospital personnel later discovered consumed high quantities of vitamin A. Carotene, on the other hand, is practically nontoxic.

VITAMIN A THERAPY FOR ORAL CANCER.   Chewing tobacco or dipping snuff may be "in" in certain groups, but it can also destroy the user's life through oral cancer. In recent years, researchers have begun testing vitamin A as a way to reduce the risk of oral cancer. Studies among chewers have found that vitamin A taken orally not only caused remission of precancerous areas but also prevented new lesions from forming.[85]

More recently, researchers found that taking 200,000 international units (IU) of vitamin A a week caused leukoplakia shrinkage in 12 of 21 study participants given the vitamin alone.[86] (The U.S. minimum daily allowance is 5,000 IU. Two hundred thousand IU a week may be toxic.) A smaller percentage showed remission after being treated with a combination of vitamin A and beta carotene, or with beta carotene alone. These prevented new leukoplakias from developing.[87]

Vitamin B_1 (Thiamine)   This vitamin is water-soluble, as are all vitamins in the B complex. It is required for normal digestion, growth, fertility, lactation, the normal functioning of nerve tissue, and carbohydrate metabolism. B_1 can be found in abundant quantities in pork, soybeans, beans, peas, nuts, and enriched and whole-grain breads and cereals.

A deficiency of vitamin B_1 can cause beriberi, a dysfunctioning of the nervous system. Other deficiency effects include loss of appetite, body swelling (edema), heart problems, nausea, vomiting, and spastic muscle contractions throughout the body.

Vitamin B_6 (Pyridoxine, Pyridoxal, Pyridoxamine)   Vitamin B_6 is necessary for the utilization of protein. It is found abundantly in liver, whole-grain cereals, potatoes, red meats, green vegetables, and yellow corn. Deficiency symptoms include mouth soreness, dizziness, nausea, weight loss, and severe nervous disturbances.

Vitamin B_{12} (Cyanocobalamin)   Vitamin B_{12} is necessary for the normal development of red blood cells, as well as the functioning of all cells, particularly in the bone marrow, nervous system, and intestines. Good sources of this vitamin are organ meats, lean meats, fish, milk, eggs, and shellfish. Since most vegetables do not contain any measurable amounts of B_{12} strict vegetarians should supplement their diets with this vitamin. A deficiency can cause pernicious anemia and, if the deficiency is prolonged, degeneration of the spinal cord.

Vitamin C (Ascorbic Acid)   This least stable of the vitamins promotes growth and tissue repair, including the healing of wounds. It also aids in tooth and bone formation and when used as a food additive acts as a preservative. Vitamin C can be found in turnip greens, green pepper, kale, broccoli, mustard greens, citrus fruits, strawberries, currants, tomatoes, and other vegetables. Just one 3-to-4 ounce serving of any of these foods will supply all your daily vitamin C needs.

Lack of vitamin C can cause one of the oldest diseases known to humans—scurvy. Signs of scurvy include lassitude, weakness, bleeding of the gums, loss of weight, irritability, and ease of bruising.

Vitamin D (Calciferol)   Vitamin D is necessary for bone formation: It aids in the absorption of calcium and phosphorus. To accomplish this work, the body—through the liver and kidneys—converts the vitamin to a hormone-like material.

Abundant sources of vitamin D include canned and fresh fish (particularly the saltwater varieties), egg yolk, and vitamin D–fortified foods such as milk and margarine. People who regularly expose their skin to the sun can get vitamin D that way, since it is formed in the skin by ultraviolet rays. The daily requirement is very small, and excess amounts are stored in the body.

Too much vitamin D can cause nausea, weight loss, weakness, excessive urination, and the more serious conditions of hypertension and calcification of soft tissue, including the blood vessels and kidneys. Bone deformities and multiple fractures are also common. Too little vitamin D can cause rickets, a bone-deforming disease that can result in bowed legs, a deformed spine, "potbelly" appearance, flat feet, or stunted growth.

Vitamin E (The Tocopherols)   Vitamin E is one of the most talked about vitamins, and to some extent the exaggerated and unsubstantiated claims made for it result from a combination of hope and misinterpretation. In actuality, vitamin E helps to prevent oxygen from destroying other substances. In other words, it is a preservative, protecting the activity of other compounds such as vitamin A and polyunsaturated fat. Abundant sources of vitamin E are vegetable oils, beans, eggs, whole grains (the germ), liver, fruits, and vegetables.

MYTH: Organic (natural) vitamins are nutritionally superior to synthetic vitamins.

FACT: Synthetic vitamins, manufactured in the laboratory, are identical to the natural vitamins found in foods. The body cannot tell the difference and gets the same benefits from both sources. Statements that "nature cannot be imitated" and "natural vitamins have the essence of life" are without meaning.

MYTH: Vitamins give you "pep" and "energy."

FACT: Vitamins yield no calories. By themselves they provide no extra pep or vitality, nor an unusual level of well-being.

MYTH: The more vitamins the better.

FACT: Taking more vitamins than necessary is a waste of money and time. In the case of some vitamins, excess amounts can be harmful.

MYTH: You cannot get enough vitamins from the conventional foods you eat.

FACT: Anyone who eats a reasonably varied diet should not need supplemental vitamins under normal circumstances.

MEGAVITAMIN MADNESS

Because people vary in nutritional needs, it is difficult to know the exact amount of vitamins that is "too much." Some individuals, however, take extremely large doses of vitamins, and evidence is accumulating that such megavitamins can be harmful:

[Mega] vitamins are being used . . . to treat everything from schizophrenia and cancer to the common cold. . . . Most scientists agree that massive doses of vitamins do have pharmacological effects on the body. They act like drugs and have drug-like effects. . . . [They also have] hazardous long-term effects. Vitamin C at 500 mg. actually destroys vitamin B_{12}, which is necessary to prevent red blood cell abnormalities and pernicious anemia. Excessive vitamin C falsifies blood sugar levels in testing diabetes. Prolonged use of large doses can be implicated in gout, hemorrhaging of ulcers, formation of kidney stones, severe diarrhea, and liver and genetic abnormalities.[88]

There are times when a person may legitimately require high doses of a particular vitamin or mineral.[89] We have seen that vitamins and minerals are used to treat medically diagnosed deficiencies among alcoholics, the elderly, pregnant or lactating women, and individuals with poor intestinal absorption. High doses of vitamins may also be used in the treatment of certain conditions. Generally, people who do not have these deficiencies or conditions do not need vitamins and minerals in high doses.

THE ELDERLY AND OTC DRUGS

The elderly population of the United States is subscribing more to the use of self-care products and therefore are self-medicating themselves for more illnesses and physical complaints.[90] Because of age-related impairments, many elderly are not able to diagnose their ailments correctly, select appropriate OTC agents, or follow directions for their use. Doctors and pharmacists alike should be very careful to question elderly people in great depth about their use of such OTC drugs before prescribing any medication or suggesting the use of any medication because when some of the drugs are combined, they have a synergistic effect.[91]

DIET PILLS

Phenylpropanolamine (PPA) is the appetite suppressant found in most diet pills. It is also one of the main drugs found in nasal decongestants such as Sineoff and Vick's Day Care. Although manufacturers of diet pills claim PPA to be safe and effective, many organizations, physicians, and public agencies have expressed concern about the safety of OTC drugs containing it. The results of studies of PPA's biological effects have been conflicting, but reports have surfaced of adverse reactions in some people.

In the United States an estimated $110 million is spent annually on OTC diet aids.[92] Many of these aids contain PPA. A less potent amphetamine, this drug acts on the central nervous system. "The pills should be continued only as long as weight loss continues without side effects or the need for increased dosages, usually four to six weeks."[93]

Approximately one quarter of the U.S. population is clinically obese. Obesity causes a considerable number of problems, among which is the stigma this country attaches to being obese. Due to this stigma, there is a lot of pressure in our society to lose weight, and one way to achieve this end is by taking diet pills containing PPA in combination with caffeine.[94] This stimulates the central nervous system. These diet pills, in addition, have vasoconstrictive properties.

Theoretically, PPA depresses the appetite and mimics the effect of amphetamines by stimulating the central nervous system.[95] Cardiac stimulation, high blood pressure, nervousness, headache, and insomnia are some of the common side effects. PPA also appears to pass into the breast milk of nursing mothers.[96] Acute temporary mental derangement is another side effect. A number of studies have indicated that PPA may cause anxiety, dizziness, hallucinations, and acute psychotic episodes.[97] Some individuals are taking OTC drugs containing PPA as amphetamines to get high.

Another safety consideration is the possible synergistic effects of PPA taken with other drugs. Over 50 percent of the diet pills in the United States OTC market contain both PPA and caffeine, which have synergistic effects on cardiac stimulation.[98] Imagine taking the recommended dosage of your favorite diet pill, which contains 50 milligrams of PPA and 200 milligrams of caffeine. You take the pill after getting up, so you won't want breakfast. In addition, you consume your usual two to three cups of coffee before going to work. After about two hours you have 50 milligrams of PPA and 380 to 500 milligrams of caffeine in your system! This level can continue throughout the day if more caffeine is consumed during coffee breaks and the lunch hour. Stimulation of the CNS to this degree can bring tachycardia (fast heart rate) and aggravate hypertension (high blood pressure), not to mention having lesser effects such as headaches and insomnia. Most people who are taking diet pills are overweight, a condition associated with cardiac problems and high blood pressure, so taking PPA and caffeine together is a threat to a person's health.

FOOD LABELS

The FDA has proposed lifting its 82-year ban on health claims on food labels.[99] This would allow companies to make a connection between food and various health benefits. The FDA hopes the public will thereby become better educated on how to eat more healthfully.

The FDA began regulating labels in 1906 because so many manufacturers were making outrageous health claims. In 1973 it began requiring companies to list nutritional information on food labels if they have added one or more nutrients to the product or made nutritional claims about it on the label.

The new FDA proposal would allow companies to make health claims provided they (1) are truthful and not misleading, (2) are backed by scientific proof, and (3) state that the product is best eaten as part of a well-balanced diet.

SUMMARY

OTC drugs account for over $15 billion in sales every year. In general, they may provide relief, but many feel these drugs are used too often and may have serious side effects or complications.

The most popular OTC drug is aspirin, which helps to eliminate headache, reduce pain in general, and lessen inflammation in arthritis sufferers. It may eventually prove effective in reducing heart attacks. Unfortunately, aspirin often has undesirable side effects and may also hinder platelet production. Acetaminophen may be used as an alternative, but it is more expensive, lacks aspirin's antiinflammatory capability, and may damage the liver. Ibuprofen is another aspirin substitute that has made its way into the marketplace. It should also be stressed that ibuprofen may cause harmful side effects in some users.

Laxatives are another popular OTC product. Though their use is largely unnecessary if proper foods, adequate fluids, and regular exercise are taken, many people employ them almost habitually.

Cough relievers are still another high-selling OTC drug. The most effective of these suppressants are codeine-based, but these also cause dependence if used regularly. Antihistamines are also potent medicines and should be taken with caution. Some antihistamines are effective in cold and allergy treatment and in the prevention of motion sickness.

The use of phenylpropanolamine (PPA) has increased in the form of diet pills. Its help in reducing appetite makes it a very popular drug in our weight-conscious society. However, caution must be practiced in its use because there is some concern about its safety.

Over-The-Counter Drugs
N O T E S

1. Richard Hall et al., "Psychiatric and Physiological Reactions Produced by Over-the-Counter Drugs," *Journal of Psychedelic Drugs* 10, no. 3 (July/September 1978):423–26.

2. Lawrence R. Krupka and Arthur M. Vener, "Drug Knowledge (Prescription, Over-the-Counter, Social): Young Adult Consumer at Risk?" *Journal of Drug Education* 17, no. 2 (1987):139–42.

3. Sidney Cohen, *The Substance Abuse Problems,* Vol. 2: *New Issues for the 1980s* (New York: Haworth Press, 1985).

4. Ibid.

5. Glyn N. Volans, "Monitoring the Safety of Over the Counter Drugs," *British Medical Journal* 295 (1987):797–98.

6. Stephen J. Coons and William G. McGhan, "The Role of Drugs in Self-Care," *Journal of Drug Issues* 18, No. 2 (Spring 1988):175–83.

7. P. Callahan, "A Pill For This . . . . Are We Writing Our Own Prescription for Trouble?" *Self,* October 1989.

8. Jeanie Wilson, "Hooked on Over-the-Counter Drugs," *Reader's Digest,* no. 133:July 1988:27–32; Marian Segal, "Should You Take Aspirin to Help Prevent a Heart Attack?" *FDA Consumer* 22, no. 5 (June 1988):19–21; Gale Maleskey, "Thin Your Blood and Live Longer," *Prevention,* May 1987, pp. 89–93.

9. Food and Drug Administration, *Current and Useful Information from the Food and Drug Administration: Self Medication* (Washington, D.C.: Department of Health, Education and Welfare, 1973).

10. Louis DeBakey, "Happiness Is Only a Pill Away: Madison Avenue Rhetoric without Reason," *Addictive Diseases* 3, no. 2 (1977):274.

11. W. H. Post and J. H. McGrath, "Patients and Potions," *Journal of Drug Issues* (Winter 1972):54.

12. "White Rabbit," *Drug Information Center (DIC)* (Eugene: University of Oregon, 1975).

13. Edward M. Brecher et al., *Licit and Illicit Drugs* (Boston: Little, Brown, 1972), p. 3.

14. Post and McGrath, "Patients and Potions," p. 52.

15. Hall et al., "Psychiatric and Physiological Reactions," p. 423.

16. Virginia P. Shands, Linda D. Goff, and David H. Goff, "Rx for OTC Users: Improved Health Education," *Consumer Health,* March 1990, pp. 125–28.

17. Cynthia Marks, "Drugstore Dangers: The Dope on Over-the-Counter Drugs," *Mademoiselle,* 96 (August 1990):30.

18. "OTC Review Milestone," *FDA Consumer,* February 1984, p. 32.

19. Zachary Schiller, "Can Procter and Gamble Commandeer More Shelves in the Medicine Chest?" *Business Week,* April 10, 1989, pp. 64–67.

20. Ibid.

21. Annabel Hecht, "OTC Drug Labels: Must Reading," *FDA Consumer* 19, no. 8 (October 1985), p. 2.

22. Ibid.

23. Melinda Beck, "Peddling Youth Over-the-Counter," *Newsweek,* March 5, 1990, pp. 50–52.

24. Martin Gross and Leon Greenberg, *The Salicylates: A Critical Bibliographic Review* (New Haven: Hillhouse Press, 1948), p. 5.

25. Gerald Weissman, "Aspirin," *Scientific American,* January 1991, pp. 84–90.

26. Ann Ranard, "Much Ado about Aspirin," *Health,* 1988, pp. 54–57, 73.

27. Ibid.

28. Ibid.

29. "White Rabbit," p. 10.

30. "Acetylsalicylic Acid (Aspirin): Alcohol and Drug Fact Sheet," *Drug Information Center (DIC)* (Eugene: University of Oregon, 1980).

31. Howard A. Pearson, "Comparative Effects of Aspirin and Acetaminophen on Homeostasis," *Pediatrics,* November 1977.

32. Geoffrey Crowley, "Some Counter Intelligence," *Newsweek,* March 12, 1990, pp. 82–84.

33. Ibid.

34. Stuart L. Nightingale, "New Warning Label for Over-the-Counter Aspirin," *Journal of the American Medical Association* 264, no. 6 (August 1990):677.

35. Quoted in Gross and Greenberg, *The Salicylates,* p. 5.

36. Dan Shapiro, "Aspirin Flunks a Coronary Test," *Newsweek,* February 18, 1980, p. 11.

37. Cited in John C. Krantz, "The Jury Is Still Out: Aspirin Medication for Heart Attack Prevention," *American Pharmacy* n.s. 19, no. 1 (January 1979):14–15.

38. Paul E. Schindler, "Aspirin: Marvel Drug," *Science Digest* 84 (December 1978):14. From *Aspirin Therapy: Cutting the Risk of Heart Disease* by Paul E. Schindler, Jr. Copyright © 1978 by Paul E. Schindler, Jr. Used with permission from the publisher, Walker and Company, New York.

39. Ranard, "Much Ado about Aspirin."

40. Joan Hamilton et al., "Miracle Drug Aspirin," *Business Week,* August 29, 1988, pp. 56–61.

41. Don L. Boroughs, "The Pill That Fits the Bill," *U.S. News & World Report,* April 2, 1990.

42. Cited in "Should You Take More Aspirin?" *Consumer Research* 71, no. 3 (March 1988):36–37.

43. David R. Zimmerman, *The Essential Guide to Non-Prescription Drugs* (New York: Harper & Row, 1983).

44. M. J. H. Smith and Paul K. Smith, eds., *The Salicylates: A Critical Bibliographic Review* (New York: Interscience Publishers, 1966), p. 215.

45. Hugh H. Hussey, "Aspirin Can Be Dangerous," *Journal of the American Medical Association* 228 (April 29, 1974):609.

46. Harvey J. Weiss, "Aspirin: A Dangerous Drug?" *Journal of the American Medical Association* 229 (August 26, 1974):1221.

47. Hussey, "Aspirin Can Be Dangerous," p. 609.

48. Gross and Greenberg, *The Salicylates,* p. 5.

49. "Drug Induced Diseases," p. 70.

50. K. A. Fackleman, "Low Dose of Aspirin Keeps Migraine Away," *Science News* 137 (February 17, 1989):103.

51. Ibid.

52. Hamilton et al., "Miracle Drug Aspirin," pp. 56–61.

53. Ibid.

54. Ibid.

55. Ibid.

56. Pearson, "Comparative Effects of Aspirin and Acetaminophen."

57. Jan Koch-Weser, "Acetaminophen," *New England Journal of Medicine* 295, no. 23 (December 2, 1976):1297.

58. "Is Tylenol (et al.) Any Better Than Aspirin?" *Consumer Reports* 142 (October 1977).

59. William Steele, "Reaching for Over-the-Counter Relief," *Current Health 2* 15, no. 4 (December 1988):16–18.

60. Ibid.

61. Lindsay Hall, "Over-the-Counter Drugs," *Current Health 2* 13 (January 1987):13–15.

62. Amy E. Young, "Mixed Messages," *Common Cause Magazine,* September/October 1989, pp. 11–12.

63. N. Nicastro, "Over-the-Counter Ibuprofen Can Cause Visual Disturbances," *American Journal of Nursing* 90, no. 3 (March 1990):64–65.

64. "Ibuprofen May Increase Risk of Ulcers," *Register-Guard* (Eugene, Oregon), February 15, 1991, p. 3A.

65. Walter Modell, *Drugs of Choice* (St. Louis: C. V. Mosby, 1960), p. 370.

66. J. H. Cummings, "Progress Report: Laxative Abuse," *GUT* 15 (September 1974):58.

67. Jeanie Wilson, "Hooked On Over-the-Counter Drugs," *Reader's Digest,* no. 133, July 1988, pp. 27–32.

68. Charles Seifert, "Over-the-Counter Drug Abuse," *USA Today* 118 (February 1990):9.

69. Charles Beck, "Laxatives: What Does Regular Mean?" *FDA Consumer* (May 1975):1.

70. Erwin Di Cyan and Lawrence Hessman, *Without Prescription* (New York: Simon & Schuster, 1972), p. 72.

71. Quoted in ibid., p. 2.

72. J. H. Cummings, G. E. Sladen, and O. F. W. James, "Laxative Induced Diarrhea: A Continuing Clinical Problem," *British Journal of Medicine* (March 23, 1974):539.

73. Griffenhagen and Hawkins, *Handbook of Non-Prescription Drugs* (Washington, D.C.: American Pharmacological Association, 1973), p. 62.

74. Amy Bernstein, "In Sickness There Is Wealth," *U.S. News & World Report,* January 29, 1990, p. 60.

75. Ibid.

76. Hall, "Over-the-Counter Drugs," p. 15.

77. Ibid.

78. Betty S. Bergersen and Andres Goth, *Pharmacology in Nursing,* 14th ed. (St. Louis: C. V. Mosby, 1979); Corman, Malcom, and Collier, "Cathartics," p. 426.

79. Walter Modell, *Drugs of Choice: 1968–1969* (St. Louis: C. V. Mosby, 1967), p. 440.

80. Annabel Hecht, "Drugs and Driving," *FDA Consumer* 12 (September 1978):17–19.

81. *Physician's Desk Reference to Pharmacological Specialties and Biologicals,* 28th ed. (Oradell, N.J.: Medical Economics, 1974).

82. Annabel Hecht, "Vitamins Over-the-Counter: Take Only When Needed," *FDA Consumer* (April 1, 1979):17.

83. "Vitamin and Mineral Overdosage," *American Family Physician* 35 (March 1987):282.

84. Hecht, "Vitamins Over-the-Counter."

85. Diane D. Edwards, "Vitamin A Therapy Chews on Oral Cancer," *Science News* 133, no. 24 (June 11, 1988):381.

86. Ibid.

87. Ibid.; Susan Brady, "Safe or Effective," *Health* 20, no. 8 (August 1988):11–13.

88. Jean Mayer, "Megavitamin Madness: How Much Is Too Much?" *Family Health* 12, no. 2 (February 1980):48–49.

89. "The Perils of Megavitamin Therapy," *Consumer Research* 70, no. 7 (July 1987):16.

90. Peter P. Lamy, "Nonprescription Drugs and the Elderly," *American Family Physician* 39, no. 6 (June 1989):175–79.

91. "Study: Healthy or Sick, Elderly Take OTC Drugs," *Geriatrics,* 40, no. 11 (November 1985):23.

92. Jean E. Laird, "Can You Get Hooked on Over-the-Counter Drugs?" *Vibrant Life* 6, no. 1 (January/February 1990):4–6.

93. Ibid.

94. Lawrence R. Krupka and Arthur M. Vener, "Over-the-Counter Appetite Suppressants Containing Phenylpropanolamine Hydrochloride (PPA) and the Young Adult: Usage and Perceived Effectiveness," *Journal of Drug Education,* 13 (1983):141–51.

95. Albert Dietz, "Amphetamine-like Reactions to Phenylpropanolamine," *Journal of the American Medical Association* 205, no. 6 (February 13, 1981):601–2.

96. James Long, *Essential Guide to Prescription Drugs,* 3rd ed. (New York: Harper & Row, 1982).

97. Dietz, "Amphetamine-like Reactions to Phenylpropanolamine," pp. 601–2; Gunnar Norvenius, "PPA and Mental Disturbances," *Lancet* 2 (1979):1367–68.

98. APA, *Handbook of Non-Prescription Drugs,* p. 221.

99. Diana Tonnessen, "The Label Debate," *Health* 20, no. 7 (July 1988):65–68.

PRESCRIPTION AND OTHER DRUGS OF INTEREST

$5-billion-a-year investment in research and development by drug companies in America is generating a wave of breakthroughs from tension relievers and cancer therapies to baldness cures and heart-attack medications—positioning pharmaceuticals to become the glamor industry of the 1990s.[1] Approximately $30 billion is spent annually in the United States on prescriptions, and an average of seven prescriptions per person are written.[2]

The wonder medicines working their way through the research and development process will keep the pharmaceutical industry prosperous into the next century if companies can overcome several obstacles, such as the increasing costs of developing new compounds, a strict regulatory environment, and growing government pressure to hold down health costs by squeezing profit margins on drugs.

A recent survey by the FDA found that one in every three people, most of them elderly, were uninformed on the drugs they were taking.[3] They had received no written information from their doctor or pharmacist and appeared unmotivated to seek information by either asking questions or obtaining literature. They tended to be taking several medications at a time—all the more reason to keep informed. They also felt that if they trusted their doctor, there was no need to ask questions.

A second group, called the "physician-reliant," composed 40 percent of those polled. These people received counseling about the drugs they were taking and were more likely to get written information at their doctor's office. But although they were informed about the drugs, they too tended not to ask questions. They relied on their physician for information.

A third group, the "pharmacy-reliant," constituted 19 percent of the respondents. These individuals were the youngest and tended to be getting medication for others, usually their children.

Only 7 percent of those surveyed were classified as "questioners." It is those in the uninformed group who need to learn more about the drugs they are taking. They also need to recognize the symptoms resulting from polypharmacy and other improper uses of drugs.

The American Association of Retired Persons found that the differences in drug costs can range up to $30 more for a single prescription.[4] A brand-name drug in one drugstore may cost up to 22 times its generic version in another. Senior citizens spend more for prescriptions than any other health service. They spend around $9 billion a year. Americans over the age of 65 make up only 12 percent of the population, but they consume 32 percent of all drugs sold.[5]

NEW DRUG APPLICATIONS

Since 1962 a drug has had to be declared safe and effective for its intended purpose by the FDA in order to be marketed. "Promising" drugs such as AZT (an AIDS drug) must meet a certain benefit-to-risk ratio in order to qualify. A New Drug Application (NDA), once filed by the sponsor of the drug, starts a "review clock"[6] that tracks the amount of time spent by the FDA on reviewing and investigating the application. The process is supposed to take 180 days, but in actuality the average amount of time required is about two years. AZT was approved in the record time of 107 days. This amount of time can be decreased or increased depending on the speed of the required information gathering and the extensive documentation.

The White House Council on Competiveness has recommended that the Food and Drug Administration implement a series of reforms to dramatically shorten the time it takes to approve new drugs—changes expected to save more than 1 million lives by the turn of the century and reduce drug-company research and development expenses by at least $1 billion a year.[7] This change is partially being motivated by other modern, industrialized countries with shorter development times and faster licensing systems, with the result that patients abroad have access to drugs not available in the United States. In the United States, it now takes an average of 9.75 years to bring new drugs to the market.[8] Under the new system, drugs for life-threatening diseases would take 5.5 years to develop.

Shortening the Time It Takes to
Approve New Drug Applications
Source: FDA

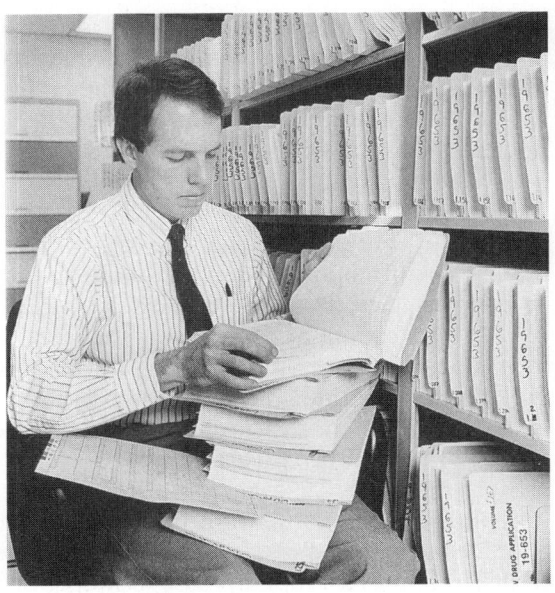

NEW MEDICINES AND DELIVERY

A revolution of scientific technology promises a wide range of new tools
for drug discovery and design. Developments in chemistry and molecular
biology provide the basis for techniques of "molecular modelling" that aim to
design drug molecules on an entirely rational basis.[9] A certain parasite's drug-
receptor molecule can be analyzed by x-ray crystallography to determine its
three-dimensional atomic arrangement. With this information and very large
computers with three-dimensional graphics, chemical molecules can be

The Pharmacist Keeping Up with
New Prescriptions
Source: Ulrike Welsh/Photo Researchers

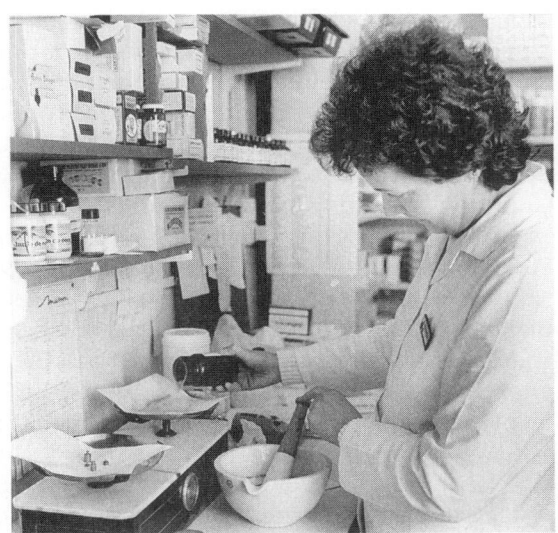

designed with a shape that binds to that receptor site and exerts the required action. For example, tiny biodegradable capsules are now available that can be embedded in a woman's thigh or arm to automatically dispense contraceptive hormones for a year.[10] Also, under development are dissolvable plastic wafers that are implanted in the brain to slowly release an antitumor drug for cancer victims. The day is not far off, either, when diabetics will be able to give themselves insulin with nasal spray.

Research is presently going on to find new drugs from the sea. About half of our drugs today, including aspirin, digitalis, morphine, and many antibiotics, come from living things, most of them land-dwelling plants. With the ocean's possessing nearly 80 percent of all life on earth, the sea is a potentially vast source of useful chemicals, including many that have never been encountered before in land organisms.[11]

PLACEBOS

INTRODUCTION

A potent analgesic such as morphine can ease the suffering of severe injuries, but it sometimes fails to relieve mild pain. Give a man a sugar pill, and his agonizing ache will vanish because he believes the doctor's medicine will help him. Bite on a bullet, receive a shot of morphine, or swallow a sugar pill—which will relieve pain best? Each can reduce pain better than the others under appropriate conditions.[12]

Placebos—substances that are used in medical treatment but have no pharmacological effect on the problem they are supposed to treat—have existed for ages. But as placebos appear in more and more medical procedures, many are questioning the validity of their use. Is the practice harmful or beneficial? Because a sugar pill can relieve a pain through the user's belief in it, should it be given? If patients do gain relief from placebo effects, perhaps placebos are a viable treatment option. But in order to formulate an answer, it is necessary to know the mechanisms of the placebo process and the possible factors in negative and positive responses to treatment.

Sometimes, a doctor may use a weak drug to achieve the placebo effect.[13] The weak drug can take the place of a stronger one, if the patient believes it will work. In this way higher and higher doses are not needed to achieve the same effect, and at the same time the patient is satisfied that the drugs are working although he may or may not know of the dosage change.

Although placebos are technically harmless substances, they can produce a wide variety of effects on the body. In some cases, the placebo is so strong that it will override the normal actions of the drug. Placebos may cause the brain to make special chemicals called endorphins.[14] These are natural pain killers. They are often made by the brain to alter an injury. Endorphins are the reason a bad injury may not hurt too much right after it happens. Hours or days later, the pain is worse because endorphins are no longer being made.

A study of the effectiveness of several products on the market made specifically for suppression of pain had interesting results.[15] One group received a placebo, one group an active, nonprescribed pain suppressant, and one group a prescribed pain suppressant. They were then monitored to see the differences in their response to questions about their level of pain.

The group given the placebo was told that they had been given a prescription pain reliever. They showed considerably less pain overall than the group that was told they had been given a nonprescription pain reliever. The placebo group showed the effects that were present in the group that had been given a prescribed drug, indicating that the thought of being given a prescribed drug elicits similar responses. The group that had been given the prescribed drug showed a considerable amount of pain relief but did not have the expectancy effect of the placebo group. The results indicated the correlation that when you expect to feel less pain, there is a drop in the pain present.[16]

However, there is also an ethical question that needs to be addressed. Is it ethical for a physician to prescribe a placebo for a patient? This has initiated considerable debate.

INDIVIDUAL DIFFERENCES

Placebos are capable of producing positive or negative effects, depending on the individual, the social milieu, and situational variables.[17] People likely to be most affected by placebos are usually those who are more open to the influence of others, are less critical of self and others, are more trusting of physicians and medicines, inhibit direct expression of hostility, and communicate socially desirable things about themselves. Individuals who are acutely distressed or anxious are also likely to experience placebo effects because of their need to obtain relief.

SOCIAL ENVIRONMENT AND SITUATIONAL VARIABLES

When a patient takes a placebo, the degree of social support he or she receives from family members for reacting positively to the placebo will influence its potency. Situational variables, such as the physician's behavior, stimulus characteristics of the placebo, and treatment milieu, exert a certain influence as well.

ADMINISTRATION, FREQUENCY, AND COST

The method by which a placebo is administered, plus the placebo's visual and sensory characteristics, affect the patient's perception of how well the "medicine" will work.[18] Many people believe that injection of a drug has a more pronounced effect than oral administration because they consider injection to be the faster method, and they therefore expect almost immediate relief from it. Also, the mechanism of injection is impressive: Invariably the patient feels that the needle coming nearer contains the much-awaited cure-all. The more impressive the visual and sensory characteristics of the placebo, the more impressive the placebo is deemed by the patient.

It is no accident that specific artificial colors and flavorings are used in brand-name drugs. Studies have indicated that if a person takes a placebo in pill form, a large brown or purple pill or a small bright red or yellow pill may produce better results than those of other colors.[19] Other studies indicate that two pills are more effective than one, and that if the pill is chewed or dissolved in the mouth, a pill with an unpleasant taste produces better effects. In one of these studies, subjects were separated into two groups and instructed to swallow a pill. Some of the pills contained lactose and some ascorbic acid. The subjects reacted negatively or had no reaction to the lactose pills, saying they felt they had been given placebos because the pills tasted so sweet. The group swallowing the pills containing ascorbic acid said they felt they had received actual medicine—a positive effect.[20]

Several other factors in placebo effectiveness are how often the dose is administered and how much the placebo costs. If a physician prescribes several doses during the day, the patient may feel a responsibility to follow the instructions and may experience greater effects. If the cost of the medicine is high, greater results are often experienced, because many believe that costlier drugs work more effectively.

In modern medicine, placebos are perceived as being limited to situations where the physician has a good feel for the medical history, current condition, and potential responses of the patient.[21] It is preferable to have a good doctor-patient relationship based on honest disclosure of medical conditions.

THE POWER OF SUGGESTION

A study of 200 subjects was conducted to determine the effectiveness of placebos.[22] In one group, half the subjects were given a placebo and the other half a low dose of amphetamine. In the second group, half were given placebos and half a lose dose of diazepam. The study hypothesized that the people with the placebo would act like the people who had actually been given the drug. All four groups were told they had been given either amphetamine or diazepam. The results both supported and contradicted the hypothesis. The subjects who were given the placebo but told they had been given amphetamine did not react as if affected by the drug. There was no evidence of a higher rate of activity, in contrast with the group given the actual drug. On the other hand the group given the placebo but told they had taken diazepam showed slower reactions and affected speech, much the same as the subjects who had taken the actual drug. The power of suggestion worked on this group.

ANTIBIOTICS

CLASSIFICATION

Antibiotics are metabolic compounds produced by microorganisms such as molds and soil bacteria that inhibit the growth of other microorganisms; their synthetic derivatives have the same effect. The three most important groups of antibiotics are penicillins, tetracyclines, and streptomycins, but there are over a dozen lesser-used antibiotics as well.[23] When at work in the body, antibiotics act either as a bacteriostatic (bacterial-growth-inhibiting) or bactericidal (bacterial-destruction) agent, or both.[24]

HISTORY

Penicillin, the first antibiotic, was discovered in 1928 by Alexander Fleming. When a culture of staphylococci was accidentally contaminated with a green mold, *Penicillin notatum,* Fleming noticed that the culture ceased to grow and was destroyed. It wasn't until 1940, however, when clinical researchers at Oxford developed a procedure for isolating and purifying the antibiotic, that its widespread use began.[25] Penicillin became known as the Wonder Drug because of its great ability to control disease-producing bacteria in the body.

EFFECTS

Antibiotics destroy or inhibit the growth of infectious bacteria in many ways. Penicillins can destroy bacteria by interfering with their production of new protective cell walls as they multiply and grow.

The three groups of antibiotics have different ranges of effectiveness. Penicillin is effective in low concentrations, though this effectiveness depends on the type of administration: Generally an oral dose is only about one fifth as effective as the same dose administered by injection. The amount of food in the stomach as well as the rate at which that organ empties also influence effectiveness, since food can slow absorption of the drug and decrease effectiveness.

Streptomycins are usually given through intramuscular injections. They lose their effectiveness if taken with milk or other dairy products.

Tetracyclines are generally considered bacteriostatic agents; they have bactericidal properties only in large doses. They are successful orally against a wide range of organisms. This family of antibiotics usually results in a modification of the infectious bacteria by slowing down or reducing their effectiveness.

Antibiotics are generally unable to affect certain regions of the body, such as the brain, the eye, and abscesses. Abscesses must be drained before antibiotic therapy will be of value.[26] Nor are antibiotics effective against viral infections, such as the common cold, influenza, measles, and mumps.

True toxic reactions to penicillin occur rarely. A number of individuals, however, do exhibit marked hypersensitivity to this drug. Symptoms of hypersensitivity include rashes, fever, skin eruptions, and more severe reactions capable of causing death. Severe symptoms may include joint pain, asthma, anaphylactic shock, and bone-marrow depression.

Though there are few toxic reactions to penicillin, toxic reactions to other antibiotics can occur with large doses. Occasional side effects may also be experienced, including hearing loss, vertigo, gastrointestinal upset, nausea, vomiting, and diarrhea. Permanent staining of developing teeth in young children and fetuses and of developed teeth in the elderly may be caused by tetracycline.

RESISTANCE TO ANTIBIOTICS

The number of antibiotic-resistant species of disease bacteria is increasing throughout the world. Penicillin, for example, used to be 100 percent effective against staphylococcus; its effectiveness has now diminished to less than 30 percent because of resistance.[27] Such growth of resistant species can be attributed to the passing on of resistance capabilities to ensuing generations of bacteria. Drug-resistant bacteria apparently manufacture a resistance-transfer chemical that enables bacteria never exposed to an antibiotic to become immune to it.[28] This resistance-transferring system is a limitation in all antibiotic therapy, and the problem will perhaps be solved only through the development of new antibiotic forms.

Resistance transferring may also be taking place outside the human body. Animals are often given antibiotics, which for unknown reasons stimulate growth in chickens, pigs, and cattle, resulting in tastier meat with more fat. Antibiotics also inhibit animal diseases that threaten when large numbers of stock are kept in close confinement. This practice may be contributing to a potentially serious health problem. Though the evidence remains inconclusive, critics of the antibiotic-feeding programs are concerned that drug-resistant bacteria within animals will transfer their resistance to human disease bacteria. In response to this possibility, British scientists have convinced the British government to place controls on the kinds of antibiotics used in their animal feeds.[29] Similar controls are also in effect in the United States.

Changes in the human body caused by antibiotics may also lead to an increase in the number of infections unresponsive to antibiotic actions. Termed *alterations in the host*, these reactions to antibiotics range from changes in the body's normal microorganism population to interference with nutrition and the development of *superinfections*. When microorganism level is changed, normal bacteria decrease and abnormal bacteria or fungi increase. When this condition becomes extreme, a superinfection develops, and organisms not affected by antibiotics are able to grow rapidly.

MISUSE

Misuse of antibiotics may involve improper dosage, improper administration, inadequate duration of treatment, or use by inappropriate patients. The patient must be sure to take the prescribed amount as well as the prescribed number of doses even though the symptoms of the infection may disappear before that number has been reached. Generally, antibiotic therapy is continued for ten days; after that time any remaining doses should be disposed of.

Proper administration is very important in antibiotic use. Penicillin can be attacked by destructive secretions in the stomach, so it should be taken before meals, when there are less such secretions. Five times as much penicillin must be taken orally as intravenously in order to have therapeutic effectiveness. But care must be taken during intravenous injection if other drugs are present; for the combination could cause a chemical reaction that would alter the effectiveness of both drugs.[30]

Age and physical condition are other important factors in antibiotics use. Since newborns do not have mature livers, they are unable to metabolize antibiotics as well as adults and should not receive them. Adults with liver or kidney damage also should not take antibiotics. Pregnant women should not be given these drugs, since they cross the placental barrier and also have been found in the mother's spinal fluid and milk. One antibiotic, strepto-mycin, has been linked to fetal abnormalities when taken during pregnancy.[31]

DRUGS FOR THE MENTALLY ILL

ANTIDEPRESSANTS

Introduction   Depression—a condition of low spirits, gloominess, dejection, and decreased activity—is a very common complaint today. It is estimated that 15 percent of the American population suffer from symptoms of depression each year.[32] Fortunately, in most cases the condition is situation-specific and of short duration. Some individuals, however, may sink into a deep pathological depression if help is not received. This state is character-ized by (1) great sadness associated with hopelessness and helplessness, and possible suicidal tendencies, (2) anxiety, and (3) inhibition.[33] Because the danger of suicide exists, chemical treatment of such depression is often nec-essary.[34]

Researchers discovered that antidepressants were able to elevate a patient's mood without also accelerating his or her heartbeat and causing insomnia or other unpleasant amphetamine side effects. Antidepressants also did not cause the relapses, confusion, and loss of memory ECT treatment often did. Antidepressant drugs soon became a "more pleasant, less traumatic form of treatment and one more suited to outpatient use."[35]

Despite the popularity of antidepressants, a great deal of controversy sur-rounds their use. A study of 51 consecutively admitted depressed patients at the National Institute of Mental Health found that many depressed patients are admitted to a hospital before they have received adequate chemotherapy as outpatients.[36] Researchers speculate that this lack of adequate drug treat-ment may result from the "physician's unfamiliarity with or bias against use of [antidepressants]."[37] But studies also show that these drugs are often pre-scribed too frequently as well.

Antidepressants should be used only when a biochemical cause for depression has been established. They are not meant for use in treating the mild and transient symptoms of depression associated with many life situa-tions.

Classification   Antidepressants fall into two categories: monoamine-oxidase inhibitors (MAOI) and tricyclics. Drugs such as amphetamines, caf-feine, barbiturates, tranquilizers, and sedatives have also been used to treat depression, but they are not classified as antidepressants.

Psychophysiological Effects   Antidepressants act on the central nervous system by increasing the availability of the chemicals (neurotrans-mitters) responsible for transmitting nerve signals at critical sites (nerve synapses) in the brain and throughout the central nervous system. The pri-mary neurotransmitter that antidepressants are thought to act on is the chem-ical norepinephrine (or noradrenaline). Research has established that when norepinephrine levels in certain portions of the brain are low, chronic depression can occur. It is thought that when a natural deficiency of norepinephrine exists in certain portions of the brain, antidepressants, by increasing the rate of norepinephrine use in the nerves, can gradually increase mood and alleviate depression.[38]

As with all drugs, however, the action of antidepressants is not entirely specific, and they may produce adverse effects, such as dry mouth, blurred vision, faintness, nasal stuffiness, chills, drowsiness, and tremors. In addition, weakened libido, confusion, gastrointestinal distress, skin eruptions, weight increase, sweating, and urinary retention may occur.

With continued use, tricyclics and MAOI drugs can impair kidney and liver functions in some individuals.[39] Tricyclics can also lower a person's seizure threshold and should therefore be used with caution in seizure-producing illnesses or disabilities. Both types of antidepressants are known to cross the placental barrier,[40] but they are not thought to produce physical or psychological dependence.

Monoamine-oxidase-inhibiting drugs increase one's chemical sensitivity to a large number of foods and other drugs, a condition that may persist for many days following MAOI discontinuation. They react unfavorably with such foods as cheese, beer, wine, pickled herring, chicken livers, and foods containing yeast extracts (tyramine-rich foods). Administration of MAOIs is especially hazardous during any drug-induced CNS depression, since it may cause an unexpected CNS-depressant overdose. Though the acute overdose level of MAOIs in humans has not been firmly established, symptoms of acute toxicity are known. They include agitation, delirium, tremors, sweating, neuromuscular irritability, and hyperthermia, which can progress to a coma and even death.

MAOIs are no longer employed routinely. Instead, almost all the antidepressants used are tricyclics. MAOIs have stronger side effects and can interact with tyramine-rich foods to dangerously increase blood pressure.

PROZAC

Prozac (fluoxetine hydrochloride), produced by Eli Lilly & Co., is the newest wonder drug on the psychiatric scene. It was the nineteenth most prescribed drug in the United States in 1990, with more than 6 million prescriptions filled.[41] Prozac is currently the most widely prescribed antidepressant in the United States partially because it produces fewer and milder side effects.[42] Prozac's low complication rate is due to its targeted chemical nature: It interacts only with serotonin. However, Prozac isn't a miracle drug; it can cause headaches, insomnia, nervousness, agitation, and the jitters.

An unexpected side effect of the drug is that it may induce suicidal thoughts in some patients. Cases of suicidal impulses arising in patients taking Prozac have been reported, and a growing number of psychiatrists are starting to warn their patients of this serious potential side effect.[43]

Researchers at Massachusetts General Hospital reviewed patient charts to determine if a higher percentage of patients treated with Prozac, in comparison to other antidepressants, became newly suicidal during treatment. Their

Prozac
The newest wonder drug on the psychiatric scene. Fluxotine, as it is also called, is the nation's most prescribed antidepressant drug. There have been some concerns about possible side effects leading to violent and suicidal behavior.

data on depressed patients treated in 1989 show that 2.8 percent of patients on Prozac became suicidal during treatment, compared with 0.7 percent on other agents.[44] Although these results suggest an association between increased suicidality and Prozac, they do not prove Prozac induces suicidal thinking. An alternative explanation is that the patients taking Prozac were more severely depressed in the first place (they had tried other antidepressants without success before Prozac).

Eli Lilly and the FDA say Prozac was tested on 5,600 patients. The FDA has detected no "worrisome patterns to date."[45] The suicide effects are attributed by the FDA to the mental illness rather than the Prozac.

CLOZAPINE (BRAND NAME CLOZARIL)

Clozapine (Brand Name Clozaril)

A new drug available for severely ill schizophrenics. There are some side effects to watch for such as convulsions and agranulocytosis, a serious blood disorder that reduces the number of white blood cells (the body's disease-fighting cells).

Clozapine is currently being used in Europe to help control schizophrenia and was approved by the Food and Drug Administration in February 1990.[46] It is a patented product, available in the United States under the brand name Clozaril. It is made by Sandoz Pharmaceuticals in New Jersey. At the present time only 5,500 Americans are in therapy with clozapine because it is so expensive; the treatment costs nearly $9,000 a year. The cost per week in the United States is approximately $172 compared to $20 or $30 in Europe. The situation has stirred outrage from patients, lawmakers, public-health professionals, insurance officials, and mental-health professionals.[47]

Some see clozapine as a miracle aid in the treatment of schizophrenia. Schizophrenia now affects over 2 million Americans and has been a concern for a long time. The FDA has approved clozapine for management of severely ill schizophrenic patients who fail to respond adequately to standard antipsychotic drug treatment. Clozapine has at least two serious side effects, however. One out of 20 patients suffers from convulsive seizures, and 1 or 2 out of 100 suffer from agranulocytosis.[48] Agranulocytosis is a serious blood disorder in which the number of white blood cells (the body's disease-fighting cells) are reduced, leaving the patient vulnerable to infection. A simple blood test can detect this decrease, and early detection along with the discontinuation of clozapine can decrease the risk of death. The rate of seizures can also be controlled. Lowering the dose of clozapine or adding an anticonvulsant drug usually controls the seizures. Clozapine has also proved to be free of other side effects typically found with the antipsychotic drugs, such as tardive dyskinesia, rigidity, masklike facial expression, or slowed movements. It must be stressed that the severity of chronic schizophrenia that may cause patients to live tormented and hopeless lives makes clozapine a drug worth the risk.

ACCUTANE

In 1982 Accutane, a derivative of vitamin A, was approved by the FDA because it was incredibly successful in treating severe cases of acne. However, a package insert warns females not to use the drug if they are pregnant or plan to become pregnant during its use. Severe birth defects can occur in babies born to women who used Accutane during pregnancy. Since Accutane hit the market, between 60 and 600 infants have been deformed because their mothers used it while they were pregnant.[49]

Because Accutane is such a powerful and potent drug, researchers are thinking about taking it off the market.[50] Accutane is intended to be a drug of last resort for acne that hasn't responded to any other type of treatment.

LITHIUM

CLASSIFICATION

Lithium is a metallic salt that can be administered as a strong antimanic tranquilizer in individuals who are suffering from a biochemical imbalance in portions of the brain that causes violent or manic behavior.

PHARMACOLOGY

Lithium helps to normalize mood and behavior in those with chronic manic-depressive illness by correcting chemical imbalances in certain nerve-impulse transmitters that can influence emotion and behavior.[51] Current thinking is that excessive levels of norepinephrine in certain sections of the brain can lead to excessive behavior characterized by emotional instability and potential violence.[52] Lithium helps reduce excessive norepinephrine firings so as to bring a person back to more normal behavior.

Lithium possesses one quality that makes it completely unlike any other drug used in psychiatry. It does not metabolize—it retains its physical integrity in the body and does not bind to any blood or tissue protein. This unique characteristic enables a physician to precisely monitor the amount of the drug in the brain or kidney. This can be done by simply determining lithium's concentration in the blood.

MEDICAL USE

Lithium's unique psychoactive qualities are of great significance in the treatment of manic depression, a disease consisting of sudden and intense mood swings. Not only does the drug inhibit depression, it curbs hyperexcitability (mania) without producing the "blanket suppressions of behavior characteristic of the standard sedatives."[53] Daily treatment with lithium brings patients to more "normal" moods and even makes it possible for some hospitalized patients to return home on only a maintenance dosage.[54]

Lithium has a very narrow margin of safe use. The level of drug required to be effective is quite close to the level that can have adverse effects. Careful dosage adjustments based on periodic measurements of blood levels are mandatory.[55]

Though lithium has many beneficial qualities, it can have adverse effects in some patients. These may include nausea, tremors, tiredness, dry mouth, and difficulty in organizing thoughts. Such effects, though, are generally mild and short-lived.[56] An overdose will affect the central nervous system, resulting in hypertonic or rigid muscles, gross contraction of skeletal muscles,[57] and possibly coma.

CONTRACEPTIVES

HISTORY

The capacity of hormones to prevent ovulation was first noted in animal experiments in 1921. Further experiments in the 1930s and 1940s clearly demonstrated that daily doses of female sex hormones, especially estrogen and progesterone, would prevent ovulation in laboratory animals.

In 1960 the first oral contraceptive, consisting of a combination of synthetic female hormones, was marketed in the United States. The Pill was heralded as a major breakthrough in the field of birth control, and was first viewed by most as the ideal contraceptive. Not only did the Pill appear to be nearly infallible as a contraceptive, but it also helped women feel secure about their birth control method. The Pill was also easy to use, and it increased independent behavior. By 1970 about 19 million women around the world were using oral contraceptives, which soon became the most popular means of birth control.[58]

Extensive controversy concerning the Pill's safety did not arise until the late 1960s, when various side effects of the drug gained worldwide prominence. Many women began to feel uneasy about taking the Pill, yet in the minds of many others the Pill's advantages still far outweighed its possible adverse effects. Today, use of oral contraceptives continues, but physicians are required to describe the drug's side effects and risks before prescribing it.

COMPOSITION AND USE

The oral contraceptive is composed of synthetic estrogens designed to prevent ovulation, thus making pregnancy impossible, and progestins, which allow the menstrual cycle to continue. The quantities of progestin and estrogen used in the various brands differ markedly, although current trends indicate a reduction in dose size to reduce the risk of blood clotting. In addition to birth control applications, oral contraceptives are used to treat certain disorders of the Fallopian tubes, menopausal stress, and menstrual irregularities.

MECHANISM

The estrogen in oral contraceptives inhibits factors involved in ovulation; progestin prevents ovulation itself and regulates the growth of the uterine lining, which is discharged as "menstrual bleeding."[59] According to Philip Corfman, director of the U.S. Center for Population Research at the Department of Health and Human Services, oral contraceptives appear to inhibit conception in six different ways:

> First, by acting on the pituitary gland, oral contraceptives inhibit the production of certain reproductive hormones. Second, [they] alter the state of the endometrium, which is the mucus coat of the uterus. Third, the progestins may alter the cervical mucus and thus create a plug to prevent the ascent of the sperm. Fourth, the oral contraceptives may alter the motility of the Fallopian tubes, again making it difficult for sperm to meet egg. Fifth, the progestogen factor may prevent capacitation, which is the ability of the

sperm to enter the egg. Sixth, the pill may have a direct inhibiting effect on the ovaries' release of eggs—apart from the effect it exercises through the pituitary hormones.[60]

Theoretically, any method having only one of these effects would prevent pregnancy. If all six actions are taken, as they are by some contraceptive preparations, the chance of pregnancy is extremely remote. Statistics show that if the Pill is taken regularly for a year, less than 1 pregnancy per 1,000 women results, making oral contraception the most effective method of birth control.[61] The failure rate of the intrauterine device (IUD) is 19 pregnancies per 1,000 women, that of the condom 26 per 1,000, and that of the diaphragm 179 per 1,000.[62]

POSSIBLE SIDE EFFECTS

Routine side effects in users of oral contraceptives include some retention of fluid with possible weight gain, spotting in the middle of the menstrual cycle, a change in the menstrual flow, breast tenderness, and an increased susceptibility to yeast infections.

Adverse reactions include pain or tenderness in the leg, which could indicate thrombophlebitis (an inflammation of a vein in the leg), with a resultant blood clot.[63] Shortness of breath, chest pain, or coughing could indicate a pulmonary embolism (the movement of a blood clot into the lungs). In some women the risk of stroke (a blood clot in the brain) is increased, so strong headaches, blackouts, sudden weakness, or paralysis of any part of the body should be immediately reported to a physician. Other rare circulatory problems with oral contraceptives can include retinal thrombosis (a blood clot in the eye), which manifests itself as a sudden impairment of vision, and heart attacks, which show up as a sudden pain in the chest, neck, or arm accompanied by weakness, sweating, and nausea. Other rare adverse reactions include a rise in blood pressure in some sensitive individuals, impairment of the liver, and depression.

The birth control pill is still a very controversial form of birth control. Three newer studies by experts relate birth control pills to cancer; however, the Food and Drug Administration said the findings from these studies were not serious enough to change the warning labels in the way they are prescribed.[64] The first study was conducted at Boston University School of Medicine to compare 400 women on the Pill with 400 others. They found that women on the Pill for less than ten years were twice as likely to develop breast cancer than the others. A second study, conducted in England, looked at 47,000 women, half of whom were on the Pill. They found no difference between the groups except for the 30–34-year-olds, where those on the Pill showed three times as much breast cancer as those not on the Pill. The third study showed that women in the high-risk group—those who menstruated before the age of 13 and those who never had children—did have a higher incidence of cancer if they were Pill users. In fact, within this group, women who had been on the Pill for 12 years or more were 12 times more likely to develop cancer than nonusers.

The experts are very concerned because breast cancer affects 130,000 American women every year, with 42,000 of those cases ending up in death.[65] Thirteen million American women use oral contraceptives and 1 in 11 develops the disease.

Effects from Smoking While Taking the Pill   The risks associated with the Pill are also affected by age, smoking, medical history, and length of use. Being over 35 increases the risks, as does smoking. "Smokers on the pill are 22 times as likely to have a blood clotting problem.[66] This large increase in risk associated with smoking extends beyond just blood-clot formation. Almost all hazards are increased when a woman on the Pill smokes. Medical history is important because a history of high blood pressure or high cholesterol increases the risk of recurrence of these negative side effects. Combining any two of these risk factors increases the user's chances of having one or more of the major problems that may accompany taking the Pill.[67]

Cancer and Tumors   Medical experts are still arguing over whether the hormones found in oral contraceptives (which create changes in the tissue lining of the uterus and cervix) cause cancer, stimulate an existing cancer, or encourage the development of a cancer. Since some cancers take as long as 15 to 20 years to develop, and since oral contraceptives were not put on the market until 1960, conclusive evidence is still unavailable. However, increased hormonal secretions may stimulate malignant growths. Regular Pap smears and breast examinations will greatly reduce the chance of such growths going undetected.

A study of the relationship between liver tumors and oral-contraceptive use in young women found that clinical symptoms of tumors were more severe among users. The study also confirmed the association between oral-contraceptive use and focal nodular hyperplasias (excessive formations of tissue due to an increase in the number of cells). These results may be somewhat subjective because of researcher interpretation, but they do appear to indicate probable relationships between tumors and oral-contraceptive use.[68]

Cancer is one of the biggest fears women have about using oral contraceptives. The probability of developing cancer varies with the individual. Developing cervical cancer depends on the woman's age and the number of years she has been on the Pill. The more sexual partners a woman has, the greater her chances of cervical cancer. Early detection is the best defense against cancer, and the only way to detect cervical cancer is a Pap smear— which is why women on the Pill should see their doctor once a year. On the other hand, the risk of breast cancer does not increase with the use of the Pill. This was proved in research by the Centers for Disease Control (CDC).[69] The reduced risk of developing epithelial ovarian cancer in women on the Pill was also proved by the CDC. The use of the Pill protects against both ovarian and uterine cancers. This effect can last up to 15 years after the last use of the Pill.

Heart Disease   In the past few years researchers have found other health benefits for women who take birth control pills. Among these are a lower risk of tubal pregnancies and less painful menstrual cramps.[70] Now it appears a lower risk of heart disease may soon be added to the list.

According to Ronald T. Burkman, chairman of the Department of Obstetrics and Gynecology at Henry Ford Hospital in Detroit, a certain type of birth control pill, Demulen, increases high-density lipoproteins and apolipoprotein A-1, two substances that help prevent coronary heart disease. Burkman says Demulen's effect on HDL levels is small—only 2 to 3 percent—but that over long periods this might be enough to benefit the cardiovascular system.

Synergism and the Pill   There are still problems with using oral contraceptives, even for a healthy young woman. A study by the Food and Drug Administration determined that the Pill does not mix well with other drugs.[71] This was first discovered in the 1970s when women on the Pill used a common medication for tuberculosis, Rifampicin. The combination of Rifampicin and the Pill diminished the effectiveness of the Pill, and women became pregnant. It turned out that the combination of the two drugs increases the metabolism of the contraceptive. This can also happen when the woman uses antibiotics such as isonaizid, ampicillin, nitrofurantoin, and griseofulvin. Also affected when a woman uses the Pill are Phenytoin and Primidone—anticonvulsants used by epileptics—and the antiinflammatory agent phenylbutazone. A more common synergistic mixture is tranquilizers, antimigraine medicine, and the Pill. There are women who are unaware of the dangers of combining oral contraceptives with certain other drugs.

A PILL FOR MALES

Chinese scientists have developed a male birth control pill that has been 99 percent effective for the 10,000 men tested so far.[72] The pill, called gossypol, is a compound extracted from cotton seed. It apparently works directly on the testes, impairing sperm production, but must be taken for at least two months before infertility occurs. The effects of the pill are reversible, with sperm counts generally returning to normal three months after the pill's discontinuation. During a 15-month study period, male sex hormone levels remained normal and little difference was observed between androgen (male hormone) levels before and after the experiment. Though some men complained of reduced sex drive, none complained of impotency. With so many apparent advantages, this contraceptive may prove to be of great value.

DEPO PROVERA

The Food and Drug Administration recently approved Depo Provera for use as an injectable contraceptive that gives three months of birth control with each shot.[73] Family planning doctors hailed the action, predicting that it would be embraced by hundreds of thousands of U.S. women eager for a long-term contraceptive that requires no maintenance except a new injection every 90 days. Depo Provera is injected into the muscle of the arm or buttock, where it is released into the bloodstream to prevent pregnancy. It is thought to be more than 99 percent effective, meaning that less than one unplanned pregnancy occurs for every hundred users each year.

Depo Provera contains the drug medroxyprogesterone acetate, a synthetic hormone similar to the natural hormone progesterone. It inhibits ovulation by suppressing the hormones secreted by the pituitary gland that stimulate the release of a mature egg. It is estimated that the cost will be $25 to $30 for each injection after the first one, which will cost more because of the need for a full examination and medical history of the patient.

NORPLANT

Norplant, the first new contraceptive approved by the U.S. government in nearly 30 years, is expected to appeal most to young women who are not ready to begin having children and older ones who want to stop.[74] It appears to be a safe method of birth control for any age woman, according to Francine Sinosky, an obstetrician-gynecologist at Robert Wood Johnson Medical School in New Brunswick, New Jersey. Norplant is a long-lasting contraceptive that is implanted under the skin. It prevents pregnancy by using the hormone progestin, which with estrogen is the active ingredient in most birth control pills. Norplant consists of six progestin-filled silicone tubes about the size of matchsticks that are inserted just beneath the skin of a woman's upper arm. Once in place, they slowly secrete the hormone and prevent pregnancy for five years.[75] The drawbacks are irregular menstrual bleeding and the cost, which will run about $500—actually less than that for five years of an oral contraceptive. The advantages are, first, that it is very reliable. During the first two years, the implant had one-tenth to one-twentieth the failure rate of oral contraceptives, which fail 3 percent of the time. Second, Norplant also requires only one birth control decision every five years, and if a woman wishes to become pregnant before the five years are up, the tubes can be removed and fertility restored within 24 hours.[76]

How Norplant Works

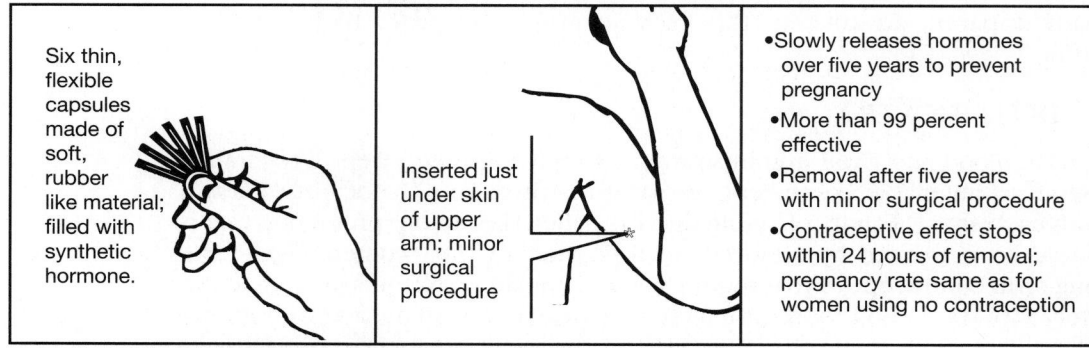

Six thin, flexible capsules made of soft, rubber like material; filled with synthetic hormone.

Inserted just under skin of upper arm; minor surgical procedure

- Slowly releases hormones over five years to prevent pregnancy
- More than 99 percent effective
- Removal after five years with minor surgical procedure
- Contraceptive effect stops within 24 hours of removal; pregnancy rate same as for women using no contraception

Source: "Norplant System Ready to Go," *Eugene-Register Guard,* December 12, 1990, p. A.

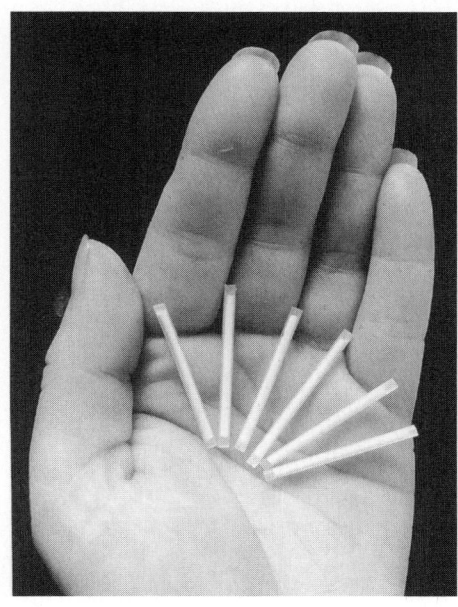

Will Norplant Be the New Form of Birth Control?
Source: Hank Morgan/Science Source/Photo Researchers

RU 486

There is now a pill called **RU 486** that, when swallowed, will cause the pregnant woman to abort her fetus within 24 hours. What some call "a remarkable breakthrough," and others "chemical warfare on unborn babies," this pill has not yet been approved for use in the United States and is causing a ruckus among activists all over the world.[77] As of right now, it is legal only in France and China.

In the United States 1.6 million abortions are performed legally each year. David Grimes and Daniel Mishell have begun testing RU 486 at the University of Southern California Medical Center and believe it is much safer than an abortion operation.[78] They also said, "It was the most exciting breakthrough in fertility in a quarter of a century." The pill has proved to work in just five weeks after conception, when it is both safe and 95 percent effective. In France more than 10,000 RU 486 abortions have taken place since the product was introduced. It is used only in designated hospitals and clinics. Women must wait a full week for assurance that this is what they want to do before they can take it.

RU 486 is an antiprogesterone steroid that destroys the uterine lining, at least in most cases, starving out the already attached fetus, which dies and is expelled.[79] The pill has been on the French market since September 1988. Meanwhile, no U.S. pharmaceutical company to date has shown the slightest interest in manufacturing or marketing it. Part of the reason for the drug industry's reluctance is probably fear of a massive boycott by the right-to-life movement of the drug company's other products. But the main reason for the hesitancy on RU 486 is undoubtedly fear of liability exposure.

RU 486

An antiprogesterone that destroys the uterine lining, at least in most cases, starving out the already attached fetus, which dies and is expelled.

FERTILITY PILLS

INTRODUCTION

Until the late 1950s, methods used to induce ovulation in women who were not ovulating remained largely unsuccessful. With the discovery of the two major fertility pills, clomiphene citrate (Clomid) and the human menopausal gonadotropin (Pergonal), the success rate improved. Clomiphene citrate is a synthetic estrogen that was originally expected to act as a contraceptive, and the human menopausal gonadotropin (HMG) is a substance originally isolated from the urine of postmenopausal nuns.[80] HMG is usually more effective in producing ovulation that clomiphene: One study found that two thirds of all anovulatory women treated with HMG become pregnant, compared with 20 to 30 percent of women who have clomiphene-citrate treatment.[81] Even so, clomiphene is often preferable: It has fewer side effects, is fairly inexpensive, and is taken for fewer days.

METHOD OF TREATMENT

Normal ovulation depends on a functioning relationship among the hypothalamus, the pituitary gland, and the ovaries. Any disturbance in this relationship may result in anovulation, the failure of an ovum to be released. When used to treat anovulation, clomiphene citrate enlarges the ovaries and increases the release of ovary-stimulating hormones. The amount of clomiphene citrate used in infertility procedures must be carefully monitored, however, because too small a dose will only supplement natural estrogens and have no evident influence on the ovaries.

When infertility treatment begins, one 50-milligram dose per day, taken orally or intravenously, is given to the patient for five days, generally from the fifth to the tenth day of the menstrual cycle. (Approximately half the drug is excreted within five days after it is taken.) After five days of treatment, instructions are given for the timing of intercourse, which for optimal results should take place every other day between the fifth and fifteenth day following the last dose of clomiphene. During this time, the basal body temperature must be carefully checked because a rise in temperature is one indication that pregnancy has taken place.[82]

If the first treatment with clomiphene is ineffective, the dose may be cautiously raised to 100 milligrams after a 30-day interval, and 5 days of doses are again administered. If this second treatment is also ineffective, one more treatment may be tried, although this decision and subsequent ones should rest solely in the hands of the patient and the physician.

Women who do not respond to three series of 100-milligram-per-day treatments may then be put on the human menopausal gonadotropin, a more powerful fertility drug. HMG doses are generally administered for 9 to 12 days and are thought to stimulate follicles that encourage the development of immature ova, though this is still uncertain.

POSSIBLE SIDE EFFECTS

Ovarian enlargement, with or without cyst formation, occurs in 14 percent of all clomiphene citrate–treated women and is considered the major side effect of the drug.[83] Pelvic tenderness or discomfort from cysts can be diminished with estrogen treatment and reduced doses of clomiphene. Women with ovarian cysts prior to treatment should not use clomiphene, and those with enlarged ovaries should take only small doses. Cysts usually subside following discontinuation of clomiphene, but if left untreated, they may burst, leading to internal hemorrhaging and death. Ovarian cysts are an even greater risk for women using Pergonal.

Hot flashes are another side effect, prevalent in 10 to 11 percent of clomiphene users; they are similar to hot flashes experienced during menopause.[84] This intermittent flushing is thought to be caused by the antiestrogen effect of clomiphene and is usually painless, dissipating once clomiphene intake ceases.

Side effects involving vision occasionally occur in clomiphene patients. Though these reactions are generally minimal, some persons have blurred vision or see spots or flashes of light. Such occurrences should be given special consideration, since they may be dangerous if experienced during activities requiring motor skills. Side effects involving sight are generally reversed once clomiphene treatment ceases.

Though most side effects of fertility-pill treatment are generally minimal, some more adverse reactions have been experienced. These include nausea, vomiting, increased nervous tension, headaches, allergic dermatitis, loss of hair, depression, fatigue, breast soreness, weight gain, increased appetite, increased urination, and heavy menstruation.

MULTIPLE BIRTHS

Though fertility-pill treatment often results in pregnancy, more than one child sometimes results from that pregnancy. Between 8 percent and 10 percent of clomiphene-treated patients give birth to two or more children in one delivery.[85]

> One theory holds that excessive dosage levels cause many ova to ripen simultaneously, but most experts agree that imprecise timing is the real problem. In natural ovulation, they say, the ovary has a way of signaling the presence of a single ripe ovum to the pituitary gland, which responds instantly by producing hormones that trigger the ovary to ovulate and cause further maturation of ova to cease. But apparently, chemicals that stimulate ovulation disrupt this delicate mechanism.[86]

The infants are not identical in drug-induced multiple births, since each child develops from a separate egg. Identical offspring are more likely to result from natural ovulation when one fertilized egg separates.

MENOPAUSE AND ESTROGEN REPLACEMENT THERAPY

Somewhere between the ages of 45 and 55, women experience a year or two of irregular periods, fluctuations in body temperature, and sleepless nights.

The good news is that approximately 70 percent of the women find relief when taking estrogen supplements; the bad news is that only 10 percent take them because of fear. Fear stories have been associated with the use of estrogen replacement therapy (ERT). In 1975 estrogen was the fifth most prescribed drug in the United States.[87] But, also in 1975, a report came out saying that estrogen use for more than 15 years increases the risk of uterine cancer.

Studies have also indicated, however, that estrogen can lower the risk of osteoporosis, cardiovascular disease, and other diseases. The question is: "Who's at risk and who is not?" Further research is needed to answer this question.

ACQUIRED IMMUNODEFICIENCY SYNDROME

Drugs for viral infections have had little success, and since the discovery of Acquired Immunodeficiency Syndrome (AIDS) the pharmacological industry has been gloomy about it. Making drugs that harm the virus but not the cell is the big challenge, for AIDS not only takes up residence but also puts its genes into cell DNA, which makes it more difficult for a drug to distinguish between cell and virus. However, more than 25 potential anti-HIV compounds are being tested, and the thought about AIDS has changed from "You will die and there is nothing we can do" to "AIDS is becoming a treatable disease."[88]

Progress has been made through understanding the virus's biology, from introduction to a cell becoming a viral factory. Cells invaded by AIDS have receptor sites called CD4 receptors on their surface. A drug developed to block the process is a synthetic CD4. It bonds to receptor sites on the virus before it can bind to real CD4; therefore the virus can't infect cells.

A few drugs for which researchers report some success with AIDS are AZT (azidothymidine or zidovudine), dextran sulfate, and Drug 566.

AZIDOTHYMIDINE

AZT acts as a vehicle for the HIV-RNA to transcribe its genetic message to the cell DNA, but the AZT was legalized by the FDA for AIDS patients before it was proved whether it was safe or not.[89] Some feel it was released prematurely because of intense pressure from AIDS lobbyers . It is felt the drug can extend the AIDS patient's life or do nothing at all. There are also those who feel this compassionate argument ends up having more to do with greed and profit than it does with real compassion. AZT treatment costs between $7,000 and $10,000 a year, although efforts are being made to lower the cost and it appears the dosage may also be able to be lowered while allowing the patient to receive the same benefits.

DEXTRAN SULFATE

Dextran sulfate is a drug that seems to block HIV virus in early Japanese tests.[90] It is a blood thinner that remains illegal in the United States, but AIDS patients are finding ways to obtain the drug. Kowa Pharmaceuticals announced it would allow dextran-sulfate imports by individuals for "personal use" but would crack down on profiteering.[91]

Dextran sulfate is a more proven drug than others. It has been used for 20 years in Japan as an anticholesterol drug. After Japanese chemists told the FDA in 1986 that the drug would stop the cell-to-cell spread of HIV virus, *in vitro* studies at the National Cancer Institute in Bethesda, Maryland, confirmed this.[92]

Another reason AIDS patients get excited about dextran sulfate is that it is inexpensive. With ten 40¢ pills a day, the standard dosage, dextran sulfate costs $1,000 a year, compared to $7,000 or more a year for AZT. Also, whereas AZT is often toxic, dextran sulfate appears safe. Americans can now buy up to 10,000 tablets of dextran sulfate a year.

DRUG 566

Burroughs Wellcome Company, the developer of AZT, has come out with a new and potentially life-saving therapy for pneumoncystis carinil pneumonia, an extremely serious respiratory infection that is the leading cause of death in AIDS patients.[93] The new drug, known as 566C80, or 566, provides an alternative for the estimated 30 to 50 percent of AIDS patients who cannot tolerate the significant side effects of the standard treatments, or for whom the other drugs are ineffective.

"The most serious side effects of 566 include severe rashes, fever, which have been experienced by a small number of patients, milder rashes, digestive problems, and minor blood abnormalities."[94]

STREPTOKINASE

Streptokinase comes from a family of drugs used as a clot-dissolving medication for people whose heart attacks are caused by blood clots. Streptokinase is called a "clot-buster." This miracle drug has been widely used in European hospitals with very significant results.[95] In one study involving over 11,000 heart-attack victims, deaths were reduced by 18 percent. When the drug was given to patients within the first hour of the attack, deaths dropped by 47 percent. In another study of 17,187 clot-buster treatments in 400 hospitals around the world, streptokinase, when used with aspirin, reduced deaths by 42 percent.[96] European doctors collectively believe that if clot-busting drugs were used in all hospitals, "several tens of thousands of deaths should be avoided each year." Jeffrey Borer of Cornell University states, "Clot-busters are the biggest advance since coronary-care units twenty-five years ago."[97]

CHOLESTEROL-LOWERING AGENTS

Numerous genetic, epidemologic, and experimental animal and clinical trials have supported the idea that there is a causal relationship between blood-cholesterol levels and coronary heart disease. There is also substantial evidence that lowering total and low-density lipoprotein-cholesterol levels will lead to reductions in the incidence of coronary heart disease.[98] For individuals who are unable to lower their cholesterol through diet and exercise, cholesterol-lowering drugs are often recommended.

There are currently eight cholesterol-lowering agents on the market. Lovastatin, a new class of drugs, was approved for marketing in the United States by the Food and Drug Administration in August 1987. Studies show that this drug has the properties of substantially lowering plasma levels of total, LDL, and very low-density lipoprotein cholesterol, triglycerides, and apoliporotein B, and of increasing plasma levels of high-density lipoprotein cholesterol.[99] Lovastatin is a chemical that can prohibit the liver from producing cholesterol, which could save millions of Americans each year from the risk of developing heart disease.[100] It won't stop people from eating bacon cheeseburgers (which can cause numerous ills besides high cholesterol), but it will probably make them feel better about it.

Retail pharmacies dispensed an estimated 4.4 million prescriptions for cholesterol-lowering drugs in the United States in 1987. This number declined to 2.6 million in 1983 and then increased dramatically to nearly 13 million in 1988.[101]

Many of these drugs are just the things doctors have been waiting for to help make their jobs a little bit easier, but one wonders if we humans will ever learn to stop relying on technological crutches and start using good habits, instead.

PEPTIDE T

Candace Pert, a neuropharmacist, focuses on brain research where she is known to be on the cutting edge of discovery and is now involved in determining the value of all peptides to drug medicine.[102] She believes peptide drugs may be the key treatment for diseases such as AIDS, schizophrenia, cancer, stroke, multiple sclerosis, Alzheimer's, asthma, and arthritis. Peptides are hormones that control communication between the brain and body cells. They are essentially a short string of amino acids. There are 60 to 70 peptides. They transmit information from the brain to the immune systems, to the organs, and to other systems in the body. Peptides may underlie all our emotions that provide a physical link between the mind and body.[103] Peptide receptors may be sites where viruses locate.

Pert maintains that a synthetic peptide called Peptide T (a drug) can block disease invasions so they do not locate on peptide receptors. She maintains that if this proves true, the drug will unlock many of the bottlenecks to curing diseases. The drug has tremendous promise but must go through further clinical trials. Peptide T may be one of the new miracle drugs of this decade. Drug technology has evolved into an exciting and fascinating field that may change the future course of various diseases and ailments.

FOOD ADDITIVES

INTRODUCTION

In a single year, people consume several kilograms of preservatives, colorings, flavorings, and other additives.[104] Yet we know very little about the effects these chemicals may have on our health. Food additives are chemicals, primarily nonnutritive ones, that are added to foods during growing or processing. These chemicals are added to maintain or improve nutritional value, to maintain freshness, to help in processing or preparation, or to make food more appealing.

> Food additives are so much a part of the American way of eating today that most of us would find it difficult to put together a meal that did not include them.
>
> Take a typical lunch, for example: sandwich, instant soup, gelatin dessert, and a cola drink. The bread has been fortified with vitamins and also contains an additive to keep it fresh. The margarine has been colored pale yellow—or, if you use salad dressing, it has been made with emulsifiers to keep it from "separating." The luncheon meat contains nitrite; the soup, an additive to keep it from becoming rancid; the gelatin, red coloring to make it pretty. Finally, the cola to wash it all down: Without coloring, flavoring, sweeteners, or artificial carbonation, the pause that refreshes is nothing more than plain water![105]

Agents that modify the appearance of foods are called thickeners, firmers, stabilizers, or emulsifiers. They are found in such products as peanut butter, in which they keep the oils from separating from the water-soluble components. Chemicals such as monoglycerides and diglycerides are used to increase volume or add uniformity and fineness to products. Antispoilants, such as calcium and sodium propionate, butylated hydroxyanisole (BHA), and butylated hydroxytoluene (BHT)—the last of which was determined to be unsafe—are used to preserve foods and lengthen their shelf life by preventing deterioration. Substances such as glycerine are added to foods to control moisture content. Other substances are added to alter natural processes; examples are ethylene, used to quick-ripen bananas, and malic hydroazide, used to prevent potatoes from sprouting.

Although chemicals with hard-to-pronounce names are common food additives, the most widely used additives are sugar, salt, and corn syrup. These three, plus such other substances as citric acid (found in oranges and lemons), baking soda, vegetable colors, mustard, and pepper, account for more than 98 percent, by weight, of all food additives used in this country.[106]

HISTORY

The use of food additives to preserve and enhance the flavor and appearance of food is not new. Salt was used to preserve meats and spices to flavor foods since early times, and it is said that the expeditions of Marco Polo and Columbus were motivated in part by the desire to find new spices for these uses. Today's additives, however, are more diverse and used more extensively, and efforts to improve and preserve foods have moved from worldwide exploration to laboratory research.

As the use of additives proliferated, concern about their effects and hazards also increased. In 1938 the Federal Food, Drug, and Cosmetic Act strengthened the 1906 Pure Food and Drug Act, authorizing potency tests for some substances and banning formaldehyde use; the act also gave the Food and Drug Administration authority to inspect processing plants. It wasn't until 1958, however, that the United States passed legislation regulating food additives. The Food Additive Amendment prohibited use of additives in amounts known to produce cancers, and required that substances be proved safe before being put into public use. To prove a product safe, manufacturers must first subject the additive to a battery of chemical tests and then feed the additive in large doses over an extended period to at least two kinds of animals, usually rodents and dogs. Manufacturers must then submit the results of all these tests to the FDA, and if they indicate the additive is safe, the agency establishes regulations for how it can be used in food. A basic rule is a 100-fold margin of safety for anything added to food. This means that the manufacturer may use in a food product only 1/100th the maximum amount of an additive that has been found not to produce any harmful effects in test animals.[107]

> Under the Food Additives Amendment two major categories of additives are exempt from the testing and approval process. The first is a group of some 700 substances "generally recognized as safe" (GRAS) by qualified experts. The idea behind what has come to be known as the GRAS List was to free FDA and manufacturers from being required to prove the safety of substances already considered harmless because of past extensive use with no known harmful effect. Their efforts, it was felt, would be better spent on new additives and on those compounds about which less is known.
>
> Also exempt from testing were "prior sanctioned substances," those that had been approved before 1958 for use in food by either FDA or the U.S. Department of Agriculture. Some prior sanctioned substances also were included on the GRAS List.
>
> These lists of exemptions are not, however, engraved in stone. As testing methods and scientific understanding of toxicology improve, new evidence and questions may arise about the safety of old standbys. To make sure these substances are judged by the latest scientific standards, FDA is reviewing all categories of food additives.[108]

In 1960 the Color Additive Amendments were passed, subjecting coloring agents used in foods, drugs, and cosmetics to rigorous premarket testing. Colors in use when the amendment was passed were placed on a provisional approval list pending further investigation or confirmation of their safety. Nearly 200 coloring agents have been on the provisional approval list at one time or another, but only 31 colors are currently fully approved for use in foods. Chemicals were dropped from the list because manufacturers were no longer interested in marketing them or because they were found to be unsafe. In 1976, for example, the FDA banned Red Dye No. 2, then the most widely used red coloring agent, because tests done on animals could not resolve whether the dye cause cancer in humans.[109]

In 1974 another piece of food additive legislation was passed—the Consumer Food Act. It was designed to close existing legal loopholes in the approval system, strengthen monitoring procedures, and extend labeling requirements.

PRESERVATIVES

This important group of additives consists of chemicals that slow food deterioration. They are particularly important in many processed meat, fish, and cheese products. Drying was one of the earliest forms of preserving food. Later, salt pickling, vinegar pickling, and smoking were used. These traditional methods are still used today, but food chemists have created an array of chemical preservatives that are more popular with the food industry. The ability to give food products longer "shelf life" is of enormous economic value to the food industry, and is of some nutritional value to consumers.[110]

Sulfiting agents are popular preservatives in the food industry. Sulfiting agents such as sodium bisulfite and sodium metabisulfite are marketed as "vegetable fresheners" or "whitening" agents. They are also used by the food-service industry—restaurant salad bars, for example—to keep lettuce, potatoes, and other vegetables "fresh," crisp, and free from discoloration when cut or peeled.[111] Sulphur dioxide and related sulfites maintain the pale color of everything from flour to sausages and beer.

Sulfites are particularly hazardous to asthmatics. Over 10 million Americans suffer from asthma, and experts estimate that up to 1 million of them have an extreme sensitivity to sulfites.

NITRITES AND NITRATES

Nitrites and nitrates have been used to preserve meats since the nineteenth century. They protect against the growth of deadly botulism spores. Unfortunately, even small amounts of nitrites and nitrates act as concentrated carcinogens when ingested.[112] But although they are two of the most carcinogenic additives known, having been linked with cancer of the liver and intestinal tract, they are also two of the most popular. They are used not only in meats but also in cheeses and canned foods.

ADVERSE EFFECTS

Additives share with all drugs the potential for precipitating allergic reactions in some individuals. Though inconclusive, evidence suggests a link between processed "convenience" foods (rich in additives) and hyperkinesis in children. Moreover, certain additives, including cyclamates, nitrates, nitrites, saccharin, and dietheyl-pyrocarbonate (DEPC), have been linked to an increased incidence of various cancers. Finally, studies have shown that food colorings Red Dye No. 2 and Red Dye No. 4 cause carcinogenic tumors in laboratory animals.[113]

Still other additives appear to have adverse effects. Nitrates and nitrites have been shown to reduce oxygen transportation by the blood, in addition to being implicated in stomach, liver, and gastrointestinal cancers. Monosodium glutamate can cause headaches, sweating, nausea, thirst, flushing, tightness in the face or chest, and abdominal pains in doses of 2 to 12 grams. It is not totally clear what effects food additives have on the fetus, but many of these substances have low molecular weights and this may allow them to cross the placental barrier.

SUCROSE (SUGAR)

Researchers have found that ingestion of sucrose leads to an increase in triglyceride production.[114] Albrink and colleagues studied men who had been put on low-cholesterol diets because of an increased risk of heart disease. They found that many of the men substituted sucrose for the fat they had to abstain from. The men who had high-sucrose diets did not experience a drop in cholesterol while on the low-fat diet, whereas those who ate very little sucrose saw their cholesterol levels plunge. Other studies have found a synergistic effect of sucrose and animal fat in increasing serum lipids, and a lowering by sucrose of high-density lipoproteins in the blood.[115]

Studies on the behavioral effects of sucrose have focused mainly on antisocial behavior and hyperactivity. A study based on anecdotal information collected by a probation officer who witnessed a plunge in recidivism rates among her probationers who had eliminated sucrose from their diets led to further investigation. Stephen Schoenthaler decided to institute dietary changes in a juvenile detention home in Virginia. The staff and residents were told that the changes were prompted by budget difficulties. Data from four months prior and three months following were compared. Age, race, gender, and arresting offense were controlled for. The results were astounding: In the months following the new diet, there was a 42 percent drop in antisocial behavior, and 82 percent reduction in assaults, a 77 percent reduction in thefts, and a 65 percent reduction in horseplay. Correctional facilities across the country are considering initiating similar diets.[116]

In a study of preschool children, half were given sucrose equivalent to that in a can of soda and half were given a control drink. Forty-five minutes after ingestion, the sugar-fed children made significantly more errors (a mean of nine versus a mean of three in a control group). The behavior of the sugar-fed children was coded and found inappropriate 29 percent of the time versus 10 percent of the time in the control group.[117] The sugar-fed children were also found to be more distractible on task-orientation tests. The subjects did not include children diagnosed as hyperactive because it was felt that hyperactive children's sensitivity to sugar was already firmly established. In spite of this evidence, the Sugar Task Force, a division of the FDA, has reported that "other than the contribution made to dental caries, there is no clear evidence in the available information that demonstrates a hazard to the public when they are used at the levels that are now current and in the manner now practiced."[118]

Sugar is an additive that may harm consumers through its contribution to obesity. At least one third of our population is overweight, and this extra weight can cause a number of health hazards. Sugar can also play a role in tooth decay.

NUTRASWEET

NutraSweet is a low-calorie sweetener made from protein products that is 180 times sweeter than sugar. It has been a boon not only to its creator, G. D. Searle and Company, but also to the makers of a growing number of consumer products. Strong demand for NutraSweet products comes from aging baby boomers who are concerned about their weight and health. Mothers like NutraSweet because it doesn't promote tooth decay.

NutraSweet, which is patented under the generic name **aspartame,** was first introduced in 1981 in Searle's tabletop sweetener Equal.[119] Now it is available in more than 60 products, including hot cocoa, pudding, chewing gum, tea, and coffee preparations. Besides General Foods, Searle's clients include Coca Cola, Pepsi Cola, Seven Up, Borden, Carnation, H. J. Heinz, and Procter and Gamble.

At the moment you cannot bake with NutraSweet because high heat removes its sweetness. But one day consumers may be able to buy cookies and cakes sweetened with it. Many soft-drink companies now sweeten their products only with NutraSweet because of increased sales from its use.

Asparatame
The generic name for the low-calorie sweetener made from protein products. It is 180 times sweeter than sugar.

SUMMARY

Approximately $30 billion is spent annually on prescription drugs in the United States. It appears that the wonder medicines working their way through the research and development process will keep the pharmaceutical industry prosperous into the next century and provide relief for many Americans.

The use of placebos in medicine is highly controversial. Should they be prescribed? The answer is still unclear. However, with proper administration, placebos do appear to be effective.

Antibiotics, the Wonder Drugs, have revolutionized our society's expectations about drugs. Penicillin, streptomycin, and tetracycline preparations have been extremely effective in fighting harmful bacteria. However, bacterial resistance to antibiotics is increasing as certain bacteria build up immunity to the drugs.

Antidepressants, such as nitrous oxide and lithium, have been used to elevate the spirits of depressed patients. Nitrous oxide may produce a dreamlike, euphoric state, but it is not metabolized, so a doctor can easily monitor the amount of it in a patient's blood.

Dimethyl sulfoxide may be the greatest drug discovery since aspirin. Arthritis sufferers and individuals with muscular ailments are apparently finding great relief through this drug. But it must undergo further testing before it is made available to the public.

Oral contraceptives can dispel the fear of pregnancy as well as enhance sexual fulfillment. However, the pills currently available sometimes lead to health problems. The current AIDS epidemic is also causing many couples to return to the condom as a safe sex practice. A male oral contraceptive called gossypol is being researched by the Chinese. In addition, there is Norplant, a new long-lasting contraceptive that is implanted under the skin, where six progestin-filled silicone tubes secrete the hormone to prevent pregnancy for five years. Also, there is now a pill called RU 486 that, when swallowed, will cause a pregnant woman to abort her fetus within 24 hours.

Fertility pills, such as clomiphene citrate and HMG, encourage ovulation and have helped many women to become pregnant. Administration of fertility pills must be monitored carefully. In some cases, multiple births result.

Food additives are another source of controversy. Though additives help foods look more appealing and add to shelf life, tests indicate that some of them may contribute to hyperkinesis, obesity, cancer, and other adverse conditions.

A whole new series of drugs are currently on the market that will reduce the severity of AIDS, control cholesterol, prevent mental illnesses, and dissolve blot clots.

NutraSweet, a low-calorie sweetener, has made a big hit in the marketplace. It offers sweetness without an increase in calories. In our weight-watching society this makes it an attractive alternative to sugar.

Prescription and Other Drugs
of Interest
N O T E S

1. Kenneth R. Sheets and Robert F. Black, "For Health and Wealth," *U.S. News & World Report,* June 6, 1988, pp. 39–44.
2. "The Safe Use of Medications," *Mayo Clinic Health Letter* 7 no. 2 (February 1989):1–2.
3. Bill Rados, "Survey Finds One in Three 'Uninformed' About Their Rx Drugs," *FDA Consumer* 20, no. 8 (October 1986):30–31.
4. Morton Paulson, "Prescription for Savings: Shop Around," *Changing Times* 44 (February 1990):102.
5. Ibid.
6. Dixie Farley, "How FDA Approves New Drugs," *FDA Consumer 21,* no. 10 (December 1987–January 1988).
7. "Council Proposing FDA Speed Up Drug Approvals," *Register-Guard* (Eugene, Oregon), November 8, 1991, p. 5A.
8. Ibid.
9. David E. Davidson, "Developing New Drugs," *World Health,* June/July 1990, pp. 28–29.
10. John Langone, "Just What the Doctor Ordered," *Science,* September 29, 1989, pp. 1511–12.
11. Ricki Lewis, "Twenty Thousand Drugs under the Sea," *Discover* 9 (May 1988):62–69.
12. Frederick J. Evans, "The Power of the Sugar Pill," *Psychology Today* 9, no. 11 (April 1974). Reprinted with permission from *Psychology Today Magazine,* Copyright © 1974 American Psychological Association (APA).
13. Greg Gregory, "The Power of Suggestion," *Current Health* 15, no. 8 (April 1989):23–25.
14. Dorice Nairns, "Placebos: Mind over Medicine," *Current Health 2* 12, no. 6 (February 1989):11–13.
15. Vance Fitzgerald and Deborah D. Goodwin, "Do Non-Prescription Pain Suppressors Work?" *Psychopharmacology* 88 (1988):1, 112–113.
16. Ibid.
17. Penny Webb, "Man, Magic and the Modern Placebo," *Health Education Journal* 37, no. 2 (June 1978):1–53.
18. Ibid., p. 23.
19. Ibid., p. 24.
20. Carol E. Gammer and Vernon L. Allen, "Note on the Use of Drugs in Psychological Research," *Psychological Reports* 18, no. 2 (January/June 1966):64.

21. Alfred Goodman Gilman, Louis S. Goodman, and Alfred Gilman, eds., *Goodman and Gilman's Pharmaceutical Basis of Therapeutics,* 6th ed. (New York: Macmillan, 1980), p. 47.

22. H. de Wit, E. H. Uhleuhuth, and L. E. Johanson, "Individual Differences in Reinforcing and Subjective Effects of Amphetamines and Diazepam," *Journal of Psychoactive Drugs* 17, no. 4 (1985):219–29.

23. "White Rabbit," *Drug Information Center (DIC)* (Eugene: University of Oregon, 1975), p. 20.

24. Richard Locscher, "Antibiotics: Use and Misuse" (lecture presented at Sacred Heart General Hospital, Eugene, Oregon, January 23, 1974).

25. William Boyd, *An Introduction to the Study of Disease* (Philadelphia: Lea & Febiger, 1971), p. 555.

26. Locscher, "Antibiotics."

27. Ibid.

28. John R. Holum, *Elements of General and Biological Chemistry,* 3rd ed. (New York: John Wiley, 1972), pp. 390–91.

29. Ibid., p. 390.

30. Locscher, "Antibiotics."

31. "White Rabbit," p. 20.

32. Ibid., p. 21.

33. Harold Himwich and Hilma S. Alpers, "Psychopharmacology," *Annual Review of Pharmacology* 10 (1970):320.

34. "Clinical Aspects of Amphetamine Abuse," *Journal of the American Medical Association* 240, no. 21 (November 17, 1978):2317.

35. "White Rabbit," p. 22.

36. Arthur K. Shapiro, "A Historical and Heuristic Definition of Placebo," *Psychiatry* 27, no. 1 (February 1964):52.

37. Joel Kotkin, Robert M. Post, and Frederick K. Goodwin, "Drug Treatment of Depressed Patients Referred for Hospitalization," *American Journal of Psychiatry* 130, no. 10 (October 1973):1141.

38. Robert Julien, *A Primer of Drug Action,* 3rd ed. (San Francisco: W. H. Freeman & Company Publishers, 1981), pp. 75–76.

39. "White Rabbit."

40. Don Mcloud et al., *Drug Information Primer* (Eugene: University of Oregon, 1980), p. 12.

41. "The Dangers of Prozac," *Health Letter,* May 1991, p. 9.

42. Cheryl Sacra, "The New Cure-Alls," *Health,* September 1990, pp. 36–37.

43. "The Dangers of Prozac."

44. Ibid.

45. Anastasia Toufexis, "Warnings about a Miracle Drug," *Time* 136, no. 5 (July 1990):54.

46. Andrew Purvis, "Way out of Reach," *Time,* October 1, 1990, p. 79.

47. Ibid.

48. Judy Folkenberg, "Balancing Hope with Safety," *FDA Consumer* 24 (June 1990):16–21.

49. Susan Brady, "Safe and Effective," *Health* 20, no. 8 (August 1988):11–13.

50. Jack Molloy, "Second Thoughts on Acne Drugs," *Self Magazine,* April 1988.

51. James W. Long, *Essential Guide to Prescription Drugs,* 4th ed. (New York: Harper & Row, 1985), p. 451.

52. Julien, *Primer of Drug Action,* pp. 75–76.

53. Samuel Gershen and Baron Shopoin, eds., *Lithium: Its Role in Psychiatric Research and Treatment* (New York: Plenum, 1973), p. 1.

54. Ibid.

55. James W. Long, *Essential Guide to Prescription Drugs,* 4th ed. (New York: Harper & Row, 1985), p. 451.

56. Joseph Mendels and Steven K. Secunda, eds., *Lithium in Medicine* (New York: Gordon & Breach, 1972), p. 11.

57. Ibid.

58. John P. Bennett, *Chemical Contraception* (New York: Columbia University Press, 1974), p. 29.

59. Ibid.

60. Quoted in Barbara Seaman, "The New Pill Scare," *MS* 3, no. 12 (June 1975):100.

61. Saltman, *The Pill,* p. 36.

62. Ibid.

63. Long, *Essential Guide to Prescription Drugs,* p. 334.

64. Geoffrey Cowley and Mary Hager, "A Scare for Pill Users," *Newsweek,* January 16, 1989, p. 62.

65. Ibid.

66. Bruce Shephard, "Update: The Pill's Risks and Benefits," *McCall's,* September 1987, p. 85.

67. Ibid.

68. Josef Vana and Gerald Murphy, "Primary Liver Tumors and Oral Contraceptives: Results of a Survey," *Journal of the American Medical Association* 238, no. 20 (November 14, 1977):2154–58.

69. L. Davis, "Pill Cleared of Breast Cancer Role," *Science News,* August 16, 1986, p. 100.

70. Ricki Lewis, "Birth Control Plus," *Health* 20, no. 6 (June 1988):29.

71. Judith Wills, "The 'Pill' May Not Mix with Other Drugs," *FDA Consumer* 21 (1987):27.

72. "Chinese 'Pill' for Men 99% Effective," *Register-Guard* (Eugene, Oregon), May 5, 1979, p. 10.

73. Jonathan Bor, "New Drug OK'd for Birth Control," *Register-Guard* (Eugene, Oregon) October 30, 1992, p. 1A.

74. "Norplant System Ready to Go," *Register-Guard* (Eugene, Oregon), December 12, 1990, p. A.

75. Andrew Purvis, "A Pill That Gets under the Skin," *Time,* December 24, 1990, p. 66.

76. "Norplant System Ready to Go."

77. Sean Segilman, Mary Hager, and Deborah Witherspoon, "Abortion in the Form of a Pill," *Newsweek,* April 1989, p. 61.

78. Ibid.

79. Charlotte Allen, "The Mysteries of RU 486," *The Human Life Review* 16, no. 1 (Winter 1990):70–79.

80. Roger Field, "Six for the Price of One: Pregnancy Pill," *Science Digest* 76, no. 6 (December 1974):44. Reprinted by permission from *Science Digest.* Copyright © 1974 The Hearst Corporation. All rights reserved.

81. Ibid., pp. 14–15.

82. Robert W. Kistner, "Induction of Ovulation with Clomiphene Citrate," in *Progress in Infertility,* 2nd ed., ed. M. D. Behrman and Robert Kistner (Boston: Little, Brown, 1975), p. 528.

83. K. D. Schulz et al., "Oestrogen-like and Antioestrogenic Potencies of Clomiphene Citrate: Biochemical Investigations," in *Fertility and Sterility,* ed. Hasegawe et al. (New York: American Elsevier, 1973), p. 524.

84. Frederick H. Meyers, Ernest Javetz, and E. Goldfein, *Review of Medical Pharmacology* (Los Altos, Calif.: Lange Medical Publications, 1968), p. 365.

85. Clinter Sotrel, Rao Ramaa, and Antonio Scommegna, "Heterotropic Pregnancy Following Clomid Treatment," *Journal of Reproductive Medicine* 16, no. 2 (February 1976):79.
86. Field, "Six for the Price of One," p. 16.
87. Lisa Davis, "The Myths of Menopause," *Hippocrates* 3, no. 3 (May/June, 1989):52.
88. Marge Petlak, "AIDS Watch: The Arsenal Gets Larger," *Discover,* April 1989, pp. 22–23.
89. B. D. Colen, "Killing with Kindness," *Health* 20 (January 1988):607.
90. Joshua Hammer, "Inside the Illegal AIDS Drug Trade," *Newsweek* 112, no. 7 (August 15, 1988):41–42.
91. Ibid.
92. Ibid.
93. "New Drug May Extend Life for Many AIDS Patients," *Register-Guard* (Eugene, Oregon), November 13, 1991, p. 7A.
94. Ibid.
95. John Pekkanen, "Drugs That Stop a Heart Attack," *Reader's Digest,* December 1990.
96. Ibid.
97. Ibid.
98. D. Wysowiski, D. Kennedy, and T. Gross, "Prescribed Use of Cholesterol-Lowering Drugs in the United States, 1978 through 1988," *Journal of the American Medical Association* 263, no. 16 (April 25, 1990):2185–88.
99. Ibid.
100. Ibid.
101. Joan Goldberg, "The Cutting Edge of Peptide Power," *American Health,* June 1990, pp. 35–41.
102. Kathleen McAuliffe, "Wonder Drugs with Hidden Dangers," *U.S. News & World Report,* September 14, 1987, p. 63.
103. Ibid.
104. Erik Millstone, "Food Additives: A Technology Out of Control?" *New Scientist* 16 (Oct. 18, 1984):20.
105. Phyllis Lehmann, "More Than You Ever Thought You Would Know about Food Additives," *FDA Consumer* (April 1979).
106. Ibid., p. 21.
107. Ibid., p. 21.
108. Ibid., p. 22.
109. Ibid., p. 23.
110. Millstone, "Food Additives," p. 24.
111. Chris Lecos, "Reacting to Sulfites," *FDA Consumer* (December 1985–January 1986).
112. Gail Vines, "Can Food Additives Damage Your Health?" *New Scientist* (October 1984).
113. Nancy Glick, "Bringing Home the (Nitrite-less) Bacon," *FDA Consumer* 13, no. 4 (May 1979):25–26.
114. Albrink et al., "Interaction of Dietary Sucrose and Fiber on Serum Lipids in Healthy Young Men Fed High Carbohydrate Diets," *American Journal of Clinical Nutrition* 43 (March 1986):419.
115. M. F. Mesquita et al., "Simple Carbohydrates in the Diet," *American Journal of Clinical Nutrition* 45 (1987):1197–1201.
116. "The Diet Connection," *Science News* 124, no. 8 (August 20, 1983):125.
117. Jane Goldman et al., "Behavioral Effects of Sucrose on Pre-School Children," *Journal of Abnormal Psychology* 14, no. 4 (1986):565–67.
118. M. D. Glinsman et al., "Report from FDA's Sugar Task Force 1986," *Journal of Nutrition Supplement* 116, no. 11 (November 1986):2.
119. "NutraSweet: How Sweet Is It?" *Register-Guard* (Eugene, Oregon), March 10, 1985, p. F6.

C H A P T E R
14

THE CONSUMER AND DRUG LEGISLATION

INTRODUCTION

How well the prescription-drug industry is regulated and functions directly affects the drug consumer. Both physicians and government regulatory agencies are involved in this supervision, as is the drug industry itself. Though all three groups are interested in safe and effective drugs, they also work to protect their own interests. To understand drug use and abuse, consumers must understand the roles physicians, business, and government play in it.

THE PHYSICIAN'S ROLE

Though most doctors are well trained in their field of practice, most do not receive adequate training in pharmacology. As doctors they are expected to prescribe drugs, but many find it difficult to understand and apply correctly the constantly increasing barrage of pharmaceutical preparations:

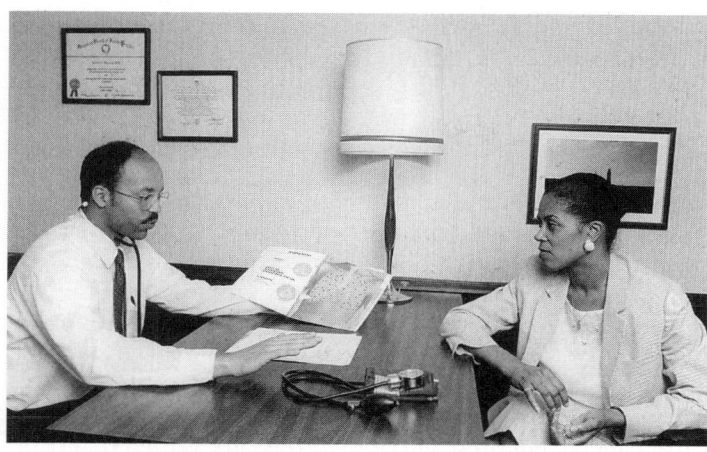

A Good Doctor and Patient
Relationship Is Important
Source: Blair Seitz/Photo Researchers

1. The physician often lacks detailed information concerning several thousand pharmaceutical products. Most doctors rely on the *Physician's Desk Reference* (PDR) for this information. "But the PDR is as much an advertising catalogue as a reference tool because the information it contains has been supplied, edited, approved and paid for by the drug manufacturers."[1]

2. By contrast, the *Medical Letter on Drugs and Therapeutics,* an authoritative, nonprofit, drug-evaluating service for physicians, is subscribed to by less than one fourth of the nation's practicing physicians.[2]

3. Surveys of physicians have indicated that drug salespeople, or "detail people," and journal or direct-mail advertisements are their "most important sources of familiarization [with] new drugs."[3] Drug companies, whose incentives are to sell their particular product, exert a marked influence on the physician, so much so that the industry spends an estimated $5,000 per year per physician on marketing and advertising.[4]

4. The American Medical Association has often called itself "the largest publisher of prescription drug advertisements in the world," with its weekly *Journal of the American Medical Association* and several specialty journals.[5]

What is the effect of most physicians' lack of understanding of pharmacology? For one thing, they may prescribe drugs they know little about. To keep up with current pharmaceutical preparations, they must follow the advice of drug companies, not sound medical information. If physicians are misled, public health may be endangered. Already, for example, the indiscriminate use of antibiotics has had the following unfortunate consequences:

1. Many bacteria that were once susceptible to these drugs have mutated, becoming highly virulent strains resistant to available chemotherapy.[6]

2. Many thousands of Americans have died from adverse drug reactions.[7]

3. Physicians have been pressured by their patients into prescribing a medication that is not indicated but is deemed psychologically necessary by the patient.

PHYSICIANS' VERSUS PHARMACISTS' DISPENSING

Increasingly, physicians have found a profit center and a marketing tool in selling the drugs they prescribe. Pharmacists cry conflict of interest but their eyes seem to be firmly on their own bottom line: Any loss to their walk-in trade means slashed profits on drugs and on sundries ranging from bunion pads to motor oil. Druggists have turned their complaint into a legislative crusade, launching lobbying efforts at state and federal levels to restrict doctors' dispensing powers.[8]

Doctors in private practice also hear the cash register ring. Squeezed by a market crowded with Health Maintenance Organizations (HMOs), group practices, and "doc-in-the-box" ambulatory-care centers, more MDs have resorted to marketing tools like late hours and convenient satellite offices. So far, doctor dispensing accounts for a mere one tenth of 1 percent of the $20-billion annual prescription drug market, says the Competitive Health Care Coalition, a trade group for the 30 to 40 repackagers.[9] The number could skyrocket.

Dispensing doctors have a few arguments of their own. They say the move will actually make the nation healthier. Since surveys show about 20 percent of prescriptions don't get filled, doctor dispensing ensures compliance—and thus recovery. Doctors answer conflict-of-interest charges with the argument that selling drugs poses no greater ethical quandries than offering medical tests and x-rays or even selling fees. While pharmacists continue to fight to restrict doctors' rights, they have expanded their own. Last year Florida pharmacists earned the right to prescribe more than 30 drugs that had previously come with only a doctor's OK. Most of the drugs are simply stronger versions of over-the-counter remedies.

For all the noise, doctors are unlikely to replace pharmacists; many prescriptions require refilling, and patients won't pay for the pleasure of a doctor's company. Also, few doctors keep pharmacy hours.

Generic Versus Name-Brand Ibuprofen
Source: Steve Goldberg/Monkmeyer Press

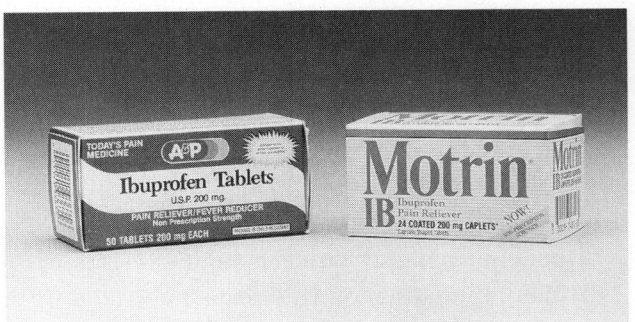

THE PATIENT'S ROLE

In addition to the problems of physicians' lack of training in pharmacology and the large-scale production and advertising of drugs, patients occasionally make mistakes with medications. Patients should carefully follow their doctor's instructions (some surveys show that a large percentage of patients receiving medication do not follow instructions) and be sure to ask for clarification of any points about the drug that are confusing or difficult to understand. On occasion it might even be a good idea to get instructions or special precautions in writing. Patients should promptly inform their doctors if they think they are experiencing side effects, adverse reactions, or overdose from a drug. Patients need to inquire if a particular drug from a physician can affect their driving behavior or cause dangerous reactions if mixed with a second drug they are using. Finally, special precautions apply to use of medications by patients who are pregnant or nursing, and by the elderly, who are more prone to side effects and adverse reactions because of their declining health.

CONSUMERS

Drug-store consumers of prescription drugs are starting to protest the high cost of drugs. Over the last decade the price of prescription drugs has soared 135 percent.[10] Inflation during the same period rose only 53 percent. In the United States $30 to $40 billion worth of prescription drugs is sold each year.[11] It should be noted that the cost of the same drug overseas, where drug costs are government regulated, is almost one sixth of what we pay in the United States.[12] There are many forms of pressure by consumer organizations to get costs reduced. Hospitals are now requiring doctors to consider the cost of a drug before they prescribe it. Some major corporations like General Motors are negotiating directly with pharmaceutical companies to reduce costs of drugs for their employees on group insurance plans.[13]

Millions of Americans either fail to take their medicines properly or don't take them at all. According to the National Council on Patient Information and Education, about 1.6 billion prescriptions are filled each year, but up to half of those drugs are taken improperly.[14]

Failure to take prescription medicine or taking it improperly can be dangerous. Recurrent infections, emergency hospital treatment, or serious medical complications are among possible consequences. It is estimated that nonadherence to drug regimen cost Americans about $22 billion a year in doctor visits, diagnostic tests, and additional drugs.[15]

Many factors contribute to pharmacophobia—the fear of taking drugs. Doctors and pharmacists often do not give patient enough information—why a drug is needed, how to take it, and how to minimize its side effects. Experts say that the cost, size, shape, and even color of medications affect people's attitude toward taking them. Drugs that improve one's looks, such as the antibaldness medicine minoxidil, tend to have the highest rate of **compliance,** while those that produce more subtle results, such as lowering blood pressure, have the lowest.[16] Nonadherence skyrockets with complex dosage schedules, asymptomatic diseases, psychiatric disorders, long-term illnesses and, not surprisingly, drug with complacent side effects.

Patient Compliance
Patients carefully following their doctor's instructions (some surveys show that a large percentage of patients receiving medication do not follow instructions) and asking for clarification of any confusing or difficult-to-understand points about the drug.

OVERPRESCRIBED MEDICATIONS IN NURSING HOMES?

It was shown in a major study that 58% of 850 residents in 12 Massachusetts nursing homes were prescribed sedatives, tranquilizers, or antipsychotic drugs.[17] It was also found that of these cases residents were taking excessive doses of these drugs and more than one drug at a time. In addition, on average, they were prescribed four other drugs for physical conditions, such as high blood pressure. This polydrug use can have an effect of its own.

(Findlay, Steven. "Is Grandma Drowsy, or Is She Drugged?" *U.S. News and World Report* 106, No. 23, June 12, 1989, p. 68).

The issue of drug-misuse in nursing homes was a big topic in the mid-1970s, after public attention was directed to the problem. Since then, the issue has again slipped away from the focus of public attention.

When studying the causes of these problems, researchers found that the main contributing reason to the aging problem in nursing homes, with more residents in their eighties and nineties who suffer from dementia and mental confusion, continued to be understaffing and poor mental-health care.[18] Another reason for overprescribed drugs in nursing homes is that many times in these homes the nurses are given "blank-check" prescriptions. This is where nurses can file prescriptions as they see fit. It is widely thought that this practice lends to abuses, but nursing home officials deny it.

An excellent way to combat misuse in a long-term care facility is by having a pharmacist as a consultant.[19] The cost associated with adverse reactions decreases. In one nursing home it was estimated that $163,000 was saved due to consultant pharmacist recommendations.[20]

A five-year study looked at the increase in drug-related errors in cases where a pharmacist was terminated.[21] The results showed an increase in death, hospitalization, and the number of drugs used by each patient. When the consultant was rehired, drug cost and related problems were reduced.

THE DRUG INDUSTRY

Every year approximately 1.5 billion prescriptions (or an average of 20 per family) are filled in this country. For these prescriptions, Americans pay $33 per year per person. In 1973 pharmaceutical companies made $5 billion; another $2 billion was garnered by middlemen such as distributors and pharmacists.[22] In 1978 the pharmaceutical industry made $10.5 billion, and an estimated $18 billion was spent in 1985 on research to develop new drugs.[23] In 1992 consumers spent close to $40 billion on prescription drugs.

The following are 10 questions a person can and should ask their pharmacist:[24]

1. What is the name of the drug, and what is it supposed to do? Find out how long the drug takes to work so you can tell if it is working.

2. When and how do I take it? In what doses? If label says, "Take four times a day," it is not telling you enough. When I wake up? Bedtime? Before or after meals? Full or empty stomach?

3. For how long should I take it, and do I need a refill?

4. Does it contain anything that can cause an allergic reaction? Penicillin and aspirin are common drugs to which people may be allergic.

5. Should I avoid foods, activities, or other drugs? Synergism is something to be aware of. Dietary changes might be needed to include extra vitamins or minerals if your medication causes your body to excrete nutrients.

6. What if I miss a dose? Some medications might require making up a missed dose. Others may advise continuing the regular schedule after an omission.

7. Is it safe to become pregnant and/or breast feed while taking this medication? Some drugs can cross the placenta barrier into the fetus's bloodstream, and some can be secreted in breast milk.

8. Can I take a generic drug instead of a brand name? Generally the generic brand name can cost 50 percent less than the name brand.

9. Will there be any side effects? If a medication causes an upset stomach, rash, or worse, should I discontinue using the medication, or will it pass?

10. Are there any special services that can help me feel more comfortable about taking this medication?

PROFIT AND PRODUCTION

The pharmaceutical industry is one of the most profitable of all industries. Profitability is maintained even though drug prices haven't climbed as rapidly as other consumer prices. This continued profitability is attributed to a high degree of automation, the absence of price competition, and the inelastic demand for prescription drugs.

MARKETING AND ADVERTISING

Many authorities believe that drug companies spend excessive amounts on marketing and advertising and too little on research and development. Most pharmaceutical houses do spend one out of every four dollars on advertising but only one quarter of that amount on research and development. In addition to the money they spend on salespeople, magazine and journal advertising, and other means of promotion, many pharmaceutical houses offer physicians and pharmacists prizes (freezers, color TV sets, camping equipment, all-expense-paid tours) and free samples of their products.[25]

Advertisers use tricks to make the product they are advertising look very appealing. One thing they do is rely on brand loyalty. That is, they figure that once we try something we like, we will keep using it.

Advertisers target their ads to different groups.[26] They try to make alcohol, for instance, look attractive at younger ages. An example of this kind of advertising ploy is the ad showing Spuds McKenzie. Advertisers do this in hopes that when you turn 21, you will remember their product and drink more of it. Advertisers try to get well-known people to speak for their products. They play mind games with you!

The trend lately has been advertisements for prescription drugs.[27] This selling tactic has both drawbacks and benefits. Companies that produce these drugs feel that many consumers aren't aware of all the medicines available to them. They claim that these ads educate patients and help them to be involved in deciding the medicines for themselves. Due to the nature of the subject advertised, however, there are strict government regulations if the drug's name is mentioned; in such an instance, the ad must also include and print adverse reactions and contraindictions.

The view doctors take on the issue seems to be quite the opposite of the drug companies. Patients may feel they know better than their doctor, or they may fail to realize that there may be other factors that would not make them appropriate candidates to use the drug. Yet a definite influence is exerted on doctors to issue these advertised drugs to patients. Most people agree that the advertising can be beneficial, however; there simply need to be stricter restrictions regarding the ad content.[28]

RESEARCH AND DEVELOPMENT

Though the drug industry has spent up to $500 million a year on research and development, the return on research investments has shown a steady decline. A number of new drugs for treating hypertension, angina pectoris, and cardiac arrhythmias have recently been introduced on the market. In a Council of Economic Priorities study, 16 companies submitted 185 new-drug applications to the **Federal Drug Administration.** Only 33 of the drugs (18 percent) were found to be significant; the rest were simply new "packages" or minor chemical variations of existing drugs.[29] Though drug companies are spending more money, they are exhibiting less productivity.

THE HIGH COST OF PRESCRIPTION DRUGS

To many observers, profits from the sale of drugs have depended too little on whether the drugs are beneficial and too much on whether they are successfully promoted.[30] This emphasis on promotion is part of the reason prescription-drug costs are so high; buying brand names rather than generic medicines may cost the American consumer $1 billion per year.

American employers will spend $22 billion on prescription drugs for their employees, retirees, and dependents, and that is not a figure companies are taking lightly.[31] Some companies have opened their own corporate pharmacies where there are enough employees to justify the volume sales. Work-

Federal Drug Administration (FDA)

A federal agency that classifies and approves drugs for medical use. It is also involved in the regulation of laws pertaining to safe drugs such as over-the-counter drugs.

ers at Rockwell's Avionics Group in Cedar Rapids, Iowa, drop off their prescriptions at the company drug store when they arrive at work.[32] The prescription is delivered to them at the worksite. The company saved $1.2 million by running its own pharmacy. Rockwell employees still may go to commercial pharmacies if they prefer, and an estimated 3 percent of employees, retirees, and dependents go outside of the company pharmacy. The use of generics is a cornerstone of many employer cost-reduction efforts. A typical 90-day supply of a brand-name drug might cost $55 or $60, whereas the same supply of generic would cost $16 or $18.

BRAND-NAME VERSUS GENERIC DRUGS

Generic drug is a term used for prescription drugs that are the same as brand names but cost a lot less. Generic drugs may be sold by competing drug companies only after the patent for the brand name has run out, generally about 17 years after the drug was discovered. Some facts about generic drugs:[33]

1. They have to meet FDA requirements.
2. They have to meet the same standards as brand-name drugs.
3. They contain the same active ingredients as brand-name drugs, must be the same dosage and strength, and must be administered by the same route.
4. They are just as potent as brand-name drugs.
5. They are just as safe as brand-name drugs. Some believe that generic drugs are made in outdated facilities. This is not so.
6. Generic-drug laboratories must meet the same standards as other pharmaceutical laboratories, and they are inspected regularly.

There are more than 8,000 generic clones of about 170 brand-name drugs.[34] Generics generally cost about half as much as the brand-name drugs. In order to introduce a generic drug a company has to carry out costly clinical trials to prove again what the innovator company had already shown: that the drug works.

Now instead of duplicating the original studies, a generic firm can show that its drug was "bioequivalent" to the brand-name product, which means it was absorbed into the bloodstream at about the same rate and it is as complete as the original drug.[35] This allows generic firms to market products quickly and inexpensively.

Today, Americans routinely received generic drugs in place of more expensive brand names ordered by doctors. To cut costs, many health maintenance organizations and private insurers, including Blue Cross and Blue Shield, now require or encourage the use of generics.[36]

For most people, most of the time this makes economic and medical sense. Generics are not exact copies of brand drugs. While the amount of the active ingredient in a generic and its brand name counterpart must be the same, the inert ingredients that bind, color, and fill the pill or capsule differ. These inactive ingredients can affect the way the drug dissolves in your stomach and thus how thoroughly it is absorbed into your blood. Some conditions

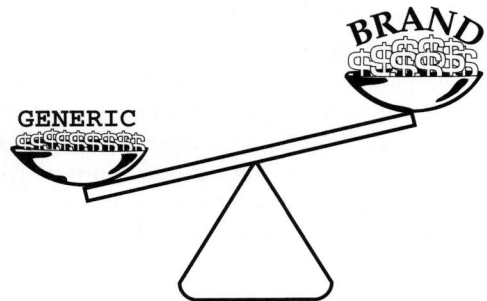

require maintaining a constant and precise level of medication in the blood over long periods. For people with epilepsy, asthma, diabetes, heart ailments, mental disorders, and thyroid problems, for example, switching drugs may upset a delicate balancing act.

One should ask the doctor whether he or she has prescribed a brand-name or a generic drug. If the prescription is for a brand name, ask whether generic substitution is a good idea. See if your doctor wants you to take the brand-name only.

CASE HISTORY—MICHAEL BURNS

Five years ago, Michael Burns seemed to have it made. A former professional policeman, he'd moved to a lucrative job as a salesman for a manufacturer of security equipment. He and his wife owned an elegant five-bedroom house in North Carolina, where they lived with their two young sons. Burns had epilepsy, but it was well under control. In fact, he'd had no seizures in the last nine years. Most people were unaware he had the disease.

But Burns's life fell apart when his pharmacist switched the brand-name epilepsy drug he'd been using for a cheaper and nearly identical-looking generic version. The pharmacist expected no problems. He didn't even bother to tell Burns or his physician of the change.

Five days later, Burn's lost control while staying overnight on business in a Raleigh hotel. "It was a nightmare," he remembers. "I woke up in the afternoon and was sore all over. I had bitten my tongue, there was blood on the pillow, I was three hours late for an appointment. I thought, Oh no, here goes my life."

Over the next three months, Burns suffered a series of violent, uncontrollable seizures. In a panic, he quit his job; soon after he sold his home and split up with his wife. "If my doctor had known from the start that my drug was switched," says Burns ruefully, "things would be a lot different now."[37]

Generic-Drug Scandal   The FDA has found that some drugs contained a different formula than initially approved. When records were demanded by the government, they were so lacking that officials believed the firms could not recall the initial drug formulas. It was found that at least two generic-drug companies substituted brand-name drugs for inspection, which the FDA approved; then the companies marketed their own generic formulas, which weren't even analyzed.[38]

A congressional investigator, when informed of the scandal, said the FDA may be "heading toward a nightmare, when we find out that almost everyone is cheating."[39] The FDA's problem with unethical behavior goes beyond the generic companies and into the brand-name firms. The FDA has since taken active measures to restore confidence to consumers on the effectiveness and other benefits of using generic drugs and has recently launched a campaign to reevaluate 30 of the most commonly prescribed generic medications.[40]

THE ORPHAN DRUG ACT

It takes an average of $70 million to bring a new drug to market.[41] To justify such expenditures, pharmaceutical companies concentrate on the "big diseases," such as heart disease, peptic ulcers, and high blood pressure. But what about the little diseases, the rare conditions, many genetically based, that afflict only a few thousand people rather than millions? Who pays for research on their causes and cures? Why, the federal government, of course.[42] Unfortunately, not until the 1980s did substantial funding for this purpose become available. In 1983 Congress passed the **Orphan Drug Act,** opening a new arena for drug research and production.

The act permits government to offer tax breaks and the exclusive right to sell the drug for seven years. This is an incentive for biotech companies to invest millions of dollars to develop a drug for a small pharmaceutical market.

Under provisions of this act, 333 new drugs have been developed for rare disorders that afflict no more than 200,000 people.[43] Forty-five have received FDA approval, including three for treating people with AIDS. Although this act has been successful, some groups want to see a change. Congressman Ron Wyden stated, "A handful of companies scam this statute."[44] AIDS patients feel they could get cheaper drugs if more companies were allowed to manufacture a drug. Some AIDS activists feel that drugs used for treating AIDS should be taken off the orphan status, but this won't guarantee that the price of the drug will decrease.

The Orphan Drug Act was intended to encourage drug companies to develop medications for rare afflictions, medications whose production would normally be considered unprofitable by these companies. To spark production of these medications, the government offered the companies tax credits and grants along with an exclusive seven-year marketing-right guarantee.[45] Interestingly, many of the drugs produced under this arrangement were more profitable than anticipated, because the drug company could take advantage of their limited monopolies on these products to charge artificially high prices to consumers. In response, the House Energy and Commerce

Orphan Drug Act
Provides drug companies with grants, tax credits, and a seven-year period of exclusive marketing, all as an incentive to develop drugs for diseases that affect fewer than 200,000 people. It allows medicines to be developed for people with rare diseases.

committees approved a bill that would reduce the huge profits being made by the pharmaceutical companies under their monopolies. This legislation expanded the Orphan Drug Act and closed the loopholes in it that allowed these companies to reap unfair profits at the expense of patients. The following are some of the provisions of the legislation.[46]

- Competing companies were able to develop and market their own version of a drug if they agreed to pay for testing and undergo the FDA approval process individually.
- The legislation provided grants for the development of medical equipment and foods needed to treat persons with rare diseases or dietary needs.
- Research funding for independent scientists developing orphan drugs was increased from $4 million in fiscal year 1987 to $10 million in 1988, $12 million in 1989, and $14 million in 1990.

DRUG USE AND THE LAW

The effect of drug legislation is, paradoxically, sometimes both considerable and minimal. It has done little to dissuade illicit use: People use the chemical of their choice regardless of existing statutes. Drug legislation therefore becomes a number of hoops that people have to go through to achieve their goal and a list of the consequences of getting caught. Legislation of morality is the key issue. It seems that morality cannot be effectively legislated and that attempts to do so are always met with hazards to the individual greater than those posed by use of the drug.

Laws are sets of standards established by society for the regulation and preservation of its stability. Based on determined values (norms) of the society, their purpose is to prevent individuals from infringing upon the rights of others. It is important to keep in mind how these social values and norms are determined and assessed, and what the individual's legal rights are.

Throughout U.S. history, most Americans have believed that solutions to problems lay in the passing of restrictive laws. "The assumption of such legislation is that it will stop or deter the particular activity, e.g., drug use, and, if it fails to do so, will punish the individual and/or protect society from such antisocial behavior by imprisoning the offender."[47] Though many laws have been passed, they have failed to greatly reduce or restrict drug use. A look at narcotics legislation provides a clue as to why these laws often fail. "One reason for the failure . . . appears obvious. They [narcotics laws] were aimed at private transactions between willing sellers and willing, usually eager, buyers. Thus there were no [complainants]."[48]

Police argue that they can't compete with a drug world that has an endless positive cash flow when they themselves are "faced with budget wars." Although the number of users of illegal drugs has decreased (14.5 million now from 23 million in 1985), there has been a 10 percent increase in crime involving violent, hard-core drug users—as well as an increase in the number of drugs people take daily.[49] It appears that the majority of the drug problems are occurring in the inner-city, low-socioeconomic classes.

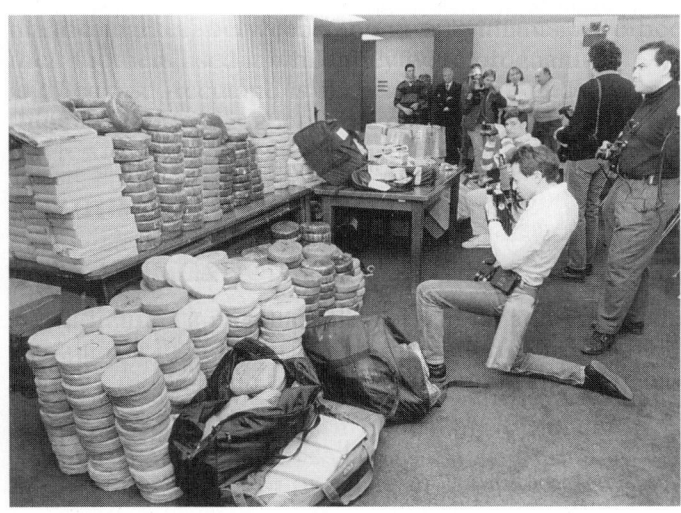

Police Bust of Illicit Drugs
Source: AP/Wide World Photos

VICTIMLESS CRIMES

It is difficult to enforce crime legislation when the crime involved has no victim. Does society have the right to interfere with an individual's right to determine his or her own actions—in this case, to use drugs? Should drug use be a crime because society at large deems it to be? The answers to these questions remain uncertain, but the mere fact that the questions arise makes it difficult to enforce legislation.

A further obstacle to narcotics-legislation enforcement is the inequitable treatment offenders often receive. Also, the types of drugs used in criminal acts are looked at in different lights. Finally, many penalties for drug use are not commensurate with the physical harm they may cause. With so many inequalities and concerns about drug-law enforcement, current regulations may be doing more harm than good.

SHOULD WE LEGALIZE DRUGS?

Recently there has been talk in the United States of treating drugs as a public health problem instead of a criminal one. Proponents—certain medical and political authorities—argue that drug-related crime damages society more than the actual drug use. These officials maintain that legalizing drugs would have a number of positive effects on society.[50] First, it would allow part of the $8 billion currently spent each year on upholding antidrug laws to be spent on education and treatment programs, which receive less than $500 million annually. Second, legalization of illicit drugs would reduce the amount of money that drug lords take in as profits (estimated at $20 billion a year). Third, legalizing drugs would improve relations with Latin American countries that depend on drug revenues as a major source of income. Finally, legalizing drugs would allow the government to tax sales and use this money.

To stop the flow of drugs through the United States, and to prevent people from selling them, there have been countless "wars" on drugs. Gary

Victimless Crime
It is difficult to enforce crime legislation when the crime involved has no victim. Does society have a right to interfere with an individual's right to determine his or her own actions—in this case, to use drugs? Should drug use be a crime because society at large deems it to be?

Becker presents the following views on this and other issues relating to decriminalization.[51]

- The "wars" on drugs have failed to stop their illegal trade and use—a situation that is often compared to Prohibition. All restrictions should be removed from the sale of marijuana, cocaine, and other drugs to adults. He says that drugs should not be available to children, but fails to specify a minimum age for purchase as an adult.

- Legalizing drugs would decrease crime. Drug users would not be compelled to steal because the cost of the drug would be cheaper if legitimate companies were allowed to produce it. Legalization would also eliminate the possibility of the drug being "cut" with a harmful ingredient.

- Studies show that with a decrease in price there would be an increase in use. To discourage people who wouldn't normally use drugs from buying them, a moderate excise tax should be levied on all legal sales of the drugs.

- Although harsh punishment has not decreased drug use thus far, it will discourage users once drugs are legalized. Users would be punished only if they had used drugs prior to engaging in activities that might harm others.

Opponents of legalization feel it would increase society's exposure to drugs and therefore to addiction.[52] They also argue that legalizing drugs would open a market for dangerous synthetic drugs or derivatives such as crack. The effects of these drugs would be unknown and therefore very dangerous. According to opponents, legalizing drugs would also increase the amount of money needed to treat drug abuse annually. Finally, opponents feel that legalization would make drug use appear to be socially acceptable. It appears that drugs will not become legalized anytime soon, and the answer must lie in more effective treatment and education efforts.

INTERVENTION PROGRAMS

It is necessary to start directing intervention and prevention programs at high-risk groups. Individuals with a particular mix of situational characteristics may be more likely to use drugs than individuals with a different mix. Such characteristics can be viewed as risk factors. The estimation of the risk of using drugs can be viewed as a two-step process.[53] The first involves assessing personal characteristics: age, sex, race, relationships with peers, and relationships with teachers. The second step is to determine high-risk geographic areas—areas where drug use is highest.

An experimental multistate correctional rehabilitation and drug treatment program for high-risk individuals is now being implemented in prisons by Narcotic and Drug Research, Inc. (NDRI).[54] During the 18-month implementation phase, states will receive technical assistance and training as needed, and up to $400,000 each to implement interventions with inmates having a history of serious drug abuse. Hawaii, New Jersey, New York, Con-

necticut, Washington, and Oregon are currently planning treatment programs with the aid of NDRI. The program shows great promise.

A WAR ON DRUGS WITH REAL TROOPS

How does the government go about decreasing the drug traffic into the
United States, and how do we go about eliminating the drug epidemic plaguing
our country today? Whereas some advocate decriminalization, others feel that
greater enforcement of drugs laws is needed to meet the nation's drug problem. Three congressmen, Jack Davis (R–Ill.), Tommy Robinson (D–Ark.), and
Duncan Hunter (R–Calif.), have been pushing for the military to take a more
aggressive role in spotting and arresting cocaine and marijuana smugglers.
According to these three, the Pentagon is "the only agency in the U.S. Government with adequate equipment . . . to establish aerial radar coverage across the
southern border of the United States."[55] Hunter says smugglers achieve a 98 percent success rate when flying across the Mexican border at night in small aircraft. He suggests using AWACS or similar aircraft to patrol at night as well as
tracking planes and helicopters to chase down suspicious aircraft.

The House liked this idea and passed an amendment to the Defense
Authorization Bill directing the secretary of defense to "substantially halt the
unlawful penetration of United States borders by aircraft and vessels carrying
narcotics." The Senate also adopted an enforcement clause. In the end, Congress softened the language of the law, asking "the military to take control of
air surveillance for drugs, but not giving them a mandate to arrest criminals or
close the border."[56] On the other side of the issue, military leaders are worried
that the military may become entangled in tedious criminal cases if it is called
upon to take an active role in drug-law enforcement.

The war on drugs, complete with military, civilian, and legislative components, has been envisioned as follows:[57]

- The Armed Services will cooperate with various civilian drug-law
  enforcement authorities under the terms of legislation signed by President Reagan in 1981.

- Two major civilian agencies involved in the fight against drugs are the
  Drug Enforcement Agency (DEA), which is "the lead Federal agency in
  enforcing narcotics and controlled substances laws and regulations," and
  the FBI, which is the "principal investigative arm of the U.S. Department
  of Justice. It is charged with gathering and reporting facts, locating wit-
  nesses, and compiling evidence in matters in which the Federal Government is, or may be, a party in interest."

- Other civilian agencies include the Narcotic and Dangerous Drug Section, the Office of National Drug Control Policy, the National Institute on
  Drug Abuse, ADAMNA, and the U.S. Customs Service.

- The new Anti-Crime Bill provides additional narcotics-control aircraft and
  aerostat radar balloons to detect air and sea shipments of illegal drugs.
  This bill also gives the Coast Guard more manpower and equipment to
  work with.

- The Anti-Crime Bill increases the penalties for illicit drug use, providing maximum penalties for the most dangerous drugs. And "if an individual intentionally engages in conduct during the course of continuing criminal enterprise and thereby knowingly causes the death of any other individual while so engaging he shall be subject to the death penalty."

DRUG VIGILANTES

In cities all over the United States, groups have been formed to combat the drug problem. Police, who have be unable to establish an effective presence, are becoming more receptive to this unorthodox source of help.

The most extreme group is the Muslims, who are found mostly in Washington and New York and who are "supremely motivated by their religion, based on self-reliance, discipline and black pride. . . . The patrollers sometimes broadcast religious slogans on loudspeakers mounted on vans or cars. Just as important, they are willing to put themselves at risk to clean up their communities—and the pushers steer clear."[58] The Muslims, with the backing of police, have succeeded in ridding many neighborhoods of drugs.

Problems can occur, however, when these groups take matters into their own hands. In Washington the normally disciplined Muslims once beat a man just for carrying a sawed-off shotgun and then injured a TV reporter who was filming the episode. Another complaint is from neighboring residents, who say the drug traffic has simply been pushed into their communities.

Some urbanologists feel that the long-term solution to the drug problem "is to create more and better jobs for ghetto young people."[59] There also need to be more effective ways of identifying drug dealers and gathering evidence against them. Laws also need to be enacted making it easier to jail gang members.

The drug problem is so bad in the inner cities that residents are willing to settle for any short-term solution. If the legal system can't take care of the problem, someone has to.

A HISTORY OF MAJOR DRUG-RELATED LEGISLATION

REGULATION OF OPIATES: 1865–1905

In the late nineteenth century, opiates were easy to obtain and could be purchased legally. They were known to be addictive yet were widely prescribed as pain killers and tranquilizers and for menstrual and menopausal discomforts, diabetes, and countless other maladies. Since there were no laws governing the labeling of ingredients on patent medicines, many preparations contained morphine, cocaine, and heroin. Manufacturers of the time were remarkably effective in preventing any congressional action that would have required disclosure of dangerous drugs in commercial preparations.[60]

THE PURE FOOD AND DRUG ACT, 1906

"The medical consensus was that morphine had been overused by the physician, addiction was a substantial possibility, and addition of narcotics to patent medicines should be minimized or stopped."[61] Also, feelings ran high that prolonged use of opiates led to criminal behavior and social decay. Lay reformers and Victorians began to take undaunted stands on the opiate issue. They looked to federal legislation as the most effective weapon against the sins of opiate use.

The first important federal regulation of opiate use was contained in the Pure Food and Drug Act of 1906. This act "prohibited interstate commerce of adulterated or misbranded food and drugs."

> In the section on misbranding, the act specifically referred to alcohol, morphine, opium, cocaine, heroin, Cannabis indica (marijuana), and several other agents. Each package was required to state how much (or what proportion) of these drugs was included in the preparation. This meant, for example, that the widely sold "cures" for morphine addiction had to indicate that they in fact contained another addicting drug.[62]

The act was a good beginning, but in 1911 a loophole was found. The law did not regulate claims of a medicine's curative powers or advertisements for the preparation. Because few people read labels if accompanying advertising promises miracles, the Pure Food and Drug Act lost much of its clout thereby.

THE SHANGHAI CONFERENCE, 1909

In 1906, in response to its growing opiate problem in the Philippines, the United States called for an international opium conference, the Shanghai Conference. But in asking for such a conference, the United States found itself in a difficult position: It had no exemplary opium laws of its own. The first attempt at such legislation grew out of the Shanghai Conference, but the bill met with defeat both at the conference and in the United States. The fight for opium legislation and international control continued. Two more international drug conferences were held—the Hague conferences of 1911 and 1914—but since the United States still had no domestic legislation, there were no exemplary laws to pattern agreements after, and thus no concerted efforts to ratify the conventions.

THE HARRISON NARCOTIC ACT, 1914

"In 1914, it was estimated that about 200,000 Americans—one in 400— were addicted to opium or its derivatives."[63] But when the Harrison Act was passed, the legal supply of opiates that led to that addiction was restricted. The Harrison Act allowed physicians to prescribe narcotics only "in the course of their professional practice," making possession of narcotics without a prescription a criminal offense. "Patent-medicine manufacturers [had to limit] themselves to preparations and remedies which do not contain more than 2 grains of opium, or more than one-fourth of a gram of morphine, or more than one-eighth of a grain of heroin . . . in one avoirdupois ounce."[64]

The law focused not on prohibition but on regulation of the marketing and sale of opium, morphine, heroin, and other drugs and the prescribing of opiates by physicians.

PROHIBITION, 1920

Alcohol-prohibition legislation, sparked by the concerted efforts of such groups as the Anti-Saloon League and the Women's Christian Temperance Union, appeared in 1919 in the form of the Volstead Act, followed in 1920 by the Eighteenth (Prohibition) Amendment to the U.S. Constitution. The idea of national prohibition had been gaining ground for over 20 years prior to the Volstead Act. Many feel World War I was what finally put Prohibition over the top. "The United States had been at war since April 1917, and the hysteria that gripped the nation in its crusade against the Kaiser extended the firm belief that liquor sapped the nation's strength and willpower, and even depleted the cereal grains that could be used in bread for the troops and starving Europeans."[65]

Prohibition outlawed the manufacture, sale, and transportation (but not the possession) of domestic and foreign liquor within the United States. But this regulation only created a thriving alcohol black market, in which adulterated and contaminated "rotgut" was easy to obtain. Some of the ingredients in these bootleg beverages occasionally led to blindness, paralysis, and even death. In addition, "the disreputable saloon was replaced by the even less savory speakeasy."[66]

Prohibition resulted not only in impure alcoholic products sold illicitly but also in a shift from weak beers and wines to hard liquors. In addition, alcohol substitutes began to fill the void. Even before Prohibition, the states that had prohibition laws of their own found that morphine sales were rising rapidly. Marijuana, which was little used prior to Prohibition, also became popular.

Despite Prohibition, alcohol remained an integral part of America's culture, as it had since the country's inception. The Eighteenth Amendment was unable to end either the use of alcohol or the problems surrounding that use, and in 1933 Prohibition was repealed. But Prohibition wasn't ended because people decided that alcohol was a harmless drug. "On the contrary, the United States learned during prohibition, even more than in prior decades, the true horrors of the drug."[67] It also learned that making a drug illegal does not end its use, but can actually encourage more adverse drug situations.

IMPORTATION OF HEROIN BANNED, 1924

Despite the passage of the Harrison Act, heroin use continued to rise. Law enforcement officials made a further attempt to eradicate the drug's use by securing legislation banning the importation of heroin, even for medicinal use. "This legislation grew out of the widespread misapprehension that, because of deteriorating health, behavior and status of addicts from morphine to heroin, heroin must be a more damaging drug than opium or morphine."[68] This, of course, is not true: the two drugs' physiological effects are not drastically different. But no matter what the reasoning was behind it, "the 1924 ban on heroin did not deter the conversion of morphine addicts to heroin."[69]

LINDER V. UNITED STATES, 1925

In 1925, in the case of *Linder v. United States,* the Supreme Court decided that drug dependency was an illness. This decision allowed physicians to once again prescribe narcotics to help cure the addict, something the Harrison Act had made illegal.

PORTER NARCOTIC FARMS BILL, 1929

Though the *Linder v. United States* decision allowed doctors to consider drug dependents as patients and prescribe opiates for them as part of their treatment, many drug dependents were in prison for violating the Harrison Act. "This . . . abundance of narcotics prisoners led, at long last, to federal hospital care for addiction."[70] Congress passed the Porter Narcotic Farms Bill in 1929, establishing "farms" in Lexington, Kentucky, and Fort Worth, Texas, for the treatment of drug-dependents convicted of breaking federal law. Despite this seeming step forward in the treatment of drug abuse, the farms, operated until 1967 by the Public Health Service and from then on by the National Institute of Mental Health, maintained a consistently low cure rate.

FEDERAL BUREAU OF NARCOTICS, 1930

In 1930 Congress reorganized the personnel responsible for opiate control into a separate enforcement body within the Treasury Department. This bureau, the Federal Bureau of Narcotics (FBN), assumed all duties previously carried out by the Federal Narcotics Control Board. In April 1968 it became the Bureau of Narcotics and Dangerous Drugs in the Department of Justice. In 1972 President Nixon further reorganized the body and changed its name to the Drug Enforcement Agency.

THE MARIJUANA TAX ACT, 1937

Once the Federal Bureau of Narcotics was formed, it began to take a hard line on drug use, including marijuana use. FBN officials and others thought that marijuana was the cause of crime, violence, mental illness, sexual deviancy, and moral degeneration, and in 1937 the Marijuana Tax Act was passed to curtail these problems. Modeled after the Harrison Act, the Marijuana Tax Act did not actually ban the use of marijuana but merely taxed physicians, druggists, growers, manufacturers, and distributors for its prescription and distribution; only the nonmedicinal untaxed possession of marijuana was illegal.

THE FOOD, DRUG AND COSMETIC ACT, 1938

In the early 1930s President Roosevelt pushed for revision of the 1906 Pure Food and Drug Act, declaring it grossly inadequate. But Congress was unresponsive. It took until 1938 for major reform to be passed, and only then mainly because of a catastrophe. A product called Elixir of Sulfanilamide was marketed to meet a demand for sulfanilamide in liquid form. The drug, whose main ingredient was similar to radiator antifreeze, killed 108 persons, mostly small children. The product had been marketed without animal testing, a situation the resultant Food, Drug and Cosmetic Act of 1938 made illegal. The law closed the legal loophole of the original Food and Drug Act, gave the Federal Trade Commission (FTC) clear powers to regulate patent-medicine advertising, and, most important, required drugs to be found safe before distribution.

THE BOGGS AMENDMENT, 1951

"Until 1951, the control of narcotics was directed toward the medical profession and their dispensing of these drugs."[71] But at the end of World War II, illegal drug traffic spiraled. Continuing to align the evils of marijuana and heroin use, Congress responded to the increased drug traffic and to pressures from the FBN by passing the Boggs Amendment to the Harrison Act. This mandatory minimum-sentence law for opiate *and* marijuana offenders reflected the country's hard-line enforcement approach by imposing severe penalties and limiting suspension of sentence and probation or parole to first-time offenders. Penalties under this act were the following:

first offense for possession: fine plus 2-to-5-year sentence, probation permitted

second offense for possession: fine plus 5-to-10-year sentence, no probation or suspended sentence

third and subsequent offenses for possession: fine plus 10-to-20-year sentence, no probation or suspended sentence

THE NARCOTIC DRUG CONTROL ACT, 1956

Though federal authorities expected a decrease in drug use after the passage of the Boggs Amendment, they saw none. Thoughts that "the laws must not be strict enough," that "drug usage is a Communist plot to demoralize and degenerate the American people" echoed throughout the land. In this emotion-laden environment, the Narcotic Drug Control Act was passed. This law increased the penalties of the Boggs bill at all levels. Fines were drastically increased, and third-time offenders were given mandatory 10-to-40-year sentences with no possibility of probation, suspension of sentence, or parole. Perhaps its most severe provision was that the death penalty could be imposed on anyone who sold, gave away, furnished, or conspired to sell heroin to a person under 18, even on the first conviction.

THE KEFAUVER-HARRIS AMENDMENTS, 1962

In 1960 a sleeping pill called Kevadon (thalidomide) was awaiting FDA approval. Though the drug had already been successfully marketed in

Europe, and despite constant pressure from the manufacturers, the FDA was not satisfied with the new drug's application and insisted on proof of the product's safety. While this proof was being awaited, West Germany announced that the drug caused birth defects when taken by pregnant women. This tragic discovery gave impetus to a new drug-reform movement, and in 1962 the Kefauver-Harris Amendments to the Pure Food and Drug Act were passed. This legislation contained the following requirements:

1. All new drug applications had to be supported by substantial evidence of the product's effectiveness as well as its safety.
2. All drugs marketed between 1938 and 1962 were to be subjected to the same efficacy demands as new products.
3. Drug advertising and other printed media seen by the physician must state drug side effects as well as contraindicated uses.[72]

ROBINSON V. CALIFORNIA, 1962

The 1925 *Linder* case affirmed that drug dependency is a medical condition that can be treated by physicians. This position was supported by the 1962 decision in *Robinson v. California.* In this case it was decided that to punish for opiate dependence was to impose cruel and unusual punishment, which is prohibited by the Bill of Rights. Since drug dependence was no longer illegal, it should not be punishable by imprisonment. Instead, states should have the right to compel drug-dependent people to undergo medical treatment.

THE COMMUNITY MENTAL HEALTH CENTERS ACT, 1963

"Although rival theories of deviance control were gaining credibility in the postwar period, the enforcement of narcotic laws did not become widely questioned and condemned until surveillance and penalties failed, even with mandatory minimum penalties and the death threat, to prevent a rapid rise in various forms of drug abuse in the 1960's."[73] At that time public officials and organizations slowly began to turn their ideas on drug abuse in the only direction afforded them—lessened penalties, medical treatment and rehabilitation, and possibly low-cost, legalized drug maintenance for drug-dependent individuals. Community mental-health centers, funded and supported by Congress, suggested that mandatory sentences and rigid controls on drug use be modified.[74] In 1963 the Community Mental Health Centers Act was passed, emphasizing decentralized treatment, rehabilitation, and reintegration of mental patients (many of whom were drug dependents) into society.

THE DRUG ABUSE CONTROL AMENDMENTS, 1965

It is ironic that at the same time rigid penalties for drug dependency began to soften, the desire for more stringent controls on nonnarcotic drug use began to grow. In 1965 the Drug Abuse Control Amendments to the 1938 Federal Food, Drug and Cosmetic Act were passed, classifying barbiturates, amphetamines, LSD, and other drugs with depressant, stimulant, or hallucinogenic effects as dangerous drugs. Penalties for possessing "dangerous drugs" were one year and/or a fine for a first offense and up to three years plus a fine for additional offenses. Penalties for selling these drugs to a minor were even greater. In 1968 a further amendment made simple possession a crime and increased maximum penalties but, strangely enough, allowed for suspension of a first offender's sentence.

> The most important aspect of [the 1965] law was its break with tradition in excluding possession for one's own use from the criminal penalties (as did the federal anti-alcohol laws) and instead concentrating on illegal manufacture and sale. The amendments, which came into effect in 1966, provide for more controls on distribution by manufacturers; limit physicians' prescription renewals of these drugs to five in any six-month period and, since 1967, bring LSD and related drugs under the same provision of control as the barbiturates and amphetamines.[75]

Exempted from parts of this act was the Native American church, which was granted the right to use peyote in its religious ceremonies on the grounds that restriction of peyote would violate the Indians' freedom of religion.

THE NARCOTIC ADDICT REHABILITATION ACT, 1966

The concept of medical treatment and rehabilitation for drug users that started in the early 1960s became more widely accepted in the mid-1960s. The Narcotic Addict Rehabilitation Act of 1966 allotted federal monies to state and local communities for treatment programs for drug abusers. The act also changed the status of the two federal narcotics "farms" (in Lexington, Kentucky, and Fort Worth, Texas) from treatment centers to research centers.[76]

THE COMPREHENSIVE DRUG ABUSE PREVENTION AND CONTROL ACT (THE CONTROLLED SUBSTANCES ACT), 1970

When this bill was originally submitted to Congress, it was a liberal one, emphasizing research, education, and rehabilitation of drug users. As a result of the prevailing law-and-order sentiment of Congress, however, the bill that finally passed both houses was more enforcement-oriented. Still, it was a major victory for those arguing for a reasonable drug law. The statute provided for the separation of law enforcement from the Department of Human Services, whose job was to scientifically evaluate which drugs to control. Other liberalizing changes from the strict 1951 and 1956 laws were the elimination of federal mandatory sentences for first-offense illegal possession, the reinstatement of the possibility of probation, and the complete erasure of conviction from public records relating to the case. "From a legal point of view, the individual is then restored to his prearrest status and can legally deny under oath that he was ever arrested on such a charge."[77]

The law's treatment of controlled drugs was divided into five dimensions called *schedules,* each carrying distinct penalties for manufacturing, distribution, and possession. A significant aspect of this law is that it focuses not on the user but on the distributor. Details about the act are provided in the following box. Controlled substances are listed in Table 14–1 (on page 398).

THE CONTROLLED SUBSTANCES ACT

Procedures for Controlling Substances

The purpose of the Federal Controlled Substances Act (CSA) is to minimize the quantity of drugs of abuse which are available to persons who are prone to abuse drugs. Procedures for controlling a substance under the CSA are set forth in Section 201 of the Act. Proceedings may be initiated by the Department of Health, Education and Welfare (HEW), by DEA, or by petition from any interested person. This may be a manufacturer, a medical society or association, a pharmacy association, a public interest group, a state or local government agency, or an individual citizen. When a petition is received by DEA, the agency begins its own investigation of the drug.

The Controlled Substances Act sets forth the findings which must be made to put a substance in any of the five schedules. These are as follows (Section 202(b)):

Schedule I

A. The drug or other substance has a high potential for abuse.
B. The drug or other substance has no currently accepted medical use in treatment in the United States.
C. There is a lack of accepted safety for use of the drug or other substance under medical supervision.

Schedule II

A. The drug or other substance has a high potential for abuse.
B. The drug or other substance has a currently accepted medical use in treatment in the United States or a currently accepted medical use with severe restrictions.
C. Abuse of the drug or other substances may lead to severe psychological or physical dependence.

Schedule III

A. The drug or other substance has a potential for abuse less than the drugs or other substances in Schedules I and II.
B. The drug or other substance has a currently accepted medical use in treatment in the United States.
C. Abuse of the drug or other substance may lead to moderate or low physical dependence or high psychological dependence.

Control Mechanisms of the CSA

Schedule	Registration	Record Keeping	Manufacturing Quotas?	Distribution Restrictions	Dispensing Limits
I	Required	Separate	Yes	Order forms	Research use only
II	Required	Separate	Yes	Order forms	Rx: written; no refills
III	Required	Readily retrievable	No *but some drugs limited by Schedule II quotas*	DEA registration number	Rx: written or oral: with medical authorization, refills up to 5 times in 6 months
IV	Required	Readily retrievable	No *but some drugs limited by Schedule II quotas*	DEA registration number	Rx: written or oral; with medical authorization, refills up to 5 times in 6 months
V	Required	Readily retrievable	No *but some drugs limited by Schedule II quotas*	DEA registration number	OTC (Rx drugs limited to MD's order)

This chart summarizes the control mechanism in a format which permits comparison between the schedules in terms of the controls imposed. Note that the distinction between Schedule III and Schedule IV is virtually nonexistent. Other than the penalties for criminal trafficking, the statute makes no distinction whatsoever. DEA, in imposing regulatory controls, has singled out narcotic drugs in Schedule III for coverage under the ARCOS system. By indirect means, some narcotics and non-narcotics in Schedule III are also under the quota system.

The differences between Schedule V and Schedules III and IV are also very small. The only practical distinction is that Schedule V drugs are generally over-the-counter, a differentiation imposed not by the CSA but by FDA.

Schedule IV

A. The drug or other substance has a low potential for abuse relative to the drugs or other substances in Schedule III.

B. The drug or other substance has a currently accepted medical use in treatment in the United States.

C. Abuse of the drug or other substance may lead to limited physical dependence or psychological dependence relative to the drugs or other substances in Schedule III.

Schedule V

A. The drug or other substance has a low potential for abuse relative to the drugs or other substances in Schedule IV.

B. The drug or other substance has a currently accepted medical use in treatment in the United States.

C. Abuse of the drug or other substance may lead to limited physical dependence or psychological dependence relative to the drugs or other substances in Schedule IV.

In making these findings, DEA and HEW are directed to consider eight specific factors (Section 201(c)):

1. its actual or relative potential for abuse;
2. scientific evidence of its pharmacological effect, if known;
3. the state of current scientific knowledge regarding the drug or other substance;
4. its history and current pattern of abuse;
5. the scope, duration, and significance of abuse;
6. what, if any, risk there is to the public health;
7. its psychic or physiological dependence liability;
8. whether the substance is an immediate precursor of a substance already controlled by this title.

A key criterion for controlling a substance, and the one which will be used most often, is the substance's potential for abuse. If the Attorney General through his designee the Administrator determines that the data gathered and the evaluations and recommendations of the Secretary of HEW constitute substantial evidence of potential for abuse, he may initiate control proceedings under this section. Final control by the Attorney General will also be based on the Administrator's findings as to the substance's potential for abuse.

Criminal Penalties for Trafficking

The most common and well-known control mechanism has not yet been mentioned: the criminal sanctions for illicit trafficking. Trafficking is defined as the unauthorized manufacture, the unauthorized distribution (i.e., delivery whether by sale, gift, or otherwise), or the possession for unauthorized manufacture or distribution of any controlled substance. The penalties for violation of this restriction are related to the schedules as well. For narcotics in Schedules I and II, a first offense is punishable by up to 15 years in prison and up to a $25,000 fine. For trafficking in a Schedule I and II non-narcotic drug or any Schedule III drug, the penalty is up to five years in prison and up to a $15,000 fine. Trafficking in a Schedule IV drug is punishable by a maximum of three years in jail and up to a $10,000 fine. And trafficking in a Schedule V substance is a misdemeanor punishable by up to one year in prison and up to a $5,000 fine. Second and subsequent offenses are punishable by up to twice the penalty imposed by the first offense.

It must be emphasized that possession for one's own use of any controlled substance is always a misdemeanor on the first offense, punishable by one year in jail and up to a $5,000 fine.[78]

THE ANTI-DRUG BILL, 1988

Anti-Drug Bill, 1988

A drug bill that includes stricter penalties in the following areas: civil penalties, user penalties, and law enforcement. It also provides for a drug czar cabinet position, more funds for education and treatment, international narcotics control, alcohol warning labels, increased penalties for child pornography, and a review of driver's licenses for those testing positive for drugs.

On November 18, 1988, President Reagan signed into law a drug bill that included the following provisions:[79]

CIVIL PENALTIES

- Allows the Justice Department to assess civil penalties of up to $10,000 for possession of "personal use" amounts of marijuana, cocaine, and other specified illegal drugs.
- Permits defendants to seek an administrative review and to appeal the penalty in federal court.
- Wipes out the records of those hit with civil fines after three years if the person remains drug-free.

USER PENALTIES

- Permits courts to deny individuals convicted of drug offenses all federal benefits except welfare, Social Security, health, disability, and some veterans' programs.
- Sets a benefit-suspension period of up to five years for first trafficking conviction and up to ten years for second trafficking conviction.
- Imposes automatic loss of benefits for third trafficking conviction.

- Sets an effective date of September 1, 1989, for the program. Requires the president to report to Congress by May 1 on implementation.
- Allows a waiver of the punishment if an individual completes a drug rehabilitation program, has otherwise been rehabilitated, or has made a good-faith effort to enter a rehabilitation program.

LAW ENFORCEMENT

- Imposes federal death penalty for drug kingpins and anyone convicted of drug-related killings.
- Allows the president to impose penalties and sanctions on foreign countries involved in money laundering.
- Regulates companies selling chemicals used to process illegal drugs.
- Stiffens penalties for convicted drug traffickers.
- Restores to federal prosecutors the ability to prosecute corrupt public officials on the theory that they deprived citizens of "intangible rights" to honest government. A Supreme Court ruling had invalidated such prosecutions.
- Establishes procedures for owners to petition the government for return of boats, planes, and other property seized for drug violations. Sets conditions for return of property if owners can show they were unaware of small amounts of drugs aboard or if owners took reasonable steps to ensure the conveyance would not be used for illegal purposes.

DRUG CZAR

- Creates a cabinet position with authority to develop national strategy for all areas of combating drug abuse.
- Makes the drug czar responsible for the entire federal drug budget.

EDUCATION AND TREATMENT

- Authorizes $900 million for additional treatment programs, although actual funding provided by the bill is far less.
- Authorizes additional money for antidrug programs for students and dropouts.
- Establishes community-based development projects for education and prevention, including programs to involve the private sector.
- Establishes a grant program for drug abuse aimed at youth-gang members.

INTERNATIONAL

- Authorizes $1 million for State Department international narcotics control programs.
- Authorizes $3 million for international and regional narcotics programs.

TABLE 14–1　CONTROLLED SUBSTANCES: USES AND EFFECTS

Drugs	Schedule*	Often Prescribed Brand Names	Medical Uses	Potential for Physical Dependence
Opium	II	Dover's Powder, Paregoric	Analgesic, antidiarrheal	High
Morphine	II	Morphine	Analgesic	High
Codeine	II,III,V	Codeine	Analgesic, antitussive	Moderate
Heroin	I	None	None	High
Meperidine (Pethidine)	II	Demerol, Pethadol	Analgesic	High
Methadone	II	Dolophine, Methadone, Methadose	Analgesic, heroin substitute	High
Other Narcotics	I,II,III,V	Dilaudid, Leritine, Numorphan, Percodan	Analgesic, antidiarrheal, antitussive	High
Chloral Hydrate	IV	Noctec, Somnos	Hypnotic	Moderate
Barbiturates	II,III,IV	Amytal, Butisol, Nembutal, Phenobarbital, Seconal, Tuinal	Anesthetic	High
Glutethimide	III	Doriden	Sedation, sleep	High
Methaqualone	II	Optimil, Parest, Quaalude, Somnafec, Sopor	Sedation, sleep	High
Tranquilizers	IV	Equanil, Librium, Miltown, Serax, Tranxene, Valium	Antianxiety, muscle relaxant, sedation	Moderate
Other	III,IV	Clonopin, Dalmane	Antianxiety, sedation, sleep	Possible
Depressants		Dormate, Noludar, Placydil, Valmid		
Cocaine†	II	Cocaine	Local anesthetic	Possible
Amphetamines	II,III	Benzedrine, Biphetamine, Desoxyn, Dexedrine	Hyperkinesis, narcolepsy, weight control	Possible
Phenmetrazine	II	Preludin	Weight control	Possible
Methylphenidate	II	Ritalin	Hyperkinesis	Possible
Other Stimulants	III,IV	Bacarate, Cylert, Didrex, Ionamin, Plegine, Pondimin, Pre-Sate, Sanorex, Voranil	Weight control	Possible
LSD	I	None	None	None
Mescaline	I	None	None	None
Psilocybin Psilocyn	I	None	None	None
MDA	I	None	None	None
PCP‡	III	Sernylan	Veterinary anesthetic	None
Other Hallucinogens	I	None	None	None
Marijuana Hashish Hashish Oil	I	None	None	Degree unknown

* Scheduling classifications vary for individual drugs, since controlled substances are often marketed in combination with other medical ingredients.

†Designated a narcotic under the Controlled Substances Act.

‡Designated a depressant under the Controlled Substances Act.

Potential for Abuse		Duration of Effects (hours)	Usual Methods of Administration	Possible Effects	Effects of Overdose	Withdrawal Syndrome
High	Yes	3 to 6	Oral, smoked	Euphoria drowsiness, respiratory depression, constricted pupils, nausea	Slow and shallow breathing, clammy skin, convulsions, coma, possible death	Watery eyes, runny nose, yawning, loss of appetite, irritability, tremors, panic chills and sweating, cramps, nausea
High	Yes	3 to 6	Injected, smoked			
Moderate	Yes	3 to 6	Oral, injected			
High	Yes	3 to 6	Injected, sniffed			
High	Yes	3 to 6	Oral, injected			
High	Yes	12 to 24	Oral, injected			
High	Yes	3 to 6	Oral, injected			
Moderate	Probable	5 to 8	Oral	Slurred speech, disorientation, drunken behavior without odor of alcohol	Shallow respiration, cold and clammy skin, dilated pupils, weak and rapid pulse, coma, possible death	Anxiety, insomnia tremors, delirium, convulsions, possible death
High	Yes	1 to 16	Oral, injected			
High	Yes	4 to 8	Oral			
High	Yes	4 to 8	Oral			
Moderate	Yes	4 to 8	Oral			
Possible	Yes	4 to 8	Oral			
High	Yes	2	Injected, sniffed	Increased alertness, excitation, euphoria, dilated pupils, increased pulse rate and blood pressure, insomnia, loss of appetite	Agitation, increase in body temperature, hallucinations, convulsions, possible death	Apathy, long periods of sleep, irritability, depression disorientation
High	Yes	2 to 4	Oral, injected			
High	Yes	2 to 4	Oral			
Possible	Yes	2 to 4	Oral			
Degree unknown	Yes	Variable	Oral	Illusions and hallucinations (with exception of MDA); poor perception of time and distance	Longer, more intense "trip" episodes, psychosis, possible death	Withdrawal syndrome not reported
Degree unknown	Yes	variable	Oral, injected			
Degree unknown	Yes	Variable	Oral			
Degree unknown	Yes	Variable sniffed	Oral, injected			
Degree unknown	Yes	Variable	Oral, injected, smoked			
Degree unknown	Yes	Variable	Oral, injected, sniffed			
Moderate	Yes	2 to 4	Oral, smoked	Euphoria, relaxed inhibitions, increased appetite, disoriented behavior	Fatigue, paranoia, possible psychosis	Insomnia, hyperactivity, and decreased appetite reported in a limited number of individuals

Source: The Controlled Substances Act (Washington D.C.: Drug Enforcement Administration, 1980).

- Authorizes $23 million for border-control programs.
- Earmarks $15 million to Mexico to fight drugs.

FINANCING

- Calls for programs that would cost an estimated $1.4 billion but provides only $500 million.

DRIVERS' LICENSES

- Establishes a one-year pilot program in four unspecified states for drug testing of new drivers' license applicants. Those testing positive would be denied licenses for at least one year.
- Allows the license to be issued after three months if the applicant agrees to regular drug testing for the remaining months.
- Authorizes $125 million to help states establish drunken driving enforcement programs that require license suspensions for those found driving under the influence of alcohol.

ALCOHOL WARNING LABELS

- Requires a health warning to be placed on all alcoholic-beverage containers.

CHILD PORNOGRAPHY

- Toughens child pornography laws, including increasing penalties for anyone who facilitates use of a child for producing sexually explicit materials.

Recently, in the Los Angeles area, there has been some controversy raised about police tactics in the war on drugs.[80] The controversy centers around one person being shot to death and another wounded during two separate drug raids that yielded no evidence of drugs. It is felt by some that police hoped to seize property under federal forfeiture laws that allow property to be confiscated before a defendent is convicted. These and other questionable raids have caused debate among legal scholars about the latitude given police in the war on drugs.

CONSUMER LEGISLATION

How well the Food and Drug Administration implements drug-related laws has been the subject of much controversy. In hearings before the Senate Health Subcommittee, Senator Edward Kennedy stated that

> on one hand, timidity and bureaucratic delay are said to be holding up approval of valuable products that already are on sale and saving lives in foreign countries. On the other hand, FDA regulations are said to often cave in to industry pressure and release dangerous and ineffective products that haven't been adequately tested.[81]

Legislation designed to help consumers cope with this and other drug-related concerns was introduced in 1973. It strengthened consumer safeguards by

1. establishing an independent federal drug-testing center, ending reliance on the FDA and drug manufacturers for drug analysis;[82]

2. requiring mandatory licensing of new drug patents at a "reasonable royalty" and keeping new brand-name product prices down while still protecting company patents;[83]

3. requiring salespeople to pass a federally approved course in pharmacology;[84]

4. providing doctors and medical students with more training in pharmacology by offering government-subsidized courses through a National Center for Clinical Pharmacology.[85]

Though the public has generally shown little interest in food and drug legislation, it is more concerned now and is becoming more involved with consumer protection.

CONSUMER DOS AND DON'TS

Consumers who self-medicate can help themselves by following a few simple rules:[86]

Don't be casual about taking drugs.

Don't take drugs you don't need.

Don't overbuy and keep drugs for long periods of time.

Don't combine drugs carelessly.

Don't continue taking OTC drugs if symptoms persist.

Don't take prescription drugs not prescribed for you.

Do read and follow directions for use.

Do be cautious when using a drug for the first time.

Do dispose of old prescription drugs and outdated OTC drugs.

Do seek professional advice when symptoms persist or return.

Do get medical check-ups regularly.

DECRIMINALIZATION

MARIJUANA

Reasons for and against the **decriminalization** of marijuana have been presented for years. In 1970 the Ledain Commission of the Canadian government urged decriminalization. After a thorough study of the nonmedical use of drugs, the commission issued the following conclusions on marijuana:

Decriminalization

An attempt to reduce the number of laws and penalties associated with drug use.

1. The use of marijuana is increasing in popularity among all age groups of the population, and particularly among the young.

2. This increase indicates that the attempt to suppress, or even to control, its use is failing and will continue to fail—that people are not deterred by the criminal law prohibiting its use.

3. The present legislative policy has not been justified by clear and unequivocal evidence of short term or long term harm caused by cannabis.

4. The individual and social harm (including the incarceration of young people and growing disrespect for law) that caused the present use of criminal law to attempt to suppress cannabis far outweighs any potential for harm which cannabis could conceivably possess, having regard for the long history of its use and the present lack of evidence.

5. The illicit status of cannabis invites exploitation by criminal elements, and abuses such as adulteration; it also brings cannabis users into contact with other criminal elements and with other drugs such as heroin, which they might not otherwise be induced to consider.[87]

Recommendations for the Future   Judging from experience, there is little likelihood that continued reliance on legal penalties will solve this nation's marijuana problem. Legislators who look to law enforcement techniques to eradicate marijuana use are failing to realize that despite every imaginable deterrent and social stigma, drug use is, and will continue to be, a part of our culture. Decriminalization may be one way to solve some of the problems marijuana use results in. More realistic attitudes toward marijuana use, as well as sound research on both short- and long-term effects, will also help resolve marijuana-related issues. Certainly, the current trend toward research and responsible drug education is a step in the right direction.

OPIATES

Introduction   The issue of opiate decriminalization, specifically the legalization of heroin for known drug-dependents, draws a negative reaction from most people. Yet proponents of heroin legalization claim that supplying morphine or heroin to users would in time reduce the size and influence of the black market in these drugs, and possibly eliminate it.

For a nominal fee, users could buy their daily doses from clinic physicians, bypassing the black market and eventually causing it to collapse because it would be unable to compete with at-cost government pricing. Furthermore, by eliminating the need to prosecute users and other opiate-related police activities, significant time and monies would be saved. With no users to prosecute, court and jail congestion would quickly be reduced. The level of drug-related crime would also likely decline, because users would no longer need to procure large amounts of money (through stealing or prostitution) to support their daily habit.

Decriminalization would help the user in another way. Clinically dispensed heroin would be pure and unadulterated, safely diluted in exact quantities in an appropriate vehicle. With proper doses, pure ingredients, and sterile packaging, needle-related diseases such as AIDS, hepatitis, and sepsis would be reduced, as well as the possibility of overdose.

Still, opponents argue that decriminalization of opiate use would be tantamount to government condonement. This, they feel, would encourage experimentation by individuals who would otherwise remain untempted. Opponents also claim that recruitment of novice users would grow as heroin was illicitly diverted from the clinics to the streets. Psychologist Thomas Szasz feels otherwise:

> The fear that free trade in narcotics would result in vast masses of our population spending their days smoking opium or mainlining heroin, rather than working and taking care of their responsibilities, is a bugaboo that does not deserve to be taken seriously. Habits of work and idleness are deep-seated cultural patterns. . . . free trade in drugs [would not] convert [industrious people] to hippies.[88]

The law has been no more effective a deterrent to opiate use than to marijuana use, and it is doubtful that it will be a significant deterrent in the future. It seems that people who wish to use opiates will do so regardless of the law. Alternatives to rigid legal penalties may need to be tried.

Opiate Maintenance   The 1970s saw a repeated call for the consideration of opiate-maintenance clinics. Perhaps the most concise and encompassing statement in this direction comes from Isador Chein, professor of psychology at New York University:

> There is an obvious expedient for reducing the demand for black market narcotics—and that is to make a better quality of narcotics more cheaply available to addicts on a legal market. There are many advocates, the present [writer] included, of one variant or another of such a plan; and the numbers seem to be increasing. No one, of course, advocates putting narcotics on the open shelves of supermarkets. The basic idea is to make it completely discretionary with the medical profession whether or not to prescribe opiate drugs to addicts for reasons having to do only with the patient's addiction. . . .
>
> We think it is high time . . . to call a policy of forcing the addict from degradation, and all in the name of concern for his welfare, just what it is—vicious, sanctimonious, and hypocritical. . . . Every addict is entitled to assessment as an individual and to be offered the best available treatment in light of his condition, situation, and his needs. No legislator, no judge, no district attorney, no directors of a narcotics bureau, no police inspector and no narcotics agent is qualified to make such an assessment. If, as a result of such an assessment and continued experience in treating the individual addict, it should be decided that the best available treatment is to continue him on narcotics . . . then he is entitled to this treatment.[89]

A study of the British narcotics system may be useful in considering the idea of opiate-maintenance clinics. In 1924 the English government formed a medical commission headed by a distinguished physician, Humphrey Rolliston, to formulate a national policy for their drug-dependence problem. In 1926 the Rolliston Commission decided that heroin could be issued to drug-dependents under several circumstances: (1) if the client was undergoing gradual detoxification at the time and was subject to review as to potential cure; (2) if it was found that prolonged attempts to cure were ill advised because of the severity of the user's withdrawal symptoms following discontinuance of opiate administration; and (3) if the individual displayed the ability to lead a useful and relatively normal lifestyle contingent upon his or her daily dose of opiates.[90]

The heroin-supply program went into effect, and British doctors were allowed to prescribe the drug. Under the program, the number of known users in England remained insignificant, usually averaging under 500 a year.[91] This low rate continued until the early 1960s, when it became apparent that a small group of doctors were overprescribing the drug. A committee was organized to review the problem and eventually a number of steps were taken. Administration of heroin was taken out of the hands of private physicians and delegated to specific doctors who were to operate in specific centers or clinics. Stricter controls on notification of the users and duties of the doctors were also established.

By the spring of 1968, 17 clinics had been authorized by the British government to dispense heroin. The clinics also offered various rehabilitation programs, and clients were consistently urged to consider detoxification and withdrawal as the final goal of their clinic experience.[92] The result of these clinics, according to one researcher, is that "in Britain, the supply of black market heroin has been almost completely eliminated—when the addict can obtain his supply for, at most, a few dollars a week, it is just not worth anyone's time to risk the penalties involved in smuggling or peddling the drug."[93] Another apparent result is that opiate-related crime is allegedly very low in England.

However, Avram Goldstein, professor of pharmacology at Stanford University and director of the Addiction Research Foundation in Palo Alto, California, feels that England's heroin black market has not substantially diminished:

> There will obviously have to be a ceiling on heroin dosage dispensed at a clinic. Then we can predict with fair confidence, on the basis of studies at the Lexington facility of the National Institute on Drug Abuse and elsewhere, that the addicts will escalate their dosage to that ceiling and will become tolerant to that dosage. . . . When their demands for more heroin are rejected, they are likely to look outside the clinic, and thus to sustain an illicit market after all. This has, indeed, happened in Britain.[94]

Joseph L. Nellis, chief counsel for the House of Representatives Select Committee on Narcotics Control, agrees:

> In Britain, approximately 300 doctors are licensed to supply heroin to certified addicts. Yet, there is a thriving black market in heroin. One reason is that certification is difficult to obtain. There are as many as five times the number of untreated addicts in England as those receiving heroin legally from doctors. Of the 10,000 heroin addicts in Britain, only 1,800 are "registered" for "treatment." The crime rate continues to increase and the opportunities for fraud in the dispensing of heroin continue to be substantial. One section of

Scotland Yard does nothing but look into abuse by doctors who are licensed to dispense heroin, and the violations are plentiful and continuous.[95]

The Future of Legalized Opiate Maintenance   From the inconclusive and varying opinions on Britain's opiate-maintenance program, it is impossible to know if that system is really working. It is also impossible to predict if such a system would work in this country. John Kaplan, of the Stanford University Law School, offers an opinion:

> I do not think that any system of heroin maintenance has yet been devised which can cope with the twin problems in that area: if the maintenance is convenient enough for the addicts . . . providing them with heroin outside secure clinics, the diversion problems, and hence the increase in use and addiction, will be substantial; . . . any method of securing clinics and checking on addicts to prevent diversion will be so inconvenient that most addicts will, in fact, prefer life on the street.[96]

Kaplan states further that even if the British system is working, running a similar program in this country would be difficult because of the greater numbers of people who would be involved. Also, Great Britain's system of nationalized health care provides more economic support and assistance to opiate-maintenance clinics than our own system of health care could provide. Finally, costs related to heroin maintenance would be substantially greater in the United States than in England. This alone could undermine any efforts to establish maintenance clinics.

Even if, despite their apparent drawbacks, maintenance clinics are given the go-ahead in this country, they will not solve the problems surrounding opiate dependency; even proponents of such clinics have never held their approach to be a curative one. Nonetheless, maintenance may be a necessary first step in the effort to reduce the personal consequences and the major social side effects of drug dependence.

SUMMARY

Historically, the United States has attempted to restrain drug consumption through legislation and judicial means. But because morality cannot be legislated and because extreme penalties do not necessarily act as a deterrent, drug use has continued, even increased. Although a new, more realistic and sensitive approach to drug abuse is in the wind, it will be slow in reaching effectiveness. In the meantime, drug abuse continues.

Changes for the better in consumer laws have also been slow in coming. Only recently were consumers able to learn about and purchase generic drugs rather than brand-name drugs, thereby often saving a lot of money. Physicians, however, are still reluctant to prescribe anything but established brand-name drugs, and pharmacists are slow to substitute generics. The drug industry has one of the most powerful lobbies in the country, as well as hard-hitting advertising campaigns, and so the slow changeover to generic drugs is not difficult to understand. Nor is the slow advance in legislation aimed at broadening and strengthening consumer rights.

While the number of new drugs on the market has grown, the physician's ability to understand and correctly prescribe many of them has not. Courses in pharmacology are sadly underemphasized in medical school, and busy physicians are rarely able to stay abreast of the new pharmaceutical options that flood their offices.

The FDA, too, has myriad problems with drug-related issues. It must determine which drugs are safe and effective, subjecting every potential product to a battery of tests. Although this long and encumbered process often protects people from the distribution of harmful or ineffective drugs, it also frequently delays for years the availability of pharmacological agents with proven effectiveness.

MILESTONES IN ATTEMPTED DRUG REGULATION

1875   City of San Francisco adopts ordinance prohibiting the smoking of opium in smoking houses.

1882   New York State bans opium smoking.

1885   Federal law limits manufacture of opium for smoking.

1906   Pure Food and Drug Act passes, regulating labeling.

1909   Opium Exclusion Act prohibits importation of opium or its derivatives for nonmedicinal use.

1909   Shanghai Conference.

1911   Hague Conference.

1912   Townsend Act penalizes opiate use.

1914   Harrison Narcotic Act passes, making possession of narcotics without a prescription a legal offense.

1919   Volstead Act.

1920   Eighteenth Amendment (Prohibition).

1924   Importation of heroin banned.

1925   *Linder v. United States* establishes drug dependency as an illness.

1929   Porter Narcotic Farms Law passes, establishing federal treatment "farms" for jailed opiate dependents.

1930   Federal Bureau of Narcotics established.

1933   Twenty-first Amendment repeals Prohibition.

1937   Marijuana Tax Act passes, taxing marijuana distributors and physicians who prescribe marijuana.

1938   Food, Drug and Cosmetic Act passes, requiring proof of product safety.

1942   Opium Exclusion Act requires domestic growers to register.

1956   Narcotic Drug Control Act.

1962   Kefauver-Harris Amendments to the Pure Food and Drug Act pass, requiring proof of product safety and effectiveness.

1963   Community Mental Health Centers Act passes, emphasizing rehabilitation of mental patients, many of whom are drug-dependents.

1965   Drug Abuse Control Amendments to the 1938 Food, Drug and Cosmetic Act pass, classifying depressant, stimulant, and hallucinogenic drugs as "dangerous drugs."

1966   National Addiction Rehabilitation Administration.

1968   Bureau of Narcotics and Dangerous Drugs established, replacing the Federal Bureau of Narcotics.

1968   1965 Drug Abuse Control Amendments further amended.

1970   Comprehensive Drug Abuse Prevention and Control Act passes, liberalizing penalties for drug-abuse offenders.

1972   Presidential Council on Marijuana and Drug Abuse recommends decriminalization of marijuana.

1972   Drug Abuse Office and Treatment Act.

1973   Oregon becomes first state to decriminalize marijuana.

1974   Narcotic Addict Treatment Act.

1974   Alcohol and Drug Abuse Education Act.

1976   Amendments to National Security Act of 1947 prohibit CIA experimentation with drugs on unknowing or unwilling human subjects. PL 94-237 establishes the Office of National Drug Control Policy within the executive office of the president.

1979   S-1075 revises FDA procedures and authority concerning new-drug introduction, testing, marketing, packaging, and recall and litigation powers.

1988   Anti-Drug Bill.

The Consumer and Drug Legislation

N O T E S

1. "Drugged," *New Republic* 169, no. 22 (December 1, 1973):9. Reprinted by permission of *The New Republic,* © 1973 The New Republic, Inc.

2. Ibid.

3. Peter J. Ognibene, "RX: Inexpensive Pills with Costly Labels," *New Republic* 168, no. 22 (June 2, 1973):12. Reprinted by permission of *The New Republic,* © 1973 The New Republic, Inc.

4. Ibid.

5. James Goddard, "The Medical Business," *Scientific American* 229, no. 3 (September 1973):92A.

6. "Clampdown on Drug Industry: Its Meaning," *U.S. News & World Report,* June 24, 1974, p. 36.

7. Ibid.

8. John Schwartz and Mary Hager, "Now, One-Stop Medicine," *Newsweek,* May 25, 1988, pp. 32–33.

9. Ibid.

10. Mary Cronin, "The Price Isn't Right," *Time,* January 8, 1990, pp. 56–58.

11. Ibid.

12. Ibid.

13. Ibid.

14. Linda J. Heller, "Playing Dice with Medicine," *New York Times,* April 16, 1989, pp. 6, 8, 10.

15. Ibid.

16. Ibid.

17. Steven Findlay, "Is Grandma Drowsy, Or Is She Drugged?" *U.S. News & World Report,* June 12, 1989, p. 68.

18. Steven Findlay, "Medicine-Chest Roulette," *U.S. News & World Report* May 9, 1988, p. 76.

19. James W. Cooper, "Medication Misuse in Nursing Homes," *Generations* 2, no. 4 (Summer 1988):56–57.

20. Ibid.

21. Ibid.

22. "Drugged," p. 9.

23. Gordon R. Trapnell, "What's the Estimated Cost of National Outpatient RX Program?" *Pharmacy Times* 46, no. 1 (January 1980):65.

24. Celia Slom, "Ten Questions to Ask Your Pharmacist," *McCall's,* February 1989, p. 96.

25. "Clampdown on Drug Industry," p. 37.

26. "The Ad Made Me Do It," *Current Health I* 14, no. 3 (November 1990):16–18.

27. Andrew Purvis, "Just What the Patient Ordered," *Time* 135 (May 1990):42.

28. Ibid.

29. "Drugged," p. 10.

30. Morton Mintz, *By Prescription Only* (Boston: Benson Press, 1967), p. 339.

31. Linda Stern, "Strategies for Managing Prescription Drug Costs," *Business and Health* June 1990, 41–43.

32. Ibid.

33. "Myths and Facts of Generic Drugs," *FDA Consumer* 21, no. 7 (September 1987):13–14.

34. "Generic Drugs: Still Safe," *Consumer Reports* 55 (May 1990):310–13.

35. Ibid.

36. Ibid.

37. Stephen Levine, "When to Worry about Generics," *Hippocrates* 3, no. 2 (March/April, 1989):28.

38. Jack Anderson and Dale Van Alta, "FDA Fears Drug Scandal Eroding Public Confidence," *The Oregonian* (Portland), October 4, 1989.

39. Christine Gorman, "A Prescription for Scandal," *Time,* August 28, 1989.

40. Ibid.

41. A. Chen, "Orphan Drug Bill Is Signed by Reagan," *Science News* 131, no. 10 (March 1983):22.

42. Ibid.; Roger W. Miller, "Rx for Orphan Drugs," *FDA Consumer* (September 1980):15–17.

43. Ann Gibbons, "Billion-Dollar Orphans: Prescription for Trouble," *Science* 248 (May 11, 1990):678–79.

44. Ibid.

45. Julie Rovner, " 'Orphan Drug' Legislation Approved by House Energy," *Congressional Quarterly Weekly Report* 45 (October 17, 1987).

46. Ibid., p. 15.

47. Joel Forte, *The Pleasure Seekers: The Drug Crisis, Youth and Society* (New York: Grove Press, 1970), p. 67. Reprinted with permission.

48. Kenneth L. Jones, Louis W. Shainberg, and Curtis O. Byer, *Drugs and Alcohol,* 2nd ed. (New York: Harper & Row, 1973), p. 109.

49. Cathy Booth et al., "A Losing Battle," *Time,* December 3, 1990, pp. 44–48.

50. George Church, "Thinking the Unthinkable," *Time,* May 30, 1988, pp. 12–19.

51. Gary S. Becker, "Should Drug Use Be Legalized?" *Business Week,* August 17, 1987, p. 22.

52. Church, "Thinking the Unthinkable."

53. Ralph Bell, "Using the Concept of Risk to Plan Drug Use Intervention Programs," *Journal of Drug Education* 18, no. 2 (1988):135–42.

54. Douglas Lipton and Harry Wexler, "Breaking the Drug-Crime Connection: Rehabilitation Projects Show Promise," *Corrections Today* 50, no. 5 (August 1988:144.

55. Quoted in Eliot Marshall, "A War on Drugs with Real Troops?" *Science* 241 (July 1, 1988):13.

56. Quoted in ibid., p. 13.

57. "Should U.S. Armed Forces Play a Major Role in Interdicting Drug Traffic into the United States?" *Congressional Digest* 65 (November 1986):259–88.

58. Kenneth T. Walsh, Ronald A. Taylor, and Ted Gest, "The New Drug Vigilantes," *U.S. News & World Report,* May 9, 1988, p. 20.

59. Ibid., p. 21.

60. David F. Musto, *The American Disease: Origins of Narcotic Control* (New Haven: Yale University Press, 1973), p. 3.

61. Jones, Shainberg, and Byer, *Drugs and Alcohol,* p. 5.

62. Ray, *Drugs, Society and Human Behavior,* p. 34.

63. Ibid., p. 20.

64. Edward M. Brecher et al., *Licit and Illicit Drugs* (Boston: Little, Brown, 1972), p. 49.

65. Musto, *The American Disease,* p. 68.

66. Brecher et al., *Licit and Illicit Drugs,* p. 265.

67. Musto, *The American Disease,* p. 254.

68. Brecher et al., *Licit and Illicit Drugs,* p. 51.

69. Ibid., p. 52.

70. Musto, *The American Disease,* p. 184.

71. Jones, Shainberg, and Byer, *Drugs and Alcohol,* p. 62.

72. Adapted from Mintz, *By Prescription Only,* pp. 93, 143.

73. Musto, *The American Disease,* p. 235.

74. Ibid.

75. Forte, *The Pleasure Seekers,* pp. 75–76.

76. Jones, Shainberg, and Byer, *Drugs and Alcohol,* p. 103.

77. Ray, *Drugs, Society and Human Behavior,* p. 42.

78. *The Controlled Substances Act* (Washington, D.C.: Drug Enforcement Administration, "Anti-Drug Bill," 1980).

79. *Register-Guard* (Eugene, Oregon), November 19, 1988, p. A8.

80. "Police Policy Questioned in Fatal Drug Raid's Wake," The *Register-Guard* (Eugene, Oregon), Sunday, November 1, 1992, p. 12A.

81. Quoted in Ognibene, "RX," p. 13.

82. Ognibene, "RX," p. 13.

83. "Clampdown on Drug Industry," p. 38.

84. Ibid.

85. "FDA's Policies and Practices for Clearing Drugs Are Criticized before Units," *Wall Street Journal,* August 26, 1974, p. 10.

86. Food and Drug Administration, *Consumer Memo* (Washington, D.C., 1987).

87. Cited in Brecher et al., *Licit and Illicit Drugs,* p. 466.

88. Thomas S. Szasz, "The Ethics of Addiction," in *Annual Editions Readings in Social Problems '73/'74* (Guilford, Conn.: Dushkin Publishing Group, 1973), p. 136.

89. Quoted in Brecher et al., *Licit and Illicit Drugs,* p. 119.

90. National Clearinghouse for Drug Abuse Information, *The British Narcotics System* (Washington, D.C., 1973), p. 2.

91. Ibid.

92. Ibid., p. 5.

93. Phillip Whitter and Ian Robertson, "A Way to Control Heroin Addiction," in *Annual Editions Readings in Social Problems, '73/'74* (Guilford, Conn.: Dushkin Publishing Group, 1973), p. 142.

94. Avram Goldstein, "Heroin Maintenance: A Medical View," *Journal of Drug Issues* 9, no. 3 (Summer 1979):343.

95. Joseph L. Nellis, "Controlling Heroin Addict Crime: Comments," *Journal of Drug Issues* 9, no. 3 (Summer 1979):318.

96. John Kaplan, "Controlling Heroin Addict Crime: Comments," *Journal of Drug Issues* 9, no. 3 (Summer 1979):331.

PREVENTION: EDUCATION AND ALTERNATIVES

INTRODUCTION

The need to address drug usse and abuse appropriately in this country is imperative. Between 9 million and 12 million of our citizens suffer from alcohol dependency, at least 500,000 to 750,000 from opiate dependency, and several million from barbiturate and tranquilizer misuse. But while these millions of citizens suffer, current laws and approaches to drug-abuse control seem inadequate to help. Instead of more and more ineffective legislation, a new perspective on drug abuse seems necessary.

President George Bush and [former] Drug Czar William Bennett are frequently quoted by the media on how the "War on Drugs" is being escalated in Columbia, Peru, Mexico, and even in the United States. This war focuses on how enforcement agencies target **suppliers** such as drug kingpins and cartels. However, there is also a tremendous amount of attention being placed on reducing the **demand** for drugs. The silent "War on Drugs" uses classrooms and community settings as their battlefields to reduce the demand for drugs through prevention/education programs.[1]

Suppliers

Kingpins and cartels that supply drugs; those who make drugs available to the public.

Demand

To ask for drugs. Prevention and education programs are designed to reduce the demand for drugs.

For years the approach to dealing with the drug problem has centered on enforcement and treatment. Recently, there has been an increasing trend to place more resources on prevention through education and intervention. Funding for promotion programs by the U.S. Department of Education increased from $3 million in 1986 to $350 million in 1989.[2]

A NEW PHILOSOPHICAL PERSPECTIVE

Physician Andrew Weil reports on the American system of drug education:

> I cannot help feeling that what we are now doing in the name of stopping the drug problem is the drug problem.. . .\t. Society, either with or without drug education, will eventually learn about the effects of a given drug, but education may facilitate this learning process and increase knowledge of the risk/benefit ratio that accompanies the use of any drug. Such knowledge will ultimately be disseminated into the community, and as a society learns of a drug's risks and benefits, a level of drug use (and abuse) that will depend upon this knowledge will become established.[3]

At the present time it looks like drug use is declining somewhat in the United States. As mentioned earlier, a federal survey brought good news about the nation's war on drugs. The 1990 National Household Survey found a 44 percent reduction in current use of any illicit drug in the past five years, down from 23 million in 1985, to 14.5 million in 1988, to 12.9 million in 1990.[4] The overall rate for current use was 6.4 percent, down from 7.3 percent in 1988. Also, during the past five years, current cocaine use has decreased 72 percent. The number of current cocaine users dropped from 5.8 million (2.9 percent of the population age 12 and older) in 1985 to 2.9 million (1.5 percent) in 1988, to 1.6 million (0.8 percent) in 1990.

While the credit for this reduction cannot go to any one program, credit should go to the collective efforts of a comprehensive program by educators, enforcement (especially educational efforts), parents, peers, counselors, and a large number of community agencies.

DRUG-EDUCATION PROGRAMS

THE ROLE OF THE SCHOOL

The School Health Education Evaluation—a three-year study of four health programs in 20 states—has shown that school health education effectively improves students' health knowledge, attitudes, and behavior.[5] The evaluation was conducted under the auspices of two federal agencies, the Centers for Disease Control and the Office of Disease Prevention. It involved teachers, parents, about 30,000 students, and others in more than 1,000 classrooms. Results showed that health education is most effective when implemented from kindergarten through high school, with administrative and pedagogic support for teacher training, integrated materials, and continuity across grades. The study supports the theory that youngsters can be taught to practice a healthful lifestyle—that educators can influence their students not to smoke; to restrict the amount of fat, sugar, and salt in their diet; to exercise; to have their blood pressure checked; and to obey speed limits and use seat belts. With adequate time (a minimum of 40 periods per year), health education leads to significant gains in knowledge, attitudes, and behavior.[6]

Drug-abuse programs have undergone radical changes in strategy within the last two decades.[7] During the 1960s the "humanistic" approach was developed. The main theme was on the development of individual self-esteem as well as general life skills in contexts irrelevant to drug abuse. Then during the 1970s and 1980s the focus shifted to the "social influences" strategy. This strategy is concerned with "social influences" that promote drug use and training in coping skills through programs designed to increase social confidence. Drug abuse prevention programs have discovered some basic findings.[8] One is that preventative intervention targeted to students in the earlier grade levels is more effective than prevention programs offered at a higher grade level. Second, "comprehensive" drug-abuse prevention programs are thought to be more effective than those based on a "one-shot" basis.

Does drug education in schools work? According to a University of Michigan Institute for Social Research report, drug use by high school students has fallen.[9] However, most experts in the field are unwilling to give full credit to school courses for that result. Indeed, the few studies that have tracked the effects of these programs show no dramatic or long-term reduction in drug use until recently.

Alcohol and drug prevention can be useful if well planned and executed.[10] Today more and more evidence indicates that educators must consider the social context of substance abuse. Among the social areas that need full attention are the following:[11]

1. *goal setting (career and life planning)*—the ability to determine long-range objectives and related activities pertaining to future job opportunities and the necessary life skills for attainment

2. *anxiety/stress-reduction skills*—the ability to recognize situations that create anxiety and stress to develop skills for eliminating and reducing the impact of their decisions.

3. *decision-making skills*—the ability to consider alternative means for dealing with problem situations and to select appropriate options based on rational criteria and judgment.

4. *self-esteem/self-concept development*—the development of perceptions concerning personal regard and personal worth

5. *communication skills*—the ability to recognize one's thoughts and ideas and to effectively share them with others

Drug education has been a long, hard road with seemingly no end. Traditionally, drug-education programs have been based on factual information, with a change in attitude and behavior as the hoped outcome. It is easy to increase knowledge in the short-term within an educational program, but it is much more difficult to change attitudes and even more difficult to change behavior. As the drug problem has not gone away, new approaches to education have been tried. These newer approaches attempt to enrich social and personal development of the student through methods designed to increase self-esteem, interpersonal skills, and participation in alternative activities. Decision-making skills are included in this new approach. Learning how to understand to make appropriate decisions is touted as being a key in prevention of substance abuse.[12] If we can teach our youth how to make good decisions, they will make good decisions about drugs.

"Schools can play a major part in the solution of student drug use by becoming involved in early prevention programming."[13] Successful prevention demands early attention to a combination of affective, attitudinal, and behavioral components in addition to disseminating accurate information.

TEACHERS

Clearly, it would be beneficial to include alcohol and drug education in teacher-preparation programs.[14] Teachers are out there to set an example and educate, along with dealing with kids with problems or kids of addicted parents. "It would be naive to expect such training to produce an abstinent group of prospective teachers." However, it would be expected that preservice training could favorably affect the alcohol and other drug attitudes of prospective teachers and certainly that these college students would be better prepared than the general college population to develop and implement prevention programs and assist in the identification of young people who have drug-abuse problems or come from chemically dependent families.

Teachers and counselors can work together to help students develop positive self-concepts.[15] Establishing a classroom atmosphere in which students are praised often, are frequently able to demonstrate their strengths, and learn ways of respecting one another and giving each other positive feedback does much to enhance student self-esteem.

A development program that complements community efforts and involves the family and peers may effectively reduce the problem of drug and alcohol experimentation and use. One way to help reduce the problem is to better target populations at whom intervention and prevention programs can be used. We should direct our programs at high-risk groups if intervention programs are to be successful.[16] The effectiveness of intervention could be increased with additional knowledge or where high-risk areas are located. Thus, the efficiency of these programs could be enhanced if we could identify in some systematic way the high-risk individuals located in high-risk areas. This information would allow decision makers to strategically locate programs where they would be most effective.

EDUCATIONAL APPROACHES

The long-term solution to the drug problem appears to lie in reducing America's seemingly insatiable demand for drugs through education, prevention, and treatment. The money should be there for every child to be exposed to a quality prevention-education program, and every addict who really wants to say no ought to have access to immediate treatment.[17] One thing for sure, drug education must start earlier, in elementary school, and must be broad-based and comprehensive, involving a cross-section of the community.

Today more and more children are faced with the intimidating problem of refusing drugs. Increasing methods are trying to be developed to help kids say no to drugs; they are being well educated and well informed, and "yet the youth succumbs." Even though a youth may be educated and informed and knows right from wrong, he or she may not have mastered the right refusal skills. "Recent work suggests that such yielding, even in the face of adequate information and motivation, may in part be a result of deficiency of refusal skills especially under real-life peer group circumstances."[18]

A variety of new approaches are being implemented in schools. A **comprehensive K–12 drug education program** that focuses on knowledge, attitude, and behavior change is a start. However, special emphasis must be placed on high-risk students. Through the use of Drug Free School federal grants, a variety of new drug-education programs, such as infusion curriculums, Children Are People Too, DARE, Here's Looking at You 2000, Health Skills for Life, skillstreaming, and Project Graduation are being implemented with favorable results.

Infusion Curriculum   The state of Texas is busy implementing "Education for Self Responsibility II: The Prevention of Drug Use."[19] This PK–12 infusion curriculum on substance abuse has several teaching-method ideas for every teacher (math, science, English) at every grade level. It is probably one of the largest and most widely used infusion curriculums ever introduced in the schools.

Children Are People Too   This K–6 program works with students to develop self-esteem, decision making, and chemical awareness. A handbook accompanies the curriculum. The attempt is to start early-prevention programs so students will be better prepared when substances are offered to them.

Drug Abuse Resistance Education   Drug Abuse Resistance Education (DARE) has been a very effective curriculum that utilizes the expertise of police and educators. It has become a national curriculum that reduces drug-abuse behavior. A short-term evaluation was designed to assess the impact of Project DARE, a joint venture of the Los Angeles Police Department and the Los Angeles Unified School District, on the knowledge, attitudes, and self-reported behavior of seventh-grade children who received a full-semester DARE curriculum during the sixth grade.[20] Compared to a control group, students who had DARE training reported significantly lower use of alcohol, cigarettes, and other drugs since graduating from the sixth grade. These findings were especially strong for boys. In response to questions for which students were to imagine friends pressuring them to use alcohol or drugs, DARE students more frequently refused the imagined offers and more often used refusal strategies that removed them from the immediate temptation. DARE seems to be increasing in popularity throughout the country.

Comprehensive K–12 Drug Education Program

A grades K–12 coordinated drug education curriculum focusing on knowledge, attitudes, and behavior change to stop drug abuse. It involves students, parents, teachers, counselors, and the community working cooperatively to curb drug abuse. School and community cooperation is essential in the fight against drugs.

Police Play a Role in Education
Source: Michael Siluk/The Image Works

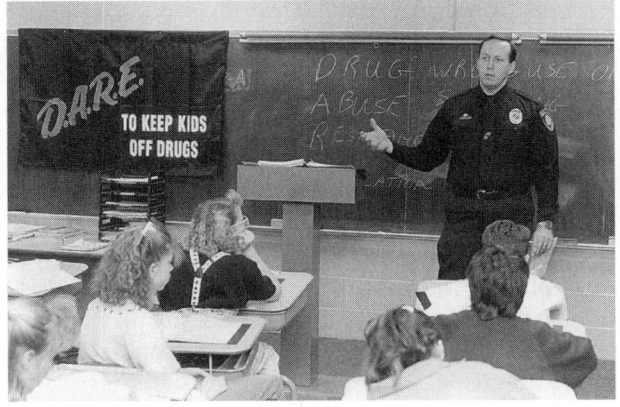

Here's Looking at You and Here's Looking at You, Part Two
Here's Looking at You and its revised programs are widely used in districts throughout the United States. The kit includes videos, puppets, games, audiotapes, and other tools. The program's objective is to increase knowledge about drug use and teach kids to resist peer pressure. Kids learn how to say no and still keep their friends.

When signing up for the curriculum Here's Looking at You, Part Two, each teacher who uses this curriculum receives 30 hours of training to make him or her a better user of the program.[21] Some of the major goals of the program include the following:

1. create in the students a higher level of self-esteem, which may result in the students' not wanting to use drugs
2. improve coping skill that will allow students to handle compromising situations
3. develop effective interpersonal decision making
4. present more facts and substantive knowledge about drug and chemical dependence

Researchers have found that the students going through Here's Looking at You, Part Two, had more knowledge; however, attitudes did not appear to change.[22]

Health Skills for Life   A national health curriculum, originating in Eugene, Oregon, which features a section on substance abuse, is Health Skills for Life. This popular, comprehensive health curriculum is a ready-made aid for teachers to teach health topics. The curriculum also includes a K–12 substance-abuse section

Skillstreaming   One approach to refusal skills is called skillstreaming. "A group approach, involving five to eight youngsters plus one or two teacher-trainers," it is used to teach the use of behaviors needed when faced with tough one-on-one situations, including those where refusal skills are needed.

The teacher teaches skillstreaming through four simple methods: The first is modeling—displaying present scenes in which the "protagonist" handles troublesome situations by employing the skill being taught. The second is role-playing, in which each peer is given the chance to role-play or practice the current skill as a rehearsal for a real situation. The third, performance feedback, is the feedback given from the other group members on the performance. And the fourth is transfer of training, in which a variety of homework and other procedures are implemented. "Skillstreaming, in its diverse but non-substance abuse utilization has been shown to be a ready learned (by trainers), effective (for trainers) and inexpensive approach, which has found very wide usage in American schools and agencies, and most frequently has been targeted to low-income and/or minority youth."[23]

Project Graduation   The state of Maine initiated Project Graduation, in which students have a drug-free graduation party. Currently 99 percent of schools in Maine have Project Graduation.[24] It is hoped that such parties will reduce the large number of fatal accidents so often associated with drinking and driving at graduation time.

COUNSELORS

Referrals to substance-abuse counselors may help intervention. In some cases students must be referred to adolescent treatment centers. It is very important to start early and offer appropriate education, intervention, treatment, and follow-up. Obviously, the school teacher can't do it all. It will take the cooperation of teachers, counselors, parents, peers, and community agencies to be successful in attacking the drug problem early.

Counseling and Prevention Programs   The New York City public schools have implemented counseling and prevention programs in which personnel use observations available to them to make essentially the same decisions trained mental-health professionals would.[25] Students most susceptible to using drugs are placed in arousal, coercion, or counseling groups. Arousal methods are aimed at enhancing the students' problem-solving skills for manageable problems and coping abilities for unmanageable one's. Coercion methods involve contingency management, in which rewards and punishments are linked closely and surely with student behavior. Counseling is of two types, A and B. Counseling A enhances self-esteem and communicates to the student new and accurate information about his or her significance. Counseling B is intended for students developing a behavior pattern that may later be termed antisocial. These counseling and prevention programs are being implemented to provide **alternatives** to drugs.

The Student Assistance Program   The Student Assistance Program (SAP) is a spin-off from the employee assistance program and is a new concept for the school system.[26] It is designed to help students with their problems, which may be drug-related or have to do with peers or family. It

Alternatives
A variety of activities, such as exercise, work, wilderness experiences, and religion to take the place of using drugs.

provides information to the students on sensitive topics. SAP offers help to students who are involved with drugs or who are living with people who use drugs and consequently are being negatively influenced by the situation.

The SAP program involves six functions: (1) early identification of the problem, (2) support, (3) referral, (4) intervention, (5) assessment, and (6) case management. The hardest part of this program is developing trust with the students because the students perceive the SAP counselor as a school official and are therefore less likely to confide. The counselor has difficulty gaining the confidence of students because he or she has not only to establish a rapport with the student but also must maintain the records and measure where change is necessary.

School districts are hiring substance-abuse specialists in intervention and counseling to work with high-risk students. In many cases these specialists have been able to keep students in school while addressing drug and other related problems.

THE ROLE OF PARENTS

Experts agree that parents are the first and best protection a child has against drug abuse, offering strong family support, positive role models, love, and guidance. But how is a parent to know if a child is abusing drugs? Be suspicious if several of these warning signals are present, suggests the Aid Association for Lutherans:[27]

- a change in friends; secrecy about new friends and activities
- withdrawal from family, old friends, school
- lots of time spent in unusual places
- mood swings; excessive anger, irritability
- changes in appearance (drug-subculture styles or sloppiness)
- increased discipline problems

Like Father, Like Son—Parent Influence
Source: Richard Hutching/Photoedit

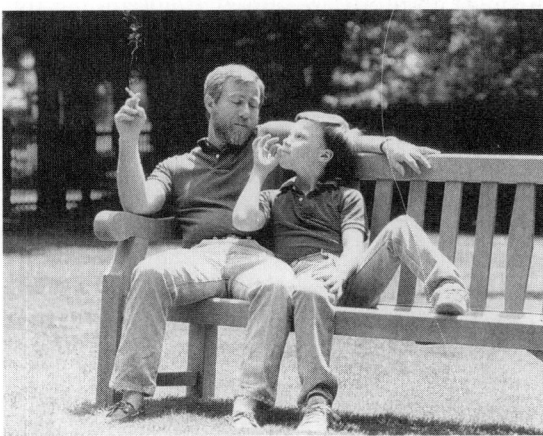

- drop in grades or other performance
- borrowing lots of money; theft
- decrease in energy and endurance
- weight loss or gain; increased or decreased hunger; increased thirst
- changes in timing and duration of sleep
- frequent use of eye drops and breath mints

Parents should not be enablers, bargaining with the abuser to stop or protecting the abuser from punishment. Nor should they point fingers haphazardly at "bad influences," or fool themselves that the solution is simple and painless. Parents should get over their initial anger before confronting the child and rehearse what they are going to say. They shouldn't be surprised if the child is defensive, denying that anything is the matter, or if he or she feigns innocence or becomes antagonistic.

For a first-time offender, the parents should increase discipline in the form of a family contract that forbids drugs, alcohol, and tobacco and sets curfews. For a second-time offender, they should seek immediate professional treatment.[28]

Parents can help keep their kids off drugs.[29] Even though drug and alcohol use by young people is all around us, parents do have some things in their favor: children are impressionable, and therefore the chances of influencing their feelings about drugs and alcohol and drugs are good. Parents should move quickly to influence their children about drugs because kids are vulnerable to peer pressure from and early age.

- Teach your children about drugs. Talk to your kids about drugs only after you have become educated yourself.
- Don't preach what you aren't willing to practice. Telling children about responsible drug use is okay only as long as you yourselves are using drugs responsibly.
- Begin drug education while your children are still young. Waiting until they reach adolescence may be a mistake.
- Take a firm stand against use of drugs and/or alcohol at an illegal age. Parents who allow minors to use are condoning criminal behavior and destroying any basis for discipline.
- Talk casually, openly, and honestly about drugs. Don't preach.
- Help your children get involved in drug-free activities. They'll learn they don't need drugs to have a good life.
- Give your children ways to say no to drugs. Role playing helps children develop the confidence to say no for real.[30]

It is estimated that one out of three U.S. families is wracked by drugs.[31] Parents have become very concerned about keeping their children off drugs. From the primary grades on, almost every child knows another who regularly uses drugs and booze. More than 4 million children between the ages of 13 and 17 said they had been offered drugs and booze. More than 4 million children between the ages of 13 and 17 said they had been offered illicit drugs.[32] Researchers say that only one weapon can start a true counterattack against chemical warfare, parents. Parents often deny their child is on drugs because it makes them look bad. Having a family pattern of drug or alcohol abuse quadruples the risk that your child will continue the cycle.

Parents need drug education as much as their children.[33] This is because if they don't receive this drug education, then they won't be able to help effectively educate their children about drugs and their harmful effects. Many parents feel they are ignorant with respect to drugs and their effects and couldn't help their children if they were to come to them with problems. In fact, many parents surveyed said that their knowledge of drugs and their effects were below what they believed their children's knowledge to be.

Many of today's drug-education programs are aimed at the school-age population, and very little has been aimed at the adult population. Parents and teachers in the early 1970s ranked very low on a drug and alcohol knowledge test with scores not much higher than would be expected of merely guessing.[34] The results of this survey concluded that more drug education programs need to be aimed at the adult population.

Parents need to begin with educating themselves about drugs before their children are exposed to them. If parents don't know how to cope with drugs, they can't very well expect their children to know.

The social learning theory implies that behavior depends on one's associates, and the parents are considered to be the primary contributors to the development of a young person. Parental influence can make the difference when the child is faced with difficult decisions.

A study was conducted in Ontario, Canada, that sampled 2,259 elementary and secondary students. The students were tested before the intervention, immediately after, and then six months later as to the peer and parental influence in cannabis use.[35] The test questions focused on infrequent, regular, and frequent use and were asked in regard to both peer and parental findings. The results of this study indicated that those children who were aware of their parents' disapproval of cannabis use were more likely not to use the substance than those who felt peer disapproval.

There are several steps that parents can take initially to help their children deal with the inevitable exposure to drugs. Keeping children's parties and other functions alcohol-free and drug-free is a good beginning in the fight against drugs.[36] Parents should obtain the phone number and address of the place where the party is being held, as well as contact the parents of the child having the party to make sure no drugs will be on the premises and that they will be personally supervising the children.

There is also a great deal of attention being paid to the amount of self-esteem a child has and his or her relation to drug use. Communication between parent and the child as well as active parent participation in the child's life all seem to have positive effects on the child's development. The key is to always keep the lines of communication open because children are continually facing crises, which deserve the respect of the parent. Don't expect them to deal with their problems as an adult would, or even expect them to recognize the seriousness of the situation. Parents, by playing an active role in the child's life, will have an easier time recognizing any problems the child might be having. If a child is taught early on to be in control of his or her life, and given the skills with which to cope with problems, then the crises will not seem unmanageable. The necessary tools for coping and living, then, don't have to be used exclusively in drug situations. If the child learns them in everyday situations, then when a serious drug situation develops, he or she will be better able to handle it when the parent is not around.[37] It can also be helpful to go over with your child some answers to give to someone offering drugs. If children are familiar with those responses, it will be easier for them to remove themselves from a negative situation. Parents themselves need to begin by educating themselves about drugs before their children are exposed to them. If parents do not know how to cope with drugs, they can't very well expect their children to cope either.

THE INFLUENCE OF PEERS

It was determined that the peer group becomes an important element when the person has already made the first step in using the drug. The peer group at this point offers support, gives access to the substance, maintains the setting, and provides reinforcement for continued usage.[38] Natural Helpers, the Drug Abuse Response Team (DART), and the Student Athletic Summer Institute (SASI) offer examples of a few peer-oriented programs to fight substance abuse and other problems.

NATURAL HELPERS

Natural Helpers is a program where students are asked to select two or three people they think could best help them with problems. A list of all these people is developed, and about 25 of the people who are most frequently mentioned are selected (representative males and females, various interest groups, and different grade levels). Those selected as the peer group are invited to a special training session so they can better help people deal with various problems. Once trained they are in a better position to help advise or refer others to specialists who may be able to provide the services needed. These select peer-group members are currently being used in middle schools, high schools, some small colleges, and even senior groups. It enables those most likely to be called on for help to learn how to advise effectively and refer when necessary.

DRUG ABUSE RESPONSE TEAM

The Drug Abuse Response Team, or DART, program was developed by the Sacred Heart Adolescent Recovery Program in Eugene, Oregon, to help students take an active position in reducing substance abuse and other negative behaviors. It is aimed at fourth and fifth graders, middle school students, high school students, and school-parent-community groups. These groups are taught how to deal with denial, provide support without becoming involved (with drugs, shop lifting, and so on), staying clear of problems, and helping oneself. Specific training is provided for each of these groups with the hope that they will help others, as well as themselves, stay out of trouble. It is an attempt to become proactive instead of just sitting around and watching problems occur.

STUDENT ATHLETIC SUMMER INSTITUTE

Another successful example of peer education is SASI—the Student Athletic Summer Institute.[39] The SASI programs has two goals: First, it was designed as an early-intervention program to reach the many student athletes involved in drugs. Second, and perhaps more important, it focused attention on training the influential students to take advantage of the power they have over their peers and by educating them against the horrors drugs can cause in a young adult's life. The pilot summer session results indicated that the program was very well received by those involved at *all levels*. Support was evident from schools, officials, and the students through their eagerness to participate in the program. The use of peer education can play a major role in supplementing classroom drug-education programs.

SCHOOL AND COMMUNITY COOPERATION

During the 1950s the community was rediscovered as a potentially effective agent for intervention, as well as a factor in mental, physical, and social problems.[40] Both alcoholism and drug use came to be viewed as legitimate concerns for community intervention. Drugs and drug use are part of our lifestyles. With this in mind, we must do the following if we are to promote community intervention and effective drug use:[41]

- define drugs and the consequences of their use
- define drug use and misuse
- define sickness, pathology, and health
- define community
- select and define reasonable criteria for success and failure of community intervention programs
- acknowledge (1) the multiplicity of factors that may reinforce, inhibit, or be irrelevant to people's chemical appetites, and (2) the state of political, economic, and social affairs at any given time

It is up to us and our communities to stop drug use and abuse through education and other means.

PROJECT IMPACT

Project Impact involves the education of administrators, teachers, and community leaders as to the nature and extent of substance abuse in their communities.[42] Training provides a heavy emphasis on communication and the importance of family systems.

Following the training, a key component remains in place. This is the "Core Team," which is composed of concerned teachers who will deal with future substance-abuse issues in that setting. The importance of this approach is that each setting is different, and not all school environments are best dealt with in the same way. Additionally, a community liaison may be trained to help coordinate referrals through out-of-school agencies.

The results of a study, which were gained through a questionnaire administered to the administrators of the schools involved, suggested that the effectiveness of Project Impact training was 5 to 20 times more effective than prior prevention strategies. Great improvement came in the understanding of available resources in intervention such as school psychologists, peer counselors, school assessment teams, and the Core Team. The most highly rated intervention strategy was parental involvement, followed by community and teacher involvement. This emphasizes the broad-based, multidisciplinary approach to successful intervention.

HAMPTON INTERVENTION AND PREVENTION PROJECT (HAMPTON, VIRGINIA)

The Hampton Intervention and Prevention Project involves not only the school system but also the police department, parent groups, and civic and human-service organizations.[43] The approach that shows the most promise targets not just drugs but a child's entire environment.

SEATTLE SCHOOL DEVELOPMENT PROJECT

A program that teaches kids to say no but also focuses on improving parenting skills and teaching methods is the Seattle School Development Project. The annual survey of high school seniors shows drug use declining slightly.[44] The war against drugs will take decades, not just months.

SOULBEAT I

In Helena, Arkansas, a new approach to the fight against drugs was undertaken by the community substance-treatment and -prevention center. The center, having difficulty reaching the black community, formed a new coalition of black (and accepted white) community leaders in order to reach the black families and youth of their community. The group began a program that would utilize the ability of local schools and churches to communicate with the black community. Soulbeat I was the devised program, consisting of various substance-abuse-center personnel as well as a "Black Task Force to provide cultural-specificity in all aspects of the project."[45] The project focused on educating the black families and their youth as to the ultimate means of substance-abuse prevention. Plays and skits were written and performed by community youths, with topics like "peer group pressures, parent-teenager communication problems, and institutional racism." Immediately following the skits a discussion was conducted with community members and church parishioners concerning "the myths associated with using alcohol." The discussion was followed by a question-and-answer period.

After the initial project, local parishioners confronted the project coordinators and expressed their own interest to continue group discussions and question-and-answer periods among community members and their own churches. The program found success in that ultimately youths found a positive community status in their association with Soulbeat I. The Soulbeaters were found to have established a group norm that discouraged drug use.

COMMUNITY TOGETHER

This is part of the Eugene-Springfield (Oregon) Community Partnership to reduce substance abuse.[46] This federally funded program is an attempt to bring together various components of the community to fight substance abuse together. This includes various educational levels, government, enforcement, public and private agencies, students, parents, and so on. The first phase was designed to create an awareness of who is available in the community to help fight substance abuse. Once identified, the second phase was an actual pulling together of over 500 representatives for a two-day conference to work together in various subgroups like family management; alienation, rebelliousness, and lack of bonding; community laws and norms; and drug availability to focus on approaches to do something positive to reduce the substance-abuse problem. This program is in the second year of a five-year plan. These subcommittees are charged with implementing a workable plan of action. Similar programs are being advanced in communities across the nation in an attempt to fight substance abuse collectively.

MASS MEDIA

Mass media can be an effective tool in reducing drug abuse. There are six key elements for successful campaigns as discovered by researchers.[47] One is the specification of a well-defined target audience; a second element is specific research to understand the target audience and pretest the materials for campaign. The third is to incorporate messages that build up from the audience's current knowledge and satisfy its preexisting needs and motives. Fourth is a media plan to ensure exposure to the campaign is needed. Fifth is the need to evaluate progress. The sixth and most important element for a campaign that works is a long-term commitment.

THE HARVARD ALCOHOL PROJECT

The Center for Health Communication of the Harvard School of Public Health conducted a research-based media campaign with the television industry to demonstrate what a public-health campaign can accomplish through advertising and public-relations strategies. The project focused on designated drivers to promote a change in the United States about the social norms associated with drinking and driving. The campaign, which was promoted through commercials as well as being incorporated as a subject in the shows themselves to reinforce the idea, appears to be very successful and is still going on. In 1989 data collected by the Gallup Organization on behalf of the project concluded that "78 percent of U.S. adults who attended social functions where alcohol is served had seen a television message promoting the designated driver concept during the previous three months."[48] In addition, it was noted, in June of 1989 the percentage of people who use designated drivers went to 72 percent, 10 percent more than just nine months previous." The percentage of people using the designated driver is almost equal to the percentage of people who actually saw the message. The messages are working, and at this time there are campaigns against marijuana, cocaine, and some other drugs with the hope they will be as successful as the ones used against alcohol.

ALTERNATIVES

When looking for appropriate alternatives to drug use, we must look for activities that fill the same needs that drugs do. As this book has shown, people take drugs for a variety of reasons:

1. to feel better
2. to obtain pleasure and reward
3. to relieve discomfort
4. to pursue an altered state of consciousness
5. to test one's maturity
6. to feel part of a group

Alternatives to drug use must therefore afford these same experiences. Though virtually any activity may be considered an alternative, some realistic alternatives are exercise, wilderness experiences, work, social and political activism, religion, biofeedback, and meditation.

One of the goals of selecting alternatives is to substitute for a negative dependency a series of positive dependencies. A positive "addiction" usually meets the following six criteria:

1. It is something noncompetitive. You choose to do it, and you can devote approximately one hour a day to it.
2. It is possible to *do it easily:* You do not need a great deal of mental effort to do it well.
3. You can *do it alone,* or rarely with others, but you do not have to depend on others in order to do it.
4. You believe that is *has some value* (physical, mental, or spiritual) for you.
5. You believe that if you persist at it *you will improve,* but this is completely subjective.
6. You can do it *without criticizing yourself.* If you can't accept yourself during this time, the activity will not be addicting.[49]

Individuals must make choices throughout their lives. The choices made regarding the use of drugs could have a dramatic impact on one's life. Drugs are extremely plentiful and people are constantly exposed to them. The following box includes a long list of alternatives a person can choose to do alone or with friends. Many of these are free or less expensive than using drugs. One can quickly observe that there are many simple alternatives to drugs. Trying new things often enables a person to overcome the temptation to try drugs.

SUGGESTED ALTERNATIVES

- Have friends over for a lunch or dinner, each bringing a course of the meal
- Work out at a gym
- Go swimming, hot tubbing or to a sauna
- Go to a movie, play, or musical
- Ride a bike
- Go for a walk
- Watch TV
- Try gardening
- Do homework
- Do volunteer work
- Play videogames
- Play cards
- Read
- Go bowling
- Listen to music
- Go to a zoo or museum

EXERCISE

Research findings indicate that exercise is likely to improve health. Depending on the intensity, exercise may aid in the decomposition of arterial cholesterol deposits that inhibit blood flow, increase cardiac efficiency by increasing blood output per beat, reduce blood pressure, aid in digestion by stimulating gastrointestinal secretion, improve respiration efficiency, stimulate production of biogenic amines (neurotransmitters that facilitate brain message sending), and stimulate production of testosterone and estrogen. Furthermore, exercise can improve muscle tone and muscle development, converts fat into caloric energy, and may aid in gradual weight reduction.

Despite all these potential physical benefits, the most important benefit of exercise may be psychological. Exercise can be an efficient way to reduce stress, develop or enhance a positive self-image, and increase personal awareness. Through intense physical movement, many people are better able to deal with daily pressure and obtain a sense of personal pride and accomplishment. Exercise's ability to produce this strong sense of self, coupled with its ability to improve strength and health, may make it a valued alternative to drug abuse.

Many people, in their efforts to survive the technocracy of our time, have forgotten, lost, or repressed the ability or desire to perceive subtle body cues, sensitive messages that tell us what's going on internally. Many people are physically out of touch. The so-called primitive people are in tune with their physiology because they have to be: It is their tool for survival. In the twentieth century, "civilized" people have placed greater emphasis on cognitive functioning, on the use of their minds, to the exclusion of body awareness. The body and its functions are an integral contributor to the understanding of the complete person.

Exercise can help a person understand his or her movement characteristics, capabilities, and limitations. Increased self-awareness enhances self-appreciation and sensitivity and therefore the possibility of understanding one's environment and fellow human beings. Accomplishment, insight and awareness, a degree of meaning, and identification of the stimulation of emotion by motion—these are some of the issues addressed by physical movement.

Jogging   Though exercise can include mountain climbing, calisthenics, walking, bicycling, canoeing, swimming, yoga, T'ai Chi, skiing, dancing, and many other forms of physical movement, jogging has become one of the more popular and successful ways to feel good and stay in shape. After initial skepticism and hesitation, millions of Americans are finding jogging to be a real source of benefit and pleasure. Joggers are also discovering that running provides "therapeutic effects for the scars caused by the stresses of modern society—including depression, nervousness, inability to sleep, inability to cope with their environment, even in some cases, schizophrenia." Jogging results in "very measurable changes in depression levels . . . stimulates the unconscious . . . , [reduces] muscular electrical activity . . . [and] nerve electrical activity,"[50] affects mental functioning in a positive way.

Jogging may work its effects by helping people to burn off the tension and frustration they encounter each day. Or it may help to reduce tension and other adverse reactions simply by providing the opportunity to physically escape the causes of those reactions.

The term *timing out,* employed by behavioral psychologists, refers to the removal of an individual from his or her immediate environment to a neutral site of seclusion. It refers to taking a break from one's present involvement. Its application to jogging is quite simple. Jogging provides a break in the pattern of mounting daily tension that people often feel on stressful days. Says one writer on the subject:

> Any measurable psychological benefits from running may come not from the act itself, but from the opportunity that act gives the runner to get away from the stresses and pressures of modern civilization. You cannot answer a jangling telephone or pay bills while circling the running track, and long runs in the woods or on back country roads may permit otherwise harassed business executives or housewives to let their minds "spin free," engage in the form of conscious daydreaming and relaxation.[51]

As early as the 1940s, Veterans Administration hospitals used running to help their clients relax. But later, as Carlyle H. Folkins of the University of California at Davis notes, "we went backwards . . . Along came tranquilizers and other forms of drugs. All the psychiatrists got out their chemistry sets and forgot about the potential benefits of exercise. It was like the old Dupont slogan: 'Better things from chemistry.' "[52] Today, however, running may be an effective alternative to chemistry.

Robert Brown of the University of Virginia is exploring natural body chemistry as it relates to exercise. Working with Fred Goodwin at the National Institute of Mental Health, he is measuring neurotransmitter metabolite levels in response to physical exercise. Blood and urine specimens are taken from subjects before exercise and at one-, two-, and three-hour intervals following exercise to determine chemical fluctuations in the body. Brown reports that people suffering from depression obtain an antidepressant factor about two hours after exercise.

Drug-treatment centers and other experts are finding that running is an effective form of therapy for drug-dependents.[53] Running is a very positive alternative to drugs because it is also a way of improving one's health. Running is so easy that anyone can take it up without having to get fancy or expensive equipment.

WILDERNESS EXPERIENCES

A wilderness environment offers a new perspective through which one may view his or her life. In such places, with positive counseling, drug users may be able to see their habits in new, more objective ways.[54] Eventually they may be able to reduce their drug consumption and perhaps eliminate it.

Though wilderness experiences may be obtained on one's own, various organizations offer opportunities to join in "risk sports" or "risk recreation." Bridge Over Troubled Waters, Inc., a drug-addiction treatment center headquartered in Berkeley, California, offers such out-of-the-ordinary experiences as river running, parachuting, skin diving, rock climbing, and skiing, and believes that participating in such adventures can address the need for risk taking that many heroin users have. The goal of the program is to show users alternative lifestyles and different ways of getting high, and to use success in an outdoor challenge as a step toward building confidence. Says one participant in the program:

> I thought it was going to be a complete bore. But then I got on that raft, and all the way down the river I felt light; I was singing, hollering. [River running] provided me with natural highs and challenges to supplant those I had been getting from involvement with heroin . . . . when we finished that run I was eager to get off on more adventures. I had enjoyed the challenge of the river more than that of running the streets looking for a fix.[55]

Confidence gained from a successful experience can spread to other areas of an individual's life. Believers in the wilderness-experience approach feel that outdoor living will help drug users develop fortitude and the drive to leave the street life. Proponents also believe that increased self-confidence will encourage increased self-esteem. A more positive self-concept, they feel, may reduce the drug-dependent's desire to escape "reality."

To bring on all these positive changes, however, wilderness experiences, like all other drug alternatives, must make the participant feel good. As one Bridge Over Troubled Waters consultant says:

> Dope makes you feel good, and unless you give drug addicts an alternative [that does the same], it's all a lot of talk. For them there's no feeling good without dope. It is a meaningless abstraction until we make the abstraction real. We are saying to them, "Hey, come do this with us. Get away from the whoring and the pimping and the buying of dope, come with us and feel good, come and get high on the 'natch.' "[56]

WORK

Many people define themselves in terms of the function they perform in society—their work. People who like what they do usually feel content and consequently treat themselves with respect. People who are out of work or have a low-paying or dissatisfying job that leaves them with no sense of worth or personal accomplishment usually are not content and may be driven to drink, take pills, or smoke to escape their unhappy state.

Meaningful work—work that is of genuine value to others and contributes to the production of quality goods or services—can do much to elevate feelings of self-worth and happiness. Such work can be fulfilling, occupy time, fill gaps, and be enjoyable and satisfying. Work can also cause fatigue, but this may actually provide an opportunity for relaxation. Finally, employment can result in paychecks, providing symbolic reinforcement of worth to society as well as purchasing power.

SOCIAL AND POLITICAL ACTIVISM

Just as work in the form of gainful employment may serve as an alternative to drug dependency, so may work in the form of political or social involvement. People can gain satisfaction by identifying with a new value system or a new political ideology, especially one that inspires hope. Working for ideological change can help drug abusers fill empty time as well as address their need for self-worth.

A case in point is the People's Republic of China. For hundreds of years, this country had great problems with opium addiction. By 1920, 25 percent of the population were believed to be using the drug. But then something happened. By 1930, the total opium-dependent population had shrunk to 10 million, and as of the late 1960s the user population was virtually nonexistent.

What caused these opium users to turn away from their drug of choice? It was ideological change. The Communist takeover in 1949 was a chance for both the nation and its youth to redefine their worth and role:

> An American who lived in a Chinese village during and after liberation explained it in terms of a meaning of a new word, "fanshen, . . . to turn the body or to turn over." To China's hundreds of millions of landless and land-poor peasants it meant to stand up to throw off the landlord yoke, to gain land, stock, implements, and houses. But, it meant much more than this. It

meant to throw off superstition and study science, to abolish "word blind-ness" and learn to read, to cease considering women as chattels and establish equality between the sexes, to do away with appointed village magistrates and replace them with elected councils. It meant to enter a new world.[57]

It also meant to help the millions of opium dependents move back into the mainstream of Chinese society. This process was effected nationwide through small street communities that offered political and cultural leader-ship as well as medical care. These small groups campaigned against opium use and were also responsible for detecting and censuring those who contin-ued to use opium. Successes and failures were reported to higher authorities, and difficult cases were referred to rehabilitation centers. A disciplined Com-munist party of six million members supported the national campaign.[58]

> Meetings about addiction . . . were part of the national action program in which all people spent an hour a day discussing political and health topics of national importance. The testimony of former addicts was important to all levels of this reformation including newspaper stories, small community groups and rehabilitation centers. Mass meetings, slogans and flags used the words of the ex-addicts. Addiction was denounced as anti-social and unhealthy because it was an imperialist and capitalist activity.[59]

In this way, current and potential drug users were separated from drug involvement by involvement in the building of a new social order—one that decried the use of opiates. Although this example shows an extreme and undesired way to achieve alternative involvement, it does show that involve-ment can bring about change. Campaigning to elect officials can give people the enjoyable sense of being on the inside, of being useful and successful. Pushing for social reform can instill a sense of self-worth and pride, as well as result in a better world. Political and social activism may not work for every-one, but for many people it can provide the highs and rewards of drug use.

RELIGION

Religion can offer the same sense of involvement and exposure to new values that political and social activism can. Adopting ideas and beliefs that others also espouse can help one develop a sense of belonging and a better understanding of oneself. The "Jesus freak" movement that began in the mid-1960s is a good example of how involvement in religion can cause change. During the late 1960s and early 1970s, hundreds of thousands of young peo-ple, many of them drug dependents, became overwhelmed by their non-establishment lifestyle and by prolonged drug use. They turned to religion, and in this straightforward and structured world they found an alternative. They found help in the form of strict adherence to a religious philosophy, which was reinforced by group demands on behavior. Specific rules and reg-ulations gave participants a clear, well-defined picture of their place in the world.

As the 1980s gave way to the 1990s, epidemic levels of vicious substance abuse have plagued the United States. This new wave of pestilence has attacked the nation with a level of violence reminiscent of that which gripped the nation during Prohibition. Current gang activity in the cocaine and crack worlds reminds us of the "Roaring '20s" in the speakeasies' world of Chicago's gangland empires. This was the world of Al Capone, Frank Nitty, and Elliot Ness of *Untouchables* fame.

The role of religion in helping those with chemical dependencies is becoming clearer. Religion, the churches of the nation, and congregations of people across the land can open the doors to the hope of a better way. Regardless of one's spiritual convictions, or lack of them, any movement away from chemical dependency is everyone's gain.

The Foursquare Gospel Fellowship of the Faith Center in Eugene, Oregon, offers such hope. A pentecostal church that believes in confronting social and moral issues, this congregation has brought in community and church professionals and paraprofessionals to provide therapy and support to individuals and families suffering from chemical dependency. The focus is on people within the church working with each other to eradicate drug and sexual problems and abuse.

There is, perhaps, no better example of the way spiritual endeavors help people to help themselves than that which the ministry of Alcoholics Anonymous (AA) provides. AA was founded in 1935, in Akron, Ohio, by Bill Wilson and Dr. Bob Smith (the topic of the May 1989 TV movie *My Name is Bill W.*). The cornerstone of AA and its sister hybrid programs Al-Anon and Narcotics Anonymous is a series of 12 simple steps. AA simply asks its members to admit powerlessness over a problem, have faith that a power greater than themselves can restore their wellness, and make a decision to turn their will and lives over to God as they understand Him. The remaining nine steps outline the process and include the importance of taking stock of oneself, confessing one's defects, being willing to atone for past wrongs, and showing a willingness and commitment to helping others in need.

BIOFEEDBACK

In the 1970s, biofeedback, the "immediate ongoing presentation of information to a person concerning his own physiologic processes,"[60] emerged as a viable means of treating drug abuse, particularly alcoholism. This alternative to drug abuse, also known as alpha training, is simple to use and capable of producing numerous benefits, including personal control of physiological functions, globular personality changes (increased ability to relax under stress, diminished overreaction to problems, reduced frustration responses), feelings of well-being, new views of one's individuality, and transcendental insights. Biofeedback encompasses a number of varied body-control techniques, the most publicized of which is the increased production of specific brain wavelengths known as alpha waves, which assist in reducing tension.

In 1924, while working with people with congenital brain openings, German psychiatrist Hans Berger first noted and recorded the electrical activity of the brain. Berger noticed that tiny cerebral voltages were being rhythmically emitted from the brain and that these waves were most visible when patients were in an alert but relaxed state. Berger continued to study the

Biofeedback to Fight Drug
Abuse
Source: Grant LeDuc/Monkmeyer
Press

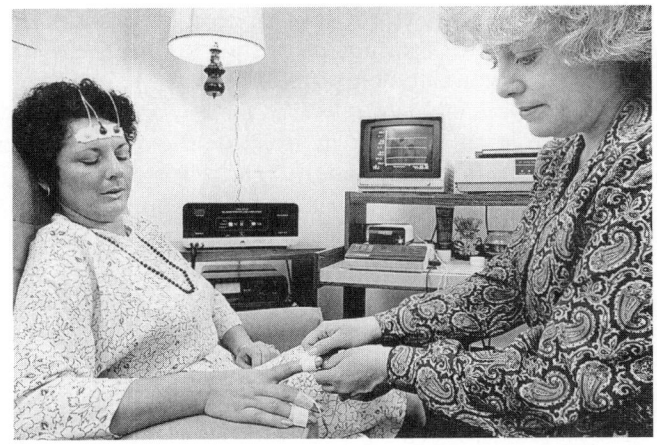

alpha waves, as they came to be known, but for many years little attention was paid to his discovery.

In 1910 Swiss psychiatrist Johannes Schultz developed the forerunner to biofeedback—autogenic training, which centered in the control of blood flow. Somewhat likened to yoga and self-hypnosis, autogenic training affects even subtle processes such as blood sugar and white-blood-cell counts, and it has become a major factor in European medicine and psychotherapy. It has been shown to be clinically effective in many patients suffering from migraine headache.[61]

Encouraged by efforts in Europe, researchers started to experiment in the United States during the late 1960s. During this time conclusive evidence documenting the ability of individuals to control autonomic processes unfolded. (Previously, the autonomic nervous system, controlling visceral or internal body organs and processes, was thought to be involuntary, or out of the realm of "voluntary," conscious control.) Research, beginning with lower-phylogenic species, has shown that animals can learn conscious control over many "involuntary" metabolic functions.

By the mid-1960s interest in alpha waves and their effects had grown. Joe Kamiya began training his students at the University of Chicago to differentiate alpha and nonalpha brain waves, and to maintain or turn off alpha-state production. He found that using a feedback device (in this case an audio tone) greatly aided skill acquisition and improved subsequent performance levels, and that the process, which is difficult to describe because of its sensory nature, helped students to detect the status of their visceral processes.[62]

Many students report that once they have learned body control through biofeedback, the minor stresses in their daily lives seem to affect them less. Though no explanation for this has been universally accepted to date, a number of theories have been postulated. Researcher Elmer Green has advanced a psychophysiological principle: "Every change in the physiological state is accompanied by an appropriate change in the mental-emotional state, conscious or unconscious . . . and conversely, every change in the mental-emotional state, conscious or unconscious, is accompanied by an appropriate change in the physiological state."[63] In other words, high levels of muscular activity cause high levels of mental anxiety and nervousness; reduced levels of muscular activity result in more relaxed mental states. Through biofeedback, a person may take note of his or her physiological state and then maintain or change that state with appropriate mental signals.

Many drug dependents will be able to use biofeedback in that way. The technique can teach these people to control the many processes that precipitate tension and stress and help them to see that they are not helpless victims of uncontrollable impulses and compulsions.

> By the time an alcoholic learns to . . . reduce his muscle tension levels to near zero, and increase his percentage of alpha rhythm, he will know, not just hope, or believe, that some processes are under his control. When that happens, he has essentially initiated a restabilization of maladjusted homeostatic processes . . . associated with total relaxation and . . . self-awareness.[64]

The alcoholic may then continue to choose biofeedback, instead of drugs, as a way to cope with tension and stress.

We are reminded that it is not life that "kills," but rather our reaction to the stress of everyday existence. We are the victims of our reactions to the frantic pace of daily life.[65] People use various coping skills according to their behavioral repertoire, experience, and knowledge. The majority of people choose to use drugs to cope with the trepidations of everyday living. If the stress becomes too great (or is perceived as such), drug use may become abuse. Biofeedback offers an alternative coping skill.

MEDITATION

Meditation is a psychological technique through which practitioners attempt to reach deep physiological relaxation. Developed several thousands of years ago by Indian philosophers and religious leaders, meditation works to exclude all thoughts from the mind through the repetition of sounds or words or through exercise or rhythmic breathing. Though there are a number of meditative techniques, transcendental meditation (TM) remains the most popular form in the United States.

TM was developed by Maharishi Mahesh Yogi, an Eastern philosopher. When using TM, followers repeat a specific phrase known only to themselves. The "objective of [this] mantra is to narrow the content of awareness to a fine point so that it may eventually break through to a higher, more intense plane [of consciousness]—as a narrow passageway might lead up toward an immense, lighted chamber."[66] The repetition of the words generates a rhythmic brain-wave pattern, which in turn quiets the sympathetic nervous branch of the autonomic nervous system. During this relaxed state, the meditator remains conscious and aware of his or her surroundings. Like a car idling, the body is functioning but expending very little energy in its effort to recharge. Meditation is an energy-restoring "time out"—the continuous repetition of a brain-wave pattern. The brain tends to respond to rhythmic stimulation, especially if it is its own source. At this moment the brain begins producing alpha waves, bearing out sensory-deprivation researcher Donald Hebb's theory that an individual must experience *varying* stimuli in order to perceive normal awareness. At the moment the incoming stimuli become uniform, the mind begins to synchronize, anesthetize, and produce alpha waves, reducing autonomic nervous system functioning.

How does this relate to the average person on the street? We might define "stress" as excitement resulting in elevated body processes. Virtually all of us are subject to stress. Publication deadlines, luncheon dates, paper-processing schedules, bills, unrequited love, economic insecurity, existential dilemma, stalled cars in an intersection, the boss who refused a raise and then increases the work load, the wife or husband who's "not in the mood"—these types of experiences generate stress. The cumulative effect of continual subjection to stress is a state that psychologists identify as the "flight or fight" phenomenon, a series of biological processes that gear up an organism in preparation to meet a threat or crisis.

The sympathetic nervous system controls this diffuse arousal reaction by constricting the arteries in the digestive tract, dilating the skeletal-muscle arteries, and diverting increased amounts of blood to locomotor muscles. Heart rate, blood pressure, respiration, and perspiration increase. Norepinephrine is released at nerve synapses, compounding these responses. With the influx of adrenalin an individual reacts quickly.

This system response is a defense reaction, mobilizing the body to accelerated states of readiness. It can become the basis of pathology when we fail to demobilize following a crisis. Some would suggest further that this 500,000-year-old machine, the human being, is in fact outmoded.

The issue is how people react to a perceived stressful situation. Studies show that meditators have greater initial arousal levels and correspondingly faster recovery periods. Daniel Coleman writes:

> People who are chronically anxious or who have a psychosomatic disorder share a specific pattern of reaction to stress; their bodies mobilize to meet the challenge, then *fail to stop reacting* when the problem is over. The initial tensing up is essential for it allows them to marshal their energy and awareness to deal with a potential threat. But bodies stay aroused for danger when they should be relaxed, recouping spent energies and gathering resources for the next brush with stress.[67]

Anxious individuals overreact, perceiving normal events as crises. Each minor occurrence increases existing tension, in turn magnifying the individual's perception of stress in the forthcoming events. Because the anxious person's body stays mobilized after an event has passed, it has a lower threshold for the next event. If the body is allowed to relax following a stress reaction, it is more likely to take the next normal occurrence in stride without becoming activated or alarmed. Those who have not learned to relax are exhausted at the end of the day. Relaxation comes in the form of four double scotches, two Valium, or a joint. Meditation can break the tension escalation of this threat-arousal-threat spiral by allowing relaxation to normalcy following a crisis. The "meditator relaxes after a challenge passes more often than the non-meditator. This makes him unlikely to see innocent occurrences as harmful. He perceives threat more accurately and reacts with arousal only when necessary. Once aroused, his rapid recovery makes him less likely than the anxious person to see the next deadline as a threat."[68]

For some, meditation may be an effective alternative to chemical dependency. This practice can often provide stress reduction and relief from the everyday tensions that precipitate destructive psychoactive substance abuse. It may also afford a means of achieving an altered state of consciousness, a "natural high" that appears initially to increase self-mastery and self-confidence. This pursuit became quite popular in the 1960s and 1970s as more and more young people began to pursue Eastern mysticism as an alternative to the western ways of civilization.

SUMMARY

During the past few years greater emphasis has been placed on education and treatment of drug abuse. It is recognized that it is much better to prevent substance abuse by starting with elementary-level education programs in schools. The schools are accepting greater responsibility for drug education, and teachers are becoming better prepared to teach in this area. In addition, several educational approaches are being applied to capture students' interest. However, schools accept all the responsibility for substance abuse education. Counselors, parents, peers, and a variety of community groups from government and private agencies are working together with the schools to combat substance abuse. This proactive campaign against substance abuse appears to be making progress. Also, media campaigns against drug use are effectively implemented.

Uninformed as well as realistic attitudes toward drug consumption seem only to increase the drug problem. Rather than assuming that all reasons for drug use are unacceptable, or that legislation will end drug use, those involved with the problem might better approach it equipped with up-to-date, unbiased drug education and a more understanding attitude. With a calm, reasonable approach, a more logical drug curriculum can be taught, with alternatives to drug use encouraged.

A variety of activities fill the same needs that drugs do. Exercise and wilderness experiences reduce stress, alter moods, and improve health. Work and social or political involvement help to build a sense of self-worth and a better set of values and beliefs. Biofeedback and meditation offer specific stress-reduction techniques as well as aid in the growth of self-confidence and self-mastery.

Prevention Education
and Alternatives

N O T E S

1. Richard G. Schlaadt, "Prevention: The Other War on Drugs," *Health Education,* May/June, 1990, pp. 58–60.
2. Mark Miller, "Teaching Kids to Say No," *Newsweek,* June 5, 1989, p. 24.
3. From *The Natural Mind* by Andrew Weil. Copyright © 1972 by Andrew Weil. Reprinted by permission of the publisher, Houghton Mifflin Company.
4. National Institute on Drug Abuse, Division of Epidemiology and Prevention Research, "National Household Survey on Drug Abuse," NIDA Capsules, CAP 21 (Rockville, Md.: U.S. Department of Health and Human Services, Public Health Service, Alcohol, Drug Abuse and Mental Health Administration, 1990).
5. The findings of the evaluation were published in L. W. Green, et al., "Thoughts from the School Health Education Advisory Panel," *Journal of School Health* 55 (October 1985):316.
6. D. B. Connel, R. R. Turner, and E. F. Mason, "Summary Findings of the School Health Education Evaluation: Health Promotion Effectiveness, Implementation, and Costs," *Journal of School Health* 55, no.4 (October 1985):316.
7. Carl Shantzis, "An Outcome Evaluation of Refusal Skills Program as a Drug Abuse Prevention Strategy," *Drug Education* 19 (1989):363–72.
8. Ibid.
9. "The High School Senior Survey," Sponsored by the National Institute of Drug Abuse (NIDA) and conducted by the University of Michigan, Institute for Social Research. HHS News, U.S. Department of Health and Human Services, News Release, January 24, 1991.
10. Nancy A. Minix, "Drug and Alcohol Prevention Education," *The Drug Abuse Clearinghouse,* December 1987, pp. 162–64.
11. Ibid.
12. Mary Rickett, "Decision Making and Young People," *Journal of Drug Education* 18, no. 2 (1988):109–13.
13. Dianne F. Bradley, "Alcohol and Drug Education in Elementary Schools," *Guidance and Counseling* 23 (December 1988):99–105.
14. Gary Fisher, Stephen J. Jenkins, and Nancy Held, "Pre-Service Teachers Use of and Attitudes toward Alcohol and Other Drugs," *Journal of Drug Education* 19, no. 4 (1989):373–84.
15. Bradley, "Alcohol and Drug Education."
16. Ralph Bell, "Using the Concept of Risk to Plan Use Intervention Programs," *Journal of Drug Education* 18 (1988):135–42.
17. Gordon Witkin, "A Modest Proposal for Dealing with Drugs," *U.S. News & World Report,* June 27, 1988, pp. 22–23.
18. Arnold B. Goldstein, "Refusal Skills: Learning to Be Positively Negative," *Journal of Drug Education* 19, no. 3 (1989):271–89.
19. Schlaadt, "Prevention."
20. "A Short-term Evaluation of Project DARE (Drug Abuse Resistance Education): Preliminary Indications of Effectiveness," *Journal of Drug Education* 17, no. 4 (1987).
21. Justin Green, "Evaluating the Effectiveness of a School Drug and Alcohol Prevention Curriculum: A New Look at 'Here's Looking at You, Two,' " *Journal of Drug Education* 19, no. 4 (1990):117–32.
22. Ibid.

23. Goldstein, "Refusal Skills."

24. Schlaadt, "Prevention."

25. Arthur P. Sullivan, "The Theoretical Model: Diagnostic Assessment and Placement in Prevention Treatment Mode by School Personnel," *Journal of Drug Education* 17, no. 1 (1987):59–67.

26. Gail G. Milgram, "Impact of a Student Assistance Program," *Journal of Drug Education* 19, no. 4 (1989):327–35.

27. Judy McDermott, "Parents Are the Best Buffer Against Drugs," *The Oregonian* (Portland), October 16, 1988.

28. Ibid.

29. Ken Barun and Philipe Bashe, "How to Keep Your Kids Off Drugs," *Reader's Digest* 133, no. 9 (September 1, 1988):85–89.

30. Ibid.

31. Joseph Shapiro, "How to Beat Drugs," *U.S. News & World Report,* September 11, 1989, pp. 69–80.

32. Ibid.

33. Terri Mulkins Manning and Kimberly Casper Banfield, "Do Parents Need Drug Education Programs as Badly as Their Parents Needed Them?" *Journal of Drug Education* 19, no. 2 (1989):97–102.

34. Ibid.

35. Margaret A. Sheppard, Michael S. Goodstadt, and Margaret Willet, "Peers and Parents: Who Has the Most Influence on Cannabis Use?" *Journal of Drug Education* 17, no. 2 (1987):123–37.

36. Ingrid Groller, "Parents vs. Drugs," *Parents* 62 (May 1987):126–28.

37. Ibid.

38. Sheppard, Goodstadt, and Willet, "Peers and Parents."

39. James Palmer et al., "High School Senior Athletes as Peer Educators and Role Models: An Innovative Approach to Drug Prevention," *Journal of Alcohol and Drug Education* 35, no. 1 (Fall 1989):23–27.

40. Stanley Einstein, "A Communication Approach to Drug Use Intervention," *International Journal of Addictions* 19, no. 8 (December 1984):925—29.

41. Ibid.

42. Barry Caudill, Brenda Kantor, and Steven Ungerleider, "Project Impact: A National Study of High School Substance Abuse Intervention Training," *Journal of Alcohol and Drug Education* 35 (Winter 1990):61–73.

43. Witkin, "A Modest Proposal."

44. Ibid.

45. Donald E. Maypole and Ruth B. Anderson, "Culture Specific Substance Abuse Prevention for Blacks," *Community Mental Health Journal* 23, no. 2 (Summer 1987):135–38.

46. Lane County Youth Development Commission/Department of Youth Services, "Community Together" (Eugene, Oregon: Grant from the Federal Office for Substance Abuse Prevention, 1991).

47. William Delong and Jay A. Winsten, "The Use of Mass Media in Substance Abuse Prevention," *Health Affairs* (Summer 1990):30–46.

48. Ibid.

49. William Glasser, *Positive Addiction* (New York: Harper & Row, 1976).

50. Hal Higdon, "Running and the Mind: Can Running Cure Mental Illness?" *Runner's World* 13, no. 1 (January 1978):36, 39.

51. Ibid., p. 38.

52. Quoted in ibid., p. 39.

53. Bob Rodale, "Regenerative Running—Running from Drugs II," *Runner's World,* February 1989, p. 24.

54. Marlene R. Ventura and Mike Durdon, "A Challenging Experience in Canoeing and Camping as a Tool in Approaching the Drug Problem," *Journal of Drug Education* 4, no 1 (Spring 1974):124.

55. Quoted in John J. Fried, "High with a Little Help from a Friend," *Sports Illustrated,* April 15, 1974, p. 88.

56. Quoted in ibid., p. 91.

57. Paul Lowinger, "How the People's Republic of China Solved the Drug Abuse Problem," *American Journal of Chinese Medicine* 1, no. 2 (1973):278.

58. Ibid.

59. Ibid., pp. 278–79.

60. Elmer Green, Alyce Green, and Dale E. Walters, "Biofeedback Training for Anxiety Tension Reduction," *Annals of the New York Academy of Sciences* 233 (1974):157.

61. Ibid.

62. Marilyn Ferguson, *The Brain Revolution: The Frontiers of Mind Research* (New York: Taplinger, 1973), p. 35.

63. Quoted in ibid., p. 38.

64. Green, Green, and Walters, "Biofeedback Training," pp. 158–59.

65. Daniel Coleman, "Meditation Helps Break the Stress Spiral," *Psychology Today* 9, no. 9 (February 1976):82. Reprinted from *Psychology Today Magazine.* Copyright © 1976 American Psychological Association (APA).

66. Ibid., p. 10. Reprinted from *Psychology Today Magazine.* Copyright © 1976 American Psychological Association (APA).

67. Ibid., p. 86. Reprinted from *Psychology Today Magazine.* Copyright © 1976 American Psychological Association (APA).

68. Maggie Scarf, "Turning Down with TM," *New York Times Magazine,* February 9, 1979.

TREATMENT OF DRUG ABUSE

INTRODUCTION

Addict

A person who has a very strong craving to use a chemical substance.

Hooked

A term often used to indicate physical and mental dependence on a drug.

The new generation has become a generation of **addicts.**[1] They are **hooked** not only on alcohol but on illegal drugs as well. This move toward a younger membership can be attributed to drugs like cocaine. Whereas alcoholism takes its toll over the course of years, coke, free-basing, and crack are causing people to bottom out in a matter of months. Most people are polydrug users; that is, they are addicted to more than one drug.

In addition to alcohol, America has an ongoing love affair with illegal drugs that costs it a fortune in death, addiction, and lost productivity, and it is getting worse every year. According to federal statistics, the United States snorts, smokes, injects, and inhales more than $110 million a year in illegal drugs.[2] America also has the highest level of teenage drug abuse of any industrialized nation in the world.

Because of the tremendous number of people experiencing drug problems in the United States, substance-abuse treatment has escalated. In fact, substance-abuse treatment centers have become a lucrative business. They have grown into a $3 billion-a-year industry and continue to grow.[3] It is estimated that 650,000 people are kicking the habit through any of the 9,000 programs available to them.

ADDICTION AND DEPENDENCY

Drug taking usually occurs in progressive and hazardous stages. Addiction or dependency is based on various components, compromised by the psychological, physiological, and social aspect of the drugs being used; dependence may occur in one of these criteria. It is a chronic, compulsive, or uncontrollable craving for and dependence on a particular substance.

Researchers now agree that addiction—whether to cocaine, heroin, amphetamines, or some other chemical substance—is a single disease.[4] According to much of the latest evidence, addicts will switch drugs when their choice is not available and will even display addictive behavior with drugs thought to be nonaddictive (such as marijuana and over-the-counter diet pills). That fact is extremely important in the way we think about drugs and addiction because it means that the chemical is not the problem, it is the individual's reaction to it that causes the difficulty.[5]

HOW DO YOU KNOW IF YOU ARE HOOKED?[6]

- Do you sometimes binge on alcohol or drugs?
- Do more people seem to be treating you unfairly and without good reason?
- Do you try to avoid family or friends while you are drinking or using drugs?
- Are you secretly irritated when family or friends discuss your drinking or drug use?
- Do you sometimes feel guilty about your drinking or drug use?
- Do you often regret things you have done or said while drunk or high?
- Have you often failed to keep the promises you have made to yourself about controlling or cutting down your drinking or drug use?
- Do you eat very little or irregularly when you are drinking or getting high?
- Do you feel low after indulging, and sometimes miss work or appointments?
- Do you use more and more to get drunk or high?

The addict is a person who has a very strong craving to use a substance. This craving is so strong that using drugs to satisfy it often becomes the central focus of the addict's life. Today it is estimated that 5.5 million people are dependent on drugs.[7] This is an astonishing number of dependents.

An addict exposed to the same amount of morphine (or any mood-altering drugs, such as cocaine or marijuana) will compulsively attempt to repeat and even intensify the feeling produced by drugs—*no matter what the circumstances.*[8] The key to diagnosing any addictive disease is in the observation that the patient persists in using drugs in spite of consequences.

INFANT ADDICTION

It should be stressed that infant addiction is 100 percent avoidable. If mothers are not using drugs, it is possible to eliminate crack babies, fetal alcohol syndrome or effect, and other negative consequences of drug taking during pregnancy. With the rise in use of addictive drugs such as (crack) cocaine, PCP, marijuana, and alcohol, we are seeing the tragic effects on infants also on the rise. The use of any drug has been identified to have some degree of effect on an unborn infant. When addictive drugs are used, the effects may be seen as violent, abusive, or lethal.

Cocaine abuse is the fastest-growing type of abuse, with alcohol still the most prevalent.[9] Fetal alcohol syndrome is described in the greatest detail, covering both the physical and psychological effects. The clear message is that no amount of drug use, even legal drugs, by an expecting mother is safe. It is essential that potential mothers be treated so they won't have babies affected by substance abuse.

INTERVENTION

The most important fact about intervention is that it works. As a consequence, most for-profit treatment facilities today can feel confident that using trained intervention specialists is a legitimate way to generate business while helping the addict. In some cases it is possible to get dependents in for early treatment instead of waiting for them to "bottom out."

TREATMENT APPROACHES

Today there is greater hope for drug addicts or dependents because treatment professionals have gained experience and new knowledge about how to deal more effectively with patients who have drug problems. Newer treatment approaches based on experience of what works most effectively, the use of chemical assistance such as methadone, and a wide range of individual and group support in intervention, treatment, aftercare, and relapse approaches have made the programs more successful.

The main reason people enter treatment centers is that they are under pressure and need a way to manage problems that arise from within (mental or physical health) or from the social environment (the law, the family, other drug users or dealers, or a sudden loss of income.[10] The effectiveness of treatment relies on the individual's ability, after detoxification or treatment, to expose him or herself to new outlooks on life, join support groups, and devise a personal path of treatment because the cure from dependency comes from within.

Treatment Programs

Treatment programs usually consist of referral, intervention, detoxification, inpatient, outpatient, counseling, nutrition, exercise, and fitness for recovering addicts.

Treatment programs usually consist of referral, intervention, detoxification, inpatient, outpatient, counseling, nutrition, exercise, and aftercare. Because of the life-threatening potential, the programs usually require hospital-like care in addition to other treatment approaches. Of course, this makes treatment very expensive. In treatment centers, dealing with the whole family is a vital factor and usually "the difference between sobriety and relapse after leaving the treatment center."

Some shocking statistics face us relating to the numbers of individuals awaiting entrance into alcohol- and drug-treatment programs. It is estimated that the number of individuals needing treatment is equal to the entire population of Santa Barbara, California; Harrisburg, Pennsylvania; or Midland, Texas.[11] A recent survey conducted by the National Association of Alcohol and Drug Abuse Directors (NASADAD) showed that "over 66,000 adult Americans are prevented from entering alcohol and drug programs because of insufficient affordable treatment slots."[12] The period of waiting varies from state to state. The demand for entrance into state-funded programs seems to be a result of the growing number of addicts who are motivated to seek recovery from their addiction(s).

In the past three years admissions across the nation have jumped 70 percent.[13] This is due, in part, to community efforts to raise public awareness about adverse long-term effects of drug abuse. A portion of these addicts are sentenced to these programs as a result of criminal drug-related offenses. Funding is the main obstacle. Nearly one third of all adults seeking care lack any legal means to pay for treatment. States are budgeting more money for these programs but still cannot keep up with the demand.

In the near future, "every addict who really wants to say no ought to have access to immediate treatment."[14] It makes it so hard for addicts to stop abusing drugs if the treatment programs are too full or too expensive. Considering how difficult it is for a cocaine addict to stop that craving, we need to have intense education programs so people do not want to use drugs.

ADOLESCENT TREATMENT

Of the millions of teenagers involved with drugs, only a few actually go through treatment. This is only because some area of their life has been disrupted or they've been referred by friends, offices, and parents. Adolescent treatment centers throughout the country follow similar programs. It is imperative that an adolescent-recovery program have a well-balanced and competent recovery staff that include physicians and nurses, mental-health staff, and a psychiatrist (preferably a child psychiatrist) who is trained in development of family systems and accepts the disease concept of alcoholism.[15]

The history of adolescent treatment for alcohol and other drug addictions is replete with unsuccessful efforts to utilize adult treatment modalities and methods with adolescents. Quality adolescent treatment requires a program design that takes into account not only special developmental needs of this population but also the reality that unless secondary emotional and behavioral problems and family-system dysfunction are addressed during treatment, treatment will be inefficacious.

Sacred Heart Adolescent Recovery Program A department of the Sacred Heart General Hospital in Eugene, Oregon, is an example of a program that stands as a model of this type of program design. Established in 1982, the Sacred Heart Adolescent Recovery Program (SHARP)[16] is the oldest acute-care facility for the treatment of adolescent chemical dependency in Oregon and one of the oldest in the country. It has received special accreditation from the Joint Commission on the Accreditation of Health Organizations (JCAHO). SHARP has also received special certification as a dual-diagnosis treatment center, for it specializes in the treatment of those teens whose substance-abuse problem has worsened or been complicated by another serious emotional or mental disorder. The following is a breakdown of discharge diagnoses:

Dual diagnosis	80 percent
Conduct disorder	63 percent
Mixed substance abuse	92 percent
Alcohol (only)	4 percent
Oppositional/defiant disorder	11 percent
Major depression	12 percent
Eating disorder	11 percent
PTSD (Post Traumatic Stress Disorder)	29 percent
Adjustment disorder	9 percent
Attention deficit disorder	9 percent

The program is a secure, locked unit with an inpatient capacity of 34 and a length of stay of four to six weeks. Following a three-to-five-day period of evaluation and testing, patients begin a highly individualized treatment regime that includes a number of innovative treatment elements like video-feedback therapy, community building, on-site challenge course (low-element-ropes course), thinking-errors group, fun-in-recovery group, anger management, grief group, and gender group in addition to the more traditional group psychotherapy and family therapy.

Patients are placed in one of two tracks based on whether they present as "externalizers" (oppositional, conduct-disordered, victimizers, etc.) or as "internalizers" (depressed, abused, self-destructive, etc.). Both groups benefit from the behavioral, milieu, family, and group therapies, but the separation, especially for group therapy, allows the therapists and counselors to approach issues in a manner more likely to be helpful to each. Moreover, the externalizers, who tend to act out, are not inhibiting to or distracted by their internalizers peers, who are prone to present themselves as victims and who require greater assurance of safety.

Outcome studies indicate an extraordinary recovery rate by graduates from programs such as SHARP. Evaluation of abstinence, commitment to sobriety, family function, parent-teen relationships, and the positive impact of treatment on siblings is most encouraging.

St. Luke's Adolescent Recovery Unit   Another example of an adolescent program is St. Luke's Adolescent Recovery Unit in Denver.[17] The teenager and his or her family must go through assessment with a counselor. The staff then determines the extent of the problem and decides if the teen can be motivated to change. Once admitted to the 45-day program (some are 21–30 days), the young person becomes a "candidate" and loses his or her street clothes and instead wears pajamas for a few days. Candidates are assigned a buddy patient (or group), but there is no contact with friends or family. Then they must write a paper on why they are in treatment, what their problem is, and why they want to be promoted to the treatment phase. This is read by them in front of their peers on the unit, after which everyone else decides if the candidate is honestly ready to begin the work of getting better. A typical day of treatment includes exercise, school work, recreational therapy, addiction education, and small-group therapy. In the evening candidates go to guest lecturers or Alcoholics Anonymous (AA) and Narcotics Anonymous (NA) meetings. The family is asked to participate in a week-long treatment with counseling sessions, since everyone in the family is affected. The reentry phase gets candidates ready for the outside world again, but they must continue AA and NA meetings. It is estimated that one third of the adolescents who go through the inpatient drug-treatment program are thoroughly treated.

Straight   Straight is a somewhat controversial adolescent-treatment program. Backers feel it is very successful; however, critics feel its tough regimen of intense discussions, separation from home, and severe penalties is abusive, and some parents want to see the group closed.[18]

Of the 5,000 youths aged 12 to 25 who have participated in the program since 1976, about 3,200 have completed treatment. Of the graduates, 75 percent have remained drug-free and sober for two years, a figure compared with the 20 to 30 percent rate typical of more conventional drug-treatment centers.[19]

The program isolates clients from outside influences during the initial treatment phase. A newcomer is prohibited from receiving mail or phone calls, and most live with the family of another youth involved in a later stage of treatment. At night, those new to the program go to the homes of their assigned old-comers, whose parents must provide short-term bed and board for two or three other clients. In addition to holding treatments down to about $11,000 a year, this exchange gives parents new to the program a chance to cool off and rebuild the family that was strained by the drug-abusing youth, according to Straight's philosophy, which considers both the parent and the child to be in treatment.

By the time the client completes the program, typically 10 to 24 months after enrollment, he or she may have stayed with dozens of host families, who in turn have housed an endless parade of youngsters. One mother says she has had about 150 youths in her home during the past 12 months. Until children reach the middle portion of treatment, parents do not know where they spend the night, and youths are not allowed to call home. Some parents feel this is too harsh and don't feel comfortable with the stress associated with such a treatment program. Drug-abuse experts stress that Straight's confrontational, group-oriented approach may be unsuitable for some youths. They urge care in choosing among the many treatment programs available.

Outward Bound   A program that is having some success with adolescents and young adults is the Outward Bound Program. Outward Bound was created in the 1940s in response to the lack of stamina and strength of the Aberdovey seamen during World War II. Kurt Hahn and fellow mate, Lawrence Hold, designed a ropes course that later became a major component of the Outward Bound Program.[20] Originating in Europe, Outward Bound programs are now located throughout the world. Many college graduates and those in transition are frequently the participants of this program to "find themselves" and to prove their capabilities. Other activities in Outward Bound include swimming, hiking, canoeing, and rock climbing. These are not all easy activities, and they involve group decision making as to the safest and most effective route while utilizing their resources. The program helps improve the attitudes and behavior of those participating. Participants achieve success, such as adapting to change, managing stress and leisure time, making informed decisions, and learning to appreciate the culture and nature around them. Those going through the program find a decrease in personal problems, an increase in the Rosenberg Self-Esteem Scale, and a slight decrease in "self-reported" frequency of drunkenness.[21]

ADULT-TREATMENT PROGRAMS

Adult programs usually last 28 days and involve detoxification, individual and small-group counseling, drug-education classes, exercise, nutritional analysis, NA and/or AA meetings and family counseling. The cost of the program ranges from $6,000 to $100,000 depending on the treatment selected. Many drug experts claim there is no substantial difference between the

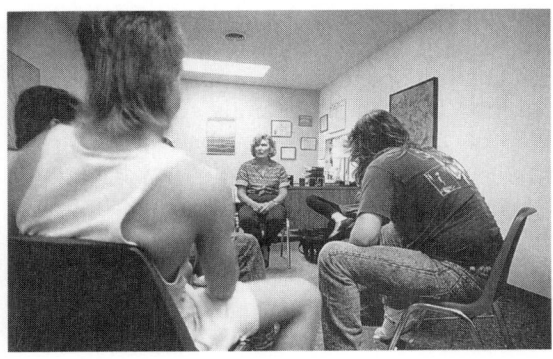

Counselling Sessions Help Drug Abusers
Source: Mulvehill/The Image Works

lower-cost program and the high-cost program. There is growing controversy regarding the extreme variation in fees for much of the same treatment. Some feel a single cap of $6,000 per treatment for drug addiction would save not only billions of dollars in lost tax revenues but countless lives as well.[22] For example, the Betty Ford Center, in Rancho Mirage, California, where Elizabeth Taylor, Lisa Minnelli, and Robert Mitchum "graduated," charges only $6,000 for treatment.

EMPLOYERS

Under a little-noticed provision of the antidrug law Congress adopted, companies and institutions will risk losing future federal contracts and grants if they do not make a "good-faith effort" to institute programs that assure a drug-free workplace.[23]

The regulations say that if "a number of employees" have been convicted of drug violations in the workplace, "the contract could be suspended or terminated" if those violations "indicate that the contractor has failed to make good faith efforts to provide a drug-free workplace." The importance of eliminating drugs in the workplace was discussed previously in Chapter 3, The Drug Scene.

KEY COMPONENTS

Inpatient Versus Outpatient   Inpatient programs are treatment programs usually offered at clinics or hospitals that require the patient to remain on the premises for a given period of time. On the other hand, an outpatient treatment programs allow the patient to live at home during the rehabilitation process. Many companies seem to be taking a long, critical look at the standard 28-day inpatient treatment benefit for substance abuse.[24] A program such as this can cost anywhere from $8,000 upward. A solid inpatient program may be essential for those patients with severe addiction problems. The specialized care and counseling provided helps remove patients from the depths of dependency. However, many employers (insurance) may prefer to spend only $2,000 to $3,000 for a well-structured, medically supervised outpatient program. Not only is the cost of this form of treatment an advantage but also workers can stay on the job. For those individuals who can handle it, and who have a good support unit, outpatient treatment may be an acceptable option.

However, outpatient treatment may not be suited for every individual. It is therefore essential to get a full evaluation of the person so his or her special needs and capacities can be taken into account. The family situation should be looked at as well. People most likely to benefit from outpatient treatment are young, healthy patients; patients with supportive family environments; patients who report past periods of success in stopping use; and patients who are highly motivated by their work.[25]

Dual Diagnosis

A combination of drug abuse and mental illness.

Dual Diagnosis   There are nearly 1 million people in America who have an added disadvantage when it comes to chemical dependency. In the past few years, psychiatrists in the United States have come to realize that drug abuse among the mentally ill can be devastating. A recent study by the Alcohol, Drug Abuse and Mental Health Administration cited that there is no such thing as recreational drug use or a social drink for someone with a severe psychiatric illness.[26] According to the study, unbalanced people are twice as likely to commit suicide as their counterparts who abstain from drug use.

Self-Help Groups   Memberships are rapidly increasing among self-help groups such as AA, NA, and Cocaine Anonymous (CA). Many of these new members are younger people. According to a 1986 AA survey, 21 percent of AA members are under 30, with 38 percent also addicted to other drugs.[27] Alcoholics Anonymous, Narcotics Anonymous, and Cocaine Anonymous have become frequent phrases in everyday conversations.

The move toward a younger membership can largely be attributed to other drugs such as cocaine. While alcoholism takes its toll over the course of years, coke, free-basing, and crack are causing people to bottom out in a matter of months.[28] In the past four years, the number of CA groups nationwide has increased from 169 to 1,043. Internationally, the number of NA groups has gone from 2,000 in early 1983 to 14,000 in 1988—with most of the increase in the United States.[29]

The new generation is full of literally thousands of groups of people who are banding together to fight their addictions. The self-help groups help fill the gaps left by the shortage of space available in publicly financed treatment programs. The success of self-help groups lies in the 12-step program. The "12 Steps to a New Life" that are recommended by AA include the following:

1. We admitted we were powerless over alcohol—that our lives had become unmanageable.
2. Came to believe that a Power greater than ourselves could restore us to sanity.
3. Made a decision to turn our will and our lives over to the care of God *as we understood Him.*
4. Made a searching and fearless moral inventory of ourselves.
5. Admitted to God, to ourselves, and to another human being the exact nature of our wrongs.
6. Were entirely ready to have God remove all these defects of character.
7. Humbly asked Him to remove our shortcomings.
8. Made a list of all persons we had harmed, and became willing to make amends to them all.
9. Made direct amends to such people wherever possible, except when to do so would injure them or others.
10. Continued to take personal inventory and when we were wrong promptly admitted it.
11. Sought through prayer and meditation to improve our conscious contact with God, *as we understood Him,* praying only for knowledge of His will for us and the power to carry that out.

12. Having had a spiritual awakening as the result of these Steps, we tried to carry this message to alcoholics and to practice these principles in all our affairs.[30]

Twelve-step programs help define the problem—addiction—in a meaningful way and enforce honesty with oneself and others. They maintain a focus in realistic goals, and they provide the support of the community of friends and peers with special understanding and empathy.

A study of 100 impaired physicians who were successfully treated in a program that combined professional, directed, psychotherapeutic treatment and peer-led self-help were still abstinent 33.4 months after admission, and they all rated AA as more important to their recovery than some of the professionals who helped.[31]

Therapeutic Recreation

Utilization of relaxation techniques, assertiveness training, social-skill development, exercise/fitness, and implementation of organized activities to help clients maintain leisure lifestyles and to choose satisfying and joyful experiences they can control.

Therapeutic Recreation   Another approach that is obtaining some success with drug-dependents is **therapeutic recreation.**[32] It is often found that people with addictive behaviors frequently occupy unsatisfying or stressful positions in society. Their occupations offer no worthwhile social rewards. The drugs simply ameliorate the feeling of unmet needs. Peele and others feel self-reliance and conscious choice are necessary for lifelong sobriety. The therapeutic-recreation professional can help enhance self-confidence and choice of substance abusers. The therapeutic-recreation specialists can also assist clients in developing and maintaining leisure lifestyles and choosing satisfying and joyful experiences they can control. Relaxation techniques, assertiveness training, social-skill development, exercise/fitness, and implementation of organized activities are some of the tools used by therapeutic-recreation specialists to allow the substance abuser to learn about him or herself.

According to 1984 Olympic gold medalist Joan Samuelson, running enhances a good drug-rehabilitation program.[33] Running opens the spirit, giving new hope. That is the one common factor linking systems that fight addiction. In her home state of Maine, Samuelson became involved with DARE (Drug Abuse Resistance Education), an antidrug course targeted at school-age children (police-sponsored) that began in Los Angeles and has since spread all over the country. She met and spoke with Portland (Maine) DARE organizers numerous times to learn more about the program and then appeared in a DARE television commercial that demonstrated "Ways to Say No." Samuelson's contribution was particularly appropriate, because the DARE program suggests running as one way to resist drug use.

Nutritional Intervention   All drug dependencies create toxicity within the body; this toxicity creates physical and mental damage as well as malnutrition, thereby impairing eating behaviors and nutritional status.[34] Drug abuse increases an individual's nutritional needs beyond normal requirements. The detoxification and metabolism of drugs, inactivation of vitamins for energy metabolism, inability of the liver to store nutrients, malabsorption and decreased utilization of nutrients, muscle and organ dysfunction, and presence of diarrhea and diuresis are additional factors that further drain nutrient fuel. Any rehabilitation effort must address the marked nutritional deficiencies occurring within the individual by providing nutritional care. This care should include an evaluation of nutritional status and supervision of nutritional rehabilitation by providing meals and by providing nutrition education and counseling to integrate new eating behaviors into the addict's new life.

Elderly   The federal government has been contemplating the idea of providing an outpatient drug benefit to Medicare beneficiaries and has focused attention on prescription drugs and the elderly as never before.[35] The misuse of medications by older Americans reflects a persistent problem with the delivery of medical services to vulnerable populations throughout the country. An increase of evidence shows previously unknown risks and benefits of medications among the elderly, which has helped stir up some controversy about pharmaceutical use among concerned consumers, public-interest organizations, private insurers, and the pharmaceutical industry, whose profit is at stake.

EXAMPLES OF ADULT-TREATMENT PROGRAMS

Serenity Lane Alcohol- and Drug-Treatment Program   The Serenity Lane program for the treatment of alcohol and drug abuse offers the following nine programs or components to meet the needs of its patients:[36]

1. PRE-SCREENING.   Serenity Lane is available for assistance and screening services that range from answering questions about admission to advice about the availability of other services in the community. Interventions, a process whereby patients are motivated to accept treatment and which are time consuming and complex, are also provide at no cost and without obligation to Serenity Lane.

2. EVALUATION AND ASSESSMENT.   This is the process (study) of defining the prospective patient's needs (diagnosis) and determining the appropriate corrective or rehabilitative steps needed (treatment). Various areas of the patient's lifestyle and environment are analyzed to determine exactly what problems need primary attention and what may be secondary. The patient's marital, vocational, economic, occupational, spiritual, physical, and psychological needs are analyzed and evaluated in order to match the patient and his or her family with exactly the right program. An extensive addiction history and Minnesota Multiphasic Personality Inventory are also used as part of the evaluation process. The medical component is performed by a licensed physician and may involve laboratory testing. Outside corroborative information (other treatment agencies, family physician, family) will be used whenever possible to maximize results and minimize costs.

The end result of the evaluation and assessment is the formulation of a professional treatment plan. This plan defines what the patient needs to do (modality and supportive activities) to achieve a drug-free lifestyle (sobriety). Each plan is cognizant of the patient's needs, quality of care, and overall costs to both third-party payors and the patient.

3. INTENSIVE CARE UNIT.   Serenity Lane maintains an intensive care unit (ICU) licensed by the Health Division to provide quality medical services to patients needing withdrawal from alcohol or other drugs or to treat other attendant physical problems commonly associated with addictions and/or the detoxification process. Commonly associated problems are liver damage, heart and pulmonary disease, pancreatitis, and abdominal complications. The major goal of Serenity Lane medical staff is to withdraw the patient safely, without seizures or other complications, and to bring the patient to a state of current health that will allow subsequent residential or outpatient treatment of the addiction problem. Because the staff can begin to establish a helping relationship while the patient is in ICU, it is often easier to motivate this same patient for treatment than it is if the patient transfers in from other programs.

4. SHORT-TERM RESIDENTIAL.   This is a newer program designed with society's current emphasis on reducing residential time and consequently costs. It is recommended only for those patients whose general motivation is better than that of the usual 28-day patient, that is, above the average, and whose ability to use intensive outpatient care is also above average. Basically, this program is designed for eight additional days beyond detoxification, or just eight days if detoxification is not needed, and then is preliminary to the utilization of a six-week intensive outpatient program followed by five months of weekly aftercare. The initial residential phase is to assist the patient to break through denial and attain a valid first-step experience. It is also designed for maximum family experience. Patients failing this program by relapse or inability to complete the program without abstinence are placed in the more intensive residential programs.

5. INTENSIVE RESIDENTIAL.   This program is Serenity Lane's most well known, and it also the most comprehensive and all-inclusive of its plans. The program includes detoxification, evaluation and assessment, a first-step program, a 28-day residential program, an integrated family program, a fourth-step program, an aftercare preparation program, an 11-month aftercare program, and a courtesy relapse program if needed. This intensive rehabilitation program is designed for the alcohol- and drug-dependent person whose disease is well advanced and who needs the maximum of care for best results.

6. INTENSIVE OUTPATIENT.   Serenity Lane offers an intensive outpatient program designed to give the maximum care possible without residential requirement. It is six weeks in duration, four hours per night, with weekend assignments. It includes participation with the spouse. Participation in a five-month aftercare program sustains the sobriety or drug-free skills. A family component is also built into the program. Since alcoholism usually involves

the whole family, it is felt that the whole family should be involved in the after-care program. It consists of group meetings and counseling.

7. GENERAL OUTPATIENT SERVICES. Patients needing general counseling regarding problems attendant to addiction are encouraged to use these services. Alcohol problems, vocational problems, adjustment problems, and parent-child problems are often associated with new sobriety, so Serenity Lane offers professional counseling in this area. These services are *not* designed to assist or obtain sobriety per se, but to assist in maintaining sobriety or a drug-free lifestyle.

8. LONG-TERM REHABILITATION. Some patients have a difficult time remaining drug-free or sober after treatment because of a difficult living situation or a difficult time in adjusting to daily living or vocational stresses. They require a supportive living environment while learning how to manage money, be more productive on the job (or even find a job), adjust to a marriage partner, or learn how to relate to people on a functional and enjoyable basis. Therefore, Serenity Lane has designed a program where patients can live in a structured residence and receive generalized counseling, work supervision and therapy, and still participate in maintenance aftercare programs. This program is available from 1 month to 18 months maximum. The patient's progress is monitored carefully monthly.

9. AFTERCARE PROGRAM. Serenity Lane's motto is "With Maintenance Sobriety Will Prevail." This simply means that after treatment is over, the process of being drug-free and sober in the everyday world is difficult without support. The organization therefore provides a two-hour group experience once weekly for a duration after graduation from the program. The minimum period is 5 months, and 11 months is standard with the intensive residential option. What's more, aftercare is provided where the patient resides, not only at the Eugene site. There is no additional charge for this program.

Crossroads Another example of adult treatment is the Crossroads program. Guinan is the director of an outpatient substance abuse treatment center in the Midwest called Crossroads, which has developed a "total" treatment program that addresses all aspects of an addict's world.[37] Rather than treat the addict with individual and "co-addict" self-help counseling alone, this program considers the particular habit as a function of many systems and defines a person's world as being comprised of three family groups: the *close* family, the *vocational* family, and the *social* family. All three groups are included in treatment.

The close family includes the traditional nuclear family members and is also comprised of people who see each other at least weekly in or around living quarters and who usually meet in random or non-goal-directed activities.

The second group is the vocational family, which is comprised of friends, colleagues, and acquaintances from the workplace or school. Many times this group is on more intimate terms with the addict than the close family. It's possible for someone to leave for work in the morning with a hangover without the spouse catching on; it's doubtful that the hangover would go unnoticed by the person at the next desk. Also, work and school are the places where many drug deals and drinking plans are made.

The third family group is the social family, which includes teammates, fellow church members, club members, and even "drinking buddies." Many times a member of the social family is also a member of the close or vocational family.

When an addict comes to Crossroads for an initial consultation, an assessment is made of the level of treatment necessary. The client is then advised of the program's "extended" treatment and given guidelines under which treatment takes place.

A Treatment Program for Inmates   A penitentiary at the Westchester County correctional complex is attempting to help inmates break the cycle of drug dependency and crime through a new 28-day program of intensive alcohol and drug rehabilitation before their release.[38] The program is treating its first group of 45 men and 15 women, and 250 to 300 inmates are expected to take part in the first year. The men are housed together in one area, separated from the rest of the prison population. The women have yet to receive a dormitory space separated from the women's prison. The program combines educational information about alcohol and drugs, group therapy, and referral to outside treatment groups. The group therapy is especially important because many inmates have a drug problem.

The average inmate stays in the prison for six months, so an attempt is made to produce some effective treatment for inmates while they are still incarcerated because once they are released, they return to the same environment that produced their drug problem in the first place. When they get out, they often face the same pressures, people, and stress that made them chemically dependent and led to crime.

Key factors that should be offered by correction facilities are the following:[39]

1. Give treatment a chance. Provide it, and leave it up to the addict to choose.
2. Support AA/NA involvement in the institution, and self-help groups within the community.
3. Subsidize the purchase of literature dealing with addiction, and become part of the recovery process.
4. At times, mandate an addict's attendance to self-help groups.
5. Require adequate substance-abuse training for the professional staff.

The recovery process should be initiated in the institutional setting before the inmate's release into society.

The Key Extended Entry Program   Estimates indicate there are about 200,000 heroin addicts in New York City. About 30,000 of them are currently enrolled in methadone programs and 1,600 are in drug-free programs.[40] The remaining addicts are not treated and are generally dependent on illegal drugs. In 1988, for the first time, the number of inmates serving in New York prisons for drug-related offenses surpassed those imprisoned for any other type of crime. The Key Extended Entry Program (KEEP) was established in March 1987 to address the needs of arrested addicts. The eventual hope was to reduce drug-related crime, crowding in the jails, and the transmission of the acquired immunodeficiency syndrome (AIDS) virus.

KEEP differs from the detoxification program used in that incarcerated narcotic addicts are maintained on methadone (30 or 40 milligrams per day) instead of being detoxified. If the individual is to be maintained in the community, the number of community-based programs should be increased for continued methadone treatment and evaluation for long-term care after their release from jail.[41]

When released from jail, inmates report within 24 hours to a community-based KEEP facility; they are continued on methadone and evaluated for up to six months. Former inmates are then referred for continuous treatment in methadone programs or drug-free therapeutic communities, as well as support groups such as outpatient clinics, Narcotics Anonymous, Cocaine Anonymous, or Alcoholic Anonymous.

KEEP has the potential to reduce the high probability of relapse to drugs after release from jail; to reduce drug-related crime; and to reduce use of contaminated needles that can lead to contracting or transmitting the AIDS virus. Eligible inmates can either start treatment in jail, which they continue upon release, or if they can, continue treatment and counseling in jail.

KEEP is a successful, innovative program that brings treatment into a new site to deal with the phenomenon emerging from or closely related to addiction: crime as well as medical and social pathology. It also represents a model of effective cooperation among agencies. The program is effective in reducing jail crowding, reducing risk behavior that transmits the AIDS virus, and inducting addicted offenders into long-term treatment.

Rational Recovery   Rational Recovery (RR) from addiction is the application of Rational Emotive Therapy (RET) to problems of self-control in the consumption of alcohol and other chemicals.[42] RET is a cognitive-behavioral psychotherapy that addresses the cognitive, behavioral, and emotional components of human behavior and disturbance. RET stresses the effects of cognitions (or thoughts) on individual behavior. Thus, Rational Recovery helps people who want to stop using drugs or to moderate their use by uncovering and disputing irrational thoughts that maintain addiction. For example, individuals who think "I can't stand discomfort" are highly likely during times of stress to give in to the desire to use a substance they have committed themselves not to consume. RET characterizes this type of belief as low frustration tolerance. The RR program helps individuals increase their frustration of doing without the substance they would otherwise use.

Rational disruption is employed to overcome low frustration tolerance. For example, an individual would forcefully state to him or herself, "There's no evidence that I can't stand discomfort. So tough luck! I'll feel uncomfortable for a short period until the desire to use goes away. I CAN stand it, and I had better if I want to get over this addiction." RET emphasizes this sort of rational disputation as an active therapeutic exercise because the mere recognition of, or insight to, irrational beliefs is insufficient. It is necessary to act against them cognitively and behaviorally.

Through practice at disputing irrational ideas one can reduce their frequency and intensity and thereby liberate oneself to opportunities and lifestyles that are more rewarding. Because people with something better to do with their time are least likely to abuse themselves with drugs, Rational Recovery assists individuals in learning how to take the risks of developing interests and activities that are incompatible with drug abuse. Therefore RET and RR employ trainings to initiate or enhance general coping skills such as relaxation, interpersonal communication, problem solving, and conflict resolution. These skills equip individuals to take the necessary risks of initiating new behaviors that are unrelated to drug use. If an individual in Rational Recovery persists at developing new interests and social circles, he or she will likely find such pursuits to be self-reinforcing and more rewarding than the short term gain and long term pain that characterizes addiction.

Rational Recovery takes three forms: an RR study group, individual study of the book *Rational Recovery from Alcoholism,* or outpatient counseling with a mental health professional trained in Rational Recovery and RET. The study groups exist in most large cities in the United States and are free and open to the public. Unlike AA meetings, they do not require lifelong attendance and the labeling of oneself, for example, as an alcoholic. According to RR proponents, drinking problems are learned behavior and so can be unlearned. It should be stressed that Rational Recovery is quite a departure from the traditional programs and is often met with resistance from these groups.

FIGHTING DRUGS WITH DRUGS

Drugs such as crack cocaine and ice are hitting the market with resounding effect, and the approach to fighting addiction is moving from the moral to the medical. The National Institute on Drug Abuse (NIDA) is heading a spending bill for fighting drug addiction. Starting with $27 million in 1989 and double that in 1990, NIDA projects spend in the upward range of $100 million or more in the 1990s.[43] Program director Marvin Snyder states that NIDA is developing medications that can interfere with drug-taking behavior and restore some degree of normalcy to a drug addict's brain function. Some drugs, such as methadone, have already been used with partial success against heroin.

ALCOHOL TREATMENT

In addition to the treatment for alcohol addiction discussed in Chapter 8, some treatment programs have incorporated the use of lithium and Prozac into the treatment regime.[44]

HEROIN TREATMENT

Considerable detail was given in the discussion of methadone and its effect on heroin in Chapter 9. Because of the great increase in drug addiction, everyone is trying to find cures and remedies to save the people. Years ago a drug called methadone was introduced. This drug was thought to be a solution to the addictive drug heroin. Yet this drug is a form of treatment and definitely not a cure. It offers relief to 100,000 heroin addicts out of the half million currently in the United States.[45] Now with our country's new addiction—cocaine—many researchers are trying to find some more relief.

Buprenorphine   Now NIDA, a federal research agency, is trying to develop drugs that can supplement or replace methadone as a more effective treatment for heroin addiction. A drug called buprenorphine has been approved by the U.S. Food and Drug Administration as an analgesic for acute, chronic pain.[46] It is an opioid that comes in two forms, an injectable liquid and a tablet. Although methadone has been very effective, withdrawal from methadone lasts a long time—about two weeks instead of five to six days, as on buprenorphine. Some investigators think this extended withdrawal prevents many addicts from attaining what should be their ultimate goal: a totally drug-free existence.

Buprenorphine is said to be as effective as methadone as a heroin substitute. It satisfies the craving of addicts; it also dulls the high of other opioids and thus discourages backsliding into heroin. It is the most promising drug being studied at this time. The drug is a pain reliever that produces a feeling of comfort rather than the harsh rush that drugs such as heroin seem to produce. This drug does not contain any addictive substances and is almost virtually impossible to overdose. In fact, the Drug Enforcement Agency gave it a Schedule V rating—compared with Schedule IV for Valium, Schedule II for methadone, and Schedule I for heroin.[47] It looks as if there might now be some competition for methadone in heroin-treatment programs, providing the pharmaceutical companies give their support.

Clonidine and Naltrexone   A study reported that combined Clonidine and naltrexone treatment allowed 38 of 40 patients addicted to methadone to withdraw completely in four to five days.[48] Clonidine reduced the intensity of naltrexone-induced withdrawal symptoms. Clonidine significantly decreased blood pressure without producing syncope (swooning or fainting) and caused sedation but no other clinical problems. Clonidine-naltrexone treatment should succeed with patients receiving methadone doses up to 50 milligrams per day, facilitate naltrexone maintenance, and apply to many clinical settings. In other words, the Clonidine and naltrexone treatment proved to be highly effective and well tolerated.

Naltrexone Maintenance   Many opiate addicts genuinely want to become opiate-free, but traditional withdrawal techniques result in high rates of dropout and early relapse. Acute methadone detoxification was induced by intravenous administration of Naloxone during simultaneous intravenous sedation with midazolam, a fully reversible short-acting benzodiazepine, in seven patients addicted to opiates.[49] Within hours the patients tolerated full doses of naltrexone. This technique enables patients to transfer easily, quickly, and safely from methadone to naltrexone maintenance.[50]

This rapid and safe approach permits opiate detoxification to be greatly accelerated without any damage; it is also economical in terms of treatment costs and time away from work. In the future, very long acting opiate antagonists should be used after rapid detoxification to block opiate receptor sites for a longer time so as to interrupt the vicious circle of addiction.

Acetorphan   The recent availability of acetorphan—an active enkephalinase inhibitor that does not produce a drug dependence and the safety of which has now been established in several hundred patients—made it feasible to test the enkephalinase-inhibitor hypothesis in human beings for the first time. A 1991 study compared the effects of acetorphan with those of Clonidine for the treatment of opioid withdrawal syndrome.[51] Nineteen patients addicted to heroin or synthetic opiates who were undergoing drug withdrawal and displayed a withdrawal symptom were studied for five days in a hospital setting. In a double-bind trial, ten subjects were given acetorphan intravenously and nine were given Clonidine; objective signs and subjective symptoms were recorded. The results indicated that on several objective signs, the effect of acetorphan was more marked than that of Clonidine; whereas the two drugs exhibited similar efficacy with respect to the subjective components of withdrawal. No side effect was noted in the subjects who received acetorphan. This study concluded that enkephalinase inhibition may constitute a novel and safe therapeutic approach to the opioid-withdrawal syndrome.

COCAINE TREATMENT

Although most treatment programs follow the models used for alcohol and heroin (opiates), there are some differences that apply to cocaine. The new therapeutic drugs that have been under development since the mid-1960s are intended, not to replace cocaine, but to help addicts past the initial depression and difficulty of going cold turkey and to give psychotherapy a chance to work. The agents that have shown success so far include antidepressants, believed to restore a brain chemical depleted by cocaine that carries signals from one nerve to another, and antiepileptic drugs that block the erratic nerve-cell firing that results from cocaine use.

Methadone for Cocaine   Serious-minded public officials have recently suggested that what is needed to bring drug abuse under control is a methadonelike medication for crack addicts and other cocaine users. Others feel that calling for the rapid development of a "methadone clone" is turning away from drug-free treatment.

Cocaine, "or coke," is certainly a tougher problem, as it is more addictive than heroin. Give a monkey free access to heroin, food, water, and monkeys of the opposite sex, and the monkey will enjoy all four. Switch the drug to cocaine, and the monkey will ignore food, water, and potential mate and take cocaine until it dies.[52]

To understand how drugs fight coke, we have to remember that the use of cocaine or crack seems to deplete the brain's synapses of dopamine and possibly other neurotransmitters.[53] The use of drugs in therapy is therefore like using chemical, not psychological, warfare. Antidepressant drugs, such as despiramine (Norpramin or Pertofane), form a chemical bond with the sites in the brain where the neurotransmitters are pumped back into the nerve cells and stored for future use. The drugs seem to act as natural antidotes to cocaine, and within a few weeks the users just do not want it. Some of the following are drugs being experimented with to help stop cocaine addiction.

Amantadine   In many cocaine-treatment clinics, the difficult task of treating the addicts is worsened by the continuing withdrawal symptoms. These symptoms seem to be of a more persistent type than those experienced by other drug addicts. Cocaine addicts have difficulty entering or staying on a recovery program because of appetite changes, irritability, depression, lack of motivation, shaking, nausea, psychomotor retardation, and irregular sleep patterns. Ronald Pike from Ad Care Hospital of Worchester, Massachusetts, has used amantadine with patients who had severe depression and other withdrawal symptoms.[54]

Bromocriptine   Researchers will also soon test bromocriptine, which increases the uptake of the neurotransmitter dopamine in the brain. Bromocriptine is now sold for several disorders, including Parkinson's disease, which is caused by a lack of dopamine in the brain.

A study was done on six cocaine addicts with a mean age of 33.[55] The bromocriptine was prescribed for four to eight weeks. The study was to see if bromocriptine reduced the amount of cocaine used by the group, and if it reduced the craving for cocaine. The patients were monitored through urine tests, and a rating system for cocaine craving was used.

Almost immediately four of the patients reported a decrease in cravings and usage of cocaine. The other two patients were hospitalized for cocaine treatment. Nausea and headaches were side effects reported by three patients. The side effects were decreased with lower doses of bromocriptine. It is felt that bromocriptine, with methadone, could reduce the number of cocaine users.

Buprenorphine   Researchers are extremely excited about buprenorphine's possibilities of treatment for heroin and cocaine addiction. The effectiveness of this drug was discussed in the heroin treatment section of this chapter.

Carbamozepine   James Halikas tested the antiepilepsy drug carbamozepine on a few dozen people at the University of Minnesota. Carbamozepine plus psychotherapy dramatically reduced cocaine usage in 13 of 21 patients.[56]

Desipramine   The antidepressant studies are the first indication that cocaine cravings can be eased by medications, and researchers are now testing several other drugs. Researchers Frank Gawin and Herbert Kleber of University School of Medicine tested desipramine on a group of chronic cocaine abusers and showed that 60 percent of those receiving desipramine were able to stop taking cocaine for three weeks or more.[57]

Phenelzine   Phenelzine is believed to correct biochemical defects caused by cocainelike depletion of serotonin, dopamine, and norepinephrine. Phenelzine increases the neurotransmitters dopamine, serotonin, and norepinephrine and therefore may help during withdrawal to reduce craving symptoms.[58]

Phenelzine is dangerous when taken in conjunction with cocaine and may assist addicts in increasing their fear of using cocaine by knowing the dangerous side effects, which include headaches, increase in blood pressure, palpitations, and chest tightness. It should be used only under the care of a physician and only when all other forms of treatment have failed.

Given the growing number of new drugs, it appears that methadonelike drugs will probably become available. Each new drug will have to be evaluated carefully to determine its effectiveness.

RELAPSE

Relapse

A return to using a drug after a person has gone through treatment. Aftercare programs are often necessary to help patients overcome periods of relapse.

A small percentage of those who suffer from addictive diseases suffer greatly. Part of the reason is **relapse.** Relapse is a serious problem in the treatment of chemical dependency. A study conducted in 1988 by the Comprehensive Care Corporation evaluated 723 patients from 50 different Care Unit facilities.[59] At one year following discharge, 57 percent of the patients had relapsed. One third of all relapses were short term and had low consequences. Two thirds were long term and had high consequences. Of these patients, 30 to 40 percent had been previously treated for their addiction on at least one occasion. On a more positive note, "one-third to one-half of all relapse-prone persons eventually find permanent abstinence."[60] The American Medical Association includes in its definition of alcoholism the fact that the disease is "characterized by a tendency to relapse."[61] (The same is true of addiction to any other drug.) Of those who are treated, one half to two thirds relapse within two years, whatever their method of treatment. Yet few treatment facilities address that issue, either before or during treatment, and few programs provide the long-term therapy necessary to give the patient the best chance against relapse.[62] The reason is simple: Treatment costs money. And most insurance policies cover only 28 days of treatment in hospital and extremely limited follow-up and outpatient treatment.

When relapse occurs, it seems to come out of the blue, blanking all reason, all experience, all logic. But there are warning signs. It may begin as anger or depression. It may begin as a sense of well-being, confidence, a warm glow of pride at how well everything is going. As one AA member said, "In my 30 years, no one ever called me to ask to be prevented from taking a drink. I myself never called for help at the threshold of relapse, probably because I did not want to be stopped."[63]

Some of the following recovery strategies are necessary to prevent relapse after undergoing treatment for chemical dependency.[64]

1. Nearly every recovering alcoholic or drug user has made at least one unsuccessful attempt to quit.

2. Of cocaine users who have received inpatient treatment, nearly half will experience at least one relapse during the first six months after leaving the rehabilitation center.

3. Although the incidence of relapse drops dramatically after the addict's being free for a year, the recovering addict will continue to feel fragile. Often it takes two to five years to feel confident and comfortable in the new life. In the meantime addicts must cope with guilt, social stigma, fear of recurrence, and a pervasive sense that life will never be safe again.

To deal with this pattern, many treatment centers have instituted aftercare programs on the assumption that almost no one stays straight by going it alone. Aftercare may include psychotherapy in both individual and group sessions, attendance at self-help meetings, or a combination of the three. Alcoholics Anonymous and groups for drug users patterned after AA, such as NA and CA, are the most widespread self-help programs in the country.

Aftercare is critical to recovery because most inpatient programs focus on what the addict has already been through, not on a practical day-to-day plan for remaining drug-free in the outside world.

A closely structured life, one providing support and activity when an addict is most likely to relapse, is essential during the first year. A good aftercare program concentrates on practical steps people can take to keep their lives in order.

Another area for concern to recovering addicts is how to deal with friends or colleagues who have drug and drinking problems.[65] Addicts must learn to dissociate themselves from people who use while realizing that not everyone is a drunk or druggie. It is essential for many that they not expose themselves to unnecessary temptation during the first year of sobriety. A good aftercare program will enable recovering addicts to learn coping strategies for dealing with situations where exposure to alcohol or drug consumption is unavoidable.

SUMMARY

Because of the tremendous number of people in the United States experiencing drug problems, substance abuse treatment has escalated. It is estimated that 650,000 people are kicking the habit through the 9000 programs available to them.

Drug addiction is a chronic, compulsive, and uncontrollable craving for and dependence on a particular substance. It can have an effect on the psychological, physiological, or social aspects of a person's life. Drug treatment programs have screening tests to determine if a person is truly dependent on drugs.

Today there is greater hope for drug addicts or dependents because treatment professionals have gained experience and knowledge about how to deal more effectively with patients who have drug problems. Newer approaches based on experience of what works most effectively, the use of chemical assistance (such as methadone), and a wide range of individual and group support in intervention, treatment, aftercare, and relapse have made the programs more successful.

Specialized treatment is available for adults as well as adolescents. A variety of inpatient and outpatient programs are available. In addition, self help groups like AA, NA, and CA are available. The traditional 12 step AA model plus some other approaches are being implemented. There is a search for new methadone-type drugs that could be used for people with chemical dependence on other drugs—in other words, fighting drugs with drugs. The chemical dependency treatment field appears to be maturing as a profession and offers new hope for those suffering from chemical dependence.

Treatment of Drug Abuse
N O T E S

1. Phoebe Hoban, "A New Generation Fights Addiction," *New York Magazine,* February 20, 1989, pp. 39–45.
2. "The 110,000,000 Problem," *USA Today* 117 (November 1988):8–9.
3. Steven Findlay, "Treatment," *U.S. News & World Report,* September 11, 1989, pp. 74–79.
4. "Addiction and Rehabilitation," *Playboy,* May 1987, pp. 149–52, 182, 184–85, 189–90, 1994, 1996, and 1998.
5. Ibid.
6. David Gelman, et al. "Roots of Addiction," *Newsweek,* February 20, 1990. p. 52.
7. Dean R. Gerstein and Lawrence S. Lewin, "Treating Drug Problems," *New England Journal of Medicine* 323, no. 12 (September 20, 1990):844–48.
8. "Addiction and Rehabilitation."
9. B. Patricia Mutch, "Infant Addicts: A Preventable Rage," *Vibrant Life* 6 (May/June 1990):16–27.
10. Gerstein and Lewin, "Treating Drug Problems."
11. National Association of State Alcohol and Drug Directors, "Waiting for Treatment," *Addiction and Recovery,* June, 1990, pp. 21–22.
12. Ibid.
13. Ibid.
14. G. Witkin, "A Modest Proposal for Dealing with Drugs," *U.S. News & World Report* June 27, 1988, p. 22.

15. Paul King, "Treatment for Chemically Dependent Adolescents," *Professional Counselor,* March/April 1988, pp. 41–44.

16. Based on an interview with Michael Goldrick, Director, Sacred Heart Adolescent Recovery Program (SHARP), Eugene, Oregon.

17. Kay M. Porterfield, "Teen Drug Rehab," *Current Health 2* 15, no. 6 (February 1989):19–21.

18. Kathryn Hudson, "Drug Therapy for Abusers, but Stress for Some Families," *Insight,* December 5, 1988, pp. 18–20.

19. Ibid.

20. Skip Gaus and Brother Gilbert Henderson, "Support Life Skills Programs for Court-Committed Adolescent Substance Abusers," Treatment Services for Adolescent Substance Abusers (Rockville, Md.: U.S. Department of Health and Human Services, 1985), pp. 204–15.

21. Ibid.

22. Tony Cohen, "Why Subsidize Expensive Private Drug Care," *New York Times,* June 6, 1988, p. 19.

23. Richard L. Berke, "Anti-Drug Steps Imposed on U.S. Contractors," *New York Times,* March 18, 1989, p. A7.

24. Judith Frabotta, "How to Weigh Drug Treatment Options," *Business and Health,* February 1989, pp. 37–38.

25. Ibid.

26. Christie Gorman, "Bad Trips for the Doubly Troubled," *Time,* August 3, 1987, p. 58.

27. Phoebe Hoban, "A New Generation Fights Addiction," *New York,* February 20, 1989, pp. 39–45.

28. Ibid.

29. Christine Bohlen, "Support Groups Are Offering Embrace to Cocaine's Victims," *New York Times,* January 29, 1991, p. A1.

30. Alcoholics Anonymous World Services, Inc.

31. Marc Galanter, "Combined Alcoholics Anonymous and Professional Care for Addicted Physicians," *American Journal of Psychiatry* 147 (January 1990):64–68.

32. R. Kunstler, "A New Analysis of Substance Abuse and the Role of Therapeutic Recreation," *Leisure Information Quarterly* 15, no. 1:6–7.

33. Bob Rodale, "Running for Drugs II," *Runner's World,* February 1989, p. 24.

34. "Position of the American Dietetic Association: Nutrition Intervention in Treatment and Recovery for Chemical Dependency," *Journal of the American Dietetics Association* 90, no. 9 (September 1990):1274–77.

35. Steven B. Soumeral and Dennis Ross-Degnan, "Experience of State Drug Benefit Programs," *Health Affairs* 9, no. 3 (Fall 1990).

36. Based on an interview with Neal McNaughton, Director, Serenity Lane Alcohol and Drug Treatment Center, Eugene, Oregon.

37. James F. Guinan, "Extending the System for the Treatment of Chemical Dependencies," *Journal of Strategic and Systematic Therapies* 9, no. 1 (Spring 1990):11–20.

38. Tom Callahan, "A Drug Program for Inmates," *New York Times,* August 7, 1988, p. 8.

39. E. M. Read, "Attitude Adjustment: The First Step in Treating Addiction," *Corrections Today* 51, no. 3:104–6.

40. Herman Joseph et al., "Heroin Addicts in Jail: New York Tries Methadone Treatment Program," *Corrections Today,* August 1989, pp. 124, 126, 130–31.

41. Ibid.

42. Based on an interview with Kevin Hornbuckle, Director of Clinical Services for the Oregon Institute for Rational Recovery, Eugene, Oregon.

43. M. Mitchell Waldrop, "NIDA Aims to Fight Drugs with Drugs," *Science* 245 (September 29, 1989):1443–44.

44. Based on an interview with Carol Peak, a nurse at Serenity Lane Alcohol and Drug Treatment Program, Eugene, Oregon.

45. Andrew Purvis, "Can Drugs Cure Drug Addiction?" *Time,* December 11, 1989, p. 104.

46. John Harold, "Lukewarm Turkey," *Scientific American* 260, no. 2 (March 1989):32–36.

47. Kathleen McAuliffe, "Getting Off the High Horse," *OMNI* 13 (December 1990):20.

48. Dennis S. Charney, George R. Heninger, and Herbert D. Kleber, "The Combined Use of Clonidine and Naltrexone as a Rapid, Safe, and Effective Treatment of Abrupt Withdrawal from Methadone," *American Journal of Psychiatry* 143 (1986):831–37.

49. Norbert Loimer et al., "Technique for Greatly Shortening the Transition from Methadone to Naltrexone Maintenance of Patients Addicted to Opiates," *American Journal of Psychiatry* 148 (1991):933–35.

50. Ibid.

51. Francois Hartman et al., "Comparison of Acetorphan with Clonidine for Opiate Withdrawal Symptoms," *American Journal of Psychiatry* 148 (May 1991):627–29.

52. Joanne Silberner, "A Technical Fix for Cocaine Addiction," *U.S. News & World Report,* April 17, 1989, p. 61.

53. Robert Wilbur, "Drugs That Fight Coke," *American Health* (June 1988):44–47.

54. Ronald F. Pike, "Cocaine Withdrawal—An Effective Three-Day Regimen," *Post Graduate Medicine* 85, no. 4 (March 1989):115–16, 121.

55. T. R. Kosten et al., "Bromocriptine Treatment of Cocaine Abuse in Patients Maintained on Methadone," *American Journal of Psychiatry,* March 1988, no. 145:381–82.

56. James Halikas and Nancy Stesin, "Dr. James Halikas Finds That Pill Made for Seizures May Help Cocaine Addicts to Just Say No," *People Weekly* 33, no. 3:81–82.

57. Deborah M. Barnes, "Breaking the Cycle of Addiction," *Science* 24 (August 26, 1988):1029–30.

58. Daniel H. Golwyn, "Cocaine Abuse Treated with Phenelzine," *International Journal of Addictions* 23, no. 9 (1988):897–905.

59. Terrance T. Gorski, "Relapse—Issues and Answers," *Alcohol and Addiction,* November 1989, p. 21.

60. Ibid.

61. "Addiction and Rehabilitation."

62. Ibid.

63. Ibid.

64. Susan Jacoby, "The Long Road Back from Addiction: The Hardest Part Isn't Getting Straight, It's Staying Straight," *Glamour,* July 1988, pp. 58–66.

65. Ibid.

GLOSSARY

Addict A person who has a very strong craving to use a chemical substance.

AIDS Acquired Immunodeficiency Syndrome This life-threatening disease is often spread by sharing syringes while injecting various drugs.

Alternatives A variety of activities, such as, exercise, work, wilderness experiences and religion to take the place of using drugs.

Amphetamine Psychosis A condition where a user of amphetamines starts having fear and suspicion and an uneasy feeling. The fear soon becomes intense, causing paranoia and a specific delusion. This amphetamine-induced paranoia causes a high rate of violence among amphetamine (speed) users.

Anti-Drug Bill, 1988 A drug bill that includes stricter penalties in the following areas: civil penalties, user penalties, and law enforcement. It also provides for a drug czar cabinet position, more funds for education and treatment, international narcotics control, alcohol warning labels, increased penalties for child pornography, and a review of driver's licenses for those testing positive for drugs.

Antihistamines Combat the effects of the naturally occurring hormone named histamine, which helps protect the body by increasing secretions that cause sneezing, running nose and eyes, congestion, itching, and nausea. Antihistamines offer relief by temporarily reducing histamine release.

Asparatame The generic name for the low-calory sweetner made from protein products. It is 180 times sweeter than sugar.

Attention-Deficit Hyperactive Disorder A recent term used to describe hyperactivity.

Biochemical Theory The concept that drug dependency from all psychoactive substances can be explained in biochemical terms.

Biofeedback The immediate ongoing presentation of information to a person concerning his or her own physiologic processes. This alternative to drug use, also known as alpha training, is simple to use and capable of producing numerous benefits, including personal control of physiological functions, globular personality changes, feelings of well-being, new views on one's individuality, and transcendental insights.

Blotter Diluted drops of LSD are placed on blotter paper and this is referred to as blotter acid. Small sections or squares are torn off and consumed by a user.

Bruxism A grinding of the teeth that often occurs in heavy methamphetamine users.

Caffeinism Is characterized by a "withdrawal headache" from a decrease in caffeine consumption and by a temporary depression.

Cannabis Sativa The scientific name for marijuana (pot, weed, dope).

Carbon Monoxide An odorless, colorless, and poisonous gas possessing an affinity for hemoglobin 250 times that of oxygen. It is one of the gases given off in cigarette smoke, and it literally drives oxygen out of body cells.

Children of Alcoholics Children who are victims of an alcoholic, dysfunctional family. They are more likely to become drinkers than children who are not from a dysfunctional family. They experience more problems because they have traits of the alcoholic personality and many of them become social outcasts, which causes them to drink even more.

"Chippers" A term applied to the periodic user of drugs, for example, an individual who periodically uses a drug such as heroin but is not using it regularly.

Chronic Bronchitis Inflammation of the bronchial tubes often caused by smoking tobacco cigarettes.

Cirrhosis After the ingestion of relatively small amounts of alcohol, the accumulation of fat in the liver can be detected. Alcohol is thought to be toxic to the liver and interferes with acetaldehyde, the intermediate by-product of alcohol metabolism. In heavy drinkers the continued use of alcohol leads to cirrhosis of the liver, which can be fatal.

Clozapin (Brand Name Clozril) A new drug available for severely ill schizophrenics. There are some side effects to watch for such as convulsions and agranulocytosis, a serious blood disorder that reduces the number of white blood cells (the body's disease-fighting cells).

Co-Dependent Family and friends of the alcoholic are often referred to as co-dependent because without realizing it they help the alcoholic to continue living his or her life with the problem. They offer excuses for the alcoholic's behavior and may even provide money to bail the alcoholic out of jail.

Comprehensive K–12 Drug Education Program A grades K–12 coordinated drug education curriculum focusing on knowledge, attitudes, and behavior change to stop drug abuse. It involves students, parents, teachers, counselors, and the community working cooperatively to curb drug abuse. School and community cooperation is essential in the fight against drugs.

Constipation A condition in which the feces become hard and dry because fluid is not absorbed quickly enough to produce softer stools.

Crack Cocaine mixed with baking soda and water over a hot flame. The substance is then dried. The soapy-looking substance that results can be broken up into rocks and smoked. These rocks are approximately five times as strong as cocaine in powder form. Crack is normally smoked, and because it is such a pure drug, it takes much less time to achieve the desired high. One puff of a pebble-sized rock produces an intense high that lasts 20 minutes.

Decriminalization An attempt to reduce the number of laws and penalties associated with drug use.

Delta-9-Tetrahydracannabinol (THC) The psychoactive ingredient in the marijuana plant that determines its potency.

Demand To ask for drugs. Prevention and education programs are designed to reduce the demand for drugs.

Detoxification A medical program designed to assist the dependent with withdrawal symptoms and help restore his or her general health with good nutrition and hygiene instructions. Proper detoxification allows the patient to start a treatment program in improved health. It is difficult for treatment to be successful when the patient is still ill.

Diazepam (Valium) An antianxiety agent and muscle relaxant that produces antiepileptic effects without sedation.

Dipping Snuff dipping consists of placing a pinch of powder tobacco (which is sold in cans) between the cheek and gum.

Drug Interactions A drug interaction occurs when two or more drugs are administered concomitantly; the responses are unexpected, unusual, or amplified.

Drug Testing It has been introduced to reduce illicit drug use. A urine test is required to determine whether or not drugs are present in the employee. Some say it is an infringement of one's rights, but others support it to ensure that performance, mental or physical, is not impaired. The test is used to keep employees off drugs so a safe work environment can be maintained.

Dual Diagnosis A combination of drug abuse and mental illness.

Ecstasy An amphetaminelike drug that is an analogue of MDA. Street names include MDMA, MDA, Adam, Ecstasy, XTC. It produces LSD effects (minus hallucinations) such as increased self-awareness, removes communication barriers, and seems to remove the fear response.

Emphysema A lung disease in which the lungs lose their normal elasticity and retain abnormal amounts of air. Smoking destroys the tiny air sacs in the lungs, where oxygen is absorbed into the body, resulting in a loss of oxygen absorption and subsequent loss of breath.

Employee Assistance Programs A formal broad-based approach to helping maintain a healthy workplace. It has been established to assist with employees' personal problems that affect the work situation. Drug problems and drug testing are a major focus of most employee assistance programs.

Enkephalins and Endorphins Enkephalins are neurotransmitters of specific neuronal systems in the brain that mediate the integration of sensory information having to do with pain and emotional behavior. The body's own natural morphinelike pain killer, endorphin, centers in the numerous pleasurable sensations associated with the body's natural secretion of this "magical" hormone. Endorphins, or their receptors, are responsible not only for their widely known anesthetic effect but also for the intensity of other emotional states, such as happiness, depression, compulsiveness, masochism, excitation, sexual satisfaction, and hunger.

Fat-Soluble Drugs that are stored in fatty tissue. THC is fat-soluble and some of it is stored in fatty tissue, where it may stay for a month or more.

FDA The Federal Drug Administration, a government agency that overlooks the production of over-the-counter drugs and prescription drugs to determine their safety and effectiveness.

Federal Drug Administration A federal agency that classifies and approves drugs for medical use. It is also involved in the regulation of laws pertaining to safe drugs such as over-the-counter drugs.

Fentanyl An intravenous analgesic-anesthetic that is a favored preanesthetic medication, anesthetic, and postsurgical analgesic. Fentanyl analogs are now being used as designer drugs like China White and synthetic heroin. They are extremely potent and make overdose a serious risk.

Fetal Alcohol Syndrome (FAS) A pattern of growth retardation, physical defects, and mental retardation found in infants born to women who drink heavily and extensively during pregnancy. The severe cases are called FAS, while the milder cases are referred to as Fetal Alcohol Effect (FAE).

Fibrocystic Breasts Lumps, nodules, and thickenings in the breast tissue of women. Caffeine and related substances are suspected of increasing the supply of Camp, a growth-promoting compound in breast tissue. Women with fibrocystic breasts have an increased risk of developing breast cancer.

Flashback A spontaneous reoccurrence of feelings that may have been experienced during an LSD trip (and with some other drugs also) weeks, months, or even years earlier. It has been estimated that flashbacks occur in approximately 5 percent of LSD users.

Gray Area A combination of fact and fiction the listener must sort through in the drug field. Research reports are often conflicting or contrary. Half truths and sensationalism distort drug-related discussions and make accurate assessments of the drug scene difficult. Wide variation in drug use and its effects on the individual further obscures attempts to clarify the issues surrounding drug use.

Hashish Hash is the resin from the leaves and flowers of the marijuana plant. This resin (hashish) is pressed into cakes or slabs.

High-Risk Factors An individual who has high potential for substance abuse may have the following high-risk factors: unconventionality (a need or tendency to rebel), uncontrolled emotions (expressed as impulsiveness), intrapsychic functioning (depression), interpersonal relations (when expressed in terms of aggression), and nonachievement (described not as a lack of ability but as a lack of motivation).

Homeostasis Refers to the body's need to keep its biological systems in balance.

Hooked A term often used to indicate physical and mental dependence on a drug.

Hypnotic Drug used to bring on sleep.

Hypersensitive Drugs interact with bodily chemicals to produce allergic reactions. The initial sign of hypersensitivity may be a skin rash or development of an asthmatic condition.

Ibuprofen Acts similarly to aspirin in that it blocks prostaglandin effects; however, it does not cause stomach upset or gastric ulcers.

ICE A stronger form of amphetamine. It is a pure form of methamphetamine hydrochloride, more dangerous than cocaine because of its purity and because the effects last for hours compared to minutes with cocaine use.

Intervention Refers to a process where an attempt is made by family, friends, and an alcohol- and drug-treatment counselor to stop substance abuse before a person bottoms out with the illness. It is a carefully executed process wherein friends, in a loving and caring manner, express their concern about the dependent's problem and cite specific examples of behaviors they have observed while the dependent was under the influence of alcohol or other drugs. It is the goal of the intervention to get the dependent into a treatment center for help.

Legalization Treating drugs as a public-health problem instead of as a criminal issue. Proponents argue that drug-related crime damages society more than actual drug use.

Lithium A metalic salt that can be administered as a strong antimanic tranquilizer in individuals who are suffering from a biochemical imbalance in portions of the brain that causes violent or manic behavior.

Mainstream Smoke Smoke that is inhaled from the burning tobacco by the user.

Major Tranquilizers Antipsychotics grouped on the basis of their widespread medical use: treatment and management of certain acute psychological disorders, notably schizophrenia and other severe conditions.

Methadone A synthetic narcotic classified as a CNS depressant. Its effects are similar to those of morphine, though they develop more slowly and persist longer. Methadone blocks the high given by heroin and has been used in treatment of heroin dependency. The heroin user substitutes methadone for heroin until he or she can be gradually withdrawn from heroin. This removes the heroin high and the withdrawal symptoms caused when heroin is no longer used.

Minor Tranquilizers Drugs used to help relieve anxiety or tension.

Narcolepsy A condition or disease causing an individual to keep falling asleep.

Natural High This refers to getting high on life without the use of drugs.

Noncompliance Patients themselves may contribute markedly to the high rates of adverse drug reactions and drug-induced death. Noncompliance with a physician's instructions can bring about serious consequences ranging from the failure of the drug to affect the disease to intensification of the disease and even death.

Nostrum A consumer product that is promoted by its maker. It may, or may not, be of any value.

Opiates Drugs, sometimes called narcotics, which are derived from opium (the thickened juice of the opium poppy), that are used to induce sleep and remove pain.

Orphan Drug Provides drug companies with grants, tax credits, and a seven-year period of exclusive marketing, all as an incentive to develop drugs for diseases that affect fewer than 200,000 people. It allows medicines to be developed for people with rare diseases.

Overdose Taking an excessive amount of a drug, such as heroin, or a combination of several drugs and adulterants that may lead to death.

Patient Compliance Patients carefully following their doctor's instructions (some surveys show that a large percentage of patients receiving medication do not follow instructions) and asking for clarification of any confusing or difficult-to-understand points about the drug.

Peer Pressure We copy the activities and behavior of our peers as a way of learning social behavior and gaining acceptance. In gaining entrance to a group, we prove ourselves to the group and to ourselves. Once individuals have been accepted to the group, socialization continues. It determines an individual's behavior, dress, skill acquisition, interests, speech, and so on.

Peer Support Student-to-student support.

Peyote Ritual Native Americans regard the peyote cactus as God's special gift to the Indians and equate its effects with the workings of the divine spirit. Slices of peyote have replaced the sacramental bread used in other services, and the use is limited to healing religious services only; the drug is not to be used for recreational purposes. Several states have made it legal for Native Americans to use peyote.

Phantasticant A substance capable of exercising its chemical power on all senses, but particularly the visual and auditory spheres as well as the general sensibility.

Phenylpropanolamine (PPA) The appetite suppressant found in most diet pills.

Physical Dependence When certain drugs, in higher concentrations made necessary by tolerance, cause various biochemical transformations that in turn cause the system to become dependent on the presence of these drugs.

Polypharmacy A term applied to the use of several drugs at the same time. A person may be taking several prescriptions from several doctors.

Positive Addiction Selecting alternatives to substitute for negative dependency and replacing them with positive dependencies. These are usually noncompetitive, done easily, done alone, have some value, allow for improvement, and can be without criticism.

Propoxyphene Hydrochloride (Darvon) A white crystalline powder that is water-soluble and usually combined with aspirin or acetaminophen to relieve mild pain. It was considered a medical breakthrough because it had the potency of codeine but not the side effects or potential for dependency. Unfortunately, this initial optimism was short-lived, since research later proved that Darvon was structurally related to methadone and could cause psychological dependency.

Prozac The newest wonder drug on the psychiatric scene. Fluxotine, as it is also called, is the nation's most prescribed antidepressant drug. There have been some concerns about possible side effects leading to violent and suicidal behavior.

Relapse A return to using a drug after a person has gone through treatment. Aftercare programs are often necessary to help patients overcome periods of relapse.

Reye's Syndrome A rare liver disease associated with taking aspirin while having chicken pox or flu. It is most common in children.

Risk Sports/Recreation Experiences such as river running, parachuting, skin diving, rock climbing, and skiing that can address the need for risk taking that many drug users have.

RU 486 An antiprogesterone that destroys the uterine lining, at least in most cases, starving out the already attached fetus, which dies and is expelled.

Sedative Drug used to induce a milder degree of CNS depression, such as anxiety relief.

Self-Care Taking care of oneself in lieu of going to a physician.

Sensory Deprivation Where stimuli are constant, uniform, and never changing. This may lead to boredom or a negative feeling produced by a lack of change in the environment.

Sensory Numbing Heightened and exciting experiences become increasingly difficult to achieve as people build up tolerance to sensation and need new regions to explore. Sensory bombardment through high technology has led to sensory numbing.

Shroomers People who collect mushrooms for use and sale. Selection of the right kind of mushrooms is very important because many mushrooms are poisonous and ingestion could lead to death.

Sidestream Smoke Smoke that rises from the cigarette, cigar, or pipe as it burns. Since each individual has a particular technique of smoking, different concentrations are found in exhaled mainstream smoke, depending on the tobacco product, the composition of the tobacco, and the degree of inhalation by the smoker. These concentrations, together with the harmful sidestream smoke, put the nonsmoker in a dangerous position when exposed to another person's smoke.

Speed Freak A heavy amphetamine user who may "shoot up" every three or four hours for five or six days before crashing from lack of exhaustion or lack of sleep.

Steroids Anabolic steroids are synthetic derivatives of the male hormone testosterone. They stimulate a building up, or anabolic, process in the body through synthesis of protein for muscle growth and tissue repair. Athletes have discovered that anabolic steroids allow them to recover more quickly from workout sessions, which in turn makes more intense training possible.

Suppliers Kingpins and cartels that supply drugs. Those who make drugs available for the public.

Synanon A drug-free therapeutic community where a dependent individual lives and attempts to gain control over his or her actions and become responsible. No drugs are allowed in this community.

Synergistic When a combination of two or more drugs are taken and may have geometric rather than arithmetic effects.

Synesthesia The ingestion of hallucinogenic drugs may lead to a blending of the senses where one perceives one is smelling noises or tasting sounds. Administration of hallucinogens changes the serotonin in the brain, and serotonin further triggers a multitude of changes involving the complexity of the brain.

Tachycardia A fast heartbeat. This is a common condition in amphetamine users and increases the concern for heart damage.

Tetrahydraisoquardrelone (THIQ) Most of alcohol is transformed and eliminated by the body; however, approximately 1 percent of it is diverted to an alternative fate. It is this fate that results in biochemical dependency. This very small percentage of residual alcohol combines with the neurotransmitter dopamine to form an addictive alkaloid called tetrahydraisoquardrelone (THIQ). This substance is closely related to the opium family, especially morphine. THIQ combines with other neurotransmitters in the central nervous system to form other similarly addictive alcoholoids.

Therapeutic Recreation Utilization of relaxation techniques, assertiveness training, social-skill development, exercise/fitness, and implementation of organized activities to help clients maintain leisure lifestyles and choose satisfying and joyful experiences they can control.

Timing Out A term, employed by behavioral psychologists, that refers to the removal of an individual from his or her immediate environment to a neutral site of seclusion. It focuses on taking a break from one's present involvement.

Tolerance The body's ability to adapt to existing drug dosage, thereby reducing or eliminating the desired effects; dose increases are then needed to produce these effects.

Transcendental Meditation (TM) A psychological technique through which practitioners attempt to reach deep physiological relaxation. TM followers repeat a specific phrase (mantra) known only to themselves. The objective of this is to narrow the content of awareness to a fine point so that it may eventually break through to a higher, more intense plane of consciousness.

Treatment Programs Provide a range of services, which may include some or all of the following: referral, intervention, detoxification, inpatient care, outpatient care, counseling, nutrition, exercise and fitness for recovering addicts.

Victimless Crime It is difficult to enforce crime legislation when the crime involved has no victim. Does society have a right to interfere with an individual's right to determine his or her own actions—in this case, to use drugs? Should drug use be a crime because society at large deems it to be?

Withdrawal Symptoms such as muscle twitching, insomnia, headache, fever, nausea, vomiting, abdominal cramps, sweating, convulsions, and even death when the drug is withdrawn from a dependent user.

INDEX

A

Absorption, 72
Accidental abuse of drugs, 62
Accutane, 350-51
Acetaminophen, 323
Acetorphan, as heroin treatment, 456
Acetylcholine (ACH), 77
Acetylsalicylic acid. *See* Salicylates (aspirin)
Acquired immunodeficiency syndrome (AIDS), 360-61
  AZT (azidothymidine/zidovudine), 360
  dextran sulfate, 360-61
  Drug 566, 361
  and heroin, 249
  and intravenous cocaine shooters, 105
  and salicylates (aspirin), 322
Action potential, defined, 76
Adam. *See* MDMA (3,4 methylenedioxymetham-phetamine)
Addict, defined, 445
Addicted smokers, 149
Addiction:
  and dependency, 440-41
  infants, 441
  predilection for, 26-27
ADH (alcoholdehydrogenase), 216
Adlerian theory of ego compensation, 27
Adolescents:
  and alcohol, 39, 42
  and caffeine (Xanthines), 126
  and cocaine, 42
  and crack, 40, 115
    sale of crack by, 111
  and drug use, 38-39
  and marijuana use, phases of, 299-300
  and psychological effects of smoking, 151
  and steroids, 40-41
  and tobacco, 39, 41
  treatment programs, 442-44
    Outward Bound, 445
    Sacred Heart Adolescent Recovery Program, 445-46
    St. Luke's Adolescent Recovery Unit, 444
    Straight program, 444-45
  See also Children; Youth drug scene
Adrenergic neurons, 77

Adult children of alcoholics (ACoA), 233
Adult drug scene, 52-60
  alcohol, 53
  amphetamines, 55
  aspirin, 54-55
  caffeine, 54
  drugs in the workplace, 55-57
  drug testing, 57-60
  major drug groups used by, 52
  marijuana, 55
  nicotine, 54
  opiates, 55
  sedative-hypnotics, 53-54
  tranquilizers, 53-54
  See also specific drugs
Adult treatment programs, 445-54
  alcohol treatment, 454
  cocaine treatment, 456-58
  for the elderly, 449
  employers, 446
  examples of, 449-54
    Crossroads program, 451-52
    inmate treatment program, 452
    Key Extended Entry Program (KEEP), 452-53
    Rational Recovery (RR), 453-54
    Serenity Lane Alcohol- and Drug-Treatment Program, 449-51
  heroin treatment, 455-56
  key components of, 446-49
    dual diagnosis, 446-47
    inpatient vs. outpatient programs, 446
    nutritional intervention, 448-49
    self-help groups, 447-48
    therapeutic recreation, 448
  See also Drug abuse, treatment of
Adverse drug reactions (ADRs), 61
Advertising, 377-78
  and alcohol, 198
  and over-the-counter (OTC) drugs, 12
  as sociological factor of drug use, 25
  and tobacco, 148-49
Age of Anxiety, 4
Aggression:
  and alcohol, 219-20
  and marijuana, 301

AIDS. *See* Acquired immunodeficiency syndrome (AIDS)
Alcohol, 4, 7, 16, 21, 32, 84, 174, 192-237
  and adult drug scene, 53
  and cancer, 208
  combining with other drugs, 209-10
  consumption in U.S., 194-97
    adults, 195-96
    elderly, 196-97
    youth, 194-95
  fetal alcohol effect (FAE), 207-8
  fetal alcohol syndrome (FAS), 207-8
  history of, 197
  and marijuana, 304
  Mothers Against Drunk Drivers (MADD), 234
  physiological effects of, 200-210
    body temperature, 207
    circulatory system/blood, 200-203
    digestive system, 206-7
    kidneys, 207
    liver, 205-6
    nervous system, 203-5
  reasons for drinking, 197-200
    advertising, 198
    changing sex roles, 199
    family influence, 200
    peer acceptance, 199
    recreation/enjoyment, 199
    sex, 199-200
  responsible drinking, 234-35
  societal/individual effects of, 210-14
    adolescent drinking, 212
    crime, 213
    economic costs, 210-12
    by ethnic group/race, 212-13
    homelessness, 213
    suicide, 214
    violence, 213
  Students Against Driving Drunk (SADD), 234
  and testosterone level, 208-9
  and tobacco, 147
  warning labels, 214
  and women, 209
  and youth drug scene, 39-40, 42
Alcoholic blackout, 205
Alcoholics Anonymous (AA), 226, 228, 231, 431, 444, 447-48

Alcoholics Anonymous (*cont.*)
  twelve-step program, 44–48
Alcoholism, 214–33
  adult children of alcoholics (ACoA), 233
  Al-Anon, 228
  Al-a-teen, 228
  alcohol addiction:
    irreversible damage, 218
    physiological changes, 218
  alcoholics, types of, 224–25
  Alcoholics Anonymous (AA), 226, 228, 231,
    431, 444, 447–48
  B-endorphins, 223
  biological marker, 224
  blackouts (alcoholic amnesia), 218
  blood enzymes, 223
  brain, 224
  causes, 221–22
  children of alcoholics, 232–33
  cognitive-behavioral indicators, 218–21
  defined, 214–21
  episodic excessive drinker, 227
  and the family, 231–33
  general hospital admission for, 226
  habitual excessive drinker, 227
  halfway houses, 226–27
  hereditary factors, 216, 222
  increased tolerance, 218
  stages in, 217–18
  symptomatic drinking, 218
  treatment approaches, 227–31
    abstinence, 231
    crisis intervention, 230–31
    detoxification, 228
    drug treatment, 227
    group therapy, 231
    lithium, 227, 454
    Prozac, 454
    Rational Recovery (RR), 229–30
    self-help programs, 228
  treatment/rehabilitation services, 226–27
  and women, 225–26
Allergic reactions, 2
  potential for, 74–75
Altered states, as psychological factor of drug
  use, 20–21
Alternatives to drug use, 425–35
  biofeedback, 431–33
  exercise, 426–28
  meditation, 433–35
  religion, 430–31
  social and political activism, 429–30
  wilderness experiences, 428–29
  work, 429
Amantadine, and cocaine treatment programs,
  457
Amateur athletics, drug use in, 47
American drug-use pattern, 4–5
Amotivational syndrome, and marijuana, 302
Amphetamine psychosis, 93–94
Amphetamines, 3, 4, 8, 55, 89–97, 398–99
  and adult drug scene, 55
  Benzedrine, 82, 90–91
  defined, 89
  Dexedrine (Dextroamphetamine), 82, 91, 92
  history of, 89–91
  medical use of, 92
  methamphetamines (crank, speed, meth), 8,
    25, 82, 93–97
  misuse/abuse of, 92

physical/psychological effects of, 91–92
  as prescription drugs, 90
Amytal. *See* Barbiturates
Anabolic steroids, 48–50
Anatomy and physiology, 75–87
  nervous system, 75–77
    central nervous system, 77–81
    peripheral nervous system, 81–87
Anorexia nervosa, and marijuana, 304
Antabuse, and alcohol treatment programs, 227
Antibiotics, 345–48
  classification, 345
  effects of, 346
  history of, 346
  misuse of, 347–48
  resistance to, 346–47
Antidepressants, 348–49
  and alcohol treatment programs, 227
  classification, 348
  psychophysiological effects of, 348–49
Anti-Drug Bill (1988), 396–400
  alcohol warning labels, 400
  child pornography, 400
  civil penalties, 396
  drivers' licenses, 400
  drug czar, 397
  education and treatment, 397
  financing, 400
  international, 397–400
  law enforcement, 397
  user penalties, 396–97
Antihistamines, 326–27
Antipsychotics. *See* Major tranquilizers
  (antipsychotics)
Antitussives, 325–26
Ascending reticular activating system. *See*
  Reticular formation
Ascorbic acid (vitamin C), 332
Asians, and alcohol, 212–13
Aspirin. *See* Salicylates (aspirin)
Asthma, and marijuana, 304
Athletics, and drugs, 46–52
Attention-deficit hyperactive disorder (ADHD),
  and Ritalin, 98–99
Autogenic training, 432
AZT (azidiothymidine/zidovudine), 360

B

Bacarate, 398–99
Bacterial infections, and marijuana, 304
Barbiturates, 54, 83, 175–77, 398–99
  abuse, 177
  classification, 175
  history, 175–76
  medical use of, 176–77
  physical effects of, 176
B-endorphins, and alcoholism, 223
Benzedrine, 82, 90–91, 398–99
"Bilious Pills," 314
Biofeedback, as alternative to drug use, 431–33
Biological perspectives, drug dependency, 28
Biphetamine, 398–99
Birth control pill, 352–54
  and cigarette smoking, 354
  for males, 355
Birth defects, and caffeine (Xanthines), 123–24
Blood-brain barrier, 72
Blood enzymes, and alcoholism, 223
Body temperature, and alcohol, 207

Boggs Amendment (1951), 390
Brain, 79
  and marijuana, physiological effects on,
    296–97
  prehistoric. *See* Hypothalamus
Brand-name vs. generic drugs, 341, 379–81
Bridge Over Troubled Waters, Inc., 428–29
Bromocriptine, and cocaine treatment
  programs, 457
Bruxism, 90
Buddhism, 20–21
Buprenorphine, 251
  and cocaine treatment programs, 457
  and heroin treatment programs, 455
Butisol. *See* Barbiturates

C

Caffeine (Xanthines), 7, 116–27
  and adult drug scene, 54
  caffeinism, 125–26
  and cardiovascular disease, 121
  and children, 126
  and cholesterol, 121–22
  content:
    in beverages, 117, 119
    in prescription/over-the-counter drugs,
      118, 119
  decaffeinated coffee, 126–27
  decreasing use of, suggestions for, 127
  diuretic action of, 126
  and fibrocystic breast disease, 126
  and gastric upset, 126
  history of, 120
  and liver, 125–26
  and pancreas, 125–26
  physical effects of, 119, 122–25
    alertness/wakefulness, 123
    on central nervous system, 123
    ergogenic aid, 124
    infertility, 124–25
    and pregnant women, 123–24
    weight loss, 124
  research findings on, 120–22
  and skeletal muscles, 126
  social acceptability of, 116
Caffeinism, 125–26
Calciferol (vitamin D), 332
Cancer:
  and alcohol, 208
  and cigarette smoking, 142–43
  and contraceptives, 354
  and marijuana, 305
  oral, vitamin A therapy for, 331
  and salicylates (aspirin), 322
  uterine, and estrogen use, 350
Cannabis sativa:
  defined, 288
  See also Marijuana
Carbamozepine, and cocaine treatment
  programs, 457–58
Cardiovascular disease. *See* Heart disease
Cardiovascular system, and marijuana, 292–93
Central nervous system, 77–81
  and caffeine (Xanthines), 123
  cerebral cortex, 80–81
  hypothalamus, 77–79
  medial forebrain bundle, 79
  medulla, 80
  periventricular system, 79

Central nervous system (cont.)
  pituitary gland, 77
  raphae nuclei, 80
  reticular formation, 79-80
Cerebral cortex, 80-81
Chancing It: Why We Take Risks, 19
Children:
  of alcoholics, 232-33
  hyperactive, and Ritalin, 98-99
  See also Adolescents; Youth drug scene
Children Are People Too program, 415
Chloral hydrate, 398-99
Cholesterol:
  and caffeine (Xanthines), 121-22
  -lowering agents, 361-62
Cholinergic neurons, 77
Chronic bronchitis, and cigarette smoking, 142
Cigarette smoking:
  alternatives to, 151-52
  and birth control pills, 354
  low-nicotine brands, 151
  nicotine gum, 152
  nicotine skin patch, 152
  nonsmokers' rights, 163-64
  quitting, 152-61
    behavioral programs, 154
    benefits of, 154-56
    company programs, 154
    elements for success, 153
    government support, 154
    process, 153
    seven-day plan, 155
  See also Nicotine; Tobacco
Cirrhosis:
  and alcohol, 205-6
  defined, 205
Clonidine and naltrexone, as combined heroin
       treatment, 455
Clonopin, 398-99
Clove cigarettes, 161
Clozapine (Clozaril), 350
Cocaine, 3, 25, 32, 82, 85, 101-16, 398-99
  administration, methods of, 105
  as an aphrodisiac, 108
  Coca-Cola and, 102
  Cocaine Anonymous (CA), 115
  cost of, 101-2
  crack, 108-15
  and crime, 111
  defined, 101
  dependency, 107-8
  and dopamine, 108
  free-base, 105-6
  history of, 102-3
  and infant addiction, 441
  injection of, 105
  medical use of, 116
  overdose, 106
  physical dependence, potential for, 75
  physiological/pharmacological effects of,
       103-8
  popularity of, 101
  in professional sports arena, 51-52
  sales estimates, 6
  sniffing, 105
  treatment programs, 456-58
    amantadine, 457
    bromocriptine, 457
    buprenorphine, 457
    carbamozepine, 457-58

desipramine, 458
methadone, 456-57
phenelzine, 458
use in the workplace, 56
young people's use of, 42
  See also Crack cocaine
Cocaine Anonymous (CA), 447, 459
Codeine, 250, 326
Co-dependents, defined, 230-31
Coffee. See Caffeine (Xanthines)
College athletics, drug use in, 47
College students, and drugs, 42-44
Color Additive Amendments (1960), 364
Commercial drugs, 13
Community Health Centers Act (1963), 391
Comprehensive Drug Abuse Prevention and
       Control Act (1970). See Controlled
       Substances Act (1970)
Comprehensive K-12 drug education program,
       414-17
  Children Are People Too, 415
  DARE (Drug Abuse Resistance Education),
       415, 448
  Health Skills for Life, 416
  Here's Looking at You, 416
  infusion curriculum, 415
  Project Graduation, 417
  skillstreaming, 416-17
Constipation, defined, 250, 324
Consumer and drug legislation, 372-410
  Anti-Drug Bill (1988), 396-400
  Boggs Amendment (1951), 390
  Community Health Centers Act (1963), 391
  Controlled Substances Act (1970), 392-96
  decriminalization, 401-5
    marijuana, 401-2
    opiates, 402-4
  Drug Abuse Control Amendments (1965),
       391-92
  drug industry, 376
    brand-name vs. generic drugs, 341, 379
    high cost of prescription drugs, 378-79
    marketing and advertising, 377-78
    profit and production, 377
    research and development, 378
  drug vigilantes, 386
  effect of, 382-86
  Federal Bureau of Narcotics (FBN), 389
  Food, Drug and Cosmetic Act (1938), 390
  Harrison Narcotic Act (1914), 102, 254,
       387-88
  heroin, ban of importation of (1924), 388-89
  intervention programs, 384-85
  Kefauver-Harris Amendments (1962), 390-91
  legalization, 383-85
  Linder v. United States (1925), 389
  Marijuana Tax Act (1937), 389
  Narcotic Addict Rehabilitation Act (1966),
       392
  Narcotic Drug Control Act (1956), 390
  opiates, regulation of (1865-1905), 386
  Orphan Drug Act, 381-82
  patient's role, 375-76
  physician's role, 372-74
  Porter Narcotic Farms Bill (1929), 389
  Prohibition, 388
  Pure Food and Drug Act (1906), 102, 387
  Robinson v. California (1962), 391
  Shanghai Conference (1909), 387
  and victimless crimes, 383

war on drugs, 385-86
Consumer safety, 70-75
  allergic reactions, potential for, 74-75
  chemical considered, 70-71
  dosage, 71-73
  drug interactions, 74
  method of administration, 73
  physical dependence, potential for, 75
  receptor mechanisms affected, 71
  tolerance, potential for, 75
Contraceptives, 352-55
  birth control pill, 352-54
    for males, 355
    and smoking, 354
    synergism and, 355
  and cancer, 354
  composition and use, 352
  Depo Provera, 355-56
  and heart disease, 354-55
  history of, 352
  mechanism, 352-53
  Norplant, 356-57
  possible side effects of, 353-54
  RU 486, 357
  and tumors, 354
Controlled Substances Act (1970), 392-96
  control mechanisms of, 394
  criminal penalties for trafficking, 396
  procedures for controlling substance, 393
  schedules, 393-95
Cosmetics, 13
Cough relievers (antitussives), 325-26
Counselors, 417-18
Crack cocaine, 8, 108-15
  animal experiments, 110-11
  and children, 115
    sale of cocaine by, 111
  compared to methamphetamines/ice, 97
  crack houses, 112-13
  and crime, 111
  defined, 108-9
  "easy access"/"press," 109
  gangs, 111-12
  and heroin, 115
  and homicide, 112
  and hospital admissions, 115
  and infant addiction, 441
  medical consequences of, 111
  mixtures of, 109
  physical/mental consequences of taking, 40
  physiological/psychological effects of, 110
  and pregnancy, 113-15
    crack babies, 114
    fetal hazards, 113-14
  problems with, 111-16
  snorting vs. smoking free-base, 109
  and women, 113-15
  young people's use of, 40-41
  See also Cocaine
Crack houses, 112-13
Crank laboratories, 94
Crime:
  and alcohol, 213
  and cocaine, 111
Crossroads program, 451-52
Crystal, 93
Cyanocobalamin (vitamin B12), 331-32
Cylert, 398-99

D

Dalmane, 21, 398–99
DARE (Drug Abuse Resistance Education), 415, 448
Darvon, 85, 252–53
Daytop, 258
Decriminalization. *See* Legalization
Delaney Amendment (1958), 13
Deliriants (volatile substances), 10, 174, 185–87
  classification, 185
  history of, 185–86
  physical effects of, 186
  psychological effects of, 186
Demand, defined, 411
Demerol, 29, 85, 398–99
Dependency, 26–33
  and addiction, 440–41
  biological perspectives of, 28
  cocaine, 75, 107–8
  dependency, defined, 26
  dependency pain, 28–32
  genetic factors, 32
  pain, 28–32
    biochemical theory of, 29
    enkephalins and endorphins, 29–32
    sources of, 29
  psychological perspectives of, 26–27
  sociological perspectives of, 27–28
Depo Provera, 355–56
Depressants, 174–91
  alcohol, 4, 7, 16, 21, 32, 84, 174, 192–237
  deliriants (volatile substances), 174, 185–87
  designer drugs, 9, 187–88
  opiates, 10, 29, 85, 174
  sedative-hypnotics, 53–54, 83, 174, 175–77
  tranquilizers, 53–54, 84, 174, 177–85, 398–99
    major, 183–85
    minor, 84, 177–83
Designer drugs, 9, 187–88
  fentanyl, 9, 188
  MDMA (3,4 methylenedioxymetham-phetamine), 187–88
  meperidine, 9, 188
  testing problems, 188
Desipramine, and cocaine treatment programs, 458
Desoxyn, 398–99
Detoxification:
  alcoholics, 228
  opiate addicts, 255–57
Dexedrine (Dextroamphetamine), 82, 91, 92, 398–99
Dextran sulfate, 360–61
Didrex, 398–99
Diet pills, 334
Digestive system, and alcohol, 206–7
Dilaudid, 29, 85, 398–99
Dispensing doctors, 374
Distribution, and absorption, 72
Disulfiram (Antabuse), and alcohol treatment programs, 227
Dolophine. *See* Methadone
Dopamine, 75, 77, 110
  and cocaine, 108
Doriden, 398–99
Dormate, 398–99
Dose-response curve, 72–73
Dose-time curve, 72–73
Dover's powder. *See* Opium

Drug abuse:
  defined, 4
  treatment of, 413, 439–62
    addiction and dependency, 440–41
    admissions, 442
    adolescent treatment programs, 442–44
    adult treatment programs, 445–54
    infant addiction, 441
    intervention, 441
    relapse, 458–59
    See also Drug-education programs
  treatment programs, defined, 442
  trends in, 5–6
Drug Abuse Control Amendments (1965), 391–92
Drug Abuse Response Team (DART), 421–22
Drug-education programs, 412–21
  comprehensive K-12 drug education program, 414–17
  counselors, 417–18
  parents' role, 418–21
  school's role, 412–14
  teachers, 414
Drug Enforcement Agency (DEA), 389
Drug 566, 361
Drug-Free Workplace Act (1988), 57
Drug industry, 376
  brand-name vs. generic drugs, 341, 379
  high cost of prescription drugs, 378–79
  marketing and advertising, 377–78
  profit and production, 377
  research and development, 378
Drug information, summary of, 82–86
Drug interactions, 74
Drug legislation. *See* Consumer and drug legislation
Drug misuse, defined, 4
Drugs:
  and athletics, 46–52
    professional sports, 51–52
    steroids, 47–51
  on campus, 42–44
  in the military, 44–46
  perspective on, 4–10
  potency, 3
  purity, 3
  ranking by addiction level, 33
  sales estimates of, 6–7
  in the workplace:
    drug testing, 55–60
    employee-assistance programs (EAPs), 57
Drug scene, 36–67
  adults, 52–60
  older Americans, 60–68
  youths, 38–52
Drug technology, 10–14
  commercial drugs, 13
  herbal preparations, 14
  illegal drugs, 14
  over-the-counter drugs, 12–13
  prescription drugs, 10–12
  recreational drugs, 13–14
Drug testing, 55–60
Drug use, 16–35
  and children, 38–39
  defined, 4
  dependency states, 26–33
  and infants/toddlers, 38–39
  psychological factors, 17–23

  sociological factors of, 23–25
Drug vigilantes, 386

E

Ecstasy, 9, 187–88
Ego compensation, Adlerian theory of, 27
Elderly drug scene. *See* Older American drug scene
Emphysema, and cigarette smoking, 142
Employee-assistance programs (EAPs), 57
Employee drug use, 59
Employers, and adult treatment programs, 446
Endocrine, and marijuana, 293–94
Endorphins, 29–32, 69–70, 343
Enkephalins, 29–32
Epilepsy, and marijuana, 304
Equanil, 398–99
Eskimos, and alcohol, 212
Estrogen replacement therapy (ERT), 359–60
Estrogen use, and uterine cancer, 350
Exercise, as alternative to drug use, 426–28
Existential view, of drug dependency, 26–27
Expectorants, 326

F

Family, as sociological factor of drug use, 23–24
Fat soluble, defined, 288
Federal Bureau of Narcotics (FBN), 389
Federal Drug Administration (FDA):
  defined, 314, 378
  and drug research and development, 378
  and generic drugs, 381
  New Drug Applications (NDAs), 341–43
  and OTC labels, 316
Fentanyl, 9, 188
Fertility pills, 358–59
  and multiple births, 359
  possible side effects of, 359
  treatment methods, 358
Fetal alcohol effect (FAE), 207–8
Fetal alcohol syndrome (FAS), 207–8, 441
Fibrocystic breast disease, and caffeine (Xanthines), 126
Flashbacks:
  LSD, 273
  marijuana, 302
Fluoxetine hydrochloride. *See* Prozac
Food additives, 13, 362–67
  adverse effects of, 365
  history of, 363–64
  nitrites and nitrates, 365
  NutraSweet, 366–67
  preservatives, 364–65
  sucrose (sugar), 365–66
Food and Drug Administration (FDA):
  drug-related definitions, 4
  and quality control, 2
Food, Drug and Cosmetic Act (1938), 390
Food labels, 334–35
Free-base cocaine, 105–6
Freewheeling junkies, 249

G

Gastric upset, and caffeine (Xanthines), 126
Gastrointestinal bleeding, and salicylates (aspirin), 321

Generic drugs vs. brand-name drugs, 341, 379-81
Genetic damage, from marijuana, 295-96
Genetic factors, drug dependency, 32
Glaucoma, and marijuana, 305
Glue, 21
Glutethimide, 398-99
Grabowski, John, 26
Gray area, 1-4
  individual differences, 2
  legality, 4
  quality control, 2-3
  set, 3-4
  setting, 4
Group structure, as sociological factor of drug use, 24-25

H

Habitual smokers, 149
Hallucinogens, 4, 270-84, 398-99
  defined, 271
  LSD (lysergic acid diethylamide-25), 9, 25, 85, 271-76
  mescaline (peyote), 9, 85, 276-78
  PCP (phencyclidine), 21, 41, 85, 279-82
  psilocybin, 9, 85, 278-79
  psychophysiological effects of, 270
  site of action, 271
Hampton (Va.) Intervention and Prevention Project, 423
Hangover, 205
Harrison Narcotic Act (1914), 102, 254, 387-88
Harvard Alcohol Project, 424-25
Hashish, 288
  See also Marijuana
Health Skills for Life program, 416
Heart disease:
  and aspirin, 320-21
  and caffeine (Xanthines), 121
  and contraceptives, 354-55
  and marijuana, 292-93
  and salicylates (aspirin), 320-21
Herbal preparations, 14
Here's Looking at You program, 416
Heroin, 10, 25, 29, 85, 245-52
  addicts' lifestyles, 248
  and AIDS, 249
  ban of importation of (1924), 388-89
  Cocaine Anonymous (CA), 115
  and crack, 115
  dependency:
    nonphysical dependence, 246
    stages of, 248-49
  freewheeling junkies, 249
  medical uses of, 249-50
  occasional users, 248
  -related deaths, 247-48
  sales estimates of, 6
  stabilized junkies, 249
  street junkies, 249
  treatment, 455-56
    acetorphan, 456
    buprenorphine, 455
    Clonidine and naltrexone, 455
    naltrexone maintenance, 455-56
    withdrawal symptoms, 245-46
HGH hormone, 69
High-risk factors, 19, 21-22
Hindu religion, and ganja (bhang), 20

Homelessness, and alcohol, 213
Homicide, and crack, 112
Hooked, defined, 445
Household chemicals, 13
Huichol Indians (Mexico), and peyote cactus, 20
Hyperactive children:
  alternative treatments for, 99-101
  and Ritalin, 98-99
Hypersensitivity reactions, 74-75
  and antipsychotics, 184
  and salicylates (aspirin), 322
Hyposensitivity, 75
Hypothalamus, 77-79

I

Ibuprofen, 323
Ice (methamphetamine), 8, 25, 95-97
  compared to methamphetamines (speed) and crack, 97
Illegal drugs, 14
  drop in sales of, 6-7
Immune system, and marijuana, 293
Individual differences, 2
Industrial chemicals, 13
Infant addiction, 441
Infertility, and caffeine (Xanthines), 124-25
Infusion curriculum, 415
Ingestion of drugs, 73
Inhalants, 10
Inhalation of drugs, 73
Injection of drugs, 73-74
  intravenous (IV), 73-74
  inunction, 74
Inmate treatment program, 452
Inorganic wastes, 13
Inpatient vs. outpatient treatment programs, 446
Interpersonal relations, as high-risk factor, 19, 22
Intervention, 441
  crisis, and alcoholism, 230-31
  defined, 230
  nutritional, 448-49
  programs, 384-85
Intramuscular (IM) injection of drugs, 74
Intrapsychic functioning, as high-risk factor, 19, 21-22
Intravenous (IV) injection of drugs, 73-74
Inunction, administering drugs by, 74
Ionamin, 398-99

J

Jogging, as alternative to drug use, 427-28
Journal of the American Medical Association, 373

K

Kefauver-Harris Amendments (1962), 390-91
Key Extended Entry Program (KEEP), 452-53
Khantziank, Edward, 26
Kidneys, and alcohol, 207

L

Laxatives, 324-25
  constipation, defined, 250, 324

Leary, Timothy, 21, 273
Legality, drugs, 4
Legalization, 383-85, 401-5
  of heroin, 402-5
  of marijuana, 305-6, 401-2
  of opiates, 402-5
Leritine, 398-99
Liberty Park Village, 258
Librium (chlordiazepoxide), 8, 84, 183, 398-99
Linder v. *United States* (1925), 389
Lithium, 351
  and alcohol treatment programs, 227, 454
  classification, 351
  medical use of, 351
  overdose, 351
  pharmacology of, 351
Liver:
  and alcohol, 205-6
  and caffeine (Xanthines), 125-26
Lovastatin, 362
LSD (lysergic acid diethylamide-25), 9, 25, 85, 271-76, 398-99
  blotter, 274
  defined, 271-72
  flashbacks, 273
  and medical research, 275-76
  microdots, 274
  and mind-control research, 275
  psychophysiological effects of, 272-73
  revival of, 274
  and society, 273-74
  windowpanes, 274
Lung cancer, and cigarette smoking, 142-43
Lung function, and marijuana, 290-92

M

Mainstream smoke, defined, 161
Major tranquilizers (antipsychotics), 183-85
  classification, 183-84
  current use, 184
  defined, 183
  physical effects of, 184-85
Marijuana, 4, 9, 16, 21, 25, 85, 285-310
  and adult drug scene, 55
  economics, 304-5
    marijuana crops, 304-5
    workplace, 304
  hashish, 288
  history of, 285-86
  legalization of, 305-6
    opponents, 306
    proponents, 306
  Marijuana Tax Act (1937), 389
  pharmacological classification of, 288
  physiological effects of, 288-98
    brain, 296-97
    cardiovascular system, 292-93
    endocrine functioning, 293-94
    extent of, 289-90
    genetic damage, 295-96
    immune system, 293
    lung function, 290-92
    memory, 297-98
    psychomotor impairment, 294-95
    tolerance, 290, 298
  popularity of, decrease in, 287
  psychological effects of, 298-302
    adolescents' perceptions, 300

Marijuana (*cont.*)
  aggression, 301
  amotivational syndrome, 302
  family cohesiveness, 301
  flashbacks, 302
  peer influences, 300
  psychopathology, 301–2
  school performance, 300–301
  social conversation, 301
  sales estimates of, 6
  THC (delta-9-tetrahydracannabinol), 292
    defined, 288
  therapeutic/medical uses of, 302–4
    in cancer, 305
    in glaucoma, 305
    medical applications, 305–6
  U.S. consumption of, 286–87
  withdrawal symptoms of, 290
  in the workplace, 56
  world-wide use of, 285–86
  and youth drug scene, 41
Marijuana Tax Act (1937), 389
MDMA (3,4
    methylenedioxymethamphetamine),
    9, 187–88, 398–99
Medial forebrain bundle, 79
Medical Letter on Drugs and Therapeutics, 373
Meditation, as alternative to drug use, 433–35
Medulla, 80
Memory:
  and alcohol, 205
  and marijuana, 297–98
Menopause, and estrogen replacement therapy
    (ERT), 359–60
Mental illness, drugs for, 348–50
  antidepressants, 348–49
  clozapine (Clozaril), 350
  Prozac, 349–50
Meperidine (Demerol), 9, 85, 188
Mescaline (peyote), 9, 85, 276–78, 398–99
  defined, 276
  history of, 276
  and Native American church, 276–77
  psychophysiological effects of, 277–78
Methadone, 10, 250–52
  for cocaine, 456–57
  defined, 250–51
  maintenance programs, 85, 259–65
    interim methadone clinic, 260–61
    possible hazards/side effects of, 261–62
    process, 262–63
    rate of success, 263–64
    social implications of, 265
  overdose of, 252
  physical effects of, 251–52
  withdrawal in infants, 252
Methadrine, 82
Methamphetamines (crank, speed, meth), 8, 25,
    82, 93–97
  adverse effects, 94
  amphetamine psychosis, 93–94
  availability of, 95
  crank laboratories, 94
  crystal, 93
  ice, 8, 25, 95–97
  laboratory wastes, dumping, 95
  price of, 95
  speed freaks, 93
  speed-taking ritual, 93–94
  treatment for, 94

Methaqualone, 21, 398–99
Methylphenidate. *See* Ritalin
Migraine headaches, and salicylates (aspirin),
    322
Military, drugs in, 44–46
Miltown, 84, 398–99
Mind-control research, and LSD, 275
Minerals. *See* Vitamins and minerals
Minorities, and psychological effects of
    smoking, 150–51
Minor tranquilizers, 84, 177–83
  classification, 177
  history of, 178
  Librium (chlordiazepoxide), 8, 84, 183
  physical effects of, 178–79
  Valium (diazepam), 8, 21, 84, 179–83
MKULTRA, 275
Monoamine-oxidase inhibitors (MAOI), 348
Morphine, 29, 85, 243–44
Mothers Against Drunk Drivers (MADD), 234
Mothers' milk, nicotine in, 145
Motor-vehicle accidents, and alcohol, 210–11
Multiple births, and fertility pills, 359
Muscle cramps, and marijuana, 304

N

Naloxone, 30
Naltrexone maintenance, and heroin, 455–56
Narcolepsy, and amphetamines, 92
Narcotic Addict Rehabilitation Act (1966), 392
Narcotic and Drug Research, Inc. (NDRI),
    384–85
Narcotic Drug Control Act (1956), 390
Narcotics. *See* Opiates
Narcotics Anonymous (NA), 444, 447, 459
National Addiction Rehabilitation
    Administration (NARA), 253–54
National Institute on Drug Abuse (NIDA), 251,
    454, 455
National trends, as sociological factor of drug
    use, 25
Native Americans:
  and alcohol, 212
  and peyote cactus, 20
Natural Helpers, 421
Negative-effect smokers, 149
Nembutal, 83, 398–99
  See also Barbiturates
Neonatal deaths, and cigarette smoking, 144–45
Nervous system, 75–77
  and alcohol, 203–5
  central nervous system, 77–81
  neurons, 75–76
  peripheral nervous system, 81–87
Neurons, 75–76
Neurotransmitters, 77
New Drug Applications (NDAs), 341–43
Nicotine, 7–8
  and adult drug scene, 54
  and coffee intake, 147
  and oral contraceptives, 146
  See also Cigarette smoking; Tobacco
Nicotine gum, 152
Nicotine skin patch, 152
Nitrites and nitrates, 365
Noctec, 398–99
Noludar, 398–99
Nonachievement, as high-risk factor, 19, 22
Nonsmokers' rights, 163–64

Nonsynthetic opiates, 242–50
  codeine, 250
  heroin, 10, 25, 85, 245–52
  morphine, 29, 85, 243–44
  opium, 29, 242–43, 398–99
  See also Opiates; Synthetic opiates
Nonvehicle accidents, and alcohol, 212, 213
Norepinephrine, 110
Norplant, 356–57
Nostrums, 317
Numorphan, 398–99
Nursing homes:
  overprescribed medications in, 376
  and Valium (diazepam), 182
NutraSweet, 366–67
Nutritional intervention, 448–49

O

Odyssey House, 258
Older American drug scene, 60–63
  over-the-counter (OTC) drugs, 333
  treatment programs for the elderly, 449
  types of drug use, 61–63
    accidental abuse of drugs, 62
    misuse of drugs, 61–62
    proper use, 61
    purposeful use of dependency-causing
      drugs, 62–63
One Flew Over the Cuckoo's Nest (Kesey), 20
Opiate-receptor mechanisms, identification of,
    29–31
Opiates, 10, 29, 85, 174, 242–69
  and adult drug scene, 55
  decriminalization, 402–5
  detoxification, 255–57
  drug-abuse related legislation, 253–55
  general effects of, 256–57
  maintenance, 403–4
    future of, 405
  methadone maintenance, 259–65
  nonsynthetic, 242–50
  regulation of (1865–1905), 386
  synthetic, 250–53
  therapeutic approaches, 257–59
    personal responsibility/ commitment,
      258–59
    small-group support, 257–58
    therapeutic communities, 258
    young users, 259
  withdrawal, and marijuana, 304
Opium, 29, 242–43, 398–99
Optimil, 398–99
Oral cancer, vitamin A therapy for, 331
Orphan Drug Act, 381–82
Outward Bound, 445
Over-the-counter (OTC) drugs, 12–13, 311–39
  antihistamines, 326–27
  cough relievers (antitussives), 325–26
  defined, 311
  development of, in U.S., 314
  diet pills, 334
  the elderly and, 333
  food labels, 334–35
  labels, 316
  laxatives, 324–25
  nostrums, 317
  prescription vs. nonprescription drugs,
    315–16
  promotion techniques, 313–14

Over-the-counter (OTC) drugs (*cont.*)
  reform, 315
  salicylates (aspirin), 317–23
  self-monitoring/self-care, 312–14
  and television advertising, 12
  vitamins and minerals, 327–23
  See also Prescription drugs

P

Paleospinothalmic pain, 30
Pancreas, and caffeine (Xanthines), 125–26
Paregoric. *See* Opium
Parest, 398–99
Patient compliance, defined, 375
PCP (phencyclidine), 21, 41, 85, 279–82,
  398–99
  defined, 279–80
  forms of, 280
  psychophysiological effects of, 281–82
    hazards, 282
    long-term effects, 282
  and society, 280–81
Peer clusters, 25
Peer-group influence, 421–22
  Drug Abuse Response Team (DART), 421–22
  Natural Helpers, 421
  Student Athletic Summer Institute, 422
Peer-group pressure, as sociological factor of
  drug use, 23–25
Penicillins, 345–47
  effects of, 346
Peptide T, 362
Percodan, 29, 398–99
Peripheral nervous system, 81–87
Periventricular system, 79
Personal habits, as psychological factor of drug
  use, 22–23
Personality, and drug dependency, 26–27
Personality traits, as psychological
  factors of drug use, 21–22
Pethadol. *See* Meperidine (Demerol)
Peyote. *See* Mescaline (peyote)
Peyote ritual, 277
Pharmacist, dispensing by, 374
Pharmacology, 68–88
  anatomy and physiology, 75–87
  consumer safety, 70–75
    allergic reactions, potential for, 74–75
    chemical considered, 70–71
    dosage, 71–73
    drug interactions, 74
    method of administration, 73
    physical dependence, potential for, 75
    receptor mechanisms affected, 71
    tolerance, potential for, 75
  endorphins, 69–70
  hGH hormone, 69
  theories and discoveries, 68–70
Phencyclidine. *See* PCP (phencyclidine)
Phenelzine, and cocaine treatment programs,
  458
Phenmetrazine, 398–99
Phenobarbital. *See* Barbiturates
Phenothiazines, 21
Phenylpropanolamine (PPA), 334
Phoenix House, 458
Physical dependence, potential for, 75
Physician's Desk Reference (PDR), 11, 373
Pituary gland, 77

Placebos, 343–45
  administration/frequency/cost, 344–45
  individual differences, 344
  power of suggestion, 345
  social environment/situational variables, 344
Placydil, 398–99
Plegine, 398–99
Political activism, as alternative to drug use,
  429–30
Polypharmacy, 11, 60
Pondimin, 398–99
Porter Narcotic Farms Bill (1929), 389
Positive-effect smokers, 149
Potency, drugs, 3
Preaddiction, 26–27
Pregnant women:
  and caffeine (Xanthines) use, 123–24
  and crack, 113–15
    crack babies, 114
    fetal hazards, 113–14
  and salicylates (aspirin), 319
  and tobacco, 144–45
    anomalies, 145
    mother's milk, 145
    spontaneous abortion, 144
    stillbirth and neonatal deaths, 144–45
  See also Women
Prehistoric brain. *See* Hypothalamus
Preludin, 398–99
Pre-Sate, 398–99
Prescription drugs, 10–12, 340–71
  accutane, 350–51
  advertisements for, 378
  and AIDS, 360–61
  antibiotics, 345–48
  antidepressants, 348–49
  brand name vs. generic drugs, 341
  cholesterol-lowering agents, 361–62
  clozapine (Clozaril), 350
  contraceptives, 352–55
  estrogen replacement therapy, 359–60
  fertility pills, 358–59
  high cost of, 378–79
  labels, 315–16
  lithium, 351
  mental illness, drugs for, 348–50
  New Drug Applications (NDAs), 341–43
  nonprescription drugs vs., 315–16
  Peptide T, 362
  placebos, 343–45
  Prozac, 349–50
  streptokinase, 361
  See also Over-the-counter (OTC) drugs
Preservatives, 364–65
Prevention, 411–38
  alternatives to drug use, 425–35
  drug-education programs, 412–21
  mass media, 424–25
  peer group influence, 421–22
  school and community cooperation, 422–24
Professional sports, drug use in, 51–52
Prohibition, 388
Project Graduation, 417
Project Impact, 422–23
Prolixin, 21
Propoxyphene hydrochloride (Darvon), 85,
  252–53
Prozac, 349–50
  and alcohol treatment programs, 454
Psilocybin, 9, 85, 278–79, 398–99

defined, 278
  psychophysiological effects of, 278–79
  "shroomers," 279
Psychedelics. *See* Hallucinogens
Psychoanalytic view, of drug dependency,
  26–27
Psychological factors of drug use, 17–23
  altered states, 20–21
  personal habits, 22–23
  personality traits, 21–22
  rebellion and alienation, 21
  recreation and social facilitation, 17–18
  religious and spiritual factors, 20
  sensation seeking and risk taking, 18–19
Psychological perspectives, drug dependency,
  26–27
Psychomotor impairment, from marijuana,
  294–95
Pure Food and Drug Act (1906), 102, 387
Purity, drugs, 3
Pyridoxine (pyridoxal, pyridoxamine, vitamin
  B2), 331

Q

Quaaludes, 83, 398–99
Quality control, 2–3

R

Raphae nuclei, 80
Rational Recovery (RR), 453–54
Rebellion, as psychological factor of drug use,
  21
Receptor sites, 76–77
Recreation, as psychological factor of drug use,
  17–18
Recreational drugs, 13–14
  in grades 4, 5, and 6, 39
Relapse, 458–59
Religion:
  as alternative to drug use, 430–31
  as psychological factor of drug use, 20
Resistance transferring, antibiotics, 347
Responsible drinking, 234–35
Reticular formation, 79–80
Retinol (vitamin A), 330–31
Reye's syndrome, and salicylates (aspirin), 321
Rheumatoid arthritis, and salicylates (aspirin),
  319–20
Risk taking, as psychological factor of drug use,
  18–19
Ritalin, 82, 97–101, 398–99
  dependence, 98
  and hyperactive children, 98–101
  side effects of, 97
  tolerance, 97–98
Robinson v. *California* (1962), 391
RU 486, 357

S

Sacred Heart Adolescent Recovery Program
  (SHARP), 445–46
St. Luke's Adolescent Recovery Unit, 444
Salicylate poisoning, 54
Salicylates (aspirin), 317–23
  acetaminophen, 323
  and adult drug scene, 54–55

Salicylates (*cont.*)
  history of, 317
  ibuprofen, 323
  intoxication from, 318
  as miracle drug, 322
  physical effects of, 317–18
  side effects of, 318–19
  therapeutic effectiveness, 319–21
    heart attacks and strokes, 320–21
    rheumatoid arthritis, 319–20
  toxicology, 321–22
    bleeding tendency, 321
    gastrointestinal bleeding, 321
    hypersensitivity reactions, 322
    migraine headaches, 322
    Reye's syndrome, 321
Sanorex, 398–99
Seattle (Wa.) School Development Project, 423
Seconal, 21, 83
  See also Barbiturates
Sedative-hypnotics, 53–54, 83, 174, 175–77
  and adult drug scene, 53–54
  barbiturates, 54, 83, 175–77
  classification of, 175
  physical effects of, 175
Sedatives, 8–9
Self-help groups, 447–48
Sensation seeking, as psychological factor of
    drug use, 18–19
Serax, 84, 398–99
Serenity Lane Alcohol- and Drug-Treatment
    Program, 449–51
Sernylan, 398–99
Serotonin, 77, 110
Set, 3–4
Setting, 4
Shanghai Conference (1909), 387
"Shroomers," 279
Sidestream smoke, defined, 161
Sinequan, 21
Skeletal muscles, and caffeine (Xanthines), 126
Skillstreaming, 416–17
Smokeless tobacco, 159–61
Snuff dipping, 159–61
Social activism, as alternative to drug use,
    429–30
Social facilitation, as psychological factor of
    drug use, 17–18
Sociological factors of drug use, 23–25
  advertising, 25
  family, 23–24
  group structure, 24–25
  national trends, 25
  peer-group pressure, 23
Sociological perspectives, drug dependency,
    27–28
Somatropin (hGH), 69
Sometimes a Great Notion (Kesey), 20
Somnafec, 398–99
Somnos, 398–99
Sopor, 398–99
Soulbeat I, 423–24
Speed. *See* Methamphetamines
    (crank, speed, meth)
Speed freaks, 93
Speed-taking ritual, 93–94
Spontaneous abortion, and cigarette smoking,
    144
Stabilized junkies, 249
Steroids, 40–41, 47–51

anabolic, 48–50
side effects of abuse, 50
Stillbirth, and cigarette smoking, 144–45
Stimulants, 8, 82, 89–134, 398–99
  amphetamines, 3, 4, 8, 55, 89–97
  caffeine (Xanthines), 7, 54, 116–27
  cocaine, 3, 25, 32, 82, 85, 101–16
  Ritalin, 97–101
Straight program, 444–45
Street junkies, 249
Streptokinase, 361
Streptomycins, 345–46
  effects of, 346
Strokes:
  and salicylates (aspirin), 320–21
  and tobacco, 141
Student Assistance Program (SAP), 417–18
Student Athletic Summer Institute (SASI), 422
Students Against Driving Drunk (SADD), 234
Subcutaneous injection of drugs, 74
Substance-abuse counselors, 417–18
Sucrose (sugar), 365–66
Sudden infant death syndrome (SIDS), and
    cigarette smoking, 144
Suicide:
  and alcohol, 214
  and Valium (diazepam), 183
Superinfections, 347
Suppliers, defined, 411
Symptomatic drinking, 218
Synanon, 258
Synapse, 76
Synergistic, defined, 75
Synergistic response, 75
Synthetic opiates, 250–53
  and acetorphan, 456
  methadone, 250–52
  propoxyphene hydrochloride (Darvon),
    252–53
  See also Nonsynthetic opiates; Opiates

T

Tachycardia, and Ritalin, 97
Talwin, 85
Tarahumara Indians (Mexico), and peyote
    cactus, 20
Tardive dyskinesia, 184
Testosterone level:
  and alcohol, 208–9
  and marijuana, 294
Tetracyclines, 345–46
  effects of, 346
Tetrahydraisoquardrelone (THIQ), 215
Thalidomide, 2
THC (delta-9-tetrahydracannabinol), 288, 292
Therapeutic recreation, 448
Thiamine (vitamin B$_1$), 331
Timing out, 427
Tobacco, 4, 7–8, 135–73
  addicted smokers, 149
  and adult drug scene, 54
  and alcohol, 147
  chemistry, 136–37
  and children, 39, 41
    selling to, 164–65
  chronic disease, 140–43
    cancer, 142–43
    cardiovascular disease, 140–41
    lung cancer, 142–43

respiratory disease, 141–42
strokes, 141
cigar smoking, 156–59
clove cigarettes as substitute for, 161
and coffee intake, 147
diversification in industry, 167
exporting, 165–67
habitual smokers, 149
history of, 136
and medication effectiveness, 146
negative-effect smokers, 149
and oral contraceptives, 146
and periodontal disease, 146
physiological effects of, 138–40
  gases, 139–40
pipe smoking, 156–59
positive-effect smokers, 149
psychological effects of, 147–51
  adolescents, 151
  advertising, 148–49
  minorities, 150–51
  reasons for smoking/not smoking, 147–48
  smoking habit, 147
  types of smokers, 149
  women, 149–50
risks of smoking/benefits of quitting (table),
    157–58
side effects, 143–47
  appetite reduction, 143–44
  metabolism, 143
  physical performance, 145
  pregnancy/fetal nutrition, 144–45
  sexual activity, 145–46
smoke, effects on nonsmokers, 161–63
smokeless tobacco, 159–61
Surgeon General's report (1979), 138
and vitamins, 147
Tocopherols (vitamin E), 332–33
Tolerance:
  marijuana, 290, 298
  potential for, 75
Tranquilizers, 53–54, 84, 174, 177–85, 398–99
  and adult drug scene, 53–54
  and alcohol treatment programs, 227
  major, 183–85
  minor, 84, 177–83
Transcendental meditation (TM), as alternative
    to drug use, 433
Tranxene, 398–99
Tricyclics, 348
Tuinal, 83
  See also Barbiturates
Tumors, and marijuana, 304
Twelve-step programs, 447–48

U

Uncontrolled emotions, as high-risk factor, 19,
    21
Unconventionality, as high-risk factor, 19, 21
U.S. servicemen in Vietnam, drug use by, 44–45
Uterine cancer, and estrogen use, 350

V

Valium (diazepam), 8, 21, 84, 179–83, 398–99
  dependence/withdrawal, 181–82
  and drugged drivers, 182–83
  history of, 179–80

Valium (*cont.*)
  and nursing home use, 182
  physical effects of, 180–81
    cognitive processes, 181
    long-term memory loss, 181
    visual-motor reaction time, 180–81
  and suicide attempts, 183
  synergism, 181
Valmid, 398–99
Ventrical fibrillation, and cocaine, 104
Victimless crimes, 383
Vietnam, drug use in, 43
Violence. *See* Aggression
Vitamins and minerals, 327–23
  excessive, adverse effects, 329
  megavitamin intake, 333
  specific use, 330
  U.S. recommended allowances, 328
  vitamin A (retinol), 330–31
  vitamin B_1 (thiamine), 331
  vitamin B_2 (pyridoxine, pyridoxal, pyridoxamine), 331

vitamin B_{12} (cyanocobalamin), 331–32
vitamin C (ascorbic acid), 332
vitamin D (calciferol), 332
vitamin E (tocopherols), 332–33
Volatile substances. *See* Deliriants (volatile substances)
Voranil, 398–99

W

War on drugs, 385–86, 411
  in American companies, 56–57
Wilderness experiences, as alternatives to drug use, 428–29
Women:
  and alcohol, 209
  and alcoholism, 225–26
  and crack, 113–15
  and drug interactions, 74
  and marijuana, 294
  psychological effects of smoking, 149–50
  See also Pregnant women

Work, as alternative to drug use, 429

X

Xanthines. *See* Caffeine (Xanthines)
XTC. *See* MDMA (3,4 methylenedioxy-methamphetamine)

Y

Youth drug scene, 38–52
  background, 38–44
  drugs and athletics, 46–52
  drugs on campus, 42–44
  drugs in the military, 44–46

Z

Zidovudine. *See* AZT (azidiothymidine/zidovudine)
Zinberg, Norman E., 25

Customer Support Information

The Almanac of American Employers 2009

Please register your book immediately...

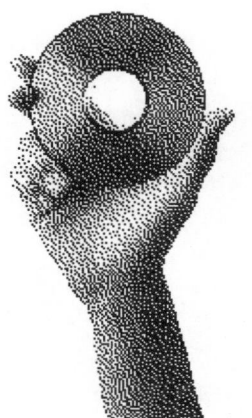

if you did not purchase it directly from Plunkett Research, Ltd. This will enable us to fulfill your replacement request if you have a damaged product, or your requests for assistance. Also it will enable us to notify you of future editions, so that you may purchase them from the source of your choice.

If you are an actual, original purchaser but did not receive a FREE CD-ROM version with your book...*

you may request it by returning this form.

_____ YES, please register me as a purchaser of the book.
I did not buy it directly from Plunkett Research, Ltd.

_____ YES, please send me a free CD-ROM version of the book.
I am an actual purchaser, but I did not receive one with my book. (Proof of purchase may be required.)

Customer Name _____

Title_____

Organization _____

Address _____

City_____State_____Zip_____

Country (if other than USA) _____

Phone_____Fax _____

E-mail _____

Mail or Fax to: **Plunkett Research, Ltd.**
Attn: FREE CD-ROM and/or Registration
P.O. Drawer 541737, Houston, TX 77254-1737 USA
713.932.0000 · Fax 713.932.7080 · www.plunkettresearch.com

* Purchasers of used books are not eligible to register. Use of CD-ROMs is subject to the terms of their end user license agreements.

THE ALMANAC OF AMERICAN EMPLOYERS 2009

The Only Guide to America's Hottest, Fastest-Growing Major Corporations

Jack W. Plunkett

Published by:
Plunkett Research, Ltd., Houston, Texas
www.plunkettresearch.com

THE ALMANAC OF AMERICAN EMPLOYERS 2009

Editor and Publisher:
Jack W. Plunkett

Executive Editor and Database Manager:
Martha Burgher Plunkett

Senior Editors and Researchers:
Brandon Brison
Addie K. FryeWeaver
Christie Manck
John Peterson

Editors, Researchers and Assistants:
Michelle Dotter
Austin Hansell
Brannon Larson
Nolan Merchan
Kathi Mestousis
Lindsey Meyn
Mandy Moench
Holly Scarpinato
Jana Sharooni
Michael Sheehan
Kyle Wark
Suzanne Zarosky

Information Technology Manager:
Wenping Guo

E-Commerce Managers:
Mark Cassells
Heather M. Cook
Emily Hurley
Lynne Zarosky

Cover Design:
Kim Paxson, Just Graphics
Junction, TX

Special Thanks to:
U.S. Department of Labor
Bureau of Labor Statistics
U.S. Department of Commerce
*Bureau of Economic Analysis, National Technical
Information Service*

Plunkett Research, Ltd.
P. O. Drawer 541737, Houston, Texas 77254 USA
Phone: 713.932.0000   Fax: 713.932.7080
www.plunkettresearch.com

Published by:
Plunkett Research, Ltd.
P. O. Drawer 541737
Houston, Texas 77254-1737

Phone: 713.932.0000
Fax: 713.932.7080
Internet: www.plunkettresearch.com

ISBN10 # 1-59392-143-8
ISBN13 # 978-1-59392-143-9

Disclaimer of liability
for use and results of use:

THE ALMANAC OF AMERICAN EMPLOYERS 2009

CONTENTS

Introduction   1
How To Use This Book   3
Chapter 1: **Major Trends Affecting Job Seekers**   7
  1) U.S. Job Market Overview   7
  2) Downsizing, Consolidation through Mergers, Layoffs and Acquisitions by Private Equity   9
  3) Continued Growth in Outsourcing, Including Supply Chain and Logistics Services   10
  4) Millions Working as Temps   11
  5) Rapid Growth in Offshoring and the Globalization of Business   12
  6) Senior Citizens Are a Hot Commodity with Many Employers—Baby Boomers Are Retiring   12
  7) Employment Sectors that Will Offer an Above-Average Number of Job Opportunities in 2009   13
Chapter 2: Statistics   15
  U.S. Employment Overview: 2008   16
  U.S. Civilian Labor Force: 1997-2008   17
  Number of People Employed, U.S.: 2007   18
  Unemployed Jobseekers by Sex, Reason for Unemployment & Active Job Search Methods Used: 2007   19
  U.S. Labor Force Ages 16 to 24 Years Old by School Enrollment, Educational Attainment, Sex, Race
    & Ethnicity: October 2007   20
  Top 20 U.S. Occupations by Numerical Change in Job Growth: 2006-2016   21
  Top 20 U.S. Occupations Percent Change in Job Growth: 2006-2016   22
  Jobs with the Largest Expected Employment Increases, U.S.: 2006-2016   23
  Jobs with the Largest Expected Employment Decreases, U.S.: 2006-2016   24
  Mean Hourly Earnings & Weekly Hours, Private Industry & State & Local Government: 2007   25
  Percent of U.S. Workers with Access to Retirement & Healthcare Benefits, Private Industry: 2007   26
  Percent of U.S. Private Industry Employers Offering Retirement & Healthcare Benefits: 2007   27
Chapter 3: Research: 7 Keys for Job Seekers   29
  1) Financial Stability   29
  2) Growth Plans   29
  3) Research & Development Programs   29
  4) Product Launch & Production   29
  5) Marketing & Distribution Methods   29
  6) Employee Benefits   29
  7) Quality of Work Factors   30
  Other Considerations   30
Chapter 4: Important Contacts for Job Seekers   37
  Addresses, Telephone Numbers and Internet Sites
Chapter 5: THE AMERICAN EMPLOYERS 500:
Who They Are and How They Were Chosen   67
  20 Largest Employers of the AMERICAN EMPLOYERS 500, By Number of Employees   69
  20 Largest Employers of the AMERICAN EMPLOYERS 500, By Revenues   70
  20 Largest Employers of the AMERICAN EMPLOYERS 500, By Profits   71
  Industry List, With Codes   72
  Index of Rankings Within Industry Groups   75
    (The AMERICAN EMPLOYERS 500 grouped by industry and ranked for sales and profits)
Continued on the next page

Continued from the previous page

Alphabetical Index   **90**
Index of Headquarters Location by U.S. State   **93**
Index by Regions of the U.S. Where the Firms Have Locations   **97**
Index of Firms with Operations Outside the U.S.   **109**
Individual Data Profiles on each of THE AMERICAN EMPLOYERS 500   **113**
<u>Additional Indexes</u>
Index of Firms Noted as Hot Spots for Advancement for Women & Minorities   **624**
Index of Subsidiaries, Brand Names and Selected Affiliations   **627**
Index by Companies for Specific Types of Job Seekers   **654**
   Information Systems   **654**
   Liberal Arts   **663**
   Management   **673**
   Professionals   **687**
   Sales/Marketing   **703**
   Technical/Scientific   **714**

INTRODUCTION

THE ALMANAC OF AMERICAN EMPLOYERS, 2009 is an easy-to-use solution to what would otherwise be a complicated problem: How can you tell, among all of America's giant companies, which firms are most likely to be hiring? Among those firms, which are the best to work for? No other source provides this book's easy-to-understand comparisons of growth, treatment of employees, salaries, benefits, pension plans, profit sharing and many other items of great importance to job seekers.

Especially helpful is the way in which THE ALMANAC OF AMERICAN EMPLOYERS enables readers with no business background to readily compare the growth potential and benefit plans of large employers. You'll see the mid-term financial record of each firm, along with the impact of earnings, sales and growth plans on each company's potential to provide employment opportunities.

Information is presented in a way that addresses the differing interests of individual employees. You'll find separate listings for dozens of categories of data that you may want to consider. While this book is aimed primarily at job seekers, it will also be of tremendous value to researchers, marketing executives and personnel professionals. THE ALMANAC OF AMERICAN EMPLOYERS is the premier guide to the most successful employers in the nation, their policies and their performance.

THE ALMANAC OF AMERICAN EMPLOYERS is your opportunity to gain valuable knowledge in a matter of minutes. Five hundred of the biggest, most successful corporate employers in America are analyzed in this book. Tens of thousands of pieces of information, gathered from a wide variety of sources, have been researched for these corporations and are presented here in a form that can be easily understood by job seekers of all types.

Thanks to THE ALMANAC OF AMERICAN EMPLOYERS' exclusive data system, potentially confusing considerations have been reduced to simple groups of focused data. By scanning the data groups and the long list of unique indexes, you can find the best employer to fit your personal needs.

The AMERICAN EMPLOYERS 500 are among the best major growth companies to work for in America. Which companies offer the best benefits, are the biggest employers or earn the most profits? Where are these companies operating? All of these things and more are made easy for the reader to determine.

Thousands of observations are made that will be of great interest to prospective employees. For many of the firms, you'll find comments about such items as plans for growth, increases or decreases in the number of employees and charitable programs. You'll also find notes about corporate culture and special programs for the convenience of employees, such as health and recreation facilities, on-site child care, job training or career paths. Finally, you'll find basic information on each company, including the home office address and telephone number; regional, national and international locations; a description of the business; and a list of selected subsidiaries and trade names. In addition, you will find fax numbers and Internet addresses.

Whether you are currently employed by one of these corporate giants or are considering applying for a job with one, you will be able to see how each company compares with the others, even if you don't have the slightest understanding of accounting, finance or employee benefits.

Whatever your purpose for researching corporate employers, you'll find this book to be an indispensable guide. Nonetheless, as is true with all resources, this volume has limitations that the reader should be aware of:

- Financial data and other corporate information can change quickly. A book of this type can be no more current than the data that was available as of the time of editing. Consequently, the financial picture, management and ownership of the firm(s) you are studying may have changed since the date of this book. For example, this almanac includes the most up-to-date sales figures and profits available to the editors as of mid-2008 That means that we have typically used corporate financial data as of the end of 2007

- Corporate mergers, changes in corporate financial ratings or stability, acquisitions and downsizing are occurring at a very rapid rate. Such events may have created significant change, subsequent to the publishing of this book, within a company you are studying.

- Some of the companies in THE AMERICAN EMPLOYERS 500 are so large in scope and in variety of business endeavors conducted within a parent organization that we have been unable to completely list all subsidiaries, affiliations, divisions and activities within a firm's corporate structure.

- This volume is intended to be a general guide to major employers in numerous industries. That means that researchers should look to this book

for an overview and, when conducting in-depth research, should contact the specific corporations and related industry associations in question for the very latest changes and data. Where possible, we have listed contact information, telephone numbers and Internet addresses for pertinent companies, government agencies and industry associations so that the reader may get further details without unnecessary delay.

- We have used exhaustive efforts to locate and fairly present accurate and complete data. However, when using this book or any other source for business and industry information, the reader should use caution and due diligence by conducting further research where it seems appropriate. We wish you success in your endeavors, and we trust that your experience with this book will be both satisfactory and productive.

- To obtain the best results and to best understand the fields in the company profiles, you should first read the chapter titled "How to Use This Book."

Good luck in your job search. Be patient, do your research and use this book as an important start in the right direction.

Jack W. Plunkett
Houston, Texas
September 2008

HOW TO USE THIS BOOK

Dozens of excellent books already exist to help you choose a career, write a resume, apply for a job and so on. That is not the purpose of THE ALMANAC OF AMERICAN EMPLOYERS. Instead, this book's job is to help you sort through America's giant corporate employers to determine which may be the best for you, or to see how your current employer compares to others. Whether you are entering the job market and looking for your first position, or you are thinking about switching companies in mid-career to find more promising vistas, this book will be a valuable guide.

The two primary sections of the book are devoted first to general information for job seekers (trends analysis and advice on conducting employer research, along with resources, statistics and contacts) and then to the "Individual Data Listings" for THE AMERICAN EMPLOYERS 500. If time permits, you should begin your research in the front chapters of this book. Also, you will find lengthy indexes in Chapter 5 and in the back of the book.

GENERAL INFORMATION FOR JOB SEEKERS

Chapter 1: Major Trends Affecting Job Seekers.
This chapter presents an encapsulated view of the major trends in business and the economy that are creating rapid changes in the employment picture at major corporations.

Chapter 2: Statistics.
This chapter presents in-depth statistics on employment by education level, sex, race, unemployment rates, fastest-growing occupations and more.

Chapter 3: Research–7 Keys for Job Seekers.
This chapter provides a definitive list of items that job seekers should look for when conducting research into major corporate employers.

Chapter 4: Important Contacts for Job Seekers.
This chapter covers contacts for important government agencies, organizations, job banks, reference sources and more. Included are Internet sites and contact addresses for a wide variety of job search uses.

THE AMERICAN EMPLOYERS 500

Chapter 5: THE AMERICAN EMPLOYERS 500: Who They Are and How They Were Chosen.
The companies compared in this book were chosen from nearly all industries, on a nationwide basis. They were individually chosen from the largest U.S. employers, based on selected types of business and industry sectors. For a complete description, see Chapter 5.

Individual Data Listings:
Look at one of the companies in THE AMERICAN EMPLOYERS 500's Individual Data Listings. You'll find the following information fields:

Company Name:

The company profiles are in alphabetical order by company name. If you don't find the company you are seeking, it may be a subsidiary or division of one of the firms covered in this book. Try looking it up in the Index by Subsidiaries, Brand Names and Selected Affiliations in the back of the book.

Ranks:

Industry Group Code: An NAIC code used to group companies within like segments. (See Chapter 5 for a list of codes.)

Ranks Within This Company's Industry Group: Ranks, within this firm's segment only, for annual sales and annual profits, with 1 being the highest rank.

Suggested Career Paths:

A grid arranged into six major career categories and several sub-categories. A "Y" indicates that the firm is suggested for certain types of employees, by job discipline.

Types of Business:

A listing of the primary types of business specialties conducted by the firm.

Brands/Divisions/Affiliations:

Major brand names, operating divisions or subsidiaries of the firm, as well as major corporate affiliations—such as another firm that owns a significant portion of the company's stock. A complete Index by Subsidiaries, Brand Names and Selected Affiliations is in the back of the book.

Contacts:

The names and titles up to 27 top officers of the company are listed, including human resources contacts.

Address:

The firm's full headquarters address, the headquarters telephone, plus toll-free and fax numbers where available. Also provided is the Internet site address.

Financials:

Annual Sales (2007 or the latest fiscal year available to the editors, plus up to four previous years): These are stated in thousands of dollars (add three zeros if you want the full number). This figure represents consolidated worldwide sales from all operations. 2007 figures may be estimates.

Annual Profits (2007 or the latest fiscal year available to the editors, plus up to four previous years): These are stated in thousands of dollars (add three zeros if you want the full number). This figure represents consolidated, after-tax net profit from all operations. 2007 figures may be estimates.

Stock Ticker, International Exchange, Parent Company: When available, the unique stock market symbol used to identify this firm's common stock for trading and tracking purposes is indicated. Where appropriate, this field may contain "private" or "subsidiary" rather than a ticker symbol. If the firm is a subsidiary, its parent company is listed.

Total Number of Employees: The approximate total number of employees, worldwide, as of the end of 2007 (or the latest data available to the editors).

Apparent Salaries/Benefits:

(The following descriptions generally apply to U.S. employers only.)

A "Y" in appropriate fields indicates "Yes."

Due to wide variations in the manner in which corporations report benefits to the U.S. Government's regulatory bodies, not all plans will have been uncovered or correctly evaluated during our effort to research this data. Also, the availability to employees of such plans will vary according to the qualifications that employees must meet to become eligible. For example, some benefit plans may be available only to salaried workers—others only to employees who work more than 1,000 hours yearly. Benefits that are available to employees of the main or parent company may not be available to employees of the subsidiaries. In addition, employers frequently alter the nature and terms of plans offered.

NOTE: Generally, employees covered by wealth-building benefit plans do not *fully* own ("vest in") funds contributed on their behalf by the employer until as many as five years of service with that employer have passed. All pension plans are voluntary—that is, employers are not obligated to offer pensions.

Pension Plan: The firm offers a pension plan to qualified employees. In this case, in order for a "Y" to appear, the editors believe that the employer offers a defined benefit or cash balance pension plan (see discussions below). The type and generosity of these plans vary widely from firm to firm. Caution: Some employers refer to plans as "pension" or "retirement" plans when they are actually 401(k) savings plans that require a contribution by the employee.

- Defined Benefit Pension Plans: Pension plans that do not require a contribution from the employee are infrequently offered. However, a few companies, particularly larger employers in high-profit-margin industries, offer defined benefit pension plans where the employee is guaranteed to receive a set pension benefit upon retirement. The amount of the benefit is determined by the years of service with the company and the employee's salary during the later years of employment. The longer a person works for the employer, the higher the retirement benefit. These defined benefit plans are funded entirely by the employer. The benefits, up to a reasonable limit, are guaranteed by the Federal Government's Pension Benefit Guaranty Corporation. These plans are not portable—if you leave the company, you cannot transfer your benefits into a different plan. Instead, upon retirement you will receive the benefits that vested during your service with the company. If your employer offers a pension plan, it must give you a summary plan description within 90 days of the date you join the plan. You can also request a summary annual report of the plan, and once every 12 months you may request an individual benefit statement accounting of your interest in the plan.

- Defined Contribution Plans: These are quite different. They do not guarantee a certain amount of pension benefit. Instead, they set out circumstances under which the employer will make a contribution to a plan on your behalf. The most common example is the 401(k) savings plan. Pension benefits are not guaranteed under these plans.

- Cash Balance Pension Plans: These plans were recently invented. These are hybrid plans—part defined benefit and part defined contribution. Many employers have converted their older defined benefit plans into cash balance plans. The employer makes deposits (or credits a given amount of money) on the employee's behalf, usually based on a percentage of pay. Employee accounts grow based on a predetermined interest benchmark, such as the interest rate on Treasury Bonds. There are some advantages to these plans, particularly for younger workers: a) The benefits, up to a reasonable limit, are guaranteed by the Pension Benefit Guaranty Corporation. b) Benefits are portable—they can be moved to another plan when the employee changes companies. c) Younger workers and those who spend a shorter number of years with an employer may receive higher benefits than they would under a traditional defined benefit plan.

ESOP Stock Plan (Employees' Stock Ownership Plan): This type of plan is in wide use. Typically, the plan borrows money from a bank and uses those funds to purchase a large block of the corporation's stock. The corporation makes contributions to the plan over a period of time, and the stock purchase loan is eventually paid off. The value of the plan grows significantly as long as the market price of the stock holds up. Qualified employees are allocated a share of the plan based on their length of service and their level of salary. Under federal regulations, participants in ESOPs are allowed to diversify their account holdings in set percentages that rise as the employee ages and gains years of service with the company. In this manner, not all of the employee's assets are tied up in the employer's stock.

Savings Plan, 401(k): Under this type of plan, employees make a tax-deferred deposit into an account. In the best plans, the company makes annual matching donations to the employees' accounts, typically in some proportion to deposits made by the employees themselves. A good plan will match one-half of employee deposits of up to 6% of wages. For example, an employee earning $30,000 yearly might deposit $1,800 (6%) into the plan. The company will match one-half of the employee's deposit, or $900. The plan grows on a tax-deferred basis, similar to an IRA. A very generous plan will match 100% of employee deposits. However, some plans do not call for the employer to make a matching deposit at all. Other plans call for a matching contribution to be made at the discretion of the firm's board of directors. Actual terms of these plans vary widely from firm to firm. Generally, these savings plans allow employees to deposit as much as 15% of salary into the plan on a tax-deferred basis. However, the portion that the company uses to calculate its matching deposit is generally limited to a maximum of 6%. Employees should take care to diversify the holdings in their 401(k) accounts, and most people should seek professional guidance or investment management for their accounts.

Stock Purchase Plan: Qualified employees may purchase the company's common stock at a price below its market value under a specific plan. Typically, the employee is limited to investing a small percentage of wages in this plan. The discount may range from 5 to 15%. Some of these plans allow for deposits to be made through regular monthly payroll deductions. However, new accounting rules for corporations, along with other factors, are leading many companies to curtail these plans—dropping the discount allowed, cutting the maximum yearly stock purchase or otherwise making the plans less generous or appealing.

Profit Sharing: Qualified employees are awarded an annual amount equal to some portion of a company's profits. In a very generous plan, the pool of money awarded to employees would be 15% of profits. Typically, this money is deposited into a long-term retirement account. Caution: Some employers refer to plans as "profit sharing" when they are actually 401(k) savings plans. True profit sharing plans are rarely offered.

Highest Executive Salary: The highest executive salary paid, typically a 2007 amount (or the latest year available to the editors) and typically paid to the Chief Executive Officer.

Highest Executive Bonus: The apparent bonus, if any, paid to the above person.

Second Highest Executive Salary: The next-highest executive salary paid, typically a 2007 amount (or the latest year available to the editors) and typically paid to the President or Chief Operating Officer.

Second Highest Executive Bonus: The apparent bonus, if any, paid to the above person.

Other Thoughts:

Apparent Women Officers or Directors: It is difficult to obtain this information on an exact basis, and employers generally do not disclose the data in a public way. However, we have indicated what our best efforts reveal to be the apparent number of women who either are in the posts of corporate officers or sit on the board of directors. There is a wide variance from company to company.

Hot Spot for Advancement for Women/Minorities: A "Y" in appropriate fields indicates "Yes." These are firms that appear either to have posted a substantial number of women and/or minorities to high posts or that appear to have a good record of going out of their way to recruit, train, promote and retain women or minorities. (See the Index of Hot Spots For Women and Minorities in the back of the book.) This information may change frequently and can be difficult to obtain and verify. Consequently, the reader should use caution and conduct further investigation where appropriate.

Growth Plans/ Special Features:

Listed here are observations regarding the firm's strategy, hiring plans, plans for growth and product development, along with general information regarding a company's business and prospects.

Locations:

A "Y" in the appropriate field indicates "Yes."

Primary locations outside of the headquarters, categorized by regions of the United States and by international locations. A complete index by locations is also in the front of this chapter.

Chapter 1

MAJOR TRENDS AFFECTING JOB SEEKERS

Major trends sweeping through business and the economy that affect job seekers of all types:
1) U.S. Job Market Overview
2) Downsizing, Consolidation through Mergers, Layoffs and Acquisitions by Private Equity
3) Continued Growth in Outsourcing, Including Supply Chain and Logistics Services
4) Millions Working as Temps
5) Rapid Growth in Offshoring and the Globalization of Business
6) Senior Citizens Are a Hot Commodity with Many Employers—Baby Boomers Are Retiring
7) Employment Sectors that Will Offer an Above-Average Number of Job Opportunities in 2009:
- Biotechnology, Including Agricultural Biotechnology
- Coal Producers
- Computer Products—Selected Computer, Server, Storage and Accessories Makers, as well as Wireless Network Makers and Distributors
- Consulting—Selected Fields where Consultants May Be Able to Effect Cost-Savings for Clients
- Consumer Products Manufacturers
- Cosmetics Manufacturers
- Data Processing Services Providers
- Defense Contractors
- Education
- Elder Care, Home Health Care, Nursing Homes and Assisted Living Communities
- Energy Conservation Products and Services
- Entertainment, Including Electronic Games
- Guard Services, Investigation and Surveillance
- Health Care Services, Including Managed Care
- Health Foods, Organic Foods, Enhanced Foods
- Health Products

- Health Technology, Including Computerized Patient Records
- Insurance Providers
- Internet Access
- Logistics, Distribution and Supply Chain Services
- Nanotechnology and MEMS
- Oil and Gas Exploration and Production
- Oil Field Services
- Online Search Services with Advertising Revenues
- Online-based Business and Consumer Services
- Outsourcing
- Pharmaceuticals—Generics
- Radio Frequency ID Tags (RFID)
- Renewable Energy, Especially Solar and Wind Power
- Restaurants
- Retailing—Basic, Including Drugstores and Selected Specialty Stores
- Retailing—Catalogs and Other Non-Store Outlets
- Retailing—Discount and Warehouse Clubs
- Wireless and Cellular Communications, including WiMax

1) U.S. Job Market Overview

Job seekers in 2009 will find the toughest hiring climate since 2002, when the economy was suffering broadly due to 9/11 and the end of the dotcom boom. Many types of employers are restructuring and downsizing thanks to the deep financial crisis of 2007-2008. Job seekers who want good positions will be forced to be better prepared and to do better research than in the boom years of the recent past. They will also have to work harder to find a good job.

The general outlook is that 2009's job market will be slow. Employers will be very cautious about hiring new people or investing in new facilities. There will be large numbers of layoffs.

In the 2007 edition of this guide, we warned of "a slowing housing market that may become very soft in 2007." Unfortunately, we were right. Job seekers in 2008 felt the effect. Job seekers in 2009 should be prepared for the fact that nearly all industry sectors will suffer some ill effects from economic and financial market problems that originated when the housing bubble finally popped in mid-2007 and the financial meltdown accelerated in 2008.

The good news is that a select set of employers and growth companies will offer good job opportunities during 2009. Meanwhile, America's unemployment rate grew steadily through 2008, and unemployment will remain high in 2009, relative to recent years.

In this period of challenges and opportunities, some companies will enjoy booming business. For example, it's a terrific time to be in the business of oil field services. Many sectors such as solar energy, education and health care are booming. Today's high price of gasoline will further boost many firms that sell goods and services online, offering PC-based alternatives to a trip in the car. Other employers will hire only limited numbers of employees, while some will continue to downsize due to a variety of factors. For example, the automotive sector will remain very slow.

However, some types of manufacturing may continue to get a boost from the relatively low value of the U.S. dollar. In fact, savvy job seekers will be alert to changes in the value of the dollar. Through mid-2008, many U.S.-based manufacturers were enjoying good growth in sales to overseas customers thanks to the low value of the dollar relative to foreign currencies.

Most firms that specialize in manufacturing or selling luxury items and discretionary items will find business to be slow.

Many companies will continue to wrestle with challenges such as intense competition and high energy costs. Americans who find themselves in the market for a job will need to understand the changes surging through the economy in order to determine which companies to pursue and which to avoid. The U.S. employment market is evolving quickly, and job seekers must be both knowledgeable and nimble in order to position themselves to find promising careers.

Job seekers in 2009 will continue to hear a lot of conflicting and sometimes confusing information about the state of the job market and the state of the economy overall. In order to create a robust job market, corporate investment, profits, productivity and revenues must align themselves correctly. Fortunately, many of these economic indicators were positive during the 2004 to mid-2007 period, and millions of new American jobs were created. As 2007 was winding down, the residential real estate crash, higher financing costs and difficult corporate credit markets were combining to restrain the economy and put a damper on the creation of new jobs. Unfortunately, 2008 saw these problems begin to spread throughout most U.S. business sectors and into the global economy as well.

During 2009, chief executives will continue to find themselves under intense pressure to maintain profitability while keeping their staffs and investment needs lean. The uncertainty created by the financial crisis and high energy costs will make corporate executives cautious.

New grads may find it extremely difficult to land their dream jobs. Nonetheless, there will still be great opportunities for those who are diligent in seeking good employers in stronger business sectors.

Many people who would prefer to be hired as permanent employees will find work as temps instead. Other employees will find that their jobs have been eliminated because work has been outsourced to another firm.

Economic Factors Affecting the Job Market

Business Productivity: Productivity has been rising at desirable rates in recent years. That is, more business can be produced—whether it is goods or services—by utilizing fewer workers than before. This will be extremely beneficial to the U.S. economy in the long run, but it can hurt the job market over the short term. Productivity is boosted by new technologies, improved management methods and other factors. It can also receive a quick boost from restrained corporate hiring. If rising productivity occurs along with rapidly rising sales and profits, then the job market will improve.

Corporate Sales: For 2009, many sectors, particularly those directly affected by housing and financial markets, will find revenue growth difficult to come by. This will make many employers much less likely to hire new people, and it will lead to layoffs at some firms.

Corporate Profits: When profits increase sharply, companies are inclined to increase business investment and hiring. Fortunately, 2004 through 2006 saw steady growth in corporate profits as the economy rebounded. As a result, large numbers of new jobs were created during that period, and the national unemployment rate was extremely low through mid 2007. Profitability took a downturn in 2008, and profits will be disappointing for many business sectors in 2009. The jobs market will suffer as a result.

The employment market during most of the 1990s was exceptionally strong. In April 2000, the unemployment rate dropped to 3.9%, a 30-year record low, and 24 million new jobs had been created in the U.S. during the then nine-year-long economic boom. (Like all boom times, the boom of the '90s finally came to a close; likewise the unprecedented job market and stock market wound down as well.)

By late 2001, as the tech boom tapered off, the national unemployment in America rate shot up to 6%, representing just under 9 million people seeking jobs.

The unemployment rate in August 2007 was only 4.6%. By August 2008, the unemployment rate shot up to

6.1%, and could easily go higher in 2009. To put this unemployment level in hard numbers, the U.S. civilian labor force was 155.3 million in August 2008 (up from 153.4 million a year earlier). The number of people considered "unemployed" was 9.4 million, up from 7.0 million a year earlier.

Meanwhile, America's 78 million Baby Boomers are hoping to retire soon and leave the job market—this will make prospects more promising for younger workers. However, this trend will be tempered to some extent by the weak financial markets of late 2008. Many people over the age of 60 who want to retire will be reluctant (or unable) to do so because the value of their investments in real estate, stocks, bonds and/or funds is down considerably, and they have lost confidence in financial markets at the same time that they lost retirement dollars. Some would-be retirees will be working later into life than they had planned.

In order to compete effectively in today's job market, one of the most important things you can do is arm yourself with knowledge. It is vital for the knowledgeable job seeker to use the best reference tools possible in order to seek out employers that offer a reasonable balance of financial stability, coupled with opportunities for advancement and monetary incentives. Excellent job opportunities exist if you know where to look. Many of America's most successful firms currently need multitudes of new employees.

For example, the health care sector continues to create large numbers of job openings yearly. There is a critical shortage of nurses and other health care specialists. Leading companies in biotechnology, renewable energy, accounting, online services and education will greatly expand their businesses over the mid term. Thousands of additional companies, in technical and non-technical sectors, will need large numbers of new hires. In particular, companies that offer products or services that save time and/or money will prosper—for example, many types of discount retailers, along with companies that offer services that help businesses operate more efficiently. Meanwhile, large companies that are not increasing their overall numbers of employees will be hiring on a regular basis due to normal attrition—that is, the loss of employees due to retirement, relocation or other personal circumstances. For example, a company the size of Walgreen's typically needs to hire tens of thousands of workers yearly due to normal attrition.

2) Downsizing, Consolidation through Mergers, Layoffs and Acquisitions by Private Equity

Mergers, consolidations, the movement of both manufacturing and office tasks to cheaper foreign locations, and other factors (including today's very high energy costs) will continue to have a major impact on the job market and, in some cases, will lead to large layoffs. Large mergers have been taking place at a steady rate in nearly all types of industries. Many mergers are initiated because of a desire to consolidate the companies involved,

combining customer bases, administrative or sales offices and production facilities, while cutting thousands of employees who hold duplicated jobs, in hopes of thereby creating more efficient, more profitable firms.

A powerful source of financing is creating a vast new wave of mergers and acquisitions. This financing comes from "private equity" firms. These companies pool billions of dollars from private investors and then use that money to seek out and acquire companies that they believe can be made more efficient and effective, and therefore more valuable.

In the case of U.S. manufacturing in particular, the loss of large numbers of jobs in recent years has sometimes been a sign of strength rather than a sign of weakness. Factories are running with fewer people thanks to immense investments in technology. Manufacturing output in the U.S. has not, as you might suspect, declined. Instead, output per employee is up spectacularly—to the extent that millions of manufacturing jobs were cut due to the rise in productivity, while total manufacturing activity soared thanks to productivity-creating technologies. Fewer employees, as a percentage of a factory's total workers, are now needed to manage non-production functions, such as engineering, logistics, administration and marketing. (Meanwhile, the much-written-about drop in America's manufacturing employment has been exaggerated by the fact that manufacturing firms now outsource a good deal of their non-manufacturing operations to services companies. For example, many computer departments, company cafeterias, distribution centers and engineering needs are outsourced to outside companies that specialize in such work, thus reducing the number of in-house jobs at manufacturing companies.)

Another extremely important factor in the loss of U.S. manufacturing jobs is the movement of production to foreign nations where costs are lower. (See "Rapid Growth in Offshoring and the Globalization of Business".)

Companies in both manufacturing and service sectors have caught on to management by teams, vastly enhanced supply chain technology (such as the use of the Internet for ordering and tracking components), along with networked management and manufacturing systems, which all add up to the fact that fewer mid-management, white-collar types are needed to communicate with the people doing the day-to-day work. Production workers have been encouraged to communicate among themselves. In many cases, workers are taking on unprecedented responsibilities, setting their own goals and schedules, tracking costs and output and boosting profits. Twenty-five years ago, these were the tasks of middle managers. Today, vast numbers of those management jobs have been eliminated.

Businesses without factories are also undergoing re-engineering and leaps in productivity. For example, by upgrading software and linking desktop computers to central databases, a major U.S. insurance firm was able to go from 3,000 employees issuing new policies to only 700. At the same time, it was able to reduce the time necessary to write a new policy from 15 days to only five.

Technology Continues to Create Sweeping Changes in the Workplace:

Technology has introduced vast changes throughout industries of all types, greatly boosting productivity and reallocating (or eliminating) workers. A major cause of change for employees, and therefore job seekers, is the tidal wave of new technologies revolutionizing the workplace at all levels. Prospering companies are using new technologies to communicate with customers, automate back-office tasks and industrial operations, and push ahead with research and development. There is a never-ending stream of technological innovation. For example, major companies have already harnessed the power of networked computers. Today, they are rapidly adopting the use Internet-based telephone systems and video conferencing technologies.

The trend of using new practices and technologies while cutting layers of management is largely about communication. This is true whether it is communication between the top offices and the factory floor, communication with customers, communication between the computers in one corporate office with those in another or communication from desk-to-desk in massive service businesses.

These new technologies mean continuous retraining for much of the workforce. Job seekers who want the best posts must have the training and skills that will let them utilize new technologies effectively. Jobs are remaining unfilled at many companies because of a shortage of technically qualified people. Workforce development is a critical need nationwide.

Jobs in America are shifting to new categories of work based on technologies that didn't exist 20 years ago. For example, the job title "webmaster" was coined in the 1990s to describe the employee in charge of a firm's Internet sites and intranet operations. Services firms, as well as manufacturers, are placing more and more employees in recently created technical and service positions, while many of the tasks once performed in-house are now provided by outsourced services providers. In the telecommunications industry, phone companies have migrated to digital switches that require far less manpower to operate, along with voice-recognition equipment that has eliminated much of the need for "information" operators. In the meantime, tens of thousands of jobs have been created at cellular telephone companies. Now, Internet-based telephony (Voice Over Internet Protocol, or VOIP), competition from cable providers, fiber to the premises and wireless networks such as WiMax are poised to revolutionize the telecommunications industry yet again.

Another excellent example: Retailing, shipping and warehousing are about to see a technology revolution due to the introduction of Radio Frequency Identification Tags (RFID). This breakthrough in inventory management is based on the placement of microchips in product packaging, combined with the use of special sensors in stores and warehouses that alert a central inventory management system of product purchases and the need to restock inventory. From loading docks to shelves to cash registers to parking lots, radio frequency readers will track the movement of each and every item. Many bar codes will eventually be replaced by RFIDs, with electronic product codes stored on these microchips. The chips even eliminate the need to scan each item at checkout. Checkout stations will be equipped with readers that automatically calculate purchases. No shoplifting, no manual count inventory errors. Another benefit is that manufacturers will be able to reduce overall inventory thanks to greater efficiency.

As online ordering, tracking and inventory management continue to become more sophisticated and cost-effective, purchasing executives at firms of all types and sizes will accelerate the use of Internet-based systems for management of their supply chains. There are significant opportunities here for e-commerce services and software companies. Likewise, there is great promise for third-party logistics (3PL) companies that combine the power of Internet-based information with strategically located warehouses to fulfill the inventory needs of manufacturers.

Massive Layoffs Become an Everyday Occurrence:

Very high numbers of layoffs have become commonplace. Here again, corporate restructuring, mergers and re-engineering are driving vast changes in businesses of all types. Even during an upturn in the economy, major job cuts are announced as corporate mergers and restructuring continue.

3) Continued Growth in Outsourcing, Including Supply Chain and Logistics Services

Part of the re-engineering process at employers has been a boom in "outsourcing," or the use of outside specialty firms to do chores that firms formerly performed through in-house departments. For example, Pitney Bowes takes over the mailrooms and copier rooms at major corporations. As part of a turnkey service, Pitney Bowes supplies its own copiers and then buys toner and paper by the truckload at the best possible price. It trains its employees to keep track of every single copy so its clients can control costs. Copy department employees are transferred from the client firm to Pitney Bowes, the outsourcing firm. There, these employees learn that the head of a Pitney Bowes copy department can rise to be a regional manager, a vice president or an even higher position within the company. The client firm's costs are lowered and its profits increase. The outsourcing provider makes a tidy profit through its focused expertise.

The greatest area of outsourcing growth has long been in computer departments. IBM, Accenture, Hewlett-Packard and Perot Systems are among the global leaders in this field. However, several other business functions are commonly outsourced. For example, ServiceMaster takes over janitorial tasks, building management and maintenance functions for giant corporate office campuses and industrial facilities. Another company outsources all of the food warehousing and distribution for nationwide restaurant chains. Why? Because it can run trucks and warehouses more efficiently while its clients concentrate on running restaurants.

While the 1960s, '70s and '80s saw many firms frantically trying to do all tasks in-house, the '90s were different. As a decade noted for rising productivity and efficiency, the '90s was an era of specialization and focus. That trend continues today. Outsourcing, which rapidly gained popularity in this period, will persist in leading the way to higher efficiency and profits. Outsourced services companies continue to grow rapidly, and they will continue to create (and displace) large numbers of jobs.

Some companies combine outsourcing services with temporary workers. For example, Spherion, a major temporary help firm and one of America's largest employers, is also a leading outsourcing company. Spherion's outsourcing division takes over all human resources administration functions for large clients. This means that Spherion's employees do all of the recruiting, employee records management, benefits management and so on for its client companies. This is a logical extension of Spherion's human resources expertise and good cross-marketing to its roster of corporate clients.

One of the fastest-growing fields in outsourcing is supply chain and logistics. Companies offering services in this field include giant transportation companies like UPS. "Supply chain" refers to the entire set of supplies and service providers involved in creating and delivering a component or end product. For example, for an automobile manufacturer like Ford, the supply chain includes companies that make tires, batteries, interior components and engine parts, as well as the trucks and trains that ship these parts and the warehouses that hold them (along with the engineering team that designs them). Further along Ford's supply chain lie the automobile dealers that receive completed cars and deliver them to the end customer. Another example: For a clothing store chain like The Gap, the supply chain includes clothing designers, clothing manufacturers and the warehouses and transportation systems that deliver completed clothes to the stores.

Logistics is the art of moving goods through the supply chain. Supply chains are so complex and so critical to a company's operations that there are countless ways to automate, improve efficiencies and cut costs. Many manufacturers and retailers are outsourcing all or part of their logistics needs to firms that specialize in creating efficiencies and saving costs. Logistics and supply chain companies are growing rapidly and creating large numbers of jobs. A concept you should be familiar with is Third Party Logistics ("3PL"), a system whereby a specialist firm in logistics provides a variety of transportation, warehousing and logistics-related services to its clients. These tasks were previously performed in-house by the client. When 3PL services are provided within the client's own facilities, it can also be referred to as "Insourcing." In other words, you might find yourself working for UPS at a site within a distribution company that has no other ties to UPS.

4)   Millions Working as Temps

More and more, major firms are using temporary workers to fill short-term needs, cutting overall employment costs since temps usually do not receive extensive benefits, bonuses or continuing training. The number of people working for temporary help agencies in the U.S. has jumped from about 500,000 in 1985 to about 2.5 to 3 million today, or a bit less than 2% of the total workforce. In addition to employees who are placed in temporary jobs by agencies, there are millions of people employed as "independent contractors" and "contract workers." Temporary staffing companies operate offices throughout the U.S., in cities small and large. To a growing extent, they hire and place workers via their sophisticated Internet sites.

The largest temporary help agencies tend to have vast global operations. For example, Adecco is a Swiss firm with extensive operations in the U.S., Europe and elsewhere, employing hundreds of thousands of people. Manpower, based in the U.S., does a major part of its business in dozens of nations worldwide.

Demand for temporary workers slows dramatically during economic downturns. The use of temps enables employers to increase the workforce quickly when orders from customers increase and to reduce it rapidly when revenues decrease. Temporary workers are also an extremely efficient way to meet needs for one-time projects, to fill the slots of permanent employees who are on leave and to screen potential candidates for full-time positions by first hiring them on a temporary basis.

In addition, some Americans prefer to work as temporary employees, feeling that this gives them more flexibility in their working lives. About one-third of temp employees state that they prefer this lifestyle. Unfortunately, many people who end up working in temporary positions would greatly prefer to be employed full-time. Many of these workers hold significant skills as well as college degrees. In fact, through the years, the temp business has become increasingly technical in nature.

A large percentage of temps work in professional specialties, such as law or accounting. Interestingly, the number of information technology temps has increased dramatically in the past several years. As shortages of certain types of IT workers occurred, many highly skilled workers were able to demand very lucrative pay for temporary assignments. Some temporary workers have gotten the most out of the system by moving readily from shrinking industries to those that are expanding as the economy evolves. Others found excellent permanent work when they were introduced to new companies as temps.

Internet Research Tip:
For data on the temporary staffing industry and the temporary workforce in the U.S., see the American Staffing Association (www.americanstaffing.net).

5) Rapid Growth in Offshoring and the Globalization of Business

Competition from workers in the Third World, in such nations as Mexico, Indonesia, Thailand, South Korea and particularly China, where a major portion of all exports to the U.S. are manufactured, means that fewer pure manufacturing jobs will be available in the U.S., where pay is high and employee benefit costs are immense. In fact, the costs of Social Security taxes, Medicare taxes, employer-sponsored health care, vacations, holidays, retirement plans and other benefits have risen so high (an amount typically equal to 38% to 45% of wages) that they provide considerable incentive for firms to hold down the number of employees working in U.S. locations. Instead, companies are utilizing workers in other nations. A typical factory worker in Mexico makes $250 to $300 monthly, while the same worker in China makes $100 to $150 monthly for a much longer work week. Employee benefit costs in such nations are nominal.

"Offshoring" is the word now used to describe the movement of jobs of all types away from industrialized nations, like America, to less developed countries, like India, the Philippines, Indonesia and China. For example, U.S. financial services companies are sending hundreds of thousands of jobs overseas, in such areas as call centers and financial analysis. Moving jobs to countries such as India, China and the Philippines pose serious job displacement problems in the U.S. (At the same time, there is a positive factor to the growth of these emerging economies: Increasing exports to these nations of U.S. goods and services of all types, thereby creating jobs and profits in America.)

Globalization has a profound effect on Americans— consumer prices become lower, while the base of U.S. manufacturing jobs shrinks. Consumer goods are quite inexpensive due to the vast variety of items the U.S. imports from other nations, and prices for many categories of these goods are declining rapidly. For example, Americans can purchase consumer electronics like DVD players and color televisions at increasingly lower prices, and the average price of many types of apparel is much lower thanks to globalization.

More than ever before, the world is one vast marketplace. Globalization of business supply and service chains is a strong trend today and will grow even stronger in the early 21st Century. For example, consider the rapid globalization of the automobile industry. The entire global automobile industry is dominated by only a handful of companies, including Toyota, GM, Ford, Daimler, Honda, Nissan, Hyundai, Volkswagen and Nissan.

American companies have been merging and consolidating on a national basis at a rapid clip. That consolidation will continue and will tend to become more global in nature. In addition, U.S. firms will enter into foreign markets through acquisitions and pure expansion.

Trade is not necessarily always stable. While global economies are undeniably linked, they do not march hand-in-hand. For example, the nose-dive taken by many Asian economies in the late 1990s occurred during one of the biggest economic booms in U.S. history. The strength of America as a consumer market was a platform that helped to stabilize and regenerate Asian businesses that were having difficulties.

The U.S. has incredible superiority in several key products needed by the rest of the world, including the hot growth areas of health products, computers, e-commerce, financial expertise, software and entertainment of all types. The message is clear: America can rapidly build millions of additional jobs through trade, and barrier-breaking agreements like NAFTA are of the greatest importance for the creation of future jobs, although, here again, some current jobs will be displaced.

A rapidly growing middle class in India and China is creating demand for goods exported from the U.S., including consumer products bearing desirable brands as well as luxury automobiles. Also, U.S.-based firms are enjoying great success in franchising and licensing their methods to startup businesses in China and India, in everything from hotels to fast food to services.

Meanwhile, the U.S. is also exporting its newfound expertise in the booming superstore and discount retailing sectors. For instance, hundreds of Wal-Mart's stores are in foreign locations such as Argentina, Brazil, Canada, China, Korea, Mexico, Puerto Rico and the U.K. Eventually, Wal-Mart may bring its brand of retailing to virtually all of the world's major markets. Likewise, Starbucks has rolled out to locations around the world with great success. Watch for a swiftly escalating expansion of the most successful U.S. retailers into overseas markets on all continents.

A study of 2006 results showed that a U.S. corporation listed in the Standard & Poor's 500 created, on average, 49% of its sales in foreign nations, up from 30% in 2001. Today, exports account for more than 11% of the U.S. Gross Domestic Product (GDP). You can readily see how important exporting is. Meanwhile, America remains an economic and technological giant, accounting for about 23% of the world's economic output.

6) Senior Citizens Are a Hot Commodity with Many Employers—Baby Boomers Are Retiring

Certain large employers, particularly national retail chains, have discovered that senior citizens are a terrific pool of potential employees. This is partly because Americans of 55 years or older are the fastest-growing segment of the population. For example, Home Depot typically makes up to 30,000 new hires yearly, and many of those new workers are seniors. In fact, nearly 20% of Home Depot's workforce consists of people over 50 years of age. This trend is powerful enough that the AARP is forming job link partnerships with national firms such as Anheuser-Busch, Barnes & Noble and Sears.

Meanwhile, 2006 marked the year that the first Baby Boomers turned 60, meaning that many will take early retirement. When they leave their jobs, openings will result for younger workers.

Baby boomer generally refers to people born from 1946 to 1964. The term evolved to include the children of soldiers and war industry workers who were involved in World War II. When those veterans and workers returned to civilian life, they started or added to families in large numbers. As a result, the baby boom generation is one of the largest demographic segments in the U.S. According to MetLife, the Baby Boomers make up about 27% of the U.S. population. Based on projections within the 2000 national census of the population, these people numbered an astonishing 77.7 million as of 2003.

By 2011, millions will begin turning traditional retirement age (65), resulting in extremely rapid growth in the senior portion of the population. Many Baby Boomers will leave their traditional, long-term jobs and turn to part-time work.

7) Employment Sectors that Will Offer an Above-Average Number of Job Opportunities in 2009

Job seekers should remain keenly aware of the fact that certain industries will have an above-average likelihood to offer large numbers of job openings during 2009. This is due to a number of circumstances, including shifts in consumer tastes and requirements, normal employee turnover and attrition, structural changes within industries, global economic conditions and national policies and priorities.

Below is a list of the industries on which job seekers should concentrate their efforts. Companies from this list of business sectors are the focus of the American Employers 500 profiled within the ALMANAC OF AMERICAN EMPLOYERS 2009:

- Biotechnology, Including Agricultural Biotechnology
- Coal Producers
- Computer Products—Selected Computer, Server, Storage and Accessories Makers, as well as Wireless Network Makers and Distributors
- Consulting—Selected Fields where Consultants May Be Able to Effect Cost-Savings for Clients
- Consumer Products Manufacturers
- Cosmetics Manufacturers
- Data Processing Services Providers
- Defense Contractors
- Education
- Elder Care, Home Health Care, Nursing Homes and Assisted Living Communities
- Energy Conservation Products and Services
- Entertainment, Including Electronic Games
- Guard Services, Investigation and Surveillance
- Health Care Services, Including Managed Care

- Health Foods, Organic Foods, Enhanced Foods
- Health Products
- Health Technology, Including Computerized Patient Records
- Insurance Providers
- Internet Access
- Logistics, Distribution and Supply Chain Services
- Nanotechnology and MEMS
- Oil and Gas Exploration and Production
- Oil Field Services
- Online Search Services with Advertising Revenues
- Online-based Business and Consumer Services
- Outsourcing
- Pharmaceuticals—Generics
- Radio Frequency ID Tags (RFID)
- Renewable Energy, Especially Solar and Wind Power
- Restaurants
- Retailing—Basic, Including Drugstores and Selected Specialty Stores
- Retailing—Catalogs and other Non-Store Outlets
- Retailing—Discount and Warehouse Clubs
- Wireless and Cellular Communications, including WiMax

Chapter 2

STATISTICS

Contents:	
U.S. Employment Overview: 2008	**16**
U.S. Civilian Labor Force: 1997-2008	**17**
Number of People Employed, U.S.: 2007	**18**
Unemployed Jobseekers by Sex, Reason for Unemployment & Active Job Search Methods Used: 2007	**19**
U.S. Labor Force Ages 16 to 24 Years Old by School Enrollment, Educational Attainment, Sex, Race & Ethnicity: October 2007	**20**
Top 20 U.S. Occupations by Numerical Change in Job Growth: 2006-2016	**21**
Top 20 U.S. Occupations Percent Change in Job Growth: 2006-2016	**22**
Jobs with the Largest Expected Employment Increases, U.S.: 2006-2016	**23**
Jobs with the Largest Expected Employment Decreases, U.S.: 2006-2016	**24**
Mean Hourly Earnings & Weekly Hours, Private Industry & State & Local Government: 2007	**25**
Percent of U.S. Workers with Access to Retirement & Healthcare Benefits, Private Industry: 2007	**26**
Percent of U.S. Private Industry Employers Offering Retirement & Healthcare Benefits: 2007	**27**

U.S. Employment Overview: 2008

(As of August 2008; Labor Counts In Thousands)

Civilian Labor Force, Total	154,853
Employed	145,477
Unemployed	9,376
Not in Labor Force	79,253
Unemployment Rate	6.1%
Average Hourly Earnings*[P]	$18.14
Weekly Earnings*[P]	$611.32
Average Work Week (Hours)	33.7
Nonfarm Employment[P]	137,473
Goods-Producing	21,386
Construction	7,168
Manufacturing	13,428
Service-Providing	116,087
Retail Trade	15,286
Professional & Business Services	17,857
Education & Health Services	18,997
Leisure & Hospitality	13,670
Government	22,486

P = Preliminary.

* Data relate to private production and nonsupervisory workers.

Source: U.S. Bureau of Labor Statistics
Plunkett Research, Ltd.
www.plunkettresearch.com

Plunkett Research, Ltd.

U.S. Civilian Labor Force:
1997-2008

(Persons 16 & Older; In Thousands)

Year	Civilian Workforce Level
1997	136,297
1998	137,673
1999	139,368
2000	142,583
2001	143,734
2002	144,863
2003	146,510
2004	147,401
2005	149,320
2006	151,428
2007	153,124
2008*	154,853

* As of August; seasonally adjusted.

Note: The labor force includes all persons classified as employed or unemployed. Employed persons include people 16 years and over in the civilian noninstitutional population who, during a reference week, (a) did any work at all (at least 1 hour) as paid employees, worked in their own business, profession, or on their own farm, or worked 15 hours or more as unpaid workers in an enterprise operated by a member of the family, and (b) all those who were not working but who had jobs or businesses from which they were temporarily absent because of vacation, illness, bad weather, childcare problems, maternity or paternity leave, labor-management dispute, job training, or other family or personal reasons, whether or not they were paid for the time off or were seeking other jobs. Each employed person is counted only once, even if he or she holds more than one job. Excluded are persons whose only activity consisted of work around their own house (painting, repairing, or own home housework) or volunteer work for religious, charitable, and other organizations.

Source: U.S. Bureau of Labor Statistics
Plunkett Research, Ltd.
www.plunkettresearch.com

Number of People Employed, U.S.: 2007

(Persons 16 & Older; In Thousands)

Occupational Group*	Civilian	Private Industry	State & Local Gov't
All workers	**129,370.0**	**110,620.0**	**18,753.4**
Management, professional & related	34,907.8	24,756.8	10,151.0
Management, business & financial	10,099.2	8,510.2	1,589.0
Professional & related	24,808.6	16,246.7	8,561.9
Service	26,919.9	22,836.0	4,083.9
Sales & office	34,458.1	31,689.5	2,768.6
Sales & related	13,009.0	12,900.1	108.9
Office & administrative support	21,449.1	18,789.4	2,659.7
Natural resources, construction & maintenance	11,966.7	10,982.4	984.2
Construction & extraction	6,619.1	6,087.8	531.2
Installation, maintenance & repair	5,187.9	4,751.3	436.7
Production, transportation & material moving	21,117.6	20,351.8	765.8
Production	10,328.0	10,185.3	142.7
Transportation & material moving	10,789.6	10,166.6	623.1

* A classification system including about 800 individual occupations is used to cover all workers in the civilian economy.

Source: U.S. Bureau of Labor Statistics
Plunkett Research, Ltd.
www.plunkettresearch.com

Unemployed Jobseekers by Sex, Reason for Unemployment & Active Job Search Methods Used: 2007

Sex and reason	Thousands of persons		Methods used as a percent of total jobseekers							Average number of methods used
	Total unemployed	Total jobseekers	Employer directly	Sent out resumes or filled out applications	Placed or answered ads	Friends or relatives	Public employment agency	Private employment agency	Other	
Total, 16 years and over	7,078	6,102	57.4	50.7	16.0	21.7	17.7	7.6	12.9	1.84
Job losers and persons who completed temporary jobs*	3,515	2,539	59.4	49.8	19.3	26.4	23.6	10.6	14.4	2.04
Job leavers	793	793	61.8	51.8	17.3	20.8	15.8	7.4	12.2	1.88
Reentrants	2,142	2,142	54.6	50.9	13.2	18.1	13.6	5.4	12.7	1.69
New entrants	627	627	53.1	52.3	9.8	16.8	9.9	3.3	8.2	1.54
Men, 16 years and over	3,882	3,266	58.3	48.5	15.7	23.2	17.8	7.8	13.1	1.85
Job losers and persons who completed temporary jobs	2,175	1,559	60.3	47.5	18.4	27.7	22.8	10.3	14.7	2.02
Job losers and persons who completed temporary jobs[1]	408	408	62.9	50.9	15.9	21.0	14.3	7.1	12.4	1.85
Reentrants	956	956	55.3	47.5	13.4	18.8	13.7	5.4	12.9	1.67
New entrants	343	343	52.0	52.8	9.9	17.7	10.4	3.7	7.7	1.54
Women, 16 years and over	3,196	2,836	56.3	53.3	16.2	20.0	17.6	7.4	12.6	1.84
Job losers and persons who completed temporary jobs*	1,340	980	58.0	53.4	20.8	24.2	25.0	11.0	13.9	2.07
Job leavers	385	385	60.5	52.7	18.8	20.7	17.3	7.7	12.0	1.91
Reentrants	1,186	1,186	54.0	53.7	13.1	17.4	13.6	5.4	12.6	1.70
New entrants	285	285	54.5	51.7	9.8	15.9	9.3	2.8	8.8	1.53

Note: The jobseekers total is less than the total unemployed because it does not include persons on temporary layoff. The percent using each method will always total more than 100 because many jobseekers use more than one method.

* Data on the number of jobseekers and the jobsearch methods used exclude persons on temporary layoff.

Source: U.S. Bureau of Labor Statistics
Plunkett Research, Ltd.
www.plunkettresearch.com

U.S. Labor Force Ages 16 to 24 Years Old by School Enrollment, Educational Attainment, Sex, Race & Ethnicity: October 2007

(Numbers in Thousands)	Civilian non-institutional population	Total	Percent of Populace	Employed Total	Employed % of Populace	Unemployed Number	Unemployed Rate (%)	Not in Labor Force
Total, 16 to 24 years	37,480	22,243	59.3	19,921	53.2	2,322	10.4	15,237
Enrolled in school	21,061	8,979	42.6	8,181	38.8	798	8.9	12,083
Enrolled in high school[1]	9,724	2,855	29.4	2,421	24.9	434	15.2	6,869
Men	5,118	1,431	28.0	1,203	23.5	227	15.9	3,687
Women	4,607	1,425	30.9	1,218	26.4	206	14.5	3,182
White	7,370	2,371	32.2	2,053	27.9	318	13.4	4,999
Black or African American	1,590	294	18.5	222	14.0	72	24.6	1,296
Asian	352	72	20.3	58	16.3	14	-2.0	281
Hispanic or Latino ethnicity	1,659	368	22.2	302	18.2	66	17.9	1,291
Enrolled in college	11,337	6,124	54.0	5,760	50.8	364	5.9	5,213
Enrolled in 2-year college	3,217	2,066	64.2	1,946	60.5	121	5.8	1,151
Enrolled in 4-year college	8,120	4,057	50.0	3,814	47.0	243	6.0	4,063
Full-time students	9,659	4,693	48.6	4,398	45.5	295	6.3	4,966
Part-time students	1,678	1,431	85.3	1,362	81.2	69	4.8	247
Men	5,226	2,664	51.0	2,508	48.0	156	5.9	2,563
Women	6,110	3,460	56.6	3,252	53.2	208	6.0	2,651
White	8,912	5,008	56.2	4,759	53.4	249	5.0	3,904
Black or African American	1,423	674	47.4	607	42.7	67	9.9	749
Asian	668	240	35.9	223	33.4	17	7.0	428
Hispanic or Latino ethnicity	1,414	836	59.1	800	56.6	36	4.3	578
Not enrolled in school	16,419	13,264	80.8	11,740	71.5	1,524	11.5	3,155
16 to 19 years	3,269	2,356	72.1	1,905	58.3	451	19.1	914
20 to 24 years	13,149	10,908	83.0	9,835	74.8	1,073	9.8	2,241
Men	8,595	7,554	87.9	6,628	77.1	926	12.3	1,042
Less than a high school diploma	1,859	1,496	80.5	1,261	67.8	236	15.7	362
High school graduates, no college[3]	4,073	3,544	87.0	3,069	75.3	475	13.4	529
Some college or associate degree	1,768	1,662	94.0	1,509	85.4	152	9.2	106
Bachelor's degree and higher[4]	895	852	95.1	789	88.1	63	7.4	44
Women	7,823	5,710	73.0	5,112	65.3	598	10.5	2,113
Less than a high school diploma	1,419	689	48.6	558	39.3	131	19.0	730
High school graduates, no college[3]	3,340	2,371	71.0	2,077	62.2	294	12.4	969
Some college or associate degree	1,884	1,527	81.1	1,416	75.1	112	7.3	357
Bachelor's degree and higher[4]	1,180	1,122	95.1	1,061	90.0	61	5.4	58
White	12,740	10,441	82.0	9,441	74.1	1,000	9.6	2,299
Black or African American	2,542	1,938	76.2	1,521	59.8	417	21.5	604
Asian	462	379	82.1	342	74.0	37	9.9	83
Hispanic or Latino ethnicity	3,559	2,655	74.6	2,349	66.0	305	11.5	904

Note: Detail for the above race groups do not sum to totals because data are not presented for all races. Persons whose ethnicity is identified as Hispanic or Latino may be of any race. Because of rounding, sums of individual items may not equal totals.
[1] Includes a small number of persons who are in grades below high school.
[2] Data not shown where base is less than 75,000.
[3] Includes persons with a high school diploma or equivalent.
[4] Includes persons with a bachelor's, master's, professional, and doctoral degrees.
Source: U.S. Bureau of Labor Statistics
Plunkett Research, Ltd.
www.plunkettresearch.com

Top 20 U.S. Occupations by Numerical Change in Job Growth: 2006-2016

(By Thousands of Employees)

Occupation	Employment		Change		Training*
	2006	2016	Number	Percent	
Registered nurses	2,505	3,092	587	23.5	Associate degree
Retail salespersons	4,477	5,034	557	12.4	Short-term on-the-job training
Customer service representatives	2,202	2,747	545	24.8	Moderate-term on-the-job training
Combined food preparation & serving workers, including fast food	2,503	2,955	452	18.1	Short-term on-the-job training
Office clerks, general	3,200	3,604	404	12.6	Short-term on-the-job training
Personal & home care aides	767	1,156	389	50.6	Short-term on-the-job training
Home health aides	787	1,171	384	48.7	Short-term on-the-job training
Postsecondary teachers	1,672	2,054	382	22.9	Doctoral degree
Janitors & cleaners, except maids & housekeeping cleaners	2,387	2,732	345	14.5	Short-term on-the-job training
Nursing aides, orderlies & attendants	1,447	1,711	264	18.2	Postsecondary vocational award
Bookkeeping, accounting & auditing clerks	2,114	2,377	263	12.5	Moderate-term on-the-job training
Waiters & waitresses	2,361	2,615	255	10.8	Short-term on-the-job training
Child care workers	1,388	1,636	248	17.8	Short-term on-the-job training
Executive secretaries & administrative assistants	1,618	1,857	239	14.8	Work experience in a related occupation
Computer software engineers, applications	507	733	226	44.6	Bachelor's degree
Accountants & auditors	1,274	1,500	226	17.7	Bachelor's degree
Landscaping & groundskeeping workers	1,220	1,441	221	18.1	Short-term on-the-job training
Elementary school teachers, except special education	1,540	1,749	209	13.6	Bachelor's degree
Receptionists & information clerks	1,173	1,375	202	17.2	Short-term on-the-job training
Truck drivers, heavy & tractor-trailer	1,860	2,053	193	10.4	Moderate-term on-the-job training

* An occupation is placed into 1 of 11 categories that best describes the postsecondary education or training needed by most workers to become fully qualified in that occupation. For more information about the categories, see Occupational Projections and Training Data, 2006-07 edition, Bulletin 2602 (Bureau of Labor Statistics, February 2006) and Occupational Projections and Training Data, 2008-09 edition, Bulletin 2702 (Bureau of Labor Statistics, forthcoming).

Source: U.S. Bureau of Labor Statistics

Plunkett Research, Ltd.

www.plunkettresearch.com

Top 20 U.S. Occupations by Percent Change in Job Growth: 2006-2016

(Employment in Thousands)

Occupation	Employment		Change		Training*
	2006	2016	Number	Percent	
Network systems & data communications analysts	262	402	140	53.4	Bachelor's degree
Personal & home care aides	767	1,156	389	50.6	Short-term on-the-job training
Home health aids	787	1,171	384	48.7	Short-term on-the-job training
Computer software engineers, applications	507	733	226	44.6	Bachelor's degree
Veterinary technologists & technicians	71	100	29	41.0	Associate degree
Personal financial advisors	176	248	72	41.0	Bachelor's degree
Makeup artists, theatrical & performance	2	3	1	39.8	Postsecondary vocational award
Medical assistants	417	565	148	35.4	Moderate-term on-the-job training
Veterinarians	62	84	22	35.0	First professional degree
Substance abuse & behavioral disorder counselors	83	112	29	34.3	Bachelor's degree
Skin care specialists	38	51	13	34.3	Postsecondary vocational award
Financial analysts	221	295	75	33.8	Bachelor's degree
Social & human service assistants	339	453	114	33.6	Moderate-term on-the-job training
Gaming surveillance officers & gaming investigators	9	12	3	33.6	Moderate-term on-the-job training
Physical therapist assistants	60	80	20	32.4	Associate degree
Pharmacy technicians	285	376	91	32.0	Moderate-term on-the-job training
Forensic science technicians	13	17	4	30.7	Bachelor's degree
Dental hygienists	167	217	50	30.1	Associate degree
Mental health counselors	100	130	30	30.0	Master's degree
Mental health & substance abuse social workers	122	159	37	29.9	Master's degree

* An occupation is placed into 1 of 11 categories that best describes the postsecondary education or training needed by most workers to become fully qualified in that occupation. For more information about the categories, see Occupational Projections and Training Data, 2006-07 edition, Bulletin 2602 (Bureau of Labor Statistics, February 2006) and Occupational Projections and Training Data, 2008-09 edition, Bulletin 2702 (Bureau of Labor Statistics, forthcoming).

Source: U.S. Bureau of Labor Statistics

Plunkett Research, Ltd.

www.plunkettresearch.com

Jobs with the Largest Expected Employment Increases, U.S.: 2006-2016

(By Number Employed)

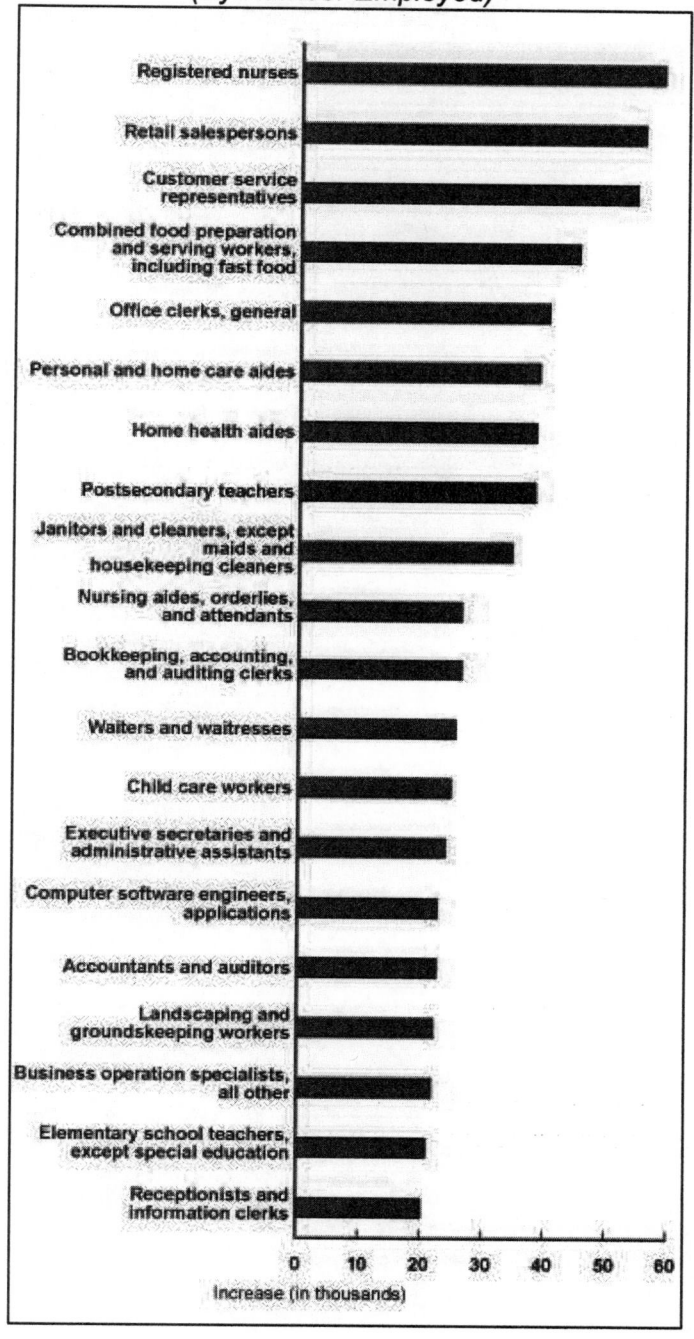

Source: U.S. Bureau of Labor Statistics
Plunkett Research, Ltd.
www.plunkettresearch.com

Jobs with the Largest Expected Employment Decreases, U.S.: 2006-2016

(By Number Employed)

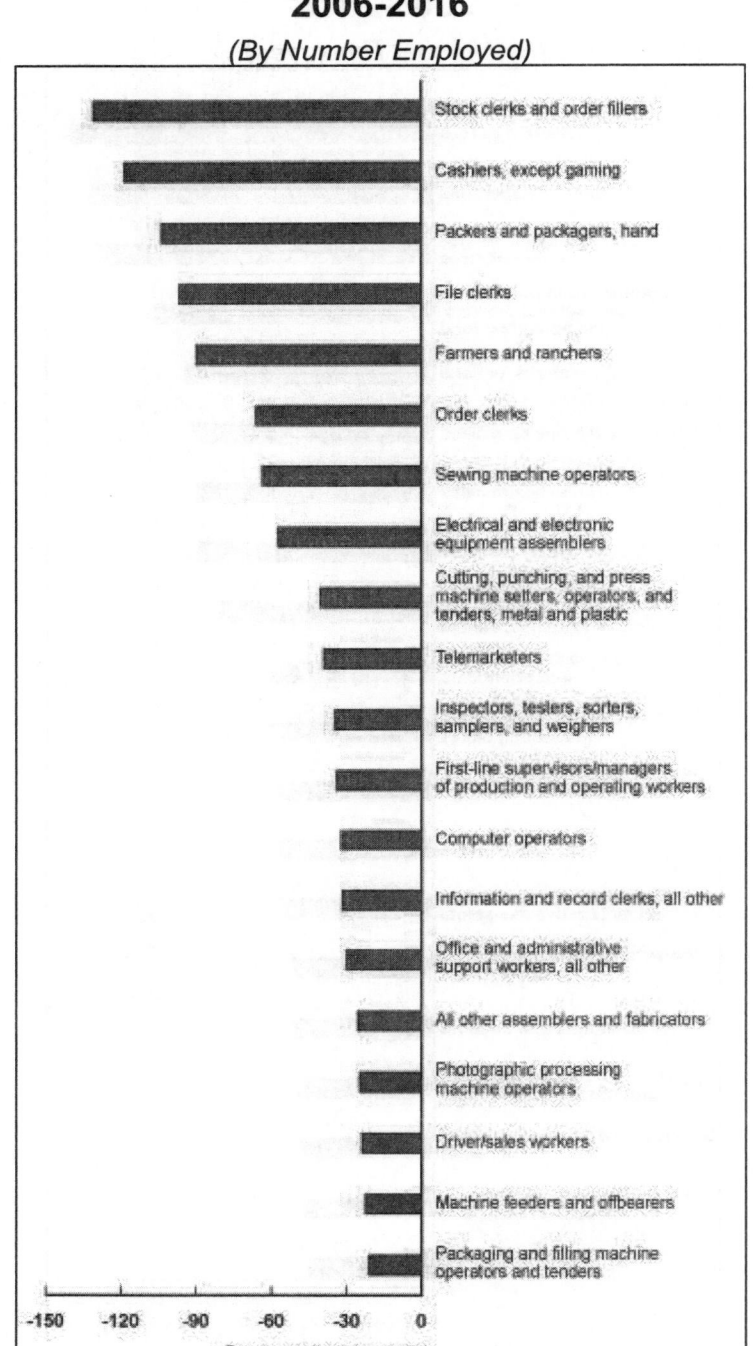

Source: U.S. Bureau of Labor Statistics
Plunkett Research, Ltd.
www.plunkettresearch.com

Mean Hourly Earnings & Weekly Hours,
Private Industry & State & Local Government: 2007

(By Worker & Establishment Characteristics)	Civilian		Private Industry		State & Local Gov't	
	Hourly Earnings[1]	Weekly Hours[2]	Hourly Earnings[1]	Weekly Hours[2]	Hourly Earnings[1]	Weekly Hours[2]
Total	**$19.88**	**35.5**	**$19.21**	**35.4**	**$24.15**	**36.3**
Worker Characteristics[3,4]						
Management, professional & related	32.38	37.1	32.96	37.5	30.63	36.0
Management, business & financial	35.97	39.6	36.54	40.0	32.65	37.5
Professional & related	30.63	36.0	30.83	36.1	30.16	35.6
Service	11.36	31.4	10.06	30.5	17.77	36.5
Sales & office	15.98	34.9	15.97	34.7	16.17	36.5
Sales & related	17.27	32.7	17.29	32.7	15.62	34.3
Office & administrative support	15.27	36.2	15.14	36.1	16.19	36.6
Natural resources, construction & maintenance	20.09	39.4	20.15	39.4	19.37	38.8
Construction & extraction	20.14	39.4	20.27	39.4	18.69	38.6
Installation, maintenance & repair	20.20	39.5	20.19	39.6	20.29	39.2
Production, transportation & material moving	15.12	37.2	15.03	37.3	18.02	34.4
Production	15.44	38.9	15.38	38.9	19.96	39.0
Transportation & material moving	14.78	35.6	14.65	35.8	17.40	33.1
Full time	21.08	39.6	20.46	39.7	24.76	38.9
Part time	11.34	20.6	11.02	20.7	15.57	18.6
Union	23.96	36.7	21.90	36.4	27.17	37.0
Nonunion	19.14	35.3	18.89	35.3	21.73	35.7
Time	19.46	35.4	18.69	35.3	24.14	36.3
Incentive	26.94	38.1	26.90	38.1	97.34	25.4
Establishment Characteristics						
Goods producing	(5)	(5)	20.79	39.5	(5)	(5)
Service Producing	(5)	(5)	18.74	34.4	(5)	(5)
1 to 49 workers	16.84	34.2	16.80	34.2	18.02	33.2
50 to 99 workers	18.06	34.9	17.99	34.9	19.24	35.8
100 to 499 workers	19.46	36.1	19.09	36.2	22.51	36.1
500 workers or more	24.75	37.0	24.30	37.1	25.71	36.7

Note: The survey covers all 50 states and the District of Columbia. Data were collected between December 2006 and January 2008. The average month of reference was July 2007.

[1] Earnings are the straight-time hourly wages or salaries paid to employees. They include incentive pay, cost-of-living adjustments, and hazard pay. Excluded are premium pay for overtime, vacations, holidays, nonproduction bonuses, and tips. The mean is computed by totaling the pay of all workers and dividing by the number of workers, weighted by hours.
[2] Mean weekly hours are the hours an employee is scheduled to work in a week, exclusive of overtime.
[3] Employees are classified as working either a full-time or a part-time schedule based on the definition used by each establishment. Union workers are those whose wages are determined through collective bargaining. Wages of time workers are based solely on hourly rate or salary; incentive workers are those whose wages are at least partially based on productivity payments such as piece rates, commissions, and production bonuses.
[4] A classification system including about 800 individual occupations is used to cover all workers in the civilian economy.
[5] Estimates for goods-producing and service-providing industries are published for private industry only. Industries are determined by the 2002 North American Industry Classification System (NAICS).

Source: U.S. Bureau of Labor Statistics

Plunkett Research, Ltd.

www.plunkettresearch,com

Percent of U.S. Workers with Access to Retirement & Healthcare Benefits, Private Industry: 2007

(By Worker Characteristics, Establishment Characteristics & Region)	Retirement Benefits			Healthcare Benefits			
	All Plans	Defined Benefit	Defined Contrib-ution	Medical Care	Dental Care	Vision Care	Outpatient Prescription Drug Coverage
All Workers	**61%**	**21%**	**55%**	**71%**	**46%**	**29%**	**68%**
Management, professional & related	76	29	71	85	62	39	82
Service	36	8	32	46	28	20	44
Sales & Office	64	19	60	71	47	27	67
Natural resources, construction & maintenance	61	26	51	76	43	31	72
Production, transportation & material moving	65	26	56	78	49	30	75
Full time	70	24	64	85	56	35	81
Part time	31	10	27	24	16	11	23
Union	84	69	49	88	68	53	85
Nonunion	58	15	56	69	44	26	66
Average wage < $15/hr.	47	11	44	57	34	20	54
Average wage > $15/hr.	76	33	69	87	61	39	84
Establishment Characteristics							
Goods-producing	70	29	62	85	54	33	81
Service-producing	58	19	53	67	44	28	64
1-to-99 workers	45	9	42	59	30	19	55
100 workers or more	78	34	70	84	64	40	81
Region							
Metropolitan areas	61	22	56	72	47	29	68
Nonmetropolitan areas	57	14	53	66	41	26	64
New England	57	21	53	68	51	23	65
Mid-Atlantic	62	27	53	72	46	34	67
East North Central	64	25	56	72	45	25	70
West North Central	63	21	56	67	43	20	66
South Atlantic	62	17	59	72	44	27	69
East South Central	66	14	64	75	52	39	73
West South Central	55	17	51	66	39	21	61
Mountain	63	18	60	70	44	28	68
Pacific	57	21	49	72	54	39	68

Source: U.S. Bureau of Labor Statistics

Plunkett Research, Ltd.

www.plunkettresearch.com

Percent of U.S. Private Industry Employers Offering Retirement & Healthcare Benefits: 2007

(By Establishment Characteristics & Region)	Retirement Benefits			Healthcare Benefits[2]
	All plans[1]	Defined Benefit	Defined Contribution	
All establishments	**46%**	**10%**	**44%**	**60%**
Establishment Characteristics				
Goods-producing	45	11	43	60
Service-producing	46	10	44	60
1-to-99 workers	44	9	42	59
100 workers or more	85	33	82	93
Region				
Metropolitan areas	48	10	46	63
Nonmetropolitan areas	37	10	37	51
New England	43	9	42	54
Middle Atlantic	49	12	47	63
East North Central	53	15	52	68
West North Central	53	14	51	56
South Atlantic	54	9	53	61
East South Central	31	5	31	68
West South Central	34	7	33	48
Mountain	38	10	35	56
Pacific	41	10	40	64

[1] Includes defined benefit pension plans and defined contribution retirement plans. The total is less than the sum of the individual items because many employers offer both types of plans.
[2] Healthcare plans may include a medical plan, or a separate dental, vision, or prescription drug plan.

Source: U.S. Bureau of Labor Statistics

Plunkett Research, Ltd.

www.plunkettresearch.com

Chapter 3

RESEARCH: 7 KEYS FOR JOB SEEKERS

**How to use your library, college placement office, the Internet and other resources
to become well-informed about a company and its industry
<u>before</u> you ask for an interview**

Research is the key to finding appropriate job openings, targeting the best possible employers and performing well when you go to job interviews. Learn what's unique about a company compared to other firms in its industry. Learn why it's prospering–or why it isn't. Where is this company going? Is it favored by stock investors? Is it privately-owned by a family, or has it been acquired by private equity investors who plan to resell it over the mid-term? What are its hottest-selling products and services? Is it investing in research and new facilities so that it may prosper in the future?

Also, as many people who have been laid off from failing startup firms have learned the hard way, determining a company's level of financial stability can be one of the most important factors in making a career decision.

The more you're willing to dig deep at the library or your college's career planning office, and the more adept you are at using the Internet for research, the better your chances of success in a job search. If you are willing to ask questions of businesspeople and of employees who currently work for your target employers, you will enhance your job search even further. The two secrets to successful job research are tenacity and focus. Know what to look for and where to find it.

Once you've landed an interview, you should research both the prospective employer and its industry even further. In this manner, you'll know what questions to ask before you agree to take the job, and you'll present yourself as a knowledgeable potential hire who is truly interested in the company and its business.

Here are the seven keys for research that can lead you to a great employer:

1) Financial Stability
Check bond ratings, credit ratings, debt level, growth in sales and growth in profits, along with the views of stock analysts and business journalists.

2) Growth Plans
Look for new plants, stores or offices to be opened; new technologies, products or divisions to be launched; or plans for strategic acquisitions. (See 3, 4 and 5 below.)

3) Research and Development Programs
How much does the firm invest in R&D? Is this research and development budget growing? For many types of companies, research is a vital investment in the future.

4) Product Launch and Production
Does the company have the ability to successfully launch new products and services (see 5 below) or to invest in and utilize cutting-edge technologies needed to maintain a competitive edge?

5) Marketing and Distribution Methods
Does the firm utilize an in-house sales force? Does it work through outside dealers and distribution partners? What are its advertising methods? Is it increasing its market share, or are competitors taking customers away? Is the company growing its international sales? Is it adept at using the Internet as a powerful sales tool? Is it successful at selling into growing international markets, such as China and India?

6) Employee Benefits
Are wealth-building benefit plans offered? Will the company match all or part of your deposits to a 401(k) savings plan? Check for tuition reimbursement, pension plans, profit sharing, ESOP stock ownership plans, discount stock purchase plans, stock options or performance-based bonuses.

7) Quality-of-Work Factors
Does the company offer continual training, wellness programs, child care, elder care support, promote-from-within policies, flexible work schedules, performance reviews, product discounts or on-site health clubs? Is it a corporate culture that fits your lifestyle?

As a serious job seeker, you should conduct in-depth research and make detailed notes about these seven key factors for each firm you are considering. Then compare each company's finances, plans and programs to others in the same industry. You'll begin to see what makes some firms outstanding and why those outstanding companies are the best places to make a career investment. For example, if you compare two discount store giants, Wal-Mart and Costco, you will find that Wal-Mart is by far the larger firm, but Costco has an outstanding record of providing superior employee pay and benefits.

Your research goal should be twofold: First, determine whether this is a firm you want to work for. Are the salaries and benefits appealing? Are layoffs likely? Is it a company with solid growth plans? A growing company will offer opportunities for you to advance when it launches new locations, services, technologies or product lines. Second, develop a personal understanding of the company and its industry so you can better sell yourself as a potential employee.

Other Considerations:

Women and Minorities:
Certain industries have a greater tendency to offer advancement opportunities for women or minorities. Historically, the banking and insurance segments have tended to promote both women and minorities, as have retailing, electric utilities, publishing and major telephone companies.

Major employers in many other industries are making serious efforts to hire, develop and promote women and minorities for top officers' positions. Some technology companies have been terrific places for women who want to advance, and a few tech companies have posted women to CEO spots, such as Margaret Whitman at eBay and Anne Mulcahy at Xerox.

Black Enterprise magazine publishes an annual list of the "Most Powerful African Americans in Corporate America," (see www.blackenterprise.com).

The Executive Leadership Council, www.elcinfo.com, a Washington, D.C.-based nonprofit group that conducts programs aimed at filling more executive posts with African-Americans, has a unique statistic to report. Its membership is composed of senior-level black executives who have jobs that are no more than three levels below the CEO spot at Fortune 500 companies. When the group was founded in 1986, it had only a handful of members. Today, its membership is about 400 people employed in high-level executive jobs at 200 major corporations. Approximately one-third of them are women.

A March 2008 study released by Catalyst, a New York-based research group that focuses on women's issues in the workplace, found that 14.8% of members of boards of directors in the *Fortune 500* firms are women, up from 9.6% in 1995. (You can access the results of Catalyst studies at www.catalyst.org.) Obviously, women are making slow progress in gaining representation in the highest ranks of corporate America, and they fall far short of parity with men in that regard. The *Fortune 1000* companies recently included 23 female CEOs, according to an August 2008 study by Catalyst.

Tips on Using Business Magazines, Newspapers and Trade Journals to Find Job Leads and Do Employer Research

Many job seekers overlook the tremendous advantages of using industry magazines (called "trade journals") and other publications to do research.

Industry-specific trade journals frequently have classified ads in the back that list job openings. An example of a great magazine to study is *American Banker,* which can be found at major libraries. Additional information is available at www.americanbanker.com.

Journalists at trade journals and business newspapers continuously interview industry-leading executives regarding their companies' growth plans. New projects and company expansion plans described in these articles provide terrific job leads.

You can also get great contact information from these publications. Read the latest business stories about companies and industries that interest you and you will learn vital information. Best of all, you can glean from stories and interviews the names and titles of executives who lead projects, divisions and subsidiaries.

There are literally hundreds of these trade journals—at least one for each industry sector and sometimes dozens covering the largest industries.

Other great resources include local business newspapers such as the *Dallas/Ft. Worth Business Journal*, *The Wall Street Journal*, the business pages of major newspapers like *The New York Times* and publications written for major investors like *Investor's Business Daily*. At www.bizjournals.com, you can gain access to news stories from business journals from all over the U.S.

Quality-of-Life Benefits:
Many companies offer benefits that help employees balance their personal and professional lives. The concept is that employees who are healthy and comfortable with their personal and family lives make better, more productive employees. To that end, many companies include fitness programs and family services such as

extended maternity leaves and child care or elder care, whether on-site or off-site in the form of referral services. Other popular family-friendly benefits include flextime, flexible benefits spending accounts, adoption assistance and telecommuting. In many cases, benefits are listed on employers' web sites.

Work-Life has become a popular phrase for family-friendly benefits and programs among major employers such as Intel, Abbott Laboratories, Baxter and Aramark. For additional information, you can study such organizations as the Alliance for Work-Life Progress at www.awlp.org.

Growth Potential and Job Stability:

A firm's growth potential should be among your top priorities. Companies are always trying to maintain or increase productivity, or the ratio of sales per employee. If a company's sales are sliding, or if it is running out of cash, the job picture starts to collapse. A little extra research into a company's finances and true potential for growth might save you from a future layoff.

Of course, employers sometimes have to resort to layoffs due to conditions outside of their control. For example, travel industry companies worldwide cut hundreds of thousands of jobs in the revenue slump following the September 11, 2001 attacks on New York City and Washington, D.C. The investment and financial services industry has been going through a period of widespread layoffs since mid-2007.

As a job seeker, you're forced to look out for your own best interests while you sort through thousands of potential employers in dozens of industries. This means that good research is vital. For example, if you put salary at the top of your list, you may have the wrong priorities. From time to time, some of the highest-paying firms have been among those cutting the largest numbers of employees. If you are looking for job stability, your biggest challenge is to pick companies that are more likely to hire now and less likely to have layoffs in the future. That's why a firm's growth outlook should be one of your guiding lights.

However, the goal is *internal* growth caused by expanding sales. Generally less appealing are firms that post a quick spike in growth through big mergers. (In many cases, merged companies lay off people who suddenly find themselves filling jobs duplicated in newly consolidated offices. Also, companies that grow excessively through acquisitions may be taking on loads of debt that can become hard to handle later. However, there are occasional exceptions to this rule, where firms are enjoying soaring demand for products or services and find it difficult to hire quickly enough to keep up.) Companies that are growing rapidly through internal expansion include those opening new stores, distribution centers or offices, developing exciting new products, moving into new markets (including international markets) and creating hot new technologies, retail formats or services. Those types of expansion frequently mean great career

opportunities, including the chance for rapid job promotion.

Where can you look for growth companies? If you're tenacious, you can find opportunities where others will find only rejection. Identifying real prospects for growth takes more than a quick glance.

Here's an extremely important point for you to remember: you should look for opportunities in growing divisions that serve special niches, even when the company as a whole is cutting jobs.

Additional key factors for strong corporate growth, and thereby the best job prospects, include:

1) Companies or divisions with a growing share of a promising market.

Management's ability to anticipate or create change in the marketplace makes for a growing company with great prospects. For example, Sam Walton revolutionized the department store business by realizing that consumers want everyday low prices on name-brand merchandise. He created Wal-Mart, while competitor Sears suffered by maintaining an old-fashioned policy of special sales events on private-label goods. Wal-Mart rapidly became one of the largest creators of new jobs in the private sector. Sears was forced to slash its ranks.

Microsoft made its way to the top with unique products serving a soaring market when it developed highly functional software for personal computers. Microsoft created thousands of millionaire employees through the immense increase in the value of its stock plans. HEB, an innovative grocer in Texas, has evolved continually over the decades, constantly introducing improvements to store layouts, and even creating an exciting new HEB Marketplace concept that is a retail industry leader. HEB has large numbers of job openings of many types on a continuous basis.

The point to these stories is that you shouldn't invest your career in a company with mediocre prospects. With perseverance, you can target your own list of employers that are posting growth due to competitive advantages or growing market demand. Your best bets are companies taking reasonable risks in order to move ahead. Those risks may include investments in advertising, research and development, new technology, improved techniques on the manufacturing floor, testing of new products and the opening of new retail store formats. For example, Chico's FAS stores scored a hit by filling a niche in the women's apparel market, and Genentech became a leader in the biotechnology field by risking vast amounts on research. Also, don't overlook the potential of the export market— many American firms find much of their growth by creating products and services that enjoy terrific demand overseas as well as in the U.S.

2) Sales and profits: past and present.

The companies most likely to move along at a good clip are those with an exciting mid-term history. Firms with an average annual growth in sales of 10% to 15% over the last three to five years are generally promising. Many small and mid-size firms grow at much faster rates and find themselves hiring continuously.

3) Beware of fads.

Unfortunately, a few companies post meteoric growth in businesses that turn out to be mere fads. The restaurant industry suffers from this problem on a regular basis. In recent years, companies selling bagels, frozen yogurt, rotisserie chicken and the like enjoyed impressive, nationwide growth only to collapse like a house of cards a couple of years later. Here's another example: the 1990s produced a rash of new dotcoms that were fueled by fad investors. Many of the biggest web-based busts were companies that planned to steal market share from traditional retail stores by selling items like pet food and living room furniture over the Internet. Most of these fad-based firms wasted valuable years in the careers of employees in addition to billions of dollars of venture capital—only a handful truly succeeded.

How to Find and Use Expert Opinions:

Superior sources used by sophisticated job researchers include reports written by: 1) stock analysts; 2) professional market research firms; and 3) journalists at business magazines and industry "trade magazines." Many major libraries have large collections of industry-specific trade magazines that can give you clues that competing job seekers will overlook. For example, *Retail Traffic Magazine*, www.retailtrafficmag.com, publishes lists of the fastest-growing retail chains. Virtually every other industry is covered by one or two trade magazines that will give you leads to growing companies. Many articles in these magazines contain the names of executives you may want to contact. Also, most industry trade magazines publish help-wanted ads in the back. The *Gale Directory of Publications and Broadcast Media* is a good index to magazines, organized by industry. You can find this directory in major libraries.

Next, move on to reports from experts. Marketing and investment professionals are looking for some of the same clues you should use as a job seeker, and reports written by full-time analysts who cover specific companies or industries can help you find firms that are growing and hiring. Reuters, www.reuters.com, is the best source for stock analysts' reports. Here, you'll find the latest business news as well as online access to industry and company coverage written by the nation's best analysts. Most of the reports have a cost, but many are free of charge, and others have prices as low as $5 to $25. Learn to use the stock research and "analyst research" features at Reuters to find exactly what you want.

Professionally written market research can be found at Marketresearch.com, www.marketresearch.com. This market research broker charges varying fees for access to the reports. However, many of the reports are reasonably priced, and the insight you gain into industries, markets

and leading companies can be extremely helpful. Web sites such as this offer the ability to search for reports by a wide variety of criteria, including company name and industry.

Other Basic Resources:

Annual Reports/10-Ks/S-1s: Companies that sell their stocks to the public, including most of the firms covered in this book, publish annual reports that contain a wealth of information. Annual reports and 10-Ks cover yearly results, financial statements, management practices and other vital information for publicly held firms. S-1s provide the same type of information on companies that are selling stock to the public for the first time. You can find copies of these reports at large libraries. Online, the best place to acquire this information is at the site of the U.S. Securities and Exchange Commission. They have a user-friendly service called EDGAR that enables you to search for companies and access their financial reports at www.sec.gov. Look especially at the five-year "summary financial statement" in the back of these reports. Also, look for growth in sales and earnings. If these are falling, dig deeper to find out why. Faltering sales or profits can lead to layoffs or to a merger with another firm (which could result in deep job cuts).

Also, you can find a wealth of financial information on publicly-traded firms at Yahoo! Finance, http://finance.yahoo.com.

See Chapter 4, "Important Contacts for Job Seekers," for additional places to get basic corporate data.

Tips on Utilizing Financial Documents Filed by Publicly Held Firms

(Access these documents at the Securities Exchange Commission, www.sec.gov.)

10-K (also called Annual Report on Form 10-K):
This is an annual filing required by federal law. It follows a standard format. Information includes a complete description of the business, risk factors, historical financial data and much more. It is vital reading for job seekers. You will find that these documents are written in dry, legal language, but they contain a wealth of information.

DEF 14A Proxy Statement:
This is an annual document that gives shareholders certain options to consider at their annual meeting. It names the firm's board of directors and top management. It also gives the dollar value and description of salaries, bonuses, pension plans, stock options and other benefits enjoyed by the company's five highest-paid officers. Job seekers can learn a great deal about a firm's management, pay and benefits from this document. Included is a list of the people or organizations that own more than 5% of the company's stock.

S-1:
This is a new registration document for companies that are going public for the first time. In other words, they are creating an IPO (initial public offering). The information includes all of the data found in the 10-K and proxy statement filed annually by companies that have been public for more than one year.

10-Q:
This is a quarterly report detailing a company's latest sales, profits and balance sheet.

More Ways to Research an Employer's Financial Stability and Growth Plans:

1) Check out its bond rating.
There's no sense in trying to become a financial analyst on your own. Instead, go to your library and turn to the *Bond Guide* published by Standard & Poor's (New York, NY). This monthly booklet rates thousands of corporate bonds, based on a company's ability to pay principal and interest when due. If you're considering a major corporation with a bond rating of less than BB (an indicator that a company's debt is riskier than "investment grade"), you should do a lot more investigating before you continue chasing a job at that company.

2) Talk to vendors and current employees.
Talk to employees who work for the employer, or talk to people who do business with it. No one knows what's really going on better than people who are on the scene. If

there are problems that are not yet known by the media, or if there are exciting new developments that have not yet been announced, you may find out a lot just by asking around. While you're at it, ask about corporate culture—how well are employees treated?

Popular Job-Search Internet Sites

HotJobs	http://hotjobs.yahoo.com/
CareerBuilder	www.careerbuilder.com
Monster	www.monster.com

Tips on Finding Information on Privately Held Employers

Study back-issue indexes and archives to major newspapers to see what journalists are reporting about a prospective employer. Many libraries have back issues of *The Wall Street Journal, The New York Times* and other important newspapers on microfilm. At major public and university libraries, you may be able to access online databases like ProQuest and InfoTrac. These databases have excellent search engines that lead you into online archives of the best publications, including *The Wall Street Journal*, as well as many trade and local publications.

For smaller firms, go online and try American Journalism Review at www.newslink.org, where you'll be able to search news sites including hometown newspapers across the nation. Likewise, search local business newspapers at www.bizjournals.com, where you'll find links to dozens of major business weeklies like the *Houston Business Journal*.

Finally, invest in a credit report. If you really want reassurance, go to Experian SmartBusinessReports, www.smartbusinessreports.com. You can use its links to order a credit report on the employer. These reports are reasonably priced from about $20 to $45, and they can help you determine whether the company is paying its bills on time or has other problems. This could be vital in helping you determine whether to accept a job at a privately-held firm.

3) Use Internet search engines.
Look up your firm and industry in an Internet search engine such as Google or a portal such as Yahoo Finance, http://finance.yahoo.com. There, you may find unusual articles that were recently written about a company's product breakthroughs, treatment of women or minorities, human interest stories, training programs or stories written from other unique slants.

4) Study other business books and guides.

Search at a library or at an online bookseller like Amazon.com for recent books regarding major companies. For example, if you want to apply to biotech leader Genentech for a job, don't fail to read *The Billion Dollar Molecule: One Company's Quest for the Perfect Drug.* With a little research, you can turn up many other excellent books about specific companies, from banks like Bank of America to publishers like Gannett.

Great Places for Industry Research

Plunkett Research, www.plunkettresearch.com. Go to the specific industry of your choice to see an overview of trends and statistics. At our subscription service, www.plunkettresearchonline.com, subscribers have access to thousands of pages of industry analysis, statistics, contacts and company profiles, along with multiple search and export tools.

Quintessentialcareers.com, www.quintessentialcareers.com. Offers a "Career Resources Toolkit."

Wetfeet.com, www.wetfeet.com. Publishes snapshots of hundreds of employers.

Vault.com, www.vault.com. This site publishes insights about careers with hundreds of leading firms.

---

5) Explore industry-specific web sites.

See Chapter 4, "Important Contacts for Job Seekers," for hundreds of sites from dozens of different industry sectors. In particular, study the industry associations for the sector you want to work in.

6) Research benefits and pension plans.

For additional information about corporate pension plans, start with the government agency charged with protecting and regulating pensions: the Pension Benefit Guaranty Corporation, 1200 K St. NW, Washington, D.C. 20005-4026, 202-326-4000, www.pbgc.gov. They can answer certain questions over the telephone.

The U.S. Department of Labor publishes a useful book titled "Protect your Pension." They can be contacted at: U.S. Department of Labor, Employee Benefits Security Administration, 200 Constitution Ave. NW, Room N5635, Washington, D.C. 20210, 866-444-3272 or 202-219-8776, www.dol.gov/ebsa/publications/main.html.

The Social Security Administration, 800-772-1213, www.ssa.gov, can provide you with information regarding your potential Social Security benefits.

NOTE: Generally, employees covered by wealth-building benefit plans do not fully own ("vest in") funds contributed on their behalf by the employer until as many as five years of service with that employer have passed.

All pension plans are voluntary—that is, employers are not obligated to offer pensions.

Pension Plans: The type and generosity of these plans vary widely from firm to firm. Caution: Some employers refer to plans as "pension" or "retirement" plans when they are actually 401(k) savings plans that require a contribution by the employee.

Defined Benefit Pension Plans: Pension plans that do not require a contribution from the employee are infrequently offered. However, a few companies, particularly larger employers in high-profit-margin industries, offer defined benefit pension plans where the employee is guaranteed to receive a set pension benefit upon retirement. The amount of the benefit is determined by the years of service with the company and the employee's salary during the later years of employment. The longer a person works for the employer, the higher the retirement benefit. These defined benefit plans are funded entirely by the employer. The benefits, up to a reasonable limit, are guaranteed by the Federal Government's Pension Benefit Guaranty Corporation. These plans are not portable—if you leave the company, you cannot transfer your benefits into a different plan. Instead, upon retirement you will receive the benefits that vested during your service with the company. If your employer offers a pension plan, it must give you a "summary plan description" within 90 days of the date you join the plan. You can also request a "summary annual report" of the plan, and once every 12 months you may request an "individual benefit statement" accounting of your interest in the plan.

Defined Contribution Plans: These are quite different. They do not guarantee a certain amount of pension benefit. Instead, they set out circumstances under which the employer will make a contribution to a plan on your behalf. The most common example is the 401(k) savings plan. Pension benefits are not guaranteed under these plans.

Cash Balance Pension Plans: These plans were recently invented. They are hybrid plans—part defined benefit and part defined contribution. Many employers have converted their older defined benefit plans into cash balance plans. The employer makes deposits (or credits a given amount of money) on the employee's behalf, usually based on a percentage of pay. Employee accounts grow based on a predetermined interest benchmark, such as the interest rate on Treasury Bonds. There are some advantages to these plans, particularly for younger workers: a) The benefits, up to a reasonable limit, are guaranteed by the Pension Benefit Guaranty Corporation. b) Benefits are portable—they can be moved to another plan when the employee changes companies. c) Younger workers and those who spend a shorter number of years with an employer may receive higher benefits than they would under a traditional defined benefit plan.

ESOP Stock Plan (Employees' Stock Ownership Plan): This type of plan is in wide use. Typically, the plan borrows money from a bank and uses those funds to purchase a large block of the corporation's stock. The corporation makes contributions to the plan over a period of time, and the stock purchase loan is eventually paid off. The value of the plan grows significantly as long as the market price of the stock holds up. Qualified employees are allocated a share of the plan based on their length of service and their level of salary. Under federal regulations, participants in ESOPs are allowed to diversify their account holdings in set percentages that rise as the employee ages and gains years of service with the company. In this manner, not all of the employee's assets are tied up in the employer's stock.

Savings Plan, 401(k): Under this type of plan, employees make a tax-deferred deposit into an account. In the best plans, the company makes annual matching donations to the employees' accounts, typically in some proportion to deposits made by the employees themselves. A good plan will match one-half of employee deposits of up to 6% of wages. For example, an employee earning $30,000 yearly might deposit $1,800 (6%) into the plan. The company will match one-half of the employee's deposit, or $900. The plan grows on a tax-deferred basis, similar to an IRA. A very generous plan will match 100% of employee deposits. However, some plans do not call for the employer to make a matching deposit at all. Other plans call for a matching contribution to be made at the discretion of the firm's board of directors. Actual terms of these plans vary widely from firm to firm. Generally, these savings plans allow employees to deposit as much as 15% of salary into the plan on a tax-deferred basis. However, the portion that the company uses to calculate its matching deposit is generally limited to a maximum of 6%. Employees should take care to diversify the holdings in their 401(k) accounts, and most people should seek professional guidance or investment management for their accounts.

Stock Purchase Plan: Qualified employees may purchase the company's common stock at a price below its market value under a specific plan. Typically, the employee is limited to investing a small percentage of wages in this plan. The discount may range from 5% to 15%. Some of these plans allow for deposits to be made through regular monthly payroll deductions. However, new accounting rules for corporations, along with other factors, are leading many companies to curtail these plans—dropping the discount allowed, cutting the maximum yearly stock purchase or otherwise making the plans less generous or appealing.

Profit Sharing: Qualified employees are awarded an annual amount equal to some portion of a company's profits. In a very generous plan, the pool of money awarded to employees would be 15% of profits. Typically, this money is deposited into a long-term retirement account. Caution: Some employers refer to plans as "profit sharing" when they are actually 401(k) savings plans. True profit sharing plans are rarely offered.

Plunkett Research Online and Plunkett's Industry Reference Books:

1) Internet-Based Services: Plunkett Research Online is a reference service that is subscribed to by the nation's leading university placement offices, libraries and information offices. You can use it to filter prospective employers by location, industry, size and more. You can then export contact information for those companies into spreadsheets or text files. In addition, you can use the site to research the latest editions of our industry analysis. Many additional tools for job seekers are included. For an extensive online tour, see www.plunkettresearch.com.

2) Printed Almanacs: Plunkett Research also publishes industry-specific almanacs for the most important industries. These are top-notch resources for job seekers.

Industry-Specific Books from Plunkett Research:

- Plunkett's Advertising & Branding Industry Almanac
- Plunkett's Airline, Hotel & Travel Industry Almanac
- Plunkett's Almanac of Middle Market Companies
- Plunkett's Apparel & Textiles Industry Almanac
- Plunkett's Automobile Industry Almanac
- Plunkett's Banking, Mortgages & Credit Industry Almanac
- Plunkett's Biotech & Genetics Industry Almanac
- Plunkett's Chemicals, Coatings & Plastics Industry Almanac
- Plunkett's Consulting Industry Almanac
- Plunkett's E-Commerce & Internet Business Almanac
- Plunkett's Energy Industry Almanac
- Plunkett's Engineering & Research Industry Almanac
- Plunkett's Entertainment & Media Industry Almanac
- Plunkett's Food Industry Almanac
- Plunkett's Health Care Industry Almanac
- Plunkett's Insurance Industry Almanac
- Plunkett's InfoTech Industry Almanac
- Plunkett's Investment & Securities Industry Almanac
- Plunkett's Nanotechnology & MEMS Industry Almanac
- Plunkett's Outsourcing & Offshoring Industry Almanac
- Plunkett's Real Estate & Construction Industry Almanac
- Plunkett's Renewable, Alternative & Hydrogen Energy Industry Almanac
- Plunkett's Retail Industry Almanac
- Plunkett's Sports Industry Almanac
- Plunkett's Telecommunications Industry Almanac

- Plunkett's Transportation, Supply Chain &
  Logistics Industry Almanac
- Plunkett's Wireless & Cellular Telephone
  Industry Almanac

**Publications from Plunkett Research Written
Especially for Job Seekers:**

- The Almanac of American Employers
- Plunkett's Companion to the Almanac of
  American Employers

Our books will give you in-depth coverage of specific industries and the leading firms in those industries, along with trends and developments in technology and services. You will find these books in public and academic libraries, college placement offices, human resources offices, corporate libraries and government agency libraries. For sample chapters and additional details, you can preview as well as purchase these books at www.plunkettresearch.com.

Plunkett's Companion to The Almanac of American Employers is our book that provides profiles on 500 additional, rapidly growing corporate employers. This companion book covers smaller firms than those in the main volume of *The Almanac of American Employers*.

Chapter 4

IMPORTANT CONTACTS
FOR JOB SEEKERS

Contents:

I. Accountants & CPAs Associations
II. Advertising/Marketing Associations
III. Aging
IV. Airline & Air Cargo Industry Associations
V. Alternative Energy-Ethanol
VI. Alternative Energy-Solar
VII. Alternative Energy-Wind
VIII. Apparel Associations
IX. Banking Industry Associations
X. Biotechnology and Biological Industry Associations
XI. Booksellers Associations
XII. Broadcasting, Cable, Radio & TV Associations
XIII. Brokers & Trading
XIV. Careers-Airlines/Flying
XV. Careers-Banking
XVI. Careers-Biotech
XVII. Careers-Computers/Technology
XVIII. Careers-First Time Jobs/New Grads
XIX. Careers-General Job Listings
XX. Careers-Health Care
XXI. Careers-Job Listings for Seniors
XXII. Careers-Job Reference Tools
XXIII. Careers-Restaurants
XXIV. Careers-Telecommunications
XXV. Communications Professional Associations

XXVI. Computer & Electronics Industry Associations
XXVII. Consulting Industry Associations
XXVIII. Corporate Information Resources
XXIX. Disabling Conditions
XXX. Economic Data & Research
XXXI. Electrical Engineering Industry Associations
XXXII. Energy Associations-Electric Power
XXXIII. Energy Associations-Natural Gas
XXXIV. Energy Associations-Other
XXXV. Energy Associations-Petroleum, Exploration, Production, etc.
XXXVI. Engineering, Research & Scientific Associations
XXXVII. Entertainment & Amusement Associations
XXXVIII. Film & Television Resources
XXXIX. Film & Theater Associations
XL. Fitness
XLI. Food Industry Associations, General
XLII. Food Processor Industry Associations
XLIII. Grocery Industry Associations
XLIV. Health Care Business & Professional Associations
XLV. Hotel/Lodging Associations
XLVI. Human Resources Industry Associations
XLVII. Industry Research/Market Research

XLVIII. Insurance, Agents & Brokers
XLIX. Insurance, Property/Casualty Associations
L. Magazines, Business & Financial
LI. MBA Resources
LII. Online Recruiting & Employment ASPs & Solutions
LIII. Pensions, Benefits & 401(k)s
LIV. Pharmaceutical Industry Associations (Drug Industry)
LV. Printers & Publishers Associations
LVI. Real Estate Industry Associations
LVII. Recording & Music Associations
LVIII. Retail Industry Associations
LIX. Satellite-Related Professional Organizations
LX. Securities Industry Associations
LXI. Software Industry Resources
LXII. Stock Market Data
LXIII. Telecommunications Industry Associations
LXIV. Temporary Staffing Firms
LXV. Testing Resources
LXVI. Textile & Fabric Associations
LXVII. Travel Business & Professional Associations
LXVIII. Travel Industry Associations

LXIX.	U.S. Government Agencies
LXX.	Waste Industry Associations
LXXI.	Water Resources Associations
LXXII.	Writers, Photographers & Editors Associations

I.   Accountants & CPAs Associations

American Institute of CPAs (AICPA)
1211 Ave. of the Americas
New York, NY 10036-8775 US
Phone: 212-596-6200
Fax: 212-596-6213
Toll Free: 888-777-7077
E-mail Address: *jmaiman@aicpa.org*
Web Address: www.aicpa.org
American Institute of CPAs (AICPA) provides information and news for CPAs, news from the organization and a search for accounting firms on its web site.

II.   Advertising/Marketing Associations

Advertising Women of New York (AWNY)
25 W. 45th St., Ste. 403
New York, NY 10036 US
Phone: 212-221-7969
Fax: 212-221-8296
E-mail Address: *awny@awny.org*
Web Address: www.awny.org
Advertising Women of New York (AWNY) provides a forum for personal and professional growth, serves as a catalyst for the advancement of women in the communications field and promotes and supports philanthropic endeavors through the AWNY Foundation. The web site also provides content from Women Executives in Public Relations (WERP), such as its a dynamic job board.

American Association of Advertising Agencies (AAAA)
405 Lexington Ave., 18th Fl.
New York, NY 10174-1801 US
Phone: 212-682-2500
Fax: 212-682-8391

E-mail Address: *kipp@aaaa.org*
Web Address: www.aaaa.org
The American Association of Advertising Agencies (AAAA) is the national trade association representing the advertising agency industry in the United States.

American Institute of Graphic Arts (AIGA)
164 5th Ave.
New York, NY 10010 US
Phone: 212-807-1990
Fax: 212-807-1799
E-mail Address: *steve_rogenstein@aiga.org*
Web Address: www.aiga.org
The American Institute of Graphic Arts (AIGA) strives to further excellence in communication design, both as a strategic tool for business and as a cultural force.

American Marketing Association (AMA)
311 S. Wacker Dr., Ste. 5800
Chicago, IL 60606 US
Phone: 312-542-9000
Fax: 312-542-9001
Toll Free: 800-262-1150
E-mail Address: *info@ama.org*
Web Address: www.marketingpower.com
The American Marketing Association (AMA) serves marketing professionals in both business and education and serves all levels of marketing practitioners, educators and students.

Cable & Telecommunications Association for Marketing (CTAM)
201 N. Union St., Ste. 440
Alexandria, VA 22314 US
Phone: 703-549-4200
E-mail Address: *info@ctam.com*
Web Address: www.ctamnetforum.com/eweb
The Cable & Telecommunications Association for Marketing (CTAM) is dedicated to the discipline and development of consumer marketing excellence in cable television, new media and telecommunications services.

Direct Marketing Association (DMA)
1120 Ave. of the Americas

New York, NY 10036-6700 US
Phone: 212-768-7277
Fax: 212-302-6714
E-mail Address: *customerservice@the-dma.org*
Web Address: www.the-dma.org
The Direct Marketing Association (DMA) is the oldest and largest trade association for users and suppliers in the direct, database and interactive marketing fields.

III.   Aging

Administration on Aging (AOA)
1 Massachusetts Ave., Stes. 4100 & 5100
Washington, DC 20201 US
Phone: 202-619-0724
Fax: 202-357-3555
E-mail Address: *aoainfo@aoa.gov*
Web Address: www.aoa.gov
The Administration on Aging (AOA) is the federal focal point and advocate agency for older persons and their concerns. In this role, AOA works to heighten awareness among other federal agencies, organizations, groups and the public.

IV.   Airline & Air Cargo Industry Associations

International Air Transport Association (IATA)
800 Place Victoria
P.O. Box 113
Montreal, QC H4Z 1M1 Canada
Phone: 514-874-0202
Fax: 514-874-9632
E-mail Address: *corpcomms@iata.org*
Web Address: www.iata.org
The International Air Transport Association (IATA) represents about 260 airlines in order to offer the highest standards of passenger and cargo service.

V.   Alternative Energy-Ethanol

Renewable Fuels Association (RFA)
1 Massachusetts Ave. NW, Ste. 820
Washington, DC 20001 US
Phone: 202-289-3835
E-mail Address: *info@ethanolrfa.org*
Web Address: www.ethanolrfa.org

The Renewable Fuels Association (RFA) is a trade organization representing the ethanol industry. It publishes a wealth of useful information, including a listing of biorefineries and monthly U.S. fuel ethanol production and demand.

VI.   Alternative Energy-Solar

Solar Energy Industries Association (SEIA)
805 15th St. NW, Ste. 510
Washington, DC 20005 US
Phone: 202-682-0556
Fax: 202-682-7779
E-mail Address: info@seia.org
Web Address: www.seia.org
Solar Energy Industries Association (SEIA) operates a web site that provides news for the solar energy industry, links to related products and companies and solar energy statistics.

VII.   Alternative Energy-Wind

American Wind Energy Association (AWEA)
1501 M St. NW, Ste. 1000
Washington, DC 20005 US
Phone: 202-383-2500
Fax: 202-383-2505
E-mail Address: windmail@awea.org
Web Address: www.awea.org
The American Wind Energy Association (AWEA) promotes wind energy as a clean source of electricity worldwide. Its website provides excellent resources for research, including an online library, discussions of legislation, and descriptions of wind technologies.

VIII.   Apparel Associations

American Apparel and Footwear Manufacturing Association (AAFA)
1601 N. Kent St., 12th Fl.
Arlington, VA 22209 US
Phone: 703-524-1864
Fax: 703-522-6741
Toll Free: 800-520-2262
E-mail Address: dvandyke@apparelandfootwear.org
Web Address: www.apparelandfootwear.org

The American Apparel and Footwear Manufacturing Association (AAFA) is the national trade association for the apparel, footwear and fashion industries and their suppliers.

IX.   Banking Industry Associations

American Bankers Association (ABA)
1120 Connecticut Ave. NW
Washington, DC 20036 US
Fax: 202-663-7578
Toll Free: 800-226-5377
E-mail Address: smarshall@aba.com
Web Address: www.aba.com
The American Bankers Association (ABA) represents banks of all sizes on issues of national importance for financial institutions and their customers. The site offers financial information and solutions, financial news and member access to further advice and content.

X.   Biotechnology and Biological Industry Associations

BioIndustry Association
14/15 Belgrave Sq.
London, SW1X 8PS UK
Phone: 44-20-7565-7190
Fax: 44-20-7565-7191
E-mail Address: admin@bioindustry.org
Web Address: www.bioindustry.org
The BioIndustry Association promotes bioscience development in the U.K. The organization operates a public affairs program, a conference and seminar program, trade missions and publications for internal and external audiences.

Biotechnology Industry Organization (BIO)
1201 Maryland Ave. SW, Ste. 900
Washington, DC 20024 US
Phone: 202-962-9200
Fax: 202-488-6301
E-mail Address: info@bio.org
Web Address: www.bio.org
The Biotechnology Industry Organization (BIO) is involved in the research and development of health care, agricultural, industrial and

environmental biotechnology products. BIO has both small and large member organizations.

XI.   Booksellers Associations

American Booksellers Association, Inc.
200 White Plains Rd., Ste. 600
Tarrytown, NY 10591 US
Fax: 914-591-2720
Toll Free: 800-637-0037
E-mail Address: info@bookweb.org
Web Address: www.bookweb.org
The American Booksellers Association is a nonprofit association representing independent bookstores in the United States.

XII.   Broadcasting, Cable, Radio & TV Associations

Academy of Television Arts and Sciences
5220 Lankershim Blvd.
North Hollywood, CA 91601-3109 US
Phone: 818-754-2800
Fax: 818-761-2827
E-mail Address: webmaster@emmys.org
Web Address: www.emmys.org
The Academy of Television Arts and Sciences is a nonprofit corporation devoted to the advancement of telecommunications arts and sciences and to fostering creative leadership in the telecommunications industry. It is one of three organizations that administer the Emmy Awards. It is responsible for prime time Emmys.

American Federation of Television and Radio Artists (AFTRA)
260 Madison Ave., 7th Fl.
New York, NY 10016-2401 US
Phone: 212-532-0800
Fax: 212-532-2242
E-mail Address: info@aftra.org
Web Address: www.aftra.org
The American Federation of Television and Radio Artists (AFTRA) represents actors and other professional performers and broadcasters in television, radio, sound recordings, non-broadcast/industrial programming and new technologies such as interactive programming and CD-ROMs.

American Women in Radio and Television, Inc. (AWRT)
1760 Old Meadow Rd., Ste. 500
McLean, VA 22102 US
Phone: 703-506-3290
Fax: 703-506-3266
E-mail Address: *info@awrt.org*
Web Address: www.awrt.org
American Women in Radio and Television (AWRT), founded in 1951, is a national nonprofit organization dedicated to advancing the role of women in electronic media and related fields.

Association of America's Public Television Stations (APTS)
2100 Crystal Dr., Ste. 700
Arlington, VA 22202 US
Phone: 202-654-4200
Fax: 202-654-4236
E-mail Address: *jeffrey@apts.org*
Web Address: www.apts.org
The Association of America's Public Television Stations (APTS) is a nonprofit membership organization formed to support the continued growth and development of strong and financially sound noncommercial television service for the American public.

Broadcast Education Association (BEA)
1771 N St. NW
Washington, DC 20036-2891 US
Phone: 202-429-3935
E-mail Address: *tbailey@nab.org*
Web Address: www.beaweb.org
The Broadcast Education Association (BEA) is the professional association for professors, industry professionals and graduate students interested in teaching and research related to electronic media and multimedia enterprises.

National Academy of Television Arts and Sciences
111 W. 57th St., Ste. 600
New York, NY 10019 US
Phone: 212-586-8424
Fax: 212-246-8129
E-mail Address: *info@emmyonline.tv*
Web Address: www.emmyonline.org
The National Academy of Television Arts and Sciences is dedicated to the advancement of the arts and sciences

of television and the promotion of creative leadership for artistic, educational and technical achievements within the television industry. It is responsible for awarding the Emmy Awards.

National Association of Broadcasters (NAB)
1771 N St. NW
Washington, DC 20036 US
Phone: 202-429-5300
Fax: 202-429-4199
E-mail Address: *nab@nab.org*
Web Address: www.nab.org
The National Association of Broadcasters (NAB) represents broadcasters for radio and television. The organization also provides benefits to employees of member companies and to individuals and companies that provide products and services to the electronic media industries.

National Association of Television Program Executives (NATPE)
5757 Wilshire Blvd., Penthouse 10
Los Angeles, CA 90036-3681 US
Phone: 310-453-4440
Fax: 310-453-5258
E-mail Address: *info@natpe.org*
Web Address: www.natpe.org
The National Association of Television Program Executives (NATPE) is the leading association for content professionals in the global television industry.

National Cable and Telecommunications Association (NCTA)
25 Massachusetts Ave. NW, Ste. 100
Washington, DC 20001 US
Phone: 202-222-2300
E-mail Address: *webmaster@ncta.com*
Web Address: www.ncta.com
The National Cable and Telecommunications Association (NCTA) is the principal trade association of the cable television industry in the United States.

Radio Television News Directors Association (RTNDA)
1600 K St. NW, Ste. 700
Washington, DC 20006-2838 US
Phone: 202-659-6510
Fax: 202-223-4007

Toll Free: 800-807-8632
E-mail Address: *rtnda@rtnda.org*
Web Address: www.rtnda.org
The Radio Television News Directors Association (RTNDA) is the world's largest professional organization exclusively committed to professionals in electronic journalism.

Satellite Broadcasting & Communications Association of America (SBCA)
1730 M St. NW, Ste. 600
Washington, DC 20036 US
Phone: 202-349-3620
Fax: 202-349-3621
Toll Free: 800-541-5981
E-mail Address: *info@sbca.org*
Web Address: www.sbca.com
The Satellite Broadcasting & Communications Association of America (SBCA) is the national trade organization representing all segments of the satellite consumer services industry.

Syndication Network Television Association (SNTA)
630 5th Ave., Ste. 2320
New York, NY 10111 US
Phone: 212-259-3740
Fax: 212-259-3770
E-mail Address: *mburg@snta.com*
Web Address: www.snta.com
The Syndication Network Television Association (SNTA) is an organization of national and independent television stations that syndicate television shows.

Women in Cable & Telecommunications (WICT)
14555 Avion Pkwy., Ste. 250
Chantilly, VA 20151 US
Phone: 703-234-9810
Fax: 703-817-1595
E-mail Address: *mnorthern@wict.org*
Web Address: www.wict.org
Women in Cable & Telecommunications (WICT) exists to advance the position and influence of women in media through leadership programs and services at both the national and local level.

XIII. Brokers & Trading

North American Securities Administrators Association, Inc. (NASAA)
750 1st St. NE, Ste. 1140
Washington, DC 20002 US
Phone: 202-737-0900
Fax: 202-783-3571
Web Address: www.nasaa.org
The North American Securities Administrators Association (NASAA) is the oldest international organization committed to investor protection. Its web site provides information on franchising and raising capital, as well as state blue sky securities laws and resources for small investment advisors.

XIV. Careers-Airlines/Flying

Aviation/Aerospace Jobs Page
NationJob, Inc.
601 SW 9th St., Stes. J&K
Des Moines, IA 50309 US
Fax: 515-283-1223
Toll Free: 888-526-5967
E-mail Address:
customerservice@nationjob.com
Web Address:
www.nationjob.com/aviation
The Aviation/Aerospace Jobs Page, a division of NationJob, Inc., features detailed aviation and aerospace job listings and company profiles.

Avjobs, Inc.
P.O. Box 630830
Littleton, CO 80163 US
Phone: 303-683-2322
Fax: 888-624-8691
E-mail Address: *info@avjobs.com*
Web Address: www.avjobs.com
Avjobs, Inc. is a group of employers dedicated to helping individuals obtain aviation, airline, aerospace and airport careers.

Flightdeck Recruitment Ltd.
82c East Hill
Colchester, Essex CO1 2QW UK
Phone: 44-1206-383730
Web Address:
www.flightdeckrecruitment.com
Flightdeck Recruitment Ltd. provides a link between aviation recruiters who are looking for flight deck crew and pilots or flight engineers who are seeking employment.

United States Air Force
Web Address: www.airforce.com
The web site of the United States Air Force offers information on basic training, careers, education, deployment, benefits and Air Force life.

XV. Careers-Banking

National Banking & Financial Service Network (NBFSN)
3075 Brickhouse Ct.
Virginia Beach, VA 23452-6860 US
Phone: 757-463-5766
Fax: 757-340-0826
E-mail Address: *susan@nbn-jobs.com*
Web Address: www.banking-financejobs.com
The National Banking & Financial Service Network (NBFSN) is made up of recruiting firms in the banking and financial services marketplace. The web site provides job listings.

XVI. Careers-Biotech

Biotechemployment.com
Phone: 561-630-5201
E-mail Address:
jobs@Biotechemployment.com
Web Address:
www.biotechemployment.com
Biotechemployment.com is an online resource for job seekers in biotechnology. The site's features includes resume posting, job search agents and employer profiles. It is part of the eJobstores.com, Inc., which includes the Health Care Job Store sites.

Chase Group (The)
10955 Lowell Ave., Ste. 500
Overland Park, KS 66210 US
Phone: 913-663-3100
Fax: 913-663-3131
E-mail Address:
chase@chasegroup.com
Web Address: www.chasegroup.com
The Chase Group is an executive search firm specializing in biomedical and pharmaceutical placement.

RPh on the Go
5510 Howard St.
Skokie, IL 60077-2620 US
Fax: 847-588-7060
Toll Free: 800-553-7359
E-mail Address: *rph@rphonthego.com*
Web Address: www.rphonthego.com
RPh on the Go places temporary and permanent qualified professionals in the pharmacy community.

XVII. Careers-Computers/Technology

Computerjobs.com, Inc.
280 Interstate N. Cir. SE, Ste. 300
Atlanta, GA 30339-2411 US
Toll Free: 800-850-0045
E-mail Address:
michael@marketingmax.com
Web Address: www.computerjobs.com
Computerjobs.com, Inc. is an employment web site that offers users a link to computer-related job opportunities organized by skill and market.

Dice
4101 NW Urbandale Dr.
Urbandale, IA 50322 US
Phone: 515-280-1144
Fax: 515-280-1452
Toll Free: 877-386-3323
Web Address: www.dice.com
Dice provides free employment services for IT jobs. The site includes advanced job searches by geographic location and category, availability announcements and resume postings, as well as employer profiles, a recruiter's page and career links. Dice is owned by Dice Holdings, Inc., a publicly traded company.

Institute for Electrical and Electronics Engineers (IEEE) Job Site
IEEE
3 Park Ave., 17th Fl.
New York, NY 10016-5997 US
Phone: 212-419-7900
Fax: 212-752-4929
Toll Free: 800-678-4333
E-mail Address: *ieeeusa@ieee.org*
Web Address: careers.ieee.org
The Institute for Electrical and Electronics Engineers (IEEE) Job Site provides a host of employment

services for technical professionals, employers and recruiters. The site offers job listings by geographic area, a resume bank and links to employment services.

Pencom Systems, Inc.
40 Fulton St.
New York, NY 10038-1850 US
Phone: 212-513-7777
Fax: 212-227-1854
E-mail Address: *tom@pencom.com*
Web Address: www.pencom.com
Pencom Systems, Inc., an open systems recruiting company, offers a web site geared toward high-technology and scientific professionals, featuring an interactive salary survey, career advisor, job listings and technology resources.

SearchTech Solutions
307 Orchard City Dr., Ste. 300
Campbell, CA 95008 US
Phone: 408-540-1800
Fax: 408-540-1815
Toll Free: 888-695-4362
E-mail Address: *resumes@stecs.com*
Web Address: www.stecs.com
SearchTech Solutions is a recruiting, placement and consulting firm focused on Engineering, Product Development and Innovation, Supply Chain and IT industries. Its web site offers resume writing assistance, including editing, writing and customizing.

XVIII.   Careers-First Time Jobs/New Grads

Alumni-Network Recruitment Corporation
Phone: 905-465-2547
E-mail Address: *karen@alumni-network.com*
Web Address: www.alumni-network.com
Alumni-Network Recruitment Corporation is a professional search and recruiting firm, specializing in ERP, E-Commerce and Engineering.

Black Collegian Online (The)
140 Carondelet St.
New Orleans, LA 70130 US
Phone: 504-523-0154
Web Address: www.black-collegian.com

The Black Collegian Online features listings for job and internship opportunities, as well as other tools for students of color; it is the web site of The Black Collegian Magazine, published by IMDiversity, Inc. The site includes a list of the top 100 minority corporate employers and an assessment of job opportunities.

Canadian Association of Career Educators and Employers (CACEE)
720 Spadina Ave., Ste. 202
Toronto, ON M5S 2T9 Canada
Fax: 416-929-5256
Toll Free: 866-922-3303
E-mail Address: *janinec@cacee.com*
Web Address: www.cacee.com
The Canadian Association of Career Educators and Employers (CACEE) is a partnership of employer recruiters and career services professionals. The group provides information, advice and professional development opportunities to employers, career services professionals and students.

Collegegrad.com, Inc.
234 E. College Ave., Ste. 200
State College, PA 16801 US
Phone: 262-375-6700
Web Address: www.collegegrad.com
Collegegrad.com offers in-depth resources for college students and recent grads seeking entry-level jobs.

Job Web
Nat'l Association of Colleges & Employers (NACE)
62 Highland Ave.
Bethlehem, PA 18017-9085 US
Phone: 610-868-1421
Fax: 610-868-0208
Toll Free: 800-544-5272
E-mail Address: *editors@jobweb.com*
Web Address: www.jobweb.com
Job Web, owned and sponsored by National Association of Colleges and Employers (NACE), displays job openings and employer descriptions. The site also offers a database of career fairs, searchable by state or keyword, with contact information.

MBAjobs.net
Fax: 413-556-8849
E-mail Address: *contact@mbajobs.net*
Web Address: www.mbajobs.net

MBAjobs.net is a unique international service for MBA students and graduates, employers, recruiters and business schools. The MBAjobs.net service is provided by WebInfoCo.

MonsterTRAK
11845 W. Olympic Blvd., Ste. 500
Los Angeles, CA 90064 US
Toll Free: 800-999-8725
E-mail Address: *student.monstertrak@monster.com*
Web Address: www.monstertrak.monster.com
MonsterTRAK features links to hundreds of university and college career centers across the U.S. with entry-level job listings categorized by industry. Major companies can also utilize MonsterTRAK.

National Association of Colleges and Employers (NACE)
62 Highland Ave.
Bethlehem, PA 18017-9085 US
Phone: 610-868-1421
Fax: 610-868-0208
Toll Free: 800-544-5272
E-mail Address: *mcollins@naceweb.org*
Web Address: www.naceweb.org
The National Association of Colleges and Employers (NACE) is a premier U.S. organization representing college placement offices and corporate recruiters who focus on hiring new grads.

XIX.   Careers-General Job Listings

6FigureJobs
25 3rd St., Ste. 230
Stamford, CT 06905 US
Toll Free: 800-605-5154
Web Address: www.6figurejobs.com
6FigureJobs offers executives a database of high-level positions. Membership is free for qualified individuals.

America's Job Bank
Toll Free: 877-348-0502
E-mail Address: *info@careeronestop.org*
Web Address: www.jobsearch.org
America's Job Bank offers an extensive set of links to job banks for each of the

50 states. Additionally, it has aggregate salary information for a variety of job titles across the U.S.

Career Exposure, Inc.
805 SW Broadway, Ste. 2250
Portland, OR 97205 US
Phone: 503-221-7779
Fax: 503-221-7780
E-mail Address: *lisam@mackenzie-marketing.com*
Web Address:
www.careerexposure.com
Career Exposure, Inc. is an online career center and job placement service, with resources for employers, recruiters and job seekers.

CareerBuilder, Inc.
200 N. LaSalle St., Ste. 1100
Chicago, IL 60601 US
Phone: 773-527-3600
Toll Free: 800-638-4212
Web Address: www.careerbuilder.com
CareerBuilder, Inc. focuses on the needs of companies and also provides a database of job openings. The site has 1.5 million jobs posted by 300,000 employers, and receives an average 23 million unique visitors monthly. The company also operates online career centers for 150 newspapers, 1,400 partners and other online portals such as America Online. Resumes are sent directly to the company, and applicants can set up a special e-mail account for job-seeking purposes. CareerBuilder is primarily a joint venture between three newspaper giants: The McClatchy Company (which recently acquired former partner Knight Ridder), Gannett Co., Inc. and Tribune Company. In 2007, Microsoft acquired a minority interest in CareerBuilder, allowing the site to ally itself with MSN.

Careers Organization (The)
E-mail Address: *info@Careers.Org*
Web Address: www.careers.org
The Career Organization is a job resource center with links to jobs and pointers to other career-related web sites as well as links to associations, franchising opportunities and library resources.

Collegerecruiter.com
3109 W 50 St., Ste. 121
Minneapolis, MN 55410-2102 US
Phone: 952-848-2211
Fax: 702-537-2227
Toll Free: 800-835-4989
E-mail Address:
Steven@CollegeRecruiter.com
Web Address:
www.collegerecruiter.com
Collegerecruiter.com provides college students with internship, part-time and summer job listings. Recent graduates can search for career opportunities by category and location. The site also provides information about student loans and loan consolidation.

ContractJobHunter
C. E. Publications, Inc.
P.O. Box 3006
Bothell, WA 98041-3006 US
Phone: 425-806-5200
Fax: 425-806-5585
E-mail Address: *staff@cjhunter.com*
Web Address: www.ceweekly.wa.com
ContractJobHunter is a web-based version of the magazine Contract Employment Weekly Online. It posts job listings and links to contract firms. Libraries for reference materials and resume writing guidelines are also offered. The site is a service of C. E. Publications, Inc.

EmploymentGuide
150 Granby St.
Norfolk, VA 23510 US
Toll Free: 877-876-4039
Web Address:
www.employmentguide.com
EmploymentGuide offers general career resources along with lists of position openings, company profiles and a resume database. It also circulates a free print publication.

EscapeArtist.com Inc.
832-1245 World Trade Ctr.
Panama, WTC-0832 Republic of Panama
Fax: 786-513-3702
Web Address: www.escapeartist.com
EscapeArtist.com Inc.'s web site provides job searches for overseas positions, as well as international working condition resources and immigration information.

ExecuNet, Inc.
295 Westport Ave.
Norwalk, CT 06851 US
Toll Free: 800-637-3126
E-mail Address:
member.services@execunet.com
Web Address: www.execunet.com
ExecuNet, Inc. is an executive career management information and contact service.

Executiveagent.com
Kennedy Information, Inc.
1 Phoenix Mill Ln., 3rd Fl.
Peterborough, NH 03458 US
Phone: 603-924-1006
Fax: 603-924-4034
Toll Free: 800-531-0007
Web Address:
www.executiveagent.com
Executiveagent.com allows senior-level professionals to have their resumes sent to executive placement firms for a fee. The site is owned by Kennedy Information, Inc.

Getajob
Web Address: www.getajob.com
Getajob provides job listings, employment articles, a resume database, book titles and newsgroups for the job seeker.

Guru.com
5001 Baum Blvd., Ste. 760
Pittsburgh, PA 15213 US
Fax: 412-687-4466
Toll Free: 888-678-0136
E-mail Address: *pr@guru.com*
Web Address: www.guru.com
Guru.com is an excellent site for freelancers and contract workers, especially in the IT field.

Higheredjobs.com
328 Innovation Blvd., Ste. 300
State College, PA 16803 US
Phone: 814-861-3080
Fax: 814-861-3082
E-mail Address:
sales@HigherEdJobs.com
Web Address: www.higheredjobs.com
Higheredjobs.com lists job vacancies in colleges and universities.

IMDiversity, Inc.
140 Carondelet St.
New Orleans, LA 70130 US

Phone: 504-523-0154
Fax: 504-523-9271
Web Address: www.imdiversity.com
IMDiversity, Inc. provides job listings
and career development information.
The web site also has divisions for
particular minority groups.

Job Search USA
E-mail Address:
info@jobsearchusa.org
Web Address: www.jobsearchusa.org
Job Search USA is a major job posting
site that contains job opportunities
classified by a variety of keywords.

JobCentral
DirectEmployers Association, Inc.
9002 N. Purdue Rd., Quad III, Ste. 100
Indianapolis, IN 46268 US
Phone: 317-874-9000
Fax: 317-874-9100
Toll Free: 866-268-6206
E-mail Address: *info@jobcentral.com*
Web Address: www.jobcentral.com
JobCentral, operated by the nonprofit
DirectEmployers Association, Inc.,
links users directly to hundreds of
thousands of job opportunities posted
on the sites of participating employers,
thus bypassing the usual job search
sites. This saves employers money and
allows job seekers to access many
more job opportunities.

Jobsinthemoney.com
4101 NW Urbandale Dr.
Urbandale, IA 50322 US
Phone: 515-280-1144
Fax: 515-280-1452
Toll Free: 800-979-3423
E-mail Address:
cs@jobsinthemoney.com
Web Address:
www.jobsinthemoney.com
Jobsinthemoney.com provides
employment listings in the finance
industry as well as job tools, such as
salary surveys, resume writing
assistance and industry news. It is
owned by Dice, a part of Dice
Holdings, Inc.

LaborMarketInfo
Employment Dev. Dept., Labor Market
Info. Div.
Info. Services Div., 7000 Franklin
Blvd., Ste. 1100

Sacramento, CA 95823 US
Phone: 916-262-2162
Fax: 916-262-2352
Web Address:
www.labormarketinfo.edd.ca.gov
LaborMarketInfo, formerly the
California Cooperative Occupational
Information System, is geared to
providing job seekers and employers a
wide range of resources, namely the
ability to find, access and use labor
market information and services. It
provides demographical statistics for
employment on both a local and
regional level, as well as career
searching tools for California residents.
The web site is sponsored by
California's Employment Development
Office.

Mediabistro.com
475 Park Ave. S., 4th Fl.
New York, NY 10016 US
Phone: 212-389-2000
Fax: 212-966-8984
E-mail Address:
laurelT@mediabistro.com
Web Address: www.mediabistro.com
Mediabistro.com offers an array of
employment resources, including job
listings in the media industry.

Monster Worldwide, Inc.
622 3rd Ave., 39th Fl.
New York, NY 10017 US
Phone: 212-351-7000
Fax: 646-658-0541
Toll Free: 800-666-7837
E-mail Address:
steve.sylven@monster.com
Web Address:
www.monsterworldwide.com
Monster Worldwide, Inc. primarily
operates Monster.com, an electronic
career center that displays hundreds of
thousands of job opportunities in 36
countries worldwide. Job seekers can
build and store a resume online and
find job listings that match their
profiles. Monster.com e-mails any
resulting hits once per week. Monster
Worldwide also offers some Internet
advertising services.

NationJob, Inc.
601 SW 9th St., Ste. J&K
Des Moines, IA 50309 US
Fax: 515-283-1223

Toll Free: 888-526-5967
E-mail Address:
customerservice@nationjob.com
Web Address: www.nationjob.com
NationJob, Inc.'s web site allows users
can develop a profile of the ideal job
based on the criterion of location,
industry, salary; and, if they provide an
e-mail address, wait for appropriate
listings to be sent to them through the
firm's PJScout feature.

NETSHARE, Inc.
83 Hamilton Dr., Ste. 202
Novato, CA 94949 US
Toll Free: 800-241-5642
E-mail Address:
netshare@netshare.com
Web Address: www.netshare.com
Netshare provides access to exclusive
listings of executive jobs that pay
$70,000 and up. Job seekers pay either
$37.50/month or $395/year for the
service.

Net-Temps
55 Middlesex St., Ste. 220
North Chelmsford, MA 01863 US
Fax: 978-251-7250
Toll Free: 800-307-0062
E-mail Address: *service@net-
temps.com*
Web Address: www.net-temps.com
Net-Temps.com is operated by
professional career consultants and
features job listings and job seeking
tips.

Recruiters Online Network
947 Essex Lane
Medina, OH 44256 US
Phone: 888-364-4667
Fax: 888-237-8686
E-mail Address:
info@recruitersonline.com
Web Address:
www.recruitersonline.com
The Recruiters Online Network
provides job postings from thousands
of recruiters, Careers Online Magazine,
a resume database, as well as other
career resources.

True Careers, Inc.
Web Address: www.truecareers.com
True Careers, Inc. offers job listings
and provides an array of career
resources. The company also offers a

search of over 2 million scholarships. It is partnered with CareerBuilder.com, which powers its career information and resume posting functions.

USAJOBS
U.S. Office of Personnel Management
1900 E St. NW
Washington, DC 20415 US
Phone: 202-606-1800
Web Address: usajobs.opm.gov
USAJOBS, a program of the U.S. Office of Personnel Management, is the official job site for the U.S. Federal Government. It provides a comprehensive list of U.S. government jobs, allowing users to search for employment by location; agency; type of work, using the Federal Government's numerical identification code, the General Schedule (GS) Series; or by senior executive positions. It also has a special veterans' employment section; an information center, offering resume and interview tips and other useful information such as hiring trends and a glossary of Federal terms; and allows users to create a profile and post a resume.

Wall Street Journal - CareerJournal
Wall Street Journal
200 Liberty St.
New York, NW 10281 US
Phone: 212-416-2000
E-mail Address:
christine.mohan@dowjones.com
Web Address: online.wsj.com/careers
The Wall Street Journal's CareerJournal, an executive career site, features a job database with thousands of available positions; career news and employment related articles; and advice regarding resume writing, interviews, networking, office life and job hunting.

Yahoo! HotJobs
45 W. 18th St., 6th Fl.
New York, NY 10011 US
Phone: 646-351-5300
Web Address: hotjobs.yahoo.com
Yahoo! HotJobs, designed for experienced professionals, employers and job seekers, is a Yahoo-owned site that provides company profiles, a resume posting service and a resume

workshop. The site allows posters to block resumes from being viewed by certain companies and provides a notification service of new jobs.

XX.   Careers-Health Care

Medicalworkers.com
191 University Blvd., Ste. 252
Denver, CO 80206 US
Phone: 720-227-9364
E-mail Address:
cs@medicalworkers.com
Web Address:
www.medicalworkers.com
Medicalworkers.com is an employment site for medical and health care professionals.

Medjump.com
7119 E. Shea Blvd., Ste. 109-535
Scottsdale, AZ 85254 US
E-mail Address: *info@medjump.net*
Web Address: www.medjump.com
Medjump.com is dedicated to empowering health care and medical-related professionals with the necessary tools to market their abilities and skills.

Medzilla, Inc.
P.O. Box 1710
Marysville, WA 98270 US
Phone: 360-657-5681
Fax: 775-514-9440
E-mail Address:
mgroutage@medzilla.com
Web Address: www.medzilla.com
Medzilla, Inc.'s web site offers job searches, salary surveys, a search agent and information on health care employment.

Monster Career Advice-Healthcare
Monster Worldwide, Inc.
622 3rd Ave.
New York, NY 10017 US
Phone: 212-351-7000
Toll Free: 800-666-7837
Web Address: career-advice.monster.com/get-the-job/healthcare/home.aspx
Monster Career Advice-Healthcare, a service of Monster Worldwide, Inc., provides job listings, job searches and search agents for the medical field.

NationJob Network-Medical and Health Care Jobs Page
601 SW 9th St., Ste. J&K
Des Moines, IA 50309 US
Fax: 515-283-1223
Toll Free: 888-526-5967
E-mail Address:
customerservice@nationjob.com
Web Address:
www.nationjob.com/medical
The NationJob Network-Medical and Health Care Jobs Page offers information and listings for health care employment.

Nurse-Recruiter.com
36 Washington St., Ste. 170
Wellesley, MA 02481 US
Toll Free: 866-560-1034
E-mail Address: *info@nurse-recruiter.com*
Web Address: www.nurse-recruiter.com
Nurse-Recruiter.com is a nurse-owned, web-centric company devoted to bringing health care employers and the nursing community together.

PracticeLink
415 2nd Ave.
P.O. Box 100
Hinton, WV 25951 US
Fax: 877-847-0120
Toll Free: 800-776-8383
E-mail Address:
info@practicelink.com
Web Address: www.practicelink.com
PracticeLink is one of the largest physician employment web sites. It is a free service used by more than 18,000 practice-seeking physicians annually to quickly search and locate potential physician practice opportunities. PracticeLink is financially supported by more than 700 hospitals, medical groups, private practices and health care systems that advertise more than 5,000 opportunities.

XXI.   Careers-Job Listings for Seniors

Dinosaur Exchange
Dino-X Ltd., P.O. Box 100
Sydney Vane House Admiral Park
St Peter Port, Guernsey GY1 3EL
Channel Islands

E-mail Address:
CustomerSupport@dinosaur-exchange.com
Web Address: www.dinosaur-exchange.com
Dinosaur Exchange, opened in 2003, is a job forum for the elderly, which allows seniors to post resumes and be contacted by employers. Dino-X Ltd. owns and operates the web site.

Employment Network for Retired Government Experts (ENRGE)
Zavala, Inc.
P.O. Box 1532
N. Falmouth, MA 02556 US
Phone: 508-564-4140
Web Address: www.enrge.us
The Employment Network for Retired Government Experts (ENRGE) helps government employees to remain active in their professions after retirement. ENERGE is the business name of Zavala, Inc.

Senior Job Bank
P.O. Box 508
Marlborough, MA 01752-0508 US
Phone: 508-624-9641
Toll Free: 888-501-0804
E-mail Address:
publisher@seniorjobbank.com
Web Address: www.seniorjobbank.org
The Senior Job Bank web site offers an easy, effective and free method for senior citizens to find occasional, part-time, flexible, temporary or full-time jobs.

Seniors4Hire.org
The Forward Group
7071 Warner Ave. F466
Huntington Beach, CA 92647 US
Phone: 714-848-0996
Fax: 714-848-5445
E-mail Address:
info@seniors4hire.org
Web Address: www.seniors4hire.org
Seniors4Hire.org is an online career center with job postings, employment resources and information on community service employment programs for older workers, retirees and senior citizens.

YourEncore
20 N. Meridian St., Ste. 802
Indianapolis, IN 46204 US

Phone: 317-336-9301
E-mail Address:
webmaster@yourencore.com
Web Address: www.yourencore.com
YourEncore is a program that seeks to employ retirees by matching them with member companies. The web site utilizes retirees mainly in the areas of engineering, science and product development.

XXII.   Careers-Job Reference Tools

CareerXroads (CXR)
Mark Mehler
P.O. Box 253
Kendall Park, NJ 08824 US
Phone: 732-821-6652
E-mail Address:
mmc@careerxroads.com
Web Address: www.careerxroads.com
CareerXroads (CXR) publishes an annual guide on job and resume web sites. It was cofounded by Gerry Crispin and Mark Mehler.

Job-Hunt.org
NETability, Inc.
186 Main St.
Marlborough, MA 01752 US
Phone: 508-624-6261
E-mail Address: *info@job-hunt.org*
Web Address: www.job-hunt.org
Job-Hunt.org, rather than collecting resumes or posting job vacancies, offers a vast list of job listing web sites and links to helpful job search tools. It is owned by NETability, Inc.

JobStar
E-mail Address:
electrajobstar@earthlink.net
Web Address: www.jobstar.org
JobStar has a salary info link to over 300 different salary information and salary survey sites. It also contains job listings focused on the California market.

Joyce Lain Kennedy's Careers
Sun Features Inc.
P.O. Box 368
Cardiff, CA 92007 US
Web Address: www.sunfeatures.com
Provides links to recommended employment sites, as well as links to Joyce Lain Kennedy's books and

booklets and her well-respected career tips.

NewsVoyager
Newspaper Association of America
4401 Wilson Blvd., Ste. 900
Arlington, VA 22203-1867 US
Phone: 571-366-1000
Fax: 571-366-1195
E-mail Address: *sally.clarke@naa.org*
Web Address: www.newsvoyager.com
NewsVoyager, a service of the Newspaper Association of America (NAA), links individuals to local, national and international newspapers. Job seekers can search through thousands of classified sections.

Quintessential Careers (QC)
DeLand, Fl 32720 US
E-mail Address:
randall@quintcareers.com
Web Address: www.quintcareers.com
Quintessential Careers (QC) provides a large collection of data and links for job seekers. Includes advice, tools and job postings and offers a guide to researching companies.

Vault.com, Inc.
150 W. 22nd St., 5th Fl.
New York, NY 10011 US
Phone: 212-366-4212
E-mail Address:
feedback@staff.vault.com
Web Address: www.vault.com
Vault.com, Inc. is a comprehensive career web site for employers and employees, with job postings and valuable information on a wide variety of industries. Vault gears many of its features toward MBAs. The site has been recognized by Forbes and Fortune Magazines.

Wageweb
600 Research Rd., Ste. 8
Richmond, VA 23236 US
Phone: 804-363-1792
Fax: 804-378-7593
E-mail Address:
custserv@wageweb.com
Web Address: www.wageweb.com
Wageweb makes salary survey data available online. The web site provides access to national average salaries for a large number of positions.

Wetfeet.com
101 Howard St., Ste. 300
San Francisco, CA 94105 US
Phone: 415-284-7900
Fax: 415-284-7910
Web Address: www.wetfeet.com
Wetfeet.com provides an excellent combination of links and resources for job seekers.

What Color is Your Parachute?
E-mail Address:
rnbolles@jobhuntersbible.com
Web Address:
www.jobhuntersbible.com
This net guide to Dick Bolle's best-selling book is based on the "Job-Hunting on the Internet" chapter. Designed to aid job hunters and career changers who want to use the Internet as part of their job search, the site provides links to job listing, resume, career counseling, contacts and research sites.

XXIII. Careers-Restaurants

Foodservice.com
Phone: 678-256-8014
Toll Free: 800-896-4442
E-mail Address:
customercare@Foodservice.com
Web Address: www.foodservice.com
Foodservice.com, managed and run by Food Service Interactive, LLC, offers web site design and job search services for the food service industry.

Resources in Food, Inc. (RIF)
1007 N. Main St.
Columbia, IL 62236 US
Phone: 618-281-3100
Fax: 618-281-3110
Toll Free: 877-743-1100
E-mail Address:
rifchicago@rifood.com
Web Address: www.rifood.com
Resources in Food (RIF) provides professional management placement for the hospitality industry.

XXIV. Careers-Telecommunications

Call Center Careers
6525 Gunpark Dr.
Ste. 570, PMB 127
Boulder, CO 80301 US

Phone: 303-527-1440
Fax: 303-530-0154
Toll Free: 877-562-8588
E-mail Address:
sales@callcentercareers.com
Web Address:
www.callcentercareers.com
Call Center Careers provides recruiting and staffing services to the call center industry.

XXV. Communications Professional Associations

Association for Women In Communications (AWC)
3337 Duke St.
Alexandria, VA 22314 US
Phone: 703-370-7436
Fax: 703-370-7437
E-mail Address: *info@womcom.org*
Web Address: www.womcom.org
The Association for Women In Communications (AWC) is a professional organization that works for the advancement of women across all communications disciplines by recognizing excellence, promoting leadership and positioning its members at the forefront of the communications industry.

International Association of Business Communicators (IABC)
1 Hallidie Plaza, Ste. 600
San Francisco, CA 94102 US
Phone: 415-544-4700
Fax: 415-544-4747
Toll Free: 800-776-4222
E-mail Address: *jugalde@iabc.com*
Web Address: www.iabc.com
The International Association of Business Communicators (IABC) is the leading resource for effective business communication practices.

XXVI. Computer & Electronics Industry Associations

AeA
5201 Great America Pkwy. #400
Santa Clara, CA 95054 US
Phone: 408-987-4200
Fax: 408-987-4298
Toll Free: 800-284-4232
E-mail Address:
anne_caliguiri@aeanet.org
Web Address: www.aeanet.org

AeA, formerly the American Electronics Association, is a trade association which represents thousands of U.S. electronics firms, including electronic systems and component manufacturers, suppliers and end users. It also publishes the annual AeA Directory with geographic and product indexes.

Association of Electronics Industries of Singapore (AEIS)
1010 Dover Rd., No. 02-03, SPGG
139658 Singapore
Phone: 65-6776-1880
Fax: 65-6776-0238
E-mail Address: *hamzah@epc.com.sg*
Web Address: www.aeis.org.sg
The Association of Electronics Industries of Singapore (AEIS) is the country's representative of electronics business, covering manufacturers of industrial electronics, electronics components and consumer electronics products as well as industrial electronics companies associated with the electronics industry.

Association of the Computer and Multimedia Industry of Malaysia (PIKOM)
1106 & 1107, Block B, Phileo Damansara II
No. 15, Jalan 16/11
Petaling Jaya, Selangor Darul Ehsan
46350 Malaysia
Phone: 603-7955-2922
Fax: 603-7955-2933
E-mail Address: *info@pikom.org.my*
Web Address: www.pikom.org.my
The Association of the Computer and Multimedia Industry of Malaysia, or, in Malay, Persatuan Industri Komputer dan Multimedia Malaysia (PIKOM), is the national association representing the information and communications technology (ICT) industry in Malaysia.

Communications Industry Association of Japan (CIAJ)
3rd Fl., JEI Hamamatsucho Bldg.
2-2-12 Hamamatsucho, Minato-ku
Tokyo, 105-0013 Japan
Phone: 81-3-5403-9363
Fax: 81-3-5463-9360
E-mail Address: *webmaster@ciaj.or.jp*
Web Address: www.ciaj.or.jp

The Communications Industry Association of Japan (CIAJ) works to help the development of the communication and information network industry in Japan through the promotion of info-communication technologies.

Electronic Industries Association of India (ELCINA)
ELCINA House, 422 Okhla Industrial Estate
New Delhi, 110020 India
Phone: 91-11-2692-4597
Fax: 91-11-2692-3440
E-mail Address: *elcina@vsnl.com*
Web Address: www.elcina.com
The Electronic Industries Association of India (ELCINA) is an organization for the promotion of electronic hardware manufacturing through active representation and advice to the Indian government.

Electronics and Computer Software Export Promotion Council (ESC)
3rd Fl., PHD House
Opp. Asiad Village
New Delhi, 110016 India
Phone: 91-11-2696-5103
Fax: 91-11-2685-3412
E-mail Address: *esc@vsnl.net*
Web Address: www.escindia.in
The Electronics and Computer Software Export Promotion Council (ESC) represents the info-communication technology industry through electronics and IT trade facilitation.

Electronics Technicians Association (ETA)
5 Depot St.
Greencastle, IN 46135 US
Phone: 765-653-8262
Fax: 765-653-4287
Toll Free: 800-288-3824
E-mail Address: *eta@eta-i.org*
Web Address: www.eta-i.org
The Electronics Technicians Association (ETA) is a nonprofit professional association for electronics technicians. The firm provides recognized professional credentials for electronics technicians.

Federation of Malaysia Manufacturers (FMM)
Wisma FMM No. 3, Persiaran Dagang, PJU 9
Bandar Sri Damansara
Kuala Lumpur, 52200 Malaysia
Phone: 603-6276-1211
Fax: 603-6274-1266
E-mail Address: *webmaster@fmm.org.my*
Web Address: www.fmm.org.my
The Federation of Malaysian Manufacturers is an economic organization for the electric and electronic industry in Malaysia.

Indian Electrical & Electronics Manufacturers Association (IEEMA)
501 Kakad Chambers
132 Dr. Annie Besant Rd., Worli
Mumbai, 400018 India
Phone: 91-22-2493-0532
Fax: 91-22-2493-2705
E-mail Address: *mumbai@ieema.org*
Web Address: www.ieema.org
The Indian Electrical & Electronics Manufacturers Association (IEEMA) represents all sectors of the electrical and allied products businesses of the Indian electrical industry.

Manufacturers' Association for Information Technology (MAIT)
4th Fl., PHD House
Opp. Asian Games Village
New Delhi, 110-016 India
Phone: 91-11-2685-5487
Fax: 91-11-2685-1321
E-mail Address: *mait@vsnl.com*
Web Address: www.mait.com
The Manufacturers' Association for Information Technology (MAIT) is an organization that focuses on the promotion of the hardware, training, design/R&D and the associated services sectors of the Indian IT industry.

National Electrical Manufacturers Association (NEMA)
1300 N. 17th St., Ste. 1752
Rosslyn, VA 22209 US
Phone: 703-841-3200
Fax: 703-841-5900
E-mail Address: *communications@nema.org*
Web Address: www.nema.org

The National Electrical Manufacturers Association (NEMA) develops standards for the electrical manufacturing industry and promotes safety in the manufacture and use of electrical products.

Semiconductor & Electronics Industries in the Philippines, Inc. (SEIPI)
Unit 902, Tower 2, Ayala Ave.
Makati City, 1200 Philippines
Phone: 632-844-9028
Fax: 632-844-9037
E-mail Address: *philippine.electronics@seipi.org.ph*
Web Address: www.seipi.org.ph
The SEIPI Foundation is an organization of foreign and local semiconductor and electronics companies in the Philippines.

Semiconductor Industry Association (SIA)
181 Metro Dr., Ste. 450
San Jose, CA 95110 US
Phone: 408-436-6600
Fax: 408-436-6646
E-mail Address: *mailbox@sia-online.org*
Web Address: www.sia-online.org
The Semiconductor Industry Association (SIA) is a trade association representing the semiconductor industry in the U.S. Through its coalition of 95 companies, SIA represents more than 85% of semiconductor production in the U.S. The coalition aims to advance the competitiveness of the chip industry and shape public policy on issues particular to the industry.

Singapore Confederation of Industries
1 Science Center Rd., No. 02-02
609077 Singapore
Phone: 65-6826-3035
Fax: 65-6822-8828
E-mail Address: *JaniceKWok@SCI.org.sg*
Web Address: www.SCI.org.sg
The Singapore Confederation of Industries (SCI) represents the manufacturing industry in Singapore, and helps its members deal issues such as productivity enhancement, research and development, technological

upgrading and innovation and worker training.

Taiwan Electrical and Electronic Manufacturers' Association (TEEMA)
Min Chuan E. Rd., 6th Fl., No. 109
Taipei, 114 Taiwan
Phone: 886-2-8792-6666
Fax: 886-2-8792-6088
The Taiwan Electrical and Electronic Manufacturers' Association (TEEMA) works as an intermediary between its members and the government to help the industry to succeed.

Telecom Equipment Manufacturers Association of India (TEMA)
PHD House, 4th Fl.
New Delhi, 110016 India
Phone: 91-11-685-9621
Fax: 91-11-685-9620
E-mail Address: *TEMA@vsnl.com*
Web Address:
www.tfci.com/cni/tema.htm
The Telecom Equipment Manufacturers Association of India (TEMA) is national organization for companies in the telecommunications industry. The group disseminates and exchanges information with the Indian government, foreign agencies, embassies, trade missions, Indian missions abroad and leading international trade associations.

The Federation of Thai Industries Electrical, Electronics and Allied Industries Club (FTI)
60 New Rachadapisek Rd., 4th Fl.,
Zone C, Klongtoey.
Bangkok, 10110 Thailand
Phone: 66-2-345-1000
Fax: 66-2-345-1296-99
E-mail Address:
information@off.fti.or.th
The Federation of Thai Industries (FTI) is the organization for the Electrical, Electronics and Allied Industries in Thailand.

Vietnam Electronic Industries Association (VEIA)
11B Phan Huy Chú, Hoàn Ki?m
Hà Noi, Vietnam
Phone: 84-4-933-2845
Fax: 84-4-933-2846
E-mail Address: *veia-vn@hn.vnn.vn*

Web Address: www.VEIA.org.vn
Vietnam Electronic Industries Association (VEIA) is the representative body for the electronic businesses in Vietnam.

XXVII. Consulting Industry Associations

American Association of Healthcare Consultants (AAHC)
5938 N. Drake Ave.
Chicago, IL 60659 US
Fax: 773-463-3552
Toll Free: 888-350-2242
E-mail Address: *info@aahcmail.org*
Web Address: www.aahc.net
The American Association of Healthcare Consultants (AAHC) is a professional society for credentialed consultants practicing in health care organization and delivery.

XXVIII. Corporate Information Resources

bizjournals.com
120 W. Morehead St., Ste. 400
Charlotte, NC 28202 US
Web Address: www.bizjournals.com
Bizjournals.com is the online media division of American City Business Journals, the publisher of dozens of leading city business journals nationwide. It provides access to research into the latest news regarding companies small and large.

Business Wire
44 Montgomery St., 39th Fl.
San Francisco, CA 94104 US
Phone: 415-986-4422
Fax: 415-788-5335
Toll Free: 800-227-0845
Web Address: www.businesswire.com
Business Wire offers news releases, industry- and company-specific news, top headlines, conference calls, IPOs on the Internet, media services and access to tradeshownews.com and BW Connect On-line through its informative and continuously updated web site.

Edgar Online, Inc.
50 Washington St., 11th Fl.
Norwalk, CT 06854 US
Phone: 203-852-5666

Fax: 203-852-5667
Toll Free: 800-416-6651
E-mail Address:
dcolgren@colcomgroup.com
Web Address: www.edgar-online.com
Edgar Online, Inc. is a gateway and search tool for viewing corporate documents, such as annual reports on Form 10-K, filed with the U.S. Securities and Exchange Commission.

PR Newswire Association LLC
810 7th Ave., 32nd Fl.
New York, NY 10019 US
Phone: 201-360-6700
Toll Free: 800-832-5522
E-mail Address:
information@prnewswire.com
Web Address: www.prnewswire.com
PR Newswire Association LLC provides comprehensive communications services for public relations and investor relations professionals ranging from information distribution and market intelligence to the creation of online multimedia content and investor relations web sites. Users can also view recent corporate press releases. The Association is owned by United Business Media plc.

Silicon Investor
100 W. Main
P.O. Box 29
Freeman, MO 64746 US
E-mail Address:
admin_dave@techstocks.com
Web Address:
siliconinvestor.advfn.com
Silicon Investor is focused on providing information about technology companies. The company's web site serves as a financial discussion forum and offers quotes, profiles and charts.

XXIX. Disabling Conditions

Job Accommodation Network (JAN)
P.O. Box 6080
Morgantown, WV 26506-6080 US
Phone: 304-293-7186
Fax: 304-293-5407
Toll Free: 800-526-7234
E-mail Address: *jan@jan.wvu.edu*
Web Address: janweb.icdi.wvu.edu

The Job Accommodation Network (JAN) is a free consulting service that provides information about job accommodations, the Americans with Disabilities Act and the employability of people with disabilities.

XXX.   Economic Data & Research

STAT-USA/Internet
STAT-USA, HCHB, Rm. 4885
U.S. Department of Commerce
Washington, DC 20230 US
Phone: 202-482-1986
Fax: 202-482-2164
Toll Free: 800-782-8872
E-mail Address: *statmail@esa.doc.gov*
Web Address: www.stat-usa.gov
STAT-USA/Internet offers daily economic news, statistical releases and databases relating to export and trade, as well as the domestic economy. It is provided by STAT-USA, which is an agency in the Economics & Statistics Administration of the U.S. Department of Commerce. The site mainly consists of two main databases, the State of the Nation (SOTN), which focuses on the current state of the U.S. economy; and the Global Business Opportunities (GLOBUS) & the National Trade Data Bank (NTDB), which deals with U.S. export opportunities, global political/socio-economic conditions and other world economic issues.

XXXI.   Electrical Engineering Industry Associations

International Society for Optical Engineering (SPIE)
1000 20th St.
Bellingham, WA 98225-6705 US
Phone: 360-676-3290
Fax: 360-647-1445
Toll Free: 888-504-8171
E-mail Address: *CustomerService@SPIE.org*
Web Address: www.spie.org
The International Society for Optical Engineering (SPIE) is a nonprofit technical society aimed at the advancement and dissemination of knowledge in optics, photonics and imaging.

XXXII.   Energy Associations-Electric Power

American Public Power Association (APPA)
1875 Connecticut Ave. NW, Ste. 1200
Washington, DC 20009-5715 US
Phone: 202-467-2900
Fax: 202-467-2910
E-mail Address: *mrufe@appanet.org*
Web Address: www.appanet.org
The American Public Power Association (APPA) is a nonprofit service organization for the country's community-owned electric utilities, dedicated to advancing the public policy interests of its members and their consumers.

Edison Electric Institute (EEI)
701 Pennsylvania Ave. NW
Washington, DC 20004-2696 US
Phone: 202-508-5000
E-mail Address: *feedback@eei.org*
Web Address: www.eei.org
The Edison Electric Institute (EEI) is an association of U.S. shareholder-owned electric companies as well as worldwide affiliates and industry associates. Its web site provides energy news and a link to Electric Perspectives magazine.

Women's International Network of Utility Professionals (WINUP)
P.O. Box 817
Fergus Falls, MN 56538-0817 US
E-mail Address: *drexler@runestone.net*
Web Address: www.winup.org
The Women's International Network of Utility Professionals (WINUP) provides networking and support for women in the utility industry.

XXXIII.   Energy Associations-Natural Gas

American Gas Association (AGA)
400 N. Capitol St. NW, Ste. 450
Washington, DC 20001 US
Phone: 202-824-7000
E-mail Address: *rshelby@aga.org*
Web Address: www.aga.org
The American Gas Association (AGA) represents a large number of natural gas providers, advocating for these companies and providing a broad range of programs and services for members.

XXXIV.   Energy Associations-Other

American Association of Blacks in Energy
1625 K St. NW, Ste. 450
Washington, DC 20006 US
Phone: 202-371-9530
Fax: 202-371-9218
E-mail Address: *info@aabe.org*
Web Address: www.aabe.org
The American Association of Blacks in Energy is dedicated to ensuring the input of African Americans and other minorities in discussions and developments of energy policies, regulations, research and development technologies and environmental issues.

Council of Petroleum Accountants Societies, Inc. (COPAS)
3900 E. Mexico Ave., Ste. 602
Denver, CO 80210 US
Phone: 303-300-1131
Fax: 303-300-3733
Toll Free: 877-992-6727
E-mail Address: *Execdir@copas.org*
Web Address: www.copas.org
The Council of Petroleum Accountants Societies, Inc. (COPAS) provides a forum for discussing and solving the variety of problems related to accounting for oil and gas. COPAS also provides valuable educational materials related to oil and gas accounting.

Society of Energy Professionals International
300-425 Bloor St. E
Toronto, ON M4W 3R4 Canada
Phone: 416-979-2709
Fax: 416-979-5794
E-mail Address: *society@society.on.ca*
Web Address: www.thesociety.ca
The Society of Energy Professionals International is an independent trade union representing professionals in the energy industry within Ontario, Canada.

XXXV. Energy Associations-Petroleum, Exploration, Production, etc.

American Association of Professional Landmen (AAPL)
4100 Fossil Creek Blvd.
Fort Worth, TX 76137 US
Phone: 817-847-7700
Fax: 817-847-7704
E-mail Address: *aapl@landman.org*
Web Address: www.landman.org
The American Association of Professional Landmen (AAPL) promotes the highest standards of performance for all land professionals and seeks to advance their stature and to encourage sound stewardship of energy and mineral resources.

American Petroleum Institute (API)
1220 L St. NW
Washington, DC 20005-4070 US
Phone: 202-682-8000
Web Address: www.api.org
American Petroleum Institute (API) represents U.S. oil and gas industries and its web site includes in-depth sections for energy consumers and energy professionals.

Independent Petroleum Association of America (IPAA)
1201 15th St. NW, Ste. 300
Washington, DC 20005 US
Phone: 202-857-4722
Fax: 202-857-4799
E-mail Address: *rcarter@ipaa.org*
Web Address: www.ipaa.org
The Independent Petroleum Association of America (IPAA) provides a forum for the exploration and production segment of the independent oil and natural gas business. It also provides information on the domestic exploration and production industry.

International Association of Drilling Contractors (IADC)
10370 Richmond Ave., Ste. 760
Houston, TX 77042 US
Phone: 713-292-1945
Fax: 713-292-1946
E-mail Address: *info@iadc.org*
Web Address: www.iadc.org
The International Association of Drilling Contractors (IADC) represents the worldwide oil and gas drilling industry and promotes commitment to safety, preservation of the environment and advances in drilling technology.

XXXVI. Engineering, Research & Scientific Associations

American Association of Petroleum Geologists (AAPG)
1444 S. Boulder Ave.
Tulsa, OK 74119 US
Phone: 918-584-2555
Fax: 918-560-2665
Toll Free: 800-364-2274
E-mail Address: *lnation@aapg.org*
Web Address: www.aapg.org
The American Association of Petroleum Geologists (AAPG) is an international geological organization that supports educational and scientific programs and projects related to geosciences.

American Chemical Society (ACS)
1155 16th St. NW
Washington, DC 20036 US
Phone: 202-872-4600
Fax: 202-776-8258
Toll Free: 800-227-5558
E-mail Address: *service@acs.org*
Web Address: portal.acs.org/portal/acs/corg/content
The American Chemical Society (ACS) is a nonprofit organization aimed at promoting the understanding of chemistry and chemical sciences. It represents a wide range of disciplines including chemistry, chemical engineering and other technical fields.

American Institute of Aeronautics and Astronautics (AIAA)
1801 Alexander Bell Dr., Ste. 500
Reston, VA 20191-4344 US
Phone: 703-264-7500
Fax: 703-264-7551
Toll Free: 800-639-2422
E-mail Address: *klausd@aiaa.org*
Web Address: www.aiaa.org
The American Institute of Aeronautics and Astronautics (AIAA) is a nonprofit society aimed at advancing the arts, sciences and technology of aeronautics and astronautics. The institute represents the U.S. in the International Astronautical Federation and the International Council on the Aeronautical Sciences.

American Institute of Chemical Engineers (AIChE)
3 Park Ave.
New York, NY 10016-5991 US
Phone: 203-702-7660
Fax: 203-775-5177
Toll Free: 800-242-4363
E-mail Address: *xpress@aiche.org*
Web Address: www.aiche.org
The American Institute of Chemical Engineers (AIChE) provides leadership in advancing the chemical engineering profession. The organization, which is comprised of 40,000 members from 93 countries, provides informational resources to chemical engineers.

American Society for Healthcare Engineering (ASHE)
1 N. Franklin, 28th Fl.
Chicago, IL 60606 US
Phone: 312-422-3800
Fax: 312-422-4571
E-mail Address: *ashe@aha.org*
Web Address: www.ashe.org
The American Society for Healthcare Engineering (ASHE) is the advocate and resource for continuous improvement in the health care engineering and facilities management professions.

American Society of Agricultural and Biological Engineers (ASABE)
2950 Niles Rd.
St. Joseph, MI 49085 US
Phone: 269-429-0300
Fax: 269-429-3852
E-mail Address: *hq@asabe.org*
Web Address: www.asabe.org
The American Society of Agricultural and Biological Engineers (ASABE) is a nonprofit professional and technical organization interested in engineering knowledge and technology for food and agriculture and associated industries.

American Society of Civil Engineers (ASCE)
1801 Alexander Bell Dr.
Reston, VA 20191-4400 US
Phone: 703-295-6300
Fax: 703-295-6222
Toll Free: 800-548-2723

Web Address: www.asce.org
The American Society of Civil Engineers (ASCE) is a leading professional organization serving civil engineers. It ensures safer buildings, water systems and other civil engineering works by developing technical codes and standards.

American Society of Mechanical Engineers (ASME)
3 Park Ave.
New York, NY 10016-5990 US
Phone: 973-882-1170
Fax: 973-882-1717
Toll Free: 800-843-2763
E-mail Address: *infocentral@asme.org*
Web Address: www.asme.org
The American Society of Mechanical Engineers (ASME) offers quality programs and activities in mechanical engineering. It also facilitates the development and application of technology in areas of interest to the mechanical engineering profession.

American Society of Safety Engineers (ASSE)
Customer Service
1800 E. Oakton St.
Des Plaines, IL 60018 US
Phone: 847-699-2929
Fax: 847-768-3434
E-mail Address: *customerservice@asse.org*
Web Address: www.asse.org
The American Society of Safety Engineers (ASSE) is the world's oldest and largest professional safety organization. It manages, supervises and consults on safety, health and environmental issues in industry, insurance, government and education.

Association of Federal Communications Consulting Engineers (AFCCE)
Web Address: www.afcce.org
The Association of Federal Communications Consulting Engineers (AFCCE) is a professional organization of individuals who regularly assist clients on technical issues before the Federal Communications Commission (FCC).

Institute of Industrial Engineers (IIE)
3577 Parkway Ln., Ste. 200
Norcross, GA 30092 US
Phone: 770-449-0460
Fax: 770-441-3295
Toll Free: 800-494-0460
E-mail Address: *execoffice@iienet.org*
Web Address: www.iienet.org
The Institute of Industrial Engineers (IIE) is dedicated to the professional needs of industrial engineers.

Institute of Structural Engineers (IStructE)
11 Upper Belgrave St.
London, SW1X 8BH UK
Phone: 44-20-7235-4535
Fax: 44-20-7235-4294
Web Address: www.istructe.org.uk
The Institute of Structural Engineers (IStructE) is a professional organization, headquartered in the U.K., that sets and maintains standards for professional structural engineers.

National Society of Professional Engineers (NSPE)
1420 King St.
Alexandria, VA 22314-2794 US
Phone: 703-684-2800
Fax: 703-836-4875
E-mail Address: *pr@nspe.org*
Web Address: www.nspe.org
The National Society of Professional Engineers (NSPE) represents individual engineering professionals and licensed engineers across all disciplines. NSPE serves 50,000 members and has more than 500 chapters.

Society of Automotive Engineers (SAE)
755 W. Big Beaver, Ste. 1600
Troy, MA 48084 US
Phone: 248-273-2455
Fax: 248-273-2494
Toll Free: 877-606-7323
E-mail Address: *automotive_hq@sae.org*
Web Address: www.sae.org
The Society of Automotive Engineers (SAE) is a resource for technical information and expertise used in designing, building, maintaining and operating self-propelled vehicles for use on land, sea, air or space.

Society of Broadcast Engineers, Inc. (SBE)
9102 N. Meridian St., Ste. 150
Indianapolis, IN 46260 US
Phone: 317-846-9000
Fax: 317-846-9120
E-mail Address: *mclappe@sbe.org*
Web Address: www.sbe.org
The Society of Broadcast Engineers (SBE) exists to increase knowledge of broadcast engineering and promote its interests, as well as to continue the education of professionals in the industry.

Society of Cable Telecommunications Engineers (SCTE)
140 Philips Rd.
Exton, PA 19341-1318 US
Phone: 610-363-6888
Fax: 610-363-5898
Toll Free: 800-542-5040
E-mail Address: *scte@scte.org*
Web Address: www.scte.org
The Society of Cable Telecommunications Engineers (SCTE) is a nonprofit professional association dedicated to advancing the careers and serving the industry of telecommunications professionals by providing technical training, certification and standards.

Society of Hispanic Professional Engineers (SHPE)
5400 E. Olympic Blvd., Ste. 210
Los Angeles, CA 90022 US
Phone: 323-725-3970
Fax: 323-725-0316
E-mail Address: *shpenational@shpe.org*
Web Address: www.shpe.org
The Society of Hispanic Professional Engineers (SHPE) is a national nonprofit organization that promotes Hispanics in science, engineering and math.

Society of Manufacturing Engineers (SME)
1 SME Dr.
Dearborn, MI 48121 US
Phone: 313-425-3000
Fax: 313-425-3412
Toll Free: 800-733-4763
E-mail Address: *communications@sme.org*

Web Address: www.sme.org
The Society of Manufacturing Engineers (SME) a leading professional organization serving engineers in the manufacturing industries.

Society of Motion Picture and Television Engineers (SMPTE)
3 Barker Ave.
White Plains, NY 10601 US
Phone: 914-761-1100
Fax: 914-761-3115
E-mail Address: *htomko@smpte.org*
Web Address: www.smpte.org
The Society of Motion Picture and Television Engineers (SMPTE) is the leading technical society for the motion imaging industry. The firm publishes recommended practice and engineering guidelines, as well the SMPTE Journal.

Society of Petroleum Engineers (SPE)
222 Palisades Creek Dr.
Richardson, TX 75080-2040 US
Phone: 972-952-9393
Fax: 972-952-9435
Toll Free: 800-456-6863
E-mail Address: *spedal@spe.org*
Web Address: www.spe.org
The Society of Petroleum Engineers (SPE) helps connect engineers in the oil and gas industry with ideas, answers, resources and technological information.

Society of Women Engineers (SWE)
230 E. Ohio St., Ste. 400
Chicago, IL 60611 US
Phone: 312-596-5223
E-mail Address: *hq@swe.org*
Web Address: www.swe.org
The Society of Women Engineers (SWE) is a nonprofit educational and service organization of female engineers.

XXXVII.   Entertainment & Amusement Associations

International Association of Amusement Parks and Attractions (IAAPA)
1448 Duke St.
Alexandria, VA 22314 US

Phone: 703-836-4800
Fax: 703-836-6742
E-mail Address: *dmandt@iaapa.org*
Web Address: www.iaapa.org
The International Association of Amusement Parks and Attractions (IAAPA) is dedicated to the preservation and prosperity of the amusement industry.

International Special Events Society (ISES)
401 N. Michigan Ave.
Chicago, IL 60611-4267 US
Phone: 312-321-6853
Fax: 312-673-6953
Toll Free: 800-688-4737
E-mail Address: *info@ises.com*
Web Address: www.ises.com
The International Special Events Society (ISES) is a society of special events professionals representing the industry's diverse disciplines.

XXXVIII.   Film & Television Resources

SCREENSite
E-mail Address: *webmaster@screensite.org*
Web Address: www.screensite.org
SCREENSite is a resource center for film and TV scholarship with an archive of course syllabi, e-mail listings of media scholars, conference information, school listings and job list.

XXXIX.   Film & Theater Associations

Academy of Motion Picture Arts and Sciences (AMPAS)
8949 Wilshire Blvd.
Beverly Hills, CA 90211-1972 US
Phone: 310-247-3000
Fax: 310-859-9619
Web Address: www.oscars.org
The Academy of Motion Picture Arts and Sciences (AMPAS) is a professional honorary organization, founded to advance the arts and sciences of motion pictures. Besides hosting the Academy Awards and selecting the winners of the Oscars, AMPAS organizes smaller events highlighting the art of filmmaking, including lectures and seminars, and is

currently building the Academy Museum of Motion Pictures.

Alliance of Motion Picture and Television Producers (AMPTP)
15301 Ventura Blvd.
Encino, CA 91403 US
Toll Free: 818-995-3600
Web Address: www.amptp.org
The Alliance of Motion Picture and Television Producers (AMPTP) is the primary trade association with respect to labor issues in the motion picture and television industry.

American Cinema Editors, Inc. (ACE)
100 Universal City Plz.
Verna Fields Bldg. 2282, Rm. 190
Universal City, CA 91608 US
Phone: 818-777-2900
Fax: 818-733-5023
E-mail Address:
amercinema@earthlink.net
Web Address: www.ace-filmeditors.org
American Cinema Editors (ACE) is an honorary society of motion picture editors that seeks to advance the art and science of the editing profession.

American Society of Cinematographers (ASC)
1782 N. Orange Dr.
Hollywood, CA 90028 US
Phone: 323-969-4333
Fax: 323-882-6391
Toll Free: 800-448-0145
E-mail Address: *office@theasc.com*
Web Address: www.theasc.com
The American Society of Cinematographers (ASC) is a trade association for cinematographers in the motion picture industry.

Art Directors Guild (ADG)
11969 Ventura Blvd., 2nd Fl.
Studio City, CA 91604 US
Phone: 818-762-9995
Fax: 818-762-9997
E-mail Address: *nick@artdirectors.org*
Web Address: www.artdirectors.org
The Art Directors Guild (ADG) represents the creative talents that conceive and manage the background and settings for most films and television projects.

Association of Cinema and Video Laboratories (ACVL)
Chip Wilkinson, Pres., ACVL
630 9th Ave.
New York, NY 10036 US
Phone: 212-586-4822
Fax: 212-582-3744
E-mail Address: *cfw2447@rcn.com*
Web Address: www.acvl.org
The Association of Cinema and Video Laboratories (ACVL) is an international organization whose members are pledged to the highest possible standards of service to the film and video industries.

Independent Film & Television Alliance (IFTA)
10850 Wilshire Blvd., 9th Fl.
Los Angeles, CA 90024-4321 US
Phone: 310-446-1000
Fax: 310-446-1600
E-mail Address: *info@ifta-online.org*
Web Address: www.ifta-online.org
The Independent Film & Television Alliance (IFTA), formerly the American Film Marketing Association (AFMA), is a trade association whose mission is to provide the independent film and television industry with high-quality, market-oriented services and worldwide representation.

International Alliance of Theatrical Stage Employees (IATSE)
1430 Broadway, 20th Fl.
New York, NY 10018 US
Phone: 212-730-1770
Fax: 212-921-7699
E-mail Address: *webmaster@iatse-intl.org*
Web Address: www.iatse-intl.org
The International Alliance of Theatrical Stage Employees (IATSE) is the labor union representing technicians, artisans and crafts workers in the entertainment industry, including live theater, film and television production and trade shows.

International Animated Film Society (ASIFA-Hollywood)
2114 W. Burbank Blvd.
Burbank, CA 91506 US
Phone: 818-842-4691
E-mail Address: *info@asifa-hollywood.org*

Web Address: www.asifa-hollywood.org
International Animated Film Society (ASIFA-Hollywood) is a nonprofit organization dedicated to the advancement of the art of animation.

International Documentary Association (IDA)
1201 W. 5th St., Ste. M270
Los Angeles, CA 90017 US
Phone: 213-534-3600
Fax: 213-534-3610
E-mail Address: *amina@documentary.org*
Web Address: www.documentary.org
The International Documentary Association (IDA) is a nonprofit member service organization, providing publications, benefits and a public forum to its members for issues regarding nonfiction film, video and multimedia.

Motion Picture Association of America (MPAA)
15301 Ventura Blvd., Bldg. E
Sherman Oaks, CA 91403 US
Phone: 818-995-6600
Fax: 818-285-4403
Web Address: www.mpaa.org
The Motion Picture Association of America (MPAA) serves as the voice and advocate of the U.S. motion picture, home video and television industries.

Motion Picture Editors Guild (MPEG)
7715 Sunset Blvd., Ste. 200
Hollywood, CA 90046 US
Phone: 323-876-4770
Fax: 323-876-0861
Toll Free: 800-705-8700
E-mail Address: *mail@editorsguild.com*
Web Address: www.editorsguild.com
The Motion Picture Editors Guild's (MPEG) web site provides an online directory of editors, a discussion forum and links to related magazines and other organizations that serve the motion picture industry.

Producers Guild of America (PGA)
8530 Wilshire Blvd., Ste. 450
Beverly Hills, CA 90211 US
Phone: 310-358-9020

Fax: 310-358-9520
E-mail Address: *info@producersguild.org*
Web Address: www.producersguild.org
The Producers Guild of America (PGA) is a nonprofit organization for career professionals who initiate, create, coordinate, supervise and control all aspects of the motion picture and television production processes.

Screen Actors Guild (SAG)
5757 Wilshire Blvd., 7th Fl.
Los Angeles, CA 90036-3600 US
Phone: 323-954-1600
Fax: 323-549-6603
Toll Free: 800-724-0767
E-mail Address: *saginfo@sag.org*
Web Address: www.sag.org
The Screen Actors Guild (SAG) represents its members through negotiation and enforcement of collective bargaining agreements that establish equitable levels of compensation, benefits and working conditions for performers. Established in 1933, the guild has 20 branches that represent 120,000 actors nationwide.

Women In Film (WIF)
8857 W. Olympic Blvd., Ste. 201
Beverly Hills, CA 90211-3605 US
Phone: 310-657-5144
Fax: 310-657-5154
E-mail Address: *info@wif.org*
Web Address: www.wif.org
Women In Film (WIF) strives to empower, promote and mentor women in the entertainment, communication and media industries through a network of contacts, educational programs and events.

XL. Fitness

American Fitness Professionals and Associates (AFPA)
P.O. Box 214
Ship Bottom, NJ 08008 US
Phone: 609-978-7583
Fax: 609-978-7582
E-mail Address: *afpa@afpafitness.com*
Web Address: www.afpafitness.com
American Fitness Professionals and Associates (AFPA) offers health and fitness professionals certification

programs, continuing education courses, home correspondence courses and regional conventions.

XLI. Food Industry Associations, General

Institute of Food Technologies (IFT)
525 W. Van Buren, Ste. 1000
Chicago, IL 60607 US
Phone: 312-782-8424
Fax: 312-782-8348
Toll Free: 800-438-3663
E-mail Address: *info@ift.org*
Web Address: www.ift.org
The Institute of Food Technologies (IFT) is devoted to the advancement of the science and technology of food through the exchange of knowledge. The site provides information and resources for job seekers in the food industry. Members work in food science, food technology and related professions in industry, academia and government.

United Food and Commercial Workers International Union (UFCW)
1775 K St. NW
Washington, DC 20006 US
Phone: 202-223-3111
Web Address: www.ufcw.org
The United Food and Commercial Workers International Union (UFCW) is a union for members who are employed in many different industries but are concentrated in retail food, meatpacking, poultry and other food processing industries.

XLII. Food Processor Industry Associations

Grocery Manufacturers Association (GMA)
1350 I St. NW, Ste. 300
Washington, DC 20005 US
Phone: 202-639-5900
Fax: 202-639-5932
E-mail Address: *info@gmaonline.org*
Web Address: www.gmaonline.org
The Grocery Manufacturers Association (GMA), formerly the National Food Products Association (NFPA), is the voice of the food, beverage and consumer products industry on scientific and public policy

issues involving food safety, food security, nutrition, technical and regulatory matters and consumer affairs.

XLIII. Grocery Industry Associations

Food Marketing Institute (FMI)
2345 Crystal Dr., Ste. 800
Arlington, VA 22202 US
Phone: 202-452-8444
Fax: 202-429-4519
E-mail Address: *fmi@fmi.org*
Web Address: www.fmi.org
The Food Marketing Institute (FMI) is a nonprofit association conducting programs in research, education, industry relations and public affairs on behalf of its 1,500 members.

XLIV. Health Care Business & Professional Associations

Advanced Medical Technology Association (AdvaMed)
701 Pennsylvania Ave. NW, Ste. 800
Washington, DC 20004-2654 US
Phone: 202-783-8700
Fax: 202-783-8750
E-mail Address: *info@advamed.org*
Web Address: www.advamed.org
The Advanced Medical Technology Association (AdvaMed) strives to be the advocate for a legal, regulatory and economic climate that advances global health care by assuring worldwide access to the benefits of medical technology.

America's Health Insurance Plans (AHIP)
601 Pennsylvania Ave. NW, Ste. 500
Washington, DC 20004 US
Phone: 202-778-3200
Fax: 202-331-7487
E-mail Address: *ahip@ahip.org*
Web Address: www.ahip.org
America's Health Insurance Plans (AHIP) is a prominent trade association representing the private health care system.

American Academy of Medical Administrators (AAMA)
701 Lee St., Ste. 600
Des Plaines, IL 60016-4516 US
Phone: 847-759-8601

Fax: 847-759-8602
E-mail Address: *info@aameda.org*
Web Address: www.aameda.org
The American Academy of Medical Administrators (AAMA) is an association for health care leaders to enhance their profession and community health.

American Academy of Nursing (AAN)
888 17th St. NW, Ste. 800
Washington, DC 20006 US
Phone: 202-777-1170
Fax: 202-777-0107
E-mail Address: *info@aannet.org*
Web Address: www.aannet.org
The American Academy of Nursing (AAN) works to help nursing leaders transform the health care system in order to optimize public well-being.

American Association of Medical Assistants (AAMA)
20 N. Wacker Dr., Ste. 1575
Chicago, IL 60606 US
Phone: 312-899-1500
Fax: 312-899-1259
Web Address: www.aama-ntl.org
The American Association of Medical Assistants (AAMA) seeks to promote the professional identity and stature of its members and the medical assisting profession through education and credentialing.

American College of Health Care Administrators (ACHCA)
12100 Sunset Hills Rd., Ste. 130
Reston, VA 20190 US
Phone: 703-739-7900
Fax: 703-435-4390
E-mail Address: *candrews@achca.org*
Web Address: www.achca.org
The American College of Health Care Administrators (ACHCA) offers educational programming and career development for health care administrators.

American College of Healthcare Executives (ACHE)
1 N. Franklin, Ste. 1700
Chicago, IL 60606-3529 US
Phone: 312-424-2800
Fax: 312-424-0023
E-mail Address: *geninfo@ache.org*
Web Address: www.ache.org

The American College of Healthcare Executives (ACHE) is an international professional society of health care executives that offers certification and educational programs.

American Dental Association (ADA)
211 E. Chicago Ave.
Chicago, IL 60611-2678 US
Phone: 312-440-2500
E-mail Address: *online@ada.org*
Web Address: www.ada.org
The American Dental Association (ADA) is a professional association of dentists committed to the public's oral health, ethics, science and professional advancement.

American Dietetic Association (ADA)
120 S. Riverside Plz., Ste. 2000
Chicago, IL 60606-6995 US
Fax: 312-899-4899
Toll Free: 800-877-1600
E-mail Address: *rmoen@eatright.org*
Web Address: www.eatright.org
The American Dietetic Association (ADA) is the world's largest organization of food and nutrition professionals, with nearly 65,000 members. In addition to services for its professional members, this organization's web site offers consumers a Nutrition Knowledge Center and a Healthy Lifestyle Center.

American Health Information Management Association (AHIMA)
233 N. Michigan Ave., 21st Fl.
Chicago, IL 60601-5800 US
Phone: 312-233-1100
Fax: 312-233-1090
E-mail Address: *info@ahima.org*
Web Address: www.ahima.org
The American Health Information Management Association (AHIMA) is a professional association that consists of specially educated health information management professionals who work throughout the health care industry.

American Medical Informatics Association (AMIA)
4915 St. Elmo Ave., Ste. 401
Bethesda, MD 20814 US
Phone: 301-657-1291
Fax: 301-657-1296

E-mail Address: *mail@amia.org*
Web Address: www.amia.org
The American Medical Informatics Association (AMIA) is a membership organization of individuals, institutions and corporations dedicated to developing and using information technologies to improve health care.

American Medical Technologists (AMT)
10700 W. Higgins Rd., Ste. 150
Rosemont, IL 60018 US
Phone: 847-823-5169
Fax: 847-823-0458
Toll Free: 800-275-1268
Web Address: www.amt1.com
American Medical Technologists (AMT) is a nonprofit certification agency and professional membership association representing individuals in health care.

American Medical Women's Association (AMWA)
100 N. 200th St., 4th Fl.
Philadelphia, PA 19103 US
Phone: 215-320-3716
Fax: 215-564-2175
Toll Free: 866-564-2483
E-mail Address: *info@amwa-doc.org*
Web Address: www.amwa-doc.org
The American Medical Women's Association (AMWA) is an organization of women physicians and medical students dedicated to serving as the unique voice for women's health and the advancement of women in medicine.

American Occupational Therapy Association, Inc. (AOTA)
4720 Montgomery Ln.
P.O. Box 31220
Bethesda, MD 20824-1220 US
Phone: 301-652-2682
Fax: 301-652-7711
Web Address: www.aota.org
The American Occupational Therapy Association, Inc. (AOTA) advances the quality, availability, use and support of occupational therapy through standard-setting, advocacy, education and research on behalf of its members and the public.

American Organization of Nurse Executives (AONE)
Liberty Place, 325 7th St. NW
Washington, DC 20004 US
Phone: 202-626-2240
Fax: 202-638-5499
E-mail Address: *aone@aha.org*
Web Address: www.aone.org
The American Organization of Nurse Executives (AONE) is a national organization of nurses who design, facilitate and manage health care.

American Public Health Association (APHA)
800 I St. NW
Washington, DC 20001-3710 US
Phone: 202-777-2742
Fax: 202-777-2534
E-mail Address: *comments@apha.org*
Web Address: www.apha.org
The American Public Health Association (APHA) is an association of individuals and organizations working to improve the public's health and to achieve equity in health status for all.

American School Health Association (ASHA)
7263 State Rte. 43
P.O. Box 708
Kent, OH 44240 US
Phone: 330-678-1601
Fax: 330-678-4526
E-mail Address: *asha@ashaweb.org*
Web Address: www.ashaweb.org
The American School Health Association (ASHA) advocates high-quality school health instruction, health services and a healthy school environment.

College of Healthcare Information Management Executives (CHIME)
3300 Washtenaw Ave., Ste. 225
Ann Arbor, MI 48104 US
Phone: 734-665-0000
Fax: 734-665-4922
E-mail Address: *staff@cio-chime.org*
Web Address: www.cio-chime.org
College of Healthcare Information Management Executives (CHIME) was formed with the dual objective of serving the professional development needs of health care CIOs and advocating the more effective use of

information management within health care.

Dental Trade Alliance (DTA)
2300 Clarendon Blvd., Ste. 1003
Arlington, VA 22201 US
Phone: 703-379-7755
Fax: 703-931-9429
E-mail Address:
info@dentaltradealliance.org
Web Address:
www.dentaltradealliance.org
The Dental Trade Alliance (DTA)
represents dental manufacturers, dental
dealers and dental laboratories.

Health and Science Communications Association (HeSCA)
39 Wedgewood Dr., Ste. A
Jewett City, CT 06351 US
Phone: 860-376-5915
Fax: 860-376-6621
E-mail Address: *hesca@hesca.org*
Web Address: www.hesca.org
The Health and Science
Communications Association (HeSCA)
is an association of communications
professionals committed to sharing
knowledge and resources in the health
sciences arena.

Health Industry Business Communications Council (HIBCC)
2525 E. Arizona Biltmore Cir., Ste. 127
Phoenix, AZ 85016 US
Phone: 602-381-1091
Fax: 602-381-1093
E-mail Address: *info@hibcc.org*
Web Address: www.hibcc.org
The Health Industry Business
Communications Council (HIBCC)
seeks to facilitate electronic
communications by developing
appropriate standards for information
exchange among all health care trading
partners.

Health Industry Distributors Association (HIDA)
310 Montgomery St.
Alexandria, VA 22314-1516 US
Phone: 703-549-4432
Fax: 703-549-6495
E-mail Address: *sandler@hida.org*
Web Address: www.hida.org
The Health Industry Distributors
Association (HIDA) is the international

trade association representing medical
products distributors.

Healthcare Financial Management Association (HFMA)
2 Westbrook Corporate Ctr., Ste. 700
Westchester, IL 60154 US
Phone: 708-531-9600
Fax: 708-531-0032
Toll Free: 800-252-4362
Web Address: www.hfma.org
The Healthcare Financial Management
Association (HFMA) is one of the
nation's leading personal membership
organizations for health care financial
management executives and leaders.

Healthcare Information and Management Systems Society (HIMSS)
230 E. Ohio St., Ste. 500
Chicago, IL 60611-3270 US
Phone: 312-664-4467
Fax: 312-664-6143
E-mail Address: *himss@himss.org*
Web Address: www.himss.org
The Healthcare Information and
Management Systems Society
(HIMSS) provides leadership in the
optimal use of technology, information
and management systems for the
betterment of health care.

Hearing Industries Association (HIA)
1444 I St., NW., Ste. 700
Washington, DC 20005 US
Phone: 202-449-1090
Fax: 202-216-9646
E-mail Address:
mspangler@bostrom.com
Web Address: www.hearing.org
The Hearing Industries Association
(HIA) represents and unifies the many
aspects of the hearing industry.

Medical Device Manufacturers Association (MDMA)
1350 I St. NW, Ste. 540
Washington, DC 20005 US
Phone: 202-354-7171
Web Address:
www.medicaldevices.org
The Medical Device Manufacturers
Association (MDMA) is a national
trade association that represents
independent manufacturers of medical

devices, diagnostic products and health
care information systems.

Medical Group Management Association (MGMA)
104 Inverness Ter. E.
Englewood, CO 80112-5306 US
Phone: 303-799-1111
Fax: 303-643-4439
Toll Free: 877-275-6462
E-mail Address: *service@mgma.com*
Web Address: www.mgma.com
Medical Group Management
Association (MGMA) is one of the
nation's principal voices for medical
group practice.

National Association of Health Services Executives (NAHSE)
1140 Connecticut Ave., NW Ste. 505
Washington, DC 20036 US
Phone: 202-429-6060
Fax: 301-429-6767
E-mail Address: *nahsehq@nahse.org*
Web Address: www.nahse.org
The National Association of Health
Services Executives (NAHSE) is a
nonprofit association of black health
care executives who promote the
advancement and development of
black health care leaders and elevate
the quality of health care services
rendered to minority and underserved
communities.

Regulatory Affairs Professionals Society (RAPS)
5635 Fishers Ln., Ste. 550
Rockville, MD 20852 US
Phone: 301-770-2920
Fax: 301-770-2924
E-mail Address: *raps@raps.org*
Web Address: www.raps.org
The Regulatory Affairs Professionals
Society (RAPS) is an international
professional society representing the
health care regulatory affairs
profession and individual professionals
worldwide.

XLV.	Hotel/Lodging Associations

American Hotel and Lodging Association
1201 New York Ave. NW, Ste. 600
Washington, DC 20005-3931 US
Phone: 202-289-3100

Fax: 202-289-3199
E-mail Address: info@ahla.com
Web Address: www.ahla.com
The American Hotel and Lodging
Association is a federation of state
lodging associations throughout the
U.S.

XLVI.   Human Resources Industry Associations

Society of Human Resource Management (SHRM)
1800 Duke St.
Alexandria, VA 22314 US
Phone: 703-548-3440
Fax: 703-535-6490
Toll Free: 800-283-7476
E-mail Address: shrm@shrm.org
Web Address: www.shrm.org
The Society of Human Resource
Management (SHRM) addresses the
interests and needs of HR professionals
through its resource materials.

XLVII.   Industry Research/Market Research

Forrester Research
400 Technology Sq.
Cambridge, MA 02139 US
Phone: 617-613-6000
Fax: 617-613-5200
Toll Free: 866-367-7378
E-mail Address: press@forrester.com
Web Address: www.forrester.com
Forrester Research identifies and
analyzes emerging trends in
technology and their impact on
business. Among the firm's specialties
are the financial services, retail, health
care, entertainment, automotive and
information technology industries.

Marketresearch.com
11200 Rockville Pike, Ste. 504
Rockville, MD 20852 US
Phone: 240-747-3000
Fax: 240-747-3004
Toll Free: 800-298-5699
E-mail Address:
customerservice@marketresearch.com
Web Address:
www.marketresearch.com
Marketresearch.com is a leading
broker for professional market research
and industry analysis. Users are able to
search the company's database of

research publications including data on
global industries, companies, products
and trends.

Plunkett Research, Ltd.
P.O. Drawer 541737
Houston, TX 77254-1737 US
Phone: 713-932-0000
Fax: 713-932-7080
E-mail Address:
info@plunkettresearch.com
Web Address:
www.plunkettresearch.com
Plunkett Research, Ltd. is a leading
provider of market research, industry
trends analysis and business statistics.
Since 1985, it has served clients
worldwide, including corporations,
universities, libraries, consultants and
government agencies. At the firm's
web site, visitors can view product
information and pricing and access a
great deal of basic market information
on industries such as financial services,
InfoTech, e-commerce, health care and
biotech.

XLVIII.   Insurance, Agents & Brokers

Council of Insurance Agents & Brokers (CIAB)
701 Pennsylvania Ave. NW, Ste. 750
Washington, DC 20004 US
Phone: 202-783-4400
Fax: 202-783-4410
E-mail Address: ciab@ciab.com
Web Address: www.ciab.com
The Council of Insurance Agents &
Brokers (CIAB) is an association for
commercial insurance and employee
benefits intermediaries in the U.S. and
abroad.

Independent Insurance Agents & Brokers of America, Inc. (IIABA)
127 S. Peyton St.
Alexandria, VA 22314 US
Fax: 703-683-7556
Toll Free: 800-221-7917
E-mail Address: info@iiaba.org
Web Address:
www.independentagent.com
Independent Insurance Agents &
Brokers of America (IIABA)
represents its over 300,000 members
who are independent insurance agents
and brokers.

Professional Insurance Agents (PIA)
25 Chamberlain St.
P.O. Box 997
Glenmont, NY 12077 US
Fax: 888-225-6935
Toll Free: 800-424-4244
E-mail Address: pia@pia.org
Web Address: www.piaonline.org
Professional Insurance Agents (PIA) is
a group of voluntary, membership-
based trade associations representing
professional, independent property and
casualty insurance agents.

XLIX.   Insurance, Property/Casualty Associations

American Insurance Association (AIA)
1130 Connecticut Ave. NW, Ste. 1000
Washington, DC 20036 US
Phone: 202-828-7100
Fax: 202-293-1219
E-mail Address: info@aiadc.org
Web Address: www.aiadc.org
The American Insurance Association
(AIA) is a leading property and
casualty insurance trade organization,
representing companies that offer all
types of property and casualty
insurance.

L.   Magazines, Business & Financial

BusinessWeek Online
P.O. Box 8418
Red Oak, IA 51591-1418 US
Fax: 712-623-5229
Toll Free: 800-635-1200
E-mail Address:
bwzcustserv@cdsfulfillment.com
Web Address: www.businessweek.com
Business Week Online offers an
investor service, global business
advice, technology news, small
business guides, career information,
business school advice, daily news
briefs and more.

Forbes Online
90 5th Ave.
New York, NY 10011 US
Phone: 212-366-8900
E-mail Address: dweathers@forbes.net
Web Address: www.forbes.com

Forbes Online offers varied stock information, news and commentary on business, technology and personal finance, as well as financial calculators and advice.

Fortune
Time & Life Bldg.
Rockefeller Ctr.
New York, NY 10020-1393 US
Phone: 212-522-6724
Fax: 212-522-6412
Toll Free: 800-777-1444
E-mail Address:
Katy_Reitz@timeinc.com
Web Address:
money.cnn.com/magazines/fortune
Fortune, one of the world's premiere business magazines, contains news, business profiles and information on investing, careers, small business, technology and other details of U.S. and international business. Fortune is a publication of Cable News Network (CNN), a Time Warner company.

Investor's Business Daily (IBD)
12655 Beatrice St.
Los Angeles, CA 90066 US
Phone: 310-448-6600
Toll Free: 800-831-2525
E-mail Address:
ibdnews@investors.com
Web Address: www.investors.com
Investor's Business Daily (IBD) offers subscribers information and articles on the stock market, educational resources, advice from analyst William O'Neil, personal portfolios and updates on events and workshops.

Wall Street Journal Online (The)
200 Liberty St.
New York, NY 10281 US
Phone: 212-416-2000
E-mail Address: *feedback@wsj.com*
Web Address: www.wsj.com
The outstanding resources of The Wall Street Journal are available online for a nominal fee.

LI. MBA Resources

MBA Depot
Phone: 512-499-8728
Web Address: www.mbadepot.com
MBA Depot is an online community for MBA professionals.

LII. Online Recruiting & Employment ASPs & Solutions

Authoria, Inc.
300 5th Ave.
Waltham, MA 02451 US
Phone: 781-530-2000
Fax: 781-530-2001
Toll Free: 877-422-1114
E-mail Address: *info@authoria.com*
Web Address: www.authoria.com
Authoria, Inc.'s web site offers companies and job seekers a variety of human resources content. The site includes recruiting management, performance management, incentive management, compensation management, succession planning and benefit and policy communication services.

Insala
1331 Airport Fwy., Ste. 313
Euless, TX 76040 US
Phone: 817-355-0939
Fax: 817-355-0746
E-mail Address: *info@insala.com*
Web Address: www.insala.com
Insala provides job search software solutions for the outplacement industry.

Kenexa
650 E. Swedesford Rd., 2nd Fl.
Wayne, PA 19087 US
Phone: 877-971-9171
Fax: 610-971-9181
Toll Free: 800-391-9557
E-mail Address:
contactus@kenexa.com
Web Address: www.kenexa.com
Kenexa is a back-end recruiting and job-posting service that is used by many companies in building a workforce. Products and services include recruitment software solutions, talent consulting and recruitment process management.

Workstream
2600 Lake Lucien Dr., Ste. 410
Maitland, FL 32751 US
Phone: 407-475-5500
Toll Free: 866-953-8800
E-mail Address:
info@workstreaminc.com

Web Address:
www.workstreaminc.com
Workstream creates workforce management solutions through a combination of technology and services designed to integrate an organization.

LIII. Pensions, Benefits & 401(k)s

Employee Benefits Security Administration (EBSA)
200 Constitution Ave. NW
Washington, DC 20210 US
Phone: 202-693-8700
Fax: 202-693-8736
Toll Free: 866-444-3272
Web Address: www.dol.gov/ebsa
The Employee Benefits Security Administration (EBSA) is a division of the U.S. Department of Labor, whose web site features a wealth of benefits information for both employers and employees. Included are the answers to such questions as to how a company's bankruptcy will affect its employees and what one should know about pension rights.

Pension Benefit Guarantee Corporation (PBGC)
1200 K St. NW
Washington, DC 20005-4026 US
Phone: 202-326-4343
Fax: 202-326-4344
Toll Free: 800-400-7242
E-mail Address: *Webmaster@pbgc.gov*
Web Address: www.pbgc.gov
The Pension Benefit Guarantee Corporation (PBGC) is a U.S. Government agency that guarantees a portion of the retirement incomes of about 44.1 million American workers in about 30,330 private defined benefit pension plans. Its web site contains information regarding this guarantee, along with information on retirement planning and links to several related organizations.

Profit Sharing/401(k) Council of America (PSCA)
20 N. Wacker Dr., Ste. 3700
Chicago, IL 60606 US
Phone: 312-419-1863
Fax: 312-419-1864
E-mail Address: *psca@psca.org*

Web Address: www.psca.org
The Profit Sharing/401(k) Council of America (PSCA) is a national nonprofit association of 1,200 companies and its 6 million employees. The group expresses its members' interests to federal policymakers and offers practical, cost-effective assistance with profit sharing and 401(k) plan design, administration, investment, compliance and communication. Its web site offers a thorough glossary, statistics and educational material.

LIV. Pharmaceutical Industry Associations (Drug Industry)

American Pharmaceutical Association (APhA)
1100 15th St. NW, Ste. 400
Washington, DC 20005-1707 US
Phone: 202-628-4410
Fax: 202-783-2351
Toll Free: 800-237-2742
E-mail Address: *infocenter@aphanet.org*
Web Address: www.aphanet.org
American Pharmaceutical Association (APhA) is a national professional society that provides news and information to pharmacists.

Pharmaceutical Research and Manufacturers of America (PhRMA)
950 F St. NW, Ste. 300
Washington, DC 20004 US
Phone: 202-835-3400
Fax: 202-835-3414
Web Address: www.phrma.org
Pharmaceutical Research and Manufacturers of America (PhRMA) represents the nation's leading research-based pharmaceutical and biotechnology companies.

LV. Printers & Publishers Associations

International Publishing Management Association (IPMA)
710 Regency Dr., Ste. 6
Kearney, MO 64060 US
Phone: 816-902-4762
Fax: 816-902-4766
E-mail Address: *ipmainfo@ipma.org*

Web Address: www.ipma.org
The International Publishing Management Association (IPMA) is an exclusive not-for-profit organization dedicated to assisting in-house corporate publishing and distribution professionals.

Magazine Publishers of America, Inc.
810 7th Ave., 24th Fl.
New York, NY 10019 US
Phone: 212-872-3700
E-mail Address: *mpa@magazine.org*
Web Address: www.magazine.org
Magazine Publishers of America is the industry association for consumer magazines.

National Association of Printers & Lithographers (NAPL)
75 W. Century Rd., Ste. 100
Paramus, NJ 07652 US
Phone: 201-634-9600
Fax: 201-634-0234
Toll Free: 800-642-6275
E-mail Address: *dlospaluto@napl.org*
Web Address: www.napl.org
The National Association of Printers & Lithographers (NAPL) focuses on helping graphic arts professionals increase their expertise.

Newspaper Association of America (NAA)
4401 Wilson Blvd., Ste. 900
Arlington, VA 22203-1867 US
Phone: 571-366-1000
Fax: 571-366-1195
E-mail Address: *webmaster@naa.org*
Web Address: www.naa.org
The Newspaper Association of America (NAA) is a nonprofit organization representing the newspaper industry.

LVI. Real Estate Industry Associations

Institute of Real Estate Management (IREM)
430 N. Michigan Ave.
Chicago, IL 60611 US
Fax: 800-338-4736
Toll Free: 800-837-0706
E-mail Address: *custserv@irem.org*
Web Address: www.irem.org

The Institute of Real Estate Management (IREM) seeks to educate real estate managers, certify their competence and professionalism, serve as an advocate on issues affecting the real estate management industry and enhance its members' professional competence so they can better identify and meet the needs of those who use their services.

National Association of Real Estate Brokers (NAREB)
9831 Greenbelt Rd., Ste. 309
Lanham, MD 20706 US
Phone: 301-552-9340
Fax: 301-552-9216
E-mail Address: *ctbroker1@aol.com*
Web Address: www.nareb.com
The National Association of Real Estate Brokers (NAREB) is a national trade organization dedicated to bringing together the nation's minority professionals in the real estate industry.

National Association of Real Estate Companies (NAREC)
Kim Klein
216 W. Jackson Blvd., Ste. 625
Chicago, IL 60606 US
Phone: 312-263-1755
Fax: 312-750-1203
E-mail Address: *info@narec.org*
Web Address: www.narec.org
The National Association of Real Estate Companies (NAREC) is composed of representatives of publicly and privately owned real estate companies, significant subsidiaries of publicly owned companies and public accounting firms.

National Association of Realtors (NAR)
430 N. Michigan Ave.
Chicago, IL 60611-4087 US
Phone: 202-383-1176
Toll Free: 800-874-6500
E-mail Address: *lsalvant@realtors.org*
Web Address: www.realtor.org
The National Association of Realtors (NAR) is composed of realtors involved in residential and commercial real estate as brokers, salespeople, property managers, appraisers and counselors and in other areas of the

industry. NAR also sponsors Realtor.com, operated by Move, Inc.

Women's Council of Realtors (WCR)
430 N. Michigan Ave.
Chicago, IL 60611 US
Toll Free: 800-245-8512
E-mail Address: *wcr@wcr.org*
Web Address: www.wcr.org
The Women's Council of Realtors (WCR) is a community of female real estate professionals.

LVII.   Recording & Music Associations

American Federation of Musicians (AFM)
1501 Broadway, Ste. 600
New York, NY 10036 US
Phone: 212-869-1330
Fax: 212-764-6134
E-mail Address: *sam@afm.org*
Web Address: www.afm.org
The American Federation of Musicians (AFM) is the largest union in the world for music professionals.

American Society of Composers, Authors & Publishers (ASCAP)
1 Lincoln Plaza
New York, NY 10023 US
Phone: 212-621-6000
Fax: 212-724-9064
E-mail Address: *info@ascap.com*
Web Address: www.ascap.com
American Society of Composers, Authors & Publishers (ASCAP) is a membership association of U.S. composers, songwriters and publishers of every kind of music with hundreds of thousands of members worldwide.

Content Delivery & Storage Association (CDSA)
182 Nassau St., Ste. 204
Princeton, NJ 08542-7005 US
Phone: 609-279-1700
Fax: 609-279-1999
E-mail Address: *mbevel@contentdeliveryandstorage.or g*
Web Address: www.contentdeliveryandstorage.org
The Content Delivery & Storage Association (CDSA), formerly the International Recording Media

Association, is a worldwide trade association encompassing organizations involved in every facet of recording media, including entertainment, information and software content storage.

International Association of Audio Information Services (IAAIS)
3920 Willshire Dr.
Lawrence, KS 66049
Toll Free: 800-280-5325
E-mail Address: *Stuart.Holland@state.mn.us*
Web Address: www.iaais.org
International Association of Audio Information Services (IAAIS) is an organization that provides audio access to information for people who are print-disabled.

Music Publisher's Association of the United States (MPA)
243 5th Ave., Ste. 236
New York, NY 10016 US
Phone: 212-327-4044
E-mail Address: *admin@mpa.org*
Web Address: mpa.org
The Music Publisher's Association of the United States (MPA) serves as a forum for publishers to deal with the music industry's vital issues and is actively involved in supporting and advancing compliance with copyright law, combating copyright infringement and exploring the need for further reform.

Recording Industry Association of America (RIAA)
1025 F St. NW, 10th Fl.
Washington, DC 20004 US
Phone: 202-775-0101
E-mail Address: *webmaster@riaa.com*
Web Address: www.riaa.com
The Recording Industry Association of America (RIAA) is the trade group that represents the U.S. recording industry.

Society of Professional Audio Recording Services (SPARS)
9 Music Sq. S., Ste. 222
Nashville, TN 37203 US
Fax: 616-296-0386
Toll Free: 800-771-7727
E-mail Address: *spars@spars.com*
Web Address: www.spars.com

The Society of Professional Audio Recording Services (SPARS) is an organization for members of the recording industry to share practical business information about audio and multimedia facility ownership, management and operations.

Songwriters Guild of America
209 10th Ave. S, Ste. 321
Nashville, TN 37203 US
Phone: 615-742-9945
Fax: 615-742-9948
E-mail Address: *corporate@songwritersguild.com*
Web Address: www.songwritersguild.com
The Songwriters Guild of America is the nation's largest and oldest songwriters' organization, serving its members with information and programs to further their careers and understanding of the music industry.

LVIII.   Retail Industry Associations

National Retail Federation (NRF)
325 7th St. NW, Ste. 1100
Washington, DC 20004 US
Phone: 202-783-7971
Fax: 202-737-2849
Toll Free: 800-673-4692
E-mail Address: *gattim@nrf.com*
Web Address: www.nrf.com
The National Retail Federation (NRF) is one of the world's largest retail trade organizations. Its membership includes the leading department, specialty, independent, discount and mass merchandise stores in the United States and 50 nations worldwide.

LIX.   Satellite-Related Professional Organizations

Society of Satellite Professionals International (SSPI)
The New York Information Technology Ctr.
55 Broad St., 14th Fl.
New York, NY 10004 US
Phone: 212-809-5199
Fax: 212-825-0075
E-mail Address: *rbell@sspi.org*
Web Address: www.sspi.org

The Society of Satellite Professionals International (SSPI) is a nonprofit member-benefit society that serves satellite professionals worldwide throughout the span of their careers.

LX.   Securities Industry Associations

Securities Industry and Financial Markets Association (SIFMA)
120 Broadway, 35th Fl.
New York, NY 10271-0080 US
Phone: 212-313-1200
Fax: 212-313-1301
E-mail Address: CMartin@sifma.org
Web Address: www.sifma.org
The Securities Industry and Financial Markets Association (SIFMA), formed by the recent merger of the Securities Industry Association (SIA) and the Bond Market Association, brings together the shared interests of more than 650 securities and bond industry firms to accomplish common goals.

LXI.   Software Industry Resources

Software Engineering Institute (SEI)-Carnegie Mellon
Customer Relations
4500 Fifth Ave.
Pittsburgh, PA 15213-2612 US
Phone: 412-268-5800
Fax: 412-268-6257
Toll Free: 888-201-4479
E-mail Address: customer-relations@sei.cmu.edu
Web Address: www.sei.cmu.edu
The Software Engineering Institute (SEI) is a federally funded research and development center at Carnegie Mellon University, sponsored by the U.S. Department of Defense through the Office of the Under Secretary of Defense for Acquisition, Technology, and Logistics [OUSD (AT&L)]. The SEI's core purpose is to help users make measured improvements in their software engineering capabilities.

LXII.   Stock Market Data

MSN Money Central
Web Address: moneycentral.msn.com

MSN Money Central features daily announcements, special reports, highlights from financial providers and a wealth of links and other financial information.

Reuters.com
Thompson Reuters Headquarters
3 Times Sq.
New York, NY 10036 US
Phone: 646-223-4000
Toll Free: 800-738-8377
Web Address: www.reuters.com
Reuters.com, a service of Thompson Reuters, offers information on business and world markets, political and international news and company-specific stock information.

Yahoo! Finance
Yahoo! Inc.
701 1st Ave.
Sunnyvale, CA 94089 US
Phone: 408-349-5070
Web Address: finance.yahoo.com
Yahoo! Finance provides a wealth of links and a supreme search guide. Users can find just about any financial information concerning both U.S. and world markets. Tax, insurance information, financial news and community research can be conducted through this site, as can searches for other aspects of the financial world.

LXIII.   Telecommunications Industry Associations

National Association of Telecommunications Officers and Advisors (NATOA)
1800 Diagonal Rd., Ste. 495
Alexandria, VA 22314 US
Phone: 703-519-8035
Fax: 703-519-8036
E-mail Address: info@natoa.org
Web Address: www.natoa.org
The National Association of Telecommunications Officers and Advisors (NATOA) works to support and serve the telecommunications interests and needs of local governments.

LXIV.   Temporary Staffing Firms

Adecco
Saegereistrasse 10
Glattbrugg, CH-8152 Switzerland
Phone: 41-44-878-88-88
Fax: 41-44-829-89-24
E-mail Address: investor.relations@adecco.com
Web Address: www.adecco.com
Adecco maintains human resources and staffing services offices in 70 countries. It provides temporary and permanent personnel.

Kelly Services, Inc.
999 W. Big Beaver Rd.
Troy, MI 48084-4782 US
Phone: 248-362-4444
E-mail Address: kfirst@kellyservices.com
Web Address: www.kellyservices.com
Kelly Services is a staffing solutions company providing approximately 700,000 employees to more than 150,000 client companies in 26 countries.

Kforce, Inc.
1001 E. Palm Ave.
Tampa, FL 33605 US
Phone: 813-552-5000
Toll Free: 877-453-6723
Web Address: www.kforce.com
Kforce, Inc. is one of the country's largest, fastest-growing temporary placement firms, with more than 70 offices in 44 cities across the U.S. It specializes in employees for the following types of jobs: finance and accounting, scientific, technology, health care, clinical research, mortgages, title insurance and real estate.

Manpower, Inc.
100 Manpower Pl.
Milwaukee, WI 53212 US
Phone: 414-961-1000
Web Address: www.manpower.com
One of the largest temporary staffing providers in the world, Manpower places approximately 2 million workers annually in a variety of positions around the world.

Robert Half International (RHI)
2884 Sand Hill Rd., Ste. 200
Menlo Park, CA 94025 US
Phone: 650-234-6000
E-mail Address: webmaster@rhi.com
Web Address: www.rhi.com

Specializing in accounting and finance positions, Robert Half International (RHI) also places workers in administrative, information technology, legal, advertising and marketing positions on temporary or permanent bases.

Spherion Corporation
2050 Spectrum Blvd.
Fort Lauderdale, FL 33309 US
Phone: 954-308-7600
Fax: 954-308-7600
E-mail Address: help@spherion.com
Web Address: www.spherion.com
Spherion, which was Interim Services, provides temporary staffing, recruitment and employee consulting. The company has more than 900 offices throughout the world.

Volt Information Sciences
560 Lexington Ave., 15th Fl.
New York, NY 10022 US
Phone: 212-704-2400
Web Address: www.volt.com
Volt Information Sciences maintains 300 temporary staffing offices in North America and in the U.K.

LXV. Testing Resources

CPP, Inc.
1055 Joaquin Rd., 2nd Fl.
Mountain View, CA 94043 US
Phone: 650-969-8901
Fax: 650-969-8608
Toll Free: 800-624-1765
E-mail Address: custserv@cpp.com
Web Address: www.cpp.com
CPP, Inc. (formerly known as Consulting Psychologists Press) publishes the Meyers-Briggs Type Indicator, Strong Inventory Test and other psychological assessment-related products. CPP also provides information about the tests and, through division Davies-Black Publishing, offers business-related books and services, including those covering career management and leadership development.

LXVI. Textile & Fabric Associations

International Textile and Apparel Association (ITAA)
6060 Sunrise Vista Dr., Ste. 1300
Citrus Heights, CA 95610 US
Phone: 916-723-1628
Fax: 719-722-8149
E-mail Address: info@itaaonline.org
Web Address: www.itaaonline.org
The International Textile and Apparel Association (ITAA) is a nonprofit educational and scientific corporation dedicated to providing opportunities to scholars in the retail, textile and apparel industries.

LXVII. Travel Business & Professional Associations

American Society of Travel Agents (ASTA)
1101 King St., Ste. 200
Alexandria, VA 22314 US
Fax: 703-739-3268
Toll Free: 800-275-2782
E-mail Address: askasta@astahq.com
Web Address: www.astanet.com
The American Society of Travel Agents (ASTA) is one of the world's largest associations of travel professionals.

Association of Corporate Travel Executives (ACTE)
515 King St., Ste. 440
Alexandria, VA 22314 US
Phone: 703-683-5322
Fax: 703-683-2720
E-mail Address: info@acte.org
Web Address: www.acte.org
The Association of Corporate Travel Executives (ACTE) serves the specialized travel interests of corporate purchasers and travel service suppliers from nearly 50 countries.

Association of Retail Travel Agents (ARTA)
c/o Travel Destinations, Inc.
4320 North Miller Rd.
Scottsdale, AZ 85251 US
Fax: 615-985-0600
Toll Free: 800-969-6069
E-mail Address: info@artaonline.com
Web Address: www.artaonline.com

The Association of Retail Travel Agents (ARTA) is one of the largest nonprofit associations in North America to exclusively represent travel agents.

Association of Travel Marketing Executives (ATME)
P.O. Box 3176
West Tisbury, MA 02575 US
Phone: 508-693-0550
Fax: 508-693-0115
E-mail Address: admin@atme.org
Web Address: www.atme.org
The Association of Travel Marketing Executives (ATME) is a global professional association of senior-level travel marketing executives dedicated to providing cutting-edge information, education and opportunities for meaningful networking with peers.

National Society of Minorities in Hospitality
107 S. West St., PMB 119
Alexandria, VA 22314 US
Phone: 703-549-9899
Fax: 703-997-7795
E-mail Address: hq@nsmh.org
Web Address: www.nsmh.org
The National Society of Minorities in Hospitality strives to establish a working relationship between the hospitality industry and minority students.

Network of Executive Women in Hospitality
P.O. Box 322
Shawano, WI 54166 US
Fax: 800-693-6394
Toll Free: 800-593-6394
Web Address: www.newh.org
The Network of Executive Women in Hospitality brings together professionals from all facets of the hospitality industry by providing opportunities for education, professional development and networking.

LXVIII. Travel Industry Associations

Destination Marketing Association International
2025 M St. NW, Ste. 500
Washington, DC 20036 US

Phone: 202-296-7888
Fax: 202-296-7889
Toll Free: 888-275-3140
E-mail Address:
info@destinationmarketing.org
Web Address:
www.destinationmarketing.org
The Destination Marketing Association
International, formerly the
International Association of
Convention & Visitor Bureaus, strives
to enhance the professionalism,
effectiveness and image of destination
management organizations worldwide.

International Association of Conference Centers (IACC)

243 N. Lindbergh Blvd.
St. Louis, MO 63141 US
Phone: 314-993-8575
Fax: 314-993-8919
E-mail Address: *info@iacconline.org*
Web Address: www.iacconline.com
The International Association of
Conference Centers (IACC) is a
nonprofit, facilities-based organization
founded to promote a greater
awareness and understanding of the
unique features of conference centers
around the world.

National Tour Association (NTA)

546 E. Main St.
Lexington, KY 40508 US
Phone: 859-226-4444
Fax: 859-226-4414
Toll Free: 800-682-8886
E-mail Address:
questions@ntastaff.com
Web Address: www.ntaonline.com
The National Tour Association (NTA)
is an association for travel
professionals who have an interest in
the packaged travel sector of the
industry.

Society of Incentive and Travel Executives

401 N. Michigan Ave.
Chicago, IL 60611 US
Phone: 312-321-5148
Fax: 312-527-6783
E-mail Address: *hq@site-intl.org*
Web Address: www.site-intl.org
The Society of Incentive and Travel
Executives is a worldwide organization
of business professionals dedicated to
the recognition and development of

motivational and performance
improvement strategies in the travel
industry.

Travel Industry Association of America

1100 New York Ave. NW, Ste. 450
Washington, DC 20005-3934 US
Phone: 202-408-8422
Fax: 202-408-1255
E-mail Address: *feedback@tia.org*
Web Address: www.tia.org
The Travel Industry Association of
America is a nonprofit association that
represents and speaks for the common
interests and concerns of all
components of the U.S. travel industry.

LXIX. U.S. Government Agencies

Bureau of Economic Analysis (BEA)

1441 L St. NW
Washington, DC 20230 US
Phone: 202-606-9900
E-mail Address:
customerservice@bea.gov
Web Address: www.bea.gov
The Bureau of Economic Analysis
(BEA), an agency of the U.S.
Department of Commerce, is the
nation's economic accountant,
preparing estimates that illuminate key
national, international and regional
aspects of the U.S. economy.

Bureau of Labor Statistics (BLS)

Postal Squre Bldg.
2 Massachusetts Ave. NE
Washington, DC 20212-0001 US
Phone: 202-691-5200
Web Address: stats.bls.gov
The Bureau of Labor Statistics (BLS)
is the principal fact-finding agency for
the Federal Government in the field of
labor economics and statistics. It is an
independent national statistical agency
that collects, processes, analyzes and
disseminates statistical data to the
American public, U.S. Congress, other
federal agencies, state and local
governments, business and labor. The
BLS also serves as a statistical
resource to the Department of Labor.

Equal Employment Opportunity Commission (EEOC)

1801 L St. NW

Washington, DC 20507 US
Phone: 202-663-4900
Toll Free: 800-669-4000
E-mail Address: *info@eeoc.gov*
Web Address: www.eeoc.gov
The Equal Employment Opportunity
Commission (EEOC) is a Federal
Government agency focused on
practices and programs that foster
equal opportunity at work and
elsewhere. Its web site features details
about various protective laws regarding
employment. It also provides
information on how to file a
discrimination claim.

FedStats

Web Address: www.fedstats.gov
FedStats compiles information for
statistics from over 100 U.S. federal
agencies. Visitors can sort the
information by agency, geography and
topic, as well as perform searches.

Government Printing Office (GPO)

732 N. Capitol St. NW
Washington, DC 20401 US
Phone: 202-512-0000
Fax: 202-512-2104
E-mail Address:
contactcenter@gpo.gov
Web Address: www.gpo.gov
The U.S. Government Printing Office
(GPO) is the primary information
source concerning the activities of
Federal agencies. GPO gathers,
catalogues, produces, provides,
authenticates and preserves published
information.

National Labor Relations Board (NLRB)

1099 14th St. NW
Washington, DC 20570-0001 US
Phone: 202-208-3000
Fax: 202-208-3013
Toll Free: 866-667-6572
Web Address: www.nlrb.gov
The National Labor Relations Board
(NLRB) provides case reports on labor
disputes, searchable by company or
union.

U.S. Business Advisor

Business Gateway Program
Management Office
U.S. Small Business Administration,
409 3rd St. SW

Washington, DC 20416 US
Phone: 202-205-6564
E-mail Address:
dennis.byrne@sba.gov
Web Address: www.business.gov
U.S. Business Advisor offers a
searchable directory of business-
specific government information.
Topics include taxes, regulations,
international trade, financial assistance
and business development. U.S.
Business Advisor was created by the
U.S. Small Business Administration
(SBA) in a partnership with 21 other
federal agencies. This partnership is
known as the Business Gateway.

U.S. Census Bureau
4700 Silver Hill Rd.
Washington, DC 20233-8800 US
Phone: 301-763-3030
Fax: 301-457-3670
E-mail Address: *pio@census.gov*
Web Address: www.census.gov
The U.S. Census Bureau is the official
collector of data about the people and
economy of the U.S. Founded in 1790,
it provides official social, demographic
and economic information.

**U.S. Department of Commerce
(DOC)**
1401 Constitution Ave. NW
Washington, DC 20230 US
Phone: 202-482-2000
E-mail Address: *cgutierrez@doc.gov*
Web Address: www.doc.gov
The U.S. Department of Commerce
(DOC) regulates trade and provides
valuable economic analysis of the
economy.

U.S. Department of Labor (DOL)
Frances Perkins Bldg.
200 Constitution Ave. NW
Washington, DC 20210 US
Toll Free: 866-487-2365
Web Address: www.dol.gov
The U.S. Department of Labor (DOL)
is the government agency responsible
for labor regulations. This site provides
tools to help citizens find out whether
companies are complying with family
and medical-leave requirements.

**U.S. Securities and Exchange
Commission (SEC)**
100 F St. NE

Washington, DC 20549 US
Phone: 202-942-8088
Toll Free: 800-732-0330
E-mail Address: *help@sec.gov*
Web Address: www.sec.gov
The U.S. Securities and Exchange
Commission (SEC) is a nonpartisan,
quasi-judicial regulatory agency
responsible for administering federal
securities laws. These laws are
designed to protect investors in
securities markets and ensure that they
have access to disclosure of all
material information concerning
publicly traded securities. Visitors to
the web site can access the EDGAR
database of corporate financial and
business information.

LXX.   Waste Industry Associations

**Air & Waste Management
Association**
1 Gateway Ctr., 3rd Fl.
420 Fort Duquesne Blvd.
Pittsburgh, PA 15222-1435 US
Phone: 412-232-3444
Fax: 412-232-3450
Toll Free: 800-270-3444
E-mail Address: *info@awma.org*
Web Address: www.awma.org
The Air & Waste Management
Association provides training,
information and networking
opportunities to environmental
professionals worldwide.

LXXI.   Water Resources Associations

**American Water Resources
Association (AWRA)**
P.O. Box 1626
Middleburg, VA 20118 US
Phone: 540-687-8390
Fax: 540-687-8395
E-mail Address: *info@awra.org*
Web Address: www.awra.org
The American Water Resources
Association (AWRA) represents the
interests of professionals involved in
water resources.

LXXII.   Writers, Photographers & Editors Associations

**American Society of Journalists and
Authors, Inc. (ASJA)**
1501 Broadway, Ste. 302
New York, NY 10036 US
Phone: 212-997-0947
Fax: 212-937-2315
E-mail Address: *director@asja.org*
Web Address: www.asja.org
The American Society of Journalists
and Authors (ASJA) is of the nation's
leading organizations of independent
nonfiction writers.

**American Society of Magazine
Editors (ASME)**
Magazine Publishers of America
(MPA)
810 7th Ave., 24th Fl.
New York, NY 10019 US
Phone: 212-872-3736
E-mail Address: *asme@magazine.org*
Web Address:
www.magazine.org/asme
The American Society of Magazine
Editors (ASME) is a professional
organization for editors of print and
online magazines. ASME is part of the
Magazine Publishers of America
(MPA).

**American Society of Newspaper
Editors (ASNE)**
11690B Sunrise Valley Dr.
Reston, VA 20191-1409 US
Phone: 703-453-1122
Fax: 703-453-1133
E-mail Address: *asne@asne.org*
Web Address: www.asne.org
The American Society of Newspaper
Editors (ASNE) is an association that
brings together editors of daily
newspapers and people directly
involved with developing content for
daily newspapers.

**International Women's Writing
Guild (IWWG)**
P.O. Box 810, Gracie Station
New York, NY 10028-0082 US
Phone: 212-737-7536
Fax: 212-737-9469
E-mail Address: *dirhahn@iwwg.org*
Web Address: www.iwwg.com
The International Women's Writing
Guild (IWWG) is a network for the

personal and professional empowerment of women through writing.

Media Communications Association International (MCAI)
2810 Crossroads Dr., Ste. 3800
Madison, WI 53718 US
Phone: 608-443-2464
Fax: 608-443-2474
E-mail Address: *execdirect@mca-i.org*
Web Address: www.mca-i.org
The Media Communications Association International (MCAI) is the leading global community for media communications professionals seeking to drive the convergence of communications and technology for the growth of the profession.

National Association of Hispanic Journalists (NAHJ)
1000 National Press Bldg.
529 14th St. NW
Washington, DC 20045-2001 US
Phone: 202-662-7145
Fax: 202-662-7144
Toll Free: 888-346-6245
E-mail Address: *nahj@nahj.org*
Web Address: www.nahj.org
The National Association of Hispanic Journalists (NAHJ) is dedicated to the recognition and professional advancement of Hispanics in the news industry.

National Association of Science Writers, Inc. (NASW)
P.O. Box 890
Hedgesville, WV 25427 US
Phone: 304-754-5077
Fax: 304-754-5076
E-mail Address: *director@nasw.org*
Web Address: www.nasw.org
The National Association of Science Writers (NASW) exists to foster the dissemination of accurate information regarding science through all media devoted to informing the public.

National Conference of Editorial Writers (NCEW)
3899 N. Front St.
Harrisburg, PA 17110 US
Phone: 717-703-3015
Fax: 717-703-3014
E-mail Address: *ncew@pa-news.org*
Web Address: www.ncew.org

The National Conference of Editorial Writers (NCEW) strives to stimulate the conscience and quality of editorial writing.

National Federation of Press Women (NFPW)
P.O. Box 5556
Arlington, VA 22205 US
Fax: 703-812-4555
Toll Free: 800-780-2715
E-mail Address: *presswomen@aol.com*
Web Address: www.nfpw.org
The National Federation of Press Women (NFPW) is an organization of professional journalists and communicators.

National Writers Union (NWU)
113 University Pl., 6th Fl.
New York, NY 10003 US
Phone: 212-254-0279
Fax: 212-254-0673
E-mail Address: *nwu@nwu.org*
Web Address: www.nwu.org
The National Writers Union (NWU) is a labor union that represents freelance writers in all genres, formats and media. It is committed to improving the economic and working conditions of freelance writers.

Society of Children's Book Writers and Illustrators (SCBWI)
8271 Beverly Blvd.
Los Angeles, CA 90048 US
Phone: 323-782-1010
Fax: 323-782-1892
E-mail Address: *scbwi@scbwi.org*
Web Address: www.scbwi.org
The Society of Children's Book Writers and Illustrators (SCBWI) serves people who write, illustrate or share a vital interest in children's literature.

Chapter 5

THE AMERICAN EMPLOYERS 500:
WHO THEY ARE AND
HOW THEY WERE CHOSEN

Note: financial data given for each of the AMERICAN EMPLOYERS 500 firms is for the year ended December 31, 2007, a fiscal year ended in 2007 or the latest figures available to the editors. Telephone numbers, addresses, contact names, Internet addresses and other vital facts were collected in the summer of 2008.

The companies chosen to be listed in THE ALMANAC OF AMERICAN EMPLOYERS are not the same as the "Fortune 500" or any other list of corporations. The AMERICAN EMPLOYERS 500 were chosen specifically for their likelihood to provide new job openings to the greatest number of employees. Complete information about each firm can be found in the "Individual Data Listings," beginning about the middle of this book. They are in alphabetical order.

THE AMERICAN EMPLOYERS 500 includes companies from all parts of the United States and from nearly all industry segments: selected banks, retailers, service companies, wholesalers and distributors, insurance companies and others, as well as industrial companies, technology firms and manufacturers.

Simply stated, the list contains 500 of the largest, most successful, employers in the United States today. In particular, the list contains companies that we have hand-selected to have qualities that we feel will be of greatest interest to job seekers of today

who are looking for opportunities to obtain employment with major corporations.

Job seekers in America will find a face a tough market in 2009. Many industry sectors are undergoing structural changes that will be long lasting and will reduce their number of job openings. Virtually all business sectors are facing challenges due to the global financial crisis of late 2008.

In order to make this reference guide as useful as possible, we have altered, in this and the most recent editions of this book, the company selection criteria that were used in early editions. Rather than focusing largely on mid-term growth histories, we are instead focusing more on type of business, industry sector served and competitive advantage. This is because some sectors may not offer good career prospects today. Consequently, we have deleted some well known companies due to the state of their particular markets.

Fortunately, in the prior 2007 and 2008 editions of this book, we had already eliminated most employers that had deep connections to mortgage brokerage or residential construction, because we were predicting a significant correction in the housing market. This remains true in this 2009 edition. Likewise, we have long been avoiding listing America's Big Three automakers in this book, and we have been avoiding most airlines for years. This 2009 edition lists only two banking firms, and does not list any of the hard-hit investment firms.

Although we expect 2009 to be a difficult year for retailers and for hotel companies, we do list a selected group of employers in these sectors that we feel will tend to have an above-average number of good job openings.

However, job seekers should always bear in mind the fact that firms of many types will continue to restrain hiring. In addition, frequent layoffs have become standard in corporate America. (See Chapter 1 "Trends" for further thoughts about layoffs and other trends.)

To be included in our list, the firms were selected on the following criteria:

1) U.S.-based companies. (However, a small number of companies may be subsidiaries of foreign-based firms. Also, one firm, Accenture, is a major U.S. employer that uses a headquarters address in Bermuda.)

2) 2,500 employees or more.

3) These are almost exclusively for-profit companies. However, a small number are major, non-profit health care companies.

4) Selected Type of Business and/or Industry Sector: Companies were chosen based on our analysis of the business potential of their products, services and industrial sectors in light of today's economy.

The companies were chosen in this manner for the following reasons:

500 COMPANIES (the actual count is 508 companies) so there is a broad base among which to make comparisons and from which you can study potential employers.

LARGER EMPLOYERS (2,500 or more employees) so the information can pertain to as many employees as reasonably possible, and so the companies ranked will tend to create large numbers of job openings. Also, large companies historically have offered significantly higher wages, better benefits and better training than small employers

FOR-PROFIT so that job seekers using THE ALMANAC OF AMERICAN EMPLOYERS can choose positions in the profit-seeking, private sector, where incentive plans are available to motivate and reward them, such as profit sharing, stock ownership, bonuses, stock options and the high pay and prestige of top executive posts.

COMPANIES THAT OPERATE IN PROMISING BUSINESS SECTORS because:

1) Companies that are stable or enjoying growing business are much more likely to have job openings. Corporate stability is more important to job seekers today than ever before due to the wave of layoffs and downsizing that continues to sweep through the U.S. business world. (See Chapter 1, "Trends.")

2) These companies are much more likely to offer advancement opportunities. Current employees will benefit from promote-from-within policies when new plants, new stores, new product lines or new offices are opened.

A low score in any part of this book should not be taken as a slur against the company so ranked; it should be taken as evidence of the obvious: some companies are better to work for than others, depending, of course, on what you value. It is not easy to get into the AMERICAN EMPLOYERS 500, and the mere presence of a company on the list can be taken as evidence that it has excelled in many ways. To start with, it has to have generated enough business to employ thousands of people–never a simple task.

20 Largest Employers of the American Employers 500,
By Number of Employees

Company	City	State	No. of Employees	Primary Line of Business
WAL-MART STORES INC	Bentonville	AR	1,900,000	Discount Department Stores
KELLY SERVICES INC	Troy	MI	750,000	Staffing & Temporary Help
UNITED PARCEL SERVICE INC (UPS)	Atlanta	GA	425,300	Express Delivery Service
MCDONALD'S CORP	Oak Brook	IL	390,000	Fast Food Restaurants
INTERNATIONAL BUSINESS MACHINES CORP (IBM)	Armonk	NY	386,558	Computer Hardware
TARGET CORPORATION	Minneapolis	MN	366,000	Discount Department Stores
HOME DEPOT INC	Atlanta	GA	331,000	Home Centers, Retail
GENERAL ELECTRIC CO (GE)	Fairfield	CT	327,000	Business Leasing & Finance
KROGER CO (THE)	Cincinnati	OH	310,000	Grocery Stores
AT&T INC	San Antonio	TX	309,050	Telephone Service
YUM! BRANDS INC	Louisville	KY	301,000	Fast Food Restaurants
ARAMARK CORPORATION	Philadelphia	PA	250,000	Food Service Contractor
VERIZON COMMUNICATIONS	New York	NY	235,000	Local Telephone Service
BERKSHIRE HATHAWAY INC	Omaha	NE	233,000	Direct Property & Casualty Insurance & Reinsurance
UNITED TECHNOLOGIES CORPORATION	Hartford	CT	225,600	Aerospace Technology
BANK OF AMERICA CORP	Charlotte	NC	210,000	Banking
LOWE'S COMPANIES INC	Mooresville	NC	210,000	Home Centers, Retail
SAFEWAY INC	Pleasanton	CA	201,000	Grocery Stores
CVS CAREMARK CORPORATION	Woonsocket	RI	200,000	Drug Stores
SUPERVALU INC	Eden Prairie	MN	191,400	Grocery Stores

20 Largest Employers of the American Employers 500, By Revenues

Company	City	State	2007 Sales (in thousands of dollars)	Primary Line of Business
EXXON MOBIL CORPORATION (EXXONMOBIL)	Irving	TX	390,328,000	Oil & Gas Exploration & Production
WAL-MART STORES INC	Bentonville	AR	344,992,000	Discount Department Stores
CHEVRON CORPORATION	San Ramon	CA	220,904,000	Oil & Gas Exploration & Production
CONOCOPHILLIPS COMPANY	Houston	TX	187,437,000	Oil & Gas Exploration & Production
GENERAL ELECTRIC CO (GE)	Fairfield	CT	172,738,000	Business Leasing & Finance
BANK OF AMERICA CORP	Charlotte	NC	124,321,000	Banking
AT&T INC	San Antonio	TX	118,928,000	Telephone Service
BERKSHIRE HATHAWAY INC	Omaha	NE	118,245,000	Direct Property & Casualty Insurance & Reinsurance
WILLIAMS COMPANIES INC (THE)	Tulsa	OK	105,558,000	Gas Exploration & Production
INTERNATIONAL BUSINESS MACHINES CORP (IBM)	Armonk	NY	98,786,000	Computer Hardware
KOCH INDUSTRIES INC	Wichita	KS	98,000,000	Petroleum Refining
VALERO ENERGY CORP	San Antonio	TX	95,327,000	Petroleum Refineries & Retail Marketing
VERIZON COMMUNICATIONS	New York	NY	93,469,000	Local Telephone Service
MCKESSON CORPORATION	San Francisco	CA	92,977,000	Pharmaceutical Solutions
CARGILL INC	Wayzata	MN	88,266,000	Crop Production, Milling and Distribution
SHELL OIL CO	Houston	TX	87,548,000	Oil & Gas Exploration & Production
CARDINAL HEALTH INC	Dublin	OH	86,852,000	Healthcare Products & Services
HOME DEPOT INC	Atlanta	GA	79,022,000	Home Centers, Retail
PROCTER & GAMBLE CO	Cincinnati	OH	76,476,000	Household Products Manufacturing
CVS CAREMARK CORPORATION	Woonsocket	RI	76,329,500	Drug Stores

20 Largest Employers of the American Employers 500, By Profits

Company	City	State	2007 Profits (in thousands of dollars)	Primary Line of Business
EXXON MOBIL CORPORATION (EXXONMOBIL)	Irving	TX	40,610,000	Oil & Gas Exploration & Production
GENERAL ELECTRIC CO (GE)	Fairfield	CT	22,208,000	Business Leasing & Finance
CHEVRON CORPORATION	San Ramon	CA	18,688,000	Oil & Gas Exploration & Production
JP MORGAN CHASE & CO INC	New York	NY	15,365,000	Banking
BANK OF AMERICA CORP	Charlotte	NC	14,982,000	Banking
MICROSOFT CORP	Redmond	WA	14,065,000	Computer Software
BERKSHIRE HATHAWAY INC	Omaha	NE	13,213,000	Direct Property & Casualty Insurance & Reinsurance
AT&T INC	San Antonio	TX	11,951,000	Telephone Service
CONOCOPHILLIPS COMPANY	Houston	TX	11,891,000	Oil & Gas Exploration & Production
WAL-MART STORES INC	Bentonville	AR	11,284,000	Discount Department Stores
JOHNSON & JOHNSON	New Brunswick	NJ	10,576,000	Personal Health Care & Hygiene Products
INTERNATIONAL BUSINESS MACHINES CORP (IBM)	Armonk	NY	10,418,000	Computer Hardware
PROCTER & GAMBLE CO	Cincinnati	OH	10,340,000	Household Products Manufacturing
ALTRIA GROUP INC	New York	NY	9,786,000	Tobacco Products
PFIZER INC	New York	NY	8,144,000	Pharmaceutical Drugs
CISCO SYSTEMS INC	San Jose	CA	7,333,000	Computer Networking Equipment
INTEL CORP	Santa Clara	CA	6,976,000	Microprocessors
COCA COLA COMPANY (THE)	Atlanta	GA	5,981,000	Soft Drink Manufacturing
HOME DEPOT INC	Atlanta	GA	5,761,000	Home Centers, Retail
PEPSICO INC	Purchase	NY	5,658,000	Soft Drink Manufacturing

INDUSTRY LIST, WITH CODES

This book refers to the following list of unique industry codes, based on the 1997 NAIC code system (NAIC is used by many analysts as a replacement for older SIC codes because NAIC is more specific to today's industry sectors). Companies profiled in this book are given a primary NAIC code, reflecting the main line of business of each firm.

Agriculture

Farming
112000	Meat Production
112300	Poultry Production

Apparel

Apparel & Shoe Manufacturing
315000	Apparel Manufacturing-General
315000A	Apparel Manufacturing-Athletic Clothes
316213	Shoe Manufacturing-Men's
316219	Shoe Manufacturing-Athletic Shoes & Misc. Shoes, Incl. Children's

Entertainment

Publishing
511140	Databases & Directories, Publishing

Broadcasting
513111	Radio Broadcasting
513120	Television Broadcasting
513210	Cable TV Networks
513220	Cable & Satellite TV & Data Service

Gambling & Recreation
713290	Gambling Equipment
713910	Golf Courses & Country Clubs
713940	Fitness Centers/Health Clubs

Hotels & Accommodations
721110	Hotels/Resorts/Motels
721120	Casino Resorts

Energy

Fuel Mining & Extraction
211111	Oil & Natural Gas Exploration & Production
212110	Coal Mining
213111	Petroleum-Drilling Oil & Gas Wells Support

Utilities
221000	Utilities-Electric & Gas
221000A	Utilities-Electric
221000B	Utilities-Gas

Petroleum-Refining & Manufacturing
324110	Petroleum Refineries
324110A	Petroleum Refineries & Retail Marketing

325110	Petrochemicals Manufacturing
325120	Industrial Gas Manufacturing

Manufacturing, Electrical
335910	Battery Manufacturing

Financial Services

Financial Data
514100	Financial Data Publishing- Print & Online

Banking, Credit & Finance
522110	Banking
522210	Credit Card Issuing
522220A	Financing--Business
522298	Pawn Shops
522320	Payment & Transaction Processing Services
522320A	Payment & Transaction Processing--Benefits Management

Insurance
524113	Insurance-Life
524114	Insurance-Health, HMO's & PPO's
524114A	Insurance--Health Supplemental & Specialty
524126	Insurance-Property & Casualty
524210	Insurance Brokerage, Agencies & Exchanges

Professional Services, Financial
541210	Accounting Services

Credit Bureaus
561450	Credit Bureaus

Food & Restaurants

Food Service
722110	Restaurants
722310	Food Service Contractors

Health Care

Health Products, Manufacturing
325412	Drugs (Pharmaceuticals), Discovery & Manufacturing
325413	Diagnostic Services and Substances Manufacturing
325416	Drugs (Pharmaceuticals), Generic Manufacturing
339113	Medical/Dental/Surgical Equipment & Supplies, Manufacturing

Health Products, Wholesale Distribution
421450	Medical/Dental/Surgical Equipment & Supplies, Distribution
422210	Drugs, Distribution

Health Care-Clinics, Labs and Organizations
524298	Disease Management & Utilization Management
621490	Clinics--Outpatient Clinics & Surgery
621511	Laboratories & Diagnostic Services--Medical
621610	Home Health Care

Hospitals
622110 Hospitals/Clinics--General & Specialty Hospitals
622210 Hospitals/Clinics--Psychiatric Clinics
Nursing
623110 Long-Term Health Care & Assisted Living
Veterinary Care
541940 Veterinary Clinics

InfoTech

Computers & Electronics Manufacturing
334110 Computer Networking & Related Equipment, Manufacturing
334111 Computer Hardware, Manufacturing
334112 Computer Storage Equipment & Misc Parts, Manufacturing
334119 Computer Accessories, Monitors, Printers Manufacturing
334413 Semiconductors (Microchips)/Integrated Circuits/Components, Manufacturing
334419 Contract Electronics Manufacturing
334500 Instrument Manufacturing, including Measurement, Control, Test & Navigational
Computers & Electronics, Distribution
421430 Computer & Telecommunications Equipment Distribution
Software
511201 Computer Software, Accounting, Banking & Financial
511203 Computer Software, Sales & Customer Relationship Management
511204 Computer Software, Operating Systems, Languages & Development Tools
511207 Computer Software, Business Management & ERP
511208 Computer Software, Games & Entertainment
511209 Computer Software, Multimedia, Graphics & Publishing
511211 Computer Software, Security & Anti-Virus
511215 Computer Software, Product Lifecycle, Engineering, Design & CAD
Information & Data Processing Services
514199 Online Publishing, Services & Niche Portals
514199B Search Engine Portals
514210 Data Processing Services
Information Services-Professional
541512 Consulting--Computer, Telecommunications & Internet

Manufacturing

Food Products Manufacturing
311000 Food Products, Manufacturing
311210 Grain Distribution, Milling & Oilseed Processing
311230 Breakfast Cereal Manufacturing
311300 Sugar & Confectionery Product Manufacturing
311330 Chocolate & Confectionery Manufacturing
311420 Fruit & Vegetable Growing & Processing
311500 Dairy Products, Manufacturing
311800 Bakeries & Tortilla Manufacturing
Beverage & Tobacco Manufacturing
312111 Beverages--Soft Drinks & Juices Manufacturing
312140 Beverages--Distilleries
312220 Tobacco, Manufacturing
Paper Products/Forest Products
322000 Forest Products/Paper, Manufacturing
322210 Packaging, Manufacturing
Printing Services
323000 Printing
Chemicals
325510 Paints & Coatings, Manufacturing
325600 Soaps, Cleaners, Cosmetics & Toiletries, Manufacturing
Machinery & Manufacturing Equipment
333000 Machinery, Manufacturing
333130 Machinery-Mining & Oil & Gas Field, Manufacturing
333313 Business Machines, Manufacturing
Electrical Equipment, Appliances, Tools
335000 Electrical Equipment, Manufacturing
Jewelry, Watch & Other Manufacturing
334518 Watch & Clock Manufacturing

Nanotechnology

Nanotechnology
541710 Research and Development/Physical, Engineering and Life Sciences

Retailing

Textiles
421220 Carpet & Flooring, Retail
Automobiles & Parts Stores
441110 Auto Dealers, Retail
441300 Tire Stores
441310 Auto Parts Stores
Furniture & Home Furnishings Stores
442110 Furniture Stores
442299 Linens/Housewares/Art/Framing Stores
Computers & Electronics Stores
443110 Electronics, Audio & Appliance Stores
443120A Computers & Software-Direct Selling
Building Materials & Garden Supplies Stores
444110 Home Centers, Retail
444120 Paint & Wallpaper Stores
Food & Beverage Stores
445110 Grocery Stores/Supermarkets
445120 Convenience Stores
Drug Stores, Beauty Supply & Health Items Stores
446110 Pharmacies & Drug Stores
446110A Pharmacies-Specialty
446120 Cosmetics, Beauty Supplies & Perfume Stores

446191A	Personal Items, Cosmetics, Health Supplements by Direct Selling

Apparel & Accessories Stores
448000	Apparel Stores, General
448000A	Apparel, Direct Selling
448110	Apparel Stores, Men's
448120	Apparel Stores, Women's
448130	Apparel Stores, Children's
448210	Shoes & Accessories Stores
448310	Jewelry Stores

Sporting Goods, Hobbies, Books & Music Stores
451110	Sporting Goods Stores
451120	Toys/Hobbies/Games Stores
451211	Book Stores
451211E	Book Stores-Online

Department & Discount Stores
452110	Department Stores
452910	Discount Stores
452910A	Warehouse Clubs

Miscellaneous Retailers
453210	Office Supplies Stores
453910	Pets/Pet Supplies Stores
453998E	Auctions, Retail-Online

Nonstore Retailers
454110B	TV Shopping

Rental & Leasing Outlets
532200	Rental Stores, Consumer Goods

Personal Services & Salons
446190	Other Health & Personal Care Stores/Weight Management
812110	Hair, Nail & Skin Care Salons

Services

Agriculture
115112	Agricultural Crop Production Support, Seeds, Fertilizers

Construction
234000	Construction, Heavy & Civil Engineering
234920	Construction, Power & Communication Line

Real Estate
525930	Real Estate Investment Trusts - REITs
531100	Real Estate Rental, Leasing & Management

Consulting & Professional Services
541330	Engineering & Facilities Support Services
541611	Consulting--Management & Business
541612	Consulting-Human Resources
541613	Consulting--Marketing
541800	Marketing Agencies & Related Services
541810	Advertising Services/Agencies
541910	Market Research

Management
551110	Management of Companies & Enterprises

Personnel, Administrative & Support Services
561300	Staffing or Outsourcing
561320	Temporary Help/Staffing

Call Centers
561422	Call Centers

Travel Agencies
561500A	Travel Services-Online

Waste Management
562000	Waste Disposal, Waste Management

Educational
611410	Business Training, Distance Learning

Security Services
561610	Security, Protection, Armored Car & Investigation Services

Automotive Services
811100	Automotive Repair & Maintenance

Telecommunications

Telecommunications Equipment
334200	Communications Equipment, Manufacturing
334210	Telecommunications Equipment Manufacturing

Telecommunications
513300A	Telephone Service-Local Exchange Carrier & Diversified
513322	Telephone Service-Cellular, U.S. & Non-U.S.
513390C	Telecommunications-Private Data Networks & Network Services

Transportation

Transportation-Manufacturing of Equipment
336120	Trucks, RVs & Misc. Automotive, Manufacturing
336300	Automobile Parts Manufacturing

Aerospace
336410	Aerospace & Aircraft Related Manufacturing

Air
481000	Air Transportation-Major Carriers

Rail
482110	Railroad Transportation

Ships
483111	Shipping-Deep Sea
483112	Cruise Lines

Truck
484122	Truck Transportation-Less Than Truckload
488510	Freight Forwarding & Support Services
492110	Courier/Express Delivery Service
532111	Automobile, Rental/Leasing
532120	Trucks, Rental/Leasing

Wholesale Distribution-Other

Distribution-Durable Goods
421800	Machinery, Equipment & Supplies, Distribution
423110	Automobile & Other Motor Vehicle Merchant, Wholesale Distribution

Distribution-Nondurable Goods
422410	Food Distribution

INDEX OF RANKINGS WITHIN INDUSTRY GROUPS

Company	Industry Code	2007 Sales (U.S. $ thousands)	Sales Rank	2007 Profits (U.S. $ thousands)	Profits Rank
Accounting Services					
BDO SEIDMAN LLP	541210	659,000	5		
DELOITTE & TOUCHE USA LLP	541210	9,850,000	3		
ERNST & YOUNG LLP	541210	21,100,000	2		
GRANT THORNTON LLP	541210	1,075,000	4		
KPMG LLP	541210				
PRICEWATERHOUSECOOPERS	541210	25,150,000	1		
Advertising Services/Agencies					
OMNICOM GROUP INC	541810	12,700,000	1	975,700	1
Aerospace & Aircraft Related Manufacturing					
BOEING COMPANY	336410	66,387,000	1	4,074,000	2
CUBIC CORP	336410	889,870	9	41,586	9
GENERAL DYNAMICS CORP	336410	27,240,000	6	2,072,000	6
HONEYWELL INTERNATIONAL	336410	34,589,000	4	2,444,000	5
LOCKHEED MARTIN CORP	336410	41,862,000	3	3,033,000	3
NORTHROP GRUMMAN CORP	336410	32,018,000	5	1,790,000	7
RAYTHEON CO	336410	21,301,000	7	2,578,000	4
TELEDYNE TECHNOLOGIES INC	336410	1,622,300	8	98,500	8
UNITED TECHNOLOGIES CORP	336410	54,759,000	2	4,224,000	1
Agricultural Crop Production Support, Seeds, Fertilizers					
SCOTTS MIRACLE GROW CO	115112	2,871,800	1	113,400	1
Air Transportation-Major Carriers					
SOUTHWEST AIRLINES CO	481000	9,860,000	1	645,000	1
Apparel Manufacturing & Design-General					
POLO RALPH LAUREN CORP	315000	4,295,400	1	400,900	1
Apparel Manufacturing-Athletic Clothes					
QUIKSILVER INC	315000A	2,426,035	1	-121,119	1
RUSSELL CORP	315000A	561,800	2		
Apparel Stores, Children's					
TWEEN BRANDS INC	448130	883,683	1	64,821	1
Apparel Stores, General					
ABERCROMBIE & FITCH CO	448000	3,318,158	3	422,186	2
AMERICAN EAGLE OUTFITTERS	448000	2,794,409	4	387,359	3
BUCKLE INC	448000	530,074	9	55,726	7
GUESS? INC	448000	1,252,664	6	131,172	5
HOT TOPIC INC	448000	751,558	8	13,626	9
PACIFIC SUNWEAR OF CALIFORNIA INC	448000	1,447,204	5	39,621	8
ROSS STORES INC	448000	5,570,210	2	241,634	4
TJX COMPANIES INC	448000	17,404,637	1	776,756	1
URBAN OUTFITTERS INC	448000	1,224,717	7	116,206	6
Apparel Stores, Men's					
MEN'S WEARHOUSE INC	448110	1,882,064	1	148,575	1
Apparel Stores, Women's					
AEROPOSTALE INC	448120	1,413,208	7	160,647	3
ANNTAYLOR STORES CORP	448120	2,342,907	3	142,982	4

Company	Industry Code	2007 Sales (U.S. $ thousands)	Sales Rank	2007 Profits (U.S. $ thousands)	Profits Rank
BEBE STORES INC	448120	670,912	9	77,278	7
CHARLOTTE RUSSE HOLDING	448120	740,939	8	36,304	8
CHARMING SHOPPES INC	448120	3,067,517	2	108,923	5
CHICO'S FAS INC	448120	1,646,482	5	166,636	2
CHRISTOPHER & BANKS CORP	448120	547,317	10	33,686	9
DRESS BARN INC	448120	1,426,607	6	101,182	6
INTIMATE BRANDS INC	448120				
LIMITED BRANDS INC	448120	10,671,000	1	676,000	1
TALBOTS INC	448120	2,231,033	4	31,576	10
Apparel, Direct Selling					
COLDWATER CREEK INC	448000A	1,054,611	1	55,372	1
Auctions, Retail-Online					
EBAY INC	453998E	7,672,329	1	348,251	1
Auto Dealers, Retail					
CARMAX GROUP	441110	8,199,600	1	182,000	1
Auto Parts Stores					
ADVANCE AUTO PARTS INC	441310	4,844,404	2	238,317	2
AUTOZONE INC	441310	6,169,804	1	595,672	1
O'REILLY AUTOMOTIVE INC	441310	2,522,319	3	193,988	3
Automobile Parts Manufacturing					
CUMMINS INC	336300	13,048,000	2	739,000	3
EATON CORP	336300	13,033,000	3	994,000	2
JOHNSON CONTROLS INC	336300	34,524,000	1	1,252,000	1
LKQ CORP	336300	1,126,825	4	65,901	4
Automobile, Rental/Leasing					
AVIS BUDGET GROUP INC	532111	5,986,000	3	-916,000	3
DOLLAR THRIFTY AUTOMOTIVE GROUP INC	532111	1,760,791	4	1,215	2
ENTERPRISE RENT-A-CAR	532111	9,500,000	1		
HERTZ GLOBAL HOLDINGS INC	532111	8,685,600	2	264,500	1
Automobile, Used Car Distribution					
ADESA INC	423110				
Automotive Repair & Maintenance					
MONRO MUFFLER BRAKE INC	811100	417,226	1	21,921	1
Bakeries & Tortilla Manufacturing					
SARA LEE CORP	311800	12,278,000	1	504,000	1
Banking					
BANK OF AMERICA CORP	522110	124,321,000	1	14,982,000	2
JP MORGAN CHASE & CO INC	522110	71,372,000	2	15,365,000	1
Battery Manufacturing					
AMERICAN POWER CONVERSION CORP	335910				
Beverages--Distilleries					
FORTUNE BRANDS INC	312140	8,563,100	1	762,600	1
Beverages--Soft Drinks, Bottled Water & Juices Manufacturing					
COCA COLA COMPANY	312111	28,857,000	2	5,981,000	1
COCA COLA ENTERPRISES INC	312111	20,936,000	3	711,000	3
PEPSI BOTTLING GROUP INC	312111	13,591,000	4	532,000	4
PEPSICO INC	312111	39,474,000	1	5,658,000	2

Company	Industry Code	2007 Sales (U.S. $ thousands)	Sales Rank	2007 Profits (U.S. $ thousands)	Profits Rank
Book Stores					
BARNES & NOBLE COLLEGE BOOKSTORES	451211				
BARNES & NOBLE INC	451211	5,261,254	1	150,527	1
Book Stores-Online					
AMAZON.COM INC	451211E	14,835,000	1	476,000	1
Breakfast Cereal Manufacturing					
GENERAL MILLS INC	311230	12,442,000	1	2,058,000	1
KELLOGG CO	311230	11,776,000	2	1,103,000	2
Business Machines, Manufacturing					
PITNEY BOWES INC	333313	6,129,795	2	366,781	2
XEROX CORP	333313	17,228,000	1	1,135,000	1
Business Training, Distance Learning					
APOLLO GROUP INC	611410	2,723,793	1	408,810	1
DEVRY INC	611410	933,473	2	76,188	2
Cable & Satellite TV & Data Service					
CABLEVISION SYSTEMS CORP	513220	6,484,481	7	218,456	5
COMCAST CORP	513220	30,895,000	2	2,587,000	2
COX COMMUNICATIONS INC	513220	8,300,000	6		
DIRECTV GROUP INC	513220	17,246,000	3	1,451,000	3
ECHOSTAR CORP	513220	11,090,375	4	756,054	4
LIBERTY GLOBAL INC	513220	9,000,000	5	-420,000	6
TIME WARNER INC	513220	46,482,000	1	4,387,000	1
Cable TV Networks					
VIACOM INC	513210	13,423,100	2	1,838,100	2
WALT DISNEY COMPANY	513210	35,510,000	1	4,687,000	1
Call Centers and Support Services Outsourcing					
SYKES ENTERPRISES INC	561422	710,120	3	39,859	2
TELETECH HOLDINGS INC	561422	1,369,632	2	53,103	1
WEST CORPORATION	561422	2,099,492	1	5,382	3
Casino Resorts					
HARRAH'S ENTERTAINMENT INC	721120	10,825,200	1	619,400	2
LAS VEGAS SANDS CORP (THE VENETIAN)	721120	3,104,422	3	116,688	4
MGM MIRAGE	721120	7,691,637	2	1,584,419	1
WYNN RESORTS LIMITED	721120	2,687,519	4	258,148	3
Chemicals, Manufacturing					
E I DU PONT DE NEMOURS & CO (DUPONT)	325000	29,378,000	1	2,988,000	1
GEORGIA GULF CORPORATION	325000	3,157,270	2	-266,027	4
SENSIENT TECHNOLOGIES	325000	1,212,561	4	111,243	3
SIGMA-ALDRICH CORP	325000	2,038,700	3	311,100	2
Chocolate & Confectionery Manufacturing					
MARS INC	311330	25,000,000	1		
Clinics--Outpatient Clinics & Surgery					
DAVITA INC	621490	5,264,151	1	381,778	1
Coal Mining					
CONSOL ENERGY INC	212110	3,762,197	2	267,782	1
MASSEY ENERGY COMPANY	212110	2,413,523	3	94,098	3
PEABODY ENERGY CORP	212110	4,574,712	1	264,285	2

Company	Industry Code	2007 Sales (U.S. $ thousands)	Sales Rank	2007 Profits (U.S. $ thousands)	Profits Rank
Communications Equipment, Manufacturing					
HARRIS CORPORATION	334200	4,243,000	2	480,400	2
L-3 COMMUNICATIONS HOLDINGS INC	334200	13,960,500	1	756,100	1
PLANTRONICS INC	334200	800,154	3	50,143	3
Computer & Telecommunications Equipment Distribution					
ARROW ELECTRONICS INC	421430	15,984,992	3	407,792	1
INGRAM MICRO INC	421430	35,047,089	1	275,908	2
TECH DATA CORP	421430	21,440,445	2	-96,981	3
Computer Accessories, Monitors, Printers Manufacturing					
LEXMARK INTERNATIONAL INC	334119	4,973,900	1	300,800	1
MOLEX INC	334119	3,265,874	2	240,768	2
PAXAR CORP	334119				
Computer Hardware, Manufacturing					
APPLE INC	334111	24,006,000	1	3,496,000	1
DIEBOLD INC	334111	2,953,000	3		
SUN MICROSYSTEMS INC	334111	13,873,000	2	473,000	2
Computer Networking & Related Equipment, Manufacturing					
CISCO SYSTEMS INC	334110	34,922,000	1	7,333,000	1
JUNIPER NETWORKS INC	334110	2,836,100	2	360,800	2
Computer Software, Accounting, Banking & Financial					
INTUIT INC	511201	2,672,947	2	440,003	1
SUNGARD DATA SYSTEMS INC	511201	4,901,000	1	-60,000	2
Computer Software, Business Management & ERP					
ORACLE CORP	511207	17,996,000	1	4,274,000	1
SAS INSTITUTE INC	511207	2,150,000	2		
Computer Software, Electronic Games & Entertainment					
ELECTRONIC ARTS INC	511208	3,091,000	1	76,000	1
Computer Software, Multimedia, Graphics & Publishing					
ADOBE SYSTEMS INC	511209	3,157,881	1	723,807	1
Computer Software, Operating Systems, Languages & Development Tools					
MICROSOFT CORP	511204	51,122,000	1	14,065,000	1
Computer Software, Product Lifecycle, Engineering, Design & CAD					
PARAMETRIC TECHNOLOGY	511215	941,279	2	143,656	1
SYNOPSYS INC	511215	1,212,469	1	130,491	2
Computer Software, Sales & Customer Relationship Management					
ACXIOM CORP	511203	1,395,136	1	70,740	1
Computer Software, Security & Anti-Virus					
MCAFEE INC	511211	1,308,220	3	166,980	2
SYMANTEC CORP	511211	5,199,370	1	404,380	1
VERISIGN INC	511211	1,496,000	2	-145,000	3
Computer Storage Equipment & Misc. Parts, Manufacturing					
EMC CORP	334112	13,230,205	1	1,665,668	1
NETWORK APPLIANCE INC	334112	2,804,282	3	297,735	3
WESTERN DIGITAL CORP	334112	5,468,000	2	564,000	2
Computers & Software-Direct Selling					
CDW CORPORATION	443120A	8,145,000	1		

Company	Industry Code	2007 Sales (U.S. $ thousands)	Sales Rank	2007 Profits (U.S. $ thousands)	Profits Rank
Construction, Heavy & Civil Engineering					
AECOM TECHNOLOGY CORP	234000	4,237,270	6	100,297	4
BECHTEL GROUP INC	234000	27,000,000	1		
FLUOR CORP	234000	16,691,000	2	533,300	1
FOSTER WHEELER LTD	234000	5,107,243	5	393,874	2
JACOBS ENGINEERING GROUP	234000	8,473,970	3	287,130	3
PARSONS BRINCKERHOFF INC	234000				
SHAW GROUP INC	234000	5,723,712	4	-19,000	5
Construction, Power & Communication Line					
DYCOM INDUSTRIES INC	234920	1,137,812	1	41,884	1
Consulting--Computer, Telecommunications & Internet					
ACCENTURE LTD	541512	21,452,747	2	1,243,148	2
AFFILIATED COMPUTER SERVICES INC	541512	5,772,479	4	253,090	5
CACI INTERNATIONAL INC	541512	1,937,972	7	78,532	7
CIBER INC	541512	1,081,975	10	29,026	10
COGNIZANT TECHNOLOGY SOLUTIONS CORP	541512	2,135,577	6	350,133	4
IGATE CORPORATION	541512	307,258	12	15,585	11
INTERNATIONAL BUSINESS MACHINES CORP (IBM)	541512	98,786,000	1	10,418,000	1
KEANE INC	541512	1,100,000	9		
L-3 TITAN GROUP	541512				
PEROT SYSTEMS CORP	541512	2,612,000	5	115,000	6
SAIC INC	541512	8,294,000	3	391,000	3
SRA INTERNATIONAL INC	541512	1,268,872	8	63,430	8
SYNTEL INC	541512	337,673	11	62,860	9
Consulting-Human Resources					
HEWITT ASSOCIATES	541612	2,990,326	2	-175,080	2
MERCER INC	541612	3,368,000	1		
TOWERS PERRIN	541612				
WATSON WYATT WORLDWIDE	541612	1,486,523	3	116,275	1
Consulting--Management & Business					
BOOZ ALLEN HAMILTON	541611	4,000,000	3		
DELOITTE CONSULTING LLP	541611	5,200,000	1		
MCKINSEY & COMPANY INC	541611	4,500,000	2		
Consulting--Marketing					
INVENTIV HEALTH INC	541613	977,300	1	47,484	1
Contract Electronics Manufacturing					
BENCHMARK ELECTRONICS	334419	2,915,919	2	93,282	1
CTS CORP	334419	685,945	4	25,412	4
JABIL CIRCUIT INC	334419	12,290,592	1	73,236	2
PLEXUS CORP	334419	1,546,264	3	65,718	3
Convenience Stores					
7-ELEVEN INC	445120	15,797,590	1	133,694	1
PANTRY INC	445120	6,911,163	2	26,732	2
Cosmetics, Beauty Supplies & Perfume Stores					
ALBERTO-CULVER COMPANY	446120	1,541,581	1	78,264	1

Company	Industry Code	2007 Sales (U.S. $ thousands)	Sales Rank	2007 Profits (U.S. $ thousands)	Profits Rank
Courier/Express Delivery Service					
FEDEX CORPORATION	492110	35,214,000	2	2,016,000	1
UNITED PARCEL SERVICE INC (UPS)	492110	49,700,000	1	447,000	2
Credit Bureaus					
EXPERIAN AMERICAS	561450	1,994,000	1		
FAIR ISAAC CORPORATION	561450	822,236	2	104,650	1
Credit Card Issuing					
AMERICAN EXPRESS CO	522210	27,731,000	1	4,012,000	1
Cruise Lines					
CARNIVAL CORPORATION	483112	13,033,000	1	2,408,000	1
ROYAL CARIBBEAN CRUISES	483112	6,149,139	2	603,405	2
Dairy Products, Manufacturing					
DEAN FOODS CO	311500	11,821,903	1	131,353	1
Data Processing Services					
AUTOMATIC DATA PROCESSING	514210	7,800,000	1	1,138,700	1
PAYCHEX INC	514210	1,886,964	2	515,447	2
Databases & Directories, Publishing					
INFOUSA INC	511140	688,773	1	40,942	1
Department Stores					
J C PENNEY COMPANY INC	452110	19,903,000	2	1,153,000	1
MACY'S INC	452110	26,970,000	1	995,000	2
NEIMAN MARCUS GROUP INC	452110	4,419,700	4	111,900	4
NORDSTROM INC	452110	8,560,698	3	667,999	3
Diagnostic Services and Substances Manufacturing					
IDEXX LABORATORIES INC	325413	922,555	1	94,014	1
Discount Stores					
DOLLAR GENERAL CORP	452910	9,169,800	4	137,900	5
FAMILY DOLLAR STORES INC	452910	6,834,305	5	242,854	4
FRED'S INC	452910	1,767,239	6	26,746	6
KOHL'S CORP	452910	15,596,910	3	1,108,681	3
TARGET CORPORATION	452910	63,367,000	2	2,849,000	2
WAL-MART STORES INC	452910	344,992,000	1	11,284,000	1
Disease Management & Utilization Management					
HEALTHWAYS INC	524298	615,586	1	45,121	1
Drugs (Pharmaceuticals), Discovery & Manufacturing					
ABBOTT LABORATORIES	325412	25,914,200	3	3,606,300	4
ALLERGAN INC	325412	3,938,900	11	499,300	10
AMGEN INC	325412	14,771,000	8	3,166,000	6
BRISTOL MYERS SQUIBB CO	325412	19,348,000	6	2,165,000	9
CEPHALON INC	325412	1,772,638	13	-191,704	13
ELI LILLY & COMPANY	325412	18,633,500	7	2,953,000	7
FOREST LABORATORIES INC	325412	3,183,324	12	454,103	11
GENENTECH INC	325412	11,724,000	10	2,769,000	8
JOHNSON & JOHNSON	325412	61,095,000	1	10,576,000	1
KENDLE INTERNATIONAL INC	325412	568,818	14	18,687	12
MERCK & CO INC	325412	24,197,700	4	3,275,400	5
PFIZER INC	325412	48,418,000	2	8,144,000	2

Company	Industry Code	2007 Sales (U.S. $ thousands)	Sales Rank	2007 Profits (U.S. $ thousands)	Profits Rank
SCHERING-PLOUGH CORP	325412	12,690,000	9	-1,473,000	14
WYETH	325412	22,399,798	5	4,615,960	3
Drugs (Pharmaceuticals), Distribution					
AMERISOURCEBERGEN CORP	422210	66,074,312	3	469,167	3
CARDINAL HEALTH INC	422210	86,852,000	2	1,931,100	1
MCKESSON CORPORATION	422210	92,977,000	1	913,000	2
Drugs (Pharmaceuticals), Generic Manufacturing					
PERRIGO CO	325416	1,447,428	2	73,797	2
WATSON PHARMACEUTICALS	325416	2,496,651	1	141,030	1
Electrical Equipment, Manufacturing					
BLACK & DECKER CORP	335000	6,563,200	2	518,100	2
DANAHER CORP	335000	11,025,917	1	1,369,904	1
Electronics, Audio & Appliance Stores					
BEST BUY CO INC	443110	35,934,000	1	1,377,000	1
Engineering & Facilities Support Services					
URS CORPORATION	541330	5,383,007	1	132,243	1
Financial Data Publishing-Print & Online					
BLOOMBERG LP	514100	5,400,000	1		
Financing--Business					
GENERAL ELECTRIC CO (GE)	522220A	172,738,000	1	22,208,000	1
Fitness Centers/Health Clubs					
HEALTH FITNESS CORP	713940	69,958	1	910	1
Food Distribution					
SYSCO CORP	422410	35,042,075	1	1,001,076	1
UNITED NATURAL FOODS INC	422410	2,754,280	2	50,153	2
Food Products, Manufacturing					
CONAGRA FOODS INC	311000	12,028,200	2	764,600	2
JM SMUCKER CO	311000	2,148,017	3	157,219	3
KRAFT FOODS INC	311000	37,241,000	1	2,590,000	1
Food Service Contractors					
ARAMARK CORPORATION	722310	12,384,300	1	30,900	2
CINTAS CORP	722310	3,706,900	2	334,538	1
Forest Products/Paper, Manufacturing					
KIMBERLY-CLARK CORP	322000	18,266,000	1	1,822,900	1
Freight Forwarding & Support Services					
CATERPILLAR LOGISTICS	488510				
CH ROBINSON WORLDWIDE	488510	7,316,223	1	324,261	1
EXEL TRANSPORTATION SERVICES INC (DHL EXEL)	488510				
EXPEDITORS INTERNATIONAL OF WASHINGTON INC	488510	5,235,171	2	269,154	2
UPS SUPPLY CHAIN SOLUTIONS	488510				
Fruit & Vegetable Growing & Processing					
DOLE FOOD COMPANY INC	311420	6,931,000	1		
Furniture Stores					
COST PLUS INC	442110	1,040,309	1	-22,536	1
Gambling Equipment					
GTECH HOLDINGS CORP	713290	1,206,846	1		

Company	Industry Code	2007 Sales (U.S. $ thousands)	Sales Rank	2007 Profits (U.S. $ thousands)	Profits Rank
SCIENTIFIC GAMES CORP	713290	1,046,704	2	65,367	1
Golf Courses & Country Clubs					
CLUBCORP INC	713910	1,000,000	1		
Grain Distribution, Milling & Oilseed Processing					
ARCHER DANIELS MIDLAND CO	311210	44,018,000	2	2,162,000	2
BUNGE LTD	311210	37,842,000	3	778,000	3
CARGILL INC	311210	88,266,000	1	2,343,000	1
Grocery Stores/Supermarkets					
HE BUTT GROCERY CO (HEB)	445110	13,500,000	6		
KROGER CO	445110	66,111,000	1	1,115,000	2
MEIJER INC	445110	13,900,000	5		
PUBLIX SUPER MARKETS INC	445110	23,016,568	4	1,183,925	1
SAFEWAY INC	445110	42,286,000	2	888,400	3
SUPERVALU INC	445110	37,406,000	3	452,000	4
WHOLE FOODS MARKET INC	445110	6,591,773	7	182,740	5
Hair, Nail & Skin Care Salons					
REGIS CORPORATION	812110	2,626,588	1	83,170	1
Home Centers, Retail					
HOME DEPOT INC	444110	79,022,000	1	5,761,000	1
LOWE'S COMPANIES INC	444110	46,927,000	2	3,105,000	2
Home Health Care					
AMEDISYS INC	621610	697,934	3	65,113	2
CHEMED CORPORATION	621610	1,100,058	2	63,976	3
LINCARE HOLDINGS INC	621610	1,595,990	1	226,077	1
ODYSSEY HEALTHCARE INC	621610	404,872	4	12,111	4
Hospitals/Clinics--General & Specialty Hospitals					
CATHOLIC HEALTH INITIATIVES	622110	7,731,500	3		
HCA INC	622110	26,900,000	2		
HEALTH MANAGEMENT ASSOCIATES INC	622110	4,392,086	4	119,879	2
KAISER PERMANENTE	622110	37,800,000	1	1,700,000	1
SELECT MEDICAL CORP	622110	1,991,666	6	35,430	4
SISTERS OF MERCY HEALTH SYSTEMS	622110	3,653,898	5	67,667	3
Hospitals/Clinics--Psychiatric Clinics					
PSYCHIATRIC SOLUTIONS INC	622210	1,481,952	1	76,208	1
RES CARE INC	622210	1,433,298	2	43,891	2
Hotels/Resorts/Motels					
GLOBAL HYATT CORPORATION	721110	3,750,000	5		
HILTON HOTELS CORP	721110	8,090,000	2	121,000	4
LODGIAN INC	721110	278,079	7	-8,446	6
MARRIOTT INTERNATIONAL INC	721110	12,990,000	1	696,000	1
RITZ-CARLTON HOTEL CO LLC	721110	1,576,000	6	72,000	5
STARWOOD HOTELS & RESORTS WORLDWIDE INC	721110	6,153,000	3	542,000	2
WYNDHAM WORLDWIDE	721110	4,360,000	4	403,000	3
Industrial Gas Manufacturing					
AIR PRODUCTS & CHEMICALS	325120	10,037,800	1	1,035,600	2
PRAXAIR INC	325120	9,402,000	2	1,177,000	1

Company	Industry Code	2007 Sales (U.S. $ thousands)	Sales Rank	2007 Profits (U.S. $ thousands)	Profits Rank
Instrument Manufacturing, including Measurement, Control, Test & Navigational					
AGILENT TECHNOLOGIES INC	334500	5,420,000	2	638,000	2
EMERSON ELECTRIC CO	334500	22,572,000	1	2,136,000	1
MILLIPORE CORP	334500	1,531,555	3	136,472	3
TEKTRONIX INC	334500	1,105,172	4	90,408	4
Insurance Brokerages, Agencies & Exchanges					
ARTHUR J GALLAGHER & CO	524210	1,623,300	2	138,800	3
BROWN & BROWN INC	524210	959,667	3	190,959	2
HILB ROGAL & HOBBS CO	524210	799,664	4	78,125	4
MARSH & MCLENNAN COMPANIES INC	524210	11,350,000	1	2,475,000	1
Insurance--Health Supplemental & Specialty					
AFLAC INC	524114A	15,393,000	1	1,634,000	1
Insurance--Health, HMO's & PPO's					
AETNA INC	524114	27,599,600	3	1,831,000	3
COVENTRY HEALTH CARE INC	524114	9,879,531	6	626,094	5
HEALTH NET INC	524114	14,108,271	5	193,697	6
HUMANA INC	524114	25,289,989	4	833,684	4
UNITEDHEALTH GROUP INC	524114	75,431,000	1	4,654,000	1
WELLPOINT INC	524114	61,134,300	2	3,345,400	2
Insurance--Life					
AXA FINANCIAL INC	524113				
GENWORTH FINANCIAL INC	524113	11,125,000	4	1,154,000	5
HARTFORD FINANCIAL SERVICES GROUP INC	524113	25,916,000	3	2,949,000	3
LINCOLN NATIONAL CORP	524113	10,594,000	6	1,215,000	4
METLIFE INC	524113	53,070,000	1	4,317,000	1
PRINCIPAL FINANCIAL GROUP	524113	10,906,500	5	860,300	6
PRUDENTIAL FINANCIAL INC	524113	34,401,000	2	3,704,000	2
Insurance--Property & Casualty					
ALLSTATE CORPORATION	524126	36,769,000	1	4,636,000	1
CHUBB CORPORATION	524126	14,107,000	6	2,807,000	3
LOEWS CORPORATION	524126	18,380,000	3	2,489,000	4
PROGRESSIVE CORPORATION	524126	14,686,800	4	1,182,500	6
SAFECO CORP	524126	6,208,800	7	707,800	8
TRAVELERS COMPANIES INC	524126	26,017,000	2	4,601,000	2
USAA	524126	14,417,900	5	1,855,500	5
W R BERKLEY CORPORATION	524126	4,575,989	8	743,646	7
Jewelry Stores					
TIFFANY & CO	448310	2,560,734	1	253,927	1
Laboratories & Diagnostic Services--Medical					
LABORATORY CORP OF AMERICA HOLDINGS	621511	4,068,200	2	476,800	1
QUEST DIAGNOSTICS INC	621511	6,704,907	1	339,939	2
Linens/Housewares/Art/Framing Stores					
BED BATH & BEYOND INC	442299	6,617,429	1	594,244	1
CONTAINER STORE	442299				
WILLIAMS SONOMA INC	442299	3,727,513	2	208,868	2

Company	Industry Code	2007 Sales (U.S. $ thousands)	Sales Rank	2007 Profits (U.S. $ thousands)	Profits Rank
Long-Term Health Care & Assisted Living					
CAPITAL SENIOR LIVING CORP	623110	189,052	5	4,360	2
EMERITUS CORP	623110	545,639	4	-48,741	4
KINDRED HEALTHCARE INC	623110	4,220,266	1	-46,870	3
MANOR CARE INC	623110				
SUN HEALTHCARE GROUP	623110	1,587,307	3	57,510	1
SUNRISE SENIOR LIVING	623110	1,652,550	2	-70,275	5
Machinery, Equipment & Supplies, Distribution					
WW GRAINGER INC	421800	6,418,014	1	420,120	1
Machinery, Manufacturing					
CATERPILLAR INC	333000	44,958,000	1	3,541,000	1
DEERE & CO	333000	24,082,200	2	1,821,700	2
Machinery, Mining & Oil & Gas Field, Manufacturing					
CAMERON INTERNATIONAL	333130	4,666,368	1	500,860	1
Management of Companies & Enterprises					
BERKSHIRE HATHAWAY INC	551110	118,245,000	1	13,213,000	1
Market Research					
IMS HEALTH INC	541910	2,192,571	1	234,040	1
Marketing Agencies & Related Services					
ICT GROUP INC	541800	453,621	1	-11,809	1
Meat Production					
SMITHFIELD FOODS INC	112000	11,911,100	1	166,800	1
Medical/Dental/Surgical Equipment & Supplies, Distribution					
HENRY SCHEIN INC	421450	5,920,190	2	215,173	1
OWENS & MINOR INC	421450	6,800,466	1	72,710	3
PATTERSON COMPANIES INC	421450	2,798,398	3	208,336	2
Medical/Dental/Surgical Equipment & Supplies, Manufacturing					
3M COMPANY	339113	24,462,000	1	4,096,000	1
BAXTER INTERNATIONAL INC	339113	11,263,000	3	1,707,000	3
BECKMAN COULTER INC	339113	2,761,300	9	211,300	11
BECTON DICKINSON & CO	339113	6,359,700	5	890,000	5
BIO RAD LABORATORIES INC	339113	1,461,052	12	92,994	13
BOSTON SCIENTIFIC CORP	339113	8,357,000	4	-495,000	16
COOPER COMPANIES INC	339113	950,641	16	-11,192	15
CR BARD INC	339113	2,202,000	10	406,400	8
DJO INC	339113				
MEDTRONIC INC	339113	12,299,000	2	2,802,000	2
RESPIRONICS INC	339113	1,195,035	14	122,285	12
ST JUDE MEDICAL INC	339113	3,779,277	8	559,038	7
STERIS CORP	339113	1,197,407	13	82,155	14
STRYKER CORP	339113	6,000,500	6	1,017,400	4
VARIAN MEDICAL SYSTEMS	339113	1,776,600	11	239,500	10
WATERS CORP	339113	1,072,864	15	268,072	9
ZIMMER HOLDINGS INC	339113	3,897,500	7	773,200	6
Office Supplies Stores					
OFFICE DEPOT INC	453210	15,527,537	2	395,615	2
STAPLES INC	453210	18,160,789	1	973,677	1

Company	Industry Code	2007 Sales (U.S. $ thousands)	Sales Rank	2007 Profits (U.S. $ thousands)	Profits Rank
Oil & Natural Gas Exploration & Production					
ANADARKO PETROLEUM CORP	211111	11,230,000	11	3,780,000	6
APACHE CORP	211111	9,977,858	12	2,812,358	9
CHESAPEAKE ENERGY CORP	211111	7,800,000	13	1,451,000	11
CHEVRON CORPORATION	211111	220,904,000	2	18,688,000	2
CONOCOPHILLIPS COMPANY	211111	187,437,000	3	11,891,000	3
DEVON ENERGY CORP	211111	11,362,000	10	3,606,000	7
EXXON MOBIL CORPORATION (EXXONMOBIL)	211111	390,328,000	1	40,610,000	1
HELMERICH & PAYNE INC	211111	1,629,658	15	449,261	14
HESS CORPORATION	211111	31,647,000	7	1,832,000	10
MARATHON OIL CORP	211111	64,552,000	6	3,956,000	5
MURPHY OIL CORPORATION	211111	18,423,771	9	766,529	13
OCCIDENTAL PETROLEUM	211111	18,784,000	8	5,400,000	4
SHELL OIL CO	211111	87,548,000	5		
TRANSOCEAN INC	211111	6,377,000	14	3,131,000	8
WILLIAMS COMPANIES INC	211111	105,558,000	4	990,000	12
Online Publishing, Services & Niche Portals					
FIRST ADVANTAGE CORP	514199	842,902	1	138,107	1
Other Health & Personal Care Stores/Weight Management					
WEIGHT WATCHERS INTERNATIONAL INC	446190	1,467,167	1	201,180	1
Packaging, Manufacturing					
WEST PHARMACEUTICAL SERVICES INC	322210	1,020,100	1	70,700	1
Paint & Wallpaper Stores					
SHERWIN WILLIAMS CO	444120	8,005,000	1	616,000	1
Paints & Coatings, Manufacturing					
VALSPAR CORPORATION	325510	3,249,287	1	172,115	1
Pawn Shops					
CASH AMERICA INTERNATIONAL INC	522298	929,394	1	79,346	1
Payment & Transaction Processing Services					
ALLIANCE DATA SYSTEMS	522320	2,291,189	5	164,061	5
CONVERGYS CORPORATION	522320	2,844,300	4	169,500	4
FIRST DATA CORP	522320	8,051,400	1	-907,200	7
FISERV INC	522320	3,922,000	3	439,000	2
GLOBAL PAYMENTS INC	522320	1,061,523	7	142,985	6
TOTAL SYSTEM SERVICES INC (TSYS)	522320	1,805,836	6	237,443	3
WESTERN UNION COMPANY	522320	4,900,200	2	857,300	1
Payment & Transaction Processing--Benefits Management					
EXPRESS SCRIPTS INC	522320A	18,273,600	2	567,800	2
MEDCO HEALTH SOLUTIONS	522320A	44,506,200	1	912,000	1
Personal Items, Cosmetics, Health Supplements by Direct Selling					
AVON PRODUCTS INC	446191A	9,938,700	1	530,700	1
MARY KAY INC	446191A	2,400,000	2		
Petrochemicals Manufacturing					
CHEVRON PHILLIPS CHEMICAL	325110	12,534,000	1	719,000	1
Petroleum Refineries					
KOCH INDUSTRIES INC	324110	98,000,000	1		

Company	Industry Code	2007 Sales (U.S. $ thousands)	Sales Rank	2007 Profits (U.S. $ thousands)	Profits Rank
Petroleum Refineries & Retail Marketing					
SUNOCO INC	324110A	44,470,000	2	891,000	2
TESORO CORP	324110A	21,915,000	3	566,000	3
VALERO ENERGY CORP	324110A	95,327,000	1	5,234,000	1
Petroleum--Drilling Oil & Gas Wells Support					
BAKER HUGHES INC	213111	10,428,200	3	1,513,900	3
BJ SERVICES COMPANY	213111	4,802,409	7	753,640	9
DIAMOND OFFSHORE DRILLING	213111	2,567,723	10	846,541	7
FMC TECHNOLOGIES INC	213111	4,615,400	8	302,800	12
HALLIBURTON COMPANY	213111	15,264,000	2	3,499,000	2
NATIONAL OILWELL VARCO INC	213111	9,789,000	4	1,337,100	4
NOBLE CORPORATION	213111	2,995,311	9	1,206,011	5
OCEANEERING INTERNATIONAL	213111	1,743,080	14	180,374	14
OIL STATES INTERNATIONAL	213111	2,088,235	12	203,372	13
PATTERSON-UTI ENERGY INC	213111	2,114,194	11	438,639	11
PRIDE INTERNATIONAL INC	213111	2,043,800	13	784,300	8
SCHLUMBERGER LIMITED	213111	23,777,000	1	5,177,000	1
SMITH INTERNATIONAL INC	213111	8,764,330	5	647,051	10
WEATHERFORD INTERNATIONAL LTD	213111	7,832,062	6	1,070,606	6
Pets/Pet Supplies Stores					
PETCO ANIMAL SUPPLIES INC	453910				
PETSMART INC	453910	4,233,857	1	185,069	1
Pharmacies & Drug Stores					
CVS CAREMARK CORP	446110	76,329,500	1	2,637,000	1
RITE AID CORPORATION	446110	17,507,719	3	26,826	3
WALGREEN CO	446110	53,762,000	2	2,041,300	2
Pharmacies-Specialty					
OMNICARE INC	446110A	6,220,010	1	114,056	1
Poultry Production					
TYSON FOODS INC	112300	26,900,000	1	268,000	1
Printing					
AVERY DENNISON CORP	323000	6,307,800	2	303,500	1
R R DONNELLEY & SONS CO	323000	11,587,100	1	-48,900	2
Radio Broadcasting					
CLEAR CHANNEL COMMUNICATIONS INC	513111	6,816,909	1	938,507	1
Railroad Transportation					
BURLINGTON NORTHERN SANTA FE CORP	482110	15,802,000	2	1,829,000	2
CSX CORP	482110	10,030,000	3	1,226,000	5
CSX TRANSPORTATION INC	482110	8,591,000	5	1,697,000	3
NORFOLK SOUTHERN CORP	482110	9,432,000	4	1,464,000	4
UNION PACIFIC CORP	482110	16,283,000	1	1,855,000	1
Real Estate Investment Trusts - REITs					
PUBLIC STORAGE INC	525930	1,816,371	1	457,527	1
Real Estate Rental, Leasing & Management					
ABM INDUSTRIES INC	531100	2,842,811	1	52,440	1
Rental Stores, Consumer Goods					
AARON RENTS INC	532200	1,494,911	2	80,275	1

Company	Industry Code	2007 Sales (U.S. $ thousands)	Sales Rank	2007 Profits (U.S. $ thousands)	Profits Rank
RENT-A-CENTER INC	532200	2,906,121	1	76,268	2
Research & Development--Physical, Engineering & Life Sciences					
CH2M HILL COMPANIES LTD	541710	4,376,200	1		
COVANCE INC	541710	1,631,516	2	175,929	1
PAREXEL INTERNATIONAL	541710	741,955	4	37,289	3
PHARMACEUTICAL PRODUCT DEVELOPMENT INC	541710	1,414,465	3	163,401	2
Restaurants					
BRINKER INTERNATIONAL INC	722110	4,376,904	4	230,049	3
BURGER KING HOLDINGS INC	722110	2,234,000	8	148,000	6
CBRL GROUP INC	722110	2,351,576	7	162,065	5
DARDEN RESTAURANTS INC	722110	5,567,100	3	201,400	4
DENNY'S CORPORATION	722110	939,368	10	34,713	9
DINEEQUITY INC	722110	484,559	11	-480	11
JACK IN THE BOX INC	722110	2,875,978	5	126,304	7
LANDRY'S RESTAURANTS INC	722110	1,171,923	9	18,112	10
MCDONALD'S CORP	722110	22,786,600	1	2,395,100	1
OSI RESTAURANT PARTNERS	722110				
WENDYS INTERNATIONAL INC	722110	2,450,244	6	87,896	8
YUM! BRANDS INC	722110	10,416,000	2	909,000	2
Search Engine Portals					
GOOGLE INC	514199B	16,593,986	1	4,203,720	1
YAHOO! INC	514199B	6,969,274	2	660,000	2
Security, Protection, Armored Car & Investigation Services					
BRINKS COMPANY	561610	3,219,000	1	137,300	1
GEO GROUP INC	561610	1,024,832	2	41,845	2
Semiconductors (Microchips)/Integrated Circuits/Components, Manufacturing					
ADVANCED MICRO DEVICES INC (AMD)	334413	6,013,000	3	-3,379,000	7
ANALOG DEVICES INC	334413	2,546,117	6	496,907	3
BROADCOM CORP	334413	3,776,395	5	213,342	5
INTEL CORP	334413	38,334,000	1	6,976,000	1
MAXIM INTEGRATED PRODUCTS INC	334413				
MICROCHIP TECHNOLOGY INC	334413	1,039,671	7	357,029	4
MICRON TECHNOLOGY INC	334413	5,688,000	4	-320,000	6
QUALCOMM INC	334413	8,871,000	2	3,303,000	2
Shipping-Deep Sea					
SEACOR HOLDINGS INC	483111	1,359,230	1	241,648	1
Shoe Manufacturing-Athletic Shoes & Misc. Shoes, Incl. Children's					
NIKE INC	316219	16,325,900	1	1,491,500	1
Shoe Manufacturing-Men's					
GENESCO INC	316213	1,460,478	1	67,646	1
Shoes & Accessories Stores					
COACH INC	448210	2,612,456	1	663,665	1
FINISH LINE INC	448210	1,331,959	2	40,264	2
Soaps, Cleaners, Cosmetics & Toiletries, Manufacturing					
COLGATE PALMOLIVE CO	325600	13,789,700	2	1,737,400	2
ESTEE LAUDER COMPANIES	325600	7,037,500	3	449,700	3
PROCTER & GAMBLE CO	325600	76,476,000	1	10,340,000	1

Company	Industry Code	2007 Sales (U.S. $ thousands)	Sales Rank	2007 Profits (U.S. $ thousands)	Profits Rank
Sporting Goods Stores					
ACADEMY SPORTS & OUTDOORS LTD	451110				
BASS PRO SHOPS INC	451110	3,000,000	2		
CABELA'S INC	451110	2,349,599	3	87,879	2
DICK'S SPORTING GOODS INC	451110	3,114,162	1	112,611	1
HIBBETT SPORTS INC	451110	512,094	4	38,073	3
Staffing or Outsourcing					
STARTEK INC	561300	245,304	1	-2,831	1
Sugar & Confectionery Product Manufacturing					
WM WRIGLEY JR COMPANY	311300	5,389,100	1	632,005	1
Telecommunications Equipment Manufacturing					
ADC TELECOMMUNICATIONS	334210	1,322,200	1	113,300	1
Telecommunications-Private Data Networks & Network Services					
LEVEL 3 COMMUNICATIONS INC	513390C	4,269,000	1	-1,114,000	2
TW TELECOM INC	513390C	1,083,679	2	-40,269	1
Telephone Service-Cellular, U.S. & Non-U.S.					
CELLCO PARTNERSHIP (VERIZON WIRELESS)	513322	43,900,000	1		
NII HOLDINGS INC	513322	3,296,295	4	378,418	2
T-MOBILE USA	513322	19,288,000	2	5,350,000	1
UNITED STATES CELLULAR	513322	3,946,264	3	314,734	3
Telephone Service--Local Exchange Carrier & Diversified					
AT&T INC	513300A	118,928,000	1	11,951,000	1
EMBARQ CORP	513300A	6,365,000	3	683,000	3
FRONTIER COMMUNICATIONS	513300A	2,288,015	5	214,654	5
TELEPHONE AND DATA SYSTEMS INC (TDS)	513300A	4,829,000	4	386,100	4
VERIZON COMMUNICATIONS	513300A	93,469,000	2	5,521,000	2
Television Broadcasting					
FOX ENTERTAINMENT GROUP	513120				
NEWS CORP	513120	28,655,000	1	3,426,000	1
UNIVISION COMMUNICATIONS	513120	2,196,000	2	-314,900	2
Temporary Help/Staffing					
KELLY SERVICES INC	561320	5,667,589	2	61,016	3
MANPOWER INC	561320	20,500,300	1	484,700	1
ROBERT HALF INTERNATIONAL	561320	4,645,666	3	296,212	2
VOLT INFORMATION SCIENCES	561320	2,353,082	4	39,332	4
Tire Stores					
TBC CORPORATION	441300	1,779,400	1		
Tobacco, Manufacturing					
ALTRIA GROUP INC	312220	73,801,000	1	9,786,000	1
Toys, Manufacturing					
MATTEL INC	339932	5,970,090	1	599,993	1
Toys/Hobbies/Games Stores					
BUILD-A-BEAR WORKSHOP INC	451120	474,361	2	22,509	2
GAMESTOP CORP	451120	5,318,900	1	158,250	1
Travel Services-Online					
SABRE HOLDINGS CORP	561500A				

Company	Industry Code	2007 Sales (U.S. $ thousands)	Sales Rank	2007 Profits (U.S. $ thousands)	Profits Rank
Truck Transportation-Less Than Truckload					
OLD DOMINION FREIGHT LINE	484122	1,401,542	1	71,832	1
Trucks, Rental/Leasing					
RYDER SYSTEM INC	532120	6,565,995	1	253,861	1
Trucks, RVs & Misc. Automotive, Manufacturing					
OSHKOSH CORPORATION	336120	6,307,300	1	268,100	1
TV Shopping					
IAC/INTERACTIVECORP	454110B	6,373,410	1	-144,069	1
Utilities-Electric					
AMERICAN ELECTRIC POWER COMPANY INC (AEP)	221000A	13,380,000	3	1,089,000	6
EDISON INTERNATIONAL	221000A	13,113,000	4	1,098,000	5
ENTERGY CORP	221000A	11,484,398	6	1,134,849	4
FIRSTENERGY CORP	221000A	12,802,000	5	1,309,000	3
FPL GROUP INC	221000A	15,263,000	2	1,312,000	2
HAWAIIAN ELECTRIC INDUSTRIES INC	221000A	2,536,400	7	84,779	7
SOUTHERN COMPANY	221000A	15,353,000	1	1,734,000	1
Utilities-Electric & Gas					
AES CORPORATION	221000	13,588,000	2	-95,000	9
BALTIMORE GAS AND ELECTRIC COMPANY	221000				
CONSOLIDATED EDISON INC	221000	13,120,000	4	929,000	6
DTE ENERGY COMPANY	221000	8,506,000	8	971,000	5
DUKE ENERGY CORP	221000	12,720,000	5	1,500,000	2
EXELON CORPORATION	221000	18,916,000	1	2,736,000	1
PG&E CORPORATION	221000	13,237,000	3	1,006,000	4
RELIANT ENERGY INC	221000	11,209,000	7	365,000	7
SCANA CORPORATION	221000	4,621,000	9	320,000	8
SEMPRA ENERGY	221000	11,438,000	6	1,099,000	3
Utilities-Gas					
ONEOK INC	221000B	13,488,027	1	304,921	1
Veterinary Clinics					
VCA ANTECH INC	541940	1,156,145	1	121,012	1
Warehouse Clubs					
BJ'S WHOLESALE CLUB INC	452910A	8,303,496	3	72,016	3
COSTCO WHOLESALE CORP	452910A	63,087,601	1	1,082,772	2
SAM'S CLUB	452910A	41,582,000	2	1,480,000	1
Waste Disposal, Waste Management					
WASTE MANAGEMENT INC	562000	13,310,000	1	1,163,000	1
Watch & Clock Manufacturing					
FOSSIL INC	334518	1,432,984	1	123,261	1

ALPHABETICAL INDEX

3M COMPANY
7-ELEVEN INC
AARON RENTS INC
ABBOTT LABORATORIES
ABERCROMBIE & FITCH CO
ABM INDUSTRIES INC
ACADEMY SPORTS & OUTDOORS
LTD
ACCENTURE LTD
ACXIOM CORP
ADC TELECOMMUNICATIONS INC
ADESA INC
ADOBE SYSTEMS INC
ADVANCE AUTO PARTS INC
ADVANCED MICRO DEVICES INC
(AMD)
AECOM TECHNOLOGY
CORPORATION
AEROPOSTALE INC
AES CORPORATION (THE)
AETNA INC
AFFILIATED COMPUTER SERVICES
INC
AFLAC INC
AGILENT TECHNOLOGIES INC
AIR PRODUCTS & CHEMICALS INC
ALBERTO-CULVER COMPANY
ALLERGAN INC
ALLIANCE DATA SYSTEMS
CORPORATION
ALLSTATE CORPORATION (THE)
ALTRIA GROUP INC
AMAZON.COM INC
AMEDISYS INC
AMERICAN EAGLE OUTFITTERS INC
AMERICAN ELECTRIC POWER
COMPANY INC (AEP)
AMERICAN EXPRESS CO
AMERICAN POWER CONVERSION
CORP
AMERISOURCEBERGEN CORP
AMGEN INC
ANADARKO PETROLEUM
CORPORATION
ANALOG DEVICES INC
ANNTAYLOR STORES CORP
APACHE CORP
APOLLO GROUP INC
APPLE INC
ARAMARK CORPORATION
ARCHER DANIELS MIDLAND CO
ARROW ELECTRONICS INC
ARTHUR J GALLAGHER & CO
AT&T INC
AUTOMATIC DATA PROCESSING INC
AUTOZONE INC
AVERY DENNISON CORP
AVIS BUDGET GROUP INC
AVON PRODUCTS INC
AXA FINANCIAL INC
BAKER HUGHES INC

BALTIMORE GAS AND ELECTRIC
COMPANY
BANK OF AMERICA CORP
BARNES & NOBLE COLLEGE
BOOKSTORES
BARNES & NOBLE INC
BASS PRO SHOPS INC
BAXTER INTERNATIONAL INC
BDO SEIDMAN LLP
BEBE STORES INC
BECHTEL GROUP INC
BECKMAN COULTER INC
BECTON DICKINSON & CO
BED BATH & BEYOND INC
BENCHMARK ELECTRONICS INC
BERKSHIRE HATHAWAY INC
BEST BUY CO INC
BIO RAD LABORATORIES INC
BJ SERVICES COMPANY
BJ'S WHOLESALE CLUB INC
BLACK & DECKER CORP
BLOOMBERG LP
BOEING COMPANY (THE)
BOOZ ALLEN HAMILTON
BOSTON SCIENTIFIC CORP
BRINKER INTERNATIONAL INC
BRINKS COMPANY (THE)
BRISTOL MYERS SQUIBB CO
BROADCOM CORP
BROWN & BROWN INC
BUCKLE INC (THE)
BUILD-A-BEAR WORKSHOP INC
BUNGE LTD
BURGER KING HOLDINGS INC
BURLINGTON NORTHERN SANTA FE
CORP
CABELA'S INC
CABLEVISION SYSTEMS CORP
CACI INTERNATIONAL INC
CAMERON INTERNATIONAL
CORPORATION
CAPITAL SENIOR LIVING CORP
CARDINAL HEALTH INC
CARGILL INC
CARMAX GROUP
CARNIVAL CORPORATION
CASH AMERICA INTERNATIONAL
INC
CATERPILLAR INC
CATERPILLAR LOGISTICS
CATHOLIC HEALTH INITIATIVES
CBRL GROUP INC
CDW CORPORATION
CELLCO PARTNERSHIP (VERIZON
WIRELESS)
CEPHALON INC
CH ROBINSON WORLDWIDE INC
CH2M HILL COMPANIES LTD
CHARLOTTE RUSSE HOLDING
CHARMING SHOPPES INC
CHEMED CORPORATION
CHESAPEAKE ENERGY CORP
CHEVRON CORPORATION
CHEVRON PHILLIPS CHEMICAL
COMPANY LLC

CHICO'S FAS INC
CHRISTOPHER & BANKS CORP
CHUBB CORPORATION (THE)
CIBER INC
CINTAS CORP
CISCO SYSTEMS INC
CLEAR CHANNEL
COMMUNICATIONS INC
CLUBCORP INC
COACH INC
COCA COLA COMPANY (THE)
COCA COLA ENTERPRISES INC
COGNIZANT TECHNOLOGY
SOLUTIONS CORP
COLDWATER CREEK INC
COLGATE PALMOLIVE CO
COMCAST CORP
CONAGRA FOODS INC
CONOCOPHILLIPS COMPANY
CONSOL ENERGY INC
CONSOLIDATED EDISON INC
CONTAINER STORE (THE)
CONVERGYS CORPORATION
COOPER COMPANIES INC
COST PLUS INC
COSTCO WHOLESALE CORP
COVANCE INC
COVENTRY HEALTH CARE INC
COX COMMUNICATIONS INC
CR BARD INC
CSX CORP
CSX TRANSPORTATION INC
CTS CORP
CUBIC CORP
CUMMINS INC
CVS CAREMARK CORPORATION
DANAHER CORP
DARDEN RESTAURANTS INC
DAVITA INC
DEAN FOODS CO
DEERE & CO
DELOITTE & TOUCHE USA LLP
DELOITTE CONSULTING LLP
DENNY'S CORPORATION
DEVON ENERGY CORPORATION
DEVRY INC
DIAMOND OFFSHORE DRILLING INC
DICK'S SPORTING GOODS INC
DIEBOLD INC
DINEEQUITY INC
DIRECTV GROUP INC (THE)
DJO INC
DOLE FOOD COMPANY INC
DOLLAR GENERAL CORPORATION
DOLLAR THRIFTY AUTOMOTIVE
GROUP INC
DRESS BARN INC (THE)
DTE ENERGY COMPANY
DUKE ENERGY CORP
DYCOM INDUSTRIES INC
E I DU PONT DE NEMOURS & CO
(DUPONT)
EATON CORP
EBAY INC
ECHOSTAR CORP

EDISON INTERNATIONAL
ELECTRONIC ARTS INC
ELI LILLY & COMPANY
EMBARQ CORP
EMC CORP
EMERITUS CORP
EMERSON ELECTRIC CO
ENTERGY CORP
ENTERPRISE RENT-A-CAR
ERNST & YOUNG LLP
ESTEE LAUDER COMPANIES INC (THE)
EXEL TRANSPORTATION SERVICES INC (DHL EXEL)
EXELON CORPORATION
EXPEDITORS INTERNATIONAL OF WASHINGTON INC
EXPERIAN AMERICAS
EXPRESS SCRIPTS INC
EXXON MOBIL CORPORATION (EXXONMOBIL)
FAIR ISAAC CORPORATION
FAMILY DOLLAR STORES INC
FEDEX CORPORATION
FINISH LINE INC (THE)
FIRST ADVANTAGE CORPORATION
FIRST DATA CORP
FIRSTENERGY CORP
FISERV INC
FLUOR CORP
FMC TECHNOLOGIES INC
FOREST LABORATORIES INC
FORTUNE BRANDS INC
FOSSIL INC
FOSTER WHEELER LTD
FOX ENTERTAINMENT GROUP INC
FPL GROUP INC
FRED'S INC
FRONTIER COMMUNICATIONS CORPORATION
GAMESTOP CORP
GENENTECH INC
GENERAL DYNAMICS CORP
GENERAL ELECTRIC CO (GE)
GENERAL MILLS INC
GENESCO INC
GENWORTH FINANCIAL INC
GEO GROUP INC
GEORGIA GULF CORPORATION
GLOBAL HYATT CORPORATION
GLOBAL PAYMENTS INC
GOOGLE INC
GRANT THORNTON LLP
GTECH HOLDINGS CORP
GUESS? INC
HALLIBURTON COMPANY
HARRAH'S ENTERTAINMENT INC
HARRIS CORPORATION
HARTFORD FINANCIAL SERVICES GROUP INC (THE)
HAWAIIAN ELECTRIC INDUSTRIES INC
HCA INC
HE BUTT GROCERY COMPANY (HEB)
HEALTH FITNESS CORP

HEALTH MANAGEMENT ASSOCIATES INC
HEALTH NET INC
HEALTHWAYS INC
HELMERICH & PAYNE INC
HENRY SCHEIN INC
HERTZ GLOBAL HOLDINGS INC
HESS CORPORATION
HEWITT ASSOCIATES
HIBBETT SPORTS INC
HILB ROGAL & HOBBS CO
HILTON HOTELS CORP
HOME DEPOT INC
HONEYWELL INTERNATIONAL INC
HOT TOPIC INC
HUMANA INC
IAC/INTERACTIVECORP
ICT GROUP INC
IDEXX LABORATORIES INC
IGATE CORPORATION
IMS HEALTH INC
INFOUSA INC
INGRAM MICRO INC
INTEL CORP
INTERNATIONAL BUSINESS MACHINES CORP (IBM)
INTIMATE BRANDS INC
INTUIT INC
INVENTIV HEALTH INC
J C PENNEY COMPANY INC
JABIL CIRCUIT INC
JACK IN THE BOX INC
JACOBS ENGINEERING GROUP INC
JM SMUCKER CO
JOHNSON & JOHNSON
JOHNSON CONTROLS INC
JP MORGAN CHASE & CO INC
JUNIPER NETWORKS INC
KAISER PERMANENTE
KEANE INC
KELLOGG CO
KELLY SERVICES INC
KENDLE INTERNATIONAL INC
KIMBERLY-CLARK CORP
KINDRED HEALTHCARE INC
KOCH INDUSTRIES INC
KOHL'S CORP
KPMG LLP
KRAFT FOODS INC
KROGER CO (THE)
L-3 COMMUNICATIONS HOLDINGS INC
L-3 TITAN GROUP
LABORATORY CORP OF AMERICA HOLDINGS
LANDRY'S RESTAURANTS INC
LAS VEGAS SANDS CORP (THE VENETIAN)
LEVEL 3 COMMUNICATIONS INC
LEXMARK INTERNATIONAL INC
LIBERTY GLOBAL INC
LIMITED BRANDS INC
LINCARE HOLDINGS INC
LINCOLN NATIONAL CORPORATION
LKQ CORP

LOCKHEED MARTIN CORP
LODGIAN INC
LOEWS CORPORATION
LOWE'S COMPANIES INC
MACY'S INC
MANOR CARE INC
MANPOWER INC
MARATHON OIL CORP
MARRIOTT INTERNATIONAL INC
MARS INC
MARSH & MCLENNAN COMPANIES INC
MARY KAY INC
MASSEY ENERGY COMPANY
MATTEL INC
MAXIM INTEGRATED PRODUCTS INC
MCAFEE INC
MCDONALD'S CORP
MCKESSON CORPORATION
MCKINSEY & COMPANY INC
MEDCO HEALTH SOLUTIONS
MEDTRONIC INC
MEIJER INC
MEN'S WEARHOUSE INC (THE)
MERCER INC
MERCK & CO INC
METLIFE INC
MGM MIRAGE
MICROCHIP TECHNOLOGY INC
MICRON TECHNOLOGY INC
MICROSOFT CORP
MILLIPORE CORP
MOLEX INC
MONRO MUFFLER BRAKE INC
MURPHY OIL CORPORATION
NATIONAL OILWELL VARCO INC
NEIMAN MARCUS GROUP INC (THE)
NETWORK APPLIANCE INC
NEWS CORP
NII HOLDINGS INC
NIKE INC
NOBLE CORPORATION
NORDSTROM INC
NORFOLK SOUTHERN CORP
NORTHROP GRUMMAN CORP
OCCIDENTAL PETROLEUM CORP
OCEANEERING INTERNATIONAL INC
ODYSSEY HEALTHCARE INC
OFFICE DEPOT INC
OIL STATES INTERNATIONAL INC
OLD DOMINION FREIGHT LINE INC
OMNICARE INC
OMNICOM GROUP INC
ONEOK INC
ORACLE CORP
O'REILLY AUTOMOTIVE INC
OSHKOSH CORPORATION
OSI RESTAURANT PARTNERS INC
OWENS & MINOR INC
PACIFIC SUNWEAR OF CALIFORNIA INC
PANTRY INC (THE)
PARAMETRIC TECHNOLOGY CORP
PAREXEL INTERNATIONAL CORP
PARSONS BRINCKERHOFF INC

PATTERSON COMPANIES INC
PATTERSON-UTI ENERGY INC
PAXAR CORP
PAYCHEX INC
PEABODY ENERGY CORP
PEPSI BOTTLING GROUP INC
PEPSICO INC
PEROT SYSTEMS CORP
PERRIGO CO
PETCO ANIMAL SUPPLIES INC
PETSMART INC
PFIZER INC
PG&E CORPORATION
PHARMACEUTICAL PRODUCT
DEVELOPMENT INC
PITNEY BOWES INC
PLANTRONICS INC
PLEXUS CORP
POLO RALPH LAUREN CORP
PRAXAIR INC
PRICEWATERHOUSECOOPERS
PRIDE INTERNATIONAL INC
PRINCIPAL FINANCIAL GROUP (THE)
PROCTER & GAMBLE CO
PROGRESSIVE CORPORATION (THE)
PRUDENTIAL FINANCIAL INC
PSYCHIATRIC SOLUTIONS INC
PUBLIC STORAGE INC
PUBLIX SUPER MARKETS INC
QUALCOMM INC
QUEST DIAGNOSTICS INC
QUIKSILVER INC
R R DONNELLEY & SONS CO
RAYTHEON CO
REGIS CORPORATION
RELIANT ENERGY INC
RENT-A-CENTER INC
RES CARE INC
RESPIRONICS INC
RITE AID CORPORATION
RITZ-CARLTON HOTEL COMPANY
LLC (THE)
ROBERT HALF INTERNATIONAL INC
ROSS STORES INC
ROYAL CARIBBEAN CRUISES
RUSSELL CORP
RYDER SYSTEM INC
SABRE HOLDINGS CORP
SAFECO CORP
SAFEWAY INC
SAIC INC
SAM'S CLUB
SARA LEE CORP
SAS INSTITUTE INC
SCANA CORPORATION
SCHERING-PLOUGH CORP
SCHLUMBERGER LIMITED
SCIENTIFIC GAMES CORPORATION
SCOTTS MIRACLE GROW CO
SEACOR HOLDINGS INC
SELECT MEDICAL CORPORATION
SEMPRA ENERGY
SENSIENT TECHNOLOGIES
CORPORATION
SHAW GROUP INC (THE)

SHELL OIL CO
SHERWIN WILLIAMS COMPANY
(THE)
SIGMA-ALDRICH CORP
SISTERS OF MERCY HEALTH
SYSTEMS
SMITH INTERNATIONAL INC
SMITHFIELD FOODS INC
SOUTHERN COMPANY (THE)
SOUTHWEST AIRLINES CO
SRA INTERNATIONAL INC
ST JUDE MEDICAL INC
STAPLES INC
STARTEK INC
STARWOOD HOTELS & RESORTS
WORLDWIDE INC
STERIS CORP
STRYKER CORP
SUN HEALTHCARE GROUP
SUN MICROSYSTEMS INC
SUNGARD DATA SYSTEMS INC
SUNOCO INC
SUNRISE SENIOR LIVING
SUPERVALU INC
SYKES ENTERPRISES INC
SYMANTEC CORP
SYNOPSYS INC
SYNTEL INC
SYSCO CORP
TALBOTS INC (THE)
TARGET CORPORATION
TBC CORPORATION
TECH DATA CORP
TEKTRONIX INC
TELEDYNE TECHNOLOGIES
INCORPORATED
TELEPHONE AND DATA SYSTEMS
INC (TDS)
TELETECH HOLDINGS INC
TESORO CORP
TIFFANY & CO
TIME WARNER INC
TJX COMPANIES INC (THE)
T-MOBILE USA
TOTAL SYSTEM SERVICES INC
(TSYS)
TOWERS PERRIN
TRANSOCEAN INC
TRAVELERS COMPANIES INC (THE)
TW TELECOM INC
TWEEN BRANDS INC
TYSON FOODS INC
UNION PACIFIC CORP
UNITED NATURAL FOODS INC
UNITED PARCEL SERVICE INC (UPS)
UNITED STATES CELLULAR CORP
UNITED TECHNOLOGIES
CORPORATION
UNITEDHEALTH GROUP INC
UNIVISION COMMUNICATIONS INC
UPS SUPPLY CHAIN SOLUTIONS
URBAN OUTFITTERS INC
URS CORPORATION
USAA
VALERO ENERGY CORP

VALSPAR CORPORATION (THE)
VARIAN MEDICAL SYSTEMS INC
VCA ANTECH INC
VERISIGN INC
VERIZON COMMUNICATIONS
VIACOM INC
VOLT INFORMATION SCIENCES INC
W R BERKLEY CORPORATION
WALGREEN CO
WAL-MART STORES INC
WALT DISNEY COMPANY (THE)
WASTE MANAGEMENT INC
WATERS CORP
WATSON PHARMACEUTICALS INC
WATSON WYATT WORLDWIDE INC
WEATHERFORD INTERNATIONAL
LTD
WEIGHT WATCHERS
INTERNATIONAL INC
WELLPOINT INC
WENDYS INTERNATIONAL INC
WEST CORPORATION
WEST PHARMACEUTICAL SERVICES
INC
WESTERN DIGITAL CORP
WESTERN UNION COMPANY (THE)
WHOLE FOODS MARKET INC
WILLIAMS COMPANIES INC (THE)
WILLIAMS SONOMA INC
WM WRIGLEY JR COMPANY
WW GRAINGER INC
WYETH
WYNDHAM WORLDWIDE
WYNN RESORTS LIMITED
XEROX CORP
YAHOO! INC
YUM! BRANDS INC
ZIMMER HOLDINGS INC

INDEX OF HEADQUARTERS LOCATION BY U.S. STATE

To help you locate members of THE AMERICAN EMPLOYERS 500 geographically, the city and state of the headquarters of each company are in the following index.

ALABAMA
HIBBETT SPORTS INC; Birmingham

ARIZONA
APOLLO GROUP INC; Phoenix
MICROCHIP TECHNOLOGY INC; Chandler
PETSMART INC; Phoenix

ARKANSAS
ACXIOM CORP; Little Rock
MURPHY OIL CORPORATION; El Dorado
SAM'S CLUB; Bentonville
TYSON FOODS INC; Springdale
WAL-MART STORES INC; Bentonville

CALIFORNIA
ADOBE SYSTEMS INC; San Jose
ADVANCED MICRO DEVICES INC (AMD); Sunnyvale
AECOM TECHNOLOGY CORPORATION; Los Angeles
AGILENT TECHNOLOGIES INC; Santa Clara
ALLERGAN INC; Irvine
AMGEN INC; Thousand Oaks
APPLE INC; Cupertino
AVERY DENNISON CORP; Pasadena
BEBE STORES INC; Brisbane
BECHTEL GROUP INC; San Francisco
BECKMAN COULTER INC; Fullerton
BIO RAD LABORATORIES INC; Hercules
BROADCOM CORP; Irvine
CHARLOTTE RUSSE HOLDING; San Diego
CHEVRON CORPORATION; San Ramon
CISCO SYSTEMS INC; San Jose
COOPER COMPANIES INC; Pleasanton
COST PLUS INC; Oakland
CUBIC CORP; San Diego
DAVITA INC; El Segundo
DINEEQUITY INC; Glendale
DIRECTV GROUP INC (THE); El Segundo
DJO INC; Vista
DOLE FOOD COMPANY INC; Westlake Village
EBAY INC; San Jose
EDISON INTERNATIONAL; Rosemead
ELECTRONIC ARTS INC; Redwood City
EXPERIAN AMERICAS; Costa Mesa

FOX ENTERTAINMENT GROUP INC; Los Angeles
GENENTECH INC; South San Francisco
GOOGLE INC; Mountain View
GUESS? INC; Los Angeles
HEALTH NET INC; Woodland Hills
HILTON HOTELS CORP; Beverly Hills
HOT TOPIC INC; City of Industry
INGRAM MICRO INC; Santa Ana
INTEL CORP; Santa Clara
INTUIT INC; Mountain View
JACK IN THE BOX INC; San Diego
JACOBS ENGINEERING GROUP INC; Pasadena
JUNIPER NETWORKS INC; Sunnyvale
KAISER PERMANENTE; Oakland
KEANE INC; San Ramon
MATTEL INC; El Segundo
MAXIM INTEGRATED PRODUCTS INC; Sunnyvale
MCAFEE INC; Santa Clara
MCKESSON CORPORATION; San Francisco
NETWORK APPLIANCE INC; Sunnyvale
NORTHROP GRUMMAN CORP; Los Angeles
OCCIDENTAL PETROLEUM CORP; Los Angeles
ORACLE CORP; Redwood Shores
PACIFIC SUNWEAR OF CALIFORNIA INC; Anaheim
PETCO ANIMAL SUPPLIES INC; San Diego
PG&E CORPORATION; San Francisco
PLANTRONICS INC; Santa Cruz
PUBLIC STORAGE INC; Glendale
QUALCOMM INC; San Diego
QUIKSILVER INC; Huntington Beach
ROBERT HALF INTERNATIONAL INC; Menlo Park
ROSS STORES INC; Pleasanton
SAFEWAY INC; Pleasanton
SAIC INC; San Diego
SEMPRA ENERGY; San Diego
SUN HEALTHCARE GROUP; Irvine
SUN MICROSYSTEMS INC; Santa Clara
SYMANTEC CORP; Cupertino
SYNOPSYS INC; Mountain View
TELEDYNE TECHNOLOGIES INCORPORATED; Thousand Oaks
URS CORPORATION; San Francisco
VARIAN MEDICAL SYSTEMS INC; Palo Alto
VCA ANTECH INC; Los Angeles
VERISIGN INC; Mountain View
WALT DISNEY COMPANY (THE); Burbank
WATSON PHARMACEUTICALS INC; Corona
WESTERN DIGITAL CORP; Lake Forest
WILLIAMS SONOMA INC; San Francisco
YAHOO! INC; Sunnyvale

COLORADO
CATHOLIC HEALTH INITIATIVES; Denver
CH2M HILL COMPANIES LTD; Englewood
CIBER INC; Greenwood Village
ECHOSTAR CORP; Englewood
FIRST DATA CORP; Greenwood Village
LEVEL 3 COMMUNICATIONS INC; Broomfield
LIBERTY GLOBAL INC; Englewood
STARTEK INC; Denver
TELETECH HOLDINGS INC; Englewood
TW TELECOM INC; Littleton
WESTERN UNION COMPANY (THE); Englewood

CONNECTICUT
AETNA INC; Hartford
FRONTIER COMMUNICATIONS CORPORATION; Stamford
GENERAL ELECTRIC CO (GE); Fairfield
HARTFORD FINANCIAL SERVICES GROUP INC (THE); Hartford
IMS HEALTH INC; Norwalk
PITNEY BOWES INC; Stamford
PRAXAIR INC; Danbury
TOWERS PERRIN; Stamford
UNITED NATURAL FOODS INC; Dayville
UNITED TECHNOLOGIES CORPORATION; Hartford
W R BERKLEY CORPORATION; Greenwich
XEROX CORP; Norwalk

DELAWARE
E I DU PONT DE NEMOURS & CO (DUPONT); Wilmington

DISTRICT OF COLUMBIA
DANAHER CORP; Washington

FLORIDA
BROWN & BROWN INC; Daytona Beach
BURGER KING HOLDINGS INC; Miami
CARNIVAL CORPORATION; Miami
CHICO'S FAS INC; Fort Myers
CSX CORP; Jacksonville
CSX TRANSPORTATION INC; Jacksonville
DARDEN RESTAURANTS INC; Orlando
DYCOM INDUSTRIES INC; Palm Beach Gardens
FIRST ADVANTAGE CORPORATION; St. Petersburg
FPL GROUP INC; Juno Beach
GEO GROUP INC; Boca Raton
HARRIS CORPORATION; Melbourne
HEALTH MANAGEMENT ASSOCIATES INC; Naples
JABIL CIRCUIT INC; St. Petersburg
LINCARE HOLDINGS INC; Clearwater
OFFICE DEPOT INC; Delray Beach

OSI RESTAURANT PARTNERS INC;
Tampa
PUBLIX SUPER MARKETS INC;
Lakeland
ROYAL CARIBBEAN CRUISES; Miami
RYDER SYSTEM INC; Miami
SEACOR HOLDINGS INC; Ft.
Lauderdale
SYKES ENTERPRISES INC; Tampa
TBC CORPORATION; Palm Beach
Gardens
TECH DATA CORP; Clearwater

GEORGIA
AARON RENTS INC; Atlanta
AFLAC INC; Columbus
COCA COLA COMPANY (THE); Atlanta
COCA COLA ENTERPRISES INC;
Atlanta
COX COMMUNICATIONS INC; Atlanta
GEORGIA GULF CORPORATION;
Atlanta
GLOBAL PAYMENTS INC; Atlanta
HOME DEPOT INC; Atlanta
LODGIAN INC; Atlanta
RUSSELL CORP; Atlanta
SOUTHERN COMPANY (THE); Atlanta
TOTAL SYSTEM SERVICES INC
(TSYS); Columbus
UNITED PARCEL SERVICE INC (UPS);
Atlanta
UPS SUPPLY CHAIN SOLUTIONS;
Alpharetta

HAWAII
HAWAIIAN ELECTRIC INDUSTRIES
INC; Honolulu

IDAHO
COLDWATER CREEK INC; Sandpoint
MICRON TECHNOLOGY INC; Boise

ILLINOIS
ABBOTT LABORATORIES; Abbott Park
ALBERTO-CULVER COMPANY;
Melrose Park
ALLSTATE CORPORATION (THE);
Northbrook
ARCHER DANIELS MIDLAND CO;
Decatur
ARTHUR J GALLAGHER & CO; Itasca
BAXTER INTERNATIONAL INC;
Deerfield
BDO SEIDMAN LLP; Chicago
BOEING COMPANY (THE); Chicago
CATERPILLAR INC; Peoria
CATERPILLAR LOGISTICS; Morton
CDW CORPORATION; Vernon Hills
DEERE & CO; Moline
DEVRY INC; Oakbrook Terrace
EXELON CORPORATION; Chicago
FORTUNE BRANDS INC; Deerfield
GLOBAL HYATT CORPORATION;
Chicago
GRANT THORNTON LLP; Chicago

HEWITT ASSOCIATES; Lincolnshire
KRAFT FOODS INC; Northfield
LKQ CORP; Chicago
MCDONALD'S CORP; Oak Brook
MOLEX INC; Lisle
R R DONNELLEY & SONS CO; Chicago
SARA LEE CORP; Downers Grove
TELEPHONE AND DATA SYSTEMS
INC (TDS); Chicago
UNITED STATES CELLULAR CORP;
Chicago
WALGREEN CO; Deerfield
WM WRIGLEY JR COMPANY; Chicago
WW GRAINGER INC; Lake Forest

INDIANA
ADESA INC; Carmel
CTS CORP; Elkhart
CUMMINS INC; Columbus
ELI LILLY & COMPANY; Indianapolis
FINISH LINE INC (THE); Indianapolis
WELLPOINT INC; Indianapolis
ZIMMER HOLDINGS INC; Warsaw

IOWA
PRINCIPAL FINANCIAL GROUP (THE);
Des Moines

KANSAS
EMBARQ CORP; Overland Park
KOCH INDUSTRIES INC; Wichita

KENTUCKY
HUMANA INC; Louisville
KINDRED HEALTHCARE INC;
Louisville
LEXMARK INTERNATIONAL INC;
Lexington
OMNICARE INC; Covington
RES CARE INC; Louisville
YUM! BRANDS INC; Louisville

LOUISIANA
AMEDISYS INC; Baton Rouge
ENTERGY CORP; New Orleans
SHAW GROUP INC (THE); Baton Rouge

MAINE
IDEXX LABORATORIES INC;
Westbrook

MARYLAND
BALTIMORE GAS AND ELECTRIC
COMPANY; Baltimore
BLACK & DECKER CORP; Towson
COVENTRY HEALTH CARE INC;
Bethesda
LOCKHEED MARTIN CORP; Bethesda
MARRIOTT INTERNATIONAL INC;
Bethesda
RITZ-CARLTON HOTEL COMPANY
LLC (THE); Chevy Chase

MASSACHUSETTS
ANALOG DEVICES INC; Norwood

BJ'S WHOLESALE CLUB INC; Natick
BOSTON SCIENTIFIC CORP; Natick
EMC CORP; Hopkinton
MILLIPORE CORP; Billerica
PARAMETRIC TECHNOLOGY CORP;
Needham
PAREXEL INTERNATIONAL CORP;
Waltham
RAYTHEON CO; Waltham
STAPLES INC; Framingham
TALBOTS INC (THE); Hingham
TJX COMPANIES INC (THE);
Framingham
WATERS CORP; Milford

MICHIGAN
DTE ENERGY COMPANY; Detroit
KELLOGG CO; Battle Creek
KELLY SERVICES INC; Troy
MEIJER INC; Grand Rapids
PERRIGO CO; Allegan
STRYKER CORP; Kalamazoo
SYNTEL INC; Troy

MINNESOTA
3M COMPANY; St. Paul
ADC TELECOMMUNICATIONS INC;
Eden Prairie
BEST BUY CO INC; Richfield
CARGILL INC; Wayzata
CH ROBINSON WORLDWIDE INC;
Eden Prairie
CHRISTOPHER & BANKS CORP;
Plymouth
FAIR ISAAC CORPORATION;
Minneapolis
GENERAL MILLS INC; Minneapolis
HEALTH FITNESS CORP; Minneapolis
MEDTRONIC INC; Minneapolis
PATTERSON COMPANIES INC; St. Paul
REGIS CORPORATION; Edina
ST JUDE MEDICAL INC; St. Paul
SUPERVALU INC; Eden Prairie
TARGET CORPORATION; Minneapolis
TRAVELERS COMPANIES INC (THE);
St. Paul
UNITEDHEALTH GROUP INC;
Minnetonka
VALSPAR CORPORATION (THE);
Minneapolis

MISSOURI
BASS PRO SHOPS INC; Springfield
BUILD-A-BEAR WORKSHOP INC; St.
Louis
EMERSON ELECTRIC CO; St. Louis
ENTERPRISE RENT-A-CAR; St. Louis
EXPRESS SCRIPTS INC; St. Louis
O'REILLY AUTOMOTIVE INC;
Springfield
PEABODY ENERGY CORP; St. Louis
SIGMA-ALDRICH CORP; St. Louis
SISTERS OF MERCY HEALTH
SYSTEMS; Chesterfield

NEBRASKA
BERKSHIRE HATHAWAY INC; Omaha
BUCKLE INC (THE); Kearney
CABELA'S INC; Sidney
CONAGRA FOODS INC; Omaha
INFOUSA INC; Omaha
UNION PACIFIC CORP; Omaha
WEST CORPORATION; Omaha

NEVADA
HARRAH'S ENTERTAINMENT INC; Las Vegas
LAS VEGAS SANDS CORP (THE VENETIAN); Las Vegas
MGM MIRAGE; Las Vegas
WYNN RESORTS LIMITED; Las Vegas

NEW JERSEY
AUTOMATIC DATA PROCESSING INC; Roseland
AVIS BUDGET GROUP INC; Parsippany
BARNES & NOBLE COLLEGE BOOKSTORES; Basking Ridge
BECTON DICKINSON & CO; Franklin Lakes
BED BATH & BEYOND INC; Union
CELLCO PARTNERSHIP (VERIZON WIRELESS); Basking Ridge
CHUBB CORPORATION (THE); Warren
COGNIZANT TECHNOLOGY SOLUTIONS CORP; Teaneck
COVANCE INC; Princeton
CR BARD INC; Murray Hill
FOSTER WHEELER LTD; Clinton
HERTZ GLOBAL HOLDINGS INC; Park Ridge
HONEYWELL INTERNATIONAL INC; Morristown
INVENTIV HEALTH INC; Somerset
JOHNSON & JOHNSON; New Brunswick
MEDCO HEALTH SOLUTIONS; Franklin Lakes
MERCK & CO INC; Whitehouse Station
PRUDENTIAL FINANCIAL INC; Newark
QUEST DIAGNOSTICS INC; Madison
SCHERING-PLOUGH CORP; Kenilworth
WYETH; Madison
WYNDHAM WORLDWIDE; Parsippany

NEW YORK
ABM INDUSTRIES INC; New York
AEROPOSTALE INC; New York
ALTRIA GROUP INC; New York
AMERICAN EXPRESS CO; New York
ANNTAYLOR STORES CORP; New York
ARROW ELECTRONICS INC; Melville
AVON PRODUCTS INC; New York
AXA FINANCIAL INC; New York
BARNES & NOBLE INC; New York
BLOOMBERG LP; New York
BRISTOL MYERS SQUIBB CO; New York
BUNGE LTD; White Plains

CABLEVISION SYSTEMS CORP; Bethpage
COACH INC; New York
COLGATE PALMOLIVE CO; New York
CONSOLIDATED EDISON INC; New York
DELOITTE & TOUCHE USA LLP; New York
DELOITTE CONSULTING LLP; New York
DRESS BARN INC (THE); Suffern
ERNST & YOUNG LLP; New York
ESTEE LAUDER COMPANIES INC (THE); New York
FOREST LABORATORIES INC; New York
HENRY SCHEIN INC; Melville
HESS CORPORATION; New York
IAC/INTERACTIVECORP; New York
INTERNATIONAL BUSINESS MACHINES CORP (IBM); Armonk
JP MORGAN CHASE & CO INC; New York
KPMG LLP; New York
L-3 COMMUNICATIONS HOLDINGS INC; New York
LOEWS CORPORATION; New York
MARSH & MCLENNAN COMPANIES INC; New York
MCKINSEY & COMPANY INC; New York
MERCER INC; New York
METLIFE INC; New York
MONRO MUFFLER BRAKE INC; Rochester
NEWS CORP; New York
OMNICOM GROUP INC; New York
PARSONS BRINCKERHOFF INC; New York
PAXAR CORP; White Plains
PAYCHEX INC; Rochester
PEPSI BOTTLING GROUP INC; Somers
PEPSICO INC; Purchase
PFIZER INC; New York
POLO RALPH LAUREN CORP; New York
PRICEWATERHOUSECOOPERS; New York
SCIENTIFIC GAMES CORPORATION; New York
STARWOOD HOTELS & RESORTS WORLDWIDE INC; White Plains
TIFFANY & CO; New York
TIME WARNER INC; New York
UNIVISION COMMUNICATIONS INC; New York
VERIZON COMMUNICATIONS; New York
VIACOM INC; New York
VOLT INFORMATION SCIENCES INC; New York
WEIGHT WATCHERS INTERNATIONAL INC; New York

NORTH CAROLINA
BANK OF AMERICA CORP; Charlotte
DUKE ENERGY CORP; Charlotte
FAMILY DOLLAR STORES INC; Charlotte
LABORATORY CORP OF AMERICA HOLDINGS; Burlington
LOWE'S COMPANIES INC; Mooresville
OLD DOMINION FREIGHT LINE INC; Thomasville
PANTRY INC (THE); Sanford
PHARMACEUTICAL PRODUCT DEVELOPMENT INC; Wilmington
SAS INSTITUTE INC; Cary

OHIO
ABERCROMBIE & FITCH CO; New Albany
AMERICAN ELECTRIC POWER COMPANY INC (AEP); Columbus
CARDINAL HEALTH INC; Dublin
CHEMED CORPORATION; Cincinnati
CINTAS CORP; Cincinnati
CONVERGYS CORPORATION; Cincinnati
DIEBOLD INC; North Canton
EATON CORP; Cleveland
FIRSTENERGY CORP; Akron
INTIMATE BRANDS INC; Columbus
JM SMUCKER CO; Orrville
KENDLE INTERNATIONAL INC; Cincinnati
KROGER CO (THE); Cincinnati
LIMITED BRANDS INC; Columbus
MACY'S INC; Cincinnati
MANOR CARE INC; Toledo
PROCTER & GAMBLE CO; Cincinnati
PROGRESSIVE CORPORATION (THE); Mayfield Village
SCOTTS MIRACLE GROW CO; Marysville
SHERWIN WILLIAMS COMPANY (THE); Cleveland
STERIS CORP; Mentor
TWEEN BRANDS INC; New Albany
WENDYS INTERNATIONAL INC; Dublin

OKLAHOMA
CHESAPEAKE ENERGY CORP; Oklahoma City
DEVON ENERGY CORPORATION; Oklahoma City
DOLLAR THRIFTY AUTOMOTIVE GROUP INC; Tulsa
HELMERICH & PAYNE INC; Tulsa
ONEOK INC; Tulsa
WILLIAMS COMPANIES INC (THE); Tulsa

OREGON
NIKE INC; Beaverton
TEKTRONIX INC; Beaverton

PENNSYLVANIA
AIR PRODUCTS & CHEMICALS INC; Allentown
AMERICAN EAGLE OUTFITTERS INC; Pittsburgh
AMERISOURCEBERGEN CORP; Chesterbrook
ARAMARK CORPORATION; Philadelphia
CEPHALON INC; Frazer
CHARMING SHOPPES INC; Bensalem
COMCAST CORP; Philadelphia
CONSOL ENERGY INC; Pittsburgh
DICK'S SPORTING GOODS INC; Pittsburgh
ICT GROUP INC; Newtown
IGATE CORPORATION; Pittsburgh
LINCOLN NATIONAL CORPORATION; Philadelphia
RESPIRONICS INC; Murrysville
RITE AID CORPORATION; Camp Hill
SELECT MEDICAL CORPORATION; Mechanicsburg
SUNGARD DATA SYSTEMS INC; Wayne
SUNOCO INC; Philadelphia
URBAN OUTFITTERS INC; Philadelphia
WEST PHARMACEUTICAL SERVICES INC; Lionville

RHODE ISLAND
AMERICAN POWER CONVERSION CORP; West Kingston
CVS CAREMARK CORPORATION; Woonsocket
GTECH HOLDINGS CORP; Providence

SOUTH CAROLINA
DENNY'S CORPORATION; Spartanburg
SCANA CORPORATION; Columbia

TENNESSEE
AUTOZONE INC; Memphis
CBRL GROUP INC; Lebanon
DOLLAR GENERAL CORPORATION; Goodlettsville
EXEL TRANSPORTATION SERVICES INC (DHL EXEL); Memphis
FEDEX CORPORATION; Memphis
FRED'S INC; Memphis
GENESCO INC; Nashville
HCA INC; Nashville
HEALTHWAYS INC; Nashville
PSYCHIATRIC SOLUTIONS INC; Franklin

TEXAS
7-ELEVEN INC; Dallas
ACADEMY SPORTS & OUTDOORS LTD; Katy
AFFILIATED COMPUTER SERVICES INC; Dallas
ALLIANCE DATA SYSTEMS CORPORATION; Dallas

ANADARKO PETROLEUM CORPORATION; The Woodlands
APACHE CORP; Houston
AT&T INC; San Antonio
BAKER HUGHES INC; Houston
BENCHMARK ELECTRONICS INC; Angleton
BJ SERVICES COMPANY; Houston
BRINKER INTERNATIONAL INC; Dallas
BURLINGTON NORTHERN SANTA FE CORP; Fort Worth
CAMERON INTERNATIONAL CORPORATION; Houston
CAPITAL SENIOR LIVING CORP; Dallas
CASH AMERICA INTERNATIONAL INC; Fort Worth
CHEVRON PHILLIPS CHEMICAL COMPANY LLC; The Woodlands
CLEAR CHANNEL COMMUNICATIONS INC; San Antonio
CLUBCORP INC; Dallas
CONOCOPHILLIPS COMPANY; Houston
CONTAINER STORE (THE); Coppell
DEAN FOODS CO; Dallas
DIAMOND OFFSHORE DRILLING INC; Houston
EXXON MOBIL CORPORATION (EXXONMOBIL); Irving
FLUOR CORP; Irving
FMC TECHNOLOGIES INC; Houston
FOSSIL INC; Richardson
GAMESTOP CORP; Grapevine
HALLIBURTON COMPANY; Houston
HE BUTT GROCERY COMPANY (HEB); San Antonio
J C PENNEY COMPANY INC; Plano
KIMBERLY-CLARK CORP; Irving
LANDRY'S RESTAURANTS INC; Houston
MARATHON OIL CORP; Houston
MARY KAY INC; Dallas
MEN'S WEARHOUSE INC (THE); Houston
NATIONAL OILWELL VARCO INC; Houston
NEIMAN MARCUS GROUP INC (THE); Dallas
NOBLE CORPORATION; Sugar Land
OCEANEERING INTERNATIONAL INC; Houston
ODYSSEY HEALTHCARE INC; Dallas
OIL STATES INTERNATIONAL INC; Houston
PATTERSON-UTI ENERGY INC; Houston
PEROT SYSTEMS CORP; Plano
PRIDE INTERNATIONAL INC; Houston
RELIANT ENERGY INC; Houston
RENT-A-CENTER INC; Plano
SABRE HOLDINGS CORP; Southlake
SCHLUMBERGER LIMITED; Houston
SHELL OIL CO; Houston

SMITH INTERNATIONAL INC; Houston
SOUTHWEST AIRLINES CO; Dallas
SYSCO CORP; Houston
TESORO CORP; San Antonio
TRANSOCEAN INC; Houston
USAA; San Antonio
VALERO ENERGY CORP; San Antonio
WASTE MANAGEMENT INC; Houston
WEATHERFORD INTERNATIONAL LTD; Houston
WHOLE FOODS MARKET INC; Austin

VIRGINIA
ADVANCE AUTO PARTS INC; Roanoke
AES CORPORATION (THE); Arlington
BOOZ ALLEN HAMILTON; McLean
BRINKS COMPANY (THE); Richmond
CACI INTERNATIONAL INC; Arlington
CARMAX GROUP; Richmond
GENERAL DYNAMICS CORP; Falls Church
GENWORTH FINANCIAL INC; Richmond
HILB ROGAL & HOBBS CO; Glen Allen
L-3 TITAN GROUP; Reston
MARS INC; McLean
MASSEY ENERGY COMPANY; Richmond
NII HOLDINGS INC; Reston
NORFOLK SOUTHERN CORP; Norfolk
OWENS & MINOR INC; Mechanicsville
SMITHFIELD FOODS INC; Smithfield
SRA INTERNATIONAL INC; Fairfax
SUNRISE SENIOR LIVING; McLean
WATSON WYATT WORLDWIDE INC; Arlington

WASHINGTON
AMAZON.COM INC; Seattle
COSTCO WHOLESALE CORP; Issaquah
EMERITUS CORP; Seattle
EXPEDITORS INTERNATIONAL OF WASHINGTON INC; Seattle
MICROSOFT CORP; Redmond
NORDSTROM INC; Seattle
SAFECO CORP; Seattle
T-MOBILE USA; Bellevue

WISCONSIN
FISERV INC; Brookfield
JOHNSON CONTROLS INC; Milwaukee
KOHL'S CORP; Menomonee Falls
MANPOWER INC; Milwaukee
OSHKOSH CORPORATION; Oshkosh
PLEXUS CORP; Neenah
SENSIENT TECHNOLOGIES CORPORATION; Milwaukee

OTHER
ACCENTURE LTD; Hamilton

INDEX BY REGIONS OF THE U.S. WHERE THE FIRMS HAVE LOCATIONS

WEST

3M COMPANY
7-ELEVEN INC
AARON RENTS INC
ABBOTT LABORATORIES
ABERCROMBIE & FITCH CO
ABM INDUSTRIES INC
ACCENTURE LTD
ACXIOM CORP
ADESA INC
ADOBE SYSTEMS INC
ADVANCED MICRO DEVICES INC
(AMD)
AECOM TECHNOLOGY
CORPORATION
AEROPOSTALE INC
AES CORPORATION (THE)
AETNA INC
AFFILIATED COMPUTER SERVICES
INC
AFLAC INC
AGILENT TECHNOLOGIES INC
AIR PRODUCTS & CHEMICALS INC
ALBERTO-CULVER COMPANY
ALLERGAN INC
ALLSTATE CORPORATION (THE)
ALTRIA GROUP INC
AMAZON.COM INC
AMERICAN EAGLE OUTFITTERS INC
AMERICAN EXPRESS CO
AMERISOURCEBERGEN CORP
AMGEN INC
ANADARKO PETROLEUM
CORPORATION
ANALOG DEVICES INC
ANNTAYLOR STORES CORP
APOLLO GROUP INC
APPLE INC
ARAMARK CORPORATION
ARCHER DANIELS MIDLAND CO
ARROW ELECTRONICS INC
ARTHUR J GALLAGHER & CO
AT&T INC
AUTOMATIC DATA PROCESSING INC
AUTOZONE INC
AVERY DENNISON CORP
AVIS BUDGET GROUP INC
AVON PRODUCTS INC
AXA FINANCIAL INC
BAKER HUGHES INC
BANK OF AMERICA CORP
BARNES & NOBLE COLLEGE
BOOKSTORES
BARNES & NOBLE INC
BASS PRO SHOPS INC
BAXTER INTERNATIONAL INC
BDO SEIDMAN LLP
BEBE STORES INC
BECHTEL GROUP INC

BECKMAN COULTER INC
BECTON DICKINSON & CO
BED BATH & BEYOND INC
BENCHMARK ELECTRONICS INC
BERKSHIRE HATHAWAY INC
BEST BUY CO INC
BIO RAD LABORATORIES INC
BJ SERVICES COMPANY
BLACK & DECKER CORP
BLOOMBERG LP
BOEING COMPANY (THE)
BOOZ ALLEN HAMILTON
BOSTON SCIENTIFIC CORP
BRINKER INTERNATIONAL INC
BRINKS COMPANY (THE)
BRISTOL MYERS SQUIBB CO
BROADCOM CORP
BROWN & BROWN INC
BUCKLE INC (THE)
BUILD-A-BEAR WORKSHOP INC
BURGER KING HOLDINGS INC
BURLINGTON NORTHERN SANTA FE
CORP
CABELA'S INC
CACI INTERNATIONAL INC
CAMERON INTERNATIONAL
CORPORATION
CAPITAL SENIOR LIVING CORP
CARDINAL HEALTH INC
CARGILL INC
CARMAX GROUP
CARNIVAL CORPORATION
CASH AMERICA INTERNATIONAL
INC
CATERPILLAR INC
CATERPILLAR LOGISTICS
CATHOLIC HEALTH INITIATIVES
CBRL GROUP INC
CELLCO PARTNERSHIP (VERIZON
WIRELESS)
CEPHALON INC
CH ROBINSON WORLDWIDE INC
CH2M HILL COMPANIES LTD
CHARLOTTE RUSSE HOLDING
CHARMING SHOPPES INC
CHEMED CORPORATION
CHEVRON CORPORATION
CHEVRON PHILLIPS CHEMICAL
COMPANY LLC
CHICO'S FAS INC
CHRISTOPHER & BANKS CORP
CHUBB CORPORATION (THE)
CIBER INC
CINTAS CORP
CISCO SYSTEMS INC
CLEAR CHANNEL
COMMUNICATIONS INC
CLUBCORP INC
COACH INC
COCA COLA COMPANY (THE)
COCA COLA ENTERPRISES INC
COGNIZANT TECHNOLOGY
SOLUTIONS CORP
COLDWATER CREEK INC
COLGATE PALMOLIVE CO

COMCAST CORP
CONAGRA FOODS INC
CONOCOPHILLIPS COMPANY
CONSOL ENERGY INC
CONTAINER STORE (THE)
CONVERGYS CORPORATION
COOPER COMPANIES INC
COST PLUS INC
COSTCO WHOLESALE CORP
COVANCE INC
COX COMMUNICATIONS INC
CR BARD INC
CSX CORP
CTS CORP
CUBIC CORP
CUMMINS INC
CVS CAREMARK CORPORATION
DANAHER CORP
DARDEN RESTAURANTS INC
DAVITA INC
DEAN FOODS CO
DEERE & CO
DELOITTE & TOUCHE USA LLP
DELOITTE CONSULTING LLP
DENNY'S CORPORATION
DEVRY INC
DICK'S SPORTING GOODS INC
DIEBOLD INC
DINEEQUITY INC
DIRECTV GROUP INC (THE)
DJO INC
DOLE FOOD COMPANY INC
DOLLAR THRIFTY AUTOMOTIVE
GROUP INC
DRESS BARN INC (THE)
DYCOM INDUSTRIES INC
E I DU PONT DE NEMOURS & CO
(DUPONT)
EATON CORP
EBAY INC
ECHOSTAR CORP
EDISON INTERNATIONAL
ELECTRONIC ARTS INC
ELI LILLY & COMPANY
EMC CORP
EMERITUS CORP
EMERSON ELECTRIC CO
ENTERPRISE RENT-A-CAR
ERNST & YOUNG LLP
EXEL TRANSPORTATION SERVICES
INC (DHL EXEL)
EXPEDITORS INTERNATIONAL OF
WASHINGTON INC
EXPERIAN AMERICAS
EXPRESS SCRIPTS INC
EXXON MOBIL CORPORATION
(EXXONMOBIL)
FAIR ISAAC CORPORATION
FAMILY DOLLAR STORES INC
FEDEX CORPORATION
FINISH LINE INC (THE)
FIRST ADVANTAGE CORPORATION
FIRST DATA CORP
FISERV INC
FLUOR CORP

FMC TECHNOLOGIES INC
FOSSIL INC
FOSTER WHEELER LTD
FOX ENTERTAINMENT GROUP INC
FPL GROUP INC
FRONTIER COMMUNICATIONS
CORPORATION
GAMESTOP CORP
GENENTECH INC
GENERAL DYNAMICS CORP
GENERAL ELECTRIC CO (GE)
GENERAL MILLS INC
GENESCO INC
GENWORTH FINANCIAL INC
GEO GROUP INC
GEORGIA GULF CORPORATION
GLOBAL HYATT CORPORATION
GLOBAL PAYMENTS INC
GOOGLE INC
GRANT THORNTON LLP
GTECH HOLDINGS CORP
GUESS? INC
HALLIBURTON COMPANY
HARRAH'S ENTERTAINMENT INC
HARTFORD FINANCIAL SERVICES
GROUP INC (THE)
HAWAIIAN ELECTRIC INDUSTRIES
INC
HCA INC
HEALTH FITNESS CORP
HEALTH MANAGEMENT
ASSOCIATES INC
HEALTH NET INC
HEALTHWAYS INC
HELMERICH & PAYNE INC
HENRY SCHEIN INC
HERTZ GLOBAL HOLDINGS INC
HESS CORPORATION
HEWITT ASSOCIATES
HILB ROGAL & HOBBS CO
HILTON HOTELS CORP
HOME DEPOT INC
HONEYWELL INTERNATIONAL INC
HOT TOPIC INC
HUMANA INC
IAC/INTERACTIVECORP
ICT GROUP INC
IDEXX LABORATORIES INC
IGATE CORPORATION
IMS HEALTH INC
INGRAM MICRO INC
INTEL CORP
INTERNATIONAL BUSINESS
MACHINES CORP (IBM)
INTIMATE BRANDS INC
INTUIT INC
INVENTIV HEALTH INC
J C PENNEY COMPANY INC
JABIL CIRCUIT INC
JACK IN THE BOX INC
JACOBS ENGINEERING GROUP INC
JM SMUCKER CO
JOHNSON & JOHNSON
JOHNSON CONTROLS INC
JP MORGAN CHASE & CO INC

JUNIPER NETWORKS INC
KAISER PERMANENTE
KEANE INC
KELLOGG CO
KELLY SERVICES INC
KENDLE INTERNATIONAL INC
KIMBERLY-CLARK CORP
KINDRED HEALTHCARE INC
KOCH INDUSTRIES INC
KOHL'S CORP
KPMG LLP
KRAFT FOODS INC
KROGER CO (THE)
L-3 COMMUNICATIONS HOLDINGS
INC
L-3 TITAN GROUP
LABORATORY CORP OF AMERICA
HOLDINGS
LANDRY'S RESTAURANTS INC
LAS VEGAS SANDS CORP (THE
VENETIAN)
LEVEL 3 COMMUNICATIONS INC
LEXMARK INTERNATIONAL INC
LIBERTY GLOBAL INC
LIMITED BRANDS INC
LINCARE HOLDINGS INC
LINCOLN NATIONAL CORPORATION
LKQ CORP
LOCKHEED MARTIN CORP
LODGIAN INC
LOEWS CORPORATION
LOWE'S COMPANIES INC
MACY'S INC
MANOR CARE INC
MANPOWER INC
MARATHON OIL CORP
MARRIOTT INTERNATIONAL INC
MARS INC
MARSH & MCLENNAN COMPANIES
INC
MARY KAY INC
MATTEL INC
MAXIM INTEGRATED PRODUCTS INC
MCAFEE INC
MCDONALD'S CORP
MCKESSON CORPORATION
MCKINSEY & COMPANY INC
MEDCO HEALTH SOLUTIONS
MEDTRONIC INC
MEN'S WEARHOUSE INC (THE)
MERCER INC
MERCK & CO INC
METLIFE INC
MGM MIRAGE
MICROCHIP TECHNOLOGY INC
MICRON TECHNOLOGY INC
MICROSOFT CORP
MILLIPORE CORP
MOLEX INC
MURPHY OIL CORPORATION
NEIMAN MARCUS GROUP INC (THE)
NETWORK APPLIANCE INC
NEWS CORP
NIKE INC
NORDSTROM INC

NORTHROP GRUMMAN CORP
OCCIDENTAL PETROLEUM CORP
OCEANEERING INTERNATIONAL INC
ODYSSEY HEALTHCARE INC
OFFICE DEPOT INC
OLD DOMINION FREIGHT LINE INC
OMNICARE INC
OMNICOM GROUP INC
ORACLE CORP
O'REILLY AUTOMOTIVE INC
OSHKOSH CORPORATION
OSI RESTAURANT PARTNERS INC
OWENS & MINOR INC
PACIFIC SUNWEAR OF CALIFORNIA
INC
PARAMETRIC TECHNOLOGY CORP
PAREXEL INTERNATIONAL CORP
PARSONS BRINCKERHOFF INC
PATTERSON COMPANIES INC
PATTERSON-UTI ENERGY INC
PAXAR CORP
PAYCHEX INC
PEABODY ENERGY CORP
PEPSI BOTTLING GROUP INC
PEPSICO INC
PEROT SYSTEMS CORP
PETCO ANIMAL SUPPLIES INC
PETSMART INC
PFIZER INC
PG&E CORPORATION
PHARMACEUTICAL PRODUCT
DEVELOPMENT INC
PITNEY BOWES INC
PLANTRONICS INC
PLEXUS CORP
POLO RALPH LAUREN CORP
PRICEWATERHOUSECOOPERS
PRINCIPAL FINANCIAL GROUP (THE)
PROCTER & GAMBLE CO
PROGRESSIVE CORPORATION (THE)
PRUDENTIAL FINANCIAL INC
PSYCHIATRIC SOLUTIONS INC
PUBLIC STORAGE INC
QUALCOMM INC
QUEST DIAGNOSTICS INC
QUIKSILVER INC
R R DONNELLEY & SONS CO
RAYTHEON CO
REGIS CORPORATION
RELIANT ENERGY INC
RENT-A-CENTER INC
RES CARE INC
RESPIRONICS INC
RITE AID CORPORATION
RITZ-CARLTON HOTEL COMPANY
LLC (THE)
ROBERT HALF INTERNATIONAL INC
ROSS STORES INC
ROYAL CARIBBEAN CRUISES
RUSSELL CORP
SABRE HOLDINGS CORP
SAFECO CORP
SAFEWAY INC
SAIC INC
SAM'S CLUB

SARA LEE CORP
SAS INSTITUTE INC
SCHERING-PLOUGH CORP
SCHLUMBERGER LIMITED
SCIENTIFIC GAMES CORPORATION
SCOTTS MIRACLE GROW CO
SEACOR HOLDINGS INC
SELECT MEDICAL CORPORATION
SEMPRA ENERGY
SENSIENT TECHNOLOGIES
CORPORATION
SHAW GROUP INC (THE)
SHELL OIL CO
SHERWIN WILLIAMS COMPANY
(THE)
SIGMA-ALDRICH CORP
SMITH INTERNATIONAL INC
SRA INTERNATIONAL INC
ST JUDE MEDICAL INC
STAPLES INC
STARTEK INC
STARWOOD HOTELS & RESORTS
WORLDWIDE INC
STERIS CORP
STRYKER CORP
SUN HEALTHCARE GROUP
SUN MICROSYSTEMS INC
SUNGARD DATA SYSTEMS INC
SUNOCO INC
SUNRISE SENIOR LIVING
SUPERVALU INC
SYKES ENTERPRISES INC
SYMANTEC CORP
SYNOPSYS INC
SYNTEL INC
SYSCO CORP
TALBOTS INC (THE)
TARGET CORPORATION
TBC CORPORATION
TECH DATA CORP
TEKTRONIX INC
TELEDYNE TECHNOLOGIES
INCORPORATED
TELEPHONE AND DATA SYSTEMS
INC (TDS)
TELETECH HOLDINGS INC
TESORO CORP
TIME WARNER INC
TJX COMPANIES INC (THE)
T-MOBILE USA
TOTAL SYSTEM SERVICES INC
(TSYS)
TOWERS PERRIN
TRAVELERS COMPANIES INC (THE)
TW TELECOM INC
TWEEN BRANDS INC
TYSON FOODS INC
UNION PACIFIC CORP
UNITED NATURAL FOODS INC
UNITED PARCEL SERVICE INC (UPS)
UNITED STATES CELLULAR CORP
UNITED TECHNOLOGIES
CORPORATION
UNITEDHEALTH GROUP INC
UNIVISION COMMUNICATIONS INC

UPS SUPPLY CHAIN SOLUTIONS
URBAN OUTFITTERS INC
URS CORPORATION
USAA
VALERO ENERGY CORP
VALSPAR CORPORATION (THE)
VARIAN MEDICAL SYSTEMS INC
VCA ANTECH INC
VERISIGN INC
VERIZON COMMUNICATIONS
VIACOM INC
VOLT INFORMATION SCIENCES INC
W R BERKLEY CORPORATION
WALGREEN CO
WAL-MART STORES INC
WALT DISNEY COMPANY (THE)
WASTE MANAGEMENT INC
WATERS CORP
WATSON PHARMACEUTICALS INC
WATSON WYATT WORLDWIDE INC
WEATHERFORD INTERNATIONAL
LTD
WEIGHT WATCHERS
INTERNATIONAL INC
WELLPOINT INC
WENDYS INTERNATIONAL INC
WEST CORPORATION
WESTERN DIGITAL CORP
WESTERN UNION COMPANY (THE)
WHOLE FOODS MARKET INC
WILLIAMS COMPANIES INC (THE)
WILLIAMS SONOMA INC
WW GRAINGER INC
WYETH
WYNDHAM WORLDWIDE
WYNN RESORTS LIMITED
XEROX CORP
YAHOO! INC
YUM! BRANDS INC
ZIMMER HOLDINGS INC

SOUTHWEST
3M COMPANY
7-ELEVEN INC
AARON RENTS INC
ABBOTT LABORATORIES
ABERCROMBIE & FITCH CO
ABM INDUSTRIES INC
ACADEMY SPORTS & OUTDOORS
LTD
ACCENTURE LTD
ACXIOM CORP
ADESA INC
ADVANCE AUTO PARTS INC
ADVANCED MICRO DEVICES INC
(AMD)
AECOM TECHNOLOGY
CORPORATION
AEROPOSTALE INC
AES CORPORATION (THE)
AETNA INC
AFFILIATED COMPUTER SERVICES
INC
AFLAC INC
AIR PRODUCTS & CHEMICALS INC

ALBERTO-CULVER COMPANY
ALLERGAN INC
ALLIANCE DATA SYSTEMS
CORPORATION
ALLSTATE CORPORATION (THE)
ALTRIA GROUP INC
AMAZON.COM INC
AMEDISYS INC
AMERICAN EAGLE OUTFITTERS INC
AMERICAN ELECTRIC POWER
COMPANY INC (AEP)
AMERICAN EXPRESS CO
AMERICAN POWER CONVERSION
CORP
AMERISOURCEBERGEN CORP
ANADARKO PETROLEUM
CORPORATION
ANALOG DEVICES INC
ANNTAYLOR STORES CORP
APACHE CORP
APOLLO GROUP INC
APPLE INC
ARAMARK CORPORATION
ARCHER DANIELS MIDLAND CO
ARROW ELECTRONICS INC
ARTHUR J GALLAGHER & CO
AT&T INC
AUTOMATIC DATA PROCESSING INC
AUTOZONE INC
AVERY DENNISON CORP
AVIS BUDGET GROUP INC
AVON PRODUCTS INC
AXA FINANCIAL INC
BAKER HUGHES INC
BANK OF AMERICA CORP
BARNES & NOBLE COLLEGE
BOOKSTORES
BARNES & NOBLE INC
BASS PRO SHOPS INC
BAXTER INTERNATIONAL INC
BDO SEIDMAN LLP
BEBE STORES INC
BECHTEL GROUP INC
BECTON DICKINSON & CO
BED BATH & BEYOND INC
BENCHMARK ELECTRONICS INC
BERKSHIRE HATHAWAY INC
BEST BUY CO INC
BJ SERVICES COMPANY
BLOOMBERG LP
BOEING COMPANY (THE)
BOOZ ALLEN HAMILTON
BOSTON SCIENTIFIC CORP
BRINKER INTERNATIONAL INC
BRINKS COMPANY (THE)
BRISTOL MYERS SQUIBB CO
BROADCOM CORP
BROWN & BROWN INC
BUCKLE INC (THE)
BUILD-A-BEAR WORKSHOP INC
BURGER KING HOLDINGS INC
BURLINGTON NORTHERN SANTA FE
CORP
CABELA'S INC
CACI INTERNATIONAL INC

CAMERON INTERNATIONAL CORPORATION
CAPITAL SENIOR LIVING CORP
CARDINAL HEALTH INC
CARGILL INC
CARMAX GROUP
CASH AMERICA INTERNATIONAL INC
CATERPILLAR INC
CATERPILLAR LOGISTICS
CATHOLIC HEALTH INITIATIVES
CBRL GROUP INC
CELLCO PARTNERSHIP (VERIZON WIRELESS)
CH ROBINSON WORLDWIDE INC
CH2M HILL COMPANIES LTD
CHARLOTTE RUSSE HOLDING
CHARMING SHOPPES INC
CHEMED CORPORATION
CHESAPEAKE ENERGY CORP
CHEVRON CORPORATION
CHEVRON PHILLIPS CHEMICAL COMPANY LLC
CHICO'S FAS INC
CHRISTOPHER & BANKS CORP
CHUBB CORPORATION (THE)
CIBER INC
CINTAS CORP
CISCO SYSTEMS INC
CLEAR CHANNEL COMMUNICATIONS INC
CLUBCORP INC
COACH INC
COCA COLA COMPANY (THE)
COCA COLA ENTERPRISES INC
COGNIZANT TECHNOLOGY SOLUTIONS CORP
COLDWATER CREEK INC
COLGATE PALMOLIVE CO
COMCAST CORP
CONAGRA FOODS INC
CONOCOPHILLIPS COMPANY
CONSOLIDATED EDISON INC
CONTAINER STORE (THE)
CONVERGYS CORPORATION
COST PLUS INC
COSTCO WHOLESALE CORP
COVANCE INC
COX COMMUNICATIONS INC
CR BARD INC
CSX CORP
CTS CORP
CUMMINS INC
CVS CAREMARK CORPORATION
DANAHER CORP
DARDEN RESTAURANTS INC
DAVITA INC
DEAN FOODS CO
DEERE & CO
DELOITTE & TOUCHE USA LLP
DELOITTE CONSULTING LLP
DENNY'S CORPORATION
DEVON ENERGY CORPORATION
DEVRY INC
DIAMOND OFFSHORE DRILLING INC

DICK'S SPORTING GOODS INC
DIEBOLD INC
DINEEQUITY INC
DIRECTV GROUP INC (THE)
DJO INC
DOLE FOOD COMPANY INC
DOLLAR GENERAL CORPORATION
DOLLAR THRIFTY AUTOMOTIVE GROUP INC
DRESS BARN INC (THE)
DYCOM INDUSTRIES INC
E I DU PONT DE NEMOURS & CO (DUPONT)
EATON CORP
EBAY INC
EDISON INTERNATIONAL
ELECTRONIC ARTS INC
ELI LILLY & COMPANY
EMERITUS CORP
EMERSON ELECTRIC CO
ENTERGY CORP
ENTERPRISE RENT-A-CAR
ERNST & YOUNG LLP
EXEL TRANSPORTATION SERVICES INC (DHL EXEL)
EXPEDITORS INTERNATIONAL OF WASHINGTON INC
EXPERIAN AMERICAS
EXPRESS SCRIPTS INC
EXXON MOBIL CORPORATION (EXXONMOBIL)
FAIR ISAAC CORPORATION
FAMILY DOLLAR STORES INC
FEDEX CORPORATION
FINISH LINE INC (THE)
FIRST ADVANTAGE CORPORATION
FIRST DATA CORP
FISERV INC
FLUOR CORP
FMC TECHNOLOGIES INC
FOSSIL INC
FOSTER WHEELER LTD
FPL GROUP INC
FRED'S INC
FRONTIER COMMUNICATIONS CORPORATION
GAMESTOP CORP
GENERAL DYNAMICS CORP
GENERAL ELECTRIC CO (GE)
GENERAL MILLS INC
GENESCO INC
GENWORTH FINANCIAL INC
GEO GROUP INC
GEORGIA GULF CORPORATION
GLOBAL HYATT CORPORATION
GLOBAL PAYMENTS INC
GOOGLE INC
GRANT THORNTON LLP
GTECH HOLDINGS CORP
GUESS? INC
HALLIBURTON COMPANY
HARRAH'S ENTERTAINMENT INC
HARTFORD FINANCIAL SERVICES GROUP INC (THE)
HCA INC

HE BUTT GROCERY COMPANY (HEB)
HEALTH FITNESS CORP
HEALTH MANAGEMENT ASSOCIATES INC
HEALTH NET INC
HEALTHWAYS INC
HELMERICH & PAYNE INC
HENRY SCHEIN INC
HERTZ GLOBAL HOLDINGS INC
HESS CORPORATION
HEWITT ASSOCIATES
HIBBETT SPORTS INC
HILB ROGAL & HOBBS CO
HILTON HOTELS CORP
HOME DEPOT INC
HONEYWELL INTERNATIONAL INC
HOT TOPIC INC
HUMANA INC
IAC/INTERACTIVECORP
ICT GROUP INC
IDEXX LABORATORIES INC
IGATE CORPORATION
INGRAM MICRO INC
INTEL CORP
INTERNATIONAL BUSINESS MACHINES CORP (IBM)
INTIMATE BRANDS INC
INTUIT INC
INVENTIV HEALTH INC
J C PENNEY COMPANY INC
JACK IN THE BOX INC
JACOBS ENGINEERING GROUP INC
JOHNSON & JOHNSON
JOHNSON CONTROLS INC
JP MORGAN CHASE & CO INC
JUNIPER NETWORKS INC
KELLOGG CO
KELLY SERVICES INC
KIMBERLY-CLARK CORP
KINDRED HEALTHCARE INC
KOCH INDUSTRIES INC
KOHL'S CORP
KPMG LLP
KRAFT FOODS INC
KROGER CO (THE)
L-3 COMMUNICATIONS HOLDINGS INC
L-3 TITAN GROUP
LABORATORY CORP OF AMERICA HOLDINGS
LANDRY'S RESTAURANTS INC
LEVEL 3 COMMUNICATIONS INC
LIMITED BRANDS INC
LINCARE HOLDINGS INC
LINCOLN NATIONAL CORPORATION
LKQ CORP
LOCKHEED MARTIN CORP
LODGIAN INC
LOEWS CORPORATION
LOWE'S COMPANIES INC
MACY'S INC
MANOR CARE INC
MANPOWER INC
MARATHON OIL CORP
MARRIOTT INTERNATIONAL INC

MARS INC
MARSH & MCLENNAN COMPANIES INC
MARY KAY INC
MATTEL INC
MAXIM INTEGRATED PRODUCTS INC
MCAFEE INC
MCDONALD'S CORP
MCKESSON CORPORATION
MCKINSEY & COMPANY INC
MEDCO HEALTH SOLUTIONS
MEDTRONIC INC
MEN'S WEARHOUSE INC (THE)
MERCER INC
MERCK & CO INC
METLIFE INC
MICROCHIP TECHNOLOGY INC
MICRON TECHNOLOGY INC
MICROSOFT CORP
MILLIPORE CORP
MURPHY OIL CORPORATION
NATIONAL OILWELL VARCO INC
NEIMAN MARCUS GROUP INC (THE)
NEWS CORP
NIKE INC
NOBLE CORPORATION
NORDSTROM INC
NORFOLK SOUTHERN CORP
NORTHROP GRUMMAN CORP
OCCIDENTAL PETROLEUM CORP
OCEANEERING INTERNATIONAL INC
ODYSSEY HEALTHCARE INC
OFFICE DEPOT INC
OIL STATES INTERNATIONAL INC
OLD DOMINION FREIGHT LINE INC
OMNICARE INC
OMNICOM GROUP INC
ONEOK INC
ORACLE CORP
O'REILLY AUTOMOTIVE INC
OSI RESTAURANT PARTNERS INC
OWENS & MINOR INC
PACIFIC SUNWEAR OF CALIFORNIA INC
PARAMETRIC TECHNOLOGY CORP
PARSONS BRINCKERHOFF INC
PATTERSON COMPANIES INC
PATTERSON-UTI ENERGY INC
PAXAR CORP
PAYCHEX INC
PEPSI BOTTLING GROUP INC
PEPSICO INC
PEROT SYSTEMS CORP
PETCO ANIMAL SUPPLIES INC
PETSMART INC
PFIZER INC
PHARMACEUTICAL PRODUCT DEVELOPMENT INC
PITNEY BOWES INC
POLO RALPH LAUREN CORP
PRICEWATERHOUSECOOPERS
PRIDE INTERNATIONAL INC
PRINCIPAL FINANCIAL GROUP (THE)
PROCTER & GAMBLE CO
PROGRESSIVE CORPORATION (THE)

PRUDENTIAL FINANCIAL INC
PSYCHIATRIC SOLUTIONS INC
PUBLIC STORAGE INC
QUALCOMM INC
QUEST DIAGNOSTICS INC
R R DONNELLEY & SONS CO
RAYTHEON CO
REGIS CORPORATION
RELIANT ENERGY INC
RENT-A-CENTER INC
RES CARE INC
RESPIRONICS INC
RITE AID CORPORATION
RITZ-CARLTON HOTEL COMPANY LLC (THE)
ROBERT HALF INTERNATIONAL INC
ROSS STORES INC
SABRE HOLDINGS CORP
SAFECO CORP
SAFEWAY INC
SAIC INC
SAM'S CLUB
SARA LEE CORP
SAS INSTITUTE INC
SCHERING-PLOUGH CORP
SCHLUMBERGER LIMITED
SCIENTIFIC GAMES CORPORATION
SCOTTS MIRACLE GROW CO
SEACOR HOLDINGS INC
SELECT MEDICAL CORPORATION
SEMPRA ENERGY
SHAW GROUP INC (THE)
SHELL OIL CO
SHERWIN WILLIAMS COMPANY (THE)
SIGMA-ALDRICH CORP
SISTERS OF MERCY HEALTH SYSTEMS
SMITH INTERNATIONAL INC
SMITHFIELD FOODS INC
SOUTHWEST AIRLINES CO
SRA INTERNATIONAL INC
ST JUDE MEDICAL INC
STAPLES INC
STARTEK INC
STARWOOD HOTELS & RESORTS WORLDWIDE INC
STERIS CORP
STRYKER CORP
SUN HEALTHCARE GROUP
SUN MICROSYSTEMS INC
SUNGARD DATA SYSTEMS INC
SUNOCO INC
SUNRISE SENIOR LIVING
SUPERVALU INC
SYKES ENTERPRISES INC
SYMANTEC CORP
SYNOPSYS INC
SYNTEL INC
SYSCO CORP
TALBOTS INC (THE)
TARGET CORPORATION
TBC CORPORATION
TECH DATA CORP
TEKTRONIX INC

TELEDYNE TECHNOLOGIES INCORPORATED
TELEPHONE AND DATA SYSTEMS INC (TDS)
TELETECH HOLDINGS INC
TESORO CORP
TIME WARNER INC
TJX COMPANIES INC (THE)
T-MOBILE USA
TOTAL SYSTEM SERVICES INC (TSYS)
TOWERS PERRIN
TRANSOCEAN INC
TRAVELERS COMPANIES INC (THE)
TW TELECOM INC
TWEEN BRANDS INC
TYSON FOODS INC
UNION PACIFIC CORP
UNITED PARCEL SERVICE INC (UPS)
UNITED STATES CELLULAR CORP
UNITED TECHNOLOGIES CORPORATION
UNITEDHEALTH GROUP INC
UNIVISION COMMUNICATIONS INC
UPS SUPPLY CHAIN SOLUTIONS
URBAN OUTFITTERS INC
URS CORPORATION
USAA
VALERO ENERGY CORP
VALSPAR CORPORATION (THE)
VCA ANTECH INC
VERISIGN INC
VERIZON COMMUNICATIONS
W R BERKLEY CORPORATION
WALGREEN CO
WAL-MART STORES INC
WALT DISNEY COMPANY (THE)
WASTE MANAGEMENT INC
WATSON WYATT WORLDWIDE INC
WEATHERFORD INTERNATIONAL LTD
WEIGHT WATCHERS INTERNATIONAL INC
WELLPOINT INC
WENDYS INTERNATIONAL INC
WEST CORPORATION
WEST PHARMACEUTICAL SERVICES INC
WESTERN UNION COMPANY (THE)
WHOLE FOODS MARKET INC
WILLIAMS COMPANIES INC (THE)
WILLIAMS SONOMA INC
WW GRAINGER INC
WYETH
WYNDHAM WORLDWIDE
XEROX CORP
YAHOO! INC
YUM! BRANDS INC
ZIMMER HOLDINGS INC

MIDWEST
3M COMPANY
7-ELEVEN INC
AARON RENTS INC
ABBOTT LABORATORIES

ABERCROMBIE & FITCH CO
ABM INDUSTRIES INC
ACADEMY SPORTS & OUTDOORS LTD
ACCENTURE LTD
ACXIOM CORP
ADC TELECOMMUNICATIONS INC
ADESA INC
ADVANCE AUTO PARTS INC
ADVANCED MICRO DEVICES INC (AMD)
AECOM TECHNOLOGY CORPORATION
AEROPOSTALE INC
AES CORPORATION (THE)
AETNA INC
AFFILIATED COMPUTER SERVICES INC
AFLAC INC
AIR PRODUCTS & CHEMICALS INC
ALBERTO-CULVER COMPANY
ALLIANCE DATA SYSTEMS CORPORATION
ALLSTATE CORPORATION (THE)
ALTRIA GROUP INC
AMAZON.COM INC
AMEDISYS INC
AMERICAN EAGLE OUTFITTERS INC
AMERICAN ELECTRIC POWER COMPANY INC (AEP)
AMERICAN EXPRESS CO
AMERICAN POWER CONVERSION CORP
AMERISOURCEBERGEN CORP
ANALOG DEVICES INC
ANNTAYLOR STORES CORP
APOLLO GROUP INC
APPLE INC
ARAMARK CORPORATION
ARCHER DANIELS MIDLAND CO
ARROW ELECTRONICS INC
ARTHUR J GALLAGHER & CO
AT&T INC
AUTOMATIC DATA PROCESSING INC
AUTOZONE INC
AVERY DENNISON CORP
AVIS BUDGET GROUP INC
AVON PRODUCTS INC
AXA FINANCIAL INC
BAKER HUGHES INC
BANK OF AMERICA CORP
BARNES & NOBLE COLLEGE BOOKSTORES
BARNES & NOBLE INC
BASS PRO SHOPS INC
BAXTER INTERNATIONAL INC
BDO SEIDMAN LLP
BEBE STORES INC
BECHTEL GROUP INC
BECTON DICKINSON & CO
BED BATH & BEYOND INC
BERKSHIRE HATHAWAY INC
BEST BUY CO INC
BJ SERVICES COMPANY
BJ'S WHOLESALE CLUB INC

BLOOMBERG LP
BOEING COMPANY (THE)
BOOZ ALLEN HAMILTON
BOSTON SCIENTIFIC CORP
BRINKER INTERNATIONAL INC
BRINKS COMPANY (THE)
BRISTOL MYERS SQUIBB CO
BROADCOM CORP
BROWN & BROWN INC
BUCKLE INC (THE)
BUILD-A-BEAR WORKSHOP INC
BUNGE LTD
BURGER KING HOLDINGS INC
BURLINGTON NORTHERN SANTA FE CORP
CABELA'S INC
CACI INTERNATIONAL INC
CAMERON INTERNATIONAL CORPORATION
CAPITAL SENIOR LIVING CORP
CARDINAL HEALTH INC
CARGILL INC
CARMAX GROUP
CARNIVAL CORPORATION
CASH AMERICA INTERNATIONAL INC
CATERPILLAR INC
CATERPILLAR LOGISTICS
CATHOLIC HEALTH INITIATIVES
CBRL GROUP INC
CDW CORPORATION
CELLCO PARTNERSHIP (VERIZON WIRELESS)
CEPHALON INC
CH ROBINSON WORLDWIDE INC
CH2M HILL COMPANIES LTD
CHARLOTTE RUSSE HOLDING
CHARMING SHOPPES INC
CHEMED CORPORATION
CHESAPEAKE ENERGY CORP
CHEVRON CORPORATION
CHEVRON PHILLIPS CHEMICAL COMPANY LLC
CHICO'S FAS INC
CHRISTOPHER & BANKS CORP
CHUBB CORPORATION (THE)
CIBER INC
CINTAS CORP
CISCO SYSTEMS INC
CLEAR CHANNEL COMMUNICATIONS INC
CLUBCORP INC
COACH INC
COCA COLA COMPANY (THE)
COCA COLA ENTERPRISES INC
COGNIZANT TECHNOLOGY SOLUTIONS CORP
COLDWATER CREEK INC
COLGATE PALMOLIVE CO
COMCAST CORP
CONAGRA FOODS INC
CONOCOPHILLIPS COMPANY
CONSOLIDATED EDISON INC
CONTAINER STORE (THE)
CONVERGYS CORPORATION

COST PLUS INC
COSTCO WHOLESALE CORP
COVANCE INC
COX COMMUNICATIONS INC
CR BARD INC
CSX CORP
CTS CORP
CUBIC CORP
CUMMINS INC
CVS CAREMARK CORPORATION
DANAHER CORP
DARDEN RESTAURANTS INC
DAVITA INC
DEAN FOODS CO
DEERE & CO
DELOITTE & TOUCHE USA LLP
DELOITTE CONSULTING LLP
DENNY'S CORPORATION
DEVRY INC
DICK'S SPORTING GOODS INC
DIEBOLD INC
DINEEQUITY INC
DIRECTV GROUP INC (THE)
DJO INC
DOLE FOOD COMPANY INC
DOLLAR GENERAL CORPORATION
DOLLAR THRIFTY AUTOMOTIVE GROUP INC
DRESS BARN INC (THE)
DTE ENERGY COMPANY
DUKE ENERGY CORP
DYCOM INDUSTRIES INC
E I DU PONT DE NEMOURS & CO (DUPONT)
EATON CORP
EBAY INC
EDISON INTERNATIONAL
ELECTRONIC ARTS INC
ELI LILLY & COMPANY
EMBARQ CORP
EMERITUS CORP
EMERSON ELECTRIC CO
ENTERPRISE RENT-A-CAR
ERNST & YOUNG LLP
ESTEE LAUDER COMPANIES INC (THE)
EXEL TRANSPORTATION SERVICES INC (DHL EXEL)
EXELON CORPORATION
EXPEDITORS INTERNATIONAL OF WASHINGTON INC
EXPERIAN AMERICAS
EXPRESS SCRIPTS INC
EXXON MOBIL CORPORATION (EXXONMOBIL)
FAIR ISAAC CORPORATION
FAMILY DOLLAR STORES INC
FEDEX CORPORATION
FINISH LINE INC (THE)
FIRST ADVANTAGE CORPORATION
FIRST DATA CORP
FIRSTENERGY CORP
FISERV INC
FLUOR CORP
FMC TECHNOLOGIES INC

FOREST LABORATORIES INC
FORTUNE BRANDS INC
FOSSIL INC
FOSTER WHEELER LTD
FPL GROUP INC
FRED'S INC
FRONTIER COMMUNICATIONS
CORPORATION
GAMESTOP CORP
GENERAL DYNAMICS CORP
GENERAL ELECTRIC CO (GE)
GENERAL MILLS INC
GENESCO INC
GENWORTH FINANCIAL INC
GEO GROUP INC
GEORGIA GULF CORPORATION
GLOBAL HYATT CORPORATION
GLOBAL PAYMENTS INC
GRANT THORNTON LLP
GTECH HOLDINGS CORP
GUESS? INC
HARRAH'S ENTERTAINMENT INC
HARRIS CORPORATION
HARTFORD FINANCIAL SERVICES
GROUP INC (THE)
HCA INC
HEALTH FITNESS CORP
HEALTH MANAGEMENT
ASSOCIATES INC
HEALTHWAYS INC
HELMERICH & PAYNE INC
HENRY SCHEIN INC
HERTZ GLOBAL HOLDINGS INC
HESS CORPORATION
HEWITT ASSOCIATES
HIBBETT SPORTS INC
HILB ROGAL & HOBBS CO
HILTON HOTELS CORP
HOME DEPOT INC
HONEYWELL INTERNATIONAL INC
HOT TOPIC INC
HUMANA INC
IAC/INTERACTIVECORP
ICT GROUP INC
IDEXX LABORATORIES INC
INFOUSA INC
INGRAM MICRO INC
INTEL CORP
INTERNATIONAL BUSINESS
MACHINES CORP (IBM)
INTIMATE BRANDS INC
INTUIT INC
INVENTIV HEALTH INC
J C PENNEY COMPANY INC
JABIL CIRCUIT INC
JACK IN THE BOX INC
JACOBS ENGINEERING GROUP INC
JM SMUCKER CO
JOHNSON & JOHNSON
JOHNSON CONTROLS INC
JP MORGAN CHASE & CO INC
JUNIPER NETWORKS INC
KAISER PERMANENTE
KELLOGG CO
KELLY SERVICES INC

KENDLE INTERNATIONAL INC
KIMBERLY-CLARK CORP
KINDRED HEALTHCARE INC
KOCH INDUSTRIES INC
KOHL'S CORP
KPMG LLP
KRAFT FOODS INC
KROGER CO (THE)
L-3 COMMUNICATIONS HOLDINGS
INC
L-3 TITAN GROUP
LABORATORY CORP OF AMERICA
HOLDINGS
LANDRY'S RESTAURANTS INC
LEXMARK INTERNATIONAL INC
LIMITED BRANDS INC
LINCARE HOLDINGS INC
LINCOLN NATIONAL CORPORATION
LKQ CORP
LOCKHEED MARTIN CORP
LODGIAN INC
LOEWS CORPORATION
LOWE'S COMPANIES INC
MACY'S INC
MANOR CARE INC
MANPOWER INC
MARATHON OIL CORP
MARRIOTT INTERNATIONAL INC
MARS INC
MARSH & MCLENNAN COMPANIES
INC
MARY KAY INC
MATTEL INC
MAXIM INTEGRATED PRODUCTS INC
MCAFEE INC
MCDONALD'S CORP
MCKESSON CORPORATION
MCKINSEY & COMPANY INC
MEDCO HEALTH SOLUTIONS
MEDTRONIC INC
MEIJER INC
MEN'S WEARHOUSE INC (THE)
MERCER INC
MERCK & CO INC
METLIFE INC
MGM MIRAGE
MICROCHIP TECHNOLOGY INC
MICRON TECHNOLOGY INC
MICROSOFT CORP
MILLIPORE CORP
MOLEX INC
MONRO MUFFLER BRAKE INC
MURPHY OIL CORPORATION
NEIMAN MARCUS GROUP INC (THE)
NEWS CORP
NIKE INC
NORDSTROM INC
NORFOLK SOUTHERN CORP
NORTHROP GRUMMAN CORP
OCCIDENTAL PETROLEUM CORP
ODYSSEY HEALTHCARE INC
OFFICE DEPOT INC
OIL STATES INTERNATIONAL INC
OLD DOMINION FREIGHT LINE INC
OMNICARE INC

OMNICOM GROUP INC
ONEOK INC
ORACLE CORP
O'REILLY AUTOMOTIVE INC
OSHKOSH CORPORATION
OSI RESTAURANT PARTNERS INC
OWENS & MINOR INC
PACIFIC SUNWEAR OF CALIFORNIA
INC
PANTRY INC (THE)
PARAMETRIC TECHNOLOGY CORP
PARSONS BRINCKERHOFF INC
PATTERSON COMPANIES INC
PATTERSON-UTI ENERGY INC
PAXAR CORP
PAYCHEX INC
PEABODY ENERGY CORP
PEPSI BOTTLING GROUP INC
PEPSICO INC
PEROT SYSTEMS CORP
PETCO ANIMAL SUPPLIES INC
PETSMART INC
PFIZER INC
PHARMACEUTICAL PRODUCT
DEVELOPMENT INC
PITNEY BOWES INC
PLEXUS CORP
POLO RALPH LAUREN CORP
PRICEWATERHOUSECOOPERS
PRINCIPAL FINANCIAL GROUP (THE)
PROCTER & GAMBLE CO
PROGRESSIVE CORPORATION (THE)
PRUDENTIAL FINANCIAL INC
PSYCHIATRIC SOLUTIONS INC
PUBLIC STORAGE INC
QUALCOMM INC
QUEST DIAGNOSTICS INC
R R DONNELLEY & SONS CO
RAYTHEON CO
REGIS CORPORATION
RELIANT ENERGY INC
RENT-A-CENTER INC
RES CARE INC
RITE AID CORPORATION
RITZ-CARLTON HOTEL COMPANY
LLC (THE)
ROBERT HALF INTERNATIONAL INC
ROYAL CARIBBEAN CRUISES
RUSSELL CORP
SAFECO CORP
SAFEWAY INC
SAIC INC
SAM'S CLUB
SARA LEE CORP
SAS INSTITUTE INC
SCHERING-PLOUGH CORP
SCHLUMBERGER LIMITED
SCIENTIFIC GAMES CORPORATION
SCOTTS MIRACLE GROW CO
SEACOR HOLDINGS INC
SELECT MEDICAL CORPORATION
SEMPRA ENERGY
SENSIENT TECHNOLOGIES
CORPORATION
SHAW GROUP INC (THE)

SHELL OIL CO
SHERWIN WILLIAMS COMPANY
(THE)
SIGMA-ALDRICH CORP
SISTERS OF MERCY HEALTH
SYSTEMS
SMITH INTERNATIONAL INC
SMITHFIELD FOODS INC
SOUTHWEST AIRLINES CO
SRA INTERNATIONAL INC
ST JUDE MEDICAL INC
STAPLES INC
STARTEK INC
STARWOOD HOTELS & RESORTS
WORLDWIDE INC
STERIS CORP
STRYKER CORP
SUN HEALTHCARE GROUP
SUN MICROSYSTEMS INC
SUNGARD DATA SYSTEMS INC
SUNOCO INC
SUNRISE SENIOR LIVING
SUPERVALU INC
SYKES ENTERPRISES INC
SYMANTEC CORP
SYNOPSYS INC
SYNTEL INC
SYSCO CORP
TALBOTS INC (THE)
TARGET CORPORATION
TECH DATA CORP
TELEDYNE TECHNOLOGIES
INCORPORATED
TELEPHONE AND DATA SYSTEMS
INC (TDS)
TELETECH HOLDINGS INC
TESORO CORP
TIME WARNER INC
TJX COMPANIES INC (THE)
T-MOBILE USA
TOTAL SYSTEM SERVICES INC
(TSYS)
TOWERS PERRIN
TRAVELERS COMPANIES INC (THE)
TW TELECOM INC
TWEEN BRANDS INC
TYSON FOODS INC
UNION PACIFIC CORP
UNITED NATURAL FOODS INC
UNITED PARCEL SERVICE INC (UPS)
UNITED STATES CELLULAR CORP
UNITED TECHNOLOGIES
CORPORATION
UNITEDHEALTH GROUP INC
UNIVISION COMMUNICATIONS INC
UPS SUPPLY CHAIN SOLUTIONS
URBAN OUTFITTERS INC
URS CORPORATION
VALERO ENERGY CORP
VALSPAR CORPORATION (THE)
VCA ANTECH INC
VERISIGN INC
VERIZON COMMUNICATIONS
VIACOM INC
W R BERKLEY CORPORATION

WALGREEN CO
WAL-MART STORES INC
WALT DISNEY COMPANY (THE)
WASTE MANAGEMENT INC
WATSON PHARMACEUTICALS INC
WATSON WYATT WORLDWIDE INC
WEATHERFORD INTERNATIONAL
LTD
WEIGHT WATCHERS
INTERNATIONAL INC
WELLPOINT INC
WENDYS INTERNATIONAL INC
WEST CORPORATION
WEST PHARMACEUTICAL SERVICES
INC
WESTERN UNION COMPANY (THE)
WHOLE FOODS MARKET INC
WILLIAMS COMPANIES INC (THE)
WILLIAMS SONOMA INC
WM WRIGLEY JR COMPANY
WW GRAINGER INC
WYETH
WYNDHAM WORLDWIDE
XEROX CORP
YAHOO! INC
YUM! BRANDS INC
ZIMMER HOLDINGS INC

SOUTHEAST
3M COMPANY
7-ELEVEN INC
AARON RENTS INC
ABERCROMBIE & FITCH CO
ABM INDUSTRIES INC
ACADEMY SPORTS & OUTDOORS
LTD
ACCENTURE LTD
ACXIOM CORP
ADESA INC
ADVANCE AUTO PARTS INC
ADVANCED MICRO DEVICES INC
(AMD)
AECOM TECHNOLOGY
CORPORATION
AEROPOSTALE INC
AETNA INC
AFFILIATED COMPUTER SERVICES
INC
AFLAC INC
AIR PRODUCTS & CHEMICALS INC
ALBERTO-CULVER COMPANY
ALLSTATE CORPORATION (THE)
ALTRIA GROUP INC
AMEDISYS INC
AMERICAN EAGLE OUTFITTERS INC
AMERICAN ELECTRIC POWER
COMPANY INC (AEP)
AMERICAN EXPRESS CO
AMERICAN POWER CONVERSION
CORP
AMERISOURCEBERGEN CORP
AMGEN INC
ANADARKO PETROLEUM
CORPORATION

ANALOG DEVICES INC
ANNTAYLOR STORES CORP
APACHE CORP
APOLLO GROUP INC
APPLE INC
ARAMARK CORPORATION
ARCHER DANIELS MIDLAND CO
ARROW ELECTRONICS INC
ARTHUR J GALLAGHER & CO
AT&T INC
AUTOMATIC DATA PROCESSING INC
AUTOZONE INC
AVERY DENNISON CORP
AVIS BUDGET GROUP INC
AVON PRODUCTS INC
AXA FINANCIAL INC
BAKER HUGHES INC
BANK OF AMERICA CORP
BARNES & NOBLE COLLEGE
BOOKSTORES
BARNES & NOBLE INC
BASS PRO SHOPS INC
BAXTER INTERNATIONAL INC
BDO SEIDMAN LLP
BEBE STORES INC
BECHTEL GROUP INC
BECKMAN COULTER INC
BECTON DICKINSON & CO
BED BATH & BEYOND INC
BENCHMARK ELECTRONICS INC
BERKSHIRE HATHAWAY INC
BEST BUY CO INC
BJ SERVICES COMPANY
BJ'S WHOLESALE CLUB INC
BLACK & DECKER CORP
BLOOMBERG LP
BOEING COMPANY (THE)
BOOZ ALLEN HAMILTON
BOSTON SCIENTIFIC CORP
BRINKER INTERNATIONAL INC
BRINKS COMPANY (THE)
BRISTOL MYERS SQUIBB CO
BROADCOM CORP
BROWN & BROWN INC
BUCKLE INC (THE)
BUILD-A-BEAR WORKSHOP INC
BURGER KING HOLDINGS INC
BURLINGTON NORTHERN SANTA FE
CORP
CABELA'S INC
CACI INTERNATIONAL INC
CAMERON INTERNATIONAL
CORPORATION
CAPITAL SENIOR LIVING CORP
CARDINAL HEALTH INC
CARGILL INC
CARMAX GROUP
CARNIVAL CORPORATION
CASH AMERICA INTERNATIONAL
INC
CATERPILLAR INC
CATERPILLAR LOGISTICS
CATHOLIC HEALTH INITIATIVES
CBRL GROUP INC

CELLCO PARTNERSHIP (VERIZON WIRELESS)
CH ROBINSON WORLDWIDE INC
CH2M HILL COMPANIES LTD
CHARLOTTE RUSSE HOLDING
CHARMING SHOPPES INC
CHEMED CORPORATION
CHESAPEAKE ENERGY CORP
CHEVRON CORPORATION
CHEVRON PHILLIPS CHEMICAL COMPANY LLC
CHICO'S FAS INC
CHRISTOPHER & BANKS CORP
CHUBB CORPORATION (THE)
CIBER INC
CINTAS CORP
CISCO SYSTEMS INC
CLEAR CHANNEL COMMUNICATIONS INC
CLUBCORP INC
COACH INC
COCA COLA COMPANY (THE)
COCA COLA ENTERPRISES INC
COLDWATER CREEK INC
COLGATE PALMOLIVE CO
COMCAST CORP
CONAGRA FOODS INC
CONOCOPHILLIPS COMPANY
CONTAINER STORE (THE)
CONVERGYS CORPORATION
COST PLUS INC
COSTCO WHOLESALE CORP
COVANCE INC
COX COMMUNICATIONS INC
CR BARD INC
CSX CORP
CSX TRANSPORTATION INC
CUBIC CORP
CUMMINS INC
CVS CAREMARK CORPORATION
DANAHER CORP
DARDEN RESTAURANTS INC
DAVITA INC
DEAN FOODS CO
DEERE & CO
DELOITTE & TOUCHE USA LLP
DELOITTE CONSULTING LLP
DENNY'S CORPORATION
DEVRY INC
DIAMOND OFFSHORE DRILLING INC
DICK'S SPORTING GOODS INC
DIEBOLD INC
DINEEQUITY INC
DIRECTV GROUP INC (THE)
DJO INC
DOLE FOOD COMPANY INC
DOLLAR GENERAL CORPORATION
DOLLAR THRIFTY AUTOMOTIVE GROUP INC
DRESS BARN INC (THE)
DUKE ENERGY CORP
DYCOM INDUSTRIES INC
E I DU PONT DE NEMOURS & CO (DUPONT)
EATON CORP

EDISON INTERNATIONAL
ELECTRONIC ARTS INC
ELI LILLY & COMPANY
EMERITUS CORP
EMERSON ELECTRIC CO
ENTERGY CORP
ENTERPRISE RENT-A-CAR
ERNST & YOUNG LLP
EXEL TRANSPORTATION SERVICES INC (DHL EXEL)
EXELON CORPORATION
EXPEDITORS INTERNATIONAL OF WASHINGTON INC
EXPERIAN AMERICAS
EXPRESS SCRIPTS INC
EXXON MOBIL CORPORATION (EXXONMOBIL)
FAIR ISAAC CORPORATION
FAMILY DOLLAR STORES INC
FEDEX CORPORATION
FINISH LINE INC (THE)
FIRST ADVANTAGE CORPORATION
FIRST DATA CORP
FISERV INC
FMC TECHNOLOGIES INC
FOSSIL INC
FOSTER WHEELER LTD
FPL GROUP INC
FRED'S INC
FRONTIER COMMUNICATIONS CORPORATION
GAMESTOP CORP
GENERAL DYNAMICS CORP
GENERAL ELECTRIC CO (GE)
GENERAL MILLS INC
GENESCO INC
GENWORTH FINANCIAL INC
GEO GROUP INC
GEORGIA GULF CORPORATION
GLOBAL HYATT CORPORATION
GLOBAL PAYMENTS INC
GRANT THORNTON LLP
GTECH HOLDINGS CORP
GUESS? INC
HALLIBURTON COMPANY
HARRAH'S ENTERTAINMENT INC
HARRIS CORPORATION
HARTFORD FINANCIAL SERVICES GROUP INC (THE)
HCA INC
HEALTH FITNESS CORP
HEALTH MANAGEMENT ASSOCIATES INC
HEALTHWAYS INC
HELMERICH & PAYNE INC
HENRY SCHEIN INC
HERTZ GLOBAL HOLDINGS INC
HESS CORPORATION
HEWITT ASSOCIATES
HIBBETT SPORTS INC
HILB ROGAL & HOBBS CO
HILTON HOTELS CORP
HOME DEPOT INC
HONEYWELL INTERNATIONAL INC
HOT TOPIC INC

HUMANA INC
IAC/INTERACTIVECORP
ICT GROUP INC
IDEXX LABORATORIES INC
INGRAM MICRO INC
INTEL CORP
INTERNATIONAL BUSINESS MACHINES CORP (IBM)
INTIMATE BRANDS INC
INTUIT INC
INVENTIV HEALTH INC
J C PENNEY COMPANY INC
JABIL CIRCUIT INC
JACK IN THE BOX INC
JACOBS ENGINEERING GROUP INC
JM SMUCKER CO
JOHNSON & JOHNSON
JOHNSON CONTROLS INC
JP MORGAN CHASE & CO INC
JUNIPER NETWORKS INC
KAISER PERMANENTE
KELLOGG CO
KELLY SERVICES INC
KIMBERLY-CLARK CORP
KINDRED HEALTHCARE INC
KOCH INDUSTRIES INC
KOHL'S CORP
KPMG LLP
KRAFT FOODS INC
KROGER CO (THE)
L-3 COMMUNICATIONS HOLDINGS INC
L-3 TITAN GROUP
LABORATORY CORP OF AMERICA HOLDINGS
LANDRY'S RESTAURANTS INC
LEVEL 3 COMMUNICATIONS INC
LIMITED BRANDS INC
LINCARE HOLDINGS INC
LINCOLN NATIONAL CORPORATION
LKQ CORP
LOCKHEED MARTIN CORP
LODGIAN INC
LOEWS CORPORATION
LOWE'S COMPANIES INC
MACY'S INC
MANOR CARE INC
MANPOWER INC
MARATHON OIL CORP
MARRIOTT INTERNATIONAL INC
MARS INC
MARY KAY INC
MATTEL INC
MAXIM INTEGRATED PRODUCTS INC
MCAFEE INC
MCDONALD'S CORP
MCKESSON CORPORATION
MCKINSEY & COMPANY INC
MEDCO HEALTH SOLUTIONS
MEDTRONIC INC
MEN'S WEARHOUSE INC (THE)
MERCER INC
MERCK & CO INC
METLIFE INC
MGM MIRAGE

MICROCHIP TECHNOLOGY INC
MICRON TECHNOLOGY INC
MICROSOFT CORP
MILLIPORE CORP
MOLEX INC
MURPHY OIL CORPORATION
NEIMAN MARCUS GROUP INC (THE)
NEWS CORP
NIKE INC
NOBLE CORPORATION
NORDSTROM INC
NORFOLK SOUTHERN CORP
NORTHROP GRUMMAN CORP
OCCIDENTAL PETROLEUM CORP
OCEANEERING INTERNATIONAL INC
ODYSSEY HEALTHCARE INC
OFFICE DEPOT INC
OIL STATES INTERNATIONAL INC
OLD DOMINION FREIGHT LINE INC
OMNICARE INC
OMNICOM GROUP INC
ORACLE CORP
O'REILLY AUTOMOTIVE INC
OSHKOSH CORPORATION
OSI RESTAURANT PARTNERS INC
OWENS & MINOR INC
PACIFIC SUNWEAR OF CALIFORNIA INC
PANTRY INC (THE)
PARAMETRIC TECHNOLOGY CORP
PARSONS BRINCKERHOFF INC
PATTERSON COMPANIES INC
PATTERSON-UTI ENERGY INC
PAXAR CORP
PAYCHEX INC
PEPSI BOTTLING GROUP INC
PEPSICO INC
PEROT SYSTEMS CORP
PETCO ANIMAL SUPPLIES INC
PETSMART INC
PFIZER INC
PHARMACEUTICAL PRODUCT DEVELOPMENT INC
PITNEY BOWES INC
PLEXUS CORP
POLO RALPH LAUREN CORP
PRICEWATERHOUSECOOPERS
PRIDE INTERNATIONAL INC
PRINCIPAL FINANCIAL GROUP (THE)
PROCTER & GAMBLE CO
PROGRESSIVE CORPORATION (THE)
PRUDENTIAL FINANCIAL INC
PSYCHIATRIC SOLUTIONS INC
PUBLIC STORAGE INC
PUBLIX SUPER MARKETS INC
QUALCOMM INC
QUEST DIAGNOSTICS INC
R R DONNELLEY & SONS CO
RAYTHEON CO
REGIS CORPORATION
RELIANT ENERGY INC
RENT-A-CENTER INC
RES CARE INC
RESPIRONICS INC
RITE AID CORPORATION

RITZ-CARLTON HOTEL COMPANY LLC (THE)
ROBERT HALF INTERNATIONAL INC
ROSS STORES INC
ROYAL CARIBBEAN CRUISES
RUSSELL CORP
RYDER SYSTEM INC
SABRE HOLDINGS CORP
SAFECO CORP
SAIC INC
SAM'S CLUB
SARA LEE CORP
SAS INSTITUTE INC
SCANA CORPORATION
SCHERING-PLOUGH CORP
SCIENTIFIC GAMES CORPORATION
SCOTTS MIRACLE GROW CO
SEACOR HOLDINGS INC
SELECT MEDICAL CORPORATION
SEMPRA ENERGY
SHAW GROUP INC (THE)
SHELL OIL CO
SHERWIN WILLIAMS COMPANY (THE)
SIGMA-ALDRICH CORP
SISTERS OF MERCY HEALTH SYSTEMS
SMITH INTERNATIONAL INC
SMITHFIELD FOODS INC
SOUTHERN COMPANY (THE)
SRA INTERNATIONAL INC
ST JUDE MEDICAL INC
STAPLES INC
STARTEK INC
STARWOOD HOTELS & RESORTS WORLDWIDE INC
STERIS CORP
STRYKER CORP
SUN HEALTHCARE GROUP
SUN MICROSYSTEMS INC
SUNGARD DATA SYSTEMS INC
SUNOCO INC
SUNRISE SENIOR LIVING
SUPERVALU INC
SYKES ENTERPRISES INC
SYMANTEC CORP
SYNOPSYS INC
SYSCO CORP
TALBOTS INC (THE)
TARGET CORPORATION
TBC CORPORATION
TECH DATA CORP
TELEDYNE TECHNOLOGIES INCORPORATED
TELEPHONE AND DATA SYSTEMS INC (TDS)
TELETECH HOLDINGS INC
TIME WARNER INC
TJX COMPANIES INC (THE)
T-MOBILE USA
TOTAL SYSTEM SERVICES INC (TSYS)
TOWERS PERRIN
TRAVELERS COMPANIES INC (THE)
TW TELECOM INC

TWEEN BRANDS INC
TYSON FOODS INC
UNION PACIFIC CORP
UNITED NATURAL FOODS INC
UNITED PARCEL SERVICE INC (UPS)
UNITED STATES CELLULAR CORP
UNITED TECHNOLOGIES CORPORATION
UNITEDHEALTH GROUP INC
UNIVISION COMMUNICATIONS INC
UPS SUPPLY CHAIN SOLUTIONS
URBAN OUTFITTERS INC
URS CORPORATION
USAA
VALERO ENERGY CORP
VALSPAR CORPORATION (THE)
VCA ANTECH INC
VERISIGN INC
VERIZON COMMUNICATIONS
W R BERKLEY CORPORATION
WALGREEN CO
WAL-MART STORES INC
WALT DISNEY COMPANY (THE)
WASTE MANAGEMENT INC
WATSON PHARMACEUTICALS INC
WATSON WYATT WORLDWIDE INC
WEATHERFORD INTERNATIONAL LTD
WEIGHT WATCHERS INTERNATIONAL INC
WELLPOINT INC
WENDYS INTERNATIONAL INC
WEST CORPORATION
WEST PHARMACEUTICAL SERVICES INC
WESTERN UNION COMPANY (THE)
WHOLE FOODS MARKET INC
WILLIAMS COMPANIES INC (THE)
WILLIAMS SONOMA INC
WM WRIGLEY JR COMPANY
WW GRAINGER INC
WYETH
WYNDHAM WORLDWIDE
XEROX CORP
YAHOO! INC
YUM! BRANDS INC
ZIMMER HOLDINGS INC

NORTHEAST
3M COMPANY
7-ELEVEN INC
AARON RENTS INC
ABBOTT LABORATORIES
ABERCROMBIE & FITCH CO
ABM INDUSTRIES INC
ACCENTURE LTD
ADESA INC
ADOBE SYSTEMS INC
ADVANCE AUTO PARTS INC
ADVANCED MICRO DEVICES INC (AMD)
AECOM TECHNOLOGY CORPORATION
AEROPOSTALE INC

AES CORPORATION (THE)
AETNA INC
AFFILIATED COMPUTER SERVICES INC
AFLAC INC
AGILENT TECHNOLOGIES INC
AIR PRODUCTS & CHEMICALS INC
ALBERTO-CULVER COMPANY
ALLIANCE DATA SYSTEMS CORPORATION
ALLSTATE CORPORATION (THE)
ALTRIA GROUP INC
AMAZON.COM INC
AMEDISYS INC
AMERICAN EAGLE OUTFITTERS INC
AMERICAN ELECTRIC POWER COMPANY INC (AEP)
AMERICAN EXPRESS CO
AMERICAN POWER CONVERSION CORP
AMERISOURCEBERGEN CORP
AMGEN INC
ANALOG DEVICES INC
ANNTAYLOR STORES CORP
APOLLO GROUP INC
APPLE INC
ARAMARK CORPORATION
ARCHER DANIELS MIDLAND CO
ARROW ELECTRONICS INC
ARTHUR J GALLAGHER & CO
AT&T INC
AUTOMATIC DATA PROCESSING INC
AUTOZONE INC
AVERY DENNISON CORP
AVIS BUDGET GROUP INC
AVON PRODUCTS INC
AXA FINANCIAL INC
BAKER HUGHES INC
BALTIMORE GAS AND ELECTRIC COMPANY
BANK OF AMERICA CORP
BARNES & NOBLE COLLEGE BOOKSTORES
BARNES & NOBLE INC
BASS PRO SHOPS INC
BAXTER INTERNATIONAL INC
BDO SEIDMAN LLP
BEBE STORES INC
BECHTEL GROUP INC
BECTON DICKINSON & CO
BED BATH & BEYOND INC
BENCHMARK ELECTRONICS INC
BERKSHIRE HATHAWAY INC
BEST BUY CO INC
BIO RAD LABORATORIES INC
BJ SERVICES COMPANY
BJ'S WHOLESALE CLUB INC
BLACK & DECKER CORP
BLOOMBERG LP
BOEING COMPANY (THE)
BOOZ ALLEN HAMILTON
BOSTON SCIENTIFIC CORP
BRINKER INTERNATIONAL INC
BRINKS COMPANY (THE)
BRISTOL MYERS SQUIBB CO

BROADCOM CORP
BROWN & BROWN INC
BUCKLE INC (THE)
BUILD-A-BEAR WORKSHOP INC
BUNGE LTD
BURGER KING HOLDINGS INC
CABELA'S INC
CABLEVISION SYSTEMS CORP
CACI INTERNATIONAL INC
CAMERON INTERNATIONAL CORPORATION
CAPITAL SENIOR LIVING CORP
CARDINAL HEALTH INC
CARMAX GROUP
CARNIVAL CORPORATION
CASH AMERICA INTERNATIONAL INC
CATERPILLAR INC
CATERPILLAR LOGISTICS
CATHOLIC HEALTH INITIATIVES
CBRL GROUP INC
CELLCO PARTNERSHIP (VERIZON WIRELESS)
CEPHALON INC
CH ROBINSON WORLDWIDE INC
CH2M HILL COMPANIES LTD
CHARLOTTE RUSSE HOLDING
CHARMING SHOPPES INC
CHEMED CORPORATION
CHEVRON CORPORATION
CHEVRON PHILLIPS CHEMICAL COMPANY LLC
CHICO'S FAS INC
CHRISTOPHER & BANKS CORP
CHUBB CORPORATION (THE)
CIBER INC
CINTAS CORP
CISCO SYSTEMS INC
CLEAR CHANNEL COMMUNICATIONS INC
CLUBCORP INC
COACH INC
COCA COLA COMPANY (THE)
COCA COLA ENTERPRISES INC
COGNIZANT TECHNOLOGY SOLUTIONS CORP
COLDWATER CREEK INC
COLGATE PALMOLIVE CO
COMCAST CORP
CONAGRA FOODS INC
CONOCOPHILLIPS COMPANY
CONSOL ENERGY INC
CONSOLIDATED EDISON INC
CONTAINER STORE (THE)
CONVERGYS CORPORATION
COOPER COMPANIES INC
COST PLUS INC
COSTCO WHOLESALE CORP
COVANCE INC
COVENTRY HEALTH CARE INC
COX COMMUNICATIONS INC
CR BARD INC
CSX CORP
CSX TRANSPORTATION INC
CTS CORP

CUBIC CORP
CUMMINS INC
CVS CAREMARK CORPORATION
DANAHER CORP
DARDEN RESTAURANTS INC
DAVITA INC
DEAN FOODS CO
DEERE & CO
DELOITTE & TOUCHE USA LLP
DELOITTE CONSULTING LLP
DENNY'S CORPORATION
DEVRY INC
DICK'S SPORTING GOODS INC
DIEBOLD INC
DINEEQUITY INC
DIRECTV GROUP INC (THE)
DJO INC
DOLE FOOD COMPANY INC
DOLLAR GENERAL CORPORATION
DOLLAR THRIFTY AUTOMOTIVE GROUP INC
DRESS BARN INC (THE)
DYCOM INDUSTRIES INC
E I DU PONT DE NEMOURS & CO (DUPONT)
EATON CORP
EBAY INC
EDISON INTERNATIONAL
ELECTRONIC ARTS INC
ELI LILLY & COMPANY
EMC CORP
EMERITUS CORP
EMERSON ELECTRIC CO
ENTERPRISE RENT-A-CAR
ERNST & YOUNG LLP
ESTEE LAUDER COMPANIES INC (THE)
EXEL TRANSPORTATION SERVICES INC (DHL EXEL)
EXELON CORPORATION
EXPEDITORS INTERNATIONAL OF WASHINGTON INC
EXPERIAN AMERICAS
EXPRESS SCRIPTS INC
EXXON MOBIL CORPORATION (EXXONMOBIL)
FAIR ISAAC CORPORATION
FAMILY DOLLAR STORES INC
FEDEX CORPORATION
FINISH LINE INC (THE)
FIRST ADVANTAGE CORPORATION
FIRST DATA CORP
FIRSTENERGY CORP
FISERV INC
FLUOR CORP
FMC TECHNOLOGIES INC
FOREST LABORATORIES INC
FOSSIL INC
FOSTER WHEELER LTD
FPL GROUP INC
FRED'S INC
FRONTIER COMMUNICATIONS CORPORATION
GAMESTOP CORP
GENERAL DYNAMICS CORP

GENERAL ELECTRIC CO (GE)
GENERAL MILLS INC
GENESCO INC
GENWORTH FINANCIAL INC
GEO GROUP INC
GEORGIA GULF CORPORATION
GLOBAL HYATT CORPORATION
GLOBAL PAYMENTS INC
GOOGLE INC
GRANT THORNTON LLP
GTECH HOLDINGS CORP
GUESS? INC
HARRAH'S ENTERTAINMENT INC
HARRIS CORPORATION
HARTFORD FINANCIAL SERVICES
GROUP INC (THE)
HCA INC
HEALTH FITNESS CORP
HEALTH MANAGEMENT
ASSOCIATES INC
HEALTH NET INC
HEALTHWAYS INC
HENRY SCHEIN INC
HERTZ GLOBAL HOLDINGS INC
HESS CORPORATION
HEWITT ASSOCIATES
HIBBETT SPORTS INC
HILB ROGAL & HOBBS CO
HILTON HOTELS CORP
HOME DEPOT INC
HONEYWELL INTERNATIONAL INC
HOT TOPIC INC
HUMANA INC
IAC/INTERACTIVECORP
ICT GROUP INC
IDEXX LABORATORIES INC
IGATE CORPORATION
IMS HEALTH INC
INGRAM MICRO INC
INTEL CORP
INTERNATIONAL BUSINESS
MACHINES CORP (IBM)
INTIMATE BRANDS INC
INTUIT INC
INVENTIV HEALTH INC
J C PENNEY COMPANY INC
JABIL CIRCUIT INC
JACK IN THE BOX INC
JACOBS ENGINEERING GROUP INC
JM SMUCKER CO
JOHNSON & JOHNSON
JOHNSON CONTROLS INC
JP MORGAN CHASE & CO INC
JUNIPER NETWORKS INC
KAISER PERMANENTE
KEANE INC
KELLOGG CO
KELLY SERVICES INC
KENDLE INTERNATIONAL INC
KIMBERLY-CLARK CORP
KINDRED HEALTHCARE INC
KOCH INDUSTRIES INC
KOHL'S CORP
KPMG LLP
KRAFT FOODS INC

KROGER CO (THE)
L-3 COMMUNICATIONS HOLDINGS
INC
L-3 TITAN GROUP
LABORATORY CORP OF AMERICA
HOLDINGS
LANDRY'S RESTAURANTS INC
LAS VEGAS SANDS CORP (THE
VENETIAN)
LEVEL 3 COMMUNICATIONS INC
LIMITED BRANDS INC
LINCARE HOLDINGS INC
LINCOLN NATIONAL CORPORATION
LKQ CORP
LOCKHEED MARTIN CORP
LODGIAN INC
LOEWS CORPORATION
LOWE'S COMPANIES INC
MACY'S INC
MANOR CARE INC
MANPOWER INC
MARATHON OIL CORP
MARRIOTT INTERNATIONAL INC
MARS INC
MARSH & MCLENNAN COMPANIES
INC
MARY KAY INC
MASSEY ENERGY COMPANY
MATTEL INC
MAXIM INTEGRATED PRODUCTS INC
MCAFEE INC
MCDONALD'S CORP
MCKESSON CORPORATION
MCKINSEY & COMPANY INC
MEDCO HEALTH SOLUTIONS
MEDTRONIC INC
MEN'S WEARHOUSE INC (THE)
MERCER INC
MERCK & CO INC
METLIFE INC
MGM MIRAGE
MICROCHIP TECHNOLOGY INC
MICRON TECHNOLOGY INC
MICROSOFT CORP
MILLIPORE CORP
MOLEX INC
MONRO MUFFLER BRAKE INC
MURPHY OIL CORPORATION
NEIMAN MARCUS GROUP INC (THE)
NETWORK APPLIANCE INC
NEWS CORP
NII HOLDINGS INC
NIKE INC
NORDSTROM INC
NORFOLK SOUTHERN CORP
NORTHROP GRUMMAN CORP
OCCIDENTAL PETROLEUM CORP
OCEANEERING INTERNATIONAL INC
ODYSSEY HEALTHCARE INC
OFFICE DEPOT INC
OLD DOMINION FREIGHT LINE INC
OMNICARE INC
OMNICOM GROUP INC
ORACLE CORP
O'REILLY AUTOMOTIVE INC

OSHKOSH CORPORATION
OSI RESTAURANT PARTNERS INC
OWENS & MINOR INC
PACIFIC SUNWEAR OF CALIFORNIA
INC
PANTRY INC (THE)
PARAMETRIC TECHNOLOGY CORP
PAREXEL INTERNATIONAL CORP
PARSONS BRINCKERHOFF INC
PATTERSON COMPANIES INC
PATTERSON-UTI ENERGY INC
PAXAR CORP
PAYCHEX INC
PEPSI BOTTLING GROUP INC
PEPSICO INC
PEROT SYSTEMS CORP
PERRIGO CO
PETCO ANIMAL SUPPLIES INC
PETSMART INC
PFIZER INC
PHARMACEUTICAL PRODUCT
DEVELOPMENT INC
PITNEY BOWES INC
PLEXUS CORP
POLO RALPH LAUREN CORP
PRAXAIR INC
PRICEWATERHOUSECOOPERS
PRINCIPAL FINANCIAL GROUP (THE)
PROCTER & GAMBLE CO
PROGRESSIVE CORPORATION (THE)
PRUDENTIAL FINANCIAL INC
PSYCHIATRIC SOLUTIONS INC
PUBLIC STORAGE INC
QUALCOMM INC
QUEST DIAGNOSTICS INC
R R DONNELLEY & SONS CO
RAYTHEON CO
REGIS CORPORATION
RELIANT ENERGY INC
RENT-A-CENTER INC
RES CARE INC
RESPIRONICS INC
RITE AID CORPORATION
RITZ-CARLTON HOTEL COMPANY
LLC (THE)
ROBERT HALF INTERNATIONAL INC
ROSS STORES INC
RUSSELL CORP
SABRE HOLDINGS CORP
SAFECO CORP
SAFEWAY INC
SAIC INC
SAM'S CLUB
SARA LEE CORP
SAS INSTITUTE INC
SCANA CORPORATION
SCHERING-PLOUGH CORP
SCHLUMBERGER LIMITED
SCIENTIFIC GAMES CORPORATION
SCOTTS MIRACLE GROW CO
SEACOR HOLDINGS INC
SELECT MEDICAL CORPORATION
SEMPRA ENERGY
SENSIENT TECHNOLOGIES
CORPORATION

SHAW GROUP INC (THE)
SHELL OIL CO
SHERWIN WILLIAMS COMPANY
(THE)
SIGMA-ALDRICH CORP
SMITH INTERNATIONAL INC
SMITHFIELD FOODS INC
SOUTHWEST AIRLINES CO
SRA INTERNATIONAL INC
ST JUDE MEDICAL INC
STAPLES INC
STARTEK INC
STARWOOD HOTELS & RESORTS
WORLDWIDE INC
STERIS CORP
STRYKER CORP
SUN HEALTHCARE GROUP
SUN MICROSYSTEMS INC
SUNGARD DATA SYSTEMS INC
SUNOCO INC
SUNRISE SENIOR LIVING
SUPERVALU INC
SYKES ENTERPRISES INC
SYMANTEC CORP
SYNOPSYS INC
SYNTEL INC
SYSCO CORP
TALBOTS INC (THE)
TARGET CORPORATION
TECH DATA CORP
TEKTRONIX INC
TELEDYNE TECHNOLOGIES
INCORPORATED
TELEPHONE AND DATA SYSTEMS
INC (TDS)
TELETECH HOLDINGS INC
TIFFANY & CO
TIME WARNER INC
TJX COMPANIES INC (THE)
T-MOBILE USA
TOTAL SYSTEM SERVICES INC
(TSYS)
TOWERS PERRIN
TRAVELERS COMPANIES INC (THE)
TW TELECOM INC
TWEEN BRANDS INC
TYSON FOODS INC
UNITED NATURAL FOODS INC
UNITED PARCEL SERVICE INC (UPS)
UNITED STATES CELLULAR CORP
UNITED TECHNOLOGIES
CORPORATION
UNITEDHEALTH GROUP INC
UNIVISION COMMUNICATIONS INC
UPS SUPPLY CHAIN SOLUTIONS
URBAN OUTFITTERS INC
URS CORPORATION
USAA
VALERO ENERGY CORP
VALSPAR CORPORATION (THE)
VARIAN MEDICAL SYSTEMS INC
VCA ANTECH INC
VERISIGN INC
VERIZON COMMUNICATIONS
VIACOM INC

VOLT INFORMATION SCIENCES INC
W R BERKLEY CORPORATION
WALGREEN CO
WAL-MART STORES INC
WALT DISNEY COMPANY (THE)
WASTE MANAGEMENT INC
WATERS CORP
WATSON PHARMACEUTICALS INC
WATSON WYATT WORLDWIDE INC
WEATHERFORD INTERNATIONAL
LTD
WEIGHT WATCHERS
INTERNATIONAL INC
WELLPOINT INC
WENDYS INTERNATIONAL INC
WEST CORPORATION
WEST PHARMACEUTICAL SERVICES
INC
WESTERN UNION COMPANY (THE)
WHOLE FOODS MARKET INC
WILLIAMS COMPANIES INC (THE)
WILLIAMS SONOMA INC
WM WRIGLEY JR COMPANY
WW GRAINGER INC
WYETH
WYNDHAM WORLDWIDE
XEROX CORP
YAHOO! INC
YUM! BRANDS INC
ZIMMER HOLDINGS INC

INDEX OF FIRMS WITH OPERATIONS OUTSIDE THE U.S.

3M COMPANY
7-ELEVEN INC
AARON RENTS INC
ABBOTT LABORATORIES
ABERCROMBIE & FITCH CO
ABM INDUSTRIES INC
ACCENTURE LTD
ACXIOM CORP
ADC TELECOMMUNICATIONS INC
ADESA INC
ADOBE SYSTEMS INC
ADVANCE AUTO PARTS INC
ADVANCED MICRO DEVICES INC
(AMD)
AECOM TECHNOLOGY
CORPORATION
AEROPOSTALE INC
AES CORPORATION (THE)
AFFILIATED COMPUTER SERVICES
INC
AFLAC INC
AGILENT TECHNOLOGIES INC
AIR PRODUCTS & CHEMICALS INC
ALBERTO-CULVER COMPANY
ALLERGAN INC
ALLIANCE DATA SYSTEMS
CORPORATION
ALLSTATE CORPORATION (THE)
ALTRIA GROUP INC
AMAZON.COM INC
AMERICAN EAGLE OUTFITTERS INC
AMERICAN EXPRESS CO
AMERICAN POWER CONVERSION
CORP
AMGEN INC
ANADARKO PETROLEUM
CORPORATION
ANALOG DEVICES INC
ANNTAYLOR STORES CORP
APACHE CORP
APOLLO GROUP INC
APPLE INC
ARAMARK CORPORATION
ARCHER DANIELS MIDLAND CO
ARROW ELECTRONICS INC
ARTHUR J GALLAGHER & CO
AT&T INC
AUTOMATIC DATA PROCESSING INC
AUTOZONE INC
AVERY DENNISON CORP
AVIS BUDGET GROUP INC
AVON PRODUCTS INC
AXA FINANCIAL INC
BAKER HUGHES INC
BANK OF AMERICA CORP
BARNES & NOBLE COLLEGE
BOOKSTORES
BASS PRO SHOPS INC
BAXTER INTERNATIONAL INC

BDO SEIMAN LLP
BEBE STORES INC
BECHTEL GROUP INC
BECKMAN COULTER INC
BECTON DICKINSON & CO
BED BATH & BEYOND INC
BENCHMARK ELECTRONICS INC
BERKSHIRE HATHAWAY INC
BEST BUY CO INC
BIO RAD LABORATORIES INC
BJ SERVICES COMPANY
BLACK & DECKER CORP
BLOOMBERG LP
BOEING COMPANY (THE)
BOOZ ALLEN HAMILTON
BOSTON SCIENTIFIC CORP
BRINKER INTERNATIONAL INC
BRINKS COMPANY (THE)
BRISTOL MYERS SQUIBB CO
BROADCOM CORP
BROWN & BROWN INC
BUILD-A-BEAR WORKSHOP INC
BUNGE LTD
BURGER KING HOLDINGS INC
BURLINGTON NORTHERN SANTA FE
CORP
CABELA'S INC
CACI INTERNATIONAL INC
CAMERON INTERNATIONAL
CORPORATION
CARDINAL HEALTH INC
CARGILL INC
CARNIVAL CORPORATION
CASH AMERICA INTERNATIONAL
INC
CATERPILLAR INC
CATERPILLAR LOGISTICS
CDW CORPORATION
CEPHALON INC
CH ROBINSON WORLDWIDE INC
CH2M HILL COMPANIES LTD
CHARLOTTE RUSSE HOLDING
CHARMING SHOPPES INC
CHEMED CORPORATION
CHEVRON CORPORATION
CHEVRON PHILLIPS CHEMICAL
COMPANY LLC
CHICO'S FAS INC
CHUBB CORPORATION (THE)
CIBER INC
CINTAS CORP
CISCO SYSTEMS INC
CLEAR CHANNEL
COMMUNICATIONS INC
CLUBCORP INC
COACH INC
COCA COLA COMPANY (THE)
COCA COLA ENTERPRISES INC
COGNIZANT TECHNOLOGY
SOLUTIONS CORP
COLGATE PALMOLIVE CO
COMCAST CORP
CONAGRA FOODS INC
CONOCOPHILLIPS COMPANY
CONSOL ENERGY INC

CONVERGYS CORPORATION
COOPER COMPANIES INC
COSTCO WHOLESALE CORP
COVANCE INC
CR BARD INC
CSX CORP
CSX TRANSPORTATION INC
CTS CORP
CUBIC CORP
CUMMINS INC
DANAHER CORP
DARDEN RESTAURANTS INC
DEAN FOODS CO
DEERE & CO
DELOITTE & TOUCHE USA LLP
DELOITTE CONSULTING LLP
DENNY'S CORPORATION
DEVON ENERGY CORPORATION
DEVRY INC
DIAMOND OFFSHORE DRILLING INC
DIEBOLD INC
DINEEQUITY INC
DIRECTV GROUP INC (THE)
DJO INC
DOLE FOOD COMPANY INC
DOLLAR THRIFTY AUTOMOTIVE
GROUP INC
DUKE ENERGY CORP
E I DU PONT DE NEMOURS & CO
(DUPONT)
EATON CORP
EBAY INC
EDISON INTERNATIONAL
ELECTRONIC ARTS INC
ELI LILLY & COMPANY
EMC CORP
EMERSON ELECTRIC CO
ENTERPRISE RENT-A-CAR
ERNST & YOUNG LLP
ESTEE LAUDER COMPANIES INC
(THE)
EXEL TRANSPORTATION SERVICES
INC (DHL EXEL)
EXPEDITORS INTERNATIONAL OF
WASHINGTON INC
EXPRESS SCRIPTS INC
EXXON MOBIL CORPORATION
(EXXONMOBIL)
FAIR ISAAC CORPORATION
FEDEX CORPORATION
FIRST ADVANTAGE CORPORATION
FIRST DATA CORP
FISERV INC
FLUOR CORP
FMC TECHNOLOGIES INC
FOREST LABORATORIES INC
FORTUNE BRANDS INC
FOSSIL INC
FOSTER WHEELER LTD
GAMESTOP CORP
GENENTECH INC
GENERAL DYNAMICS CORP
GENERAL ELECTRIC CO (GE)
GENERAL MILLS INC
GENESCO INC

GENWORTH FINANCIAL INC
GEO GROUP INC
GEORGIA GULF CORPORATION
GLOBAL HYATT CORPORATION
GLOBAL PAYMENTS INC
GOOGLE INC
GTECH HOLDINGS CORP
GUESS? INC
HALLIBURTON COMPANY
HARRAH'S ENTERTAINMENT INC
HARRIS CORPORATION
HARTFORD FINANCIAL SERVICES
GROUP INC (THE)
HCA INC
HE BUTT GROCERY COMPANY (HEB)
HEALTH FITNESS CORP
HEALTHWAYS INC
HELMERICH & PAYNE INC
HENRY SCHEIN INC
HERTZ GLOBAL HOLDINGS INC
HESS CORPORATION
HEWITT ASSOCIATES
HILB ROGAL & HOBBS CO
HILTON HOTELS CORP
HOME DEPOT INC
HONEYWELL INTERNATIONAL INC
HOT TOPIC INC
HUMANA INC
IAC/INTERACTIVECORP
ICT GROUP INC
IDEXX LABORATORIES INC
IGATE CORPORATION
IMS HEALTH INC
INFOUSA INC
INGRAM MICRO INC
INTEL CORP
INTERNATIONAL BUSINESS
MACHINES CORP (IBM)
INTIMATE BRANDS INC
INTUIT INC
J C PENNEY COMPANY INC
JABIL CIRCUIT INC
JACOBS ENGINEERING GROUP INC
JM SMUCKER CO
JOHNSON & JOHNSON
JOHNSON CONTROLS INC
JP MORGAN CHASE & CO INC
JUNIPER NETWORKS INC
KEANE INC
KELLOGG CO
KELLY SERVICES INC
KENDLE INTERNATIONAL INC
KIMBERLY-CLARK CORP
KOCH INDUSTRIES INC
KRAFT FOODS INC
L-3 COMMUNICATIONS HOLDINGS
INC
L-3 TITAN GROUP
LABORATORY CORP OF AMERICA
HOLDINGS
LAS VEGAS SANDS CORP (THE
VENETIAN)
LEVEL 3 COMMUNICATIONS INC
LEXMARK INTERNATIONAL INC
LIBERTY GLOBAL INC

LIMITED BRANDS INC
LINCOLN NATIONAL CORPORATION
LOCKHEED MARTIN CORP
LODGIAN INC
LOEWS CORPORATION
LOWE'S COMPANIES INC
MACY'S INC
MANPOWER INC
MARATHON OIL CORP
MARRIOTT INTERNATIONAL INC
MARS INC
MARSH & MCLENNAN COMPANIES INC
MARY KAY INC
MATTEL INC
MAXIM INTEGRATED PRODUCTS INC
MCAFEE INC
MCDONALD'S CORP
MCKESSON CORPORATION
MCKINSEY & COMPANY INC
MEDTRONIC INC
MEN'S WEARHOUSE INC (THE)
MERCER INC
MERCK & CO INC
METLIFE INC
MGM MIRAGE
MICROCHIP TECHNOLOGY INC
MICRON TECHNOLOGY INC
MICROSOFT CORP
MILLIPORE CORP
MOLEX INC
MURPHY OIL CORPORATION
NATIONAL OILWELL VARCO INC
NETWORK APPLIANCE INC
NEWS CORP
NII HOLDINGS INC
NIKE INC
NOBLE CORPORATION
NORDSTROM INC
NORFOLK SOUTHERN CORP
NORTHROP GRUMMAN CORP
OCCIDENTAL PETROLEUM CORP
OCEANEERING INTERNATIONAL INC
OFFICE DEPOT INC
OIL STATES INTERNATIONAL INC
OMNICARE INC
OMNICOM GROUP INC
ORACLE CORP
OSHKOSH CORPORATION
OSI RESTAURANT PARTNERS INC
PACIFIC SUNWEAR OF CALIFORNIA INC
PARAMETRIC TECHNOLOGY CORP
PAREXEL INTERNATIONAL CORP
PARSONS BRINCKERHOFF INC
PATTERSON COMPANIES INC
PATTERSON-UTI ENERGY INC
PAXAR CORP
PAYCHEX INC
PEABODY ENERGY CORP
PEPSI BOTTLING GROUP INC
PEPSICO INC
PEROT SYSTEMS CORP
PERRIGO CO
PETSMART INC

PFIZER INC
PHARMACEUTICAL PRODUCT DEVELOPMENT INC
PITNEY BOWES INC
PLANTRONICS INC
PLEXUS CORP
POLO RALPH LAUREN CORP
PRAXAIR INC
PRICEWATERHOUSECOOPERS
PRIDE INTERNATIONAL INC
PRINCIPAL FINANCIAL GROUP (THE)
PROCTER & GAMBLE CO
PRUDENTIAL FINANCIAL INC
QUALCOMM INC
QUEST DIAGNOSTICS INC
QUIKSILVER INC
R R DONNELLEY & SONS CO
RAYTHEON CO
REGIS CORPORATION
RENT-A-CENTER INC
RES CARE INC
RESPIRONICS INC
RITZ-CARLTON HOTEL COMPANY LLC (THE)
ROBERT HALF INTERNATIONAL INC
ROSS STORES INC
ROYAL CARIBBEAN CRUISES
RUSSELL CORP
RYDER SYSTEM INC
SABRE HOLDINGS CORP
SAFEWAY INC
SAIC INC
SAM'S CLUB
SARA LEE CORP
SAS INSTITUTE INC
SCHERING-PLOUGH CORP
SCHLUMBERGER LIMITED
SCIENTIFIC GAMES CORPORATION
SCOTTS MIRACLE GROW CO
SEACOR HOLDINGS INC
SELECT MEDICAL CORPORATION
SEMPRA ENERGY
SENSIENT TECHNOLOGIES CORPORATION
SHAW GROUP INC (THE)
SHELL OIL CO
SHERWIN WILLIAMS COMPANY (THE)
SIGMA-ALDRICH CORP
SISTERS OF MERCY HEALTH SYSTEMS
SMITH INTERNATIONAL INC
SMITHFIELD FOODS INC
ST JUDE MEDICAL INC
STAPLES INC
STARTEK INC
STARWOOD HOTELS & RESORTS WORLDWIDE INC
STERIS CORP
STRYKER CORP
SUN MICROSYSTEMS INC
SUNGARD DATA SYSTEMS INC
SUNOCO INC
SUNRISE SENIOR LIVING
SYKES ENTERPRISES INC

SYMANTEC CORP
SYNOPSYS INC
SYNTEL INC
SYSCO CORP
TALBOTS INC (THE)
TARGET CORPORATION
TBC CORPORATION
TECH DATA CORP
TEKTRONIX INC
TELEDYNE TECHNOLOGIES INCORPORATED
TELETECH HOLDINGS INC
TESORO CORP
TIME WARNER INC
TJX COMPANIES INC (THE)
TOTAL SYSTEM SERVICES INC (TSYS)
TOWERS PERRIN
TRANSOCEAN INC
TRAVELERS COMPANIES INC (THE)
TWEEN BRANDS INC
TYSON FOODS INC
UNITED PARCEL SERVICE INC (UPS)
UNITED TECHNOLOGIES CORPORATION
UNIVISION COMMUNICATIONS INC
UPS SUPPLY CHAIN SOLUTIONS
URBAN OUTFITTERS INC
URS CORPORATION
USAA
VALERO ENERGY CORP
VALSPAR CORPORATION (THE)
VARIAN MEDICAL SYSTEMS INC
VERISIGN INC
VERIZON COMMUNICATIONS
VIACOM INC
VOLT INFORMATION SCIENCES INC
W R BERKLEY CORPORATION
WALGREEN CO
WAL-MART STORES INC
WALT DISNEY COMPANY (THE)
WATERS CORP
WATSON PHARMACEUTICALS INC
WATSON WYATT WORLDWIDE INC
WEATHERFORD INTERNATIONAL LTD
WEIGHT WATCHERS INTERNATIONAL INC
WENDYS INTERNATIONAL INC
WEST CORPORATION
WEST PHARMACEUTICAL SERVICES INC
WESTERN DIGITAL CORP
WESTERN UNION COMPANY (THE)
WILLIAMS COMPANIES INC (THE)
WILLIAMS SONOMA INC
WM WRIGLEY JR COMPANY
WW GRAINGER INC
WYETH
WYNDHAM WORLDWIDE
WYNN RESORTS LIMITED
XEROX CORP
YAHOO! INC
YUM! BRANDS INC
ZIMMER HOLDINGS INC

Individual Data
Profiles
On Each Of
The AMERICAN EMPLOYERS 500

3M COMPANY

www.mmm.com

Industry Group Code: 339113 Ranks within this company's industry group: Sales: 1 Profits: 1

Management:		Sales/Marketing:		Liberal Arts:		Information Systems:		Professionals:		Technical/Scientific:	
Mgmt. Trainees:		Mktg. Professionals:	Y	Gen. Writing/Editing:	Y	Info. Management:	Y	Finance/Accounting:	Y	Engineers, Elec.:	Y
Experienced Mgmt.:	Y	Retail Sales:		Technical Writing:	Y	Software Dev.:	Y	Law:	Y	Engineers, Other:	Y
Int'l Business:	Y	Commercial/Industrial:	Y	Graphic Arts/Photog.:	Y	Hardware Dev.:	Y	HR/Other:	Y	Health/Lab:	Y
MBA Graduates:	Y	Sales Trainees:		Music:		Systems Integration:		Training:	Y	Scientists/Research:	Y
		Advertising Pros.:	Y	Broadcasting:		Consulting/Other:		Health Care:	Y	Petroleum/Chemicals:	
				Other:	Y			Consulting:		Math/Other:	Y

TYPES OF BUSINESS:

Health Care Products
Specialty Materials & Textiles
Industrial Products
Safety, Security & Protection Products
Display & Graphics Products
Consumer & Office Products
Electronics & Communications Products
Fuel-Cell Technology

BRANDS/DIVISIONS/AFFILIATES:

Lingualcare
Accuspray Application Technologies
Innovative Paper Technologies
Powell
Venture Tape
Bondo
Aearo Technologies Inc
3M eStore

CONTACTS: *Note: Officers with more than one job title may be intentionally listed here more than once.*

George W. Buckley, CEO
George W. Buckley, Pres.
Patrick D. Campbell, CFO/Sr. VP
Robert D. MacDonald, Sr. VP-Mktg. & Sales
Angela S. Lalor, Sr. VP-Human Resources
Frederick J. Palensky, Exec. VP-R&D
Marschall I. Smith, General Counsel/Sr. VP-Legal Affairs
Brad T. Sauer, Exec. VP-Health Care Bus.
Hak Cheol (H.C.) Shin, Exec. VP-Industrial & Transportation Bus.
Joe E. Harlan, Exec. VP-Electro & Comm. Bus.
Moe S. Nozari, Exec. VP-Consumer & Office Bus.
George W. Buckley, Chmn.
Inge Thulin, Exec. VP-Int'l Oper.
John K. Woodworth, Sr. VP-Corp. Supply Chain Oper.

Phone: 651-733-1110	Fax: 651-733-9973
Toll-Free: 800-364-3577	
Address: 3M Center, Bldg. 220-11W-02, St. Paul, MN 55144-1000 US	

GROWTH PLANS/SPECIAL FEATURES:

3M Company, founded in 1902, is involved in the research, manufacturing and marketing of a variety of products. The firm is organized into six segments: health care; consumer and office; display and graphics; electronics and communications; industrial and transportation; and safety, security and protection. The health care segment's products include medical and surgical supplies, skin infection prevention products, pharmaceuticals, drug delivery systems, orthodontic products, health information systems and microbiology products. The consumer and office segment includes office supply, stationery, construction, home improvement, protective material and visual systems products. The display and graphics segment's products include optical film and lenses for electronic displays; touch screens and monitors; screen filters; reflective sheeting; and commercial graphics systems. The electronics and communications segment's products include packaging and interconnection devices (used in circuits); fluids used in computer chips; high-temperature and display tapes; pressure-sensitive tapes and resins; and products for telecommunications systems. The industrial and transportation segment's products include vinyl, polyester, tapes, a variety of non-woven abrasives, adhesives, specialty materials, supply chain execution software, filtration systems, paint finishing products, engineering fluids and components for catalytic converters. The safety, security and protection services segment provides products for personal protection, safety and security, energy control, commercial cleaning and protection, passports and secure cards. During 2007, 3M acquired 15 companies, including Lingualcare, Accuspray Application Technologies, Innovative Paper Technologies, Powell, Venture Tape and Bondo. In November 2007, 3M agreed to acquire Aearo Technologies, a manufacturer of personal protection equipment, for $1.2 billion. In July 2007, the company launched its 3M eStore, providing easy access to its line of industrial products.

3M offers its employees tuition reimbursement; an employee assistance program; adoption assistance; onsite fitness centers; a Work and Personal Life Resource Center; educational opportunities; domestic partner benefits; health and dependent care reimbursement accounts; and medical, dental, disability and life insurance.

FINANCIALS: Sales and profits are in thousands of dollars—add 000 to get the full amount. 2007 Note: Financial information for 2007 was not available for all companies at press time.

2007 Sales: $24,462,000	2007 Profits: $4,096,000	**U.S. Stock Ticker:** MMM
2006 Sales: $22,923,000	2006 Profits: $3,851,000	**Int'l Ticker:** Int'l Exchange:
2005 Sales: $21,167,000	2005 Profits: $3,111,000	Employees: 76,239
2004 Sales: $20,011,000	2004 Profits: $2,841,000	Fiscal Year Ends: 12/31
2003 Sales: $18,232,000	2003 Profits: $2,403,000	Parent Company:

SALARIES/BENEFITS:

Pension Plan: Y	ESOP Stock Plan: Y	Profit Sharing:	Top Exec. Salary: $1,600,000	Bonus: $7,448,240
Savings Plan: Y	Stock Purch. Plan:		Second Exec. Salary: $714,595	Bonus: $778,328

OTHER THOUGHTS:

Apparent Women Officers or Directors: 4
Hot Spot for Advancement for Women/Minorities: Y

LOCATIONS: ("Y" = Yes)

West:	Southwest:	Midwest:	Southeast:	Northeast:	International:
Y	Y	Y	Y	Y	Y

7-ELEVEN INC
www.7-eleven.com

Industry Group Code: 445120 Ranks within this company's industry group: Sales: Profits:

Management:		Sales/Marketing:		Liberal Arts:		Information Systems:		Professionals:		Technical/Scientific:	
Mgmt. Trainees:	Y	Mktg. Professionals:	Y	Gen. Writing/Editing:		Info. Management:	Y	Finance/Accounting:	Y	Engineers, Elec.:	
Experienced Mgmt.:	Y	Retail Sales:	Y	Technical Writing:		Software Dev.:		Law:	Y	Engineers, Other:	
Int'l Business:	Y	Commercial/Industrial:		Graphic Arts/Photog.:	Y	Hardware Dev.:		HR/Other:	Y	Health/Lab:	
MBA Graduates:	Y	Sales Trainees:	Y	Music:		Systems Integration:		Training:	Y	Scientists/Research:	
		Advertising Pros.:	Y	Broadcasting:		Consulting/Other:		Health Care:		Petroleum/Chemicals:	
				Other:				Consulting:		Math/Other:	

TYPES OF BUSINESS:
Convenience Stores
Gas Stations

BRANDS/DIVISIONS/AFFILIATES:
Seven & I Holdings Co Ltd
Cafe Select
Big Gulp
Big Bite
Go-Go Taquitos
World Ovens Bakery
Slurpee
White Hen Pantry, Inc.

CONTACTS: *Note: Officers with more than one job title may be intentionally listed here more than once.*
Joseph DePinto, CEO
Masaaki Asakura, COO/Exec. VP
Joseph DePinto, Pres.
Stanley Reynolds, CFO/Exec. VP
Kevin Elliott, Sr. VP-Mktg.
Krystin Mitchell, Sr. VP-Human Resources
Sharon Stufflebeme, CIO/Sr. VP
Kevin Elliott, Sr. VP-Merch.
Dave Fenton, General Counsel/Sr. VP/Corp. Sec.
Darren Rebelez, Sr. VP-Store Oper.
Carole Davidson, Sr. VP-Strategic Planning
Don Thomas, Chief Acct. Officer/VP/Controller
Jeffrey Schenck, Sr. VP-National Franchise
Shiro Ozeki, VP/Treas.
David Seltzer, VP-Bus. Dev.
Mark Wise, VP-New Store Dev.
Bob Jenkins, VP-Int'l. & Domestic Licensing
Kevin Elliott, Sr. VP-Logistics

Phone: 214-828-7011	Fax: 214-828-7848
Toll-Free:	
Address: 2711 N. Haskell Ave., Dallas, TX 75204-2906 US	

GROWTH PLANS/SPECIAL FEATURES:

7-Eleven, Inc., the North American subsidiary for Seven & I Holdings Co, Ltd., franchises and licenses a total of 7,500 7-Eleven convenience stores throughout the U.S. and Canada. The company's convenience stores are extended-hour retail stores, emphasizing convenience and providing beverages, candy, fresh take-out foods, groceries, tobacco items, beer, wine, self-serve gasoline, magazines, specialty items, lottery tickets and certain financial services. 7-Eleven, Inc. also operates a number of additional store chains, including Garb-Ko, Inc. and White Hen Pantry, Inc. in the Midwest, Handee Marts, Inc. in Pennsylvania and Ohio, Resort Retailers in Utah, Prima Marketing in West Virginia and Southwest Convenience Stores, Inc. in Texas and New Mexico. The company continues to focus on its point-of-sale automated retail information system, the first of its kind in use in a major convenience store chain. The firm also continues to seek new store sites, both freestanding and in-line, for development. Annual sales are affected by seasonality and weather, because many of the company's traditional products attract more shoppers during warm, dry weather and during the summer months, when leisure time activities are more prevalent. With regard to merchandising programs, 7-Eleven offers Vcom kiosks in many of its locations. These computerized, interactive kiosks offer self service financial transactions including wire transfers, money orders and check cashing, in addition to standard ATM services. Through a partnership with Citibank, the company also offers free ATM access to Citibank customers in more than 5,500 of its stores.

The firm offers its employees a benefits package that includes a stock purchase plan, 401(k) program, an employee assistance program, tuition reimbursement, adoption assistance, same-sex domestic partner benefits and a company vehicle or car allowance for field consultants.

FINANCIALS: Sales and profits are in thousands of dollars—add 000 to get the full amount. 2007 Note: Financial information for 2007 was not available for all companies at press time.

2007 Sales: $15,797,590	2007 Profits: $133,694	**U.S. Stock Ticker: Subsidiary**
2006 Sales: $15,373,770	2006 Profits: $130,200	**Int'l Ticker:** Int'l Exchange:
2005 Sales: $14,000,000	2005 Profits: $110,000	Employees: 32,000
2004 Sales: $12,121,000	2004 Profits: $96,500	Fiscal Year Ends: 2/28
2003 Sales: $10,784,700	2003 Profits: $64,100	Parent Company: SEVEN & I HOLDINGS CO LTD

SALARIES/BENEFITS:

Pension Plan:	ESOP Stock Plan:	Profit Sharing:	Top Exec. Salary: $748,750	Bonus: $870,422
Savings Plan: Y	Stock Purch. Plan: Y		Second Exec. Salary: $418,750	Bonus: $324,531

OTHER THOUGHTS:
Apparent Women Officers or Directors: 7
Hot Spot for Advancement for Women/Minorities: Y

LOCATIONS: ("Y" = Yes)

West:	Southwest:	Midwest:	Southeast:	Northeast:	International:
Y	Y	Y	Y	Y	Y

Note: Financial information, benefits and other data can change quickly and may vary from those stated here.

AARON RENTS INC

www.aaronrents.com

Industry Group Code: 532200 Ranks within this company's industry group: Sales: 2 Profits: 2

Management:		Sales/Marketing:		Liberal Arts:		Information Systems:		Professionals:		Technical/Scientific:	
Mgmt. Trainees:	Y	Mktg. Professionals:	Y	Gen. Writing/Editing:		Info. Management:	Y	Finance/Accounting:	Y	Engineers, Elec.:	
Experienced Mgmt.:	Y	Retail Sales:	Y	Technical Writing:		Software Dev.:	Y	Law:	Y	Engineers, Other:	
Int'l Business:	Y	Commercial/Industrial:	Y	Graphic Arts/Photog.:	Y	Hardware Dev.:		HR/Other:	Y	Health/Lab:	
MBA Graduates:	Y	Sales Trainees:	Y	Music:		Systems Integration:		Training:	Y	Scientists/Research:	
		Advertising Pros.:	Y	Broadcasting:		Consulting/Other:		Health Care:		Petroleum/Chemicals:	
				Other:				Consulting:		Math/Other:	

TYPES OF BUSINESS:

Furniture Stores, Rental
Home & Office Accessories Rental
Consumer Electronics Rental
Household Appliances Rental
Business Equipment Rental
Furniture Manufacturing
Rent-to-Own Contracts

BRANDS/DIVISIONS/AFFILIATES:

MacTavish Furniture Industries

CONTACTS: *Note: Officers with more than one job title may be intentionally listed here more than once.*

Robert C. Loudermilk, Jr., CEO
William K. Butler, Jr., COO
Robert C. Loudermilk, Jr., Pres.
Gilbert L. Danielson, CFO/Exec. VP
B. Lee Landers, Jr., CIO/VP
Mitchell S. Paull, Sr. VP-Merch.
Elizabeth L. Gibbs, General Counsel/VP
Robert P. Sinclair, Jr., Controller/VP
William K. Butler, Jr., Pres., Aarons Sales & Lease Ownership Div.
Eduardo Quinones, Pres., Aaron Rents' Rent-to-Rent Div.
K. Todd Evans, VP-Franchising
R. Charles Loudermilk, Sr., Chmn.
Mitchell S. Paull, Sr. VP-Logistics

Phone: 404-231-0011	Fax: 404-240-6584
Toll-Free:	
Address: 309 E. Paces Ferry Rd., NE, Atlanta, GA 30305-2377 US	

GROWTH PLANS/SPECIAL FEATURES:

Aaron Rents, Inc. operates in the lease ownership, rental and specialty retailing businesses. The firm's major operating divisions are the sales and lease Ownership division; the corporate furnishings division; and the MacTavish Furniture Industries division. Aaron's sales and lease ownership division has approximately 1,014 company-operated sales and lease ownership stores in 33 states and Canada, and 484 franchised stores in 45 states and Canada. This division provides household goods such as furniture, household appliances, electronics and accessories, for consumers with limited or no access to traditional credit sources. The company offers monthly and semi-monthly payments, in contrast to of weekly payments required by many of its competitors, and also offers a rent-to-own option that leads to ownership within one-year as opposed to the 18-24 months some company's require. Its rental products are serviced or replaced free of charge. A typical sales & lease ownership store combines a showroom and warehouse, averages 9,000 square feet and is often located in working class neighborhoods and communities. Aaron's corporate furnishings division, which rents residential and office furniture to businesses, operates 62 company-owned stores in 16 states. It primarily rents new and rental return furniture often to provide furniture for relocated employees, or for start-up companies. A typical corporate furnishings store is also a combination showroom and warehouse and is 19,000 square feet. The MacTavish Furniture Industries division manufactures more than half of the furniture for the company's rental purchase stores through its seven furniture manufacturing plants, five bedding facilities and one lamp manufacturing facility. Aaron Rents is one of the only rental companies in the U.S. that manufactures its own furniture. In October 2007, the firm acquired all Prime Time Rentals stores.

Aaron's offers its employees 401(k) savings plans, tuition reimbursement and Aaron's University, an on-the-job training program.

FINANCIALS: Sales and profits are in thousands of dollars—add 000 to get the full amount. 2007 Note: Financial information for 2007 was not available for all companies at press time.

2007 Sales: $1,494,911	2007 Profits: $80,275	**U.S. Stock Ticker: RNT**
2006 Sales: $1,326,592	2006 Profits: $78,635	**Int'l Ticker:** Int'l Exchange:
2005 Sales: $1,125,505	2005 Profits: $57,993	Employees: 8,400
2004 Sales: $946,480	2004 Profits: $52,616	Fiscal Year Ends: 12/31
2003 Sales: $766,797	2003 Profits: $36,426	Parent Company:

SALARIES/BENEFITS:

Pension Plan:	ESOP Stock Plan:	Profit Sharing:	Top Exec. Salary: $454,000	Bonus: $1,259,722
Savings Plan: Y	Stock Purch. Plan:		Second Exec. Salary: $450,000	Bonus: $243,120

OTHER THOUGHTS:

Apparent Women Officers or Directors: 1
Hot Spot for Advancement for Women/Minorities:

LOCATIONS: ("Y" = Yes)

West:	Southwest:	Midwest:	Southeast:	Northeast:	International:
Y	Y	Y	Y	Y	Y

Note: Financial information, benefits and other data can change quickly and may vary from those stated here.

ABBOTT LABORATORIES

www.abbott.com

Industry Group Code: 325412 Ranks within this company's industry group: Sales: 2   Profits: 4

Management:		Sales/Marketing:		Liberal Arts:		Information Systems:		Professionals:		Technical/Scientific:	
Mgmt. Trainees:	Y	Mktg. Professionals:	Y	Gen. Writing/Editing:		Info. Management:	Y	Finance/Accounting:	Y	Engineers, Elec.:	Y
Experienced Mgmt.:	Y	Retail Sales:		Technical Writing:	Y	Software Dev.:	Y	Law:	Y	Engineers, Other:	Y
Int'l Business:	Y	Commercial/Industrial:	Y	Graphic Arts/Photog.:	Y	Hardware Dev.:		HR/Other:	Y	Health/Lab:	Y
MBA Graduates:	Y	Sales Trainees:	Y	Music:		Systems Integration:		Training:	Y	Scientists/Research:	Y
		Advertising Pros.:	Y	Broadcasting:		Consulting/Other:		Health Care:	Y	Petroleum/Chemicals:	
				Other:				Consulting:		Math/Other:	Y

TYPES OF BUSINESS:

Pharmaceuticals Manufacturing
Nutritional Products
Diagnostics
Consumer Health Products
Medical & Surgical Devices
Pharmaceutical Products
Animal Health

BRANDS/DIVISIONS/AFFILIATES:

Vysis Inc
I-Stat Corp
KOS Pharmaceuticals Inc
Experimental & Applied Sciences Inc
Humira
Simcor
Similac
Ensure

CONTACTS: *Note: Officers with more than one job title may be intentionally listed here more than once.*

Miles D. White, CEO
Richard A. Gonzalez, COO
Thomas C. Freyman, CFO
Stephen R. Fussell, Sr. VP-Human Resources
John C. Landgraf, Sr. VP-Global Pharmaceutical Mgmt. & Supply
Laura J. Schumacher, General Counsel/Exec. VP/Corp. Sec.
Richard Ashley, Exec. VP-Corp. Dev.
Melissa Brotz, VP-External Comm.
Thomas C. Freyman, Exec. VP-Finance
William G. Dempsey, Exec. VP-Pharmaceutical Group
Holger Liepmann, Exec. VP-Global Nutrition
John M. Capek, Exec. VP-Medical Devices
Edward L. Michael, Exec. VP-Diagnostics
Miles D. White, Chmn.
Olivier Bohuon, Sr. VP-Int'l Oper.

Phone: 847-937-6100	Fax: 847-937-9555

Toll-Free:

Address: 100 Abbott Park Rd., Abbott Park, IL 60064 US

GROWTH PLANS/SPECIAL FEATURES:

Abbott Laboratories' principal business is to discover, develop, manufacture and sell health care products and technologies ranging from pharmaceuticals, animal health products and medical devices. The pharmaceutical segment deals with adult and pediatric conditions such as rheumatoid arthritis, HIV, epilepsy and manic depression. The diagnostic instruments and test segment deals with a range of medical tests to diagnose infectious diseases, cancer, diabetes and genetic conditions. The nutritional products segment offers consumer products such as Similac, Ensure, Glucerna and AdvantEdge, as well as medical nutritional products and feeding devices. The medical and surgical devices segment includes minimally invasive treatment options that improve the care of people with vascular disease and spinal conditions. Vascular offerings include vessel closure devices, carotid and coronary stents, catheters and other interventional tools and devices. This segment also produces minimally invasive spinal fixation products. The animal health segment serves the veterinarian market with products that include anesthetic and wound care products, nutritional supplements, and intravenous sets and solutions. The company operates internationally in Europe, Asia, Africa, Latin and South America and the Middle East. Abbott's holds a 50% share in TAP Pharmaceutical Products, which makes the prostate cancer drug, Lupron, and Prevacid (Ogastro), a proton pump inhibitor for the short-term treatment of gastroesophageal reflux disease. In 2008, the firm received FDA approval for Humira, a medication for polyarticular juvenile idiopathic arthritis, as well as Simcor, a combination medicine for comprehensive cholesterol management.

Employee benefits include medical, dental and vision coverage; flexible spending accounts; profit sharing; 401(k); retirement pension; employee assistance program; tuition assistance; paternity leave; and life and AD&D insurance.

FINANCIALS: Sales and profits are in thousands of dollars—add 000 to get the full amount. 2007 Note: Financial information for 2007 was not available for all companies at press time.

2007 Sales: $25,914,200	2007 Profits: $3,606,300	**U.S. Stock Ticker: ABT**
2006 Sales: $22,476,322	2006 Profits: $1,716,755	**Int'l Ticker:** Int'l Exchange:
2005 Sales: $22,337,808	2005 Profits: $3,372,065	Employees: 68,000
2004 Sales: $19,680,016	2004 Profits: $3,235,851	Fiscal Year Ends: 12/31
2003 Sales: $19,680,600	2003 Profits: $2,753,200	Parent Company:

SALARIES/BENEFITS:

Pension Plan: Y	ESOP Stock Plan:	Profit Sharing: Y	Top Exec. Salary: $1,661,973	Bonus: $4,050,000
Savings Plan: Y	Stock Purch. Plan:		Second Exec. Salary: $973,931	Bonus: $1,535,000

OTHER THOUGHTS:

Apparent Women Officers or Directors: 11
Hot Spot for Advancement for Women/Minorities: Y

LOCATIONS: ("Y" = Yes)

West:	Southwest:	Midwest:	Southeast:	Northeast:	International:
Y	Y	Y		Y	Y

ABERCROMBIE & FITCH CO   www.abercrombie.com

Industry Group Code: 448000 Ranks within this company's industry group: Sales: 3   Profits: 2

Management:		Sales/Marketing:		Liberal Arts:		Information Systems:		Professionals:		Technical/Scientific:	
Mgmt. Trainees:	Y	Mktg. Professionals:	Y	Gen. Writing/Editing:	Y	Info. Management:	Y	Finance/Accounting:	Y	Engineers, Elec.:	
Experienced Mgmt.:	Y	Retail Sales:	Y	Technical Writing:		Software Dev.:	Y	Law:	Y	Engineers, Other:	
Int'l Business:	Y	Commercial/Industrial:	Y	Graphic Arts/Photog.:	Y	Hardware Dev.:		HR/Other:	Y	Health/Lab:	
MBA Graduates:	Y	Sales Trainees:	Y	Music:		Systems Integration:		Training:	Y	Scientists/Research:	
		Advertising Pros.:	Y	Broadcasting:		Consulting/Other:		Health Care:		Petroleum/Chemicals:	
				Other:	Y			Consulting:		Math/Other:	

TYPES OF BUSINESS:
Casual Apparel-Young Adults, Retail
Catalog & Online Sales
Children's Apparel
Casual Adult Apparel, Retail
Lingerie Stores

BRANDS/DIVISIONS/AFFILIATES:
Abercrombie & Fitch
Gilly Hicks
Hollister Co.
RUEHL
A&F Film
Abercrombie.com
AbercrombieKids.com
HollisterCo.com

CONTACTS: Note: Officers with more than one job title may be intentionally listed here more than once.
Michael S. Jeffries, CEO
Michael Nuzzo, Principal Financial Officer
Kristen Blum, CIO/Sr. VP
David S. Cupps, General Counsel/Sr. VP/Sec.
Leslee K. Herro, Sr. VP-Planning & Allocation
Michael Nuzzo, Principal Acct. Officer
Jeffrey Sinkey, Sr. VP-Real Estate
Michael S. Jeffries, Chmn.
Diane Chang, Sr. VP-Sourcing

Phone: 614-283-6500	Fax: 614-283-6710
Toll-Free: 888-856-4480	
Address: 6301 Fitch Path, New Albany, OH 43054 US	

GROWTH PLANS/SPECIAL FEATURES:
Abercrombie & Fitch Company retails upscale casual American clothing and accessories. The Abercrombie & Fitch brand was established in 1892, and the firm became well known as a supplier of rugged, high-quality outdoor gear, outfitting expeditions, including those of Theodore Roosevelt, Ernest Hemingway, Charles Lindbergh and Richard Byrd. However, to boost sales and focus on a high-growth market segment, the company shifted its focus from outdoor gear and accessories to fashion-oriented casual wear. Abercrombie & Fitch operated 1,035 stores in the U.S., U.K. and Canada at the beginning of 2008, running five store brands. Abercrombie & Fitch (359 branches known as A&F), the company's main store, targets 18-22 year-old men and women, offering casual clothing. The firm's 201 abercrombie stores offer A&F-style clothing for ages 7-14. The Hollister Co., with 450 stores, markets to teenagers aged 14-18. One of the company's newer brands, RUEHL, with 22 stores, markets to those aged 22-35. RUEHL sells casual sportswear and fashion clothing. Abercrombie & Fitch also sells through its catalog magazine and its four web sites, one each for A&F, Abercrombie, Hollister and RUEHL. The web sites also contain an e-mail newsletter, screen savers, MP3 downloads and A&F Film. Gilly Hicks is a new lingerie and loungewear store, with three locations. The company has high hopes for this concept, projecting that it could eventually grow to 1,000 locations. Abercrombie & Fitch is currently planning a European expansion to Italy, France, Germany, Spain, Denmark and Sweden as well as Japan. The Copenhagen, Denmark and Tokyo, Japan locations will open in 2009.

Abercrombie & Fitch features an extensive manager-in-training (MIT) program for new hires, specifically college seniors and graduates. It also offers a corporate training program, providing merchandising, corporate finance, sourcing, allocation and IT (Information Technology) on-the-job training and assistantship programs.

FINANCIALS: Sales and profits are in thousands of dollars—add 000 to get the full amount. 2007 Note: Financial information for 2007 was not available for all companies at press time.

2007 Sales: $3,318,158	2007 Profits: $422,186	**U.S. Stock Ticker:** ANF
2006 Sales: $2,784,711	2006 Profits: $333,986	**Int'l Ticker:** Int'l Exchange:
2005 Sales: $2,021,253	2005 Profits: $216,376	Employees: 76,100
2004 Sales: $1,707,810	2004 Profits: $205,102	Fiscal Year Ends: 1/31
2003 Sales: $1,595,800	2003 Profits: $194,900	Parent Company:

SALARIES/BENEFITS:
Pension Plan:	ESOP Stock Plan:	Profit Sharing:	Top Exec. Salary: $1,494,321	Bonus: $2,228,400
Savings Plan: Y	Stock Purch. Plan:		Second Exec. Salary: $826,058	Bonus: $756,728

OTHER THOUGHTS:
Apparent Women Officers or Directors: 3
Hot Spot for Advancement for Women/Minorities: Y

LOCATIONS: ("Y" = Yes)
West:	Southwest:	Midwest:	Southeast:	Northeast:	International:
Y	Y	Y	Y	Y	Y

Note: Financial information, benefits and other data can change quickly and may vary from those stated here.

ABM INDUSTRIES INC

www.abm.com

Industry Group Code: 531100 Ranks within this company's industry group: Sales: 1 Profits: 2

Management:		Sales/Marketing:		Liberal Arts:		Information Systems:		Professionals:		Technical/Scientific:	
Mgmt. Trainees:	Y	Mktg. Professionals:	Y	Gen. Writing/Editing:		Info. Management:	Y	Finance/Accounting:	Y	Engineers, Elec.:	
Experienced Mgmt.:	Y	Retail Sales:		Technical Writing:		Software Dev.:	Y	Law:	Y	Engineers, Other:	
Int'l Business:	Y	Commercial/Industrial:	Y	Graphic Arts/Photog.:		Hardware Dev.:		HR/Other:	Y	Health/Lab:	
MBA Graduates:	Y	Sales Trainees:		Music:		Systems Integration:		Training:	Y	Scientists/Research:	
		Advertising Pros.:		Broadcasting:		Consulting/Other:		Health Care:		Petroleum/Chemicals:	
				Other:				Consulting:		Math/Other:	

TYPES OF BUSINESS:

Janitorial Services
Parking Facilities
Maintenance Personnel
Security Services
Lighting Services
Billing & Accounting Services
Supplier Management
Call Center Services

BRANDS/DIVISIONS/AFFILIATES:

ABM Janitorial Services
American Building Maintenance
ABM Security Services
Security Services of America
Silverhawk Security Specialists
Elite Protection Services
ABM Engineering Services
Amtech Lighting Services

CONTACTS: *Note: Officers with more than one job title may be intentionally listed here more than once.*

Henrik C. Slipsager, CEO
Henrik C. Slipsager, Pres.
James Lusk, CFO/Exec. VP
Gary R. Wallace, Chief Mktg. Officer
Erin M. Andre, Sr. VP-Human Resources
Linda S. Auwers, General Counsel/Sr. VP/Corp. Sec.
Gary R. Wallace, Sr. VP-Bus. Dev.
Joe Yospe, Chief Acct. Officer/Controller/Sr. VP
James P. McClure, Pres., ABM Janitorial Svcs./Exec. VP
Steven M. Zaccagnini, Pres., ABM Facility Svcs./Exec. VP
David L. Farwell, Sr. VP/Chief-Staff
Maryellen C. Herringer, Chmn.

Phone: 212-297-0200	Fax: 415-733-7333
Toll-Free:	
Address: 551 5th Ave., Ste. 300, New York, NY 10176 US	

GROWTH PLANS/SPECIAL FEATURES:

ABM Industries, Inc. is one of the country's largest facility services providers. Founded in California in 1909 as a one-man window cleaning business, today the firm provides janitorial, parking, engineering, security, lighting and mechanical services to commercial, industrial, institutional and retail facilities throughout the U.S. and Canada. ABM operates through a number of subsidiaries which are grouped into five segments: janitorial, parking, security, engineering and lighting. The company's janitorial services companies include ABM Janitorial Services and American Building Maintenance. Services provided include floor cleaning and finishing; window washing; furniture polishing; and carpet cleaning and dusting. ABM's security services subsidiaries include ABM Security Services, SSA Security, Security Services of America, Silverhawk Security Specialists and Elite Protection Services. Security services offered by these subsidiaries include security officers; investigative services; electronic monitoring of fire, life safety systems and access control devices; and security consulting. ABM Engineering Services is the company's primary engineering subsidiary, offering on-site engineers to operate and maintain mechanical, electrical and plumbing systems at such facilities as high-rise office buildings, schools, computer centers, shopping malls, manufacturing facilities, museums and universities. The engineering segment also provides facility services through ABM Facility Services, which provides streamlined, centralized control and coordination of multiple facility service needs. ABM's primary lighting subsidiary is Amtech Lighting Services, providing relamping, fixture cleaning, energy retrofits and lighting maintenance services. In November 2007, the company acquired OneSource Services, Inc. for $365 million. In January 2008, AMB acquired the remaining 50% stake in Southern Management Company, a Tennessee based facilities services company acquired by ABM with OneSource, for $24 million.

ABM offers its employees a tuition reimbursement program, credit union membership, an employee assistance program and medical, dental, vision, life, AD&D and disability insurance.

FINANCIALS: Sales and profits are in thousands of dollars—add 000 to get the full amount. 2007 Note: Financial information for 2007 was not available for all companies at press time.

2007 Sales: $2,842,811	2007 Profits: $52,440	U.S. Stock Ticker: ABM
2006 Sales: $2,792,668	2006 Profits: $93,205	Int'l Ticker: Int'l Exchange:
2005 Sales: $2,587,761	2005 Profits: $57,941	Employees: 107,000
2004 Sales: $2,375,149	2004 Profits: $30,473	Fiscal Year Ends: 10/31
2003 Sales: $2,222,367	2003 Profits: $90,920	Parent Company:

SALARIES/BENEFITS:

Pension Plan:	ESOP Stock Plan:	Profit Sharing:	Top Exec. Salary: $700,000	Bonus: $728,000
Savings Plan: Y	Stock Purch. Plan:		Second Exec. Salary: $450,000	Bonus: $343,980

OTHER THOUGHTS:

Apparent Women Officers or Directors: 4
Hot Spot for Advancement for Women/Minorities: Y

LOCATIONS: ("Y" = Yes)

West:	Southwest:	Midwest:	Southeast:	Northeast:	International:
Y	Y	Y	Y	Y	Y

Note: Financial information, benefits and other data can change quickly and may vary from those stated here.

ACADEMY SPORTS & OUTDOORS LTD   www.academy.com

Industry Group Code: 451110 Ranks within this company's industry group: Sales: Profits:

Management:		Sales/Marketing:		Liberal Arts:		Information Systems:		Professionals:		Technical/Scientific:	
Mgmt. Trainees:	Y	Mktg. Professionals:	Y	Gen. Writing/Editing:	Y	Info. Management:	Y	Finance/Accounting:	Y	Engineers, Elec.:	
Experienced Mgmt.:	Y	Retail Sales:	Y	Technical Writing:		Software Dev.:	Y	Law:	Y	Engineers, Other:	
Int'l Business:		Commercial/Industrial:	Y	Graphic Arts/Photog.:	Y	Hardware Dev.:		HR/Other:	Y	Health/Lab:	
MBA Graduates:	Y	Sales Trainees:	Y	Music:		Systems Integration:		Training:	Y	Scientists/Research:	
		Advertising Pros.:	Y	Broadcasting:		Consulting/Other:		Health Care:		Petroleum/Chemicals:	
				Other:				Consulting:		Math/Other:	

TYPES OF BUSINESS:

Sporting Goods Stores
Apparel
Footwear
Outdoor Sports Gear
Hunting Licenses

BRANDS/DIVISIONS/AFFILIATES:

CONTACTS: *Note: Officers with more than one job title may be intentionally listed here more than once.*

David Gochman, CEO
Arthur Gochman, Pres.
Robert Frennea, Exec. VP-Apparel
David Gochman, Chmn.

Phone: 281-646-5200	Fax: 281-646-5000
Toll-Free: 888-922-2336	
Address: 1800 N. Mason Rd., Katy, TX 77449 US	

GROWTH PLANS/SPECIAL FEATURES:

Academy Sports & Outdoors, Ltd. is one of the largest sporting goods retailers in the U.S. The company operates over 90 stores in Alabama, Arkansas, Florida, Georgia, Louisiana, Mississippi, Missouri, Oklahoma, Tennessee and Texas, with plans for further expansion in the Southeast in the near future. Academy Sports offers a broad selection of sporting equipment, apparel and footwear. The stores, which range in size from 50,000 to 80,000 square feet, are laid out in a racetrack format with athletic, casual and seasonal apparel on the inside and camping, hunting, fishing, marine, golf, fitness, team sports and footwear products on the outside. The firm also offers recipes for wild game, online applications for hunting and fishing licenses, a propane exchange service, sports tips, corporate incentives and various contests. Academy Sports has experienced steady sales growth over the past decade at an average of 17% a year. The company supplies its stores through a 1 million square foot distribution center out of Katy, Texas. The center utilizes radio frequency devices (RFD), automated inventory and replenishment systems and a state-of-the-art warehouse management system to smoothly operate its large processing and inventory space.

The company offers its employees a 401(k) plan; medical, dental and vision insurance; life insurance; short- and long-term disability benefits; tuition reimbursement; merchandise discounts; continuing education benefits; and business travel accident insurance.

FINANCIALS: Sales and profits are in thousands of dollars—add 000 to get the full amount. 2007 Note: Financial information for 2007 was not available for all companies at press time.

2007 Sales: $	2007 Profits: $	U.S. Stock Ticker: Private
2006 Sales: $1,840,000	2006 Profits: $	Int'l Ticker: Int'l Exchange:
2005 Sales: $1,215,100	2005 Profits: $65,000	Employees: 11,000
2004 Sales: $1,059,000	2004 Profits: $	Fiscal Year Ends: 1/31
2003 Sales: $1,000,000	2003 Profits: $	Parent Company:

SALARIES/BENEFITS:

Pension Plan:	ESOP Stock Plan:	Profit Sharing:	Top Exec. Salary: $	Bonus: $
Savings Plan: Y	Stock Purch. Plan:		Second Exec. Salary: $	Bonus: $

OTHER THOUGHTS:

Apparent Women Officers or Directors:
Hot Spot for Advancement for Women/Minorities:

LOCATIONS: ("Y" = Yes)

West:	Southwest:	Midwest:	Southeast:	Northeast:	International:
	Y	Y	Y		

ACCENTURE LTD

www.accenture.com

Industry Group Code: 541512 Ranks within this company's industry group: Sales: 2   Profits: 2

Management:		Sales/Marketing:		Liberal Arts:		Information Systems:		Professionals:		Technical/Scientific:	
Mgmt. Trainees:	Y	Mktg. Professionals:	Y	Gen. Writing/Editing:	Y	Info. Management:	Y	Finance/Accounting:	Y	Engineers, Elec.:	Y
Experienced Mgmt.:	Y	Retail Sales:		Technical Writing:	Y	Software Dev.:	Y	Law:	Y	Engineers, Other:	
Int'l Business:	Y	Commercial/Industrial:	Y	Graphic Arts/Photog.:	Y	Hardware Dev.:		HR/Other:	Y	Health/Lab:	
MBA Graduates:	Y	Sales Trainees:		Music:		Systems Integration:	Y	Training:	Y	Scientists/Research:	Y
		Advertising Pros.:	Y	Broadcasting:		Consulting/Other:	Y	Health Care:		Petroleum/Chemicals:	
				Other:				Consulting:	Y	Math/Other:	

TYPES OF BUSINESS:

Technology Consulting Services
Computer Operations Outsourcing
Supply Chain Management
Technology Research
Software Development
Human Resources Consulting
Management Consulting
Research & Development

BRANDS/DIVISIONS/AFFILIATES:

Digiplug S.A.S.
Mediasenz
H.B. Maynard and Co., Inc.
Corliant, Inc.
MAXIM Systems, Inc.
Gestalt, LLC
Maxamine
SOPIA Corporation

CONTACTS: *Note: Officers with more than one job title may be intentionally listed here more than once.*

William D. Green, CEO
Stephen J. Rohleder, COO
Pamela J. Craig, CFO
Roxanne Taylor, Chief Mktg. Officer
Jill B. Smart, Chief Human Resources Officer
Gianfranco Casati, Group CEO-Prod.
Douglas G. Scrivner, General Counsel/Corp. Sec./Compliance Officer
David C. Thomlinson, Sr. Managing Dir.-Geographic Strategy & Oper.
R. Timothy Breene, Chief Strategy & Corp. Dev. Officer
Roxanne Taylor, Chief Comm. Officer
David P. Rowland, Sr. VP-Finance
Karl-Heinz Floether, Group CEO-Systems Integration, Tech. & Delivery
Martin I. Cole, Group CEO-Comm. & High Tech.
Kevin M. Campbell, Group CEO-Outsourcing
Mark Foster, Group CEO-Mgmt. Consulting & Integrated Mkts.
William D. Green, Chmn.
Diego Visconti, Chmn.-Int'l
Basilio Rueda, Sr. Managing Dir.-Global Delivery Network

Phone: 441-296-8262	Fax: 441-296-4245
Toll-Free:	
Address: Canon Court, 22 Victoria St., Hamilton, HM12 Bermuda	

GROWTH PLANS/SPECIAL FEATURES:

Accenture, Ltd. is a leading provider of management consulting, technology and outsourcing services and solutions, with operations in over 150 offices in 49 countries. Clients include AT&T; Microsoft; Sony; Bank of America; and the U.S. Department of Commerce. The firm delivers services through five operating groups, which together comprise 17 industry groups. The operating groups are communications and high-tech; financial services; products; resources; and public services. Accenture's communications and high-tech group offers technology, consulting and systems integration to the electronics, communications and media industries. Its financial services group provides consulting and outsourcing strategies to the insurance, capital markets and banking industries. Accenture's products group serves the automotive; health and life sciences; consumer goods; industrial equipment; retail; and transportation and travel services industries. The company's resources group works with the chemicals; energy; forest products; metals and mining; and utilities industries. Finally, its public service group works with local, state, provincial and national governments in the areas of defense; revenue; human services; health; justice; and postal and education authorities. Accenture offers management consulting services including customer relationship management; supply chain management; human performance; finance and performance management; and strategy. The firm's systems integration and technology services include enterprise resource planning; service-oriented architecture; mobility solutions; Microsoft solutions; IT strategy and transformation services; enterprise architecture; infrastructure consulting services; research and development services; and e-commerce solutions. Accenture also offers business process outsourcing, application outsourcing and infrastructure outsourcing. During 2007, Accenture acquired Digiplug S.A.S.; Mediasenz; H.B. Maynard and Co., Inc.; Corliant, Inc.; and MAXIM Systems, Inc. In January 2008, the company acquired defense consulting firm Gestalt, LLC. In February 2008, Accenture acquired Maxamine, a provider of testing and optimization services. In April 2008, the company agreed to acquire SOPIA Corporation, a consulting and IT solutions company specializing in Oracle systems integration.

FINANCIALS: Sales and profits are in thousands of dollars—add 000 to get the full amount. 2007 Note: Financial information for 2007 was not available for all companies at press time.

2007 Sales: $21,452,747	2007 Profits: $1,243,148	U.S. Stock Ticker: ACN
2006 Sales: $18,228,366	2006 Profits: $973,329	Int'l Ticker: Int'l Exchange:
2005 Sales: $17,094,400	2005 Profits: $940,500	Employees: 170,000
2004 Sales: $15,113,582	2004 Profits: $690,828	Fiscal Year Ends: 8/31
2003 Sales: $13,397,200	2003 Profits: $498,200	Parent Company:

SALARIES/BENEFITS:

Pension Plan:	ESOP Stock Plan:	Profit Sharing:	Top Exec. Salary: $2,547,750	Bonus: $2,191,400
Savings Plan:	Stock Purch. Plan:		Second Exec. Salary: $2,439,183	Bonus: $1,799,236

OTHER THOUGHTS:

Apparent Women Officers or Directors: 8
Hot Spot for Advancement for Women/Minorities: Y

LOCATIONS: ("Y" = Yes)

West:	Southwest:	Midwest:	Southeast:	Northeast:	International:
Y	Y	Y	Y	Y	Y

Note: Financial information, benefits and other data can change quickly and may vary from those stated here.

ACXIOM CORP

www.acxiom.com

Industry Group Code: 511203 Ranks within this company's industry group: Sales: 1   Profits: 1

Management:		Sales/Marketing:		Liberal Arts:		Information Systems:		Professionals:		Technical/Scientific:	
Mgmt. Trainees:	Y	Mktg. Professionals:	Y	Gen. Writing/Editing:		Info. Management:	Y	Finance/Accounting:	Y	Engineers, Elec.:	Y
Experienced Mgmt.:	Y	Retail Sales:		Technical Writing:	Y	Software Dev.:	Y	Law:	Y	Engineers, Other:	
Int'l Business:	Y	Commercial/Industrial:	Y	Graphic Arts/Photog.:		Hardware Dev.:		HR/Other:	Y	Health/Lab:	
MBA Graduates:	Y	Sales Trainees:		Music:		Systems Integration:		Training:	Y	Scientists/Research:	Y
		Advertising Pros.:		Broadcasting:		Consulting/Other:		Health Care:		Petroleum/Chemicals:	
				Other:				Consulting:		Math/Other:	

TYPES OF BUSINESS:

Consumer Data Management
Database Products
Consulting and Analytics
IT Outsourcing
Analytics
Privacy Leadership
Risk Mitigation
CDI Technology

BRANDS/DIVISIONS/AFFILIATES:

PersonicX
InfoBase
Acxiom Access-X Express
Acxiom Digital
InsightIdentify
Acxiom Information Security Services

CONTACTS: *Note: Officers with more than one job title may be intentionally listed here more than once.*

John A. Meyer, CEO
John A. Meyer, Pres.
Christopher W. Wolf, CFO
Richard K. Howe, Mktg. Organization Leader
Cindy K. Childers, Organizational Dev. Leader, Human Resources
Terry M. Talley, Chief Tech. Leader
Alex Dietz, Info. Prod. Div. Leader
Rodger S. Kline, Chief Admin. Leader
Catherine L. Hughes, Corp. Governance Officer/Sec.
Holly Marr, Oper. Mgmt. Organization Leader
Jerry C. Jones, Bus. Dev. & Legal Leader
Cindy K. Childers, Organizational Dev. Leader, Corp. Comm.
Dathan A. Gaskill, Corp. Finance Leader/Treas.
Timothy Christin, Risk Organization Leader
Mike Cool, Bus. Unit Leader, Acxiom Info. Security Svcs.
Lee Hodges, Svcs. Div. Leader
Scott D. Hambuchen, Traditional Svcs. Organization Leader, Svcs. Div.
Michael Durham, Chmn.
James T. Womble, Global Dev. Leader
Michael J. Lloyd, Delivery Ctr. Organization Leader, Svcs. Div.

Phone: 501-342-1000	**Fax:** 501-342-3913
Toll-Free: 800-322-9466	
Address: 1 Information Way, Little Rock, AR 72202 US	

GROWTH PLANS/SPECIAL FEATURES:

Acxiom Corp. mainly offers customer information management. It has nine core solutions. Customer data integration (CDI) solutions include analyzing, optimizing, expanding and protecting a client's existing customer data. Data solutions include InfoBase, a database of U.S. telephone and consumer data, and products that customize InfoBase, such as PersonicX, which divides InfoBase into 70 segments based on demographics and consumer behavior; Acxiom Access-X Express, an data management tool for InfoBase; and others. Database solutions include developing, designing and hosting custom or packaged databases for clients. Consulting and analytics solutions include diagnostic software, analytic consulting and other professional services to support existing customer information. Privacy leadership solutions consist mainly of privacy policy and compliance consultations. IT infrastructure management solutions include IT outsourcing, network management and other services, such as IT security. Direct marketing solutions include campaign and database management; direct mail and e-mail services; creative consultations; and CDI and analytics. Digital solutions, provided by Acxiom Digital, include web site personalization; e-mail and search engine marketing; agency services; and customer acquisition assistance. Lastly, risk mitigation solutions include identification products, such as InsightIdentify, to assist banks, investigators and credit unions prevent fraud loss, and meet U.S.A. P.A.T.R.I.O.T. Act regulations; and investigation tools, as for debt collection or law enforcement agencies. Additionally, Acxiom Information Security Services (AISS) provides criminal, civil and driving record background searches. Acxiom's clients are mostly of Fortune 1000 finance, insurance, information services, direct marketing, publishing, retail and telecommunications companies.

Employees of Acxiom receive AD&D, dependent life, pet, vision and life insurance; paternity and adoption leave; employee assistance; health and spending care accounts; paid holidays; and paid days off.

FINANCIALS: Sales and profits are in thousands of dollars—add 000 to get the full amount. 2007 Note: Financial information for 2007 was not available for all companies at press time.

2007 Sales: $1,395,136	2007 Profits: $70,740	**U.S. Stock Ticker: ACXM**
2006 Sales: $1,332,568	2006 Profits: $64,128	**Int'l Ticker:** Int'l Exchange:
2005 Sales: $1,223,042	2005 Profits: $69,718	Employees: 7,100
2004 Sales: $1,010,822	2004 Profits: $58,344	Fiscal Year Ends: 3/31
2003 Sales: $958,222	2003 Profits: $21,767	Parent Company:

SALARIES/BENEFITS:

Pension Plan:	ESOP Stock Plan:	Profit Sharing:	Top Exec. Salary: $796,250	Bonus: $318,500
Savings Plan: Y	Stock Purch. Plan: Y		Second Exec. Salary: $490,000	Bonus: $147,000

OTHER THOUGHTS:

Apparent Women Officers or Directors: 4
Hot Spot for Advancement for Women/Minorities: Y

LOCATIONS: ("Y" = Yes)

West:	Southwest:	Midwest:	Southeast:	Northeast:	International:
Y	Y	Y	Y		Y

ADC TELECOMMUNICATIONS INC

www.adc.com

Industry Group Code: 334210 Ranks within this company's industry group: Sales: 1 Profits: 1

Management:		Sales/Marketing:		Liberal Arts:		Information Systems:		Professionals:		Technical/Scientific:	
Mgmt. Trainees:	Y	Mktg. Professionals:	Y	Gen. Writing/Editing:		Info. Management:	Y	Finance/Accounting:	Y	Engineers, Elec.:	Y
Experienced Mgmt.:	Y	Retail Sales:		Technical Writing:	Y	Software Dev.:	Y	Law:	Y	Engineers, Other:	
Int'l Business:	Y	Commercial/Industrial:	Y	Graphic Arts/Photog.:	Y	Hardware Dev.:	Y	HR/Other:	Y	Health/Lab:	Y
MBA Graduates:	Y	Sales Trainees:		Music:		Systems Integration:		Training:	Y	Scientists/Research:	Y
		Advertising Pros.:	Y	Broadcasting:		Consulting/Other:		Health Care:		Petroleum/Chemicals:	
				Other:				Consulting:		Math/Other:	

TYPES OF BUSINESS:

Telecommunications Equipment
Networking Systems
Broadband Connectivity Products
Equipment Services
Systems Integration

BRANDS/DIVISIONS/AFFILIATES:

OmniReach FTTX Infrastructure Solutions
Fiber Guide Raceway
Century Man Communication
RF Worx
DSX1/3
ADC Krone
LGC Wireless

CONTACTS: *Note: Officers with more than one job title may be intentionally listed here more than once.*

Robert E. Switz, CEO
Robert E. Switz, Pres.
James G. Mathews, VP-CFO
Hubert Shanne, VP-EMAS, Mktg. & Customer Service
Laura N. Owen, VP-Human Resources
Christopher Jurasek, CIO
Mike Day, CTO
Laura N. Owen, VP-Chief Admin. Officer
Jeffery D. Pflaum, General Counsel/Sec./VP
Mike Day, VP-Strategy
Mike Smith, Dir.-Corp. Communications
Mark P. Borman, VP-Investor Rel./Treas.
Bradley V. Crary, VP-Tax
Kimberly Hartwell, VP-Americas Sales, Mktg. & Customer Service
Hilton Nicholson, VP/Pres., Network Solutions
Patrick D. O'Brien, Pres., Global Connectivity Solutions
Steven G. Nemitz, VP/Controller
Robert E. Switz, Chmn.

Phone: 952-938-8080	**Fax:** 952-917-1717
Toll-Free: 800-366-3889	
Address: 13625 Technology Dr., Eden Prairie, MN 55344 US	

GROWTH PLANS/SPECIAL FEATURES:

ADC Telecommunications, Inc. is a provider of global network infrastructure products and services that enable the delivery of high-speed Internet, data, video and voice services to consumers and businesses worldwide. ADC has offices in over 30 countries and sells products in over 130 countries. ADC's services exist in four categories: global connectivity, wireless, wireline and professional services. Global connectivity is by far its largest segment, accounting for 77.2% of ADC's net sales in 2007. ADC's connectivity devices are used in copper, coaxial, fiber-optic, wireless and broadcast communications networks. These products provide the physical interconnections between network components or access points into networks. These devices include: DSX and DDF products, FTTX products, fiber distribution panels and frames, radio frequency digital management products, power distribution and protection panels, modular fiber-optic cable systems, structured cabling products and broadcast and entertainment products. ADC's wireless services cover both in-building and outdoor services, and its wireline products (principally Soneplex and HiGain) enable communications service providers to deliver high capacity voice and data services over copper or optical facilities in the last mile/kilometer of communications networks. The company's professional services department helps operators plan, deploy and maintain networks, including cable, wireless and wireline networks. ADC serves markets such as broadcast and entertainment, global and local carriers, global OEM's, government and wireless. ADC subsidiary ADC Krone is a global supplier of copper-and fiber-based connectivity solutions. In October 2007, ADC acquired LGC Wireless, a specialized wireless provider. In January 2008, the company completed its acquisition of Century Man Communication, a provider of communication distribution frame products in China. In July 2008, ADC announced a new version of its InterReach Fusion in-building cellular system designated for use by Canadian cellular providers.

FINANCIALS: Sales and profits are in thousands of dollars—add 000 to get the full amount. 2007 Note: Financial information for 2007 was not available for all companies at press time.

2007 Sales: $1,322,200	2007 Profits: $113,300	**U.S. Stock Ticker: ADCT**
2006 Sales: $1,281,700	2006 Profits: $95,300	**Int'l Ticker:** Int'l Exchange:
2005 Sales: $1,128,900	2005 Profits: $98,800	Employees: 9,050
2004 Sales: $733,900	2004 Profits: $16,400	Fiscal Year Ends: 10/31
2003 Sales: $579,800	2003 Profits: $-76,700	Parent Company:

SALARIES/BENEFITS:

Pension Plan:	ESOP Stock Plan:	Profit Sharing:	Top Exec. Salary: $703,269	Bonus: $
Savings Plan:	Stock Purch. Plan:		Second Exec. Salary: $282,560	Bonus: $

OTHER THOUGHTS:

Apparent Women Officers or Directors: 2
Hot Spot for Advancement for Women/Minorities: Y

LOCATIONS: ("Y" = Yes)

West:	Southwest:	Midwest:	Southeast:	Northeast:	International:
		Y			Y

Note: Financial information, benefits and other data can change quickly and may vary from those stated here.

ADESA INC

www.adesainc.com

Industry Group Code: 423110 Ranks within this company's industry group: Sales: 1   Profits: 1

Management:		Sales/Marketing:		Liberal Arts:	Information Systems:		Professionals:		Technical/Scientific:
Mgmt. Trainees:		Mktg. Professionals:		Gen. Writing/Editing:	Info. Management:	Y	Finance/Accounting:	Y	Engineers, Elec.:
Experienced Mgmt.:	Y	Retail Sales:		Technical Writing:	Software Dev.:		Law:	Y	Engineers, Other:
Int'l Business:	Y	Commercial/Industrial:	Y	Graphic Arts/Photog.:	Hardware Dev.:		HR/Other:	Y	Health/Lab:
MBA Graduates:	Y	Sales Trainees:		Music:	Systems Integration:		Training:	Y	Scientists/Research:
		Advertising Pros.:		Broadcasting:	Consulting/Other:		Health Care:		Petroleum/Chemicals:
				Other:			Consulting:		Math/Other:

TYPES OF BUSINESS:

Vehicle Auctions-Wholesale
Salvage Vehicle Auctions
Automobile Transportation
Automobile Reconditioning
Automotive Market Analysis

BRANDS/DIVISIONS/AFFILIATES:

Dent Demon
Pennsylvania Auto Dealers' Exchange
ADESA Run Lists
ADESA Market Guide
ADESA Virtual Inventory
ADESA Notify Me
ADESA LiveBlock
Kontos Kommentary

CONTACTS: *Note: Officers with more than one job title may be intentionally listed here more than once.*

James P. Hallett, CEO
Tom Caruso, COO
James P. Hallett, Pres.
Bob Rauschenberg, Exec. VP-Mktg. & Sales
Michelle Mallon, VP-Legal
Paul Lips, Exec. VP-Oper.
Warren Byrd, VP-Corp. Dev.
Jason Ferreri, VP-e-business Sales & Oper.
Paul Lips, Exec. VP-Finance
Jeff Bescher, VP-Commercial Sales & Oper.
Mike Caggiano, Regional VP-Eastern Region
Tim DeBerry, Regional VP-Western Region
Tom Kontos, Exec. VP-Customer Strategies & Analytics
Benjamin Skuy, Exec. VP-Int'l Markets
David Vignes, Exec. VP-Logistics & Strategic Improvements

Phone: 317-815-1100	Fax: 317-249-4603
Toll-Free: 800-923-3725	
Address: 13085 Hamilton Crossing Blvd., Carmel, IN 46032 US	

GROWTH PLANS/SPECIAL FEATURES:

ADESA, Inc., a wholly-owned subsidiary of KAR Holdings, Inc., is primarily engaged in automotive auctions, transportation and cosmetic and mechanical reconditioning. The firm operates 60 used-vehicle auction sites across the U.S. and serves two main client types, institutional buyers and dealers. The firm's institutional customers include vehicle manufacturers; banks, credit unions and other financial institutions; vehicle finance companies; vehicle rental companies; and insurance companies. Dealers buying from ADESA include both licensed franchises and independent wholesale dealers. ADESA's online auction tools include ADESA LiveBlock, an online real-time bidding tool; ADESA Run Lists, a summary of consigned vehicles offered for auction sale; and ADESA DealerBlock, a bulletin board type online auction platform. The firm also offers ADESA Market Guide, a summary of wholesale auction prices, auction sales results, market data and condition reports; ADESA Virtual Inventory, a subscription-based service that allows dealers to embed ADESA Search technology into their web sites; and ADESA Notify Me, an e-mail notification service for dealers looking for particular vehicles. The firm also offers analytical services via monthly, semi-annual and annual market analysis publications including Kontos Kommentary, Pulse and Global Vehicle Remarketing. ADESA was acquired by KAR Holdings, Inc., in April 2007. ADESA acquired Dent Demon, a paintless dent repair service provider, in January 2008. In February 2008, ADESA purchased Pennsylvania Auto Dealers' Exchange (PADE), a used vehicle auction located in York, Pennsylvania. PADE will be renamed ADESA PA.

ADESA offers its employees an employee assistance plan; medical and dependent day care; flexible spending accounts; and an extensive employee orientation program.

FINANCIALS: Sales and profits are in thousands of dollars—add 000 to get the full amount. 2007 Note: Financial information for 2007 was not available for all companies at press time.

2007 Sales: $	2007 Profits: $	U.S. Stock Ticker: Private
2006 Sales: $1,103,900	2006 Profits: $126,300	Int'l Ticker: Int'l Exchange:
2005 Sales: $968,800	2005 Profits: $125,500	Employees: 11,915
2004 Sales: $931,600	2004 Profits: $105,300	Fiscal Year Ends: 12/31
2003 Sales: $911,900	2003 Profits: $115,100	Parent Company: KAR HOLDINGS INC

SALARIES/BENEFITS:

Pension Plan:	ESOP Stock Plan:	Profit Sharing:	Top Exec. Salary: $639,658	Bonus: $320,288
Savings Plan: Y	Stock Purch. Plan: Y		Second Exec. Salary: $376,508	Bonus: $157,259

OTHER THOUGHTS:

Apparent Women Officers or Directors: 4
Hot Spot for Advancement for Women/Minorities: Y

LOCATIONS: ("Y" = Yes)

West:	Southwest:	Midwest:	Southeast:	Northeast:	International:
Y	Y	Y	Y	Y	Y

ADOBE SYSTEMS INC
www.adobe.com

Industry Group Code: 511209 Ranks within this company's industry group: Sales: 1 Profits: 1

Management:		Sales/Marketing:		Liberal Arts:		Information Systems:		Professionals:		Technical/Scientific:	
Mgmt. Trainees:	Y	Mktg. Professionals:	Y	Gen. Writing/Editing:	Y	Info. Management:	Y	Finance/Accounting:	Y	Engineers, Elec.:	Y
Experienced Mgmt.:	Y	Retail Sales:		Technical Writing:	Y	Software Dev.:	Y	Law:	Y	Engineers, Other:	
Int'l Business:	Y	Commercial/Industrial:	Y	Graphic Arts/Photog.:	Y	Hardware Dev.:		HR/Other:	Y	Health/Lab:	
MBA Graduates:	Y	Sales Trainees:		Music:		Systems Integration:		Training:	Y	Scientists/Research:	Y
		Advertising Pros.:	Y	Broadcasting:		Consulting/Other:		Health Care:		Petroleum/Chemicals:	
				Other:	Y			Consulting:		Math/Other:	

TYPES OF BUSINESS:

Computer Software-Desktop & Publishing
Document Management Software
Photo Editing & Management Software
Graphic Design Software

BRANDS/DIVISIONS/AFFILIATES:

Adobe Acrobat
Adobe Flash Player
Adobe Photoshop
Adobe Creative Suite
Macromedia Flash SDK
Adobe Reader LE
Macromedia ColdFusion
Scene7 Inc

CONTACTS: *Note: Officers with more than one job title may be intentionally listed here more than once.*

Shantanu Narayen, CEO
Shantanu Narayen, Pres.
Mark Garrett, CFO/Exec. VP
Ann Lewnes, Sr. VP-Corp. Mktg.
Donna Morris, Sr. VP-Human Resources
Naresh Gupta, Managing Dir.-R&D, India
Gerri Martin-Flickinger, CIO/Sr. VP
Kevin Lynch, CTO
Digby Horner, Sr. VP-Eng. Tech. Group
Karen Cottle, General Counsel/Corp. Sec./Sr. VP
Matt Thompson, Sr. VP-Worldwide Field Oper.
Rob Tarkoff, Sr. VP-Corp. Dev.
Kevin Burr, VP-Corp. Comm.
Mike Saviage, VP-Investor Rel.
John E. Warnock, Co-Chmn.
John Brennan, Sr. VP-Platform Bus. Unit
John Loiacono, Sr. VP-Creative Solutions Bus. Unit
Naresh Gupta, Sr. VP-Print & Classic Publishing
Charles M. Geschke, Co-Chmn.

Phone: 408-536-6000	Fax: 408-537-6000
Toll-Free: 800-833-6687	
Address: 345 Park Ave., San Jose, CA 95110 US	

GROWTH PLANS/SPECIAL FEATURES:

Adobe Systems, Inc. is one of the largest software companies in the world. It offers a line of creative, business and mobile software and services used by creative professionals, designers, knowledge workers, high-end consumers, original equipment manufacturers, developers and enterprises for creating, managing, delivering and engaging with content and experiences across multiple operating systems, devices and media. The company operates in five segments: creative solutions; knowledge worker solutions (KWS); enterprise and developer solutions (EDS); mobile and device solutions (MDS); and other. Creative Solutions focuses primarily on creative professional customers such as graphic designers, production artists, writers and photographer. Products include Adobe After Effects, used to create sophisticated animation, motion graphics and visual effects; Adobe Audition, an audio editing environment; Adobe Photoshop, which provides photo design, enhancement and editing capabilities; and Macromedia Fireworks, a professional graphics design tool for building interactive web graphics. The KWS segment focuses on knowledge customers such as accountants, architects, educators, insurance underwriters and stock analysts. Products include Adobe Document Center, a hosted service enabling customers to secure and manage Adobe PDF files and other common business document files; and Create Adobe PDF Online, a web-based subscription service that converts documents to Adobe PDF. The EDS segment's products include Adobe Output Designer, a tool that creates electronic document templates; and Macromedia ColdFusion, used for building database-driven scalable applications accessible through web browsers. The MDS segment's products include Adobe Reader LE, a version of the Adobe Reader for mobile phones, and Macromedia Flash SDK, a software development kit for bringing Flash-based content to consumer electronic devices. The other segment contains products and services that address market opportunities ranging from publishing to printing.

Employee benefits include medical, dental and vision insurance.

FINANCIALS: Sales and profits are in thousands of dollars—add 000 to get the full amount. 2007 Note: Financial information for 2007 was not available for all companies at press time.

2007 Sales: $3,157,881	2007 Profits: $723,807	**U.S. Stock Ticker: ADBE**
2006 Sales: $2,575,300	2006 Profits: $505,809	**Int'l Ticker:** Int'l Exchange:
2005 Sales: $1,966,321	2005 Profits: $602,839	Employees: 6,959
2004 Sales: $1,666,581	2004 Profits: $450,398	Fiscal Year Ends: 11/30
2003 Sales: $1,294,749	2003 Profits: $266,344	Parent Company:

SALARIES/BENEFITS:

Pension Plan:	ESOP Stock Plan:	Profit Sharing: Y	Top Exec. Salary: $925,000	Bonus: $681,262
Savings Plan: Y	Stock Purch. Plan: Y		Second Exec. Salary: $575,000	Bonus: $376,925

OTHER THOUGHTS:

Apparent Women Officers or Directors: 4
Hot Spot for Advancement for Women/Minorities: Y

LOCATIONS: ("Y" = Yes)

West:	Southwest:	Midwest:	Southeast:	Northeast:	International:
Y				Y	Y

ADVANCE AUTO PARTS INC   www.advanceautoparts.com

Industry Group Code: 441310 Ranks within this company's industry group: Sales: 2 Profits: 2

Management:		Sales/Marketing:		Liberal Arts:		Information Systems:		Professionals:		Technical/Scientific:	
Mgmt. Trainees:	Y	Mktg. Professionals:	Y	Gen. Writing/Editing:	Y	Info. Management:	Y	Finance/Accounting:	Y	Engineers, Elec.:	
Experienced Mgmt.:	Y	Retail Sales:	Y	Technical Writing:		Software Dev.:	Y	Law:	Y	Engineers, Other:	
Int'l Business:	Y	Commercial/Industrial:	Y	Graphic Arts/Photog.:	Y	Hardware Dev.:		HR/Other:	Y	Health/Lab:	
MBA Graduates:	Y	Sales Trainees:	Y	Music:		Systems Integration:		Training:	Y	Scientists/Research:	
		Advertising Pros.:	Y	Broadcasting:		Consulting/Other:		Health Care:		Petroleum/Chemicals:	
				Other:				Consulting:		Math/Other:	

TYPES OF BUSINESS:
Auto Parts & Accessories Stores
Online Sales

BRANDS/DIVISIONS/AFFILIATES:
Western Auto
Advance Discount Auto Parts

CONTACTS: *Note: Officers with more than one job title may be intentionally listed here more than once.*
Darren R. Jackson, CEO
Darren R. Jackson, Pres.
Mike Norona, CFO/Exec. VP
Donna Broome, Sr. VP-Commercial Sales
Keith A. Oreson, Sr. VP-Human Resources
Rick Coro, CIO/Sr. VP-IT
Elwyn G. Murray III, Exec. VP-Tech.
Kevin Freeland, Exec. VP-Merch. & IT
Eric M. Margolin, General Counsel/Sr. VP/Sec.
Carl Hauch, Sr. VP-Oper., West
Jim L. Wade, Exec. VP-Bus. Dev.
Jill A. Livesay, Controller/Sr. VP
Jim Wade, Exec. VP/Customer Dev. Officer, Commercial
Elwyn G. Murray, Exec. VP/Customer Dev. Officer, DIY
Ken Wirth, Sr. VP/Customer Experience Officer
Mike Marolt, Sr. VP/Customer Oper. Excellence Officer
John Brouillard, Interim Chmn.
Kevin Freeland, Exec. VP-Supply Chain

Phone: 540-362-4911	Fax: 540-561-1448
Toll-Free:	
Address: 5008 Airport Rd., Roanoke, VA 24012 US	

GROWTH PLANS/SPECIAL FEATURES:

Advance Auto Parts, Inc. primarily operates within the automotive aftermarket industry, which includes replacement parts (excluding tires), accessories, maintenance items, batteries and automotive chemicals for cars and light trucks (pickup trucks, vans, minivans and sport utility vehicles). The company is the second largest specialty retailer of automotive parts, accessories and maintenance items to do-it-yourself (DIY) and do-it-for-me customers in the U.S. The firm operates in two segments: Advance Auto Parts (AAP) and Autopart International (AI). The AAP segment operates roughly 3,153 stores within the 40 U.S. states, Puerto Rico and the Virgin Islands under the Advance Discount Auto Parts trade name, which offers a broad selection of brand name and proprietary automotive replacement parts, accessories and maintenance items for domestic and imported cars and light trucks. In addition, the firm operates about 30 stores under the Western Auto and Advance Auto Parts trade names, located primarily in Puerto Rico and the Virgin Islands, which offer automotive tires and service in addition to automotive parts, accessories and maintenance items. Replacement parts sold at the firm's stores include automotive filters, radiators, brake pads, fan belts, radiator hoses, starters, alternators, batteries, shock absorbers, engines and transmissions. Advance Auto Parts offers online shopping and access to over 2 million stock keeping units (SKUs). The AI segment, which includes 108 stores throughout New England and New York, a distribution center and a wholesale distribution business, primarily serves the commercial market from its store locations. In February 2007, the company announced plans to open a new distribution facility in Indiana in 2010.

The company offers its employee medical, dental and vision insurance; life insurance; short- and long-term disability insurance; and flexible spending accounts.

FINANCIALS: Sales and profits are in thousands of dollars—add 000 to get the full amount. 2007 Note: Financial information for 2007 was not available for all companies at press time.

2007 Sales: $4,844,404	2007 Profits: $238,317	**U.S. Stock Ticker: AAP**
2006 Sales: $4,616,503	2006 Profits: $231,318	**Int'l Ticker:** Int'l Exchange:
2005 Sales: $4,264,971	2005 Profits: $234,725	Employees: 44,065
2004 Sales: $3,770,297	2004 Profits: $187,988	Fiscal Year Ends: 12/31
2003 Sales: $3,493,696	2003 Profits: $124,935	Parent Company:

SALARIES/BENEFITS:

Pension Plan:	ESOP Stock Plan:	Profit Sharing:	Top Exec. Salary: $784,625	Bonus: $
Savings Plan: Y	Stock Purch. Plan: Y		Second Exec. Salary: $496,449	Bonus: $21,699

OTHER THOUGHTS:
Apparent Women Officers or Directors: 3
Hot Spot for Advancement for Women/Minorities: Y

LOCATIONS: ("Y" = Yes)

West:	Southwest:	Midwest:	Southeast:	Northeast:	International:
	Y	Y	Y	Y	Y

Note: Financial information, benefits and other data can change quickly and may vary from those stated here.

ADVANCED MICRO DEVICES INC (AMD)

www.amd.com

Industry Group Code: 334413 Ranks within this company's industry group: Sales: 3 Profits: 8

Management:		Sales/Marketing:		Liberal Arts:		Information Systems:		Professionals:		Technical/Scientific:	
Mgmt. Trainees:	Y	Mktg. Professionals:	Y	Gen. Writing/Editing:		Info. Management:	Y	Finance/Accounting:	Y	Engineers, Elec.:	Y
Experienced Mgmt.:	Y	Retail Sales:		Technical Writing:	Y	Software Dev.:	Y	Law:	Y	Engineers, Other:	
Int'l Business:	Y	Commercial/Industrial:	Y	Graphic Arts/Photog.:	Y	Hardware Dev.:	Y	HR/Other:	Y	Health/Lab:	Y
MBA Graduates:	Y	Sales Trainees:		Music:		Systems Integration:		Training:	Y	Scientists/Research:	Y
		Advertising Pros.:	Y	Broadcasting:		Consulting/Other:		Health Care:		Petroleum/Chemicals:	
				Other:				Consulting:		Math/Other:	Y

TYPES OF BUSINESS:

Microprocessors
Semiconductors
Low-End PCs

BRANDS/DIVISIONS/AFFILIATES:

AMD Athlon 64 FX
AMD Athlon 64
AMD Athlon XP
AMD Duron
AMD Sempron
AMD Opteron

CONTACTS: Note: Officers with more than one job title may be intentionally listed here more than once.

Dirk Meyer, CEO
Robert Rivet, CFO/Exec. VP
Nigel Dessau, Chief Mktg. Officer/Sr. VP
Amhed Mahamoud, CIO
Douglas Grose, Sr. VP-Mfg.
Thomas M. McCoy, Chief Admin. Officer
Thomas M. McCoy, Exec. VP-Legal Affairs
William T. Edwards, Chief Innovation Officer/Sr. VP
Richard Bergman, Sr. VP-Graphics Product Group
Mike Uhler, VP
Mario Rivas, Exec. VP-Computing Products Group
Hector Ruiz, Exec. Chmn.
Adrian Hartog, Pres., AMD Canada
Douglas Grose, Sr. VP-Supply Chain

Phone: 408-749-4000	Fax: 408-749-4291
Toll-Free: 800-538-8450	
Address: 1 AMD Pl., Sunnyvale, CA 94088-3453 US	

GROWTH PLANS/SPECIAL FEATURES:

Advanced Micro Devices, Inc. (AMD) is a global semiconductor company that provides processing solutions for the computing, graphics and consumer electronics markets. It supplies semiconductors, 3D graphics; video and multimedia products; chipsets for PCs, including desktop and notebook PCs, professional workstations and servers; and products for consumer electronic devices such as mobile phones, digital TVs and game consoles. AMD has manufacturing operations in the U.S., Europe and Asia and sales offices throughout the U.S. The company operates through four segments: Computation Products; Embedded Products; Graphics and Chipsets; and Consumer Electronics. AMD's computation products segment encompasses microprocessor products, servers and workstations, notebook PCs and desktop PCs. Its Embedded Products segment consists of two microprocessor family groups (Geode Processor family and AMD64 Embedded Processor family), AMD development boards and Reference Design Kits (RDKs), and AMD Embedded Solutions. The Graphics and Chipsets segment consists of Discrete Desktop Products (consisting of its two major product series, ATI Radeon X1000 and the new ATI Radeon HD 2000 graphics processors), discrete notebook products (its ATI Mobility Radeon X1000 series), chipset products (motherboard solutions delivered through AMD's Radeon Xpress and Crossfire products) and home media PC products (such as its ATI Avivo technology which enables PCs to record and playback in HD). Prominent customers include Microsoft, Macintosh and Toshiba. In 2007, AMD formed a partnership with Computer Tech. Co. Ltd (TCL), a Chinese computer company, making AMD products available in seven of China's top computer manufacturers. In 2008, AMD sold its digital TV assets to Broadcom Corporation.

AMD offers perks to employees including an educational assistance program and a profit sharing plan. Additionally, it offers volunteer opportunities to employees and some locations have on-site health clubs.

FINANCIALS: Sales and profits are in thousands of dollars—add 000 to get the full amount. 2007 Note: Financial information for 2007 was not available for all companies at press time.

2007 Sales: $6,013,000	2007 Profits: $-3,379,000	U.S. Stock Ticker: AMD
2006 Sales: $5,649,000	2006 Profits: $-166,000	Int'l Ticker: Int'l Exchange:
2005 Sales: $4,973,000	2005 Profits: $165,000	Employees: 16,420
2004 Sales: $3,924,000	2004 Profits: $91,000	Fiscal Year Ends: 12/31
2003 Sales: $3,519,169	2003 Profits: $-274,490	Parent Company:

SALARIES/BENEFITS:

Pension Plan:	ESOP Stock Plan:	Profit Sharing: Y	Top Exec. Salary: $1,046,358	Bonus: $2,598,750
Savings Plan: Y	Stock Purch. Plan: Y		Second Exec. Salary: $631,759	Bonus: $662,188

OTHER THOUGHTS:

Apparent Women Officers or Directors:
Hot Spot for Advancement for Women/Minorities:

LOCATIONS: ("Y" = Yes)

West:	Southwest:	Midwest:	Southeast:	Northeast:	International:
Y	Y	Y	Y	Y	Y

Note: Financial information, benefits and other data can change quickly and may vary from those stated here.

AECOM TECHNOLOGY CORPORATION   www.aecom.com

Industry Group Code: 234000 Ranks within this company's industry group: Sales: 6 Profits: 4

Management:		Sales/Marketing:		Liberal Arts:		Information Systems:		Professionals:		Technical/Scientific:	
Mgmt. Trainees:	Y	Mktg. Professionals:	Y	Gen. Writing/Editing:		Info. Management:	Y	Finance/Accounting:	Y	Engineers, Elec.:	Y
Experienced Mgmt.:	Y	Retail Sales:		Technical Writing:	Y	Software Dev.:		Law:	Y	Engineers, Other:	Y
Int'l Business:	Y	Commercial/Industrial:	Y	Graphic Arts/Photog.:	Y	Hardware Dev.:		HR/Other:	Y	Health/Lab:	
MBA Graduates:	Y	Sales Trainees:		Music:		Systems Integration:		Training:	Y	Scientists/Research:	
		Advertising Pros.:		Broadcasting:		Consulting/Other:		Health Care:		Petroleum/Chemicals:	
				Other:				Consulting:		Math/Other:	

TYPES OF BUSINESS:
Engineering & Design Services
Transportation Projects
Environmental Projects
Power & Mining Support
Consulting
Economic Development Consulting

BRANDS/DIVISIONS/AFFILIATES:
AGS
CTE
DMJM Aviation
Faber Maunsell
Metcalf & Eddy
UMA
PADCO
AECOM Austin

CONTACTS: *Note: Officers with more than one job title may be intentionally listed here more than once.*
John M. Dionisio, CEO
James R. Royer, COO/Exec. VP
John M. Dionisio, Pres.
Michael S. Burke, CFO/Sr. VP
Bob Kelleher, Chief Human Capital Officer
Raul Cruz, CIO/Sr. VP
Stephanie Hunter, Chief Admin. Officer
Eric Chen, General Counsel
Joseph E. Brown, CEO-Global Planning, Design & Dev.
Paul J. Gennaro, Jr., Chief Communications Officer
Paul J. Gennaro, Jr., Sr. VP-Investor Rel.
Eric Chen, Sr. VP-Finance
Anthony C. K. Shum, CEO-Hong Kong, China & Asia
Glenn R. Robson, Chief Strategy Officer
Frederick W. Werner, CEO-US
Jane Chmielinski, CEO-Corp. Dev.
Richard G. Newman, Chmn.
Robert C. Weber, CEO-Global Environmental Mgmt.

Phone: 213-593-8000	Fax: 213-593-8730
Toll-Free:	
Address: 555 S. Flower St., Ste. 3700, Los Angeles, CA 90071-2300 US	

GROWTH PLANS/SPECIAL FEATURES:
AECOM Technology Corporation is a global engineering and design company engaged in facility, transportation, environment and specialty engineering projects for corporate, institutional and government clients. Certain specialized services are available in mining, power, international development, and operations and maintenance. The firm's facility design and construction projects encompass land development assignments and a wide variety of building projects. Transportation services include feasibility studies, planning, design, engineering, construction management and asset management for transit and rail, highway, bridge, port, harbor and airport projects. AECOM offers water resource, wastewater, wet weather, hazardous waste management and other environmental engineering services. The power sector offers design, construction management and commissioning services. The company operates largely through a network of subsidiaries, including AGS, AECOM's government services arm; CTE, an infrastructure engineering firm (with a wastewater treatment plant in Antarctica); DMJM Aviation, the firm's flagship aviation design and construction management company; Faber Maunsell, a European engineering consultancy firm; Metcalf & Eddy, an environmental engineering group; UMA, a Canadian division; Hayes, Seay, Mattern & Mattern, Inc., an architectural and engineering firm that merged into AECOM in January 2007; and PADCO, a firm that promotes sustainable economic development in more than 100 countries. AECOM Austin, another subsidiary, is devoted to serving engineering and development clients in a variety of sectors, including pharmaceutical, industrial and aviation companies. Recent company acquisitions include Tecsult, Inc., The Services Group (TSG), Economics Research Associates, CityMark Architects and Engineers, Gartner Lee Limited and KMK Consulting Ltd. In early 2008 the firm announced plans to acquire Earth Tech, Inc. and Boyle Engineering, both engineering firms for environmental marketplaces. AECOM also recently won a $930 million contract to serve as the prime consultant on the Twin Cities Light Rail Project.

AECOM offers employees educational assistance and full health and insurance benefits.

FINANCIALS: Sales and profits are in thousands of dollars—add 000 to get the full amount. 2007 Note: Financial information for 2007 was not available for all companies at press time.

2007 Sales: $4,237,270	2007 Profits: $100,297	U.S. Stock Ticker: ACM
2006 Sales: $3,421,492	2006 Profits: $53,686	Int'l Ticker: Int'l Exchange:
2005 Sales: $2,395,340	2005 Profits: $53,814	Employees: 32,000
2004 Sales: $2,012,000	2004 Profits: $50,400	Fiscal Year Ends: 9/30
2003 Sales: $1,914,500	2003 Profits: $36,900	Parent Company:

SALARIES/BENEFITS:

Pension Plan: Y	ESOP Stock Plan:	Profit Sharing:	Top Exec. Salary: $900,016	Bonus: $1,500,000
Savings Plan: Y	Stock Purch. Plan: Y		Second Exec. Salary: $867,514	Bonus: $1,500,000

OTHER THOUGHTS:
Apparent Women Officers or Directors: 3
Hot Spot for Advancement for Women/Minorities: Y

LOCATIONS: ("Y" = Yes)

West:	Southwest:	Midwest:	Southeast:	Northeast:	International:
Y	Y	Y	Y	Y	Y

AEROPOSTALE INC
www.aeropostale.com

Industry Group Code: 448120   Ranks within this company's industry group: Sales: 9   Profits: 6

Management:		Sales/Marketing:		Liberal Arts:		Information Systems:		Professionals:		Technical/Scientific:	
Mgmt. Trainees:	Y	Mktg. Professionals:	Y	Gen. Writing/Editing:	Y	Info. Management:	Y	Finance/Accounting:	Y	Engineers, Elec.:	
Experienced Mgmt.:	Y	Retail Sales:	Y	Technical Writing:		Software Dev.:	Y	Law:	Y	Engineers, Other:	
Int'l Business:	Y	Commercial/Industrial:	Y	Graphic Arts/Photog.:	Y	Hardware Dev.:		HR/Other:	Y	Health/Lab:	
MBA Graduates:	Y	Sales Trainees:	Y	Music:		Systems Integration:		Training:	Y	Scientists/Research:	
		Advertising Pros.:	Y	Broadcasting:		Consulting/Other:		Health Care:		Petroleum/Chemicals:	
				Other:	Y			Consulting:		Math/Other:	

TYPES OF BUSINESS:

Teen Apparel-Retail
Online Sales
Young Adult Apparel-Retail
College Campus Sales Events

BRANDS/DIVISIONS/AFFILIATES:

Aeropostale West, Inc.
aeropostale.com
Jimmy'Z Surf Co., Inc.
Woody Car Design

CONTACTS: Note: Officers with more than one job title may be intentionally listed here more than once.

Julian R. Geiger, CEO
Thomas P. Johnson, COO/Exec. VP
Mindy C. Meads, Pres.
Michael J. Cunningham, CFO/Exec. VP
Scott K. Birnbaum, Sr. VP/Dir.-Mktg.
Ann E. Joyce, CIO/Sr. VP
Mindy C. Meads, Chief Merch. Officer
Marc A. Babins, Sr. VP-Prod.
Edward M. Slezak, General Counsel/Sr. VP/ Corp. Sec.
Barbara Pindar, Sr. VP-Planning & Allocation
Olivera Lazic-Zangas, Sr. VP/Dir.-Design
Mary Jo Pile, Chief Store Officer/Sr. VP
Marc D. Miller, Sr. VP-New Bus. Dev. & Strategic Planning
Julian R. Geiger, Chmn.
Mark A. Dorwart, Sr. VP-Logistics

Phone: 646-452-6217	Fax: 646-485-5430
Toll-Free: 877-674-0624	
Address: 112 W. 34th St., 22nd Fl., New York, NY 10120 US	

GROWTH PLANS/SPECIAL FEATURES:

Aeropostale, Inc., together with its wholly-owned subsidiary, Aeropostale West, Inc., is a mall-based specialty designer, marketer and retailer of casual apparel and accessories, principally targeting 14-17 year old young men and women. In addition to its mall and web site sales, the company sells products through organized sales events on college campuses. Aeropostale maintains control over its proprietary brands by designing, sourcing, marketing and selling all of its own merchandise, both through retail locations and its online store. The company's unusual name is derived from the first transatlantic airmail carrier, Compagnie Generale Aeropostale. The firm operates over 850 stores in 47 states, Canada and Puerto Rico, as well as 11 Jimmy'Z Surf Co., Inc. stores in 11 states. The Jimmy'Z brand, which was acquired along with Woody Car Design, is a California lifestyle-oriented brand targeting trend-aware young women and men aged 18-25. Aeropostale primarily markets its products through in-store communications, promotions and advertising. However, the company does advertise via other means, such as radio promotions, during key selling periods. Aeropostale carefully controls its sourcing and branding and aims for a price point of $10 to $40. The firm has a major distribution and warehouse center in South River, New Jersey, capable of supporting over 800 stores. In 2008, the firm expanded into Puerto Rico, opening its first store in Carolina, Puerto Rico. Aeropostale has further expansion planned for Barcelonesa and San Juan, Puerto Rico.

Aeropostale offers its employees tuition reimbursement, training and career development, bonuses and a merchandise discount both to its retail and corporate employees.

FINANCIALS: Sales and profits are in thousands of dollars—add 000 to get the full amount. 2007 Note: Financial information for 2007 was not available for all companies at press time.

2007 Sales: $1,413,208	2007 Profits: $160,647	U.S. Stock Ticker: ARO
2006 Sales: $1,204,347	2006 Profits: $83,954	Int'l Ticker: Int'l Exchange:
2005 Sales: $964,200	2005 Profits: $84,100	Employees: 10,756
2004 Sales: $734,868	2004 Profits: $54,254	Fiscal Year Ends: 1/31
2003 Sales: $550,904	2003 Profits: $31,290	Parent Company:

SALARIES/BENEFITS:

Pension Plan:	ESOP Stock Plan:	Profit Sharing:	Top Exec. Salary: $945,389	Bonus: $2,380,984
Savings Plan: Y	Stock Purch. Plan:		Second Exec. Salary: $509,192	Bonus: $642,121

OTHER THOUGHTS:

Apparent Women Officers or Directors: 5
Hot Spot for Advancement for Women/Minorities: Y

LOCATIONS: ("Y" = Yes)

West:	Southwest:	Midwest:	Southeast:	Northeast:	International:
Y	Y	Y	Y	Y	Y

Note: Financial information, benefits and other data can change quickly and may vary from those stated here.

AES CORPORATION (THE)

www.aes.com

Industry Group Code: 221000 Ranks within this company's industry group: Sales: Profits:

Management:		Sales/Marketing:		Liberal Arts:		Information Systems:		Professionals:		Technical/Scientific:	
Mgmt. Trainees:	Y	Mktg. Professionals:	Y	Gen. Writing/Editing:	Y	Info. Management:	Y	Finance/Accounting:	Y	Engineers, Elec.:	Y
Experienced Mgmt.:	Y	Retail Sales:		Technical Writing:		Software Dev.:	Y	Law:	Y	Engineers, Other:	
Int'l Business:	Y	Commercial/Industrial:	Y	Graphic Arts/Photog.:		Hardware Dev.:		HR/Other:	Y	Health/Lab:	
MBA Graduates:	Y	Sales Trainees:		Music:		Systems Integration:		Training:	Y	Scientists/Research:	
		Advertising Pros.:	Y	Broadcasting:		Consulting/Other:		Health Care:		Petroleum/Chemicals:	
				Other:				Consulting:		Math/Other:	

TYPES OF BUSINESS:

Utilities-Electricity
Wind Generation
Contract Power Generation
Competitive Supply
Biomass Energy
LNG Terminals

BRANDS/DIVISIONS/AFFILIATES:

Indianapolis Power & Light
Eletropaulo Metropolitana Electricidad
La Electricidad de Caracas
IPALCO Enterprises, Inc.
AES SONEL
AES Eletropaulo
Kievoblenergo
Rivneenergo

CONTACTS: Note: Officers with more than one job title may be intentionally listed here more than once.

Paul T. Hanrahan, CEO
Andre Gluski, COO/Exec. VP
Paul T. Hanrahan, Pres.
Victoria Harker, CFO/Exec. VP
Rita Trehan, VP-People & Learning
Ahmed Pasha, CIO/VP
Scott Kicker, VP-Eng. & Construction
Brian Miller, General Counsel/Exec. VP/Corp. Sec.
Roger Naill, Sr. VP-Strategic Planning
Robin Pence, VP-Comm.
Ahmed Pasha, VP-Investor Rel.
Chip Hoagland, Treas./VP
Andrew M. Vesey, Exec. VP/Pres., Latin America
Ned Hall, Exec. VP/Pres., North America
John McLaren, Exec. VP/Pres., Europe & Africa
David Gee, Exec. VP
Richard Darman, Chmn.
Mark Woodruff, Exec. VP/Pres., Asia & Middle East

Phone: 703-522-1315	Fax: 703-528-4510
Toll-Free:	
Address: 4300 Wilson Blvd., 11th Fl., Arlington, VA 22203 US	

GROWTH PLANS/SPECIAL FEATURES:

The AES Corporation, through its subsidiaries, operates in the global power industry in 28 countries on five continents. AES operates two primary business lines, power generation and distribution/utilities. The company is in the process of developing an alternative energy business through the investiture of approximately $1 billion. The distribution/utilities business consists of 15 distribution companies in eight countries with over 11 million customers. The segment has integrated utilities in the U.S. through Indianapolis Power & Light and in Cameroon through AES SONEL; additionally, it has distribution companies in Brazil through AES Eletropaulo and AES Sul; in Argentina through Empresa Dristribuidora La Plata S.A.; in El Salvador through Compañia de Alumbrado Eléctrico de San Salvador, S.A.; and in the Ukraine through Kievoblenergo and Rivneenergo. AES's generation business generates and sells electricity to wholesale customers through 121 power generation plants in 26 countries. Typically, these facilities sell into local power pools under short-term contracts or into daily spot markets. This segment does do some long-term contracting, but generally for less than 75% of a given plant's capacity. In 2007, AES expanded its facilities through the acquisition of two 230 megawatt (MW) petroleum power facilities in Mexico; two wind farm projects totaling 186 MW from GE Energy Financial Systems; a controlling interest in the hydroelectric company, IC ICTAS Energy Group in Turkey; constructed a 50 MW wind generation joint venture in China; was declared the preferred bidder in two South African plants; and constructed a 233 MW wind farm and began a 170 MW wind farm in Texas. In April 2008, the firm acquired a 660 MW power plant in the Philippines. In May 2008, AES sold a Kazakhi power plant and coal mine in for $1.1 billion. In July 2008, the company acquired 49% of the Guohua Hulunbeier Wind Farm in China.

FINANCIALS: Sales and profits are in thousands of dollars—add 000 to get the full amount. 2007 Note: Financial information for 2007 was not available for all companies at press time.

2007 Sales: $13,588,000	2007 Profits: $-95,000	U.S. Stock Ticker: AES
2006 Sales: $11,576,000	2006 Profits: $247,000	Int'l Ticker: Int'l Exchange:
2005 Sales: $11,021,000	2005 Profits: $605,000	Employees: 32,000
2004 Sales: $9,392,000	2004 Profits: $300,000	Fiscal Year Ends: 12/31
2003 Sales: $8,413,000	2003 Profits: $-452,000	Parent Company:

SALARIES/BENEFITS:

Pension Plan: Y	ESOP Stock Plan:	Profit Sharing: Y	Top Exec. Salary: $897,667	Bonus: $4,049,800
Savings Plan: Y	Stock Purch. Plan:		Second Exec. Salary: $481,250	Bonus: $532,000

OTHER THOUGHTS:

Apparent Women Officers or Directors: 8
Hot Spot for Advancement for Women/Minorities: Y

LOCATIONS: ("Y" = Yes)

West:	Southwest:	Midwest:	Southeast:	Northeast:	International:
Y	Y	Y		Y	Y

AETNA INC

www.aetna.com

Industry Group Code: 524114 **Ranks within this company's industry group:** Sales: Profits:

Management:		Sales/Marketing:		Liberal Arts:		Information Systems:		Professionals:		Technical/Scientific:	
Mgmt. Trainees:	Y	Mktg. Professionals:	Y	Gen. Writing/Editing:	Y	Info. Management:	Y	Finance/Accounting:	Y	Engineers, Elec.:	
Experienced Mgmt.:	Y	Retail Sales:		Technical Writing:		Software Dev.:	Y	Law:	Y	Engineers, Other:	Y
Int'l Business:		Commercial/Industrial:	Y	Graphic Arts/Photog.:		Hardware Dev.:		HR/Other:	Y	Health/Lab:	
MBA Graduates:	Y	Sales Trainees:		Music:		Systems Integration:		Training:	Y	Scientists/Research:	Y
		Advertising Pros.:	Y	Broadcasting:		Consulting/Other:		Health Care:	Y	Petroleum/Chemicals:	
				Other:				Consulting:		Math/Other:	Y

TYPES OF BUSINESS:

Insurance-Medical & Health
Long-Term Care Insurance
Group Insurance
Pension Products
Dental Insurance
Disability Insurance
Life Insurance

BRANDS/DIVISIONS/AFFILIATES:

Schaller Anderson, Inc.
Goodhealth Worldwide
Aetna Global Benefits

CONTACTS: *Note: Officers with more than one job title may be intentionally listed here more than once.*

Ronald A. Williams, CEO
Mark T. Bertolini, Pres.
Joseph M. Zubretsky, CFO/Exec. VP
Robert M. Mead, Sr. VP-Strategic Mktg.
Elease E. Wright, Sr. VP-Human Resources
Troyen A. Brennan, Chief Medical Officer/Sr. VP
Meg McCarthy, CIO
Michael Mathias, CTO
William J. Casazza, General Counsel/Sr. VP
Gery J. Barry, Chief Strategy Officer
Robert M. Mead, Sr. VP-Comm. & Strategic Mktg.
Jean LaTorre, Sr. VP/Chief Investment Officer
Mohit N. Ghose, VP-Public Affairs
Rajan Parmeswar, Chief Acct. Officer/VP/Controller
Ronald A. Williams, Chmn.
Martha Temple, Pres., Aetna Global Benefits
Meg McCarthy, Sr. VP-Procurement & Real Estate

Phone: 860-273-0123	Fax: 860-273-3971
Toll-Free: 800-872-3862	
Address: 151 Farmington Ave., Hartford, CT 06156 US	

GROWTH PLANS/SPECIAL FEATURES:

Aetna, Inc. is a diversified healthcare benefits company, offering a broad range of traditional and consumer-directed health insurance products and related services, including medical, pharmacy, dental, behavioral health, group life, long-term care and disability plans and medical management capabilities. The firm operates in three segments: health care, group insurance and large case pensions. The health care segment's products consist of medical, pharmacy, benefits management, dental and vision plans offered on both a risk basis and an employee-funded basis. Medical products also include point of service, health maintenance organization, preferred provider organization and indemnity benefit plans. The group insurance segment's products consist primarily of life insurance products, including renewable life insurance; disability insurance products, which provide employee income replacement benefits for both short- and long-term disability; and long-term care insurance products, which provide befits to cover the cost of care in private home settings, adult day care, assisted living or nursing facilities. The large case pensions segment manages retirement products primarily for tax qualified pension plans. Customers include employer groups; individuals; college students; part-time and hourly workers; health plans; and government-sponsored plans. In August 2007, Aetna acquired Schaller Anderson, Inc., a provider of healthcare management services, for roughly $535 million. In September 2007, the company acquired Goodhealth Worldwide, a managing general underwriter for international private medical insurance. In June 2008, Aetna set up a representative office in Shanghai, China, beginning a two-year process towards a market expansion through Aetna' international division, Aetna Global Benefits.

The company offers its employees medical, dental and vision insurance; flexible spending accounts; life insurance; short- and long-term disability insurance; a 401(k) plan; a retirement plan; an employee stock purchase plan; and tuition assistance.

FINANCIALS: Sales and profits are in thousands of dollars—add 000 to get the full amount. 2007 Note: Financial information for 2007 was not available for all companies at press time.

2007 Sales: $27,599,600	2007 Profits: $1,831,000	U.S. Stock Ticker: AET
2006 Sales: $25,145,700	2006 Profits: $1,701,700	Int'l Ticker: Int'l Exchange:
2005 Sales: $22,491,900	2005 Profits: $1,634,500	Employees: 30,000
2004 Sales: $19,904,100	2004 Profits: $2,245,100	Fiscal Year Ends: 12/31
2003 Sales: $17,976,400	2003 Profits: $933,800	Parent Company:

SALARIES/BENEFITS:

Pension Plan: Y	ESOP Stock Plan:	Profit Sharing:	Top Exec. Salary: $1,073,077	Bonus: $7,732,500
Savings Plan: Y	Stock Purch. Plan: Y		Second Exec. Salary: $825,000	Bonus: $7,437,015

OTHER THOUGHTS:

Apparent Women Officers or Directors: 6
Hot Spot for Advancement for Women/Minorities: Y

LOCATIONS: ("Y" = Yes)

West:	Southwest:	Midwest:	Southeast:	Northeast:	International:
Y	Y	Y	Y	Y	

Note: Financial information, benefits and other data can change quickly and may vary from those stated here.

AFFILIATED COMPUTER SERVICES INC   www.acs-inc.com

Industry Group Code: 541512 Ranks within this company's industry group: Sales: 4   Profits: 4

Management:		Sales/Marketing:		Liberal Arts:		Information Systems:		Professionals:		Technical/Scientific:	
Mgmt. Trainees:	Y	Mktg. Professionals:	Y	Gen. Writing/Editing:	Y	Info. Management:	Y	Finance/Accounting:	Y	Engineers, Elec.:	Y
Experienced Mgmt.:	Y	Retail Sales:		Technical Writing:	Y	Software Dev.:	Y	Law:	Y	Engineers, Other:	
Int'l Business:	Y	Commercial/Industrial:	Y	Graphic Arts/Photog.:	Y	Hardware Dev.:		HR/Other:	Y	Health/Lab:	
MBA Graduates:	Y	Sales Trainees:		Music:		Systems Integration:	Y	Training:	Y	Scientists/Research:	
		Advertising Pros.:		Broadcasting:		Consulting/Other:	Y	Health Care:		Petroleum/Chemicals:	
				Other:				Consulting:	Y	Math/Other:	

TYPES OF BUSINESS:
IT Consulting
Loan Processing Services
Systems Integration
Human Resources Services
IT Outsourcing
Business Process Outsourcing

BRANDS/DIVISIONS/AFFILIATES:
Bowers & Associates
sds business services GmbH
Syan Holdings Limited

CONTACTS: *Note: Officers with more than one job title may be intentionally listed here more than once.*
Lynn Blodgett, CEO
Tom Burlin, COO/Exec. VP
Lynn Blodgett, Pres.
Kevin Kyser, CFO/Exec. VP
Lora Villarreal, Chief People Officer/Exec. VP
Tas Panos, General Counsel/Exec. VP
John Rexford, Exec. VP-Corp. Dev.
Ann Vezina, Exec. VP/Pres., Commercial Solutions
Tom Blodgett, Exec. VP/Pres., Bus. Process Solutions
John Rexford, Exec. VP
Darwin Deason, Chmn.

Phone: 214-841-6111	Fax: 214-821-8315
Toll-Free:	
Address: 2828 N. Haskell Ave., Bldg. 1, Dallas, TX 75204 US	

GROWTH PLANS/SPECIAL FEATURES:
Affiliated Computer Services, Inc. (ACS) provides a full range of information technology (IT) services to clients who have time-critical, transaction-intensive information processing needs. Based in Texas, the company's offices are located primarily in North America, as well as in Central America, Europe, Africa and the Middle East. The company serves two primary markets: governments and commercial. Through the commercial sector, which represents approximately 60% of its revenues, ACS provides business process outsourcing, systems integration services and technology outsourcing to a variety of clients, including retailers, local municipalities, state agencies, health care providers, telecommunications companies, wholesale distributors, manufacturers, utilities, financial institutions and insurance companies. Services in the government market, which represents approximately 40% of the company's revenues, include business process outsourcing, consisting primarily of loan processing services and human resources services; and systems integration services, such as application development and outsourcing, network implementation and maintenance, desktop services, technical staff augmentation and training under long-term contracts. The company typically receives client information in all media formats, including via the web, EDI, fax, voice, paper, microfilm, computer tape, optical disk and CD-ROM. This information is immediately digitized and sent through the firm's proprietary workflow process, which is tailored to clients' requirements. In September 2007, the company announced a $111 million Medicaid contract award with the Washington, D.C. and a $130 million contract with the state of Alaska. In early 2008, ACS acquired Bowers & Associates, a provider of healthcare data analytics, for $8 million; sds business services GmbH, a Germany-based provider of data center, infrastructure and application related solutions, for $67 million; and Syan Holdings Limited, a U.K. based provider of IT outsourcing services, for $60 million.

ACS offers its employees medical, dental, vision, life and disability insurance.

FINANCIALS: Sales and profits are in thousands of dollars—add 000 to get the full amount. 2007 Note: Financial information for 2007 was not available for all companies at press time.

		U.S. Stock Ticker: ACS
2007 Sales: $5,772,479	2007 Profits: $253,090	Int'l Ticker: Int'l Exchange:
2006 Sales: $5,353,661	2006 Profits: $358,806	Employees: 60,000
2005 Sales: $4,351,159	2005 Profits: $409,569	Fiscal Year Ends: 6/30
2004 Sales: $4,106,393	2004 Profits: $521,728	Parent Company:
2003 Sales: $3,787,200	2003 Profits: $306,800	

SALARIES/BENEFITS:

Pension Plan:	ESOP Stock Plan:	Profit Sharing:	Top Exec. Salary: $916,053	Bonus: $1,835,468
Savings Plan: Y	Stock Purch. Plan: Y		Second Exec. Salary: $698,654	Bonus: $

OTHER THOUGHTS:
Apparent Women Officers or Directors: 3
Hot Spot for Advancement for Women/Minorities: Y

LOCATIONS: ("Y" = Yes)

West:	Southwest:	Midwest:	Southeast:	Northeast:	International:
Y	Y	Y	Y	Y	Y

AFLAC INC

www.aflac.com

Industry Group Code: 524114A **Ranks within this company's industry group:** Sales: 1   Profits: 1

Management:		Sales/Marketing:		Liberal Arts:		Information Systems:		Professionals:		Technical/Scientific:	
Mgmt. Trainees:	Y	Mktg. Professionals:	Y	Gen. Writing/Editing:	Y	Info. Management:	Y	Finance/Accounting:	Y	Engineers, Elec.:	
Experienced Mgmt.:	Y	Retail Sales:		Technical Writing:	Y	Software Dev.:	Y	Law:	Y	Engineers, Other:	
Int'l Business:	Y	Commercial/Industrial:	Y	Graphic Arts/Photog.:	Y	Hardware Dev.:		HR/Other:	Y	Health/Lab:	
MBA Graduates:	Y	Sales Trainees:	Y	Music:		Systems Integration:		Training:	Y	Scientists/Research:	Y
		Advertising Pros.:	Y	Broadcasting:		Consulting/Other:		Health Care:	Y	Petroleum/Chemicals:	
				Other:				Consulting:		Math/Other:	Y

TYPES OF BUSINESS:

Insurance-Supplemental & Specialty Health
Life Insurance
Cancer Insurance
Medicare Supplement Insurance
Accident & Disability Insurance
Long-Term Care Insurance
Dental Plans

BRANDS/DIVISIONS/AFFILIATES:

AFLAC Japan
AFLAC U.S.
American Family Life Assurance Company of Columbus
Ever

CONTACTS: *Note: Officers with more than one job title may be intentionally listed here more than once.*

Daniel P. Amos, CEO
Paul S. Amos, II, COO
Kriss Cloninger, III, Pres.
Kriss Cloninger, III, CFO
Gerald Shields, CIO/Sr. VP-IT
Teresa Lynne White, Chief Admin. Officer/Exec. VP
Joey M. Loudermilk, General Counsel/Exec. VP/Corp. Sec.
Audrey Boone Tillman, Exec. VP-Corp. Svcs.
Kenneth S. Janke, Jr., Sr. VP-Investor Rel.
Ralph A. Rogers, Chief Acct. Officer/Sr. VP-Financial Svcs.
Janet Baker, Sr. VP-Client Svcs.
Paul S. Amos, II, Pres./COO-Aflac U.S.
Kermitt L. Cox, Sr. VP/Corp. Actuary
Phillip J. Friou, Sr. VP-Gov't Rel.
Daniel P. Amos, Chmn.
Charles D. Lake II, Chmn., Aflac Int'l

Phone: 706-323-3431	Fax: 706-324-6330
Toll-Free: 800-992-3522	
Address: 1932 Wynnton Rd., Columbus, GA 31999 US	

GROWTH PLANS/SPECIAL FEATURES:

AFLAC, Inc. is a holding company whose principle subsidiary, AFLAC (American Family Life Assurance Company of Columbus), insures more than 40 million people worldwide. The subsidiary is a leading writer of supplemental insurance marketed to employers in the U.S., offering policies for 400,000 payroll accounts through more than 69,000 licensed agents. AFLAC U.S. sells cancer plans and various types of health insurance, including accident and disability, fixed-benefit dental, personal sickness and hospital indemnity, hospital intensive care, long-term care, ordinary life and short-term disability plans. In addition, AFLAC offers specified health event coverage for major medical crises such as heart attack and stroke, among others. U.S. insurance products are designed to provide supplemental coverage to individuals who already have major medical or primary insurance coverage. Another subsidiary, AFLAC Japan, is the largest foreign-based insurer in that country, insuring one in four households. AFLAC Japan's insurance products are designed to help consumers pay for medical and non-medical costs that are not reimbursed under Japan's national health insurance system. Ever, a whole life medical insurance policy sold in Japan, hit the 500,000 policy sales mark the year it was introduced. AFLAC Japan sells cancer plans, care plans, general medical expense plans, medical/sickness riders to its cancer plan, a living benefit life plan, ordinary life insurance plans and annuities. AFLAC Japan accounted for about 71% of AFLAC's insurance earnings in 2007.

AFLAC offers employees on-site childcare and fitness centers; extensive training; a health clinic; employee discount programs; continuing education programs; and up to $20,000 in college tuition reimbursement for employee dependents with at least a 2.5 GPA.

FINANCIALS: Sales and profits are in thousands of dollars—add 000 to get the full amount. 2007 Note: Financial information for 2007 was not available for all companies at press time.

2007 Sales: $15,393,000	2007 Profits: $1,634,000	**U.S. Stock Ticker:** AFL
2006 Sales: $14,616,000	2006 Profits: $1,483,000	**Int'l Ticker:** Int'l Exchange:
2005 Sales: $14,363,000	2005 Profits: $1,483,000	Employees: 7,411
2004 Sales: $13,281,000	2004 Profits: $1,266,000	Fiscal Year Ends: 12/31
2003 Sales: $11,447,000	2003 Profits: $795,000	Parent Company:

SALARIES/BENEFITS:

Pension Plan:	ESOP Stock Plan:	Profit Sharing: Y	Top Exec. Salary: $1,242,000	Bonus: $2,208,897
Savings Plan: Y	Stock Purch. Plan: Y		Second Exec. Salary: $796,000	Bonus: $1,109,027

OTHER THOUGHTS:

Apparent Women Officers or Directors: 6
Hot Spot for Advancement for Women/Minorities: Y

LOCATIONS: ("Y" = Yes)

West:	Southwest:	Midwest:	Southeast:	Northeast:	International:
Y	Y	Y	Y	Y	Y

AGILENT TECHNOLOGIES INC

www.agilent.com

Industry Group Code: 334500 Ranks within this company's industry group: Sales: 2 Profits: 1

Management:		Sales/Marketing:		Liberal Arts:		Information Systems:		Professionals:		Technical/Scientific:	
Mgmt. Trainees:	Y	Mktg. Professionals:	Y	Gen. Writing/Editing:	Y	Info. Management:	Y	Finance/Accounting:	Y	Engineers, Elec.:	Y
Experienced Mgmt.:	Y	Retail Sales:		Technical Writing:	Y	Software Dev.:	Y	Law:	Y	Engineers, Other:	
Int'l Business:	Y	Commercial/Industrial:	Y	Graphic Arts/Photog.:		Hardware Dev.:	Y	HR/Other:	Y	Health/Lab:	Y
MBA Graduates:	Y	Sales Trainees:		Music:		Systems Integration:	Y	Training:	Y	Scientists/Research:	Y
		Advertising Pros.:	Y	Broadcasting:		Consulting/Other:	Y	Health Care:		Petroleum/Chemicals:	
				Other:				Consulting:	Y	Math/Other:	Y

TYPES OF BUSINESS:

Test Equipment
Communications Test Equipment
Integrated Circuits Test Equipment
Optoelectronics Test Equipment
Image Sensors
Bioinstrumentation
Software Products
Informatics Products

BRANDS/DIVISIONS/AFFILIATES:

Agilent Technologies Laboratories
Stratagene Corp.

CONTACTS: Note: Officers with more than one job title may be intentionally listed here more than once.

William P. Sullivan, CEO
William P. Sullivan, Pres.
Adrian T. Dillon, CFO
Jean M. Halloran, Sr. VP-Human Resources
Darlene J. S. Solomon, CTO-Agilent Tech./VP-Agilent Laboratories
Adrian T. Dillon, Exec. VP-Admin.
G. Craig Nordlund, General Counsel/Sec./Sr. VP
Amy Flores, Mgr.-Public Rel.
Rodney Gonsalves, Dir.-Investor Rel.
Adrian T. Dillon, Exec. VP-Finance
Gooi Soon Chai, VP/Gen. Mgr.-Electronic Instruments
Ron Nersesian, VP/Gen. Mgr.-Wireless
Nick Roelofs, VP/Gen. Mgr.-Life Sciences Solutions
Michael Gasparian, VP/Gen. Mgr.-Materials Science Solutions
James G. Cullen, Chmn.

Phone: 408-348-8886	**Fax:** 408-345-8474
Toll-Free: 877-424-4536	
Address: 5301 Stevens Creek Blvd., Santa Clara, CA 95051 US	

GROWTH PLANS/SPECIAL FEATURES:

Agilent Technologies, Inc. is a diversified technology company with two main business segments: Electronic Measurement, which generated 63% of 2007 revenue; and Bio-analytical Measurement, 37%. The Electronic Measurement business operates in two markets. Its products for the communications testing market include testing equipment for fiber optic networks; broadband and data networks; and wireless communications and microwave networks. It also assists in installing, activating and maintaining optical, wireless, wireline and large-company networks. Supplying the aerospace, defense, computer and semiconductor industries, its offerings for the general purpose testing market include general purpose instruments; modular instruments and test software used as reconfigurable testing platforms; digital design products, including complex high-speed servers and logic analyzers; high-frequency electronic design automation software tools used to construct computer simulations; parametric test instruments and systems for semiconductor wafers; and electronic manufacturing test products such as automated x-ray inspection and in-circuit testing products. The Bio-analytical Measurement business serves three main life sciences markets: Pharmaceuticals, biotech, contract research and contract manufacturing; academic and government institutions; and clinical diagnostics. It also serves five main chemical analysis markets: Petroleum and chemicals; the environment; forensics and homeland security; bio-agriculture and food safety; and materials science. Its main product categories are gas chromatography, liquid chromatography, mass spectrometry, microfluidics, microarrays, atomic force microscopy, PCR (Polymerase Chain Reaction) instrumentation, software and informatics. Nano-positioning products were transferred to the materials science portion of this segment in late 2007. Agilent conducts centralized research for both segments through Agilent Technologies Laboratories, based in Santa Clara, California. Other primary research, development and manufacturing sites are located in Colorado, Delaware, Washington, China, Germany, India, Japan, Malaysia, Singapore and the U.K. In June 2007, Agilent acquired life science research and diagnostic product manufacturer Stratagene Corp. for $250 million.

FINANCIALS: Sales and profits are in thousands of dollars—add 000 to get the full amount. 2007 Note: Financial information for 2007 was not available for all companies at press time.

2007 Sales: $5,420,000	2007 Profits: $638,000	**U.S. Stock Ticker:** A
2006 Sales: $4,973,000	2006 Profits: $3,307,000	**Int'l Ticker:** Int'l Exchange:
2005 Sales: $4,685,000	2005 Profits: $327,000	Employees: 2,760
2004 Sales: $4,556,000	2004 Profits: $369,000	Fiscal Year Ends: 10/31
2003 Sales: $4,468,000	2003 Profits: $-2,058,000	Parent Company:

SALARIES/BENEFITS:

Pension Plan: Y	ESOP Stock Plan:	Profit Sharing: Y	Top Exec. Salary: $946,874	Bonus: $619,496
Savings Plan: Y	Stock Purch. Plan: Y		Second Exec. Salary: $699,996	Bonus: $848,093

OTHER THOUGHTS:

Apparent Women Officers or Directors: 3
Hot Spot for Advancement for Women/Minorities: Y

LOCATIONS: ("Y" = Yes)

West:	Southwest:	Midwest:	Southeast:	Northeast:	International:
Y				Y	Y

Note: Financial information, benefits and other data can change quickly and may vary from those stated here.

AIR PRODUCTS & CHEMICALS INC   www.airproducts.com

Industry Group Code: 325120 Ranks within this company's industry group: Sales: 1 Profits: 2

Management:		Sales/Marketing:		Liberal Arts:		Information Systems:		Professionals:		Technical/Scientific:	
Mgmt. Trainees:	Y	Mktg. Professionals:	Y	Gen. Writing/Editing:		Info. Management:	Y	Finance/Accounting:	Y	Engineers, Elec.:	Y
Experienced Mgmt.:	Y	Retail Sales:		Technical Writing:	Y	Software Dev.:		Law:	Y	Engineers, Other:	
Int'l Business:	Y	Commercial/Industrial:	Y	Graphic Arts/Photog.:		Hardware Dev.:		HR/Other:	Y	Health/Lab:	Y
MBA Graduates:	Y	Sales Trainees:		Music:		Systems Integration:		Training:	Y	Scientists/Research:	Y
		Advertising Pros.:	Y	Broadcasting:		Consulting/Other:		Health Care:		Petroleum/Chemicals:	
				Other:				Consulting:		Math/Other:	

TYPES OF BUSINESS:
Industrial Gases & Chemicals
Respiratory Therapy & Home Medical Equipment
Specialty Resins
Hydrogen Refinery
Natural Gas Liquefaction
Semiconductor Materials

BRANDS/DIVISIONS/AFFILIATES:
Air Products Asia
Air Products Europe
Air Products Japan

CONTACTS: Note: Officers with more than one job title may be intentionally listed here more than once.
John E. McGlade, CEO
John E. McGlade, Pres.
Paul E. Huck, CFO/Sr. VP
Lynn C. Minella, Sr. VP-Human Resources & Comm.
Glenn E. Beck, CIO/VP-Global Enterprise Oper.
Montgomery Alger, CTO/VP
Robert D. Conley, VP-Global Eng.
Stephen J. Jones, General Counsel/Corp. Sec./VP
Joseph M. Pietrantonio, VP-Global Oper.
Norma J. Curby, VP-Strategic Planning
Elizabeth L. Klebe, VP-Corp. Comm.
George G. Bitto, Treas./VP
Scott A. Sherman, VP-Tonnage Gases, Equipment & Energy
Diane L. Sheridan, Chief Risk Officer/VP
Patricia A. Mattimore, VP-Energy & Materials
Charles G. Stinner, VP-Taxes
John P. Jones, III, Chmn.
Wilbur W. Mok, Pres., Air Products Asia, Inc.
William J. Cantwell, VP-Supply Chain

Phone: 610-481-4911	Fax: 610-481-5900
Toll-Free:	
Address: 7201 Hamilton Blvd., Allentown, PA 18195-1501 US	

GROWTH PLANS/SPECIAL FEATURES:
Air Products and Chemicals, Inc., founded in 1940, serves global technology, energy, industrial and healthcare customers. Products and services include atmospheric gases; process and specialty gases; performance materials; and equipment and services. The company is one of the world's largest suppliers of hydrogen and helium and has built leading positions in growth markets such as semiconductor materials, refinery hydrogen, natural gas liquefaction, and advanced coatings and adhesives. The firm conducts business under six segments: merchant gasses; tonnage gases; electronics and performance materials; equipment and energy; healthcare; and chemicals. The merchant gasses segment sells industrial gases such as oxygen, nitrogen, argon, hydrogen and helium, as well as certain medical and specialty gases. Tonnage gases provides hydrogen, carbon monoxide, nitrogen, oxygen and syngas, primarily to the petroleum refining, chemical and metallurgical industries worldwide. Electronics and performance materials provides solutions to a broad range of global industries through chemical synthesis, analytical technology, process engineering and surface science. The equipment and energy segment designs and manufactures cryogenic and gas processing equipment for air separation, hydrocarbon recovery and purification, natural gas liquefaction and helium distribution. This segment is also engaged in power generation, both domestically and internationally. The healthcare segment provides respiratory therapies, home medical equipment and infusion services to over 500,000 patients in their homes. This segment provides oxygen therapy, pharmacist-managed direct-shipped respiratory medications, home nebulizer therapy, sleep management therapy, anti-infection therapy, enteral nutrition, beds and wheelchairs. The chemicals segment is comprised of a polymer emulsions business and a polyurethane intermediates business. The firm is in the process of divesting itself of its polymer emulsions business. The company has majority or wholly-owned foreign subsidiaries that operate in Canada, 17 European countries, 11 Asian countries and four Latin American countries. International subsidiaries include Air Products Asia, Air Products Europe and Air Products Japan.

FINANCIALS: Sales and profits are in thousands of dollars—add 000 to get the full amount. 2007 Note: Financial information for 2007 was not available for all companies at press time.

		U.S. Stock Ticker: APD
2007 Sales: $10,037,800	2007 Profits: $1,035,600	Int'l Ticker: Int'l Exchange:
2006 Sales: $8,752,800	2006 Profits: $723,400	Employees: 22,100
2005 Sales: $7,673,000	2005 Profits: $711,700	Fiscal Year Ends: 9/30
2004 Sales: $7,031,900	2004 Profits: $604,100	Parent Company:
2003 Sales: $6,297,300	2003 Profits: $397,000	

SALARIES/BENEFITS:
Pension Plan: Y	ESOP Stock Plan:	Profit Sharing:	Top Exec. Salary: $1,170,000	Bonus: $2,585,000
Savings Plan: Y	Stock Purch. Plan:		Second Exec. Salary: $700,000	Bonus: $937,000

OTHER THOUGHTS:
Apparent Women Officers or Directors: 11
Hot Spot for Advancement for Women/Minorities: Y

LOCATIONS: ("Y" = Yes)
West:	Southwest:	Midwest:	Southeast:	Northeast:	International:
Y	Y	Y	Y	Y	Y

Note: Financial information, benefits and other data can change quickly and may vary from those stated here.

ALBERTO-CULVER COMPANY   www.alberto.com

Industry Group Code: 446120 Ranks within this company's industry group: Sales: 1   Profits: 1

Management:		Sales/Marketing:		Liberal Arts:		Information Systems:		Professionals:		Technical/Scientific:	
Mgmt. Trainees:	Y	Mktg. Professionals:	Y	Gen. Writing/Editing:	Y	Info. Management:	Y	Finance/Accounting:	Y	Engineers, Elec.:	
Experienced Mgmt.:	Y	Retail Sales:	Y	Technical Writing:	Y	Software Dev.:		Law:	Y	Engineers, Other:	
Int'l Business:	Y	Commercial/Industrial:	Y	Graphic Arts/Photog.:	Y	Hardware Dev.:		HR/Other:	Y	Health/Lab:	Y
MBA Graduates:	Y	Sales Trainees:	Y	Music:		Systems Integration:		Training:	Y	Scientists/Research:	
		Advertising Pros.:	Y	Broadcasting:		Consulting/Other:		Health Care:		Petroleum/Chemicals:	
				Other:	Y			Consulting:		Math/Other:	

TYPES OF BUSINESS:

Beauty Supplies, Retail
Branded Consumer Products
Food Preparation Products
Beauty Supply Distribution

BRANDS/DIVISIONS/AFFILIATES:

Sally Beauty Company
Salve
Heil Beauty Supply
Alberto VO5
TRESemme
Mrs. Dash
St. Ives Swiss Formula
Cederroth International

CONTACTS: Note: Officers with more than one job title may be intentionally listed here more than once.

V. James Marino, CEO
V. James Marino, Pres.
Ralph J. Nicoletti, CFO/Sr. VP
Richard Gerstein, Chief Mktg. Officer
John R. Berschied, Jr., Group VP-Global R&D
Gary P. Schmidt, General Counsel/Sr. VP/Corp. Sec.
Richard Mewborn, VP-Global Oper.
Gina Boswell, Pres., Global Brands
Carol L. Bernick, Chmn.
Richard J. Hynes, Pres., Int'l

Phone: 708-450-3000	Fax: 708-450-3354
Toll-Free:	
Address: 2525 Armitage Ave., Melrose Park, IL 60160-1163 US	

GROWTH PLANS/SPECIAL FEATURES:

Alberto-Culver Company is a manufacturer and marketer of consumer packaged goods and beauty products. The company's two divisions are Consumer Packaged Goods, which manufactures, markets and distributes beauty care products, food and household items to the U.S. and over 100 countries worldwide; and Cederroth International, located in Sweden, primarily involved with beauty care and health products marketed in Scandinavia and Europe. Consumer products include the Alberto VO5, TRESemme, Consort and Nexxus line of hair products; the St. Ives line of skin care products; FDS feminine deodorant sprays; and the Soft & Beautiful, Just For Me, Comb-Thru, TCB and Motions lines of ethnic hair care products. The division also produces the Molly McButter, Mrs. Dash and SugarTwin lines of food preparation products; as well as the Static Guard and Kleen Guard household items. Cederroth's products include Salve adhesive bandages, Seltin salt substitute, Bliw liquid soaps, Jordan toothbrushes and Pharbio natural pharmaceuticals as well as other Alberto products such as St. Ives. The company's products are also available in Australia, Asia, Africa, Canada and Latin America. At the close of the 2007 fiscal year, approximately 46.4% of the company's sales came from outside the U.S. Alberto-Culver owns Armstrong-McCall, Heil Beauty Supply, Davidson Supply Co. and B&H Supply Co., Salon Success and CosmoProf five major professional beauty products distributors; and Pro-line, a manufacturer and marketer of personal care products for the African-American market. In July 2008, Alberto-Culver sold Cederroth International to CapMan, a Nordic private equity firm.

FINANCIALS: Sales and profits are in thousands of dollars—add 000 to get the full amount. 2007 Note: Financial information for 2007 was not available for all companies at press time.

2007 Sales: $1,541,581	2007 Profits: $78,264	U.S. Stock Ticker: ACV
2006 Sales: $1,398,901	2006 Profits: $	Int'l Ticker: Int'l Exchange:
2005 Sales: $3,531,231	2005 Profits: $210,901	Employees: 3,800
2004 Sales: $3,258,000	2004 Profits: $141,770	Fiscal Year Ends: 9/30
2003 Sales: $2,891,400	2003 Profits: $162,200	Parent Company:

SALARIES/BENEFITS:

Pension Plan:	ESOP Stock Plan:	Profit Sharing:	Top Exec. Salary: $1,550,000	Bonus: $1,412,000
Savings Plan:	Stock Purch. Plan:		Second Exec. Salary: $883,333	Bonus: $275,000

OTHER THOUGHTS:

Apparent Women Officers or Directors: 3
Hot Spot for Advancement for Women/Minorities: Y

LOCATIONS: ("Y" = Yes)

West:	Southwest:	Midwest:	Southeast:	Northeast:	International:
Y	Y	Y	Y	Y	Y

ALLERGAN INC   www.allergan.com

Industry Group Code: 325412 **Ranks within this company's industry group:** Sales: 6   Profits: 9

Management:		Sales/Marketing:		Liberal Arts:		Information Systems:		Professionals:		Technical/Scientific:	
Mgmt. Trainees:	Y	Mktg. Professionals:	Y	Gen. Writing/Editing:	Y	Info. Management:	Y	Finance/Accounting:	Y	Engineers, Elec.:	
Experienced Mgmt.:	Y	Retail Sales:		Technical Writing:	Y	Software Dev.:		Law:	Y	Engineers, Other:	Y
Int'l Business:	Y	Commercial/Industrial:	Y	Graphic Arts/Photog.:	Y	Hardware Dev.:		HR/Other:	Y	Health/Lab:	Y
MBA Graduates:	Y	Sales Trainees:	Y	Music:		Systems Integration:		Training:	Y	Scientists/Research:	Y
		Advertising Pros.:	Y	Broadcasting:		Consulting/Other:		Health Care:	Y	Petroleum/Chemicals:	
				Other:				Consulting:		Math/Other:	Y

TYPES OF BUSINESS:
Pharmaceutical Development
Eye Care Supplies
Dermatological Products
Neuromodulator Products
Obesity Intervention Products
Urologic Products
Medical Aesthetics

BRANDS/DIVISIONS/AFFILIATES:
Restasis
Lumigan
Optive
Refresh
Botox
Sanctura XR
Esprit Pharma Holdings
EndoArt S.A.

CONTACTS: *Note: Officers with more than one job title may be intentionally listed here more than once.*
David Pyott, CEO
F. Michael Ball, Pres.
Jeffrey L. Edwards, CFO
Scott M. Whitcup, Exec. VP-R&D
Raymond H. Diradoorian, Exec. VP-Global Tech. Oper.
Douglas S. Ingram, Chief Admin. Officer
Douglas S. Ingram, General Counsel/Corp. Sec./Exec. VP
Jeffrey L. Edwards, Exec. VP-Bus. Dev.
Jeffrey L. Edwards, Exec. VP-Finance
Douglas S. Ingram, Chief Ethics Officer
David Pyott, Chmn.

Phone: 714-246-4500	Fax: 714-246-4971
Toll-Free:	
Address: 2525 Dupont Dr., Irvine, CA 92612 US	

GROWTH PLANS/SPECIAL FEATURES:

Allergan, Inc. is a technology-driven global health care company that develops and commercializes specialty pharmaceutical products, biologics and medical devices for the ophthalmic, neuromodulator, dermatological and other specialty markets. The company focuses on treatments for glaucoma and retinal disease, cataracts, dry eye, psoriasis, acne and neuromuscular disorders. Allergan's eye care products include Restasis ophthalmic emulsion, Lumigan ophthalmic solution, Optive lubricant eye drops and the Refresh line of artificial tears. The firm's primary neuromodulator product is Botox, which is used for the treatment of neuromuscular disorders, chronic migraine and pain management. Allergan's skin care product line is comprised of tazarotene products in cream and gel formulations for the treatment of acne, facial wrinkles and psoriasis, marketed under the name Tazorac, and Botox for the treatment of excessive sweating. Obesity intervention products include the Lap-Band, an adjustable gastric banding system and the BIB intragastric balloon system. Medical aesthetics products include the Natrelle Collection, a line of breast implants; Botox Cosmetic, for the temporary improvement of wrinkles; and the Juvederm line of dermal filler products. Products in the area of Urologics consist primarily of Sanctura XR, a medication for overactive bladder. In early 2007, Allergan acquired EndoArt S.A., a Swiss company with technology to remotely tighten or loosen a gastric band, for $97 million. In October 2007, the firm acquired Esprit Pharma Holding Company, Inc.

The firm offers employees benefits including a 401(k) plan; a defined benefit retirement contribution; adoption assistance, education assistance; before-tax flex dollars and flexible spending accounts; backup child care; company store; on-site gym and athletic fields; computer training facilities; an employee credit union; an employee assistance program; dependent scholarship awards; and U.S. savings bond deductions.

FINANCIALS: Sales and profits are in thousands of dollars—add 000 to get the full amount. 2007 Note: Financial information for 2007 was not available for all companies at press time.

2007 Sales: $3,938,900	2007 Profits: $499,300	**U.S. Stock Ticker: AGN**
2006 Sales: $3,063,300	2006 Profits: $-127,400	**Int'l Ticker:** Int'l Exchange:
2005 Sales: $2,319,200	2005 Profits: $403,900	Employees: 7,886
2004 Sales: $2,045,600	2004 Profits: $377,100	Fiscal Year Ends: 12/31
2003 Sales: $1,171,400	2003 Profits: $-52,500	Parent Company:

SALARIES/BENEFITS:

Pension Plan: Y	ESOP Stock Plan:	Profit Sharing: Y	Top Exec. Salary: $1,233,769	Bonus: $2,000,000
Savings Plan: Y	Stock Purch. Plan: Y		Second Exec. Salary: $593,613	Bonus: $571,200

OTHER THOUGHTS:
Apparent Women Officers or Directors: 2
Hot Spot for Advancement for Women/Minorities: Y

LOCATIONS: ("Y" = Yes)

West:	Southwest:	Midwest:	Southeast:	Northeast:	International:
Y	Y				Y

Note: Financial information, benefits and other data can change quickly and may vary from those stated here.

ALLIANCE DATA SYSTEMS CORPORATION
www.alliancedata.com

Industry Group Code: 522320 Ranks within this company's industry group: Sales: 4   Profits: 4

Management:		Sales/Marketing:		Liberal Arts:		Information Systems:		Professionals:		Technical/Scientific:	
Mgmt. Trainees:	Y	Mktg. Professionals:	Y	Gen. Writing/Editing:		Info. Management:	Y	Finance/Accounting:	Y	Engineers, Elec.:	
Experienced Mgmt.:	Y	Retail Sales:		Technical Writing:		Software Dev.:	Y	Law:	Y	Engineers, Other:	
Int'l Business:	Y	Commercial/Industrial:	Y	Graphic Arts/Photog.:		Hardware Dev.:		HR/Other:	Y	Health/Lab:	
MBA Graduates:	Y	Sales Trainees:		Music:		Systems Integration:		Training:	Y	Scientists/Research:	
		Advertising Pros.:	Y	Broadcasting:		Consulting/Other:	Y	Health Care:		Petroleum/Chemicals:	
				Other:				Consulting:	Y	Math/Other:	

TYPES OF BUSINESS:
Marketing Services
Credit Services
Transaction Services

BRANDS/DIVISIONS/AFFILIATES:
Epsilon
World Financial Network National Bank
World Financial Capital Bank

CONTACTS: *Note: Officers with more than one job title may be intentionally listed here more than once.*
Michael Parks, CEO
John Scullion, COO
John Scullion, Pres.
Edward Heffernan, CFO/Exec. VP
Dwayne Tucker, Exec. VP-Human Resources & Transaction Svcs.
Alan Utay, Chief Admin. Officer
Alan Utay, General Counsel/Exec. VP/Corp. Sec.
Bryan A. Pearson, Exec. VP/Pres., Loyalty Svcs.
Ivan Szeftel, Exec. VP/Pres., Retail Credit Svcs.
Michael L. Iaccarino, Exec. VP/Pres., Mktg. Svcs.
Michael Parks, Chmn.

Phone: 972-348-5100	Fax: 972-348-5335
Toll-Free:	
Address: 17655 Waterview Pkwy., Dallas, TX 75252 US	

GROWTH PLANS/SPECIAL FEATURES:

Alliance Data Systems Corp. (ADS) is a provider of loyalty and marketing solutions derived from transaction rich data. It partner with clients to develop unique insight into consumer behavior. It then uses that insight to create and manage customized solutions that helps its clients strengthen their relationship with their customers. The company operates in three segments: marketing services, credit services and transaction services. Through the marketing service segment, the firm creates and manages targeted marketing programs that result in securing more frequent and sustained customer behavior. It utilizes the information gathered through loyalty and targeted marketing programs to help clients design and implement marketing program. Subsidiary Epsilon, a part of this segment, provides integrated direct marketing solutions that combine consulting and creative services, database services, analytical services and interactive delivery services. Through the credit services division, ADS finances and operates private label and co-branded credit card programs. Through subsidiaries World Financial Network National Bank and World Financial Capital Bank, the division underwrites accounts and funds purchases for over 85 private label credit card and commercial credit clients. The transaction services segment facilitates and manages transactions between clients and their customers through its scalable processing system. The division's largest clients include Limited Brands and its retail affiliates. ADS has a client base in excess of 600 companies, consisting mostly of specialty retailers, petroleum retailers, utilities, supermarkets and financial services companies. In May 2007, the firm agreed to be acquired by The Blackstone Group for roughly $7.8 billion, including assumption of debt.

The company offers its employees medical, dental and vision insurance; flexible spending accounts; a 401(k) plan; tuition reimbursement; and an employee assistance program.

FINANCIALS: Sales and profits are in thousands of dollars—add 000 to get the full amount. 2007 Note: Financial information for 2007 was not available for all companies at press time.

2007 Sales: $2,291,189	2007 Profits: $164,061	**U.S. Stock Ticker: ADS**
2006 Sales: $1,998,742	2006 Profits: $189,605	**Int'l Ticker:** Int'l Exchange:
2005 Sales: $1,552,437	2005 Profits: $138,745	Employees: 9,800
2004 Sales: $1,257,438	2004 Profits: $120,371	Fiscal Year Ends: 12/31
2003 Sales: $1,049,100	2003 Profits: $67,300	Parent Company:

SALARIES/BENEFITS:

Pension Plan:	ESOP Stock Plan:	Profit Sharing:	Top Exec. Salary: $840,000	Bonus: $1,572,196
Savings Plan: Y	Stock Purch. Plan:		Second Exec. Salary: $549,622	Bonus: $883,476

OTHER THOUGHTS:
Apparent Women Officers or Directors:
Hot Spot for Advancement for Women/Minorities:

LOCATIONS: ("Y" = Yes)

West:	Southwest:	Midwest:	Southeast:	Northeast:	International:
	Y	Y		Y	Y

ALLSTATE CORPORATION (THE)   www.allstate.com

Industry Group Code: 524126 Ranks within this company's industry group: Sales: Profits:

Management:		Sales/Marketing:		Liberal Arts:		Information Systems:		Professionals:		Technical/Scientific:	
Mgmt. Trainees:	Y	Mktg. Professionals:	Y	Gen. Writing/Editing:	Y	Info. Management:	Y	Finance/Accounting:	Y	Engineers, Elec.:	
Experienced Mgmt.:	Y	Retail Sales:		Technical Writing:		Software Dev.:	Y	Law:	Y	Engineers, Other:	
Int'l Business:	Y	Commercial/Industrial:	Y	Graphic Arts/Photog.:		Hardware Dev.:		HR/Other:	Y	Health/Lab:	
MBA Graduates:	Y	Sales Trainees:		Music:		Systems Integration:		Training:	Y	Scientists/Research:	Y
		Advertising Pros.:	Y	Broadcasting:		Consulting/Other:		Health Care:		Petroleum/Chemicals:	
				Other:				Consulting:		Math/Other:	Y

TYPES OF BUSINESS:
Insurance, Direct Property & Casualty
Auto Insurance
Homeowners Insurance
Life Insurance
Business Insurance

BRANDS/DIVISIONS/AFFILIATES:
Allstate Insurance Co.
Allstate Life Insurance Co.
Allstate Motor Club, Inc.
Deerbrook
Encompass
Allstate
Partnership Marketing Group
Sterling Autobody Centers

CONTACTS: Note: Officers with more than one job title may be intentionally listed here more than once.
Tom Wilson, CEO
Tom Wilson, Pres.
Samuel H. Pilch, Interim CFO/VP
Jim D. DeVries, Sr. VP-Human Resources
Catherine S. Brune, CIO/Sr. VP
Michele Coleman Mayes, General Counsel/ VP
Joan H. Walker, Sr. VP-Corp. Rel.
George E. Ruebenson, Pres., Allstate Protection, Allstate Insurance Co.
Eric A. Simonson, CIO/Sr. VP-Allstate Insurance Co.
James E. Hohmann, CEO/Pres., Allstate Financial
Joan H. Walker, Interim Chief Mktg Officer-AIC
Thomas J. Wilson, Chmn.

Phone: 847-402-5000	Fax: 847-326-7519
Toll-Free: 800-574-3553	
Address: 2775 Sanders Rd., Northbrook, IL 60062 US	

GROWTH PLANS/SPECIAL FEATURES:

The Allstate Corp., a holding company for Allstate Insurance Co. through which it principally conducts its business, is primarily engaged in the personal property and casualty insurance business and the life insurance, retirement and investment products business. The firm provides insurance products to more than 17 million households through a distribution network that utilizes a total of roughly 14,900 exclusive agencies and exclusive financial specialists in the U.S. and Canada. The company conducts its business through four business segments: Allstate Protection; Allstate Financial; discounted lines and coverages; and corporate and other. Allstate Protection, which accounted for 94% of 2007 consolidated insurance premiums and contract charges, sells primarily private passenger auto and homeowners insurance, principally through agencies, under the Allstate, Encompass and Deerbrook brand names. The segment also sells a wide range of personal property and casualty insurance products such as landlords, personal umbrella, renters, condominiums, residential fire, manufactured housing, boat owners, loan protection and selected commercial property and casualty products. In addition, it operates the Allstate Motor Club, Inc., which provides emergency road service. Allstate Financial provides life insurance; retirement and investment products; and supplemental accident and health insurance to individual and institutional customers. The discontinued lines and coverages segment includes results from insurance coverage that the company no longer writes and results for certain commercial and other business in run-off. The corporate and other segment is comprised of holding company activities and certain non-insurance operations. In June 2008, Allstate agreed to acquire Partnership Marketing Group, to be combined with its Motor Club division, from General Electric Money.

The company offers its employees medical, dental, vision and life insurance; AD&D and long-term disability insurance; flexible spending accounts; a retirement plan; a profit sharing fund with 401(k) options; tuition reimbursement; and childcare discounts.

FINANCIALS: Sales and profits are in thousands of dollars—add 000 to get the full amount. 2007 Note: Financial information for 2007 was not available for all companies at press time.

2007 Sales: $36,769,000	2007 Profits: $4,636,000	U.S. Stock Ticker: ALL
2006 Sales: $35,796,000	2006 Profits: $4,993,000	Int'l Ticker: Int'l Exchange:
2005 Sales: $35,383,000	2005 Profits: $1,765,000	Employees: 38,000
2004 Sales: $33,936,000	2004 Profits: $3,181,000	Fiscal Year Ends: 12/31
2003 Sales: $32,108,000	2003 Profits: $2,705,000	Parent Company:

SALARIES/BENEFITS:
Pension Plan: Y	ESOP Stock Plan:	Profit Sharing: Y	Top Exec. Salary: $1,225,008	Bonus: $4,947,361
Savings Plan: Y	Stock Purch. Plan:		Second Exec. Salary: $957,596	Bonus: $3,551,118

OTHER THOUGHTS:
Apparent Women Officers or Directors: 5
Hot Spot for Advancement for Women/Minorities: Y

LOCATIONS: ("Y" = Yes)
West:	Southwest:	Midwest:	Southeast:	Northeast:	International:
Y	Y	Y	Y	Y	Y

Note: Financial information, benefits and other data can change quickly and may vary from those stated here.

ALTRIA GROUP INC   www.altria.com

Industry Group Code: 312220 **Ranks within this company's industry group:** Sales: Profits:

Management:		Sales/Marketing:		Liberal Arts:		Information Systems:		Professionals:		Technical/Scientific:	
Mgmt. Trainees:	Y	Mktg. Professionals:	Y	Gen. Writing/Editing:	Y	Info. Management:	Y	Finance/Accounting:	Y	Engineers, Elec.:	
Experienced Mgmt.:	Y	Retail Sales:		Technical Writing:		Software Dev.:		Law:	Y	Engineers, Other:	
Int'l Business:	Y	Commercial/Industrial:	Y	Graphic Arts/Photog.:	Y	Hardware Dev.:		HR/Other:	Y	Health/Lab:	
MBA Graduates:	Y	Sales Trainees:		Music:		Systems Integration:		Training:	Y	Scientists/Research:	
		Advertising Pros.:	Y	Broadcasting:		Consulting/Other:		Health Care:		Petroleum/Chemicals:	
				Other:				Consulting:		Math/Other:	

TYPES OF BUSINESS:

Tobacco Products
Cigarette Manufacturing
Consumer Packaged Goods
Prepared Foods
Beer Brewing
Corporate Property Leasing
Beverage Bottling & Distribution

BRANDS/DIVISIONS/AFFILIATES:

Philip Morris U.S.A., Inc.
Philip Morris International, Inc.
Philip Morris Capital Corp.
Miller Brewing Company
John Middleton, Inc.

CONTACTS: *Note: Officers with more than one job title may be intentionally listed here more than once.*

Louis C. Camilleri, CEO
Dinyar S. Devitre, CFO/Sr. VP
Charles R. Wall, General Counsel/Sr. VP
Steven C. Parrish, Sr. VP-Corp. Affairs
Amy Engel, Treas./VP
David I. Greenberg, Chief Compliance Officer/Sr. VP
G. Penn Holsenbeck, Associate General Counsel/Corp. Sec./VP
Michael E. Szymanczyk, CEO/Chmn.-Philip Morris USA, Inc.
John J. Mulligan, Pres./CEO-Phillip Morris Capital Corp.
Louis C. Camilleri, Chmn.
Andre Calantzopoulos, CEO/Pres., Philip Morris Int'l, Inc.

Phone: 917-663-4000	Fax:
Toll-Free:	
Address: 120 Park Ave., New York, NY 10017 US	

GROWTH PLANS/SPECIAL FEATURES:

Altria Group, Inc., formerly Philip Morris Companies, Inc., manufactures and sells cigarettes, foods and beverages. It operates primarily through wholly-owned subsidiaries, Philip Morris USA, Inc. (PMUS) and Philip Morris International, Inc. (PMI). PMUS is the largest cigarette company in the U.S. Its brands include Marlboro (one of the world's top-selling cigarettes, which accounts for one-third of U.S. cigarette sales), Virginia Slims, Benson & Hedges and Parliament. PMI is one of the leading non-U.S. cigarette businesses, with more than 50 manufacturing facilities worldwide. Its affiliates manufacture, market, sell and distribute cigarettes in over 160 countries, and seven of its brands rank among the 20 top-sellers outside of the U.S. PMI's key brands include Marlboro, Bond Street, Chesterfield and Lark. Another subsidiary, Philip Morris Capital Corp., is engaged in building and leasing corporate properties such as office buildings, aircraft, manufacturing facilities and power generation facilities to other corporations. Altria is also the largest shareholder (36%) in SABMiller plc, one of the largest brewers in the world. SABMiller owns and operates the Miller Brewing Company in the U.S. and is one of the largest bottlers and distributors of Coca-Cola products in the world. In 2007, the firm acquired John Middleton, Inc., a leading manufacturer of machine-made cigars. Altria also completed the spin-off of its 88.9% stake in Kraft Foods to Altria shareholders. Kraft Foods is one of the largest food companies in the U.S., with brands including Velveeta, Philadelphia, Oreo, Jell-O, Post, Maxwell House, Oscar Mayer and Kool-aid. Kraft's various branches have operations in 68 countries and sell products in more than 150 countries. In January 2008, the company announced plans to spin off Philip Morris International Inc.

FINANCIALS: Sales and profits are in thousands of dollars—add 000 to get the full amount. 2007 Note: Financial information for 2007 was not available for all companies at press time.

2007 Sales: $73,801,000	2007 Profits: $9,786,000	**U.S. Stock Ticker:** MO
2006 Sales: $67,051,000	2006 Profits: $12,022,000	**Int'l Ticker:** Int'l Exchange:
2005 Sales: $97,854,000	2005 Profits: $10,435,000	Employees: 175,000
2004 Sales: $89,610,000	2004 Profits: $9,416,000	Fiscal Year Ends: 12/31
2003 Sales: $81,832,000	2003 Profits: $9,204,000	Parent Company:

SALARIES/BENEFITS:

Pension Plan:	ESOP Stock Plan:	Profit Sharing:	Top Exec. Salary: $1,750,000	Bonus: $4,500,000
Savings Plan:	Stock Purch. Plan:		Second Exec. Salary: $1,152,000	Bonus: $2,000,000

OTHER THOUGHTS:

Apparent Women Officers or Directors: 2
Hot Spot for Advancement for Women/Minorities: Y

LOCATIONS: ("Y" = Yes)

West:	Southwest:	Midwest:	Southeast:	Northeast:	International:
Y	Y	Y	Y	Y	Y

AMAZON.COM INC
www.amazon.com

Industry Group Code: 451211E **Ranks within this company's industry group:** Sales: 1   Profits: 1

Management:		Sales/Marketing:		Liberal Arts:		Information Systems:		Professionals:		Technical/Scientific:	
Mgmt. Trainees:	Y	Mktg. Professionals:	Y	Gen. Writing/Editing:	Y	Info. Management:	Y	Finance/Accounting:	Y	Engineers, Elec.:	
Experienced Mgmt.:	Y	Retail Sales:	Y	Technical Writing:		Software Dev.:	Y	Law:	Y	Engineers, Other:	
Int'l Business:	Y	Commercial/Industrial:	Y	Graphic Arts/Photog.:	Y	Hardware Dev.:		HR/Other:	Y	Health/Lab:	
MBA Graduates:	Y	Sales Trainees:	Y	Music:		Systems Integration:		Training:	Y	Scientists/Research:	
		Advertising Pros.:	Y	Broadcasting:		Consulting/Other:		Health Care:		Petroleum/Chemicals:	
				Other:	Y			Consulting:		Math/Other:	

TYPES OF BUSINESS:
Online Retail
Online Books & Music Retail
Online Videos/DVDs Retail
Online Electronics Retail
Online Auctions
Online Household Goods Retail
E-Commerce Support & Hosting
Search Engine Technology

BRANDS/DIVISIONS/AFFILIATES:
Amazon Marketplace
Merchants@
A9.com, Inc.
Aexa.com
Fabric.com
IMDb.com
Withoutabox
ABeBooks

CONTACTS: Note: Officers with more than one job title may be intentionally listed here more than once.
Jeffrey P. Bezos, CEO
Jeffrey P. Bezos, Pres.
Thomas J. Szkutak, CFO/Sr. VP
Richard (Rick) Dalzell, CIO/Sr. VP
L. Michelle Wilson, General Counsel/Sr. VP/Sec.
Marc Onetto, Sr. VP-Worldwide Oper.
Jeffrey Blackburn, Sr. VP-Bus. Dev.
H. Brian Valentine, Sr. VP-e-commerce
Shelley Reynolds, VP-Worldwide Controller/Principal Acct. Officer
Sebastian J. Gunningham, Sr. VP-Merchant Svcs.
Andrew Jassy, Sr. VP-Web Svcs.
Steven Kessel, Sr. VP-Worldwide Digital Media
Jeff Wilke, Sr. VP-North American Retail
Jeffrey P. Bezos, Chmn.
Diego Piacentini, Sr. VP-Int'l Retail

Phone: 206-266-2171	Fax: 206-266-1355
Toll-Free:	
Address: 1200 12th Ave. S., Ste. 1200, Seattle, WA 98144-2734 US	

GROWTH PLANS/SPECIAL FEATURES:

Amazon.com, Inc. is an Internet consumer-shopping site which offers millions of new, used, refurbished and collectible items in categories such as apparel, software, consumer electronics, automotive, music, DVDs, pet supplies, office products, tools and books. The company operates several international web sites such as Amazon.co.uk and Amazon.de, serving the U.K. and Germany respectively, as well as sites for Canada, Japan, China and France. A large part of the firm's revenue comes from enabling e-commerce for others. For instance, Amazon manages online sales for Office Depot and Target. The Amazon Marketplace and Merchants@ programs allow third parties to integrate their products on Amazon web sites; allow customers to shop for products owned by third parties using Amazon's features and technologies; and allow customers to complete transactions that include multiple sellers in a single checkout process. Amazon Marketplace serves individuals and small businesses, while the Merchants@ program serves larger companies, primarily concentrating on expanding the selection of new products available on Amazon's web sites. Amazon also provides technology services and other marketing and promotional services, especially through subsidiaries, A9.com and Alexa.com. These sites focus on cutting-edge open search technology, scouring the web for image search results in addition to .html findings. The firm also operates IMDB.com, an international movie database, offering film reviews and other information. In August 2008, the company agreed to acquire AbeBooks. In June 2008, the firm acquired Fabric.com, an online fabric store. Amazon.com announced the acquisition of Audible, Inc. in March 2008. Audible provides spoken audio information and entertainment on the Internet. In January 2008, IMDb.com, a subsidiary of Amazon.com, agreed to acquire Withoutabox, which offers a fully integrated service for submitting films to festivals worldwide and assistance in promoting the films.

Amazon.com offers employees flexible spending accounts, relocation assistance and discount programs. Full-time employees also receive units of restricted stock.

FINANCIALS: Sales and profits are in thousands of dollars—add 000 to get the full amount. 2007 Note: Financial information for 2007 was not available for all companies at press time.

2007 Sales: $14,835,000	2007 Profits: $476,000	**U.S. Stock Ticker: AMZN**
2006 Sales: $10,711,000	2006 Profits: $190,000	**Int'l Ticker:** Int'l Exchange:
2005 Sales: $8,490,000	2005 Profits: $359,000	Employees: 13,900
2004 Sales: $6,921,124	2004 Profits: $588,000	Fiscal Year Ends: 12/31
2003 Sales: $5,263,699	2003 Profits: $35,282	Parent Company:

SALARIES/BENEFITS:

Pension Plan:	ESOP Stock Plan:	Profit Sharing:	Top Exec. Salary: $211,502	Bonus: $
Savings Plan: Y	Stock Purch. Plan: Y		Second Exec. Salary: $175,000	Bonus: $

OTHER THOUGHTS:
Apparent Women Officers or Directors: 4
Hot Spot for Advancement for Women/Minorities: Y

LOCATIONS: ("Y" = Yes)

West:	Southwest:	Midwest:	Southeast:	Northeast:	International:
Y	Y	Y		Y	Y

AMEDISYS INC

www.amedisys.com

Industry Group Code: 621610 Ranks within this company's industry group: Sales: 3 Profits: 3

Management:		Sales/Marketing:		Liberal Arts:		Information Systems:		Professionals:		Technical/Scientific:	
Mgmt. Trainees:		Mktg. Professionals:	Y	Gen. Writing/Editing:		Info. Management:	Y	Finance/Accounting:	Y	Engineers, Elec.:	
Experienced Mgmt.:	Y	Retail Sales:		Technical Writing:	Y	Software Dev.:		Law:	Y	Engineers, Other:	Y
Int'l Business:		Commercial/Industrial:		Graphic Arts/Photog.:		Hardware Dev.:		HR/Other:	Y	Health/Lab:	
MBA Graduates:	Y	Sales Trainees:		Music:		Systems Integration:		Training:	Y	Scientists/Research:	
		Advertising Pros.:	Y	Broadcasting:		Consulting/Other:		Health Care:	Y	Petroleum/Chemicals:	
				Other:				Consulting:		Math/Other:	

TYPES OF BUSINESS:

Home Health Care
Home Health Care
Hospice Care

BRANDS/DIVISIONS/AFFILIATES:

Partners in Wound Care Program
Heart @ Home
Diabetes @ Home
Rehab Therapy @ Home
Wound Care - A Therapy Approach
Orthopedic Recovery @ Home
Stroke Recovery @ Home
Pain Management @ Home

CONTACTS: Note: Officers with more than one job title may be intentionally listed here more than once.

William F. Borne, CEO
Larry R. Graham, COO
Larry R. Graham, Pres.
Dale E. Redman, Interim CFO
Patty Graham, Sr. VP-Mktg.
Cindy Phillips, Sr. VP-Human Resources
Alice Ann Schwartz, CIO
Jeffrey D. Jeter, Corporate Counsel/Chief Compliance Officer
Jill Cannon, Sr. VP-Oper.
John R. Nugent, Chief Dev. Officer
Tom Dolan, Sr. VP-Finance
Beth Boulet, VP-Audit
Janet Britt, Sr. VP-Billing/Collections
Thomas Fisher, Sr. VP-MIS
Scott Ginn, Sr. VP-Acct./Treas.
William F. Borne, Chmn.
Francis Mayer, Sr. VP-Contracting

Phone: 225-292-2031	Fax: 225-295-8163
Toll-Free: 800-467-2662	
Address: 5959 South Sherwood Forest Blvd., Baton Rouge, LA 70816 US	

GROWTH PLANS/SPECIAL FEATURES:

Amedisys, Inc. provides services on a multi-state basis which include both home health and hospice services with over 8,900 employees and approximately 89% of the firm's revenue derived from Medicare. As of December 2007, the firm owned and operated 325 Medicare-certified home health agencies, 29 Medicare-certified hospice agencies and managed the operations of four Medicare-certified home health and two Medicare-certified hospice agencies in 30 states. The company's services include skilled nursing; home health aides, physical therapy, occupational therapy, speech therapy, medical social workers, hospice care cardiac and diabetes care, oncology and psychiatric services. In December 2007, the company announced the acquisition of six home health agencies located in Georgia and South Carolina from Memorial Health University Medical Center of Savannah, Georgia. Amedisys also announced the acquisition of a home health agency in Carolina, Puerto Rico. In March 2008, the firm acquired TLC Health Care Services, Inc., a provider of home nursing and hospice services with 93 home health and 11 hospice agencies located in 22 states and Washington, D.C. for $395 million. In June 2008, Amedisys entered into a $43 million agreement to acquire the holding company that operates Family Home Health Care, Inc. and Comprehensive Home Healthcare Services, Inc. The two businesses operate home health locations in Kentucky and Tennessee. The company also announced in June 2008 that it had acquired five home health locations from Health Management Associates, Inc.

Amedisys offers employees a benefits package which includes a 401(K) plan, medical, dental and vision insurance, supplemental life insurance, supplemental cancer insurance, flexible spending account, stock purchase plan, tuition reimbursement, employee assistance program and paid vacation.

FINANCIALS: Sales and profits are in thousands of dollars—add 000 to get the full amount. 2007 Note: Financial information for 2007 was not available for all companies at press time.

2007 Sales: $697,934	2007 Profits: $65,113	U.S. Stock Ticker: AMED
2006 Sales: $541,148	2006 Profits: $38,255	Int'l Ticker: Int'l Exchange:
2005 Sales: $381,558	2005 Profits: $30,102	Employees: 6,892
2004 Sales: $227,100	2004 Profits: $20,500	Fiscal Year Ends: 12/31
2003 Sales: $142,500	2003 Profits: $84,800	Parent Company:

SALARIES/BENEFITS:

Pension Plan:	ESOP Stock Plan:	Profit Sharing:	Top Exec. Salary: $396,153	Bonus: $
Savings Plan: Y	Stock Purch. Plan: Y		Second Exec. Salary: $315,230	Bonus: $

OTHER THOUGHTS:

Apparent Women Officers or Directors: 7
Hot Spot for Advancement for Women/Minorities: Y

LOCATIONS: ("Y" = Yes)

West:	Southwest:	Midwest:	Southeast:	Northeast:	International:
	Y	Y	Y	Y	

AMERICAN EAGLE OUTFITTERS INC
www.ae.com

Industry Group Code: 448000 Ranks within this company's industry group: Sales: 4 Profits: 3

Management:		Sales/Marketing:		Liberal Arts:		Information Systems:		Professionals:		Technical/Scientific:	
Mgmt. Trainees:	Y	Mktg. Professionals:	Y	Gen. Writing/Editing:	Y	Info. Management:	Y	Finance/Accounting:	Y	Engineers, Elec.:	
Experienced Mgmt.:	Y	Retail Sales:	Y	Technical Writing:		Software Dev.:	Y	Law:	Y	Engineers, Other:	
Int'l Business:	Y	Commercial/Industrial:	Y	Graphic Arts/Photog.:	Y	Hardware Dev.:		HR/Other:	Y	Health/Lab:	
MBA Graduates:	Y	Sales Trainees:	Y	Music:		Systems Integration:		Training:	Y	Scientists/Research:	
		Advertising Pros.:	Y	Broadcasting:		Consulting/Other:		Health Care:		Petroleum/Chemicals:	
				Other:	Y			Consulting:		Math/Other:	

TYPES OF BUSINESS:
Casual Apparel, Retail
Online Sales
Intimates Apparel
Online Music Sales

BRANDS/DIVISIONS/AFFILIATES:
AE
aerie by American Eagle
MARTIN + OSA
77kids
ae.com
aerie.com
martinandosa.com

CONTACTS: Note: Officers with more than one job title may be intentionally listed here more than once.
James V. O'Donnell, CEO
Susan P. McGalla, Pres.
Joan Holstein Hilson, CFO/Exec. VP
Katherine J. Savitt, Chief Mktg. Officer/Exec. VP
Thomas A. DiDonato, Exec. VP-Human Resources
Susan P. McGalla, Chief Merch. Officer
Joseph E. Kerin, Exec. VP/Dir.-Store Oper.
Roger S. Markfield, Vice Chmn.
Dennis R. Parodi, Exec. VP/COO-NY Design Center
LeAnn Nealz, Chief Design Officer/Exec. VP
Jay L. Schottenstein, Chmn.

Phone: 412-432-3300	Fax: 724-776-6160
Toll-Free:	
Address: 77 Hot Metal St., Pittsburgh, PA 15203 US	

GROWTH PLANS/SPECIAL FEATURES:

American Eagle Outfitters, Inc. (AE) designs, markets and retails clothing targeting 15 to 25 year olds under the American Eagle Outfitters, aerie by American Eagle (aerie) and MARTIN + OSA brands. AE operates approximately 929 American Eagle Outfitters stores in the U.S. and Canada; 39 aerie stand-alone stores; and 19 MARTIN + OSA stores. The firm also operates ae.com, its retail website featuring an expanded offering of sizes, colors and styles of its merchandise. AE's aerie collection includes bras, underwear, camis, hoodies, robes, boxers, sweats, leggings, fitness apparel and personal care products and is sold through stand-alone aerie stores, most America Eagle Outfitters stores and at aerie.com. MARTIN + OSA sells clothing and accessories targeting 28 to 40 year old women and men. During 2007, the company opened 80 new stores, consisting of 27 U.S. AE stores, three Canadian AE stores, 36 aerie stores (including one Canadian aerie store) and 14 MARTIN + OSA stores. AE stores average approximately 3,500 to 4,500 gross square feet. In January 2008, the company announced plans to launch a new children's apparel brand, 77kids, which will provide clothing and accessories for children ages two to 10. The firm plans to begin opening 77kids stores in the U.S. during 2010. In April 2008, AE launched its e-commerce web site for MARTIN + OSA, martinandosa.com.

AE offers its employees merchandise discounts and medical, dental, life and disability insurance.

FINANCIALS: Sales and profits are in thousands of dollars—add 000 to get the full amount. 2007 Note: Financial information for 2007 was not available for all companies at press time.

2007 Sales: $2,794,409	2007 Profits: $387,359	U.S. Stock Ticker: AEO
2006 Sales: $2,321,962	2006 Profits: $294,153	Int'l Ticker: Int'l Exchange:
2005 Sales: $1,889,647	2005 Profits: $213,300	Employees: 27,600
2004 Sales: $1,519,968	2004 Profits: $60,000	Fiscal Year Ends: 1/31
2003 Sales: $1,463,100	2003 Profits: $88,700	Parent Company:

SALARIES/BENEFITS:

Pension Plan:	ESOP Stock Plan:	Profit Sharing: Y	Top Exec. Salary: $1,019,231	Bonus: $3,741,372
Savings Plan: Y	Stock Purch. Plan: Y		Second Exec. Salary: $866,346	Bonus: $2,384,744

OTHER THOUGHTS:
Apparent Women Officers or Directors: 5
Hot Spot for Advancement for Women/Minorities: Y

LOCATIONS: ("Y" = Yes)

West:	Southwest:	Midwest:	Southeast:	Northeast:	International:
Y	Y	Y	Y	Y	Y

Note: Financial information, benefits and other data can change quickly and may vary from those stated here.

AMERICAN ELECTRIC POWER COMPANY INC (AEP)

www.aep.com

Industry Group Code: 221000A Ranks within this company's industry group: Sales:　Profits:

Management:		Sales/Marketing:		Liberal Arts:		Information Systems:		Professionals:		Technical/Scientific:	
Mgmt. Trainees:	Y	Mktg. Professionals:	Y	Gen. Writing/Editing:	Y	Info. Management:	Y	Finance/Accounting:	Y	Engineers, Elec.:	Y
Experienced Mgmt.:	Y	Retail Sales:		Technical Writing:		Software Dev.:	Y	Law:	Y	Engineers, Other:	
Int'l Business:	Y	Commercial/Industrial:	Y	Graphic Arts/Photog.:		Hardware Dev.:		HR/Other:	Y	Health/Lab:	Y
MBA Graduates:	Y	Sales Trainees:		Music:		Systems Integration:		Training:	Y	Scientists/Research:	Y
		Advertising Pros.:	Y	Broadcasting:		Consulting/Other:		Health Care:		Petroleum/Chemicals:	
				Other:				Consulting:		Math/Other:	Y

TYPES OF BUSINESS:

Utilities-Electricity
Natural Gas Power Generation
Nuclear Power Generation
Coal Transport-Barge & Rail
Energy Trading
Coal Power Generation

BRANDS/DIVISIONS/AFFILIATES:

AEP Ohio
AEP Texas
Appalachian Power
Indiana Michigan Power
Kentucky Power
Public Service Company of Oklahoma
Southwestern Electric Power Company
MEMCO Barge Line, Inc.

CONTACTS: Note: Officers with more than one job title may be intentionally listed here more than once.

Michael G. Morris, CEO
Carl English, COO
Robert P. Powers, Pres.
Holly Koeppel, CFO/Exec. VP
Stephen P. Smith, Sr. VP-Human Resources
Kevin Walker, CIO
Barbara Radous, Sr. VP-Commercial Oper.
Dale Heydlauff, VP-Corp. Comm.
Charles E. Zebula, Treas./Sr. VP
Robert Powers, Pres., AEP Utilities
Susan Tomasky, Pres., AEP Transmission
Venita McCellon-Allen, Exec. VP-AEP Utilities West
Brian Tierney, Exec. VP-AEP Utilities East
Michael G. Morris, Chmn.
Stephen P. Smith, Sr. VP-Bus. Logistics & IT

Phone: 614-716-1000	Fax: 614-716-1823
Toll-Free:	
Address: 1 Riverside Plz., Columbus, OH 43215-2372 US	

GROWTH PLANS/SPECIAL FEATURES:

American Electric Power Company, Inc. (AEP) serves 5 million customers through eight utility units: AEP Ohio, AEP Texas; Appalachian Power; AEP Appalachian Power; Indiana Michigan Power; Kentucky Power; Public Service Company of Oklahoma; and Southwestern Electric Power Company.　AEP's generating and transmission facilities comprise a 39,000-mile network spanning 11 states.　The company's transmission system serves roughly 10% of the electrical demand in the Eastern Interconnection in the U.S. and eastern Canada; and approximately 11% of the electrical demand for Electric Reliability Council of Texas. AEP owns approximately 80 generating stations in the U.S., with 73% based on coal, 16% natural gas and 8% nuclear. Through MEMCO Barge Line, Inc., the company transports coal by rail car, barge and tugboat. AEP has interests in two terminal facilities: the Cook Coal Terminal on the Ohio River and the International Marine Terminal in New Orleans. In September 2007, the company signed a long-term power purchase agreement for renewable wind energy with Camp Grove Wind Farm LLC; and purchased a natural gas-fired power plant near Dresden, Ohio, from Dresden Energy. In October 2007, the company sold its 50% interest in the Sweeny Cogeneration plant (Texas) to ConocoPhillips for approximately $80 million. In December 2007, AEP entered a joint venture with MidAmerican Energy Holdings Co. to establish Electric Transmission Texas, LLC. In 2008, the firm plans to build plants and transmissions in West Virginia, Arkansas and Kansas. In February 2008, the firm sold four inactive plants in Texas. In July 2008, the joint venture between AEP and MidAmerican Energy Holdings, formed a joint venture company with OGE Energy Corp. In August 2008, the firm formed a joint venture with Duke Energy to build new electric transmission assets.

FINANCIALS: Sales and profits are in thousands of dollars—add 000 to get the full amount. 2007 Note: Financial information for 2007 was not available for all companies at press time.

2007 Sales: $13,380,000	2007 Profits: $1,089,000	**U.S. Stock Ticker: AEP**
2006 Sales: $12,622,000	2006 Profits: $1,002,000	**Int'l Ticker:** Int'l Exchange:
2005 Sales: $12,111,000	2005 Profits: $814,000	Employees: 19,630
2004 Sales: $14,245,000	2004 Profits: $1,089,000	Fiscal Year Ends: 12/31
2003 Sales: $14,833,000	2003 Profits: $110,000	Parent Company:

SALARIES/BENEFITS:

Pension Plan:	ESOP Stock Plan:	Profit Sharing:	Top Exec. Salary: $1,200,000	Bonus: $2,200,000
Savings Plan: Y	Stock Purch. Plan:		Second Exec. Salary: $500,000	Bonus: $510,000

OTHER THOUGHTS:

Apparent Women Officers or Directors: 5
Hot Spot for Advancement for Women/Minorities: Y

LOCATIONS: ("Y" = Yes)

West:	Southwest:	Midwest:	Southeast:	Northeast:	International:
	Y	Y	Y	Y	

AMERICAN EXPRESS CO

www.americanexpress.com

Industry Group Code: 522210 Ranks within this company's industry group: Sales: 1 Profits: 1

Management:		Sales/Marketing:		Liberal Arts:		Information Systems:		Professionals:		Technical/Scientific:	
Mgmt. Trainees:	Y	Mktg. Professionals:	Y	Gen. Writing/Editing:	Y	Info. Management:	Y	Finance/Accounting:	Y	Engineers, Elec.:	
Experienced Mgmt.:	Y	Retail Sales:		Technical Writing:		Software Dev.:	Y	Law:	Y	Engineers, Other:	
Int'l Business:	Y	Commercial/Industrial:	Y	Graphic Arts/Photog.:	Y	Hardware Dev.:		HR/Other:	Y	Health/Lab:	
MBA Graduates:	Y	Sales Trainees:	Y	Music:		Systems Integration:		Training:	Y	Scientists/Research:	
		Advertising Pros.:	Y	Broadcasting:		Consulting/Other:		Health Care:		Petroleum/Chemicals:	
				Other:				Consulting:		Math/Other:	

TYPES OF BUSINESS:

Credit Card Issuing
Travel-Related Services
Lending & Financing
Transaction Services
Point-of-Sale Systems
International Banking Services
Expense Management
Magazine Publishing

BRANDS/DIVISIONS/AFFILIATES:

American Express Travel Related Services Company
American Express Publishing Corporation
Food & Wine
Travel+Leisure
OPEN: The Small Business Network
Ameriprise Financial, Inc.
American Express Business Travel
Farrington American Express Travel Services Ltd.

CONTACTS: Note: Officers with more than one job title may be intentionally listed here more than once.

Kenneth I. Chenault, CEO
Alfred F. Kelly, Jr., Pres.
Daniel Henry, CFO/Exec. VP
John D. Hayes, Chief Mktg. Officer/Exec. VP-Global Advertising
L. Kevin Cox, Exec. VP-Human Resources & Quality
Stephen Squeri, CIO/Exec. VP
Louise M. Parent, General Counsel/Exec. VP
Thomas Schick, Exec. VP-Corp. Affairs & Comm.
Edward P. Gilligan, Group CEO-Business-to-Business
Ahswini Gupta, Pres., Risk, Info. Mgmt. & Banking Group
Judson C. Linville, CEO/Pres., Consumer Services
William H. Glenn, Pres., Global Establishment Svcs./Global Merchant
Kenneth I. Chenault, Chmn.
Douglas E. Buckminster, Pres., Int'l Consumer

Phone: 212-640-2000	Fax: 212-619-9802
Toll-Free:	
Address: World Financial Ctr., 200 Vesey St., New York, NY 10285 US	

GROWTH PLANS/SPECIAL FEATURES:

American Express Co. (AmEx) provides travel-related services, credit cards and international banking services. During 2007, the company reorganized their businesses into two customer-focused groups—the Global Consumer Group and the Global Business-to-Business Group. U.S. Card Services and International Card Services are aligned within the Global Consumer Group and Global Commercial Services and Global Network & Merchant Services are aligned within the Global Business-to-Business Group. The Global Consumer Group generates revenue and provides products and services including: credit cards for consumers and small businesses globally, travel services for consumers and stored value products, such as gift cards or Travelers Cheques. The Global Business-to-Business Group provides similar products services for businesses across the world, such as business travel services, corporate and expense management cards and services, network services and merchant services. American Express cards, the firm's most notable product, are issued in over 40 currencies and enable card members to purchase goods and services worldwide. The company has a wholesale travel business in the U.S. through subsidiary Travel Impressions. Another division, American Express Publishing, operates several leading magazines for affluent readers, including Food & Wine and Travel+Leisure. In July 2007, American Express Business Travel completed the acquisition of Farrington American Express Travel Services Limited in Hong Kong. In February 2008, the firm sold its international banking operations, American Express Bank Ltd., to Standard Chartered PLC for $823 million, and entered into an agreement that will allow Standard Chartered to purchase American Express International Deposit Company in 2009.

For its U.S. employees, AmEx provides health care plans; a life and disability insurance plan; travel discounts; and assistance programs covering legal advice, adoption, education and personal issues.

FINANCIALS: Sales and profits are in thousands of dollars—add 000 to get the full amount. 2007 Note: Financial information for 2007 was not available for all companies at press time.

2007 Sales: $27,731,000	2007 Profits: $4,012,000	**U.S. Stock Ticker:** AXP
2006 Sales: $25,154,000	2006 Profits: $3,707,000	**Int'l Ticker:** Int'l Exchange:
2005 Sales: $24,300,000	2005 Profits: $3,734,000	Employees: 67,700
2004 Sales: $22,000,000	2004 Profits: $3,445,000	Fiscal Year Ends: 12/31
2003 Sales: $25,866,000	2003 Profits: $2,987,000	Parent Company:

SALARIES/BENEFITS:

Pension Plan:	ESOP Stock Plan:	Profit Sharing: Y	Top Exec. Salary: $1,238,461	Bonus: $6,500,000
Savings Plan: Y	Stock Purch. Plan:		Second Exec. Salary: $771,154	Bonus: $5,039,500

OTHER THOUGHTS:

Apparent Women Officers or Directors: 5
Hot Spot for Advancement for Women/Minorities: Y

LOCATIONS: ("Y" = Yes)

West:	Southwest:	Midwest:	Southeast:	Northeast:	International:
Y	Y	Y	Y	Y	Y

Note: Financial information, benefits and other data can change quickly and may vary from those stated here.

AMERICAN POWER CONVERSION CORP   www.apcc.com

Industry Group Code: 335910 Ranks within this company's industry group: Sales: Profits:

Management:		Sales/Marketing:		Liberal Arts:		Information Systems:		Professionals:		Technical/Scientific:	
Mgmt. Trainees:	Y	Mktg. Professionals:	Y	Gen. Writing/Editing:		Info. Management:	Y	Finance/Accounting:	Y	Engineers, Elec.:	Y
Experienced Mgmt.:	Y	Retail Sales:		Technical Writing:	Y	Software Dev.:	Y	Law:	Y	Engineers, Other:	Y
Int'l Business:		Commercial/Industrial:	Y	Graphic Arts/Photog.:	Y	Hardware Dev.:	Y	HR/Other:	Y	Health/Lab:	
MBA Graduates:	Y	Sales Trainees:		Music:		Systems Integration:		Training:	Y	Scientists/Research:	Y
		Advertising Pros.:	Y	Broadcasting:		Consulting/Other:	Y	Health Care:		Petroleum/Chemicals:	
				Other:				Consulting:	Y	Math/Other:	

TYPES OF BUSINESS:
Back-Up Power Supplies
Power Protection & Management Products
Consulting Services
PC Accessories
Power Management Software

BRANDS/DIVISIONS/AFFILIATES:
InfraStruXure
Mobile Power Pack
Smart-UPS
SureArrest
PowerChute
NetworkAIR
Silcon UPS
Schneider Electric SA

CONTACTS: Note: Officers with more than one job title may be intentionally listed here more than once.
Laurent Vernerey, CEO
Laurent Vernerey, Pres.
Herve Coureil, CFO
Aaron Davis, Chief Mktg. Officer
Kevin Roche, Sr. VP-Human Resources
Jim Simonelli, CTO
Ed Machala, Sr. VP-Mfg.
Nei Rasmussen, Chief Innovation Officer
Chun Lauener, Pres., Greater China
Jean-Marc Lang, Sr. VP-Customer Care, Quality & Bus. Processes
Dave Guidette, Sr. VP-Enterprise Sys. & Svc.
Daniel Doimo, Pres., Europe, Middle East, Africa & Latin America
Ed Machala, Sr. VP-Supply Chain & Purchasing

Phone: 401-789-5735	**Fax:** 401-789-3710
Toll-Free: 800-788-2208	
Address: 132 Fairgrounds Rd., West Kingston, RI 02892 US	

GROWTH PLANS/SPECIAL FEATURES:

American Power Conversion Corp. (APC), a subsidiary of Schneider Electric SA, designs, develops, manufactures and markets power protection and management solutions for computer, communications and electronic applications worldwide. The company's products include uninterruptible power supply products, commonly known as UPSs; electrical surge protection devices; power distribution products; precision cooling equipment; power management software and accessories; racks and enclosures; and various desktop and notebook personal computer accessories. These products are primarily used with sensitive electronic devices which rely on electric utility power, such as home electronics, PCs, high-performance computer workstations, servers, networking equipment, communications equipment, Internet equipment, data centers, mainframe computers and facilities. APC's UPS products regulate the flow of utility power to the protected equipment and provide seamless back-up power during utility power interruptions. The back-up power lasts for enough time to continue computer operations, conduct an orderly shutdown, preserve data, work through short power outages or, in some cases, continue operating for several hours or longer. The company's security and environmental appliances and accessories protect against environmental or human threats and monitor valuable systems with sensors, cameras and accessories. APC's precision cooling equipment regulates temperature and humidity. In addition, the company provides power management software, consulting services and notebook and PC accessories. In 2008, APC introduced its Fuel Cell Extended Run (FCXR) product that provides hydrogen-based power backup for the firm's InfraStruXure power, cooling, environmental monitoring and management data center for modular and mobile configurations. The firm also launched an AV In-Wall Power Filter and Connection Kit designed to protect home theater components such as wall mounted TVs and ceiling mounted projectors. In 2007, the company was acquired by Schneider Electric for $6.1 billion.

APC offers employees comprehensive health coverage as well as other benefits, including flexible spending accounts, tuition assistance and a relocation program.

FINANCIALS: Sales and profits are in thousands of dollars—add 000 to get the full amount. 2007 Note: Financial information for 2007 was not available for all companies at press time.

2007 Sales: $	2007 Profits: $	**U.S. Stock Ticker: Subsidiary**
2006 Sales: $	2006 Profits: $	**Int'l Ticker:** Int'l Exchange:
2005 Sales: $1,979,532	2005 Profits: $144,081	Employees:
2004 Sales: $1,699,900	2004 Profits: $181,500	Fiscal Year Ends: 12/31
2003 Sales: $1,464,798	2003 Profits: $176,938	Parent Company: SCHNEIDER ELECTRIC SA

SALARIES/BENEFITS:

Pension Plan:	ESOP Stock Plan:	Profit Sharing:	Top Exec. Salary: $896,538	Bonus: $230,019
Savings Plan: Y	Stock Purch. Plan: Y		Second Exec. Salary: $470,596	Bonus: $122,158

OTHER THOUGHTS:
Apparent Women Officers or Directors: 1
Hot Spot for Advancement for Women/Minorities:

LOCATIONS: ("Y" = Yes)

West:	Southwest:	Midwest:	Southeast:	Northeast:	International:
	Y	Y	Y	Y	Y

Note: Financial information, benefits and other data can change quickly and may vary from those stated here.

AMERISOURCEBERGEN CORP www.amerisourcebergen.com

Industry Group Code: 422210 Ranks within this company's industry group: Sales: Profits:

Management:		Sales/Marketing:		Liberal Arts:		Information Systems:		Professionals:		Technical/Scientific:	
Mgmt. Trainees:	Y	Mktg. Professionals:	Y	Gen. Writing/Editing:	Y	Info. Management:	Y	Finance/Accounting:	Y	Engineers, Elec.:	
Experienced Mgmt.:	Y	Retail Sales:		Technical Writing:	Y	Software Dev.:	Y	Law:	Y	Engineers, Other:	
Int'l Business:	Y	Commercial/Industrial:	Y	Graphic Arts/Photog.:	Y	Hardware Dev.:		HR/Other:	Y	Health/Lab:	
MBA Graduates:	Y	Sales Trainees:	Y	Music:		Systems Integration:		Training:	Y	Scientists/Research:	
		Advertising Pros.:	Y	Broadcasting:		Consulting/Other:		Health Care:	Y	Petroleum/Chemicals:	
				Other:				Consulting:	Y	Math/Other:	

TYPES OF BUSINESS:

Drug Distribution
Pharmacy Management & Consulting Services
Packaging Solutions
Information Technology
Healthcare Equipment

BRANDS/DIVISIONS/AFFILIATES:

AmerisourceBergen Drug Corp.
AmerisourceBergen Specialty Group
AmerisourceBergen Packaging Group
American Health Packaging
Anderson Packaging
Brecon Pharmaceutical, Ltd.
Kindred Healthcare, Inc.
PharMerica Corporation

CONTACTS: Note: Officers with more than one job title may be intentionally listed here more than once.

R. David Yost, CEO
R. David Yost, Pres.
Michael D. DiCandilo, CFO/Exec. VP
David W. Neu, Sr. VP-Retail Sales & Mktg.
Jeanne Fisher, Sr. VP-Human Resources
Thomas H. Murphy, CIO/Sr. VP
John G. Chou, General Counsel/Sr. VP/Sec.
David M. Senior, Sr. VP-Strategy & Corp. Dev.
Michael Kilpatric, VP, Corp & Investor Rel.
J.F. Quinn, Treas./VP
Steven H. Collis, Exec. VP/Pres., AmerisourceBergen Specialty Group
Terrance P. Hass, Exec. VP/Chief Integration Officer
John Palumbo, Sr. VP-Health Systems Solutions
Tim G. Guttman, Corp. Controller/VP
Richard C. Gozon, Chmn.
Len DeCandia, Sr. VP-Supply Chain Mgmt.

Phone: 610-727-7000	Fax: 610-727-3600
Toll-Free: 800-829-3132	
Address: 1300 Morris Dr., Ste. 100, Chesterbrook, PA 19087 US	

GROWTH PLANS/SPECIAL FEATURES:

AmerisourceBergen Corp is one of the largest wholesale distributors of pharmaceutical products and services to a wide variety of healthcare providers and pharmacies. The firm offers brand name and generic pharmaceuticals, supplies and equipment and serves the United States, Canada and selected global markets. Operations are comprised of two reportable segments: Pharmaceutical Distribution and Other. Included in the Other segment is Long-Term Care which is a leading national dispenser of pharmaceutical products and services to long-term care and alternate healthcare facilities. The Pharmaceutical Distribution segment is currently comprised of four operating segments, which includes the operations of the AmerisourceBergen Drug Corporation (ABDC), the AmerisourceBergen Specialty Group (ABSG), Bellco Health (Bellco), and the AmerisourceBergen Packaging Group (ABPG). Servicing both healthcare providers and pharmaceutical manufacturers in the pharmaceutical supply channel, the Pharmaceutical Distribution segment's operations provide drug distribution and related services designed to reduce healthcare costs and improve patient outcomes. ABDC also provides pharmacy management, staffing and other consulting services, scalable automated pharmacy dispensing equipment, medication and supply dispensing cabinets, and supply management software to a variety of retail and institutional healthcare providers.The company excluded quarterly reporting of PMSI from its Other segment August 2008. The company agreed to sell PMSI for approximately $40 million and expects to complete the transaction by September 2008. In connection with these efforts, in May 2008, the company announced a more streamlined organizational structure in order to increase efficiency and reduce operating costs. In October 2007, the company acquired Bellco Health, a distributor of pharmaceuticals to retail pharmacies and clinics. Bellco's revenues were 2.1 billion for fiscal year 2007.

The company offers its employees medical, dental and vision insurance; a 401(k) plan; short- and long-term disability insurance; quartly reward plan, employee stock purchase plan; tuition reimbursement; and an employee assistance program.

FINANCIALS: Sales and profits are in thousands of dollars—add 000 to get the full amount. 2007 Note: Financial information for 2007 was not available for all companies at press time.

		U.S. Stock Ticker: ABC
2007 Sales: $66,074,312	2007 Profits: $469,167	Int'l Ticker: Int'l Exchange:
2006 Sales: $61,203,145	2006 Profits: $467,714	Employees: 14,700
2005 Sales: $54,577,300	2005 Profits: $264,645	Fiscal Year Ends: 9/30
2004 Sales: $53,178,954	2004 Profits: $468,390	Parent Company:
2003 Sales: $49,657,300	2003 Profits: $441,200	

SALARIES/BENEFITS:

Pension Plan:	ESOP Stock Plan:	Profit Sharing:	Top Exec. Salary: $1,081,718	Bonus: $1,585,479
Savings Plan: Y	Stock Purch. Plan: Y		Second Exec. Salary: $647,116	Bonus: $869,440

OTHER THOUGHTS:

Apparent Women Officers or Directors: 2
Hot Spot for Advancement for Women/Minorities:

LOCATIONS: ("Y" = Yes)

West:	Southwest:	Midwest:	Southeast:	Northeast:	International:
Y	Y	Y	Y	Y	

AMGEN INC

www.amgen.com

Industry Group Code: 325412 Ranks within this company's industry group: Sales: 3 Profits: 2

Management:		Sales/Marketing:		Liberal Arts:		Information Systems:		Professionals:		Technical/Scientific:	
Mgmt. Trainees:	Y	Mktg. Professionals:	Y	Gen. Writing/Editing:	Y	Info. Management:	Y	Finance/Accounting:	Y	Engineers, Elec.:	Y
Experienced Mgmt.:	Y	Retail Sales:		Technical Writing:	Y	Software Dev.:	Y	Law:	Y	Engineers, Other:	Y
Int'l Business:	Y	Commercial/Industrial:	Y	Graphic Arts/Photog.:	Y	Hardware Dev.:		HR/Other:	Y	Health/Lab:	Y
MBA Graduates:	Y	Sales Trainees:	Y	Music:		Systems Integration:		Training:	Y	Scientists/Research:	Y
		Advertising Pros.:	Y	Broadcasting:		Consulting/Other:		Health Care:	Y	Petroleum/Chemicals:	
				Other:				Consulting:		Math/Other:	Y

TYPES OF BUSINESS:

Drugs-Diversified
Oncology Drugs
Nephrology Drugs
Inflammation Drugs
Neurology Drugs
Metabolic Drugs

BRANDS/DIVISIONS/AFFILIATES:

Aranesp
EPOGEN
Neulasta
NEUPOGEN
Enbrel
Alantos
Ilypsa

CONTACTS: Note: Officers with more than one job title may be intentionally listed here more than once.

Kevin W. Sharer, CEO
Kevin W. Sharer, Pres.
Robert A. Bradway, CFO/Exec. VP
Brian McNamee, Sr. VP-Human Resources
Roger M. Perlmutter, Exec. VP-R&D
Thomas J. (Tom) Flanagan, CIO/Sr. VP
David J. Scott, General Counsel/Sr. VP/Corp. Sec.
Fabrizio Bonanni, Exec. VP-Oper.
George J. Morrow, Exec. VP-Global Commercial Oper.
Kevin W. Sharer, Chmn.

Phone: 805-447-1000	Fax: 805-447-1010
Toll-Free:	
Address: 1 Amgen Center Dr., Thousand Oaks, CA 91320-1799 US	

GROWTH PLANS/SPECIAL FEATURES:

Amgen, Inc. is a global biotechnology company that develops, manufactures and markets human therapeutics based on cellular and molecular biology. Its products are used for treatment in the fields of supportive cancer care, nephrology, inflammation and oncology. Amgen's primary products include Aranesp, EPOGEN, Neulasta, NEUPOGEN and Enbrel, which together represent 95% of the company's sales. Aranesp and EPOGEN stimulate the production of red blood cells to treat anemia and belong to a class of drugs referred to as erythropoiesis-stimulating agents. Aranesp is used for the treatment of anemia both in supportive cancer care and in nephrology. EPOGEN is used to treat anemia associated with chronic renal failure. Neulasta and NEUPOGEN selectively stimulate the production of neutrophils, one type of white blood cell that helps the body fight infections. ENBREL inhibits tumor necrosis factor (TNF), a substance induced in response to inflammatory and immunological responses, such as rheumatoid arthritis and psoriasis. Amgen maintains sales and marketing forces primarily in the U.S., Europe and Canada, and markets its products to healthcare providers including physicians, dialysis centers, hospitals and pharmacies. Amgen focuses its research and development efforts in the core areas of oncology, inflammation, bone and metabolic disorders, taking a modality-independent approach to drug discovery by choosing the best possible approach to block a specific disease process before considering the type of drug that may be required to pursue that approach. In July 2007, Amgen acquired Alantos, a developer of drugs for the treatment of diabetes and inflammatory disease; and Ilypsa, a developer of non-absorbed drugs for renal disorders. In August 2007, the firm announced a restructuring plan that will slash staff by 14% and capital expenses by $1.9 billion.

Amgen offers its employees an education reimbursement plan, a Long Term Incentive program and medical, prescription, vision and dental benefits.

FINANCIALS: Sales and profits are in thousands of dollars—add 000 to get the full amount. 2007 Note: Financial information for 2007 was not available for all companies at press time.

2007 Sales: $14,771,000	2007 Profits: $3,166,000	**U.S. Stock Ticker:** AMGN
2006 Sales: $14,268,000	2006 Profits: $2,950,000	**Int'l Ticker:** Int'l Exchange:
2005 Sales: $12,430,000	2005 Profits: $3,674,000	Employees: 20,100
2004 Sales: $10,550,000	2004 Profits: $2,363,000	Fiscal Year Ends: 12/31
2003 Sales: $8,356,000	2003 Profits: $2,259,500	Parent Company:

SALARIES/BENEFITS:

Pension Plan: Y	ESOP Stock Plan:	Profit Sharing:	Top Exec. Salary: $1,482,692	Bonus: $4,525,000
Savings Plan: Y	Stock Purch. Plan: Y		Second Exec. Salary: $928,596	Bonus: $1,720,000

OTHER THOUGHTS:

Apparent Women Officers or Directors: 1
Hot Spot for Advancement for Women/Minorities: Y

LOCATIONS: ("Y" = Yes)

West:	Southwest:	Midwest:	Southeast:	Northeast:	International:
Y			Y	Y	Y

ANADARKO PETROLEUM CORPORATION www.anadarko.com

Industry Group Code: 211111 Ranks within this company's industry group: Sales: Profits:

Management:		Sales/Marketing:		Liberal Arts:		Information Systems:		Professionals:		Technical/Scientific:	
Mgmt. Trainees:	Y	Mktg. Professionals:	Y	Gen. Writing/Editing:		Info. Management:	Y	Finance/Accounting:	Y	Engineers, Elec.:	Y
Experienced Mgmt.:	Y	Retail Sales:		Technical Writing:	Y	Software Dev.:	Y	Law:	Y	Engineers, Other:	
Int'l Business:	Y	Commercial/Industrial:	Y	Graphic Arts/Photog.:		Hardware Dev.:		HR/Other:	Y	Health/Lab:	Y
MBA Graduates:	Y	Sales Trainees:		Music:		Systems Integration:		Training:	Y	Scientists/Research:	Y
		Advertising Pros.:		Broadcasting:		Consulting/Other:		Health Care:		Petroleum/Chemicals:	Y
				Other:				Consulting:		Math/Other:	Y

TYPES OF BUSINESS:

Oil & Gas Exploration & Production
Field Services
Drilling Technology
Mineral Exploration
Coal-Bed Methane Production

BRANDS/DIVISIONS/AFFILIATES:

Anadarko Energy Services Company
Anadarko Land Corp.
Anadarko Algeria Company LLC
Headwater LLC
Howell Petroleum Corporation
Kerr-McGee Corporation
Western Gas Resources

CONTACTS: *Note: Officers with more than one job title may be intentionally listed here more than once.*

James T. Hackett, CEO
Karl F. Kurz, COO
James T. Hackett, Pres.
R. A. Walker, CFO/Sr. VP-Finance
Preston Johnson, Jr., VP-Human Resources
Mario M. Coll, III, CIO/VP-IT
Robert K. Reeves, Chief Admin. Officer/Sr. VP
Robert K. Reeves, General Counsel
Charles A. Meloy, Sr. VP-Worldwide Oper.
Albert L. Richey, VP-Corp. Dev.
Bruce W. Busmire, Chief Acct. Officer/VP
Robert G. Gwin, Sr. VP/CEO-Western Gas Holdings LP
Mark L. Pease, Sr. VP-Exploration & Production
Gregory M. Pensabene, VP-Gov't Rel.
Robert P. Daniels, Sr. VP-Worldwide Exploration
James T. Hackett, Chmn.

Phone: 832-636-7557	**Fax:** 832-636-8220
Toll-Free:	
Address: 1201 Lake Robbins Dr., The Woodlands, TX 77380 US	

GROWTH PLANS/SPECIAL FEATURES:

Anadarko Petroleum Corporation is one of the world's largest independent oil and gas exploration and production companies, holding approximately 2.43 billion barrels of oil equivalent (BOE) of proved reserves, consisting of 8.5 trillion cubic feet of natural gas and 1.0 billion barrels of crude oil, condensate and natural gas liquids (NGL). The company operates approximately 44 exploratory wells and 1,750 development wells worldwide, with production located primarily in Louisiana, Texas, the U.S. mid-continent area, Alaska, Canada and offshore in the Gulf of Mexico. The company is also active in Venezuela, Algeria, Qatar, Tunisia, West Africa, the North Atlantic Margin and the Black Sea. The firm's domestic and international operations lie in field services, producer services, market services and financial services. Field services include gathering, compression and processing operations. The company actively markets natural gas, oil and natural gas liquids and owns and operates gas-gathering systems in its core producing areas. In addition to traditional drilling, the company is engaged in carbon-dioxide-enhanced oil recovery, as well as coal-bed methane production and the production of minerals including coal and soda ash. The company has several subsidiaries, including Western Gas Holdings LLC and the recently acquired Kerr-McGee Oil and Gas Corporation. In July 2007, the company announced the formation of a joint venture with Chesapeake Energy Corporation in the Deep Haley area of the Delaware Basin in West Texas. In March 2008, Anadarko sold its 50% interest in the Peregrino field offshore Brazil and its 25% interest in the Kaskida Unit in the deepwater Gulf of Mexico to StatoilHydro. In recent news, the company's subsidiary, Western Gas Partners, LP, commenced an initial public offering. Anadarko will retain a 60-65% stake in the company.

Anadarko offers its employees an employee assistance program; adoption assistance; educational assistance; credit union membership; and medical, dental and vision insurance.

FINANCIALS: Sales and profits are in thousands of dollars—add 000 to get the full amount. 2007 Note: Financial information for 2007 was not available for all companies at press time.

2007 Sales: $11,230,000	2007 Profits: $3,780,000	**U.S. Stock Ticker: APC**
2006 Sales: $10,187,000	2006 Profits: $4,854,000	**Int'l Ticker:** Int'l Exchange:
2005 Sales: $7,100,000	2005 Profits: $2,466,000	Employees: 3,300
2004 Sales: $6,079,000	2004 Profits: $1,601,000	Fiscal Year Ends: 12/31
2003 Sales: $5,113,000	2003 Profits: $1,287,000	Parent Company:

SALARIES/BENEFITS:

Pension Plan: Y	ESOP Stock Plan:	Profit Sharing:	Top Exec. Salary: $1,316,667	Bonus: $2,043,694
Savings Plan: Y	Stock Purch. Plan:		Second Exec. Salary: $466,667	Bonus: $535,500

OTHER THOUGHTS:

Apparent Women Officers or Directors: 2
Hot Spot for Advancement for Women/Minorities:

LOCATIONS: ("Y" = Yes)

West:	Southwest:	Midwest:	Southeast:	Northeast:	International:
Y	Y		Y		Y

ANALOG DEVICES INC
www.analog.com

Industry Group Code: 334413 Ranks within this company's industry group: Sales: 6   Profits: 3

Management:		Sales/Marketing:		Liberal Arts:		Information Systems:		Professionals:		Technical/Scientific:	
Mgmt. Trainees:	Y	Mktg. Professionals:	Y	Gen. Writing/Editing:		Info. Management:	Y	Finance/Accounting:	Y	Engineers, Elec.:	Y
Experienced Mgmt.:	Y	Retail Sales:		Technical Writing:	Y	Software Dev.:	Y	Law:	Y	Engineers, Other:	
Int'l Business:	Y	Commercial/Industrial:	Y	Graphic Arts/Photog.:		Hardware Dev.:	Y	HR/Other:	Y	Health/Lab:	Y
MBA Graduates:	Y	Sales Trainees:		Music:		Systems Integration:		Training:	Y	Scientists/Research:	Y
		Advertising Pros.:	Y	Broadcasting:		Consulting/Other:		Health Care:		Petroleum/Chemicals:	
				Other:				Consulting:		Math/Other:	Y

TYPES OF BUSINESS:

Integrated Circuits-Analog & Digital
MEMS Products
DSP Products
Accelerometers & Gyroscopes

BRANDS/DIVISIONS/AFFILIATES:

CONTACTS: *Note: Officers with more than one job title may be intentionally listed here more than once.*

Jerald G. Fishman, CEO
Jerald G. Fishman, Pres.
Joseph E. McDonough, CFO/VP-Finance
Vincent Roche, VP-Worldwide Sales
William Matson, VP-Human Resources
Samuel H. Fuller, VP-R&D
Robert R. Marshall, VP-Worldwide Mfg.
Margaret K. Seif, General Counsel/VP/Sec.
Keith Rutherford, VP-Comm. Bus. Dev.
William A. Martin, Treas.
Lewis Counts, VP-Linear Prod.
Dennis Dempsey, VP/Gen. Mgr.-Limerick Mfg.
Mark Norton, VP/Gen. Mgr.-Mfg.
Ray Stata, Chmn.
Howard Cheng, VP-China Sales
Gerry Dundon, VP-Planning & Supply Chain Logistics

Phone: 781-329-4700	Fax: 781-461-4482
Toll-Free: 800-262-5643	
Address: 1 Technology Way, P.O. Box 9106, Norwood, MA 02062 US	

GROWTH PLANS/SPECIAL FEATURES:

Analog Devices, Inc. (ADI) designs, manufactures and markets a broad line of high-performance analog, mixed-signal and digital signal processing (DSP) integrated circuits (ICs). Its principal products are used in a wide variety of electronic equipment, including industrial process control, factory automation systems, smart munitions, base stations, central office equipment, wireless telephones, computers, cars, CAT scanners, digital cameras and DVD players. The company's product portfolio includes several thousand analog ICs, with as many as several hundred customers per design. ADI's analog technology base also includes an advanced IC technology known in the industry as surface micromachining, which is used to produce micro-electromechanical systems (MEMS) semiconductor products. The firm's MEMS product portfolio includes accelerometers used to sense acceleration and gyroscopes used to sense position. The majority of the ADI's current revenue from micromachined products comes from accelerometers used by automotive manufacturers in airbag applications. These accelerometers are also used in the IBM ThinkPad to protect the hard drives from drops and falls. The company offers both general-purpose and application-specific DSP products. Its application-specific DSP products typically include analog and DSP technology, with the DSPs preprogrammed to execute software for applications such as wireless telecommunications or image processing. ADI's customers include Dell, Alcatel, Lucent, Ericsson, Siemens, Sony, Philips, Ford and Volkswagen. The firm has manufacturing facilities in the U.S., Ireland and the Philippines. The company has over 1,350 U.S. patents and more than 450 non-provisional pending U.S. patent applications. In September 2007, ADI agreed to sell its baseband chipset business and related support operations to MediaTek, Inc.

The company offers its employees medical, dental and vision insurance; life and AD&D insurance; short- and long-term disability insurance; a retirement plan; and education assistance.

FINANCIALS: Sales and profits are in thousands of dollars—add 000 to get the full amount. 2007 Note: Financial information for 2007 was not available for all companies at press time.

2007 Sales: $2,546,117	2007 Profits: $496,907	U.S. Stock Ticker: ADI
2006 Sales: $2,342,919	2006 Profits: $549,482	Int'l Ticker: Int'l Exchange:
2005 Sales: $2,134,800	2005 Profits: $414,787	Employees: 9,600
2004 Sales: $2,633,800	2004 Profits: $570,738	Fiscal Year Ends: 10/31
2003 Sales: $2,047,268	2003 Profits: $298,281	Parent Company:

SALARIES/BENEFITS:

Pension Plan: Y	ESOP Stock Plan:	Profit Sharing:	Top Exec. Salary: $930,935	Bonus: $1,314,767
Savings Plan:	Stock Purch. Plan:		Second Exec. Salary: $430,219	Bonus: $334,181

OTHER THOUGHTS:

Apparent Women Officers or Directors: 2
Hot Spot for Advancement for Women/Minorities: Y

LOCATIONS: ("Y" = Yes)

West:	Southwest:	Midwest:	Southeast:	Northeast:	International:
Y	Y	Y	Y	Y	Y

Note: Financial information, benefits and other data can change quickly and may vary from those stated here.

ANNTAYLOR STORES CORP

www.anntaylor.com

Industry Group Code: 448120 Ranks within this company's industry group: Sales: 5   Profits: 7

Management:		Sales/Marketing:		Liberal Arts:		Information Systems:		Professionals:		Technical/Scientific:	
Mgmt. Trainees:	Y	Mktg. Professionals:	Y	Gen. Writing/Editing:	Y	Info. Management:	Y	Finance/Accounting:	Y	Engineers, Elec.:	
Experienced Mgmt.:	Y	Retail Sales:	Y	Technical Writing:		Software Dev.:	Y	Law:	Y	Engineers, Other:	
Int'l Business:	Y	Commercial/Industrial:	Y	Graphic Arts/Photog.:	Y	Hardware Dev.:		HR/Other:	Y	Health/Lab:	
MBA Graduates:	Y	Sales Trainees:	Y	Music:		Systems Integration:		Training:	Y	Scientists/Research:	
		Advertising Pros.:	Y	Broadcasting:		Consulting/Other:		Health Care:		Petroleum/Chemicals:	
				Other:	Y			Consulting:		Math/Other:	

TYPES OF BUSINESS:

Women's Apparel, Retail
Clothing & Accessories
Shoes
Online & Catalog Sales
Ann Taylor University
Accelerated Leadership Program

BRANDS/DIVISIONS/AFFILIATES:

Ann Taylor
Ann Taylor LOFT
Ann Taylor Factory Store

CONTACTS: *Note: Officers with more than one job title may be intentionally listed here more than once.*

Kay Krill, CEO
Kay Krill, Pres.
Michael J. Nicholson, CFO/Exec. VP
Barbara K. Eisenberg, General Counsel/Exec. VP/Corp. Sec.
Brian E. Lynch, Pres., Corp. Oper.
Christine M. Beauchamp, Pres., Ann Taylor Stores
Judith Pirro, Dir.-Investor Rel.

Phone: 212-541-3300	Fax: 212-541-3379
Toll-Free: 800-342-5266	
Address: 7 Times Sq., 15th Fl., New York, NY 10036 US	

GROWTH PLANS/SPECIAL FEATURES:

women's apparel, shoes and accessories. Its stores offer a full range of career and casual separates, weekend wear, dresses, tops, accessories and shoes, coordinated as part of a total wardrobe strategy. All of the company's merchandise is developed and designed exclusively for its own stores. The company's line is marketed in 941 stores in 46 states, the District of Columbia and Puerto Rico under three divisions, Ann Taylor, Ann Taylor Loft, and Ann Taylor Factory. Ann Taylor stores represent the firm's core merchandise line and compete in the higher-priced market. Its Located primarily in regional malls and upscale specialty retail centers, these stores cater primarily to affluent, fashion-conscious, professional women with limited time from the ages of 25-55. Ann Taylor Loft is the firm's more moderately priced operation. Loft is marketed toward more price-conscious women with a more relaxed lifestyle and work environment. The Loft stores have enjoyed terrific success recently due to consumer response to stylish designs at reasonable prices. Through the Ann Taylor Factory stores, the firm offers clearance merchandise from the other two store formats. In 2008, the firm announced plans to close 117 stores due to the slowing economy.

AnnTaylor employees receive benefits including medical, dental and vision insurance, flexible spending accounts, a transportation reimbursement incentive program, tuition assistance, an adoption assistance program, an employee assistance program, discounted merchandise, a pension plan and a 401(k) savings plan.

FINANCIALS: Sales and profits are in thousands of dollars—add 000 to get the full amount. 2007 Note: Financial information for 2007 was not available for all companies at press time.

2007 Sales: $2,342,907	2007 Profits: $142,982	U.S. Stock Ticker: ANN
2006 Sales: $2,073,146	2006 Profits: $81,872	Int'l Ticker: Int'l Exchange:
2005 Sales: $1,853,583	2005 Profits: $63,276	Employees: 17,700
2004 Sales: $1,587,700	2004 Profits: $100,900	Fiscal Year Ends: 1/31
2003 Sales: $1,381,000	2003 Profits: $80,200	Parent Company:

SALARIES/BENEFITS:

Pension Plan: Y	ESOP Stock Plan:	Profit Sharing:	Top Exec. Salary: $1,000,000	Bonus: $1,781,394
Savings Plan: Y	Stock Purch. Plan: Y		Second Exec. Salary: $570,017	Bonus: $397,636

OTHER THOUGHTS:

Apparent Women Officers or Directors: 4
Hot Spot for Advancement for Women/Minorities: Y

LOCATIONS: ("Y" = Yes)

West:	Southwest:	Midwest:	Southeast:	Northeast:	International:
Y	Y	Y	Y	Y	Y

APACHE CORP   www.apachecorp.com

Industry Group Code: 211111 Ranks within this company's industry group: Sales: Profits:

Management:	Sales/Marketing:	Liberal Arts:	Information Systems:	Professionals:	Technical/Scientific:
Mgmt. Trainees:	Mktg. Professionals:	Gen. Writing/Editing:	Info. Management:	Finance/Accounting:	Engineers, Elec.:
Experienced Mgmt.:	Retail Sales:	Technical Writing:	Software Dev.:	Law:	Engineers, Other:
Int'l Business:	Commercial/Industrial:	Graphic Arts/Photog.:	Hardware Dev.:	HR/Other:	Health/Lab:
MBA Graduates:	Sales Trainees:	Music:	Systems Integration:	Training:	Scientists/Research:
	Advertising Pros.:	Broadcasting:	Consulting/Other:	Health Care:	Petroleum/Chemicals:
		Other:		Consulting:	Math/Other:

TYPES OF BUSINESS:
Oil & Gas Exploration & Production

BRANDS/DIVISIONS/AFFILIATES:
Apache Canada Ltd.
DEK Energy Company
Apache Energy Ltd.
Apache North America, Inc.
Apache Overseas, Inc.

CONTACTS: *Note: Officers with more than one job title may be intentionally listed here more than once.*
G. Steven Farris, CEO
G. Steven Farris, COO
G. Steven Farris, Pres.
Roger B. Plank, CFO/Exec. VP
Janine J. McArdle, VP-Oil & Gas Mktg.
Margery M. Harris, VP-Human Resources
Michael S. Bahorich, Exec. VP-Exploration & Production Tech.
Kregg Olson, Sr. VP-Corp. Reservoir Eng.
P. Anthony Lannie, General Counsel/Sr. VP
John J. Christmann, IV, VP-Bus. Dev.
Anthony Lentini, Jr., VP-Public & Int'l Affairs
Robert J. Dye, VP-Investor Rel.
Matthew W. Dundrea, Treas./VP
Floyd R. Price, Exec. VP-Eurasia, Latin America & New Ventures
Jon A. Jeppesen, Sr. VP-Gulf Coast Region
Rodney J. Eichler, Exec. VP/Gen. Mgr.-Apache Egypt Companies
John A. Crum, Pres., Apache Canada
Raymond Plank, Chmn.
Floyd R. Price, Exec. VP-Eurasia, Latin America & New Ventures
Scott Byrd, Mgr.-Global Sourcing & Special Projects

Phone: 713-296-6000	Fax: 713-296-6496
Toll-Free: 800-272-2434	
Address: 2000 Post Oak Blvd., Ste. 100, Houston, TX 77056-4400 US	

GROWTH PLANS/SPECIAL FEATURES:
Apache Corp. is an independent energy company that explores, develops and produces natural gas, crude oil and natural gas liquids in North America, Argentina, the U.K., Egypt and Australia. In North America, Apache's exploration and production interests are focused on the Gulf of Mexico; the Anadarko Basin of western Oklahoma; the Permian Basin of western Texas and New Mexico; the Texas-Louisiana Gulf Coast; East Texas; and the Western Sedimentary basin of Canada. Internationally, Apache has exploration and production interests in Egypt, Australia, Argentina and the U.K. sector of the North Sea. Approximately 53% of the company's production is natural gas, and 47% oil. Although the company treats all operations as one line of business, interests in many of its properties are through subsidiaries, such as Apache Canada Ltd.; DEK Energy Company; Apache Energy Ltd.; Apache North America, Inc.; and Apache Overseas, Inc. Apache's Canadian natural gas operations have been growing significantly in recent years due to several acquisitions and discoveries. Growth strategies in the U.S. focus on exploiting and expanding established areas, while growth abroad is a mix of exploration and exploitation. In 2007, Apache acquired an additional $1 billion of producing properties in the Permian Basin of Texas. Also in 2007, the firm was the high bidder on two exploration blocks on the Chilean side of the island of Tierra del Fuego. In 2008, Apache's exploration and drilling budget rose 9% over the previous year to approximately $4.6 billion, with another $400 million allocated for gathering transmission and processing assets.

Employees of Apache receive education assistance, a gift matching program, compressed work-week options, tax-free day care spending accounts and an employee assistance plan.

FINANCIALS: Sales and profits are in thousands of dollars—add 000 to get the full amount. 2007 Note: Financial information for 2007 was not available for all companies at press time.
2007 Sales: $9,977,858	2007 Profits: $2,812,358	**U.S. Stock Ticker:** APA
2006 Sales: $8,288,779	2006 Profits: $2,552,451	**Int'l Ticker:** Int'l Exchange:
2005 Sales: $7,584,244	2005 Profits: $2,623,730	Employees: 2,806
2004 Sales: $5,332,900	2004 Profits: $1,668,800	Fiscal Year Ends: 12/31
2003 Sales: $4,190,299	2003 Profits: $1,121,885	Parent Company:

SALARIES/BENEFITS:
Pension Plan: Y	ESOP Stock Plan:	Profit Sharing:	Top Exec. Salary: $1,331,250	Bonus: $1,100,000
Savings Plan: Y	Stock Purch. Plan:		Second Exec. Salary: $1,331,250	Bonus: $1,100,000

OTHER THOUGHTS:
Apparent Women Officers or Directors: 5
Hot Spot for Advancement for Women/Minorities: Y

LOCATIONS: ("Y" = Yes)
West:	Southwest:	Midwest:	Southeast:	Northeast:	International:
	Y		Y		Y

Note: Financial information, benefits and other data can change quickly and may vary from those stated here.

APOLLO GROUP INC
www.apollogrp.edu

Industry Group Code: 611410 **Ranks within this company's industry group:** Sales: 1 Profits: 1

Management:		Sales/Marketing:		Liberal Arts:		Information Systems:		Professionals:		Technical/Scientific:	
Mgmt. Trainees:	Y	Mktg. Professionals:	Y	Gen. Writing/Editing:	Y	Info. Management:	Y	Finance/Accounting:	Y	Engineers, Elec.:	
Experienced Mgmt.:	Y	Retail Sales:		Technical Writing:		Software Dev.:	Y	Law:	Y	Engineers, Other:	
Int'l Business:	Y	Commercial/Industrial:		Graphic Arts/Photog.:		Hardware Dev.:		HR/Other:	Y	Health/Lab:	
MBA Graduates:	Y	Sales Trainees:		Music:		Systems Integration:		Training:	Y	Scientists/Research:	
		Advertising Pros.:	Y	Broadcasting:		Consulting/Other:		Health Care:	Y	Petroleum/Chemicals:	
				Other:				Consulting:		Math/Other:	

TYPES OF BUSINESS:
University-Level Education
Continuing Education
Online University Courses
Adult Education

BRANDS/DIVISIONS/AFFILIATES:
University of Phoenix, Inc. (The)
University of Phoenix Online
Institute for Professional Development
College for Financial Planning, Inc.
Western International University, Inc.
Meritus University

CONTACTS: *Note: Officers with more than one job title may be intentionally listed here more than once.*
Charles B. Edelstein, CEO
Joe D'Amico, Pres.
Joe D'Amico, CFO
Rob Wrubel, VP-Mktg.
Diane Thompson, Chief Human Resources Officer
Joe Mildenhall, CIO
John Kline, Chief Admin. Officer
Robert Moya, General Counsel/Sr. VP
Gregory W. Cappelli, Exec. VP-Global Strategy
Terri Bishop, Chief Comm. Officer/Sr. VP
James Pasinski, Investor Rel.
Brian Swartz, Sr. VP-Finance
William Pepicello, Pres., University of Phoenix
Brian Swartz, Chief Acct. Officer
Dianne Pusch, Exec. VP
Jay Goin, Exec. VP
John G. Sperling, Chmn.

Phone: 480-966-5394	Fax: 480-379-3503
Toll-Free: 800-990-2765	
Address: 4025 S. Riverpoint Pkwy., Phoenix, AZ 85040 US	

GROWTH PLANS/SPECIAL FEATURES:

Apollo Group, Inc., through its subsidiaries, is a provider of higher education programs for working adults. Its subsidiaries include the University of Phoenix, Inc.; University of Phoenix Online; the Institute for Professional Development; the College for Financial Planning; and Western International University, Inc. The consolidated enrollment in the company's educational programs is approximately 313,000 students, over 80% of whom work full-time. Apollo offers its programs and services at 102 campuses and 157 learning centers in 40 states, Puerto Rico, Mexico, Canada and the Netherlands. The University of Phoenix Online has the distinction of being the leading private, accredited university in the U.S. with undergraduate and graduate degree programs. The Institute for Professional Development, Inc. (IPD) enables private, small to medium-sized accredited colleges and universities to provide viable degree programs for working adults. IPD offers its clients services such as degree program design, curriculum development, market research, student recruitment, accounting and administrative services. The College for Financial Planning provides financial planning education, including the Certified Financial Planner Professional Education Program. Western International University offers undergraduate and graduate degree programs at campuses in Arizona and, through joint ventures, in China and India. Apollo's online programs have enrolled students from over 130 countries. In August 2007, the company acquired online advertising network Aptimus, Inc. for $48 million. In October 2007, Apollo announced a $1 billion joint venture with The Carlyle Group, called Apollo Global, to pursue investments in various international education service sectors. In May 2008, Apollo announced plans to establish Meritus University, an online university offering degree programs to working Canadian professionals, based in Fredericton, New Brunswick.

The company offers employees a college savings plan, employee assistance programs, community service leave and flexible scheduling options. Employees receive free tuition for classes at Apollo institutions, and their spouses receive discounts of 80%.

FINANCIALS: Sales and profits are in thousands of dollars—add 000 to get the full amount. 2007 Note: Financial information for 2007 was not available for all companies at press time.

2007 Sales: $2,723,793	2007 Profits: $408,810	**U.S. Stock Ticker: APOL**
2006 Sales: $2,477,533	2006 Profits: $414,833	**Int'l Ticker:** Int'l Exchange:
2005 Sales: $2,251,472	2005 Profits: $444,731	Employees: 36,418
2004 Sales: $1,798,423	2004 Profits: $277,774	Fiscal Year Ends: 8/31
2003 Sales: $1,339,517	2003 Profits: $247,010	Parent Company:

SALARIES/BENEFITS:

Pension Plan:	ESOP Stock Plan:	Profit Sharing:	Top Exec. Salary: $	Bonus: $4,462,500
Savings Plan: Y	Stock Purch. Plan: Y		Second Exec. Salary: $450,000	Bonus: $450,000

OTHER THOUGHTS:
Apparent Women Officers or Directors: 3
Hot Spot for Advancement for Women/Minorities: Y

LOCATIONS: ("Y" = Yes)

West:	Southwest:	Midwest:	Southeast:	Northeast:	International:
Y	Y	Y	Y	Y	Y

Note: Financial information, benefits and other data can change quickly and may vary from those stated here.

APPLE INC

www.apple.com

Industry Group Code: 334111 Ranks within this company's industry group: Sales: 2   Profits: 2

Management:		Sales/Marketing:		Liberal Arts:		Information Systems:		Professionals:		Technical/Scientific:	
Mgmt. Trainees:	Y	Mktg. Professionals:	Y	Gen. Writing/Editing:	Y	Info. Management:	Y	Finance/Accounting:	Y	Engineers, Elec.:	Y
Experienced Mgmt.:	Y	Retail Sales:	Y	Technical Writing:	Y	Software Dev.:	Y	Law:	Y	Engineers, Other:	
Int'l Business:	Y	Commercial/Industrial:	Y	Graphic Arts/Photog.:	Y	Hardware Dev.:	Y	HR/Other:	Y	Health/Lab:	Y
MBA Graduates:	Y	Sales Trainees:	Y	Music:	Y	Systems Integration:	Y	Training:	Y	Scientists/Research:	Y
		Advertising Pros.:	Y	Broadcasting:		Consulting/Other:	Y	Health Care:		Petroleum/Chemicals:	
				Other:	Y			Consulting:		Math/Other:	Y

TYPES OF BUSINESS:

Computer Hardware-PCs
Software
Computer Accessories
Retail Stores
Portable Music Players
Online Music Sales
Cellular Phones
Home Entertainment Software & Systems

BRANDS/DIVISIONS/AFFILIATES:

Apple Computer Inc
MacBook Pro
Xserve
Mac OS X
Intel
iPod
iPhone
Safari

CONTACTS: *Note: Officers with more than one job title may be intentionally listed here more than once.*

Steve P. Jobs, CEO
Timothy D. Cook, COO
Peter Oppenheimer, CFO/Sr. VP
Philip W. Schiller, Sr. VP-Worldwide Prod. Mktg.
Bertrand Serlet, Sr. VP-Software Eng.
Daniel Cooperman, General Counsel/Sr. VP/Sec.
Ronald B. Johnson, Sr. VP-Retail
Jonathan Ive, Sr. VP-Industrial Design
Sina Tamaddon, Sr. VP-Applications
Tony Fadell, Sr. VP-iPod Div.
Bill Campbell, Chmn.

Phone: 408-996-1010	**Fax:** 408-974-2113
Toll-Free: 800-275-2273	
Address: 1 Infinite Loop, Cupertino, CA 95014 US	

GROWTH PLANS/SPECIAL FEATURES:

Apple, Inc. designs, manufactures and markets personal computers, portable digital music players and mobile communication devices; and sells a variety of related software, services, peripherals and networking solutions. The company's hardware products include the MacBook and MacBook Pro notebook computers; Mac Pro and iMac desktop computers; Mac minis; and Xserve servers and Xserve RAID Storage Systems. The firm's Mac products feature Intel microprocessors, Mac OS X Leopard operating systems and iLife software. Software products include Mac OS X; iLife '08; iWork '08; Logic Studio; and FileMaker Pro. Additional products include the iSight digital video cameras; the iPod line of portable digital music players and accessories; the iPhone, with touch controls, phone, iPod, and Internet services; Final Cut Studio, a high-definition video production suite of applications; and the iTunes digital entertainment management software for MP3 music files, television shows and movies. Peripheral products include printers, storage devices, memory, still cameras, widescreen flat panel displays and Apple TV, which plays iTunes content wirelessly. The firm operates over 215 retail stores in Canada, China, Japan, the U.K., the U.S., Australia and Italy. Apple's retail stores average an amazing $4,000 in sales per square foot per year. The iPod has sold over 100 million units; iTunes has sold over 5 billion songs and rents and sells over 50,000 movies daily. In 2008, the company released upgraded versions of the Mac Pro, MacBook and MacBook Pro, iMac, iPod, iPhone, and introduced new products such as the MacBook Air notebook computer, which is less than an inch thick; Time Capsule, a wireless backup appliance for Mac computers; and MobileMe internet service for mobile Apple products. In June 2008, Apple previewed Mac OS X Snow Leopard for 2009. In July 2008, Apple released the iPhone 3G, available in 22 countries, selling 1 million units in three days.

FINANCIALS: Sales and profits are in thousands of dollars—add 000 to get the full amount. 2007 Note: Financial information for 2007 was not available for all companies at press time.

2007 Sales: $24,006,000	2007 Profits: $3,496,000	**U.S. Stock Ticker:** AAPL
2006 Sales: $19,315,000	2006 Profits: $1,989,000	**Int'l Ticker:** Int'l Exchange:
2005 Sales: $13,931,000	2005 Profits: $1,328,000	Employees: 23,700
2004 Sales: $8,279,000	2004 Profits: $266,000	Fiscal Year Ends: 9/30
2003 Sales: $6,207,000	2003 Profits: $69,000	Parent Company:

SALARIES/BENEFITS:

Pension Plan:	ESOP Stock Plan:	Profit Sharing:	Top Exec. Salary: $700,014	Bonus: $700,000
Savings Plan: Y	Stock Purch. Plan: Y		Second Exec. Salary: $600,012	Bonus: $600,000

OTHER THOUGHTS:

Apparent Women Officers or Directors:
Hot Spot for Advancement for Women/Minorities:

LOCATIONS: ("Y" = Yes)

West:	Southwest:	Midwest:	Southeast:	Northeast:	International:
Y	Y	Y	Y	Y	Y

Note: Financial information, benefits and other data can change quickly and may vary from those stated here.

ARAMARK CORPORATION

www.aramark.com

Industry Group Code: 722310 Ranks within this company's industry group: Sales: 1   Profits: 2

Management:		Sales/Marketing:		Liberal Arts:		Information Systems:		Professionals:		Technical/Scientific:	
Mgmt. Trainees:	Y	Mktg. Professionals:	Y	Gen. Writing/Editing:	Y	Info. Management:	Y	Finance/Accounting:	Y	Engineers, Elec.:	
Experienced Mgmt.:	Y	Retail Sales:		Technical Writing:		Software Dev.:	Y	Law:	Y	Engineers, Other:	
Int'l Business:	Y	Commercial/Industrial:	Y	Graphic Arts/Photog.:	Y	Hardware Dev.:		HR/Other:	Y	Health/Lab:	
MBA Graduates:	Y	Sales Trainees:		Music:		Systems Integration:		Training:	Y	Scientists/Research:	
		Advertising Pros.:		Broadcasting:		Consulting/Other:		Health Care:		Petroleum/Chemicals:	
				Other:				Consulting:		Math/Other:	

TYPES OF BUSINESS:

Food Service Contractor
Facilities Management
Uniforms & Career Apparel Rental
Parks & Resorts Concessions & Facilities
Health Care Support Services
Apparel Manufacturing
Clinical Equipment Maintenance

BRANDS/DIVISIONS/AFFILIATES:

ARAMARK Uniform Services
Galls
Just4U
GS Capital Partners
CCMP Capital Advisors
J.P. Morgan Partners
Thomas H. Lee Partners
Warburg Pincus LLC

CONTACTS: Note: Officers with more than one job title may be intentionally listed here more than once.

Joseph Neubauer, CEO
L. Frederick Sutherland, CFO/Exec. VP
Lynn B. McKee, Exec. VP-Human Resources
Bart J. Colli, General Counsel/Exec. VP
Ron Iori, Sr. VP-Corp. Comm. & Public Affairs
John R. Donovan, Pres., ARAMARK Bus. Sports & Entertainment
Andrew C. Kerin, Pres., Domestic Food, Hospitality & Facilities
Thomas J. Vozzo, Pres., ARAMARK Uniform & Career Apparel
Joseph Neubauer, Chmn.
Ravi K. Saligram, Sr. VP/Pres., ARAMARK Int'l

Phone: 215-238-3000	Fax: 215-238-3333
Toll-Free: 800-272-6275	
Address: ARAMARK Tower, 1101 Market St., Philadelphia, PA 19107-2988 US	

GROWTH PLANS/SPECIAL FEATURES:

ARAMARK Corporation provides outsourced services to business, educational, health care, governmental institutions and sports, recreation and entertainment facilities. The company is a leader in the food and support services and uniform and career apparel rental industries. ARAMARK provides food and support services to business and industrial clients; sports teams; convention centers; national and state parks; over 200 school districts; over 400 colleges and universities; more than 475 correctional institutions; and approximately 1,000 healthcare and senior living facilities. These services include dining halls, concessions, banquets, catering and executive dining rooms. The firm also provides many clients with facilities management services, such as housekeeping, maintenance, laundry, grounds keeping, landscaping and other facility consulting services. Its services for the health care industry include specialty services such as clinical equipment maintenance management and provision of clean room garments and disposables. ARAMARK provides services internationally to clients in 18 countries. Its uniform and career apparel segment provides both rental and direct marketing services to customers in the manufacturing, transportation, construction, restaurant, hotel, public safety and health care industries, including gear and clothing for emergency response and law enforcement under the Galls name. The firm operates a fabric cutting plant in Georgia and sewing plants in Puerto Rico and Mexico. Based on company survey results, ARAMARK has begun offering more vegan meal options to college campuses as part of its Just4U menu program. In January 2007, ARAMARK was acquired by an investor group led by Chairman and CEO Joseph Neubauer and investment funds managed by GS Capital Partners, CCMP Capital Advisors and J.P. Morgan Partners, Thomas H. Lee Partners and Warburg Pincus LLC. The deal was valued at $8.3 billion, including $2 billion in debt. In May 2007, ARAMARK acquired the Seattle office coffee service business of Caffe Pazzesco.

FINANCIALS: Sales and profits are in thousands of dollars—add 000 to get the full amount. 2007 Note: Financial information for 2007 was not available for all companies at press time.

2007 Sales: $12,384,300	2007 Profits: $30,900	U.S. Stock Ticker: Private
2006 Sales: $11,621,173	2006 Profits: $261,098	Int'l Ticker: Int'l Exchange:
2005 Sales: $10,963,360	2005 Profits: $288,475	Employees: 240,000
2004 Sales: $10,192,200	2004 Profits: $263,100	Fiscal Year Ends: 9/30
2003 Sales: $9,447,800	2003 Profits: $301,100	Parent Company:

SALARIES/BENEFITS:

Pension Plan: Y	ESOP Stock Plan:	Profit Sharing:	Top Exec. Salary: $1,000,000	Bonus: $1,600,000
Savings Plan:	Stock Purch. Plan:		Second Exec. Salary: $568,750	Bonus: $375,000

OTHER THOUGHTS:

Apparent Women Officers or Directors: 1
Hot Spot for Advancement for Women/Minorities:

LOCATIONS: ("Y" = Yes)

West:	Southwest:	Midwest:	Southeast:	Northeast:	International:
Y	Y	Y	Y	Y	Y

ARCHER DANIELS MIDLAND CO
www.admworld.com

Industry Group Code: 311210 Ranks within this company's industry group: Sales: 2 Profits: 2

Management:		Sales/Marketing:		Liberal Arts:		Information Systems:		Professionals:		Technical/Scientific:	
Mgmt. Trainees:	Y	Mktg. Professionals:	Y	Gen. Writing/Editing:	Y	Info. Management:	Y	Finance/Accounting:	Y	Engineers, Elec.:	Y
Experienced Mgmt.:	Y	Retail Sales:		Technical Writing:	Y	Software Dev.:	Y	Law:	Y	Engineers, Other:	
Int'l Business:	Y	Commercial/Industrial:	Y	Graphic Arts/Photog.:	Y	Hardware Dev.:		HR/Other:	Y	Health/Lab:	Y
MBA Graduates:	Y	Sales Trainees:		Music:		Systems Integration:		Training:	Y	Scientists/Research:	Y
		Advertising Pros.:	Y	Broadcasting:		Consulting/Other:		Health Care:		Petroleum/Chemicals:	Y
				Other:				Consulting:		Math/Other:	

TYPES OF BUSINESS:
Food Processing-Oilseeds, Corn & Wheat
Agricultural Services
Nutraceuticals
Transportation Services
Biodiesel
Natural Plastics

BRANDS/DIVISIONS/AFFILIATES:
ADM Cocoa
ADM Milling Co.

CONTACTS: Note: Officers with more than one job title may be intentionally listed here more than once.
Patricia A. Woertz, CEO
Patricia A. Woertz, Pres.
Steven R. Mills, CFO/Exec. VP
John D. Rice, Exec. VP-Global Mktg. & Risk Mgmt.
Michael D'Ambrose, Sr. VP-Human Resources
John D. Rice, Exec. VP-Commercial & Production
David J. Smith, General Counsel/Exec. VP/Sec.
Ismael Roig, VP-Planning & Bus. Dev.
Victoria A. Podesta, VP-Corp. Comm.
Vikram Luthar, VP/Treas.
Lewis W. Batchelder, Sr. VP-Toepfer/ADM Value Creation Team
Edward A. Harjehausen, Sr. VP-Global Corn
Mark J. Cheviron, VP-Security & Corp. Svcs.
Mark Bemis, VP-Cocoa & Milling.
Patricia A. Woertz, Chmn.

Phone: 217-424-5200	Fax: 217-424-6196
Toll-Free: 800-637-5843	
Address: 4666 Faries Pkwy., Decatur, IL 62525 US	

GROWTH PLANS/SPECIAL FEATURES:
Archer Daniels Midland Co. (ADM) is an agricultural processor in the world, which produces and sells oils and corn-based sweeteners. It procures, transports, stores, processes and markets oils and protein meals from soy, canola, sunflower seeds, palm, cotton, peanut and other oilseeds; uses corn to develop sweeteners, such as high fructose corn syrup, citric acid, feed additives; biofuels like ethanol; and produces a variety of other food and feed ingredients, including cocoa, wheat flour, soy concentrates and nutraceuticals. Other agricultural products include oats, bulgur, starch, beans and industrial flour used to make wallboard. These materials are processed and stored in over 480 processing plants and 600 grain elevators in the U.S. and abroad. ADM offers sourcing and distribution services for third parties, making use of the company's network of 21,000 railcars, 2,310 tractor trailers, 2,100 barges, 75 tow boats and 29 lines boats, also used for its own goods. It owns a controlling interest in Wilmar International Limited, which operates palm and other plantations. ADM also has a number of corn milling plants; and owns International Malting Co., which operates barley malting plants in the U.S., Canada, New Zealand and Australia. In September 2007, the company partnered with ConocoPhillips to develop renewable transportation fuels from biomass. In October 2007, ADM formed an industrial chemicals business to commercialize chemicals from feedstocks. In August 2008, the firm agreed to acquire Campa Sued GmbH & Co KG, including a German rapeseed crushing plant that produces oil and meal for the food, feed and BioEnergy markets.

The company's employee benefits package features flexible spending accounts, group auto and home insurance, wellness benefits, a company fitness center, employee assistance and work-life programs, adoption assistance, a pre-paid legal plan, tuition reimbursement, a company store and employee discount programs.

FINANCIALS: Sales and profits are in thousands of dollars—add 000 to get the full amount. 2007 Note: Financial information for 2007 was not available for all companies at press time.

2007 Sales: $44,018,000	2007 Profits: $2,162,000	U.S. Stock Ticker: ADM
2006 Sales: $36,596,111	2006 Profits: $1,312,070	Int'l Ticker: Int'l Exchange:
2005 Sales: $35,943,810	2005 Profits: $1,044,385	Employees: 27,300
2004 Sales: $36,151,394	2004 Profits: $494,710	Fiscal Year Ends: 6/30
2003 Sales: $30,708,033	2003 Profits: $451,145	Parent Company:

SALARIES/BENEFITS:

Pension Plan: Y	ESOP Stock Plan: Y	Profit Sharing:	Top Exec. Salary: $3,051,667	Bonus: $
Savings Plan: Y	Stock Purch. Plan:		Second Exec. Salary: $856,311	Bonus: $

OTHER THOUGHTS:
Apparent Women Officers or Directors: 4
Hot Spot for Advancement for Women/Minorities: Y

LOCATIONS: ("Y" = Yes)

West:	Southwest:	Midwest:	Southeast:	Northeast:	International:
Y	Y	Y	Y	Y	Y

ARROW ELECTRONICS INC

www.arrow.com

Industry Group Code: 421430 Ranks within this company's industry group: Sales: Profits:

Management:	Sales/Marketing:	Liberal Arts:	Information Systems:	Professionals:	Technical/Scientific:
Mgmt. Trainees:	Mktg. Professionals:	Gen. Writing/Editing:	Info. Management:	Finance/Accounting:	Engineers, Elec.:
Experienced Mgmt.:	Retail Sales:	Technical Writing:	Software Dev.:	Law:	Engineers, Other:
Int'l Business:	Commercial/Industrial:	Graphic Arts/Photog.:	Hardware Dev.:	HR/Other:	Health/Lab:
MBA Graduates:	Sales Trainees:	Music:	Systems Integration:	Training:	Scientists/Research:
	Advertising Pros.:	Broadcasting:	Consulting/Other:	Health Care:	Petroleum/Chemicals:
		Other:		Consulting:	Math/Other:

TYPES OF BUSINESS:

Electronic Components-Distributor
Computer Products-Distributor
Technical Support Services
Supply Chain Services
Design Services
Materials Planning
Assembly Services
Inventory Management

BRANDS/DIVISIONS/AFFILIATES:

ArrowDevTools.com
North American Components
Alternative Technology, Inc.
Agilysys Keylink Systems Group
Arrow ECS
Electronics Japan, GK
Universe Electron Corporation
Centia Group Limited

CONTACTS: Note: Officers with more than one job title may be intentionally listed here more than once.

William E. Mitchell, CEO
William E. Mitchell, Pres.
Paul J. Reilly, CFO/Sr. VP
John P. McMahon, Sr. VP-Human Resources
Vincent Melvin, CIO/VP
Peter S. Brown, General Counsel/Sr. VP/Sec.
Jacqueline F. Strayer, VP-Corp. Comm.
Germano Fanelli, VP/Chmn.-Arrow Electronics EMEASA
Michael J. Long, Sr. VP/Pres., Arrow Global Components
Brian P. McNally, VP/Pres., Global Alliance & Supply Chain
Kevin J. Gilroy, Sr.VP/Pres., Arrow Enterprise Computing Solutions
William E. Mitchell, Chmn.
Peter T. Kong, VP/Pres., Arrow Asia Pacific
Bhawnesh Mathur, Sr. VP/Chief Supply Chain Officer

Phone: 631-847-2000	Fax: 631-847-2222
Toll-Free: 877-237-8621	
Address: 50 Marcus Dr., Melville, NY 11747-4210 US	

GROWTH PLANS/SPECIAL FEATURES:

Arrow Electronics, Inc. is a distributor of electronic components and computer products to industrial and commercial customers. It also offers services including materials planning, programming and assembly services, inventory management, online supply chain tools and design services to the electronics industry. The company's distribution network spans the three dominant electronics markets: North America, Europe and the Asia/Pacific region. Arrow serves as a supply channel partner for over 600 suppliers and 140,000 original equipment manufacturers and commercial customers through a global network of 260 locations in 55 countries and territories. Approximately 80% of the company's consolidated sales consist of semiconductor products and related services; industrial and computer products make up 20% of sales. In order to boost profit margins and provide an avenue for growth, the company is focusing on providing value-added services for its clients, such as procurement and inventory management. These services are designed to reduce inventory problems, cut delivery times and save component costs for the clients. In 2007, Arrow completed the acquisition of Agilysys Keylink Systems Group for $485 million in cash. Soon after, Arrow Asia Pacific purchased the component distribution business of Adilam Pty. Ltd (Adilam), a leading component distributor in Australia and New Zealand. Also in 2007, the company acquired Centia Group Limited and AKS Group Nordic AB (Centia/AKS), Europe's leading specialty distributors of access infrastructure, security and virtualization software solutions, for $32 million. In October 2007, the company acquired Universe Electron Corporation. Recently, Arrow opened a new office in St. Petersburg, Russia.

The company offers a stock option plan for all North American employees. It also provides a paid 10-week sabbatical every seven years and educational assistance.

FINANCIALS: Sales and profits are in thousands of dollars—add 000 to get the full amount. 2007 Note: Financial information for 2007 was not available for all companies at press time.

2007 Sales: $15,984,992	2007 Profits: $407,792	U.S. Stock Ticker: ARW
2006 Sales: $13,577,112	2006 Profits: $388,331	Int'l Ticker: Int'l Exchange:
2005 Sales: $11,164,196	2005 Profits: $253,600	Employees: 12,000
2004 Sales: $10,646,113	2004 Profits: $207,500	Fiscal Year Ends: 12/31
2003 Sales: $8,679,313	2003 Profits: $25,700	Parent Company:

SALARIES/BENEFITS:

Pension Plan: Y	ESOP Stock Plan: Y	Profit Sharing:	Top Exec. Salary: $990,000	Bonus: $1,099,120
Savings Plan: Y	Stock Purch. Plan:		Second Exec. Salary: $494,158	Bonus: $300,000

OTHER THOUGHTS:

Apparent Women Officers or Directors:
Hot Spot for Advancement for Women/Minorities: Y

LOCATIONS: ("Y" = Yes)

West:	Southwest:	Midwest:	Southeast:	Northeast:	International:
Y	Y	Y	Y	Y	Y

ARTHUR J GALLAGHER & CO   www.ajg.com

Industry Group Code: 524210   Ranks within this company's industry group: Sales: 1   Profits: 2

Management:		Sales/Marketing:		Liberal Arts:		Information Systems:		Professionals:		Technical/Scientific:	
Mgmt. Trainees:	Y	Mktg. Professionals:	Y	Gen. Writing/Editing:		Info. Management:	Y	Finance/Accounting:	Y	Engineers, Elec.:	
Experienced Mgmt.:	Y	Retail Sales:		Technical Writing:	Y	Software Dev.:		Law:	Y	Engineers, Other:	
Int'l Business:	Y	Commercial/Industrial:	Y	Graphic Arts/Photog.:		Hardware Dev.:		HR/Other:	Y	Health/Lab:	
MBA Graduates:	Y	Sales Trainees:		Music:		Systems Integration:		Training:	Y	Scientists/Research:	
		Advertising Pros.:	Y	Broadcasting:		Consulting/Other:		Health Care:		Petroleum/Chemicals:	
				Other:				Consulting:		Math/Other:	

TYPES OF BUSINESS:

Insurance Brokerage & Management
Risk Management Services
Employee Benefit Services
Investment Operations
Claims Management
Information Management
Insurance Software
Reinsurance

BRANDS/DIVISIONS/AFFILIATES:

Arthur J. Gallagher (UK), Ltd.
CoverageFirst
Gallagher Basset Services, Inc.
Gallagher Benefit Administrators
MountainView Software Corp.
Gallagher RE
I. Arthur Yanoff & Co., Ltd.
BenefitPort Northwest

CONTACTS: Note: Officers with more than one job title may be intentionally listed here more than once.

J. Patrick Gallagher, Jr., CEO
James S. Gault, COO
J. Patrick Gallagher, Jr., Pres.
Douglas K. Howell, CFO/VP
David E. McGurn, Jr., VP/Pres., Specialty Mktg. Div.
Susan E. McGrath, Chief Human Resources Officer/Corp. VP
Walter D. Bay, General Counsel/VP/Corp. Sec.
J. Patrick Gallagher, Jr., Chmn.
David E. McGurn, Jr., Pres., Int'l Div.

Phone: 630-773-3800	Fax: 630-285-4000
Toll-Free:	
Address: 2 Pierce Pl., Itasca, IL 60143-3141 US	

GROWTH PLANS/SPECIAL FEATURES:

Arthur J. Gallagher and Co. (Gallagher) and its subsidiaries provide insurance brokerage, risk management, employee benefits and other related services through a network of more than 250 offices in the seven countries and a network of brokers and consultants in 120 countries. Some of these offices are fully staffed with sales, marketing, claims and other service personnel; others function as servicing offices for the brokerage and risk management service operations of Gallagher. The firm has numerous subsidiaries. Arthur J. Gallagher handles direct insurance and reinsurance worldwide. Canadian CoverageFirst handles niche and wholesale insurance brokerage. Gallagher Basset Services provides risk management services, claims management, loss control and information management services. Gallagher Benefit Administrators offers integrated health benefit plan administration. MountainView Software Corporation designs customized electronic claims reporting and claims management software. Recent acquisitions include Strategic Health Plans Corporation; Spanjers Insurance Agency, Inc.; Carpenter, Cammack and Associates, Inc.; Woods and Grooms, Inc.; Tropp and Company; Melton Insurance Associates, Inc.; BIS Insurance Services, Inc.; Cedar Hill Insurance Agency, Inc.; C & B Consulting Group, Inc.; Powell Insurance Agency, Inc.; Robert A. Schneider Agency, Inc.; Intermountain Financial Benefits; an equity interest in CGM Group Limited; Koster Insurance Agency, Inc.; AVRECO; Crist Elliott Machette Insurance Services, Inc.; Yanni Partners, Inc.; Petty Burton Associates, Inc.; The Commonwealth Consulting Group; Taylor Benefits; Leicht General Agency; The Splinter Group, Inc.; Bankers Financial Benefits; Providium Consulting Group, LLC; Healthcare Risk Solutions, LLC; Life Insurance Strategies; RSI; Specialty Risk, Inc.; Lance Group, LLC; Voluntary Benefits Solutions, LLC; Gale Smith & Company, Inc.; and Wm. W. George & Associates, Inc. In March 2008, Gallagher sold its U.K. reinsurance brokerage business to Aon Corporation.

The company offers employees educational expense reimbursement; employee assistance programs; a casual dress policy; and flexible work hours depending upon the division and job function.

FINANCIALS: Sales and profits are in thousands of dollars—add 000 to get the full amount. 2007 Note: Financial information for 2007 was not available for all companies at press time.

2007 Sales: $1,623,300	2007 Profits: $138,800	U.S. Stock Ticker: AJG
2006 Sales: $1,470,100	2006 Profits: $128,500	Int'l Ticker: Int'l Exchange:
2005 Sales: $1,483,900	2005 Profits: $30,800	Employees: 8,757
2004 Sales: $1,437,000	2004 Profits: $188,500	Fiscal Year Ends: 12/31
2003 Sales: $1,221,100	2003 Profits: $146,200	Parent Company:

SALARIES/BENEFITS:

Pension Plan:	ESOP Stock Plan:	Profit Sharing:	Top Exec. Salary: $925,000	Bonus: $856,849
Savings Plan: Y	Stock Purch. Plan: Y		Second Exec. Salary: $550,000	Bonus: $267,168

OTHER THOUGHTS:

Apparent Women Officers or Directors: 3
Hot Spot for Advancement for Women/Minorities: Y

LOCATIONS: ("Y" = Yes)

West:	Southwest:	Midwest:	Southeast:	Northeast:	International:
Y	Y	Y	Y	Y	Y

AT&T INC

www.att.com

Industry Group Code: 513300A **Ranks within this company's industry group:** Sales: 4   Profits: 1

Management:		Sales/Marketing:		Liberal Arts:		Information Systems:		Professionals:		Technical/Scientific:	
Mgmt. Trainees:	Y	Mktg. Professionals:	Y	Gen. Writing/Editing:	Y	Info. Management:	Y	Finance/Accounting:	Y	Engineers, Elec.:	Y
Experienced Mgmt.:	Y	Retail Sales:		Technical Writing:		Software Dev.:	Y	Law:	Y	Engineers, Other:	
Int'l Business:	Y	Commercial/Industrial:	Y	Graphic Arts/Photog.:		Hardware Dev.:		HR/Other:	Y	Health/Lab:	
MBA Graduates:	Y	Sales Trainees:		Music:		Systems Integration:		Training:	Y	Scientists/Research:	
		Advertising Pros.:	Y	Broadcasting:		Consulting/Other:		Health Care:		Petroleum/Chemicals:	
				Other:				Consulting:		Math/Other:	

TYPES OF BUSINESS:

Local Telephone Service
Wireless Telecommunications
Long-Distance Telephone Service
Corporate Telecom, Backbone & Wholesale Services
Directory Publishing
Entertainment & Television via Internet
International Telephone Services
Internet Access via DSL

BRANDS/DIVISIONS/AFFILIATES:

Edge Wireless
Ingenio
Cingular Wireless
Dobson Communications Corp.
BellSouth

CONTACTS: Note: Officers with more than one job title may be intentionally listed here more than once.

Randall L. Stephenson, CEO
Randall L. Stephenson, Pres.
Richard G. Lindner, CFO/Sr. Exec. VP
Catherine M. Coughlin, Global Mktg. Officer/Sr. Exec. VP
William A. Blase Jr., Sr. Exec. VP-Human Resources
John Donovan, CTO
Wayne Watts, General Counsel/Sr. Exec. VP
James W. Callaway, Sr. Exec. VP-Exec. Oper.
Forest Miller, Group Pres., Corp. Strategy & Dev.
Ronald E. Spears, Group Pres., Global Bus. Svcs.
John Stankey, Group Pres., Telecom Oper.
Ralph de la Vega, Pres./CEO-AT&T Mobility
Rayford Wilkins, Jr., Group Pres., Diversified Bus.
Randall L. Stephenson, Chmn.
Mary Beth Asher, Exec. Dir.-Strategic Account Management APAC

Phone: 210-821-4105	Fax: 210-351-2071
Toll-Free:	
Address: 175 E. Houston, San Antonio, TX 78205 US	

GROWTH PLANS/SPECIAL FEATURES:

AT&T, Inc. is one of the world's largest providers of diversified telecommunications services. The company and its subsidiaries deliver a portfolio of traditional and IP-based voice; broadband Internet; data transport; entertainment; networking; wireless; video services; advertising; and transport and termination of wholesale traffic services. AT&T offers Virtual Private Network (VPN), Voice over IP (VoIP), security and support services and provides interoperability with the world's five leading IP PBX vendors as well as being a top provider of broadband DSL and Wi-Fi. The firm offers one of the world's most advanced and powerful global backbone networks, carrying more than 15.9 petabytes of data traffic daily to nearly every continent and country, with up to 99.999% reliability. It is also one of the nation's largest wireless carriers, serving 71.4 million customers and with service spanning more than 200 countries worldwide. Growth over the mid term will be focused on wireless subscriptions, the sale of advertising on its cellphone, TV and Internet services, Internet-based TV subscriptions and global corporate telecom services. Over the past year, AT&T launched a 3G network and became the exclusive retailer for the Apple iPhone, which has sold approximately 10 million units since its release. In 2007, AT&T completed its acquisition of BellSouth, which gave AT&T a 100% ownership of Cingular Wireless (which now uses the AT&T brand). In 2008, the company acquired Edge Wireless, a provider of wireless communications services in Oregon, northern California, Idaho and Wyoming; and Ingenio, a leading provider of Pay Per Call technology. AT&T plans to invest $1 billion in 2008 to continue the expansion of its network and portfolio of solutions for multinational companies. By the beginning of 2008, AT&T had 70.1 million wireless customers, making it number one in the U.S., 14 million broadband subscribers, 2.3 million TV subscribers and a massive wholesale and special services business.

FINANCIALS: Sales and profits are in thousands of dollars—add 000 to get the full amount. 2007 Note: Financial information for 2007 was not available for all companies at press time.

2007 Sales: $118,928,000	2007 Profits: $11,951,000	**U.S. Stock Ticker: T**
2006 Sales: $63,055,000	2006 Profits: $7,356,000	Int'l Ticker: Int'l Exchange:
2005 Sales: $43,764,000	2005 Profits: $4,786,000	Employees: 309,050
2004 Sales: $40,733,000	2004 Profits: $5,887,000	Fiscal Year Ends: 12/31
2003 Sales: $40,498,000	2003 Profits: $8,505,000	Parent Company:

SALARIES/BENEFITS:

Pension Plan: Y	ESOP Stock Plan: Y	Profit Sharing: Y	Top Exec. Salary: $1,199,167	Bonus: $1,983,470
Savings Plan: Y	Stock Purch. Plan:		Second Exec. Salary: $1,158,583	Bonus: $4,500,000

OTHER THOUGHTS:

Apparent Women Officers or Directors: 7
Hot Spot for Advancement for Women/Minorities: Y

LOCATIONS: ("Y" = Yes)

West:	Southwest:	Midwest:	Southeast:	Northeast:	International:
Y	Y	Y	Y	Y	Y

AUTOMATIC DATA PROCESSING INC   www.adp.com

Industry Group Code: 514210 Ranks within this company's industry group: Sales: 1   Profits: 1

Management:		Sales/Marketing:		Liberal Arts:		Information Systems:		Professionals:		Technical/Scientific:	
Mgmt. Trainees:	Y	Mktg. Professionals:	Y	Gen. Writing/Editing:	Y	Info. Management:	Y	Finance/Accounting:	Y	Engineers, Elec.:	Y
Experienced Mgmt.:	Y	Retail Sales:		Technical Writing:	Y	Software Dev.:	Y	Law:	Y	Engineers, Other:	
Int'l Business:	Y	Commercial/Industrial:	Y	Graphic Arts/Photog.:	Y	Hardware Dev.:		HR/Other:	Y	Health/Lab:	
MBA Graduates:	Y	Sales Trainees:		Music:		Systems Integration:	Y	Training:	Y	Scientists/Research:	Y
		Advertising Pros.:	Y	Broadcasting:		Consulting/Other:	Y	Health Care:		Petroleum/Chemicals:	
				Other:				Consulting:		Math/Other:	Y

TYPES OF BUSINESS:
Data Processing Services
Business Outsourcing Solutions
Information Services
Payroll Processing
Automobile Dealer Services

BRANDS/DIVISIONS/AFFILIATES:
ADP TotalSource
Broadridge Financial Solutions, Inc.

CONTACTS: Note: Officers with more than one job title may be intentionally listed here more than once.
Gary C. Butler, CEO
S. Michael Martone, COO
Gary C. Butler, Pres.
Christopher R. Reidy, CFO
James B. Benson, General Counsel/VP/Sec.
Steven J. Anenen, Pres., Dealer Svcs.
Campbell B. Langdon, Pres., Employer Svcs.-Major Acct. Div.
Regina R. Lee, Pres., Employer Svcs.-National Acct. Div.
Carlos Rodriguez, Pres., Employer Svcs.-Small Bus. Svcs. Div.
Leslie A. Brun, Chmn.
George I. Stoeckert, Pres., Employer Svcs.-Int'l

Phone: 973-974-5000	Fax: 973-974-3334
Toll-Free: 800-225-5237	
Address: 1 ADP Blvd., Roseland, NJ 07068 US	

GROWTH PLANS/SPECIAL FEATURES:

Automatic Data Processing, Inc. (ADP) is one of the world's largest providers of business outsourcing solutions. The company offers a wide range of human resources, payroll, tax and benefits administration solutions from a single source. The firm also provides integrated computing solutions to automotive, heavy truck, motorcycle, marine and recreational vehicle dealers throughout the world. ADP operates in two segments: employer services and dealer services. The employer services division offers a range of human resources information, payroll processing, tax and benefits administration products and services, including traditional and web-based outsourcing solutions, that assist roughly 560,000 employers in the U.S., Canada, Europe, South America, Australia and Asia to staff, manage, pay and retain their employees. In the U.S., ADP TotalSource, the company's professional employer organization business, provides clients with employment administration outsourcing solutions through a co-employment relationship, including payroll, payroll tax filing, human resources guidance, 401(k) plan administration, benefits administration, compliance services, health and workers' compensation coverage and other supplemental benefits for employees. The dealer services division provides integrated dealer management systems and business solutions to over 25,000 automotive, heavy truck and powersports vehicle retailers in over 50 countries. In March 2007, the company completed the spin-off of its former brokerage services group business into an independent company called Broadridge Financial Solutions, Inc. In July 2007, the company sold its travel clearing business for about $116 million.

The company offers its employees medical, dental and vision insurance; life and AD&D insurance; personal accident and business travel accident insurance; a pension plan; a 401(k) plan; a stock purchase plan; a college savings plan; tuition reimbursement; a credit union; and auto and home insurance program.

FINANCIALS: Sales and profits are in thousands of dollars—add 000 to get the full amount. 2007 Note: Financial information for 2007 was not available for all companies at press time.

2007 Sales: $7,800,000	2007 Profits: $1,138,700	U.S. Stock Ticker: ADP
2006 Sales: $6,835,600	2006 Profits: $1,554,000	Int'l Ticker: Int'l Exchange:
2005 Sales: $6,131,300	2005 Profits: $1,055,400	Employees: 46,000
2004 Sales: $7,279,400	2004 Profits: $935,600	Fiscal Year Ends: 6/30
2003 Sales: $7,147,000	2003 Profits: $1,018,200	Parent Company:

SALARIES/BENEFITS:

Pension Plan: Y	ESOP Stock Plan:	Profit Sharing:	Top Exec. Salary: $850,005	Bonus: $2,330,000
Savings Plan: Y	Stock Purch. Plan: Y		Second Exec. Salary: $581,365	Bonus: $874,000

OTHER THOUGHTS:
Apparent Women Officers or Directors: 2
Hot Spot for Advancement for Women/Minorities: Y

LOCATIONS: ("Y" = Yes)

West:	Southwest:	Midwest:	Southeast:	Northeast:	International:
Y	Y	Y	Y	Y	Y

Note: Financial information, benefits and other data can change quickly and may vary from those stated here.

AUTOZONE INC

www.autozone.com

Industry Group Code: 441310 **Ranks within this company's industry group:** Sales: 1 Profits: 1

Management:		Sales/Marketing:		Liberal Arts:		Information Systems:		Professionals:		Technical/Scientific:	
Mgmt. Trainees:	Y	Mktg. Professionals:	Y	Gen. Writing/Editing:	Y	Info. Management:	Y	Finance/Accounting:	Y	Engineers, Elec.:	
Experienced Mgmt.:	Y	Retail Sales:	Y	Technical Writing:		Software Dev.:	Y	Law:	Y	Engineers, Other:	
Int'l Business:	Y	Commercial/Industrial:	Y	Graphic Arts/Photog.:	Y	Hardware Dev.:		HR/Other:	Y	Health/Lab:	
MBA Graduates:	Y	Sales Trainees:	Y	Music:		Systems Integration:		Training:	Y	Scientists/Research:	
		Advertising Pros.:	Y	Broadcasting:		Consulting/Other:		Health Care:		Petroleum/Chemicals:	
				Other:				Consulting:		Math/Other:	

TYPES OF BUSINESS:

Auto Parts, Retail
Automotive Software
Online Sales
General Automotive Service

BRANDS/DIVISIONS/AFFILIATES:

Autozone.com
ALLDATA
Loan-a-Tool

CONTACTS: Note: Officers with more than one job title may be intentionally listed here more than once.

William C. Rhodes, III, CEO
William C. Rhodes, III, Pres.
William T. Giles, CFO
James A. Shea, Exec. VP-Mktg., Merch. & Supply Chain
Timothy W. Briggs, Sr. VP-Human Resources
Jon A. Bascom, CIO/Sr. VP
Mark A. Finestone, Exec. VP-Merch.
Harry L. Goldsmith, General Counsel/Exec. VP/Corp. Sec.
Robert D. Olsen, Exec. VP-Retail & Commercial Oper.
William T. Giles, Exec. VP-Finance
William T. Giles, Exec. VP-Store Dev. & IT
Thomas B. Newbern, Sr. VP-Store Oper.
Charlie Pleas, III, Sr. VP/Controller
Lisa R. Kranc, Sr. VP-Mktg.
William C. Rhodes, III, Chmn.
Robert D. Olsen, Sr. VP-Mexico
William W. Graves, Sr. VP-Supply Chain

Phone: 901-495-6500	Fax: 901-495-8300
Toll-Free: 800-288-6966	
Address: 123 S. Front St., Memphis, TN 38103 US	

GROWTH PLANS/SPECIAL FEATURES:

AutoZone, Inc. is a leading specialty retailer of automotive parts and accessories, targeting do-it-yourself (DIY) customers. With over 3,933 stores in the U.S. and Puerto Rico and 123 in Mexico, each AutoZone store carries an extensive product line for cars, sport utility vehicles, vans and light trucks, including new and remanufactured automotive parts, maintenance items, accessories and non-automotive products. Many AutoZone stores have a commercial sales program that provides commercial credit and prompt delivery of parts and other products to local, regional and national repair garages, dealers and service stations. Stores generally carry approximately 21,000 stock keeping units (SKU), while another 750,000 SKUs are available for order. Although each of the company's stores carry the same basic product lines, the company does tailor each store's parts inventory to the makes and models of the vehicles in their trade areas. Parts not kept in stock can be ordered and delivered to the store within a few days, or they can be ordered online. AutoZone allows parts ordered online to be returned at any store location. The company also has a Loan-a-Tool program, through which customers can borrow a specialty tool, such as a steering wheel puller, for which they would have little or no use other than for a single job. AutoZone also provides other free services, including check engine light readings; battery charging and installation assistance; fluid recycling; and testing of starters, alternators, batteries, sensors and actuators. The company also offers automotive diagnostic software and repair through its ALLDATA subsidiary.

AutoZone offers its employees a comprehensive benefits package including credit union membership; adoption assistance; ASE training and certification reimbursement; tuition reimbursement; merchandise discounts; a matching gift program; wellness programs; and a scholarship award program.

FINANCIALS: Sales and profits are in thousands of dollars—add 000 to get the full amount. 2007 Note: Financial information for 2007 was not available for all companies at press time.

2007 Sales: $6,169,804	2007 Profits: $595,672	**U.S. Stock Ticker:** AZO
2006 Sales: $5,948,355	2006 Profits: $569,275	**Int'l Ticker:** Int'l Exchange:
2005 Sales: $5,710,900	2005 Profits: $571,000	**Employees:** 55,000
2004 Sales: $5,637,025	2004 Profits: $566,202	**Fiscal Year Ends:** 8/31
2003 Sales: $5,457,123	2003 Profits: $517,604	**Parent Company:**

SALARIES/BENEFITS:

Pension Plan:	ESOP Stock Plan:	Profit Sharing:	Top Exec. Salary: $618,385	Bonus: $664,764
Savings Plan: Y	Stock Purch. Plan: Y		Second Exec. Salary: $433,231	Bonus: $279,434

OTHER THOUGHTS:

Apparent Women Officers or Directors: 2
Hot Spot for Advancement for Women/Minorities:

LOCATIONS: ("Y" = Yes)

West:	Southwest:	Midwest:	Southeast:	Northeast:	International:
Y	Y	Y	Y	Y	Y

Note: Financial information, benefits and other data can change quickly and may vary from those stated here.

AVERY DENNISON CORP

www.averydennison.com

Industry Group Code: 323000 Ranks within this company's industry group: Sales: 3   Profits: 3

Management:		Sales/Marketing:		Liberal Arts:		Information Systems:		Professionals:		Technical/Scientific:	
Mgmt. Trainees:	Y	Mktg. Professionals:	Y	Gen. Writing/Editing:	Y	Info. Management:	Y	Finance/Accounting:	Y	Engineers, Elec.:	Y
Experienced Mgmt.:	Y	Retail Sales:		Technical Writing:	Y	Software Dev.:	Y	Law:	Y	Engineers, Other:	
Int'l Business:	Y	Commercial/Industrial:	Y	Graphic Arts/Photog.:	Y	Hardware Dev.:		HR/Other:	Y	Health/Lab:	
MBA Graduates:	Y	Sales Trainees:		Music:		Systems Integration:		Training:	Y	Scientists/Research:	
		Advertising Pros.:	Y	Broadcasting:		Consulting/Other:		Health Care:		Petroleum/Chemicals:	Y
				Other:				Consulting:		Math/Other:	

TYPES OF BUSINESS:

Printing-Adhesive Labels
Office Products
Labeling Systems
Adhesive Materials
Highway Safety Products
Specialty Chemicals

BRANDS/DIVISIONS/AFFILIATES:

Avery
Fasson
Marks-A-Lot
HI-LITER
JAC
Paxar Corp.

CONTACTS: Note: Officers with more than one job title may be intentionally listed here more than once.

Dean A. Scarborough, CEO
Dean A. Scarborough, Pres.
Daniel R. O'Bryant, CFO/Exec. VP-Finance
Anne Hill, Chief Human Resources Officer/Sr. VP
Kenneth A. Wolinsky, CIO/VP
David N. Edwards, CTO/VP
Susan C. Miller, General Counsel/Sr. VP
Robert M. Malchione, Sr. VP-Corp. Strategy & Tech.
Diane B. Dixon, Sr. VP-Corp. Comm. & Advertising
Mitchell R. Butier, Controller/VP/Chief Acct. Officer
Robert G. van Schoonenberg, Chief Legal Officer/Exec. VP/Sec.
Donald A. Nolan, Group VP-Roll Materials
Terrence J. Hemmelgarn, Group VP-Retail Info. Systems
Timothy G. Bond, Group VP-Office Products
Kent Kresa, Chmn.
Greg E. Temple, VP-Global Oper.
Greg E. Temple, VP-Supply Chain

Phone: 626-304-2000	Fax: 626-792-7312
Toll-Free:	
Address: 150 N. Orange Grove Blvd., Pasadena, CA 91103 US	

GROWTH PLANS/SPECIAL FEATURES:

Avery Dennison Corporation is a global leader in pressure-sensitive technology and innovative self-adhesive solutions for consumer products and label materials. The company manufactures and markets a wide range of products for consumer and industrial markets, including Avery-brand office products, Fasson-brand self-adhesive materials, peel-and-stick postage stamps, battery labels, reflective highway safety products, automated retail tag and labeling systems and specialty tapes and chemicals. Its reporting segments are pressure-sensitive materials, office and consumer products and retail information services. Pressure-sensitive materials comprise about 55% of the firm's total 2007 sales and as a segment, specialize in making papers, films and foils coated with adhesive and sold in rolls to printers under the Avery Dennison, JAC and Fasson brands. Avery's office and consumer supplies segment manufactures and sells products for office, school and home use such as printer products, filing and presentation products and ink-jet and laser printer cards. In addition, it makes notebooks, three-ring binders, markers, fasteners, business forms, tickets, tags and imprinting equipment, marketed under the brand names Avery, Marks-A-Lot and HI-LITER. Finally, the retail information services segment designs, manufactures and sells price marking and brand identification products for retailers, apparel manufacturers, distributors and industrial customers. Avery also has several businesses that produce specialty tapes and engineered labels that include radio frequency identification (RFID) inlays and other converted products. International sales accounted for 60% of 2007 sales, with newly expanded efforts in Asia, Latin America and Eastern Europe. In June 2007, the company acquired Paxar Corporation for approximately $1.34 billion.

The company offers its employees several leadership development programs including the Future Leaders Program for those interested in management opportunities and the Human Resources Leadership Development Program, a rotational program for recent graduates.

FINANCIALS: Sales and profits are in thousands of dollars—add 000 to get the full amount. 2007 Note: Financial information for 2007 was not available for all companies at press time.

2007 Sales: $6,307,800	2007 Profits: $303,500	U.S. Stock Ticker: AVY
2006 Sales: $5,575,900	2006 Profits: $373,200	Int'l Ticker: Int'l Exchange:
2005 Sales: $5,743,500	2005 Profits: $226,400	Employees: 22,700
2004 Sales: $5,317,000	2004 Profits: $279,700	Fiscal Year Ends: 12/31
2003 Sales: $4,736,800	2003 Profits: $267,900	Parent Company:

SALARIES/BENEFITS:

Pension Plan:	ESOP Stock Plan:	Profit Sharing:	Top Exec. Salary: $847,000	Bonus: $2,147,723
Savings Plan: Y	Stock Purch. Plan: Y		Second Exec. Salary: $555,533	Bonus: $987,112

OTHER THOUGHTS:

Apparent Women Officers or Directors: 5
Hot Spot for Advancement for Women/Minorities: Y

LOCATIONS: ("Y" = Yes)

West:	Southwest:	Midwest:	Southeast:	Northeast:	International:
Y	Y	Y	Y	Y	Y

AVIS BUDGET GROUP INC
www.avisbudgetgroup.com

Industry Group Code: 532111 Ranks within this company's industry group: Sales: 3 Profits: 3

Management:		Sales/Marketing:		Liberal Arts:		Information Systems:		Professionals:		Technical/Scientific:	
Mgmt. Trainees:	Y	Mktg. Professionals:	Y	Gen. Writing/Editing:	Y	Info. Management:	Y	Finance/Accounting:	Y	Engineers, Elec.:	
Experienced Mgmt.:	Y	Retail Sales:		Technical Writing:		Software Dev.:	Y	Law:	Y	Engineers, Other:	
Int'l Business:	Y	Commercial/Industrial:	Y	Graphic Arts/Photog.:	Y	Hardware Dev.:		HR/Other:	Y	Health/Lab:	
MBA Graduates:	Y	Sales Trainees:		Music:		Systems Integration:		Training:	Y	Scientists/Research:	
		Advertising Pros.:	Y	Broadcasting:		Consulting/Other:		Health Care:		Petroleum/Chemicals:	
				Other:				Consulting:		Math/Other:	

TYPES OF BUSINESS:
Automobile Rental
Franchising
Truck Rental

BRANDS/DIVISIONS/AFFILIATES:
Avis
Budget
Budget Truck
Carey International

CONTACTS: Note: Officers with more than one job title may be intentionally listed here more than once.
Ronald L. Nelson, CEO
F. Robert Salerno, COO
F. Robert Salerno, Pres.
David B. Wyshner, CFO/Exec. VP
Thomas M. Gartland, Exec. VP-Mktg. & Sales
Mark J. Servodidio, Chief Human Resources Officer/Exec. VP
Mary LeBlanc, CIO/Sr. VP
Karen Sclafani, General Counsel/Exec. VP
Larry De Shon, Exec. VP-Oper.
Scott Deaver, Exec. VP-Strategy
John Barrows, VP-Corp. Comm. & Public Affairs
Brett Weinblatt, Sr. VP/Chief Acct. Officer
Kaye E. Ceille, Sr. VP-Global Travel & Partnership Sales
Bob Lambert, Sr. VP-Commercial Sales
Edward Gitlitz, Sr. VP-Fleet Svcs.
Becky Alseth, Sr. VP-Mktg.
Ronald L. Nelson, Chmn.
Patric Siniscalchi, Exec. VP-Int'l Oper.

Phone: 973-496-4700	Fax: 973-496-0202
Toll-Free:	
Address: 6 Sylvan Way, Parsippany, NJ 07054 US	

GROWTH PLANS/SPECIAL FEATURES:

Avis Budget Group, Inc. (ABG) operates in the global vehicle rental industry through Avis and Budget. Avis is a rental car supplier to the premium commercial and leisure segments of the travel industry and Budget is a rental car supplier to the price-conscious. Its car rental operations share the same fleet, maintenance facilities, technology and administrative infrastructure. The company operates in three segments: Domestic car rental, international car rental and truck rental. The Avis, Budget and Budget Truck brands accounted for approximately 63%, 30% and 7% of ABG's vehicle rental revenue, respectively, in 2007. ABG's operations include approximately 6,900 car and truck rental locations in the U.S., Canada, Australia, New Zealand, Latin America, the Caribbean and the Pacific region. It completed more than 28 million vehicle rental transactions worldwide in 2007. Domestically, ABG derived approximately 81% of its car rental revenue from on-airport locations in 2007 and the remainder from off-airport locations, referred to as the local rental segment. In 2007, ABG expanded its presence in the local segment and plans to continue this expansion in 2008. ABG rents its fleet of approximately 28,700 Budget trucks through a network of approximately 2,500 dealer-operated, 230 company-operated and 85 franchise-operated locations throughout the continental U.S. ABG also licenses the use of the Avis and Budget trademarks to multiple licensees in areas where the company does not operate. The Avis and/or Budget vehicle rental systems in Europe, Africa, the Middle East and parts of Asia are operated at approximately 3,600 locations by subsidiaries and sub-licensees of an independent third party. As of 2007, the firm had a market share at U.S. airport locations of about 30.1%, compared to Hertz's 28.5%. In 2007, the firm opened 195 new off-airport locations. In 2007, Avis acquired a 45% stake in Carey International, a provider of chauffeured vehicles.

FINANCIALS: Sales and profits are in thousands of dollars—add 000 to get the full amount. 2007 Note: Financial information for 2007 was not available for all companies at press time.

2007 Sales: $5,986,000	2007 Profits: $-916,000	U.S. Stock Ticker: CAR
2006 Sales: $5,689,000	2006 Profits: $-1,994,000	Int'l Ticker: Int'l Exchange:
2005 Sales: $5,400,000	2005 Profits: $1,618,000	Employees: 30,000
2004 Sales: $4,820,000	2004 Profits: $2,091,000	Fiscal Year Ends: 12/31
2003 Sales: $	2003 Profits: $	Parent Company:

SALARIES/BENEFITS:

Pension Plan:	ESOP Stock Plan:	Profit Sharing:	Top Exec. Salary: $1,000,000	Bonus: $900,000
Savings Plan: Y	Stock Purch. Plan:		Second Exec. Salary: $700,000	Bonus: $420,000

OTHER THOUGHTS:
Apparent Women Officers or Directors: 7
Hot Spot for Advancement for Women/Minorities: Y

LOCATIONS: ("Y" = Yes)

West:	Southwest:	Midwest:	Southeast:	Northeast:	International:
Y	Y	Y	Y	Y	Y

Note: Financial information, benefits and other data can change quickly and may vary from those stated here.

AVON PRODUCTS INC   www.avoncompany.com

Industry Group Code: 446191A Ranks within this company's industry group: Sales: 1 Profits: 1

Management:		Sales/Marketing:		Liberal Arts:		Information Systems:		Professionals:		Technical/Scientific:	
Mgmt. Trainees:	Y	Mktg. Professionals:	Y	Gen. Writing/Editing:	Y	Info. Management:	Y	Finance/Accounting:	Y	Engineers, Elec.:	
Experienced Mgmt.:	Y	Retail Sales:	Y	Technical Writing:		Software Dev.:	Y	Law:	Y	Engineers, Other:	
Int'l Business:	Y	Commercial/Industrial:	Y	Graphic Arts/Photog.:	Y	Hardware Dev.:		HR/Other:	Y	Health/Lab:	
MBA Graduates:	Y	Sales Trainees:	Y	Music:		Systems Integration:		Training:	Y	Scientists/Research:	
		Advertising Pros.:	Y	Broadcasting:		Consulting/Other:		Health Care:		Petroleum/Chemicals:	
				Other:	Y			Consulting:		Math/Other:	

TYPES OF BUSINESS:
Cosmetics & Beauty Supplies, Direct Selling
Fragrances & Toiletries
Gift & Decorative Items
Apparel & Accessories
Fashion Jewelry
Health & Fitness Products
Online Sales
Retail Kiosks

BRANDS/DIVISIONS/AFFILIATES:
Avon Color
Beyond Color
Anew
Avon Skin-So-Soft
Naturals
Avon Fragrance
M-The Catalog for Men
Mark

CONTACTS: *Note: Officers with more than one job title may be intentionally listed here more than once.*
Andrea Jung, CEO
Gina R. Boswell, COO
Elizabeth A. Smith, Pres.
Charles Cramb, CFO/Chief Strategy Officer
Srdjan Mijuskovic, Exec. VP-Global Sales Strategy
Lucien Alziari, Sr. VP-Human Resources
Donagh Herlihy, CIO
Geralyn R. Breig, Sr. VP/Pres., Global Brand
Kim Rucker, General Counsel/Sr. VP
Nancy Glaser, Sr. VP-Global Comm.
Richard S. Foggio, Corp. Controller/Sr. VP
Charles M. Herington, Sr. VP-Latin America
John P. Higson, Sr. VP-Central & Eastern Europe
James C. Wei, Sr. VP-Asia Pacific
Andrea Jung, Chmn.
Bennett R. Gallina, Sr. VP-China, Western Europe, Middle East & Africa
John F. Owen, Sr. VP-Global Supply Chain

Phone: 212-282-5000	Fax: 212-282-6049
Toll-Free: 800-367-2866	
Address: 1345 Ave. of the Americas, New York, NY 10105-0196 US	

GROWTH PLANS/SPECIAL FEATURES:
Avon Products, Inc. is a global manufacturer and marketer of beauty and related products. The firm groups these products into three categories: Beauty, consisting of cosmetics, fragrances and toiletries; Beauty Plus, made up of jewelry, watches, apparel and accessories; and Beyond Beauty, with home products, gifts, candles and other decorative items. The company sells makeup under the Avon Color and Beyond Color brands; skincare products under Anew and Avon Solutions; bath and body products under Avon Skin-So-Soft and Naturals; hair care products under Advance Techniques; supplements and therapeutic products under Avon Wellness; and fragrance products under Avon Fragrance. It is one of the largest sellers of perfumes in the world. Additionally, Avon has launched a global business targeting teenage girls through the Mark brand name and a portfolio of products for men offered in a publication called M-The Men's Catalog. The company sells products through a combination of direct selling and marketing by more than 5.4 million independent representatives, in over 114 countries in North America, Latin America, Asia-Pacific, Africa and Europe. Avon also retails products through Avon Centers, licensed kiosks in shopping malls across the U.S., and inside J.C. Penney stores, as well as online. Avon manufactures almost all of its products in 13 manufacturing facilities located around the world. In January 2008, the company announced plans to realign certain Latin America distribution and manufacturing operations, including plans to build a new distribution center in Brazil that is expected to open in 2010. The firm will phase-out its current distribution center in Sao Paulo, Brazil by 2011. Avon will also close a manufacturing facility in Guatemala in late 2008, transferring production to an existing facility in Mexico.

FINANCIALS: Sales and profits are in thousands of dollars—add 000 to get the full amount. 2007 Note: Financial information for 2007 was not available for all companies at press time.

2007 Sales: $9,938,700	2007 Profits: $530,700	**U.S. Stock Ticker: AVP**
2006 Sales: $8,763,900	2006 Profits: $477,600	**Int'l Ticker:** Int'l Exchange:
2005 Sales: $8,149,600	2005 Profits: $847,600	Employees: 40,300
2004 Sales: $7,747,800	2004 Profits: $846,100	Fiscal Year Ends: 12/31
2003 Sales: $6,876,000	2003 Profits: $664,800	Parent Company:

SALARIES/BENEFITS:

Pension Plan: Y	ESOP Stock Plan:	Profit Sharing:	Top Exec. Salary: $1,375,000	Bonus: $3,300,000
Savings Plan: Y	Stock Purch. Plan:		Second Exec. Salary: $1,000,000	Bonus: $1,867,500

OTHER THOUGHTS:
Apparent Women Officers or Directors: 5
Hot Spot for Advancement for Women/Minorities: Y

LOCATIONS: ("Y" = Yes)

West:	Southwest:	Midwest:	Southeast:	Northeast:	International:
Y	Y	Y	Y	Y	Y

AXA FINANCIAL INC

www.axa-financial.com

Industry Group Code: 524113 **Ranks within this company's industry group:** Sales: Profits:

Management:		Sales/Marketing:		Liberal Arts:		Information Systems:		Professionals:		Technical/Scientific:	
Mgmt. Trainees:	Y	Mktg. Professionals:	Y	Gen. Writing/Editing:	Y	Info. Management:	Y	Finance/Accounting:	Y	Engineers, Elec.:	
Experienced Mgmt.:	Y	Retail Sales:		Technical Writing:		Software Dev.:	Y	Law:	Y	Engineers, Other:	
Int'l Business:	Y	Commercial/Industrial:		Graphic Arts/Photog.:	Y	Hardware Dev.:		HR/Other:	Y	Health/Lab:	
MBA Graduates:	Y	Sales Trainees:		Music:		Systems Integration:		Training:	Y	Scientists/Research:	Y
		Advertising Pros.:	Y	Broadcasting:		Consulting/Other:		Health Care:		Petroleum/Chemicals:	
				Other:				Consulting:		Math/Other:	

TYPES OF BUSINESS:

Investment Management
Mutual Funds & Pension Funds
Stock Brokerage
Investment Banking
Securities Underwriting
Annuities
Asset Management
Life Insurance

BRANDS/DIVISIONS/AFFILIATES:

AXA Advisors LLC
AXA Equitable Life Insurance Company
AXA Distributors
AllianceBernstein LP
MONY Group
MONY Life Insurance Company
MONY Life Insurance Company of America
AXA Group

CONTACTS: Note: Officers with more than one job title may be intentionally listed here more than once.

Christopher M. (Kip) Condron, CEO
Christopher M. (Kip) Condron, Pres.
Richard S. Dziadzio, CFO
Barbara Goodstein, Exec. VP-Mktg./Chief Innovation Officer
Jennifer L. Blevins, Exec. VP-Human Resources
Kevin E. Murray, CIO/Exec. VP
Barbara Goodstein, Exec. VP/Dir.-Prod. Dev.
Richard V. Silver, General Counsel/Exec. VP
Charles Marino, Sr. VP-Chief Actuary
William Whitesell, VP-Underwriting & New Business Administration
Michael Arcaro, VP-External Affairs
Christine Nigro, Pres., AXA Advisors
Kevin Molloy-, Sr. VP-Distribution Finance, AXA Equitable Life
Christopher M. (Kip) Condron, Chmn.

Phone: 212-554-1234	Fax: 212=314-4480
Toll-Free: 888-292-4492	
Address: 1290 Ave. of the Americas, New York, NY 10104 US	

GROWTH PLANS/SPECIAL FEATURES:

AXA Financial, Inc., a wholly-owned subsidiary of AXA Group, is a diversified financial services organization offering a broad spectrum of insurance, investment banking and asset management services. The company's main operating subsidiaries are AXA Advisors, AXA Equitable, AXA Distributors, AllianceBernstein and The MONY Group. AXA Advisors provides financial, retirement and estate planning; life insurance; annuities; and mutual funds to individuals and small businesses. AXA Equitable Life Insurance Company offers a variety of traditional variable and interest-sensitive life insurance products, variable and fixed-interest annuity products, mutual funds and other investment products to individuals, small groups, small and medium-size corporations, state and local governments and not-for-profit organizations. AXA Distributors, another of AXA Financial's main operating subsidiaries, distributes managed investment products and services including whole and variable life insurance and fixed and variable annuities, as well as mutual funds to affiliated and independent professional financial intermediaries like brokerages, banks and independent financial planners. AXA Distributors approximately 400 firms and represents over 17,000 individual producers. AllianceBernstein, L.P. provides investment management services and is one of the largest mutual fun sponsors, with approximately $800 billion in assets under management. The MONY Group is a financial services organization that originates and distributes protection, asset accumulation and retail brokerage products and services to individuals, corporations and institutions through advisory and wholesale distribution channels. MONY companies include MONY Life Insurance Company and MONY Life Insurance Company of America.

The company offers performance-based compensation including short- and long-term incentive compensation. Employees can build healthcare based on their own specifications, in addition, the company offers dental, vision and retirement plans.

FINANCIALS: Sales and profits are in thousands of dollars—add 000 to get the full amount. 2007 Note: Financial information for 2007 was not available for all companies at press time.

2007 Sales: $	2007 Profits: $	**U.S. Stock Ticker: Subsidiary**
2006 Sales: $	2006 Profits: $	**Int'l Ticker:** Int'l Exchange:
2005 Sales: $10,964,800	2005 Profits: $553,200	Employees: 3,994
2004 Sales: $9,644,500	2004 Profits: $944,900	Fiscal Year Ends: 12/31
2003 Sales: $7,578,000	2003 Profits: $	Parent Company: AXA GROUP

SALARIES/BENEFITS:

Pension Plan:	ESOP Stock Plan:	Profit Sharing:	Top Exec. Salary: $	Bonus: $
Savings Plan:	Stock Purch. Plan:		Second Exec. Salary: $	Bonus: $

OTHER THOUGHTS:

Apparent Women Officers or Directors: 3
Hot Spot for Advancement for Women/Minorities: Y

LOCATIONS: ("Y" = Yes)

West:	Southwest:	Midwest:	Southeast:	Northeast:	International:
Y	Y	Y	Y	Y	Y

Note: Financial information, benefits and other data can change quickly and may vary from those stated here.

BAKER HUGHES INC
www.bakerhughes.com

Industry Group Code: 213111   Ranks within this company's industry group: Sales: 3   Profits: 2

Management:		Sales/Marketing:		Liberal Arts:		Information Systems:		Professionals:		Technical/Scientific:	
Mgmt. Trainees:	Y	Mktg. Professionals:	Y	Gen. Writing/Editing:		Info. Management:	Y	Finance/Accounting:	Y	Engineers, Elec.:	Y
Experienced Mgmt.:	Y	Retail Sales:		Technical Writing:	Y	Software Dev.:	Y	Law:	Y	Engineers, Other:	Y
Int'l Business:	Y	Commercial/Industrial:	Y	Graphic Arts/Photog.:	Y	Hardware Dev.:		HR/Other:	Y	Health/Lab:	
MBA Graduates:	Y	Sales Trainees:		Music:		Systems Integration:		Training:	Y	Scientists/Research:	
		Advertising Pros.:		Broadcasting:		Consulting/Other:		Health Care:		Petroleum/Chemicals:	Y
				Other:				Consulting:		Math/Other:	

TYPES OF BUSINESS:

Oil & Gas Drilling Support Services
Specialty Chemicals
Process Equipment
Geophysical Services
Drilling Fluids
Drill Bits

BRANDS/DIVISIONS/AFFILIATES:

Baker Atlas
Baker Hughes INTEQ
Baker Hughes Drilling Fluids
Hughes Christensen
Tricone
Baker Oil Tools
Baker Petrolite
Centrilift

CONTACTS: *Note: Officers with more than one job title may be intentionally listed here more than once.*

Chad C. Deaton, CEO
James R. Clark, COO
James R. Clark, Pres.
Peter Ragauss, CFO/Sr. VP
Didier Charreton, VP-Human Resources
Joe Vandevier, Dir.-Tech.
David H. Barr, Group Pres., Completions & Production
Alan R. Crain, Jr., General Counsel/Sr. VP
David E. Emerson, VP-Corp. Dev.
Gary R. Flaharty, Dir.-Investor Rel.
Alan J. Keifer, Controller/VP
Martin S. Craighead, Group Pres., Drilling & Evaluation
Paul S. Butero, VP/Pres., INTEQ
Gary G. Rich, VP/Pres., Hughes Christensen Company
Richard Williams, VP/Pres., Baker Hughes Drilling Fluids
Chad C. Deaton, Chmn.
Tayo Akinokun, Country Dir.-Nigeria

Phone: 713-439-8600	Fax: 713-439-8699
Toll-Free: 888-408-4244	
Address: 2929 Allen Pkwy., Ste. 2100, Houston, TX 77019-2118 US	

GROWTH PLANS/SPECIAL FEATURES:

Baker Hughes, Inc. is engaged in the oilfield and process industries, through its two main segments: drilling and evaluation; and completion and production. The drilling and evaluation segment includes subsidiary Baker Atlas, a premier provider of downhole well logging technology and services, including advanced formation evaluation, production and reservoir engineering and petrophysical and geophysical data acquisition services. The division also provides perforating and completion technologies, pipe recovery and data management, processing and analysis. Baker Hughes INTEQ, another subsidiary, is a major supplier of real-time drilling and evaluation services to the oil and gas industry, providing drilling technologies, drilling fluid systems, coring, subsurface surveying and other services. Baker Hughes Drilling Fluids provides drilling and completion fluids and related services, fluids environmental services and drill-in fluids. Hughes Christensen is a leading manufacturer and marketer of Tricone roller cone drill bits and polycrystalline diamond compact fixed cutter bits for the worldwide oil, gas, mining and geothermal industries. Baker Hughes' completion and production segment includes Baker Oil Tools, a provider of downhole completion, workover and fishing equipment and services, with product lines including packers, flow control equipment and sand control systems. Baker Petrolite provides oilfield specialty chemicals and integrated chemical technology solutions for petroleum production, transportation and refining. Centrilift is a market leader for oilfield electric submersible pumping systems and downhole oil/water separation technology. As of July 2008, Baker Hughes operated 3,436 rigs worldwide. In April 2008, the firm acquired Gaffney, Cline & Associates and GeoMechanics International, both reservoir consulting firms to enhance the company's reservoir engineering, technical and managerial advisory services and reservoir geomechanics portfolios.

Baker Hughes offers its employees a benefits package that includes flexible spending accounts, tuition reimbursement and an employee assistance program. The company generally promotes from within.

FINANCIALS: Sales and profits are in thousands of dollars—add 000 to get the full amount. 2007 Note: Financial information for 2007 was not available for all companies at press time.

2007 Sales: $10,428,200	2007 Profits: $1,513,900	**U.S. Stock Ticker: BHI**
2006 Sales: $9,027,400	2006 Profits: $2,419,000	**Int'l Ticker:** Int'l Exchange:
2005 Sales: $7,185,500	2005 Profits: $878,400	Employees: 34,600
2004 Sales: $6,079,600	2004 Profits: $528,600	Fiscal Year Ends: 12/31
2003 Sales: $5,233,300	2003 Profits: $128,900	Parent Company:

SALARIES/BENEFITS:

Pension Plan:	ESOP Stock Plan:	Profit Sharing:	Top Exec. Salary: $1,001,923	Bonus: $1,915,677
Savings Plan: Y	Stock Purch. Plan: Y		Second Exec. Salary: $645,000	Bonus: $1,109,128

OTHER THOUGHTS:

Apparent Women Officers or Directors: 3
Hot Spot for Advancement for Women/Minorities: Y

LOCATIONS: ("Y" = Yes)

West:	Southwest:	Midwest:	Southeast:	Northeast:	International:
Y	Y	Y	Y	Y	Y

BALTIMORE GAS AND ELECTRIC COMPANY   www.bge.com

Industry Group Code: 221000 Ranks within this company's industry group: Sales: Profits:

Management:		Sales/Marketing:		Liberal Arts:		Information Systems:		Professionals:		Technical/Scientific:	
Mgmt. Trainees:	Y	Mktg. Professionals:	Y	Gen. Writing/Editing:		Info. Management:	Y	Finance/Accounting:	Y	Engineers, Elec.:	Y
Experienced Mgmt.:	Y	Retail Sales:		Technical Writing:	Y	Software Dev.:	Y	Law:	Y	Engineers, Other:	Y
Int'l Business:		Commercial/Industrial:	Y	Graphic Arts/Photog.:		Hardware Dev.:		HR/Other:	Y	Health/Lab:	
MBA Graduates:	Y	Sales Trainees:		Music:		Systems Integration:		Training:	Y	Scientists/Research:	
		Advertising Pros.:		Broadcasting:		Consulting/Other:		Health Care:		Petroleum/Chemicals:	Y
				Other:				Consulting:		Math/Other:	

TYPES OF BUSINESS:

Utilities-Electricity & Natural Gas
Distribution & Transmission Lines

BRANDS/DIVISIONS/AFFILIATES:

Constellation Energy Group
PJM Interconnection, LLC

CONTACTS: *Note: Officers with more than one job title may be intentionally listed here more than once.*

Kenneth W. DeFontes, Jr., CEO
Kenneth W. DeFontes, Jr., Pres.
Pat Walls, Mgr.-Human Resources
Stephen Woerner, Sr. VP-Gas & Electric Operations
Malinda Small, VP-Corp. Comm.
Anne A. Hahn, Mgr.-Finance & Acct.
Jeannette Mills, Sr. VP-Customer Relations & Account Services
A. Christopher Burton, Sr. VP-Integrated Field Services
Thomas Valenti, Sr. VP-Logistics Management Services
Mark Case, Sr. VP-Strategy & Regulatory Affairs

Phone: 410-685-0123	**Fax:** 410-712-9323
Toll-Free: 800-685-0123	
Address: 39 W. Lexington St., Baltimore, MD 21201 US	

GROWTH PLANS/SPECIAL FEATURES:

Baltimore Gas and Electric Company (BGE), a subsidiary of Constellation Energy, is a regulated electric and gas public utility serving Baltimore City and 10 central Maryland counties. It transmits and distributes electricity to over 1.2 million business and residential customers and distributes natural gas to more than 630,000 customers. Overall, the firm's electric service spans more than 2,300 square miles, and its natural gas service covers 800 square miles. The company only delivers energy produced by neighboring utility systems. The company maintains approximately 248 substations and more than 1,269 circuit miles of electrical transmission lines and over 22,500 circuit miles of overhead and underground distribution lines. Under the PJM Tariff and various agreements, BGE and other market participants can use regional transmission facilities for energy, capacity, and ancillary services transactions including emergency assistance. In addition to providing its residential natural gas customers with storage, distribution and livery services, BGE also provides customers with meter reading, billing, emergency response, regular maintenance and balancing services. The firm delivers gas through contracts with Columbia Transmission Corporation, Transcontinental Gas Pipe Line Corporation and Dominion Transmission, Inc. The company is a member of PJM Interconnection, LLC; the independent system operator in Maryland, Pennsylvania, New Jersey and Delaware. BGE also has large volumes of propane under contract for the operation of its propane air facility and is capable of liquefying sufficient volumes of natural gas during the summer months for operations of its liquefied natural gas facility during peak winter periods

The company offers its employees flexible spending accounts and educational assistance. Employees also have access to auto and home insurance discounts, adoption assistance, a travel reimbursement incentive program, alternate work schedules and onsite medical facilities.

FINANCIALS: Sales and profits are in thousands of dollars—add 000 to get the full amount. 2007 Note: Financial information for 2007 was not available for all companies at press time.

2007 Sales: $	2007 Profits: $	**U.S. Stock Ticker: Subsidiary**
2006 Sales: $	2006 Profits: $	**Int'l Ticker:** Int'l Exchange:
2005 Sales: $3,009,300	2005 Profits: $189,000	Employees:
2004 Sales: $2,724,700	2004 Profits: $166,300	Fiscal Year Ends: 12/31
2003 Sales: $2,647,600	2003 Profits: $163,200	Parent Company: CONSTELLATION ENERGY GROUP

SALARIES/BENEFITS:

Pension Plan: Y	ESOP Stock Plan:	Profit Sharing:	Top Exec. Salary: $375,000	Bonus: $475,780
Savings Plan:	Stock Purch. Plan:		Second Exec. Salary: $	Bonus: $

OTHER THOUGHTS:

Apparent Women Officers or Directors: 2
Hot Spot for Advancement for Women/Minorities:

LOCATIONS: ("Y" = Yes)

West:	Southwest:	Midwest:	Southeast:	Northeast:	International:
				Y	

Note: Financial information, benefits and other data can change quickly and may vary from those stated here.

BANK OF AMERICA CORP   www.bankofamerica.com

Industry Group Code: 522110   Ranks within this company's industry group: Sales: 2   Profits: 2

Management:		Sales/Marketing:		Liberal Arts:		Information Systems:		Professionals:		Technical/Scientific:	
Mgmt. Trainees:	Y	Mktg. Professionals:	Y	Gen. Writing/Editing:	Y	Info. Management:	Y	Finance/Accounting:	Y	Engineers, Elec.:	
Experienced Mgmt.:	Y	Retail Sales:		Technical Writing:		Software Dev.:	Y	Law:	Y	Engineers, Other:	
Int'l Business:	Y	Commercial/Industrial:	Y	Graphic Arts/Photog.:	Y	Hardware Dev.:		HR/Other:	Y	Health/Lab:	
MBA Graduates:	Y	Sales Trainees:		Music:		Systems Integration:		Training:	Y	Scientists/Research:	
		Advertising Pros.:	Y	Broadcasting:		Consulting/Other:		Health Care:		Petroleum/Chemicals:	
				Other:				Consulting:		Math/Other:	

TYPES OF BUSINESS:

Banking
Commercial Real Estate
Investment & Brokerage Services
Insurance
Mutual Funds
Venture Capital
Mortgages
Credit Cards

BRANDS/DIVISIONS/AFFILIATES:

Barnett Banks, Inc.
FleetBoston
National Processing
MBNA Corp.
China Construction Bank
Countrywide Financial Corp
LaSalle Bank Corp
U.S. Trust

CONTACTS: Note: Officers with more than one job title may be intentionally listed here more than once.

Kenneth D. Lewis, CEO
Kenneth D. Lewis, Pres.
Joe L. Price, CFO
J. Steele Alphin, Chief Admin. Officer
Walter J. Muller, Chief Investment Officer
Amy Woods Brinkley, Chief Risk Officer
Barbara J. Desoer, Pres., Mortgage, Home Equity & Insurance Svcs.
Brian Moynihan, Pres., Global Corp. & Investment Banking
Liam McGee, Pres., Consumer & Small Bus. Bank
Kenneth D. Lewis, Chmn.
Thomas White, CEO-Banc of America Securities (Global Markets)

Phone: 704-386-8486	Fax: 704-386-6699
Toll-Free: 800-432-1000	
Address: 100 N. Tryon St., 18th Fl., Charlotte, NC 28255 US	

GROWTH PLANS/SPECIAL FEATURES:

Bank of America Corp. is a global provider of a diversified range of banking and financial services. The company operates through three business segments: global consumer and small business banking; global corporate and investment banking; and global wealth and investment management. The firm's global consumer and small business banking division maintains nearly 6,100 banking centers worldwide with more than 19,000 ATMs serving 59 million consumer and small business customers. Over 24 million customers are active in Bank of America's online banking service. The global consumer and small business banking division offers a variety of services including checking and savings accounts, CDs, IRAs, debit cards, credit cards, mortgage and home equity products. The global corporate and investment banking division provides services in three areas: business lending; capital markets and advisory services; and treasury services. The global wealth and investment banking segment includes Premier Banking and Investments, which provides banking, credit, investment services to clients with less than $3 million in assets, The Private Bank for clients with greater than $3 million in assets; Columbia Management Group for intuitional customers; and other services including alternative investments and market-maker services. Bank of America's credit card business is the result of the $35 billion acquisition of MBNA. It also bought a stake in China Construction Bank for $3 billion. In 2007, the firm acquired LaSalle Bank Corp. from ABN AMRO for $21 billion. In July 2008, the firm acquired Countrywide Financial, Corp., one of the largest mortgage lenders in the U.S.

The company offers its employees educational partnerships, performance-based compensation, health care and dependent care flexible spending accounts, as well as discounts on bank products and services, including home loans.

FINANCIALS: Sales and profits are in thousands of dollars—add 000 to get the full amount. 2007 Note: Financial information for 2007 was not available for all companies at press time.

2007 Sales: $124,321,000	2007 Profits: $14,982,000	**U.S. Stock Ticker: BAC**
2006 Sales: $117,017,000	2006 Profits: $21,133,000	**Int'l Ticker:** Int'l Exchange:
2005 Sales: $83,980,000	2005 Profits: $16,465,000	Employees: 203,425
2004 Sales: $48,965,000	2004 Profits: $14,143,000	Fiscal Year Ends: 12/31
2003 Sales: $49,006,000	2003 Profits: $10,810,000	Parent Company:

SALARIES/BENEFITS:

Pension Plan: Y	ESOP Stock Plan:	Profit Sharing:	Top Exec. Salary: $1,500,000	Bonus: $6,500,000
Savings Plan: Y	Stock Purch. Plan:		Second Exec. Salary: $800,000	Bonus: $3,875,000

OTHER THOUGHTS:

Apparent Women Officers or Directors: 4
Hot Spot for Advancement for Women/Minorities: Y

LOCATIONS: ("Y" = Yes)

West:	Southwest:	Midwest:	Southeast:	Northeast:	International:
Y	Y	Y	Y	Y	Y

Note: Financial information, benefits and other data can change quickly and may vary from those stated here.

BARNES & NOBLE COLLEGE BOOKSTORES www.bkstore.com

Industry Group Code: 451211 Ranks within this company's industry group: Sales: Profits:

Management:		Sales/Marketing:		Liberal Arts:		Information Systems:		Professionals:		Technical/Scientific:	
Mgmt. Trainees:	Y	Mktg. Professionals:	Y	Gen. Writing/Editing:	Y	Info. Management:	Y	Finance/Accounting:	Y	Engineers, Elec.:	
Experienced Mgmt.:	Y	Retail Sales:	Y	Technical Writing:		Software Dev.:	Y	Law:	Y	Engineers, Other:	
Int'l Business:	Y	Commercial/Industrial:	Y	Graphic Arts/Photog.:	Y	Hardware Dev.:		HR/Other:	Y	Health/Lab:	
MBA Graduates:	Y	Sales Trainees:	Y	Music:		Systems Integration:		Training:	Y	Scientists/Research:	
		Advertising Pros.:		Broadcasting:		Consulting/Other:		Health Care:		Petroleum/Chemicals:	
				Other:				Consulting:		Math/Other:	

TYPES OF BUSINESS:
Book Stores
Online Sales
Marketing Services
College Merchandise

BRANDS/DIVISIONS/AFFILIATES:
Barnes & Noble Inc
TextBooks.com
Barnes & Noble Classics
Barnes & Noble College Marketing Network

CONTACTS: *Note: Officers with more than one job title may be intentionally listed here more than once.*
Max J. Roberts, COO
Max J. Roberts, Pres.
Jack A. Dill, CFO/Sr. VP
Bill Maloney, Exec. VP-Mktg.
Bill Maloney, Exec. VP-Planning
Patrick Maloney, Exec. VP-e-commerce
Janine von Juergensonn, VP-Mktg.
Leonard S. Riggio, Chmn.

Phone: 908-991-2665	Fax: 908-991-2846
Toll-Free:	
Address: 120 Mountain View Blvd., Basking Ridge, NJ 07920 US	

GROWTH PLANS/SPECIAL FEATURES:

Barnes & Noble College Bookstores, Inc. (BNCB) is the sister company to Barnes & Noble, which has 800 bookstores across the country. BNCB operates over 650 campus bookstores in 44 states in the U.S. The company has stores on the Columbia University, Yale University, University of Chicago and Massachusetts Institute of Technology campuses, along with many others. These stores provide textbooks, trade books, school supplies, collegiate clothing and other merchandise. Colleges, universities and medical and law schools hire BNCB to replace traditional campus cooperatives and receive a percentage of the sales. The firm's college marketing network division, B&N College Marketing Division, provides on-campus marketing opportunities to businesses. In addition, the company operates textbooks.com, an online retailer. Many of the firm's locations feature Starbucks coffee service. Leonard Riggio owns a controlling interest in BNCB. The firm recently completed major bookstore renovations on 28 campuses, including a 50,000-square-foot superstore at Georgia Tech. BNCB recently launched a line of classic books called Barnes & Noble Classics, which include a biographical summary of the author; historical context for the book; footnotes; a collection of parodies, paintings, poems and other works inspired by the book; an introduction; and other features. It also runs a division called Barnes & Noble College Marketing Network which provides retailers outlets for their products and various advertising opportunities.

The company offers employees medical, dental and vision insurance, including medical and dental insurance for employees' domestic partners; time off with pay; short and long term disability plans; and product discounts. BNCB also sends its managers to formal training classes three times a year.

FINANCIALS: Sales and profits are in thousands of dollars—add 000 to get the full amount. 2007 Note: Financial information for 2007 was not available for all companies at press time.

2007 Sales: $	2007 Profits: $	**U.S. Stock Ticker: Private**	
2006 Sales: $1,590,000	2006 Profits: $	**Int'l Ticker:** Int'l Exchange:	
2005 Sales: $1,540,000	2005 Profits: $	Employees: 12,000	
2004 Sales: $1,300,000	2004 Profits: $	Fiscal Year Ends: 4/30	
2003 Sales: $1,300,000	2003 Profits: $	Parent Company:	

SALARIES/BENEFITS:

Pension Plan:	ESOP Stock Plan:	Profit Sharing:	Top Exec. Salary: $	Bonus: $
Savings Plan: Y	Stock Purch. Plan:		Second Exec. Salary: $	Bonus: $

OTHER THOUGHTS:
Apparent Women Officers or Directors:
Hot Spot for Advancement for Women/Minorities:

LOCATIONS: ("Y" = Yes)					
West:	Southwest:	Midwest:	Southeast:	Northeast:	International:
Y	Y	Y	Y	Y	Y

BARNES & NOBLE INC   www.barnesandnobleinc.com

Industry Group Code: 451211   Ranks within this company's industry group: Sales: 1   Profits: 1

Management:		Sales/Marketing:		Liberal Arts:		Information Systems:		Professionals:		Technical/Scientific:	
Mgmt. Trainees:	Y	Mktg. Professionals:	Y	Gen. Writing/Editing:		Info. Management:	Y	Finance/Accounting:	Y	Engineers, Elec.:	
Experienced Mgmt.:	Y	Retail Sales:	Y	Technical Writing:		Software Dev.:		Law:	Y	Engineers, Other:	
Int'l Business:		Commercial/Industrial:	Y	Graphic Arts/Photog.:		Hardware Dev.:		HR/Other:	Y	Health/Lab:	
MBA Graduates:	Y	Sales Trainees:	Y	Music:		Systems Integration:		Training:	Y	Scientists/Research:	
		Advertising Pros.:	Y	Broadcasting:		Consulting/Other:		Health Care:		Petroleum/Chemicals:	
				Other:	Y			Consulting:		Math/Other:	

TYPES OF BUSINESS:

Book Stores
Music & Software Sales
In-Store Cafes
Online Sales
Book Publishing
Book Distribution

BRANDS/DIVISIONS/AFFILIATES:

B. Dalton Bookseller
Barnes & Noble Bookseller
Sterling Publishing Co., Inc.
BarnesandNoble.com Inc

CONTACTS: *Note: Officers with more than one job title may be intentionally listed here more than once.*

Stephen Riggio, CEO
Mitchell S. Klipper, COO
Joseph Lombardi, CFO
Michelle Smith, VP-Human Resources
Chris Troia, CIO
Jennifer Daniels, General Counsel/VP/Sec.
David Deason, VP-Dev.
Marie J. Toulantis, CEO-BarnesandNoble.com
Mary Ellen Keating, Sr. VP-Corp. Comm. & Public Affairs
Andy Milevoj, Mgr.-Investor Rel.
Mark Bottini, VP/Dir.-Stores
J. Alan Kahn, Pres., Publishing Group
Leonard Riggio, Chmn.
William F. Duffy, Exec. VP-Logistics & Dist.

Phone: 212-633-3300	**Fax:** 212-352-3660
Toll-Free: 800-422-7717	
Address: 122 5th Ave., New York, NY 10011 US	

GROWTH PLANS/SPECIAL FEATURES:

Barnes & Noble, Inc. (B&N) is the nation's largest bookseller, operating 801 book stores in all 50 states. Approximately 700 stores operate under the Barnes & Noble Bookseller trade name, and roughly 100 stores operate under the B. Dalton Bookseller trade name. The company conducts the online part of its business through Barnesandnoble.com. The firm is also a general trade book publisher, offering many series of books with the label Barnes and Noble Classics. This is enabled in part through the firm's acquisition of Sterling Publishing, a non-fiction trade publisher. Sterling is now a subsidiary of the firm. B&N's principal business is the sale of trade books (generally hardcover and paperback consumer titles, excluding educational textbooks and specialized religious titles), mass market paperbacks (such as mystery, romance, science fiction and other popular fiction), children's books, bargain books, magazines, music and movies direct to customers. B&N stores are designed to be reminiscent of old-world libraries, with wood fixtures; antique-style chairs and tables; ample public space; a cafe serving sandwiches and Starbucks coffee; a children's area; music, DVD, books, video and game sections; and public restrooms. In-store music departments provides over 40,000 titles in classical music, opera, jazz, blues and pop rock. While stores average 25,000 square feet each, the largest are 60,000-square-foot giants stocking up to 200,000 titles. Typical stores stock approximately 60,000 core titles within a variety of popular subject categories reflecting local interests, which are supplemented by new releases and bestsellers. In total, B&N has publishing or distribution rights to nearly 10,000 titles.

The company offers its employees medical, vision and dental insurance; life insurance; business travel insurance; short- and long-term disability; a 401(k) plan; tuition assistance; a book loan program; and merchandise discounts.

FINANCIALS: Sales and profits are in thousands of dollars—add 000 to get the full amount. 2007 Note: Financial information for 2007 was not available for all companies at press time.

2007 Sales: $5,261,254	2007 Profits: $150,527	**U.S. Stock Ticker:** BKS
2006 Sales: $5,103,004	2006 Profits: $146,681	**Int'l Ticker:** Int'l Exchange:
2005 Sales: $4,873,595	2005 Profits: $143,376	Employees: 39,000
2004 Sales: $4,372,177	2004 Profits: $151,775	Fiscal Year Ends: 1/31
2003 Sales: $	2003 Profits: $	Parent Company:

SALARIES/BENEFITS:

Pension Plan:	ESOP Stock Plan:	Profit Sharing:	Top Exec. Salary: $786,538	Bonus: $
Savings Plan: Y	Stock Purch. Plan:		Second Exec. Salary: $636,538	Bonus: $1,000,000

OTHER THOUGHTS:

Apparent Women Officers or Directors: 4
Hot Spot for Advancement for Women/Minorities: Y

LOCATIONS: ("Y" = Yes)

West:	Southwest:	Midwest:	Southeast:	Northeast:	International:
Y	Y	Y	Y	Y	

BASS PRO SHOPS INC   www.basspro.com

Industry Group Code: 451110 Ranks within this company's industry group: Sales: Profits:

Management:		Sales/Marketing:		Liberal Arts:		Information Systems:		Professionals:		Technical/Scientific:	
Mgmt. Trainees:	Y	Mktg. Professionals:	Y	Gen. Writing/Editing:	Y	Info. Management:	Y	Finance/Accounting:	Y	Engineers, Elec.:	
Experienced Mgmt.:	Y	Retail Sales:	Y	Technical Writing:		Software Dev.:	Y	Law:	Y	Engineers, Other:	
Int'l Business:	Y	Commercial/Industrial:		Graphic Arts/Photog.:	Y	Hardware Dev.:		HR/Other:	Y	Health/Lab:	
MBA Graduates:	Y	Sales Trainees:	Y	Music:		Systems Integration:	Y	Training:	Y	Scientists/Research:	
		Advertising Pros.:	Y	Broadcasting:		Consulting/Other:		Health Care:		Petroleum/Chemicals:	
				Other:	Y			Consulting:		Math/Other:	

TYPES OF BUSINESS:

Sporting Goods, Retail
Sport Boats
Hunting & Fishing Equipment
Catalog & Online Sales
Outdoor Apparel
Resort Operations
Television Production

BRANDS/DIVISIONS/AFFILIATES:

Outdoor World
RedHead
Offshore Angler
White River Fly Shops
Tracker Marine
American Rod & Gun
Big Cedar Lodge
Dogwood Canyon

CONTACTS: Note: Officers with more than one job title may be intentionally listed here more than once.

James Hagale, COO
James Hagale, Pres.
Toni Miller, CFO/VP
Katie A. Mitchell, Specialist-Comm.
Martin G. MacDonald, Dir.-Conservation
Larry L. Whiteley, Mgr.-Public Relations & Outdoor Education
Martin G. MacDonald, Dir.-Public Relations & Conservation
Jenna M. Kendall, Coordinator-Media Info.
John L. Morris, Chmn.

Phone: 417-873-5000	Fax: 417-873-5060
Toll-Free: 800-227-7776	
Address: 2500 E. Kearney St., Springfield, MO 65898 US	

GROWTH PLANS/SPECIAL FEATURES:

Bass Pro Shops, Inc. is a leader in sporting goods retail. The company markets its products through 49 sports superstores across the United States and Canada, a mail-order catalog and through Internet sites. The firm is dedicated to providing outdoor recreational products, including specialty apparel, and also aims to model and inspire environmental conservation among its customers. The sporting goods superstores operate under the Bass Pro Shop and Outdoor World brand names and range from 100,000 to 600,000 square feet. Products include boats and campers, as well as myriads of fishing, hunting, camping, automobile and marine supplies. Many of these stores sport a variety of unique features and attractions to draw more customers, including restaurants, snack bars, archery ranges, indoor fish tanks, waterfalls and video arcades. In addition to its stores, the company sells goods over the Internet and through more than 34 million mail-order catalogs under the Bass Pro Shops, RedHead, Offshore Angler and White River Fly Shops brand names. On the wholesale side, the firm owns and operates Tracker Marine, a leader in sport boat manufacturing, and American Rod & Gun, one of the largest wholesale hunting and fishing distributors in the country. In addition to offering a variety of hunting and fishing trips and contests, the Bass Pro runs Big Cedar Lodge, an outdoors-themed vacation spot in Missouri, located near the company's own nature park, Dogwood Canyon; and produces two weekly television programs on The Outdoor Channel. During 2007 and 2008, the company opened several new stores in locations across the country, including: Independence, Missouri; Pearland, Texas; Foxborough, Massachusetts; Miami, Florida; Prattville, Alabama; Rancho Cucamonga, California; Mesa, Arizona; Bolingbrook, Illinois; Portage, Indiana; and Olathe, Kansas.

FINANCIALS: Sales and profits are in thousands of dollars—add 000 to get the full amount. 2007 Note: Financial information for 2007 was not available for all companies at press time.

2007 Sales: $3,000,000	2007 Profits: $	U.S. Stock Ticker: Private
2006 Sales: $2,660,000	2006 Profits: $	Int'l Ticker: Int'l Exchange:
2005 Sales: $1,915,000	2005 Profits: $	Employees: 15,000
2004 Sales: $2,050,000	2004 Profits: $	Fiscal Year Ends: 12/31
2003 Sales: $1,600,000	2003 Profits: $	Parent Company:

SALARIES/BENEFITS:

Pension Plan:	ESOP Stock Plan:	Profit Sharing:	Top Exec. Salary: $	Bonus: $
Savings Plan:	Stock Purch. Plan:		Second Exec. Salary: $	Bonus: $

OTHER THOUGHTS:

Apparent Women Officers or Directors: 3
Hot Spot for Advancement for Women/Minorities: Y

LOCATIONS: ("Y" = Yes)

West:	Southwest:	Midwest:	Southeast:	Northeast:	International:
Y	Y	Y	Y	Y	Y

Note: Financial information, benefits and other data can change quickly and may vary from those stated here.

BAXTER INTERNATIONAL INC

www.baxter.com

Industry Group Code: 339113 Ranks within this company's industry group: Sales: Profits:

Management:		Sales/Marketing:		Liberal Arts:		Information Systems:		Professionals:		Technical/Scientific:	
Mgmt. Trainees:	Y	Mktg. Professionals:	Y	Gen. Writing/Editing:	Y	Info. Management:	Y	Finance/Accounting:	Y	Engineers, Elec.:	Y
Experienced Mgmt.:	Y	Retail Sales:		Technical Writing:	Y	Software Dev.:	Y	Law:	Y	Engineers, Other:	Y
Int'l Business:	Y	Commercial/Industrial:	Y	Graphic Arts/Photog.:	Y	Hardware Dev.:	Y	HR/Other:	Y	Health/Lab:	Y
MBA Graduates:	Y	Sales Trainees:		Music:		Systems Integration:		Training:	Y	Scientists/Research:	Y
		Advertising Pros.:	Y	Broadcasting:		Consulting/Other:		Health Care:	Y	Petroleum/Chemicals:	
				Other:				Consulting:		Math/Other:	Y

TYPES OF BUSINESS:

Medical Equipment Manufacturing
Supplies-Intravenous & Renal Dialysis Systems
Medication Delivery Products & IV Fluids
Biopharmaceutical Products
Plasma Collection & Processing
Vaccines
Software
Contract Research

BRANDS/DIVISIONS/AFFILIATES:

Medication Delivery
BioScience
Renal
Colleague CX
Enlightened
ADVATE
RenalSoft HD
BioLife Plasma Services

CONTACTS: *Note: Officers with more than one job title may be intentionally listed here more than once.*

Robert L. Parkinson, Jr., CEO
Robert L. Parkinson, Jr., Pres.
Robert M. Davis, CFO/VP
Jeanne K. Mason, VP-Human Resources
Norbert G. Riedel, Chief Scientific Officer/VP
Karenann K. Terrell, CIO/VP
James M. Gatling, VP-Mfg.
Susan R. Lichtenstein, General Counsel/VP
Michael J. Baughman, Controller/VP
Joy A. Amundson, Pres., Bioscience/VP
Bruce McGillivray, Pres., Renal/VP
Peter J. Arduini, Pres., Medication Delivery/VP
Gerald Lema, Pres., Asia Pacific/VP
Robert L. Parkinson, Jr., Chmn.
John J. Greisch, Pres., Int'l/VP

Phone: 847-948-2000	Fax: 847-948-3642
Toll-Free: 800-422-9837	
Address: 1 Baxter Pkwy., Deerfield, IL 60015-4625 US	

GROWTH PLANS/SPECIAL FEATURES:

Baxter International, Inc., founded in 1931, manufactures and markets products for the treatment of hemophilia, immune disorders, cancer, infectious diseases, kidney disease, trauma and other chronic and acute medical conditions, offering expertise in medical devices, pharmaceuticals and biotechnology. Baxter markets its offerings to hospitals; clinical and medical research labs; blood and blood dialysis centers; rehab facilities; nursing homes; doctor's offices; and patients undergoing supervised home care. The firm has manufacturing facilities in 26 countries and offers products and services in 100 countries. Baxter operates in three segments: Medication Delivery, its largest sector, provides a range of intravenous solutions and specialty products that are used in combination for fluid replenishment, nutrition therapy, pain management, antibiotic therapy and chemotherapy; BioScience, which develops biopharmaceuticals, biosurgery products, vaccines, blood collection, processing and storage products and technologies; and Renal, which develops products and provides services to treat end-stage kidney disease. Products include the Colleague CX infusion pump; the Enlightened bar-coding system for flexible IV containers; ADVATE, a coagulant for hemophilia patients; and RenalSoft HD, a software module for the management of prescription, therapy and monitoring information relating to patients suffering from kidney failure. In addition, the company provides the following services: BioLife Plasma Services, a plasma collection and processing business; BioPharma Solutions, biotechnology; Global Technical Services, providing instrument service and support for devices manufactured and marketed by Baxter; Renal Clinical Helpline; Renal Services, an education and research operation; and Training and Education, a portfolio of interactive clinical web sites. In March 2007, the firm sold its Transfusion Therapies business (now called Fenwal, Inc.) to Texas Pacific Group and Maverick Capital, Ltd. for $540 million.

Baxter offers its employees educational assistance, credit union membership, an employee assistance program, center-based child care benefits, adoption reimbursement, alternative work arrangements, reimbursement accounts and medical, dental and vision insurance.

FINANCIALS: Sales and profits are in thousands of dollars—add 000 to get the full amount. 2007 Note: Financial information for 2007 was not available for all companies at press time.

2007 Sales: $11,263,000	2007 Profits: $1,707,000	**U.S. Stock Ticker:** BAX
2006 Sales: $10,378,000	2006 Profits: $1,397,000	**Int'l Ticker:** Int'l Exchange:
2005 Sales: $9,849,000	2005 Profits: $956,000	Employees: 46,000
2004 Sales: $9,509,000	2004 Profits: $388,000	Fiscal Year Ends: 12/31
2003 Sales: $8,916,000	2003 Profits: $881,000	Parent Company:

SALARIES/BENEFITS:

Pension Plan:	ESOP Stock Plan:	Profit Sharing:	Top Exec. Salary: $1,190,769	Bonus: $3,000,000
Savings Plan: Y	Stock Purch. Plan: Y		Second Exec. Salary: $564,000	Bonus: $938,952

OTHER THOUGHTS:

Apparent Women Officers or Directors: 6
Hot Spot for Advancement for Women/Minorities: Y

LOCATIONS: ("Y" = Yes)

West:	Southwest:	Midwest:	Southeast:	Northeast:	International:
Y	Y	Y	Y	Y	Y

Note: Financial information, benefits and other data can change quickly and may vary from those stated here.

BDO SEIDMAN LLP

www.bdo.com

Industry Group Code: 541210 Ranks within this company's industry group: Sales: 5 Profits:

Management:		Sales/Marketing:		Liberal Arts:		Information Systems:		Professionals:		Technical/Scientific:	
Mgmt. Trainees:		Mktg. Professionals:	Y	Gen. Writing/Editing:	Y	Info. Management:	Y	Finance/Accounting:	Y	Engineers, Elec.:	
Experienced Mgmt.:	Y	Retail Sales:		Technical Writing:	Y	Software Dev.:		Law:	Y	Engineers, Other:	
Int'l Business:		Commercial/Industrial:		Graphic Arts/Photog.:		Hardware Dev.:		HR/Other:	Y	Health/Lab:	
MBA Graduates:	Y	Sales Trainees:		Music:		Systems Integration:	Y	Training:	Y	Scientists/Research:	
		Advertising Pros.:	Y	Broadcasting:		Consulting/Other:	Y	Health Care:		Petroleum/Chemicals:	
				Other:	Y			Consulting:	Y	Math/Other:	

TYPES OF BUSINESS:

Accounting Services
Financial Regulatory Assurance
Tax Services
Financial Consulting
Business Consulting
Insurance & Insurance Consulting
Securities Brokerage Services

BRANDS/DIVISIONS/AFFILIATES:

Seidman Private Advisors, LLC
Seidman Private Securities, LLC
Seidman Insurance Consultants, LLC
BDO Consulting Services
Trenwith Group, LLC
BDO Seidman Alliance
BDO Business Resource Network
BDO International

CONTACTS: Note: Officers with more than one job title may be intentionally listed here more than once.

Jack Weisbaum, CEO
Carl W. Pergola, Exec. Dir.-BDO Consulting
Timothy L. Mohr, Dir.-Employee Misconduct Investigations
Stephanie Giammarco, Dir.-Computer Forensics & E-Discovery
Lee Dewey, Dir.-Corporate Investigations
Wayne Kolins, Chmn.

Phone: 312-240-1236	Fax: 312-240-3311
Toll-Free:	
Address: 130 E. Randolph, Ste. 2800, 1 Prudential Pl., Chicago, IL 60601 US	

GROWTH PLANS/SPECIAL FEATURES:

BDO Seidman, LLP is a financial, tax advisory, assurance, consulting and accounting firm. Its main service branches cover assurance, taxes, private client wealth management and corporate real estate. Assurance services cover regulatory compliance, financial statement audits, access to capital markets, information systems assurance and employee benefit plan audits. Tax services cover about 15 different topics, including property, sales and international tax; mergers and acquisitions; cost segregation; family wealth planning; employee benefits; and nonprofit issues. Private client wealth management services are offered through three subsidiaries: Seidman Private Advisors, LLC, which offers financial planning, investment management and investment advisory services; Seidman Private Securities, LLC offers clients securities brokerage services; and Seidman Insurance Consultants, LLC offers insurance consulting services as well as long-term care, disability and life insurance products. Corporate real estate services include lease audits, lease consulting and analysis of and consultations regarding utilities fees. The firm also runs BDO Consulting Services, offering litigation, risk advisory, restructuring and investigations services; and offers investment banking and business valuation services through its affiliate, Trenwith Group, LLC. Additionally, the BDO Seidman Alliance is a network of independent businesses that share resources with BDO and with each other. It includes the BDO Business Resource Network, which focuses on IT related issues, and various industry groups, mainly serving construction, governmental, healthcare, nonprofit, manufacturing, energy, dealership or financial institution clients. While BDO has only 35 offices of its own in the U.S., through its alliances it offers an additional 300 independent locations nationwide. It is also the U.S. member of BDO International, which has 626 member firm offices in 110 countries, the services of which the firm can extend to its customers.

Employees of BDO receive life, medical, dental and vision insurance; paid time off; flexible spending accounts; continuing education and tuition reimbursement; and legal assistance.

FINANCIALS: Sales and profits are in thousands of dollars—add 000 to get the full amount. 2007 Note: Financial information for 2007 was not available for all companies at press time.

		U.S. Stock Ticker: Private
2007 Sales: $659,000	2007 Profits: $	Int'l Ticker: Int'l Exchange:
2006 Sales: $558,000	2006 Profits: $	Employees: 30,000
2005 Sales: $440,000	2005 Profits: $	Fiscal Year Ends: 6/30
2004 Sales: $365,000	2004 Profits: $	Parent Company:
2003 Sales: $	2003 Profits: $	

SALARIES/BENEFITS:

Pension Plan:	ESOP Stock Plan:	Profit Sharing:	Top Exec. Salary: $	Bonus: $
Savings Plan: Y	Stock Purch. Plan:		Second Exec. Salary: $	Bonus: $

OTHER THOUGHTS:

Apparent Women Officers or Directors:
Hot Spot for Advancement for Women/Minorities:

LOCATIONS: ("Y" = Yes)

West:	Southwest:	Midwest:	Southeast:	Northeast:	International:
Y	Y	Y	Y	Y	Y

Note: Financial information, benefits and other data can change quickly and may vary from those stated here.

BEBE STORES INC

www.bebe.com

Industry Group Code: 448120 Ranks within this company's industry group: Sales: 13   Profits: 9

Management:		Sales/Marketing:		Liberal Arts:		Information Systems:		Professionals:		Technical/Scientific:	
Mgmt. Trainees:	Y	Mktg. Professionals:	Y	Gen. Writing/Editing:	Y	Info. Management:	Y	Finance/Accounting:	Y	Engineers, Elec.:	
Experienced Mgmt.:	Y	Retail Sales:	Y	Technical Writing:		Software Dev.:	Y	Law:	Y	Engineers, Other:	
Int'l Business:	Y	Commercial/Industrial:	Y	Graphic Arts/Photog.:	Y	Hardware Dev.:		HR/Other:	Y	Health/Lab:	
MBA Graduates:	Y	Sales Trainees:	Y	Music:		Systems Integration:		Training:	Y	Scientists/Research:	
		Advertising Pros.:	Y	Broadcasting:		Consulting/Other:		Health Care:		Petroleum/Chemicals:	
				Other:	Y			Consulting:		Math/Other:	

TYPES OF BUSINESS:

Young Women's Apparel, Retail
Accessories
Shoes
Online Sales

BRANDS/DIVISIONS/AFFILIATES:

bebe
BEBE SPORT
bebe.com
bebe Outlet
clubbebe
Neda by bebe

CONTACTS: *Note: Officers with more than one job title may be intentionally listed here more than once.*

Gregory Scott, CEO
Walter Parks, COO
Walter Parks, CFO
Barbara Wambach, Chief Admin. Officer
Lawrence Smith, VP/Gen. Counsel
Dyan Jozwick, Exec. VP/Chief Merch. Officer-bebe Retail Div.
Susan Peterson, VP-Design, bebe
Manny Mashouf, Chmn.

Phone: 415-715-3900	Fax: 415-715-3939
Toll-Free: 877-232-3777	
Address: 400 Valley Dr., Brisbane, CA 94005 US	

GROWTH PLANS/SPECIAL FEATURES:

Bebe Stores, Inc. designs, develops and produces a line of contemporary women's apparel and accessories, marketed under the bebe, bebe O and BEBE SPORT brand names. The company operates 306 stores located in 31 states, the District of Columbia, Puerto Rico, the U.S. Virgin Islands and Canada. Of these stores, 214 are bebe stores, 64 are BEBE SPORT stores, 20 are bebe outlet stores and one is a bebe accessories store. In addition, the firm operates an online store at bebe.com and holds 13 international stores through licensees in Singapore, Indonesia, Israel, Thailand, the Middle East, Malaysia, Egypt, Turkey and Mexico. The company targets women between the ages of 21 and 35, with offerings including suits, skirts, dresses, pants, active wear, outerwear and handbags, shoes, jewelry and other accessories. Most of its merchandise is designed and developed in-house and sometimes manufactured in conjunction with third parties. The company has pursued growth through new store openings and the introduction of new product categories, including denim, leather, lingerie, swimwear and footwear. The firm's existing bebe stores are 3,800 square feet on average and are primarily located in regional shopping malls and freestanding street locations. BEBE SPORT stores average approximately 2,200 square feet.

Bebe offers its employees medical, dental and vision coverage, as well as discounts on store merchandise.

FINANCIALS: Sales and profits are in thousands of dollars—add 000 to get the full amount. 2007 Note: Financial information for 2007 was not available for all companies at press time.

2007 Sales: $670,912	2007 Profits: $77,278	U.S. Stock Ticker: BEBE	
2006 Sales: $579,073	2006 Profits: $73,807	Int'l Ticker: Int'l Exchange:	
2005 Sales: $509,527	2005 Profits: $66,332	Employees: 4,297	
2004 Sales: $372,257	2004 Profits: $33,770	Fiscal Year Ends: 6/30	
2003 Sales: $323,500	2003 Profits: $19,300	Parent Company:	

SALARIES/BENEFITS:

Pension Plan:	ESOP Stock Plan:	Profit Sharing:	Top Exec. Salary: $500,000	Bonus: $
Savings Plan: Y	Stock Purch. Plan: Y		Second Exec. Salary: $500,000	Bonus: $

OTHER THOUGHTS:

Apparent Women Officers or Directors: 6
Hot Spot for Advancement for Women/Minorities: Y

LOCATIONS: ("Y" = Yes)

West:	Southwest:	Midwest:	Southeast:	Northeast:	International:
Y	Y	Y	Y	Y	Y

BECHTEL GROUP INC

www.bechtel.com

Industry Group Code: 234000 Ranks within this company's industry group: Sales: 1 Profits:

Management:		Sales/Marketing:		Liberal Arts:		Information Systems:		Professionals:		Technical/Scientific:	
Mgmt. Trainees:	Y	Mktg. Professionals:	Y	Gen. Writing/Editing:		Info. Management:	Y	Finance/Accounting:	Y	Engineers, Elec.:	Y
Experienced Mgmt.:	Y	Retail Sales:		Technical Writing:	Y	Software Dev.:	Y	Law:	Y	Engineers, Other:	Y
Int'l Business:	Y	Commercial/Industrial:	Y	Graphic Arts/Photog.:	Y	Hardware Dev.:		HR/Other:	Y	Health/Lab:	
MBA Graduates:	Y	Sales Trainees:		Music:		Systems Integration:	Y	Training:	Y	Scientists/Research:	Y
		Advertising Pros.:		Broadcasting:		Consulting/Other:	Y	Health Care:		Petroleum/Chemicals:	Y
				Other:				Consulting:	Y	Math/Other:	Y

TYPES OF BUSINESS:

Engineering, Construction & Project Management Services
Civic Engineering
Outsourcing
Financial Services
Atomic Propulsion Systems Engineering
Airport Construction

BRANDS/DIVISIONS/AFFILIATES:

Bechtel Systems & Infrastructure, Inc.
Six Sigma
Bechtel Power Corp.

CONTACTS:
Note: Officers with more than one job title may be intentionally listed here more than once.

Riley P. Bechtel, CEO
Bill Dudley, COO
Bill Dudley, Pres.
Peter Dawson, CFO
John MacDonald, Dir.-Human Resources
Geir Ramleth, Dir.-Info. Systems & Tech.
Ed Richardson, Mgr.-Eng.
Judith Miller, General Counsel
Lee Lushbaugh, Pres., Comm.
Jim Jackson, Pres., Oil, Gas & Chemicals
Mike Adams, Pres., Civil
Scott Ogilvie, Pres., Bechtel Systems & Infrastructure, Inc.
Andy Greig, Pres., Mining & Metals
Riley P. Bechtel, Chmn.
Eli Smith, Mgr.-Contracts & Procurement

Phone: 415-768-1234	Fax: 415-768-9038

Toll-Free:

Address: 50 Beale St., San Francisco, CA 94105-1895 US

GROWTH PLANS/SPECIAL FEATURES:

Bechtel Group, Inc., started in 1906 by Warren A. Bechtel, is one of the world's largest engineering companies. The privately-owned firm offers engineering, construction and project management services, with a broad project portfolio including road and rail systems, airports and seaports, nuclear power plants, petrochemical facilities, mines, defense and aerospace facilities, environmental cleanup projects, telecommunication networks, pipelines and oil fields development. The firm has participated in such notable endeavors as the construction of the Hoover Dam, the creation of the Bay Area Rapid Transit system in San Francisco, the massive James Bay Hydroelectric Project in Quebec and the quelling of oil field fires in Kuwait following the Persian Gulf War. Bechtel also constructed the Trans-Alaska Oil Pipeline, covering 800 miles between the Prudhoe Bay oil field and Valdez. In recent years, Bechtel has been awarded two multi-million dollar contracts by the U.S. Agency for International Development for the repair and reconstruction of Iraq's infrastructure. Bechtel has also been contracted to develop the New Doha International Airport in Qatar. An 11-year, multi-billion-dollar project, the new airport will be designed to accommodate six Airbus A380-800's, the largest passenger aircraft in the world. Recently, Bechtel Power Corp., a company subsidiary and one of the largest U.S. nuclear contractors, was chosen by the TVA, the nation's largest public power provider, to lead engineering, procurement and construction for its Watts Bar Unit 2 Nuclear Plant expansion project in Spring City, Tennessee. The five-year contract is worth $2.5 billion. Other current projects include a $2.2 billion national highway project in Romania, the Autostrada Transilvania, and a $2.9 billion engineering, procurement, construction and management agreement (through Bechtel Power Corp.) with Prairie State Energy Campus in St. Louis.

FINANCIALS:
Sales and profits are in thousands of dollars—add 000 to get the full amount. 2007 Note: Financial information for 2007 was not available for all companies at press time.

2007 Sales: $27,000,000	2007 Profits: $	U.S. Stock Ticker: Private
2006 Sales: $20,500,000	2006 Profits: $	Int'l Ticker: Int'l Exchange:
2005 Sales: $18,600,000	2005 Profits: $	Employees: 40,000
2004 Sales: $17,400,000	2004 Profits: $	Fiscal Year Ends: 12/31
2003 Sales: $16,300,000	2003 Profits: $	Parent Company:

SALARIES/BENEFITS:

Pension Plan:	ESOP Stock Plan:	Profit Sharing:	Top Exec. Salary: $	Bonus: $
Savings Plan:	Stock Purch. Plan:		Second Exec. Salary: $	Bonus: $

OTHER THOUGHTS:

Apparent Women Officers or Directors: 2
Hot Spot for Advancement for Women/Minorities: Y

LOCATIONS: ("Y" = Yes)

West:	Southwest:	Midwest:	Southeast:	Northeast:	International:
Y	Y	Y	Y	Y	Y

Note: Financial information, benefits and other data can change quickly and may vary from those stated here.

BECKMAN COULTER INC   www.beckmancoulter.com

Industry Group Code: 339113 Ranks within this company's industry group: Sales: 8   Profits: 10

Management:		Sales/Marketing:		Liberal Arts:		Information Systems:		Professionals:		Technical/Scientific:	
Mgmt. Trainees:	Y	Mktg. Professionals:	Y	Gen. Writing/Editing:	Y	Info. Management:	Y	Finance/Accounting:	Y	Engineers, Elec.:	Y
Experienced Mgmt.:	Y	Retail Sales:		Technical Writing:	Y	Software Dev.:	Y	Law:	Y	Engineers, Other:	Y
Int'l Business:	Y	Commercial/Industrial:	Y	Graphic Arts/Photog.:	Y	Hardware Dev.:	Y	HR/Other:	Y	Health/Lab:	Y
MBA Graduates:	Y	Sales Trainees:		Music:		Systems Integration:		Training:	Y	Scientists/Research:	Y
		Advertising Pros.:	Y	Broadcasting:		Consulting/Other:		Health Care:	Y	Petroleum/Chemicals:	
				Other:				Consulting:		Math/Other:	Y

TYPES OF BUSINESS:

Equipment-Laboratory Instruments
Chemistry Systems
Genetic Analysis/Nucleic Acid Testing
Biomedical Research Supplies
Immunoassay Systems
Cellular Systems
Discovery & Automation Systems

BRANDS/DIVISIONS/AFFILIATES:

UniCel DxC 880i Sychrom Access Clinical System
GemomeLab GeXP
Solid Phase Reversible Immobilization (SPRI)
ProteomeLab
CyAn ADP Analyzer
Optima MAX-MP
Vi-Cell
Q-Prep Workstation

CONTACTS: *Note: Officers with more than one job title may be intentionally listed here more than once.*

Scott Garrett, CEO
Scott Garrett, Pres.
Charlie Slacik, CFO
Bob Hurley, Sr. VP-Human Resources
Russ Bell, Chief Scientific Officer/Sr. VP
Charlie Slacik, Sr. VP-IT
Arnie Pinkston, General Counsel/Sr. VP/Corp. Sec.
Paul Glyer, Sr. VP-Strategy & Bus. Dev.
Bob Hurley, Sr. VP-Comm.
Paul Glyer, Sr. VP-Investor Rel.
Carolyn D. Beaver, Chief Acct. Officer/Controller/VP
Russ Bell, Sr. VP
Bob Kleinert, Exec. VP-Worldwide Commercial Oper.
Mike Whelan, Group VP-High Sensitivity Testing Group
Cynthia Collins, Group VP-Cellular Business Group
Scott Garrett, Chmn.
Pam Miller, Sr. VP-Supply Chain Mgmt.

Phone: 714-871-4848	Fax: 714-773-8283
Toll-Free: 800-233-4685	
Address: 4300 N. Harbor Blvd., Fullerton, CA 92834-3100 US	

GROWTH PLANS/SPECIAL FEATURES:

Beckman Coulter, Inc. develops, manufactures and markets biomedical testing instrument systems, tests, and supplies that automate complex biomedical tests. Spanning the biomedical testing continuum, from pioneering medical research and clinical trials to laboratory diagnostics and point-of-care testing, the company installed base of over 200,000 systems provides essential biomedical information to enhance health care around the world. The firm's predominate customer base includes hospital clinical laboratories, physicians' offices, group practices, commercial reference laboratories, universities, medical research laboratories, pharmaceutical companies and biotechnology firms. Based on profitability, the company has four focus segments: chemistry systems, immunoassay systems, cellular systems, and discovery and automation systems. The firm's revenue is about evenly distributed inside and outside the United States. Sales to clinical laboratories represent nearly 83% of its total revenue, with the balance coming from the life sciences markets. About 78% of the company's total revenue is generated by the sale of supplies, test kits, services and operating-type lease payments. Central laboratories of mid- to large-size hospitals represent its most significant customer group. Beckman also obtained the rights to acquire the worldwide diagnostics assets of Nephromics.

The company offers health benefits, paid vacations and holidays, tuition assistance and savings and retirement plans.

FINANCIALS: Sales and profits are in thousands of dollars—add 000 to get the full amount. 2007 Note: Financial information for 2007 was not available for all companies at press time.

2007 Sales: $2,761,300	2007 Profits: $211,300	**U.S. Stock Ticker: BEC**
2006 Sales: $2,528,500	2006 Profits: $186,900	**Int'l Ticker:** Int'l Exchange:
2005 Sales: $2,443,800	2005 Profits: $150,600	Employees: 10,500
2004 Sales: $2,408,300	2004 Profits: $210,900	Fiscal Year Ends: 12/31
2003 Sales: $2,192,500	2003 Profits: $207,200	Parent Company:

SALARIES/BENEFITS:

Pension Plan: Y	ESOP Stock Plan:	Profit Sharing:	Top Exec. Salary: $730,366	Bonus: $655,000
Savings Plan: Y	Stock Purch. Plan:		Second Exec. Salary: $380,000	Bonus: $177,600

OTHER THOUGHTS:

Apparent Women Officers or Directors: 3
Hot Spot for Advancement for Women/Minorities: Y

LOCATIONS: ("Y" = Yes)

West:	Southwest:	Midwest:	Southeast:	Northeast:	International:
Y			Y		Y

BECTON DICKINSON & CO

www.bd.com

Industry Group Code: 339113 Ranks within this company's industry group: Sales: 4 Profits: 5

Management:		Sales/Marketing:		Liberal Arts:		Information Systems:		Professionals:		Technical/Scientific:	
Mgmt. Trainees:	Y	Mktg. Professionals:	Y	Gen. Writing/Editing:	Y	Info. Management:	Y	Finance/Accounting:	Y	Engineers, Elec.:	Y
Experienced Mgmt.:	Y	Retail Sales:		Technical Writing:	Y	Software Dev.:	Y	Law:	Y	Engineers, Other:	Y
Int'l Business:	Y	Commercial/Industrial:	Y	Graphic Arts/Photog.:	Y	Hardware Dev.:	Y	HR/Other:	Y	Health/Lab:	Y
MBA Graduates:	Y	Sales Trainees:		Music:		Systems Integration:		Training:	Y	Scientists/Research:	Y
		Advertising Pros.:	Y	Broadcasting:		Consulting/Other:		Health Care:	Y	Petroleum/Chemicals:	
				Other:				Consulting:		Math/Other:	Y

TYPES OF BUSINESS:
Medical Equipment-Injection/Infusion
Drug Delivery Systems
Infusion Therapy Products
Diabetes Care Products
Surgical Products
Microbiology Products
Diagnostic Products
Consulting Services

BRANDS/DIVISIONS/AFFILIATES:
Becton Dickinson Medical
Becton Dickinson Biosciences
Becton Dickinson Diagnostics
Vacutainer
Hypak
GeneOhm Sciences
TriPath Imaging

CONTACTS: Note: Officers with more than one job title may be intentionally listed here more than once.
Edward J. Ludwig, CEO
Edward J. Ludwig, Pres.
John R. Considine, CFO/Sr. VP/Vice. Chmn.
Donna M. Boles, Sr. VP-Human Resources
Jeffrey S. Sherman, General Counsel/Sr. VP
Vincent A. Forlenza, Exec. VP
Gary M. Cohen, Exec. VP
William A. Kozy, Exec. VP
A. John Hanson, Exec. VP
Edward J. Ludwig, Chmn.

Phone: 201-847-6800 | **Fax:** 201-847-6475
Toll-Free: 800-284-6845
Address: 1 Becton Dr., Franklin Lakes, NJ 07417-1880 US

GROWTH PLANS/SPECIAL FEATURES:
Becton, Dickinson & Company (BD) manufactures and sells a broad line of medical supplies, devices and diagnostic systems used by health care professionals, medical research institutions and the general public. The company operates in three segments, medical, biosciences and diagnostics. The medical segment offers hypodermic products, specially designed devices for diabetes care; prefillable drug delivery systems; and infusion therapy products. It also offers anesthesia and surgical products; ophthalmic surgery devices; critical care systems; elastic support products; and thermometers. The biosciences segment offers industrial microbiology products; cellular analysis systems; research; and clinical reagents for cellular and nucleic acid analysis; cell culture lab ware and growth media; hematology instruments; and other diagnostic systems, including immunodiagnostic test kits. The diagnostics segment offers specimen collection products and services, consulting services and customized, automated barcode systems for patient identification and point-of-care data capture. Two of BD's most popular products are Hypak prefillable syringes and Vacutainer blood-collection products. Outside of the U.S., BD's products are manufactured and sold in Europe, Japan, Mexico, Asia Pacific, Canada and Brazil. In May 2007, BD acquired all of the outstanding shares of Plasso Technology, Ltd. May 2007 also saw the company expand its manufacturing facilities in Durham, NC. In December 2007, the company acquired TriPath Imaging.

The firm offers its employees fitness centers, an employee assistance program and adoption assistance, as well as stock options and scholarship programs. Larger facilities have heath centers offering preventive health screenings and routine examinations.

FINANCIALS: Sales and profits are in thousands of dollars—add 000 to get the full amount. 2007 Note: Financial information for 2007 was not available for all companies at press time.
2007 Sales: $6,359,700 | 2007 Profits: $890,000 | **U.S. Stock Ticker: BDX**
2006 Sales: $5,738,000 | 2006 Profits: $752,300 | **Int'l Ticker:** Int'l Exchange:
2005 Sales: $5,340,800 | 2005 Profits: $722,300 | Employees: 28,000
2004 Sales: $4,934,745 | 2004 Profits: $467,402 | Fiscal Year Ends: 9/30
2003 Sales: $4,527,940 | 2003 Profits: $547,056 | Parent Company:

SALARIES/BENEFITS:
Pension Plan: Y | ESOP Stock Plan: | Profit Sharing: | Top Exec. Salary: $1,030,000 | Bonus: $1,400,000
Savings Plan: Y | Stock Purch. Plan: | | Second Exec. Salary: $643,951 | Bonus: $670,000

OTHER THOUGHTS:
Apparent Women Officers or Directors: 1
Hot Spot for Advancement for Women/Minorities:

LOCATIONS: ("Y" = Yes)
West:	Southwest:	Midwest:	Southeast:	Northeast:	International:
Y	Y	Y	Y	Y	Y

BED BATH & BEYOND INC
www.bedbathandbeyond.com

Industry Group Code: 442299 Ranks within this company's industry group: Sales: 1 Profits: 1

Management:		Sales/Marketing:		Liberal Arts:		Information Systems:		Professionals:		Technical/Scientific:	
Mgmt. Trainees:	Y	Mktg. Professionals:	Y	Gen. Writing/Editing:	Y	Info. Management:	Y	Finance/Accounting:	Y	Engineers, Elec.:	
Experienced Mgmt.:	Y	Retail Sales:	Y	Technical Writing:		Software Dev.:	Y	Law:	Y	Engineers, Other:	
Int'l Business:	Y	Commercial/Industrial:	Y	Graphic Arts/Photog.:	Y	Hardware Dev.:		HR/Other:	Y	Health/Lab:	
MBA Graduates:	Y	Sales Trainees:	Y	Music:		Systems Integration:		Training:	Y	Scientists/Research:	
		Advertising Pros.:	Y	Broadcasting:		Consulting/Other:		Health Care:		Petroleum/Chemicals:	
				Other:	Y			Consulting:		Math/Other:	

TYPES OF BUSINESS:
Linens & Housewares, Retail
Small Appliances
Home Accessories
Health & Beauty Care
Baby & Toddler Merchandise

BRANDS/DIVISIONS/AFFILIATES:
Bed Bath & Beyond Superstores
Harmon Stores, Inc.
Christmas Tree Shops
buybuy BABY

CONTACTS: Note: Officers with more than one job title may be intentionally listed here more than once.
Steven H. Temares, CEO
Arthur Stark, Pres.
Eugene A. Castagna, CFO/Treas.
Rita Little, VP-Mktg.
Concetta Van Dyke, VP-Human Resources
G. William Waltzinger, Jr., VP-Corp. Dev.
Kevin Murphy, CIO/VP
Kevin Wanner, VP-Tech. & Oper.
Arthur Stark, Chief Merch. Officer
Allan N. Rauch, Legal & General Counsel
Richard McMahon, VP-Corp. Oper.
Richard McMahon, Chief Strategy Officer
Joseph P. Rowland, VP-E-Service Oper.
Ronald Curwin, Sr. VP-Investor Rel.
Susan E. Lattmann, VP-Finance
Matthew Fiorilli, Sr. VP-Stores
Chuck Bilezikian, CEO-Christmas Tree Shops, Inc.
G. William Waltzinger, Jr., Pres., Harmon Stores, Inc.
Leonard Feinstein, Co-Chmn.
Warren Eisenberg, Co-Chmn.
Jeffrey W. Macak, VP-Supply Chain Logistics

Phone: 908-688-0888	Fax: 908-688-6483
Toll-Free: 800-462-3966	
Address: 650 Liberty Ave., Union, NJ 07083 US	

GROWTH PLANS/SPECIAL FEATURES:
Bed Bath & Beyond, Inc. (BBB) is one of the nation's largest operators of domestic superstores, with more than 971 stores in 49 states, Washington, D.C. and Puerto Rico. BBB operates four retail entities: Bed Bath and Beyond stores, Harmon stores, buybuy BABY and Christmas Tree Shops. Bed Bath and Beyond stores offer high-quality domestic merchandise and home furnishings at relatively low prices. The firm's domestic merchandise line includes items such as bed linens, bath accessories and kitchen tiles, while its home furnishings line includes cookware, dinnerware, glassware and basic housewares. Harmon stores sell beauty care products in 40 stores in New York, New Jersey and Connecticut. Buybuy BABY is a retailer of infant and toddler merchandise, with nine stores in Maryland, New Jersey, New York and Virginia. Christmas Tree Shops offer giftware, household items and furnishings in 41 stores in ten states. BBB relies on paid advertising and uses circulars and mailing pieces as its primary vehicles for paid advertising. In addition, the company only has two central distribution centers, since the majority of merchandise is shipped to each store from the firm's 4,600 vendors. BBB is engaged in an ongoing expansion program involving the opening of new stores in both existing and new markets, as well as the expansion or replacement of existing stores with larger ones. Local store managers have significant influence over the merchandise they carry. In August 2008, the company branched out into international retailing when by opening a store in Ontario, Canada.

FINANCIALS: Sales and profits are in thousands of dollars—add 000 to get the full amount. 2007 Note: Financial information for 2007 was not available for all companies at press time.

2007 Sales: $6,617,429	2007 Profits: $594,244	U.S. Stock Ticker: BBBY
2006 Sales: $5,809,562	2006 Profits: $572,847	Int'l Ticker: Int'l Exchange:
2005 Sales: $5,147,678	2005 Profits: $504,964	Employees: 3,500
2004 Sales: $4,477,981	2004 Profits: $399,470	Fiscal Year Ends: 2/25
2003 Sales: $3,665,200	2003 Profits: $302,200	Parent Company:

SALARIES/BENEFITS:

Pension Plan:	ESOP Stock Plan:	Profit Sharing:	Top Exec. Salary: $1,230,769	Bonus: $
Savings Plan: Y	Stock Purch. Plan:		Second Exec. Salary: $1,100,000	Bonus: $

OTHER THOUGHTS:
Apparent Women Officers or Directors: 9
Hot Spot for Advancement for Women/Minorities: Y

LOCATIONS: ("Y" = Yes)

West:	Southwest:	Midwest:	Southeast:	Northeast:	International:
Y	Y	Y	Y	Y	Y

Note: Financial information, benefits and other data can change quickly and may vary from those stated here.

BENCHMARK ELECTRONICS INC   www.bench.com

Industry Group Code: 334419 Ranks within this company's industry group: Sales: 2 Profits: 2

Management:		Sales/Marketing:		Liberal Arts:		Information Systems:		Professionals:		Technical/Scientific:	
Mgmt. Trainees:	Y	Mktg. Professionals:	Y	Gen. Writing/Editing:		Info. Management:	Y	Finance/Accounting:	Y	Engineers, Elec.:	Y
Experienced Mgmt.:	Y	Retail Sales:		Technical Writing:	Y	Software Dev.:	Y	Law:	Y	Engineers, Other:	Y
Int'l Business:	Y	Commercial/Industrial:	Y	Graphic Arts/Photog.:		Hardware Dev.:	Y	HR/Other:	Y	Health/Lab:	
MBA Graduates:	Y	Sales Trainees:		Music:		Systems Integration:		Training:	Y	Scientists/Research:	
		Advertising Pros.:	Y	Broadcasting:		Consulting/Other:		Health Care:		Petroleum/Chemicals:	
				Other:				Consulting:		Math/Other:	

TYPES OF BUSINESS:

Contract Manufacturing-Printed Circuit Boards
Design & Engineering

BRANDS/DIVISIONS/AFFILIATES:

Pemstar, Inc.

CONTACTS: Note: Officers with more than one job title may be intentionally listed here more than once.

Cary T. Fu, CEO
Gayla J. Delly, Pres.
Donald F. Adam, CFO
Kenneth S. Barrow, Sec.
Steven A. Barton, Exec. VP
Donald E. Nigbor, Chmn.

Phone: 979-849-6550	Fax: 979-848-5270
Toll-Free:	
Address: 3000 Technology Dr., Angleton, TX 77515 US	

GROWTH PLANS/SPECIAL FEATURES:

Benchmark Electronics, Inc. provides contract-manufacturing services for complex printed circuit boards and related electronics systems and subsystems. The firm also provides comprehensive design and manufacturing services, from initial product design to volume production and direct order fulfillment, to original equipment manufacturers of computers, medical devices, video/audio/entertainment products, industrial control equipment, testing and instrumentation products and telecommunications equipment. In addition, the company offers specialized engineering services including printed circuit board layout, prototyping and test development. Substantially all of Benchmark's manufacturing services are provided on a turnkey basis (though some is provided on consignment), whereby it purchases customer-specified components from its suppliers, assembles the components on finished printed circuit boards, performs post-production testing and provides production process and testing documentation. Sales of computer and related products account for roughly 58% of the company's revenue. Benchmark offers flexible, just-in-time delivery programs allowing product shipments to be closely coordinated with customer inventory requirements. The firm has 64 domestic manufacturing facilities in Alabama, California, Minnesota, New Hampshire, North Dakota, Oregon, Texas and Washington. The company also has 86 international manufacturing facilities in Brazil, China, Ireland, Mexico, the Netherlands, Romania, Singapore and Thailand, providing its international customers with a combination of strategic regional locations and global procurement capabilities. In early 2007, the firm acquired Pemstar, Inc., a provider of engineering, design and manufacturing services, for $300 million.

FINANCIALS: Sales and profits are in thousands of dollars—add 000 to get the full amount. 2007 Note: Financial information for 2007 was not available for all companies at press time.

2007 Sales: $2,915,919	2007 Profits: $93,282	U.S. Stock Ticker: BHE
2006 Sales: $2,907,304	2006 Profits: $111,677	Int'l Ticker: Int'l Exchange:
2005 Sales: $2,257,225	2005 Profits: $80,589	Employees: 10,920
2004 Sales: $2,001,340	2004 Profits: $70,991	Fiscal Year Ends: 12/31
2003 Sales: $1,839,800	2003 Profits: $55,400	Parent Company:

SALARIES/BENEFITS:

Pension Plan:	ESOP Stock Plan:	Profit Sharing: Y	Top Exec. Salary: $603,604	Bonus: $1,101,577
Savings Plan: Y	Stock Purch. Plan: Y		Second Exec. Salary: $422,577	Bonus: $565,197

OTHER THOUGHTS:

Apparent Women Officers or Directors: 1
Hot Spot for Advancement for Women/Minorities:

LOCATIONS: ("Y" = Yes)

West:	Southwest:	Midwest:	Southeast:	Northeast:	International:
Y	Y		Y	Y	Y

BERKSHIRE HATHAWAY INC   www.berkshirehathaway.com

Industry Group Code: 551110 Ranks within this company's industry group: Sales: 1   Profits: 1

Management:		Sales/Marketing:		Liberal Arts:		Information Systems:		Professionals:		Technical/Scientific:	
Mgmt. Trainees:	Y	Mktg. Professionals:	Y	Gen. Writing/Editing:	Y	Info. Management:	Y	Finance/Accounting:	Y	Engineers, Elec.:	Y
Experienced Mgmt.:	Y	Retail Sales:	Y	Technical Writing:	Y	Software Dev.:	Y	Law:	Y	Engineers, Other:	
Int'l Business:	Y	Commercial/Industrial:	Y	Graphic Arts/Photog.:	Y	Hardware Dev.:		HR/Other:	Y	Health/Lab:	
MBA Graduates:	Y	Sales Trainees:	Y	Music:		Systems Integration:		Training:	Y	Scientists/Research:	Y
		Advertising Pros.:	Y	Broadcasting:		Consulting/Other:		Health Care:		Petroleum/Chemicals:	
				Other:				Consulting:		Math/Other:	Y

TYPES OF BUSINESS:

Direct Property & Casualty Insurance & Reinsurance
Retail Operations
Foodservice Operations
Building Products & Services
Apparel & Footwear
Technology Training
Manufactured Housing & RVs
Business Jet Flexible Ownership Services

BRANDS/DIVISIONS/AFFILIATES:

General Re Corporation
GEICO Corporation
International Dairy Queen
Benjamin Moore & Co
Netjets Inc
Cort Business Services Corporation
Clayton Homes Inc
Russell Corp

CONTACTS: Note: Officers with more than one job title may be intentionally listed here more than once.

Warren E. Buffet, CEO
Marc D. Hamburg, CFO/VP
Forrest N. Krutter, Sec.
Marc D. Hamburg, Treas./VP
Charles T. Munger, Vice Chmn.
Jo Ellen Rieck, Dir.-Taxes
Mark D. Millard, Dir.-Financial Assets
Daniel J. Jakisch, Controller
Warren E. Buffet, Chmn.

Phone: 402-346-1400	Fax: 402-346-3375
Toll-Free:	
Address: 1440 Kiewit Plz., Omaha, NE 68131 US	

GROWTH PLANS/SPECIAL FEATURES:

Berkshire Hathaway, Inc. is a holding company that owns subsidiaries engaged in diverse business activities, most importantly insurance and reinsurance. Berkshire provides property and casualty insurance and reinsurance, as well as life accident and health reinsurance, through approximately 60 U.S. and foreign businesses. General Re Corp., through its subsidiaries, conducts global reinsurance business in 61 cities and provides reinsurance worldwide. GEICO mainly provides private passenger auto insurance to individuals in 49 states in the U.S. and Washington, D.C. The company's financial subsidiaries include Clayton Homes, a manufactured housing company; XTRA Corporation, a provider of transportation equipment leases; furniture rental company CORT Business Services Corp.; and General Re Securities. Berkshire's apparel and footwear businesses include Fruit of the Loom, Garan, Fechheimer Brothers, H.H. Brown Shoe Group and Justin Brands. The firm manufactures and distributes building products through Acme Brick Company, Benjamin Moore & Co., Johns Manville and MiTek. Subsidiary FlightSafety provides training to aircraft and ship pilots; while NetJets, Inc. offers fractional ownership programs for aircraft. In addition, subsidiary International Dairy Queen services approximately 6,000 Dairy Queen, Orange Julius and Karmelkorn stores. Other non-insurance operations include grocery and foodservice distribution, furniture retail, jewelry retail, carpet manufacturing, utilities and energy, newspapers, cleaning products, confectioneries, agricultural equipment, kitchen tools and recreational vehicles. In July 2007, Berkshire acquired jewelry manufacturers Bel-Oro International and Aurafin LLC and combined the two to form Richline Group. In March 2008, the firm acquired approximately 60% of Marmon Holdings, Inc. for $4.5 billion.

FINANCIALS: Sales and profits are in thousands of dollars—add 000 to get the full amount. 2007 Note: Financial information for 2007 was not available for all companies at press time.

2007 Sales: $118,245,000	2007 Profits: $13,213,000	U.S. Stock Ticker: BRK
2006 Sales: $98,539,000	2006 Profits: $11,015,000	Int'l Ticker: Int'l Exchange:
2005 Sales: $81,663,000	2005 Profits: $8,528,000	Employees: 217,000
2004 Sales: $74,382,000	2004 Profits: $7,308,000	Fiscal Year Ends: 12/31
2003 Sales: $64,288,000	2003 Profits: $8,151,000	Parent Company:

SALARIES/BENEFITS:

Pension Plan: Y	ESOP Stock Plan: Y	Profit Sharing:	Top Exec. Salary: $662,500	Bonus: $
Savings Plan:	Stock Purch. Plan:		Second Exec. Salary: $100,000	Bonus: $

OTHER THOUGHTS:

Apparent Women Officers or Directors: 2
Hot Spot for Advancement for Women/Minorities: Y

LOCATIONS: ("Y" = Yes)

West:	Southwest:	Midwest:	Southeast:	Northeast:	International:
Y	Y	Y	Y	Y	Y

BEST BUY CO INC

www.bestbuy.com

Industry Group Code: 443110 **Ranks within this company's industry group:** Sales: 1 Profits: 1

Management:		Sales/Marketing:		Liberal Arts:		Information Systems:		Professionals:		Technical/Scientific:	
Mgmt. Trainees:	Y	Mktg. Professionals:	Y	Gen. Writing/Editing:	Y	Info. Management:	Y	Finance/Accounting:	Y	Engineers, Elec.:	
Experienced Mgmt.:	Y	Retail Sales:	Y	Technical Writing:		Software Dev.:	Y	Law:	Y	Engineers, Other:	
Int'l Business:	Y	Commercial/Industrial:	Y	Graphic Arts/Photog.:	Y	Hardware Dev.:		HR/Other:	Y	Health/Lab:	
MBA Graduates:	Y	Sales Trainees:	Y	Music:		Systems Integration:		Training:	Y	Scientists/Research:	
		Advertising Pros.:	Y	Broadcasting:		Consulting/Other:		Health Care:		Petroleum/Chemicals:	
				Other:				Consulting:		Math/Other:	

TYPES OF BUSINESS:

Consumer Electronics Stores
Retail Music & Video Sales
Personal Computers
Office Supplies
Furniture
Appliances
Cameras
Consumer Electronics Installation & Service

BRANDS/DIVISIONS/AFFILIATES:

Geek Squad
Future Shop, Ltd.
Magnolia Audio Video
Studio D
Pacific Sales
Jiangsu Five Star Appliance Co., Ltd.
Speakeasy, Inc.
The Carphone Warehouse

CONTACTS: *Note: Officers with more than one job title may be intentionally listed here more than once.*

Bradbury H. Anderson, CEO/Vice Chmn.
Brian Dunn, COO
Brian J. Dunn, Pres.
James L. Muehlbauer, CFO/Exec. VP
Robert A. Willett, CIO
Joseph M. Joyce, General Counsel/Sr. VP/Asst. Sec.
David P. Berg, Exec. VP-Int'l Strategy & Corp. Dev.
Susan S. Grafton, Chief Acct. Officer/Controller/VP
Shari L. Ballard, Exec. VP-Retail Channel Mgmt.
Michael J. Pratt, Pres., Best Buy Canada
Kevin T. Layden, COO-Best Buy Int'l
David J. Morrish, Exec. VP-Connected Digital Solutions
Richard M. Schulze, Chmn.
Robert A. Willett, CEO-Best Buy Int'l
Michael London, Exec. VP-Global Sourcing

Phone: 612-291-1000	Fax: 612-292-4001
Toll-Free: 888-237-8289	
Address: 7601 Penn Ave. S., Richfield, MN 55423 US	

GROWTH PLANS/SPECIAL FEATURES:

Best Buy Co., Inc. is a retailer of name-brand consumer electronics, entertainment software and appliances. The company conducts business in the domestic and international markets. The domestic includes Best Buy, Best Buy Mobile, Geek Squad, Magnolia Audio Video, Pacific Sales Kitchen and Bath Centers and Speakeasy. The international segment, in Canada and China, includes Best Buy, Future Shop, Geek Squad and Five Star. The company's products include home office equipment; cameras; computer and audio/video equipment furniture; computer upgrades; and car audio and security system installation. The firm offers product service and repair through 10,000 Geek Squad agents, available in all U.S. and Canadian Best Buy stores and 12 stand-alone Geek Squad stores. Best Buy operates 923 retail stores in 49 states and Washington, D.C. and 121 Future Shop and 47 Best Buy stores in Canada. Sales per square foot per year average $940. The firm plans to open about 75 new Best Buy stores yearly, 60 in the U.S. and 15 in Canada. Much of its future growth will be in smaller cities, using the 20,000 square foot format. The eventual goal is roughly 1,000 Best Buy stores in the U.S. and 200 Best Buy and Future Shop stores in Canada. In addition, the Geek Squad will open about 50 free-standing stores in urban areas over the mid term, and Best Buy will open several consumer electronics stores in China. The firm is experimenting with a boutique store format called Studio D in Naperville, Illinois. The firm's 20 Magnolia Audio Video stores serve the upscale home electronics market. In May 2007, Best Buy acquired Speakeasy, Inc., which provides small businesses with VoIP services, for $97 million. In June 2008, Best Buy and the Carphone Warehouse Group PLC entered into a joint venture in the constantly evolving European consumer electronics field.

Qualified employees enjoy savings and stock purchase plans, insurance coverage, employee discounts and tuition assistance.

FINANCIALS: Sales and profits are in thousands of dollars—add 000 to get the full amount. 2007 Note: Financial information for 2007 was not available for all companies at press time.

2007 Sales: $35,934,000	2007 Profits: $1,377,000	**U.S. Stock Ticker: BBY**
2006 Sales: $30,848,000	2006 Profits: $1,140,000	**Int'l Ticker:** Int'l Exchange:
2005 Sales: $27,433,000	2005 Profits: $984,000	Employees: 140,000
2004 Sales: $24,547,000	2004 Profits: $704,000	Fiscal Year Ends: 2/28
2003 Sales: $20,946,000	2003 Profits: $99,000	Parent Company:

SALARIES/BENEFITS:

Pension Plan:	ESOP Stock Plan:	Profit Sharing:	Top Exec. Salary: $1,172,995	Bonus: $2,650,969
Savings Plan: Y	Stock Purch. Plan: Y		Second Exec. Salary: $746,309	Bonus: $1,271,250

OTHER THOUGHTS:

Apparent Women Officers or Directors: 2
Hot Spot for Advancement for Women/Minorities: Y

LOCATIONS: ("Y" = Yes)

West:	Southwest:	Midwest:	Southeast:	Northeast:	International:
Y	Y	Y	Y	Y	Y

Note: Financial information, benefits and other data can change quickly and may vary from those stated here.

BIO RAD LABORATORIES INC   www.bio-rad.com

Industry Group Code: 339113 Ranks within this company's industry group: Sales: 13   Profits: 12

Management:		Sales/Marketing:		Liberal Arts:		Information Systems:		Professionals:		Technical/Scientific:	
Mgmt. Trainees:	Y	Mktg. Professionals:	Y	Gen. Writing/Editing:	Y	Info. Management:	Y	Finance/Accounting:	Y	Engineers, Elec.:	Y
Experienced Mgmt.:	Y	Retail Sales:		Technical Writing:	Y	Software Dev.:	Y	Law:	Y	Engineers, Other:	Y
Int'l Business:	Y	Commercial/Industrial:	Y	Graphic Arts/Photog.:	Y	Hardware Dev.:	Y	HR/Other:	Y	Health/Lab:	Y
MBA Graduates:	Y	Sales Trainees:		Music:		Systems Integration:		Training:	Y	Scientists/Research:	Y
		Advertising Pros.:	Y	Broadcasting:		Consulting/Other:		Health Care:	Y	Petroleum/Chemicals:	
				Other:				Consulting:		Math/Other:	Y

TYPES OF BUSINESS:
Equipment-Life Sciences Research
Clinical Diagnostics Products
Analytical Instruments
Laboratory Devices
Biomaterials
Imaging Products
Assays
Software

BRANDS/DIVISIONS/AFFILIATES:
KnowItAll
BioPlex 2200
iScript
Proeton XPR36
DiaMed Holding AG

CONTACTS: *Note: Officers with more than one job title may be intentionally listed here more than once.*
Norman Schwartz, CEO
Norman Schwartz, Pres.
Christine Tsingos, CFO/VP
Colleen Corey, Dir.-Corp. Human Resources
Sanford S. Wadler, General Counsel/VP/Sec.
James R. Stark, Corp. Controller
Ronald W. Hutton, Treas.
Brad Crutchfield, VP/Group Mgr.-Life Science
John Goetz, VP/Group Mgr.-Clinical Diagnostics
Giovanni Magni, VP/Mgr.-Int'l Sales
David Schwartz, Chmn.
David Forrester, Mgr.-European Region

Phone: 510-724-7000	Fax: 510-741-5815
Toll-Free:	
Address: 1000 Alfred Nobel Dr., Hercules, CA 94547 US	

GROWTH PLANS/SPECIAL FEATURES:
Bio-Rad Laboratories, Inc. supplies the life science research, health care and analytical chemistry markets with a broad range of products and systems used to separate complex chemical and biological materials and to identify, analyze and purify components. The company operates in two industry segments: life science and clinical diagnostics. The firm's life science division develops products for applications including electrophoresis, image analysis, molecular detection, chromatography, gene transfer, sample preparation and amplification. Products include a range of laboratory instruments, apparatus and consumables used for research in genomics, proteomics and food safety. The Bio-Rad life science division provides its services to universities and medical schools, industrial research organizations, government agencies and biotechnology researchers. The company's clinical diagnostics division encompasses a broad array of technologies incorporated into a variety of tests used to detect, identify and quantify substances in blood or other body fluids and tissues. The test results are used as aids for medical diagnosis, detection, evaluation, monitoring and treatment of diseases and other medical conditions. This division is known for diabetes monitoring products, quality control systems, blood virus testing, blood typing, toxicology, genetic disorders products, molecular pathology and Internet-based software. In addition, Bio-Rad is a leading provider of bovine spongiform encephalopathy (mad cow disease) tests throughout the world. Some of Bio-Rad's numerous brand name systems include: KnowItAll, an informatics systems integrating software and database management for a variety of biological information; the BioPlex 2200 multiplex testing platform; iScript, reverse transcription reagent kits; and Proeton XPR36, a protein interaction array system. In October 2007, Bio-Rad acquired DiaMed Holding AG, which develops, manufactures and markets products used in blood typing and screening, for approximately $460 million.

FINANCIALS: Sales and profits are in thousands of dollars—add 000 to get the full amount. 2007 Note: Financial information for 2007 was not available for all companies at press time.

2007 Sales: $1,461,052	2007 Profits: $92,994	**U.S. Stock Ticker: BIO**
2006 Sales: $1,273,930	2006 Profits: $103,263	**Int'l Ticker:** Int'l Exchange:
2005 Sales: $1,180,985	2005 Profits: $81,553	Employees: 6,400
2004 Sales: $1,090,012	2004 Profits: $68,242	Fiscal Year Ends: 12/31
2003 Sales: $1,003,382	2003 Profits: $76,171	Parent Company:

SALARIES/BENEFITS:

Pension Plan:	ESOP Stock Plan:	Profit Sharing:	Top Exec. Salary: $628,465	Bonus: $560,847
Savings Plan: Y	Stock Purch. Plan:		Second Exec. Salary: $520,065	Bonus: $234,000

OTHER THOUGHTS:
Apparent Women Officers or Directors: 3
Hot Spot for Advancement for Women/Minorities: Y

LOCATIONS: ("Y" = Yes)

West:	Southwest:	Midwest:	Southeast:	Northeast:	International:
Y				Y	Y

BJ SERVICES COMPANY

www.bjservices.com

Industry Group Code: 213111 Ranks within this company's industry group: Sales: 7 Profits: 5

Management:		Sales/Marketing:		Liberal Arts:		Information Systems:		Professionals:		Technical/Scientific:	
Mgmt. Trainees:	Y	Mktg. Professionals:	Y	Gen. Writing/Editing:		Info. Management:	Y	Finance/Accounting:	Y	Engineers, Elec.:	Y
Experienced Mgmt.:	Y	Retail Sales:		Technical Writing:		Software Dev.:	Y	Law:	Y	Engineers, Other:	Y
Int'l Business:	Y	Commercial/Industrial:	Y	Graphic Arts/Photog.:		Hardware Dev.:		HR/Other:	Y	Health/Lab:	Y
MBA Graduates:	Y	Sales Trainees:		Music:		Systems Integration:		Training:	Y	Scientists/Research:	
		Advertising Pros.:		Broadcasting:		Consulting/Other:		Health Care:		Petroleum/Chemicals:	Y
				Other:				Consulting:		Math/Other:	

TYPES OF BUSINESS:

Oil & Gas Drilling Support Services
Casing & Tubular Services
Pipeline & Industrial Commissioning
Oilfield Equipment Sales
Specialty Chemical Services
Stimulation Services
Commissioning & Inspection Services
Product & Software Engineering

BRANDS/DIVISIONS/AFFILIATES:

CONTACTS: Note: Officers with more than one job title may be intentionally listed here more than once.

J. W. Stewart, CEO
David D. Dunlap, COO/Exec. VP
J. W. Stewart, Pres.
Jeffrey E. Smith, CFO/Sr. VP-Finance
Susan E. Douget, VP-Human Resources
Paul F. Yust, CIO/VP
Jeff Hibbeler, VP-Tech.
Margaret B. Shannon, General Counsel/VP/Corp. Sec.
Bret Wells, Chief Tax Officer/Treas.
Ronald F. Coleman, VP-North America Pressure Pumping Oper.
L. Scott Biar, VP/Controller
Kenneth A. Williams, VP/Pres., US Oper.
J.W. Stewart, Chmn.
Alasdair I. Buchanan, VP-Int'l Pressure Pumping Svcs.
Jeff Hibbeler, VP-Logistics

Phone: 713-462-4239	Fax: 713-895-5898
Toll-Free:	
Address: 4601 Westway Park Blvd., Houston, TX 77041 US	

GROWTH PLANS/SPECIAL FEATURES:

BJ Services Company is a leading provider of pressure pumping and other oilfield services for the petroleum industry. BJ provides its services on a 24-hour-a-day, on-call basis through facilities in approximately 200 locations worldwide. It conducts operations through four principal segments: U.S./Mexico Pressure Pumping Services, International Pressure Pumping Services, Canada Pressure Pumping Services and the Oilfield Services Group. The company's pressure pumping services include cementing and stimulation services. Cementing services seal off a wellbore to prevent fluid loss or to provide structural support. Stimulation services include fracturing, which enhances natural gas and oil production by opening up, or fracturing, a well with specialized fluids pumped in at pressures up to 20,000 p.s.i.; acidizing, which utilizes corrosives to open up a well; sand control, which utilizes gravel as a filter to keep sand out of a wellbore; nitrogen services, which displaces fluids in a well with nitrogen gas; coiled tubing services, which includes injecting a flexible steel pipe into a well for various applications such as directing fluids into a wellbore or providing a power source for downhole tools; and general downhole service tools, which the firm generally rents. The oilfield services division installs wellbore casing and production tubing; testing, cleaning, drying and inserting pipelines; production enhancing chemical production and design; downhole completion tool design, manufacturing and installation; and sells and reclaims completion fluids, which help control well pressure. Approximately 84% of BJ Services' revenue came from pressure pumping services and 16% from oilfield services, with 60% of that total revenue generated by operations in the U.S. and 40% from international operations.

FINANCIALS: Sales and profits are in thousands of dollars—add 000 to get the full amount. 2007 Note: Financial information for 2007 was not available for all companies at press time.

2007 Sales: $4,802,409	2007 Profits: $753,640	**U.S. Stock Ticker: BJS**
2006 Sales: $4,367,864	2006 Profits: $804,610	**Int'l Ticker:** Int'l Exchange:
2005 Sales: $3,243,186	2005 Profits: $453,042	Employees: 16,000
2004 Sales: $2,600,986	2004 Profits: $361,041	Fiscal Year Ends: 9/30
2003 Sales: $2,142,877	2003 Profits: $188,177	Parent Company:

SALARIES/BENEFITS:

Pension Plan: Y	ESOP Stock Plan:	Profit Sharing:	Top Exec. Salary: $987,501	Bonus: $1,750,014
Savings Plan: Y	Stock Purch. Plan: Y		Second Exec. Salary: $464,163	Bonus: $575,755

OTHER THOUGHTS:

Apparent Women Officers or Directors: 2
Hot Spot for Advancement for Women/Minorities:

LOCATIONS: ("Y" = Yes)

West:	Southwest:	Midwest:	Southeast:	Northeast:	International:
Y	Y	Y	Y	Y	Y

BJ'S WHOLESALE CLUB INC

www.bjs.com

Industry Group Code: 452910A Ranks within this company's industry group: Sales: 3 Profits: 2

Management:		Sales/Marketing:		Liberal Arts:		Information Systems:		Professionals:		Technical/Scientific:	
Mgmt. Trainees:	Y	Mktg. Professionals:	Y	Gen. Writing/Editing:	Y	Info. Management:	Y	Finance/Accounting:	Y	Engineers, Elec.:	
Experienced Mgmt.:	Y	Retail Sales:	Y	Technical Writing:		Software Dev.:	Y	Law:	Y	Engineers, Other:	
Int'l Business:		Commercial/Industrial:	Y	Graphic Arts/Photog.:	Y	Hardware Dev.:		HR/Other:	Y	Health/Lab:	
MBA Graduates:	Y	Sales Trainees:	Y	Music:		Systems Integration:	Y	Training:	Y	Scientists/Research:	
		Advertising Pros.:	Y	Broadcasting:		Consulting/Other:		Health Care:		Petroleum/Chemicals:	
				Other:	Y			Consulting:		Math/Other:	

TYPES OF BUSINESS:

Warehouse Clubs, Retail
Gas Stations
Optical Stores
Photo Labs
Travel Services
Pharmacies
Restaurant Supply

BRANDS/DIVISIONS/AFFILIATES:

Executive Choice
Berkley & Jensen
Inner Circle

CONTACTS: Note: Officers with more than one job title may be intentionally listed here more than once.

Herbert J. Zarkin, CEO
Laura Sen, COO
Laura Sen, Pres.
Frank D. Forward, CFO/Exec. VP
Allison G. Corcoran, Exec. VP-Mktg.
Paul M. Bass, Exec. VP-Merch.
Kellye L. Walker, General Counsel/Sr. VP/Corp. Sec.
Thomas F. Gallagher, Exec. VP-Store Oper.
Cathy Maloney, VP-Investor Rel.
Frank D. Forward, Accounting Officer
Alison G. Corcoran, Exec. VP-Member Insight
Herbert J. Zarkin, Chmn.

Phone: 508-651-7400	Fax: 508-651-6114
Toll-Free:	
Address: 1 Mercer Rd., Natick, MA 01760 US	

GROWTH PLANS/SPECIAL FEATURES:

BJ's Wholesale Club, Inc. sells nearly 7,300 brand-name general merchandise items and food products, with food accounting for approximately 60% of sales. General merchandise items include office supplies, electronics, media, auto accessories, jewelry, books, apparel, toys, personal care items and seasonal items. Food categories include frozen foods, canned goods, fresh produce, dairy products, fresh meat and dry grocery items. Prices are generally lower than those of typical wholesalers and supermarkets. The company operates approximately 178 warehouse clubs in 16 states and has approximately 8.7 million members. BJ's offers two types of membership, business and Inner Circle, the latter of which targets home owners with above-average incomes. Both memberships are generally $45 per year, which includes one free supplemental membership, with additional supplemental memberships for $20 each. In addition, the company has its own private labels: Executive Choice for products marketed to business members and Berkley and Jensen for products marketed to Inner Circle members. BJ's also offers its members a number of specialty services, including full-service optical stores, one-hour photo services, travel services, including member discounts on rental cars, food courts, a selection of garden sheds and gazebos, a propane tank filling service and muffler and brake services. BJ's has 100 gas stations currently located at its clubs. The company attracts potential customers by being the only major warehouse club operator that accepts manufacturers' coupons and several major credit cards. BJ's also increases customer awareness through direct mail, public relations efforts, new club marketing programs and television and radio advertising (during the holiday season), as well as the BJ's Journal, a publication sent to members throughout the year.

FINANCIALS: Sales and profits are in thousands of dollars—add 000 to get the full amount. 2007 Note: Financial information for 2007 was not available for all companies at press time.

2007 Sales: $8,303,496	2007 Profits: $72,016	U.S. Stock Ticker: BJ
2006 Sales: $7,748,184	2006 Profits: $128,533	Int'l Ticker: Int'l Exchange:
2005 Sales: $7,375,300	2005 Profits: $114,400	Employees: 20,300
2004 Sales: $6,724,219	2004 Profits: $102,866	Fiscal Year Ends: 1/31
2003 Sales: $5,859,700	2003 Profits: $130,900	Parent Company:

SALARIES/BENEFITS:

Pension Plan: Y	ESOP Stock Plan:	Profit Sharing:	Top Exec. Salary: $738,943	Bonus: $29,510
Savings Plan: Y	Stock Purch. Plan:		Second Exec. Salary: $625,961	Bonus: $

OTHER THOUGHTS:

Apparent Women Officers or Directors: 2
Hot Spot for Advancement for Women/Minorities: Y

LOCATIONS: ("Y" = Yes)

West:	Southwest:	Midwest:	Southeast:	Northeast:	International:
		Y	Y	Y	

Note: Financial information, benefits and other data can change quickly and may vary from those stated here.

BLACK & DECKER CORP

www.bdk.com

Industry Group Code: 335000 Ranks within this company's industry group: Sales: 2 Profits: 2

Management:		Sales/Marketing:		Liberal Arts:		Information Systems:		Professionals:		Technical/Scientific:	
Mgmt. Trainees:	Y	Mktg. Professionals:	Y	Gen. Writing/Editing:	Y	Info. Management:	Y	Finance/Accounting:	Y	Engineers, Elec.:	Y
Experienced Mgmt.:	Y	Retail Sales:		Technical Writing:	Y	Software Dev.:	Y	Law:	Y	Engineers, Other:	Y
Int'l Business:	Y	Commercial/Industrial:	Y	Graphic Arts/Photog.:	Y	Hardware Dev.:	Y	HR/Other:	Y	Health/Lab:	
MBA Graduates:	Y	Sales Trainees:		Music:		Systems Integration:		Training:	Y	Scientists/Research:	
		Advertising Pros.:	Y	Broadcasting:		Consulting/Other:		Health Care:		Petroleum/Chemicals:	
				Other:	Y			Consulting:		Math/Other:	

TYPES OF BUSINESS:

Power Tools & Accessories Manufacturer
Residential Security Hardware
Household Appliances
Home Improvement Products
Fastening & Assembly Systems
Plumbing Products

BRANDS/DIVISIONS/AFFILIATES:

DeWALT
Dustbuster
Price Pfister
Kwikset
SnakeLight
Vector Products, Inc.
Porter-Cable
Emhart Teknologies

CONTACTS: Note: Officers with more than one job title may be intentionally listed here more than once.

Nolan D. Archibald, CEO
Nolan D. Archibald, Pres.
Michael D. Mangan, CFO/Sr. VP
Paul F. McBride, Sr. VP-Human Resources & Corp. Initiatives
Charles E. Fenton, General Counsel/Sr. VP
Les. H. Ireland, VP/Pres., Commercial Oper.
James R. Raskin, VP-Bus. Dev.
Mark M. Rothleitner, VP-Investor Rel.
Christina M. McMullen, Controller/VP
James T. Caudill, VP/Pres., Hardware & Home Improvement Group
Bruce W. Brooks, VP/Pres., Consumer Products Group
Natalie A. Shields, Corp. Sec./VP
Michael A. Tyll, VP/Pres., Fastening & Assembly Systems Group
Nolan D. Archibald, Chmn.
Les H. Ireland, VP/Pres., Europe, Middle East & Africa

Phone: 410-716-3900	Fax: 410-716-2933
Toll-Free: 800-544-6986	
Address: 701 E. Joppa Rd., Towson, MD 21286 US	

GROWTH PLANS/SPECIAL FEATURES:

The Black & Decker Corp. is a global manufacturer and marketer of power tools and accessories; hardware and home improvement products; and technology-based fastening systems. The firm is also a global supplier of engineered fastening and assembly systems. The company's products and services are marketed in over 100 countries in hardware and home improvement stores around the globe. Black & Decker operates in three business segments: power tools and accessories; hardware and home improvement; and fastening and assembly systems with these business segments comprising approximately 73%, 15%, and 12%, respectively, of the corporation's sales for the six-month period ended June 29, 2008. The power tools and accessories segment includes consumer and industrial power tools and accessories; lawn and garden tools; electric cleaning; automotive; lightning products; and product services. In addition, the power pools and accessories segment has responsibility for the sale of security hardware to customers in Mexico, Central America, the Caribbean, and South America; for the sale of plumbing products to customers outside of the U.S. and Canada; and for sales of household products, principally in Europe and Brazil. The hardware and home improvement segment includes security hardware such as locksets keying systems and exit devices; general hardware products including hinges, door stops and kick plates; decorative hardware such as cabinet hardware, switchplates and door pulls; and plumbing products. This section of the company is also responsible for producing faucets. The fastening and assembly systems group manufactures and sells an array of metal and plastic fasteners and engineered fastening systems for commercial applications. The company's product names include DeWALT and Black and Decker, as well as Price Pfister plumbing products, Kwikset security hardware, Emhart fastening systems, Dustbuster vacuum cleaners and SnakeLight flashlights.

FINANCIALS: Sales and profits are in thousands of dollars—add 000 to get the full amount. 2007 Note: Financial information for 2007 was not available for all companies at press time.

2007 Sales: $6,563,200	2007 Profits: $518,100	U.S. Stock Ticker: BDK	
2006 Sales: $6,447,300	2006 Profits: $486,100	Int'l Ticker:	Int'l Exchange:
2005 Sales: $6,523,700	2005 Profits: $5,352,100	Employees: 25,000	
2004 Sales: $5,398,400	2004 Profits: $445,600	Fiscal Year Ends: 12/31	
2003 Sales: $4,482,700	2003 Profits: $293,000	Parent Company:	

SALARIES/BENEFITS:

Pension Plan:	ESOP Stock Plan:	Profit Sharing:	Top Exec. Salary: $1,523,077	Bonus: $
Savings Plan:	Stock Purch. Plan:		Second Exec. Salary: $563,013	Bonus: $55,000

OTHER THOUGHTS:

Apparent Women Officers or Directors: 4
Hot Spot for Advancement for Women/Minorities: Y

LOCATIONS: ("Y" = Yes)

West:	Southwest:	Midwest:	Southeast:	Northeast:	International:
Y			Y	Y	Y

Note: Financial information, benefits and other data can change quickly and may vary from those stated here.

BLOOMBERG LP

www.bloomberg.com

Industry Group Code: 514100 Ranks within this company's industry group: Sales: 1 Profits: 1

Management:		Sales/Marketing:		Liberal Arts:		Information Systems:		Professionals:		Technical/Scientific:	
Mgmt. Trainees:		Mktg. Professionals:	Y	Gen. Writing/Editing:	Y	Info. Management:	Y	Finance/Accounting:	Y	Engineers, Elec.:	Y
Experienced Mgmt.:	Y	Retail Sales:		Technical Writing:	Y	Software Dev.:	Y	Law:	Y	Engineers, Other:	
Int'l Business:	Y	Commercial/Industrial:	Y	Graphic Arts/Photog.:	Y	Hardware Dev.:		HR/Other:	Y	Health/Lab:	
MBA Graduates:	Y	Sales Trainees:		Music:		Systems Integration:	Y	Training:	Y	Scientists/Research:	
		Advertising Pros.:	Y	Broadcasting:		Consulting/Other:		Health Care:		Petroleum/Chemicals:	
				Other:	Y			Consulting:		Math/Other:	

TYPES OF BUSINESS:
Financial Data Publishing-Print & Online
Magazine Publishing
Management Software
Multimedia Presentation Services
Broadcast Television
Radio Broadcasting
Electronic Exchange Systems
Software

BRANDS/DIVISIONS/AFFILIATES:
Bloomberg Professional
Bloomberg Terminals
Bloomberg Tradebook
Bloomberg Electronic Trading Systems
Bloomberg Roadshows
Bloomberg Television
Bloomberg Magazine
Bloomberg News

CONTACTS: Note: Officers with more than one job title may be intentionally listed here more than once.
Lex Fenwick, CEO
Tom Secunda, Dir.-Worldwide Sales
Peter T. Grauer, Chmn.

Phone: 212-318-2000	**Fax:** 917-369-5000
Toll-Free:	
Address: 731 Lexington Ave., New York, NY 10022 US	

GROWTH PLANS/SPECIAL FEATURES:

Bloomberg LP is one of the world's largest information services, news and media companies, serving the financial services industry as well as government offices and agencies, corporations and news organizations in 126 countries. The firm's core business, the Bloomberg Professional service, is delivered online to Bloomberg Terminals that are rented by subscribers. The terminals provide traders and asset managers a combination of real-time, around-the-clock financial news, market data, analysis, electronic trading, multimedia report capabilities and e-mail on a single platform at an average monthly fee of about $1,500 per month per terminal. There are four primary services included with Bloomberg Professional. Bloomberg Tradebook is an electronic global agency trader offering customers the ability to trade on 65 markets in 54 countries. The Bloomberg Electronic Trading Systems allows the firm's professional services to work in conjunction with outside infrastructure and includes a global risk-management software solution and a portfolio management system. Bloomberg Data License provides access to the Bloomberg financial database and to more than 4 million financial instruments. Finally, Bloomberg Roadshows is a multimedia presentation service featuring synchronized slides, audio, streaming video and live video technology. The company also offers Bloomberg Television, broadcasting in seven languages across 10 networks into 200 million homes; Bloomberg Radio, providing business news to 750 affiliates worldwide; Bloomberg.com, offering financial news and information; and Bloomberg Magazine, specially edited for Bloomberg Professional subscribers. Bloomberg Law provides legal research tools. Finally, Bloomberg News, staffed with 1,600 reporters and editors in 94 bureaus worldwide, files more than 5,000 news stories daily.

Bloomberg offers its employees tuition reimbursement; adoption assistance; back-up childcare services; short- and long-term disability insurance; medical, dental and vision care benefits; onsite medical services at major office locations; commuter expense saving programs; and flexible spending accounts for health expenses.

FINANCIALS: Sales and profits are in thousands of dollars—add 000 to get the full amount. 2007 Note: Financial information for 2007 was not available for all companies at press time.

2007 Sales: $5,400,000	2007 Profits: $	**U.S. Stock Ticker: Private**
2006 Sales: $4,700,000	2006 Profits: $1,500,000	**Int'l Ticker:** Int'l Exchange:
2005 Sales: $4,100,000	2005 Profits: $	Employees: 9,800
2004 Sales: $3,100,000	2004 Profits: $	Fiscal Year Ends: 12/31
2003 Sales: $3,000,000	2003 Profits: $	Parent Company:

SALARIES/BENEFITS:

Pension Plan:	ESOP Stock Plan:	Profit Sharing:	Top Exec. Salary: $	Bonus: $
Savings Plan: Y	Stock Purch. Plan:		Second Exec. Salary: $	Bonus: $

OTHER THOUGHTS:

Apparent Women Officers or Directors:
Hot Spot for Advancement for Women/Minorities:

LOCATIONS: ("Y" = Yes)

West:	Southwest:	Midwest:	Southeast:	Northeast:	International:
Y	Y	Y	Y	Y	Y

BOEING COMPANY (THE)   www.boeing.com

Industry Group Code: 336410 Ranks within this company's industry group: Sales: 1   Profits: 3

Management:		Sales/Marketing:		Liberal Arts:		Information Systems:		Professionals:		Technical/Scientific:	
Mgmt. Trainees:		Mktg. Professionals:	Y	Gen. Writing/Editing:	Y	Info. Management:	Y	Finance/Accounting:	Y	Engineers, Elec.:	Y
Experienced Mgmt.:	Y	Retail Sales:		Technical Writing:	Y	Software Dev.:	Y	Law:	Y	Engineers, Other:	Y
Int'l Business:	Y	Commercial/Industrial:	Y	Graphic Arts/Photog.:	Y	Hardware Dev.:	Y	HR/Other:	Y	Health/Lab:	
MBA Graduates:	Y	Sales Trainees:		Music:		Systems Integration:	Y	Training:	Y	Scientists/Research:	Y
		Advertising Pros.:		Broadcasting:		Consulting/Other:		Health Care:		Petroleum/Chemicals:	
				Other:	Y			Consulting:		Math/Other:	Y

TYPES OF BUSINESS:

Commercial Aircraft Manufacturing
Aerospace Technology & Manufacturing
Military Aircraft
Satellite Manufacturing
Communications Products & Services
Air Traffic Management Technology
Financing Services
Research & Development

BRANDS/DIVISIONS/AFFILIATES:

Boeing Business Jets
787 Dreamliner
Integrated Defense Systems
Boeing Capital
Phantom Works
AH-64D Apache
F-15 Eagle
Air Force One

CONTACTS: Note: Officers with more than one job title may be intentionally listed here more than once.

W. James McNerney, Jr., CEO
W. James McNerney, Jr., Pres.
James A. Bell, CFO
Richard Stephens, Sr. VP-Human Resources
John J. Tracy, CTO/Sr. VP-Tech., Eng. & Oper. Bus.
Richard Stephens, Sr. VP-Admin.
J. Michael Luttig, General Counsel/Sr. VP
Michael J. Cave, Sr. VP-Bus. Dev. & Strategy
Thomas J. Downey, Sr. VP-Comm.
James A. Bell, Exec. VP-Finance
James F. Albaugh, CEO/Pres., Integrated Defense Systems/Exec. VP
Scott E. Carson, CEO/Pres., Commercial Airplanes/Exec. VP
Tod R. Hullin, Sr. VP-Public Policy
Wanda K. Denson-Low, Sr. VP-Office of Internal Governance
W. James McNerney, Jr., Chmn.
Shephard W. Hill, Pres., Boeing Int'l

Phone: 312-544-2000	Fax: 312-544-2082
Toll-Free:	
Address: 100 N. Riverside, Chicago, IL 60606 US	

GROWTH PLANS/SPECIAL FEATURES:

The Boeing Co. is one of the world's major aerospace firms. It operates in three segments: commercial airplanes (CA); integrated defense systems, which is comprised of precision engagement and mobility systems (PE&MS), network and space systems (N&SS) and support systems; and Boeing Capital Corp. CA develops, produces and markets commercial jet aircraft and provides related support services. The family of jet aircraft includes the 737 Next-Generation narrow-body model and the 747, 767, 777 and the new 787 Dreamliner wide-body models. The division also offers aviation support, aircraft modifications, training, maintenance documents and technical advice to commercial customers worldwide. The integrated defense systems segment researches, develops, produces, modifies and supports products and related systems and services such as military aircraft, including fighters, transports, tankers and helicopters; missiles; space systems; missile defense systems; satellites and satellite launch vehicles; and communications, information and battle management systems. The PE&MS subdivision oversees precision engagement and mobility products and services. The N&SS subdivision provides products and services to assist customers in transforming operations through network integration, intelligence and surveillance systems, communications and space exploration. The support systems subdivision is engaged in operations, maintenance, and logistics support functions for military platforms. Boeing Capital Corp. provides financing to CA customers. Boeing's other businesses include Connection by Boeing, a high speed broadband communications business; and Engineering, Operations and Technology, a research and development organization. The 787 Dreamliner is Boeing's exciting, new-generation aircraft. It is manufactured of extremely light components that, combined with advanced technology jet engines, will enable the aircraft to enjoy very high fuel efficiency. It will seat 210 to 250 passengers, with a maximum range of 9,266 miles. The aircraft's first deliveries have been pushed back to 2009 due to production complications.

The company offers its employees health, disability and life insurance; and an employee assistance program. It will discontinue its pension plan for new employees.

FINANCIALS: Sales and profits are in thousands of dollars—add 000 to get the full amount. 2007 Note: Financial information for 2007 was not available for all companies at press time.

2007 Sales: $66,387,000	2007 Profits: $4,074,000	U.S. Stock Ticker: BA
2006 Sales: $61,530,000	2006 Profits: $2,215,000	Int'l Ticker: Int'l Exchange:
2005 Sales: $53,621,000	2005 Profits: $2,572,000	Employees: 159,300
2004 Sales: $51,400,000	2004 Profits: $1,872,000	Fiscal Year Ends: 12/31
2003 Sales: $50,485,000	2003 Profits: $718,000	Parent Company:

SALARIES/BENEFITS:

Pension Plan:	ESOP Stock Plan:	Profit Sharing:	Top Exec. Salary: $1,750,000	Bonus: $4,025,000
Savings Plan: Y	Stock Purch. Plan:		Second Exec. Salary: $865,769	Bonus: $729,500

OTHER THOUGHTS:

Apparent Women Officers or Directors: 3
Hot Spot for Advancement for Women/Minorities: Y

LOCATIONS: ("Y" = Yes)

West:	Southwest:	Midwest:	Southeast:	Northeast:	International:
Y	Y	Y	Y	Y	Y

Note: Financial information, benefits and other data can change quickly and may vary from those stated here.

BOOZ ALLEN HAMILTON

www.boozallen.com

Industry Group Code: 541611 Ranks within this company's industry group: Sales: 3   Profits:

Management:		Sales/Marketing:		Liberal Arts:		Information Systems:		Professionals:		Technical/Scientific:	
Mgmt. Trainees:	Y	Mktg. Professionals:	Y	Gen. Writing/Editing:	Y	Info. Management:	Y	Finance/Accounting:	Y	Engineers, Elec.:	Y
Experienced Mgmt.:	Y	Retail Sales:		Technical Writing:	Y	Software Dev.:	Y	Law:	Y	Engineers, Other:	
Int'l Business:	Y	Commercial/Industrial:	Y	Graphic Arts/Photog.:	Y	Hardware Dev.:		HR/Other:	Y	Health/Lab:	
MBA Graduates:	Y	Sales Trainees:		Music:		Systems Integration:	Y	Training:	Y	Scientists/Research:	Y
		Advertising Pros.:	Y	Broadcasting:		Consulting/Other:	Y	Health Care:		Petroleum/Chemicals:	
				Other:				Consulting:	Y	Math/Other:	Y

TYPES OF BUSINESS:

Strategy Consulting
Engineering & IT Consulting
Supply Chain Management
Industry Research & Publications
War Gaming & Strategic Simulation

BRANDS/DIVISIONS/AFFILIATES:

strategy+business

CONTACTS: Note: Officers with more than one job title may be intentionally listed here more than once.

Ralph W. Shrader, CEO
Douglas G. Swenson, CFO
Barry Jaruzelski, VP/Lead Mktg. Officer
Horacio D. Rozanski, Chief Personnel Officer
Frank S. Smith, III, CIO
Samuel R. Strickland, Chief Admin. Officer
C. G. Appleby, Chief Legal Officer
Dennis O. Doughty, Pres., U.S. Gov't Bus.
Cesare R. Mainardi, Pres., North American Commercial Bus.
Joseph E. Garner, Sr. VP-Defense
Nancy Hardwick, VP/Intellectual Capital Officer
Ralph W. Shrader, Chmn.
Shumeet Banerji, Pres., Global Commercial Bus.

Phone: 703-902-5000	Fax: 703-902-3333
Toll-Free:	
Address: 8283 Greensboro Dr., McLean, VA 22102 US	

GROWTH PLANS/SPECIAL FEATURES:

Booz Allen Hamilton, founded in 1914, is a global strategy and technology consulting firm with operations on six continents. Booz Allen's major areas of expertise include corporate finance and business analysis; information technology; marketing and sales; mergers and restructuring; operations and logistics; organization and change; product and service innovation; public sector mission effectiveness; strategy and leadership; and systems engineering and integration. The company serves such market sectors as aerospace, automotive, chemicals, defense, energy, environment, financial services, government departments, health, homeland security, media, non-profits, oil, retail, technology, telecommunications and transportation. Some of Booz Allen's commercial clients have included Aetna, Boeing, BP, MTV, Pfizer, RJ Reynolds and Vodafone. The company's work with national governments around the world has included enhancing national security, economic well-being and the health and safety of citizens. Some of Booz Allen's largest clients have included the U.S. Department of Defense; the Air Force, Army, Navy and Marine Corps; the U.S. Departments of Energy, Health, Human Services, Homeland Security, Justice, Labor, Transportation and Treasury; NASA; the U.S. Centers for Disease Control and Prevention; the U.S. Environmental Protection Agency; the U.S. General Services Administration; and the U.S. Internal Revenue Service. The company's work for other governments includes assignments with the U.K. Department for Work and Pensions as well as government institutions in Abu Dhabi, Australia, Germany, Italy, Jordan and New Zealand. The company also publishes books, reports and studies on industry subjects ranging from information technology to leadership, the foremost of which is its quarterly strategy+business periodical. In March 2007, the U.S. Agency for International Development awarded a Global, Business, Trade and Investment II contract worth up to $3 billion to nine companies, including Booz Allen. In May 2008, the firm spun off all business units that do not provide consulting to the U.S. government into a new company called Booz & Company.

FINANCIALS: Sales and profits are in thousands of dollars—add 000 to get the full amount. 2007 Note: Financial information for 2007 was not available for all companies at press time.

2007 Sales: $4,000,000	2007 Profits: $	U.S. Stock Ticker: Private
2006 Sales: $3,700,000	2006 Profits: $	Int'l Ticker: Int'l Exchange:
2005 Sales: $3,500,000	2005 Profits: $	Employees: 18,000
2004 Sales: $3,300,000	2004 Profits: $	Fiscal Year Ends: 3/31
2003 Sales: $2,500,000	2003 Profits: $	Parent Company:

SALARIES/BENEFITS:

Pension Plan:	ESOP Stock Plan:	Profit Sharing: Y	Top Exec. Salary: $	Bonus: $
Savings Plan: Y	Stock Purch. Plan:		Second Exec. Salary: $	Bonus: $

OTHER THOUGHTS:

Apparent Women Officers or Directors: 2
Hot Spot for Advancement for Women/Minorities: Y

LOCATIONS: ("Y" = Yes)

West:	Southwest:	Midwest:	Southeast:	Northeast:	International:
Y	Y	Y	Y	Y	Y

BOSTON SCIENTIFIC CORP

www.bostonscientific.com

Industry Group Code: 339113 Ranks within this company's industry group: Sales: 3 Profits: 18

Management:		Sales/Marketing:		Liberal Arts:		Information Systems:		Professionals:		Technical/Scientific:	
Mgmt. Trainees:	Y	Mktg. Professionals:	Y	Gen. Writing/Editing:	Y	Info. Management:	Y	Finance/Accounting:	Y	Engineers, Elec.:	
Experienced Mgmt.:	Y	Retail Sales:		Technical Writing:	Y	Software Dev.:	Y	Law:	Y	Engineers, Other:	Y
Int'l Business:	Y	Commercial/Industrial:	Y	Graphic Arts/Photog.:		Hardware Dev.:		HR/Other:	Y	Health/Lab:	Y
MBA Graduates:	Y	Sales Trainees:		Music:		Systems Integration:		Training:	Y	Scientists/Research:	
		Advertising Pros.:	Y	Broadcasting:		Consulting/Other:		Health Care:		Petroleum/Chemicals:	
				Other:				Consulting:		Math/Other:	

TYPES OF BUSINESS:

Supplies-Surgery
Interventional Medical Products
Catheters
Guide wires
Stents
Oncology & Electrophysiology Research

BRANDS/DIVISIONS/AFFILIATES:

Advanced Bionics Corp.
IQ Guide Wire
Taxus
Advanced Stent Technologies
TriVascular
Radial Jaw
Guidant
iLab

CONTACTS: Note: Officers with more than one job title may be intentionally listed here more than once.

James R. Tobin, CEO
Paul A. LaViolette, COO
James R. Tobin, Pres.
Samuel R. Leno, CFO/Exec. VP
Lucia Luce Quinn, Exec. VP-Human Resources
Donald S. Baim, Chief Medical & Scientific Officer/Exec. VP
Samuel R. Leno, Exec. VP-Info. Sys.
Fredericus A. Colen, Exec. VP-Oper./Tech./Cardiac Rhythm Mgmt.
Timothy Pratt, General Counsel/Exec. VP/Corp. Sec.
Kenneth J. Pucel, Exec. VP-Oper.
Jim Gilbert, Exec. VP-Strategy & Bus. Dev.
Paul Donovan, Sr. VP-Corp. Comm.
Samuel R. Leno, Exec. VP-Finance
Stephen F. Moreci, Sr. VP/Group Pres., Endosurgery
Mark H. Paul, Pres., Neurovascular
John B. Pedersen, Pres., Peripheral Interventions
Brian R. Burns, Sr. VP-Quality
Peter M. Nicholas, Chmn.
David McFaul, Sr. VP-Int'l.

Phone: 508-650-8000	Fax: 508-650-8923
Toll-Free: 888-272-1001	
Address: 1 Boston Scientific Pl., Natick, MA 01760-1537 US	

GROWTH PLANS/SPECIAL FEATURES:

Boston Scientific Corp. (BSC), with offices in over 30 countries, manufactures minimally invasive medical devices intended as an alternative to major surgical procedures that reduces risk, trauma, cost, procedure time and the need for aftercare. The company's products are used in a wide range of interventional medical applications, including cardiology, electrophysiology, gastroenterology, neuro-endovascular therapy, pulmonary medicine, radiology, urology and vascular surgery. Products include steerable catheters, micro-guidewires, polypectomy snares and stents. Stents, flexible metal tubes used to open arteries, account for 20% of sales. Boston Scientific's electrophysiology division is currently investigating advanced modalities for arrhythmia diagnosis and treatment of atrial flutter and atrial fibrillation. The firm's electrophysiology products are used to map the electrical structure of a patient's heart, the map is then used as a guide for minimally invasive surgery. Additionally, the firm's oncology division is studying technologies intended to treat kidney disease and symptomatic uterine fibroids. TriVascular, a subsidiary, makes devices and treatments for abdominal aortic aneurysms. The company sells its products to over 10,000 hospitals, clinics, outpatient facilities and medical offices. Recent product developments include drug-eluting stents, which have been proven more effective than bare metal stents, and the company's LATITUDE Patient Management system which allows clinicians to access information from a patient's implanted cardiac device and store it in GE Healthcare's Centricity Electronic Medical Record as lab results. LATITUDE; CONFIENT, an implantable cardioverter defibrillator; and LIVIAN, a cardiac resynchronization therapy defibrillator, are three cardiac rhythm management products recently approved by the Food and Drug Administration. In October 2007, the firm announced plans to lay off 2,300 employees. In December 2007, the firm announced it would sell its Venous Access businesses to Avista Capital Partners, a leading private equity firm, for $425 million in cash.

Boston Scientific offers employees a complete benefits package, tuition reimbursement and adoption assistance.

FINANCIALS: Sales and profits are in thousands of dollars—add 000 to get the full amount. 2007 Note: Financial information for 2007 was not available for all companies at press time.

		U.S. Stock Ticker: BSX
2007 Sales: $8,357,000	2007 Profits: $-495,000	Int'l Ticker: Int'l Exchange:
2006 Sales: $7,821,000	2006 Profits: $-3,577,000	Employees: 27,500
2005 Sales: $6,283,000	2005 Profits: $628,000	Fiscal Year Ends: 12/31
2004 Sales: $5,624,000	2004 Profits: $1,062,000	Parent Company:
2003 Sales: $3,476,000	2003 Profits: $472,000	

SALARIES/BENEFITS:

Pension Plan:	ESOP Stock Plan: Y	Profit Sharing:	Top Exec. Salary: $922,576	Bonus: $324,100
Savings Plan: Y	Stock Purch. Plan:		Second Exec. Salary: $660,000	Bonus: $616,400

OTHER THOUGHTS:

Apparent Women Officers or Directors: 4
Hot Spot for Advancement for Women/Minorities: Y

LOCATIONS: ("Y" = Yes)

West:	Southwest:	Midwest:	Southeast:	Northeast:	International:
Y	Y	Y	Y	Y	Y

Note: Financial information, benefits and other data can change quickly and may vary from those stated here.

BRINKER INTERNATIONAL INC

www.brinker.com

Industry Group Code: 722110 Ranks within this company's industry group: Sales: 4 Profits: 4

Management:		Sales/Marketing:		Liberal Arts:		Information Systems:		Professionals:		Technical/Scientific:	
Mgmt. Trainees:	Y	Mktg. Professionals:	Y	Gen. Writing/Editing:	Y	Info. Management:	Y	Finance/Accounting:	Y	Engineers, Elec.:	
Experienced Mgmt.:	Y	Retail Sales:		Technical Writing:		Software Dev.:	Y	Law:	Y	Engineers, Other:	
Int'l Business:	Y	Commercial/Industrial:		Graphic Arts/Photog.:	Y	Hardware Dev.:		HR/Other:	Y	Health/Lab:	
MBA Graduates:	Y	Sales Trainees:		Music:		Systems Integration:		Training:	Y	Scientists/Research:	
		Advertising Pros.:	Y	Broadcasting:		Consulting/Other:		Health Care:		Petroleum/Chemicals:	
				Other:	Y			Consulting:		Math/Other:	

TYPES OF BUSINESS:
Casual Dining Restaurants
Cafes

BRANDS/DIVISIONS/AFFILIATES:
Chili's Grill and Bar
Romano's Macaroni Grill
On the Border Mexican Grill and Cantina
Maggiano's Little Italy
HMSHost Corp.
Duke Investments, LLC
Mac Acquisition LLC

CONTACTS: *Note: Officers with more than one job title may be intentionally listed here more than once.*
Douglas H. Brooks, CEO
Charles M. Sonsteby, CFO/Exec. VP
Michael B. Webberman, Exec. VP-Brand Solutions
Valerie Davisson, Exec. VP-PeopleWorks
Roger F. Thomson, Chief Admin. Officer/Exec. VP
Roger F. Thomson, General Counsel/Sec.
Todd E. Diener, Pres., Chili's Grill & Bar
Wyman Roberts, Pres., Maggiano's Little Italy
David M. Orenstein, Pres., On The Border Mexican Grill & Cantina
Douglas H. Brooks, Chmn.
Greg Walther, Pres., Global Bus. Dev.

Phone: 972-980-9917	Fax:
Toll-Free:	
Address: 6820 LBJ Fwy., Dallas, TX 75240 US	

GROWTH PLANS/SPECIAL FEATURES:
Brinker International, Inc. owns, operates, develops and franchises approximately 1,800 casual dining restaurant chains in the U.S. and in 24 countries. Chili's Grill & Bar serves lunch and dinner, also offering a To-Go menu. Entrée selections for Chili's range in price from approximately $6 to $18. Romano's Macaroni Grill is an Italian restaurant featuring brick ovens, festive string lights and a selection of wines. Entrée selections for Macaroni Grill range in price from approximately $9 to $20. On The Border is a Mexican restaurant known for its fajitas and margaritas. On The Border also offers a To-Go entrance and a catering service. Entrees for On The Border range in price from approximately $8 to $14. Maggiano's Little Italy is a classic Italian-American restaurant, featuring individual and family style menus and extensive banquet facilities. Entrée selections for Maggiano's range in price from approximately $8 to $39. Brinker also grows through franchises and joint ventures, most revolving around Chili's Grill and Bar. The firm opened over 195 restaurants in 2007 and plans to open over 150 more in 2008. In June 2007, Brinker completed a transaction with Pepper Dining, Inc. in which they established a new franchise relationship and Pepper Dining purchased 95 Chili's Grill & Bar restaurants in the Northeast and Mid-Atlantic region for approximately $155 million. In September 2007, the firm partnered with HMSHost to develop 26 restaurants over five years in its travel locations. In October 2007, the company partnered with Duke Investments, LLC to develop two Macaroni Grill Alaskan locations. In May 2008, Brinker signed with Top Down Enterprises, Inc. to develop five Chili's locations in the Toronto area. In August 2008, Brinker agreed to sell a majority interest in Macaroni Grill to Mac Acquisition LLC, an affiliate of Golden Gate Capital. Brinker will retain 19.9% interest.

FINANCIALS: Sales and profits are in thousands of dollars—add 000 to get the full amount. 2007 Note: Financial information for 2007 was not available for all companies at press time.

2007 Sales: $4,376,904	2007 Profits: $230,049	**U.S. Stock Ticker: EAT**
2006 Sales: $4,151,291	2006 Profits: $212,395	Int'l Ticker: Int'l Exchange:
2005 Sales: $3,749,291	2005 Profits: $160,219	Employees: 113,900
2004 Sales: $3,541,005	2004 Profits: $150,918	Fiscal Year Ends: 6/30
2003 Sales: $3,141,611	2003 Profits: $166,200	Parent Company:

SALARIES/BENEFITS:

Pension Plan:	ESOP Stock Plan:	Profit Sharing:	Top Exec. Salary: $900,000	Bonus: $706,667
Savings Plan:	Stock Purch. Plan:		Second Exec. Salary: $609,612	Bonus: $392,291

OTHER THOUGHTS:
Apparent Women Officers or Directors: 2
Hot Spot for Advancement for Women/Minorities: Y

LOCATIONS: ("Y" = Yes)

West:	Southwest:	Midwest:	Southeast:	Northeast:	International:
Y	Y	Y	Y	Y	Y

Note: Financial information, benefits and other data can change quickly and may vary from those stated here.

BRINKS COMPANY (THE)

www.brinkscompany.com

Industry Group Code: 561610 Ranks within this company's industry group: Sales: 1 Profits: 1

Management:		Sales/Marketing:		Liberal Arts:		Information Systems:		Professionals:		Technical/Scientific:	
Mgmt. Trainees:	Y	Mktg. Professionals:	Y	Gen. Writing/Editing:	Y	Info. Management:	Y	Finance/Accounting:	Y	Engineers, Elec.:	
Experienced Mgmt.:	Y	Retail Sales:		Technical Writing:		Software Dev.:	Y	Law:	Y	Engineers, Other:	
Int'l Business:	Y	Commercial/Industrial:	Y	Graphic Arts/Photog.:		Hardware Dev.:		HR/Other:	Y	Health/Lab:	
MBA Graduates:	Y	Sales Trainees:	Y	Music:		Systems Integration:		Training:	Y	Scientists/Research:	
		Advertising Pros.:	Y	Broadcasting:		Consulting/Other:		Health Care:		Petroleum/Chemicals:	
				Other:				Consulting:		Math/Other:	

TYPES OF BUSINESS:

Security Services
Armored Car Transport
Document Shredding Services
ATM Servicing
Safe Services
Currency & Deposit Processing
Residential Security Systems & Electronics

BRANDS/DIVISIONS/AFFILIATES:

Brink's, Inc.
Brink's Home Security, Inc.
CompuSafe
SCS Technology
Secure Data Solutions

CONTACTS: Note: Officers with more than one job title may be intentionally listed here more than once.

Michael T. Dan, CEO
Michael T. Dan, Pres.
Michael J. Cazer, CFO/VP
Frank T. Lennon, Chief Admin. Officer/VP
Austin F. Reed, General Counsel/Sec./VP
James B. Hartough, VP-Corp. Finance/Treas.
Arthur E. Wheatley, VP-Risk Mgmt. & Insurance
Matthew A.P. Schumacher, Controller
Michael T. Dan, Chmn.

Phone: 804-289-9600	Fax: 804-289-9770
Toll-Free:	
Address: 1801 Bayberry Ct., Richmond, VA 23226-1800 US	

GROWTH PLANS/SPECIAL FEATURES:

The Brink's Company operates through two major subsidiaries: Brink's, Inc. and Brink's Home Security, Inc. The company is based in Richmond, Virginia and employs 52,000, with operations in roughly 50 countries. North American operations include 182 branches in the U.S. and 52 branches in Canada. Brink's, Inc. provides armored-car transportation; automated teller machine (ATM) services; currency and deposit processing; coin sorting; check and cash processing services; guarding services, including airport security; and secure air transportation of valuable property, including its patented CompuSafe service. CompuSafe is utilized by a number of the firm's cash-intensive retail customers, including convenience stores, gas stations and restaurants. The service includes installing a specialized safe in the retail establishment that holds safeguarded cassettes. The customer's employees deposit currency into the cassettes, which can only be removed by Brink's armored car personnel. Brinks, Inc. also provides secure document destruction services through its SCS Technology, an advanced size-based shredding system, as well as Secure Data Solutions, which provides customers with domestic and international solutions for transferring, storing and destroying sensitive information. The firm's other main subsidiary, Brink's Home Security (BHS), is one of the largest providers of residential monitored security services in North America. The firm markets, sells, installs, monitors and services electronic security systems, with approximately 1,125,000 existing systems in all 50 states, the D.C. area and two provinces in Canada. BHS offers equipment that can be customized to alert intrusion, fire or medical emergencies. When an alarm is tripped, a digital or analog signal is sent to BHS' central monitoring station, which directs appropriate emergency services to the situation. In August 2007, the firm sold its U.K. cash handling operations to Loomis U.K., Ltd.

FINANCIALS: Sales and profits are in thousands of dollars—add 000 to get the full amount. 2007 Note: Financial information for 2007 was not available for all companies at press time.

2007 Sales: $3,219,000	2007 Profits: $137,300	**U.S. Stock Ticker: BCO**	
2006 Sales: $2,793,300	2006 Profits: $587,200	**Int'l Ticker:** Int'l Exchange:	
2005 Sales: $2,505,400	2005 Profits: $142,400	Employees: 53,900	
2004 Sales: $2,277,500	2004 Profits: $121,500	Fiscal Year Ends: 12/31	
2003 Sales: $3,998,600	2003 Profits: $29,400	Parent Company:	

SALARIES/BENEFITS:

Pension Plan: Y	ESOP Stock Plan:	Profit Sharing:	Top Exec. Salary: $1,027,846	Bonus: $1,350,000
Savings Plan: Y	Stock Purch. Plan:		Second Exec. Salary: $456,750	Bonus: $380,000

OTHER THOUGHTS:

Apparent Women Officers or Directors: 1
Hot Spot for Advancement for Women/Minorities:

LOCATIONS: ("Y" = Yes)

West:	Southwest:	Midwest:	Southeast:	Northeast:	International:
Y	Y	Y	Y	Y	Y

BRISTOL MYERS SQUIBB CO

www.bms.com

Industry Group Code: 325412 Ranks within this company's industry group: Sales: Profits:

Management:		Sales/Marketing:		Liberal Arts:		Information Systems:		Professionals:		Technical/Scientific:	
Mgmt. Trainees:	Y	Mktg. Professionals:	Y	Gen. Writing/Editing:	Y	Info. Management:	Y	Finance/Accounting:	Y	Engineers, Elec.:	Y
Experienced Mgmt.:	Y	Retail Sales:		Technical Writing:	Y	Software Dev.:	Y	Law:	Y	Engineers, Other:	Y
Int'l Business:	Y	Commercial/Industrial:	Y	Graphic Arts/Photog.:	Y	Hardware Dev.:		HR/Other:	Y	Health/Lab:	Y
MBA Graduates:	Y	Sales Trainees:	Y	Music:		Systems Integration:		Training:	Y	Scientists/Research:	Y
		Advertising Pros.: ·	Y	Broadcasting:		Consulting/Other:		Health Care:	Y	Petroleum/Chemicals:	
				Other:				Consulting:		Math/Other:	Y

TYPES OF BUSINESS:

Drugs-Diversified
Medical Imaging Products
Nutritional Products
Wound Care Products

BRANDS/DIVISIONS/AFFILIATES:

Convatec
Plavix
Enfamil
Bufferin
Excedrin
Reyataz
Ixempra
Natura

CONTACTS: *Note: Officers with more than one job title may be intentionally listed here more than once.*

James M. Cornelius, CEO
Lamberto Andreotti, COO/Exec. VP
Andrew R.J. Bonfield, CFO/Exec. VP
Anthony McBride, Sr. VP-Human Resources
Brian Daniels, Sr. VP-Global Dev./R&D
Sandra Leung, General Counsel/Sr. VP/Corp. Sec.
John E. Celentano, Sr. VP-Strategy & Productivity Transformation
Robert T. Zito, Chief Comm. Officer/Sr. VP-Corp. & Bus. Comm.
Anthony C. Hooper, Pres., US Pharmaceuticals
Elliott Sigal, Chief Scientific Officer/Pres., R&D/Exec. VP
James M. Cornelius, Chmn.

Phone: 212-546-4000	Fax: 212-546-4020
Toll-Free:	
Address: 345 Park Ave., New York, NY 10154 US	

GROWTH PLANS/SPECIAL FEATURES:

Bristol-Myers Squibb Co. discovers, develops, licenses, manufactures, markets, distributes and sells pharmaceuticals and other health care related products. It operates in three segments: Pharmaceuticals, nutritionals and ConvaTec. The pharmaceuticals segment manufactures drugs across multiple therapeutic classes, including cardiovascular; virology, including immunodeficiency virus infection; oncology; affective and other psychiatric disorders; and immunoscience. Products include Plavix, Avapro/Avalide, Reyataz, Sprycel and Ixempra. These products are manufactured in the U.S. and Puerto Rico and 14 foreign countries. The nutritionals segment, through Mead Johnson, manufactures, markets, distributes and sells infant formulas and other nutritional products, including the entire line of Enfamil products. Nutritional products are generally sold by wholesalers and retailers and are promoted primarily to health are professionals. The ConvaTec segment manufactures, distributes and sells ostomy and modern wound and skin care products. Principal brands of ConvaTec include Natura, Sur-Fit, Esteem, Aquacel, Duoderm and Flexi-Seal. The products are marketed worldwide, primarily to hospitals, medical professions and medical suppliers. In July 2007, Bristol-Myers completed the sale of the Bufferin and Excedrin brands in Japan, Asia and certain Oceanic countries to Lion Corp. for $247 million. In October 2007, the company acquired Adnexus Therapeutics, Inc., a developer of a new therapeutic class of biologics called Adnectins, for $415 million. In January 2008, the firm sold its medical imaging business to Avista Capital Partners LP for $525 million.

FINANCIALS: Sales and profits are in thousands of dollars—add 000 to get the full amount. 2007 Note: Financial information for 2007 was not available for all companies at press time.

2007 Sales: $19,348,000	2007 Profits: $2,165,000	U.S. Stock Ticker: BMY
2006 Sales: $17,256,000	2006 Profits: $1,585,000	Int'l Ticker: Int'l Exchange:
2005 Sales: $18,605,000	2005 Profits: $3,000,000	Employees: 42,000
2004 Sales: $19,380,000	2004 Profits: $2,388,000	Fiscal Year Ends: 12/31
2003 Sales: $20,671,000	2003 Profits: $2,952,000	Parent Company:

SALARIES/BENEFITS:

Pension Plan:	ESOP Stock Plan:	Profit Sharing:	Top Exec. Salary: $1,043,269	Bonus: $
Savings Plan:	Stock Purch. Plan:		Second Exec. Salary: $1,008,345	Bonus: $1,104,887

OTHER THOUGHTS:

Apparent Women Officers or Directors: 2
Hot Spot for Advancement for Women/Minorities: Y

LOCATIONS: ("Y" = Yes)

West:	Southwest:	Midwest:	Southeast:	Northeast:	International:
Y	Y	Y	Y	Y	Y

BROADCOM CORP

www.broadcom.com

Industry Group Code: 334413 Ranks within this company's industry group: Sales: 5 Profits: 6

Management:		Sales/Marketing:		Liberal Arts:		Information Systems:		Professionals:		Technical/Scientific:	
Mgmt. Trainees:		Mktg. Professionals:	Y	Gen. Writing/Editing:		Info. Management:	Y	Finance/Accounting:	Y	Engineers, Elec.:	Y
Experienced Mgmt.:	Y	Retail Sales:		Technical Writing:	Y	Software Dev.:	Y	Law:	Y	Engineers, Other:	
Int'l Business:	Y	Commercial/Industrial:	Y	Graphic Arts/Photog.:		Hardware Dev.:	Y	HR/Other:	Y	Health/Lab:	
MBA Graduates:	Y	Sales Trainees:		Music:		Systems Integration:	Y	Training:	Y	Scientists/Research:	
		Advertising Pros.:		Broadcasting:		Consulting/Other:		Health Care:		Petroleum/Chemicals:	
				Other:				Consulting:		Math/Other:	

TYPES OF BUSINESS:
Integrated Circuits-Broadband Transmission
Communications Products

BRANDS/DIVISIONS/AFFILIATES:
LVL7 Systems, Inc.
Octalica, Inc.
Intensi-fi
NetLink
Octal-PHY
Bladerunner
AirForce
DOCSIS 1.1

CONTACTS: Note: Officers with more than one job title may be intentionally listed here more than once.
Scott McGregor, CEO
Scott McGregor, Pres.
Eric K. Brandt, CFO/Sr. VP
Thomas F. Lagatta, Sr. VP-Worldwide Sales
Dianne Dyer-Bruggeman, Sr. VP-Global Human Resources
Edward H. Frank, VP-R&D
Kenneth Venner, CIO/Sr. VP
Henry Samueli, CTO
Neil Y. Kim, Sr. VP-Central Eng.
Vahid Manian, Sr. VP-Global Mfg. Oper.
David Dull, General Counsel/Sec.
David Dull, Sr. VP-Bus. Affairs
Bret Johnsen, Corp. Controller/Principal Accounting Officer/VP
Robert Rango, Sr. VP/Gen. Mgr.-Wireless Connectivity Group
Nariman Yousefi, Sr. VP/Gen. Mgr.-Enterprise Networking Group
Daniel Marotta, Sr. VP/Gen. Mgr.- Broadband Comm. Group
Yossi Cohen, Sr. VP/Gen. Mgr.-Mobile Platforms Group
Henry Samueli, Chmn.
Thomas F. Lagatta, VP-Worldwide Sales

Phone: 949-926-5000	Fax: 949-926-5203
Toll-Free:	
Address: 5300 California Ave., Irvine, CA 92617 US	

GROWTH PLANS/SPECIAL FEATURES:
Broadcom Corp. deals with the technology of semiconductors for wired and wireless communications. The company's products enable the delivery of voice, data and multimedia to and throughout the home, office and the mobile environment. Broadcom produces highly integrated silicon chips and software solutions to manufacturers of computing and networking equipment, digital entertainment products, broadband access products and mobile devices. The firm's product portfolio includes solutions for digital cable, satellite and Internet Protocol (IP) set-top boxes and media servers; high definition television (HDTV); high definition DVD players and personal video recording (PVR) devices; cable and DSL modems and residential gateways; high-speed transmission and switching for local, metropolitan ,wide area and storage networking; SystemI/OTM server solutions; broadband network and security processors; wireless and personal area networking; cellular communications; mobile multimedia and applications processors; mobile power management; and Voice over Internet Protocol (VoIP) gateway and telephony systems. In May 2007, the company acquired Octalica, Inc., a privately-held fabless semiconductor company that specializes in the design and development of networking technologies based on the MoCA (Multimedia over Coax Alliance) standard. In March 2008, Broadcom acquired Sunext Design, Inc., which will contribute technology for the development of a Blu-ray DVD disk platform.

Broadcom employees enjoy health, survivor's, dental and vision care benefits; disability programs; flexible spending accounts; 401(k); a credit union; and tuition reimbursement. In addition, staff are offered employee referral and employee assistance programs.

FINANCIALS: Sales and profits are in thousands of dollars—add 000 to get the full amount. 2007 Note: Financial information for 2007 was not available for all companies at press time.

2007 Sales: $3,776,395	2007 Profits: $213,342	U.S. Stock Ticker: BRCM
2006 Sales: $3,667,818	2006 Profits: $379,041	Int'l Ticker: Int'l Exchange:
2005 Sales: $2,670,788	2005 Profits: $367,089	Employees: 6,347
2004 Sales: $2,400,610	2004 Profits: $173,185	Fiscal Year Ends: 12/31
2003 Sales: $1,610,095	2003 Profits: $-959,865	Parent Company:

SALARIES/BENEFITS:
Pension Plan:	ESOP Stock Plan:	Profit Sharing:	Top Exec. Salary: $600,000	Bonus: $240,000
Savings Plan: Y	Stock Purch. Plan: Y		Second Exec. Salary: $275,712	Bonus: $100,000

OTHER THOUGHTS:
Apparent Women Officers or Directors: 1
Hot Spot for Advancement for Women/Minorities:

LOCATIONS: ("Y" = Yes)
West:	Southwest:	Midwest:	Southeast:	Northeast:	International:
Y	Y	Y	Y	Y	Y

Note: Financial information, benefits and other data can change quickly and may vary from those stated here.

BROWN & BROWN INC   www.bbinsurance.com

Industry Group Code: 524210 Ranks within this company's industry group: Sales: 2 Profits: 1

Management:		Sales/Marketing:		Liberal Arts:		Information Systems:		Professionals:		Technical/Scientific:	
Mgmt. Trainees:		Mktg. Professionals:	Y	Gen. Writing/Editing:		Info. Management:	Y	Finance/Accounting:	Y	Engineers, Elec.:	
Experienced Mgmt.:	Y	Retail Sales:		Technical Writing:	Y	Software Dev.:		Law:	Y	Engineers, Other:	
Int'l Business:		Commercial/Industrial:		Graphic Arts/Photog.:		Hardware Dev.:		HR/Other:	Y	Health/Lab:	
MBA Graduates:	Y	Sales Trainees:		Music:		Systems Integration:		Training:	Y	Scientists/Research:	Y
		Advertising Pros.:	Y	Broadcasting:		Consulting/Other:		Health Care:		Petroleum/Chemicals:	
				Other:				Consulting:		Math/Other:	

TYPES OF BUSINESS:
Insurance-Property & Casualty
Risk Management Services
Professional Liability Insurance
Third-Party Administration & Consulting
Managed Care & Utilization Management Services
Reinsurance
Life Insurance
Health Insurance

BRANDS/DIVISIONS/AFFILIATES:
Poe & Brown, Inc.
Decus Insurance Brokers, Limited

CONTACTS: *Note: Officers with more than one job title may be intentionally listed here more than once.*
J. Hyatt Brown, CEO
Jim W. Henderson, COO/Vice Chmn.
J. Powell Brown, Pres.
Cory T. Walker, CFO/Sr. VP
Laurel L. Grammig, General Counsel/VP/Sec.
Richard Freebourn, Sr., VP-Internal Oper.
Cory T. Walker, Treas.
Kenneth Kirk, Regional Pres.
Thomas Riley, Regional Pres.
Linda S. Downs, Exec. VP-Leadership Dev.
C. Roy Bridges, Regional Exec. VP
J. Hyatt Brown, Chmn.

Phone: 386-252-9601	Fax: 386-239-5729
Toll-Free:	
Address: 220 S. Ridgewood Ave., Daytona Beach, FL 32114 US	

GROWTH PLANS/SPECIAL FEATURES:
Brown & Brown, Inc., formerly Poe and Brown, Inc., is a leading diversified insurance agency. The firm markets and sells insurance products and services, primarily in the property, casualty and employee benefit areas. As an agent and broker, Brown & Brown does not assume underwriting risks. The company operates through 198 locations in 38 states and one location in London. It operates through four segments: retail, wholesale brokerage, national programs and services. The retail segment provides a range of insurance products and services to commercial, public entity, professional and individual customers. The wholesale brokerage division markets and sells excess and surplus commercial and personal insurance and reinsurance, primarily through independent agents and brokers. The national programs segments is composed of two units: professional programs, which provides professional liability and related package products for certain professionals; and special programs, which markets targeted products and services designated for specific industries, trade groups, public entities and market niches. The services division provides clients with third-party claims administration, consulting for the workers' compensation insurance markets, comprehensive medical utilization management services and Medicare Secondary Payer statute compliance-related services. During 2007, Brown & Brown acquired 41 insurance intermediary operations, including customer accounts. In March 2008, Brown & Brown launched Decus Insurance Brokers, Limited, its London-based wholesale brokerage subsidiary.

FINANCIALS: Sales and profits are in thousands of dollars—add 000 to get the full amount. 2007 Note: Financial information for 2007 was not available for all companies at press time.

2007 Sales: $959,667	2007 Profits: $190,959	U.S. Stock Ticker: BRO
2006 Sales: $878,004	2006 Profits: $172,350	Int'l Ticker: Int'l Exchange:
2005 Sales: $785,807	2005 Profits: $150,551	Employees: 4,733
2004 Sales: $646,934	2004 Profits: $128,843	Fiscal Year Ends: 12/31
2003 Sales: $551,040	2003 Profits: $110,322	Parent Company:

SALARIES/BENEFITS:
Pension Plan:	ESOP Stock Plan:	Profit Sharing:	Top Exec. Salary: $614,629	Bonus: $1,142,292
Savings Plan:	Stock Purch. Plan:		Second Exec. Salary: $439,589	Bonus: $1,013,838

OTHER THOUGHTS:
Apparent Women Officers or Directors: 4
Hot Spot for Advancement for Women/Minorities: Y

LOCATIONS: ("Y" = Yes)
West:	Southwest:	Midwest:	Southeast:	Northeast:	International:
Y	Y	Y	Y	Y	Y

BUCKLE INC (THE)

www.buckle.com

Industry Group Code: 448000 Ranks within this company's industry group: Sales: 9   Profits: 8

Management:		Sales/Marketing:		Liberal Arts:		Information Systems:		Professionals:		Technical/Scientific:	
Mgmt. Trainees:	Y	Mktg. Professionals:	Y	Gen. Writing/Editing:	Y	Info. Management:	Y	Finance/Accounting:	Y	Engineers, Elec.:	
Experienced Mgmt.:	Y	Retail Sales:	Y	Technical Writing:		Software Dev.:		Law:	Y	Engineers, Other:	
Int'l Business:		Commercial/Industrial:		Graphic Arts/Photog.:	Y	Hardware Dev.:		HR/Other:	Y	Health/Lab:	
MBA Graduates:	Y	Sales Trainees:	Y	Music:		Systems Integration:		Training:	Y	Scientists/Research:	
		Advertising Pros.:	Y	Broadcasting:		Consulting/Other:		Health Care:		Petroleum/Chemicals:	
				Other:	Y			Consulting:		Math/Other:	

TYPES OF BUSINESS:

Teen Apparel, Retail
Children's Apparel
Online Sales
Promotional Merchandise

BRANDS/DIVISIONS/AFFILIATES:

Buckle
Buckle [The]
Buckle Screenprinting
buckle.com

CONTACTS: *Note: Officers with more than one job title may be intentionally listed here more than once.*

Dennis H. Nelson, CEO
Dennis H. Nelson, Pres.
Karen B. Rhoads, CFO
Kari Smith, VP-Sales
Patricia K. Whisler, VP-Women's Merch.
Kyle L. Hanson, General Counsel
Karen B. Rhoads, VP-Finance
Brett P. Milkie, VP-Leasing
Robert M. Carlberg, VP-Men's Merch.
Daniel J. Hirschfeld, Chmn.

Phone: 308-236-8491	Fax: 308-236-4493
Toll-Free: 800-626-1255	
Address: 2407 W. 24th St., Kearney, NE 68845-4915 US	

GROWTH PLANS/SPECIAL FEATURES:

The Buckle, Inc. is a retailer of medium- to high-priced casual apparel, footwear and accessories primarily for young men and women ages 12-24. The company currently operates more than 368 stores in 39 states throughout the central, northwest, southwest and southeast U.S. These stores operate under the names Buckle and The Buckle. The majority of the stores are located in regional shopping malls, although some are located in strip centers, downtown areas and lifestyle centers. Buckle markets mostly brand-name casual apparel including denims, tops, sportswear, outerwear, accessories and footwear. Brand names such as Lucky Brand Dungarees, Big Star, Silver, Hurley, Affliction, Fossil, MEK, Billabong, Guess, Quiksilver/Roxy, 7 Diamonds, OBEY and Manchester constitute about 70% of overall sales. The remaining merchandise consists of items manufactured to the company's specifications by private labels. The firm emphasizes personalized attention to its customers by providing free alterations, free gift-wrapping and a frequent shopper program. Buckle Screenprinting offers promotional merchandising to outside athletic teams, organizations, clubs and individuals. The company tailors individual store inventories to reflect differences in customer buying patterns by shipping new merchandise daily to most stores through its transfer program. This assures that popular merchandise is in stock and reduces the need to lower the price of low-selling merchandise at a particular location.

The company offers employees merchandise discounts; medical, dental and life insurance; and performance-based bonuses.

FINANCIALS: Sales and profits are in thousands of dollars—add 000 to get the full amount. 2007 Note: Financial information for 2007 was not available for all companies at press time.

2007 Sales: $530,074	2007 Profits: $55,726	U.S. Stock Ticker: BKE	
2006 Sales: $501,101	2006 Profits: $51,906	Int'l Ticker:	Int'l Exchange:
2005 Sales: $470,937	2005 Profits: $43,229	Employees: 6,500	
2004 Sales: $422,820	2004 Profits: $33,745	Fiscal Year Ends: 1/31	
2003 Sales: $401,100	2003 Profits: $32,100	Parent Company:	

SALARIES/BENEFITS:

Pension Plan:	ESOP Stock Plan:	Profit Sharing: Y	Top Exec. Salary: $805,000	Bonus: $1,232,031
Savings Plan: Y	Stock Purch. Plan:		Second Exec. Salary: $460,000	Bonus: $616,016

OTHER THOUGHTS:

Apparent Women Officers or Directors: 2
Hot Spot for Advancement for Women/Minorities: Y

LOCATIONS: ("Y" = Yes)

West:	Southwest:	Midwest:	Southeast:	Northeast:	International:
Y	Y	Y	Y	Y	

Note: Financial information, benefits and other data can change quickly and may vary from those stated here.

BUILD-A-BEAR WORKSHOP INC

www.buildabear.com

Industry Group Code: 451120 Ranks within this company's industry group: Sales: 2 Profits: 2

Management:		Sales/Marketing:		Liberal Arts:		Information Systems:		Professionals:		Technical/Scientific:	
Mgmt. Trainees:	Y	Mktg. Professionals:	Y	Gen. Writing/Editing:	Y	Info. Management:	Y	Finance/Accounting:	Y	Engineers, Elec.:	
Experienced Mgmt.:	Y	Retail Sales:	Y	Technical Writing:		Software Dev.:	Y	Law:	Y	Engineers, Other:	
Int'l Business:	Y	Commercial/Industrial:	Y	Graphic Arts/Photog.:	Y	Hardware Dev.:		HR/Other:	Y	Health/Lab:	
MBA Graduates:	Y	Sales Trainees:	Y	Music:		Systems Integration:		Training:	Y	Scientists/Research:	
		Advertising Pros.:	Y	Broadcasting:		Consulting/Other:		Health Care:		Petroleum/Chemicals:	
				Other:	Y			Consulting:		Math/Other:	

TYPES OF BUSINESS:

Retail-Stuffed Animals
Custom Stuffed Animal Making
Custom Doll Making

BRANDS/DIVISIONS/AFFILIATES:

RidemakerZ LLC
BuildaBearville.com
Cub Condo
CubCase
Bear Bunk Trunk
Friends 2B Made
Bear Factory Limited (The)
Amsbra, Ltd.

CONTACTS: *Note: Officers with more than one job title may be intentionally listed here more than once.*

Maxine Clark, Chief Exec. Bear
Scott Seay, Chief Operating Bear
Scott Seay, Pres.
Tina Klocke, Chief Financial Bear
Teresa Kroll, Chief Mktg. Bear
Dave Finnegan, Chief Info. Bear
Eric Fencl, General Counsel
Tina Klocke, Treas./Sec.
Scott Seay, Chief Workshop Bear
Maxine Clark, Chmn.

Phone: 314-423-8000	**Fax:** 314-423-8188
Toll-Free: 877-789-2327	
Address: 1954 Innerbelt Business Ctr. Dr., St. Louis, MO 63114 US	

GROWTH PLANS/SPECIAL FEATURES:

Build-A-Bear Workshop, Inc. is a leading retail firm providing customers a chance to make, personalize and customize their stuffed animals, capitalizing on the relatively untapped demand for experience-based shopping as well as the widespread appeal of stuffed animals. The company has sold 47 million stuffed animals since the company's inception in 1997. Customers choose from between 30-35 styles of animals to customize, stuff and sew. The customer then accessorizes the stuffed animal with a wide variety of stuffed animal clothing, shoes and accessories. The company forms product licensing relationships with other brands, such as National Football League (NFL), National Basketball League (NBA) and Major League Baseball (MLB) team apparel; SKECHERS shoes; and Limited Too clothing. Build-A-Bear operates approximately 278 stores, primarily located in major malls, throughout the U.S., Puerto Rico and Canada, and 52 stores in the U.K., Ireland and France. The firm has an additional 58 franchised stores in Australia, Belgium, Denmark, Germany, India, Japan, The Netherlands, Norway, South Korea, Russia, Singapore, South Africa, Sweden, Taiwan and Thailand. Many stores host customer birthday parties and other special events for groups through the Build-A-Party service, starting at $10 per guest. In addition to the company's retail locations, Build-A-Bear markets its products through its web site and in event-based locations and sports venues. Brand names include Bearemy, Cub Condo, Beararmoire, CubCase, Bear Bunk Trunk and Corbearate Gifts. The company operates Friends 2B Made, which builds dolls instead of teddy bears, offer 14 varieties of girl dolls and three kinds of build-your-own boys. Its primary customers are 5-12 year-old girls. The company holds a minority interest in RidemakerZ, LLC, a company that allows children and families to build and customize their own personalized cars. In December 2007, the company launched BuildaBearville.com, a virtual online world for Build-A-Bear stuffed animals.

FINANCIALS: Sales and profits are in thousands of dollars—add 000 to get the full amount. 2007 Note: Financial information for 2007 was not available for all companies at press time.

2007 Sales: $474,361	2007 Profits: $22,509	**U.S. Stock Ticker:** BBW
2006 Sales: $437,072	2006 Profits: $29,490	**Int'l Ticker:** Int'l Exchange:
2005 Sales: $361,809	2005 Profits: $27,314	Employees: 6,900
2004 Sales: $301,662	2004 Profits: $20,000	Fiscal Year Ends: 12/31
2003 Sales: $213,700	2003 Profits: $8,000	Parent Company:

SALARIES/BENEFITS:

Pension Plan:	ESOP Stock Plan:	Profit Sharing:	Top Exec. Salary: $520,673	Bonus: $156,058
Savings Plan: Y	Stock Purch. Plan: Y		Second Exec. Salary: $375,000	Bonus: $301,251

OTHER THOUGHTS:

Apparent Women Officers or Directors: 3
Hot Spot for Advancement for Women/Minorities: Y

LOCATIONS: ("Y" = Yes)

West:	Southwest:	Midwest:	Southeast:	Northeast:	International:
Y	Y	Y	Y	Y	Y

BUNGE LTD

www.bunge.com

Industry Group Code: 311210 Ranks within this company's industry group: Sales: Profits:

Management:	Sales/Marketing:	Liberal Arts:	Information Systems:	Professionals:	Technical/Scientific:
Mgmt. Trainees:	Mktg. Professionals:	Gen. Writing/Editing:	Info. Management:	Finance/Accounting:	Engineers, Elec.:
Experienced Mgmt.:	Retail Sales:	Technical Writing:	Software Dev.:	Law:	Engineers, Other:
Int'l Business:	Commercial/Industrial:	Graphic Arts/Photog.:	Hardware Dev.:	HR/Other:	Health/Lab:
MBA Graduates:	Sales Trainees:	Music:	Systems Integration:	Training:	Scientists/Research:
	Advertising Pros.:	Broadcasting:	Consulting/Other:	Health Care:	Petroleum/Chemicals:
		Other:		Consulting:	Math/Other:

TYPES OF BUSINESS:

Crop Production, Soybeans
Oils & Shortening
Oilseed Processing
Ingredients & Prepared Foods
Fertilizer
Milling

BRANDS/DIVISIONS/AFFILIATES:

Serrana
Manah
Ouro Verde
IAP
Sinograin
Agroindustrial Santa Juliana

CONTACTS: *Note: Officers with more than one job title may be intentionally listed here more than once.*

Alberto Weisser, CEO
Jacqualyn A. Fouse, CFO
Archibald Gwathmey, Managing Dir.-Bunge Global Markets
Flavio Sa Carvalho, Chief Personnel Officer
Joao Fernando Kfouri, Managing Dir.-Food Products
Jorge Born, Jr., Deputy Chmn.
Mario A. Barbosa Neto, CEO-Bunge Fertilizantes
Andrew J. Burke, Co-CEO-Bunge Global Agribusiness
Carl L. Hausmann, CEO-Bunge North America
Alberto Weisser, Chmn.
Jean-Louis Gourbin, CEO-Bunge Europe

Phone: 914-684-2800	Fax: 914-684-3499
Toll-Free:	
Address: 50 Main St., 6th Fl., White Plains, NY 10606 US	

GROWTH PLANS/SPECIAL FEATURES:

Bunge, Ltd., founded in 1818, is a Bermuda-based agribusiness and food company with operations in oilseed processing; fertilizer production and supply; and bottled vegetable oil supply. Through its facilities in North and South America, the company processes and exports soybeans and soybean products; produces and supplies fertilizers to farmers in Latin America; produces edible oils and shortenings in Brazil and premium edible oils in the U.S.; mills corn and wheat in Latin America; and manufactures isolated soybean products globally. The agribusiness division includes grain origination, oilseed processing and international marketing. Agribusiness products are distributed through Bunge's international sales and marketing division, which has roughly 18 marketing and distribution offices throughout the world. The fertilizer division is engaged in all stages of the fertilizer business, from mining of raw materials to sales of mixed fertilizer formulas, with activities located primarily in Brazil. Bunge has approximately 26% of the market share of NPK (nitrogen, phosphate and potash) fertilizers in Brazil, which it markets under the Serrana, Manah, Ouro Verde and IAP brand names. Bunge's food products division produces and sells shortenings, mayonnaise, bakery mixes, baked goods and food ingredients. It is a leading provider of premium shortenings and oils to the U.S. foodservice industry; one of the world's leading producers of canola oil; one of the top makers and sellers of flours and mixes in Brazil; and a leading global corn dry miller. In April 2007, Bunge acquired a majority interest in a joint venture to operate a soybean processing plant in Tianjin, China. In July 2007, the company established a joint venture to build and operate a soybean processing plant in Dongguan, China with Sinograin, the Chinese state-owned grain company. In September 2007, Bunge agreed to acquire Agroindustrial Santa Juliana, a sugarcane mill and ethanol production facility in Brazil.

FINANCIALS: Sales and profits are in thousands of dollars—add 000 to get the full amount. 2007 Note: Financial information for 2007 was not available for all companies at press time.

2007 Sales: $37,842,000	2007 Profits: $778,000	**U.S. Stock Ticker: BG**
2006 Sales: $26,274,000	2006 Profits: $521,000	**Int'l Ticker:** Int'l Exchange:
2005 Sales: $24,377,000	2005 Profits: $530,000	Employees: 22,000
2004 Sales: $25,168,000	2004 Profits: $469,000	Fiscal Year Ends: 12/31
2003 Sales: $22,165,000	2003 Profits: $411,000	Parent Company:

SALARIES/BENEFITS:

Pension Plan: Y	ESOP Stock Plan:	Profit Sharing:	Top Exec. Salary: $1,200,000	Bonus: $1,150,000
Savings Plan: Y	Stock Purch. Plan:		Second Exec. Salary: $600,000	Bonus: $300,000

OTHER THOUGHTS:

Apparent Women Officers or Directors: 1
Hot Spot for Advancement for Women/Minorities:

LOCATIONS: ("Y" = Yes)

West:	Southwest:	Midwest:	Southeast:	Northeast:	International:
		Y		Y	Y

Note: Financial information, benefits and other data can change quickly and may vary from those stated here.

BURGER KING HOLDINGS INC   www.burgerking.com

Industry Group Code: 722110 Ranks within this company's industry group: Sales: 7   Profits: 8

Management:		Sales/Marketing:		Liberal Arts:		Information Systems:		Professionals:		Technical/Scientific:	
Mgmt. Trainees:	Y	Mktg. Professionals:	Y	Gen. Writing/Editing:	Y	Info. Management:	Y	Finance/Accounting:	Y	Engineers, Elec.:	
Experienced Mgmt.:	Y	Retail Sales:		Technical Writing:		Software Dev.:	Y	Law:	Y	Engineers, Other:	
Int'l Business:	Y	Commercial/Industrial:	Y	Graphic Arts/Photog.:	Y	Hardware Dev.:		HR/Other:	Y	Health/Lab:	
MBA Graduates:	Y	Sales Trainees:		Music:		Systems Integration:		Training:	Y	Scientists/Research:	
		Advertising Pros.:	Y	Broadcasting:		Consulting/Other:		Health Care:		Petroleum/Chemicals:	
				Other:	Y			Consulting:		Math/Other:	

TYPES OF BUSINESS:

Fast Food Restaurants
Franchising

BRANDS/DIVISIONS/AFFILIATES:

Whopper
BK Fish Filet
BK Veggie Burger
Croissan'wich
Fresh Apple Fries

CONTACTS: *Note: Officers with more than one job title may be intentionally listed here more than once.*

John W. Chidsey, CEO
James F. Hyatt, COO
Ben K. Wells, CFO
Russell B. Klein, Pres., Global Mktg. Strategy & Innovation
Peter C. Smith, Chief Human Resources Officer
Raj Rawal, CIO/Sr. VP
Anne Chwat, General Counsel/Corp. Sec.
Julio Ramirez, Exec. VP-Global Oper.
Russ Klein, Pres., Strategy & Innovation
Amy E. Wagner, Sr. VP-Global Comm.
Amy E. Wagner, Sr. VP-Investor Rel.
Ben K. Wells, Treas.
Chuck Fallon, Pres., North America
Dave Gagnon, Sr. VP-North America Co. Oper./Training
Peter Tan, Pres., Asia Pacific
Armando Jacomino, Sr. VP/Pres., Latin America & Caribbean
John W. Chidsey, Chmn.
Peter Robinson, Pres., EMEA/Exec. VP

Phone: 305-378-3000	Fax: 305-378-7262
Toll-Free:	
Address: 5505 Blue Lagoon Dr., Miami, FL 33126 US	

GROWTH PLANS/SPECIAL FEATURES:

Burger King Holdings, Inc., one of the largest fast food restaurant chains in the world, operates approximately 11,400 restaurants in 70 countries and U.S. territories and serves about 11.8 million customers daily. Approximately 90% of Burger King restaurants are owned and operated by independent franchisees. The company's products include hamburgers, chicken sandwiches and tenders, fish sandwiches, french fries, onion rings and shakes, as well as breakfast items including croissant and sourdough sandwiches, french toast sticks and hash browns. Brand names include the Whopper, BK Fish Filet, BK Veggie Burger and Croissan'wich. In an effort to provide healthier food choices, the firm has added a line of salads to its menu, low-fat versions of existing menu items and Fresh Apple Fries, red apples skinned and sliced to look like french fries. Burger King has also begun to transition to using only trans fat free oil. Burger King restaurants typically offer counter service, a dining room and drive-through service. Many franchises offer regional favorites in addition to standard menu items. These offerings include breakfast burritos in the southwestern U.S., garlic-flavored pork Bulgogi Burgers in Korea, Churrasquito steak sandwiches in Argentina and fried Green Tea Pies in Thailand. In 2008, Burger King announced the opening of the first Burger King restaurants in Curacao and Suriname.

Burger King full-time employees receive medical and dental coverage, flexible spending accounts, a 401(k) savings plan and tuition assistance.

FINANCIALS: Sales and profits are in thousands of dollars—add 000 to get the full amount. 2007 Note: Financial information for 2007 was not available for all companies at press time.

2007 Sales: $2,234,000	2007 Profits: $148,000	**U.S. Stock Ticker: BKC**	
2006 Sales: $2,048,000	2006 Profits: $27,000	**Int'l Ticker:**	Int'l Exchange:
2005 Sales: $1,940,000	2005 Profits: $47,000	Employees: 37,000	
2004 Sales: $1,754,000	2004 Profits: $5,000	Fiscal Year Ends: 6/30	
2003 Sales: $1,657,000	2003 Profits: $-868,000	Parent Company:	

SALARIES/BENEFITS:

Pension Plan:	ESOP Stock Plan:	Profit Sharing:	Top Exec. Salary: $1,021,923	Bonus: $12,421,349
Savings Plan: Y	Stock Purch. Plan:		Second Exec. Salary: $814,567	Bonus: $7,139,170

OTHER THOUGHTS:

Apparent Women Officers or Directors: 2
Hot Spot for Advancement for Women/Minorities: Y

LOCATIONS: ("Y" = Yes)

West:	Southwest:	Midwest:	Southeast:	Northeast:	International:
Y	Y	Y	Y	Y	Y

BURLINGTON NORTHERN SANTA FE CORP   www.bnsf.com

Industry Group Code: 482110 **Ranks within this company's industry group:** Sales: 2 Profits: 1

Management:		Sales/Marketing:		Liberal Arts:		Information Systems:		Professionals:		Technical/Scientific:	
Mgmt. Trainees:		Mktg. Professionals:	Y	Gen. Writing/Editing:		Info. Management:	Y	Finance/Accounting:	Y	Engineers, Elec.:	Y
Experienced Mgmt.:	Y	Retail Sales:	Y	Technical Writing:	Y	Software Dev.:	Y	Law:	Y	Engineers, Other:	Y
Int'l Business:	Y	Commercial/Industrial:	Y	Graphic Arts/Photog.:		Hardware Dev.:		HR/Other:	Y	Health/Lab:	
MBA Graduates:	Y	Sales Trainees:		Music:		Systems Integration:		Training:	Y	Scientists/Research:	
		Advertising Pros.:		Broadcasting:		Consulting/Other:		Health Care:		Petroleum/Chemicals:	
				Other:				Consulting:		Math/Other:	

TYPES OF BUSINESS:

Rail Transportation
Railroad Infrastructure Management
Locomotive Operation
Logistics Services
Intermodal Hubs
Supply Chain Management

BRANDS/DIVISIONS/AFFILIATES:

BSNF Railway Company
Diversified Freight Logistics, Inc.
BNSF Logistics
Royal Cargo Line

CONTACTS: Note: Officers with more than one job title may be intentionally listed here more than once.

Matthew K. Rose, CEO
Carl R. Ice, COO/Exec. VP
Matthew K. Rose, Pres.
Thomas N. Hund, CFO/Exec. VP
John P. Lanigan, Jr., Chief Mktg. Officer/Exec. VP
Linda Longo-Kazanova, VP-Human Resources & Medical
Jeffrey J. Campbell, CIO/VP
Jeffrey J. Campbell, VP-Tech. Svcs.
Paul R. Hoferer, General Counsel/VP
Peter J. Rickershauser, VP-Network Dev.
Mary Jo Keating, VP-Corp. Rel.
Marsha K. Morgan, VP-Investor Rel.
Linda J. Hurt, Treas.
Roger Norber, Exec. VP-Law/Sec.
Shelley J. Venick, VP/General Tax Counsel
Paul W. Bischler, Controller/VP
Matthew K. Rose, Chmn.

Phone:	Fax: 817-352-7171
Toll-Free: 800-795-2673	
Address: 2650 Lou Menk Dr., Fort Worth, TX 76131-2830 US	

GROWTH PLANS/SPECIAL FEATURES:

Burlington Northern Santa Fe Corp. (BNSF) is engaged, through its subsidiaries, in the rail transportation business. The firm's principal operating subsidiary, BNSF Railway Company, controls one of North America's largest railroad systems. The railway operates approximately 32,000 route miles of track, approximately 24,000 of which are owned route miles, through 28 states and two Canadian provinces. BNSF Railway operates various facilities and equipment to support its transportation systems, including over 6,300 locomotives. On average 220,000 freight cars are on its system at any given time. It also operates 25 intermodal hubs, as well as 23 automotive distribution facilities where automobiles are loaded or unloaded from multi-level rail cars. In addition to major cities and ports, the company serves smaller markets through partnerships with over 200 shortline partners. The railway carries both consumer and industrial freight products produced throughout the country. Examples of consumer products include food items, perishables, cotton, salt, rubber and tires. The firm is also one of the largest transporters of low-sulfur coal in the U.S. In addition, BNSF Railway transports agricultural products such as wheat, corn, bulk foods, soybeans, oil seeds, feeds, flour and mill products, oils, malt and fertilizer. As a supplement to railway revenues, subsidiary BNSF Logistics offers logistics and demurrage to third-party contractors. The logistics unit offers a comprehensive set of supply chain services, including management of supply networks. In February of 2008, BNSF Logistics acquired Diversified Freight Logistics, Inc. and Royal Cargo Line (known together as DFL), an international freight management company.

BNSF provides its employees with health and other insurance, flexible spending accounts, tuition reimbursement and an incentive compensation plan.

FINANCIALS: Sales and profits are in thousands of dollars—add 000 to get the full amount. 2007 Note: Financial information for 2007 was not available for all companies at press time.

2007 Sales: $15,802,000	2007 Profits: $1,829,000	U.S. Stock Ticker: BNI
2006 Sales: $14,985,000	2006 Profits: $1,887,000	Int'l Ticker: Int'l Exchange:
2005 Sales: $12,987,000	2005 Profits: $1,531,000	Employees: 41,000
2004 Sales: $10,946,000	2004 Profits: $791,000	Fiscal Year Ends: 12/31
2003 Sales: $9,413,000	2003 Profits: $816,000	Parent Company:

SALARIES/BENEFITS:

Pension Plan: Y	ESOP Stock Plan:	Profit Sharing:	Top Exec. Salary: $1,100,000	Bonus: $2,196,751
Savings Plan: Y	Stock Purch. Plan: Y		Second Exec. Salary: $533,450	Bonus: $715,570

OTHER THOUGHTS:

Apparent Women Officers or Directors: 7
Hot Spot for Advancement for Women/Minorities: Y

LOCATIONS: ("Y" = Yes)

West:	Southwest:	Midwest:	Southeast:	Northeast:	International:
Y	Y	Y	Y		Y

Note: Financial information, benefits and other data can change quickly and may vary from those stated here.

CABELA'S INC

www.cabelas.com

Industry Group Code: 451110 Ranks within this company's industry group: Sales: 2 Profits: 1

Management:		Sales/Marketing:		Liberal Arts:		Information Systems:		Professionals:		Technical/Scientific:	
Mgmt. Trainees:	Y	Mktg. Professionals:	Y	Gen. Writing/Editing:	Y	Info. Management:	Y	Finance/Accounting:	Y	Engineers, Elec.:	
Experienced Mgmt.:	Y	Retail Sales:	Y	Technical Writing:		Software Dev.:	Y	Law:	Y	Engineers, Other:	
Int'l Business:		Commercial/Industrial:	Y	Graphic Arts/Photog.:	Y	Hardware Dev.:		HR/Other:	Y	Health/Lab:	
MBA Graduates:	Y	Sales Trainees:	Y	Music:		Systems Integration:		Training:	Y	Scientists/Research:	
		Advertising Pros.:	Y	Broadcasting:		Consulting/Other:		Health Care:		Petroleum/Chemicals:	
				Other:				Consulting:		Math/Other:	

TYPES OF BUSINESS:
Sporting Goods Stores
Hunting & Fishing Supplies
Antique & Collectible Furniture
Outdoor Apparel
Catalog & Online Sales
Credit Cards

BRANDS/DIVISIONS/AFFILIATES:
World's Foremost Bank
Cabela's Club
SIR Warehouse Sports Store
Bargain Cave
Dunn's
VanDyke's
Wild Wings
Herters

CONTACTS: Note: Officers with more than one job title may be intentionally listed here more than once.
Dennis Highby, CEO
Dennis Highby, Pres.
Ralph W. Castner, CFO/VP
Patrick A. Snyder, Sr. VP-Mktg.
Charles Baldwin, Chief Human Resources Officer/VP
Patrick A. Snyder, Sr. VP-Merch. & Retail Oper.
Brian J. Linneman, Sr. VP-Oper.
Joe Arterburn, Media Contact
Chris Gay, Investor Rel. Contact
Ralph W. Castner, Chmn.-World's Foremost Bank
James W. Cabela, Vice Chmn.
Joseph M. Friebe, CEO-World's Foremost Bank
Richard N. Cabela, Chmn.
Brian J. Linneman, Sr. VP-Global Supply Chain

Phone: 308-254-5505   **Fax:** 308-254-4800
Toll-Free:
Address: 1 Cabela Dr., Sidney, NE 69160 US

GROWTH PLANS/SPECIAL FEATURES:
Cabela's, Inc. is a leading outdoor and hunting supply store, which mails over 140 million catalogs yearly. Through its web site, mail-order catalogs and retail stores, the company supplies hunting, marine, automobile, ATV, fishing, camping and clothing equipment. Hunting supplies include archery equipment, muzzleloaders, rifles, pistols, collectible guns, ammunition and optics. Fishing and marine supplies include trailers, engines, canoes, GPS units, fishing gear, tackle supplies and life jackets, as well as over 20,000 types of fishing lures. Camping gear includes tents, sleeping bags, stoves, backpacks, lanterns and automobile and ATV accessories. Cabela's also has a line of brand-name casual clothing and hunting and outdoors gear in a variety of camouflage and safety patterns. The company had 27 retail stores as of early 2008, in states such as Arizona, Idaho, Nebraska, Minnesota, Wisconsin, Michigan, Pennsylvania, West Virginia, South Dakota, Kansas, Utah, Washington, Nevada and Texas. In 2007, the company opened eight new stores, increasing its retail square footage by 49%. The stores, which are considered tourist attractions, receive as many as 6 million visitors per year. They are designed to communicate an outdoor lifestyle environment characterized by the outdoor feel of the lighting, wood or tile flooring, cedar wood beams, open ceilings and lodge-style atmosphere. The large-format stores contain a mountain and pond with museum-quality taxidermy and native game fish; gun libraries featuring high-quality firearms; archery training systems; virtual shooting arcades; museums or educational centers; and restaurants and banquet and meeting facilities. Additionally, the firm owns the World's Foremost Bank, a wholly-owned subsidiary managing store-branded Visa credit cards, with approximately 1 million accounts. In September 2007, the company purchased Canadian outdoors equipment retailer S.I.R. Warehouse Sports Store. Also in 2007, the company introduced in-store pick-up for web orders.

Cabela's offers its employees benefits including product discounts and health and dental coverage.

FINANCIALS: Sales and profits are in thousands of dollars—add 000 to get the full amount. 2007 Note: Financial information for 2007 was not available for all companies at press time.

2007 Sales: $2,349,599	2007 Profits: $87,879	**U.S. Stock Ticker:** CAB
2006 Sales: $2,063,524	2006 Profits: $85,785	**Int'l Ticker:** Int'l Exchange:
2005 Sales: $1,799,661	2005 Profits: $72,569	Employees: 15,000
2004 Sales: $1,555,974	2004 Profits: $64,996	Fiscal Year Ends: 12/31
2003 Sales: $1,392,400	2003 Profits: $51,400	Parent Company:

SALARIES/BENEFITS:
Pension Plan:	ESOP Stock Plan:	Profit Sharing:	Top Exec. Salary: $691,320 Bonus: $999,550
Savings Plan: Y	Stock Purch. Plan:		Second Exec. Salary: $436,061 Bonus: $300,425

OTHER THOUGHTS:
Apparent Women Officers or Directors:
Hot Spot for Advancement for Women/Minorities:

LOCATIONS: ("Y" = Yes)
West:	Southwest:	Midwest:	Southeast:	Northeast:	International:
Y	Y	Y	Y	Y	Y

Note: Financial information, benefits and other data can change quickly and may vary from those stated here.

CABLEVISION SYSTEMS CORP

www.cablevision.com

Industry Group Code: 513220 Ranks within this company's industry group: Sales: 6 Profits: 6

Management:		Sales/Marketing:		Liberal Arts:		Information Systems:		Professionals:		Technical/Scientific:	
Mgmt. Trainees:	Y	Mktg. Professionals:	Y	Gen. Writing/Editing:	Y	Info. Management:	Y	Finance/Accounting:	Y	Engineers, Elec.:	Y
Experienced Mgmt.:	Y	Retail Sales:		Technical Writing:		Software Dev.:	Y	Law:	Y	Engineers, Other:	
Int'l Business:		Commercial/Industrial:	Y	Graphic Arts/Photog.:	Y	Hardware Dev.:		HR/Other:	Y	Health/Lab:	
MBA Graduates:	Y	Sales Trainees:		Music:	Y	Systems Integration:		Training:	Y	Scientists/Research:	
		Advertising Pros.:	Y	Broadcasting:	Y	Consulting/Other:		Health Care:		Petroleum/Chemicals:	
				Other:	Y			Consulting:		Math/Other:	

TYPES OF BUSINESS:

Cable Television Service
Professional Sports Teams
Television Programming
Communications Services
Sports & Music Venues
Voice Over Internet Protocol
High-Speed Internet

BRANDS/DIVISIONS/AFFILIATES:

Rainbow Media Holdings LLC
Lightpath, Inc.
New York Rangers
New York Knickerbockers
Hartford Wolf Pack
MSG Entertainment
Madison Square Garden
Sundance Channel

CONTACTS: Note: Officers with more than one job title may be intentionally listed here more than once.

James L. Dolan, CEO
Tom Rutledge, COO
James L. Dolan, Pres.
Michael Huseby, CFO/Exec. VP
Wilt Hildenbrand, Sr. Advisor-Tech.
Wilt Hildenbrand, Sr. Advisor-Eng.
Jonathan D. Schwartz, General Counsel/Exec. VP
John Bickman, Pres., Cable & Comm.
Joshua Sapan, Pres./CEO-Rainbow Media Holdings LLC
James L. Dolan, Chmn.-MSG
Hank J. Ratner, Vice Chmn.
Charles F. Dolan, Chmn.

Phone: 516-803-2300	Fax: 516-803-3134
Toll-Free:	
Address: 1111 Stewart Ave., Bethpage, NY 11714 US	

GROWTH PLANS/SPECIAL FEATURES:

Cablevision Systems Corp. operates solely through cable operator subsidiary CSC Holdings. CSC has investments in cable programming networks, entertainment businesses and telecommunications companies. It serves about 3.1 million basic video subscribers in and around the New York City metropolitan area. Through wholly-owned subsidiary Rainbow Media Holdings, LLC, the company owns interests in and manages numerous national and regional programming networks, the Madison Square Garden sports and entertainment businesses and cable television advertising sales companies. Through wholly-owned subsidiary Lightpath, Inc., the firm provides telephone services and high-speed Internet access to the business market. CSC operates in three segments: telecommunications services, Rainbow and Madison Square Garden. The telecommunications services segment includes the cable television business, including its video, high-speed data and voice over Internet protocol (VoIP) and the operations of the telephone and high-speed data services provided by Lightpath. The Rainbow segment consists principally of interests in national programming services (AMC, WE tv, IFC, fuse and VOOM) and regional news programming businesses held by Rainbow Media Holdings. The division also includes a local advertising sales representation business. The Madison Square Garden segment owns and operates the Madison Square Garden Arena and the adjoining WaMu Theater at Madison Square Garden; the New York Knickerbockers professional basketball team; the New York Rangers professional hockey team; the New York Liberty professional women's basketball team; the Hartford Wolf Pack professional hockey team; the regional sports programming networks Madison Square Garden Network and Fox Sports Net New York; and MSG Entertainment. In May 2008, Cablevision purchased the Sundance Channel, a cable network founded by Robert Redford, for about $500 million.

FINANCIALS: Sales and profits are in thousands of dollars—add 000 to get the full amount. 2007 Note: Financial information for 2007 was not available for all companies at press time.

2007 Sales: $6,484,481	2007 Profits: $218,456	U.S. Stock Ticker: CVC
2006 Sales: $5,828,493	2006 Profits: $-126,465	Int'l Ticker: Int'l Exchange:
2005 Sales: $5,082,045	2005 Profits: $89,320	Employees: 22,935
2004 Sales: $4,750,037	2004 Profits: $-676,092	Fiscal Year Ends: 12/31
2003 Sales: $4,177,148	2003 Profits: $-297,311	Parent Company:

SALARIES/BENEFITS:

Pension Plan:	ESOP Stock Plan:	Profit Sharing:	Top Exec. Salary: $1,800,000	Bonus: $10,310,769
Savings Plan:	Stock Purch. Plan:		Second Exec. Salary: $1,600,000	Bonus: $6,360,000

OTHER THOUGHTS:

Apparent Women Officers or Directors:
Hot Spot for Advancement for Women/Minorities:

LOCATIONS: ("Y" = Yes)

West:	Southwest:	Midwest:	Southeast:	Northeast:	International:
				Y	

Note: Financial information, benefits and other data can change quickly and may vary from those stated here.

CACI INTERNATIONAL INC   www.caci.com

Industry Group Code: 541512 Ranks within this company's industry group: Sales: 6   Profits: 6

Management:		Sales/Marketing:		Liberal Arts:		Information Systems:		Professionals:		Technical/Scientific:	
Mgmt. Trainees:	Y	Mktg. Professionals:	Y	Gen. Writing/Editing:		Info. Management:	Y	Finance/Accounting:	Y	Engineers, Elec.:	Y
Experienced Mgmt.:	Y	Retail Sales:		Technical Writing:	Y	Software Dev.:	Y	Law:	Y	Engineers, Other:	Y
Int'l Business:	Y	Commercial/Industrial:	Y	Graphic Arts/Photog.:	Y	Hardware Dev.:	Y	HR/Other:	Y	Health/Lab:	
MBA Graduates:	Y	Sales Trainees:		Music:		Systems Integration:	Y	Training:	Y	Scientists/Research:	Y
		Advertising Pros.:		Broadcasting:		Consulting/Other:	Y	Health Care:		Petroleum/Chemicals:	
				Other:				Consulting:	Y	Math/Other:	Y

TYPES OF BUSINESS:
Consulting-InfoTech Related
Engineering Simulation Software
Custom Software Engineering
Managed Network Services
Information Management Tools
Marketing Systems Software

BRANDS/DIVISIONS/AFFILIATES:
CACI Limited
Institute for Quality Management, Inc.
Wexford Group International
Athena Innovative Solutions, Inc.
Dragon Development Corp.

CONTACTS: Note: Officers with more than one job title may be intentionally listed here more than once.
Paul M. Cofoni, CEO
Paul M. Cofoni, Pres.
Thomas A. Mutryn, CFO/Exec. VP
H. Robert Boehm, Chief Human Resources Officer/Exec. VP
Deborah B. Dunie, CTO/Exec. VP
Dale E. Luddeke, Exec. VP-Bus. Dev.
Jody A. Brown, Exec. VP-Public Rel. & Bus. Comm.
Thomas A. Mutryn, Treas.
William M. Fairl, Pres., U.S. Oper.
Randall C. Fuerst, COO-US Oper.
Richard F. G. Miller, Exec. VP-Corp. Dev.
Steven H. Weiss, Exec. VP-Gov't Bus. Oper.
J.P. London, Chmn.

Phone: 703-841-7800	Fax: 703-841-7882
Toll-Free:	
Address: 1100 N. Glebe Rd., Arlington, VA 22201 US	

GROWTH PLANS/SPECIAL FEATURES:

CACI International, Inc. is an information technology (IT) company that provides IT and network services to defense, intelligence and e-government departments. The company's domestic operations are divided into four categories: systems integration, managed network, knowledge management and engineering services. The systems integration offerings combine current systems with new technologies or integrate hardware and software from multiple sources. Services including planning, designing, implementing and managing solutions that resolve specific technical or business needs; extracting core business logic from existing systems and preserving it for migration to modern environments; helping clients visualize possible changes in processes and systems before implementation; and web-enabling systems and applications, bringing the power of the Internet to clients and system users. Managed network services offerings include a complete suite of solutions for total life cycle support of global communication networks. These offerings include planning and building voice, video and data networks; managing network communication infrastructure; operating network systems; and assuring that information is secure from unauthorized interception and intrusion during its storage and transmission. Knowledge management offerings encompass a range of information management tools and enabling technologies, including Internet-based user interfaces, commercial off-the-shelf software and workflow management systems. Engineering services offerings enable clients to standardize and improve the way they manage the logistical life cycles of systems, products and material assets. International operations are conducted through European subsidiary CACI Limited. In 2007, CACI acquired Institute for Quality Management, Inc.; Wexford Group International; Athena Innovative Solutions, Inc; and Dragon Development Corp.

The company offers its employees medical, dental and vision insurance; life and AD&D insurance; short- and long-term disability insurance; a 401(k) plan; an employee stock purchase plan; tuition reimbursement; and an employee assistance program.

FINANCIALS: Sales and profits are in thousands of dollars—add 000 to get the full amount. 2007 Note: Financial information for 2007 was not available for all companies at press time.

2007 Sales: $1,937,972	2007 Profits: $78,532	**U.S. Stock Ticker:** CAI
2006 Sales: $1,755,324	2006 Profits: $84,840	**Int'l Ticker:** Int'l Exchange:
2005 Sales: $1,623,062	2005 Profits: $79,725	Employees: 10,400
2004 Sales: $1,145,785	2004 Profits: $57,714	Fiscal Year Ends: 6/30
2003 Sales: $843,100	2003 Profits: $44,700	Parent Company:

SALARIES/BENEFITS:

Pension Plan:	ESOP Stock Plan:	Profit Sharing:	Top Exec. Salary: $714,600	Bonus: $219,160
Savings Plan: Y	Stock Purch. Plan: Y		Second Exec. Salary: $510,000	Bonus: $118,347

OTHER THOUGHTS:

Apparent Women Officers or Directors: 2
Hot Spot for Advancement for Women/Minorities: Y

LOCATIONS: ("Y" = Yes)

West:	Southwest:	Midwest:	Southeast:	Northeast:	International:
Y	Y	Y	Y	Y	Y

Note: Financial information, benefits and other data can change quickly and may vary from those stated here.

CAMERON INTERNATIONAL CORPORATION www.c-a-m.com

Industry Group Code: 333130 Ranks within this company's industry group: Sales: 1 Profits: 1

Management:		Sales/Marketing:		Liberal Arts:		Information Systems:		Professionals:		Technical/Scientific:	
Mgmt. Trainees:	Y	Mktg. Professionals:	Y	Gen. Writing/Editing:		Info. Management:	Y	Finance/Accounting:	Y	Engineers, Elec.:	Y
Experienced Mgmt.:	Y	Retail Sales:		Technical Writing:	Y	Software Dev.:	Y	Law:	Y	Engineers, Other:	Y
Int'l Business:	Y	Commercial/Industrial:	Y	Graphic Arts/Photog.:		Hardware Dev.:		HR/Other:	Y	Health/Lab:	
MBA Graduates:	Y	Sales Trainees:		Music:		Systems Integration:		Training:	Y	Scientists/Research:	Y
		Advertising Pros.:		Broadcasting:		Consulting/Other:		Health Care:		Petroleum/Chemicals:	Y
				Other:				Consulting:		Math/Other:	

TYPES OF BUSINESS:

Oil Field Machinery
Gas Turbines, Compressors & Engines
Oil Field Services
Pressure & Flow Control Equipment

BRANDS/DIVISIONS/AFFILIATES:

Cooper Cameron Corporation
Cameron Offshore Systems
Petreco
Cameron Valves & Measurement
Cameron Compression
NuFlo Technologies, Inc.
Grove
Wheatley

CONTACTS: *Note: Officers with more than one job title may be intentionally listed here more than once.*

Jack B. Moore, CEO
Jack B. Moore, Pres.
Charles M. Sledge, CFO/VP
Joseph H. Mongrain, VP-Human Resources
John Bartos, VP-Tech. & Dev.
William C. Lemmer, General Counsel/Corp. Sec./VP
Stephen P. Tomlinson, VP-Oper. Support
R. Scott Amann, VP-Investor Rel.
Christopher A. Krummel, VP/Chief Acct. Officer
Robert J. Rajeski, VP/Pres., Cameron Compression Systems
Jim E. Wright, VP/Pres., Cameron Valves & Measurement
John Carne, Sr. VP/Pres., Cameron Drilling & Prod. Systems
Sheldon R. Erikson, Chmn.
Erik Peyrer, VP-Bus. Dev., Asia Pacific & Middle East

Phone: 713-513-3300	Fax: 713-513-3456
Toll-Free:	
Address: 1333 West Loop S., Ste. 1700, Houston, TX 77027 US	

GROWTH PLANS/SPECIAL FEATURES:

Cameron International Corporation, based in Texas, is an international provider of flow equipment products, systems and services to oil, gas and processing industries. The firm is also a leading manufacturer of centrifugal air compressors, integral and separable gas compressors and turbochargers. The company operates in more than 100 countries and is divided into three business segments: drilling and production systems; valves and measurement; and compression systems. The drilling and production systems products include surface and subsea production systems, blowout preventers (BOPs), drilling and production control systems, oil and gas separation equipment, gate valves, actuators, chokes, wellheads, drilling riser and aftermarket parts and services. The division's products are marketed under the brand names Cameron, W-K-M, McEvoy and Willis. The valves and measurement segment's products include ball valves, butterfly valves, Orbit valves, double block and bleed valves, globe valves and aftermarket parts and services. The segment markets its products under various brand names, including WKM, Demco, Nutron, TBV, TexSteam and Wheatley. The compression systems segment produces reciprocating and integrally geared centrifugal compression equipment and aftermarket parts and services, and markets under various brand names, including Ajax, Superior, Compression Specialties and Turbine Specialties. In 2007, Cameron introduced the LoadKing riser system, a 3.5 million-pound load capacity product used for drilling in up to 10,000-foot water depths. In July 2008, the company entered a frame agreement to supply subsea production systems for a major development program off the coast of Angola, Africa. The first phase of the agreement is worth approximately $800 million, which includes orders for subsea wellheads, trees, control systems, manifolds and chokes.

The company offers its employees a benefits package that includes dependent and health care spending accounts and educational assistance.

FINANCIALS: Sales and profits are in thousands of dollars—add 000 to get the full amount. 2007 Note: Financial information for 2007 was not available for all companies at press time.

2007 Sales: $4,666,368	2007 Profits: $500,860	**U.S. Stock Ticker: CAM**	
2006 Sales: $3,742,907	2006 Profits: $317,816	**Int'l Ticker:** Int'l Exchange:	
2005 Sales: $2,517,847	2005 Profits: $171,130	Employees: 12,400	
2004 Sales: $2,092,845	2004 Profits: $94,415	Fiscal Year Ends: 12/31	
2003 Sales: $1,634,346	2003 Profits: $69,450	Parent Company:	

SALARIES/BENEFITS:

Pension Plan:	ESOP Stock Plan:	Profit Sharing: Y	Top Exec. Salary: $950,000	Bonus: $1,900,000
Savings Plan: Y	Stock Purch. Plan:		Second Exec. Salary: $420,000	Bonus: $504,000

OTHER THOUGHTS:

Apparent Women Officers or Directors:
Hot Spot for Advancement for Women/Minorities:

LOCATIONS: ("Y" = Yes)

West:	Southwest:	Midwest:	Southeast:	Northeast:	International:
Y	Y	Y	Y	Y	Y

CAPITAL SENIOR LIVING CORP   www.capitalsenior.com

Industry Group Code: 623110 Ranks within this company's industry group: Sales: 5   Profits: 4

Management:		Sales/Marketing:		Liberal Arts:		Information Systems:		Professionals:		Technical/Scientific:	
Mgmt. Trainees:		Mktg. Professionals:	Y	Gen. Writing/Editing:		Info. Management:	Y	Finance/Accounting:	Y	Engineers, Elec.:	
Experienced Mgmt.:	Y	Retail Sales:		Technical Writing:	Y	Software Dev.:		Law:	Y	Engineers, Other:	Y
Int'l Business:		Commercial/Industrial:		Graphic Arts/Photog.:		Hardware Dev.:		HR/Other:	Y	Health/Lab:	
MBA Graduates:	Y	Sales Trainees:		Music:		Systems Integration:		Training:	Y	Scientists/Research:	
		Advertising Pros.:		Broadcasting:		Consulting/Other:		Health Care:	Y	Petroleum/Chemicals:	
				Other:				Consulting:		Math/Other:	

TYPES OF BUSINESS:

Long-Term Health Care
Nursing Homes
Assisted Living Services
Home Care Services

BRANDS/DIVISIONS/AFFILIATES:

CONTACTS: *Note: Officers with more than one job title may be intentionally listed here more than once.*

Lawrence A. Cohen, CEO
Keith N. Johannessen, COO
Keith N. Johannessen, Pres.
Ralph A. Beattie, CFO/Exec. VP
David R. Brickman, General Counsel
James A. Stroud, Chmn.

Phone: 972-770-5600	Fax: 972-770-5666
Toll-Free:	
Address: 14160 Dallas Pkwy., Ste. 300, Dallas, TX 75254 US	

GROWTH PLANS/SPECIAL FEATURES:

Capital Senior Living Corporation (CSL) is one of the nation's largest operators and developers of residential communities for seniors. The firm operates 64 communities in 23 states with an aggregate capacity of 9,500 residents, including 37 communities that it owns or in which it has an ownership interest and 4 communities which it manages for third parties. 95% of the company's revenue is generated through private pay parties at these communities. The firm provides senior living services to the elderly, including independent living, assisted living, skilled nursing and home care services. Many of CSL's communities offer a continuum of care to meet its residents' needs as they change over time. This continuum of care, which integrates independent living and assisted living and is bridged by home care through independent home care agencies or the company's home care agency, sustains residents' autonomy and independence based on their physical and mental abilities. Each Capital community features social and recreational programs, maid service, restaurant-quality meals and complimentary laundry rooms.

FINANCIALS: Sales and profits are in thousands of dollars—add 000 to get the full amount. 2007 Note: Financial information for 2007 was not available for all companies at press time.

2007 Sales: $189,052	2007 Profits: $4,360	**U.S. Stock Ticker: CSU**
2006 Sales: $159,070	2006 Profits: $-2,600	**Int'l Ticker:** Int'l Exchange:
2005 Sales: $126,404	2005 Profits: $-5,354	Employees: 3,711
2004 Sales: $108,935	2004 Profits: $-6,758	Fiscal Year Ends: 12/31
2003 Sales: $66,325	2003 Profits: $4,990	Parent Company:

SALARIES/BENEFITS:

Pension Plan:	ESOP Stock Plan:	Profit Sharing:	Top Exec. Salary: $390,323	Bonus: $302,345
Savings Plan: Y	Stock Purch. Plan:		Second Exec. Salary: $325,269	Bonus: $183,001

OTHER THOUGHTS:

Apparent Women Officers or Directors:
Hot Spot for Advancement for Women/Minorities:

LOCATIONS: ("Y" = Yes)

West:	Southwest:	Midwest:	Southeast:	Northeast:	International:
Y	Y	Y	Y	Y	

Note: Financial information, benefits and other data can change quickly and may vary from those stated here.

CARDINAL HEALTH INC

www.cardinal.com

Industry Group Code: 422210 Ranks within this company's industry group: Sales: 2 Profits: 1

Management:		Sales/Marketing:		Liberal Arts:		Information Systems:		Professionals:		Technical/Scientific:	
Mgmt. Trainees:	Y	Mktg. Professionals:	Y	Gen. Writing/Editing:	Y	Info. Management:	Y	Finance/Accounting:	Y	Engineers, Elec.:	
Experienced Mgmt.:	Y	Retail Sales:		Technical Writing:	Y	Software Dev.:	Y	Law:	Y	Engineers, Other:	
Int'l Business:	Y	Commercial/Industrial:	Y	Graphic Arts/Photog.:	Y	Hardware Dev.:		HR/Other:	Y	Health/Lab:	
MBA Graduates:	Y	Sales Trainees:	Y	Music:		Systems Integration:		Training:	Y	Scientists/Research:	
		Advertising Pros.:	Y	Broadcasting:		Consulting/Other:		Health Care:	Y	Petroleum/Chemicals:	
				Other:				Consulting:		Math/Other:	

TYPES OF BUSINESS:

Healthcare Products & Services
Supply chain services
Medical products

BRANDS/DIVISIONS/AFFILIATES:

Alaris
Pyxis
MedMined, Inc.
Viasys Healthcare, Inc.
CareFusion
ChloraPrep

CONTACTS: *Note: Officers with more than one job title may be intentionally listed here more than once.*

R. Kerry Clark, CEO
R. Kerry Clark, Pres.
Jeff Henderson, CFO
Carole Watkins, Chief Human Resources Officer
Jody Davids, CIO/Exec. VP-Global Shares Svcs.
Ivan Fong, Chief Legal Officer/Sec.
Mike Duffy, Exec. VP-Oper., Supply Chain Services
Vivek Jain, Exec. VP-Strategy & Corp. Dev.
Shelley Bird, Exec. VP-Global Comm.
Gary Dolch, Exec. VP, Quality & Regulatory Affairs
Dave Schlotterbeck, CEO, Clinical and Medical Products/Vice Chmn.
Mark W. Parrish, CEO, Healthcare Supply Chain Svcs.
George Barrett, CEO, Healthcare Supply Chain Svcs.
Robert D. Walter, Exec. Chmn. Of the Board
Rudy Mareel, Pres., Int'l

Phone: 614-757-5000	Fax: 614-757-8871
Toll-Free: 800-234-8701	
Address: 7000 Cardinal Pl., Dublin, OH 43017 US	

GROWTH PLANS/SPECIAL FEATURES:

Cardinal Health, Inc. is a provider of products and services that improve the safety and productivity of healthcare. In July 2008, the company announced a consolidation of its businesses into two segments: Healthcare supply chain services, clinical and medical products. The healthcare supply chain segment provides comprehensive financial inventory and marketing services as well as specialized nuclear pharmaceuticals to hospitals and outpatient centers. The clinical and medical products segment provides services and technologies to hospitals that aid in the prevention of medication errors, the reduction of infections and the management of medications and supplies. The products in this segment include CareFusion patient identification systems, Alaris infusion devices, Pyxis medication dispensing systems, Convertors brand surgical gowns and Esteem brand medical gloves. The company completed the sale of the PTS Business during the fourth quarter of fiscal 2007. Effective the first quarter of fiscal 2008, the Medical Products Manufacturing segment was renamed Medical Products and Technologies in connection with the firm's acquisition of VIASYS Healthcare Inc., which was completed during the fourth quarter of fiscal 2007 In March 2008, the firm announced a definitive agreement to acquire the assets of privately held Enturia Inc. for $490 million. The cash transaction includes Enturia's leading line of infection prevention products sold under the ChloraPrep brand name. In July 2008, the company announced a consolidation of its businesses into two segments: Healthcare supply chain services and clinical and medical products segment as a part of the restructuring in 2008. The company is considering supporting a management recommendation to explore a potential separation of segments as separate publicly traded companies and will announce its decision later in 2008.

The company offers its employees medical, dental, vision and life insurance; a 401(k) plan; an employee assistance program; an employee stock purchase plan; business travel insurance; and tuition reimbursement.

FINANCIALS: Sales and profits are in thousands of dollars—add 000 to get the full amount. 2007 Note: Financial information for 2007 was not available for all companies at press time.

2007 Sales: $86,852,000	2007 Profits: $1,931,100	**U.S. Stock Ticker:** CAH
2006 Sales: $79,664,200	2006 Profits: $1,000,100	**Int'l Ticker:** Int'l Exchange:
2005 Sales: $72,666,000	2005 Profits: $1,050,700	Employees: 43,500
2004 Sales: $63,043,100	2004 Profits: $1,474,500	Fiscal Year Ends: 6/30
2003 Sales: $56,737,000	2003 Profits: $1,405,800	Parent Company:

SALARIES/BENEFITS:

Pension Plan:	ESOP Stock Plan:	Profit Sharing:	Top Exec. Salary: $1,065,116	Bonus: $2,911,527
Savings Plan: Y	Stock Purch. Plan:		Second Exec. Salary: $701,885	Bonus: $400,000

OTHER THOUGHTS:

Apparent Women Officers or Directors: 3
Hot Spot for Advancement for Women/Minorities: Y

LOCATIONS: ("Y" = Yes)

West:	Southwest:	Midwest:	Southeast:	Northeast:	International:
Y	Y	Y	Y	Y	Y

CARGILL INC
www.cargill.com

Industry Group Code: 311210 Ranks within this company's industry group: Sales: 1   Profits: 1

Management:		Sales/Marketing:		Liberal Arts:		Information Systems:		Professionals:		Technical/Scientific:	
Mgmt. Trainees:	Y	Mktg. Professionals:	Y	Gen. Writing/Editing:		Info. Management:	Y	Finance/Accounting:	Y	Engineers, Elec.:	Y
Experienced Mgmt.:	Y	Retail Sales:		Technical Writing:	Y	Software Dev.:	Y	Law:	Y	Engineers, Other:	
Int'l Business:	Y	Commercial/Industrial:	Y	Graphic Arts/Photog.:	Y	Hardware Dev.:		HR/Other:	Y	Health/Lab:	Y
MBA Graduates:	Y	Sales Trainees:		Music:		Systems Integration:		Training:	Y	Scientists/Research:	Y
		Advertising Pros.:		Broadcasting:		Consulting/Other:		Health Care:		Petroleum/Chemicals:	Y
				Other:				Consulting:		Math/Other:	

TYPES OF BUSINESS:
Crop Production, Milling and Distribution
Meat Processing
Food Ingredients
Fertilizers
Steel
Money Markets & Commodity Trading
Supply Chain Solutions
Risk Management & Financial Services

BRANDS/DIVISIONS/AFFILIATES:
Cargill AgHorizons U.S.
Emerald Renewable Energy LLC
Renessen Feed & Processing
Cerestar Sweeteners Europe
Black River Asset Management
Duckworth Flavors
Cargill Animal Nutrition
Truvia

CONTACTS: *Note: Officers with more than one job title may be intentionally listed here more than once.*
Gregory R. Page, CEO
Gregory R. Page, Pres.
David MacLennan, CFO
Peter Vrijsen, VP-Human Resources
Christopher P. Mallett, VP-R&D
Rita J. Heise, VP-IT
Ronald L. Christenson, CTO/VP
Steven C. Euller, General Counsel/VP/Corp. Sec.
Bonnie E. Raquet, VP-Corp. Affairs
Galen G. Johnson, Controller/VP
Frank L. Sims, VP-Transportation & Product Assurance
Jayme D. Olson, Treas./VP
Scott Portnoy, VP-Biofuels & Bioproducts Bus.
Gert Jan Vandenakker, Head-Ocean Transportation
Gregory R. Page, Chmn.

Phone: 952-742-7575	Fax: 952-742-7393
Toll-Free: 800-277-4455	
Address: 15407 McGinty Rd. W., Wayzata, MN 55391 US	

GROWTH PLANS/SPECIAL FEATURES:
Cargill, Inc. provides food, agricultural and risk management products and service in five sectors: Agriculture services; industrial; food ingredients and applications; origination and processing; and risk management and financial.   The company provides customized farm services and products and operates worldwide through its five agricultural services companies: Banks Cargill Agriculture; Cargill AgHorizons Canada; Cargill AgHorizons U.S.; Cargill Animal Nutrition; and Renessen Feed & Processing.   The company's food sector serves food manufacturers, food service companies and retailers with food and beverage ingredients and meat and poultry products.   Cargill's food ingredient subsidiaries include Cargill Dressings, Sauces and Oils North America; Cargill Cocoa; Cerestar Sweeteners Europe; Cargill Juice North America; Duckworth Flavors; Wilbur Chocolate; Sun Valley Canada; and Cargill Kitchens.   In the industrial sector, Cargill supplies customers worldwide with fertilizer through The Mosaic Co.; steel products and services through North Star Steel, and industrial applications for agricultural feedstocks through NatureWorks LLC.   The origination and processing unit connects producers and users of grain, oilseeds and other agricultural commodities through its three subsidiaries, Cargill Cotton; Cargill Grain & Oilseed Supply Chain; and Cargill Sugar, which provides origination, processing, marketing and distribution services.   In addition, the firm provides risk management and financial solutions through Black River Asset Management LLC; Cargill Risk Management; Cargill Trade & Structured Finance; Cargill Value Investments; Cargill Ventures; and Cargill Investor Services.   In 2007, the firm opened Emerald Renewable Energy, LLC, an aqua research facility in Elk River, Minnesota, and a specialty canola research farm in Aberdeen, Saskatchewan.   In May 2008, the company introduced Truvia, billed as the first natural, zero-calorie sweetener.

Cargill offers its employees tuition reimbursement, an employee assistance plan and relocation services.

FINANCIALS: Sales and profits are in thousands of dollars—add 000 to get the full amount. 2007 Note: Financial information for 2007 was not available for all companies at press time.

2007 Sales: $88,266,000	2007 Profits: $2,343,000	**U.S. Stock Ticker: Private**
2006 Sales: $75,208,000	2006 Profits: $1,537,000	**Int'l Ticker:** Int'l Exchange:
2005 Sales: $71,066,000	2005 Profits: $2,103,000	Employees: 158,000
2004 Sales: $62,907,000	2004 Profits: $1,331,000	Fiscal Year Ends: 5/31
2003 Sales: $59,894,000	2003 Profits: $1,290,000	Parent Company:

SALARIES/BENEFITS:
Pension Plan:	ESOP Stock Plan: Y	Profit Sharing:	Top Exec. Salary: $	Bonus: $
Savings Plan: Y	Stock Purch. Plan:		Second Exec. Salary: $	Bonus: $

OTHER THOUGHTS:
Apparent Women Officers or Directors: 2
Hot Spot for Advancement for Women/Minorities: Y

LOCATIONS: ("Y" = Yes)
West:	Southwest:	Midwest:	Southeast:	Northeast:	International:
Y	Y	Y	Y		Y

Note: Financial information, benefits and other data can change quickly and may vary from those stated here.

CARMAX GROUP

www.carmax.com

Industry Group Code: 441110 Ranks within this company's industry group: Sales: 2   Profits: 2

Management:		Sales/Marketing:		Liberal Arts:		Information Systems:		Professionals:		Technical/Scientific:	
Mgmt. Trainees:	Y	Mktg. Professionals:	Y	Gen. Writing/Editing:	Y	Info. Management:	Y	Finance/Accounting:	Y	Engineers, Elec.:	
Experienced Mgmt.:	Y	Retail Sales:	Y	Technical Writing:		Software Dev.:	Y	Law:	Y	Engineers, Other:	
Int'l Business:		Commercial/Industrial:	Y	Graphic Arts/Photog.:	Y	Hardware Dev.:		HR/Other:	Y	Health/Lab:	
MBA Graduates:	Y	Sales Trainees:	Y	Music:		Systems Integration:		Training:	Y	Scientists/Research:	
		Advertising Pros.:	Y	Broadcasting:		Consulting/Other:		Health Care:		Petroleum/Chemicals:	
				Other:				Consulting:		Math/Other:	

TYPES OF BUSINESS:

Used Auto Dealers, Retail
New Auto Dealers
Online Sales
Vehicle Repair Services
Financial Services

BRANDS/DIVISIONS/AFFILIATES:

CarMax Foundation

CONTACTS: Note: Officers with more than one job title may be intentionally listed here more than once.

Thomas J. Folliard, CEO
Thomas J. Folliard, Pres.
Keith D. Browning, CFO/Exec. VP
Joseph S. Kunkel, Sr. VP-Mktg. & Strategy
Roberta Douma, VP-Human Resource Dev.
Richard M. Smith, CIO/Sr. VP
Michael K. Dolan, Chief Admin. Officer/Exec. VP
Eric Margolin, General Counsel/Sr. VP/Corp. Sec.
Ed Hill, VP-Svc. Oper.
Anu Agarwal, VP-Bus. Strategy
John Montegari, Assistant VP-Media
Katharine Kenny, Assistant VP-Investor Rel.
Thomas W. Reedy, Jr., VP/Treas.
Laura Donahue, VP-Advertising
Angela S. Chattin, VP-CarMax Auto Finance
Barbara Harvill, VP-IT
Kim Orcutt, VP/Controller
William R. Tiefel, Chmn.
Dodie Fix, Assistant. VP-Procurement

Phone: 804-747-0422	Fax: 804-967-2918
Toll-Free: 800-519-1511	
Address: 12800 Tuckahoe Creek Pkwy., Richmond, VA 23238 US	

GROWTH PLANS/SPECIAL FEATURES:

CarMax Group is one of the nation's largest retailers of used cars. The firm purchases, reconditions and sells used vehicles through its 89 used car superstores in 41 metropolitan markets across the U.S. CarMax also sells new vehicles at seven of its locations under franchise agreements with four new car manufacturers. The company offers a wide selection of makes and models of both domestic and imported vehicles to appeal to diverse consumer preferences and budgets, including popular brands from manufacturers such as Daimler, Chrysler, Ford, General Motors, Honda, Mitsubishi, Subaru, Toyota and Volkswagen. Vehicles purchased through the company's in-store appraisal process that fall short of retail standards are sold at on-site wholesale auctions restricted to licensed automobile dealers. All store locations provide vehicle repair service and used-car warranty service. In addition, through the company's web site, customers can search new and used cars as well as find information on Kelley Blue Book figures, car buying tips, rebates and incentives and more. CarMax has finance operations through CarMax Auto Finance that offer revolving credit and automobile installment loans. The firm sold approximately 337,000 used vehicles retailed in 2007. CarMax recently opened stores in Augusta, Georgia and Tulsa, Oklahoma.

CarMax offers its employees a benefits package including educational assistance, a daycare savings account, life insurance, adoption assistance, an associate discount program and an employee assistance program. CarMax has been named by FORTUNE magazine as one of its 2008 100 Best Companies to Work For.

FINANCIALS: Sales and profits are in thousands of dollars—add 000 to get the full amount. 2007 Note: Financial information for 2007 was not available for all companies at press time.

2007 Sales: $8,199,600	2007 Profits: $182,000	U.S. Stock Ticker: KMX
2006 Sales: $7,465,700	2006 Profits: $198,600	Int'l Ticker: Int'l Exchange:
2005 Sales: $5,260,300	2005 Profits: $112,900	Employees: 15,637
2004 Sales: $4,597,691	2004 Profits: $116,450	Fiscal Year Ends: 4/24
2003 Sales: $3,969,900	2003 Profits: $94,800	Parent Company:

SALARIES/BENEFITS:

Pension Plan: Y	ESOP Stock Plan:	Profit Sharing:	Top Exec. Salary: $645,602	Bonus: $1,050,000
Savings Plan: Y	Stock Purch. Plan: Y		Second Exec. Salary: $554,933	Bonus: $505,197

OTHER THOUGHTS:

Apparent Women Officers or Directors: 15
Hot Spot for Advancement for Women/Minorities: Y

LOCATIONS: ("Y" = Yes)

West:	Southwest:	Midwest:	Southeast:	Northeast:	International:
Y	Y	Y	Y	Y	

Note: Financial information, benefits and other data can change quickly and may vary from those stated here.

CARNIVAL CORPORATION

www.carnivalcorp.com

Industry Group Code: 483112 Ranks within this company's industry group: Sales: 1 Profits: 1

Management:		Sales/Marketing:		Liberal Arts:		Information Systems:		Professionals:		Technical/Scientific:	
Mgmt. Trainees:	Y	Mktg. Professionals:	Y	Gen. Writing/Editing:	Y	Info. Management:	Y	Finance/Accounting:	Y	Engineers, Elec.:	Y
Experienced Mgmt.:	Y	Retail Sales:		Technical Writing:		Software Dev.:	Y	Law:	Y	Engineers, Other:	Y
Int'l Business:	Y	Commercial/Industrial:	Y	Graphic Arts/Photog.:	Y	Hardware Dev.:		HR/Other:	Y	Health/Lab:	
MBA Graduates:	Y	Sales Trainees:		Music:	Y	Systems Integration:		Training:	Y	Scientists/Research:	
		Advertising Pros.:	Y	Broadcasting:		Consulting/Other:		Health Care:	Y	Petroleum/Chemicals:	
				Other:	Y			Consulting:		Math/Other:	

TYPES OF BUSINESS:

Cruise Line
On-Board Casinos
Tours
Resort Hotels

BRANDS/DIVISIONS/AFFILIATES:

Carnival Cruise Lines
Holland America Line
P&O Cruises Australia
Seabourn Cruise Line
Princess Cruises
Costa Cruises
Cunard Line
P&O Cruises

CONTACTS: Note: Officers with more than one job title may be intentionally listed here more than once.

Micky Arison, CEO
Howard S. Frank, COO/Vice Chmn.
David Bernstein, CFO/Sr. VP
Arnaldo Perez, General Counsel/Sr. VP/Corp. Sec.
Larry Freedman, VP/Controller/Chief Acct. Officer
Richard D. Ames, Sr. VP-Shared Svcs.
Michael Thamm, Pres., AIDA Cruises
Gerald R. Cahill, CEO/Pres., Carnival Cruise Lines
Micky Arison, Chmn.
Alan B. Buckelew, CEO-P&O Princess Cruises Int'l

Phone: 305-599-2600	Fax: 305-406-4700
Toll-Free:	
Address: 3655 N.W. 87th Ave., Miami, FL 33178-2428 US	

GROWTH PLANS/SPECIAL FEATURES:

Carnival Corporation provides cruises and tours to vacation destinations worldwide. Its cruise brands include Carnival Cruise Lines, Princess Cruises, Costa Cruises, Holland America Line, P&O Cruises, Cunard, AIDA, Ibero Cruises, Seabourn Cruise Line, Ocean Village and Swan Hellenic. In total, the company operates 85 ships, representing over 158,352 berths. Carnival Cruise Lines operates 22 ships and is based in North America. Princess is a global cruise and tour company operating 17 ships. Costa Crociere is the leading cruise company in Europe and South America, operating a modern fleet of 12 ships. Holland America Line serves the industry's premium segment, with 13 ships sailing to all seven continents. P&O Cruises offers passengers destinations including the Caribbean, South America, Scandinavia, the Mediterranean, Atlantic Islands and Round the World cruises. Cunard operates the Queen Mary 2, the Queen Elizabeth 2 and Queen Victoria, though the Queen Elizabeth 2 will be leaving the fleet in November 2008. AIDA Cruises operates in the German-speaking cruise market and Ibero Cruises caters to the Spanish-speaking cruise market in Southern Europe. Seabourn Cruise Line offers luxury cruises on their combined three yachts. Ocean Village and Swan Hellenic operate informal and discovery cruises for younger, more active passengers. The company also owns Holland America Tours and Princess Tours, which are tour operators in Alaska and the Canadian Yukon. These companies offer lodging, chartered motorcoaches, rail cars, luxury day boats, and sightseeing packages. The firm has over 22 cruise ships scheduled to enter service between April 2008 and June 2012. In 2007, Carnival sold the Windstar Cruises brand to Ambassadors International, Inc. for $100 million.

Carnival offers employee benefits such as tuition reimbursement and discounted or complimentary travel.

FINANCIALS: Sales and profits are in thousands of dollars—add 000 to get the full amount. 2007 Note: Financial information for 2007 was not available for all companies at press time.

2007 Sales: $13,033,000	2007 Profits: $2,408,000	**U.S. Stock Ticker: CCL**
2006 Sales: $11,839,000	2006 Profits: $2,279,000	**Int'l Ticker:** Int'l Exchange:
2005 Sales: $11,094,000	2005 Profits: $2,253,000	Employees: 81,100
2004 Sales: $9,727,000	2004 Profits: $1,809,000	Fiscal Year Ends: 11/30
2003 Sales: $6,718,000	2003 Profits: $1,194,000	Parent Company:

SALARIES/BENEFITS:

Pension Plan:	ESOP Stock Plan:	Profit Sharing:	Top Exec. Salary: $1,244,400	Bonus: $909,840
Savings Plan: Y	Stock Purch. Plan: Y		Second Exec. Salary: $1,150,000	Bonus: $

OTHER THOUGHTS:

Apparent Women Officers or Directors: 4
Hot Spot for Advancement for Women/Minorities: Y

LOCATIONS: ("Y" = Yes)

West:	Southwest:	Midwest:	Southeast:	Northeast:	International:
Y		Y	Y	Y	Y

CASH AMERICA INTERNATIONAL INC www.cashamerica.com

Industry Group Code: 522298 Ranks within this company's industry group: Sales: 1 Profits: 1

Management:		Sales/Marketing:		Liberal Arts:		Information Systems:		Professionals:		Technical/Scientific:	
Mgmt. Trainees:	Y	Mktg. Professionals:	Y	Gen. Writing/Editing:		Info. Management:	Y	Finance/Accounting:	Y	Engineers, Elec.:	
Experienced Mgmt.:	Y	Retail Sales:	Y	Technical Writing:		Software Dev.:		Law:	Y	Engineers, Other:	
Int'l Business:		Commercial/Industrial:	Y	Graphic Arts/Photog.:		Hardware Dev.:		HR/Other:	Y	Health/Lab:	
MBA Graduates:	Y	Sales Trainees:	Y	Music:		Systems Integration:		Training:	Y	Scientists/Research:	
		Advertising Pros.:	Y	Broadcasting:		Consulting/Other:		Health Care:		Petroleum/Chemicals:	
				Other:				Consulting:		Math/Other:	

TYPES OF BUSINESS:

Pawn Shops
Check Cashing
Payday Loans
Money Orders
Money Transfers
Stored Value Cards

BRANDS/DIVISIONS/AFFILIATES:

Mr. Payroll Corp.
SuperPawn
Cashland Financial Services, Inc.
Cash America Payday Advance
CashNet USA
Cash Net Holdings, LLC
Check Giant, LLC (The)

CONTACTS: *Note: Officers with more than one job title may be intentionally listed here more than once.*

Daniel R. Feehan, CEO
Daniel R. Feehan, Pres.
Thomas A. Bessant, Jr., CFO/Exec. VP
Robert D. Brockman, Exec. VP-Admin.
J. Curtis Linscott, General Counsel/Exec. VP/Corp. Sec.
Michael D. Gaston, Exec. VP-Corp. Dev.
Jerry D. Finn, Exec. VP-Domestic Pawn Oper.
Dennis J. Weese, COO/Pres., Retail Services Division
Jerry A. Wackerhagen, Pres., Stores Division
John A. McDorman, Pres., Shared Svcs. Division
Jack R. Daugherty, Chmn.

Phone: 817-335-1100	Fax: 817-570-1225
Toll-Free:	
Address: 1600 W. 7th St., Fort Worth, TX 76102 US	

GROWTH PLANS/SPECIAL FEATURES:

Cash America International, Inc. provides pawn loans, short-term cash advances, check cashing services and other specialty financial services to individuals in the U.S. and recently the U.K.. The company also sells merchandise in its pawnshops, primarily personal property that has been forfeited in connection with its pawn lending operations. The firm provides its specialty financial services through 499 pawnshops in 22 states (including 12 pawnshops that are franchises), 295 stand-alone cash advance locations and 136 check cashing locations, and via the Internet. Most of Cash American's pawnshops operate under the Cash America trade name; 42 pawnshops (located in Arizona, California, Nevada and Washington) operate under the SuperPawn trade name. The company offers unsecured cash advances to individuals through most of its pawnshops, in 87 stand-alone Cash America Payday Advance locations, in 217 locations operated by wholly-owned subsidiary Cashland Financial Services, Inc., under the Cashland trade name, and over the internet under the trade name CashNetUSA at cashnetusa.com. Through Mr. Payroll Corp., it offers check cashing services through 134 franchised and five company-owned check cashing centers. Many of Cash America's pawn and cash advance locations also offer check cashing services and other retail financial services such as stored value cards, money orders and money transfers. During the three-year period ended December 31, 2007, the company acquired 33 operating units, established 15 locations, and combined or closed four locations for a net increase in owned pawn lending units of 44. For the three year period ended December 31, 2007, the company acquired one location, established 60 locations and combined or closed 10 locations for a net increase in cash advance locations of 51. CashNetUSA serves multiple markets through its internet distribution channel and had cash advances outstanding in 32 states and in the United Kingdom as of December 31, 2007.

.

FINANCIALS: Sales and profits are in thousands of dollars—add 000 to get the full amount. 2007 Note: Financial information for 2007 was not available for all companies at press time.

2007 Sales: $929,394	2007 Profits: $79,346	**U.S. Stock Ticker: CSH**
2006 Sales: $694,514	2006 Profits: $60,940	**Int'l Ticker:** Int'l Exchange:
2005 Sales: $594,346	2005 Profits: $45,018	Employees: 5,152
2004 Sales: $469,478	2004 Profits: $56,835	Fiscal Year Ends: 12/31
2003 Sales: $437,677	2003 Profits: $30,036	Parent Company:

SALARIES/BENEFITS:

Pension Plan:	ESOP Stock Plan:	Profit Sharing:	Top Exec. Salary: $503,571	Bonus: $246,795
Savings Plan: Y	Stock Purch. Plan:		Second Exec. Salary: $297,517	Bonus: $116,648

OTHER THOUGHTS:

Apparent Women Officers or Directors:
Hot Spot for Advancement for Women/Minorities:

LOCATIONS: ("Y" = Yes)

West:	Southwest:	Midwest:	Southeast:	Northeast:	International:
Y	Y	Y	Y	Y	Y

CATERPILLAR INC

www.cat.com

Industry Group Code: 333000 Ranks within this company's industry group: Sales: 1 Profits: 1

Management:		Sales/Marketing:		Liberal Arts:		Information Systems:		Professionals:		Technical/Scientific:	
Mgmt. Trainees:	Y	Mktg. Professionals:	Y	Gen. Writing/Editing:	Y	Info. Management:	Y	Finance/Accounting:	Y	Engineers, Elec.:	Y
Experienced Mgmt.:	Y	Retail Sales:		Technical Writing:	Y	Software Dev.:	Y	Law:	Y	Engineers, Other:	
Int'l Business:	Y	Commercial/Industrial:	Y	Graphic Arts/Photog.:	Y	Hardware Dev.:		HR/Other:	Y	Health/Lab:	
MBA Graduates:	Y	Sales Trainees:	Y	Music:		Systems Integration:		Training:	Y	Scientists/Research:	Y
		Advertising Pros.:	Y	Broadcasting:		Consulting/Other:		Health Care:		Petroleum/Chemicals:	
				Other:				Consulting:		Math/Other:	

TYPES OF BUSINESS:

Machinery-Earth Moving & Agricultural
Engines
Financing
Fuel Cell Manufacturing
Turbine Engines
Engine & Equipment Remanufacturing
Supply Chain Services

BRANDS/DIVISIONS/AFFILIATES:

Solar Turbines
Caterpillar Remanufacturing Services
Progress Rail Services, Inc.
Eurenov S.A.S.
Blount
Lovat, Inc.

CONTACTS: *Note: Officers with more than one job title may be intentionally listed here more than once.*

James W. Owens, CEO
David B. Burritt, CFO/VP
Sidney C. Banwart, VP-Human Svcs.
John S. Heller, CIO/VP
Tana L. Utley, CTO/VP
James B. Buda, General Counsel/VP/Corp. Sec.
Kevin E. Colgan, Treas.
Mark Pflederer, VP/Gen. Mgr.-Mining & Construction Equipment
Thomas A. Gales, VP-Latin America Div.
Bradley M. Halverson, Controller
Steven L. Fisher, VP-Remanufacturing Div.
James W. Owens, Chmn.
Michael J. Baunton, VP-EMEA
Daniel M. Murphy, VP-Global Purchasing

Phone: 309-675-1000	Fax: 309-675-4332
Toll-Free:	
Address: 100 NE Adams St., Peoria, IL 61629 US	

GROWTH PLANS/SPECIAL FEATURES:

Caterpillar, Inc. manufactures construction equipment. The company's three principal lines of business are machinery, engines and financial products. The machinery segment designs, manufactures and markets construction, mining, agricultural and forestry machinery, including track and wheel tractors, track and wheel loaders, pipe layers, motor graders, wheel tractor-scrapers, track and wheel excavators, backhoe loaders, mining shovels, log skidders, log loaders, off-highway trucks, articulated trucks, paving products, telescopic handlers, skid steer loaders and parts. The engines segment designs, manufactures and markets engines for Caterpillar machinery; electric power generation systems; on-highway vehicles and locomotives; marine, petroleum, construction, industrial, agricultural and other applications; and related parts. Caterpillar also manufactures fuel cells, designed to incorporate ethanol, methanol, natural gas, propane, methane, hydrogen and biomass fuels. The firm's Solar Turbines subsidiary is a world leader in industrial gas turbine power system engines. The financial products segment provides financing to customers and dealers for the purchase and lease of Caterpillar and other equipment, financing approximately 64% of equipment sold. Caterpillar has a network 53 U.S. dealers and 128 outside of the U.S. Worldwide, these dealers serve 182 countries and operate 3,645 places of business, including 1,606 dealer rental outlets. More than half of the company's sales are to overseas customers. Caterpillar's logistics business provides supply chain services to Caterpillar and over 65 other companies worldwide. The firm's mid-term goal is to grow to $50 billion in annual revenue by 2010, largely through expansion of financing and engine remanufacturing. Operations in China are also targeted for rapid growth. Caterpillar also holds Progress Rail Services, a remanufacturer of locomotives and railcars. In April 2007, the company finished the acquisition of Eurenov S.A.S., a remanufacturer of engines, transmissions and components. In November 2007, Caterpillar acquired Blount's Forestry Division. In March 2008, the firm acquired Lovat, Inc., which manufactures tunnel boring machines.

FINANCIALS: Sales and profits are in thousands of dollars—add 000 to get the full amount. 2007 Note: Financial information for 2007 was not available for all companies at press time.

2007 Sales: $44,958,000	2007 Profits: $3,541,000	U.S. Stock Ticker: CAT
2006 Sales: $41,517,000	2006 Profits: $3,537,000	Int'l Ticker: Int'l Exchange:
2005 Sales: $36,339,000	2005 Profits: $2,854,000	Employees: 97,444
2004 Sales: $30,306,000	2004 Profits: $2,035,000	Fiscal Year Ends: 12/31
2003 Sales: $22,807,000	2003 Profits: $1,099,000	Parent Company:

SALARIES/BENEFITS:

Pension Plan: Y	ESOP Stock Plan:	Profit Sharing:	Top Exec. Salary: $1,512,504	Bonus: $4,742,998
Savings Plan: Y	Stock Purch. Plan:		Second Exec. Salary: $826,177	Bonus: $1,979,081

OTHER THOUGHTS:

Apparent Women Officers or Directors: 7
Hot Spot for Advancement for Women/Minorities: Y

LOCATIONS: ("Y" = Yes)

West:	Southwest:	Midwest:	Southeast:	Northeast:	International:
Y	Y	Y	Y	Y	Y

CATERPILLAR LOGISTICS
www.catlogistics.com

Industry Group Code: 488510 Ranks within this company's industry group: Sales: Profits:

Management:		Sales/Marketing:		Liberal Arts:		Information Systems:		Professionals:		Technical/Scientific:	
Mgmt. Trainees:	Y	Mktg. Professionals:	Y	Gen. Writing/Editing:		Info. Management:	Y	Finance/Accounting:	Y	Engineers, Elec.:	
Experienced Mgmt.:	Y	Retail Sales:		Technical Writing:	Y	Software Dev.:	Y	Law:	Y	Engineers, Other:	
Int'l Business:	Y	Commercial/Industrial:	Y	Graphic Arts/Photog.:		Hardware Dev.:		HR/Other:	Y	Health/Lab:	
MBA Graduates:	Y	Sales Trainees:		Music:		Systems Integration:	Y	Training:	Y	Scientists/Research:	
		Advertising Pros.:		Broadcasting:		Consulting/Other:	Y	Health Care:		Petroleum/Chemicals:	
				Other:				Consulting:	Y	Math/Other:	Y

TYPES OF BUSINESS:

Freight Logistics
Supply Chain Management
Supply Chain Strategy & Design
Systems & Technology Services

BRANDS/DIVISIONS/AFFILIATES:

Caterpillar Inc

CONTACTS: Note: Officers with more than one job title may be intentionally listed here more than once.

Stephen Larson, Pres.
David Hoffman, CFO
John Bolden, VP-Human Resources
Richard Burritt, VP-Tech. Svcs. & Mgmt.
Mark Hynes, VP-Mfg. Logistics
Wesley Blumenshine, VP-Legal Svcs.
Liva Vosekalna, Media Rel.
Jim Owens, CEO/Pres., Caterpillar, Inc.
Jim Boehm, VP-Americas
Paul Joseph, Pres., Asia-Pacific
Stephen Larson, Chmn.
Bob Sweikert, Pres., EMEA
Dan Spellman, VP-Logistics Dev. & Supply Chain Svcs.

Phone: 309-266-3591	Fax: 309-266-4420
Toll-Free: 800-240-2126	
Address: 500 N. Morton Ave., Morton, IL 61550-0474 US	

GROWTH PLANS/SPECIAL FEATURES:

Caterpillar Logistics Services, Inc. (CLS), a subsidiary of Caterpillar, Inc., provides supply chain management services to its parent company and approximately 65 other companies worldwide, including Ford Motor Company, the U.S. Navy, Fisher Controls International, Hyundai, SAAB Cars USA and DELPHI Automotive Systems. The company serves clients in the automotive, industrial equipment, consumer durables, energy, manufacturing logistics, high-tech hardware and aerospace and defense industries. Its supply chain management services include supply chain strategy (network design, channel strategy, optimization/simulation and asset planning); supply chain design (operational design, transportation modeling and business process engineering); systems and technology (IT planning, application selection, systems integration, data warehousing and application maintenance outsourcing); and execution services (distribution, global compliance, transportation management, manufacturing logistics, order management, materials management, reverse logistics and business support). CLS offers these services through its network of over 105 offices and facilities in 25 countries on six continents, and provides customer shipments to over 200 countries, shipping more than 84 million lines annually. In recent news, the firm has expanded its facilities by building a new 975,000 square foot logistics and distribution center in Waco, Texas; a 110,300 square-foot logistics center in Moscow, Russia; and through a partnership with Mosaic Fertilizer, LLC, an 80,000 square foot state-of-the-art distribution facility in Lakeland, Florida.

CLS provides its U.S. employees with an employee assistance program (confidential counseling), a tuition assistance plan and flexible spending accounts for health care (to be used on healthcare expenses not covered by the company health plan), dependant care and paid time off. The firm's manufacturing employees receive matching 401(k) contributions and medical coverage, while office employees receive 100% matching on 401(k) contributions, a pension plan and medical, dental and vision coverage.

FINANCIALS: Sales and profits are in thousands of dollars—add 000 to get the full amount. 2007 Note: Financial information for 2007 was not available for all companies at press time.

2007 Sales: $	2007 Profits: $	U.S. Stock Ticker: Subsidiary
2006 Sales: $2,400,000	2006 Profits: $	Int'l Ticker: Int'l Exchange:
2005 Sales: $	2005 Profits: $	Employees: 12,000
2004 Sales: $	2004 Profits: $	Fiscal Year Ends: 12/31
2003 Sales: $	2003 Profits: $	Parent Company: CATERPILLAR INC

SALARIES/BENEFITS:

Pension Plan: Y	ESOP Stock Plan:	Profit Sharing:	Top Exec. Salary: $	Bonus: $
Savings Plan: Y	Stock Purch. Plan:		Second Exec. Salary: $	Bonus: $

OTHER THOUGHTS:

Apparent Women Officers or Directors: 1
Hot Spot for Advancement for Women/Minorities: Y

LOCATIONS: ("Y" = Yes)

West:	Southwest:	Midwest:	Southeast:	Northeast:	International:
Y	Y	Y	Y	Y	Y

Note: Financial information, benefits and other data can change quickly and may vary from those stated here.

CATHOLIC HEALTH INITIATIVES   www.catholichealthinit.org

Industry Group Code: 622110 Ranks within this company's industry group: Sales: 2   Profits: 2

Management:		Sales/Marketing:	Liberal Arts:		Information Systems:		Professionals:		Technical/Scientific:	
Mgmt. Trainees:		Mktg. Professionals:	Gen. Writing/Editing:	Y	Info. Management:	Y	Finance/Accounting:	Y	Engineers, Elec.:	
Experienced Mgmt.:	Y	Retail Sales:	Technical Writing:		Software Dev.:		Law:	Y	Engineers, Other:	
Int'l Business:		Commercial/Industrial:	Graphic Arts/Photog.:		Hardware Dev.:		HR/Other:	Y	Health/Lab:	
MBA Graduates:	Y	Sales Trainees:	Music:		Systems Integration:		Training:	Y	Scientists/Research:	
		Advertising Pros.:	Broadcasting:		Consulting/Other:		Health Care:	Y	Petroleum/Chemicals:	
			Other:				Consulting:		Math/Other:	

TYPES OF BUSINESS:

Hospitals
Long-Term Care
Assisted & Independent Living Facilities
Community Health Organizations
Home Care Services
Occupational Health Clinic
Cancer Prevention Institute

BRANDS/DIVISIONS/AFFILIATES:

Centura Health
Franciscan Health System
Alegant Health
Good Samaritan Health Systems
Premier Health Partners
Captive Management Initiatives

CONTACTS: Note: Officers with more than one job title may be intentionally listed here more than once.

Kevin E. Lofton, CEO
Michael T. Rowan, COO/Exec. VP
Kevin E. Lofton, Pres.
Colleen M. Blye, CFO
Herbert J. Vallier, Chief Human Resource Officer/Sr. VP
Michael O'Rourke, Interim CIO
Michael L. Fordyce, Chief Admin. Officer
Paul G. Neumann, General Counsel/Sr. VP-Legal Svcs.
Gary Campbell, Sr. VP-Oper.
John F. DiCola, Sr. VP-Strategy & Bus. Dev.
Joyce M. Ross, Sr. VP-Comm.
Colleen M. Blye, Sr. VP-Finance & Treasury
A. Michelle Cooper, VP-Corp. Responsibility
Mitch H. Merlfi, Chief Risk Officer/Sr. VP
Susan E. Peach, Sr. VP-Performance Mgmt.
Kathy Sanford, Chief Nursing Officer/Sr. VP
Phillip W. Mears, Sr. VP-Supply Chain

Phone: 303-298-9100	Fax: 303-298-9690
Toll-Free:	
Address: 1999 Broadway, Ste. 2600, Denver, CO 80202 US	

GROWTH PLANS/SPECIAL FEATURES:

Catholic Health Initiatives is a national nonprofit health care organization focused on strengthening and advancing the Catholic health ministry. The organization encompasses approximately 77 hospitals; more than 40 long-term care, assisted and independent living residential facilities; and two community health organizations, across 20 states. The group's major affiliates include Centura Health, Alegent Health, Good Samaritan Health Systems, Premier Health Partners and Franciscan Health System. Altogether, CHI has over 10,000 beds. Catholic Health is the second largest Catholic health system in the U.S. Centura Health, jointly operated between CHI and PorterCare Adventist Health Care, has 12 hospitals and seven senior residences and home care and hospice services. Alegent Health, jointly operated with Immanuel Healthcare System, is made up of nine acute care hospitals with 1,800 beds, two long-term care facilities and a primary care physician network. Good Samaritan Health Systems is a network of hospitals and services serving more than 350,000 customers in its region. Premier Health Partners, jointly operated with MedAmerica Health Systems, includes four hospitals, one assisted living community, a home health care service and a cancer prevention institute. The Franciscan Health System includes four full-service hospitals, a long-term care facility, a women's health center and midwife service and an occupational health clinic, among other services. In recent news, the Good Samaritan Hospital of Dayton, Ohio, will acquire the assets of Dayton Heart Hospital for $55 million. CHI also launched Captive Management Initiatives, a wholly-owned subsidiary that provides management services for the captive insurance industry.

FINANCIALS: Sales and profits are in thousands of dollars—add 000 to get the full amount. 2007 Note: Financial information for 2007 was not available for all companies at press time.

2007 Sales: $7,731,500	2007 Profits: $	U.S. Stock Ticker: Nonprofit
2006 Sales: $7,636,233	2006 Profits: $693,701	Int'l Ticker: Int'l Exchange:
2005 Sales: $7,091,448	2005 Profits: $498,374	Employees: 65,070
2004 Sales: $6,659,711	2004 Profits: $538,295	Fiscal Year Ends:
2003 Sales: $6,071,600	2003 Profits: $202,900	Parent Company:

SALARIES/BENEFITS:

Pension Plan:	ESOP Stock Plan:	Profit Sharing:	Top Exec. Salary: $	Bonus: $
Savings Plan:	Stock Purch. Plan:		Second Exec. Salary: $	Bonus: $

OTHER THOUGHTS:

Apparent Women Officers or Directors: 8
Hot Spot for Advancement for Women/Minorities: Y

LOCATIONS: ("Y" = Yes)

West:	Southwest:	Midwest:	Southeast:	Northeast:	International:
Y	Y	Y	Y	Y	

Note: Financial information, benefits and other data can change quickly and may vary from those stated here.

CBRL GROUP INC

www.cbrlgroup.com

Industry Group Code: 722110 Ranks within this company's industry group: Sales: Profits:

Management:		Sales/Marketing:		Liberal Arts:		Information Systems:		Professionals:		Technical/Scientific:	
Mgmt. Trainees:	Y	Mktg. Professionals:	Y	Gen. Writing/Editing:		Info. Management:	Y	Finance/Accounting:	Y	Engineers, Elec.:	
Experienced Mgmt.:	Y	Retail Sales:		Technical Writing:		Software Dev.:		Law:	Y	Engineers, Other:	
Int'l Business:		Commercial/Industrial:		Graphic Arts/Photog.:		Hardware Dev.:		HR/Other:	Y	Health/Lab:	
MBA Graduates:	Y	Sales Trainees:		Music:		Systems Integration:		Training:	Y	Scientists/Research:	
		Advertising Pros.:	Y	Broadcasting:		Consulting/Other:		Health Care:		Petroleum/Chemicals:	
				Other:				Consulting:		Math/Other:	

TYPES OF BUSINESS:

Restaurants-Country Cooking, Food Service
Retail Gifts and Food Products

BRANDS/DIVISIONS/AFFILIATES:

Cracker Barrel Old Country Store

CONTACTS: Note: Officers with more than one job title may be intentionally listed here more than once.

Michael A. Woodhouse, CEO
Doug Barber, COO/Exec. VP
N. B. Forrest Shoaf, Interim CFO
Robert J. Harig, Sr. VP-Human Resources
N. B. Forrest Shoaf, General Counsel
Edward A. Greene, Sr. VP-Strategic Initiatives
Diana S. Wynne, Sr. VP-Corp. Affairs
Lawrence E. White, Sr. VP-Finance
Terry Maxwell, Sr. VP-Retail
Michael A. Woodhouse, Chmn.

Phone: 615-444-5533	Fax: 615-443-9399
Toll-Free:	
Address: 305 Hartmann Dr., Lebanon, TN 37088 US	

GROWTH PLANS/SPECIAL FEATURES:

CBRL Group, Inc. is primarily a restaurant chain operator, with 565 Cracker Barrel Old Country Store restaurants in 41 states. In 1999, CBRL Group underwent restructuring, transforming itself into a holding company in order to accommodate plans to expand into new business areas. Cracker Barrel Old Country Store restaurants resemble turn-of-the-century country stores and are famous throughout the southern portion of the U.S. for country cooking and early 20th century decor. Restaurants also feature small retail areas where customers can purchase various products reminiscent of turn-of-the century goods typically found at old-fashioned general stores, such as rocking chairs, seasonal gifts, apparel, toys, music CDs, cookware, old-fashioned-looking ceramics, figurines, a book-on-audio sale-and-exchange program and various other gift items, as well as various candies, preserves, syrups and other food items. Cracker Barrel's Books-on-Audio program allows customers to purchase an audio book at any location, listen to it and then return it for full price minus a small exchange fee. The company's restaurant operations generated approximately 78% of total revenue in 2007. The retail operations generated approximately 22% of Cracker Barrel's total revenue in 2007.

FINANCIALS: Sales and profits are in thousands of dollars—add 000 to get the full amount. 2007 Note: Financial information for 2007 was not available for all companies at press time.

2007 Sales: $2,351,576	2007 Profits: $162,065	U.S. Stock Ticker: CBRL
2006 Sales: $2,219,475	2006 Profits: $116,291	Int'l Ticker: Int'l Exchange:
2005 Sales: $2,190,866	2005 Profits: $126,640	Employees: 65,192
2004 Sales: $1,595,244	2004 Profits: $113,262	Fiscal Year Ends: 7/31
2003 Sales: $2,198,200	2003 Profits: $106,500	Parent Company:

SALARIES/BENEFITS:

Pension Plan:	ESOP Stock Plan:	Profit Sharing:	Top Exec. Salary: $700,000	Bonus: $1,640,625
Savings Plan: Y	Stock Purch. Plan: Y		Second Exec. Salary: $500,000	Bonus: $781,250

OTHER THOUGHTS:

Apparent Women Officers or Directors: 1
Hot Spot for Advancement for Women/Minorities:

LOCATIONS: ("Y" = Yes)

West:	Southwest:	Midwest:	Southeast:	Northeast:	International:
Y	Y	Y	Y	Y	

CDW CORPORATION   www.cdw.com

Industry Group Code: 443120A Ranks within this company's industry group: Sales: 1   Profits: 1

Management:		Sales/Marketing:		Liberal Arts:		Information Systems:		Professionals:		Technical/Scientific:	
Mgmt. Trainees:	Y	Mktg. Professionals:	Y	Gen. Writing/Editing:	Y	Info. Management:	Y	Finance/Accounting:	Y	Engineers, Elec.:	
Experienced Mgmt.:	Y	Retail Sales:	Y	Technical Writing:	Y	Software Dev.:	Y	Law:	Y	Engineers, Other:	
Int'l Business:	Y	Commercial/Industrial:	Y	Graphic Arts/Photog.:	Y	Hardware Dev.:		HR/Other:	Y	Health/Lab:	
MBA Graduates:	Y	Sales Trainees:	Y	Music:		Systems Integration:		Training:	Y	Scientists/Research:	
		Advertising Pros.:	Y	Broadcasting:		Consulting/Other:		Health Care:		Petroleum/Chemicals:	
				Other:				Consulting:		Math/Other:	

TYPES OF BUSINESS:
Computer Products, Direct Selling
Catalog Sales
Online Sales
Retail Showrooms
Support Services

BRANDS/DIVISIONS/AFFILIATES:
CDW Government Inc
CDW Canada Inc
Berbee Information Networks Corp
Madison Dearborn Partners, LLC
Providence Equity Partners Inc.

CONTACTS: *Note: Officers with more than one job title may be intentionally listed here more than once.*
John A. Edwardson, CEO
Ann E. Ziegler, CFO/Sr. VP
Mark J. Gambill, VP-Mktg.
Dennis G. Berger, Sr. VP/Chief Coworker Services Officer
Jonathan J. Stevens, CIO/Sr. VP
Christine A. Leahy, General Counsel/Sr. VP/Sec.
Douglas E. Eckrote, Sr. VP-Oper.
Anne B. Ireland, Sales Planning & Operations
Gary Ross, Sr. Mgr.-Corp. Communications
Cindy Thorson Klimstra, VP-Investor Rel.
Virginia L. Seggerman, Controller
Kevin P. Adams, VP-Program Mgmt., CDW Government, Inc.
Kenneth B. Grimsley, VP-Strategic Sales, CDW Government, Inc.
Harry J. Harczak, Jr., Exec. VP
Matthew A. Troka, VP-Prod. & Partner Mgmt.
John A. Edwardson, Chmn.

Phone: 847-465-6000	Fax: 847-465-6800
Toll-Free: 800-750-4239	
Address: 200 N. Milwaukee Ave., Vernon Hills, IL 60061 US	

GROWTH PLANS/SPECIAL FEATURES:
CDW Corp. is a provider of multi-branded information technology products and services to business, government and education customers in the U.S. and Canada. The company operates in three segments, corporate sector, public sector and Berbee. The firm offers more than 80,000 microcomputer products include hardware and peripherals; software; accessories; and other products. CDW offers customers a broad range of technology products from brands such as Acer, Adobe, APS, Apple, Cisco, Fujitsu, Hewlett-Packard, IBM, Lenovo, Microsoft, Panasonic, Quantum, Samsung, Sony, Symantec and ViewSonic, among others. The company manages its inventory with a proprietary information technology system combined with a 450,000-square-foot distribution center, shipping approximately 15,000 items daily. The firm focuses on selling to small and medium-sized businesses through catalogs, direct mailings, advertisements in trade magazines, web sites and various other web advertising vehicles. Additionally, it promotes the CDW brand nationally through its branding campaign, which includes television, print media and other activities. CDW offers customers free access to over 140 support technicians with over 400 manufacturer certifications, in addition to direct links to manufacturers' tech support web sites. CDW Government, Inc. subsidiary provides specialized product offerings and services to federal, state and local governments, as well as the educational sector. CDW Canada, Inc. serves business and public sector customers in Canada. In October 2007, CDW Corporation was acquired by an entity controlled by investment funds affiliated with Madison Dearborn Partners, LLC and Providence Equity Partners Inc.

The company offers its employees medical, dental and vision insurance; a 401(k) plan; a profit sharing plan; an employee stock purchase plan; life and AD&D insurance; short- and long-term disability insurance; and an employee assistance program.

FINANCIALS: Sales and profits are in thousands of dollars—add 000 to get the full amount. 2007 Note: Financial information for 2007 was not available for all companies at press time.

2007 Sales: $8,145,000	2007 Profits: $	U.S. Stock Ticker: Private
2006 Sales: $6,785,473	2006 Profits: $266,080	Int'l Ticker: Int'l Exchange:
2005 Sales: $6,291,845	2005 Profits: $272,092	Employees: 5,500
2004 Sales: $5,737,800	2004 Profits: $241,400	Fiscal Year Ends: 12/31
2003 Sales: $4,664,616	2003 Profits: $175,186	Parent Company:

SALARIES/BENEFITS:
Pension Plan:	ESOP Stock Plan: Y	Profit Sharing: Y	Top Exec. Salary: $760,000	Bonus: $1,055,629
Savings Plan: Y	Stock Purch. Plan:		Second Exec. Salary: $320,000	Bonus: $783,564

OTHER THOUGHTS:
Apparent Women Officers or Directors: 7
Hot Spot for Advancement for Women/Minorities: Y

LOCATIONS: ("Y" = Yes)
West:	Southwest:	Midwest:	Southeast:	Northeast:	International:
		Y			Y

CELLCO PARTNERSHIP (VERIZON WIRELESS)
www.verizonwireless.com

Industry Group Code: 513322 **Ranks within this company's industry group:** Sales: 2 Profits:

Management:		Sales/Marketing:		Liberal Arts:		Information Systems:		Professionals:		Technical/Scientific:	
Mgmt. Trainees:	Y	Mktg. Professionals:	Y	Gen. Writing/Editing:		Info. Management:	Y	Finance/Accounting:	Y	Engineers, Elec.:	Y
Experienced Mgmt.:	Y	Retail Sales:	Y	Technical Writing:		Software Dev.:	Y	Law:	Y	Engineers, Other:	
Int'l Business:		Commercial/Industrial:	Y	Graphic Arts/Photog.:		Hardware Dev.:		HR/Other:	Y	Health/Lab:	
MBA Graduates:	Y	Sales Trainees:	Y	Music:		Systems Integration:		Training:	Y	Scientists/Research:	
		Advertising Pros.:	Y	Broadcasting:		Consulting/Other:		Health Care:		Petroleum/Chemicals:	
				Other:				Consulting:		Math/Other:	

TYPES OF BUSINESS:
Cellular Phone Service
Retail Sales
Wireless Internet
Media & Ringtones

BRANDS/DIVISIONS/AFFILIATES:
Verizon Wireless
Verizon Communications, Inc.
Vodafone Group PLC
SureWest Communications
Rural Cellular Corp.
Ramcell
LiMo Foundation
West Virginia Wireless

CONTACTS: Note: Officers with more than one job title may be intentionally listed here more than once.
Lowell McAdam, CEO
Jack Plating, COO/Exec. VP
Lowell McAdam, Pres.
John Townsend, CFO/VP
Mike Lanman, Chief Mktg. Officer/VP
Martha Delehanty, VP-Human Resources
Ajay Waghray, CIO
Anthony Melone, CTO/Sr. VP
Steve Zipperstein, VP-Legal & External Affairs
Margaret Feldman, VP-Bus. Dev.
Jim Gerace, VP-Corp. Comm.
Michael Maiorana, VP-Gov't Sales & Oper.
Charlie Falco, VP-Customer Service Oper.
Rose Kirk, VP-Enterprise Sales & Distribution
Anthony Lewis, VP-Open Dev.

Phone: 908-559-7000	Fax:
Toll-Free: 800-922-0204	
Address: 1 Verizon Way, Basking Ridge, NJ 07920 US	

GROWTH PLANS/SPECIAL FEATURES:

Cellco Partnership, doing business as Verizon Wireless, is a joint venture between Verizon Communications and Vodafone; the former owns 55% of Cellco, while the latter owns 45%. Verizon Wireless was formed in 2000 when Vodafone and Bell Atlantic merged their U.S. wireless holdings. The company then acquired the U.S. wireless assets of GTE, when Bell Atlantic bought GTE to create Verizon Communications. The firm operates over 2,400 company stores and kiosks and 175 switching centers and serves over 67 million customers. It continues to expand its network, with recent growth in service areas including Indiana, Kentucky, South Carolina, Colorado, Montana and Ohio. The company offers BroadbandAccess and NationalAccess for coast-to-coast laptop, personal digital assistants (PDAs) and handset connectivity; VCAST Music service for downloading music, music videos, VCAST video clips, 3D games and other multimedia services; and Get It Now for text and picture messaging, downloading ringtones, ringback tones, games and news alerts on a mobile handset. In February 2007, the company purchased the operating assets of West Virginia Wireless, owned by Key Communications LLC, to aid expansion into new West Virginia markets. In June 2007, the firm agreed to acquire Rural Cellular Corp., with presence in 16 states, and in August, the company purchased the operating assets of Ramcell, active in Kentucky and Oregon. In May 2008, Verizon Wireless signed a five-year agreement with Qwest Communications International Inc. for Qwest to market and sell Verizon service. Also in May, the company purchased the wireless assets of SureWest Communications in the Sacramento, California area. In May 2008, the firm joined the LiMo Foundation, a global alliance based around open handset platform development.

The company provides its employees with medical and dental insurance; vision care; life insurance; prescription drug benefits; adoption assistance; health and dependant care spending accounts; phone discounts; childcare discounts; and tuition assistance.

FINANCIALS: Sales and profits are in thousands of dollars—add 000 to get the full amount. 2007 Note: Financial information for 2007 was not available for all companies at press time.

2007 Sales: $43,900,000	2007 Profits: $	U.S. Stock Ticker: Joint Venture
2006 Sales: $38,000,000	2006 Profits: $	Int'l Ticker: Int'l Exchange:
2005 Sales: $32,300,000	2005 Profits: $6,152,000	Employees: 69,000
2004 Sales: $27,662,000	2004 Profits: $4,698,000	Fiscal Year Ends: 12/31
2003 Sales: $22,489,000	2003 Profits: $3,083,000	Parent Company:

SALARIES/BENEFITS:

Pension Plan:	ESOP Stock Plan:	Profit Sharing: Y	Top Exec. Salary: $2,100,000	Bonus: $4,252,500
Savings Plan: Y	Stock Purch. Plan:		Second Exec. Salary: $1,200,000	Bonus: $1,824,000

OTHER THOUGHTS:
Apparent Women Officers or Directors: 3
Hot Spot for Advancement for Women/Minorities: Y

LOCATIONS: ("Y" = Yes)

West:	Southwest:	Midwest:	Southeast:	Northeast:	International:
Y	Y	Y	Y	Y	

Note: Financial information, benefits and other data can change quickly and may vary from those stated here.

CEPHALON INC

www.cephalon.com

Industry Group Code: 325412 Ranks within this company's industry group: Sales: 8 Profits: 7

Management:		Sales/Marketing:		Liberal Arts:		Information Systems:		Professionals:		Technical/Scientific:	
Mgmt. Trainees:		Mktg. Professionals:	Y	Gen. Writing/Editing:		Info. Management:	Y	Finance/Accounting:	Y	Engineers, Elec.:	Y
Experienced Mgmt.:	Y	Retail Sales:		Technical Writing:	Y	Software Dev.:	Y	Law:	Y	Engineers, Other:	Y
Int'l Business:	Y	Commercial/Industrial:	Y	Graphic Arts/Photog.:	Y	Hardware Dev.:		HR/Other:	Y	Health/Lab:	Y
MBA Graduates:	Y	Sales Trainees:	Y	Music:		Systems Integration:	Y	Training:	Y	Scientists/Research:	Y
		Advertising Pros.:		Broadcasting:		Consulting/Other:		Health Care:	Y	Petroleum/Chemicals:	Y
				Other:				Consulting:		Math/Other:	Y

TYPES OF BUSINESS:

Pharmaceutical Discovery & Development
Neurological Disorder Treatments
Cancer Treatments
Pain Medications
Addiction Treatment

BRANDS/DIVISIONS/AFFILIATES:

Provigil
Actiq
Fentora
Trisenox
Vivitrol
Nuvigil
Treanda for Injection
AMRIX

CONTACTS: Note: Officers with more than one job title may be intentionally listed here more than once.

Frank Baldino, Jr., CEO
J. Kevin Buchi, CFO/Exec. VP
Jeffry L. Vaught, Exec. VP-R&D
Peter E. Grebow, Sr. VP-Worldwide Tech. Oper.
Carl A. Savini, Chief Admin. Officer/Exec. VP
Gerald J. Pappert, General Counsel/Exec. VP
Lesley Russell, Exec. VP-Worldwide Medical & Regulatory Oper.
Valli F. Baldassano, Chief Compliance Officer/Exec. VP
Frank Baldino, Jr., Chmn.
Robert P. Roche, Jr., Sr. VP-Worldwide Pharmaceutical Oper.

Phone: 610-344-0200	Fax: 610-738-6590
Toll-Free:	
Address: 41 Moores Rd., Frazer, PA 19355 US	

GROWTH PLANS/SPECIAL FEATURES:

Cephalon, Inc. is a biopharmaceutical company focused on the discovery, development and marketing of products in four core areas: Central nervous system (CNS) disorders, pain, oncology (the study of cancer) and addiction. It conducts research and development as well as marketing its products in the U.S. and Europe. Cephalon's technology principally focuses on understanding the class of enzymes known as kinases and the role they play in cellular survival and proliferation. The company's CNS products include its most significant product, Provigil Tablets, which generated 49% of 2007 sales. Based on the stimulant modafinil, Provigil is indicated for extreme sleepiness associated with narcolepsy and other sleep disorders. The firm's other CNS medication is Gabitril, indicated for partial seizures in epileptic patients. The firm's two pain management products, Actiq (oral transmucosal fentanyl citrate) and Fentora (fentanyl buccal tablet), comprise Cephalon's next most significant products; together they generated 29% of 2007 sales. Approximately 94% of Provigil sales, as well as 92% of Actiq and Fentora sales, were generated in the U.S. Cephalon's oncology products include Trisenox (an arsenic salt), which is marketed in the U.S. and Europe to treat patients with relapsed acute promyelocytic leukemia (APL). Vivitrol is the firm's only approved addiction treatment. It is an injectable form of the drug naltrexone, indicated for the treatment of alcohol dependant patients. The more than 30 products sold in Europe generated 15% of 2007 sales. In June 2007, Cephalon's modafinil-based Nuvigil tablets, which treat the same indications as Provigil, received FDA approval. In March 2008, the firm received FDA approval for Treanda for Injection, which treats chronic lymphocytic leukemia (CLL). In August 2007, the firm acquired the North American distribution rights for muscle relaxant AMRIX from E. Claiborne Robins Company, Inc. (doing business as ECR Pharmaceuticals) for $100.1 million.

FINANCIALS: Sales and profits are in thousands of dollars—add 000 to get the full amount. 2007 Note: Financial information for 2007 was not available for all companies at press time.

2007 Sales: $1,772,638
2006 Sales: $1,764,069
2005 Sales: $1,211,892
2004 Sales: $1,015,400
2003 Sales: $714,800

2007 Profits: $-191,704
2006 Profits: $144,816
2005 Profits: $-174,954
2004 Profits: $-73,800
2003 Profits: $83,900

U.S. Stock Ticker: CEPH
Int'l Ticker: Int'l Exchange:
Employees: 2,796
Fiscal Year Ends: 12/31
Parent Company:

SALARIES/BENEFITS:

Pension Plan:	ESOP Stock Plan:	Profit Sharing: Y	Top Exec. Salary: $1,196,700	Bonus: $2,213,900
Savings Plan: Y	Stock Purch. Plan:		Second Exec. Salary: $509,300	Bonus: $356,500

OTHER THOUGHTS:

Apparent Women Officers or Directors: 1
Hot Spot for Advancement for Women/Minorities:

LOCATIONS: ("Y" = Yes)

West:	Southwest:	Midwest:	Southeast:	Northeast:	International:
Y		Y		Y	Y

Note: Financial information, benefits and other data can change quickly and may vary from those stated here.

CH ROBINSON WORLDWIDE INC
www.chrobinson.com

Industry Group Code: 488510 Ranks within this company's industry group: Sales: 1 Profits: 1

Management:		Sales/Marketing:		Liberal Arts:		Information Systems:		Professionals:		Technical/Scientific:	
Mgmt. Trainees:	Y	Mktg. Professionals:	Y	Gen. Writing/Editing:		Info. Management:	Y	Finance/Accounting:	Y	Engineers, Elec.:	
Experienced Mgmt.:	Y	Retail Sales:		Technical Writing:	Y	Software Dev.:	Y	Law:	Y	Engineers, Other:	
Int'l Business:	Y	Commercial/Industrial:	Y	Graphic Arts/Photog.:		Hardware Dev.:		HR/Other:	Y	Health/Lab:	
MBA Graduates:	Y	Sales Trainees:		Music:		Systems Integration:		Training:	Y	Scientists/Research:	
		Advertising Pros.:		Broadcasting:		Consulting/Other:		Health Care:		Petroleum/Chemicals:	
				Other:				Consulting:		Math/Other:	Y

TYPES OF BUSINESS:

Freight Logistics
Produce Sourcing
Expedited Services
Fuel Purchasing Management Services
3PL Third Party Logistics
Warehouse & Distribution Services

BRANDS/DIVISIONS/AFFILIATES:

CHREX
T-Check Systems, Inc.
Fresh 1 (The)

CONTACTS: Note: Officers with more than one job title may be intentionally listed here more than once.

John P. Wiehoff, CEO
Chad M. Lindbloom, CFO/VP
Linda U. Feuss, General Counsel/Corp. Sec./VP
Thomas K. Mahlke, Corp. Controller
James E. Butts, VP-Transportation
Mark A. Walker, VP-Transportation
Scott A. Satterlee, VP-Produce
John P. Wiehoff, Chmn.

Phone: 952-937-8500	Fax: 952-937-6714
Toll-Free:	
Address: 8100 Mitchell Rd., Eden Prairie, MN 55344-2248 US	

GROWTH PLANS/SPECIAL FEATURES:

C.H. Robinson Worldwide, Inc. (CHRW) is one of North America's largest third-party logistics (3PL) providers and a global provider of multimodal transportation services. It operates through 218 offices in 42 states across the U.S., as well as in Canada, Mexico, Europe, South America and Asia. CHRW operates in three sectors: multimodal transportation services, which account for 87% of the firm's gross profits; fresh produce sourcing, 9%; and information services, 4%. In the multimodal transportation services sector, the company (which does not own any of its own equipment) maintains one of the largest networks of motor carrier capacity in the world through contracts with approximately 48,000 carriers. CHRW serves more than 25,000 customers and handles approximately 5.2 million shipments annually. Subsidiary CHREX provides expedited services and is one of the largest capacity providers in the expedited market. The group also contracts air carriers and specialty motor carriers that provide temperature-controlled and less-than-truckload services. The sourcing sector was the firm's original business when it was founded in 1905, and today focuses on procuring fresh produce for retailers, wholesalers and foodservice operators nationwide. CHRW has its own brand of produce called The Fresh 1, which is sourced through various growers and packed through contract agreements with other packaging firms. The information services segment operates primarily through subsidiary T-Check Systems, Inc., which offers fuel purchasing management services for motor carriers.

The company offers its employees a 401(k) plan, discretionary profit sharing, an employee stock purchase plan and an employee assistance program.

FINANCIALS: Sales and profits are in thousands of dollars—add 000 to get the full amount. 2007 Note: Financial information for 2007 was not available for all companies at press time.

2007 Sales: $7,316,223	2007 Profits: $324,261	**U.S. Stock Ticker: CHRW**
2006 Sales: $6,556,194	2006 Profits: $266,925	**Int'l Ticker:** Int'l Exchange:
2005 Sales: $5,688,948	2005 Profits: $203,358	Employees: 7,300
2004 Sales: $4,341,500	2004 Profits: $137,300	Fiscal Year Ends: 12/31
2003 Sales: $3,613,645	2003 Profits: $114,123	Parent Company:

SALARIES/BENEFITS:

Pension Plan:	ESOP Stock Plan:	Profit Sharing: Y	Top Exec. Salary: $400,000	Bonus: $1,030,000
Savings Plan: Y	Stock Purch. Plan: Y		Second Exec. Salary: $260,000	Bonus: $210,000

OTHER THOUGHTS:

Apparent Women Officers or Directors: 1
Hot Spot for Advancement for Women/Minorities: Y

LOCATIONS: ("Y" = Yes)

West:	Southwest:	Midwest:	Southeast:	Northeast:	International:
Y	Y	Y	Y	Y	Y

CH2M HILL COMPANIES LTD   www.ch2m.com

Industry Group Code: 541710 Ranks within this company's industry group: Sales: 1   Profits:

Management:		Sales/Marketing:		Liberal Arts:		Information Systems:		Professionals:		Technical/Scientific:	
Mgmt. Trainees:		Mktg. Professionals:	Y	Gen. Writing/Editing:	Y	Info. Management:	Y	Finance/Accounting:	Y	Engineers, Elec.:	Y
Experienced Mgmt.:	Y	Retail Sales:		Technical Writing:		Software Dev.:	Y	Law:	Y	Engineers, Other:	Y
Int'l Business:	Y	Commercial/Industrial:	Y	Graphic Arts/Photog.:		Hardware Dev.:	Y	HR/Other:	Y	Health/Lab:	
MBA Graduates:	Y	Sales Trainees:		Music:		Systems Integration:	Y	Training:	Y	Scientists/Research:	
		Advertising Pros.:		Broadcasting:		Consulting/Other:		Health Care:		Petroleum/Chemicals:	
				Other:				Consulting:	Y	Math/Other:	

TYPES OF BUSINESS:

Engineering Services-Consultation
Environmental Engineering & Consulting
Nuclear Management Services
Water & Electrical Utility Services
Decommissioning & Decontamination
Facilities Design & Construction
Project Financing & Procurement
Nanotechnology Research

BRANDS/DIVISIONS/AFFILIATES:

Operations Management International
CH2M HILL Canada, Ltd.
Lockwood Greene
Industrial Design and Construction
CH2M-IDC China
Wade & Assoicates, Inc.
Goldston Engineering, Inc.
VECO

CONTACTS: Note: Officers with more than one job title may be intentionally listed here more than once.

Ralph R. Peterson, CEO
Lee A. McIntire, COO
Lee A. McIntire, Pres.
M. Catherine Santee, CFO
Donald S. Evans, Chief Mktg. Officer
Bob Allen, Chief Human Resource Officer/Sr. VP
Mike Szomjassy, Dir.-Global Bus. Oper.
John Corsi, Dir.-Public Rel.
Catherine Santee, Sr. VP-Finance
Thomas G. Searle, Pres., CH2M HILL Int'l
Mike McKelvy, Pres., CH2M HILL Industrial
Robert G. Card, Chmn.-CH2M HILL Int'l
Nancy Tuor, Pres., CH2M HILL Federal
Ralph R. Peterson, Chmn.
Greg Turner, Mgr.- Bus. Dev. & Planning, Southeast Asia & India

Phone: 303-771-0900	Fax: 720-286-9250
Toll-Free: 888-242-6445	
Address: 9191 S. Jamaica St., Englewood, CO 80112 US	

GROWTH PLANS/SPECIAL FEATURES:

CH2M HILL Companies, Ltd. is an employee-owned firm that offers engineering, consulting, design, construction, procurement, operations, maintenance and program and project management services to clients in the public and private sectors. CH2M Hill has approximately 493 offices worldwide from which it conducts business in more than 40 countries. The company's environmental services division offers its clients ecological and natural resource damage assessments, environmental consulting for remediation projects and treatment systems for properties that have been contaminated by toxic or radioactive waste. The nuclear services segment manages the decontamination and demolition of weapons production facilities and designs nuclear waste treatment and handling facilities. CH2M HILL's Operations Management International subsidiary provides water, wastewater and electrical utility services to private and public clients. CH2M HILL Canada, Ltd. is the Canadian division of the company. Lockwood Greene is a major engineering and construction firm focused on national and multinational industrial and power clients worldwide. Industrial Design and Construction (IDC) is a high-technology facilities design, construction, maintenance and operations company serving process-intensive technology clients. IDC also has interests in nanotechnology research and manufacturing. CH2M-IDC China provides full-service solution to manufacturing companies that are building or have plants in China. Recent acquisitions include Texas-based Goldston Engineering, Inc.; Trigon EPC, a leading engineering and field service company; and VECO, an Alaskan engineering company that serves oil and gas, mining and power clients, for approximately $463 million. Also in 2007, the company was awarded a $5.25 billion program management contract by the Panama Canal Authority (ACP) for its Panama Canal Expansion program.

In 2008, CH2M IDC was ranked 54 on FORTUNE Magazine's 11th annual list of the 100 Best Companies to Work For.

FINANCIALS: Sales and profits are in thousands of dollars—add 000 to get the full amount. 2007 Note: Financial information for 2007 was not available for all companies at press time.

2007 Sales: $4,376,200	2007 Profits: $	U.S. Stock Ticker: Private
2006 Sales: $4,000,000	2006 Profits: $	Int'l Ticker: Int'l Exchange:
2005 Sales: $3,152,200	2005 Profits: $81,600	Employees: 22,000
2004 Sales: $2,715,400	2004 Profits: $32,300	Fiscal Year Ends: 12/31
2003 Sales: $2,154,300	2003 Profits: $23,800	Parent Company:

SALARIES/BENEFITS:

Pension Plan:	ESOP Stock Plan:	Profit Sharing:	Top Exec. Salary: $	Bonus: $
Savings Plan:	Stock Purch. Plan:		Second Exec. Salary: $	Bonus: $

OTHER THOUGHTS:

Apparent Women Officers or Directors: 4
Hot Spot for Advancement for Women/Minorities: Y

LOCATIONS: ("Y" = Yes)

West:	Southwest:	Midwest:	Southeast:	Northeast:	International:
Y	Y	Y	Y	Y	Y

CHARLOTTE RUSSE HOLDING www.charlotte-russe.com

Industry Group Code: 448120 Ranks within this company's industry group: Sales: 11 Profits: 12

Management:		Sales/Marketing:		Liberal Arts:		Information Systems:		Professionals:		Technical/Scientific:	
Mgmt. Trainees:	Y	Mktg. Professionals:	Y	Gen. Writing/Editing:	Y	Info. Management:	Y	Finance/Accounting:	Y	Engineers, Elec.:	
Experienced Mgmt.:	Y	Retail Sales:	Y	Technical Writing:		Software Dev.:	Y	Law:	Y	Engineers, Other:	
Int'l Business:	Y	Commercial/Industrial:	Y	Graphic Arts/Photog.:	Y	Hardware Dev.:		HR/Other:	Y	Health/Lab:	
MBA Graduates:	Y	Sales Trainees:	Y	Music:		Systems Integration:		Training:	Y	Scientists/Research:	
		Advertising Pros.:	Y	Broadcasting:		Consulting/Other:		Health Care:		Petroleum/Chemicals:	
				Other:	Y			Consulting:		Math/Other:	

TYPES OF BUSINESS:

Women's Apparel, Retail

BRANDS/DIVISIONS/AFFILIATES:

Charlotte Russe
Rampage Clothing Co.
blu chic
Refuge

CONTACTS: *Note: Officers with more than one job title may be intentionally listed here more than once.*

Leonard Mogil, Interim CEO
Mark A. Hoffman, Pres.
Leonard Mogil, Interim CFO
Patti Shields, Exec. VP/Gen. Merch. Mgr.
Leonard Mogil, Sr. VP-Store Oper.
Bernard Zeichner, Chmn.
Edward Wong, Exec. VP/Chief Supply Chain Officer

Phone: 858-587-1500	Fax: 858-587-0902
Toll-Free: 877-266-9327	
Address: 4645 Morena Blvd., San Diego, CA 92117 US	

GROWTH PLANS/SPECIAL FEATURES:

Charlotte Russe Holding, Inc. is a mall-based specialty retailer of fashionable, value-priced apparel and accessories targeting young women between ages 15-35. The stores offer a broad assortment of merchandise centered on styles that are affordable and feminine and reflect the latest fashion trends. There are approximately 430 Charlotte Russe stores located in 45 states and Puerto Rico. These stores reflect established fashion trends and rely on exciting in-store graphics and window displays to convey a fashion-forward orientation, and offer ready-to-wear apparel such as tops, dresses, shorts, pants and skirts, as well as seasonal items such as prom dresses and outerwear. The majority of merchandise sold at the Charlotte Russe stores is under the company's proprietary labels, which has the symbols of a heart, moon and star, and includes Charlotte Russe, Refuge and blu Chic. The company markets this merchandise to both younger career women and to teenagers, building brand awareness through a national print marketing campaign. Charlotte Russe stores are located predominantly in high-visibility, center court mall locations in spaces that average 7,100 square feet. The company has two distribution facilities located in San Diego and Ontario, California.

Charlotte Russe employees enjoy a stock purchase plan, a 401k plan with a 25% employer contribution, as well as a merchandise discount and a tuition reimbursement program.

FINANCIALS: Sales and profits are in thousands of dollars—add 000 to get the full amount. 2007 Note: Financial information for 2007 was not available for all companies at press time.

2007 Sales: $740,939	2007 Profits: $36,304	**U.S. Stock Ticker:** CHIC
2006 Sales: $681,504	2006 Profits: $25,138	**Int'l Ticker:** **Int'l Exchange:**
2005 Sales: $511,259	2005 Profits: $10,801	Employees: 8,961
2004 Sales: $449,035	2004 Profits: $15,084	Fiscal Year Ends: 9/30
2003 Sales: $456,622	2003 Profits: $11,013	Parent Company:

SALARIES/BENEFITS:

Pension Plan:	ESOP Stock Plan:	Profit Sharing:	Top Exec. Salary: $612,206	Bonus: $492,349
Savings Plan: Y	Stock Purch. Plan: Y		Second Exec. Salary: $324,154	Bonus: $238,500

OTHER THOUGHTS:

Apparent Women Officers or Directors: 2
Hot Spot for Advancement for Women/Minorities: Y

LOCATIONS: ("Y" = Yes)

West:	Southwest:	Midwest:	Southeast:	Northeast:	International:
Y	Y	Y	Y	Y	Y

CHARMING SHOPPES INC　　www.charmingshoppes.com

Industry Group Code: 448120　**Ranks within this company's industry group:** Sales: 4　Profits: 4

Management:		Sales/Marketing:		Liberal Arts:		Information Systems:		Professionals:		Technical/Scientific:	
Mgmt. Trainees:	Y	Mktg. Professionals:	Y	Gen. Writing/Editing:	Y	Info. Management:	Y	Finance/Accounting:	Y	Engineers, Elec.:	
Experienced Mgmt.:	Y	Retail Sales:	Y	Technical Writing:		Software Dev.:	Y	Law:	Y	Engineers, Other:	
Int'l Business:	Y	Commercial/Industrial:	Y	Graphic Arts/Photog.:	Y	Hardware Dev.:		HR/Other:	Y	Health/Lab:	
MBA Graduates:	Y	Sales Trainees:	Y	Music:		Systems Integration:		Training:	Y	Scientists/Research:	
		Advertising Pros.:	Y	Broadcasting:		Consulting/Other:		Health Care:		Petroleum/Chemicals:	
				Other:	Y			Consulting:		Math/Other:	

TYPES OF BUSINESS:

Women's Apparel, Retail
Plus-Size Women's Apparel
Fashion Accessories
Food & Gifts

BRANDS/DIVISIONS/AFFILIATES:

Lane Bryant
Venezia
Cacique
Lane Bryant Outlet
Petite Sophisticate Outlet
Fashion Bug
Catherine's Plus Sizes
Figi's

CONTACTS: *Note: Officers with more than one job title may be intentionally listed here more than once.*

Alan Rosskamm, CEO
Joseph M. Baron, COO/Exec. VP
Dorrit J. Bern, Pres.
Eric M. Specter, CFO/Exec. VP
Tim M. White, Chief Mkt. Officer/Exec. VP
Gale H. Varma, Exec. VP-Human Resources
James G. Bloise, VP-Tech. & Bus. Svcs.
Colin D. Stern, General Counsel/Exec. VP/Sec.
Lori Twomey, Pres., Direct-to-Consumer
Anthony A. DeSabato, Exec. VP-Corp. & Labor Rel.
Gayle M. Coolick, VP-Investor Rel.
John J. Sullivan, VP/Corp. Controller
Michel Bourlon, Exec. VP-Sourcing
Alan Rosskamm, Chmn.
James G. Bloise, Exec. VP-Supply Chain

Phone: 215-245-9100	Fax: 215-633-4640
Toll-Free:	
Address: 450 Winks Ln., Bensalem, PA 19020 US	

GROWTH PLANS/SPECIAL FEATURES:

Charming Shoppes, Inc. operates women's plus size specialty apparel stores, including Lane Bryant, Fashion Bug and Catherines. Charming Shoppes maintains 795 Lane Bryant stores, catering to women ages 25-45, in forty-six states and averaging about 5,800 square feet. Through private labels, such as Venezia, Cacique, and Lane Bryant, the company offers fashionable and sophisticated apparel in sizes 14-28, including intimate apparel, wear-to-work, and casual sportswear, as well as accessories. Lane Bryant Outlet operates 101 stores in 35 states, and is the only national chain offering women's plus-size apparel in the outlet sales channel. The 52 Petite Sophisticate Outlet stores, averaging 2,700 square feet, target women 35-55 years-old, offering traditional, updated classic and contemporary apparel, sizes 0-14, in casual and career assortments, tailored to women 4'11"-5'4". The company's 989 Fashion Bug and Fashion stores specialize in selling a wide variety of plus size, misses and junior apparel, accessories, intimate apparel, and footwear. It targets customers 20-49 years old who shop in the low-to-moderate price range. Fashion Bug's stores are located in 44 states, primarily in strip shopping centers, and average approximately 8,800 square feet. The firm's 468 Catherine's stores, catering primarily to women ages 40-65, specialize in plus-sized classic apparel and accessories for career and casual lifestyles. The chain is well known for its extended sizes (over size 28) and its petite plus-sizes. Located in 44 states, the stores, averaging approximately 4,100 square feet, are primarily in strip shopping centers in the Southeast, Mid-Atlantic, and Eastern Central U.S. Some of Charming Shoppes' products are sold online or through catalogues. Its Figi's catalog offers food and gifts. In August 2008, entered into a definitive agreement to sell its non-core misses apparel catalogs (collectively, \"Crosstown Traders\") to Orchard Brands, a portfolio company of Golden Gate Capital, for a purchase price of $35 million in cash.

The company offers employees a 40% discount on company merchandise; medical, dental and vision insurance; on-site childcare at headquarters; dependant care spending account; membership in a credit union and fitness centers; adoption assistance; prescription drug coverage; parenting education resources; and tuition reimbursement.

FINANCIALS: Sales and profits are in thousands of dollars—add 000 to get the full amount. 2007 Note: Financial information for 2007 was not available for all companies at press time.

2007 Sales: $3,067,517	2007 Profits: $108,923	**U.S. Stock Ticker: CHRS**
2006 Sales: $2,755,725	2006 Profits: $99,391	Int'l Ticker:　Int'l Exchange:
2005 Sales: $2,332,334	2005 Profits: $64,526	Employees:　30,000
2004 Sales: $2,285,680	2004 Profits: $40,639	Fiscal Year Ends: 1/31
2003 Sales: $2,412,400	2003 Profits: $-2,800	Parent Company:

SALARIES/BENEFITS:

Pension Plan:	ESOP Stock Plan:	Profit Sharing: Y	Top Exec. Salary: $1,250,000	Bonus: $1,197,501
Savings Plan: Y	Stock Purch. Plan: Y		Second Exec. Salary: $516,672	Bonus: $247,486

OTHER THOUGHTS:

Apparent Women Officers or Directors: 1
Hot Spot for Advancement for Women/Minorities: Y

LOCATIONS: ("Y" = Yes)

West:	Southwest:	Midwest:	Southeast:	Northeast:	International:
Y	Y	Y	Y	Y	Y

Note: Financial information, benefits and other data can change quickly and may vary from those stated here.

CHEMED CORPORATION

www.chemed.com

Industry Group Code: 621610 Ranks within this company's industry group: Sales: 2 Profits: 2

Management:		Sales/Marketing:		Liberal Arts:		Information Systems:		Professionals:		Technical/Scientific:	
Mgmt. Trainees:	Y	Mktg. Professionals:	Y	Gen. Writing/Editing:		Info. Management:	Y	Finance/Accounting:	Y	Engineers, Elec.:	Y
Experienced Mgmt.:	Y	Retail Sales:		Technical Writing:		Software Dev.:		Law:	Y	Engineers, Other:	
Int'l Business:	Y	Commercial/Industrial:	Y	Graphic Arts/Photog.:		Hardware Dev.:		HR/Other:	Y	Health/Lab:	Y
MBA Graduates:	Y	Sales Trainees:		Music:		Systems Integration:		Training:	Y	Scientists/Research:	
		Advertising Pros.:		Broadcasting:		Consulting/Other:		Health Care:	Y	Petroleum/Chemicals:	
				Other:				Consulting:		Math/Other:	

TYPES OF BUSINESS:

Hospice & Home Health Care Services
Drain Cleaning Services
Water Lines/Pipework
In-Home Care
Hospice Care

BRANDS/DIVISIONS/AFFILIATES:

Roto-Rooter Group, Inc.
Vitas Group
Vitas Healthcare Corp.

CONTACTS: *Note: Officers with more than one job title may be intentionally listed here more than once.*

Kevin McNamara, CEO
Kevin McNamara, Pres.
David P. Williams, CFO/Exec. VP
Lisa A. Reinhard, Chief Admin. Officer
Naomi C. Dallob, Sec./VP
Arthur V. Tucker, Controller/VP
Tim S. O'Toole, Exec. VP
Spencer S. Lee, Exec. VP
Thomas J. Reilly, VP
Thomas C. Hutton, VP
Edward L. Hutton, Chmn.

Phone: 513-726-6900	Fax: 513-762-6919
Toll-Free:	
Address: 2600 Chemed Ctr., 255 E. 5th St., Cincinnati, OH 45202-4726 US	

GROWTH PLANS/SPECIAL FEATURES:

Chemed Corporation primarily does business through two segments: Roto-Rooter Group, Inc., and VITAS Group (Vitas). Founded in 1935, Roto-Rooter provides plumbing, sewer, drain and pipe cleaning, pipe rehabilitation, drain cleaning equipment and drain cleaning products, supporting the maintenance needs of the residential, industrial, commercial and municipal markets. One of the largest businesses of its type in North America, Roto-Rooter runs businesses in more than 100 company-owned branch and contractor territories as well as approximately 500 franchisees, serving almost 90% of the U.S. Additionally, the company operates franchises in Japan, the Philippines, Mexico, U.K., China, Indonesia, Singapore and Canada. VITAS is one of the largest national provider of hospice care and end-of-life services. The company operates 42 hospice programs in 16 states. In excess of 90% of Vitas' net patient service revenue consists of payments from the Medicare and Medicaid programs. In April 2008, the company acquired a Roto-Rooter franchise in Topeka, Kansas.

FINANCIALS: Sales and profits are in thousands of dollars—add 000 to get the full amount. 2007 Note: Financial information for 2007 was not available for all companies at press time.

2007 Sales: $1,100,058	2007 Profits: $63,976	U.S. Stock Ticker: CHE	
2006 Sales: $1,018,587	2006 Profits: $50,651	Int'l Ticker: Int'l Exchange:	
2005 Sales: $915,970	2005 Profits: $35,817	Employees: 11,621	
2004 Sales: $734,877	2004 Profits: $27,512	Fiscal Year Ends: 12/31	
2003 Sales: $260,776	2003 Profits: $-3,435	Parent Company:	

SALARIES/BENEFITS:

Pension Plan: Y	ESOP Stock Plan: Y	Profit Sharing:	Top Exec. Salary: $625,000	Bonus: $900,000
Savings Plan: Y	Stock Purch. Plan:		Second Exec. Salary: $435,750	Bonus: $225,000

OTHER THOUGHTS:

Apparent Women Officers or Directors: 2
Hot Spot for Advancement for Women/Minorities: Y

LOCATIONS: ("Y" = Yes)

West:	Southwest:	Midwest:	Southeast:	Northeast:	International:
Y	Y	Y	Y	Y	Y

CHESAPEAKE ENERGY CORP   www.chkenergy.com

Industry Group Code: 211111 Ranks within this company's industry group: Sales: Profits:

Management:	Sales/Marketing:	Liberal Arts:	Information Systems:	Professionals:	Technical/Scientific:
Mgmt. Trainees:	Mktg. Professionals:	Gen. Writing/Editing:	Info. Management:	Finance/Accounting:	Engineers, Elec.:
Experienced Mgmt.:	Retail Sales:	Technical Writing:	Software Dev.:	Law:	Engineers, Other:
Int'l Business:	Commercial/Industrial:	Graphic Arts/Photog.:	Hardware Dev.:	HR/Other:	Health/Lab:
MBA Graduates:	Sales Trainees:	Music:	Systems Integration:	Training:	Scientists/Research:
	Advertising Pros.:	Broadcasting:	Consulting/Other:	Health Care:	Petroleum/Chemicals:
		Other:		Consulting:	Math/Other:

TYPES OF BUSINESS:
Oil & Gas Exploration & Production

BRANDS/DIVISIONS/AFFILIATES:

CONTACTS: *Note: Officers with more than one job title may be intentionally listed here more than once.*
Aubrey K. McClendon, CEO
Steven C. Dixon, COO
Marcus C. Rowland, CFO/Exec. VP
Martha A. Burger, Sr. VP-Human & Corp. Resources.
Jeffrey L. Mobley, Sr. VP-Research
Cathy L. Tompkins, Sr. VP-IT
Henry J. Hood, General Counsel/Sr. VP-Land & Legal
Steven C. Dixon, Exec. VP-Oper.
Thomas S. Price, Jr., Sr. VP-Corp. Dev.
Jeffrey L. Mobley, Sr. VP-Investor Rel.
Jennifer M. Grigsby, Treas./Sr. VP/Corp. Sec.
J. Mark Lester, Exec. VP-Exploration
Douglas J. Jacobson, Exec. VP-Acquisitions & Divestitures
Jeffrey A. Fisher, Sr. VP-Production
Michael A. Johnson, Chief Acct. Officer/Controller/Sr. VP-Acct.
Aubrey K. McClendon, Chmn.

Phone: 405-848-8000	**Fax:** 405-843-0573
Toll-Free:	
Address: 6100 N. Western Ave., Oklahoma City, OK 73118 US	

GROWTH PLANS/SPECIAL FEATURES:

Chesapeake Energy Corp. is one of the top independent producers of natural gas in the U.S. The company owns interests in about 38,500 producing oil and natural gas wells that are currently producing roughly 2.2 billion cubic feet equivalent (bcfe), 92% of which is natural gas. The firm's operations are located in the Mid-continent region, which includes Oklahoma, Arkansas, southwestern Kansas and the Texas Panhandle; the Fort Worth Basin in north-central Texas; the Appalachian Basin, principally in West Virginia, eastern Kentucky, eastern Ohio and southern New York; the Permian and Delaware Basins of west Texas and eastern New Mexico; the Ark-La-Tex area of east Texas and northern Louisiana; and the south Texas and Texas Gold Coast regions. Chesapeake Energy has about 10.879 trillion cubic feet equivalent of proved reserves, of which 93% are natural gas and all of which is onshore. During 2007, the company produced an average of 1.957 bcfe per day. During 2007, through its drilling activities, which utilized about 138 operated rigs and 77 non-operated rigs, the company drilled over 1,992 gross operated wells and participated in over 1,679 wells operated by other companies. The success rate was 99% for operates wells and 97% for non-operated wells. In 2007, the firm shifted its acquisition strategy from significant stock and asset acquisitions to targeted leasehold and property acquisitions needed for planned oil and natural gas development. In March 2008, the firm announced new natural gas discoveries and five new unconventional oil projects. In September 2008, the firm and BP America announced intent to form a joint venture in Fayetteville Shale assets. Also in 2008, it closed the sale of its Arkoma Basin Woodford Shale assets to BP America Inc. and entered into a Haynesville Shale joint venture with Plains Exploration and Production.

The company offers its employees medical, dental and vision insurance; a 401(k) plan; life insurance; short- and long-term disability insurance; and an employee assistance program.

FINANCIALS: Sales and profits are in thousands of dollars—add 000 to get the full amount. 2007 Note: Financial information for 2007 was not available for all companies at press time.

2007 Sales: $7,800,000	2007 Profits: $1,451,000	**U.S. Stock Ticker: CHK**
2006 Sales: $7,325,595	2006 Profits: $2,003,323	**Int'l Ticker:** Int'l Exchange:
2005 Sales: $4,665,290	2005 Profits: $948,302	Employees: 2,885
2004 Sales: $2,709,268	2004 Profits: $515,155	Fiscal Year Ends: 12/31
2003 Sales: $1,717,432	2003 Profits: $312,981	Parent Company:

SALARIES/BENEFITS:

Pension Plan:	ESOP Stock Plan:	Profit Sharing:	Top Exec. Salary: $975,000	Bonus: $1,581,000
Savings Plan: Y	Stock Purch. Plan:		Second Exec. Salary: $675,000	Bonus: $1,051,000

OTHER THOUGHTS:
Apparent Women Officers or Directors: 4
Hot Spot for Advancement for Women/Minorities: Y

LOCATIONS: ("Y" = Yes)

West:	Southwest:	Midwest:	Southeast:	Northeast:	International:
	Y	Y	Y		

CHEVRON CORPORATION

www.chevron.com

Industry Group Code: 211111 Ranks within this company's industry group: Sales: 2 Profits: 2

Management:		Sales/Marketing:		Liberal Arts:		Information Systems:		Professionals:		Technical/Scientific:	
Mgmt. Trainees:	Y	Mktg. Professionals:	Y	Gen. Writing/Editing:	Y	Info. Management:	Y	Finance/Accounting:	Y	Engineers, Elec.:	Y
Experienced Mgmt.:	Y	Retail Sales:		Technical Writing:	Y	Software Dev.:	Y	Law:	Y	Engineers, Other:	
Int'l Business:	Y	Commercial/Industrial:	Y	Graphic Arts/Photog.:	Y	Hardware Dev.:		HR/Other:	Y	Health/Lab:	Y
MBA Graduates:	Y	Sales Trainees:		Music:		Systems Integration:		Training:	Y	Scientists/Research:	Y
		Advertising Pros.:	Y	Broadcasting:		Consulting/Other:		Health Care:		Petroleum/Chemicals:	Y
				Other:				Consulting:		Math/Other:	Y

TYPES OF BUSINESS:

Oil & Gas Exploration & Production
Power Generation
Petrochemicals
Gasoline Retailing
Coal Mining
Fuel & Oil Additives
Convenience Stores
Pipelines

BRANDS/DIVISIONS/AFFILIATES:

Texaco
Energy Technology Company
Chevron Technology Ventures
Diamondoids
Caltex
Texaco Nederland B.V.

CONTACTS: Note: Officers with more than one job title may be intentionally listed here more than once.

David J. O'Reilly, CEO
Stephen J. Crowe, CFO/VP
John E. Bethancourt, Exec. VP-Tech. & Svcs.
Charles A. James, General Counsel/VP
John S. Watson, Exec. VP-Strategy & Dev.
George L. Kirkland, Exec. VP-Global Upstream & Gas
Michael K. Wirth, Exec. VP-Global Downstream
David J. O'Reilly, Chmn.

Phone: 925-842-1000	Fax: 925-842-3530
Toll-Free:	
Address: 6001 Bollinger Canyon Rd., San Ramon, CA 94583 US	

GROWTH PLANS/SPECIAL FEATURES:

Chevron Corp. is an integrated energy company that conducts petroleum operations, chemical operations, mining operations, power generation and energy services. The company conducts business activities in the U.S. and approximately 180 other countries. Petroleum operations consist of the exploration, development and production of crude oil and natural gas; refining crude oil into finished petroleum products; marketing crude oil, natural gas and petroleum products; and transporting oil, gas and petroleum products by pipeline, marine vessels, trucks and railroad. Chemical operations include the manufacturing and marketing of fuel and lubricating oil additives and commodity petrochemicals for industrial uses by Chevron's affiliates and subsidiaries. The firm has a global refining capacity of 2.6 million oil barrels per day; a marketing network that supports approximately 26,500 retail locations; and interests in 16 power-generating assets in the U.S. and Asia. Chevron owns or franchises 16,700 global service stations under the brand names Chevron, Texaco and Caltex. In addition, the company's subsidiary, Energy Technology Company, identifies, grows and commercializes emerging technologies in energy production with the use of biofuels, hydrogen infrastructure, advanced batteries, nano-materials and renewable energy applications. In nanotechnology, Chevron's MolecularDiamond Technologies (MDT) business unit recently isolated a new class of carbon based nanomaterials called higher diamondoids from petroleum. Diamondoids possess the same internal carbon structure as a diamond and can easily be derivatized and polymerized for a variety of applications within the petrochemical market. In March 2007, Chevron's subsidiary, Texaco Nederland B.V., signed an agreement to sell its Netherlands manufacturing business to BP.

The company offers its employees medical and dental insurance; disability benefits; life and accident insurance; domestic partner benefits; a retirement plan; a 401(k) plan; and auto and home insurance.

FINANCIALS: Sales and profits are in thousands of dollars—add 000 to get the full amount. 2007 Note: Financial information for 2007 was not available for all companies at press time.

2007 Sales: $220,904,000	2007 Profits: $18,688,000	U.S. Stock Ticker: CVX
2006 Sales: $210,118,000	2006 Profits: $17,138,000	Int'l Ticker: Int'l Exchange:
2005 Sales: $198,200,000	2005 Profits: $14,099,000	Employees: 65,000
2004 Sales: $155,300,000	2004 Profits: $13,328,000	Fiscal Year Ends: 12/31
2003 Sales: $121,761,000	2003 Profits: $7,230,000	Parent Company:

SALARIES/BENEFITS:

Pension Plan: Y	ESOP Stock Plan:	Profit Sharing:	Top Exec. Salary: $1,620,833	Bonus: $3,500,000
Savings Plan: Y	Stock Purch. Plan:		Second Exec. Salary: $935,417	Bonus: $1,500,000

OTHER THOUGHTS:

Apparent Women Officers or Directors: 1
Hot Spot for Advancement for Women/Minorities:

LOCATIONS: ("Y" = Yes)

West:	Southwest:	Midwest:	Southeast:	Northeast:	International:
Y	Y	Y	Y	Y	Y

Note: Financial information, benefits and other data can change quickly and may vary from those stated here.

CHEVRON PHILLIPS CHEMICAL COMPANY LLC

www.cpchem.com

Industry Group Code: 325110 Ranks within this company's industry group: Sales: 1   Profits: 1

Management:		Sales/Marketing:		Liberal Arts:		Information Systems:		Professionals:		Technical/Scientific:	
Mgmt. Trainees:	Y	Mktg. Professionals:	Y	Gen. Writing/Editing:		Info. Management:	Y	Finance/Accounting:	Y	Engineers, Elec.:	Y
Experienced Mgmt.:	Y	Retail Sales:		Technical Writing:	Y	Software Dev.:	Y	Law:	Y	Engineers, Other:	
Int'l Business:	Y	Commercial/Industrial:	Y	Graphic Arts/Photog.:		Hardware Dev.:		HR/Other:	Y	Health/Lab:	Y
MBA Graduates:	Y	Sales Trainees:		Music:		Systems Integration:		Training:	Y	Scientists/Research:	Y
		Advertising Pros.:		Broadcasting:		Consulting/Other:		Health Care:		Petroleum/Chemicals:	
				Other:				Consulting:		Math/Other:	

TYPES OF BUSINESS:

Petrochemical & Plastics Manufacturing
Olefins & Polyolefins
Aromatics & Styrenics
Specialty Chemicals

BRANDS/DIVISIONS/AFFILIATES:

K-Resin
Aromax
Ryton
TrackTek
Soltex
Marlex
MarFlex
Scentinel

CONTACTS: Note: Officers with more than one job title may be intentionally listed here more than once.

Greg Garland, CEO
Greg Garland, Pres.
Greg Maxwell, CFO/Sr. VP/Controller
Don Kremer, VP-Human Resources
Larry Frazier, CIO
Mary Jane Hagenson, VP-Tech.
Rick Roberts, Sr. VP-Mfg.
Craig Glidden, General Counsel/Sr. VP/Corp. Sec.
Mark Lashier, VP-Corp. Planning & Dev.
Joe McKee, VP/Treas.
Mark Haney, Sr. VP-Specialties, Aromatics & Styrenics
Tim Taylor, Sr. VP-Olefins & Polyolefins
Greg Hanggi, VP-Environment, Health & Safety
Dave Smith, VP-Polyethylene
Bob Patel, Mgr.-Asia Region

Phone: 832-813-4100	Fax:
Toll-Free: 800-231-1212	
Address: 10001 Six Pines Dr., The Woodlands, TX 77380 US	

GROWTH PLANS/SPECIAL FEATURES:

Chevron Phillips Chemical Company LLC (CPChem) is the combined petrochemical businesses of Chevron Corporation and ConocoPhillips, both 50% owners. With 36 plants and six research centers in nine countries, CPChem is an international producer of olefins and polyolefins and is also a supplier of aromatics, alpha olefins, styrenics, specialty chemicals, polyethylene pipe and proprietary plastics. The company manufactures chemical products that are vital in the various production processes of 70,000 consumer and industrial products. Its mix of petrochemical and plastics businesses is segmented into three divisions: olefins and polyolefins; aromatics and styrenics; and specialty products. Products in the olefins and polyolefins family consist of ethylene, propylene and their polymer derivatives; olefins and polyalpha olefins; and high-density polyethylene pipe, conduit and pipe fitting. These products are sold as building blocks for other chemicals and as ingredients for use in a variety of end-products including motor oils, lubricants, plastics, coatings, textiles and packaging. CPChem's aromatics and styrenics include cyclohexane, paraxylene, benzene, styrene, polystyrene and K-Resin SBC, a unique type of copolymer. Aromax, the company's proprietary benzene production process, is considered the most cost-effective available. The aromatics and styrenics are used in the manufacturing of insulation products, housewares, food packaging, electronic parts and media enclosures. Its specialty chemicals are used in various applications, including electronics, automobiles, oil and gas well drilling, appliances, agriculture and pharmaceuticals. This division sells TrackTek brand racing fuels and Soltex drill mud additive. Olefins and polyolefins account for 67% of sales; aromatics and styrenics for 28%; and specialty products for 5%. In 2007, CPChem began building a new Ryton brand polyphenylene sulfide plant. In 2008, the firm's joint venture with The Dow Chemical Company, Americas Styrenics LLC, began operations.

CPChem offers employees 80% reimbursement for education costs after successful completion of approved college level courses.

FINANCIALS: Sales and profits are in thousands of dollars—add 000 to get the full amount. 2007 Note: Financial information for 2007 was not available for all companies at press time.

2007 Sales: $12,534,000	2007 Profits: $719,000	**U.S. Stock Ticker: Joint Venture**	
2006 Sales: $11,839,000	2006 Profits: $1,349,000	**Int'l Ticker:** Int'l Exchange:	
2005 Sales: $11,038,000	2005 Profits: $853,000	Employees:	
2004 Sales: $9,558,000	2004 Profits: $605,000	Fiscal Year Ends: 12/31	
2003 Sales: $7,018,000	2003 Profits: $7,000	Parent Company:	

SALARIES/BENEFITS:

Pension Plan:	ESOP Stock Plan:	Profit Sharing:	Top Exec. Salary: $	Bonus: $
Savings Plan:	Stock Purch. Plan:		Second Exec. Salary: $	Bonus: $

OTHER THOUGHTS:

Apparent Women Officers or Directors: 1
Hot Spot for Advancement for Women/Minorities:

LOCATIONS: ("Y" = Yes)

West:	Southwest:	Midwest:	Southeast:	Northeast:	International:
Y	Y	Y	Y	Y	Y

CHICO'S FAS INC

www.chicos.com

Industry Group Code: 448120 **Ranks within this company's industry group:** Sales: 7 Profits: 3

Management:		Sales/Marketing:		Liberal Arts:		Information Systems:		Professionals:		Technical/Scientific:	
Mgmt. Trainees:	Y	Mktg. Professionals:	Y	Gen. Writing/Editing:	Y	Info. Management:	Y	Finance/Accounting:	Y	Engineers, Elec.:	
Experienced Mgmt.:	Y	Retail Sales:	Y	Technical Writing:		Software Dev.:	Y	Law:	Y	Engineers, Other:	
Int'l Business:	Y	Commercial/Industrial:	Y	Graphic Arts/Photog.:	Y	Hardware Dev.:		HR/Other:	Y	Health/Lab:	
MBA Graduates:	Y	Sales Trainees:	Y	Music:		Systems Integration:		Training:	Y	Scientists/Research:	
		Advertising Pros.:	Y	Broadcasting:		Consulting/Other:		Health Care:		Petroleum/Chemicals:	
				Other:	Y			Consulting:		Math/Other:	

TYPES OF BUSINESS:
Women's Apparel, Retail
Online & Catalog Sales
Franchising

BRANDS/DIVISIONS/AFFILIATES:
Chico's
White House/Black Market
Soma by Chico's
Fitigues
Passport Club
Chico's Outlet

CONTACTS: Note: Officers with more than one job title may be intentionally listed here more than once.
Scott Edmonds, CEO
Chuck Nesbit, COO/Exec. VP
Scott Edmonds, Pres.
Kent Kleeberger, CFO/Treas./Exec. VP
Judd Harner, Chief Mktg. Officer/Sr. VP-Chico's brand
Manuel Jessup, Chief Human Resources Officer/Exec. VP
Linda Costello, Sr. VP-Prod. Dev.
Gary King, CIO/Exec. VP
Linda Costello, Sr. VP-Prod. Dev.
Sandy Rhodes, General Counsel/Corp. Sec./Sr. VP
Elaine Boltz, Sr. VP-Strategy & Consumer Research
Michael Kincaid, Sr. VP-Finance/Chief Acct. Officer
Sher Canada, Sr. VP-Chico's Stores
Mike Elleman, Sr. VP-Real Estate
Mori MacKenzie, Exec. VP/Chief Stores Officer
Scott Edmonds, Chmn.

Phone: 239-277-6200	Fax: 239-277-5237
Toll-Free: 888-550-5559	
Address: 11215 Metro Pkwy., Fort Myers, FL 33966 US	

GROWTH PLANS/SPECIAL FEATURES:

Chico's FAS, Inc. retails exclusively designed, private label, sophisticated, casual-to-dressy clothing, complementary accessories and gift items under the Chico's, White House/Black Market and Soma by Chico's. Chico's currently operates 1,045 retail stores in 49 states, Washington, D.C., the U.S. Virgin Islands and Puerto Rico. The Chico's brand primarily targets women aged 35 and over with moderate and high income levels. All of Chico's products are designed and developed by its Product Development Team, headquartered in Fort Myers, Florida. Chico's mails a monthly catalog. To increase its customer base, the company advertises in national fashion and home and garden magazines such as Martha Stewart Living, Vogue and Vanity Fair. The company offers Passport Club membership to women who have spent at least $500 over time, allowing them perks, such as a permanent 5% discount on future purchases. There are 606 Chico's front-line stores and 37 Chico's outlet stores. Chico's also operates the White House/Black Market chain of 313 women's clothing stores and 19 outlet locations that focuses on women aged 25 and older who lead active work and social lives with moderate to high income levels. White House/Black Market offers clothes in shades of white and black, although the stores do offer a line of denim jeans as well. The Soma intimate wear line currently consists of 69 boutique-style stores and one outlet location. Soma by Chico's offers foundation products in intimate apparel, sleepwear, bodywear and active wear that the firm hopes could ultimately appeal to a broader customer base than Chico's. In 2007, the company acquired the franchise rights for Minnesota from Intraco Inc. At the close of fiscal 2007, the firm ceased all Fitigues operations.

Chico's employee benefits include merchandise discounts, a retirement savings plan and a stock purchase plan.

FINANCIALS: Sales and profits are in thousands of dollars—add 000 to get the full amount. 2007 Note: Financial information for 2007 was not available for all companies at press time.

2007 Sales: $1,646,482	2007 Profits: $166,636	**U.S. Stock Ticker:** CHS
2006 Sales: $1,404,575	2006 Profits: $193,981	**Int'l Ticker:** Int'l Exchange:
2005 Sales: $1,066,882	2005 Profits: $141,206	Employees: 12,500
2004 Sales: $768,499	2004 Profits: $100,230	Fiscal Year Ends: 1/31
2003 Sales: $531,100	2003 Profits: $66,800	Parent Company:

SALARIES/BENEFITS:

Pension Plan:	ESOP Stock Plan:	Profit Sharing:	Top Exec. Salary: $996,153	Bonus: $2,400,000
Savings Plan: Y	Stock Purch. Plan: Y		Second Exec. Salary: $621,154	Bonus: $1,312,500

OTHER THOUGHTS:
Apparent Women Officers or Directors: 12
Hot Spot for Advancement for Women/Minorities: Y

LOCATIONS: ("Y" = Yes)

West:	Southwest:	Midwest:	Southeast:	Northeast:	International:
Y	Y	Y	Y	Y	Y

CHRISTOPHER & BANKS CORP
www.christopherandbanks.com
Industry Group Code: 448120 **Ranks within this company's industry group:** Sales: 14 Profits: 11

Management:		Sales/Marketing:		Liberal Arts:		Information Systems:		Professionals:		Technical/Scientific:	
Mgmt. Trainees:	Y	Mktg. Professionals:	Y	Gen. Writing/Editing:	Y	Info. Management:	Y	Finance/Accounting:	Y	Engineers, Elec.:	
Experienced Mgmt.:	Y	Retail Sales:	Y	Technical Writing:		Software Dev.:	Y	Law:	Y	Engineers, Other:	
Int'l Business:		Commercial/Industrial:	Y	Graphic Arts/Photog.:	Y	Hardware Dev.:		HR/Other:	Y	Health/Lab:	
MBA Graduates:	Y	Sales Trainees:	Y	Music:		Systems Integration:		Training:	Y	Scientists/Research:	
		Advertising Pros.:	Y	Broadcasting:		Consulting/Other:		Health Care:		Petroleum/Chemicals:	
				Other:	Y			Consulting:		Math/Other:	

TYPES OF BUSINESS:
Women's Business Apparel, Retail
Private-Label Merchandise
Accessories

BRANDS/DIVISIONS/AFFILIATES:
C.J. Banks
Acorn
Braun's

CONTACTS: Note: Officers with more than one job title may be intentionally listed here more than once.
Lorna Nagler, CEO
Lorna Nagler, Pres.
Andrew K. Moller, CFO/Exec. VP
Jillian May, VP-Mktg.
Kipp Sassaman, VP-Human Resources
Steve Danker, VP-Info. Sys.
Susan Connell, Chief Merch. Officer
Luke R. Komarek, General Counsel/Sr. VP
Gary Thompson, Sr. VP-Store Oper.
Steve Danker, VP-Strategy
Monica Dahl, Sr. VP-Planning & Allocation/E-Commerce
Dustin Henry, Mktg. Coordinator
Larry Barenbaum, Chmn.

Phone: 763-551-5000	Fax: 763-551-5198
Toll-Free:	
Address: 2400 Xenium Ln. N., Plymouth, MN 55441 US	

GROWTH PLANS/SPECIAL FEATURES:
Christopher & Banks Corporation (C&B) is a Minneapolis-based specialty retailer of women's specialty apparel. The company operates 837 stores in 46 states under the names Christopher & Banks (543 stores), C.J. Banks (257) and Acorn (36). The stores are generally mall-based and located in small to mid-sized markets. Sportswear and sweaters account for the bulk of the company's sales, though the firm has been shifting merchandise focus away from sweaters and expanding its offering of novelty jackets and fashion-knit tops. Sweaters comprised 23% of the company's sales in 2007, down from previous years. The principal store concept, Christopher & Banks, emphasizes style, quality and value in casual sportswear and sweaters exclusively designed for working women ages 40-60. The company's plus size store concept, C.J. Banks, offers similar apparel in sizes 14-24, and is often paired with an existing C&B store. Acorn is a small women's specialty retailer selling accessories and apparel appealing to the more affluent woman aged 35-60 with an upscale fashion taste. C&B uses carefully designed front-of-store displays to attract customers. To keep its fashions fresh, it introduces a new color palette from month to month. The company is also upgrading customer service, offering merchandise on wooden hangers, receipts placed in envelopes and purchases wrapped in tissue and placed in drawstring bags. In February 2008, the company launched separate e-commerce websites for its Christopher & Banks and C.J. Banks brands. In July 2008, C&B announced plans to close its 36 Acorn stores and exit its Acorn business division by December 2008.

The firm offers employees medical, dental and vision plans, a cafeteria flex plan that includes daycare, merchandise discounts and a 401(k) savings plan.

FINANCIALS: Sales and profits are in thousands of dollars—add 000 to get the full amount. 2007 Note: Financial information for 2007 was not available for all companies at press time.

2007 Sales: $547,317	2007 Profits: $33,686	**U.S. Stock Ticker:** CBK	
2006 Sales: $490,508	2006 Profits: $30,413	**Int'l Ticker:** Int'l Exchange:	
2005 Sales: $438,862	2005 Profits: $27,015	Employees: 6,900	
2004 Sales: $390,723	2004 Profits: $39,340	Fiscal Year Ends: 2/28	
2003 Sales: $338,800	2003 Profits: $38,500	Parent Company:	

SALARIES/BENEFITS:
Pension Plan:	ESOP Stock Plan:	Profit Sharing:	Top Exec. Salary: $536,058	Bonus: $140,000
Savings Plan: Y	Stock Purch. Plan:		Second Exec. Salary: $530,000	Bonus: $

OTHER THOUGHTS:
Apparent Women Officers or Directors: 5
Hot Spot for Advancement for Women/Minorities: Y

LOCATIONS: ("Y" = Yes)
West:	Southwest:	Midwest:	Southeast:	Northeast:	International:
Y	Y	Y	Y	Y	

Note: Financial information, benefits and other data can change quickly and may vary from those stated here.

CHUBB CORPORATION (THE)

www.chubb.com

Industry Group Code: 524126 Ranks within this company's industry group: Sales: Profits:

Management:		Sales/Marketing:		Liberal Arts:		Information Systems:		Professionals:		Technical/Scientific:	
Mgmt. Trainees:	Y	Mktg. Professionals:	Y	Gen. Writing/Editing:	Y	Info. Management:	Y	Finance/Accounting:	Y	Engineers, Elec.:	
Experienced Mgmt.:	Y	Retail Sales:		Technical Writing:		Software Dev.:	Y	Law:	Y	Engineers, Other:	
Int'l Business:	Y	Commercial/Industrial:	Y	Graphic Arts/Photog.:		Hardware Dev.:		HR/Other:	Y	Health/Lab:	
MBA Graduates:	Y	Sales Trainees:		Music:		Systems Integration:		Training:	Y	Scientists/Research:	Y
		Advertising Pros.:	Y	Broadcasting:		Consulting/Other:		Health Care:		Petroleum/Chemicals:	
				Other:				Consulting:		Math/Other:	Y

TYPES OF BUSINESS:

Insurance, Direct Property & Casualty
Reinsurance Services
Consulting Services
Claims Administration Services
Real Estate
Computer Training & Staffing
Luxury Items Insurance

BRANDS/DIVISIONS/AFFILIATES:

Chubb Commercial Insurance
Chubb Specialty Insurance
Chubb Personal Insurance
Federal Insurance Company
Pacific Indemnity Company
Vigilant Insurance Company
Chubb Custom Insurance Company
Executive Risk Indemnity, Inc

CONTACTS: Note: Officers with more than one job title may be intentionally listed here more than once.

John D. Finnegan, CEO
John J. Degnan, COO/Vice Chmn.
John D. Finnegan, Pres.
Michael O'Reilly, CFO/Vice Chmn.
James P. Knight, CIO/Exec. VP-Chubb & Son
Dino E. Robusto, Chief Admin. Officer/Exec. VP
Maureen Brundage, General Counsel/Exec. VP
Paul J. Krump, Exec. VP/Chief Underwriting Officer
Robert C. Cox, Exec. VP-Chubb & Son/COO-Chubb Specialty Insurance
Andrew A. McElwee, Jr., Exec. VP-Chubb & Son/COO-Chubb Personal Insurance
Janice M. Tomlinson, Exec. VP/Int'l Field Oper. Mgr.-Chubb & Son
John D. Finnegan, Chmn.
Harold L. Morrison, Jr., Chief Global Field Officer/Exec. VP

Phone: 908-903-2000	Fax: 908-903-2027
Toll-Free:	
Address: 15 Mountain View Rd., Warren, NJ 07061 US	

GROWTH PLANS/SPECIAL FEATURES:

The Chubb Corporation is a holding company whose subsidiaries provide property and casualty insurance in the U.S., Canada, Europe, Australia and parts of Latin America and Asia. Headquartered in New Jersey, the firm has $51 billion in assets and more than 120 offices in 29 countries around the globe. The firm's property and casualty group is divided into three units: Chubb Commercial Insurance, which offers a range of commercial insurance products; Chubb Specialty Insurance, which offers a variety of specialized professional liability products for privately and publicly owned companies, financial institutions, professional firms and healthcare organizations; and Chubb Personal Insurance, which offers products for individuals who require more coverage choices and higher limits than standard insurance policies. The firm's property and casualty insurance group includes, among others, Federal Insurance Company; Pacific Indemnity Company; Vigilant Insurance Company; Chubb Custom Insurance Company; and Executive Risk Indemnity, Inc. The group underwrites mostly lines of property and casualty insurance and writes non-participating policies. Several members also write participating policies, particularly in the workers' compensation class of business. The firm's other operations include commercial real estate development activities, primarily in New Jersey; residential development activities, primarily in central Florida; consulting and claims administration services; computer training and staffing; and reinsurance services. Chubb offers insurance for primary vacation homes and contents; city homes; valuable possessions including much of the world's individually owned precious jewelry, automobiles and watercraft; and personal liability for some of the wealthiest people in the U.S. In March 2007, the company launched a new product, My Loss Scenarios, which provides over 150 professional and management liability loss scenarios through an online library.

Chubb offers its employees flexible spending accounts and medical, dental, vision, life, business travel and disability insurance.

FINANCIALS: Sales and profits are in thousands of dollars—add 000 to get the full amount. 2007 Note: Financial information for 2007 was not available for all companies at press time.

2007 Sales: $14,107,000	2007 Profits: $2,807,000	U.S. Stock Ticker: CB
2006 Sales: $14,003,000	2006 Profits: $2,528,000	Int'l Ticker: Int'l Exchange:
2005 Sales: $14,082,300	2005 Profits: $1,825,900	Employees: 10,800
2004 Sales: $13,177,200	2004 Profits: $1,548,400	Fiscal Year Ends: 12/31
2003 Sales: $11,394,000	2003 Profits: $808,800	Parent Company:

SALARIES/BENEFITS:

Pension Plan:	ESOP Stock Plan:	Profit Sharing:	Top Exec. Salary: $1,275,000	Bonus: $3,242,850
Savings Plan:	Stock Purch. Plan:		Second Exec. Salary: $715,001	Bonus: $1,502,500

OTHER THOUGHTS:

Apparent Women Officers or Directors: 6
Hot Spot for Advancement for Women/Minorities: Y

LOCATIONS: ("Y" = Yes)

West:	Southwest:	Midwest:	Southeast:	Northeast:	International:
Y	Y	Y	Y	Y	Y

CIBER INC
www.ciber.com

Industry Group Code: 541512 Ranks within this company's industry group: Sales: 9 Profits: 12

Management:		Sales/Marketing:		Liberal Arts:		Information Systems:		Professionals:		Technical/Scientific:	
Mgmt. Trainees:	Y	Mktg. Professionals:	Y	Gen. Writing/Editing:	Y	Info. Management:	Y	Finance/Accounting:	Y	Engineers, Elec.:	Y
Experienced Mgmt.:	Y	Retail Sales:		Technical Writing:	Y	Software Dev.:	Y	Law:	Y	Engineers, Other:	
Int'l Business:	Y	Commercial/Industrial:	Y	Graphic Arts/Photog.:	Y	Hardware Dev.:	Y	HR/Other:	Y	Health/Lab:	
MBA Graduates:	Y	Sales Trainees:		Music:		Systems Integration:	Y	Training:	Y	Scientists/Research:	
		Advertising Pros.:		Broadcasting:		Consulting/Other:	Y	Health Care:		Petroleum/Chemicals:	
				Other:				Consulting:	Y	Math/Other:	

TYPES OF BUSINESS:
IT Consulting
Equipment Reselling
Application Development
Enterprise Integrations
Application Management Outsourcing
Global Security Solutions

BRANDS/DIVISIONS/AFFILIATES:
CIBER Europe
Metamor Enterprise Solutions, LLC
Condevor AB

CONTACTS: Note: Officers with more than one job title may be intentionally listed here more than once.
Mac J. Slingerlend, CEO
Mac J. Slingerlend, Pres.
Peter H. Cheesbrough, CFO/Exec. VP
Robin Caputo, VP-Mktg.
Susan Keesen, General Counsel/VP
Robin Caputo, VP-Public Rel.
Jennifer J. Matuschek, VP-Investor Rel.
Chris Loffredo, Chief Acct. Officer/VP
Russ Wheeler, Pres., CIBER Enterprise Solutions
Joe Mancuso, Sr. VP-US Commercial Oper.
Ed Burns, Pres., State Gov't Solutions
Shashank Joshi, Pres., CIBER (India), Ltd.
Bobby G. Stevenson, Chmn.
Terje Laugerund, CEO-Ciber Europe

Phone: 303-220-0100	Fax: 303-220-7100
Toll-Free: 800-242-3799	
Address: 5251 DTC Pkwy., Ste. 1400, Greenwood Village, CO 80111 US	

GROWTH PLANS/SPECIAL FEATURES:
CIBER, Inc. provides information technology (IT) system integration consulting and other IT services. To a small extent, it also resells certain IT hardware and software products. The company operates in five segments: commercial solutions; federal government solutions; state and local solutions; U.S. package solutions; and European operations. The commercial, federal government and state and local solutions segments offer services including application development, enterprise integrations, application management outsourcing and global security. Application development services provide analysis, design, development, testing, implementation and maintenance of business applications. The enterprise integration services integrate data and applications for companies and organizations to deliver functional business solutions. The application management outsourcing service assumes responsibility for a client's specific IT operation and provides ongoing application support. The U.S. package solutions segment operates as the CIBER Enterprise Solutions (CES) division. With over 400 consultants, CES provides consulting services to support software from enterprise solutions vendors including Oracle, SAP and Lawson, as well as several supply chain and higher education management products. Services include package software assessment, selection, planning and implementation. The European operations segment provides a broad range of business and technical consulting services that include package implementation, application development, systems integration and support services, as well as the firm's own Customer Relationship Management software products. CIBER Europe has over 1,300 consultants in more than 10 European countries, plus China, Australia and New Zealand. Partner relationships in Europe include SAP, Sage, Microsoft and Oracle. In September 2007, CIBER acquired the SAP Practice of Headstrong Corp., which was operated under Metamor Enterprise Solutions, LLC. In October 2007, the company acquired Condevor AB, a Swedish company focused on SAP consultancy.

The company offer its employees medical, dental and vision insurance; disability insurance; life insurance; a 401(k) plan; an employee stock purchase plan; and tuition assistance.

FINANCIALS: Sales and profits are in thousands of dollars—add 000 to get the full amount. 2007 Note: Financial information for 2007 was not available for all companies at press time.

2007 Sales: $1,081,975	2007 Profits: $29,026	U.S. Stock Ticker: CBR
2006 Sales: $995,837	2006 Profits: $24,735	Int'l Ticker: Int'l Exchange:
2005 Sales: $956,009	2005 Profits: $24,707	Employees: 8,400
2004 Sales: $843,021	2004 Profits: $29,701	Fiscal Year Ends: 12/31
2003 Sales: $691,987	2003 Profits: $19,984	Parent Company:

SALARIES/BENEFITS:
Pension Plan:	ESOP Stock Plan:	Profit Sharing:	Top Exec. Salary: $565,000	Bonus: $220,699
Savings Plan: Y	Stock Purch. Plan: Y		Second Exec. Salary: $416,000	Bonus: $172,755

OTHER THOUGHTS:
Apparent Women Officers or Directors: 4
Hot Spot for Advancement for Women/Minorities: Y

LOCATIONS: ("Y" = Yes)
West:	Southwest:	Midwest:	Southeast:	Northeast:	International:
Y	Y	Y	Y	Y	Y

Note: Financial information, benefits and other data can change quickly and may vary from those stated here.

CINTAS CORP

www.cintas-corp.com

Industry Group Code: 722310   Ranks within this company's industry group: Sales: 2   Profits: 1

Management:		Sales/Marketing:		Liberal Arts:	Information Systems:		Professionals:		Technical/Scientific:	
Mgmt. Trainees:	Y	Mktg. Professionals:	Y	Gen. Writing/Editing:	Info. Management:	Y	Finance/Accounting:	Y	Engineers, Elec.:	
Experienced Mgmt.:	Y	Retail Sales:		Technical Writing:	Software Dev.:	Y	Law:	Y	Engineers, Other:	
Int'l Business:	Y	Commercial/Industrial:	Y	Graphic Arts/Photog.:	Hardware Dev.:		HR/Other:	Y	Health/Lab:	
MBA Graduates:	Y	Sales Trainees:		Music:	Systems Integration:		Training:	Y	Scientists/Research:	
		Advertising Pros.:	Y	Broadcasting:	Consulting/Other:		Health Care:		Petroleum/Chemicals:	
				Other:			Consulting:		Math/Other:	

TYPES OF BUSINESS:

Linen & Uniform Supply
Uniform Rental, Sales & Cleaning
Uniform Design & Manufacturing
Outsourcing Services
Dust Control Services
Restroom Cleaning Services
Document Shredding & Management
First Aid & Safety Products

BRANDS/DIVISIONS/AFFILIATES:

CONTACTS: *Note: Officers with more than one job title may be intentionally listed here more than once.*

Scott D. Farmer, CEO
J. Phillip Holloman, COO
J. Phillip Holloman, Pres.
William C. Gale, CFO/Sr. VP
Thomas Frooman, General Counsel/VP/Corp. Sec.
Michael L. Thompson, Treas./VP
Richard T. Farmer, Chmn.

Phone: 513-459-1200	Fax: 513-573-4130
Toll-Free:	
Address: 6800 Cintas Blvd., Cincinnati, OH 45262-5737 US	

GROWTH PLANS/SPECIAL FEATURES:

Cintas Corp., a leading uniform supplier in the U.S., designs, manufactures and implements corporate identity uniform programs. The company's products include entrance mats, restroom supplies, hygiene service supplies, first aid and safety products, fire protection products, document shredding and storage, cleanroom resources and flame resistant clothing. Cintas supplies products and services to approximately 800,000 businesses of all types. The company's products and services are designed to enhance its customers' images and brand identification as well as provide a safe and efficient workplace. The firm operates through two segments: Rental Uniforms and Ancillary Products and Other Services. The rentals segment, accounting for approximately 72% of the company's revenue, reflects the rental and servicing of uniforms and other garments, mats, mops, shop towels and restroom and hygiene products and services. Rental services include the cleaning of uniforms as well as providing on-going uniform replacements as required to each customer. The other services unit, accounting for approximately 28% of the company's revenue, consists of the direct sale of uniforms and related items, first aid, safety and fire protection products and services, document management services and branded promotional products. The company also has specialized services tailored to the requirements of a number of additional industries, including automotive, casino, food processing, healthcare, lawn & garden, lodging, pest control, restaurant, supermarket and veterinary. The firm operates ten manufacturing plants and eight distribution centers across North America, as well as more than 400 other facilities. Cintas provides its products and services through a distribution network and approximately 7,300 local delivery routes. In June 2008, following the opening of service offices in Hong Kong and Macau, the company announced plans to launch services in various other international markets, led by Cintas' new Global Accounts and Strategic Markets Division.

FINANCIALS: Sales and profits are in thousands of dollars—add 000 to get the full amount. 2007 Note: Financial information for 2007 was not available for all companies at press time.

2007 Sales: $3,706,900	2007 Profits: $334,538	U.S. Stock Ticker: CTAS
2006 Sales: $3,403,608	2006 Profits: $323,382	Int'l Ticker: Int'l Exchange:
2005 Sales: $3,067,283	2005 Profits: $292,547	Employees: 34,000
2004 Sales: $2,814,059	2004 Profits: $300,518	Fiscal Year Ends: 5/31
2003 Sales: $2,686,585	2003 Profits: $249,253	Parent Company:

SALARIES/BENEFITS:

Pension Plan:	ESOP Stock Plan: Y	Profit Sharing: Y	Top Exec. Salary: $630,000	Bonus: $236,000
Savings Plan: Y	Stock Purch. Plan:		Second Exec. Salary: $500,000	Bonus: $

OTHER THOUGHTS:

Apparent Women Officers or Directors:
Hot Spot for Advancement for Women/Minorities:

LOCATIONS: ("Y" = Yes)

West:	Southwest:	Midwest:	Southeast:	Northeast:	International:
Y	Y	Y	Y	Y	Y

Note: Financial information, benefits and other data can change quickly and may vary from those stated here.

CISCO SYSTEMS INC

www.cisco.com

Industry Group Code: 334110 Ranks within this company's industry group: Sales: 1   Profits: 1

Management:		Sales/Marketing:		Liberal Arts:		Information Systems:		Professionals:		Technical/Scientific:	
Mgmt. Trainees:	Y	Mktg. Professionals:	Y	Gen. Writing/Editing:	Y	Info. Management:	Y	Finance/Accounting:	Y	Engineers, Elec.:	Y
Experienced Mgmt.:	Y	Retail Sales:		Technical Writing:	Y	Software Dev.:	Y	Law:	Y	Engineers, Other:	
Int'l Business:	Y	Commercial/Industrial:	Y	Graphic Arts/Photog.:		Hardware Dev.:	Y	HR/Other:	Y	Health/Lab:	
MBA Graduates:	Y	Sales Trainees:		Music:		Systems Integration:	Y	Training:	Y	Scientists/Research:	
		Advertising Pros.:	Y	Broadcasting:		Consulting/Other:	Y	Health Care:		Petroleum/Chemicals:	
				Other:				Consulting:		Math/Other:	

TYPES OF BUSINESS:

Computer Networking Equipment
Routers & Switches
Adapters & Hubs
Router Management Software
Data Storage Products
Security Products

BRANDS/DIVISIONS/AFFILIATES:

Scientific Atlanta Inc
Cognio, Inc.
Navini Networks, Inc.
Latigent, LLC
Securent, Inc.
Tivella, Inc.
NeoPath Networks
Webex Communications Inc

CONTACTS: Note: Officers with more than one job title may be intentionally listed here more than once.

John T. Chambers, CEO
Dennis D. Powell, CFO/Exec. VP
Susan Bostrom, Chief Mktg. Officer
Brian Schipper, Sr. VP-Human Resources
Rebecca J. Jacoby, CIO/Sr. VP
Padmasree Warrior, CTO
Angel L. Mendez, Sr. VP-Worldwide Mfg.
Mark Chandler, General Counsel/Sr. VP-Legal Svcs./Sec.
Richard J. Justice, Exec. VP-Worldwide Oper. & Bus. Dev.
Ned Hooper, Sr. VP-Bus. Dev.
Susan Bostrom, Exec. VP-Global Policy & Gov't Affairs
Jonathan Chadwick, Principal Acct. Officer/Controller/Sr. VP
Alan Baratz, Sr. VP-Network Software & Systems Tech. Group
Frank Calderoni, Sr. VP-Costumer Solutions Finance
David K. Holland, Treas./Sr. VP
Randy Pond, Exec. VP-Oper., Processes & Systems
John T. Chambers, Chmn.
Chris Dedicoat, Pres., European Markets

Phone: 408-526-4000	Fax: 408-526-4100
Toll-Free: 800-553-6387	
Address: 170 W. Tasman Dr., San Jose, CA 95134 US	

GROWTH PLANS/SPECIAL FEATURES:

Cisco Systems, Inc. designs, manufactures and sells Internet protocol (IP)-based networking and other products related to the communications and information technology industry; and provides services associated with these products and their use. The company provides a broad line of products for transporting data, voice and video within buildings, across campuses and around the world. The firm's products, which include routers, switches and advanced technologies, are installed at large enterprises, public institutions, telecommunications companies, commercial businesses and personal residences. Advanced technologies operations involve emerging technologies such as application networking services, home networking, hosted small business systems, security and wireless technology. Application networking services help IT departments integrate hardware and software. Security products include embedded security devices, firewalls and virtual private networks. Wireless offerings provide a broad variety of in-building wireless LAN and outdoor wireless bridging products. In addition to its product offerings, Cisco provides a range of services, including technical support and training. The firm's business is divided into five segments based on region: the U.S. and Canada, European Markets, Emerging Markets, Asia Pacific and Japan. In 2007, Cisco acquired Tivella, Inc., which offers digital signage software and systems; Reactivity, Inc., an eXtensible Markup Language gateway provider; NeoPath Networks, a provider of file storage management solutions; WebEx Communications, Inc., a provider of on-demand collaboration applications; and Broadway Technologies, which offers IP-based video surveillance software. The firm also acquired Cognio, Inc., involved in the wireless spectrum analysis and management for wireless network; Latigent, LLC, a provider of web-based business intelligence and analytics reporting solutions; Securent, Inc., which officer policy management solutions; and Navini Networks, Inc., a provider in the mobile WiMAX broadband wireless industry. In July 2008, Cisco announced plans to acquire Pure Networks, a Seattle-based manufacturer of networking equipment and software for the home, for $120 million.

FINANCIALS: Sales and profits are in thousands of dollars—add 000 to get the full amount. 2007 Note: Financial information for 2007 was not available for all companies at press time.

2007 Sales: $34,922,000	2007 Profits: $7,333,000	**U.S. Stock Ticker:** CSCO
2006 Sales: $28,484,000	2006 Profits: $5,580,000	**Int'l Ticker:** Int'l Exchange:
2005 Sales: $24,801,000	2005 Profits: $5,741,000	Employees: 61,535
2004 Sales: $22,045,000	2004 Profits: $4,401,000	Fiscal Year Ends: 7/31
2003 Sales: $18,878,000	2003 Profits: $3,578,000	Parent Company:

SALARIES/BENEFITS:

Pension Plan:	ESOP Stock Plan:	Profit Sharing:	Top Exec. Salary: $451,154	Bonus: $2,329,875
Savings Plan:	Stock Purch. Plan:		Second Exec. Salary: $451,154	Bonus: $1,980,394

OTHER THOUGHTS:

Apparent Women Officers or Directors: 6
Hot Spot for Advancement for Women/Minorities: Y

LOCATIONS: ("Y" = Yes)

West:	Southwest:	Midwest:	Southeast:	Northeast:	International:
Y	Y	Y	Y	Y	Y

Note: Financial information, benefits and other data can change quickly and may vary from those stated here.

CLEAR CHANNEL COMMUNICATIONS INC
www.clearchannel.com

Industry Group Code: 513111   **Ranks within this company's industry group:**   Sales: 1   Profits: 1

Management:		Sales/Marketing:		Liberal Arts:		Information Systems:		Professionals:		Technical/Scientific:	
Mgmt. Trainees:		Mktg. Professionals:	Y	Gen. Writing/Editing:	Y	Info. Management:	Y	Finance/Accounting:	Y	Engineers, Elec.:	Y
Experienced Mgmt.:	Y	Retail Sales:		Technical Writing:		Software Dev.:	Y	Law:	Y	Engineers, Other:	
Int'l Business:	Y	Commercial/Industrial:	Y	Graphic Arts/Photog.:	Y	Hardware Dev.:		HR/Other:	Y	Health/Lab:	
MBA Graduates:	Y	Sales Trainees:		Music:	Y	Systems Integration:	Y	Training:	Y	Scientists/Research:	
		Advertising Pros.:	Y	Broadcasting:	Y	Consulting/Other:		Health Care:		Petroleum/Chemicals:	
				Other:	Y			Consulting:		Math/Other:	

TYPES OF BUSINESS:
Radio Station Owner/Operator
Outdoor Advertising

BRANDS/DIVISIONS/AFFILIATES:
Thomas H Lee Partners LP
Bain Capital LLC
CC Media Holdings
Katz Media
Katz Group of Companies (The)
Providence Equity Partners
Clear Channel Independent
Newport Television, LLC

CONTACTS: *Note: Officers with more than one job title may be intentionally listed here more than once.*
Mark P. Mays, CEO
Randall T. Mays, Pres.
Randall T. Mays, CFO/Exec. VP
Bill Hamersly, Sr. VP-Human Resources
David Wilson, CIO/Sr. VP
Joe Shannon, CTO/VP
Andrew W. Levin, Chief Legal Officer/Exec. VP/Corp. Sec.
John T. Tippit, Sr. VP-Strategic Dev.
Lisa Dollinger, Chief Comm. Officer
Randy Palmer, Sr. VP-Investor Rel.
Herb Hill, Chief Acct. Officer
Jessica Marventano, Sr. VP-Gov't Affairs
Chad Dan, Sr. VP-Real Estate
Paul Meyer, CEO/Pres., Clear Channel Outdoor
John Hogan, CEO/Pres., Radio
L. Lowry Mays, Chmn.

Phone: 210-822-2828	Fax: 210-822-2299
Toll-Free:	
Address: 200 E. Basse Rd., San Antonio, TX 78209 US	

GROWTH PLANS/SPECIAL FEATURES:
Clear Channel Communications, Inc. is a diversified media company with operations in radio broadcasting, domestic outdoor advertising and international outdoor advertising. The company agreed to be acquired by a group led by Thomas H. Lee Partners and Bain Capital Partners, LLC for approximately $18.7 billion and $8 billion in acquired debt in late 2006. The transaction is expected to close during 2008, at which point Clear Channel will become a subsidiary of CC Media Holdings. The company owns 717 core radio stations and 288 non-core radio stations which are being marketed for sale. 275 of its stations operate in the top 50 markets. It also owns a leading national radio network and holds equity interests in various international radio broadcasting companies. Clear Channel's radio network produces, distributes and represents approximately 70 syndicated radio programs and services for roughly 5,000 radio stations. Some of the company's more popular syndicated programs include Rush Limbaugh, Steve Harvey, Ryan Seacrest and Jeff Foxworthy. Its radio broadcasting segment represents 50% of its revenue. Clear Channel owns and operates approximately 209,000 outdoor advertising displays throughout North America, which represent 21% of its revenue, and approximately 687,000 international outdoor advertising display faces, which represent 26% of its revenue. Clear Channel's other businesses represent 3% of its revenue and include subsidiary Katz Media, which sells national spot advertising time for roughly 3,200 clients in the radio industry and 380 clients in the television industry. In April 2007, the firm sold 56 TV and 161 radio stations to Providence Equity Partners and other parties for $1.5 billion. In January 2008, the company agreed to sell its equity investment in Clear Channel Independent, an out-of-home advertising company headquartered in South Africa. In March 2008, Clear Channel sold its television group to Newport Television, LLC for $1.1 billion.

FINANCIALS: Sales and profits are in thousands of dollars—add 000 to get the full amount. 2007 Note: Financial information for 2007 was not available for all companies at press time.

2007 Sales: $6,816,909	2007 Profits: $938,507	**U.S. Stock Ticker: CCU**
2006 Sales: $6,457,435	2006 Profits: $691,517	**Int'l Ticker:** Int'l Exchange:
2005 Sales: $6,019,029	2005 Profits: $935,662	Employees: 28,900
2004 Sales: $6,600,954	2004 Profits: $-4,038,169	Fiscal Year Ends: 12/31
2003 Sales: $8,930,899	2003 Profits: $1,145,591	Parent Company:

SALARIES/BENEFITS:

Pension Plan:	ESOP Stock Plan:	Profit Sharing:	Top Exec. Salary: $750,000	Bonus: $157,500
Savings Plan: Y	Stock Purch. Plan: Y		Second Exec. Salary: $695,000	Bonus: $

OTHER THOUGHTS:
Apparent Women Officers or Directors: 8
Hot Spot for Advancement for Women/Minorities: Y

LOCATIONS: ("Y" = Yes)

West:	Southwest:	Midwest:	Southeast:	Northeast:	International:
Y	Y	Y	Y	Y	Y

CLUBCORP INC
www.clubcorp.com

Industry Group Code: 713910 Ranks within this company's industry group: Sales: Profits:

Management:	Sales/Marketing:	Liberal Arts:	Information Systems:	Professionals:	Technical/Scientific:
Mgmt. Trainees:	Mktg. Professionals:	Gen. Writing/Editing:	Info. Management:	Finance/Accounting:	Engineers, Elec.:
Experienced Mgmt.:	Retail Sales:	Technical Writing:	Software Dev.:	Law:	Engineers, Other:
Int'l Business:	Commercial/Industrial:	Graphic Arts/Photog.:	Hardware Dev.:	HR/Other:	Health/Lab:
MBA Graduates:	Sales Trainees:	Music:	Systems Integration:	Training:	Scientists/Research:
	Advertising Pros.:	Broadcasting:	Consulting/Other:	Health Care:	Petroleum/Chemicals:
		Other:		Consulting:	Math/Other:

TYPES OF BUSINESS:
Golf Courses & Country Clubs
Business/Sports Clubs
Resorts

BRANDS/DIVISIONS/AFFILIATES:
Mission Hills Country Club
Firestone Country Club
Indian Wells Country Club
Homestead (The)
Boston College Club
Metropolitan Club
Ocean Edge Resort & Golf Club (The)
KSL Capital LLC

CONTACTS: *Note: Officers with more than one job title may be intentionally listed here more than once.*
Eric L. Affeldt, CEO
Eric L. Affeldt, Pres.
Frank C. Gore, Exec. VP-Sales
John H. Longstreet, Exec. VP-People Strategy
Daniel T. Tilley, CIO/Exec. VP
Ingrid Keiser, Chief Legal Officer/Corp. Sec.
Douglas T. Howe, Exec. VP-New Bus. Dev.
Angela A. Stephens, Exec. VP-Finance
Mark Burnett, Exec. VP-Golf & Country Club Div.
Mark Murphy, Sr. VP-Integrated Revenue
David B. Woodyard, Exec. VP-Bus. & Sports Div.
William T. Walden, Sr. VP-Purchasing

Phone: 972-243-6191	Fax: 972-888-7558
Toll-Free:	
Address: 3030 LBJ Freeway, Ste. 600, Dallas, TX 75234 US	

GROWTH PLANS/SPECIAL FEATURES:
ClubCorp, Inc. is an owner and operator of nearly 200 golf courses, country clubs, private clubs and golf resorts in the U.S., with additional operations in Australia, Europe and Asia. The company has approximately 200,000 memberships and 170 operations in 29 states and 3 foreign countries (Australia, China and Mexico), including 73 private country clubs, 12 semi-private golf clubs, 9 public golf facilities, 3 destination golf resorts (Firestone Country Club, the Homestead and Barton Creek Resort and Spa) and 69 business/sports clubs (including 42 business clubs, 14 business/sports clubs and 3 sports clubs). The firm's operations include nationally recognized golf courses and country clubs such as the Firestone Country Club in Akron, Ohio; the Indian Wells Country Club in Indian Wells, California; The Homestead in Hot Springs, Virginia, the oldest resort in America; and the Mission Hills Country Club in Rancho Mirage, California. Additionally, the company's business and sports clubs can be found in major metropolitan areas, including the City Club on Bunker Hill in Los Angeles; the Citrus Club in Orlando, Florida; the Columbia Tower Club in Seattle; the Metropolitan Club in Chicago; the Tower Club in Dallas; the Boston College Club; and the City Club in Washington, D.C. The firm owns The Ocean Edge Resort & Golf Club in Cape Cod, Massachusetts, which is located on 400 acres of property and features a romantic beach and boardwalk as well as 336 guest accommodations. The firm is owned by Denver-based KSL Capital, a private-equity investor.

The company offers internship programs for training in the areas of kitchen and catering; golf course operations and maintenance; accounting; and member relations.

FINANCIALS: Sales and profits are in thousands of dollars—add 000 to get the full amount. 2007 Note: Financial information for 2007 was not available for all companies at press time.

2007 Sales: $1,000,000	2007 Profits: $	**U.S. Stock Ticker: Private**
2006 Sales: $1,020,000	2006 Profits: $	**Int'l Ticker:** Int'l Exchange:
2005 Sales: $1,028,088	2005 Profits: $70,754	Employees: 16,000
2004 Sales: $938,802	2004 Profits: $-6,242	Fiscal Year Ends: 12/31
2003 Sales: $892,709	2003 Profits: $-105,246	Parent Company:

SALARIES/BENEFITS:
Pension Plan:	ESOP Stock Plan:	Profit Sharing:	Top Exec. Salary: $500,000	Bonus: $281,250
Savings Plan:	Stock Purch. Plan:		Second Exec. Salary: $500,000	Bonus: $235,000

OTHER THOUGHTS:
Apparent Women Officers or Directors: 2
Hot Spot for Advancement for Women/Minorities: Y

LOCATIONS: ("Y" = Yes)
West:	Southwest:	Midwest:	Southeast:	Northeast:	International:
Y	Y	Y	Y	Y	Y

COACH INC
www.coach.com

Industry Group Code: 448210 Ranks within this company's industry group: Sales: 1   Profits: 1

Management:		Sales/Marketing:		Liberal Arts:		Information Systems:		Professionals:		Technical/Scientific:	
Mgmt. Trainees:	Y	Mktg. Professionals:	Y	Gen. Writing/Editing:	Y	Info. Management:	Y	Finance/Accounting:	Y	Engineers, Elec.:	
Experienced Mgmt.:	Y	Retail Sales:	Y	Technical Writing:		Software Dev.:	Y	Law:	Y	Engineers, Other:	
Int'l Business:	Y	Commercial/Industrial:	Y	Graphic Arts/Photog.:	Y	Hardware Dev.:		HR/Other:	Y	Health/Lab:	
MBA Graduates:	Y	Sales Trainees:	Y	Music:		Systems Integration:		Training:	Y	Scientists/Research:	
		Advertising Pros.:	Y	Broadcasting:		Consulting/Other:		Health Care:		Petroleum/Chemicals:	
				Other:	Y			Consulting:		Math/Other:	

TYPES OF BUSINESS:
Leather Accessories-Retail
Online & Catalog Sales
Outlet Stores

BRANDS/DIVISIONS/AFFILIATES:
Coach.com
Coach Japan, Inc.
Coach Legacy
ImagineX
Jamilco

CONTACTS: *Note: Officers with more than one job title may be intentionally listed here more than once.*
Lew Frankfort, CEO
Jerry Stritzke, COO/Pres.
Reed Krakoff, Pres./Exec. Creative Dir.
Micheal F. Devine, III, CFO/Exec. VP
Sarah Dunn, Sr. VP-Human Resources
Todd Kahn, Gen. Counsel/Sr. VP/Sec.
Lew Frankfort, Chmn.

Phone: 212-594-1850	Fax: 212-594-1682
Toll-Free: 1-888-262-6224	
Address: 516 W. 34th St., New York, NY 10001-1394 US	

GROWTH PLANS/SPECIAL FEATURES:
Coach, Inc. is a designer, producer and marketer of fine accessories and gifts for men and women, including handbags, women's and men's accessories, footwear, outerwear, business luggage and travel accessories, cases, eyewear, watches, jewelry and fragrance. The firm also licenses its name for watches, shoes and eyewear. The company sells its products through a number of direct channels, accounting for approximately 80% of its sales. As of the 2007 fiscal year end, the Coach brand was made available at over 900 department store locations in the U.S., 140 international department stores, retail store and duty free shop locations in 21 countries, 137 department store shop-in-shops and retail and factory store locations operated by Coach Japan, Inc. and through the company's corporate sales program. At the June 2008 fiscal year end, 62% of the company's sales came from handbags, accessories (wristlets, cosmetic cases, money pieces, etc.) represented 29% of sales and the final 9% of sales derived from all other products(sunglasses, watches, fragrance, etc.). Over the last several years, Coach has successfully transformed itself from a manufacturer of classic leather products to a marketer of more modern, fashionable handbags and accessories, using a broader range of fabrics and materials. In January 2008, the firm announced plans to enter the Russian market through an agreement with Jamilco, a domestic distributor. Coach plans to open 15 locations in Russia over a five year time frame. In May 2008, the company announced that it acquired the Coach domestic retail businesses in Hong Kong, Macau and mainland China from its current distributor, ImagineX group.

FINANCIALS: Sales and profits are in thousands of dollars—add 000 to get the full amount. 2007 Note: Financial information for 2007 was not available for all companies at press time.

2007 Sales: $2,612,456	2007 Profits: $663,665	U.S. Stock Ticker: COH
2006 Sales: $2,035,085	2006 Profits: $494,277	Int'l Ticker: Int'l Exchange:
2005 Sales: $1,651,704	2005 Profits: $358,612	Employees: 10,100
2004 Sales: $1,316,300	2004 Profits: $261,700	Fiscal Year Ends: 6/30
2003 Sales: $953,226	2003 Profits: $146,528	Parent Company:

SALARIES/BENEFITS:

Pension Plan:	ESOP Stock Plan:	Profit Sharing:	Top Exec. Salary: $1,875,000	Bonus: $5,295,625
Savings Plan:	Stock Purch. Plan:		Second Exec. Salary: $971,667	Bonus: $1,931,673

OTHER THOUGHTS:
Apparent Women Officers or Directors: 1
Hot Spot for Advancement for Women/Minorities: Y

LOCATIONS: ("Y" = Yes)

West:	Southwest:	Midwest:	Southeast:	Northeast:	International:
Y	Y	Y	Y	Y	Y

Note: Financial information, benefits and other data can change quickly and may vary from those stated here.

# COCA COLA COMPANY (THE)		www.coca-cola.com

Industry Group Code: 312111 Ranks within this company's industry group: Sales: 2 Profits: 2

Management:		Sales/Marketing:		Liberal Arts:		Information Systems:		Professionals:		Technical/Scientific:	
Mgmt. Trainees:	Y	Mktg. Professionals:	Y	Gen. Writing/Editing:	Y	Info. Management:	Y	Finance/Accounting:	Y	Engineers, Elec.:	Y
Experienced Mgmt.:	Y	Retail Sales:		Technical Writing:		Software Dev.:		Law:	Y	Engineers, Other:	
Int'l Business:	Y	Commercial/Industrial:	Y	Graphic Arts/Photog.:	Y	Hardware Dev.:		HR/Other:	Y	Health/Lab:	
MBA Graduates:	Y	Sales Trainees:		Music:		Systems Integration:		Training:	Y	Scientists/Research:	
		Advertising Pros.:	Y	Broadcasting:		Consulting/Other:		Health Care:		Petroleum/Chemicals:	
				Other:				Consulting:		Math/Other:	

TYPES OF BUSINESS:
Soft Drink Manufacturing
Concentrates & Syrups
Sports Drinks
Bottled Water
Fruit Juices

BRANDS/DIVISIONS/AFFILIATES:
Dasani
Odwalla
Powerade
Sprite
Minute Maid Company (The)
Canada Dry
Beverage Partners Worldwide
Energy Brands, Inc.

CONTACTS: *Note: Officers with more than one job title may be intentionally listed here more than once.*
E. Neville Isdell, CEO
Muhtar Kent, COO
Muhtar Kent, Pres.
Gary P. Fayard, CFO/Exec. VP
Joseph V. Tripodi, Chief Mktg. & Commercial Officer/Sr. VP
Cynthia P. McCague, Sr. VP-Human Resources
Jean-Michel R. Ares, CIO/Sr. VP
Danny L. Strickland, CTO/Chief Innovation Officer
Geoffrey J. Kelly, General Counsel/Sr. VP
Thomas G. Mattia, Sr. VP-Worldwide Public Affairs & Comm.
David M. Taggart, Treas./VP
Alexander B. Cummings, Pres./COO-Africa Group
J. Alexander M. Douglas, Jr., Pres./COO-North America Group
Glenn G. Jordan S., Pres./COO-Pacific Group
Carol Crofoot Hayes, Corp. Sec.
E. Neville Isdell, Chmn.
Ahmet C. Bozer, Pres./COO-Eurasia Group
Irial Finan, Exec. VP-Bottling Investments & Supply Chain

Phone: 404-676-2121	Fax:
Toll-Free:	
Address: 1 Coca-Cola Plaza, Atlanta, GA 30313 US	

GROWTH PLANS/SPECIAL FEATURES:
The Coca-Cola Co. manufactures, distributes and markets nonalcoholic beverage concentrates and syrups, selling its products in more than 200 countries. It is divided into six regional operating segments in addition to a corporate and a bottling operations segment. The company sells concentrates and syrups for bottled and canned beverages; and concentrates in powder form for purified water products such as Dasani to authorized bottling and canning operations. Authorized bottlers and canners either combine the syrups with sparkling water or combine the concentrates with sweeteners, water and sparkling water to produce finished sparkling beverages. The finished sparkling beverages are packaged in authorized containers bearing Coca-Cola's trademarks and are then sold to retailers or wholesalers. Beverage products include Coca-Cola Classic, Cherry Coke, Diet Coke, Fanta, Sprite, Pibb Extra, Mello Yello, Fresca, Barq's, Powerade, Dasani, Kinley, Schweppes, Canada Dry, Dr. Pepper and Crush. The firm also produces, distributes and markets juice and juice-drink products including Minute Maid Premium juice and juice drinks; Simply juices and juice drinks; Odwalla nourishing health beverages; Five Alive refreshment beverages; Bacardi mixers concentrate; and Hi-C ready-to-serve juice drinks. Coca-Cola also has a license to manufacture and sell concentrates for Seagram's mixers, a line of sparkling drinks. The company is the exclusive master distributor of Evian bottled water in North America and of Rockstar, an energy drink. Multon, a Russian juice business operated as a joint venture with Coca-Cola Hellenic Bottling Company S.A., markets juice products under various trademarks, including Dobriy, Rich and Nico, in Russia, Ukraine and Belarus. Beverage Partners Worldwide, a joint venture with Nestlé S.A., markets tea products under trademarks including Enviga, Gold Peak, Nestea, Heaven and Earth, Frestea, Ten Ren, Modern Tea Workshop and Tian Tey; and coffee products under Nescafé, Taster's Choice and Georgia Club. In mid-2007, Coca-Cola acquired Energy Brands, Inc., known as glaceau, a vitamin water producer.

FINANCIALS: Sales and profits are in thousands of dollars—add 000 to get the full amount. 2007 Note: Financial information for 2007 was not available for all companies at press time.

2007 Sales: $28,857,000	2007 Profits: $5,981,000	**U.S. Stock Ticker: KO**
2006 Sales: $24,088,000	2006 Profits: $5,080,000	**Int'l Ticker:** Int'l Exchange:
2005 Sales: $23,104,000	2005 Profits: $4,872,000	Employees: 71,000
2004 Sales: $21,962,000	2004 Profits: $4,847,000	Fiscal Year Ends: 12/31
2003 Sales: $21,044,000	2003 Profits: $4,347,000	Parent Company:

SALARIES/BENEFITS:

Pension Plan:	ESOP Stock Plan:	Profit Sharing:	Top Exec. Salary: $1,500,000	Bonus: $5,550,000
Savings Plan: Y	Stock Purch. Plan:		Second Exec. Salary: $773,077	Bonus: $1,809,962

OTHER THOUGHTS:
Apparent Women Officers or Directors: 7
Hot Spot for Advancement for Women/Minorities: Y

LOCATIONS: ("Y" = Yes)

West:	Southwest:	Midwest:	Southeast:	Northeast:	International:
Y	Y	Y	Y	Y	Y

COCA COLA ENTERPRISES INC

www.cokecce.com

Industry Group Code: 312111 Ranks within this company's industry group: Sales: Profits:

Management:		Sales/Marketing:		Liberal Arts:		Information Systems:		Professionals:		Technical/Scientific:	
Mgmt. Trainees:	Y	Mktg. Professionals:	Y	Gen. Writing/Editing:		Info. Management:	Y	Finance/Accounting:	Y	Engineers, Elec.:	Y
Experienced Mgmt.:	Y	Retail Sales:		Technical Writing:		Software Dev.:		Law:	Y	Engineers, Other:	
Int'l Business:	Y	Commercial/Industrial:	Y	Graphic Arts/Photog.:		Hardware Dev.:		HR/Other:	Y	Health/Lab:	
MBA Graduates:	Y	Sales Trainees:	Y	Music:		Systems Integration:		Training:	Y	Scientists/Research:	
		Advertising Pros.:	Y	Broadcasting:		Consulting/Other:		Health Care:		Petroleum/Chemicals:	
				Other:				Consulting:		Math/Other:	

TYPES OF BUSINESS:

Soft Drink Bottling
Production, Marketing & Distribution-Coca-Cola Products
Vending Machines

BRANDS/DIVISIONS/AFFILIATES:

Coca Cola Co

CONTACTS: *Note: Officers with more than one job title may be intentionally listed here more than once.*

John F. Brock, CEO
John F. Brock, Pres.
William W. Douglas III, CFO/Sr. VP
Greg A. Lee, Sr. VP-Human Resources
Esat Sezer, CIO/Sr. VP
Vicki R. Palmer, Exec. VP-Admin. & Financial Svcs.
John J. Culhane, General Counsel/Exec. VP
Brian E. Wynne, VP-Bus. Dev. & Revenue Growth Mgmt.
John H. Downs, Jr., Sr. VP-Public Affairs & Comm.
Joseph D. Heinrich, Chief Acct. Officer/Controller/VP
Terrance M. Marks, Exec. VP/Pres., North American Group
Scott Anthony, CFO/VP-North American Group
Joyce King-Lavinder, Treas./VP
William T. Plybon, Corp. Sec./VP
Lowry F. Kline, Chmn.
Steve Cahillane, Exec. VP/Pres., European Group
Edward L. Sutter, VP-Supply Chain

Phone: 770-989-3000	Fax: 770-989-3788
Toll-Free:	
Address: 2500 Windy Ridge Pkwy., Atlanta, GA 30339 US	

GROWTH PLANS/SPECIAL FEATURES:

Coca-Cola Enterprises, Inc. (CCE) is one of the largest marketers, distributors and producers of bottled and canned non-alcoholic beverages in the world. CCE serves a market of approximately 412 million consumers in North America, Great Britain, France, Belgium, the Netherlands, Luxembourg and Monaco, selling around 42 billion bottles and cans in its territories. It is also the largest marketer, producer and distributor of Coca-Cola products, representing approximately 21% of Coca-Cola product volume worldwide. The Coca-Cola Company in turn owns 38% of CCE. The firm sells 80% of The Coca-Cola Company's bottle and can volumes in North America and has operations in 46 U.S. states and all 10 provinces in Canada. The firm also distributes Dr Pepper, Sprite, A&W, Canada Dry, Nestea, Fanta, Schweppes, bottled water, juices, coffee-based drinks and sports drinks. Products are manufactured from syrups and concentrates purchased from The Coca-Cola Company and other licensors. The firm delivers most of its products directly to retailers, but some drink brands, in some territories, are distributed through wholesalers who then deliver to retailers. About 54% of the company's North American bottle and can volume and 43% of its European bottle and can volume are sold through in supermarkets. CCE has 431 facilities, 54,000 vehicles and 2.4 million vending machines, beverage dispensers and coolers in operation. Approximately 94% of company sales are Coca-Cola products.

The company offers its employees a 401(k) plan, a pension plan, life insurance, an employee assistance program and educational assistance.

FINANCIALS: Sales and profits are in thousands of dollars—add 000 to get the full amount. 2007 Note: Financial information for 2007 was not available for all companies at press time.

2007 Sales: $20,936,000	2007 Profits: $711,000	**U.S. Stock Ticker: CCE**
2006 Sales: $19,804,000	2006 Profits: $-1,143,000	**Int'l Ticker:** Int'l Exchange:
2005 Sales: $18,743,000	2005 Profits: $514,000	Employees: 74,000
2004 Sales: $18,158,000	2004 Profits: $596,000	Fiscal Year Ends: 12/31
2003 Sales: $17,330,000	2003 Profits: $676,000	Parent Company:

SALARIES/BENEFITS:

Pension Plan: Y	ESOP Stock Plan:	Profit Sharing:	Top Exec. Salary: $751,667	Bonus: $1,038,261
Savings Plan: Y	Stock Purch. Plan:		Second Exec. Salary: $859,500	Bonus: $811,368

OTHER THOUGHTS:

Apparent Women Officers or Directors: 6
Hot Spot for Advancement for Women/Minorities: Y

LOCATIONS: ("Y" = Yes)

West:	Southwest:	Midwest:	Southeast:	Northeast:	International:
Y	Y	Y	Y	Y	Y

COGNIZANT TECHNOLOGY SOLUTIONS CORP
www.cognizant.com

Industry Group Code: 541512 Ranks within this company's industry group: Sales: 7　Profits: 5

Management:		Sales/Marketing:		Liberal Arts:		Information Systems:		Professionals:		Technical/Scientific:	
Mgmt. Trainees:	Y	Mktg. Professionals:	Y	Gen. Writing/Editing:		Info. Management:	Y	Finance/Accounting:	Y	Engineers, Elec.:	
Experienced Mgmt.:	Y	Retail Sales:		Technical Writing:	Y	Software Dev.:	Y	Law:	Y	Engineers, Other:	
Int'l Business:	Y	Commercial/Industrial:	Y	Graphic Arts/Photog.:	Y	Hardware Dev.:		HR/Other:	Y	Health/Lab:	
MBA Graduates:	Y	Sales Trainees:		Music:		Systems Integration:	Y	Training:	Y	Scientists/Research:	Y
		Advertising Pros.:		Broadcasting:		Consulting/Other:		Health Care:		Petroleum/Chemicals:	
				Other:				Consulting:	Y	Math/Other:	

TYPES OF BUSINESS:
Consulting-IT & Systems
Outsourcing Services
Software Engineering

BRANDS/DIVISIONS/AFFILIATES:
Q*VIEW

CONTACTS: Note: Officers with more than one job title may be intentionally listed here more than once.
Fransisco D'Souza, CEO
Gordon Coburn, COO
Fransisco D'Souza, Pres.
Gordon Coburn, CFO
Gordon Coburn, Sec.
Chandra Sekaran, Pres./Managing Dir.-Global Delivery
Rajeev Mehta, COO-Global Client Svcs.
John E. Klein, Chmn.

Phone: 201-801-0233	**Fax:** 201-801-0243
Toll-Free: 888-937-3277	
Address: 500 Glenpointe Ctr. W., Teaneck, NJ 07666 US	

GROWTH PLANS/SPECIAL FEATURES:
Cognizant Technology Solutions Corporation is a leading provider of custom IT design, development, integration and maintenance services, primarily for Global 2000 companies located in the U.S., Europe and Asia. The company's core competencies include Technology Strategy Consulting, Complex Systems Development, Enterprise Software Package Implementation and Maintenance, Data Warehousing & Business Intelligence, Application Testing, Application Maintenance, Infrastructure Management and Vertically-Oriented Business Process Outsourcing (V-BPO). Cognizant provides its IT services using an integrated on-site/offshore business model. This business model combines technical and account management teams located on-site at the customer location and offshore at dedicated development centers located primarily in India. Cognizant operates in four business segments: financial services, which provides services to customers in the capital markets, banking and insurance industries; healthcare, which provides services to healthcare and life science industries; manufacturing, retail and logistics, which provides services to those industries; and other, which covers telecommunications, information services, media and high technology. The firm has developed proprietary methodologies for integrating on-site and offshore teams, including Cognizant's Q*VIEW software engineering process, which is available to all on-site and offshore programmers. For most projects, Q*VIEW is used as part of an initial assessment that allows the firm to define the scope and risks of the project and subdivide the project into smaller phases with frequent deliverables and feedback from customers. The company also uses its Q*VIEW process to detect, mitigate and correct possible quality defects and to establish appropriate contingencies for each project. Cognizant has offices in the U.S., Canada, and throughout Asia and Europe. In April 2007, the firm announced plans to double the size of its Japanese operations located in Tokyo, and offshore near Shanghai.

The company provides its U.S. employees with benefits including stock purchase plan; employee stock options; medical, dental and vision coverage; and life insurance.

FINANCIALS: Sales and profits are in thousands of dollars—add 000 to get the full amount. 2007 Note: Financial information for 2007 was not available for all companies at press time.

2007 Sales: $2,135,577	2007 Profits: $350,133	**U.S. Stock Ticker:** CTSH
2006 Sales: $1,424,267	2006 Profits: $232,795	**Int'l Ticker:**　Int'l Exchange:
2005 Sales: $885,830	2005 Profits: $166,266	Employees: 55,400
2004 Sales: $586,673	2004 Profits: $100,243	Fiscal Year Ends: 12/31
2003 Sales: $365,656	2003 Profits: $57,365	Parent Company:

SALARIES/BENEFITS:

Pension Plan:	ESOP Stock Plan: Y	Profit Sharing:	Top Exec. Salary: $360,000	Bonus: $491,520
Savings Plan: Y	Stock Purch. Plan: Y		Second Exec. Salary: $324,000	Bonus: $442,368

OTHER THOUGHTS:
Apparent Women Officers or Directors:
Hot Spot for Advancement for Women/Minorities:

LOCATIONS: ("Y" = Yes)

West:	Southwest:	Midwest:	Southeast:	Northeast:	International:
Y	Y	Y		Y	Y

Note: Financial information, benefits and other data can change quickly and may vary from those stated here.

COLDWATER CREEK INC

www.coldwatercreek.com

Industry Group Code: 448000A   Ranks within this company's industry group: Sales: 1   Profits: 1

Management:		Sales/Marketing:		Liberal Arts:		Information Systems:		Professionals:		Technical/Scientific:	
Mgmt. Trainees:	Y	Mktg. Professionals:	Y	Gen. Writing/Editing:	Y	Info. Management:	Y	Finance/Accounting:	Y	Engineers, Elec.:	
Experienced Mgmt.:	Y	Retail Sales:		Technical Writing:		Software Dev.:	Y	Law:	Y	Engineers, Other:	
Int'l Business:		Commercial/Industrial:		Graphic Arts/Photog.:	Y	Hardware Dev.:		HR/Other:	Y	Health/Lab:	
MBA Graduates:	Y	Sales Trainees:		Music:		Systems Integration:		Training:	Y	Scientists/Research:	
		Advertising Pros.:	Y	Broadcasting:		Consulting/Other:		Health Care:		Petroleum/Chemicals:	
				Other:	Y			Consulting:		Math/Other:	

TYPES OF BUSINESS:

Upscale Apparel-Women's
Catalog Sales
Gifts, Jewelry & Accessories
Retail & Outlet Stores
Online Sales

BRANDS/DIVISIONS/AFFILIATES:

Coldwatercreek.com
Gifts-To-Go
Northcountry
Spirit

CONTACTS: Note: Officers with more than one job title may be intentionally listed here more than once.

Daniel Griesemer, CEO/Pres.
Georgia Shonk-Simmons, Pres.
Tim Martin, CFO/Exec. VP
Peter Prandato, VP-Creative
Brett Avner, Sr. VP-Human Resources
Dan Moen, CIO/Sr. VP
Mike Carper, VP-Tech. Oper.
Georgia Shonk-Simmons, Chief Merch. Officer
Jeffrey Parisian, VP-Admin.
Gerard El Chaar, Sr. VP-Oper.
Michael Feurer, Pres., New Strategic Concepts Div.
Christine Laczai, VP-Internet Div.
David Gunter, Dir.-Corp. Comm.
David Gunter, Dir.-Investor Rel.
Tim Martin, VP-Finance
Joe Gravitt, VP-Retail Oper.
Arthur (Skip) Jones, VP-Outlet Stores
Patricia Sikorsky, VP-Sourcing Dev.
Ann Kasper, VP-Channel Merch.
Dennis Pence, Chmn.
Ronn Hall, VP-Sourcing & Production

GROWTH PLANS/SPECIAL FEATURES:

Coldwater Creek, Inc. retails women's apparel, jewelry, footwear, gift items and home merchandise through three sales channels: a traditional catalog business, an e-commerce business and retail stores. The company targets professional women who are 35 years of age and older, with household incomes in excess of $75,000. Approximately 60% of its customers live on the East Coast. The firm's primary catalog titles and merchandise lines are Northcountry and Spirit. Northcountry is the firm's most established and popular line, offering a broad selection of casual merchandise at price points between $20 and $120. Spirit offers a more upscale assortment of apparel, including dresses, jackets and sportswear appropriate for office wear. Recently the company introduced its Coldwater Creek catalog, which exclusively features merchandise available in the company's stores and is designed to encourage customers to shop at its stores. Coldwater Creek also sends periodic specialty mailings, such as the Gifts-To-Go holiday catalog. The company's e-commerce business is its most profitable segment, representing over 25% of the company's total profits. The firm's web site features its entire full-priced, first-line merchandise collection. Coldwater Creek's fastest-growing segment is its retail store business, for which it opened 65 additional stores in fiscal 2007. The company currently has 306 full-line stores and 30 merchandise clearance outlet stores across the U.S. To remove customers' reluctance about buying online or through a catalog, the company has an all-inclusive return policy. The firm's long-range plan is to have as many as 550 stores by 2011.

Employees of Coldwater Creek enjoy an employee assistance program, a smoking cessation program, travel accident insurance, adoption reimbursement, a founder's scholarship program, jury leave and flexible spending accounts.

Phone: 208-263-2266	**Fax:** 208-263-1582
Toll-Free: 800-510-2808	
Address: 1 Coldwater Creek Dr., Sandpoint, ID 83864 US	

FINANCIALS: Sales and profits are in thousands of dollars—add 000 to get the full amount. 2007 Note: Financial information for 2007 was not available for all companies at press time.

2007 Sales: $1,054,611	2007 Profits: $55,372	**U.S. Stock Ticker:** CWTR
2006 Sales: $779,663	2006 Profits: $41,570	**Int'l Ticker:** Int'l Exchange:
2005 Sales: $590,310	2005 Profits: $29,130	Employees: 11,577
2004 Sales: $518,800	2004 Profits: $12,500	Fiscal Year Ends: 1/31
2003 Sales: $473,200	2003 Profits: $9,400	Parent Company:

SALARIES/BENEFITS:

Pension Plan:	ESOP Stock Plan:	Profit Sharing:	Top Exec. Salary: $1,000,000	Bonus: $323,720
Savings Plan: Y	Stock Purch. Plan:		Second Exec. Salary: $600,000	Bonus: $302,648

OTHER THOUGHTS:

Apparent Women Officers or Directors: 8
Hot Spot for Advancement for Women/Minorities: Y

LOCATIONS: ("Y" = Yes)

West:	Southwest:	Midwest:	Southeast:	Northeast:	International:
Y	Y	Y	Y	Y	

Note: Financial information, benefits and other data can change quickly and may vary from those stated here.

COLGATE PALMOLIVE CO   www.colgate.com

Industry Group Code: 325600 Ranks within this company's industry group: Sales: 2 Profits: 2

Management:		Sales/Marketing:		Liberal Arts:		Information Systems:		Professionals:		Technical/Scientific:	
Mgmt. Trainees:	Y	Mktg. Professionals:	Y	Gen. Writing/Editing:	Y	Info. Management:	Y	Finance/Accounting:	Y	Engineers, Elec.:	Y
Experienced Mgmt.:	Y	Retail Sales:		Technical Writing:	Y	Software Dev.:	Y	Law:	Y	Engineers, Other:	Y
Int'l Business:	Y	Commercial/Industrial:	Y	Graphic Arts/Photog.:	Y	Hardware Dev.:		HR/Other:	Y	Health/Lab:	Y
MBA Graduates:	Y	Sales Trainees:	Y	Music:		Systems Integration:		Training:	Y	Scientists/Research:	
		Advertising Pros.:	Y	Broadcasting:		Consulting/Other:		Health Care:		Petroleum/Chemicals:	
				Other:	Y			Consulting:		Math/Other:	

TYPES OF BUSINESS:

Toothpaste & Oral Care Products Manufacturer
Household Cleaning Products
Soap Products
Baby Care Products
Pet Food
Hair Products
Shaving Products

BRANDS/DIVISIONS/AFFILIATES:

Softsoap
Palmolive
Ajax
Irish Spring
Tom's of Maine
Lady Speed Stick
Hill's Pet Nutrition
Science Diet

CONTACTS: Note: Officers with more than one job title may be intentionally listed here more than once.

Ian M. Cook, CEO
Ian M. Cook, Pres.
Stephen C. Patrick, CFO
Stephen J. Fogarty, VP-Worldwide Shopper Mktg.
Daniel B. Marsili, VP-Global Human Resources
Constantina Christopoulou, VP-Global R&D
Tom Greene, CIO/VP
Derrick E. M. Samuel, Pres., Global Tech.
Andrew D. Hendry, General Counsel/Sr. VP/Sec.
Franck J. Moison, Pres., Global Bus. Dev. & Tech.
Jack J. Haber, VP-e-bus. & Global Advertising
Jan Guifarro, VP-Corp. Comm.
Bina H. Thompson, VP-Investor Rel.
Edward J. Filusch, Corp. Treas./VP
Nigel B. Burton, Pres., Global Oral Care
Hector I. Erezuma, VP-Taxation
Thomas M. Chappell, CEO-Tom's of Maine
Robert C. Wheeler, CEO-Hill's Pet Nutrition
Reuben Mark, Chmn.
Michael J. Tangney, COO-Colgate-Europe, Greater Asia & Africa
David R. Groener, VP-Global Supply Chain

Phone: 212-310-2000	Fax: 212-310-2475
Toll-Free: 800-468-6502	
Address: 300 Park Ave., New York, NY 10022 US	

GROWTH PLANS/SPECIAL FEATURES:

Colgate-Palmolive Co. (Colgate), founded in 1806, is a consumer products company whose products are marketed in over 200 countries and territories throughout the world. The company manages its business in two product segments: oral, personal and home care; and pet nutrition. Colgate oral care products include toothbrushes, toothpaste, tooth whitener, mouth rinses, dental floss and pharmaceutical products for dentists and other oral health professionals. The segment also markets bar and liquid hand soaps; shower gels, shampoos; conditioners; deodorants; antiperspirants; and shave products. The firm's Softsoap and Palmolive brands are two U.S. market leaders in liquid soaps. Other major products include household care products such as Ajax and Palmolive dishwashing liquids, Murphy's Oil Soap and Fabuloso laundry detergent. Additional oral, personal and home care brands include Mennen, Irish Spring, Tom's of Maine and Lady Speed Stick. Sale of oral, personal and home care products accounted for 40%, 23% and 24%, respectively, of total worldwide sales in 2007. Colgate also supplies specialty pet nutrition products for dogs and cats through subsidiary Hill's Pet Nutrition, with products marketed in over 90 countries. Pet foods are marketed primarily under the Science Diet and Prescription Diet trademarks. Science Diet is sold by authorized pet supply retailers, breeders and veterinarians for everyday nutritional needs, while Prescription Diet includes a range of therapeutic products sold by veterinarians to help nutritionally manage disease conditions in dogs and cats. Sales of pet nutrition products generated approximately 13% of Colgate's worldwide sales in 2007.

Colgate offers its employees tuition assistance, relocation assistance, back-up childcare centers, flexible spending accounts and medical, dental, disability and life insurance.

FINANCIALS: Sales and profits are in thousands of dollars—add 000 to get the full amount. 2007 Note: Financial information for 2007 was not available for all companies at press time.

2007 Sales: $13,789,700	2007 Profits: $1,737,400	U.S. Stock Ticker: CL
2006 Sales: $12,237,700	2006 Profits: $1,353,400	Int'l Ticker: Int'l Exchange:
2005 Sales: $11,396,900	2005 Profits: $1,351,400	Employees: 34,700
2004 Sales: $10,584,200	2004 Profits: $1,327,100	Fiscal Year Ends: 12/31
2003 Sales: $9,903,400	2003 Profits: $1,421,300	Parent Company:

SALARIES/BENEFITS:

Pension Plan: Y	ESOP Stock Plan:	Profit Sharing: Y	Top Exec. Salary: $1,871,750	Bonus: $4,465,125
Savings Plan: Y	Stock Purch. Plan:		Second Exec. Salary: $891,250	Bonus: $1,977,188

OTHER THOUGHTS:

Apparent Women Officers or Directors: 36
Hot Spot for Advancement for Women/Minorities: Y

LOCATIONS: ("Y" = Yes)

West:	Southwest:	Midwest:	Southeast:	Northeast:	International:
Y	Y	Y	Y	Y	Y

COMCAST CORP

www.comcast.com

Industry Group Code: 513220 Ranks within this company's industry group: Sales: 2 Profits: 2

Management:		Sales/Marketing:		Liberal Arts:		Information Systems:		Professionals:		Technical/Scientific:	
Mgmt. Trainees:	Y	Mktg. Professionals:	Y	Gen. Writing/Editing:	Y	Info. Management:	Y	Finance/Accounting:	Y	Engineers, Elec.:	Y
Experienced Mgmt.:	Y	Retail Sales:	Y	Technical Writing:		Software Dev.:	Y	Law:	Y	Engineers, Other:	
Int'l Business:	Y	Commercial/Industrial:	Y	Graphic Arts/Photog.:	Y	Hardware Dev.:		HR/Other:	Y	Health/Lab:	
MBA Graduates:	Y	Sales Trainees:	Y	Music:		Systems Integration:		Training:	Y	Scientists/Research:	
		Advertising Pros.:	Y	Broadcasting:	Y	Consulting/Other:		Health Care:		Petroleum/Chemicals:	
				Other:	Y			Consulting:		Math/Other:	

TYPES OF BUSINESS:
Cable Television
VoIP Service
Cable Network Programming
High-Speed Internet Service
Video-on-Demand
Advertising Services
Interactive Program Schedules
Wireless Services

BRANDS/DIVISIONS/AFFILIATES:
Fandango Inc
Philadelphia Flyers
Philadelphia 76ers
Global Spectrum LP
E! Channel
Golf Channel (The)
Comcast Interactive Media
Comcast Spectator

CONTACTS: *Note: Officers with more than one job title may be intentionally listed here more than once.*
Brian L. Roberts, CEO
Stephen B. Burke, COO
Michael J. Angelakis, CFO/Exec. VP
Charisse Lillie, VP-Human Resources
Karen D. Buchholz, VP-Admin.
Arthur R. Block, General Counsel/Sr. VP/Corp. Sec.
Mark A. Coblitz, Sr. VP-Strategic Planning
D'Arcy F. Rudnay, Sr. VP-Corp. Comm.
Marlene S. Dooner, Sr. VP-Investor Rel.
Lawrence J. Salva, Chief Acct. Officer/Controller/Sr. VP
Stephen B. Burke, Pres., Comcast Cable Comm.
Robert S. Victor, Sr. VP-Strategic & Financial Planning
Amy L. Banse, Pres., Comcast Interactive Media/Sr. VP
Robert S. Pick, Sr. VP-Corp. Dev.
Brian L. Roberts, Chmn.

Phone: 215-286-1700	Fax:
Toll-Free: 800-266-2278	
Address: 1 Comcast Ctr., Philadelphia, PA 19103 US	

GROWTH PLANS/SPECIAL FEATURES:

Comcast Corp. is one of the largest cable operators in the U.S. and offers a variety of entertainment and communications products and services. Its cable systems serve roughly 24.1 million video subscribers, 13.2 million high-speed Internet subscribers and 4.6 million phone subscribers and pass about 48.5 million homes in 39 states and Washington, D.C. The company operates in two segments, cable and programming. The cable segments, which generates approximately 95% of revenue, manages and operates the firm's cable systems, including video, high-speed Internet and phone services, as well as the regional sports and news networks. The programming segment consists primarily of consolidated national programming networks, including E!, The Golf Channel, VERSUS, G4 and Style. Comcast's other business interests include Comcast Spectacor and Comcast Interactive Media. Comcast Spectacor owns the Philadelphia Flyers, the Philadelphia 76ers and two large, multipurpose arenas in Philadelphia, in addition to managing other facilities for sporting events, concerts and other events. Comcast Interactive Media develops and operates the company's Internet businesses focused on entertainment, information and communication, including comcast.net, Fancast, thePlatform and Fandango. Recent acquisitions include Fandango, an online entertainment site and movie-ticket service; the cable system of Patriot Media; and Rainbow Media Holdings' 60% interest in Bay Area SportsNet and 50% interest in Sports Channel New England. In 2007, Comcast announced its fancast.com online entertainment site. Fancast has made a deal with CBS Interactive to provide CBS programming via the Fancast site, which will allow users to search for programming that is then downloaded to a DVR for viewing. In 2007, Comcast Interactive Media and Yahoo! entered into a multi-year strategic partnership for online display and video advertising services on comcast.net.

The company offers its employees health and life insurance; disability benefits; an employee assistance program; educational assistance; a 401(k) plan; and an employee stock purchase plan.

FINANCIALS: Sales and profits are in thousands of dollars—add 000 to get the full amount. 2007 Note: Financial information for 2007 was not available for all companies at press time.

2007 Sales: $30,895,000	2007 Profits: $2,587,000	**U.S. Stock Ticker: CMCSA**	
2006 Sales: $24,966,000	2006 Profits: $2,533,000	**Int'l Ticker:** Int'l Exchange:	
2005 Sales: $23,556,000	2005 Profits: $928,000	Employees: 100,000	
2004 Sales: $20,307,000	2004 Profits: $970,000	Fiscal Year Ends: 12/31	
2003 Sales: $18,348,000	2003 Profits: $3,240,000	Parent Company:	

SALARIES/BENEFITS:

Pension Plan:	ESOP Stock Plan:	Profit Sharing:	Top Exec. Salary: $2,638,500	Bonus: $7,770,068
Savings Plan: Y	Stock Purch. Plan: Y		Second Exec. Salary: $2,113,500	Bonus: $5,070,000

OTHER THOUGHTS:
Apparent Women Officers or Directors: 5
Hot Spot for Advancement for Women/Minorities: Y

LOCATIONS: ("Y" = Yes)

West:	Southwest:	Midwest:	Southeast:	Northeast:	International:
Y	Y	Y	Y	Y	Y

Note: Financial information, benefits and other data can change quickly and may vary from those stated here.

CONAGRA FOODS INC

www.conagrafoods.com

Industry Group Code: 311000 **Ranks within this company's industry group:** Sales: Profits:

Management:		Sales/Marketing:		Liberal Arts:		Information Systems:		Professionals:		Technical/Scientific:	
Mgmt. Trainees:	Y	Mktg. Professionals:	Y	Gen. Writing/Editing:	Y	Info. Management:	Y	Finance/Accounting:	Y	Engineers, Elec.:	Y
Experienced Mgmt.:	Y	Retail Sales:		Technical Writing:	Y	Software Dev.:	Y	Law:	Y	Engineers, Other:	
Int'l Business:	Y	Commercial/Industrial:	Y	Graphic Arts/Photog.:	Y	Hardware Dev.:		HR/Other:	Y	Health/Lab:	Y
MBA Graduates:	Y	Sales Trainees:		Music:		Systems Integration:		Training:	Y	Scientists/Research:	
		Advertising Pros.:	Y	Broadcasting:		Consulting/Other:		Health Care:		Petroleum/Chemicals:	
				Other:				Consulting:		Math/Other:	

TYPES OF BUSINESS:

Food Products Manufacturing
Food Ingredients
Meat Processing
Foodservice Supply

BRANDS/DIVISIONS/AFFILIATES:

Marie Callender's
Healthy Choice
Hunt's
Chef Boyardee
Peter Pan
Slim Jim
Orville Redenbacher's
Alexia Foods, Inc.

CONTACTS: *Note: Officers with more than one job title may be intentionally listed here more than once.*

Gary Rodkin, CEO
Andre J. Hawaux, CFO/Exec. VP
Joan K. Chow, Chief Mktg. Officer/Exec. VP
Peter M. Perez, Exec. VP-Human Resources
Al Bolles, Exec. VP-Research, Quality & Innovation
Owen Johnson, Chief Admin. Officer/Exec. VP
Robert F. Sharpe, Jr., Exec. VP-Legal & External Affairs
King Pouw, Exec. VP-Bus. Transformation
Doug Knudsen, Pres., ConAgra Food Sales
Jim Hardy, Jr., Exec. VP-Prod. Supply
Greg Heckman, Pres./COO-Commercial Prod.
Steven F. Goldstone, Chmn.

Phone: 402-595-4000	Fax: 402-595-4707
Toll-Free:	
Address: 1 ConAgra Dr., Omaha, NE 68102 US	

GROWTH PLANS/SPECIAL FEATURES:

ConAgra Foods, Inc. is a packaged food company serving grocery retailers, as well as restaurants and other food service establishments. It operates in four segments: consumer foods; food and ingredients; trading and merchandising; and international foods. The consumer foods segment includes branded, private label and customized food products that are sold in various retail and foodservice channels. Products include a variety of categories (meals, entrees, condiments, sides, snacks and desserts) across frozen, refrigerated and shelf-stable temperature classes. Brands include Chef Boyardee, Healthy Choice, Marie Callender's, Orville Redenbacher's, Slim Jim, Hebrew National, Kid Cuisine, Reddi-Wip, VanCamp, Libby's, LaChoy, The Max, David's, Angela Mia, Wesson, Swiss Miss, Egg Beaters, Blue Bonnet and Rosarita. The foods and ingredients segment includes commercially branded foods and ingredients that are sold principally to foodservice, food manufacturing and industrial customers. The division's primary products include specialty potato products, milled grain ingredients, dehydrated vegetables and seasonings, blends and flavors that are sold under brands such as Lamb Weston, Gilroy Foods and Spicetec to food processors. The trading and merchandising segment includes the sourcing, merchandising, marketing and distribution of agricultural and energy commodities. The international foods segment includes branded food products that are sold principally in retail channels in North America, Europe and Asia. Recently, the firm completed the divestitures of its packaged meats business, packaged cheese business, oat milling business and the refrigerated pizza business. In July 2007, ConAgra Foods acquired Alexia Foods, Inc., a New York-based private natural food company.

FINANCIALS: Sales and profits are in thousands of dollars—add 000 to get the full amount. 2007 Note: Financial information for 2007 was not available for all companies at press time.

2007 Sales: $12,028,200	2007 Profits: $764,600	U.S. Stock Ticker: CAG
2006 Sales: $11,482,000	2006 Profits: $533,800	Int'l Ticker: Int'l Exchange:
2005 Sales: $11,383,800	2005 Profits: $641,500	Employees: 24,500
2004 Sales: $10,926,300	2004 Profits: $811,300	Fiscal Year Ends: 5/31
2003 Sales: $19,839,000	2003 Profits: $774,800	Parent Company:

SALARIES/BENEFITS:

Pension Plan:	ESOP Stock Plan:	Profit Sharing:	Top Exec. Salary: $1,000,000	Bonus: $3,600,000
Savings Plan: Y	Stock Purch. Plan:		Second Exec. Salary: $600,000	Bonus: $1,350,000

OTHER THOUGHTS:

Apparent Women Officers or Directors: 2
Hot Spot for Advancement for Women/Minorities: Y

LOCATIONS: ("Y" = Yes)

West:	Southwest:	Midwest:	Southeast:	Northeast:	International:
Y	Y	Y	Y	Y	Y

Note: Financial information, benefits and other data can change quickly and may vary from those stated here.

CONOCOPHILLIPS COMPANY
www.conocophillips.com

Industry Group Code: 211111 Ranks within this company's industry group: Sales: 3 Profits: 3

Management:		Sales/Marketing:		Liberal Arts:		Information Systems:		Professionals:		Technical/Scientific:	
Mgmt. Trainees:	Y	Mktg. Professionals:	Y	Gen. Writing/Editing:	Y	Info. Management:	Y	Finance/Accounting:	Y	Engineers, Elec.:	Y
Experienced Mgmt.:	Y	Retail Sales:		Technical Writing:	Y	Software Dev.:	Y	Law:	Y	Engineers, Other:	
Int'l Business:	Y	Commercial/Industrial:	Y	Graphic Arts/Photog.:	Y	Hardware Dev.:		HR/Other:	Y	Health/Lab:	Y
MBA Graduates:	Y	Sales Trainees:		Music:		Systems Integration:		Training:	Y	Scientists/Research:	Y
		Advertising Pros.:	Y	Broadcasting:		Consulting/Other:		Health Care:		Petroleum/Chemicals:	Y
				Other:				Consulting:		Math/Other:	Y

TYPES OF BUSINESS:
Oil & Gas Exploration & Production
Natural Gas Distribution
Refining
Pipelines
Gasoline Retailing
Chemical Production
Technology Investment
Oil Sands Operations

BRANDS/DIVISIONS/AFFILIATES:
Duke Energy Field Services LLC
Conoco
Phillips 66
JET
Chevron Phillips Chemical Company LLC
LUKOIL
Kendall
76

CONTACTS: Note: Officers with more than one job title may be intentionally listed here more than once.
James J. Mulva, CEO
James J. Mulva, Pres.
John A. Carrig, CFO
James L. Gallogly, Exec. VP-Mktg.
Carin S. Knickel, VP-Human Resources
Gene L. Batchelder, CIO/Sr. VP-Svcs.
Stephen R. Brand, Sr. VP-Tech.
Luc J. Messier, Sr. VP-Prod. Dev.
Janet Langford Kelly, Sr. VP-Legal/General Counsel/Corp. Sec.
Sigmund L. Cornelius, Sr. VP-Planning & Strategy
Sigmund L. Cornelius, Sr. VP-Corp. Affairs
John A. Carrig, Exec. VP-Finance
Robert A. Ridge, VP-Health, Safety & Environment
John E. Lowe, Exec. VP-Exploration & Prod.
W.C.W Chiang, Sr. VP-Commercial
James J. Mulva, Chmn.
Ryan M. Lance, Pres., Exploration & Prod. Europe

Phone: 281-293-1000	Fax: 281-293-2819
Toll-Free: 800-840-1208	
Address: 600 N. Dairy Ashford Rd., Houston, TX 77079-1175 US	

GROWTH PLANS/SPECIAL FEATURES:

ConocoPhillips is an integrated global energy company. Its five business segments are: exploration and production, midstream, refining and marketing, chemicals and emerging businesses. The exploration and production segment focuses on crude oil, natural gas and natural gas liquids. It also mines oil sands to extract bitumen which it upgrades into synthetic crude oil. The midstream division gathers and processes natural gas, while the refining and marketing segment delivers brands like Phillips 66 and JET. The chemicals group manufactures petrochemicals and plastics, and the emerging businesses segment oversees businesses such as technologies related to carbon fibers, which are beyond the company's traditional operations. In March 2007, ConocoPhillips and EnCana Corporation agreed to create an integrated North American oil business consisting of two 50/50 operating partnerships, one Canadian upstream and one U.S. downstream. In 2008, the company acquired 50% ownership interest in Transcanada's Keystone Oil Pipeline, a project capable of producing 590,000 barrels of crude oil per day, scheduled to begin deliveries in 2009. The company is also seeking to advance negotiations with the state of Alaska to move forward with the Alaska North Slope gas pipeline project. The pipeline would transport approximately four billion cubic feet per day of natural gas from the Alaska North Slope to markets in Canada and the United States. Additionally, ConocoPhillips and Peabody Energy recently announced plans to begin development on a major commercial scale coal-to-gas facility in Kentucky.

ConocoPhillips' employees receive benefits including spending accounts, insurance, a retirement plan, paid time off, scholarships and tuition reimbursement.

FINANCIALS: Sales and profits are in thousands of dollars—add 000 to get the full amount. 2007 Note: Financial information for 2007 was not available for all companies at press time.

2007 Sales: $187,437,000	2007 Profits: $11,891,000	U.S. Stock Ticker: COP
2006 Sales: $183,650,000	2006 Profits: $15,550,000	Int'l Ticker: Int'l Exchange:
2005 Sales: $179,442,000	2005 Profits: $13,529,000	Employees: 32,600
2004 Sales: $135,076,000	2004 Profits: $8,129,000	Fiscal Year Ends: 12/31
2003 Sales: $105,097,000	2003 Profits: $4,735,000	Parent Company:

SALARIES/BENEFITS:
Pension Plan: Y	ESOP Stock Plan: Y	Profit Sharing:	Top Exec. Salary: $1,500,000	Bonus: $4,800,276
Savings Plan: Y	Stock Purch. Plan:		Second Exec. Salary: $695,000	Bonus: $1,176,761

OTHER THOUGHTS:
Apparent Women Officers or Directors: 2
Hot Spot for Advancement for Women/Minorities: Y

LOCATIONS: ("Y" = Yes)
West:	Southwest:	Midwest:	Southeast:	Northeast:	International:
Y	Y	Y	Y	Y	Y

Note: Financial information, benefits and other data can change quickly and may vary from those stated here.

CONSOL ENERGY INC
www.consolenergy.com

Industry Group Code: 212110 Ranks within this company's industry group: Sales: 2 Profits: 2

Management:		Sales/Marketing:		Liberal Arts:		Information Systems:		Professionals:		Technical/Scientific:	
Mgmt. Trainees:	Y	Mktg. Professionals:	Y	Gen. Writing/Editing:		Info. Management:	Y	Finance/Accounting:	Y	Engineers, Elec.:	Y
Experienced Mgmt.:	Y	Retail Sales:		Technical Writing:		Software Dev.:		Law:	Y	Engineers, Other:	
Int'l Business:	Y	Commercial/Industrial:		Graphic Arts/Photog.:		Hardware Dev.:		HR/Other:	Y	Health/Lab:	Y
MBA Graduates:	Y	Sales Trainees:		Music:		Systems Integration:		Training:	Y	Scientists/Research:	
		Advertising Pros.:		Broadcasting:		Consulting/Other:		Health Care:		Petroleum/Chemicals:	Y
				Other:				Consulting:		Math/Other:	

TYPES OF BUSINESS:
Coal Mining
Energy Services
Gas Exploration & Production

BRANDS/DIVISIONS/AFFILIATES:
CNX Gas Corporation
CNX Land Resources Inc

CONTACTS: Note: Officers with more than one job title may be intentionally listed here more than once.
J. Brett Harvey, CEO
J. Brett Harvey, Pres.
William J. Lyons, CFO
James L. McCaffrey, VP-Mktg. Services
Albert A. Aloila, Sr. VP-Human Resources
Steven E. Winberg, VP-R&D
George F. Rosato, VP-IT
Robert P. King, Sr. VP-Admin.
P. Jerome Richey, General Counsel/Chief Legal Officer/VP/Corp. Sec.
Thomas F. Hoffman, VP-Public Rel.
Thomas F. Hoffman, VP-Investor Rel.
John M. Reilly, VP/Treas.
Jack A. Holt, Sr. VP-Safety
Nicholas J. Deluliis, CEO/Pres., Gas Corp.
Peter B. Lilly, COO-Coal
Ronald E. Smith, COO-Gas Corp.
John L. Whitmire, Chmn.
James D. Kingsley, VP-Purchasing

Phone: 412-831-4000	**Fax:** 412-831-4103
Toll-Free:	
Address: Consol Plaza, 1800 Washington Rd., Pittsburgh, PA 15241-1421 US	

GROWTH PLANS/SPECIAL FEATURES:

CONSOL Energy, Inc. is a multi-fuel energy producer and energy services provider, primarily serving the U.S. electric power generation industry. It produces high-BTU bituminous coal from 17 mining complexes in the U.S., as well as pipeline-quality coalbed methane gas from coal properties in Pennsylvania, Virginia and West Virginia, and conventional gas from Tennessee and Virginia. The company's mining complexes contain an approximate reserve base of 4.3 billion tons of coal. CONSOL is the largest producer of bituminous coal in the U.S., as well as the largest coal producer from underground mines, the largest coal producer east of the Mississippi River and the largest coal exporter. The company owns five towboats and a fleet of approximately 300 barges, and it employs transportation specialists who negotiate freight and equipment agreements with railroads, barge lines, terminal operators, ocean vessel brokers and trucking companies. CONSOL's gas operations involve producing coalbed methane and natural gas. The company owns over 2,980 wells, primarily in Virginia, and has estimated proved reserves of approximately 1.3 trillion cubic feet of oil equivalent. Through its subsidiary, CNX Land Resources, Inc., the firm has timber and farming operations, as well as commercial development ventures. CNX Gas Corp., a wholly-owned subsidiary, produces pipeline-quality coalbed methane gas from coal properties in the Northern and Central Appalachian basin. In addition, the firm provides industrial supply services, terminal services, river and dock services and coal waste disposal services. In July 2008, the company announced a joint venture with Synthesis Energy Systems Inc., a global industrial gasification company, to develop a coal gasification and liquefaction plant in West Virginia.

CONSOL offers an employee compensation package which includes incentive compensation, employee assistance, relocation assistance, an employee credit union, on-going training options and an educational assistance program.

FINANCIALS: Sales and profits are in thousands of dollars—add 000 to get the full amount. 2007 Note: Financial information for 2007 was not available for all companies at press time.

2007 Sales: $3,762,197	2007 Profits: $267,782	**U.S. Stock Ticker: CNX**	
2006 Sales: $3,715,171	2006 Profits: $408,882	**Int'l Ticker:** Int'l Exchange:	
2005 Sales: $3,810,449	2005 Profits: $580,861	Employees: 7,253	
2004 Sales: $2,776,749	2004 Profits: $198,582	Fiscal Year Ends: 12/31	
2003 Sales: $2,222,466	2003 Profits: $-7,798	Parent Company:	

SALARIES/BENEFITS:

Pension Plan: Y	ESOP Stock Plan:	Profit Sharing:	Top Exec. Salary: $956,192	Bonus: $1,450,000
Savings Plan: Y	Stock Purch. Plan:		Second Exec. Salary: $541,346	Bonus: $111,505

OTHER THOUGHTS:
Apparent Women Officers or Directors:
Hot Spot for Advancement for Women/Minorities: Y

LOCATIONS: ("Y" = Yes)

West:	Southwest:	Midwest:	Southeast:	Northeast:	International:
Y				Y	Y

Note: Financial information, benefits and other data can change quickly and may vary from those stated here.

CONSOLIDATED EDISON INC

www.conedison.com

Industry Group Code: 221000 Ranks within this company's industry group: Sales: Profits:

Management:		Sales/Marketing:		Liberal Arts:		Information Systems:		Professionals:		Technical/Scientific:	
Mgmt. Trainees:	Y	Mktg. Professionals:	Y	Gen. Writing/Editing:	Y	Info. Management:	Y	Finance/Accounting:	Y	Engineers, Elec.:	Y
Experienced Mgmt.:	Y	Retail Sales:		Technical Writing:	Y	Software Dev.:	Y	Law:	Y	Engineers, Other:	
Int'l Business:	Y	Commercial/Industrial:	Y	Graphic Arts/Photog.:		Hardware Dev.:		HR/Other:	Y	Health/Lab:	
MBA Graduates:	Y	Sales Trainees:		Music:		Systems Integration:		Training:	Y	Scientists/Research:	
		Advertising Pros.:	Y	Broadcasting:		Consulting/Other:		Health Care:		Petroleum/Chemicals:	
				Other:				Consulting:		Math/Other:	

TYPES OF BUSINESS:

Utilities-Electricity & Natural Gas
Steam Utility
Electric Generation
Energy Consulting
Energy Marketing

BRANDS/DIVISIONS/AFFILIATES:

Orange and Rockland Utilities, Inc.
Consolidated Edison Company of New York, Inc.
Consolidated Edison Development
Consolidated Edison Solutions
Consolidated Edison Energy

CONTACTS: Note: Officers with more than one job title may be intentionally listed here more than once.

Kevin Burke, CEO
Kevin Burke, Pres.
Robert N. Hoglund, CFO/Sr. VP
Charles E. McTiernan, Jr., General Counsel
Gurudatta Nadkarni, VP-Strategic Planning
Jan C. Childress, Dir.-Investor Rel.
Edward J. Rasmussen, Controller/Chief Acct. Officer/VP
James P. O'Brien, Treas./VP
Carole Sobin, Corp. Sec.
Louis L. Rana, COO/Pres., Consolidated Energy Co. of NY, Inc.
John D. McMahon, CEO/Pres., Orange & Rockland Utilities, Inc.
Kevin Burke, Chmn.

Phone: 212-460-4600	Fax: 212-982-7816
Toll-Free:	
Address: 4 Irving Pl., Room 1618 S, New York, NY 10003 US	

GROWTH PLANS/SPECIAL FEATURES:

Consolidated Edison, Inc. (Con Edison) principally operates through the regulated electric, gas and steam utility segments of its two main subsidiaries, Consolidated Edison Company of New York, Inc. and Orange and Rockland Utilities, Inc. (O&R). Con Edison of New York provides electric services to New York City and most of Westchester County, a service area covering approximately 660 square miles with a population of over 9 million. The company provides gas services in Manhattan, the Bronx and parts of Queens and Westchester, and steam services in parts of Manhattan. The firm purchases all its electricity and gas from other suppliers. O&R and its subsidiaries provide electricity to southeastern New York, northern New Jersey and eastern Pennsylvania, an approximately 1,350-square-mile service area. The firm's non-utilities subsidiaries include Consolidated Edison Energy, Inc.; Consolidated Edison Development; and Consolidated Edison Solutions. Consolidated Edison Energy supplies wholesale energy and specialized energy supply services to customers in the electric and gas markets in the Northeast and Mid-Atlantic regions. Consolidated Edison Development owns, leases or operates energy and infrastructure projects, principally in the United States, and sells capacity and energy in wholesale markets administered by independent system operators in New England and New York and to other utilities through Consolidated Edison Energy. The segment currently owns the equivalent of 1,739 megawatts (MW) of capacity. Consolidated Edison Solutions is a leading non-residential retail energy and services provider, primarily selling electricity to industrial and large commercial customer and also to residential customers in 11 states and Washington D.C., serving approximately 48,300 customers, not including 176,000 served under a single aggregation agreement in Massachusetts. Con Edison Solutions sold 12.2 million megawatt hours (MWH) of electricity in 2007. In December 2007, Con Edison Development agreed to sell 1,706 megawatts of generation projects for $1.477 billion.

FINANCIALS: Sales and profits are in thousands of dollars—add 000 to get the full amount. 2007 Note: Financial information for 2007 was not available for all companies at press time.

2007 Sales: $13,120,000	2007 Profits: $929,000	U.S. Stock Ticker: ED
2006 Sales: $11,962,000	2006 Profits: $737,000	Int'l Ticker: Int'l Exchange:
2005 Sales: $11,641,000	2005 Profits: $719,000	Employees: 14,537
2004 Sales: $9,730,000	2004 Profits: $537,000	Fiscal Year Ends: 12/31
2003 Sales: $9,827,000	2003 Profits: $528,000	Parent Company:

SALARIES/BENEFITS:

Pension Plan: Y	ESOP Stock Plan:	Profit Sharing:	Top Exec. Salary: $1,000,000	Bonus: $755,000
Savings Plan: Y	Stock Purch. Plan: Y		Second Exec. Salary: $665,000	Bonus: $500,000

OTHER THOUGHTS:

Apparent Women Officers or Directors: 3
Hot Spot for Advancement for Women/Minorities: Y

LOCATIONS: ("Y" = Yes)

West:	Southwest:	Midwest:	Southeast:	Northeast:	International:
	Y	Y		Y	

CONTAINER STORE (THE)
www.containerstore.com

Industry Group Code: 442299 **Ranks within this company's industry group:** Sales: Profits:

Management:		Sales/Marketing:		Liberal Arts:		Information Systems:		Professionals:		Technical/Scientific:	
Mgmt. Trainees:	Y	Mktg. Professionals:	Y	Gen. Writing/Editing:	Y	Info. Management:	Y	Finance/Accounting:	Y	Engineers, Elec.:	
Experienced Mgmt.:	Y	Retail Sales:	Y	Technical Writing:		Software Dev.:	Y	Law:	Y	Engineers, Other:	
Int'l Business:		Commercial/Industrial:	Y	Graphic Arts/Photog.:	Y	Hardware Dev.:		HR/Other:	Y	Health/Lab:	
MBA Graduates:	Y	Sales Trainees:	Y	Music:		Systems Integration:		Training:	Y	Scientists/Research:	
		Advertising Pros.:	Y	Broadcasting:		Consulting/Other:		Health Care:		Petroleum/Chemicals:	
				Other:	Y			Consulting:		Math/Other:	

TYPES OF BUSINESS:
Home Organization Products, Retail
Luggage
Packing Materials
Specialty Boxes
Online Sales

BRANDS/DIVISIONS/AFFILIATES:
Elfa
Leonard Green & Partners

CONTACTS: Note: Officers with more than one job title may be intentionally listed here more than once.
Kip Tindell, CEO
Melissa Reiff, Pres.
Kip Tindell, Chmn.

Phone: 972-538-6000	Fax: 972-538-7623
Toll-Free: 800-733-3532	
Address: 500 Freeport Pkwy., Coppell, TX 75019 US	

GROWTH PLANS/SPECIAL FEATURES:

The Container Store is a national retailer known for its unique organizational and storage products and its commitment to customer service. The company sells drawer and cabinet organizers, luggage, tool racks, packing materials, specialty and shipping boxes and locker organizers, among many other household objects designed to manage space efficiently. Store interiors have an open layout, which is divided into sections with brightly colored banners such as Closet, Kitchen, Closet and Laundry. The firm's stores average 25,000 square feet and carry more than 10,000 items, with the company's Elfa brand of wire shelving making up nearly one-fifth of sales. The majority of the Container Store's 40 stores are located in large cities, including locations in Atlanta, Chicago, Houston, Miami, New York and San Diego. The Container Store processes and ships its entire product line from its 725,000-square-foot distribution center near Dallas, Texas. The distribution center uses state-of-the-art warehouse and inventory systems to increase profitability and response time. The company's web site allows customers to view and order store products, plan organizational and storage projects and receive free customized assistance from in-store space planning experts. In July 2007, the company was acquired by Leonard Green & Partners, a private investment firm.

The company offers its employees a benefits package that includes a 40% discount on merchandise, flexible spending plans, a 401(k) savings plan and special schedules for employees with children. Each full-time employee receives about 240 hours of training during his or her first year and almost one-half of new hires come from employee recommendations.

FINANCIALS: Sales and profits are in thousands of dollars—add 000 to get the full amount. 2007 Note: Financial information for 2007 was not available for all companies at press time.

2007 Sales: $	2007 Profits: $	U.S. Stock Ticker: Private
2006 Sales: $491,000	2006 Profits: $	Int'l Ticker: Int'l Exchange:
2005 Sales: $425,000	2005 Profits: $	Employees: 3,994
2004 Sales: $350,000	2004 Profits: $	Fiscal Year Ends: 3/31
2003 Sales: $300,000	2003 Profits: $	Parent Company: LEONARD GREEN & PARTNERS

SALARIES/BENEFITS:

Pension Plan:	ESOP Stock Plan:	Profit Sharing:	Top Exec. Salary: $	Bonus: $
Savings Plan: Y	Stock Purch. Plan:		Second Exec. Salary: $	Bonus: $

OTHER THOUGHTS:
Apparent Women Officers or Directors: 1
Hot Spot for Advancement for Women/Minorities:

LOCATIONS: ("Y" = Yes)

West:	Southwest:	Midwest:	Southeast:	Northeast:	International:
Y	Y	Y	Y	Y	

CONVERGYS CORPORATION

www.convergys.com

Industry Group Code: 522320 Ranks within this company's industry group: Sales: 3 Profits: 5

Management:		Sales/Marketing:		Liberal Arts:		Information Systems:		Professionals:		Technical/Scientific:	
Mgmt. Trainees:	Y	Mktg. Professionals:	Y	Gen. Writing/Editing:	Y	Info. Management:	Y	Finance/Accounting:	Y	Engineers, Elec.:	
Experienced Mgmt.:	Y	Retail Sales:		Technical Writing:		Software Dev.:	Y	Law:	Y	Engineers, Other:	
Int'l Business:	Y	Commercial/Industrial:	Y	Graphic Arts/Photog.:		Hardware Dev.:		HR/Other:	Y	Health/Lab:	
MBA Graduates:	Y	Sales Trainees:		Music:		Systems Integration:		Training:	Y	Scientists/Research:	
		Advertising Pros.:	Y	Broadcasting:		Consulting/Other:		Health Care:		Petroleum/Chemicals:	
				Other:				Consulting:		Math/Other:	

TYPES OF BUSINESS:

Outsourced Customer Care Services
Professional & Consulting Services
Information Management Solutions & Software
Human Resource Business Process Outsourcing Solutions

BRANDS/DIVISIONS/AFFILIATES:

Infinys
Wizard
ICOMS

CONTACTS: Note: Officers with more than one job title may be intentionally listed here more than once.

David F. Dougherty, CEO
David F. Dougherty, Pres.
Earl C. Shanks, CFO
Clark D. Handy, Sr. VP-Human Resources
Karen R. Bowman, General counsel/Corp. Sec.
Philip A. Odeen, Chmn.

Phone: 513-723-7000	Fax: 513-421-8624
Toll-Free: 800-284-9900	
Address: 201 E. 4th St., Cincinnati, OH 45202 US	

GROWTH PLANS/SPECIAL FEATURES:

Convergys Corp. is a global provider of customer care, billing and human resources services. It operates through three segments: customer care, information management and employee care. The customer care segment provides outsourced customer care services and professional and consulting services to in-house customer care operations. The division manages customer relationships on behalf of clients through multi-channel customer care contact centers and through consulting engagements. Phone and web-based agent-assisted service channels provide customers with assistance across the entire customer lifecycle. The company delivers these services using a variety of tools including computer telephony integration, interactive voice response, advanced speech recognition, knowledge-based management and the Internet through agent-assisted and self-service channels. The information management segment serves clients principally by providing and managing complex bulling and information software that addresses all segments of the communications industry, including wireless, wireline, cable, cable telephony, broadband, direct broadcast satellite and the Internet. The division's component-based framework supports the creation of billing and customer care solutions ranging from a single application to the combination of applications to a complete, end-to-end billing system. Products include the Infinys software; the ICOMS solution designed for the broadband convergent vide, high-speed data and telephony markets; and the Wizard solution designed to serve multimedia operators. The employee care segment provides human resource business process outsourcing solutions. Services include recruiting and resources; compensation; human resource administration; payroll administration; benefits administration; organizational development; learning; and business intelligence.

The company offers its employees medical, dental and vision insurance; life and AD&D insurance; disability insurance; tuition reimbursement; a 401(k) plan; a pension plan; and an employee stock purchase plan.

FINANCIALS: Sales and profits are in thousands of dollars—add 000 to get the full amount. 2007 Note: Financial information for 2007 was not available for all companies at press time.

2007 Sales: $2,844,300	2007 Profits: $169,500	**U.S. Stock Ticker: CVG**
2006 Sales: $2,789,800	2006 Profits: $166,200	**Int'l Ticker:** Int'l Exchange:
2005 Sales: $2,582,100	2005 Profits: $122,600	Employees: 75,000
2004 Sales: $2,487,700	2004 Profits: $111,500	Fiscal Year Ends: 12/31
2003 Sales: $2,288,800	2003 Profits: $171,600	Parent Company:

SALARIES/BENEFITS:

Pension Plan: Y	ESOP Stock Plan:	Profit Sharing:	Top Exec. Salary: $964,000	Bonus: $1,326,271
Savings Plan: Y	Stock Purch. Plan: Y		Second Exec. Salary: $563,333	Bonus: $738,365

OTHER THOUGHTS:

Apparent Women Officers or Directors: 1
Hot Spot for Advancement for Women/Minorities:

LOCATIONS: ("Y" = Yes)

West:	Southwest:	Midwest:	Southeast:	Northeast:	International:
Y	Y	Y	Y	Y	Y

Note: Financial information, benefits and other data can change quickly and may vary from those stated here.

COOPER COMPANIES INC

www.coopercos.com

Industry Group Code: 339113 Ranks within this company's industry group: Sales: 16　Profits: 15

Management:		Sales/Marketing:		Liberal Arts:		Information Systems:		Professionals:		Technical/Scientific:	
Mgmt. Trainees:	Y	Mktg. Professionals:	Y	Gen. Writing/Editing:		Info. Management:	Y	Finance/Accounting:	Y	Engineers, Elec.:	
Experienced Mgmt.:	Y	Retail Sales:		Technical Writing:	Y	Software Dev.:	Y	Law:	Y	Engineers, Other:	Y
Int'l Business:	Y	Commercial/Industrial:	Y	Graphic Arts/Photog.:		Hardware Dev.:		HR/Other:	Y	Health/Lab:	Y
MBA Graduates:	Y	Sales Trainees:		Music:		Systems Integration:		Training:	Y	Scientists/Research:	
		Advertising Pros.:		Broadcasting:		Consulting/Other:		Health Care:	Y	Petroleum/Chemicals:	
				Other:				Consulting:		Math/Other:	

TYPES OF BUSINESS:

Medical Devices
Contact Lenses
Gynecological Instruments
Diagnostic Products

BRANDS/DIVISIONS/AFFILIATES:

CooperVision, Inc.
CooperSurgical, Inc.
Cerveillance Scope
Lone Star Medical Products, Inc.
Wallach Surgical Decives Inc

CONTACTS: Note: Officers with more than one job title may be intentionally listed here more than once.

A. Thomas Bender, CEO
Robert S. Weiss, COO/Exec. VP/Pres., CooperVision
A. Thomas Bender, Pres.
Eugene J. Midlock, CFO/Sr. VP
Carol R. Kaufman, Chief Admin. Officer/Sr. VP-Legal Affairs/Sec.
Daniel G. McBride, General Counsel/VP
B. Norris Battin, VP-Comm.
Albert G. White, III, VP-Investor Rel.
Albert G. White, III, Treas.
John A. Weber, Pres.-CooperVision Inc.
Paul L. Remmell, Pres./COO-CooperSurgical, Inc.
Nicholas J. Pichotta, CEO-CooperSurgical, Inc.
Rodney E. Folden, Corp. Controller
A. Thomas Bender, Chmn.
Andrew Sedgwick, Pres.-EMEA, CooperVision, Inc.

Phone: 925-460-3600	Fax: 925-460-3649
Toll-Free: 800-538-7850	
Address: 6140 Stoneridge Mall Road, Pleasanton, CA 94588 US	

GROWTH PLANS/SPECIAL FEATURES:

Cooper Companies, Inc. develops, manufactures and markets healthcare products, primarily medical devices. The company operates through two business units: CooperVision, Inc. (CVI) and CooperSurgical, Inc. (CSI). CooperVision manufactures and markets a broad range of contact lenses for the worldwide vision correction market. CVI has two segments: spherical lenses and specialty lenses. CVI's core product lines include silicone hydrogel spherical lenses, single-use lenses and PC Technology brand spherical lenses. PC Technology products include Biomedics XC, Proclear 1 Day and Biofinity. Cooper's Proclear line of spherical, multifocal and toric lenses, are manufactured with omafilcon A, a material that incorporates a proprietary phosphorylcholine technology that helps enhance tissue-device compatibility. CooperVision's products are primarily manufactured at its facilities located in the U.K., Puerto Rico, Virginia and New York. CooperSurgical develops, manufactures and markets medical devices, diagnostic products and surgical instruments and accessories for the women's healthcare market used primarily by gynecologists and obstetricians. CSI has produced a number of products for in-office practices where physicians screen, diagnose and treat commonly occurring gynecological conditions. One such product is the digital colposcopy system, Cerveillance Scope. Using Cerveillance Scope, physicians can examine the cervix and then document, store and recall digital images of their findings. CooperSurgical's products are primarily manufactured and distributed at its facility in Connecticut. In February 2007, CSI acquired all of the outstanding shares of Wallach Surgical Devices Inc. for $20.0 million. Wallach's products consist of various diagnostic and therapeutic medical instruments primarily for in-office use in women's healthcare and other specialty instruments relating to dermatology, ophthalmology, anesthesiology, dentistry and veterinary medicine.

FINANCIALS: Sales and profits are in thousands of dollars—add 000 to get the full amount. 2007 Note: Financial information for 2007 was not available for all companies at press time.

2007 Sales: $950,641	2007 Profits: $-11,192	U.S. Stock Ticker: COO
2006 Sales: $858,960	2006 Profits: $66,234	Int'l Ticker:　Int'l Exchange:
2005 Sales: $806,617	2005 Profits: $91,722	Employees: 7,500
2004 Sales: $490,176	2004 Profits: $92,825	Fiscal Year Ends: 10/31
2003 Sales: $411,790	2003 Profits: $68,770	Parent Company:

SALARIES/BENEFITS:

Pension Plan:	ESOP Stock Plan:	Profit Sharing:	Top Exec. Salary: $725,000	Bonus: $95,156
Savings Plan:	Stock Purch. Plan:		Second Exec. Salary: $462,500	Bonus: $52,609

OTHER THOUGHTS:

Apparent Women Officers or Directors: 2
Hot Spot for Advancement for Women/Minorities:

LOCATIONS: ("Y" = Yes)

West:	Southwest:	Midwest:	Southeast:	Northeast:	International:
Y				Y	Y

COST PLUS INC

www.worldmarket.com

Industry Group Code: 442110 Ranks within this company's industry group: Sales: 1 Profits: 1

Management:		Sales/Marketing:		Liberal Arts:		Information Systems:		Professionals:		Technical/Scientific:	
Mgmt. Trainees:	Y	Mktg. Professionals:	Y	Gen. Writing/Editing:	Y	Info. Management:	Y	Finance/Accounting:	Y	Engineers, Elec.:	
Experienced Mgmt.:	Y	Retail Sales:	Y	Technical Writing:		Software Dev.:	Y	Law:	Y	Engineers, Other:	
Int'l Business:		Commercial/Industrial:	Y	Graphic Arts/Photog.:	Y	Hardware Dev.:		HR/Other:	Y	Health/Lab:	
MBA Graduates:	Y	Sales Trainees:	Y	Music:		Systems Integration:		Training:	Y	Scientists/Research:	
		Advertising Pros.:	Y	Broadcasting:		Consulting/Other:		Health Care:		Petroleum/Chemicals:	
				Other:	Y			Consulting:		Math/Other:	

TYPES OF BUSINESS:

Retail-Furniture
Housewares
Gifts
Accessories
Gourmet Foods
Wine
Imports

BRANDS/DIVISIONS/AFFILIATES:

World Market
World Market Stores
Cost Plus World Market
Cost Plus

CONTACTS: Note: Officers with more than one job title may be intentionally listed here more than once.

Barry J. Feld, CEO
Barry J. Feld, Pres.
Jane L. Baughman, CFO/Exec. VP
George K. Whitney, Sr. VP-Merchandising
Jane L. Baughman, Corp. Sec.
Michael J. Allen, Exec. VP-Store Oper.
Julie Joy, Senior National Wine Buyer
Fredric M. Roberts, Chmn.
Rayford K. whitley, Sr. VP-Supply Chain

Phone: 510-893-7300	Fax: 510-893-3681
Toll-Free: 877-967-5362	
Address: 200 Fourth St., Oakland, CA 94607 US	

GROWTH PLANS/SPECIAL FEATURES:

Cost Plus, Inc. is a specialty retailer of casual home furnishings and entertainment products. The company's 290 plus World Market stores in 34 states imports and features a selection of casual home furnishings, house wares, gifts, decorative accessories and gourmet foods and beverages imported from around the world. The firm's product offerings are designed to provide solutions to customers' casual living and home entertaining needs and are imported from more than 50 countries. The company purchases its merchandise from approximately 2,000 suppliers. Decorative items for the home include furniture, rugs, pillows, lamps, window coverings, frames and baskets. In addition, the company sells a number of tabletop and kitchen items such as glassware, ceramics, textiles and cooking utensils. As of February 2008, 61% of the company's sales were derived from home furnishings and 39% of sales were from consumables. Many of the firm's products are proprietary or private-label, often incorporating the firm's own designs, World Market brand name, quality standards and specifications. The average selling space of a Cost Plus World Market store is 15,700 square feet. The firm's stores have a twofold design. They attempt to evoke the feeling of a world marketplace through colorful and creative visual displays and merchandise presentations, including goods in open barrels and crates and cooking demonstrations. However, through concrete floors, open ceilings, and simple wooden fixtures, the stores' appearance is also meant to indicate that it is a low-price outlet. The company's expansion strategy is to open stores primarily in metropolitan and suburban markets that can support multiple stores.

Cost Plus offers its employees a 401(k) plan; a flexible spending account; employee assistance programs; health and wellness programs; a prescription drug plan; and medical, dental and vision coverage.

FINANCIALS: Sales and profits are in thousands of dollars—add 000 to get the full amount. 2007 Note: Financial information for 2007 was not available for all companies at press time.

2007 Sales: $1,040,309	2007 Profits: $-22,536	U.S. Stock Ticker: CPWM
2006 Sales: $970,441	2006 Profits: $16,589	Int'l Ticker: Int'l Exchange:
2005 Sales: $908,560	2005 Profits: $28,179	Employees: 6,741
2004 Sales: $801,566	2004 Profits: $32,988	Fiscal Year Ends: 2/3
2003 Sales: $692,300	2003 Profits: $28,400	Parent Company:

SALARIES/BENEFITS:

Pension Plan:	ESOP Stock Plan:	Profit Sharing:	Top Exec. Salary: $375,000	Bonus: $
Savings Plan: Y	Stock Purch. Plan:		Second Exec. Salary: $309,615	Bonus: $

OTHER THOUGHTS:

Apparent Women Officers or Directors: 2
Hot Spot for Advancement for Women/Minorities: Y

LOCATIONS: ("Y" = Yes)

West:	Southwest:	Midwest:	Southeast:	Northeast:	International:
Y	Y	Y	Y	Y	

COSTCO WHOLESALE CORP

www.costco.com

Industry Group Code: 452910A Ranks within this company's industry group: Sales: 1 Profits: 1

Management:		Sales/Marketing:		Liberal Arts:		Information Systems:		Professionals:		Technical/Scientific:	
Mgmt. Trainees:	Y	Mktg. Professionals:	Y	Gen. Writing/Editing:	Y	Info. Management:	Y	Finance/Accounting:	Y	Engineers, Elec.:	
Experienced Mgmt.:	Y	Retail Sales:	Y	Technical Writing:		Software Dev.:	Y	Law:	Y	Engineers, Other:	
Int'l Business:	Y	Commercial/Industrial:	Y	Graphic Arts/Photog.:	Y	Hardware Dev.:		HR/Other:	Y	Health/Lab:	
MBA Graduates:	Y	Sales Trainees:	Y	Music:		Systems Integration:		Training:	Y	Scientists/Research:	
		Advertising Pros.:	Y	Broadcasting:		Consulting/Other:		Health Care:		Petroleum/Chemicals:	
				Other:	Y			Consulting:		Math/Other:	

TYPES OF BUSINESS:

Warehouse Clubs, Retail
Food
Health & Beauty Products
Electronics
Furniture
Apparel
Automotive Supplies
Gasoline Sales

BRANDS/DIVISIONS/AFFILIATES:

Costco Wholesale Industries

CONTACTS: Note: Officers with more than one job title may be intentionally listed here more than once.

James D. Sinegal, CEO
W. Craig Jelinek, COO
James D. Sinegal, Pres.
Richard A. Galanti, CFO/Exec. VP
John Matthews, Sr. VP-Human Resources
Don Burdick, Sr. VP-Info. Sys.
W. Craig Jelinek, Exec. VP-Merch.
Joel Benoliel, Sr. VP-Admin.
Joel Benoliel, Chief Legal Officer
Richard D. DiCerchio, COO-Global Oper.
Richard C. Chavez, Sr. VP-Bus. Dev.
Ginnie M. Roeglin, Sr. VP-e-Commerce & Publishing
David S. Petterson, Corp. Controller/Sr. VP
Charles V. Burnett, Sr. VP-Pharmacy
Jaime Gonzalez, Sr. VP/Gen. Mgr.-Mexico
Joseph P. Portera, Exec. VP/COO-Eastern & Canadian Div.
Thomas K. Walker, Exec. VP-Construction & Dist.
Jeffrey H. Brotman, Chmn.
James P. Murphy, Sr. VP-Int'l Oper.
Richard D. DiCerchio, COO-Distribution/Sr. Exec. VP

Phone: 425-313-8100	Fax: 425-313-8103
Toll-Free:	
Address: 999 Lake Dr., Issaquah, WA 98027 US	

GROWTH PLANS/SPECIAL FEATURES:

Costco Wholesale Corp. operates membership warehouses based on the concept that offering members very low prices on a limited selection of branded and private-label products will produce high sales volumes and rapid inventory turnover. This rapid turnover, combined with volume purchasing, efficient distribution and reduced handling of merchandise in self-service warehouse facilities, allows the firm to operate at significantly lower margins than traditional discount retailers. Costco buys the majority of its merchandise directly from manufacturers for shipment to warehouses or to consolidation points, minimizing freight and handling costs. Products include health and beauty aids, cleaning supplies, foods, alcohol, appliances, electronics, tools, office supplies, furniture, automotive supplies, apparel, cameras, housewares and books. Stores contain other features, including pharmacies, print shops, photo labs and gas stations. Memberships are designed to build customer loyalty and cost between $40 and $100 per year. Costco has approximately 5.4 million business members and approximately 18.6 million Gold Star (individual) members. The firm operates 543 stores in the U.S., U.K., Canada, Mexico, Korea, Taiwan and Japan. The stores average approximately 140,000 square feet and stock around 4,000 distinct products, including upscale items such as jewelry and wines. Costco Wholesale Industries, a division of the company, operates manufacturing businesses, including special food packaging, optical laboratories, meat processing and jewelry distribution.

Costco offers employee benefits including employee assistance, free store memberships, a pharmacy program and many other benefits. It promotes the majority of its management from within.

FINANCIALS: Sales and profits are in thousands of dollars—add 000 to get the full amount. 2007 Note: Financial information for 2007 was not available for all companies at press time.

2007 Sales: $63,087,601	2007 Profits: $1,082,772	U.S. Stock Ticker: COST
2006 Sales: $58,963,180	2006 Profits: $1,103,215	Int'l Ticker: Int'l Exchange:
2005 Sales: $51,789,080	2005 Profits: $1,063,092	Employees: 127,000
2004 Sales: $47,148,627	2004 Profits: $882,393	Fiscal Year Ends: 8/31
2003 Sales: $41,694,561	2003 Profits: $721,000	Parent Company:

SALARIES/BENEFITS:

Pension Plan:	ESOP Stock Plan:	Profit Sharing:	Top Exec. Salary: $535,096	Bonus: $200,000
Savings Plan: Y	Stock Purch. Plan: Y		Second Exec. Salary: $535,096	Bonus: $81,917

OTHER THOUGHTS:

Apparent Women Officers or Directors: 1
Hot Spot for Advancement for Women/Minorities:

LOCATIONS: ("Y" = Yes)

West:	Southwest:	Midwest:	Southeast:	Northeast:	International:
Y	Y	Y	Y	Y	Y

COVANCE INC

www.covance.com

Industry Group Code: 541710 Ranks within this company's industry group: Sales: 2 Profits: 2

Management:		Sales/Marketing:		Liberal Arts:		Information Systems:		Professionals:		Technical/Scientific:	
Mgmt. Trainees:	Y	Mktg. Professionals:	Y	Gen. Writing/Editing:		Info. Management:	Y	Finance/Accounting:	Y	Engineers, Elec.:	
Experienced Mgmt.:	Y	Retail Sales:		Technical Writing:	Y	Software Dev.:	Y	Law:	Y	Engineers, Other:	Y
Int'l Business:	Y	Commercial/Industrial:	Y	Graphic Arts/Photog.:	Y	Hardware Dev.:		HR/Other:	Y	Health/Lab:	Y
MBA Graduates:	Y	Sales Trainees:		Music:		Systems Integration:	Y	Training:	Y	Scientists/Research:	Y
		Advertising Pros.:	Y	Broadcasting:		Consulting/Other:	Y	Health Care:	Y	Petroleum/Chemicals:	
				Other:				Consulting:	Y	Math/Other:	Y

TYPES OF BUSINESS:

Pharmaceutical Research & Development
Drug Preclinical/Clinical Trials
Laboratory Testing & Analysis
Approval Assistance
Health Economics & Outcomes Services
Online Tools

BRANDS/DIVISIONS/AFFILIATES:

LabLink
Study Tracker
Trial Tracker

CONTACTS: *Note: Officers with more than one job title may be intentionally listed here more than once.*

Joseph L. Herring, CEO
Wendel Barr, COO/Exec. VP
William Klitgaard, CFO/Sr. VP
Donald Kraft, Sr. VP-Human Resources
James W. Lovett, General Counsel/Sr. VP
Joseph L. Herring, Chmn.
Anthony Cork, Sr. VP/Pres., Early Dev. Europe

Phone: 609-452-4440	Fax: 609-452-9375
Toll-Free: 888-268-2623	
Address: 210 Carnegie Ctr., Princeton, NJ 08540 US	

GROWTH PLANS/SPECIAL FEATURES:

Covance, Inc. is a leading drug development services company and contract research organization. It provides a wide range of product development services to pharmaceutical, biotechnology and medical device industries across the globe. The company also provides laboratory testing services for clients in the chemical, agrochemical and food businesses. The firm operates two business segments: Early development services and late-stage development services. Covance's early development services include preclinical services (such as toxicology, pharmaceutical development, research products and a bioanalytical testing service) and Phase I clinical services. Its late-stage development services cover clinical development and support; clinical trials; periapproval and market access; and central laboratory operations. Covance has also introduced several Internet-based products: Study Tracker is an Internet-based client access product, which permits customers of toxicology services to review study data and schedules on a near real-time basis; LabLink is a client access program that allows customers of central laboratory services to review and query lab data on a near real-time basis; and Trial Tracker is a web-enabled clinical trial project management and tracking tool intended to allow both employees and customers of its late-stage clinical business to review and manage all aspects of clinical-trial projects. In November 2007, the company sold its ECG business (which had been part of the late stage development segment) to eResearch Technology, Inc. for roughly $35 million.

Covance offers its employees benefits such as medical, dental and vision plans; a range of insurance benefits; employee assistance; financial planning services; and tuition reimbursement.

FINANCIALS: Sales and profits are in thousands of dollars—add 000 to get the full amount. 2007 Note: Financial information for 2007 was not available for all companies at press time.

2007 Sales: $1,631,516	2007 Profits: $175,929	**U.S. Stock Ticker: CVD**
2006 Sales: $1,406,058	2006 Profits: $144,998	**Int'l Ticker:** Int'l Exchange:
2005 Sales: $1,250,400	2005 Profits: $119,600	Employees: 8,700
2004 Sales: $1,056,397	2004 Profits: $97,947	Fiscal Year Ends: 12/31
2003 Sales: $974,210	2003 Profits: $76,136	Parent Company:

SALARIES/BENEFITS:

Pension Plan:	ESOP Stock Plan:	Profit Sharing:	Top Exec. Salary: $591,667	Bonus: $1,347,475
Savings Plan: Y	Stock Purch. Plan: Y		Second Exec. Salary: $308,646	Bonus: $219,854

OTHER THOUGHTS:

Apparent Women Officers or Directors: 2
Hot Spot for Advancement for Women/Minorities: Y

LOCATIONS: ("Y" = Yes)

West:	Southwest:	Midwest:	Southeast:	Northeast:	International:
Y	Y	Y	Y	Y	Y

COVENTRY HEALTH CARE INC   www.coventryhealth.com

Industry Group Code: 524114 Ranks within this company's industry group: Sales: 4 Profits: 4

Management:		Sales/Marketing:		Liberal Arts:		Information Systems:		Professionals:		Technical/Scientific:	
Mgmt. Trainees:	Y	Mktg. Professionals:	Y	Gen. Writing/Editing:	Y	Info. Management:	Y	Finance/Accounting:	Y	Engineers, Elec.:	
Experienced Mgmt.:	Y	Retail Sales:		Technical Writing:	Y	Software Dev.:	Y	Law:	Y	Engineers, Other:	Y
Int'l Business:		Commercial/Industrial:	Y	Graphic Arts/Photog.:	Y	Hardware Dev.:		HR/Other:	Y	Health/Lab:	
MBA Graduates:	Y	Sales Trainees:		Music:		Systems Integration:		Training:	Y	Scientists/Research:	Y
		Advertising Pros.:	Y	Broadcasting:		Consulting/Other:		Health Care:	Y	Petroleum/Chemicals:	
				Other:				Consulting:		Math/Other:	

TYPES OF BUSINESS:
Health Plans
Insurance
Managed Care Products

BRANDS/DIVISIONS/AFFILIATES:
Altius Health Plans
Carelink Health Plans
HealthAmerica
HealthAssurance
OmniCare
PersonalCare
WellPath
Southern Health

CONTACTS: *Note: Officers with more than one job title may be intentionally listed here more than once.*
Dale B. Wolf, CEO
Thomas P. McDonough, Pres.
Shawn M. Guertin, CFO/Exec. VP
Patrisha L. Davis, Sr. VP-Chief Human Resources
Thomas Zielinski, General Counsel/Exec. VP
John J. Ruhlmann, Sr. VP/Corp. Controller
Harvey C. DeMovick, Jr., Exec. VP
Francis S. Soistman, Jr., Exec. VP-Health Plan Oper.
Vishu Jhaveri, Exec. VP
E. Harry (Skip) Creasey, Sr. VP
John H. Austin, Chmn.

Phone: 301-581-0600	Fax: 301-493-0742
Toll-Free:	
Address: 6705 Rockledge Dr., Ste. 900, Bethesda, MD 20817 US	

GROWTH PLANS/SPECIAL FEATURES:
Coventry Healthcare Inc. is a diversified national managed healthcare company operating health plans, insurance companies, network rental and workers' compensation services companies. The firm provides a full range of risk and fee-based managed care products and services to a broad cross section of individuals, employer and government-funded groups, government agencies, and other insurance carriers. The firm operates three divisions: commercial business, individual consumer and government business, and specialty business divisions. The commercial business division provides products to a cross section of employer groups of all sizes including health maintenance organization (HMO), preferred provider organizations (PPO), and point of service (POS) products. The company offers these products on an underwritten or risk basis where they receive a monthly premium in exchange for assuming underwriting risks including all medical and administrative costs. The individual consumer & government division provides comprehensive health benefits to members participating in the Medicare Advantage HMO, Medicare Advantage PPO, Medicare Advantage Private-Fee-For-Service, Medicare Prescription Drug, and Medicaid programs and receives premium payments from federal and state governments. The specialty business division provides workers' compensation managed care services on a fee-based basis, with products that include access to a provider network, pharmacy benefits management, field case management, telephonic case management, and independent medical exam and bill review capabilities. The firm's health plans are operated under the names; Altius Health Plans; Carelink Health Plans; Coventry Health Care; Coventry Health and Life; Group Health Plan; HealthAmerica; HealthAssurance; HealthCare USA; OmniCare; PersonalCare, Southern Health; Vista and WellPath. In September 2007, the firm acquired Florida Health Plan Administrators, LLC,. In February 13, 2008, the company acquired Mental Health Network Institutional Services, Inc.

The company offers its employees medical, dental and vision insurance; flexible spending accounts; a 401(k) plan; tuition assistance; and an employee assistance plan.

FINANCIALS: Sales and profits are in thousands of dollars—add 000 to get the full amount. 2007 Note: Financial information for 2007 was not available for all companies at press time.

2007 Sales: $9,879,531	2007 Profits: $626,094	**U.S. Stock Ticker:** CVH
2006 Sales: $7,733,756	2006 Profits: $560,045	**Int'l Ticker:** Int'l Exchange:
2005 Sales: $6,611,246	2005 Profits: $501,639	Employees: 10,250
2004 Sales: $5,311,969	2004 Profits: $337,117	Fiscal Year Ends: 12/31
2003 Sales: $4,535,143	2003 Profits: $250,145	Parent Company:

SALARIES/BENEFITS:
Pension Plan:	ESOP Stock Plan:	Profit Sharing:	Top Exec. Salary: $850,000	Bonus: $3,532,047
Savings Plan: Y	Stock Purch. Plan:		Second Exec. Salary: $850,000	Bonus: $3,076,985

OTHER THOUGHTS:
Apparent Women Officers or Directors: 1
Hot Spot for Advancement for Women/Minorities:

LOCATIONS: ("Y" = Yes)
West:	Southwest:	Midwest:	Southeast:	Northeast:	International:
				Y	

COX COMMUNICATIONS INC

www.cox.com

Industry Group Code: 513220 Ranks within this company's industry group: Sales: Profits:

Management:		Sales/Marketing:		Liberal Arts:		Information Systems:		Professionals:		Technical/Scientific:	
Mgmt. Trainees:	Y	Mktg. Professionals:	Y	Gen. Writing/Editing:	Y	Info. Management:	Y	Finance/Accounting:	Y	Engineers, Elec.:	Y
Experienced Mgmt.:	Y	Retail Sales:		Technical Writing:		Software Dev.:	Y	Law:	Y	Engineers, Other:	
Int'l Business:	Y	Commercial/Industrial:	Y	Graphic Arts/Photog.:	Y	Hardware Dev.:		HR/Other:	Y	Health/Lab:	
MBA Graduates:	Y	Sales Trainees:		Music:		Systems Integration:		Training:	Y	Scientists/Research:	
		Advertising Pros.:	Y	Broadcasting:	Y	Consulting/Other:		Health Care:		Petroleum/Chemicals:	
				Other:	Y			Consulting:		Math/Other:	

TYPES OF BUSINESS:

Cable TV Service
Digital Cable TV Service
Cable-Based Internet Access
Local & Long-Distance Phone Service
Video-On-Demand
VOIP Service
Commercial Telecommunications Services

BRANDS/DIVISIONS/AFFILIATES:

Cox Enterprises, Inc.
Cox Cable
Cox Digital Cable
Cox High Speed
Cox Digital Telephone
Cox Business Services
Phone Tools

CONTACTS: Note: Officers with more than one job title may be intentionally listed here more than once.

James O. Robbins, CEO
Patrick J. Esser, Pres.
Jimmy W. Hayes, CFO/Exec. VP/Pres., Admin.
Joseph J. Rooney, Chief Mktg. Officer/Sr. VP
Mae A. Douglas, Chief People Officer/Sr. VP
Scott A. Hatfield, CIO/Sr. VP
Christopher J. Bowick, CTO/Sr. VP
Steve M. Gorman, VP-Prod. Mgmt.
Christopher J. Bowick, Sr. VP-Eng.
James A. Hatcher, Sr. VP-Legal & Regulatory Affairs
Jill Campbell, Sr. VP-Oper.
Dallas S. Clement, Sr. VP-Strategy & Dev.
Steve M. Gorman, VP-Internet Mktg.
James Ashurst, VP-Comm.
J. Lacey Lewis, VP-Investor Rel.
Jimmy W. Hayes, Pres., Finance
Susan W. Coker, VP/Treas.
Robert C. Wilson, Sr. VP-Programming
Sheila Crosby, VP-Sales & Dist.
William J. Fitzsimmons, Chief Acct. Officer/VP-Acct. & Financial Planning
James Cox Kennedy, Chmn.

Phone: 404-843-5000	Fax: 404-843-5939
Toll-Free:	
Address: 1400 Lake Hearn Dr. NE, Atlanta, GA 30319 US	

GROWTH PLANS/SPECIAL FEATURES:

Cox Communications, Inc., owned by Cox Enterprises, Inc. is the U.S.'s third-largest cable broadband communications company, with cable systems in 20 states serving over six million customers nationwide. Cox offers a variety of residential services through its subsidiaries, including cable television under the Cox Cable brand; advanced digital video programming services under the Cox Digital Cable brand; high-speed Internet access via Cox High Speed; local and long-distance telephone services under the Cox Digital Telephone brand; and commercial voice, video and data services via Cox Business Services. The firm invests in telecommunications companies such as Sprint PCS, as well as programming networks, including the Discovery Channel and TV Works, a provider of software for digital cable systems. Cable television services include basic cable, expanded cable, broadband Internet-supported VoIP service, pay-per-view and entertainment-on-demand packages. Cox has a joint venture with Sprint, Time Warner, Comcast, Nextel and Andvance/Newhouse that offers a combined package of cable TV, high-speed Internet access, VOIP and cellular service for a single price. In addition, the firm owns and operates the Travel Channel. In 2007, Cox extended its On DEMAND service to its Gainesville/Ocala and Pensacola/Fort Walton, Florida markets. Also in 2007, the company entered into an agreement with Discovery Communications to significantly expand its HD line-up with four high-definition (HD) networks: Discovery Channel; TLC; Animal Planet; and The Science Channel, to be launched on a market-by-market basis. Cox then furthered its HD offering with Turner Networks by adding CNN and TBS.

Cox employees receive discounted cable television, health club discounts and free tickets to cultural and sporting events. It offers tuition reimbursement, 150 free online courses and discounts through Dell, Sprint, GM, Ford and Phillips Electronics. Other benefits include adoption assistance, an employee assistance program, a pension plan, a 401(k) savings plan and an employee stock purchase plan.

FINANCIALS: Sales and profits are in thousands of dollars—add 000 to get the full amount. 2007 Note: Financial information for 2007 was not available for all companies at press time.

2007 Sales: $8,300,000	2007 Profits: $	U.S. Stock Ticker: Subsidiary
2006 Sales: $7,300,000	2006 Profits: $	Int'l Ticker: Int'l Exchange:
2005 Sales: $7,054,300	2005 Profits: $-230,700	Employees:
2004 Sales: $6,106,100	2004 Profits: $-2,375,300	Fiscal Year Ends: 12/31
2003 Sales: $5,458,800	2003 Profits: $-137,801	Parent Company: COX ENTERPRISES INC

SALARIES/BENEFITS:

Pension Plan: Y	ESOP Stock Plan:	Profit Sharing:	Top Exec. Salary: $1,322,900	Bonus: $1,166,798
Savings Plan: Y	Stock Purch. Plan: Y		Second Exec. Salary: $760,000	Bonus: $574,560

OTHER THOUGHTS:

Apparent Women Officers or Directors: 12
Hot Spot for Advancement for Women/Minorities: Y

LOCATIONS: ("Y" = Yes)

West:	Southwest:	Midwest:	Southeast:	Northeast:	International:
Y	Y	Y	Y	Y	

Note: Financial information, benefits and other data can change quickly and may vary from those stated here.

CR BARD INC

www.crbard.com

Industry Group Code: 339113 **Ranks within this company's industry group:** Sales: 9   Profits: 7

Management:		Sales/Marketing:		Liberal Arts:		Information Systems:		Professionals:		Technical/Scientific:	
Mgmt. Trainees:	Y	Mktg. Professionals:	Y	Gen. Writing/Editing:	Y	Info. Management:	Y	Finance/Accounting:	Y	Engineers, Elec.:	Y
Experienced Mgmt.:	Y	Retail Sales:		Technical Writing:	Y	Software Dev.:	Y	Law:	Y	Engineers, Other:	Y
Int'l Business:	Y	Commercial/Industrial:	Y	Graphic Arts/Photog.:	Y	Hardware Dev.:	Y	HR/Other:	Y	Health/Lab:	Y
MBA Graduates:	Y	Sales Trainees:	Y	Music:		Systems Integration:		Training:	Y	Scientists/Research:	Y
		Advertising Pros.:	Y	Broadcasting:		Consulting/Other:		Health Care:	Y	Petroleum/Chemicals:	
				Other:				Consulting:		Math/Other:	Y

TYPES OF BUSINESS:

Equipment-Urological Catheters
Diagnostic and Interventional Products
Minimally Invasive Vascular Products
Surgical Specialty Products
Supply Chain and Business Services

BRANDS/DIVISIONS/AFFILIATES:

Specialized Health Products International, Inc
LifeStent
Bard Medical Systems
Bard Peripheral Vascular-Biopsy
Bard Peripheral Vascular-Interventional
Genyx Medical, Inc.
Salute Fixation
Davol, Inc.

CONTACTS: Note: Officers with more than one job title may be intentionally listed here more than once.

Timothy M. Ring, CEO
John H. Weiland, COO
John H. Weiland, Pres.
Todd C. Schermerhorn, CFO/Sr. VP
Bronwen K. Kelly, VP-Human Resources
John A. DeFord, VP-Science, Tech. & Clinical Affairs
Vincent J. Gurnari, Jr., VP-IT
Stephen J. Long, General Counsel/Sec./VP
Joseph A. Cherry, VP-Oper.
Holly Glass, VP-Gov't & Public Rel.
Eric J. Shick, VP-Investor Rel.
Scott T. Lowry, VP/Treas.
Amy S. Paul, Group VP
Brian P. Kelly, Group VP
James M. Howard, VP-Regulatory Sciences
Christopher D. Ganser, VP-Quality, Environmental Sciences & Safety
Timothy M. Ring, Chmn.
Sharon M. Alterio, Group VP-Int'l

Phone: 908-277-8000	Fax: 908-277-8240
Toll-Free: 800-367-2273	
Address: 730 Central Ave., Murray Hill, NJ 07974 US	

GROWTH PLANS/SPECIAL FEATURES:

C.R. Bard, Inc. designs, manufactures, packages, distributes and sells medical, surgical and diagnostic devices. The company's line of minimally invasive vascular products includes peripheral angioplasty stents, catheters, guidewires, introducers and accessories, vena cava filters and biopsy devices. Additional products include cardiac mapping and electrophysiology laboratory systems, as well as diagnostic and temporary pacing electrode catheters; fabrics and meshes; and implantable blood vessel replacements. The firm's surgical specialty products include meshes for vessel and hernia repair; irrigation devices for orthopedic, laparoscopic and gynecological procedures; and products for topical hemostasis. These products include the PerFix plug, Kugel patch, Composix sheet, HydroFlex Multi-Application Irrigation Pump System, Avitene and Avifoam. Hernia operations using these products can be done in an outpatient setting in as little as 20 minutes. The company's products are distributed in the U.S. directly to hospitals and other health care institutions, as well as through numerous hospital/surgical supply and other medical specialty distributors. Internationally, C.R. Bard markets its products through 20 subsidiaries and a joint venture. About 62% of C.R. Bard's international sales are products manufactured in the U.S., Puerto Rico or Mexico. In November 2007, the firm's Agento IC silver-coated endotracheal tube was cleared for sale by the FDA. In January 2008, C.R. Bard acquired the assets of the LifeStent family of products from Edwards Lifesciences Corporation. In June 2008, C.R. Bard Inc. finalized the acquisition of the remaining shares of Specialized Health Products International, Inc.

FINANCIALS: Sales and profits are in thousands of dollars—add 000 to get the full amount. 2007 Note: Financial information for 2007 was not available for all companies at press time.

2007 Sales: $2,202,000	2007 Profits: $406,400	U.S. Stock Ticker: BCR	
2006 Sales: $1,979,600	2006 Profits: $272,100	Int'l Ticker:	Int'l Exchange:
2005 Sales: $1,771,300	2005 Profits: $337,100	Employees: 9,400	
2004 Sales: $1,656,100	2004 Profits: $302,800	Fiscal Year Ends: 12/31	
2003 Sales: $1,433,100	2003 Profits: $233,000	Parent Company:	

SALARIES/BENEFITS:

Pension Plan: Y	ESOP Stock Plan:	Profit Sharing:	Top Exec. Salary: $900,000	Bonus: $1,389,420
Savings Plan: Y	Stock Purch. Plan:		Second Exec. Salary: $726,500	Bonus: $905,502

OTHER THOUGHTS:

Apparent Women Officers or Directors: 4
Hot Spot for Advancement for Women/Minorities: Y

LOCATIONS: ("Y" = Yes)

West:	Southwest:	Midwest:	Southeast:	Northeast:	International:
Y	Y	Y	Y	Y	Y

Note: Financial information, benefits and other data can change quickly and may vary from those stated here.

CSX CORP

www.csx.com

Industry Group Code: 482110 Ranks within this company's industry group: Sales: 3 Profits: 4

Management:		Sales/Marketing:		Liberal Arts:		Information Systems:		Professionals:		Technical/Scientific:	
Mgmt. Trainees:		Mktg. Professionals:	Y	Gen. Writing/Editing:		Info. Management:	Y	Finance/Accounting:	Y	Engineers, Elec.:	Y
Experienced Mgmt.:	Y	Retail Sales:		Technical Writing:	Y	Software Dev.:	Y	Law:	Y	Engineers, Other:	Y
Int'l Business:	Y	Commercial/Industrial:	Y	Graphic Arts/Photog.:		Hardware Dev.:		HR/Other:	Y	Health/Lab:	
MBA Graduates:	Y	Sales Trainees:		Music:		Systems Integration:	Y	Training:	Y	Scientists/Research:	
		Advertising Pros.:	Y	Broadcasting:		Consulting/Other:	Y	Health Care:		Petroleum/Chemicals:	
				Other:				Consulting:		Math/Other:	

TYPES OF BUSINESS:

Railroad Transportation
Intermodal Services
Logistics Software & Services
Real Estate
Resort Operations
Automotive Distribution & Storage

BRANDS/DIVISIONS/AFFILIATES:

CSX Transportation, Inc.
CSX Intermodal, Inc.
CSX Real Property, Inc.
CSX Hotels, Inc.
Greenbrier (The)
CSX Technology
TRANSFLO
Total Distribution Services, Inc.

CONTACTS: Note: Officers with more than one job title may be intentionally listed here more than once.

Michael J. Ward, CEO
Michael J. Ward, Pres.
Oscar Munoz, CFO/Exec. VP
Clarence W. Gooden, Exec. VP-Mktg. & Sales
Robert J. Haulter, Sr. VP-Human Resources & Labor Rel.
Ellen M. Fitzsimmons, General Counsel/Corp. Sec.
Lester M. Passa, Sr. VP-Strategic Planning
David A. Boor, VP-Tax/Treas.
Ellen M. Fitzsimmons, Sr. VP-Law & Public Affairs
Michael J. Ruehling, VP-Federal Legislation
Clarence W. Gooden, Chief Commercial Officer
Carolyn T. Sizemore, Controller/VP
Michael J. Ward, Chmn.

Phone: 904-359-3200	Fax: 904-633-3450
Toll-Free:	
Address: 500 Water St., 15th Fl., Jacksonville, FL 32202 US	

GROWTH PLANS/SPECIAL FEATURES:

CSX Corporation is a leading rail and intermodal transportation company. The company's largest business unit, CSX Transportation, Inc. (CSXT), is a leading railroad company in the U.S. The division covers over 21,000 route miles in 23 states in the eastern half of the U.S. and two Canadian provinces. CSXT provides transportation for customers in a wide variety of industries, such as coal, chemicals, automobiles, minerals, agricultural products, food and consumer goods, metals, forest and paper products and phosphates and fertilizer. The firm's intermodal segment, operated through subsidiary CSX Intermodal, Inc., combines rail and truck services with a domestic container fleet to provide a network of intermodal facilities across North America. Other major company subsidiaries include CSX Real Property, Inc., an organization responsible for the management, sale, lease, acquisition and development of company properties; CSX Hotels, Inc., a resort doing business as The Greenbrier, located in White Sulphur Springs, West Virginia; CSX Technology, a company providing software applications for various shipping needs such as scheduling, tracking and monitoring of freight, data resource management, system architecture and resource management; TRANSFLO, which handles intermodal bulk transportation and materials services; and Total Distribution Services, Inc., which operates value added distribution and storage services to the automotive industry. In November 2007, the firm signed a $491 million agreement with the Florida Department of Transportation to bring a commuter rail system to central Florida, spanning a 61-mile corridor from DeLand in Volusia County to Poinciana in Osceola County.

FINANCIALS: Sales and profits are in thousands of dollars—add 000 to get the full amount. 2007 Note: Financial information for 2007 was not available for all companies at press time.

2007 Sales: $10,030,000	2007 Profits: $1,226,000	U.S. Stock Ticker: CSX
2006 Sales: $9,566,000	2006 Profits: $1,310,000	Int'l Ticker: Int'l Exchange:
2005 Sales: $8,618,000	2005 Profits: $1,145,000	Employees: 36,005
2004 Sales: $8,040,000	2004 Profits: $339,000	Fiscal Year Ends: 12/31
2003 Sales: $7,793,000	2003 Profits: $246,000	Parent Company:

SALARIES/BENEFITS:

Pension Plan: Y	ESOP Stock Plan:	Profit Sharing:	Top Exec. Salary: $995,833	Bonus: $2,031,500
Savings Plan: Y	Stock Purch. Plan:		Second Exec. Salary: $595,833	Bonus: $836,000

OTHER THOUGHTS:

Apparent Women Officers or Directors: 4
Hot Spot for Advancement for Women/Minorities: Y

LOCATIONS: ("Y" = Yes)

West:	Southwest:	Midwest:	Southeast:	Northeast:	International:
Y	Y	Y	Y	Y	Y

CSX TRANSPORTATION INC

www.csxt.com

Industry Group Code: 482110 Ranks within this company's industry group: Sales: Profits:

Management:		Sales/Marketing:		Liberal Arts:		Information Systems:		Professionals:		Technical/Scientific:	
Mgmt. Trainees:		Mktg. Professionals:	Y	Gen. Writing/Editing:		Info. Management:	Y	Finance/Accounting:	Y	Engineers, Elec.:	Y
Experienced Mgmt.:	Y	Retail Sales:		Technical Writing:	Y	Software Dev.:		Law:	Y	Engineers, Other:	Y
Int'l Business:	Y	Commercial/Industrial:	Y	Graphic Arts/Photog.:		Hardware Dev.:		HR/Other:	Y	Health/Lab:	
MBA Graduates:	Y	Sales Trainees:		Music:		Systems Integration:		Training:	Y	Scientists/Research:	
		Advertising Pros.:		Broadcasting:		Consulting/Other:		Health Care:		Petroleum/Chemicals:	
				Other:				Consulting:		Math/Other:	

TYPES OF BUSINESS:
Railroad

BRANDS/DIVISIONS/AFFILIATES:
CSX Corp

GROWTH PLANS/SPECIAL FEATURES:

CSX Transportation, Inc. (CSXT) is one of the largest rail networks in the eastern U.S., providing rail freight transportation over a network of more than 22,000 route miles in 23 states, Washington, D.C. and two Canadian provinces. The network connects over 70 ocean, lake and river ports and includes over 200 short-line railroads. Based in Jacksonville, Florida, the company is the principal operating subsidiary of CSX Corp. The firm carries freight including chemicals, agricultural and food products, forest and industrial products, phosphates and fertilizer, automotive products and coal, coke and iron ore. Parent company CSX also operates road carriers, freight terminal operations and ocean container shipping operations.

CONTACTS: Note: Officers with more than one job title may be intentionally listed here more than once.
Michael J. Ward, CEO
Tony L. Ingram, COO/Exec. VP
Michael J. Ward, Pres.
Oscar Munoz, CFO/Exec. VP

Phone: 904-359-3100	Fax: 904-359-2459
Toll-Free:	
Address: 500 Water St., 15th Fl., Jacksonville, FL 32202 US	

FINANCIALS: Sales and profits are in thousands of dollars—add 000 to get the full amount. 2007 Note: Financial information for 2007 was not available for all companies at press time.

2007 Sales: $8,591,000	2007 Profits: $1,697,000	U.S. Stock Ticker: Subsidiary
2006 Sales: $8,140,000	2006 Profits: $1,598,000	Int'l Ticker: Int'l Exchange:
2005 Sales: $7,256,000	2005 Profits: $1,086,000	Employees:
2004 Sales: $6,694,000	2004 Profits: $841,000	Fiscal Year Ends: 12/31
2003 Sales: $6,182,000	2003 Profits: $196,000	Parent Company: CSX CORP

SALARIES/BENEFITS:

Pension Plan:	ESOP Stock Plan:	Profit Sharing:	Top Exec. Salary: $	Bonus: $
Savings Plan:	Stock Purch. Plan:		Second Exec. Salary: $	Bonus: $

OTHER THOUGHTS:

Apparent Women Officers or Directors:
Hot Spot for Advancement for Women/Minorities:

LOCATIONS: ("Y" = Yes)

West:	Southwest:	Midwest:	Southeast:	Northeast:	International:
			Y	Y	Y

CTS CORP

www.ctscorp.com

Industry Group Code: 334419 **Ranks within this company's industry group:** Sales: 4   Profits: 4

Management:		Sales/Marketing:		Liberal Arts:		Information Systems:		Professionals:		Technical/Scientific:	
Mgmt. Trainees:		Mktg. Professionals:	Y	Gen. Writing/Editing:		Info. Management:	Y	Finance/Accounting:	Y	Engineers, Elec.:	Y
Experienced Mgmt.:	Y	Retail Sales:		Technical Writing:	Y	Software Dev.:	Y	Law:	Y	Engineers, Other:	
Int'l Business:	Y	Commercial/Industrial:	Y	Graphic Arts/Photog.:		Hardware Dev.:	Y	HR/Other:	Y	Health/Lab:	
MBA Graduates:	Y	Sales Trainees:		Music:		Systems Integration:	Y	Training:	Y	Scientists/Research:	
		Advertising Pros.:		Broadcasting:		Consulting/Other:		Health Care:		Petroleum/Chemicals:	
				Other:				Consulting:		Math/Other:	

TYPES OF BUSINESS:

Electronic Components
Components & Sensors
Manufacturing & Assembly Services
Interconnect Systems
Supply Chain Services
Electronics Manufacturing Services

BRANDS/DIVISIONS/AFFILIATES:

CTS Electronics Manufacturing Solutions
Alpha Ceramics Inc

CONTACTS: *Note: Officers with more than one job title may be intentionally listed here more than once.*

Vinod M. Khilnani, CEO
Vinod M. Khilnani, Pres.
Matthew W. Long, CFO/Treas.
James L. Cummins, Sr. VP-Admin.
Richard G. Cutter, General Counsel/Sec./VP
Rohit Rai, VP-Strategy & Corp. Dev.
Mitchell J. Walorski, Dir.-Investor Rel. & Planning
Thomas A. Kroll, Controller/VP
Donald R. Schroeder, Exec. VP/Pres., CTS Electronics Mfg. Solutions
H. Tyler Buchanan, Sr. VP
Roger R. Hemminghaus, Chmn.

Phone: 574-293-7511	Fax: 574-293-6146
Toll-Free:	
Address: 905 West Blvd. N., Elkhart, IN 46514 US	

GROWTH PLANS/SPECIAL FEATURES:

CTS Corp. designs, manufactures and sells electronic components and custom electronic assemblies for the automotive, computer, communications, medical, industrial and defense and aerospace markets. The company operates manufacturing facilities throughout North America, Asia and Europe. Its product lines serve major markets worldwide, focused primarily on the needs of original equipment manufacturers. The company operates through two business segments: components and sensors, and electronics manufacturing services (EMS). The components and sensors segment consists primarily of automotive sensors and actuators used in commercial or consumer vehicles; electronic components used in communications infrastructure and computer markets; terminators, used in computer and other high speed applications; switches, resistor networks and potentiometers used to serve multiple markets; and fabricated piezoelectric materials and substrates used primarily in medical and industrial markets. CTS' EMS segment offers high-level assembly of electronic and mechanical components into finished subassemblies, including printed circuit assembly, as well as final assembly of products performed under a contract manufacturing agreement. In addition, this segment designs interconnect systems and complex backplanes and offers global supply chain management and other outsourcing, support and logistical services. In November 2007, the company announced plans to realign certain manufacturing operations and eliminate approximately 103 net positions. In December 2007, the firm acquired the technology, manufacturing process and certain other assets of Alpha Ceramics Inc., a privately held company. The acquisition expands the company's portfolio of piezoceramic offerings.

Employee benefits include medical and dental coverage; life insurance and dependant life insurance; 401(k); and tuition reimbursement.

FINANCIALS: Sales and profits are in thousands of dollars—add 000 to get the full amount. 2007 Note: Financial information for 2007 was not available for all companies at press time.

2007 Sales: $685,945	2007 Profits: $25,412	**U.S. Stock Ticker:** CTS
2006 Sales: $655,614	2006 Profits: $24,197	**Int'l Ticker:** Int'l Exchange:
2005 Sales: $617,484	2005 Profits: $20,756	Employees: 4,746
2004 Sales: $531,316	2004 Profits: $19,956	Fiscal Year Ends: 12/31
2003 Sales: $462,987	2003 Profits: $12,575	Parent Company:

SALARIES/BENEFITS:

Pension Plan:	ESOP Stock Plan:	Profit Sharing:	Top Exec. Salary: $766,022	Bonus: $62,346
Savings Plan: Y	Stock Purch. Plan:		Second Exec. Salary: $357,808	Bonus: $54,550

OTHER THOUGHTS:

Apparent Women Officers or Directors: 1
Hot Spot for Advancement for Women/Minorities:

LOCATIONS: ("Y" = Yes)

West:	Southwest:	Midwest:	Southeast:	Northeast:	International:
Y	Y	Y		Y	Y

CUBIC CORP

www.cubic.com

Industry Group Code: 336410 Ranks within this company's industry group: Sales: 9 Profits: 9

Management:		Sales/Marketing:		Liberal Arts:		Information Systems:		Professionals:		Technical/Scientific:	
Mgmt. Trainees:	Y	Mktg. Professionals:	Y	Gen. Writing/Editing:		Info. Management:	Y	Finance/Accounting:	Y	Engineers, Elec.:	Y
Experienced Mgmt.:	Y	Retail Sales:		Technical Writing:	Y	Software Dev.:	Y	Law:	Y	Engineers, Other:	Y
Int'l Business:	Y	Commercial/Industrial:	Y	Graphic Arts/Photog.:	Y	Hardware Dev.:	Y	HR/Other:	Y	Health/Lab:	
MBA Graduates:	Y	Sales Trainees:		Music:		Systems Integration:	Y	Training:	Y	Scientists/Research:	Y
		Advertising Pros.:	Y	Broadcasting:		Consulting/Other:	Y	Health Care:		Petroleum/Chemicals:	
				Other:				Consulting:		Math/Other:	

TYPES OF BUSINESS:
Communications & Surveillance Systems
Military Training Systems
Automated Ticketing Systems

BRANDS/DIVISIONS/AFFILIATES:
Cubic Transportation Systems,Ltd.
Cubic Defense Systems, Inc.
Cubic Defence New Zealand, Ltd.
Cubic Fiend Services, Ltd.
Cubic Applications, Inc.
Cubic Advanced Tactical Systems, LLC

CONTACTS: *Note: Officers with more than one job title may be intentionally listed here more than once.*
Walter J. Zable, CEO
Walter J. Zable, Pres.
William W. Boyle, CFO
Bernard A. Kulchin, VP-Human Resources
John A. Minteer, VP-IT
William L. Hoesee, Gen. Counsel/VP/Corp. Sec.
John D. Thomas, VP-Corp. Dev./Fin.
Mark A. Harrison, VP/Corp. Controller
Raymond L. deKozan, Sr. Group VP
Richard A. Efland, Pres., Transportation Systems Group
Daniel A. Kacobsen, VP-Ethics/Compliance
Kenneth A. Kopf, Chief Legal Officer/VP
Walter J. Zable, Chmn.

Phone: 858-277-6780	Fax: 858-277-1878
Toll-Free: 800-818-8303	
Address: 9333 Balboa Ave., San Diego, CA 92123 US	

GROWTH PLANS/SPECIAL FEATURES:

Cubic Corporation designs, develops, manufactures and installs products for military defense and mass transit networks. The company has two primary segments: Defense and Transportation Systems. The Defense segment has three main business units: Readiness Systems, Mission Support Services, and Communications & Electronics. The company's products include customized military range instrumentation systems, tactical engagement simulation systems, firearm simulation systems, communications and surveillance systems, surveillance receivers, power amplifiers, and avionics systems. Services offered within the Defense segment include training mission support, computer simulation training, distributed interactive simulation, development of military training doctrine, and field operations and maintenance. The firm markets its capabilities directly to various U.S. government departments and agencies and foreign governments. The company also frequently contracts or teams with other defense suppliers. In addition to the three business units, Cubic formed a joint venture with Rafael Armament Development Authority Ltd., an Israeli company, to produce certain Rafael defense systems in the U.S. for Israel and for U.S. customers. The Transportation Systems segment designs, produces, installs and services electronic revenue collection systems for mass transit projects, including bus, bus rapid transit, light rail, commuter rail, heavy rail, ferry and parking markets. Its products include contactless smart cards, magnetic stripe cards, device software, central computer systems, passenger gates, card readers and ticket vending machines. The company's transportation segment has been awarded over 400 projects in 40 major markets on 5 continents. Active projects include London, the New York / New Jersey region, the Washington, D.C. / Baltimore / Virginia region, the Los Angeles region, the San Diego region, San Francisco, Minneapolis/St. Paul, Chicago, Atlanta, Brisbane, Australia, and Sweden. In July 2008 Cubic expanded its defense training services business with the acquisition of Omega Training Group, Inc.

FINANCIALS: Sales and profits are in thousands of dollars—add 000 to get the full amount. 2007 Note: Financial information for 2007 was not available for all companies at press time.

2007 Sales: $889,870	2007 Profits: $41,586	**U.S. Stock Ticker: CUB**
2006 Sales: $821,386	2006 Profits: $24,133	**Int'l Ticker:** Int'l Exchange:
2005 Sales: $804,372	2005 Profits: $11,628	Employees: 6,000
2004 Sales: $722,012	2004 Profits: $36,911	Fiscal Year Ends: 9/30
2003 Sales: $634,061	2003 Profits: $36,519	Parent Company:

SALARIES/BENEFITS:
Pension Plan: Y	ESOP Stock Plan:	Profit Sharing: Y	Top Exec. Salary: $686,400	Bonus: $250,000
Savings Plan:	Stock Purch. Plan:		Second Exec. Salary: $462,800	Bonus: $160,000

OTHER THOUGHTS:
Apparent Women Officers or Directors:
Hot Spot for Advancement for Women/Minorities:

LOCATIONS: ("Y" = Yes)
West:	Southwest:	Midwest:	Southeast:	Northeast:	International:
Y		Y	Y	Y	Y

CUMMINS INC

www.cummins.com

Industry Group Code: 336300 Ranks within this company's industry group: Sales: 3 Profits: 3

Management:		Sales/Marketing:		Liberal Arts:		Information Systems:		Professionals:		Technical/Scientific:	
Mgmt. Trainees:	Y	Mktg. Professionals:	Y	Gen. Writing/Editing:		Info. Management:	Y	Finance/Accounting:	Y	Engineers, Elec.:	Y
Experienced Mgmt.:	Y	Retail Sales:		Technical Writing:	Y	Software Dev.:	Y	Law:	Y	Engineers, Other:	Y
Int'l Business:	Y	Commercial/Industrial:	Y	Graphic Arts/Photog.:	Y	Hardware Dev.:	Y	HR/Other:	Y	Health/Lab:	
MBA Graduates:	Y	Sales Trainees:		Music:		Systems Integration:		Training:	Y	Scientists/Research:	
		Advertising Pros.:	Y	Broadcasting:		Consulting/Other:		Health Care:		Petroleum/Chemicals:	
				Other:				Consulting:		Math/Other:	

TYPES OF BUSINESS:

Automotive Products, Motors & Parts Manufacturing
Engines
Filtration Systems
Power Generation Systems
Alternators
Air Handling Systems
Filtration & Emissions Solutions
Fuel Systems

BRANDS/DIVISIONS/AFFILIATES:

Cummins Power Generation
Onan

CONTACTS: Note: Officers with more than one job title may be intentionally listed here more than once.

Theodore M. Solso, CEO
Tom Linebarger, COO
Tom Linebarger, Pres.
Pat Ward, CFO/VP
John C. Wall, CTO/VP
Mark Gerstle, Chief Admin. Officer/ VP-Corp. Quality
Marya M. Rose, General Counsel/VP/Sec.
Richard J. Freeland
Tony Satterthwaite, VP/Pres., Components Group
J. D. Kelly, VP/Pres., Engine Bus.
Steven M. Chapman, VP-Emerging Markets & Bus.
Theodore M. Solso, Chmn.

Phone: 812-377-5000	Fax: 812-377-3334
Toll-Free:	
Address: 500 Jackson St., Columbus, IN 47202 US	

GROWTH PLANS/SPECIAL FEATURES:

Cummins, Inc. designs, manufactures, distributes and services diesel and natural gas engines; electric power generation systems; and engine-related component products, including filtration and emissions solutions, fuel systems, controls and air handling systems. The engine segment, which generated 52% of 2007 sales, manufactures and markets diesel and natural gas-powered engines, parts, and services under the Cummins brand name for the heavy- and medium-duty truck, bus, recreational vehicle, light-duty automotive, agricultural, construction, mining, marine, oil and gas, rail and governmental equipment markets. The power generation segment generated 19% of 2007 revenue, and designs and manufactures components of power generation systems, including engines, controls, alternators, transfer switches and switchgear. Products are marketed principally under the Cummins Power Generation and Onan brands and include diesel and alternative-fuel electrical generator sets for commercial, institutional and consumer applications, such as office buildings, hospitals, factories, municipalities, utilities, universities, boats and homes. The components segment, which accounted for 19% of 2007 net sales, produces filters, silencers and intake and exhaust systems and commercial turbochargers. The distribution segment, producing 10% of revenue, consists of 17 company-owned and 15 joint ventures that distribute the company's products and services in over 70 countries and territories. Cummins serves customers through a network of more than 500 company-owned and independent distributor locations and roughly 5,200 dealer locations in more than 190 countries and territories. In 2007, the firm's North American heavy-duty truck engine market declined 50% due to new emissions regulations; over half of 2007 sales came from countries outside the U.S. In January 2008, Cummins entered into an agreement with Elmarco s.ro., a Czech nanotechnology designer, to develop nanofiber filtration technologies. In July 2008, the company concluded joint ventures with CNH Global N.V. and Iveco N.V.; Cummins will make Consolidated Diesel Company a subsidiary, and sell its interest in European Engine Alliance.

FINANCIALS: Sales and profits are in thousands of dollars—add 000 to get the full amount. 2007 Note: Financial information for 2007 was not available for all companies at press time.

2007 Sales: $13,048,000	2007 Profits: $739,000	U.S. Stock Ticker: CMI
2006 Sales: $11,362,000	2006 Profits: $715,000	Int'l Ticker: Int'l Exchange:
2005 Sales: $9,918,000	2005 Profits: $550,000	Employees: 37,800
2004 Sales: $8,438,000	2004 Profits: $350,000	Fiscal Year Ends: 12/31
2003 Sales: $6,296,000	2003 Profits: $50,000	Parent Company:

SALARIES/BENEFITS:

Pension Plan:	ESOP Stock Plan:	Profit Sharing: Y	Top Exec. Salary: $1,110,000	Bonus: $6,274,000
Savings Plan: Y	Stock Purch. Plan: Y		Second Exec. Salary: $812,500	Bonus: $2,840,750

OTHER THOUGHTS:

Apparent Women Officers or Directors: 3
Hot Spot for Advancement for Women/Minorities: Y

LOCATIONS: ("Y" = Yes)

West:	Southwest:	Midwest:	Southeast:	Northeast:	International:
Y	Y	Y	Y	Y	Y

Note: Financial information, benefits and other data can change quickly and may vary from those stated here.

CVS CAREMARK CORPORATION

www.cvs.com

Industry Group Code: 446110 **Ranks within this company's industry group:** Sales: 2 Profits: 2

Management:		Sales/Marketing:		Liberal Arts:		Information Systems:		Professionals:		Technical/Scientific:	
Mgmt. Trainees:	Y	Mktg. Professionals:	Y	Gen. Writing/Editing:	Y	Info. Management:	Y	Finance/Accounting:	Y	Engineers, Elec.:	
Experienced Mgmt.:	Y	Retail Sales:	Y	Technical Writing:		Software Dev.:	Y	Law:	Y	Engineers, Other:	Y
Int'l Business:		Commercial/Industrial:	Y	Graphic Arts/Photog.:	Y	Hardware Dev.:		HR/Other:	Y	Health/Lab:	
MBA Graduates:	Y	Sales Trainees:	Y	Music:		Systems Integration:		Training:	Y	Scientists/Research:	
		Advertising Pros.:	Y	Broadcasting:		Consulting/Other:		Health Care:	Y	Petroleum/Chemicals:	
				Other:				Consulting:		Math/Other:	

TYPES OF BUSINESS:

Drug Stores
Pharmacy Benefits Management
Online Pharmacy Services

BRANDS/DIVISIONS/AFFILIATES:

MinuteClinic
Caremark Rx., Inc.
CVS Corp.
CVS/pharmacy
PharmaCare Pharmacy
Caremark Pharmacy Services
PharmaCare Management Services
SilverScript Insurance, Co.

CONTACTS: *Note: Officers with more than one job title may be intentionally listed here more than once.*

Thomas M. Ryan, CEO
Thomas M. Ryan, Pres.
David B. Rickard, CFO/Exec. VP
V. Michael Ferdinandi, Sr. VP-Human Resources
Jonathan C. Roberts, CIO/Sr. VP
David B. Rickard, Chief Admin. Officer
Douglas A. Sgarro, Chief Legal Officer/Exec. VP/Pres., CVS Realty Co.
V. Michael Ferdinandi, Sr. VP-Corp. Comm.
David M. Denton, Chief Acct. Officer/Controller/Sr. VP
Chris W. Bodine, Pres., CVS Caremark Health Care Svcs./Exec. VP
Larry J. Merlo, Pres., CVS/pharmacy-Retail/Exec. VP
Howard A. McLure, Pres., Caremark Pharmacy Svcs./Exec. VP
Helena B. Foulkes, Sr. VP-Health Svcs.-CVS Pharmacy, Inc.
Thomas M. Ryan, Chmn.

Phone: 401-765-1500	Fax: 401-762-9227
Toll-Free: 888-607-4287	
Address: 1 CVS Dr., Woonsocket, RI 02895 US	

GROWTH PLANS/SPECIAL FEATURES:

CVS Caremark Corp., the result of the 2007 merger of CVS Corp. and Caremark RX, Inc., is one of the largest providers of prescription and related healthcare services in the U.S., filling more than 1 billion prescriptions annually. It operates in two segments: retail pharmacy and pharmacy services. The retail pharmacy services segment includes over 6,200 retail drugstores, of which over 6,150 operate a pharmacy; the online retail web site, CVS.com; and retail healthcare clinics. The retail drugstores are located in 40 states and Washington, D.C. operating under the CVS or CVS/pharmacy names. CVS/pharmacy stores sell prescription drugs and a wide assortment of general merchandise, including over-the-counter drugs, beauty products and cosmetics, photo finishing, seasonal merchandise, greeting cards and convenience foods. Existing stores generally range in size from 8,000 to 18,000 square feet, although most stores range in size from roughly 10,000 to 13,000 square feet and typically include a drive-through pharmacy. The division operates over 460 retail healthcare clinics in 25 states under the MinuteClinic name, of which about 435 are located within CVS retail drug stores. The clinics diagnose and treat minor health conditions and are staffed by board-certified nurse practitioners and physician assistants. The pharmacy service segment provides a full range of prescription benefit management services, including mail order pharmacy services, specialty pharmacy services, plan design and administration, formulary management and claims processing. It also offers health management programs. Through subsidiary SilverScript Insurance Co., the division is a national provider of drug benefits. The segment operates a national retail pharmacy network with over 60,000 participating pharmacies; 56 retail specialty pharmacy stores; 20 specialty mail order pharmacies; and nine mail services pharmacies located in 26 states and Washington, D.C. Specialty pharmacy stores average 2,000 square feet in size. In March 2007, CVS Corp. merged with Caremark Rx, Inc., with a total of $75 billion in annual revenues.

FINANCIALS: Sales and profits are in thousands of dollars—add 000 to get the full amount. 2007 Note: Financial information for 2007 was not available for all companies at press time.

2007 Sales: $76,329,500	2007 Profits: $2,637,000	**U.S. Stock Ticker:** CVS	
2006 Sales: $43,821,400	2006 Profits: $1,368,900	**Int'l Ticker:** Int'l Exchange:	
2005 Sales: $37,006,200	2005 Profits: $1,224,700	Employees: 176,000	
2004 Sales: $30,594,300	2004 Profits: $918,800	Fiscal Year Ends: 12/31	
2003 Sales: $26,588,000	2003 Profits: $847,300	Parent Company:	

SALARIES/BENEFITS:

Pension Plan:	ESOP Stock Plan:	Profit Sharing:	Top Exec. Salary: $1,150,000	Bonus: $8,172,600
Savings Plan:	Stock Purch. Plan:		Second Exec. Salary: $713,750	Bonus: $2,413,200

OTHER THOUGHTS:

Apparent Women Officers or Directors: 4
Hot Spot for Advancement for Women/Minorities: Y

LOCATIONS: ("Y" = Yes)

West:	Southwest:	Midwest:	Southeast:	Northeast:	International:
Y	Y	Y	Y	Y	

Note: Financial information, benefits and other data can change quickly and may vary from those stated here.

DANAHER CORP

www.danaher.com

Industry Group Code: 335000 Ranks within this company's industry group: Sales: 1   Profits: 1

Management:		Sales/Marketing:		Liberal Arts:		Information Systems:		Professionals:		Technical/Scientific:	
Mgmt. Trainees:	Y	Mktg. Professionals:	Y	Gen. Writing/Editing:		Info. Management:	Y	Finance/Accounting:	Y	Engineers, Elec.:	Y
Experienced Mgmt.:	Y	Retail Sales:		Technical Writing:	Y	Software Dev.:		Law:	Y	Engineers, Other:	Y
Int'l Business:	Y	Commercial/Industrial:	Y	Graphic Arts/Photog.:		Hardware Dev.:		HR/Other:	Y	Health/Lab:	Y
MBA Graduates:	Y	Sales Trainees:		Music:		Systems Integration:		Training:		Scientists/Research:	
		Advertising Pros.:	Y	Broadcasting:		Consulting/Other:		Health Care:		Petroleum/Chemicals:	
				Other:				Consulting:		Math/Other:	

TYPES OF BUSINESS:

Power Tools Manufacturing
Test & Calibration Equipment
Controls
Bar Code Equipment

BRANDS/DIVISIONS/AFFILIATES:

VIDEOJET
ACCU-SORT
Delta Consolidated Industries
Hennessy Industries
Jacobs Chuck Manufacturing Company
Jacobs Vehicle Systems
Craftsman
ChemTreat, Inc.

CONTACTS: *Note: Officers with more than one job title may be intentionally listed here more than once.*

H. Lawrence Culp, Jr., CEO
H. Lawrence Culp, Jr., Pres.
Daniel L. Comas, CFO/Exec. VP
Jonathan P. Graham, General Counsel/Sr. VP
Daniel A. Raskas, VP-Corp. Dev.
Robert S. Lutz, Chief Acct. Officer/VP
James H. Ditkoff, Sr. VP-Finance & Tax
Mitchell P. Rales, Chmn.-Exec. Committee
Phillip W. Knisely, Exec. VP
Thomas P. Joyce, Exec. VP
Steven M. Rales, Chmn.

Phone: 202-828-0850	Fax: 202-828-0860
Toll-Free:	
Address: 2099 Pennsylvania Ave., Washington, DC 20006-1813 US	

GROWTH PLANS/SPECIAL FEATURES:

Danaher Corp., through its subsidiaries, designs, manufactures and markets industrial and consumer products, which are typically characterized by strong brand names, proprietary technology and major market positions, in four business segments: Professional Instrumentation; Medical Technologies; Industrial Technologies; and Tools & Components. Businesses in the Professional Instrumentation segment, which accounted for 32% of 2007 revenue, offer professional and technical customers products and services in connection with the performance of their work. Danaher's Medical Technologies segment, accounting for 27%, caters to dentists, doctors and hospital, research and scientific professionals. The Industrial Technologies segment, accounting for 29%, manufactures products and sub-systems that are typically incorporated by customers and systems integrators into production and packaging lines and by original equipment manufacturers into various end-products and systems. Industries served include motion, with products including standard and custom motors; product identification, with products marketed under such brands as VIDEOJET and ACCU-SORT; aerospace and defense, with products including smoke detection systems and submarine periscopes; sensors and controls; and power quality. The Tools & Components segment, accounting for 12%, produces mechanic's hand tools, and contains four niche businesses: Delta Consolidated Industries, Hennessy Industries, Jacobs Chuck Manufacturing Company and Jacobs Vehicle Systems. The mechanics' hand tools platform is the principal manufacturer of Sears' Craftsman line of hand tools and the primary supplier of automotive service tools to the National Automotive Parts Association (NAPA). In July 2007 Danaher sold its Power Quality business to Thomas & Betts Corp. for approximately $280 million and acquired ChemTreat, Inc., a leading provider of industrial water treatment solutions. Danaher has a goal of growing to $25 billion in revenues by 2012. Much of that growth will come through continued acquisitions. As of 2007, the firm owned about 600 subsidiaries. In November 2007, Danaher, through Raven Acquisition Corp., acquired 90% of Tektronix, Inc.'s common stock.

FINANCIALS: Sales and profits are in thousands of dollars—add 000 to get the full amount. 2007 Note: Financial information for 2007 was not available for all companies at press time.

2007 Sales: $11,025,917	2007 Profits: $1,369,904	**U.S. Stock Ticker: DHR**
2006 Sales: $9,466,056	2006 Profits: $1,122,029	**Int'l Ticker:** Int'l Exchange:
2005 Sales: $7,984,704	2005 Profits: $897,800	Employees: 45,000
2004 Sales: $6,889,301	2004 Profits: $746,000	Fiscal Year Ends: 12/31
2003 Sales: $5,293,900	2003 Profits: $536,800	Parent Company:

SALARIES/BENEFITS:

Pension Plan: Y	ESOP Stock Plan:	Profit Sharing:	Top Exec. Salary: $1,100,000	Bonus: $3,525,000
Savings Plan:	Stock Purch. Plan:		Second Exec. Salary: $610,000	Bonus: $1,000,000

OTHER THOUGHTS:

Apparent Women Officers or Directors:
Hot Spot for Advancement for Women/Minorities:

LOCATIONS: ("Y" = Yes)

West:	Southwest:	Midwest:	Southeast:	Northeast:	International:
Y	Y	Y	Y	Y	Y

DARDEN RESTAURANTS INC   www.dardenrestaurants.com

Industry Group Code: 722110 Ranks within this company's industry group: Sales: 3 Profits: 3

Management:		Sales/Marketing:		Liberal Arts:		Information Systems:		Professionals:		Technical/Scientific:	
Mgmt. Trainees:	Y	Mktg. Professionals:	Y	Gen. Writing/Editing:	Y	Info. Management:	Y	Finance/Accounting:	Y	Engineers, Elec.:	
Experienced Mgmt.:	Y	Retail Sales:		Technical Writing:		Software Dev.:	Y	Law:	Y	Engineers, Other:	
Int'l Business:	Y	Commercial/Industrial:		Graphic Arts/Photog.:	Y	Hardware Dev.:		HR/Other:	Y	Health/Lab:	
MBA Graduates:	Y	Sales Trainees:		Music:		Systems Integration:		Training:	Y	Scientists/Research:	
		Advertising Pros.:	Y	Broadcasting:		Consulting/Other:		Health Care:		Petroleum/Chemicals:	
				Other:	Y			Consulting:		Math/Other:	

TYPES OF BUSINESS:
Restaurants-Casual Dining

BRANDS/DIVISIONS/AFFILIATES:
Red Lobster
Olive Garden
Olive Garden Cafe
Bahama Breeze
LongHorn Steakhouse
Seasons 52
The Capital Grille

CONTACTS: *Note: Officers with more than one job title may be intentionally listed here more than once.*
Clarence Otis, Jr., CEO
Andrew H. Madsen, COO
Andrew H. Madsen, Pres.
C. Bradford (Brad) Richmond, CFO/Sr. VP
Ronald Bojalad, Sr. VP-Group Human Resources
Paula J. Shives, General Counsel/Sr. VP/Corp./Sec.
J.J. Buettgen, Sr. VP-Bus. Dev.
Valerie K. Collins, Corp. Controller
David T. Pickens, Sr. VP/Pres., Olive Garden
Laurie B. Burns, Sr. VP/Pres., Bahama Breeze
Kim A. Lopdrup, Sr. VP/Pres., Red Lobster
Stephen Judge, Sr. VP/Pres., Seasons 52
Clarence Otis, Jr., Chmn.
Barry B. Moullet, Sr. VP-Supply Chain & Dev.

Phone: 407-245-4000	Fax: 407-245-5389
Toll-Free:	
Address: 5900 Lake Ellenor Dr., Orlando, FL 32809 US	

GROWTH PLANS/SPECIAL FEATURES:
Darden Restaurants, Inc. is one of the largest publicly held casual dining companies in the U.S. It owns and operates over 1,700 restaurants throughout the U.S. and Canada. Darden operates six restaurant chains: Red Lobster, Olive Garden, LongHorn Steakhouse, The Capital Grille, Bahama Breeze and Seasons 52. Red Lobster, with 651 restaurants, is seafood-specialty restaurant in the U.S. Its menu features fresh fish, shrimp, crab, lobster, scallops and other seafood, as well as non-seafood entrees, appetizers and desserts. Olive Garden, with 647 restaurants, is a casual dining Italian restaurants in the U.S. Its menu includes a variety of Italian foods, including antipasti; soups, salad and garlic breadsticks; baked pastas; sauteed specialties with chicken, seafood and fresh vegetables; grilled meats; and a variety of desserts. It also offers an expanded wine list that includes a broad selection of imported Italian wines, as well as coffee imported from Italy for its espresso and cappuccino. LongHorn Steakhouse restaurants, with 305 locations, are full service establishments serving both lunch and dinner in an attractive and inviting atmosphere reminiscent of the American West. The Capital Grille features relaxed elegance and style. The restaurant dry-ages its steaks on premises and flies in fresh seafood daily to its 32 locations. Bahama Breeze, which has 23 restaurants, is a Caribbean-themed restaurant that offers guests an island dining experience with a menu featuring Caribbean-style beef, pork, chicken and seafood. Seasons 52, with seven restaurants, is a fresh grill and wine bar with seasonally inspired menus, offering nutritionally balanced meals lower in calories than comparable restaurant meals. In December 2007, Darden sold its Smokey Bones restaurant operations. In October 2007, Darden Restaurants acquired RARE Hospitality International, Inc., owner of restaurant chains LongHorn Steakhouse and Capital Grille, for $1.19 billion.

FINANCIALS: Sales and profits are in thousands of dollars—add 000 to get the full amount. 2007 Note: Financial information for 2007 was not available for all companies at press time.

2007 Sales: $5,567,100	2007 Profits: $201,400	**U.S. Stock Ticker: DRI**
2006 Sales: $5,353,600	2006 Profits: $338,194	**Int'l Ticker:** Int'l Exchange:
2005 Sales: $4,977,600	2005 Profits: $290,606	Employees: 156,500
2004 Sales: $5,003,355	2004 Profits: $231,462	Fiscal Year Ends: 5/31
2003 Sales: $4,654,571	2003 Profits: $232,260	Parent Company:

SALARIES/BENEFITS:

Pension Plan: Y	ESOP Stock Plan:	Profit Sharing:	Top Exec. Salary: $804,113	Bonus: $1,094,200
Savings Plan: Y	Stock Purch. Plan: Y		Second Exec. Salary: $675,356	Bonus: $909,500

OTHER THOUGHTS:
Apparent Women Officers or Directors: 3
Hot Spot for Advancement for Women/Minorities: Y

LOCATIONS: ("Y" = Yes)

West:	Southwest:	Midwest:	Southeast:	Northeast:	International:
Y	Y	Y	Y	Y	Y

DAVITA INC

www.davita.com

Industry Group Code: 621490 **Ranks within this company's industry group:** Sales: 1 Profits: 1

Management:		Sales/Marketing:		Liberal Arts:		Information Systems:		Professionals:		Technical/Scientific:	
Mgmt. Trainees:	Y	Mktg. Professionals:	Y	Gen. Writing/Editing:		Info. Management:	Y	Finance/Accounting:	Y	Engineers, Elec.:	
Experienced Mgmt.:	Y	Retail Sales:		Technical Writing:	Y	Software Dev.:		Law:	Y	Engineers, Other:	Y
Int'l Business:		Commercial/Industrial:	Y	Graphic Arts/Photog.:		Hardware Dev.:		HR/Other:	Y	Health/Lab:	Y
MBA Graduates:	Y	Sales Trainees:		Music:		Systems Integration:		Training:	Y	Scientists/Research:	Y
		Advertising Pros.:		Broadcasting:		Consulting/Other:		Health Care:	Y	Petroleum/Chemicals:	
				Other:				Consulting:		Math/Other:	

TYPES OF BUSINESS:

Renal Care Services
Clinical Research

BRANDS/DIVISIONS/AFFILIATES:

DaVita Rx
DaVita Clinical Research

CONTACTS: *Note: Officers with more than one job title may be intentionally listed here more than once.*

Kent J. Thiry, CEO
Joseph C. Mello, COO
Richard K. Whitney, CFO
Joseph Schohl, General Counsel/VP/Sec.
LeAnne Zumwalt, VP-Investor Rel.
Thomas O. Usilton, Sr. VP
Charlie McAllister, Chief Medical Officer
Kent J. Thiry, Chmn.

Phone: 310-536-2400	**Fax:** 310-536-2675
Toll-Free: 800-310-4872	
Address: 601 Hawaii St., El Segundo, CA 90245 US	

GROWTH PLANS/SPECIAL FEATURES:

DaVita, Inc. is a provider of dialysis services in the United States for patients suffering from chronic kidney failure, also known as end stage renal disease, or ESRD. The company operates or provides administrative services to roughly 1,359 outpatient dialysis centers located in 43 states and Washington D.C., serving approximately 107,000 patients. The firm also provides acute inpatient dialysis services in approximately 700 hospitals and related laboratory services. The firm's dialysis services include hemodialysis, peritoneal dialysis, acute dialysis and pre-ESRD education. DaVita also provides training, supplies and on-call support services to peritoneal dialysis patients. In addition, the company provides certain patients the option of home-based hemodialysis. The firm owns two licensed clinical laboratories, located in Florida, specialized in ERSD patient testing. These specialized laboratories provide routine laboratory tests covered by the Medicare composite payment rate for dialysis and other physician-prescribed laboratory tests for ESRD patients. DaVita Rx is a wholly-owned pharmacy that provides oral medications to DaVita's patients with chronic kidney disease and ERSD. DaVita Clinical Research conducts research trials with dialysis patients and provides administrative support for research conducted by DaVita-affiliated nephrology practices. Other ancillary services provided by DaVita include management and administrative services to physician-owned vascular access clinics; and advanced care management services to employers, health plans and government agencies for employees/members diagnosed with chronic kidney disease.

The company provides its employees medical, dental and vision insurance; short- and long-term disability insurance; flexible spending accounts; life insurance; a 401(k) plan; a stock purchase program; and tuition reimbursement.

FINANCIALS: Sales and profits are in thousands of dollars—add 000 to get the full amount. 2007 Note: Financial information for 2007 was not available for all companies at press time.

2007 Sales: $5,264,151	2007 Profits: $381,778	**U.S. Stock Ticker:** DVA
2006 Sales: $4,880,662	2006 Profits: $289,691	**Int'l Ticker:** Int'l Exchange:
2005 Sales: $2,973,918	2005 Profits: $228,643	Employees: 28,900
2004 Sales: $2,177,330	2004 Profits: $222,254	Fiscal Year Ends: 12/31
2003 Sales: $2,016,418	2003 Profits: $175,791	Parent Company:

SALARIES/BENEFITS:

Pension Plan:	ESOP Stock Plan:	Profit Sharing:	Top Exec. Salary: $885,079	Bonus: $1,800,000
Savings Plan: Y	Stock Purch. Plan: Y		Second Exec. Salary: $630,768	Bonus: $1,200,000

OTHER THOUGHTS:

Apparent Women Officers or Directors: 1
Hot Spot for Advancement for Women/Minorities: Y

LOCATIONS: ("Y" = Yes)

West:	Southwest:	Midwest:	Southeast:	Northeast:	International:
Y	Y	Y	Y	Y	

DEAN FOODS CO

www.deanfoods.com

Industry Group Code: 311500 Ranks within this company's industry group: Sales: Profits:

Management:		Sales/Marketing:		Liberal Arts:	Information Systems:		Professionals:		Technical/Scientific:	
Mgmt. Trainees:	Y	Mktg. Professionals:	Y	Gen. Writing/Editing:	Info. Management:	Y	Finance/Accounting:	Y	Engineers, Elec.:	
Experienced Mgmt.:	Y	Retail Sales:		Technical Writing:	Software Dev.:		Law:	Y	Engineers, Other:	Y
Int'l Business:	Y	Commercial/Industrial:	Y	Graphic Arts/Photog.:	Hardware Dev.:		HR/Other:	Y	Health/Lab:	
MBA Graduates:	Y	Sales Trainees:		Music:	Systems Integration:		Training:	Y	Scientists/Research:	
		Advertising Pros.:	Y	Broadcasting:	Consulting/Other:		Health Care:		Petroleum/Chemicals:	
				Other:			Consulting:		Math/Other:	

TYPES OF BUSINESS:

Dairy Products, Manufacturing
Milk Processing & Distribution
Organic Dairy Products
Soy-Based Products
Juices
Coffee Creamers
Powdered Ingredients

BRANDS/DIVISIONS/AFFILIATES:

WhiteWave Foods Company
Creamland
Hershey's
LAND O'LAKES
Silk
Horizon Organic
International Delight
Rachel's Organic

CONTACTS: Note: Officers with more than one job title may be intentionally listed here more than once.

Gregg L. Engles, CEO
Jack F. Callahan, CFO/Exec. VP
Paul Moskowitz, Exec. VP-Human Resources
Arthur F. Fino, CIO/Sr. VP
Michelle P. Goolsby, Chief Admin. Officer
Michelle P. Goolsby, General Counsel/Exec. VP
Ronald L. McCrummen, Chief Acct. Officer/Sr. VP
Debbie Carosella, Sr. VP-Innovation
Joseph E. Scalzo, CEO/Pres., WhiteWave Foods
Bill Tinklepaugh, Sr. VP-Gov't & Industry Rel.
Steven J. Kemps, Deputy General Counsel/Sr. VP/Corp. Sec.
Gregg L. Engles, Chmn.
Gregg A. Tanner, Chief Supply Chain Officer/Exec. VP

Phone: 214-303-3400	Fax: 214-303-2850
Toll-Free: 800-431-9214	
Address: 2515 McKinney Ave. LB 30, Ste. 1200, Dallas, TX 75201 US	

GROWTH PLANS/SPECIAL FEATURES:

Dean Foods Co. is a leading food and beverage company, which operates through two business segments, the dairy group and WhiteWave Foods. Generating approximately 87% of the company's net sales, Dean's dairy group manufactures, markets and distributes a variety of branded and private-label dairy-case products to retailers, distributors, foodservice outlets, schools and government entities across the U.S, with 98 manufacturing facilities in 34 states. Products sold by the dairy group include fresh milk, ice cream, flavored milks, buttermilk, half-and-half, whipping cream, coffee creamers, yogurt, cottage cheese, sour cream and dairy based dips, under its more than 50 proprietary and licensed brands, including Berkeley Farms, Brown Cow, Chug, Country Charm, Creamland, Dairy Fresh, Dean's, Hershey's, LAND O'LAKES, Meadow Brook, Mountain High, Nature's Pride, Oak Farms, Shenandoah's Pride and Swiss Pride. Dean purchases its raw milk primarily from farmers' cooperatives. Generating approximately 13% of Dean's net sales, subsidiary White Wave Foods Company develops, manufactures, markets and sells a variety of nationally branded soy, dairy and dairy-related products, such as Silk soymilk and cultured soy products; Horizon Organic dairy products; International Delight coffee creamers; Rachel's Organic dairy products; The Organic Cow organic dairy products; White Wave and Tofu Town branded tofu; and Hershey's milks and milkshakes. Roughly 25% of White Wave's products are manufactured by third-party manufacturers under processing agreements. It purchases organic raw milk from a network of over 360 dairy farmers across the U.S., as well as producing certain of its own organic raw milk in at two organic farms that it owns and one organic farm that it leases and manages. WhiteWave Foods sells its products to a variety of customers, including grocery stores, club stores, natural foods stores, mass merchandisers, convenience stores and foodservice outlets. The segment's largest customer is Wal-Mart and its subsidiary, Sam's Club.

FINANCIALS: Sales and profits are in thousands of dollars—add 000 to get the full amount. 2007 Note: Financial information for 2007 was not available for all companies at press time.

2007 Sales: $11,821,903	2007 Profits: $131,353	U.S. Stock Ticker: DF
2006 Sales: $10,098,555	2006 Profits: $225,414	Int'l Ticker: Int'l Exchange:
2005 Sales: $10,174,718	2005 Profits: $308,654	Employees: 26,348
2004 Sales: $10,822,300	2004 Profits: $324,100	Fiscal Year Ends: 12/31
2003 Sales: $9,184,616	2003 Profits: $355,703	Parent Company:

SALARIES/BENEFITS:

Pension Plan:	ESOP Stock Plan:	Profit Sharing:	Top Exec. Salary: $1,200,000	Bonus: $2,220,480
Savings Plan: Y	Stock Purch. Plan:		Second Exec. Salary: $620,000	Bonus: $860,157

OTHER THOUGHTS:

Apparent Women Officers or Directors: 5
Hot Spot for Advancement for Women/Minorities: Y

LOCATIONS: ("Y" = Yes)

West:	Southwest:	Midwest:	Southeast:	Northeast:	International:
Y	Y	Y	Y	Y	Y

Note: Financial information, benefits and other data can change quickly and may vary from those stated here.

DEERE & CO

www.deere.com

Industry Group Code: 333000 **Ranks within this company's industry group:** Sales: 2   Profits: 2

Management:		Sales/Marketing:		Liberal Arts:		Information Systems:		Professionals:		Technical/Scientific:	
Mgmt. Trainees:	Y	Mktg. Professionals:	Y	Gen. Writing/Editing:	Y	Info. Management:	Y	Finance/Accounting:	Y	Engineers, Elec.:	Y
Experienced Mgmt.:	Y	Retail Sales:	Y	Technical Writing:	Y	Software Dev.:	Y	Law:	Y	Engineers, Other:	Y
Int'l Business:	Y	Commercial/Industrial:	Y	Graphic Arts/Photog.:	Y	Hardware Dev.:		HR/Other:	Y	Health/Lab:	
MBA Graduates:	Y	Sales Trainees:	Y	Music:		Systems Integration:		Training:	Y	Scientists/Research:	
		Advertising Pros.:	Y	Broadcasting:		Consulting/Other:		Health Care:		Petroleum/Chemicals:	
				Other:				Consulting:		Math/Other:	

TYPES OF BUSINESS:

Construction & Agricultural Equipment
Commercial & Consumer Equipment
Forestry Equipment
Financing
Health Care Plans-HMO

BRANDS/DIVISIONS/AFFILIATES:

John Deere
John Deere Health Plan, Inc.
John Deere Construction & Forestry Company
John Deere Credit Company
John Deere Agricultural Holdings, Inc.
John Deere Construction Holdings, Inc.
John Deere Lawn & Grounds Care Holdings, Inc.
John Deere Commercial Worksite Products, Inc.

CONTACTS: Note: Officers with more than one job title may be intentionally listed here more than once.

Robert W. Lane, CEO
Michael J. Mack, Jr., CFO/Sr. VP
Metroe B. Hornbuckle, VP-Human Resources
James R. Jabanoski, VP-IT
Klaus G. Hoehn, VP-Advanced Tech.
Klaus G. Hoehn, VP-Eng.
James R. Jenkins, General Counsel/Sr. VP
Ganesh Jayaram, VP-Corp. Bus. Dev.
H.J. Markley, VP-Corp. Comm.
Marie Z. Ziegler, VP-Investor Rel.
James A. Davlin, VP/Treas.
Kenneth C. Huhn, VP-Industrial Rel.
Thomas K. Jarrett, VP-Taxes
Dennis R. Schwartz, VP-Pension Fund & Investments
Linda E. Newborn, VP/Chief Compliance Officer
Robert W. Lane, Chmn.
Markwart von Pentz, Pres., Agriculture-Europe, Africa & South America
H.J. Markley, Exec. VP-Global Supply Mgmt. & Logistics

Phone: 309-765-8000	Fax: 309-765-5671
Toll-Free:	
Address: 1 John Deere Pl., Moline, IL 61265-8098 US	

GROWTH PLANS/SPECIAL FEATURES:

Deere & Co., better known by its John Deere brand name, conduct business in four divisions: Agricultural equipment; commercial and consumer equipment; construction and forestry; and credit. The agricultural equipment segment manufactures and distributes farm equipment and service parts including tractors; combines and harvesters; tillage, seeding and soil preparation machinery; sprayers; hay and forage equipment; material handling equipment; integrated agricultural management systems technology; and precision agricultural irrigation equipment. The commercial and consumer equipment segment manufactures and distributes equipment and service parts, including small tractors for lawn, garden, commercial and utility purposes; riding and walk-behind mowers; golf course equipment; utility vehicles; landscape and irrigation equipment; and other outdoor power products. The construction and forestry segment manufactures and distributes machines and service parts used in construction, earthmoving, material handling and timber harvesting, including backhoe loaders; crawler dozers and loaders; four-wheel-drive loaders; excavators; motor graders; articulated dump trucks; landscape loaders; skid-steer loaders; and log skidders, loaders, forwarders and harvesters. The credit segment finances sales and leases by John Deere dealers of agricultural, commercial and consumer, and construction and forestry equipment. In addition, it provides wholesale financing to dealers of the foregoing equipment, provides operating loans and finances retail revolving charge accounts. In 2007, Deere & Co. acquired Ningbo Benye Tractor & Automobile Manufacture Co. Ltd. of China. Deere entered into a joint-venture agreement with Xuzhou Bohui Science and Technology Development CO. Ltd., to expand its construction equipment presence in China. In April 2008, the company announced plans for a new facility in Russia. In May 2008, the firm acquired T-Systems International, Inc., a Californian drip irrigation company, followed by the acquisition of the Israel-based Plastro Irrigation Systems, Ltd. in June 2008.

Deere & Co. offers its employees tuition reimbursement, fitness centers, flexible work arrangements, parent resources, day care services, company discounts and membership in a credit union.

FINANCIALS: Sales and profits are in thousands of dollars—add 000 to get the full amount. 2007 Note: Financial information for 2007 was not available for all companies at press time.

2007 Sales: $24,082,200	2007 Profits: $1,821,700	U.S. Stock Ticker: DE
2006 Sales: $22,147,800	2006 Profits: $1,693,800	Int'l Ticker: Int'l Exchange:
2005 Sales: $21,190,800	2005 Profits: $1,446,800	Employees: 52,000
2004 Sales: $19,204,200	2004 Profits: $1,406,100	Fiscal Year Ends: 10/31
2003 Sales: $15,535,600	2003 Profits: $643,100	Parent Company:

SALARIES/BENEFITS:

Pension Plan: Y	ESOP Stock Plan:	Profit Sharing:	Top Exec. Salary: $1,306,280	Bonus: $6,393,070
Savings Plan: Y	Stock Purch. Plan: Y		Second Exec. Salary: $551,465	Bonus: $1,898,567

OTHER THOUGHTS:

Apparent Women Officers or Directors: 7
Hot Spot for Advancement for Women/Minorities: Y

LOCATIONS: ("Y" = Yes)

West:	Southwest:	Midwest:	Southeast:	Northeast:	International:
Y	Y	Y	Y	Y	Y

Note: Financial information, benefits and other data can change quickly and may vary from those stated here.

DELOITTE & TOUCHE USA LLP

www.deloitte.com

Industry Group Code: 541210 Ranks within this company's industry group: Sales: 2 Profits:

Management:		Sales/Marketing:		Liberal Arts:		Information Systems:		Professionals:		Technical/Scientific:	
Mgmt. Trainees:	Y	Mktg. Professionals:	Y	Gen. Writing/Editing:	Y	Info. Management:	Y	Finance/Accounting:	Y	Engineers, Elec.:	
Experienced Mgmt.:	Y	Retail Sales:		Technical Writing:	Y	Software Dev.:	Y	Law:	Y	Engineers, Other:	
Int'l Business:	Y	Commercial/Industrial:	Y	Graphic Arts/Photog.:	Y	Hardware Dev.:		HR/Other:	Y	Health/Lab:	
MBA Graduates:	Y	Sales Trainees:		Music:		Systems Integration:	Y	Training:	Y	Scientists/Research:	Y
		Advertising Pros.:	Y	Broadcasting:		Consulting/Other:	Y	Health Care:		Petroleum/Chemicals:	
				Other:				Consulting:	Y	Math/Other:	Y

TYPES OF BUSINESS:

Accounting Services
Management Consulting
Risk Management Services
Financial Advisory Services
Outsourcing Services
Legal & Compliance Advisory Services

BRANDS/DIVISIONS/AFFILIATES:

Deloitte Touche Tohmatsu
Deloitte & Touche LLP
Deloitte Consulting
Deloitte Financial Advisory Services
Deloitte Tax
Xcelicor, Inc.
Iditarod Systems, Inc.
TI Consulting

CONTACTS: Note: Officers with more than one job title may be intentionally listed here more than once.

Barry Salzberg, CEO
Jeff Rohr, CFO
Sigmund Jamison,, Dir.-Infrastructure
Stacy Janiak, Vice Chmn.-US Retail Leader, Deloitte & Touche LLP
John Hagel, Co-Chmn.-Center for Strategy & Tech.
John Seely-Brown, Co-Chmn.-Center for Strategy & Tech.
Sharon Allen, Chmn.

Phone: 212-489-1600	Fax: 212-489-1687
Toll-Free:	
Address: 1633 Broadway, New York, NY 10019-6754 US	

GROWTH PLANS/SPECIAL FEATURES:

Deloitte & Touche USA LLP (D&T), the U.S. division of global accounting firm Deloitte Touche Tohmatsu, offers a variety of financial and consulting services. The firm operates through several subsidiaries, including Deloitte & Touche LLP; Deloitte Consulting; Deloitte Financial Advisory Services; and Deloitte Tax. The largest portion of the firm's revenue comes from audit and enterprise risk services. The firm also offers consulting, tax advice and other financial advisory services. Additionally, the firm has expertise in offering complementary services such as legal and compliance advisory services involving litigation, ethics, management and disclosure issues. Industries served by D&T include aviation and transport; financial services; the public sector (federal services, education and nonprofit); retail; health care; real estate; energy (petroleum and utilities); manufacturing; and communications. The firm also funds the Deloitte Foundation, created 75 years ago and dedicated to supporting accounting, business and related fields of study in the U.S. The foundation funds the Deloitte Doctoral Fellowship Program and Trueblood Seminars for Professors, among other higher education initiatives. The firm also conducts and publishes research concerning consumer spending patterns and economic growth, and maintains offices in 148 countries. Recent acquisitions include certain assets of Barrasso Consulting LLC (Barrasso); Xcelicor, Inc.; Iditarod Systems, Inc.; and TI Consulting.

Employees of the firm are offered child care and adoption assistance; flexible work arrangements; educational programs based on past experience, future goals and area of specialty. In 2008, for the ninth year, Deloitte & Touche was named to FORTUNE magazine's list of 100 Best Companies to Work For; in 2007, the firm was named to Working Mother magazine's 100 Best Companies for the fourteenth consecutive year.

FINANCIALS: Sales and profits are in thousands of dollars—add 000 to get the full amount. 2007 Note: Financial information for 2007 was not available for all companies at press time.

2007 Sales: $9,850,000	2007 Profits: $	U.S. Stock Ticker: Subsidiary
2006 Sales: $8,769,000	2006 Profits: $	Int'l Ticker: Int'l Exchange:
2005 Sales: $7,814,000	2005 Profits: $	Employees: 37,118
2004 Sales: $6,876,000	2004 Profits: $	Fiscal Year Ends: 5/31
2003 Sales: $6,511,000	2003 Profits: $	Parent Company: DELOITTE TOUCHE TOHMATSU

SALARIES/BENEFITS:

Pension Plan: Y	ESOP Stock Plan:	Profit Sharing:	Top Exec. Salary: $	Bonus: $
Savings Plan: Y	Stock Purch. Plan:		Second Exec. Salary: $	Bonus: $

OTHER THOUGHTS:

Apparent Women Officers or Directors: 4
Hot Spot for Advancement for Women/Minorities: Y

LOCATIONS: ("Y" = Yes)

West:	Southwest:	Midwest:	Southeast:	Northeast:	International:
Y	Y	Y	Y	Y	Y

DELOITTE CONSULTING LLP

www.deloitte.com

Industry Group Code: 541611 Ranks within this company's industry group: Sales: 1 Profits:

Management:		Sales/Marketing:		Liberal Arts:		Information Systems:		Professionals:		Technical/Scientific:	
Mgmt. Trainees:	Y	Mktg. Professionals:	Y	Gen. Writing/Editing:	Y	Info. Management:	Y	Finance/Accounting:	Y	Engineers, Elec.:	
Experienced Mgmt.:	Y	Retail Sales:		Technical Writing:	Y	Software Dev.:	Y	Law:	Y	Engineers, Other:	
Int'l Business:	Y	Commercial/Industrial:	Y	Graphic Arts/Photog.:	Y	Hardware Dev.:		HR/Other:	Y	Health/Lab:	
MBA Graduates:	Y	Sales Trainees:		Music:		Systems Integration:	Y	Training:	Y	Scientists/Research:	Y
		Advertising Pros.:	Y	Broadcasting:		Consulting/Other:		Health Care:		Petroleum/Chemicals:	
				Other:				Consulting:	Y	Math/Other:	

TYPES OF BUSINESS:

Management Consulting
Technology Integration Consulting
Human Resources Consulting
Business Strategy Consulting
Outsourcing Services
Strategic Consulting
Software

BRANDS/DIVISIONS/AFFILIATES:

Deloitte Touche Tohmatsu
J.D. Edwards
Oracle Corp
PeopleSoft
SAP AG
Xcelicor, Inc.
Oracle Human Capital Management

CONTACTS: *Note: Officers with more than one job title may be intentionally listed here more than once.*

Ainar D. Aijala Jr., Global Managing Partner
John Kocjan, National Managing Dir.-Financial Svcs.
Bruce Westbrook, National Managing Dir.-Consumer Bus.
Douglas J. Lattner, Chmn.

Phone: 212-618-4000	Fax: 212-618-4500
Toll-Free:	
Address: 25 Broadway, New York, NY 10004 US	

GROWTH PLANS/SPECIAL FEATURES:

Deloitte Consulting LLC, the largest subsidiary of Deloitte Touche Tohmatsu, offers a range of expert consulting services from offices in 40 countries worldwide. It operates five main service categories: enterprise applications; human capital; outsourcing; strategy and operations; and technology integration. Enterprise applications are software tools that help companies coordinate information, talk with business partners and utilize customer data better. The company maintains partnerships with business software developers (including J.D. Edwards, Oracle, PeopleSoft and SAP) that give Deloitte Consulting's consultants the information necessary to help customers implement technological and organizational changes. The firm's human capital expertise provides ways to measure and manage employee productivity, change organizational structure, improve human resource functions and manage isolated groups of employees. Deloitte Consulting's outsourcing services help companies make outsourcing decisions in IT and noncore business functions. The company also analyzes and revises its clients' customer strategies, merger and acquisition strategies, supply chain operations, investment priorities and IT strategies. Lastly, Deloitte Consulting provides technology integration. Since businesses are beginning to integrate desktop and laptop PCs, the firm's consultants help its clients to figure out the how to use their computerized assets. In December 2007, Deloitte Consulting acquired Xcelicor, Inc., a leading North American Oracle Human Capital Management systems integrator.

Deloitte Consulting offers its employees tuition assistance; flexible work arrangements; an employee assistance program; adoption assistance and reimbursement; emergency backup daycare; a lactation support program; flexible spending accounts; medical, dental, prescription and vision plans; and a professional development program.

FINANCIALS: Sales and profits are in thousands of dollars—add 000 to get the full amount. 2007 Note: Financial information for 2007 was not available for all companies at press time.

2007 Sales: $5,200,000	2007 Profits: $	**U.S. Stock Ticker: Subsidiary**
2006 Sales: $4,500,000	2006 Profits: $	**Int'l Ticker:** Int'l Exchange:
2005 Sales: $4,300,000	2005 Profits: $	Employees: 25,000
2004 Sales: $3,900,000	2004 Profits: $	Fiscal Year Ends: 5/31
2003 Sales: $2,278,850	2003 Profits: $	Parent Company: DELOITTE TOUCHE TOHMATSU

SALARIES/BENEFITS:

Pension Plan: Y	ESOP Stock Plan:	Profit Sharing:	Top Exec. Salary: $	Bonus: $
Savings Plan: Y	Stock Purch. Plan:		Second Exec. Salary: $	Bonus: $

OTHER THOUGHTS:

Apparent Women Officers or Directors:
Hot Spot for Advancement for Women/Minorities: Y

LOCATIONS: ("Y" = Yes)					
West:	Southwest:	Midwest:	Southeast:	Northeast:	International:
Y	Y	Y	Y	Y	Y

DENNY'S CORPORATION

www.dennys.com

Industry Group Code: 722110 Ranks within this company's industry group: Sales: 9   Profits: 7

Management:		Sales/Marketing:		Liberal Arts:		Information Systems:		Professionals:		Technical/Scientific:	
Mgmt. Trainees:	Y	Mktg. Professionals:	Y	Gen. Writing/Editing:	Y	Info. Management:	Y	Finance/Accounting:	Y	Engineers, Elec.:	
Experienced Mgmt.:	Y	Retail Sales:		Technical Writing:		Software Dev.:	Y	Law:	Y	Engineers, Other:	
Int'l Business:	Y	Commercial/Industrial:		Graphic Arts/Photog.:	Y	Hardware Dev.:		HR/Other:	Y	Health/Lab:	
MBA Graduates:	Y	Sales Trainees:		Music:		Systems Integration:	Y	Training:	Y	Scientists/Research:	
		Advertising Pros.:	Y	Broadcasting:		Consulting/Other:		Health Care:		Petroleum/Chemicals:	
				Other:	Y			Consulting:		Math/Other:	

TYPES OF BUSINESS:
Restaurants-Casual Dining

BRANDS/DIVISIONS/AFFILIATES:
Denny's, Inc.
Denny's Holdings, Inc.
Meat Lover's Breakfast
Original Grand Slam
Meadowbrook Meat Company

CONTACTS: *Note: Officers with more than one job title may be intentionally listed here more than once.*
Nelson J. Marchioli, CEO
Samuel M. Wilensky, Acting Head-Oper./Sr. VP
Nelson J. Marchioli, Pres.
F. Mark Wolfinger, CFO/Exec. VP-Growth Initiatives
Louis Laguardia, VP-Human Resources & Diversity
Susan L. Mirdamadi, CIO/VP-IT
Rhonda J. Parish, Exec. VP/Chief Legal Officer/Sec.
Janis S. Emplit, Sr. VP-Oper.
Steve Dunn, VP-Dev.
S. Alex Lewis, VP-Investor Rel./Treas.
Jay C. Gilmore, Chief Acct. Officer/Controller
Mark E. Chmiel, Sr. VP-Concept Innovation
Timothy E. Fleming, General Counsel/VP
Michael J. Jank, VP-Risk Mgmt.
Enrique Mayor-Mora, VP-Planning & Analysis
Debra Smithart-Oglesby, Chmn.
Mark C. Smith, VP-Procurement & Dist.

Phone: 864-597-8000	Fax: 864-597-8780
Toll-Free: 800-733-6697	
Address: 203 E. Main St., Spartanburg, SC 29319-9966 US	

GROWTH PLANS/SPECIAL FEATURES:

Denny's Corporation, through its wholly-owned subsidiaries Denny's Holdings, Inc. and Denny's, Inc., owns and operates the Denny's restaurant brand, one of America's largest family-style restaurant chains. The company consists of approximately 1,545 restaurants, 521 of which are company-owned and operated and 1,024 of which are franchised/licensed restaurants. Denny's restaurants operate in 49 states, Washington, D.C., two U.S. territories and five foreign countries. The company offers traditional American-style food, and is known for serving breakfast around the clock, including its Meat Lover's Breakfast and Original Grand Slam. Denny's restaurants are open 24-hours-a-day, seven-days-a-week. Denny's employs both unit managers and regional/area managers to ensure brand consistency in all of its company restaurants. A network of regional franchise operations managers provides the same function for franchised restaurants. Denny's franchise system requires franchisees to meet minimum liquidity and net worth requirements and to have appropriate operational experience. The initial fee for a single 20-year Denny's franchise agreement is $40,000 and the royalty payment is 4% of gross sales. Franchisees are also required to contribute up to 4% of gross sales for advertising. The company uses a centralized purchasing program that is designed to ensure uniform product quality as well as to minimize food, beverage and supply costs. Approximately 85% of Denny's products are purchased and distributed through the Meadowbrook Meat Company under a long-term distribution contract.

Denny's offers its employees tuition reimbursement, an employee assistance plan, a student loan program, service awards, internal promotional opportunities, referral bonuses, free meals and medical, dental, vision, life, accident and disability insurance.

FINANCIALS: Sales and profits are in thousands of dollars—add 000 to get the full amount. 2007 Note: Financial information for 2007 was not available for all companies at press time.

2007 Sales: $939,368	2007 Profits: $34,713	U.S. Stock Ticker: DENN
2006 Sales: $994,044	2006 Profits: $30,338	Int'l Ticker: Int'l Exchange:
2005 Sales: $978,725	2005 Profits: $-7,328	Employees: 27,000
2004 Sales: $960,006	2004 Profits: $-37,675	Fiscal Year Ends: 12/31
2003 Sales: $	2003 Profits: $	Parent Company:

SALARIES/BENEFITS:

Pension Plan:	ESOP Stock Plan:	Profit Sharing:	Top Exec. Salary: $734,616	Bonus: $772,600
Savings Plan: Y	Stock Purch. Plan:		Second Exec. Salary: $430,192	Bonus: $285,698

OTHER THOUGHTS:
Apparent Women Officers or Directors: 7
Hot Spot for Advancement for Women/Minorities: Y

LOCATIONS: ("Y" = Yes)

West:	Southwest:	Midwest:	Southeast:	Northeast:	International:
Y	Y	Y	Y	Y	Y

DEVON ENERGY CORPORATION
www.devonenergy.com

Industry Group Code: 211111 Ranks within this company's industry group: Sales: Profits:

Management:	Sales/Marketing:	Liberal Arts:	Information Systems:	Professionals:	Technical/Scientific:
Mgmt. Trainees:	Mktg. Professionals:	Gen. Writing/Editing:	Info. Management:	Finance/Accounting:	Engineers, Elec.:
Experienced Mgmt.:	Retail Sales:	Technical Writing:	Software Dev.:	Law:	Engineers, Other:
Int'l Business:	Commercial/Industrial:	Graphic Arts/Photog.:	Hardware Dev.:	HR/Other:	Health/Lab:
MBA Graduates:	Sales Trainees:	Music:	Systems Integration:	Training:	Scientists/Research:
	Advertising Pros.:	Broadcasting:	Consulting/Other:	Health Care:	Petroleum/Chemicals:
		Other:		Consulting:	Math/Other:

TYPES OF BUSINESS:
Oil & Gas Exploration & Production
Pipelines
Gas Storage & Processing

BRANDS/DIVISIONS/AFFILIATES:
Dana Petroleum plc
Afren plc
Oranje-Nassau Energie B.V.
GEPetrol
Jackfish
Barnett Shale

CONTACTS: *Note: Officers with more than one job title may be intentionally listed here more than once.*
J. Larry Nichols, CEO
John Richels, Pres.
Darryl G. Smette, Sr. VP-Mktg. & Midstream
Frank W. Rudolph, Sr. VP-Human Resources
R. Alan Marcum, Sr. VP-Admin.
Lyndon C. Taylor, General Counsel/Sr. VP
K. Earl Reynolds, VP-Strategic Planning
Chip Minty, Supervisor, External Comm.
Vincent W. White, VP-Investor Rel.
Jeff A. Agosta, VP-Corp. Finance/Treas.
Don D. DeCarlo, VP/Gen. Mgr., Western Div.
Janice A. Dobbs, Mgr.-Corp. Governance/Corp. Sec.
Bradley A. Foster, VP/Gen. Mgr.-Central Div.
Stephen J. Hadden, Sr. VP-Exploration & Production
J. Larry Nichols, Chmn.
Joseph P. Ash, VP/Gen. Mgr.-Int'l Div.

Phone: 405-235-3611	Fax: 405-552-4550
Toll-Free:	
Address: 20 N. Broadway, Oklahoma City, OK 73102-8260 US	

GROWTH PLANS/SPECIAL FEATURES:

Devon Energy Corporation is an independent energy company engaged primarily in oil and gas exploration, development and production; the transportation of oil, gas and natural gas liquids (NGL); and the processing of natural gas. In addition to its oil and gas operations, the company has marketing and midstream operations primarily in North America. Devon's U.S. onshore operations include the Barnett Shale in north Texas; the Carthage, Groesbeck and Permian Basin areas in Texas; the Washakie area in southern Wyoming; and the Permian Basin in New Mexico. Barnett Shale is Devon's largest property, consisting of 727,000 net acres. The company's U.S. offshore operations include deepwater productions in the Gulf of Mexico, deepwater development and deepwater exploration. Deepwater production properties include Magnolia, Merganser, Nansen and Red Hawk, totaling approximately 46,000 net acres. Devon's Canadian operations include its 100% owned Jackfish thermal heavy oil project in central Alberta; its Deep Basin properties in Alberta and British Columbia; its Lloydminster properties in Alberta and Saskatchewan; its Peace River Arch properties in Alberta; and its northeast British Columbia properties. The company's international operations include its Azeri-Chirag-Gunashli (ACG) oil field offshore Azerbaijan; its Panyu field in the South China Sea; and its Polvo field offshore Brazil. In October 2007, Devon completed the sale of its Egyptian oil and gas operations to Dana Petroleum plc. In March 2008, the company agreed to sell its Cote d'Ivoire oil and gas business to Afren plc. In May 2008, Devon completed the sale of its Gabon operations to Oranje-Nassau Energie B.V., and in June completed the sale of its Equatorial Guinea oil and gas business to GEPetrol for $2.2 billion.

Devon Energy offers its U.S. employees a flexible spending account; an employee assistance program; a tuition reimbursement program; business travel insurance; and medical, dental and vision insurance.

FINANCIALS: Sales and profits are in thousands of dollars—add 000 to get the full amount. 2007 Note: Financial information for 2007 was not available for all companies at press time.

2007 Sales: $11,362,000	2007 Profits: $3,606,000	U.S. Stock Ticker: DVN
2006 Sales: $9,767,000	2006 Profits: $2,846,000	Int'l Ticker: Int'l Exchange:
2005 Sales: $10,741,000	2005 Profits: $2,920,000	Employees: 4,075
2004 Sales: $9,189,000	2004 Profits: $2,176,000	Fiscal Year Ends: 12/31
2003 Sales: $7,352,000	2003 Profits: $1,747,000	Parent Company:

SALARIES/BENEFITS:

Pension Plan: Y	ESOP Stock Plan:	Profit Sharing:	Top Exec. Salary: $1,200,000	Bonus: $2,600,600
Savings Plan: Y	Stock Purch. Plan:		Second Exec. Salary: $825,000	Bonus: $1,500,600

OTHER THOUGHTS:
Apparent Women Officers or Directors: 3
Hot Spot for Advancement for Women/Minorities: Y

LOCATIONS: ("Y" = Yes)

West:	Southwest:	Midwest:	Southeast:	Northeast:	International:
	Y				Y

DEVRY INC   www.devryinc.com

Industry Group Code: 611410 Ranks within this company's industry group: Sales: 2   Profits: 2

Management:		Sales/Marketing:		Liberal Arts:		Information Systems:		Professionals:		Technical/Scientific:	
Mgmt. Trainees:		Mktg. Professionals:	Y	Gen. Writing/Editing:	Y	Info. Management:	Y	Finance/Accounting:	Y	Engineers, Elec.:	
Experienced Mgmt.:	Y	Retail Sales:		Technical Writing:		Software Dev.:	Y	Law:	Y	Engineers, Other:	
Int'l Business:	Y	Commercial/Industrial:		Graphic Arts/Photog.:		Hardware Dev.:		HR/Other:	Y	Health/Lab:	
MBA Graduates:	Y	Sales Trainees:		Music:		Systems Integration:		Training:	Y	Scientists/Research:	
		Advertising Pros.:	Y	Broadcasting:		Consulting/Other:		Health Care:	Y	Petroleum/Chemicals:	
				Other:				Consulting:		Math/Other:	

TYPES OF BUSINESS:
Higher Education
Online Education
Medical School
Nursing School
Veterinary School
Accounting School

BRANDS/DIVISIONS/AFFILIATES:
DeVry University
Ross University
Keller Graduate School of Management
Becker Professional Review
Chamberlain College of Nursing
Stalla Review

CONTACTS: *Note: Officers with more than one job title may be intentionally listed here more than once.*
Daniel Hamburger, CEO
Daniel Hamburger, Pres.
Richard M. Gunst, CFO/Sr. VP
Donna M. Jennings, VP-Human Resources
Eric Dirst, CIO/VP
Gregory S. Davis, General Counsel/Sr. VP/Sec.
John P. Roselli, VP-Corp. Dev. & Planning
Steven P. Riehs, VP/General Manager-DeVry University Online
Richard M. Gunst, Treas.
David J. Pauldine, Exec. VP/Pres., DeVry University
Thomas C. Shepherd, Exec. VP/Pres., Ross University
Thomas J. Vucinic, Pres., Becker Professional Review
Sharon Thomas Parrott, Sr. VP-Gov. & Reg. Affairs-Chief Compliance Office
Harold T. Shapiro, Chmn.

Phone: 630-571-7700	Fax: 630-571-0317
Toll-Free:	
Address: 1 Tower Ln., Ste. 1000, Oakbrook Terrace, IL 60181 US	

GROWTH PLANS/SPECIAL FEATURES:
DeVry, Inc. is a publicly held higher-education company in North America, operating DeVry University, Ross University, Chamberlain College of Nursing and Becker CPA Review. DeVry University provides career-oriented, business- and technology-based education to students and graduates at 91 locations in the US and Canada both in traditional classrooms and online. The university offers undergraduate and graduate degree programs in technology; undergraduate and graduate degree programs in business and healthcare technology; and graduate degree programs in management offered through the university's Keller Graduate School of Management. Ross University operates two schools. The Ross University School of Medicine confers the Doctor of Medicine (MD) degree and The Ross University School of Veterinary Medicine confers the Doctor of Veterinary Medicine (DVM) degree. Nearly 6,000 graduates have received MD degrees and over 2,000 have received DVM degrees since the university's inception. The Chamberlain College of Nursing offers programs in nursing education. The Becker Professional Review is a provider of professional education and training serving the accounting and finance professions. Becker served more than 47,000 students in 2007. In November 2007, DeVry acquired Advanced Academics Inc. In 2008, the firm announced it will acquire U.S. Education Corporation, which is the parent company of Apollo College and Western Career College in Mission Viejo California. These two colleges operate 17 campus locations in the U.S. and serve 8,700 healthcare students. Becker announced an exclusive provider agreement between its Stalla Review and the CFA Society of the U.K. to provide Chartered Financial Analyst review courses. On February 29, 2008, DeVry University announced a sale and leaseback its 98,000 square foot Houston campus for approximately $14.5 million. DeVry will leaseback approximately 60 percent of the original space.

FINANCIALS: Sales and profits are in thousands of dollars—add 000 to get the full amount. 2007 Note: Financial information for 2007 was not available for all companies at press time.

2007 Sales: $933,473	2007 Profits: $76,188	**U.S. Stock Ticker: DV**
2006 Sales: $839,513	2006 Profits: $43,053	**Int'l Ticker:** Int'l Exchange:
2005 Sales: $780,662	2005 Profits: $18,011	Employees: 5,400
2004 Sales: $784,885	2004 Profits: $58,061	Fiscal Year Ends: 6/30
2003 Sales: $679,579	2003 Profits: $61,148	Parent Company:

SALARIES/BENEFITS:

Pension Plan:	ESOP Stock Plan:	Profit Sharing:	Top Exec. Salary: $900,000	Bonus: $810,113
Savings Plan:	Stock Purch. Plan:		Second Exec. Salary: $400,000	Bonus: $272,880

OTHER THOUGHTS:
Apparent Women Officers or Directors: 5
Hot Spot for Advancement for Women/Minorities: Y

LOCATIONS: ("Y" = Yes)

West:	Southwest:	Midwest:	Southeast:	Northeast:	International:
Y	Y	Y	Y	Y	Y

Note: Financial information, benefits and other data can change quickly and may vary from those stated here.

DIAMOND OFFSHORE DRILLING INC
www.diamondoffshore.com

Industry Group Code: 213111 Ranks within this company's industry group: Sales: 12 Profits: 7

Management:		Sales/Marketing:		Liberal Arts:		Information Systems:		Professionals:		Technical/Scientific:	
Mgmt. Trainees:	Y	Mktg. Professionals:	Y	Gen. Writing/Editing:		Info. Management:	Y	Finance/Accounting:	Y	Engineers, Elec.:	Y
Experienced Mgmt.:	Y	Retail Sales:		Technical Writing:		Software Dev.:		Law:	Y	Engineers, Other:	Y
Int'l Business:	Y	Commercial/Industrial:	Y	Graphic Arts/Photog.:		Hardware Dev.:		HR/Other:	Y	Health/Lab:	Y
MBA Graduates:	Y	Sales Trainees:		Music:		Systems Integration:		Training:	Y	Scientists/Research:	
		Advertising Pros.:		Broadcasting:		Consulting/Other:		Health Care:		Petroleum/Chemicals:	Y
				Other:				Consulting:		Math/Other:	

TYPES OF BUSINESS:
Oil & Gas Drilling
Contract Drilling

BRANDS/DIVISIONS/AFFILIATES:

CONTACTS: Note: Officers with more than one job title may be intentionally listed here more than once.
Lawrence R. Dickerson, CEO
Lawrence R. Dickerson, Pres.
Gary T. Krenek, CFO/Sr. VP
John L. Gabriel, Sr. VP-Contracts & Mktg.
R. Lynn Charles, VP-Human Resources
John M. Vecchio, Sr. VP-Tech. Svcs.
Karl S. Sellers, VP-Eng.
Mark F. Baudoin, Sr. VP-Admin. & Oper. Svcs.
William C. Long, General Counsel/Sr. VP/Sec.
Lyndol L. Dew, Sr. VP-Worldwide Oper.
Scott L. Kornblau, Treas.
Steven A. Nelson, VP-Domestic Oper.
Glen E. Merrifield, VP-Oper. Mgmt. Systems & Marine Dept.
Beth G. Gordon, Controller
Bodley P. Thornton, VP-Mktg.
James S. Tisch, Chmn.
Morrison R. Plaisance, VP-Int'l Oper.

Phone: 281-492-5300	Fax: 281-492-5378
Toll-Free: 800-848-1980	
Address: 15415 Katy Fwy., Ste. 100, Houston, TX 77094-1810 US	

GROWTH PLANS/SPECIAL FEATURES:
Diamond Offshore Drilling, Inc. is a leading deepwater drilling contractor. Diamond operates one of the world's largest fleets of offshore drilling units, consisting of 30 semi-submersibles, 13 jack-ups and one drill ship. Its semi-submersible rigs float with their lower hulls between 55 and 90 feet below the water line and are held in position partly with anchors and partly through a special hull characteristic known as wave transparency; three of the rigs also have a special computer-controlled thruster system known as dynamic-positioning. Nine of Diamond's semi-submersibles are high-specification, which means that they are capable of drilling in harsh environments and water depths greater than 4,000 feet; and the other 21 rigs may only work in depths up to 4,000 feet. The company operates in many geographic areas, including the Gulf of Mexico, including the U.S. and Mexico; Europe, principally in the U.K. and Norway; the Mediterranean Basin, including Egypt, Libya, Tunisia and other parts of Africa; South America, principally in Brazil; Australia and Asia, including Malaysia, Indonesia and Vietnam; and the Middle East, including Kuwait, Qatar and Saudi Arabia.

Diamond provides employees with life, accidental death and dismemberment insurance; dependant life insurance for spouses and children; medical, dental and prescription drug coverage; an employee assistance plan; and flexible spending accounts.

FINANCIALS: Sales and profits are in thousands of dollars—add 000 to get the full amount. 2007 Note: Financial information for 2007 was not available for all companies at press time.

2007 Sales: $2,567,723	2007 Profits: $846,541	**U.S. Stock Ticker: DO**	
2006 Sales: $2,052,572	2006 Profits: $706,847	Int'l Ticker:	Int'l Exchange:
2005 Sales: $1,221,002	2005 Profits: $260,337	Employees: 4,800	
2004 Sales: $814,662	2004 Profits: $-7,243	Fiscal Year Ends: 12/31	
2003 Sales: $680,941	2003 Profits: $-48,414	Parent Company:	

SALARIES/BENEFITS:

Pension Plan:	ESOP Stock Plan:	Profit Sharing: Y	Top Exec. Salary: $627,747	Bonus: $460,000
Savings Plan: Y	Stock Purch. Plan:		Second Exec. Salary: $368,456	Bonus: $255,000

OTHER THOUGHTS:
Apparent Women Officers or Directors: 1
Hot Spot for Advancement for Women/Minorities:

LOCATIONS: ("Y" = Yes)

West:	Southwest:	Midwest:	Southeast:	Northeast:	International:
	Y		Y		Y

Note: Financial information, benefits and other data can change quickly and may vary from those stated here.

DICK'S SPORTING GOODS INC www.dickssportinggoods.com

Industry Group Code: 451110 Ranks within this company's industry group: Sales: 1 Profits: 2

Management:		Sales/Marketing:		Liberal Arts:		Information Systems:		Professionals:		Technical/Scientific:	
Mgmt. Trainees:		Mktg. Professionals:	Y	Gen. Writing/Editing:	Y	Info. Management:	Y	Finance/Accounting:	Y	Engineers, Elec.:	
Experienced Mgmt.:	Y	Retail Sales:	Y	Technical Writing:		Software Dev.:	Y	Law:	Y	Engineers, Other:	
Int'l Business:		Commercial/Industrial:	Y	Graphic Arts/Photog.:	Y	Hardware Dev.:		HR/Other:	Y	Health/Lab:	
MBA Graduates:	Y	Sales Trainees:	Y	Music:		Systems Integration:		Training:	Y	Scientists/Research:	
		Advertising Pros.:	Y	Broadcasting:		Consulting/Other:		Health Care:		Petroleum/Chemicals:	
				Other:				Consulting:		Math/Other:	

TYPES OF BUSINESS:

Sporting Goods Stores
Outdoor Apparel
Footwear
Hunting & Fishing Supplies
Golf Supplies
Bicycles
Online Sales

BRANDS/DIVISIONS/AFFILIATES:

Golf Galaxy
Chick's Sporting Goods

CONTACTS: *Note: Officers with more than one job title may be intentionally listed here more than once.*

Edward W. Stack, CEO
Joseph H. Schmidt, COO/Exec. VP
Timothy E. Kullman, CFO
Kathy Sutter, Sr. VP-Human Resources
Matthew J. Lynch, CIO/Sr. VP
Jeffrey R. Hennion, Chief Merch. Officer/Exec. VP
Timothy E. Kullman, Exec. VP-Admin.
Timothy E. Kullman, Exec. VP-Finance
Gwen Manto, Chief Merch. Officer/Exec. VP
Douglas Walrod, Sr. VP-Real Estate & Dev.
Edward W. Stack, Chmn.
Lee Belitsky, Sr. VP-Distribution & Transportation

Phone: 724-273-3400	Fax: 724-227-1904
Toll-Free:	
Address: 300 Industry Dr., RIDC Park W., Pittsburgh, PA 15275 US	

GROWTH PLANS/SPECIAL FEATURES:

Dick's Sporting Goods, Inc. is a retail sporting goods chain with 340 stores in 36 states, primarily in the eastern half of the U.S. The company offers a broad assortment of sporting goods and fitness equipment, apparel and footwear under national and private-brand labels, including its own Ativa, PowerBolt, Fitness Gear, DBX, Acuity and Northeast Outfitters brands. Each Dick's location typically contains five store-within-a-store specialty stores. The company seeks to create a distinct look and feel for each specialty department to heighten the customer's interest in the products offered. A typical facility has the following in-store specialty shops: the Pro Shop, a golf shop with a putting green and hitting area and video monitors featuring golf tournaments and instruction on the Golf Channel or other sources; the Footwear Center, featuring hardwood floors, a track for testing athletic shoes or in-line skates and a bank of video monitors playing sporting events; the Cycle Shop, designed to sell and service bikes, complete with a mechanics' work area and equipment on the sales floor; the Sportsman's Lodge for the hunting and fishing customer, designed to have the look of an authentic bait and tackle shop; and Total Sports, a seasonal sports area displaying sports equipment and athletic apparel associated with specific seasonal sports. Dick's stores offer a variety of maintenance, repair and support services in all departments, as well as an e-commerce site. The company also owns Golf Galaxy, a specialty golf retailer acquired in 2007, with 77 locations in 29 states, catalog operations and e-commerce web sites. In late 2007, the firm agreed to acquire Chick's Sporting Goods for about $40 million.

FINANCIALS: Sales and profits are in thousands of dollars—add 000 to get the full amount. 2007 Note: Financial information for 2007 was not available for all companies at press time.

2007 Sales: $3,114,162	2007 Profits: $112,611	**U.S. Stock Ticker: DKS**
2006 Sales: $2,624,987	2006 Profits: $72,980	**Int'l Ticker:** Int'l Exchange:
2005 Sales: $2,109,400	2005 Profits: $68,905	Employees: 10,400
2004 Sales: $1,470,800	2004 Profits: $52,408	Fiscal Year Ends: 1/31
2003 Sales: $1,272,600	2003 Profits: $38,300	Parent Company:

SALARIES/BENEFITS:

Pension Plan:	ESOP Stock Plan:	Profit Sharing:	Top Exec. Salary: $662,500	Bonus: $2,650,000
Savings Plan:	Stock Purch. Plan:		Second Exec. Salary: $629,808	Bonus: $944,712

OTHER THOUGHTS:

Apparent Women Officers or Directors: 2
Hot Spot for Advancement for Women/Minorities: Y

LOCATIONS: ("Y" = Yes)

West:	Southwest:	Midwest:	Southeast:	Northeast:	International:
Y	Y	Y	Y	Y	

Note: Financial information, benefits and other data can change quickly and may vary from those stated here.

DIEBOLD INC
www.diebold.com

Industry Group Code: 334111 Ranks within this company's industry group: Sales: 4 Profits: 3

Management:		Sales/Marketing:		Liberal Arts:		Information Systems:		Professionals:		Technical/Scientific:	
Mgmt. Trainees:	Y	Mktg. Professionals:	Y	Gen. Writing/Editing:	Y	Info. Management:	Y	Finance/Accounting:	Y	Engineers, Elec.:	Y
Experienced Mgmt.:	Y	Retail Sales:		Technical Writing:	Y	Software Dev.:	Y	Law:	Y	Engineers, Other:	
Int'l Business:	Y	Commercial/Industrial:	Y	Graphic Arts/Photog.:	Y	Hardware Dev.:	Y	HR/Other:	Y	Health/Lab:	
MBA Graduates:	Y	Sales Trainees:	Y	Music:		Systems Integration:	Y	Training:	Y	Scientists/Research:	Y
		Advertising Pros.:	Y	Broadcasting:		Consulting/Other:	Y	Health Care:		Petroleum/Chemicals:	
				Other:				Consulting:		Math/Other:	Y

TYPES OF BUSINESS:
Computer Hardware-Automated Teller Machines
Self-Service Terminals
Security Systems
Technical Services
Software
Electronic Voting Machines

BRANDS/DIVISIONS/AFFILIATES:
Diebold North America
Diebold International
Diebold Elections Systems, Inc.
Procomp Industria Electronica S.A.
Opteva
Diebold 450 ATM

CONTACTS: Note: Officers with more than one job title may be intentionally listed here more than once.
Thomas W. Swidarski, CEO
Thomas W. Swidarski, Pres.
Kevin J. Krakora, CFO/Exec. VP
Sheila M. Rutt, Chief Human Resources Officer/VP
Sean F. Forrester, CIO/VP
Warren W. Dettinger, General Counsel./VP
George S. Mayes, Jr., Exec. VP-Global Oper.
Robert J. Warren, VP-Corp. Dev. & Finance
John D. Kristoff, Chief Comm. Officer/VP
Timothy J. McDannold, VP/Treas.
David Bucci, Sr. VP-Customer Solutions Group
M. Scott Hunter, Chief Tax Officer/VP
Dennis M. Moriarty, Sr. VP-Global Security Div.
M. Scott Hunter, VP/Chief Tax Officer
John N. Lauer, Chmn.
James L.M. Chen, Sr. VP-EMEA & Asia Pacific Divisions
George S. Mayes, Jr., Sr. VP-Global Mfg. & Supply Chain

Phone: 330-490-4000	**Fax:** 330-490-3794
Toll-Free: 800-999-3600	
Address: 5995 Mayfair Rd., North Canton, OH 44720-8077 US	

GROWTH PLANS/SPECIAL FEATURES:

Diebold, Inc., incorporated in 1876, develops, manufactures, sells and services self-service transaction systems; electronic and physical security systems; software; and various products used to equip bank facilities and electronic voting terminals. The company's primary customers include banks and financial institutions, as well as public libraries, government agencies, utilities and various retail outlets. The company is comprised of three segments, Diebold North America (DNA), Diebold International (DI) and Diebold Elections Systems, Inc. (DESI), which comprise its main sales channels. DNA sells financial and retail systems and also services them in the U.S. and Canada. The DI segment sells and services financial and retail systems in 90 countries worldwide. DESI manufactures and supplies electronic voting terminals and solutions, and is a leading producer of touch-screen-voting systems. Diebold's Self-Service Product division provides self-service banking products and is a leading global supplier of ATMs. The firm's Physical Security and Facility Products division designs and manufactures several financial service solutions offerings, including the proprietary Remote Teller System (RTS), vaults, safes, safe deposit boxes and drive-up banking equipment. The Election Systems division, supplied by both DESI and Procomp Industria Electronica S.A., is one of the largest electronic voting system providers in the world. The Integrated Security Solutions division provides global sales, service, installation, project management and monitoring of electronic security products. The Software Solutions and Services division offers solutions consisting of multiple applications that process events and transactions. In August 2008, Diebold announced the closure of a 100-employee manufacturing plant in Newark, Ohio for early 2009. In August 2008, Diebold stated its plan to leave the German market and close its subsidiary there, Diebold Germany GmbH.

Diebold offers its employees educational assistance, long term disability plan, employee assistance program, adoption assistance, flexible spending accounts and a college scholarship program.

FINANCIALS: Sales and profits are in thousands of dollars—add 000 to get the full amount. 2007 Note: Financial information for 2007 was not available for all companies at press time.

2007 Sales: $2,953,000	2007 Profits: $	**U.S. Stock Ticker:** DBD
2006 Sales: $2,906,232	2006 Profits: $86,547	**Int'l Ticker:** Int'l Exchange:
2005 Sales: $2,587,049	2005 Profits: $96,746	Employees: 15,451
2004 Sales: $2,357,108	2004 Profits: $183,797	Fiscal Year Ends: 12/31
2003 Sales: $2,109,700	2003 Profits: $174,800	Parent Company:

SALARIES/BENEFITS:

Pension Plan:	ESOP Stock Plan:	Profit Sharing:	Top Exec. Salary: $550,000	Bonus: $392,500
Savings Plan: Y	Stock Purch. Plan: Y		Second Exec. Salary: $320,000	Bonus: $171,273

OTHER THOUGHTS:
Apparent Women Officers or Directors: 3
Hot Spot for Advancement for Women/Minorities: Y

LOCATIONS: ("Y" = Yes)

West:	Southwest:	Midwest:	Southeast:	Northeast:	International:
Y	Y	Y	Y	Y	Y

Note: Financial information, benefits and other data can change quickly and may vary from those stated here.

DINEEQUITY INC

www.dineequity.com

Industry Group Code: 722110 Ranks within this company's industry group: Sales: Profits:

Management:	Sales/Marketing:	Liberal Arts:	Information Systems:	Professionals:	Technical/Scientific:
Mgmt. Trainees:	Mktg. Professionals:	Gen. Writing/Editing:	Info. Management:	Finance/Accounting:	Engineers, Elec.:
Experienced Mgmt.:	Retail Sales:	Technical Writing:	Software Dev.:	Law:	Engineers, Other:
Int'l Business:	Commercial/Industrial:	Graphic Arts/Photog.:	Hardware Dev.:	HR/Other:	Health/Lab:
MBA Graduates:	Sales Trainees:	Music:	Systems Integration:	Training:	Scientists/Research:
	Advertising Pros.:	Broadcasting:	Consulting/Other:	Health Care:	Petroleum/Chemicals:
		Other:		Consulting:	Math/Other:

TYPES OF BUSINESS:
Restaurants

BRANDS/DIVISIONS/AFFILIATES:
International House of Pancakes
IHOP Restaurant Training Program
Applebee's International Inc

CONTACTS: Note: Officers with more than one job title may be intentionally listed here more than once.
Julia Stewart, CEO
Greggory Calvin, Interim CFO/Controller
John Jakubek, VP-Human Resources
Patrick J. Piccininno, VP-IT
Mark D. Weisberger, General Counsel/VP-Legal/Corp. Sec.
Michael Mendelsohn, VP-Finance
Dustin Dixon, VP-Quality Assurance
Richard C. Celio, Chief Restaurant Support Officer
Des Hague, Pres., IHOP Restaurants
Mike Archer, Pres., Applebee's International, Inc.
Julia Stewart, Chmn.
David Parsley, Sr. VP-Supply Chain

Phone: 818-240-6055	Fax: 818-637-3131
Toll-Free:	
Address: 450 N. Brand Blvd., 7rd Fl., Glendale, CA 91203-1903 US	

GROWTH PLANS/SPECIAL FEATURES:
DineEquity, Inc., formerly IHOP Corp., owns and operates two restaurant concepts in the casual dining and family dining niches: Applebee's Neighborhood Grill and Bar, or Applebee's, and International House of Pancakes, or IHOP. The company develops, franchises and operates roughly 1,300 IHOP restaurants in North America. IHOP restaurants offer a selection of pancakes, omelets and other breakfast items, as well as lunch, dinner and snack items. Most of the restaurants additionally offer special items for children and seniors at reduced prices. In recognition of local tastes, IHOP restaurants typically offer regional specialties that complement the IHOP core menu. Applebee's restaurants operate in the bar and grill segment of the casual dining industry. DineEquity currently controls nearly 2,000 Applebee's restaurants across the U.S. The company operates in four categories: franchise operations, rental operations, company restaurant operations and financing operations. The franchise operations segment consists of restaurant operated by the firm's franchisees and area licensees in the U.S. and Canada, with revenue consisting primarily of royalty revenues, sales of proprietary products, advertising fees and the portion of the franchise fees allocated to the company's intellectual property. Rental operations revenue consists of revenue from operating leases and interest income from direct financing leases. The company restaurant operations segment consists of company-operated restaurants. Financing operations revenue consists of the portion of franchise fees not allocated to DineEquity's intellectual property and sales of equipment. In November 2007, IHOP acquired Applebee's International, Inc. for $2.1 billion, which included more than 3,250 restaurants. The company intends to franchise the majority of Applebee's company-owned restaurants by 2010. In March 2008, DineEquity reached an agreement to sell 41 company-operated Applebee's restaurants located in California and Nevada.

FINANCIALS: Sales and profits are in thousands of dollars—add 000 to get the full amount. 2007 Note: Financial information for 2007 was not available for all companies at press time.

2007 Sales: $484,559	2007 Profits: $- 480	U.S. Stock Ticker: DIN
2006 Sales: $349,560	2006 Profits: $44,553	Int'l Ticker: Int'l Exchange:
2005 Sales: $348,023	2005 Profits: $43,937	Employees: 32,300
2004 Sales: $	2004 Profits: $	Fiscal Year Ends: 12/31
2003 Sales: $	2003 Profits: $	Parent Company:

SALARIES/BENEFITS:

Pension Plan:	ESOP Stock Plan:	Profit Sharing:	Top Exec. Salary: $630,625	Bonus: $1,952,025
Savings Plan: Y	Stock Purch. Plan:		Second Exec. Salary: $368,127	Bonus: $249,752

OTHER THOUGHTS:
Apparent Women Officers or Directors: 2
Hot Spot for Advancement for Women/Minorities: Y

LOCATIONS: ("Y" = Yes)

West:	Southwest:	Midwest:	Southeast:	Northeast:	International:
Y	Y	Y	Y	Y	Y

Note: Financial information, benefits and other data can change quickly and may vary from those stated here.

DIRECTV GROUP INC (THE)

www.directv.com

Industry Group Code: 513220 Ranks within this company's industry group: Sales: 3 Profits: 3

Management:		Sales/Marketing:		Liberal Arts:		Information Systems:		Professionals:		Technical/Scientific:	
Mgmt. Trainees:		Mktg. Professionals:	Y	Gen. Writing/Editing:	Y	Info. Management:	Y	Finance/Accounting:	Y	Engineers, Elec.:	
Experienced Mgmt.:	Y	Retail Sales:		Technical Writing:		Software Dev.:	Y	Law:	Y	Engineers, Other:	
Int'l Business:	Y	Commercial/Industrial:		Graphic Arts/Photog.:	Y	Hardware Dev.:		HR/Other:	Y	Health/Lab:	
MBA Graduates:	Y	Sales Trainees:		Music:		Systems Integration:	Y	Training:	Y	Scientists/Research:	
		Advertising Pros.:	Y	Broadcasting:	Y	Consulting/Other:		Health Care:		Petroleum/Chemicals:	
				Other:	Y			Consulting:		Math/Other:	

TYPES OF BUSINESS:

Satellite Broadcasting
Commercial Satellite Fleet
Satellite-Based Internet Services
Digital Television

BRANDS/DIVISIONS/AFFILIATES:

Liberty Media Corp
DIRECTV U.S.
DIRECTV Latin America
PanAmericana
Sky Brasil Servicos Ltda.
Innova, S. de R.L. de C.V.
Sat-Go

CONTACTS: Note: Officers with more than one job title may be intentionally listed here more than once.

Chase Carey, CEO
Chase Carey, Pres.
Romulo G. Pontual, CTO/Exec. VP
Larry D. Hunter, General Counsel/Corp. Sec./Exec. VP
Michael W. Palkovic, Exec. VP-Oper.
J. William Little, Sr. VP-Bus. Dev./Treas.
Robert Mercer, Press Contact
John F. Murphy, Chief Acct. Officer/Controller/Sr. VP
Bruce B. Churchill, Pres., New Ventures/Exec. VP
John C. Malone, Chmn.
Bruce B. Churchill, CEO/Pres., Latin America & New Enterprises

Phone: 212-462-5200	Fax: 310-535-5225
Toll-Free:	
Address: 2230 E. Imperial Hwy., El Segundo, CA 90245-0956 US	

GROWTH PLANS/SPECIAL FEATURES:

The DIRECTV Group, Inc. is one of the world's top providers of digital television entertainment and wireless systems. The company's two business segments, DIRECTV U.S. and DIRECTV Latin America (DTVLA), are engaged in acquiring, promoting, selling and distributing digital entertainment programming via satellite to residential and commercial subscribers. DIRECTV U.S. is the one of the largest providers of direct-to-home digital television services, as well as in the multi-channel video programming distribution industry, with over 16.8 million subscribers and about 1,800 digital video and audio channels, including satellite radio and specialty networks. DIRECTV U.S. currently broadcasts its service from 11 geosynchronous satellites, 10 owned and one leased, and has plans to launch one more in 2008. DTVLA comprises PanAmericana, which provides services in Venezuela, Argentina, Chile, Colombia, Puerto Rico and certain other countries through wholly-owned subsidiary DIRECTV Latin America, LLC. PanAmericana also operates through 74%-owned subsidiary Sky Brasil Servicos Ltda. (Sky Brazil); and 41%-owned subsidiary Innova, S. de R.L. de C.V. (Sky Mexico). PanAmericana has approximately 1.7 million subscribers; Sky Brazil, 1.5 million; and Sky Mexico, 1.6 million. The firm is considering the launch of a massive wireless voice and data network, probably based on WiMax, which would offer bundled services including TV, phone and Internet access. In May 2007, the firm announced the launch of the world's first portable satellite system, Sat-Go. In October 2007, the company launched its HD service, which now offers over 90 channels. In February 2008, Liberty Media Corp. acquired majority control of DIRECTV, exchanging its 16.3%-interest in News Corp. for News Corp.'s 41% stake in DIRECTV (valued at $12.5 billion), $465 million in cash and News Corp.'s interests in three regional sports networks. In April 2008, Liberty increased its stake in DIRECTV to 48%.

DIRECTV's employees receive medical and dental insurance; educational assistance; and free products.

FINANCIALS: Sales and profits are in thousands of dollars—add 000 to get the full amount. 2007 Note: Financial information for 2007 was not available for all companies at press time.

2007 Sales: $17,246,000	2007 Profits: $1,451,000	**U.S. Stock Ticker:** DTV	
2006 Sales: $14,755,500	2006 Profits: $1,420,100	**Int'l Ticker:** Int'l Exchange:	
2005 Sales: $13,164,500	2005 Profits: $335,900	**Employees:** 11,300	
2004 Sales: $11,360,000	2004 Profits: $-1,944,000	**Fiscal Year Ends:** 12/31	
2003 Sales: $10,121,200	2003 Profits: $-361,800	**Parent Company:**	

SALARIES/BENEFITS:

Pension Plan: Y	ESOP Stock Plan:	Profit Sharing:	Top Exec. Salary: $2,213,822	Bonus: $4,200,000
Savings Plan: Y	Stock Purch. Plan:		Second Exec. Salary: $1,091,242	Bonus: $1,350,000

OTHER THOUGHTS:

Apparent Women Officers or Directors: 1
Hot Spot for Advancement for Women/Minorities:

LOCATIONS: ("Y" = Yes)

West:	Southwest:	Midwest:	Southeast:	Northeast:	International:
Y	Y	Y	Y	Y	Y

Note: Financial information, benefits and other data can change quickly and may vary from those stated here.

DJO INC

www.djortho.com

Industry Group Code: 339113 Ranks within this company's industry group: Sales: 18 Profits: 17

Management:		Sales/Marketing:		Liberal Arts:		Information Systems:		Professionals:		Technical/Scientific:	
Mgmt. Trainees:		Mktg. Professionals:	Y	Gen. Writing/Editing:		Info. Management:	Y	Finance/Accounting:	Y	Engineers, Elec.:	Y
Experienced Mgmt.:	Y	Retail Sales:		Technical Writing:	Y	Software Dev.:		Law:	Y	Engineers, Other:	Y
Int'l Business:	Y	Commercial/Industrial:	Y	Graphic Arts/Photog.:	Y	Hardware Dev.:		HR/Other:	Y	Health/Lab:	Y
MBA Graduates:	Y	Sales Trainees:		Music:		Systems Integration:		Training:	Y	Scientists/Research:	
		Advertising Pros.:		Broadcasting:		Consulting/Other:		Health Care:		Petroleum/Chemicals:	
				Other:				Consulting:		Math/Other:	

TYPES OF BUSINESS:

Orthopedic Device Manufacturing
Bone Growth Stimulators
Rehabilitation Products
Pain Management Products
Soft Goods-Braces & Fracture Boots
Regeneration Products

BRANDS/DIVISIONS/AFFILIATES:

DonJoy
Regentek
KD Innovation
ProCare
OfficeCare
SpinaLogic
Orthologic
Aircast, Inc.

CONTACTS: Note: Officers with more than one job title may be intentionally listed here more than once.

Leslie H. Cross, CEO
Luke T. Faulstick, COO
Vickie L. Capps, CFO
Louis T. Ruggiero, Sr. VP-Mktg. & Sales
Tom Capizzi, Exec. VP-Global Human Resources
Donald M. Roberts, General Counsel/Exec. VP/Sec.
Luke T. Faulstick, Sr. VP-Oper.
Mark Francois, Dir-Investor Rel.
Vickie L. Capps, Treas.
Kenneth W. Davidson, Chmn.
Vickie L. Capps, Exec. VP-Int'l Sales & Mktg.

Phone: 760-727-1280	Fax: 760-734-3595
Toll-Free: 800-321-9549	
Address: 1430 Decision St, Vista, CA 92081 US	

GROWTH PLANS/SPECIAL FEATURES:

DJO, Inc. is a global medical device company specializing in rehabilitation and regeneration products for the non-operative orthopedic and spine markets. The firm has a broad portfolio of over 600 products, marketed under the DonJoy and ProCare brands. Products include rigid knee braces, soft goods and pain management products, all of which are used to prevent injury, treat chronic conditions, and aid in recovery after surgery or injury. Sales of rigid knee braces represented approximately 21% of DJO's revenues during 2007. DJO's soft goods product line consists of over 500 products that offer immobilization and support from head to toe. DJO's portfolio of pain management products primarily includes cold therapy products, which help reduce pain and swelling. The firm also offers a system that employs ambulatory infusion pumps for the delivery of local anesthetic to a surgical site. DJO sells its products domestically and in over 70 other countries through a network of agents, distributors and the company's direct sales force. The firm's customers include orthopedic and spine surgeons, podiatrists, orthopedic and prosthetic centers, third-party distributors, hospitals, surgery centers, physical therapists, athletic trainers and other healthcare professionals. The company's brands include Defiance, dj Ortho, FourcePoint, IceMan, OfficeCare, SpinaLogic, Velocity, Knee Guarantee and others. In July 2007, the firm was acquired by acquired by ReAble Therapeutics, Inc. for $1.18 billion. ReAble is owned by the Blackstone Group, which is financing the acquisition. In March 2008, the company launched the Aircast Cryo/Cuff IC Cryo-compression system, which uses cold therapy and focused compression to control hemathrosis, edema, and pain.

DJO offers its employees a fitness room, income protection, flexible spending accounts, tuition reimbursement, 401(k), and a credit union membership.

FINANCIALS: Sales and profits are in thousands of dollars—add 000 to get the full amount. 2007 Note: Financial information for 2007 was not available for all companies at press time.

2007 Sales: $	2007 Profits: $	U.S. Stock Ticker: Subsidiary
2006 Sales: $413,058	2006 Profits: $12,641	Int'l Ticker: Int'l Exchange:
2005 Sales: $286,167	2005 Profits: $29,198	Employees: 3,000
2004 Sales: $255,999	2004 Profits: $14,015	Fiscal Year Ends: 12/31
2003 Sales: $197,939	2003 Profits: $12,071	Parent Company: REABLE THERAPEUTICS INC

SALARIES/BENEFITS:

Pension Plan:	ESOP Stock Plan:	Profit Sharing:	Top Exec. Salary: $499,167	Bonus: $236,554
Savings Plan: Y	Stock Purch. Plan: Y		Second Exec. Salary: $301,667	Bonus: $111,639

OTHER THOUGHTS:

Apparent Women Officers or Directors: 1
Hot Spot for Advancement for Women/Minorities:

LOCATIONS: ("Y" = Yes)

West:	Southwest:	Midwest:	Southeast:	Northeast:	International:
Y	Y	Y	Y	Y	Y

DOLE FOOD COMPANY INC

www.dole.com

Industry Group Code: 311420 Ranks within this company's industry group: Sales: 1   Profits: 1

Management:		Sales/Marketing:		Liberal Arts:	Information Systems:		Professionals:		Technical/Scientific:	
Mgmt. Trainees:	Y	Mktg. Professionals:	Y	Gen. Writing/Editing:	Info. Management:	Y	Finance/Accounting:	Y	Engineers, Elec.:	
Experienced Mgmt.:	Y	Retail Sales:		Technical Writing:	Software Dev.:		Law:	Y	Engineers, Other:	
Int'l Business:	Y	Commercial/Industrial:	Y	Graphic Arts/Photog.:	Hardware Dev.:		HR/Other:	Y	Health/Lab:	
MBA Graduates:	Y	Sales Trainees:		Music:	Systems Integration:		Training:	Y	Scientists/Research:	
		Advertising Pros.:		Broadcasting:	Consulting/Other:		Health Care:		Petroleum/Chemicals:	
				Other:			Consulting:		Math/Other:	

TYPES OF BUSINESS:

Fruit Farming
Fresh-Cut Flowers
Fresh Produce
Packaged Foods
Imports

BRANDS/DIVISIONS/AFFILIATES:

DHM Holding Company
JP Fruit Distributors Ltd.
5 A Day for Better Health

CONTACTS: *Note: Officers with more than one job title may be intentionally listed here more than once.*

David DeLorenzo, CEO
David DeLorenzo, Pres.
Roberta Wieman, Chief of Staff/Exec. VP
Scott A. Griswold, Exec. VP-Corp. Dev.
David H. Murdock, Chmn.

Phone: 818-879-6600	Fax: 818-879-6615
Toll-Free: 800-356-3111	
Address: 1 Dole Dr., Westlake Village, CA 91362 US	

GROWTH PLANS/SPECIAL FEATURES:

Dole Food Company, Inc. is engaged in the growing, processing, packaging, distribution and marketing of fresh produce, packaged foods (value-added products) and fresh-cut flowers. It sources or sells over 200 products in more than 90 countries. The company operates through four primary segments: fresh fruit, fresh vegetables, packaged foods and fresh-cut flowers. Its fully integrated operations include sourcing, growing, processing, distributing and marketing products. The firm's products benefit from the focus on research and development in the areas of harvesting, processing, packing and cooling of fresh produce. Dole has offices in California and Florida, as well as offices worldwide that sell its products to companies involved in the wholesale, retail and institutional markets. The firm is one of the world's leading producers of bananas and pineapples and an importer of fresh-cut flowers in the U.S. These flowers are grown on Dole-owned land in Latin America and subsequently imported to the U.S. where they are distributed to retail flower stores and grocery chains. DHM Holding Company, a company entirely owned by David Murdoch, owns all of Dole's stock. Recently, the firm inaugurated a new organic banana facility in Columbia and acquired JP Fruit Distributors Ltd. from the Jamaica Producers Group Ltd. for roughly $41.9 million.

The company offers its employees medical, dental and vision insurance; life and AD&D insurance; business travel accident and long-term disability insurance; flexible spending accounts; a 401(k) plan; and an employee assistance program.

FINANCIALS: Sales and profits are in thousands of dollars—add 000 to get the full amount. 2007 Note: Financial information for 2007 was not available for all companies at press time.

2007 Sales: $6,931,000	2007 Profits: $	**U.S. Stock Ticker: Private**
2006 Sales: $6,171,500	2006 Profits: $89,000	Int'l Ticker: Int'l Exchange:
2005 Sales: $5,870,600	2005 Profits: $	Employees: 47,000
2004 Sales: $5,316,200	2004 Profits: $134,400	Fiscal Year Ends: 12/31
2003 Sales: $4,773,100	2003 Profits: $83,900	Parent Company:

SALARIES/BENEFITS:

Pension Plan:	ESOP Stock Plan:	Profit Sharing:	Top Exec. Salary: $950,000	Bonus: $285,000
Savings Plan: Y	Stock Purch. Plan:		Second Exec. Salary: $750,000	Bonus: $225,000

OTHER THOUGHTS:

Apparent Women Officers or Directors: 1
Hot Spot for Advancement for Women/Minorities:

LOCATIONS: ("Y" = Yes)

West:	Southwest:	Midwest:	Southeast:	Northeast:	International:
Y	Y	Y	Y	Y	Y

Note: Financial information, benefits and other data can change quickly and may vary from those stated here.

DOLLAR GENERAL CORPORATION   www.dollargeneral.com

Industry Group Code: 452910 **Ranks within this company's industry group:** Sales: 4   Profits: 4

Management:		Sales/Marketing:		Liberal Arts:		Information Systems:		Professionals:		Technical/Scientific:	
Mgmt. Trainees:	Y	Mktg. Professionals:	Y	Gen. Writing/Editing:	Y	Info. Management:	Y	Finance/Accounting:	Y	Engineers, Elec.:	
Experienced Mgmt.:	Y	Retail Sales:	Y	Technical Writing:		Software Dev.:	Y	Law:	Y	Engineers, Other:	
Int'l Business:		Commercial/Industrial:	Y	Graphic Arts/Photog.:	Y	Hardware Dev.:		HR/Other:	Y	Health/Lab:	
MBA Graduates:	Y	Sales Trainees:	Y	Music:		Systems Integration:		Training:	Y	Scientists/Research:	
		Advertising Pros.:	Y	Broadcasting:		Consulting/Other:		Health Care:		Petroleum/Chemicals:	
				Other:				Consulting:		Math/Other:	

TYPES OF BUSINESS:
Discount Stores
Dollar Stores

BRANDS/DIVISIONS/AFFILIATES:
KKR & Co LP (Kohlberg Kravis Roberts & Co)

CONTACTS: *Note: Officers with more than one job title may be intentionally listed here more than once.*
Richard W. (Rick) Dreiling, CEO
David L. Bere, Pres.
David M. Tehle, CFO/Exec. VP
Challis M. Lowe, Exec. VP-Human Resources
Susan S. Lanigan, General Counsel/Exec. VP
Kathleen Guion, Pres., Store Oper. & Dev.
David L. Bere, Chief Strategy Officer
David A. Perdue, Chmn.

Phone: 615-855-4000	Fax: 615-855-5252
Toll-Free:	
Address: 100 Mission Ridge, Goodlettsville, TN 37072 US	

GROWTH PLANS/SPECIAL FEATURES:
Dollar General Corporation, a subsidiary of KKR & Co., owns and operates more than 8,300 discount merchandise stores in 35 states, serving primarily low- and fixed-income families. The traditional Dollar General store has, on average, approximately 6,900 square feet of selling space, which is attractive to the company's target customers who live within five miles of the store. Roughly half of the company's stores serve communities with populations of 20,000 or less. Dollar General stores offer such products as health and beauty aids; packaged food and refrigerated products; home cleaning supplies; housewares; stationery; seasonal goods; basic apparel; and domestics. The majority of Dollar General's products are priced at $10 or less, with nearly a third of the products priced at $1 or less. The most expensive items generally cost $20. The company operates nine distribution facilities located in Oklahoma, Virginia, Ohio, South Carolina, Mississippi, Kentucky, Missouri, Florida and Indiana. In July 2007, Dollar General was acquired by a private equity investment group led by KKR & Co. for approximately $7.3 billion.

Dollar General offers its employees flexible spending accounts, wellness programs, a homebuyer assistance program, an employee assistance program and medical, dental, vision, prescription, business travel accident, AD&D, life and disability insurance.

FINANCIALS: Sales and profits are in thousands of dollars—add 000 to get the full amount. 2007 Note: Financial information for 2007 was not available for all companies at press time.

2007 Sales: $9,169,800	2007 Profits: $137,900	**U.S. Stock Ticker:** Private
2006 Sales: $8,582,237	2006 Profits: $350,155	**Int'l Ticker:** Int'l Exchange:
2005 Sales: $7,660,927	2005 Profits: $344,190	Employees: 69,500
2004 Sales: $6,871,992	2004 Profits: $301,000	Fiscal Year Ends: 1/31
2003 Sales: $6,100,400	2003 Profits: $264,900	Parent Company: KKR & CO LP (KOHLBERG KRAVIS ROBERTS & CO)

SALARIES/BENEFITS:
Pension Plan:	ESOP Stock Plan:	Profit Sharing:	Top Exec. Salary: $1,037,540	Bonus: $
Savings Plan: Y	Stock Purch. Plan:		Second Exec. Salary: $404,182	Bonus: $133,250

OTHER THOUGHTS:
Apparent Women Officers or Directors: 2
Hot Spot for Advancement for Women/Minorities: Y

LOCATIONS: ("Y" = Yes)
West:	Southwest:	Midwest:	Southeast:	Northeast:	International:
	Y	Y	Y	Y	

DOLLAR THRIFTY AUTOMOTIVE GROUP INC   www.dtag.com

Industry Group Code: 532111 Ranks within this company's industry group: Sales: 4 Profits: 2

Management:		Sales/Marketing:		Liberal Arts:		Information Systems:		Professionals:		Technical/Scientific:	
Mgmt. Trainees:	Y	Mktg. Professionals:	Y	Gen. Writing/Editing:	Y	Info. Management:	Y	Finance/Accounting:	Y	Engineers, Elec.:	
Experienced Mgmt.:	Y	Retail Sales:	Y	Technical Writing:		Software Dev.:	Y	Law:	Y	Engineers, Other:	
Int'l Business:	Y	Commercial/Industrial:	Y	Graphic Arts/Photog.:	Y	Hardware Dev.:		HR/Other:	Y	Health/Lab:	
MBA Graduates:	Y	Sales Trainees:	Y	Music:		Systems Integration:		Training:	Y	Scientists/Research:	
		Advertising Pros.:	Y	Broadcasting:		Consulting/Other:		Health Care:		Petroleum/Chemicals:	
				Other:				Consulting:		Math/Other:	

TYPES OF BUSINESS:
Automobile Rental
Used Car Sales
Financial Services

BRANDS/DIVISIONS/AFFILIATES:
Dollar Rent A Car, Inc.
Thrifty, Inc.
Thrifty Car Sales, Inc.
Thrifty Canada, Ltd.
Rental Car Finance Corp.
Dollar Thrifty Funding Corp.
Thrifty Rent-A-Car System, Inc.
DTG Operations, Inc.

CONTACTS: *Note: Officers with more than one job title may be intentionally listed here more than once.*
Gary L. Paxton, CEO
Gary L. Paxton, Pres.
Scott L. Thompson, CFO/Sr. Exec. VP
Scott Anderson, Chief Mktg. Officer/Sr. Exec. VP
Rick Morris, CIO/Exec. VP
Richard Halbrook, Exec. VP-Admin.
Vicki Vaniman, General Counsel/Sec./Exec. VP
John J. Foley, Chief Oper. Officer/Sr. Exec. VP
Thomas P. Capo, Chmn.

Phone: 918-660-7700	Fax: 918-669-3912
Toll-Free:	
Address: 5330 E. 31st St., Tulsa, OK 74135 US	

GROWTH PLANS/SPECIAL FEATURES:
Dollar Thrifty Automotive Group, Inc. (the group) is involved in many aspects of renting and selling vehicles. The firm owns DTG Operations, Inc.; Dollar Rent A Car, Inc. (Dollar); and Thrifty, Inc. (Thrifty). Thrifty owns Thrifty Car Sales, Inc., which operates a franchised retail used car sales network, and Thrifty Rent-A-Car System, Inc., which owns Dollar Thrifty Automotive Group Canada, Inc. DTG Operations operates company-owned stores under the Dollar and Thrifty brands; provides vehicle leasing to franchisees; and operates reservation centers for both brands. Thrifty Rent-A-Car System, Inc. and Dollar Rent A Car, Inc. conduct franchising, sales and marketing activities for their respective brands. The group has two additional subsidiaries, Rental Car Finance Corp. and Dollar Thrifty Funding Corp., which are special purpose financing companies. Dollar, Thrifty and their respective independent franchisees operate the Dollar and Thrifty vehicle rental systems. The Dollar and Thrifty brands are primarily utilized by leisure customers, including foreign tourists, and to small businesses, government business and independent business travelers. The Dollar brand's main focus is serving the airport and retail market, with most locations either at or near an airport. The brand has 111 in-terminal locations in the U.S., and 359 total locations in the U.S. and Canada. The Thrifty brand serves both the airport, with 80% of revenue derived, and local markets, with 20% of revenue. The brand has 472 total retail locations in the U.S. and Canada, with 115 of those being in-terminal U.S. locations. The company is highly focused on expanding its holdings through acquiring other rent-a-car franchises. In 2007, Chrysler vehicles represented approximately 88% of the total U.S. fleet purchases by DTG Operations. In August 2007, the group commenced a reorganization that will eliminate approximately 25% of management positions at the company headquarters.

FINANCIALS: Sales and profits are in thousands of dollars—add 000 to get the full amount. 2007 Note: Financial information for 2007 was not available for all companies at press time.

2007 Sales: $1,760,791	2007 Profits: $1,215	**U.S. Stock Ticker:** DTG
2006 Sales: $1,660,677	2006 Profits: $51,692	**Int'l Ticker:** Int'l Exchange:
2005 Sales: $1,507,554	2005 Profits: $76,355	Employees: 8,500
2004 Sales: $1,403,847	2004 Profits: $66,473	Fiscal Year Ends: 12/31
2003 Sales: $1,227,886	2003 Profits: $19,840	Parent Company:

SALARIES/BENEFITS:

Pension Plan:	ESOP Stock Plan:	Profit Sharing: Y	Top Exec. Salary: $695,017	Bonus: $
Savings Plan: Y	Stock Purch. Plan:		Second Exec. Salary: $379,461	Bonus: $

OTHER THOUGHTS:
Apparent Women Officers or Directors: 2
Hot Spot for Advancement for Women/Minorities: Y

LOCATIONS: ("Y" = Yes)

West:	Southwest:	Midwest:	Southeast:	Northeast:	International:
Y	Y	Y	Y	Y	Y

DRESS BARN INC (THE)   www.dressbarn.com

Industry Group Code: 448120 Ranks within this company's industry group: Sales: 8   Profits: 8

Management:		Sales/Marketing:		Liberal Arts:		Information Systems:		Professionals:		Technical/Scientific:	
Mgmt. Trainees:	Y	Mktg. Professionals:	Y	Gen. Writing/Editing:	Y	Info. Management:	Y	Finance/Accounting:	Y	Engineers, Elec.:	
Experienced Mgmt.:	Y	Retail Sales:	Y	Technical Writing:		Software Dev.:		Law:	Y	Engineers, Other:	
Int'l Business:		Commercial/Industrial:		Graphic Arts/Photog.:	Y	Hardware Dev.:		HR/Other:	Y	Health/Lab:	
MBA Graduates:	Y	Sales Trainees:	Y	Music:		Systems Integration:		Training:	Y	Scientists/Research:	
		Advertising Pros.:	Y	Broadcasting:		Consulting/Other:		Health Care:		Petroleum/Chemicals:	
				Other:				Consulting:		Math/Other:	

TYPES OF BUSINESS:

Women's Apparel, Retail
Teen Fashion Stores
Fashion Accessories
Private-Label Credit Cards

BRANDS/DIVISIONS/AFFILIATES:

Maurice's
Atrium
Westport, Ltd.
Princeton Club
SBX
Dress Barn Woman
Studio Y
Industrial Exchange

CONTACTS: Note: Officers with more than one job title may be intentionally listed here more than once.

David R. Jaffe, CEO
David R. Jaffe, Pres.
Armand Correia, CFO/Sr. VP
Vivian Behrens, Chief Mktg. Officer/Sr. VP
Gene L. Wexler, General Counsel/Sr. VP/Assist. Sec.
Elliot S. Jaffe, Chmn.

Phone: 845-369-4500	**Fax:** 845-369-4829
Toll-Free: 1-800-373-7722	
Address: 30 Dunnigan Dr., Suffern, NY 10901 US	

GROWTH PLANS/SPECIAL FEATURES:

The Dress Barn, Inc. operates a national chain, primarily located in strip malls, of value-priced specialty stores offering in-season, moderate- to better-quality career apparel and accessories, primarily to working women in their mid-30's to mid-50's. The company has three store formats: dressbarn stores, which carry junior and misses sizes; dressbarn woman stores, which feature larger sizes; and combination stores, which carry both. The combination stores are more prevalent, though the company does have some locations that are only either dressbarn or dressbarn women. Dress Barn's subsidiary, maurices, offers moderately priced, up-to-date fashions designed to appeal to a younger female consumer than the dressbarn and dressbarn woman brands. From its Duluth, Minnesota headquarters, maurices operates primarily within smaller cities of 25,000 to 100,000 in population. Maurice's merchandise is sold under three brand names: maurices, Studio Y and Industrial Exchange. As of July 2008, Dress Barn operated 821 Dress Barn stores in 48 states and the District of Columbia and 607 maurices stores in 42 states. The company offers a dressbarn credit card operated by World Financial Network National Bank, as well as personal and corporate gift cards in a variety of values. Holders of the dressbarn credit card receive targeted promotions including directed mailings and special coupons. Dressbarn plans to open approximately 106 stores in 2008, consisting of 65 maurices locations and 41 dressbarn locations with a focus on the economically successfully combination dressbarn stores. The company will also continue converting existing stores into combination stores as well as closing or relocating under-performing locations.

The company offers its employees short term disability, life and accidental death and dismemberment insurance, paid time off, 30% merchandise discount, career training, merchandise discounts, tuition reimbursement and medical, dental and vision coverage.

FINANCIALS: Sales and profits are in thousands of dollars—add 000 to get the full amount. 2007 Note: Financial information for 2007 was not available for all companies at press time.

2007 Sales: $1,426,607	2007 Profits: $101,182	**U.S. Stock Ticker:** DBRN
2006 Sales: $1,300,277	2006 Profits: $78,954	**Int'l Ticker:** Int'l Exchange:
2005 Sales: $1,000,264	2005 Profits: $52,560	Employees: 13,200
2004 Sales: $754,903	2004 Profits: $30,141	Fiscal Year Ends: 7/31
2003 Sales: $707,100	2003 Profits: $8,000	Parent Company:

SALARIES/BENEFITS:

Pension Plan:	ESOP Stock Plan:	Profit Sharing:	Top Exec. Salary: $750,000	Bonus: $750,000
Savings Plan: Y	Stock Purch. Plan: Y		Second Exec. Salary: $640,000	Bonus: $640,000

OTHER THOUGHTS:

Apparent Women Officers or Directors: 4
Hot Spot for Advancement for Women/Minorities: Y

LOCATIONS: ("Y" = Yes)

West:	Southwest:	Midwest:	Southeast:	Northeast:	International:
Y	Y	Y	Y	Y	

DTE ENERGY COMPANY

www.dteenergy.com

Industry Group Code: 221000   Ranks within this company's industry group: Sales: 4   Profits: 4

Management:		Sales/Marketing:		Liberal Arts:		Information Systems:		Professionals:		Technical/Scientific:	
Mgmt. Trainees:	Y	Mktg. Professionals:	Y	Gen. Writing/Editing:	Y	Info. Management:	Y	Finance/Accounting:	Y	Engineers, Elec.:	Y
Experienced Mgmt.:	Y	Retail Sales:		Technical Writing:	Y	Software Dev.:	Y	Law:	Y	Engineers, Other:	Y
Int'l Business:		Commercial/Industrial:	Y	Graphic Arts/Photog.:	Y	Hardware Dev.:		HR/Other:	Y	Health/Lab:	
MBA Graduates:	Y	Sales Trainees:		Music:		Systems Integration:		Training:	Y	Scientists/Research:	
		Advertising Pros.:	Y	Broadcasting:		Consulting/Other:		Health Care:		Petroleum/Chemicals:	
				Other:				Consulting:		Math/Other:	

TYPES OF BUSINESS:

Utilities-Electricity & Natural Gas
Energy Management
Wholesale Energy Trading
Fuel Supply Services
Hydroelectric Power
Nuclear Power
Coal Shipping-Rail & Boat
Consulting Services

BRANDS/DIVISIONS/AFFILIATES:

Detroit Edison Company (The)
Michigan Consolidated Gas (MichCon)
Midwest Energy Resources
DTE Biomass Energy
DTE Coal Services
DTE Energy Services
Citizen's Gas Fuel Corp.

CONTACTS: Note: Officers with more than one job title may be intentionally listed here more than once.

Anthony F. Earley, Jr., CEO
Gerard M. Anderson, COO
Gerard M. Anderson, Pres.
David E. Meador, CFO/Exec. VP
Trevor F. Lauer, VP-Retail Mktg.
Larry Steward, VP-Human Resources
Lynne Ellyn, CIO/Sr. VP
Bruce Peterson, General Counsel/Sr. VP
Paul Hillegonds, Sr. VP-Corp. Affairs
Peter Oleksiak, Controller/VP
Robert Buckler, Pres./COO-Detroit Edison
Jerry Norcia, Pres./COO-MichCon
Ron A. May, Sr. VP
Michael Porter, VP-Corp. Comm.
Anthony F. Earley, Jr., Chmn.

Phone: 313-235-4000	Fax: 313-235-8055
Toll-Free: 866-966-5555	
Address: 2000 2nd Ave., Detroit, MI 48226-1279 US	

GROWTH PLANS/SPECIAL FEATURES:

DTE Energy Company is a leading energy and energy technology provider that develops merchant power and industrial energy projects and works in energy trading, selling electricity, natural gas, coal, chilled water, landfill gas and steam. DTE is one of the nation's largest purchasers, transporters and marketers of coal. The company's principal operating segments include its Electric Utility division, which consists of The Detroit Edison Company, an electric utility in southeastern Michigan that has a generating capacity of 11,000 megawatts and serves 2.2 million customers; and its Gas Utilities division, which is represented by Michigan Consolidated Gas (MichCon), one of the nation's largest natural gas distributors, distributing gas to 1.3 million customers. The firm's Non-Utility Operations division includes: Coal and Gas Midstream, which is made up of the company's gas pipelines, its marketing and transportation of coal, its rail management services, and its storage services; Power and Industrial Projects, primarily consisting of on-site energy services, steel-related projects and power generation; Unconventional Gas Production, primarily consisting of unconventional gas project development and production; DTE Energy Trading, which buys, sells and trades electricity, coal and natural gas and provides risk management services consisting of energy marketing and trading operations; and Synthetic Fuel, consisting of the operations of the company's nine synthetic fuel plants and landfill gas-to-energy projects. In addition to these segments the company also operates the following wholly-owned subsidiaries: Midwest Energy Resources, a wholly-owned subsidiary of Detroit Edison, transports and delivers low-sulfur western coal by rail and ship; Edison Development Corporation funds venture capital investments in new energy technologies; and Citizen's Gas Fuel Corporation distributes natural gas to customers in Lenawee County, Michigan. In April 2007, MichCon began a two-year project to install a 16.3 mile long natural gas pipeline in West Michigan that will be able to help meet future market demand.

FINANCIALS: Sales and profits are in thousands of dollars—add 000 to get the full amount. 2007 Note: Financial information for 2007 was not available for all companies at press time.

2007 Sales: $8,506,000	2007 Profits: $971,000	U.S. Stock Ticker: DTE
2006 Sales: $8,159,000	2006 Profits: $433,000	Int'l Ticker: Int'l Exchange:
2005 Sales: $9,021,000	2005 Profits: $537,000	Employees: 10,527
2004 Sales: $7,071,000	2004 Profits: $431,000	Fiscal Year Ends: 12/31
2003 Sales: $7,005,000	2003 Profits: $521,000	Parent Company:

SALARIES/BENEFITS:

Pension Plan: Y	ESOP Stock Plan:	Profit Sharing:	Top Exec. Salary: $1,125,000	Bonus: $1,964,191
Savings Plan: Y	Stock Purch. Plan:		Second Exec. Salary: $700,000	Bonus: $1,012,075

OTHER THOUGHTS:

Apparent Women Officers or Directors: 4
Hot Spot for Advancement for Women/Minorities: Y

LOCATIONS: ("Y" = Yes)

West:	Southwest:	Midwest:	Southeast:	Northeast:	International:
		Y			

Note: Financial information, benefits and other data can change quickly and may vary from those stated here.

DUKE ENERGY CORP

www.duke-energy.com

Industry Group Code: 221000 Ranks within this company's industry group: Sales: 2 Profits: 1

Management:		Sales/Marketing:		Liberal Arts:		Information Systems:		Professionals:		Technical/Scientific:	
Mgmt. Trainees:	Y	Mktg. Professionals:	Y	Gen. Writing/Editing:		Info. Management:	Y	Finance/Accounting:	Y	Engineers, Elec.:	Y
Experienced Mgmt.:	Y	Retail Sales:		Technical Writing:	Y	Software Dev.:	Y	Law:	Y	Engineers, Other:	Y
Int'l Business:	Y	Commercial/Industrial:	Y	Graphic Arts/Photog.:		Hardware Dev.:		HR/Other:	Y	Health/Lab:	
MBA Graduates:	Y	Sales Trainees:		Music:		Systems Integration:		Training:	Y	Scientists/Research:	
		Advertising Pros.:		Broadcasting:		Consulting/Other:		Health Care:		Petroleum/Chemicals:	
				Other:				Consulting:		Math/Other:	

TYPES OF BUSINESS:

Utilities-Electricity & Natural Gas
Merchant Power Generation
Natural Gas Transportation & Storage
Electricity Transmission
Energy Marketing
Real Estate
Telecommunications
Facility & Plant Services

BRANDS/DIVISIONS/AFFILIATES:

Franchised Electric & Gas Service
Crescent Resources, LLC
Duke Energy Generation Services
Duke Energy International, LLC
National Methanol Company
Attiki Gas Supply S.A.

CONTACTS: Note: Officers with more than one job title may be intentionally listed here more than once.

James E. Rogers, CEO
James E. Rogers, Pres.
David L. Hauser, CFO/Group Exec.
Christopher Rolfe, VP-Human Resources
David W. Mohler, CTO/VP
Christopher C. Rolfe, Chief Admin. Officer/Group Exec.
Marc Manly, Chief Legal Officer/Group Exec.
B. Keith Trent, Chief Strategy, Policy & Regulatory. Officer
Cathy S. Roche, Chief Comm. Officer/Sr. VP
R. Sean Trauschke, VP-Investor Rel.
Stephen D. De May, Treas./VP
James L. Turner, COO/Pres., U.S. Franchised Electric & Gas
Ellen T. Ruff, Pres., Duke Energy Carolinas
Dhiaa M. Jamil, Chief Nuclear Officer/Group Exec.
Julia S. Janson, Sr. VP-Ethics & Compliance/Corp. Sec.
James E. Rogers, Chmn.

Phone: 704-594-6200	Fax: 704-382-3814
Toll-Free: 800-873-3853	
Address: 526 S. Church St., Charlotte, NC 28202-1802 US	

GROWTH PLANS/SPECIAL FEATURES:

Duke Energy Corp. is an integrated energy and energy services provider that offers delivery and management of electricity and natural gas throughout the U.S. The company operates four principle business segments: U.S. franchised electric & gas service; commercial power; international energy; and the company's 50% interest in the Crescent Resources joint venture. The franchised electric & gas service segment can generate 32,000 megawatts of electricity, has 4 million customers, including 515,000 retail gas customers, and has locations in Ohio, Indiana, Kentucky and the Carolinas, covering approximately 47,000 square miles. This segment operates three nuclear power plants; fifteen coal-fire plants; thirty-one hydroelectric stations; fifteen combustion turbines that burn natural gas, oil or other fuels; and two combine cycle stations that burn natural or synthetic gas. The commercial power segment owns, operates and manages non-regulated power plants and engages in the marketing and procurement of electric power, fuel and emissions allowances related to the plants. Its plants utilize a variety of fuels such as natural gas, waste coal and wood, and can generate approximately 8,020 megawatts of power primarily in the Midwestern U.S. Duke Energy International, LLC, operates power generation plants primarily in Latin America. It also has investments in National Methanol Company, a regional producer of methanol in Saudi Arabia; and Attiki Gas Supply S.A., a natural gas distributor located in Athens, Greece. The Crescent Resources joint venture develops and manages commercial, residential and multi-family real estate projects, and manages land holdings, primarily in the Southeastern and Southwestern U.S. The venture owns 900,000 square feet of real estate, with an additional 500,000 under construction. In September 2008, the company announced plans to begin installing solar electric panels at 850 locations in North Carolina, capable of generating 16 megawatts of electricity, enough to power 2,600 homes for one year.

FINANCIALS: Sales and profits are in thousands of dollars—add 000 to get the full amount. 2007 Note: Financial information for 2007 was not available for all companies at press time.

2007 Sales: $12,720,000	2007 Profits: $1,500,000	U.S. Stock Ticker: DUK
2006 Sales: $10,607,000	2006 Profits: $1,863,000	Int'l Ticker: Int'l Exchange:
2005 Sales: $16,297,000	2005 Profits: $1,824,000	Employees: 25,600
2004 Sales: $19,596,000	2004 Profits: $1,490,000	Fiscal Year Ends: 12/31
2003 Sales: $22,529,000	2003 Profits: $-1,323,000	Parent Company:

SALARIES/BENEFITS:

Pension Plan: Y	ESOP Stock Plan:	Profit Sharing:	Top Exec. Salary: $755,496	Bonus: $797,747
Savings Plan: Y	Stock Purch. Plan:		Second Exec. Salary: $549,996	Bonus: $543,396

OTHER THOUGHTS:

Apparent Women Officers or Directors: 4
Hot Spot for Advancement for Women/Minorities: Y

LOCATIONS: ("Y" = Yes)

West:	Southwest:	Midwest:	Southeast:	Northeast:	International:
		Y	Y		Y

Note: Financial information, benefits and other data can change quickly and may vary from those stated here.

DYCOM INDUSTRIES INC

www.dycomind.com

Industry Group Code: 234920 **Ranks within this company's industry group:** Sales: 1   Profits: 1

Management:		Sales/Marketing:		Liberal Arts:		Information Systems:		Professionals:		Technical/Scientific:	
Mgmt. Trainees:	Y	Mktg. Professionals:	Y	Gen. Writing/Editing:		Info. Management:	Y	Finance/Accounting:	Y	Engineers, Elec.:	Y
Experienced Mgmt.:	Y	Retail Sales:		Technical Writing:	Y	Software Dev.:		Law:	Y	Engineers, Other:	Y
Int'l Business:		Commercial/Industrial:	Y	Graphic Arts/Photog.:	Y	Hardware Dev.:		HR/Other:	Y	Health/Lab:	
MBA Graduates:	Y	Sales Trainees:		Music:		Systems Integration:		Training:	Y	Scientists/Research:	
		Advertising Pros.:		Broadcasting:		Consulting/Other:		Health Care:		Petroleum/Chemicals:	
				Other:				Consulting:		Math/Other:	

TYPES OF BUSINESS:
Construction, Maintenance & Installation Services
Engineering Services
Utility Maintenance Services

BRANDS/DIVISIONS/AFFILIATES:

CONTACTS:
Note: Officers with more than one job title may be intentionally listed here more than once.
Steven E. Nielsen, CEO
Timothy R. Estes, COO/Exec. VP
Steven E. Nielsen, Pres.
H. Andrew DeFerrari, CFO
Richard B. Vilsoet, General Counsel/VP/Corp. Sec.
Steven E. Nielsen, Chmn.

Phone: 561-627-7171	Fax: 561-627-7709
Toll-Free:	
Address: 11770 U.S. Highway 1, Ste. 101, Palm Beach Gardens, FL 33408 US	

GROWTH PLANS/SPECIAL FEATURES:

Dycom Industries, Inc. is a leading provider of specialty contracting services. Dycom provides services throughout the U.S. and on a limited basis in Canada, including engineering, construction, maintenance and installation services to telecommunications providers; underground locating services to various utilities including telecommunications providers; and other construction and maintenance services to electric utilities and others. During 2007, the company generated approximately 74.7% of its total revenues from specialty contracting services related to the telecommunications industry; approximately 18.9% from underground utility locating; and approximately 6.4% from electric and other construction and maintenance services to electric utilities and others. Dycom provides outside plant engineers and drafters to telecommunication providers, who design aerial, underground and buried optic, copper and coaxial cable systems that extend from the telephone company central office, or cable operator headend, to the consumer's home or business. Engineering services the company provides to telephone companies include fiber cable routing and design; the design of service area concept boxes, terminals, drops and transmission and central office equipment; and the proper administration of feeder and distribution cable pairs. For cable television multiple system operators, Dycom performs make-ready studies, strand mapping, field walk-out, computer-aided radio frequency design and fiber cable routing and design. The firm's construction, maintenance and installation services include placing and splicing fiber, copper and coaxial cables; excavating trenches in which to place cables; placing related structures such as poles, anchors, conduits, manholes, cabinets and closures; placing drop lines from main distribution lines to the consumer's home or business; and maintaining and removing these facilities. It also provides premise wiring services to various corporations and state and local governments, predominantly limited to the installation, repair and maintenance of telecommunications infrastructure within improved structures.

FINANCIALS:
Sales and profits are in thousands of dollars—add 000 to get the full amount. 2007 Note: Financial information for 2007 was not available for all companies at press time.

2007 Sales: $1,137,812	2007 Profits: $41,884	**U.S. Stock Ticker:** DY
2006 Sales: $1,023,673	2006 Profits: $18,180	**Int'l Ticker:** Int'l Exchange:
2005 Sales: $986,627	2005 Profits: $24,314	Employees: 9,352
2004 Sales: $872,700	2004 Profits: $58,600	Fiscal Year Ends: 7/31
2003 Sales: $618,200	2003 Profits: $17,100	Parent Company:

SALARIES/BENEFITS:

Pension Plan:	ESOP Stock Plan:	Profit Sharing:	Top Exec. Salary: $680,000	Bonus: $821,618
Savings Plan:	Stock Purch. Plan:		Second Exec. Salary: $460,000	Bonus: $460,000

OTHER THOUGHTS:
Apparent Women Officers or Directors: 1
Hot Spot for Advancement for Women/Minorities:

LOCATIONS: ("Y" = Yes)

West:	Southwest:	Midwest:	Southeast:	Northeast:	International:
Y	Y	Y	Y	Y	

Note: Financial information, benefits and other data can change quickly and may vary from those stated here.

E I DU PONT DE NEMOURS & CO (DUPONT) www.dupont.com

Industry Group Code: 325000 Ranks within this company's industry group: Sales: Profits:

Management:		Sales/Marketing:		Liberal Arts:		Information Systems:		Professionals:		Technical/Scientific:	
Mgmt. Trainees:	Y	Mktg. Professionals:	Y	Gen. Writing/Editing:	Y	Info. Management:	Y	Finance/Accounting:	Y	Engineers, Elec.:	Y
Experienced Mgmt.:	Y	Retail Sales:		Technical Writing:	Y	Software Dev.:		Law:	Y	Engineers, Other:	
Int'l Business:	Y	Commercial/Industrial:	Y	Graphic Arts/Photog.:		Hardware Dev.:		HR/Other:	Y	Health/Lab:	Y
MBA Graduates:	Y	Sales Trainees:		Music:		Systems Integration:		Training:	Y	Scientists/Research:	
		Advertising Pros.:		Broadcasting:		Consulting/Other:		Health Care:		Petroleum/Chemicals:	
				Other:				Consulting:		Math/Other:	

TYPES OF BUSINESS:

Chemicals Manufacturing
Polymers
Performance Coatings
Nutrition & Health Products
Electronics Materials
Agricultural Seeds
Fuel-Cell, Biofuels & Solar Panel Technology
Contract Research & Development

BRANDS/DIVISIONS/AFFILIATES:

Pioneer
Teflon
Corian
Kevlar
Tyvek
Process Dynamic
IsoTherming Technology
Chemtura Corporation

CONTACTS: *Note: Officers with more than one job title may be intentionally listed here more than once.*

Charles O. Holliday, Jr., CEO
Richard R. Goodmanson, COO/Exec. VP
Jeffrey L. Keefer, CFO/Exec. VP
David G. Bills, Chief Mktg. & Sales Officer
W. Donald Johnson, Sr. VP-Human Resources
Uma Chowdhry, Chief Science Officer
Phuong Tram, CIO/VP-IT
Uma Chowdhry, CTO/Sr. VP
James B. Porter, Jr., Chief Eng./VP-Eng. & Oper.
Stacey J. Mobley, General Counsel/Sr. VP/ Chief Admin. Officer
Mathieu Vrijsen, Sr. VP-Oper. & Eng.
William J. Harvey, VP-Planning
Kathleen H. Forte, VP-Public Affairs
Carl J. Lukach, VP-Investor Rel.
Susan M. Stalnecker, Treas./VP-Finance
Ellen J. Kullman, Exec. VP
Diane H. Gulyas, VP-Performance Materials
Terry Caloghiris, VP-Coatings & Color Tech.
Charles O. Holliday, Jr., Chmn.
Ian Hudson, Pres., EMEA & Du Pont de Nemours Int'l SA Geneva
Jeffrey A. Coe, Chief Procurement Officer/VP-Sourcing & Logistics

Phone: 302-774-1000	Fax: 302-773-2631
Toll-Free: 800-441-7515	
Address: 1007 Market St., Wilmington, DE 19898 US	

GROWTH PLANS/SPECIAL FEATURES:

E. I. du Pont de Nemours & Co. (DuPont), founded in 1802, develops and manufactures products in the biotechnology, electronics, materials science, synthetic fibers and safety and security sectors. DuPont operates in five segments: Agriculture and nutrition (A&N); coatings and color technologies (C&CT); electronic and communication technologies (E&C); performance materials (PM); and safety and protection (S&P). A&N delivers Pioneer brand seed products, insecticides, fungicides, herbicides, soy-based food ingredients, food quality diagnostic testing equipment and liquid food packaging systems. The C&CT segment supplies automotive coatings, titanium dioxide white pigments and pigment and dye-based inks for ink-jet digital printing. E&C provides a range of advanced materials for the electronics industry, flexographic printing, color communication systems and a range of fluoropolymer and fluorochemical products. PM manufactures polymer-based materials, which include engineered polymers, specialized resins and films for use in food packaging, sealants, adhesives, sporting goods and laminated safety glass. The S&P segment provides protective materials and safety consulting services. Significant brands include Teflon fluoropolymers, films, fabric protectors, fibers and dispersions; Corian surfaces; Kevlar high strength material; and Tyvek protective material. Recent acquisitions include Process Dynamic's IsoTherming Technology for reducing motor fuel sulfur content in August 2007 and Chemtura Corporation's fluorine chemicals business in February 2008. Recent divestitures include DuPont Cotoran fluometuron herbicide in September 2007; its terbacil herbicide assets in December 2007; DuPont Super Boll and FreeFall brand cotton products in February 2008; and its 8th Continent soy milk joint venture with General Mills in February 2008. In March 2008, DuPont launched a new research and greenhouse facility equipped with cutting-edge robotics, imaging and the capacity to accelerate the growth rate of test plants.

DuPont offers its employees tuition assistance, ongoing training programs, flexible work practices, adoption assistance, an employee resource program, an emergency backup childcare resource and dependent care spending accounts.

FINANCIALS: Sales and profits are in thousands of dollars—add 000 to get the full amount. 2007 Note: Financial information for 2007 was not available for all companies at press time.

2007 Sales: $29,378,000	2007 Profits: $2,988,000	U.S. Stock Ticker: DD
2006 Sales: $27,421,000	2006 Profits: $3,148,000	Int'l Ticker: Int'l Exchange:
2005 Sales: $26,639,000	2005 Profits: $2,053,000	Employees: 60,000
2004 Sales: $27,340,000	2004 Profits: $1,780,000	Fiscal Year Ends: 12/31
2003 Sales: $26,996,000	2003 Profits: $973,000	Parent Company:

SALARIES/BENEFITS:

Pension Plan: Y	ESOP Stock Plan:	Profit Sharing:	Top Exec. Salary: $1,293,000	Bonus: $2,103,000
Savings Plan: Y	Stock Purch. Plan:		Second Exec. Salary: $811,000	Bonus: $850,000

OTHER THOUGHTS:

Apparent Women Officers or Directors: 17
Hot Spot for Advancement for Women/Minorities: Y

LOCATIONS: ("Y" = Yes)

West:	Southwest:	Midwest:	Southeast:	Northeast:	International:
Y	Y	Y	Y	Y	Y

EATON CORP

www.eaton.com

Industry Group Code: 336300 **Ranks within this company's industry group:** Sales: 2 Profits: 2

Management:		Sales/Marketing:		Liberal Arts:		Information Systems:		Professionals:		Technical/Scientific:	
Mgmt. Trainees:	Y	Mktg. Professionals:	Y	Gen. Writing/Editing:		Info. Management:	Y	Finance/Accounting:	Y	Engineers, Elec.:	Y
Experienced Mgmt.:	Y	Retail Sales:		Technical Writing:	Y	Software Dev.:	Y	Law:	Y	Engineers, Other:	
Int'l Business:	Y	Commercial/Industrial:	Y	Graphic Arts/Photog.:	Y	Hardware Dev.:	Y	HR/Other:	Y	Health/Lab:	Y
MBA Graduates:	Y	Sales Trainees:	Y	Music:		Systems Integration:		Training:	Y	Scientists/Research:	Y
		Advertising Pros.:	Y	Broadcasting:		Consulting/Other:		Health Care:		Petroleum/Chemicals:	
				Other:				Consulting:		Math/Other:	Y

TYPES OF BUSINESS:

Hydraulic Products
Electrical Power Distribution & Control Equipment
Truck Transmissions & Axles
Engine Components
Aerospace & Military Components

BRANDS/DIVISIONS/AFFILIATES:

Senyuan International Holdings Limited
Catalytica Energy Systems, Inc.
Schreder-Hazemeyer
Ronningen-Petter
Marina Power Lighting
Synflex
Arrow Hose & Tubing, Inc.
Babco Electric Group

CONTACTS: Note: Officers with more than one job title may be intentionally listed here more than once.

Alexander M. Cutler, CEO
Alexander M. Cutler, Pres.
Richard H. Fearon, CFO
Jeffrey M. Krakowiak, Sr. VP-Mktg. & Sales
Susan J. Cook, Exec. VP-Human Resources
William W. Blausey, Jr., CIO/VP
Yannis P. Tsavalas, CTO/VP
Mark M. McGuire, General Counsel/VP
Richard H. Fearon, Chief Planning Officer/Exec. VP
William B. Doggett, Sr. VP-Comm. & Public Affairs
William C. Hartman, Sr. VP-Investor Rel.
Billie K. Rawot, Sr. VP/Controller
Joseph P. Palchak, CEO-Automotive
James E. Sweetnam, CEO-Truck
Craig Arnold, CEO-Fluid Power
Randy W. Carson, CEO-Electrical
Alexander M. Cutler, Chmn.
Jean-Pierre Lacombe, Pres., Europe

Phone: 216-523-5000	Fax: 216-523-4787
Toll-Free: 800-386-1911	
Address: 1111 Superior Ave., Cleveland, OH 44114-2584 US	

GROWTH PLANS/SPECIAL FEATURES:

Eaton Corporation designs, manufactures, markets and services electrical systems and components in four business segments: fluid power, electrical, automotive and truck. The fluid power segment, the firm's largest segment, develops and sells fluid power products to industrial, mobile equipment and aerospace customers worldwide. The segment also handles Eaton's aerospace business, which serves commercial and military aviation, space, military weapon systems, marine, off-road and other severe environment applications. The electrical segment distributes electrical power and control equipment for industrial, commercial and residential markets. The automotive segment focuses on the powertrain and specialized sensor and actuator areas of passenger cars and light trucks. Its primary products include mirror and engine management controls, as well as engine air management systems, including superchargers, cylinder head modules, engine valves and lifters. The truck segment features drivetrain systems and components for medium-duty and heavy-duty commercial vehicles. Its products include manual and automatic transmissions, clutches, driveshafts, steering, drive and trailer axles, brakes, chassis control systems, and collision warning systems. During 2007, the company acquired Arrow Hose & Tubing Inc.; MGE small systems UPS business from Schneider Electric; Babco Electric Group; Pulizzi Engineering; Technology and related assets of SMC Electrical Products, Inc.'s industrial medium-voltage adjustable frequency drive business; Fuel components division of Saturn Electronics & Engineering, Inc.; Aphel Technologies Limited; Argo-Tech Corporation; and Power Protection Business of Power Products Ltd. In the first half of 2008, the firm acquired the engine valves business of Kirloskar Oil Engines Ltd.; The Moeller Group; and Phoenixtec Power Company Ltd. In August 2008, Eaton agreed to a joint-venture with Nittan Valve Co. Ltd. for engine valve products in Japan and Korea.

Eaton offers employees benefits including flexible spending accounts, a personal investment plan, employee assistance, tuition reimbursements, adoption assistance and work/life programs.

FINANCIALS: Sales and profits are in thousands of dollars—add 000 to get the full amount. 2007 Note: Financial information for 2007 was not available for all companies at press time.

2007 Sales: $13,033,000	2007 Profits: $994,000	**U.S. Stock Ticker: ETN**
2006 Sales: $12,232,000	2006 Profits: $950,000	**Int'l Ticker:** Int'l Exchange:
2005 Sales: $10,874,000	2005 Profits: $805,000	Employees: 64,000
2004 Sales: $9,712,000	2004 Profits: $648,000	Fiscal Year Ends: 12/31
2003 Sales: $8,061,000	2003 Profits: $386,000	Parent Company:

SALARIES/BENEFITS:

Pension Plan: Y	ESOP Stock Plan:	Profit Sharing:	Top Exec. Salary: $1,069,305	Bonus: $9,520,197
Savings Plan: Y	Stock Purch. Plan:		Second Exec. Salary: $511,695	Bonus: $2,894,807

OTHER THOUGHTS:

Apparent Women Officers or Directors: 2
Hot Spot for Advancement for Women/Minorities:

LOCATIONS: ("Y" = Yes)

West:	Southwest:	Midwest:	Southeast:	Northeast:	International:
Y	Y	Y	Y	Y	Y

Note: Financial information, benefits and other data can change quickly and may vary from those stated here.

EBAY INC

www.ebay.com

Industry Group Code: 453998E Ranks within this company's industry group: Sales: 1   Profits: 1

Management:		Sales/Marketing:		Liberal Arts:		Information Systems:		Professionals:		Technical/Scientific:	
Mgmt. Trainees:	Y	Mktg. Professionals:	Y	Gen. Writing/Editing:	Y	Info. Management:	Y	Finance/Accounting:	Y	Engineers, Elec.:	
Experienced Mgmt.:	Y	Retail Sales:	Y	Technical Writing:	Y	Software Dev.:	Y	Law:	Y	Engineers, Other:	
Int'l Business:	Y	Commercial/Industrial:	Y	Graphic Arts/Photog.:	Y	Hardware Dev.:		HR/Other:	Y	Health/Lab:	
MBA Graduates:	Y	Sales Trainees:	Y	Music:		Systems Integration:	Y	Training:	Y	Scientists/Research:	
		Advertising Pros.:	Y	Broadcasting:		Consulting/Other:		Health Care:		Petroleum/Chemicals:	
				Other:				Consulting:		Math/Other:	

TYPES OF BUSINESS:

Online Retail-Auctions
Online Payment Processing
Memorabilia & Collectibles
E-Commerce Services
VoIP Telecommunications Services

BRANDS/DIVISIONS/AFFILIATES:

eBay Express
Skype
PayPal
Rent.com
Shopping.com
Kijiji
VeriSign
StumbleUpon

CONTACTS: *Note: Officers with more than one job title may be intentionally listed here more than once.*

John Donahoe, CEO
John Donahoe, Pres.
Bob Swan, CFO
Elizabeth Axelrod, Sr. VP-Human Resources
Michael Jacobson, General Counsel/Sr. VP
Michael van Swaaij, Chief Strategy Officer
Alan Marks, Sr. VP-Corp. Comm.
Bob Swan, Sr. VP-Finance
Scott Thompson, Pres., PayPal
Lorrie Norrington,, Pres., eBay Marketplaces
Pierre M. Omidyar, Chmn.

Phone: 408-376-7400	Fax: 408-376-7401
Toll-Free:	
Address: 2145 Hamilton Ave., San Jose, CA 95125 US	

GROWTH PLANS/SPECIAL FEATURES:

eBay, Inc. is an online auction venue that brings together millions of buyers and sellers every day locally, nationally and internationally through its array of websites. eBay provides online marketplaces for the sale of goods and services, online payments services and online communication offerings. It currently has three primary businesses: the eBay Marketplaces, payments and communications. eBay Marketplaces provides the infrastructure to enable online commerce in various formats, including the traditional auction platform that the original eBay site is based on. Other online platforms include Rent.com, Shopping.com, Kijiji, Gumtree.com, LoQUo.com, Intoko, Marktplaats.nl and mobile.de. eBay Express is a new fixed-price, rather than auction, service aimed at buyers who want to purchase immediately. The payments business, PayPal, enables individuals or businesses to securely, easily and quickly send and receive payments online. The VeriSign payment gateway business allows merchants to authorize, process, and manage online payments. Subsidiary Skype enables VoIP calls between Skype users and fixed-line and mobile telephones, and also provides Skype users the ability to connect to other users directly. In October 2007, eBay acquired ViA-Online GmbH, a German-based auction management company that operates Afterbuy.com.

eBay offers its employees adoption assistance, a pet insurance plan, tuition reimbursement, employee training courses, referral bonuses and on-site services such as dry cleaning and chiropractic care. The firm also provides a wide range of insurance benefits such as medical, dental, vision, life and accidental death and dismemberment, short and long term disability and business travel accident insurance.

FINANCIALS: Sales and profits are in thousands of dollars—add 000 to get the full amount. 2007 Note: Financial information for 2007 was not available for all companies at press time.

2007 Sales: $7,672,329	2007 Profits: $348,251	**U.S. Stock Ticker: EBAY**
2006 Sales: $5,969,741	2006 Profits: $1,125,639	**Int'l Ticker:** Int'l Exchange:
2005 Sales: $4,552,401	2005 Profits: $1,082,043	Employees: 13,200
2004 Sales: $3,271,309	2004 Profits: $778,223	Fiscal Year Ends: 12/31
2003 Sales: $2,165,096	2003 Profits: $441,771	Parent Company:

SALARIES/BENEFITS:

Pension Plan:	ESOP Stock Plan:	Profit Sharing:	Top Exec. Salary: $995,016	Bonus: $1,134,692
Savings Plan: Y	Stock Purch. Plan: Y		Second Exec. Salary: $790,385	Bonus: $1,271,536

OTHER THOUGHTS:

Apparent Women Officers or Directors: 4
Hot Spot for Advancement for Women/Minorities: Y

LOCATIONS: ("Y" = Yes)

West:	Southwest:	Midwest:	Southeast:	Northeast:	International:
Y	Y	Y		Y	Y

ECHOSTAR CORP

www.echostar.com

Industry Group Code: 513220 Ranks within this company's industry group: Sales: 4 Profits: 5

Management:		Sales/Marketing:		Liberal Arts:		Information Systems:		Professionals:		Technical/Scientific:	
Mgmt. Trainees:	Y	Mktg. Professionals:	Y	Gen. Writing/Editing:	Y	Info. Management:	Y	Finance/Accounting:	Y	Engineers, Elec.:	Y
Experienced Mgmt.:	Y	Retail Sales:		Technical Writing:	Y	Software Dev.:	Y	Law:	Y	Engineers, Other:	
Int'l Business:	Y	Commercial/Industrial:	Y	Graphic Arts/Photog.:	Y	Hardware Dev.:		HR/Other:	Y	Health/Lab:	
MBA Graduates:	Y	Sales Trainees:		Music:		Systems Integration:		Training:	Y	Scientists/Research:	
		Advertising Pros.:	Y	Broadcasting:	Y	Consulting/Other:		Health Care:		Petroleum/Chemicals:	
				Other:				Consulting:		Math/Other:	

TYPES OF BUSINESS:

Digital Set-Top Boxes & Related Products
Fixed Satellite Services

BRANDS/DIVISIONS/AFFILIATES:

DISH Network Corp.
EchoStar Holding Corp.

CONTACTS: *Note: Officers with more than one job title may be intentionally listed here more than once.*

Charles W. Ergen, CEO
Charles W. Ergen, Pres.
Bernard L. Han, CFO/Exec. VP
R. Stanton Dodge, General Counsel/Exec. VP/Corp. Sec.
Mark W. Jackson, Pres., EchoStar Technologies, LLC
Dean A. Olmstead, Pres., EchoStar Satellite Services, LLC
Charles W. Ergen, Chmn.
Steven B. Schaver, Pres., EchoStar International Corp.

Phone: 303-706-4444	Fax:
Toll-Free:	
Address: 90 Inverness Cir. E., Englewood, CO 80112 US	

GROWTH PLANS/SPECIAL FEATURES:

EchoStar Corp., formerly known as EchoStar Holding Corp., is a newly formed entity that had not conducted any operations prior to its spin-off from DISH Network in January 2008. It has historically operated a digital set-top box business that comprises substantially all of its historical revenue. The company intends to develop a fixed satellite services business using its fleet of owned and leased in-orbit satellites. The firm operates in two segments: Digital set-top boxes and fixed satellite services. The set-top box business designs, develops and distributes set-top boxes and related products for direct-to-home satellite service providers. Most of EchoStar's set-top boxes are sold to DISH Network, but it also sells a significant number of set-top boxes to BellExpressVu and other international customers. The company intends to develop its fixed satellite services business using its nine owned or leased in-orbit satellites and related Federal Communication Commission (FCC) licenses, a network of seven full service digital broadcast centers and leased fiber optic capacity with points of presence in roughly 150 cities. The firm expects that its primary customer initially will be DISH Network, but it also expects to leave capacity in the spot market and to government and enterprise customers. EchoStar has entered into commercial agreements with DISH Network pursuant to which it will have the obligation to sell set-top boxes and related products and provide fixed satellite services to DISH Network at set prices for a period of two years. However, DISH Network is under no obligation to purchase its set-top boxes and related products during or after this two-year period; additionally, DISH Network may terminate the agreements to receive fixed satellite services upon 60 days notice.

FINANCIALS: Sales and profits are in thousands of dollars—add 000 to get the full amount. 2007 Note: Financial information for 2007 was not available for all companies at press time.

2007 Sales: $11,090,375	2007 Profits: $756,054	**U.S. Stock Ticker:** SATS
2006 Sales: $9,818,486	2006 Profits: $608,272	**Int'l Ticker:** Int'l Exchange:
2005 Sales: $8,447,175	2005 Profits: $1,514,540	Employees: 23,000
2004 Sales: $7,158,471	2004 Profits: $214,769	Fiscal Year Ends: 12/31
2003 Sales: $5,739,296	2003 Profits: $707,548	Parent Company:

SALARIES/BENEFITS:

Pension Plan:	ESOP Stock Plan:	Profit Sharing:	Top Exec. Salary: $592,308	Bonus: $
Savings Plan:	Stock Purch. Plan:		Second Exec. Salary: $400,000	Bonus: $20,000

OTHER THOUGHTS:

Apparent Women Officers or Directors:
Hot Spot for Advancement for Women/Minorities:

LOCATIONS: ("Y" = Yes)

West:	Southwest:	Midwest:	Southeast:	Northeast:	International:
Y					

Note: Financial information, benefits and other data can change quickly and may vary from those stated here.

EDISON INTERNATIONAL

www.edison.com

Industry Group Code: 221000A Ranks within this company's industry group: Sales: Profits:

Management:		Sales/Marketing:		Liberal Arts:		Information Systems:		Professionals:		Technical/Scientific:	
Mgmt. Trainees:	Y	Mktg. Professionals:	Y	Gen. Writing/Editing:	Y	Info. Management:	Y	Finance/Accounting:	Y	Engineers, Elec.:	Y
Experienced Mgmt.:	Y	Retail Sales:		Technical Writing:		Software Dev.:	Y	Law:	Y	Engineers, Other:	
Int'l Business:	Y	Commercial/Industrial:	Y	Graphic Arts/Photog.:		Hardware Dev.:		HR/Other:	Y	Health/Lab:	
MBA Graduates:	Y	Sales Trainees:		Music:		Systems Integration:		Training:	Y	Scientists/Research:	
		Advertising Pros.:	Y	Broadcasting:		Consulting/Other:		Health Care:		Petroleum/Chemicals:	
				Other:				Consulting:		Math/Other:	

TYPES OF BUSINESS:

Utilities-Electricity & Natural Gas
Financial Services
Operations Services
Energy Trading

BRANDS/DIVISIONS/AFFILIATES:

Southern California Edison Company
Edison Mission Energy
Edison Capital

CONTACTS: Note: Officers with more than one job title may be intentionally listed here more than once.

Theodore F. Craver Jr., CEO
Theodore F. Craver Jr., Pres.
Jim Scilacci, CFO/Exec. VP
Diane L. Featherstone, Sr. VP-Human Resources
Mahvash Yazdi, CIO/Sr. VP-Bus. Integration
Robert L. Adler, General Counsel/Exec. VP
Barbara J. Parsky, Sr. VP-Corp. Comm.
Scott Cunningham, VP-Investor Rel.
Thomas R. McDaniel, Treas.
Polly Gault, Exec. VP-Public Affairs
Jeff Barnett, VP-Tax
Barbara E. Matthews, Corp. Sec./VP/Chief Governance Officer
Linda G. Sullivan, Controller/VP
Theodore F. Craver Jr., Chmn.

Phone: 626-302-2222	Fax: 626-302-2517
Toll-Free: 800-655-4555	
Address: 2244 Walnut Grove Ave., Rosemead, CA 91770 US	

GROWTH PLANS/SPECIAL FEATURES:

Edison International is a California-based holding company with subsidiaries operating primarily in the U.S., with some investments abroad. Major subsidiaries include Southern California Edison Company (SCE), a utility corporation, and non-utility companies Edison Mission Energy (EME) and Edison Capital. SCE is one of the nation's largest electric utilities, providing electric service to a 50,000-square-mile area of California, including 430 cities and communities, serving over 13 million customers. The energy provided is developed from a range of different kinds of power plants including coal-burning, nuclear, hydroelectric and diesel-burning facilities. SCE also owns over 71,550 circuit miles of overhead lines and about 40,000 circuit miles of underground lines. SCE has assets of over $27.5 billion. EME is an independent power producer engaged in the business of developing, acquiring, owning or leasing, operating and selling energy and capacity from independent power production facilities. These operations consist in owning or leasing interests in 28 domestic operating power plants with a capacity of over 10,600 megawatts. EME also conducts price risk management and energy trading activities in power markets open to competition. Edison Capital invests in energy and infrastructure projects, including power generation; electric transmission and distribution; transportation; affordable housing; and telecommunications. In March 2008, SCE began constructing the largest wind transmission project in the U.S., projected to deliver over 4,500 megawatts of power. Also in March, SCE began the U.S.'s largest solar panel installation, covering 65 million square feet on commercial building roofs in Southern California and is projected to power 162,000 homes.

FINANCIALS: Sales and profits are in thousands of dollars—add 000 to get the full amount. 2007 Note: Financial information for 2007 was not available for all companies at press time.

2007 Sales: $13,113,000	2007 Profits: $1,098,000	**U.S. Stock Ticker: EIX**
2006 Sales: $12,622,000	2006 Profits: $1,181,000	**Int'l Ticker:** Int'l Exchange:
2005 Sales: $11,852,000	2005 Profits: $1,137,000	Employees: 15,838
2004 Sales: $10,199,000	2004 Profits: $916,000	Fiscal Year Ends: 12/31
2003 Sales: $10,732,000	2003 Profits: $821,000	Parent Company:

SALARIES/BENEFITS:

Pension Plan: Y	ESOP Stock Plan:	Profit Sharing:	Top Exec. Salary: $1,210,308	Bonus: $1,936,000
Savings Plan: Y	Stock Purch. Plan:		Second Exec. Salary: $643,238	Bonus: $684,000

OTHER THOUGHTS:

Apparent Women Officers or Directors: 6
Hot Spot for Advancement for Women/Minorities: Y

LOCATIONS: ("Y" = Yes)

West:	Southwest:	Midwest:	Southeast:	Northeast:	International:
Y	Y	Y	Y	Y	Y

Note: Financial information, benefits and other data can change quickly and may vary from those stated here.

ELECTRONIC ARTS INC   www.ea.com

Industry Group Code: 511208   Ranks within this company's industry group: Sales: 1   Profits: 1

Management:		Sales/Marketing:		Liberal Arts:		Information Systems:		Professionals:		Technical/Scientific:	
Mgmt. Trainees:	Y	Mktg. Professionals:	Y	Gen. Writing/Editing:	Y	Info. Management:	Y	Finance/Accounting:	Y	Engineers, Elec.:	Y
Experienced Mgmt.:	Y	Retail Sales:		Technical Writing:	Y	Software Dev.:	Y	Law:	Y	Engineers, Other:	
Int'l Business:	Y	Commercial/Industrial:	Y	Graphic Arts/Photog.:	Y	Hardware Dev.:		HR/Other:	Y	Health/Lab:	
MBA Graduates:	Y	Sales Trainees:		Music:	Y	Systems Integration:		Training:	Y	Scientists/Research:	
		Advertising Pros.:	Y	Broadcasting:		Consulting/Other:		Health Care:		Petroleum/Chemicals:	
				Other:	Y			Consulting:		Math/Other:	

TYPES OF BUSINESS:
Computer Software-Video Games
Online Interactive Games
E-Commerce Sales
Mobile Games

BRANDS/DIVISIONS/AFFILIATES:
EA GAMES
EA SPORTS
EA Casual Entertainment
Sims (The)
Madden NFL
Pogo.com
TheSimsOnStage.ea.com
BioWare Corp.

CONTACTS: *Note: Officers with more than one job title may be intentionally listed here more than once.*
John S. Riccitiello, CEO
John Pleasants, COO
Eric Brown, CFO/Exec. VP
Gabrielle Toledano, Exec. VP-Human Resources
Warren C. Jenson, Chief Admin. Officer
Stephen G. Bene, General Counsel/Sec./Sr. VP
Tammy Schachter, Sr. Dir.-Public Rel.
Ken Barker, Chief Acct. Officer/Sr. VP
Peter Moore, Pres., EA Sports Label
Frank Gibeau, Pres., EA Games Label
Nancy Smith, Pres., The Sims Label
Kathy Vrabeck, Pres., EA Casual Entertainment Label
Lawrence F. Probst, III, Exec. Chmn.
Gerhard Florin, Exec. VP/Gen. Manager-Int'l Publishing

Phone: 650-628-1500	Fax: 650-628-1415
Toll-Free:	
Address: 209 Redwood Shores Pkwy., Redwood City, CA 94065-1175 US	

GROWTH PLANS/SPECIAL FEATURES:
Electronic Arts, Inc. (EA) creates, markets and distributes entertainment software. In 2007, the firm reorganized, dividing its business into four labels: EA SPORTS, EA Games, EA Casual Entertainment and The Sims. EA SPORTS is responsible for many of the company's flagship franchises including Madden NFL, NBA Live, FIFA Soccer, Tiger Woods PGA TOUR, NHL Hockey and NASCAR. EA Games handles Need for Speed, Medal of Honor, SPORE, Battlefield, Burnout, Command & Conquer and The Simpsons; and will also be home to the EA Partners publishing business. EA Casual Entertainment focuses on lighter, more accessible games for families and new consumers, including EA franchises and games such as Harry Potter and Boogie, as well as EA Mobile and EA's casual suite of online games, Pogo.com. The Sims upcoming releases include: MySims for the Wii and Nintendo DS, SimCity Societies, Rail Sim and The Sims Castaway Stories and many more. The firm develops products for 11 main hardware platforms including the Xbox 360, PlayStation 3, Nintendo Wii, Nintendo DS, Game Boy Advance, PCs, PSP and cellular handsets. It also generates revenue from co-publication and distribution; licensing; and subscription services for its Internet games, including Ultima Online and the upcoming Warhammer Online. In 2007, EA acquired Singshot Media, an online karaoke community now available at TheSimsOnStage. In March 2007, online mobile phone service EA SPORTS Link launched, allowing U.S. Cingular customers to trade sports game information and challenge one another to live, networked games. In January 2008, EA acquired VG Holding Corp., owner of leading action, adventure and role-paying game development studios BioWare Corp. and Pandemic Studios, LLC (now part of the EA Games Label), for $780 million.

EA offers its employees on-site fitness facilities; discounts on game systems; education reimbursement; a company store; and full-time employees receive a paid week off at Christmas.

FINANCIALS: Sales and profits are in thousands of dollars—add 000 to get the full amount. 2007 Note: Financial information for 2007 was not available for all companies at press time.

2007 Sales: $3,091,000	2007 Profits: $76,000	**U.S. Stock Ticker: ERTS**
2006 Sales: $2,951,000	2006 Profits: $236,000	**Int'l Ticker:** Int'l Exchange:
2005 Sales: $3,129,000	2005 Profits: $504,000	Employees: 7,900
2004 Sales: $2,957,141	2004 Profits: $577,292	Fiscal Year Ends: 3/31
2003 Sales: $2,482,200	2003 Profits: $317,100	Parent Company:

SALARIES/BENEFITS:
Pension Plan:	ESOP Stock Plan:	Profit Sharing:	Top Exec. Salary: $738,462	Bonus: $993,517
Savings Plan: Y	Stock Purch. Plan: Y		Second Exec. Salary: $591,648	Bonus: $639,020

OTHER THOUGHTS:
Apparent Women Officers or Directors: 4
Hot Spot for Advancement for Women/Minorities: Y

LOCATIONS: ("Y" = Yes)
West:	Southwest:	Midwest:	Southeast:	Northeast:	International:
Y	Y	Y	Y	Y	Y

ELI LILLY & COMPANY

www.lilly.com

Industry Group Code: 325412 Ranks within this company's industry group: Sales: Profits:

Management:		Sales/Marketing:		Liberal Arts:		Information Systems:		Professionals:		Technical/Scientific:	
Mgmt. Trainees:	Y	Mktg. Professionals:	Y	Gen. Writing/Editing:	Y	Info. Management:	Y	Finance/Accounting:	Y	Engineers, Elec.:	Y
Experienced Mgmt.:	Y	Retail Sales:		Technical Writing:	Y	Software Dev.:	Y	Law:	Y	Engineers, Other:	Y
Int'l Business:	Y	Commercial/Industrial:	Y	Graphic Arts/Photog.:	Y	Hardware Dev.:		HR/Other:	Y	Health/Lab:	Y
MBA Graduates:	Y	Sales Trainees:	Y	Music:		Systems Integration:		Training:	Y	Scientists/Research:	Y
		Advertising Pros.:	Y	Broadcasting:		Consulting/Other:		Health Care:	Y	Petroleum/Chemicals:	
				Other:				Consulting:		Math/Other:	Y

TYPES OF BUSINESS:

Pharmaceuticals Discovery & Development
Veterinary Products

BRANDS/DIVISIONS/AFFILIATES:

Zyprexa
Prozac
Humalog
Gemzar
Coban
Applied Molecular Evolution Inc
Icos Corporation
Hypnion, Inc.

CONTACTS: *Note: Officers with more than one job title may be intentionally listed here more than once.*

Sidney Taurel, CEO
John Lechleiter, COO
John Lechleiter, Pres.
Derica Rice, CFO/Sr. VP
Richard Pilnik, Chief Mktg. Officer/VP
Anthony Murphy, Sr. VP-Human Resources
Thomas Verhoeven, VP-Prod. R&D
Michael Heim, CIO/VP-IT
Bryce Carmine, Pres., Global Prod. Dev.
Robert A. Cole, VP-Global Eng. & Environmental Health & Safety
Frank Deane, Pres., Mfg.
Robert A. Armitage, General Counsel/Sr. VP
Peter Johnson, Exec. Dir.-Corp. Strategic Planning
Alex M. Azar II, Sr. VP-Corp. Affairs & Comm.
Thomas W. Grein, Treas./VP
Deirdre Connelly, Pres., Lilly USA
Newton F. Crenshaw, Pres./Gen. Mgr.-Lilly Japan
Alecia A. DeCoudreaux, General Counsel/VP
Tim Garnett, Chief Medical Officer/VP-Medical
Sidney Taurel, Chmn.

Phone: 317-276-2000	Fax:
Toll-Free:	
Address: Lilly Corporate Ctr., Indianapolis, IN 46285 US	

GROWTH PLANS/SPECIAL FEATURES:

Eli Lilly & Co. researches, develops, manufactures and sells pharmaceuticals designed to treat a variety of conditions. Most of Eli Lilly's products are developed by its in-house research staff, which primarily directs its research efforts towards the search for products to prevent and treat cancer and diseases of the central nervous, endocrine and cardiovascular systems. The firm's other research lies in anti-infectives and products to treat animal diseases. Major brands include neuroscience products Zyprexa, Strattera, Prozac, Cymbalta and Permax; endocrine products Humalog, Humulin and Actos; oncology products Gemzar and Alimta; animal health products Tylan, Rumensin and Coban; cardiovascular products ReoPro and Xigris; anti-infectives Ceclor and Vancocin; and Cialis, for erectile dysfunction. In the U.S., the company distributes pharmaceuticals primarily through independent wholesale distributors. Marketing is through an in-house sales force that calls upon physicians, hospitals and managed care providers directly. Outside of the U.S., Eli Lilly products are primarily marketed either through this direct sales force or by way of standing partnerships with several companies, including Takeda Chemical Industries; ICOS Corp.; Quintiles Transnational; and Boehringer Ingelheim. The company manufactures and distributes its products through facilities in the U.S., Puerto Rico and 25 other countries, which are then sold to markets in 135 countries throughout the world. In April 2008, the firm acquired Hypnion, Inc., a neuroscience drug discovery company focused on sleep disorder research.

Eli Lilly offers its employees domestic partner benefits and an employee assistance program, as well as up to 10 weeks of paid maternity leave. The firm also offers an on-site fitness center, flexible hours or telecommuting, parenting and dependant care leaves, adoption assistance and tuition reimbursement, among many other things.

FINANCIALS: Sales and profits are in thousands of dollars—add 000 to get the full amount. 2007 Note: Financial information for 2007 was not available for all companies at press time.

2007 Sales: $18,633,500	2007 Profits: $2,953,000	**U.S. Stock Ticker: LLY**	
2006 Sales: $15,691,000	2006 Profits: $2,662,700	**Int'l Ticker:** Int'l Exchange:	
2005 Sales: $14,645,300	2005 Profits: $1,979,600	Employees: 40,600	
2004 Sales: $13,857,900	2004 Profits: $1,810,100	Fiscal Year Ends: 12/31	
2003 Sales: $12,582,500	2003 Profits: $2,560,800	Parent Company:	

SALARIES/BENEFITS:

Pension Plan: Y	ESOP Stock Plan:	Profit Sharing:	Top Exec. Salary: $1,717,417	Bonus: $4,035,929
Savings Plan: Y	Stock Purch. Plan:		Second Exec. Salary: $1,149,083	Bonus: $2,160,277

OTHER THOUGHTS:

Apparent Women Officers or Directors: 10
Hot Spot for Advancement for Women/Minorities: Y

LOCATIONS: ("Y" = Yes)

West:	Southwest:	Midwest:	Southeast:	Northeast:	International:
Y	Y	Y	Y	Y	Y

EMBARQ CORP

www.embarq.com

Industry Group Code: 513300A **Ranks within this company's industry group:** Sales: 3   Profits: 3

Management:		Sales/Marketing:		Liberal Arts:		Information Systems:		Professionals:		Technical/Scientific:	
Mgmt. Trainees:		Mktg. Professionals:	Y	Gen. Writing/Editing:		Info. Management:	Y	Finance/Accounting:	Y	Engineers, Elec.:	Y
Experienced Mgmt.:	Y	Retail Sales:		Technical Writing:	Y	Software Dev.:	Y	Law:	Y	Engineers, Other:	
Int'l Business:		Commercial/Industrial:	Y	Graphic Arts/Photog.:		Hardware Dev.:		HR/Other:	Y	Health/Lab:	
MBA Graduates:	Y	Sales Trainees:		Music:		Systems Integration:	Y	Training:	Y	Scientists/Research:	
		Advertising Pros.:	Y	Broadcasting:		Consulting/Other:		Health Care:		Petroleum/Chemicals:	
				Other:				Consulting:		Math/Other:	

TYPES OF BUSINESS:

Local & Long-Distance Phone Services
High-Speed Internet Access
Satellite Video Services
Wireless Services

BRANDS/DIVISIONS/AFFILIATES:

Sprint Nextel Corp

CONTACTS: Note: Officers with more than one job title may be intentionally listed here more than once.

Thomas A. (Tom) Gerke, CEO
Thomas A. (Tom) Gerke, Pres.
Gene M. Betts, CFO
E.J. Holland, Jr., Sr. VP-Human Resources
Vercie L. Lark, CIO
Dennis G. Huber, CTO
Claudia S. Toussaint, General Counsel/Corp. Sec./Chief Ethics Officer
Dennis G. Huber, Sr. VP-Corp. Strategy & Dev.
E.J. Holland, Jr., Sr. VP-Comm.
Les Meredith, Treas.
William E. (Bill) Cheek, Pres., Wholesale Markets
Harrison S. Campbell, Pres., Consumer Markets
Thomas J. McEvoy, Pres., Bus. Markets
James C. Mayfield, Pres., EMBARQ Logistics
William A. Owens, Chmn.

Phone: 913-323-4637	Fax: 913-523-9120
Toll-Free:	
Address: 5454 W. 110th St., Overland Park, KS 66211 US	

GROWTH PLANS/SPECIAL FEATURES:

Embarq Corporation is a provider of local and long-distance voice, data, high-speed Internet, satellite, video, wireless and other communication-related products and services to consumer and business customers in 18 states. It also provides access to its local network and other wholesale communications services for customers, including other carriers. Through its Logistics segment, the firm provides wholesale product distribution, logistics and configuration services. Embarq has a significant presence in Florida, North Carolina, Nevada and Ohio, which together represent approximately 66% of all its access lines. The company offers six general categories of products and services through its Telecommunications segment: Voice, data, high-speed Internet, wireless, product and other. As of December 2007, Embarq had approximately 4.3 million local service consumer access lines and 2 million business access lines. It offers long-distance voice and data services through a wholesale agreement with Sprint Nextel. The company's most significant data service is special access, which consists of dedicated circuits used to connect the customer's business sites or network to its network; to connect the customer's networks directly to their customers' locations, or, in the case of wireless carriers, to connect their cell sites with their mobile switching centers. As of December 2007, Embarq provided high-speed Internet access to approximately 1.3 million subscribers. The company offers wireless services through a wholesale arrangement involving a mobile virtual network operator relationship with Sprint Nextel. Embarq sells and services a range of customer premises equipment and wireless handsets and sells video services through its sales agency relationship with DISH Network Corporation and DIRECTV. The firm's Logistics segment operates seven distribution centers throughout the U.S., stocking over 20,000 items.

Embarq offers its employees tuition assistance, employee discount, employee assistance, service awards, adoption assistance and wellness programs; reimbursement accounts; and medical, dental, vision, prescription, life, AD&D and disability insurance.

FINANCIALS: Sales and profits are in thousands of dollars—add 000 to get the full amount. 2007 Note: Financial information for 2007 was not available for all companies at press time.

2007 Sales: $6,365,000	2007 Profits: $683,000	U.S. Stock Ticker: EQ
2006 Sales: $6,363,000	2006 Profits: $784,000	Int'l Ticker: Int'l Exchange:
2005 Sales: $6,254,000	2005 Profits: $878,000	Employees: 18,000
2004 Sales: $6,139,000	2004 Profits: $917,000	Fiscal Year Ends: 12/31
2003 Sales: $	2003 Profits: $	Parent Company:

SALARIES/BENEFITS:

Pension Plan: Y	ESOP Stock Plan:	Profit Sharing:	Top Exec. Salary: $1,026,822	Bonus: $
Savings Plan: Y	Stock Purch. Plan:		Second Exec. Salary: $472,907	Bonus: $508,935

OTHER THOUGHTS:

Apparent Women Officers or Directors: 3
Hot Spot for Advancement for Women/Minorities: Y

LOCATIONS: ("Y" = Yes)

West:	Southwest:	Midwest:	Southeast:	Northeast:	International:
		Y			

Note: Financial information, benefits and other data can change quickly and may vary from those stated here.

EMC CORP   www.emc.com

Industry Group Code: 334112 **Ranks within this company's industry group:** Sales: 1 Profits: 1

Management:		Sales/Marketing:		Liberal Arts:		Information Systems:		Professionals:		Technical/Scientific:	
Mgmt. Trainees:	Y	Mktg. Professionals:	Y	Gen. Writing/Editing:		Info. Management:	Y	Finance/Accounting:	Y	Engineers, Elec.:	Y
Experienced Mgmt.:	Y	Retail Sales:		Technical Writing:	Y	Software Dev.:	Y	Law:	Y	Engineers, Other:	
Int'l Business:	Y	Commercial/Industrial:	Y	Graphic Arts/Photog.:	Y	Hardware Dev.:	Y	HR/Other:	Y	Health/Lab:	Y
MBA Graduates:	Y	Sales Trainees:		Music:		Systems Integration:		Training:	Y	Scientists/Research:	Y
		Advertising Pros.:	Y	Broadcasting:		Consulting/Other:		Health Care:		Petroleum/Chemicals:	
				Other:				Consulting:		Math/Other:	

TYPES OF BUSINESS:

Computer Storage Equipment-Mainframe Disk Memory
Network Storage Systems
Management Protection Software
Consulting Services
Storage Management Services

BRANDS/DIVISIONS/AFFILIATES:

Symmetrix
CLARiiON
Celera
Documentum
Captiva
VMware Inc
Verid
Berkeley Data Systems

CONTACTS: *Note: Officers with more than one job title may be intentionally listed here more than once.*

Joseph M. Tucci, CEO
Joseph M. Tucci, Pres.
David I. Goulden, CFO/Exec. VP
Frank M. Hauck, Exec. VP-Global Mktg. & Customer Quality
John T. Mollen, Exec. VP-Human Resources
Jeffrey M. Nick, CTO/Sr. VP
Paul T. Dacier, General Counsel/Exec. VP
Louise O'Brien, Exec. VP-Corp. Strategy & Dev.
Irina Simmons, Treas./Sr. VP
William J. Teuber, Jr., Vice Chmn.
Arthur W. Coviello, Jr., Pres., RSA Security Div.
David A. Donatelli, Pres., Storage Div.
Mark S. Lewis, Pres., Content Mgmt. & Archiving
Joseph M. Tucci, Chmn.
Howard D. Elias, Pres., Global Svcs. & Resource Mgmt. Software

Phone: 508-435-1000	Fax: 508-497-6912
Toll-Free: 877-362-6973	
Address: 176 South St., Hopkinton, MA 01748-9103 US	

GROWTH PLANS/SPECIAL FEATURES:

EMC Corporation, along with its subsidiaries, develops, delivers and supports systems, software and services for the storage, management and protection of electronic information. EMC operates in four segments: information storage; content management and archiving; RSA information security; and VMware virtual infrastructure. The information storage segment is composed of storage systems, platform-based and multi-platform software and services. EMC's storage systems are the foundation of an information infrastructure and can be deployed in a storage area network (SAN), network attached storage (NAS), content addressed storage (CAS) or direct attached storage environment. Product lines include the Symmetrix, CLARiiON, Celera, Centera and Connectrix systems. EMC's content management and archiving software includes the Documentum family, the Captiva family and the e-Discovery Solution. The RSA information security segment includes RSA Key Manager software, enabling businesses to effectively manage the lifecycle of encryption keys. VMware, Inc., a subsidiary of EMC, provides virtual infrastructure solutions and services to over 20,000 enterprises for server consolidation; disaster recovery and business continuity; capacity planning and development; enterprise desktop hosting; test optimization; and software distribution. VMware's products include Infrastructure 3, Virtual Desktop Infrastructure, VMware Lab Manager, VMware Converter 3, VMware Server and the Virtual Appliance Marketplace. During 2007, the company acquired Verid, a private information security technology company; Berkeley Data Systems, provider of Mozy, an online information backup and recovery service; and Voyence, a provider of network configuration and change management solutions. In December 2007, EMC agreed to acquire Document Sciences Corporation for roughly $85 million. In 2008, the firm agreed to acquire Iomega Corp. for $213 million.

EMC offers its employees tuition assistance; a domestic partner program; adoption assistance; a dependent care flexible spending account; on-site daycare; credit union membership; a group legal plan; employee discount programs; behavioral health benefits; a health care flexible spending account; and medical, dental, prescription and vision insurance.

FINANCIALS: Sales and profits are in thousands of dollars—add 000 to get the full amount. 2007 Note: Financial information for 2007 was not available for all companies at press time.

2007 Sales: $13,230,205	2007 Profits: $1,665,668	**U.S. Stock Ticker:** EMC
2006 Sales: $11,155,090	2006 Profits: $1,227,601	**Int'l Ticker:** Int'l Exchange:
2005 Sales: $9,663,955	2005 Profits: $1,133,165	Employees: 37,700
2004 Sales: $8,229,488	2004 Profits: $871,189	Fiscal Year Ends: 12/31
2003 Sales: $6,236,808	2003 Profits: $496,108	Parent Company:

SALARIES/BENEFITS:

Pension Plan:	ESOP Stock Plan:	Profit Sharing:	Top Exec. Salary: $1,000,000	Bonus: $1,440,000
Savings Plan: Y	Stock Purch. Plan: Y		Second Exec. Salary: $600,000	Bonus: $450,000

OTHER THOUGHTS:

Apparent Women Officers or Directors: 3
Hot Spot for Advancement for Women/Minorities: Y

LOCATIONS: ("Y" = Yes)

West:	Southwest:	Midwest:	Southeast:	Northeast:	International:
Y				Y	Y

EMERITUS CORP
www.emeritus.com

Industry Group Code: 623110   Ranks within this company's industry group: Sales: 4   Profits: 5

Management:		Sales/Marketing:		Liberal Arts:		Information Systems:		Professionals:		Technical/Scientific:	
Mgmt. Trainees:	Y	Mktg. Professionals:	Y	Gen. Writing/Editing:		Info. Management:	Y	Finance/Accounting:		Engineers, Elec.:	
Experienced Mgmt.:	Y	Retail Sales:		Technical Writing:		Software Dev.:		Law:	Y	Engineers, Other:	Y
Int'l Business:	Y	Commercial/Industrial:		Graphic Arts/Photog.:		Hardware Dev.:		HR/Other:	Y	Health/Lab:	
MBA Graduates:	Y	Sales Trainees:		Music:		Systems Integration:		Training:	Y	Scientists/Research:	
		Advertising Pros.:		Broadcasting:		Consulting/Other:		Health Care:		Petroleum/Chemicals:	
				Other:				Consulting:		Math/Other:	

TYPES OF BUSINESS:
Long-Term Health Care
Assisted Living Communities

BRANDS/DIVISIONS/AFFILIATES:
Arbor Place at Silverlake

CONTACTS: *Note: Officers with more than one job title may be intentionally listed here more than once.*
Daniel R. Baty, Co-CEO
Justin Hutchens, COO
Granger Cobb, Pres./Co-CEO
Raymond R. Brandstrom, CFO/Exec. VP-Finance
John Cincotta, Sr. VP-Sales & Mktg.
Melanie Werdel, Exec. VP-Admin.
Raymond R. Brandstrom, Corp. Sec.
Justin Hutchens, Exec. VP-Oper.
Eric Mendelsohn, Sr. VP-Corp. Dev.
Jim L. Hanson, Sr. VP-Financial Svcs./Controller
Budgie Amparo, Sr. VP-Quality & Risk Mgmt.
Martin D. Roffe, Sr. VP-Financial Planning
Daniel R. Baty, Chmn.

Phone: 206-298-2909	Fax: 206-301-4500
Toll-Free: 800-429-4828	
Address: 3131 Elliott Ave., Ste. 500, Seattle, WA 98121 US	

GROWTH PLANS/SPECIAL FEATURES:
Emeritus Corp. operates assisted living residential communities in the U.S. It operates or has an interest in 287 communities across 35 states, totaling approximately 25,000 units with a capacity for roughly 30,000 residents. These communities cater to senior citizens who need help with daily living, but do not require the intensive care provided in skilled nursing facilities. Assisted living generally provides housing and 24-hour personal support services. Seniors reside in a private or semi-private residential unit for a monthly fee based on each resident's individual service needs. Emeritus's specialty is in Alzheimer's and dementia related care, for which the company has developed a program that links memory training, familiar environments and personalized care services. Accessing the market for Alzheimer's care is one of the firm's key business strategies. In its other assisted living programs, Emeritus business strategy calls for customer service that addresses both physical and social health. The firm's target customers are middle to upper-middle income seniors living in smaller cities (50,000 to 150,000 persons). Emeritus attempts to generate growth through increases in residential occupancy rates and revenue per occupied unit as well as through investments in IT infrastructure and through the selective acquisition of assisted living communities. In recent years, the company has sought to increase the number of communities it owns and decrease the number it merely manages. In March 2007, the firm purchased three communities that it had previously leased for roughly $28.7 million. In September 2007, Emeritus acquired Summerville Senior Living, Inc., a California-based operator of 81 communities comprising 7,935 units in 13 states.

The company offers its employees health care benefits, a retirement savings plan and a stock purchase plan.

FINANCIALS: Sales and profits are in thousands of dollars—add 000 to get the full amount. 2007 Note: Financial information for 2007 was not available for all companies at press time.

2007 Sales: $545,639	2007 Profits: $-48,741	**U.S. Stock Ticker: ESC**
2006 Sales: $421,865	2006 Profits: $-14,618	**Int'l Ticker:** Int'l Exchange:
2005 Sales: $387,732	2005 Profits: $11,703	Employees: 16,205
2004 Sales: $316,866	2004 Profits: $-40,540	Fiscal Year Ends: 12/31
2003 Sales: $206,657	2003 Profits: $-8,081	Parent Company:

SALARIES/BENEFITS:

Pension Plan:	ESOP Stock Plan:	Profit Sharing:	Top Exec. Salary: $300,000	Bonus: $
Savings Plan: Y	Stock Purch. Plan: Y		Second Exec. Salary: $207,083	Bonus: $

OTHER THOUGHTS:
Apparent Women Officers or Directors: 1
Hot Spot for Advancement for Women/Minorities:

LOCATIONS: ("Y" = Yes)

West:	Southwest:	Midwest:	Southeast:	Northeast:	International:
Y	Y	Y	Y	Y	

Note: Financial information, benefits and other data can change quickly and may vary from those stated here.

EMERSON ELECTRIC CO
www.gotoemerson.com

Industry Group Code: 334500 Ranks within this company's industry group: Sales: 1 Profits: 2

Management:		Sales/Marketing:		Liberal Arts:		Information Systems:		Professionals:		Technical/Scientific:	
Mgmt. Trainees:		Mktg. Professionals:	Y	Gen. Writing/Editing:		Info. Management:	Y	Finance/Accounting:	Y	Engineers, Elec.:	Y
Experienced Mgmt.:	Y	Retail Sales:		Technical Writing:	Y	Software Dev.:	Y	Law:	Y	Engineers, Other:	Y
Int'l Business:	Y	Commercial/Industrial:	Y	Graphic Arts/Photog.:	Y	Hardware Dev.:	Y	HR/Other:	Y	Health/Lab:	
MBA Graduates:	Y	Sales Trainees:		Music:		Systems Integration:	Y	Training:	Y	Scientists/Research:	Y
		Advertising Pros.:	Y	Broadcasting:		Consulting/Other:		Health Care:		Petroleum/Chemicals:	
				Other:				Consulting:		Math/Other:	Y

TYPES OF BUSINESS:
Engineering & Technology Products & Services
Industrial Automation Products
Power Products
Air Conditioning & Refrigeration Products
Appliances & Tools

BRANDS/DIVISIONS/AFFILIATES:
PlantWeb Digital Plant Architecture
Process Management
Industrial Automation
Network Power
Knurr AG
Artesyn Technologies
Damcos Holding A/S
Lionville Systems, Inc.

CONTACTS: Note: Officers with more than one job title may be intentionally listed here more than once.
David N. Farr, CEO
Edward L. Monser, COO
David N. Farr, Pres.
Walter J. Galvin, CFO/Sr. Exec. VP
Frank L. Steeves, General Counsel/Sec.
Charles A. Peters, Sr. Exec. VP
John M. Berra, Exec. VP-Emerson Process Mgmt.
Thomas E. Bettcher, Exec. VP-Emerson Climate Tech.
Ed Feeney, Exec. VP-Emerson Network Power
David N. Farr, Chmn.

Phone: 314-553-2000	Fax: 314-553-3527
Toll-Free:	
Address: 8000 W. Florissant Ave., P.O. Box 4100, St. Louis, MO 63136 US	

GROWTH PLANS/SPECIAL FEATURES:
Emerson Electric Co. designs and supplies technology products and engineering services, serving a wide range of industrial, commercial and consumer markets worldwide. The company is organized into five business segments. The Process Management segment provides measurement, control and diagnostic capabilities for automated industrial processes producing items such as foods, medicines, power and fuels. As part of this segment, Emerson offers PlantWeb Digital Plant Architecture, a platform designed to open communication between industrial plant devices and, with its accompanying software, collect and analyze information concerning plant assets and processes. These capabilities give customers the ability to predict changes in equipment and process performance and the impact they can have on plant operations. The Industrial Automation segment assists clients in automating production lines. Products for this group include motors, transmissions, alternators, fluid controls and materials joining equipment. The Network Power segment provides power and environmental conditioning systems to help ensure telecommunication systems, data networks and critical business applications operate continuously. The Climate Technologies segment primarily focuses on household and commercial air-conditioning and refrigeration technologies for comfort and food safety. Lastly, the Appliances and Tools segment provides motors for a broad range of applications, appliances and integrated appliance solutions; tools for homeowners and professionals; and home and commercial storage systems. Emerson operates approximately 100 manufacturing locations in the U.S. and 165 overseas, evenly divided between Europe, Asia and other locations. It recently acquired Knurr AG, German developer of enclosure systems and cooling technologies for telecommunication and data applications; and Artesyn Technologies, designer of power conversion and embedded information technology products. In January 2007, it acquired Damcos Holding A/S, developer of automated tank and valve systems. In March 2007, Emerson acquired Lionville Systems, Inc. a manufacturer of medication management systems. In September 2007, Emerson agreed to acquire Motorola's Embedded Communications Computing business for $350 million.

FINANCIALS: Sales and profits are in thousands of dollars—add 000 to get the full amount. 2007 Note: Financial information for 2007 was not available for all companies at press time.

2007 Sales: $22,572,000	2007 Profits: $2,136,000	U.S. Stock Ticker: EMR
2006 Sales: $20,133,000	2006 Profits: $1,845,000	Int'l Ticker: Int'l Exchange:
2005 Sales: $17,305,000	2005 Profits: $1,422,000	Employees: 137,700
2004 Sales: $15,615,000	2004 Profits: $1,257,000	Fiscal Year Ends: 9/30
2003 Sales: $13,958,000	2003 Profits: $1,089,000	Parent Company:

SALARIES/BENEFITS:

Pension Plan: Y	ESOP Stock Plan:	Profit Sharing:	Top Exec. Salary: $1,150,000	Bonus: $2,700,000
Savings Plan:	Stock Purch. Plan:		Second Exec. Salary: $680,000	Bonus: $1,025,000

OTHER THOUGHTS:
Apparent Women Officers or Directors:
Hot Spot for Advancement for Women/Minorities:

LOCATIONS: ("Y" = Yes)

West:	Southwest:	Midwest:	Southeast:	Northeast:	International:
Y	Y	Y	Y	Y	Y

Note: Financial information, benefits and other data can change quickly and may vary from those stated here.

ENTERGY CORP

www.entergy.com

Industry Group Code: 221000A Ranks within this company's industry group: Sales: Profits:

Management:		Sales/Marketing:		Liberal Arts:		Information Systems:		Professionals:		Technical/Scientific:	
Mgmt. Trainees:	Y	Mktg. Professionals:	Y	Gen. Writing/Editing:	Y	Info. Management:	Y	Finance/Accounting:	Y	Engineers, Elec.:	Y
Experienced Mgmt.:	Y	Retail Sales:		Technical Writing:		Software Dev.:	Y	Law:	Y	Engineers, Other:	
Int'l Business:	Y	Commercial/Industrial:	Y	Graphic Arts/Photog.:		Hardware Dev.:		HR/Other:	Y	Health/Lab:	
MBA Graduates:	Y	Sales Trainees:		Music:		Systems Integration:		Training:	Y	Scientists/Research:	
		Advertising Pros.:	Y	Broadcasting:		Consulting/Other:		Health Care:		Petroleum/Chemicals:	
				Other:				Consulting:		Math/Other:	

TYPES OF BUSINESS:

Utilities-Electric
Energy Management
Energy Trading
Nuclear Generation
Hydroelectric Generation
Wind Generation

BRANDS/DIVISIONS/AFFILIATES:

Entergy Arkansas
Entergy Louisiana
Entergy Mississipi
Entergy Texas
Entergy New Orleans
Enexus Energy Corporation

CONTACTS: Note: Officers with more than one job title may be intentionally listed here more than once.

J. Wayne Leonard, CEO
Richard Smith, COO
Richard Smith, Pres.
Leo Denault, CFO/Exec. VP
Terry Seamons, Sr. VP-Human Resources
Terry Seamons, Sr. VP-Admin.
Robert Sloan, General Counsel/Exec. VP
Mark T. Savoff, Exec. VP-Oper.
Michele Lopiccolo, Sr. VP-Investor Rel.
Curt L. Hebert, Jr., Exec. VP-External Affairs
Gary Taylor, Pres., Utility Oper.
Michael D. Bakewell, Sr. VP-Fossil Oper.
Steven Agresta, Exec. VP-Enexus Energy Corp.
J. Wayne Leonard, Chmn.

Phone: 504-576-4000	Fax: 504-576-4428
Toll-Free:	
Address: 639 Loyola Ave., New Orleans, LA 70113 US	

GROWTH PLANS/SPECIAL FEATURES:

Entergy Corp. is an integrated energy company engaged primarily in the electric power production and retail electric distribution operations. The company owns and operates power plants with roughly 30,000 megawatts of electric general capacity, making it one of the largest nuclear power generators in the U.S. The firm operates in two primary segments, utility and non-utility nuclear. The utility segment, which generated 80% of revenue in 2007, generates, transmits, distributes and sells electric power in a four-state service territory that includes portions of Arkansas, Mississippi, Texas and Louisiana, including New Orleans. The division also operates a small natural gas distribution system. The non-utility nuclear segment, responsible for 18% of revenue in 2007, owns and operates five nuclear power plants located in the northeastern U.S. and sells the electric power produced by those plants primarily to wholesale customers. The division also provides services to other nuclear power plant owners. In addition to these two segments, Entergy also operates a non-nuclear wholesale assets business, which sells to wholesale customers the electric power produced by power plants that it owns while it focuses on improving performance and exploring sales or restructuring opportunities for its power plants. The firm has six main regional subsidiaries, all falling under the U.S. utility segment: Entergy Arkansas, Entergy Gulf States of Louisiana, Entergy Louisiana, Entergy Mississippi, Entergy New Orleans and System Energy Resources. Entergy New Orleans is in the process of reorganization under Chapter 11. In August 2008, the firm announced Enexus Energy Corporation will be the independent, publicly traded nuclear power company that it plans to spin-off later in 2008 and EquaGen L.L.C. as the new joint venture between Entergy and Enexus, which will operate the six nuclear reactors.

FINANCIALS: Sales and profits are in thousands of dollars—add 000 to get the full amount. 2007 Note: Financial information for 2007 was not available for all companies at press time.

2007 Sales: $11,484,398	2007 Profits: $1,134,849	U.S. Stock Ticker: ETR
2006 Sales: $10,932,158	2006 Profits: $1,132,602	Int'l Ticker: Int'l Exchange:
2005 Sales: $10,106,247	2005 Profits: $923,758	Employees: 13,814
2004 Sales: $9,685,521	2004 Profits: $933,049	Fiscal Year Ends: 12/31
2003 Sales: $9,032,714	2003 Profits: $950,467	Parent Company:

SALARIES/BENEFITS:

Pension Plan: Y	ESOP Stock Plan:	Profit Sharing:	Top Exec. Salary: $1,168,577	Bonus: $2,235,870
Savings Plan: Y	Stock Purch. Plan:		Second Exec. Salary: $538,493	Bonus: $722,358

OTHER THOUGHTS:

Apparent Women Officers or Directors: 4
Hot Spot for Advancement for Women/Minorities: Y

LOCATIONS: ("Y" = Yes)

West:	Southwest:	Midwest:	Southeast:	Northeast:	International:
	Y		Y		

Note: Financial information, benefits and other data can change quickly and may vary from those stated here.

ENTERPRISE RENT-A-CAR   www.enterprise.com

Industry Group Code: 532111 Ranks within this company's industry group: Sales: 1   Profits:

Management:		Sales/Marketing:		Liberal Arts:		Information Systems:		Professionals:		Technical/Scientific:	
Mgmt. Trainees:	Y	Mktg. Professionals:	Y	Gen. Writing/Editing:	Y	Info. Management:	Y	Finance/Accounting:	Y	Engineers, Elec.:	
Experienced Mgmt.:	Y	Retail Sales:	Y	Technical Writing:		Software Dev.:	Y	Law:	Y	Engineers, Other:	
Int'l Business:	Y	Commercial/Industrial:	Y	Graphic Arts/Photog.:	Y	Hardware Dev.:		HR/Other:	Y	Health/Lab:	
MBA Graduates:	Y	Sales Trainees:	Y	Music:		Systems Integration:		Training:	Y	Scientists/Research:	
		Advertising Pros.:	Y	Broadcasting:		Consulting/Other:		Health Care:		Petroleum/Chemicals:	
				Other:				Consulting:		Math/Other:	

TYPES OF BUSINESS:
Automobile Rental
Fleet Management Services
Used Vehicle Sales
Commuter Services

BRANDS/DIVISIONS/AFFILIATES:
Enterprise Rent-a-Car
Enterprise Car Sales
Enterprise Fleet Services
Enterprise Rent-a-Truck
Vanguard Car Rental USA Inc
National Car Rental
Alamo Rental

CONTACTS: *Note: Officers with more than one job title may be intentionally listed here more than once.*
Andrew C. Taylor, CEO
Pamela M. Nicholson, COO/Exec. VP
Donald L. Ross, Pres./Vice. Chmn.
William W. Snyder, CFO/Exec. VP
Edward Adams, Sr. VP-Human Resources
Craig Kennedy, CIO/Sr. VP
Lee Kaplan, Sr. VP/Chief Admin. Officer
Rose Langhorst, Treas./VP
Matthew G. Darrah, Sr. VP-North American Oper.
Jim Runnels, Sr. VP-Rental
Andrew C. Taylor, Chmn.
James Burrell, Sr. VP-European Oper.

Phone: 314-512-5000	**Fax:** 314-512-4706
Toll-Free:	
Address: 600 Corporate Park Dr., St. Louis, MO 63105 US	

GROWTH PLANS/SPECIAL FEATURES:

Enterprise Rent-A-Car is a car rental company with over 728,000 rental and fleet vehicles through more than 7,000 locations in the U.S. and 900 in Canada, Germany, Ireland and the U.K. The firm markets to visitors from other cities, and people whose cars are in repair shops or who want luxury cars or convertibles for special occasions. The company serves the most-traveled airports in the U.S. and several of the largest airports in Canada and the U.K. Enterprise's services also include fleet management, used car sales, the California Vanpool Services and Rent-A-Truck. Enterprise Fleet Services (EFS) provides a number of services, including acquisition, insurance services, registration, funding, fuel management, maintenance and disposal. Enterprise Car Sales (ECS) sells used vehicles directly to local franchised dealers, independent used car dealers and auto auctions. Customers are offered an inventory of over 120 makes and models, most of which are low-mileage cars. The Enterprise Rideshare division, also known as the California Vanpool Service, operates over 700 vehicles, which are used to transport commuters in Northern and Southern California. Enterprise Rent-a-Truck has over 90 locations across the nation specializing in commercial truck rentals. In August 2007, Enterprise acquired Vanguard Car Rental and its National Car Rental and Alamo Rental Businesses from private equity group Cerberus Capital Management LP. The acquisition gives Enterprise a total of 27% market share at U.S. airport locations, compared to its previous 8%. This will put it head-to-head with Hertz's 28.5% share at airports and the Avis Budget Group's 30.1%. The firm anticipates that acquisition will increase total revenues to about $12 billion yearly. In 2008, Enterprise initiated various environmentally friendly efforts, including E85/flexfuel locations, increased hybrid and fuel-efficient vehicles, carbon offset programs and car sharing services.

Employee benefits include adoption assistance and employee discounts.

FINANCIALS: Sales and profits are in thousands of dollars—add 000 to get the full amount. 2007 Note: Financial information for 2007 was not available for all companies at press time.

		U.S. Stock Ticker: Private
2007 Sales: $9,500,000	2007 Profits: $	**Int'l Ticker:** Int'l Exchange:
2006 Sales: $9,000,000	2006 Profits: $	Employees: 66,700
2005 Sales: $8,230,000	2005 Profits: $	Fiscal Year Ends: 7/31
2004 Sales: $7,400,000	2004 Profits: $	Parent Company:
2003 Sales: $6,900,000	2003 Profits: $	

SALARIES/BENEFITS:

Pension Plan:	ESOP Stock Plan:	Profit Sharing: Y	Top Exec. Salary: $	Bonus: $
Savings Plan: Y	Stock Purch. Plan:		Second Exec. Salary: $	Bonus: $

OTHER THOUGHTS:
Apparent Women Officers or Directors: 3
Hot Spot for Advancement for Women/Minorities: Y

LOCATIONS: ("Y" = Yes)

West:	Southwest:	Midwest:	Southeast:	Northeast:	International:
Y	Y	Y	Y	Y	Y

Note: Financial information, benefits and other data can change quickly and may vary from those stated here.

ERNST & YOUNG LLP

www.ey.com

Industry Group Code: 541210 Ranks within this company's industry group: Sales: Profits:

Management:		Sales/Marketing:		Liberal Arts:		Information Systems:		Professionals:		Technical/Scientific:	
Mgmt. Trainees:	Y	Mktg. Professionals:	Y	Gen. Writing/Editing:	Y	Info. Management:	Y	Finance/Accounting:	Y	Engineers, Elec.:	
Experienced Mgmt.:	Y	Retail Sales:		Technical Writing:	Y	Software Dev.:	Y	Law:	Y	Engineers, Other:	
Int'l Business:	Y	Commercial/Industrial:	Y	Graphic Arts/Photog.:	Y	Hardware Dev.:		HR/Other:	Y	Health/Lab:	
MBA Graduates:	Y	Sales Trainees:		Music:		Systems Integration:	Y	Training:	Y	Scientists/Research:	Y
		Advertising Pros.:	Y	Broadcasting:		Consulting/Other:	Y	Health Care:		Petroleum/Chemicals:	
				Other:				Consulting:	Y	Math/Other:	Y

TYPES OF BUSINESS:

Accounting
Risk Management
Tax Preparation Services
Human Resources Management
IT Services
Transaction Support Services
Industry Publications

BRANDS/DIVISIONS/AFFILIATES:

Ernst & Young International
Ernst & Young Online
Entrepreneur of the Year Award

CONTACTS: *Note: Officers with more than one job title may be intentionally listed here more than once.*

James S. Turley, CEO
John Ferraro, COO
Pierre Hurstel, Global Managing Partner-People
Jeffrey Dworken, Global Managing Partner-Oper.
Beth Brooke, Global Vice Chair-Strategy & Regulatory Affairs
Jeffrey Dworken, Global Managing Partner-Finance
Dave Read, Global Vice Chair-Transaction Advisory Svcs.
Steve Howe, Area Managing Partner-Americas
Herman Hulst, Global Managing Partner-Client Service & Accts.
Sam Fouad, Global Vice Chair-Tax
James S. Turley, Chmn.
James Millar, Area Managing Partner-Oceania

Phone: 212-773-3000	Fax: 212-773-6350
Toll-Free:	
Address: 5 Times Sq., New York, NY 10036 US	

GROWTH PLANS/SPECIAL FEATURES:

Ernst & Young, LLP (EY), the U.S. branch of the global accounting firm Ernst & Young International, is a provider of audit, tax, transaction and risk-related services. The firm has offices throughout the U.S. and Puerto Rico. In addition to providing accounting advisory and tax preparation services, the firm offers a number of complementary services such as human resource programs and online/IT services. EY serves companies in a number of industry sectors, including the financial services, automotive, consumer products, oil/gas, health care, technology, real estate, retail, communications and entertainment industries. In addition, the company publishes a variety of industry-specific publications and studies providing expertise in quickly-changing markets. Ernst & Young Online is a personalized client portal that provides news and information relating to specific customer needs, a reference library and links to other web resources, as well as access to EY staff for answers to direct questions. Additionally, the firm oversees the Entrepreneur of the Year Award, a prestigious award given to one individual each year for exceptional business acumen and ability.

FINANCIALS: Sales and profits are in thousands of dollars—add 000 to get the full amount. 2007 Note: Financial information for 2007 was not available for all companies at press time.

2007 Sales: $21,100,000	2007 Profits: $	U.S. Stock Ticker: Subsidiary
2006 Sales: $18,000,000	2006 Profits: $	Int'l Ticker: Int'l Exchange:
2005 Sales: $	2005 Profits: $	Employees:
2004 Sales: $	2004 Profits: $	Fiscal Year Ends: 6/30
2003 Sales: $	2003 Profits: $	Parent Company: ERNST & YOUNG INTERNATIONAL

SALARIES/BENEFITS:

Pension Plan:	ESOP Stock Plan:	Profit Sharing:	Top Exec. Salary: $	Bonus: $
Savings Plan:	Stock Purch. Plan:		Second Exec. Salary: $	Bonus: $

OTHER THOUGHTS:

Apparent Women Officers or Directors: 2
Hot Spot for Advancement for Women/Minorities: Y

LOCATIONS: ("Y" = Yes)

West:	Southwest:	Midwest:	Southeast:	Northeast:	International:
Y	Y	Y	Y	Y	Y

ESTEE LAUDER COMPANIES INC (THE) www.elcompanies.com

Industry Group Code: 325600 Ranks within this company's industry group: Sales: 3 Profits: 3

Management:		Sales/Marketing:		Liberal Arts:		Information Systems:		Professionals:		Technical/Scientific:	
Mgmt. Trainees:	Y	Mktg. Professionals:	Y	Gen. Writing/Editing:	Y	Info. Management:	Y	Finance/Accounting:	Y	Engineers, Elec.:	
Experienced Mgmt.:	Y	Retail Sales:	Y	Technical Writing:	Y	Software Dev.:		Law:	Y	Engineers, Other:	
Int'l Business:	Y	Commercial/Industrial:	Y	Graphic Arts/Photog.:	Y	Hardware Dev.:		HR/Other:	Y	Health/Lab:	Y
MBA Graduates:	Y	Sales Trainees:	Y	Music:		Systems Integration:		Training:	Y	Scientists/Research:	Y
		Advertising Pros.:	Y	Broadcasting:		Consulting/Other:		Health Care:		Petroleum/Chemicals:	
				Other:	Y			Consulting:		Math/Other:	

TYPES OF BUSINESS:

Cosmetics & Toiletries Manufacturing
Cosmetic & Fragrance Sales
Retail Cosmetics Stores
Hair Care Products

BRANDS/DIVISIONS/AFFILIATES:

Aveda
La Mer
Clinique
Prescriptivees
Bobbie Brown
M.A.C
Origins
Aramis

CONTACTS: *Note: Officers with more than one job title may be intentionally listed here more than once.*

William P. Lauder, CEO
Fabrizio Freda, COO
Fabrizio Freda, Pres.
Richard W. Kunes, CFO/Exec. VP
Amy DiGeso, Exec. VP-Human Resources
Harvey Gedeon, Exec. VP-Global R&D
Sara E. Moss, General Counsel/Exec. VP/Sec.
Malcolm Bond, Exec. VP-Global Oper.
Alexandra C. Trower, Exec. VP-Global Comm.
John Demsey, Group Pres.
Harvey Gedeon, Exec. VP-Global R&D
Evelyn H. Lauder, Sr. Corp. VP
Leonard A. Lauder, Chmn.
Cedric Prouve, Group Pres., Int'l
Gregory Polcer, Exec. VP-Global Supply Chain

Phone: 212-572-4200	Fax: 212-572-3941
Toll-Free:	
Address: 767 Fifth Ave., New York, NY 10153 US	

GROWTH PLANS/SPECIAL FEATURES:

The Estee Lauder Companies, Inc. is a global manufacturer and marketer of skin care, cosmetics, fragrance and hair care products. The company's products are sold in over 140 countries and territories under brand names such as Estee Lauder, Aramis, Clinique, Prescriptives, Lab Series, Origins, M.A.C., Bobbi Brown, La Mer, Aveda, Jo Malone, Bumble and bumble, Darphin, American Beauty, Flirt!, Good Skin and Grassroots. The firm is also the global licensee for fragrances and cosmetics sold under the Tommy Hilfiger, Donna Karan, Michael Kors, Sean John, Missoni, Daisy Fuentes and Tom Ford brand names. Estee Lauder sells its products principally through 20,000 points of sale including upscale department stores, specialty retailers, upscale perfumeries and pharmacies and prestige salons and spas, as well as freestanding company-owned stores and spas, authorized retailer web sites, stores on cruise ships, television direct marketing, in-flight and duty-free shops and self-select outlets. Estee Lauder has 15 manufacturing factories in six countries and 450 scientists working in research and development in seven principle facilities. The founding Lauder family still controls roughly 90% of the company's voting shares. The company operates on a global basis, with approximately 59% of its 2008 sales generated outside the U.S. In July 2008, the company acquired a minority stake in a privately held Indian company that manufactures, markets and sells beauty products.

FINANCIALS: Sales and profits are in thousands of dollars—add 000 to get the full amount. 2007 Note: Financial information for 2007 was not available for all companies at press time.

2007 Sales: $7,037,500	2007 Profits: $449,700	**U.S. Stock Ticker:** EL
2006 Sales: $6,463,800	2006 Profits: $244,200	**Int'l Ticker:** Int'l Exchange:
2005 Sales: $6,336,300	2005 Profits: $406,100	Employees: 26,200
2004 Sales: $5,790,400	2004 Profits: $342,100	Fiscal Year Ends: 6/30
2003 Sales: $5,117,600	2003 Profits: $319,800	Parent Company:

SALARIES/BENEFITS:

Pension Plan:	ESOP Stock Plan:	Profit Sharing:	Top Exec. Salary: $1,500,000	Bonus: $1,521,100
Savings Plan:	Stock Purch. Plan:		Second Exec. Salary: $1,440,000	Bonus: $1,369,000

OTHER THOUGHTS:

Apparent Women Officers or Directors: 4
Hot Spot for Advancement for Women/Minorities: Y

LOCATIONS: ("Y" = Yes)

West:	Southwest:	Midwest:	Southeast:	Northeast:	International:
		Y		Y	Y

Note: Financial information, benefits and other data can change quickly and may vary from those stated here.

EXEL TRANSPORTATION SERVICES INC (DHL EXEL)
www.exel.com/cl/home/
Industry Group Code: 488510 Ranks within this company's industry group: Sales: Profits:

Management:		Sales/Marketing:		Liberal Arts:		Information Systems:		Professionals:		Technical/Scientific:	
Mgmt. Trainees:		Mktg. Professionals:	Y	Gen. Writing/Editing:		Info. Management:	Y	Finance/Accounting:	Y	Engineers, Elec.:	
Experienced Mgmt.:	Y	Retail Sales:		Technical Writing:	Y	Software Dev.:	Y	Law:	Y	Engineers, Other:	
Int'l Business:	Y	Commercial/Industrial:	Y	Graphic Arts/Photog.:		Hardware Dev.:		HR/Other:	Y	Health/Lab:	
MBA Graduates:	Y	Sales Trainees:	Y	Music:		Systems Integration:	Y	Training:	Y	Scientists/Research:	
		Advertising Pros.:	Y	Broadcasting:		Consulting/Other:		Health Care:		Petroleum/Chemicals:	
				Other:				Consulting:		Math/Other:	Y

TYPES OF BUSINESS:
Freight Transportation Arrangement
Contract Logistics Services
Sub-Assembly & Secondary Packaging
Warehousing
Fleet Management Services

BRANDS/DIVISIONS/AFFILIATES:
Exel plc
Consumer Delivery Network
DHL Worldwide Network
Deutsche Post
Innogistics
Industrial Transport

CONTACTS: Note: Officers with more than one job title may be intentionally listed here more than once.
James Damman, CEO
James Damman, Pres.
Andrew Hadland, CFO
Andrew Hadland, Sr. VP-Oper.
Todd Thompson, Sr. VP-Bus. Dev.

Phone: 901-767-4455	Fax: 901-767-1929
Toll-Free:	
Address: 965 Ridge Lake Blvd., Ste. 103, Memphis, TN 38120 US	

GROWTH PLANS/SPECIAL FEATURES:
Exel Transportation Services, Inc. (ETS), a recently acquired subsidiary of DHL Worldwide Network, itself a subsidiary of Deutsche Post World Net group, is a non-asset-based logistics business that arranges for the domestic and international transportation of its customers' freight throughout the U.S., Latin America and Canada. ETS and its affiliates also provide contract logistics services such as private fleet management, warehousing and distribution. It focuses its business in six core service areas: contract logistics services, global forwarding, consultancy services, information services, specialist services and minority business enterprise. Consultancy logistics services include the design, implementation and delivery of dedicated and multi-user facilities and distribution. Global forwarding, which includes time-definite and flexible schedule operations, is offered through a variety of multi-modal transportation services, including air, ground, rail and water, as well as fully integrated systems, to customers in nine focused industries, including hospitality, gaming and furniture. Information services are offered even when Exel is not acting as the physical logistics provider and include information management, order management, systems integration and document management. Specialist services are individually designed to meet client supply chain needs and include procurement and logistics, property and real estate, supply chain consultancy and inventory optimization. Finally, minority business enterprise is run through Innogistics, which is jointly owned with Industrial Transport. Innogistics focuses on strategies for sequencing, sub-assembly and secondary packaging. ETS operates more than 150 agent network locations throughout North America. The firm's Consumer Delivery Network is an organized national network of concurring carriers that provide home delivery services throughout the U.S.

FINANCIALS: Sales and profits are in thousands of dollars—add 000 to get the full amount. 2007 Note: Financial information for 2007 was not available for all companies at press time.
2007 Sales: $	2007 Profits: $	U.S. Stock Ticker: Subsidiary
2006 Sales: $4,600,000	2006 Profits: $	Int'l Ticker: Int'l Exchange:
2005 Sales: $	2005 Profits: $	Employees: 40,000
2004 Sales: $	2004 Profits: $	Fiscal Year Ends: 12/31
2003 Sales: $	2003 Profits: $	Parent Company: DHL WORLDWIDE NETWORK SA/NV

SALARIES/BENEFITS:
Pension Plan:	ESOP Stock Plan:	Profit Sharing:	Top Exec. Salary: $	Bonus: $
Savings Plan:	Stock Purch. Plan:		Second Exec. Salary: $	Bonus: $

OTHER THOUGHTS:
Apparent Women Officers or Directors:
Hot Spot for Advancement for Women/Minorities:

LOCATIONS: ("Y" = Yes)
West:	Southwest:	Midwest:	Southeast:	Northeast:	International:
Y	Y	Y	Y	Y	Y

Note: Financial information, benefits and other data can change quickly and may vary from those stated here.

EXELON CORPORATION

www.exeloncorp.com

Industry Group Code: 221000 Ranks within this company's industry group: Sales: Profits:

Management:		Sales/Marketing:		Liberal Arts:		Information Systems:		Professionals:		Technical/Scientific:	
Mgmt. Trainees:	Y	Mktg. Professionals:	Y	Gen. Writing/Editing:	Y	Info. Management:	Y	Finance/Accounting:	Y	Engineers, Elec.:	Y
Experienced Mgmt.:	Y	Retail Sales:		Technical Writing:		Software Dev.:	Y	Law:	Y	Engineers, Other:	
Int'l Business:		Commercial/Industrial:	Y	Graphic Arts/Photog.:		Hardware Dev.:		HR/Other:	Y	Health/Lab:	
MBA Graduates:	Y	Sales Trainees:		Music:		Systems Integration:		Training:	Y	Scientists/Research:	
		Advertising Pros.:	Y	Broadcasting:		Consulting/Other:		Health Care:		Petroleum/Chemicals:	
				Other:				Consulting:		Math/Other:	

TYPES OF BUSINESS:
Utilities-Electricity & Natural Gas
Nuclear Generation
Energy Marketing

BRANDS/DIVISIONS/AFFILIATES:
Commonwealth Edison Company
PECO Energy Company
Exelon Generation Company, LLC

CONTACTS: Note: Officers with more than one job title may be intentionally listed here more than once.
John W. Rowe, CEO
John W. Rowe, Pres.
John F. Young, CFO
Andrea I. Zopp, Exec. VP-Human Resources
William A. Von Hoene, Jr., Exec. VP/General Counsel
Elizabeth A. Moler, Exec. VP-Gov't & Environmental Affairs
Ian P. McLean, Exec. VP-Finance & Markets
Frank M. Clark, Chmn./CEO-ComEd
J. Barry Mitchell, COO/Pres., ComEd
Mark Schiavoni, Sr. VP-Exelon Generation/Pres., Exelon Power
Ruth Ann M. Gillis, Pres., Exelon Bus. Svcs. Co./Sr. VP
John W. Rowe, Chmn.

Phone: 312-394-7398	Fax: 312-394-7945
Toll-Free: 800-483-3220	
Address: 10 S. Dearborn St., 48th Fl., Chicago, IL 60680 US	

GROWTH PLANS/SPECIAL FEATURES:
Exelon Corporation is a utility services company that operates through subsidiaries Exelon Generation Company, LLC; Commonwealth Edison Company (ComEd); and PECO Energy Company. Exelon Generation's business consists of its owned and contracted electric generating facilities; its wholesale energy marketing operations; and its retail sales operations. The subsidiary owns generation assets, which include nuclear, fossil and hydropower, with an aggregate net capacity of more than 25,000 megawatts (MW), including over 16,500 MW of nuclear capacity. Additionally, Generation controls over 7,500 MW of capacity through long-term contracts. ComEd's energy delivery business consists of the purchase and regulated retail and wholesale sale of electricity; and the provision of distribution and transmission services to retail and wholesale customers in northern Illinois, including Chicago. The subsidiary's retail service territory has an area of roughly 11,300 square miles and an estimated population of 8 million. PECO's energy delivery business consists of the purchase and regulated retail sale of electricity; and the provision of distribution and transmission services to retail customers in southeastern Pennsylvania, including Philadelphia, as well as surrounding counties. The subsidiary's retail service territory has an area of about 2,100 square miles and an estimated population of 3.8 million. PECO delivers electricity to roughly 1.6 million customers and natural gas to approximately 480,000 customers.

The company offers its employees medical, dental, vision and hearing insurance; paid time off, life and AD&D insurance; short- and long-term disability insurance; flexible spending accounts; and tuition reimbursement.

FINANCIALS: Sales and profits are in thousands of dollars—add 000 to get the full amount. 2007 Note: Financial information for 2007 was not available for all companies at press time.

2007 Sales: $18,916,000	2007 Profits: $2,736,000	U.S. Stock Ticker: EXC
2006 Sales: $15,655,000	2006 Profits: $1,592,000	Int'l Ticker: Int'l Exchange:
2005 Sales: $15,357,000	2005 Profits: $923,000	Employees: 17,200
2004 Sales: $14,515,000	2004 Profits: $1,864,000	Fiscal Year Ends: 12/31
2003 Sales: $15,812,000	2003 Profits: $905,000	Parent Company:

SALARIES/BENEFITS:

Pension Plan:	ESOP Stock Plan:	Profit Sharing:	Top Exec. Salary: $1,291,918	Bonus: $1,851,800
Savings Plan: Y	Stock Purch. Plan: Y		Second Exec. Salary: $630,959	Bonus: $616,744

OTHER THOUGHTS:
Apparent Women Officers or Directors: 5
Hot Spot for Advancement for Women/Minorities: Y

LOCATIONS: ("Y" = Yes)

West:	Southwest:	Midwest:	Southeast:	Northeast:	International:
		Y	Y	Y	

EXPEDITORS INTERNATIONAL OF WASHINGTON INC
www.expeditors.com
Industry Group Code: 488510 Ranks within this company's industry group: Sales: 2 Profits: 2

Management:		Sales/Marketing:		Liberal Arts:		Information Systems:		Professionals:		Technical/Scientific:	
Mgmt. Trainees:	Y	Mktg. Professionals:	Y	Gen. Writing/Editing:		Info. Management:	Y	Finance/Accounting:	Y	Engineers, Elec.:	
Experienced Mgmt.:	Y	Retail Sales:		Technical Writing:		Software Dev.:	Y	Law:	Y	Engineers, Other:	
Int'l Business:	Y	Commercial/Industrial:	Y	Graphic Arts/Photog.:		Hardware Dev.:		HR/Other:	Y	Health/Lab:	
MBA Graduates:	Y	Sales Trainees:		Music:		Systems Integration:	Y	Training:	Y	Scientists/Research:	
		Advertising Pros.:		Broadcasting:		Consulting/Other:		Health Care:		Petroleum/Chemicals:	
				Other:				Consulting:		Math/Other:	

TYPES OF BUSINESS:
Freight Logistics Services
Online Services
Logistics Software

BRANDS/DIVISIONS/AFFILIATES:
exp.o
Sn@p
Quota Monitor
TRACE
TradeFlow

CONTACTS: *Note: Officers with more than one job title may be intentionally listed here more than once.*
Peter J. Rose, CEO
R. Jordan Gates, COO
R. Jordan Gates, Pres.
R. Jordan Gates, CFO/Exec. VP
Timothy C. Barber, Pres., Global Sales & Mktg.
Jeffery S. Musser, CIO/Sr. VP
Amy Jo Tangeman, General Counsel/VP/Sec.
Charles J. Lynch, Corp. Controller
Robert L. Villanueva, Pres., The Americas
Rosanne Esposito, Exec. VP-Global Customs
Sandy K.Y. Liu, COO-Asia
Jean-Claude Carcaillet, Sr. VP-Australasia
Peter J. Rose, Chmn.
Rommel C. Saber, Pres., EMEA & Indian Subcont.

Phone: 206-674-3400	Fax: 206-682-9777
Toll-Free:	
Address: 1015 3rd Ave., 12th Fl., Seattle, WA 98104 US	

GROWTH PLANS/SPECIAL FEATURES:
Expeditors International of Washington, Inc. provides global logistics services through an international network spanning six continents. The company's services include consolidation or forwarding of air and ocean freight, customs brokerage, distribution management, vendor consolidation, cargo insurance, purchase order management and customized logistics information. Expeditors International does not compete for domestic freight, overnight courier or small parcel business and does not own aircraft or steamships. The company provides many services over the Internet. Expeditors' web-based tracking system, exp.o, possesses query capabilities to find the status of inbound shipments or orders and to view customs details. Linked to exp.o, Sn@p is the company's web-based electronic booking tool that provides notifications, pick-up arrangements, shipment tracking and document generation. Quota Monitor translates complex U.S. textile and apparel data into easy-to-understand quota status reports. Subscribers can research and monitor quota categories for specific countries; multi-country agreements such as AGOA, CBTPA and ATPDEA; or across regions online or by scheduled e-mail reports. The company's TRACE application gives real-time global access to insurance certificate creation, claims filing, claim status viewing and insurance document maintenance. Through web access to international tariff data and rules, TradeFlow helps international companies to reduce the risks and manage the costs associated with importing and exporting.

Expeditors International offers its employees competitive benefits, including medical, dental and vision insurance; a 401(k) program; and an employee stock purchase plan.

FINANCIALS: Sales and profits are in thousands of dollars—add 000 to get the full amount. 2007 Note: Financial information for 2007 was not available for all companies at press time.

2007 Sales: $5,235,171	2007 Profits: $269,154	U.S. Stock Ticker: EXPD
2006 Sales: $4,633,987	2006 Profits: $235,094	Int'l Ticker: Int'l Exchange:
2005 Sales: $3,901,800	2005 Profits: $190,436	Employees: 12,310
2004 Sales: $3,317,499	2004 Profits: $129,949	Fiscal Year Ends: 12/31
2003 Sales: $2,624,941	2003 Profits: $121,952	Parent Company:

SALARIES/BENEFITS:
Pension Plan:	ESOP Stock Plan:	Profit Sharing:	Top Exec. Salary: $110,000	Bonus: $4,608,619
Savings Plan: Y	Stock Purch. Plan: Y		Second Exec. Salary: $105,879	Bonus: $4,348,131

OTHER THOUGHTS:
Apparent Women Officers or Directors: 3
Hot Spot for Advancement for Women/Minorities: Y

LOCATIONS: ("Y" = Yes)
West:	Southwest:	Midwest:	Southeast:	Northeast:	International:
Y	Y	Y	Y	Y	Y

EXPERIAN AMERICAS

www.experian.com

Industry Group Code: 561450 Ranks within this company's industry group: Sales: Profits:

Management:		Sales/Marketing:		Liberal Arts:		Information Systems:		Professionals:		Technical/Scientific:	
Mgmt. Trainees:		Mktg. Professionals:	Y	Gen. Writing/Editing:	Y	Info. Management:	Y	Finance/Accounting:	Y	Engineers, Elec.:	
Experienced Mgmt.:	Y	Retail Sales:		Technical Writing:		Software Dev.:	Y	Law:	Y	Engineers, Other:	
Int'l Business:		Commercial/Industrial:	Y	Graphic Arts/Photog.:	Y	Hardware Dev.:		HR/Other:	Y	Health/Lab:	
MBA Graduates:	Y	Sales Trainees:		Music:		Systems Integration:		Training:	Y	Scientists/Research:	Y
		Advertising Pros.:		Broadcasting:		Consulting/Other:		Health Care:		Petroleum/Chemicals:	
				Other:				Consulting:		Math/Other:	

TYPES OF BUSINESS:

Credit Bureau
Customer Relationship Software & Solutions
Marketing Software & Solutions
Vehicle Database
Online Services
Business & Consumer Internet Sites

BRANDS/DIVISIONS/AFFILIATES:

Experian Information Solutions, Inc.
Advanced Select
Credit Migration Solutions
Experian Group
Precise ID
ScoreRight
QAS
CheetahMail

CONTACTS: Note: Officers with more than one job title may be intentionally listed here more than once.

Michael DeVico, Exec. VP-Experian North America
Cindy Thomas, Sr. VP-Corp. Mktg.
Paul Brooks, CFO-Experian plc
Kerry Williams, Pres., Credit Svcs. & Decisions Analytics, N. Amer
Donald A. Robert, CEO-Experian plc

Phone: 714-830-7000	Fax: 714-830-2444
Toll-Free:	
Address: 475 Anton Blvd., Costa Mesa, CA 92626 US	

GROWTH PLANS/SPECIAL FEATURES:

Experian Americas, formerly Experian Information Solutions, Inc., is a subsidiary of Experian plc, formerly Experian Group Limited. Experian Americas is a leading credit-reporting agency in the U.S. It also helps organizations find, develop and manage customer relationships by providing information, decision-making solutions and processing services. Experian operates through four segments: credit solutions, marketing solutions, automotive solutions and Experian Interactive. The credit solutions unit provides clients with solutions that optimize processes in acquiring new customers (Advanced Select), maximize customer relationships (Credit Migration Solutions), improve collections (Credit Profile Report), prevent fraud losses (Precise ID), analyze critical data (ScoreRight) and improve business-to-business results (Business credit reports). The marketing solutions unit improves customer relations for marketers in the catalog, retail, financial services, nonprofit, media, consumer products and mid-tier/reseller markets. Subsidiaries in this segment include Simmons, a marketing research firm; QAS, an address verification software company; and CheetahMail, an e-mail marketing firm. The automotive solutions unit provides vehicle, credit, consumer and business information to manufacturers, dealers, finance and insurance companies and consumers. Its National Vehicle Database houses more than 450 million vehicles, while its credit, consumer and business information assets analyze and store buyer data. Experian Interactive offers consumers access to their credit histories through various web tools, including Triple Advantage, Experian 3 Bureau Online Credit Report and VantageScore. In May 2008, Experian plc launched Account Monitoring Service, a credit monitoring system for businesses, with credit-based alerts.

Experian offers its employees flexible spending accounts, education assistance, credit union membership, employee assistance, referral bonuses, recreational activities, adoption assistance and fitness reimbursement.

FINANCIALS: Sales and profits are in thousands of dollars—add 000 to get the full amount. 2007 Note: Financial information for 2007 was not available for all companies at press time.

2007 Sales: $1,994,000	2007 Profits: $	U.S. Stock Ticker: Subsidiary
2006 Sales: $1,804,000	2006 Profits: $	Int'l Ticker: Int'l Exchange:
2005 Sales: $	2005 Profits: $	Employees:
2004 Sales: $	2004 Profits: $	Fiscal Year Ends: 3/31
2003 Sales: $	2003 Profits: $	Parent Company: EXPERIAN PLC

SALARIES/BENEFITS:

Pension Plan:	ESOP Stock Plan:	Profit Sharing:	Top Exec. Salary: $	Bonus: $
Savings Plan: Y	Stock Purch. Plan:		Second Exec. Salary: $	Bonus: $

OTHER THOUGHTS:

Apparent Women Officers or Directors: 2
Hot Spot for Advancement for Women/Minorities: Y

LOCATIONS: ("Y" = Yes)

West:	Southwest:	Midwest:	Southeast:	Northeast:	International:
Y	Y	Y	Y	Y	

Note: Financial information, benefits and other data can change quickly and may vary from those stated here.

EXPRESS SCRIPTS INC
www.express-scripts.com

Industry Group Code: 522320A Ranks within this company's industry group: Sales: 3   Profits: 3

Management:		Sales/Marketing:		Liberal Arts:		Information Systems:		Professionals:		Technical/Scientific:	
Mgmt. Trainees:	Y	Mktg. Professionals:	Y	Gen. Writing/Editing:	Y	Info. Management:	Y	Finance/Accounting:	Y	Engineers, Elec.:	
Experienced Mgmt.:	Y	Retail Sales:		Technical Writing:	Y	Software Dev.:	Y	Law:	Y	Engineers, Other:	Y
Int'l Business:	Y	Commercial/Industrial:	Y	Graphic Arts/Photog.:	Y	Hardware Dev.:		HR/Other:	Y	Health/Lab:	
MBA Graduates:	Y	Sales Trainees:		Music:		Systems Integration:		Training:	Y	Scientists/Research:	
		Advertising Pros.:	Y	Broadcasting:		Consulting/Other:		Health Care:	Y	Petroleum/Chemicals:	
				Other:				Consulting:		Math/Other:	

TYPES OF BUSINESS:

Pharmacy Benefits Management
Mail & Internet Pharmacies
Formulary Management
Integrated Drug & Medical Data Analysis
Market Research Programs
Medical Information Management
Workers' Compensation Programs
Informed-Decision Counseling

BRANDS/DIVISIONS/AFFILIATES:

CuraScript, Inc.
Phoenix Marketing Group LLC

CONTACTS: *Note: Officers with more than one job title may be intentionally listed here more than once.*

George Paz, CEO
George Paz, Pres.
Edward B. Ignaczak, Exec. VP-Sales & Acct. Mgmt.
Thomas M. Boudreau, General Counsel/Exec. VP-Law
Thomas M. Boudreau, Exec. VP-Strategy
George Paz, Chmn.

Phone: 314-996-0900	Fax: 314-770-0303
Toll-Free:	
Address: 1 Express Way, St. Louis, MO 63121 US	

GROWTH PLANS/SPECIAL FEATURES:

Express Scripts, Inc. is one of the nation's largest independent pharmacy benefit managers, providing pharmacy service and pharmacy benefit plan design consultation for clients including HMOs, unions and government health care plans. The company's core services include pharmacy network management, mail and Internet pharmacies, formulary management, targeted clinical programs, integrated drug and medical data analysis, market research programs, medical information management, workers' compensation programs and informed-decision counseling. Express Scripts provides progressive health care management by leveraging expertise in pharmacy benefit management (PBM) in order to positively impact clients' total health care benefits. The firm combines pharmacy and medical claims data to develop new strategies for decreasing total health care spending and improving health outcomes. The PBM business provides managed prescription drug services to members in the U.S. and Canada. Services from the specialty and ancillary services segment, which consists of the specialty operations of CuraScript, Inc., and the specialty distribution services and Phoenix Marketing Group LLC lines of business, include delivery of injectible biopharmaceutical products to patients' homes, physician offices and certain associated patient care services; third party logistics services for contracted pharma clients; distribution of sample units to physicians and verification of practitioner licensure; and biopharma services. Through pharmacy network management, the firm contracts with retail pharmacies to provide prescription drugs to members of the pharmacy benefit plans it manages. Express Scripts also provides a number of Internet-based services, including disease tracking, consumer prescription drug information and electronic claims processing. The company has over 60,000 participating pharmacies nationwide, and fills over 430 million prescriptions a year.

The company offers its employees health and dental insurance; flexible spending accounts; a 401(k) plan; an employee stock purchase program; life insurance; tuition assistance; short- and long-term disability insurance; prescription drug insurance; and an employee assistance program.

FINANCIALS: Sales and profits are in thousands of dollars—add 000 to get the full amount. 2007 Note: Financial information for 2007 was not available for all companies at press time.

2007 Sales: $18,273,600	2007 Profits: $567,800	**U.S. Stock Ticker: ESRX**
2006 Sales: $17,554,000	2006 Profits: $474,400	**Int'l Ticker:** Int'l Exchange:
2005 Sales: $16,212,000	2005 Profits: $400,100	Employees: 11,820
2004 Sales: $15,114,700	2004 Profits: $278,200	Fiscal Year Ends: 12/31
2003 Sales: $13,294,517	2003 Profits: $249,600	Parent Company:

SALARIES/BENEFITS:

Pension Plan:	ESOP Stock Plan:	Profit Sharing:	Top Exec. Salary: $882,308	Bonus: $2,124,000
Savings Plan: Y	Stock Purch. Plan: Y		Second Exec. Salary: $492,231	Bonus: $

OTHER THOUGHTS:

Apparent Women Officers or Directors: 1
Hot Spot for Advancement for Women/Minorities:

LOCATIONS: ("Y" = Yes)

West:	Southwest:	Midwest:	Southeast:	Northeast:	International:
Y	Y	Y	Y	Y	Y

EXXON MOBIL CORPORATION (EXXONMOBIL)

www.exxonmobil.com

Industry Group Code: 211111 Ranks within this company's industry group: Sales: 1   Profits: 1

Management:		Sales/Marketing:		Liberal Arts:		Information Systems:		Professionals:		Technical/Scientific:	
Mgmt. Trainees:	Y	Mktg. Professionals:	Y	Gen. Writing/Editing:	Y	Info. Management:	Y	Finance/Accounting:	Y	Engineers, Elec.:	Y
Experienced Mgmt.:	Y	Retail Sales:		Technical Writing:	Y	Software Dev.:	Y	Law:	Y	Engineers, Other:	Y
Int'l Business:	Y	Commercial/Industrial:	Y	Graphic Arts/Photog.:	Y	Hardware Dev.:		HR/Other:	Y	Health/Lab:	Y
MBA Graduates:	Y	Sales Trainees:		Music:		Systems Integration:		Training:	Y	Scientists/Research:	Y
		Advertising Pros.:	Y	Broadcasting:		Consulting/Other:		Health Care:		Petroleum/Chemicals:	Y
				Other:				Consulting:		Math/Other:	Y

TYPES OF BUSINESS:

Oil & Gas Exploration & Production
Gas Refining & Supply
Fuel Marketing
Power Generation
Coal & Mineral Exploration
Chemicals
Fuel Cell Research
Convenience Stores

BRANDS/DIVISIONS/AFFILIATES:

ExxonMobil Chemica
Exxon Neftegas Limited

CONTACTS: *Note: Officers with more than one job title may be intentionally listed here more than once.*

Rex W. Tillerson, CEO
Lucille J. Cavanaugh, VP-Human Resources
C. W. Matthews, General Counsel/VP
R. A. Luxbacher, Gen. Mgr.-Corp. Planning
K.P. Cohen, VP-Public Affairs
Henry H. Hubble, VP-Investor Rel./Sec.
Donald D. Humphreys, Treas./Sr. VP
P. T. Mulva, Controller/VP
S. R. LaSala, VP/General Tax Counsel
J. Stephen Simon, Sr. VP
A.Tim Cejka, Sr. VP
Rex W. Tillerson, Chmn.

Phone: 972-444-1000	Fax: 972-444-1350
Toll-Free:	
Address: 5959 Las Colinas Blvd., Irving, TX 75039 US	

GROWTH PLANS/SPECIAL FEATURES:

Exxon Mobil Corporation (ExxonMobil) is one of the largest global petroleum and natural gas exploration and production companies in the world. ExxonMobil's various divisions and affiliated companies operate and market products in the U.S. and about 200 other countries and territories. Its principal business is energy, involving exploration and production crude oil and natural gas; manufacture of petroleum products; and transportation and sale of crude oil, natural gas and petroleum products. The company has a resource base of over 70 billion oil equivalent barrels of discovered resources and produces more than 4 million oil equivalent barrels of oil and gas each day. The firm is also a major manufacturer and marketer of commodity petrochemicals, including olefins, aromatics, polyethylene and polypropylene plastics and a wide variety of specialty products. In addition, Exxon Mobil has interests in electric power generation facilities. Moreover, the firm has a chemical company and a coal and minerals company. The company has several divisions and hundreds of affiliates, many with names that include ExxonMobil, Exxon or Mobil. Overall, the firm has 11 separate global business units. The five global upstream businesses undertake exploration, development, production, gas marketing and upstream research. The four global downstream businesses carry out refining and supply, fuels marketing, lubricants and petroleum technology operations. Exxon Mobil spends more than $700 million annually towards research in new technologies, including developments in synthetic lubricants, catalyst research, nanotechnology, biomedical services and hydro-carbon-based fuel cells. In 2007, the firm announced that subsidiary Exxon Neftegas Limited completed drilling of the longest measured depth, extended-reach drilling well in the world offshore of Eastern Russia with a depth of 37,016 feet (over seven miles).

FINANCIALS: Sales and profits are in thousands of dollars—add 000 to get the full amount. 2007 Note: Financial information for 2007 was not available for all companies at press time.

2007 Sales: $390,328,000	2007 Profits: $40,610,000	**U.S. Stock Ticker: XOM**
2006 Sales: $365,467,000	2006 Profits: $39,500,000	**Int'l Ticker:** Int'l Exchange:
2005 Sales: $358,955,000	2005 Profits: $36,130,000	Employees: 80,800
2004 Sales: $291,252,000	2004 Profits: $25,330,000	Fiscal Year Ends: 12/31
2003 Sales: $213,199,000	2003 Profits: $21,510,000	Parent Company:

SALARIES/BENEFITS:

Pension Plan: Y	ESOP Stock Plan:	Profit Sharing:	Top Exec. Salary: $1,500,000	Bonus: $2,800,000
Savings Plan:	Stock Purch. Plan:		Second Exec. Salary: $935,000	Bonus: $2,150,000

OTHER THOUGHTS:

Apparent Women Officers or Directors: 2
Hot Spot for Advancement for Women/Minorities: Y

LOCATIONS: ("Y" = Yes)

West:	Southwest:	Midwest:	Southeast:	Northeast:	International:
Y	Y	Y	Y	Y	Y

Note: Financial information, benefits and other data can change quickly and may vary from those stated here.

FAIR ISAAC CORPORATION

www.fairisaac.com

Industry Group Code: 561450 Ranks within this company's industry group: Sales: 1 Profits: 1

Management:		Sales/Marketing:		Liberal Arts:	Information Systems:		Professionals:		Technical/Scientific:	
Mgmt. Trainees:	Y	Mktg. Professionals:	Y	Gen. Writing/Editing:	Info. Management:	Y	Finance/Accounting:	Y	Engineers, Elec.:	
Experienced Mgmt.:	Y	Retail Sales:		Technical Writing:	Software Dev.:	Y	Law:	Y	Engineers, Other:	
Int'l Business:	Y	Commercial/Industrial:	Y	Graphic Arts/Photog.:	Hardware Dev.:		HR/Other:	Y	Health/Lab:	
MBA Graduates:	Y	Sales Trainees:		Music:	Systems Integration:		Training:	Y	Scientists/Research:	Y
		Advertising Pros.:		Broadcasting:	Consulting/Other:		Health Care:		Petroleum/Chemicals:	
				Other:			Consulting:		Math/Other:	

TYPES OF BUSINESS:

Credit Scoring Systems
Data Management Systems & Services
Marketing Services & Support
Personal Lines Insurance Industry Services
Financial Risk Management
Computer-Related Services
Strategic Application Processing Systems
Customer Relationship Management

BRANDS/DIVISIONS/AFFILIATES:

Fair, Isaac & Company, Inc.
North American Financial Services
TRIAD
myfico.com
myFICO
FICO Score Simulator
Braun Consulting, Inc.

CONTACTS: *Note: Officers with more than one job title may be intentionally listed here more than once.*

Mark N. Greene, CEO
Michael H. Campbell, COO/Exec. VP
Charles M. Osborne, CFO/Exec. VP
Laurent Pacalin, Chief Mktg. Officer/Sr. VP
Richard S. Deal, Chief Human Resources Officer/Sr. VP
Larry E. Rosenberger, VP-R&D
Mark R. Scadina, General Counsel/Corp. Sec./Sr. VP
John D. Emerick, Jr., VP-Corp. Dev./Treas.
Michael J. Pung, VP-Finance
Richard A. Stewart, VP-Professional Svcs.
George Battle, Chmn.
Greg Corgan, VP-Global Sales

Phone: 612-758-5200	Fax: 415-446-6191
Toll-Free: 800-999-2955	
Address: 901 Marquette Ave., Ste. 3200, Minneapolis, MN 55402 US	

GROWTH PLANS/SPECIAL FEATURES:

Fair Isaac Corporation, formerly Fair, Isaac and Company, Inc., is a leading developer of credit scoring systems for the consumer credit industry. Over 2,600 companies in more than 60 countries use Fair Isaac technology to acquire customers more efficiently, increase customer value and retention, reduce fraud and credit losses, lower operating costs and enter new markets more profitably. Its principal products are statistically derived, rule-based analytic tools designed to help businesses make more profitable decisions. The company's signature products are North American Financial Services, used throughout the credit card, mortgage, retail, auto lending and other industries; TRIAD, the world's leading credit account management system; and the leading scoring systems for granting small business credit. Regular clients include hundreds of the world's leading credit card and travel card issuers, retailers, telecommunications service providers and consumer and commercial lenders. Through alliances with all three major credit bureaus, and firms such as Equifax, the firm serves a large and growing number of middle-market credit grantors, primarily by providing direct-mail solicitation screening, application scoring and account management services on a usage-fee basis. Through the myfico.com web site, consumers use the company's FICO scores, the standard measure of credit risk, to manage their financial health. FICO Score Simulator, an enhancement of the myFICO service, provides free interest rate information based upon the client's individual score. The company increased its international presence in 2008 by expanding its product offerings to France and Russia via partnerships with EURODECISION and National Bureau of Credit Histories. In 2008, the company acquired U.K.-based Dash Optimization, makers of Xpress-MP, the world's leading software product for decision modeling and optimization.

The company offers tuition reimbursement, business casual attire, commuter benefits, flexible work schedules and some health benefits.

FINANCIALS: Sales and profits are in thousands of dollars—add 000 to get the full amount. 2007 Note: Financial information for 2007 was not available for all companies at press time.

2007 Sales: $822,236	2007 Profits: $104,650	U.S. Stock Ticker: FIC
2006 Sales: $825,365	2006 Profits: $103,486	Int'l Ticker: Int'l Exchange:
2005 Sales: $798,671	2005 Profits: $134,548	Employees: 2,824
2004 Sales: $706,200	2004 Profits: $102,800	Fiscal Year Ends: 9/30
2003 Sales: $629,295	2003 Profits: $107,157	Parent Company:

SALARIES/BENEFITS:

Pension Plan: Y	ESOP Stock Plan:	Profit Sharing:	Top Exec. Salary: $653,269	Bonus: $660,000
Savings Plan: Y	Stock Purch. Plan: Y		Second Exec. Salary: $390,385	Bonus: $100,000

OTHER THOUGHTS:

Apparent Women Officers or Directors:
Hot Spot for Advancement for Women/Minorities:

LOCATIONS: ("Y" = Yes)

West:	Southwest:	Midwest:	Southeast:	Northeast:	International:
Y	Y	Y	Y	Y	Y

FAMILY DOLLAR STORES INC
www.familydollar.com

Industry Group Code: 452910 Ranks within this company's industry group: Sales: 5 Profits: 5

Management:		Sales/Marketing:		Liberal Arts:		Information Systems:		Professionals:		Technical/Scientific:	
Mgmt. Trainees:	Y	Mktg. Professionals:	Y	Gen. Writing/Editing:	Y	Info. Management:	Y	Finance/Accounting:	Y	Engineers, Elec.:	
Experienced Mgmt.:	Y	Retail Sales:	Y	Technical Writing:		Software Dev.:	Y	Law:	Y	Engineers, Other:	
Int'l Business:		Commercial/Industrial:	Y	Graphic Arts/Photog.:	Y	Hardware Dev.:		HR/Other:	Y	Health/Lab:	
MBA Graduates:	Y	Sales Trainees:	Y	Music:		Systems Integration:		Training:	Y	Scientists/Research:	
		Advertising Pros.:	Y	Broadcasting:		Consulting/Other:		Health Care:		Petroleum/Chemicals:	
				Other:				Consulting:		Math/Other:	

TYPES OF BUSINESS:
Discount Stores
Dollar Stores

BRANDS/DIVISIONS/AFFILIATES:

CONTACTS: *Note: Officers with more than one job title may be intentionally listed here more than once.*
Howard R. Levine, CEO
R. James Kelly, COO
R. James Kelly, Pres.
Kenneth T. Smith, CFO/Sr. VP
John J. Scanlon, Sr. VP-Mktg. & Hardlines
Kathi S. Child, Sr. VP-Human Resources
Joshua R. Jewett, CIO/Sr. VP-IT & Procurement
Robert George, Chief Merch. Officer/Exec. VP
Janet G. Kelley, General Counsel/Corp. Sec./Sr. VP
Barry Sullivan, Sr. VP-Store Oper.
Dorlisa K. Flur, Sr. VP-Bus. Dev. & Strategy
C. Martin Sowers, Sr. VP-Finance
Bryan P. Causey, Sr. VP-Planning, Allocation & Replenishment
Keith M. Gehl, Sr. VP-Construction & Facilities Management
Mike Kvitko, Sr. VP-Softlines
Wook Lee, Sr. VP-Global Sourcing
Howard R. Levine, Chmn.
Charles S. Gibson, Jr., Exec. VP-Supply Chain

Phone: 704-847-6961	Fax:
Toll-Free:	
Address: 10401 Old Monroe Rd., Charlotte, NC 28201-1017 US	

GROWTH PLANS/SPECIAL FEATURES:
Family Dollar Stores, Inc. operates a chain of more than 6,400 general merchandise retail discount stores across 44 states, providing primarily low to lower-middle income consumers with a wide range of competitively priced basic merchandise in convenient neighborhood stores. The goods offered by Family Dollar generally have price points that range from under $1to $10 and include apparel, food, cleaning products, paper products, home decor, beauty products, health aids, toys, pet products, automotive products, domestics, seasonal goods and electronics. The company purchases its merchandise from approximately 1,250 suppliers. Approximately 58% of its products are manufactured in the U.S., and substantially all such merchandise is purchased directly from the manufacturer. Family Dollar owns and operates nine distribution centers. Nationally advertised brand name merchandise accounts for approximately 40% of Family Dollar's sales, with the company's private label merchandise accounting for approximately 4%. The company supplements its basic assortment of merchandise with the purchase of certain Treasure Hunt items designed to create more excitement in stores and attract customers throughout the year, with particular emphasis on the holiday seasons. Approximately 5,100 stores include refrigerated coolers for a perishable food section. In the fiscal 2007 year, consumables, such as household chemicals, paper products, food, health and beauty items, hardware, automotive supplies and pet supplies accounted for 58.8% of sales; followed by home products; apparel and accessories; and seasonal and electronics with 15.1%, 14.4% and 11.7% respectively.

Family Dollar Stores offers its employees medical and dental insurance, prescription drug benefits, military and bereavement leave, service awards and a 401(k) savings plan.

FINANCIALS: Sales and profits are in thousands of dollars—add 000 to get the full amount. 2007 Note: Financial information for 2007 was not available for all companies at press time.

2007 Sales: $6,834,305	2007 Profits: $242,854	U.S. Stock Ticker: FDO
2006 Sales: $6,394,772	2006 Profits: $195,111	Int'l Ticker: Int'l Exchange:
2005 Sales: $5,824,808	2005 Profits: $217,509	Employees: 44,000
2004 Sales: $5,281,888	2004 Profits: $262,685	Fiscal Year Ends: 8/31
2003 Sales: $4,750,200	2003 Profits: $247,500	Parent Company:

SALARIES/BENEFITS:
Pension Plan:	ESOP Stock Plan:	Profit Sharing:	Top Exec. Salary: $728,585	Bonus: $857,537
Savings Plan: Y	Stock Purch. Plan: Y		Second Exec. Salary: $465,774	Bonus: $408,950

OTHER THOUGHTS:
Apparent Women Officers or Directors: 3
Hot Spot for Advancement for Women/Minorities: Y

LOCATIONS: ("Y" = Yes)
West:	Southwest:	Midwest:	Southeast:	Northeast:	International:
Y	Y	Y	Y	Y	

FEDEX CORPORATION

www.fedex.com

Industry Group Code: 492110 Ranks within this company's industry group: Sales: 2 Profits: 2

Management:		Sales/Marketing:		Liberal Arts:		Information Systems:		Professionals:		Technical/Scientific:	
Mgmt. Trainees:	Y	Mktg. Professionals:	Y	Gen. Writing/Editing:	Y	Info. Management:	Y	Finance/Accounting:	Y	Engineers, Elec.:	Y
Experienced Mgmt.:	Y	Retail Sales:		Technical Writing:	Y	Software Dev.:	Y	Law:	Y	Engineers, Other:	
Int'l Business:	Y	Commercial/Industrial:	Y	Graphic Arts/Photog.:	Y	Hardware Dev.:		HR/Other:	Y	Health/Lab:	
MBA Graduates:	Y	Sales Trainees:		Music:		Systems Integration:		Training:	Y	Scientists/Research:	Y
		Advertising Pros.:	Y	Broadcasting:		Consulting/Other:		Health Care:		Petroleum/Chemicals:	
				Other:				Consulting:	Y	Math/Other:	Y

TYPES OF BUSINESS:

Express Delivery Services
Ground Delivery Services
Freight Services
Document Solutions & Business Services
International Trade Services

BRANDS/DIVISIONS/AFFILIATES:

FedEx Ground Package System Inc
FedEx Freight Corp
FedEx Express Corp
FedEx Custom Critical Inc
FedEx Trade Networks Inc
FedEx Supply Chain Services Inc
FedEx Kinkos Office And Print Services Inc
Prakash Air Freight Pvt. Ltd.

CONTACTS: Note: Officers with more than one job title may be intentionally listed here more than once.

Frederick W. Smith, CEO
Frederick W. Smith, Pres.
Alan B. Graf, Jr., CFO/Exec. VP
Robert B. Carter, CIO/Exec. VP-Info. Svcs.
Christine P. Richards, General Counsel/Exec. VP/Corp. Sec.
T. Michael Glenn, Exec. VP-Corp. Comm. & Market Dev.
David J. Bronczek, CEO/Pres., FedEx Express
David F. Rebholz, CEO/Pres., FedEx Ground
Kenneth A. May, CEO/Pres., FedEx Kinko's
Douglas G. Duncan, CEO/Pres., FedEx Freight
Frederick W. Smith, Chmn.
Michael L. Ducker, Pres., FedEx Express Int'l

Phone: 901-818-7500	Fax: 901-395-2000
Toll-Free:	
Address: 942 S. Shady Grove Rd., Memphis, TN 38120 US	

GROWTH PLANS/SPECIAL FEATURES:

FedEx Corporation provides transportation, e-commerce and business services and operates through Federal Express Corp. (FedEx Express); FedEx Ground Package System, Inc. (FedEx Ground); FedEx Freight Corp. (FedEx Freight); and FedEx Kinko's Office & Print Services, Inc. (FedEx Kinko's). FedEx Express is an express transportation company, offering time-certain delivery within one to three business days. The division also includes FedEx Trade Networks, Inc., which provides international trade services, specializing in custom brokerage and global cargo distribution. FedEx Ground offers small-package ground delivery service. It provides service to almost every business address in the U.S., Canada and Puerto Rico, as well as residential delivery to nearly 100% of U.S. residents through FedEx Home Delivery. The segment also includes FedEx SmartPost, Inc., which specializes in the consolidation and delivery of high volumes of low-weight, less time-sensitive business-to-consumer packages using the U.S. Postal Service for final delivery to residences. FedEx Freight provides less-than-truckload (LTL) freight services through the FedEx Freight business (regional next-day and second-day and interregional LTL freight services) and the FedEx National LTL business (long-haul LTL freight services). The division also includes FedEx Custom Critical, Inc., a time-specific, critical shipment carrier; and Caribbean Transportation Services, Inc., a provider of airfreight forwarding services between the U.S. and Puerto Rico. FedEx Kinko's offers business services, including access to technology for copying and printing, professional finishing, document creation, Internet access, computer rentals, videoconferencing, signs and graphics, direct mail, web-based printing and the full range of FedEx day-definite ground shipping and time-definite global express shipping services, in addition to a variety of other retail services and products. In 2007, FedEx began offering day-definite deliveries to over 200 cities in China from its new operations base at the Hangzhou Xiaoshan International Airport in Zhejiang Province; and acquired Prakash Air Freight Pvt. Ltd., headquartered in Mumbai, India.

FINANCIALS: Sales and profits are in thousands of dollars—add 000 to get the full amount. 2007 Note: Financial information for 2007 was not available for all companies at press time.

2007 Sales: $35,214,000	2007 Profits: $2,016,000	U.S. Stock Ticker: FDX
2006 Sales: $32,294,000	2006 Profits: $1,806,000	Int'l Ticker: Int'l Exchange:
2005 Sales: $29,363,000	2005 Profits: $1,449,000	Employees: 143,000
2004 Sales: $24,710,000	2004 Profits: $838,000	Fiscal Year Ends: 5/31
2003 Sales: $22,487,000	2003 Profits: $830,000	Parent Company:

SALARIES/BENEFITS:

Pension Plan: Y	ESOP Stock Plan:	Profit Sharing:	Top Exec. Salary: $1,393,931	Bonus: $4,772,851
Savings Plan: Y	Stock Purch. Plan: Y		Second Exec. Salary: $908,305	Bonus: $2,203,193

OTHER THOUGHTS:

Apparent Women Officers or Directors: 2
Hot Spot for Advancement for Women/Minorities: Y

LOCATIONS: ("Y" = Yes)

West:	Southwest:	Midwest:	Southeast:	Northeast:	International:
Y	Y	Y	Y	Y	Y

Note: Financial information, benefits and other data can change quickly and may vary from those stated here.

FINISH LINE INC (THE)

www.finishline.com

Industry Group Code: 448210 Ranks within this company's industry group: Sales: 2   Profits: 2

Management:		Sales/Marketing:		Liberal Arts:		Information Systems:		Professionals:		Technical/Scientific:	
Mgmt. Trainees:	Y	Mktg. Professionals:	Y	Gen. Writing/Editing:	Y	Info. Management:	Y	Finance/Accounting:	Y	Engineers, Elec.:	
Experienced Mgmt.:	Y	Retail Sales:	Y	Technical Writing:		Software Dev.:	Y	Law:	Y	Engineers, Other:	
Int'l Business:		Commercial/Industrial:	Y	Graphic Arts/Photog.:	Y	Hardware Dev.:		HR/Other:	Y	Health/Lab:	
MBA Graduates:	Y	Sales Trainees:	Y	Music:		Systems Integration:		Training:	Y	Scientists/Research:	
		Advertising Pros.:	Y	Broadcasting:		Consulting/Other:		Health Care:		Petroleum/Chemicals:	
				Other:				Consulting:		Math/Other:	

TYPES OF BUSINESS:

Athletic Shoes, Retail
Activewear
Athletic Accessories

BRANDS/DIVISIONS/AFFILIATES:

Finish Line
Man Alive
Genesco, Inc.

CONTACTS: Note: Officers with more than one job title may be intentionally listed here more than once.

Alan H. Cohen, CEO
Steven J. Schneider, COO
Glenn S. Lyon, Pres.
Kevin S. Wampler, CFO/Exec. VP/Asst. Sec.
Kevin G. Flynn, Sr. VP-Mktg.
Donald E. Courtney, CIO/Exec. VP/Asst. Sec.
Samuel M. Sato, Chief Merch. Officer/Exec. VP
Gary D. Cohen, General Counsel/Exec. VP/Corp. Sec.
Michael L. Marchetti, Exec. VP-Store Oper.
George S. Sanders, Exec. VP-Store Dev. & Real Estate
David I. Klapper, Sr. Exec. VP
Larry J. Sablosky, Sr. Exec. VP
Roger C. Underwood, Sr. VP-Info. Systems
Michael J. Smith, Sr. VP-Loss Prevention
Alan H. Cohen, Chmn.
Robert A. Edwards, Sr. VP-Dist.

Phone: 317-899-1022	Fax:
Toll-Free: 888-777-3949	
Address: 3308 N. Mitthoeffer Rd., Indianapolis, IN 46235 US	

GROWTH PLANS/SPECIAL FEATURES:

Finish Line, Inc. is a mall-based specialty retailer of men's, women's and children's brand-name athletic, outdoor and casual footwear, activewear and accessories in the U.S. Finish Line does business under the Finish Line and Man Alive names. The company owns and operates 700 Finish Line stores in 47 states, which average approximately 5,530 square feet. Brand names offered by these stores include Nike, adidas, Puma, Reebok, Skechers, K-Swiss, New Balance, Timberland, Asics and Converse. Softgoods account for approximately 17% of the store's net sales. Finish Line owns and operates 94 Man Alive stores in 19 states, which average approximately 3,472 square feet. Man Alive is stocked with a wide variety of brands such as L.R.G., Miskeen, Rocawear, Enyce, Girbaud, Akademiks, Sean John, Parish, Baby Phat, Apple Bottoms, Ecko and Dickies. Softgoods account for approximately 91% of the store's net sales. In June 2007, Finish Line agreed to acquire Genesco, Inc. for $1.5 billion. In August 2007, Finish Line agreed to close all 15 Paiva stores.

The Finish Line offers its employees an education reimbursement plan, employee discounts, paid time off, basic life insurance and medical, dental and vision coverage plans.

FINANCIALS: Sales and profits are in thousands of dollars—add 000 to get the full amount. 2007 Note: Financial information for 2007 was not available for all companies at press time.

2007 Sales: $1,331,959	2007 Profits: $40,264	**U.S. Stock Ticker: FINL**
2006 Sales: $1,306,045	2006 Profits: $61,049	**Int'l Ticker:** Int'l Exchange:
2005 Sales: $1,166,767	2005 Profits: $61,263	Employees: 13,000
2004 Sales: $985,891	2004 Profits: $47,270	Fiscal Year Ends: 2/28
2003 Sales: $757,200	2003 Profits: $25,000	Parent Company:

SALARIES/BENEFITS:

Pension Plan:	ESOP Stock Plan:	Profit Sharing: Y	Top Exec. Salary: $570,000	Bonus: $28,500
Savings Plan: Y	Stock Purch. Plan:		Second Exec. Salary: $450,000	Bonus: $18,000

OTHER THOUGHTS:

Apparent Women Officers or Directors: 1
Hot Spot for Advancement for Women/Minorities:

LOCATIONS: ("Y" = Yes)

West:	Southwest:	Midwest:	Southeast:	Northeast:	International:
Y	Y	Y	Y	Y	

FIRST ADVANTAGE CORPORATION

www.fadv.com

Industry Group Code: 514199 Ranks within this company's industry group: Sales: 1 Profits: 1

Management:		Sales/Marketing:		Liberal Arts:		Information Systems:		Professionals:		Technical/Scientific:	
Mgmt. Trainees:		Mktg. Professionals:	Y	Gen. Writing/Editing:	Y	Info. Management:	Y	Finance/Accounting:	Y	Engineers, Elec.:	
Experienced Mgmt.:	Y	Retail Sales:		Technical Writing:	Y	Software Dev.:	Y	Law:	Y	Engineers, Other:	
Int'l Business:	Y	Commercial/Industrial:	Y	Graphic Arts/Photog.:		Hardware Dev.:		HR/Other:	Y	Health/Lab:	
MBA Graduates:	Y	Sales Trainees:		Music:		Systems Integration:	Y	Training:	Y	Scientists/Research:	
		Advertising Pros.:		Broadcasting:		Consulting/Other:		Health Care:		Petroleum/Chemicals:	
				Other:				Consulting:		Math/Other:	

TYPES OF BUSINESS:

Employee Screening Services
Computer Forensics
Legal & Criminal Records Investigation
Tax Consulting
Credit Information
Supply Chain Services

BRANDS/DIVISIONS/AFFILIATES:

Fiserv Inc
CredStar
R E Austin Ltd.
Lender Services
Data Services
Dealer Services
Employer Services
Multifamily Services

CONTACTS: Note: Officers with more than one job title may be intentionally listed here more than once.

Anand K. Nallathambi, CEO
Anand K. Nallathambi, Pres.
John Lamson, CFO/Exec. VP
Anita Tefft, VP-Human Resources
Alan Missen, CIO
Julie Waters, General Counsel/VP
Akshaya Mehta, Exec. VP-Oper.
Andrew MacDonald, Sr. VP-Corp. Dev.
Thomas Milligan, Treas./VP
Isabell Theisen, Chief Security Officer
Todd L. Mavis, Exec. VP-Oper.
Lisa Steinbach, Controller/VP
Parker S. Kennedy, Chmn.

Phone: 727-214-3411	Fax: 727-214-3410
Toll-Free:	
Address: 100 Carillon Pkwy., St. Petersburg, FL 33716 US	

GROWTH PLANS/SPECIAL FEATURES:

First Advantage Corporation is a provider of risk mitigation and business solutions. The company is divided into six business segments: Lender Services, Data Services, Dealer Services, Employer Services, Multifamily Services, and Investigative and Litigation Support Services. Lender Services, generating roughly 23% of the company's service revenue, provides specialized credit reports for mortgage lenders. Data Services, generating about 19% of First Advantage's service revenue, offers motor vehicle records; transportation industry credit reporting; supply chain theft and damage mitigation consulting; consumer location; criminal records reselling; subprime credit reporting; consumer credit reporting services; and lead generation. Dealer Services, accounting for approximately 16% of the company's service revenue, provides specialized credit reports, credit automation software and lead generation services to auto dealers and lenders. First Advantage's Employer Services segment, generating roughly 25% of the company's service revenue, helps companies manage risk with its employment screening, occupational health, tax incentive and services hiring solutions. The Multifamily Services segment, generating approximately 9% of the company's service revenue, provides resident screening services, including information about a prospective renter's eviction record, lease and payment performance history. Investigative and Litigation Support Services, generating roughly 8% of the company's service revenue, provides surveillance services, field interviews, computer forensics, electronic discovery and other high level investigations. In January 2007, First Advantage acquired Fiserv, Inc.'s mortgage credit reporting business unit, CredStar. In February 2007, the company acquired R E Austin Ltd., an employment screening company based outside of London in Colchester, expanding First Advantage's international market share.

First Advantage offers its employees tuition reimbursement; e-learning programs; banking discounts; an employee assistance program; flexible spending accounts; and medical, dental, vision, prescription, life and disability insurance.

FINANCIALS: Sales and profits are in thousands of dollars—add 000 to get the full amount. 2007 Note: Financial information for 2007 was not available for all companies at press time.

2007 Sales: $842,902	2007 Profits: $138,107	U.S. Stock Ticker: FADV
2006 Sales: $797,801	2006 Profits: $66,161	Int'l Ticker: Int'l Exchange:
2005 Sales: $643,749	2005 Profits: $58,426	Employees: 4,400
2004 Sales: $516,741	2004 Profits: $42,333	Fiscal Year Ends: 12/31
2003 Sales: $420,361	2003 Profits: $37,885	Parent Company:

SALARIES/BENEFITS:

Pension Plan:	ESOP Stock Plan:	Profit Sharing:	Top Exec. Salary: $600,000	Bonus: $703,125
Savings Plan: Y	Stock Purch. Plan: Y		Second Exec. Salary: $525,000	Bonus: $615,235

OTHER THOUGHTS:

Apparent Women Officers or Directors: 6
Hot Spot for Advancement for Women/Minorities: Y

LOCATIONS: ("Y" = Yes)

West:	Southwest:	Midwest:	Southeast:	Northeast:	International:
Y	Y	Y	Y	Y	Y

Note: Financial information, benefits and other data can change quickly and may vary from those stated here.

FIRST DATA CORP

www.firstdatacorp.com

Industry Group Code: 522320 Ranks within this company's industry group: Sales: 1   Profits: 1

Management:		Sales/Marketing:		Liberal Arts:		Information Systems:		Professionals:		Technical/Scientific:	
Mgmt. Trainees:	Y	Mktg. Professionals:	Y	Gen. Writing/Editing:		Info. Management:	Y	Finance/Accounting:	Y	Engineers, Elec.:	
Experienced Mgmt.:	Y	Retail Sales:		Technical Writing:	Y	Software Dev.:	Y	Law:	Y	Engineers, Other:	
Int'l Business:	Y	Commercial/Industrial:	Y	Graphic Arts/Photog.:	Y	Hardware Dev.:		HR/Other:	Y	Health/Lab:	
MBA Graduates:	Y	Sales Trainees:		Music:		Systems Integration:		Training:	Y	Scientists/Research:	
		Advertising Pros.:	Y	Broadcasting:		Consulting/Other:		Health Care:		Petroleum/Chemicals:	
				Other:				Consulting:		Math/Other:	

TYPES OF BUSINESS:

Credit Card Processing
Electronic Payment Processing
Check Verification
Prepaid Card Services
Private-Label Credit Card Services
ATMs

BRANDS/DIVISIONS/AFFILIATES:

eONE Global, LP
First Data Resources
PaySys International, Inc.
TeleCheck Services, Inc.
AIB Merchant Services
Merchant Solutions
Kohlberg Kravis Roberts & Co.

CONTACTS:
Note: Officers with more than one job title may be intentionally listed here more than once.

Michael Capellas, CEO
Kimberly Patmore, CFO/Exec. VP
Grace Chen Trent, Exec. VP-Mktg.
Peter Boucher, Exec. VP-Human Resources
David Dibble, CTO/Exec. VP
David Money, General Counsel/Exec. VP
Thomas R. Bell, Jr., Chief Strategy Officer/Exec. VP
Grace Chen Trent, Exec. VP-Corp. Comm.
David Yates, Pres., First Data Int'l
Ed Labry, Pres., First Data USA
Michael Capellas, Chmn.

Phone: 303-488-8000	Fax: 303-967-6701
Toll-Free: 800-735-3362	
Address: 6200 S. Quebec St., Greenwood Village, CO 80111 US	

GROWTH PLANS/SPECIAL FEATURES:

First Data Corp. is a payment services company that processes and safeguards every type of electronic payment method, including credit cards, debit cards, stored-value cards and electronic checks.   Through ValueLink, it also develops, implements and manages prepaid stored-value card services for retailers (i.e., gift cards) and provides prepaid phone top-up services.   First Data's card issuing services segment, operating through First Data Resources, First Data Europe and PaySys International, Inc., provides processing and related services to financial institutions issuing credit and debit cards and to issuers of oil and private-label retail credit cards.   Services include account maintenance, transaction authorizing and posting, card embossing, fraud and risk management services and settlement.   The firm's merchant services segment comprises First Data Merchant Services and TeleCheck Services, Inc. and provides merchants with credit and debit card transaction processing services, including authorization, transaction capture, Internet-based transaction processing, check verification and guarantee services, as well as operating an ATM network.   The emerging payments segment consists of a majority interest in eONE Global, LP, a leader in identifying, developing, commercializing and operating emerging payment technologies that support government payments, mobile payments and enterprise payments.   In September 2007, First Data was acquired by Kohlberg Kravis Roberts & Co., a private equity firm, for $29 billion. As a result, First Data Corp. combined its commercial and financial institution services segments.   In late 2007, First Data Corp. and Standard Chartered PLC launched Merchant Solutions, a joint venture headquartered in Singapore that provides acquiring services to merchants across Asia, with plans to further expand around the world.   The company also partnered with Allied Irish Banks p.l.c. (AIB) and the Republic of Ireland to establish AIB Merchant Services in Ireland.   The new joint venture, based in Dublin, provides card acquiring services in the Republic of Ireland, the U.K. and Europe.

FINANCIALS:
Sales and profits are in thousands of dollars—add 000 to get the full amount. 2007 Note: Financial information for 2007 was not available for all companies at press time.

2007 Sales: $8,051,400	2007 Profits: $-907,200	**U.S. Stock Ticker: Private**
2006 Sales: $7,076,400	2006 Profits: $1,513,400	**Int'l Ticker:** Int'l Exchange:
2005 Sales: $6,526,100	2005 Profits: $1,717,400	Employees: 29,000
2004 Sales: $6,633,400	2004 Profits: $1,908,300	Fiscal Year Ends: 12/31
2003 Sales: $8,400,200	2003 Profits: $1,408,700	Parent Company: KKR & CO LP (KOHLBERG KRAVIS ROBERTS & CO)

SALARIES/BENEFITS:

Pension Plan:	ESOP Stock Plan:	Profit Sharing:	Top Exec. Salary: $750,000	Bonus: $655,000
Savings Plan: Y	Stock Purch. Plan: Y		Second Exec. Salary: $591,667	Bonus: $1,200,000

OTHER THOUGHTS:

Apparent Women Officers or Directors: 2
Hot Spot for Advancement for Women/Minorities: Y

LOCATIONS: ("Y" = Yes)

West:	Southwest:	Midwest:	Southeast:	Northeast:	International:
Y	Y	Y	Y	Y	Y

Note: Financial information, benefits and other data can change quickly and may vary from those stated here.

FIRSTENERGY CORP

www.firstenergycorp.com

Industry Group Code: 221000A Ranks within this company's industry group: Sales: Profits:

Management:		Sales/Marketing:		Liberal Arts:		Information Systems:		Professionals:		Technical/Scientific:	
Mgmt. Trainees:	Y	Mktg. Professionals:	Y	Gen. Writing/Editing:	Y	Info. Management:	Y	Finance/Accounting:	Y	Engineers, Elec.:	Y
Experienced Mgmt.:	Y	Retail Sales:		Technical Writing:		Software Dev.:	Y	Law:	Y	Engineers, Other:	
Int'l Business:		Commercial/Industrial:	Y	Graphic Arts/Photog.:		Hardware Dev.:		HR/Other:	Y	Health/Lab:	
MBA Graduates:	Y	Sales Trainees:		Music:		Systems Integration:		Training:	Y	Scientists/Research:	
		Advertising Pros.:	Y	Broadcasting:		Consulting/Other:		Health Care:		Petroleum/Chemicals:	
				Other:				Consulting:		Math/Other:	

TYPES OF BUSINESS:

Utilities-Electricity & Natural Gas
Power Generation
Energy Management
Telecommunications

BRANDS/DIVISIONS/AFFILIATES:

Ohio Edison Co.
Cleveland Electric Illuminating Co. (The)
Toledo Edison Co. (The)
Pennsylvania Electric Co.
American Transmission Systems, Inc.
Jersey Central Power & Light Co.
Metropolitan Edison Co.
Pennsylvania Power Co.

CONTACTS: Note: Officers with more than one job title may be intentionally listed here more than once.

Anthony J. Alexander, CEO
Richard R. Grigg, COO/Exec. VP
Anthony J. Alexander, Pres.
Richard H. Marsh, CFO/Sr. VP
Leila L. Vespoli, General Counsel/Sr. VP
Michael J. Dowling, VP-Communications
James F. Pearson, Treas./VP
Harvey L. Wagner, Controller/Chief Acct. Officer/VP
Rhonda S. Ferguson, Corp. Sec.
George M. Smart, Chmn.

Phone: 330-761-4245	Fax: 330-384-3866
Toll-Free: 800-736-3402	
Address: 76 S. Main St., Akron, OH 44308 US	

GROWTH PLANS/SPECIAL FEATURES:

FirstEnergy Corporation is a diversified energy services holding company involved in the generation, transmission and distribution of electricity, energy management and other energy-related services. The firm operates eight principal electric utility subsidiaries: Ohio Edison Co.; The Cleveland Electric Illuminating Co.; The Toledo Edison Co.; Pennsylvania Electric Co.; American Transmission Systems, Inc.; Jersey Central Power & Light Co.; Metropolitan Edison Co.; and Pennsylvania Power Co. FirstEnergy is one of the largest investor-owned electric systems, serving 4.5 million customers in a service area that ranges over 36,100 square miles of Ohio, Pennsylvania and New Jersey. It has more than 14,127 megawatts (MW) of generating capacity and around 15,014 miles of transmissions lines. Generation is conducted through a variety of methods including coal, nuclear power, gas and oil and hydroelectric generation. Through its subsidiaries, the firm also offers a wide range of energy-related products and services, including ventilating, heating, refrigeration, air conditioning, process piping, electrical plumbing, building controls and systems and facility management. FirstEnergy also has subsidiaries in the telecommunications market. . In addition, FirstEnergy holds all of the outstanding common stock of other direct subsidiaries including: FirstEnergy Properties, Inc., FirstEnergy Ventures Corp., FENOC, FirstEnergy Securities Transfer Company, GPU Diversified Holdings, LLC, GPU Telecom Services, Inc., GPU Nuclear, Inc. and FESC. In July 2008, the firm entered into a joint venture with the Boich Companies, to acquire a majority stake in the Bull Mountain Mine Operations near Roundup, Montana. In August 2008, FirstEnergy Solutions expanded its service territory to include Illinois.

FINANCIALS: Sales and profits are in thousands of dollars—add 000 to get the full amount. 2007 Note: Financial information for 2007 was not available for all companies at press time.

2007 Sales: $12,802,000	2007 Profits: $1,309,000	U.S. Stock Ticker: FE
2006 Sales: $11,501,000	2006 Profits: $1,254,000	Int'l Ticker: Int'l Exchange:
2005 Sales: $11,358,000	2005 Profits: $861,000	Employees: 13,739
2004 Sales: $11,600,000	2004 Profits: $878,200	Fiscal Year Ends: 12/31
2003 Sales: $11,325,000	2003 Profits: $422,764	Parent Company:

SALARIES/BENEFITS:

Pension Plan:	ESOP Stock Plan:	Profit Sharing:	Top Exec. Salary: $1,216,923	Bonus: $2,000,000
Savings Plan: Y	Stock Purch. Plan:		Second Exec. Salary: $749,154	Bonus: $874,086

OTHER THOUGHTS:

Apparent Women Officers or Directors: 4
Hot Spot for Advancement for Women/Minorities: Y

LOCATIONS: ("Y" = Yes)

West:	Southwest:	Midwest:	Southeast:	Northeast:	International:
		Y		Y	

Note: Financial information, benefits and other data can change quickly and may vary from those stated here.

FISERV INC

www.fiserv.com

Industry Group Code: 522320 **Ranks within this company's industry group:** Sales: 2   Profits: 2

Management:		Sales/Marketing:		Liberal Arts:		Information Systems:		Professionals:		Technical/Scientific:	
Mgmt. Trainees:	Y	Mktg. Professionals:	Y	Gen. Writing/Editing:	Y	Info. Management:	Y	Finance/Accounting:	Y	Engineers, Elec.:	
Experienced Mgmt.:	Y	Retail Sales:		Technical Writing:	Y	Software Dev.:	Y	Law:	Y	Engineers, Other:	
Int'l Business:	Y	Commercial/Industrial:	Y	Graphic Arts/Photog.:	Y	Hardware Dev.:		HR/Other:	Y	Health/Lab:	
MBA Graduates:	Y	Sales Trainees:		Music:		Systems Integration:		Training:	Y	Scientists/Research:	
		Advertising Pros.:	Y	Broadcasting:		Consulting/Other:		Health Care:		Petroleum/Chemicals:	
				Other:				Consulting:		Math/Other:	

TYPES OF BUSINESS:

Financial Services
Investment Services
Online Banking
Electronic Billing & Payment
Software Applications & Investment Management Solutions

BRANDS/DIVISIONS/AFFILIATES:

Avidyn Inc
CheckFree Corp.
NetEconomy, B.V.
WorkingRx Holding Co.
BancIntelligence.com, Inc.

CONTACTS: *Note: Officers with more than one job title may be intentionally listed here more than once.*

Jeffery W. Yabuki, CEO
Jeffery W. Yabuki, Pres.
Thomas J. Hirsch, CFO/Exec. VP
Bridie A. Fanning, Exec. VP-Human Resources
Richard K. Jones, CIO/Exec. VP
Charles W. Sprague, Chief Admin. Officer/Exec. VP
Charles W. Sprague, General Counsel/Corp. Sec.
Douglas J. Craft, Exec. VP-Oper.
James W. Cox, Exec. VP-Corp. Dev.
Thomas J. Hirsch, Treas.
Rahul Gupta, Pres., Payments & Industry Prod.
Thomas A. Neill, Pres., Depository Institutions
Thomas E. Warsop, III, Pres., Financial Institutions
Norman Balthasar, Sr. Exec. VP
Donald F. Dillon, Chmn.

Phone: 262-879-5000	Fax: 262-879-5013
Toll-Free: 800-872-7882	
Address: 255 Fiserv Dr., Brookfield, WI 53045 US	

GROWTH PLANS/SPECIAL FEATURES:

Fiserv, Inc. provides integrated data processing and information management systems to more than 18,000 financial services providers, including banks, credit unions, financial planners, investment advisers and insurance companies. It operates in three segments. The financial segment provides account and transaction processing systems and services to financial institutions, such as banks, thrifts and credit unions, and other financial intermediaries. The insurance segment provides a wide range of services to insurance carriers, agents and distributors. The CreckFree segment provides online banking, electronic billing and payment, software applications and investment management solutions to financial institutions and financial services organizations. The company operates centers nationwide for full-service data processing, software development, item processing and check imaging, technology support and related product businesses, and additionally has support centers in Argentina, Australia, Canada, Colombia, China, Costa Rica, France, India, Indonesia, Luxembourg, Malaysia, Mexico, the Netherlands, the Philippines, Puerto Rico, Oland, Poland, Singapore and the U.K. In 2007, the firm acquired NetEconomy, B.V.; BancIntelligence.com, Inc.; and WorkingRx Holding Co. In December 2007, Fiserv acquired CheckFree Corp., an electronic commerce services and products provider, for roughly $4.4 billion. That same month, it sold CredStar, a mortgage credit reporting unit. In early 2008, the company sold Fiserv Health, Inc. to UnitedHealthcare Services, Inc. for $721 million. The firm also sold the majority of its Fiserv Investment support Services business to Ameritrade Online Holdings, Inc. for $225 million; and Del Mar Database, a provider of loan broker management products.

The company offers its employees medical and dental insurance; life and AD&D insurance; short- and long-term disability plans; an employee stock purchase plan; a 401(k) plan; education assistance; and an employee assistance plan.

FINANCIALS: Sales and profits are in thousands of dollars—add 000 to get the full amount. 2007 Note: Financial information for 2007 was not available for all companies at press time.

2007 Sales: $3,922,000	2007 Profits: $439,000	**U.S. Stock Ticker: FISV**
2006 Sales: $3,566,000	2006 Profits: $450,000	**Int'l Ticker:** Int'l Exchange:
2005 Sales: $4,059,478	2005 Profits: $516,438	Employees: 23,000
2004 Sales: $3,729,746	2004 Profits: $377,642	Fiscal Year Ends: 12/31
2003 Sales: $3,033,700	2003 Profits: $315,000	Parent Company:

SALARIES/BENEFITS:

Pension Plan:	ESOP Stock Plan:	Profit Sharing:	Top Exec. Salary: $840,000	Bonus: $888,720
Savings Plan: Y	Stock Purch. Plan: Y		Second Exec. Salary: $730,000	Bonus: $620,500

OTHER THOUGHTS:

Apparent Women Officers or Directors: 2
Hot Spot for Advancement for Women/Minorities: Y

LOCATIONS: ("Y" = Yes)

West:	Southwest:	Midwest:	Southeast:	Northeast:	International:
Y	Y	Y	Y	Y	Y

FLUOR CORP

www.fluor.com

Industry Group Code: 234000 **Ranks within this company's industry group:** Sales: 2 Profits: 1

Management:		Sales/Marketing:		Liberal Arts:		Information Systems:		Professionals:		Technical/Scientific:	
Mgmt. Trainees:	Y	Mktg. Professionals:	Y	Gen. Writing/Editing:		Info. Management:	Y	Finance/Accounting:	Y	Engineers, Elec.:	Y
Experienced Mgmt.:	Y	Retail Sales:		Technical Writing:		Software Dev.:		Law:	Y	Engineers, Other:	Y
Int'l Business:	Y	Commercial/Industrial:	Y	Graphic Arts/Photog.:		Hardware Dev.:		HR/Other:	Y	Health/Lab:	Y
MBA Graduates:	Y	Sales Trainees:		Music:		Systems Integration:		Training:		Scientists/Research:	Y
		Advertising Pros.:	Y	Broadcasting:		Consulting/Other:	Y	Health Care:	Y	Petroleum/Chemicals:	Y
				Other:				Consulting:		Math/Other:	Y

TYPES OF BUSINESS:

Construction, Heavy & Civil Engineering
Power Plant Construction
Facilities Management
Procurement Services
Consulting Services
Project Management
Asset Management
Staffing Services

BRANDS/DIVISIONS/AFFILIATES:

Fluor Construction Company
Department of Energy
Department of Homeland Security
Department of Defense
Kuwait Oil Company
LDK Solar Co

CONTACTS: Note: Officers with more than one job title may be intentionally listed here more than once.

Alan L. Boeckmann, CEO
D. Michael Steuert, CFO/Sr. VP
H. Steven Gilbert, Sr. VP-Human Resources
Ray Barnard, CIO
Carlos M. Hernandez, Chief Legal Officer/Corp. Sec.
Lee Tashjian, VP-Corp. Comm.
Kenneth H. Lockwood, VP-Investor Rel. & Corp. Finance
Victor L. Prechtl, Controller/VP
Stephen B. Dobbs, Pres., Industrial, Infrastructure, Gov't & Global
Jeff L. Faulk, Pres., Energy, Chemicals & Power
Garry Flowers, Sr. VP-Health, Safety & Environment
Wendy Hallgren, VP-Corp. Compliance
Alan L. Boeckmann, Chmn.
J. Robert Fluor II, VP-Global Public Affairs

Phone: 469-398-7000	Fax: 469-398-7255
Toll-Free:	
Address: 6700 Las Colinas Blvd., Irving, TX 75039 US	

GROWTH PLANS/SPECIAL FEATURES:

Fluor Corp., founded in 1912 as Fluor Construction Company, is a privately-held, global provider of engineering, procurement, construction and maintenance services. As well as being a primary service provider to the U.S. federal government, Fluor serves a diverse set of industries including oil and gas; chemical and petrochemicals; transportation; mining and metals; power; life sciences; and manufacturing. Fluor operates in five business segments: Oil and gas; industrial and infrastructure; government; global services; and power. The oil and gas segment offers design, engineering, procurement, construction and project management services to energy-related industries. The industrial and infrastructure segment provides design, engineering and construction services to the transportation, mining, life sciences, telecommunications, manufacturing, commercial, institutional, microelectronics and healthcare sectors. The government segment provides project management services, including environmental restoration, engineering, construction, site operations and maintenance, to the U.S. government, particularly to the Department of Energy, the Department of Homeland Security and the Department of Defense. The global services segment provides operations, maintenance and construction services, as well as industrial fleet outsourcing, plant turnaround services, temporary staffing, procurement services and construction-related support. The power segment provides such services as engineering, procurement, construction, program management, start-up, commissioning and maintenance to the gas, solid fuel, nuclear and plant betterment marketplaces. In early 2007, Fluor created a new business line within the power group dedicated to the nuclear new build power market. In January 2008, the company was awarded a $334 million consultancy services contract to provide overall program management for the Kuwait Oil Company. In April 2008, Fluor was awarded an engineering, procurement and construction management contract by LDK Solar Co., Ltd. for the world's largest new polysilicon facility in Xinyu City, China.

Fluor offers its employees education assistance, an employee assistance program and medical, dental, life and disability insurance.

FINANCIALS: Sales and profits are in thousands of dollars—add 000 to get the full amount. 2007 Note: Financial information for 2007 was not available for all companies at press time.

2007 Sales: $16,691,000	2007 Profits: $533,300	**U.S. Stock Ticker:** FLR
2006 Sales: $14,078,500	2006 Profits: $263,500	**Int'l Ticker:** Int'l Exchange:
2005 Sales: $13,161,100	2005 Profits: $227,300	Employees: 41,260
2004 Sales: $9,380,300	2004 Profits: $186,700	Fiscal Year Ends: 12/31
2003 Sales: $8,805,703	2003 Profits: $157,450	Parent Company:

SALARIES/BENEFITS:

Pension Plan: Y	ESOP Stock Plan:	Profit Sharing:	Top Exec. Salary: $1,153,335	Bonus: $5,220,000
Savings Plan: Y	Stock Purch. Plan:		Second Exec. Salary: $732,598	Bonus: $2,265,600

OTHER THOUGHTS:

Apparent Women Officers or Directors: 4
Hot Spot for Advancement for Women/Minorities: Y

LOCATIONS: ("Y" = Yes)

West:	Southwest:	Midwest:	Southeast:	Northeast:	International:
Y	Y	Y		Y	Y

Note: Financial information, benefits and other data can change quickly and may vary from those stated here.

FMC TECHNOLOGIES INC

www.fmctechnologies.com

Industry Group Code: 213111 Ranks within this company's industry group: Sales: 8   Profits: 12

Management:		Sales/Marketing:		Liberal Arts:		Information Systems:		Professionals:		Technical/Scientific:	
Mgmt. Trainees:	Y	Mktg. Professionals:	Y	Gen. Writing/Editing:		Info. Management:	Y	Finance/Accounting:	Y	Engineers, Elec.:	Y
Experienced Mgmt.:	Y	Retail Sales:		Technical Writing:	Y	Software Dev.:	Y	Law:	Y	Engineers, Other:	Y
Int'l Business:	Y	Commercial/Industrial:	Y	Graphic Arts/Photog.:	Y	Hardware Dev.:		HR/Other:	Y	Health/Lab:	
MBA Graduates:	Y	Sales Trainees:		Music:		Systems Integration:		Training:	Y	Scientists/Research:	Y
		Advertising Pros.:		Broadcasting:		Consulting/Other:		Health Care:		Petroleum/Chemicals:	Y
				Other:				Consulting:		Math/Other:	

TYPES OF BUSINESS:

Oil & Gas Production & Processing Equipment
Airport & Airline Equipment
Food Handling & Processing Systems

BRANDS/DIVISIONS/AFFILIATES:

Jetway
Technisys, Inc.
John Bean Technologies Corporation

CONTACTS: Note: Officers with more than one job title may be intentionally listed here more than once.

Peter D. Kinnear, CEO
Peter D. Kinnear, Pres.
William H. Schumann, III, CFO/Exec. VP
Randall S. Ellis, CIO/VP
Maryann T. Seaman, VP-Admin.
Jeffrey W. Carr, General Counsel/VP/Corp. Sec.
Jeffrey S. Beyersdorfer, Treas.
Jay A. Nutt, Controller
John T. Gremp, Exec. VP-Energy Systems
Tore Halvorsen, VP-Global Subsea Prod. Systems
Robert L. Potter, Sr. VP-Energy Processing & Global Surface Wellhead
Joseph H. Netherland, Chmn.

Phone: 281-591-4000	Fax: 281-591-4102
Toll-Free:	
Address: 1803 Gears Rd., Houston, TX 77067 US	

GROWTH PLANS/SPECIAL FEATURES:

FMC Technologies, Inc., formerly John Bean Manufacturing Co., designs, manufactures and services technologically sophisticated systems and products such as subsea production and processing systems, surface wellhead production systems, high pressure fluid control equipment, measurement solutions and marine loading equipment for the oil and gas industry. The company's business segments are: Energy Systems, FoodTech and Airport Systems. The Energy Systems business segment comprises Energy Production Systems and Energy Processing Systems. The Energy Production Systems division designs and manufactures systems and provides services used by the oil and gas companies involved in land and offshore, including deepwater, exploration and production of crude oil gas. The Energy Processing Systems division designs, manufactures and supplies technologically advanced high pressure valves and fittings for oilfield service customers, as well as manufacturing liquid and gas measurement and transportation equipment and systems to customers involved in the production, transportation and processing of crude oil, natural gas and petroleum-based refined products. The FoodTech division designs, manufactures and services technologically sophisticated food processing and handling systems used primarily for fruit juice production, frozen food production, shelf-stable food production and convenience food preparation for the food industry. The Airport Systems division is a global supplier of passenger boarding bridges, cargo loaders and other ground support products, as well as airport management services. The company's Jetway passenger boarding bridges provide passengers access from the aircraft to the terminal. In June 2007, FMC acquired Technisys, Inc., an electrical integration company. In August 2008, FMC completed the transition of its FoodTech and Airport Systems segment into an independent publicly-traded company, John Bean Technologies Corporation.

FMC Technologies offers its employees a benefits package that includes legal services, educational assistance, an employee assistance program, dependent care reimbursement and savings account plans, a Dollars for Doers volunteer program and a Matching Gift Plan.

FINANCIALS: Sales and profits are in thousands of dollars—add 000 to get the full amount. 2007 Note: Financial information for 2007 was not available for all companies at press time.

2007 Sales: $4,615,400	2007 Profits: $302,800	**U.S. Stock Ticker: FTI**
2006 Sales: $3,755,600	2006 Profits: $276,300	**Int'l Ticker:** Int'l Exchange:
2005 Sales: $3,107,000	2005 Profits: $106,100	Employees: 13,000
2004 Sales: $2,767,700	2004 Profits: $116,700	Fiscal Year Ends: 12/31
2003 Sales: $2,307,100	2003 Profits: $75,600	Parent Company:

SALARIES/BENEFITS:

Pension Plan: Y	ESOP Stock Plan:	Profit Sharing:	Top Exec. Salary: $918,677	Bonus: $2,500,000
Savings Plan: Y	Stock Purch. Plan:		Second Exec. Salary: $523,022	Bonus: $755,085

OTHER THOUGHTS:

Apparent Women Officers or Directors: 1
Hot Spot for Advancement for Women/Minorities:

LOCATIONS: ("Y" = Yes)

West:	Southwest:	Midwest:	Southeast:	Northeast:	International:
Y	Y	Y	Y	Y	Y

FOREST LABORATORIES INC   www.frx.com

Industry Group Code: 325412 Ranks within this company's industry group: Sales: 7 Profits: 6

Management:		Sales/Marketing:		Liberal Arts:		Information Systems:		Professionals:		Technical/Scientific:	
Mgmt. Trainees:	Y	Mktg. Professionals:	Y	Gen. Writing/Editing:	Y	Info. Management:	Y	Finance/Accounting:	Y	Engineers, Elec.:	Y
Experienced Mgmt.:	Y	Retail Sales:		Technical Writing:	Y	Software Dev.:	Y	Law:	Y	Engineers, Other:	Y
Int'l Business:	Y	Commercial/Industrial:	Y	Graphic Arts/Photog.:	Y	Hardware Dev.:		HR/Other:	Y	Health/Lab:	Y
MBA Graduates:	Y	Sales Trainees:	Y	Music:		Systems Integration:		Training:	Y	Scientists/Research:	Y
		Advertising Pros.:		Broadcasting:		Consulting/Other:		Health Care:	Y	Petroleum/Chemicals:	
				Other:				Consulting:		Math/Other:	Y

TYPES OF BUSINESS:
Drugs, Manufacturing
Over-the-Counter Pharmaceuticals
Generic Pharmaceuticals
Antidepressants
Asthma Medications
Cardiovascular Products
OB/Gyn Products
Endocrinology

BRANDS/DIVISIONS/AFFILIATES:
Lexapro
Namenda
Benicar
Forest Research Institute
Forest Pharmaceuticals, Inc.
Forest Laboratories Europe
Inwood Laboratories
Cerexa, Inc.

CONTACTS: Note: Officers with more than one job title may be intentionally listed here more than once.
Howard Solomon, CEO
Lawrence S. Olanoff, COO
Lawrence S. Olanoff, Pres.
Francis I. Perier, Jr., CFO
Elaine Hochberg, Sr. VP-Mktg.
Ivan Gergel, Sr. VP-Scientific Affairs
William J. Candee, III, Sec.
Charles E. Triano, VP-Investor Rel.
Francis I. Perier, Jr., Sr. VP-Finance
Ivan Gergel, Pres., Forest Research Institute
Howard Solomon, Chmn.

Phone: 212-421-7850	Fax:
Toll-Free: 800-947-5227	
Address: 909 3rd Ave., New York, NY 10022 US	

GROWTH PLANS/SPECIAL FEATURES:

Forest Laboratories, Inc. identifies, develops and delivers pharmaceutical products. It currently covers six therapeutic areas, developing treatments for respiratory, pain management, ob/gyn, endocrinology, central nervous system and cardiovascular conditions. Forest's three principal brands are Lexapro, an antidepressant; Benicar, a hypertension treatment; and Namenda, a therapy for moderate or severe Alzheimer's disease. Other products include Aerobid, an asthma medication; AeroChamber Plus, an inhalant delivery system for asthma medications; Infasurf, used to prevent respiratory distress syndrome (RDS), a condition caused by a lack of surfactant, found mainly in premature infants; Campral, which helps reduce withdrawals for those seeking to eliminate alcohol dependence; Armour Thyroid, Levothroid and Thyrolar, for treating hypothyroidism; Cervidil, used to prepare the cervix before inducing labor; and Combunox, a pain medication combining both opioids and non-steroidal anti-inflammatory drugs. Forest markets directly to physicians who have the most potential for growth and are agreeable to the introduction of new products. Forest Research Institute, Forest's scientific division, maintains labs on Long Island and in New Jersey. St. Louis, MO based subsidiary Forest Pharmaceuticals, Inc. manufactures and distributes Forest's branded prescription products in the U.S. and Puerto Rico. Subsidiary Forest Laboratories Europe has two manufacturing sites in Dublin, Ireland and one in Bexley, Kent (in the U.K.); it also distributes prescription and over-the-counter drugs in Europe, the Middle East, Australia and Asia. Subsidiary Inwood Laboratories manufactures and supplies generic versions of Forest's medications. In January 2007, the firm acquired Cerexa, Inc., a biopharmaceutical development company based in Alameda, CA. In February 2007, Forest began collaborating with Bangalore-based discovery services company Aurigene to discover small-molecule drug candidates for a novel obesity and metabolic disorders target.

Employees at Forest receive financial assistance for adoption and fertility treatments; medical, dental and life insurance; flexible spending accounts; child-care resources; and a commuter benefit program.

FINANCIALS: Sales and profits are in thousands of dollars—add 000 to get the full amount. 2007 Note: Financial information for 2007 was not available for all companies at press time.

		U.S. Stock Ticker: FRX
2007 Sales: $3,183,324	2007 Profits: $454,103	Int'l Ticker: Int'l Exchange:
2006 Sales: $2,793,934	2006 Profits: $708,514	Employees: 5,126
2005 Sales: $3,052,408	2005 Profits: $838,805	Fiscal Year Ends: 3/31
2004 Sales: $2,650,432	2004 Profits: $735,874	Parent Company:
2003 Sales: $2,206,700	2003 Profits: $622,000	

SALARIES/BENEFITS:
Pension Plan:	ESOP Stock Plan:	Profit Sharing: Y	Top Exec. Salary: $1,105,000	Bonus: $600,000
Savings Plan: Y	Stock Purch. Plan: Y		Second Exec. Salary: $556,500	Bonus: $385,000

OTHER THOUGHTS:
Apparent Women Officers or Directors: 3
Hot Spot for Advancement for Women/Minorities: Y

LOCATIONS: ("Y" = Yes)
West:	Southwest:	Midwest:	Southeast:	Northeast:	International:
		Y		Y	Y

Note: Financial information, benefits and other data can change quickly and may vary from those stated here.

FORTUNE BRANDS INC

www.fortunebrands.com

Industry Group Code: 312140   Ranks within this company's industry group: Sales: 1   Profits: 1

Management:		Sales/Marketing:		Liberal Arts:		Information Systems:		Professionals:		Technical/Scientific:	
Mgmt. Trainees:	Y	Mktg. Professionals:	Y	Gen. Writing/Editing:	Y	Info. Management:	Y	Finance/Accounting:	Y	Engineers, Elec.:	Y
Experienced Mgmt.:	Y	Retail Sales:		Technical Writing:		Software Dev.:		Law:	Y	Engineers, Other:	Y
Int'l Business:	Y	Commercial/Industrial:	Y	Graphic Arts/Photog.:	Y	Hardware Dev.:		HR/Other:	Y	Health/Lab:	
MBA Graduates:	Y	Sales Trainees:	Y	Music:		Systems Integration:		Training:	Y	Scientists/Research:	
		Advertising Pros.:	Y	Broadcasting:		Consulting/Other:		Health Care:		Petroleum/Chemicals:	
				Other:				Consulting:		Math/Other:	

TYPES OF BUSINESS:

Home & Hardware Products
Spirits & Wine
Golf Products

BRANDS/DIVISIONS/AFFILIATES:

MasterBrand Cabinets, Inc.
Moen, Inc.
Simonton Holdings, Inc.
Beam Global Spirits & Wine, Inc.
Acushnet Co.
Aristokraft
Omega
FootJoy

CONTACTS: *Note: Officers with more than one job title may be intentionally listed here more than once.*

Bruce A. Carbonari, CEO
Bruce A. Carbonari, Pres.
Craig P. Omtvedt, CFO/Sr. VP
Mark A. Roche, General Counsel/Sr. VP/Sec.
Christopher J. Klein, Sr. VP-Strategy & Corp. Dev.
C. Clarkson Hine, VP-Corp. Comm.
Anthony J. Diaz, VP-Investor Rel.
Mark Hausberg, Sr. VP-Finance/Treas.
Elizabeth R. Lane, VP-Compensation & Benefits
Charlie Ryan, VP-Taxes
Allan J. Snape, VP-Bus. Dev.
Edward Wiertel, Controller/VP
Norman H. Wesley, Chmn.

Phone: 847-484-4400	Fax: 847-478-0073
Toll-Free:	
Address: 520 Lake Cook Rd., Deerfield, IL 60015 US	

GROWTH PLANS/SPECIAL FEATURES:

Fortune Brands, Inc. is a holding company with subsidiaries engaged in the manufacture, production and sale of home and hardware products, spirits and wine, and golf products. Home and hardware subsidiaries include MasterBrand Cabinets, Inc., which manufactures custom, semi-custom, stock and ready-to-assemble cabinetry for the kitchen, bath and home sold under brands including Aristokraft, Omega, Kitchen Craft, Schrock, Diamond, Decora and Kemper; Moen, Inc., which manufactures faucets, bath furnishings, accessories, parts and kitchen sinks in North America and China; Therma-Thru Corp., which manufactures fiberglass and steel residential entry door and patio door systems; Simonton Holdings, Inc., whose brands include Simonton Windows, a vinyl-framed windows and patio doors brand; and Fortune Brands Storage and Security, LLC, which manufactures tool storage products and safety and security devices. The spirits and wine business operates through holding company Beam Global Spirits & Wine, Inc., whose subsidiaries include Jim Beam Brands Co.; Future Brands, LLC; Jim Brands Australia Pty. Ltd.; Beam Global Espanol S.A.; Beam Global Spirits & Wine (U.K.) Ltd.; Tequila Sauza S.A. de C.F.; Canadian Club Canada, Inc.; Maker's Mark Distillery, Inc.; Courvoisier S.A.S.; and Beam Wine Estates, Inc. The company has significant positions in categories including tequila, cognac, Scotch whisky and Canadian whisky. It also has significant business in regional and national spirits categories such as German liqueurs and Spanish brandies; a large portfolio of premium, super-premium and ultra-premium U.S. wines; and an agency relationship for the importation and marketing of New Zealand and Australian wines of the Lion Nathan Wine Group. The golf business operates through Acushnet Co., a manufacturer and marketer of golf balls, clubs, shoes and gloves. Other products include golf bags, outwear and accessories. Brands include Titleist, Pinnacle, Scotty Cameron, Vokey and FootJoy. In November 2007, Fortune Brands agreed to sell its U.S. wine business to Constellation Brands, Inc. for $885 million.

FINANCIALS: Sales and profits are in thousands of dollars—add 000 to get the full amount. 2007 Note: Financial information for 2007 was not available for all companies at press time.

2007 Sales: $8,563,100	2007 Profits: $762,600	U.S. Stock Ticker: FO
2006 Sales: $8,769,000	2006 Profits: $830,100	Int'l Ticker: Int'l Exchange:
2005 Sales: $7,061,200	2005 Profits: $621,100	Employees: 36,251
2004 Sales: $7,320,900	2004 Profits: $783,800	Fiscal Year Ends: 12/31
2003 Sales: $6,214,500	2003 Profits: $579,200	Parent Company:

SALARIES/BENEFITS:

Pension Plan:	ESOP Stock Plan:	Profit Sharing:	Top Exec. Salary: $1,166,000	Bonus: $1,553,200
Savings Plan: Y	Stock Purch. Plan:		Second Exec. Salary: $575,000	Bonus: $522,200

OTHER THOUGHTS:

Apparent Women Officers or Directors: 5
Hot Spot for Advancement for Women/Minorities: Y

LOCATIONS: ("Y" = Yes)

West:	Southwest:	Midwest:	Southeast:	Northeast:	International:
		Y			Y

FOSSIL INC
www.fossil.com

Industry Group Code: 334518 Ranks within this company's industry group: Sales: 1 Profits: 1

Management:		Sales/Marketing:		Liberal Arts:		Information Systems:		Professionals:		Technical/Scientific:	
Mgmt. Trainees:	Y	Mktg. Professionals:	Y	Gen. Writing/Editing:		Info. Management:	Y	Finance/Accounting:	Y	Engineers, Elec.:	Y
Experienced Mgmt.:	Y	Retail Sales:	Y	Technical Writing:	Y	Software Dev.:	Y	Law:	Y	Engineers, Other:	
Int'l Business:	Y	Commercial/Industrial:	Y	Graphic Arts/Photog.:	Y	Hardware Dev.:	Y	HR/Other:	Y	Health/Lab:	
MBA Graduates:	Y	Sales Trainees:	Y	Music:		Systems Integration:		Training:	Y	Scientists/Research:	
		Advertising Pros.:	Y	Broadcasting:		Consulting/Other:		Health Care:		Petroleum/Chemicals:	
				Other:	Y			Consulting:		Math/Other:	

TYPES OF BUSINESS:
Watch Manufacturing
Accessories
Online Sales
Leather Goods
Belts
Handbags
Jewelry
Retail Stores

BRANDS/DIVISIONS/AFFILIATES:
Fossil
Relic
Zodiac
Abacus
MW
MW Michele
Big Tic
Fifty-Four by Fossil

CONTACTS: Note: Officers with more than one job title may be intentionally listed here more than once.
Kosta N. Kartsotis, CEO
Michael W. Barnes, COO
Michael W. Barnes, Pres.
Mike L. Kovar, CFO/Sr. VP
Mike L. Kovar, Treas.
Livio Galanti, Exec. VP
Jennifer Pritchard, Pres., Retail Div.
Tom Kartsotis, Chmn.

Phone: 972-234-2525	Fax: 972-234-4669
Toll-Free:	
Address: 2280 N. Greenville Ave., Richardson, TX 75082 US	

GROWTH PLANS/SPECIAL FEATURES:
Fossil, Inc. designs, develops, markets and distributes fashion accessories. The company's principal offerings include a line of men's and women's watches and jewelry sold under proprietary and licensed brands, handbags, leather goods, sunglasses, and apparel. In the watch and jewelry product category, Fossil has a diverse portfolio of globally recognized brands such as Fossil, Relic, MW, MW Michele, Abacus Wrist Net, Abacus Wrist PDA and Zodiac. Also, through license agreements, the company utilizes prestigious brand names such as Burberry, DKNY, Michael Kors, Marc Jacobs, Jacobs and Emporio Armani. The company distributes products through various channels including wholesale, export and direct to the consumer. Domestically, the company sells its products through a distribution network that includes Neiman Marcus, Nordstrom, Macy's, Dillard's, JCPenney, Kohl's, Sears, Wal-Mart and Target. The firm also sells its products through a network of company-owned stores, which includes 96 retail and 74 outlet stores. Additionally, the company offers an extensive collection of Fossil brand products through its catalog and website as well as proprietary and licensed watch and jewelry brands through other managed and affiliate websites. Internationally, products are sold to department stores and specialty stores in over 90 countries through 23 company-owned foreign sales subsidiaries and through approximately 56 independent distributors. Fossil products are offered on airlines, cruise ships and in international company-owned retail stores, which included 55 accessory retail stores, 13 multi-brand stores and 6 outlet stores in select international markets. At the end of 2007, the company operated 244 stores, including 113 full price accessory stores, 55 of which are outside the U.S., 80 outlets, including 6 outside the U.S.; 33 apparel stores; and 18 multi-brand stores. In 2008, the firm plans to open 80 to 85 stores, concentrating on the full price accessory concept with equal distribution between U.S. and international locations.

FINANCIALS: Sales and profits are in thousands of dollars—add 000 to get the full amount. 2007 Note: Financial information for 2007 was not available for all companies at press time.

2007 Sales: $1,432,984	2007 Profits: $123,261	U.S. Stock Ticker: FOSL
2006 Sales: $1,213,965	2006 Profits: $77,582	Int'l Ticker: Int'l Exchange:
2005 Sales: $1,043,120	2005 Profits: $75,670	Employees: 7,400
2004 Sales: $957,309	2004 Profits: $89,545	Fiscal Year Ends: 12/31
2003 Sales: $781,175	2003 Profits: $68,335	Parent Company:

SALARIES/BENEFITS:

Pension Plan:	ESOP Stock Plan:	Profit Sharing:	Top Exec. Salary: $436,538	Bonus: $100,000
Savings Plan:	Stock Purch. Plan:		Second Exec. Salary: $411,154	Bonus: $200,000

OTHER THOUGHTS:
Apparent Women Officers or Directors: 4
Hot Spot for Advancement for Women/Minorities: Y

LOCATIONS: ("Y" = Yes)

West:	Southwest:	Midwest:	Southeast:	Northeast:	International:
Y	Y	Y	Y	Y	Y

FOSTER WHEELER LTD

www.fwc.com

Industry Group Code: 234000 Ranks within this company's industry group: Sales: 5 Profits: 2

Management:		Sales/Marketing:		Liberal Arts:		Information Systems:		Professionals:		Technical/Scientific:	
Mgmt. Trainees:		Mktg. Professionals:	Y	Gen. Writing/Editing:		Info. Management:	Y	Finance/Accounting:	Y	Engineers, Elec.:	Y
Experienced Mgmt.:	Y	Retail Sales:		Technical Writing:	Y	Software Dev.:	Y	Law:	Y	Engineers, Other:	Y
Int'l Business:	Y	Commercial/Industrial:	Y	Graphic Arts/Photog.:	Y	Hardware Dev.:		HR/Other:	Y	Health/Lab:	
MBA Graduates:	Y	Sales Trainees:		Music:		Systems Integration:	Y	Training:	Y	Scientists/Research:	
		Advertising Pros.:		Broadcasting:		Consulting/Other:	Y	Health Care:		Petroleum/Chemicals:	
				Other:				Consulting:	Y	Math/Other:	

TYPES OF BUSINESS:

Engineering & Construction
Industrial Plant Design & Development
Energy & Methanol Equipment
Power Systems Manufacturer
Cogeneration Electric Plant Operation
Independent Power Plant Operation
Renewable Energy Technology
Fluidized Bed & Conventional Boilers

BRANDS/DIVISIONS/AFFILIATES:

Foster Wheeler Power Machinery Co., Ltd.
Foster Wheeler International Corp.
Foster Wheeler Energy, Ltd.
Foster Wheeler Constructors
Steril S.p.A.
Foster Wheeler Review

CONTACTS: *Note: Officers with more than one job title may be intentionally listed here more than once.*

Raymond J. Milchovich, CEO
Umberto della Sala, COO
Umberto della Sala, Pres.
Franco Baseotto, CFO/Exec. VP
Peter J. Ganz, General Counsel/Exec. VP
Thierry Desmaris, VP-Corp. Dev.
W. Scott Lamb, VP-Investor Rel.
Lisa Z. Wood, VP/Controller
Troy Roder, VP/Corp. Treasurer
Rakesh K. Jindal, VP-Tax
David Wardlaw, VP-Project Risk Mgmt. Group
Raymond J. Milchovich, Chmn.

Phone: 908-730-4000	Fax: 908-730-5315
Toll-Free:	
Address: Perryville Corp. Park, Clinton, NJ 08809-4000 US	

GROWTH PLANS/SPECIAL FEATURES:

Foster Wheeler, Ltd. provides services in the petroleum and gas, petrochemical, pharmaceutical, biotechnology, health care, chemical processing, engineering and construction, energy equipment and power systems industries. The company operates through its numerous subsidiaries, including Foster Wheeler Power Machinery Co., Ltd.; Foster Wheeler International Corp.; Foster Wheeler Energy, Ltd.; Foster Wheeler Constructors; and Steril S.p.A. The firm's engineering services include industrial plant construction, water treatment plant engineering, and petroleum, chemical and alternative fuel facilities construction. Other services include manufacturing energy equipment, pollution control equipment and steam generation services. Foster Wheeler operates under two business groups: the Global Engineering and Construction (E&C) Group, which designs, engineers and constructs leading-edge processing facilities and related infrastructure for upstream oil and gas, LNG and gas-to-liquids, refining, chemicals and petrochemicals, pharmaceuticals, biotechnology and healthcare, environmental and power industries; and the Global Power Group, which offers energy solutions to customers around the world. The company has engineered and built process, power and industrial facilities in over 125 countries. Additionally, Foster Wheeler produces technical papers and a quarterly newsletter, Foster Wheeler Review, concerning the company's global project developments. Foster Wheeler Energy has long-term contracts with several prominent companies, including ExxonMobil and Shell. In 2008, the company strengthened its foothold in the biotech and pharmaceutical markets with the acquisition of Biokinetics Inc., a leading U.S. biopharmaceutical process design company, from MPA Holdings LP.

FINANCIALS: Sales and profits are in thousands of dollars—add 000 to get the full amount. 2007 Note: Financial information for 2007 was not available for all companies at press time.

2007 Sales: $5,107,243	2007 Profits: $393,874	**U.S. Stock Ticker:** FWLT
2006 Sales: $3,495,048	2006 Profits: $261,984	**Int'l Ticker:** Int'l Exchange:
2005 Sales: $2,199,955	2005 Profits: $-109,749	Employees: 13,859
2004 Sales: $2,661,324	2004 Profits: $-285,294	Fiscal Year Ends: 12/31
2003 Sales: $3,723,800	2003 Profits: $-157,100	Parent Company:

SALARIES/BENEFITS:

Pension Plan: Y	ESOP Stock Plan:	Profit Sharing:	Top Exec. Salary: $992,250	Bonus: $2,484,500
Savings Plan: Y	Stock Purch. Plan:		Second Exec. Salary: $516,189	Bonus: $828,765

OTHER THOUGHTS:

Apparent Women Officers or Directors: 1
Hot Spot for Advancement for Women/Minorities: Y

LOCATIONS: ("Y" = Yes)

West:	Southwest:	Midwest:	Southeast:	Northeast:	International:
Y	Y	Y	Y	Y	Y

FOX ENTERTAINMENT GROUP INC
www.fox.com

Industry Group Code: 513120 Ranks within this company's industry group: Sales: Profits:

Management:		Sales/Marketing:		Liberal Arts:		Information Systems:		Professionals:		Technical/Scientific:	
Mgmt. Trainees:	Y	Mktg. Professionals:	Y	Gen. Writing/Editing:	Y	Info. Management:	Y	Finance/Accounting:	Y	Engineers, Elec.:	Y
Experienced Mgmt.:	Y	Retail Sales:		Technical Writing:		Software Dev.:	Y	Law:	Y	Engineers, Other:	
Int'l Business:	Y	Commercial/Industrial:	Y	Graphic Arts/Photog.:	Y	Hardware Dev.:		HR/Other:	Y	Health/Lab:	
MBA Graduates:	Y	Sales Trainees:		Music:	Y	Systems Integration:		Training:	Y	Scientists/Research:	
		Advertising Pros.:	Y	Broadcasting:	Y	Consulting/Other:		Health Care:		Petroleum/Chemicals:	
				Other:	Y			Consulting:		Math/Other:	

TYPES OF BUSINESS:
Broadcast Television
Film Distribution and Production
Television Programming
Online Communities and Game Sites
Professional Sports
Electronic Games
Cable TV Programming
Online Entertainment

BRANDS/DIVISIONS/AFFILIATES:
News Corp
Fox Filmed Entertainment
Twentieth Century Fox Television
Fox Television Studios
Fox Interactive Media
National Geographic Channel

CONTACTS: Note: Officers with more than one job title may be intentionally listed here more than once.
Rupert Murdoch, CEO
Peter Chernin, COO
Peter Chernin, Pres.
David DeVoe, CFO/Sr. Exec. VP
K. Rupert Murdoch, Chmn.
Mitsy Wilson, Sr. VP-Diversity Dev.

Phone: 310-369-1000	Fax: 310-969-3300
Toll-Free:	
Address: 10201 W. Pico Blvd., Bldg. 100, Ste. 3220, Los Angeles, CA 90035 US	

GROWTH PLANS/SPECIAL FEATURES:
Fox Entertainment Group, Inc. (FEG), a wholly-owned subsidiary of The News Corporation, is an entertainment conglomerate that operates through four business segments: filmed entertainment, television stations, television broadcast network and cable network programming. The company engages in feature film and television production and distribution principally through the following businesses: Fox Filmed Entertainment, a leading producer and distributor of feature films; Twentieth Century Fox Television, a producer of network television programming; Fox Television Studios, a leading producer of U.S. broadcast, cable and international programming; and Fox Interactive Media, a network of integrated Internet sites including Myspace.com, which has more than 60 million users worldwide. Twentieth Century Fox Home Entertainment, Inc. distributes motion pictures and other programming produced by units of Fox Entertainment and its affiliates in all home media formats, including digital media available for download from Apple's iTunes Music Store. The company's motion picture and television library consists of varying rights to well over 3,000 previously released motion pictures and many television programs. In television, Fox Television Stations owns and operates 27 located in nine of the 10 largest designated market areas. Its television broadcast network consists of approximately 200 affiliated stations, including the full-power stations that are owned by subsidiaries of Fox. The company produces television programs through Twentieth Century Fox Television, Fox Television Studios, Fox News Channel, Fox Sports Networks, FX Network, SPEED Channel, FUEL TV, Fox College Sports, Fox Movie Channel, Fox Sports International, National Geographic Channel, Fox Movie Channel and several foreign subsidiaries. The company also owns a 14.6% limited partnership interest in the Colorado Rockies, the baseball franchise in Denver, Colorado. In December 2007, FEG acquired Beliefnet, a web site that assists consumers better understand various faiths.

FINANCIALS: Sales and profits are in thousands of dollars—add 000 to get the full amount. 2007 Note: Financial information for 2007 was not available for all companies at press time.

2007 Sales: $	2007 Profits: $	U.S. Stock Ticker: Subsidiary
2006 Sales: $	2006 Profits: $	Int'l Ticker: Int'l Exchange:
2005 Sales: $	2005 Profits: $	Employees:
2004 Sales: $12,175,000	2004 Profits: $1,353,000	Fiscal Year Ends: 6/30
2003 Sales: $11,002,000	2003 Profits: $1,031,000	Parent Company: NEWS CORP

SALARIES/BENEFITS:
Pension Plan:	ESOP Stock Plan:	Profit Sharing:	Top Exec. Salary: $4,508,694	Bonus: $21,175,000
Savings Plan:	Stock Purch. Plan:		Second Exec. Salary: $8,100,008	Bonus: $21,175,000

OTHER THOUGHTS:
Apparent Women Officers or Directors:
Hot Spot for Advancement for Women/Minorities:

LOCATIONS: ("Y" = Yes)
West:	Southwest:	Midwest:	Southeast:	Northeast:	International:
Y					

FPL GROUP INC

www.fplgroup.com

Industry Group Code: 221000A Ranks within this company's industry group: Sales: 1 Profits: 2

Management:		Sales/Marketing:		Liberal Arts:		Information Systems:		Professionals:		Technical/Scientific:	
Mgmt. Trainees:	Y	Mktg. Professionals:	Y	Gen. Writing/Editing:		Info. Management:	Y	Finance/Accounting:	Y	Engineers, Elec.:	Y
Experienced Mgmt.:	Y	Retail Sales:		Technical Writing:	Y	Software Dev.:	Y	Law:	Y	Engineers, Other:	Y
Int'l Business:		Commercial/Industrial:		Graphic Arts/Photog.:	Y	Hardware Dev.:		HR/Other:	Y	Health/Lab:	
MBA Graduates:	Y	Sales Trainees:		Music:		Systems Integration:		Training:	Y	Scientists/Research:	
		Advertising Pros.:		Broadcasting:		Consulting/Other:		Health Care:		Petroleum/Chemicals:	
				Other:				Consulting:		Math/Other:	

TYPES OF BUSINESS:

Utilities-Electricity & Natural Gas
Fiber-Optic Services
Financial Services
Nuclear Power
Energy Trading & Marketing
Wind Power

BRANDS/DIVISIONS/AFFILIATES:

Florida Power & Light Company
FPL Energy, LLC
FPL FiberNet, LLC
FPL Group Capitol
FPL Energy Power Marking, Inc.
Duane Arnold Energy Center
Interstate Power and Light Company

CONTACTS: *Note: Officers with more than one job title may be intentionally listed here more than once.*

Lewis Hay, III, CEO
James L. Robo, COO
James L. Robo, Pres.
Armando Pimentel, Jr., CFO/VP
Mary Lou Kromer, VP-Mktg.
Robert Escoto, VP-Human Resources
Robert L. McGrath, VP-Eng., Construction & Corp. Svcs.
Edward F. Tancer, General Counsel/VP
Christopher A. Bennett, VP/Chief Strategy, Policy & Bus. Officer
Mary Lou Kromer, VP-Comm.
K. Michael Davis, Chief Acct. Officer/Controller
Carmen Perez, Pres., FPL FiberNet
F. Mitchell Davidson, Pres., FPL Energy, LLC
Armando J. Olivera, Pres., Florida Power & Light Company
Antonio Rodriguez, VP-Power Generation Div.
Lewis Hay, III, Chmn.

Phone: 561-694-3715	Fax: 561-694-4620
Toll-Free:	
Address: 700 Universe Blvd., Juno Beach, FL 33408-0420 US	

GROWTH PLANS/SPECIAL FEATURES:

FPL Group, Inc. is a public utility holding company. Its primary subsidiary, Florida Power & Light Company (FPL), generates, transmits, distributes, buys and sells electricity with a supply capacity of approximately 25,100 megawatts (mw). FPL supplies electric service to over 8.7 million people throughout the east and lower west coasts of Florida, and has 4.5 million customer accounts. Approximately 54% of its 2007 sales were from residential customers, 39% from commercial customers, 3% from industrial customers and 4% others. Approximately 52% of the company's 2007 power was produced by natural gas fueled plants, 19% by nuclear plants, 8% by oil plants, 6% by coal plants and 15% of the company's power was purchased from other companies. In all, FPL operates 83 plants that burn natural gas, oil or a combination of both; three coal plants; and four nuclear plants. Besides FPL, the group operates FPL Energy, LLC, and FPL FiberNet, LLC, both of which are owned by subsidiary FPL Group Capitol. FPL Energy has a capacity of 15,543 mw, utilizing 42% natural gas, 33% wind, 16% nuclear, 5% oil, 2% hydro and 2% other energy sources. FPL Energy Power Marking, Inc., a subsidiary of FPL Energy, buys and sells wholesale energy commodities, such as natural gas, oil and electricity. FPL FiberNet leases wholesale fiber-optic network capacity and dark fiber to various clients. In October 2007, FPL Energy, LLC acquired a two-unit 1,035 mw nuclear power plant in Wisconsin. In March 2008, FPL Energy, LLC applied to build, own and operate a 250 mw solar plant in California's Mojave Desert. In July 2008, FPL was approved to construct three new solar projects in Florida for 110 mw of total power.

FPL offers some medical, dental and vision benefits; paid vacations; life insurance and dependant life insurance; and education and adoption assistance.

FINANCIALS: Sales and profits are in thousands of dollars—add 000 to get the full amount. 2007 Note: Financial information for 2007 was not available for all companies at press time.

2007 Sales: $15,263,000	2007 Profits: $1,312,000	**U.S. Stock Ticker: FPL**
2006 Sales: $15,710,000	2006 Profits: $1,281,000	**Int'l Ticker:** Int'l Exchange:
2005 Sales: $11,846,000	2005 Profits: $901,000	Employees: 10,400
2004 Sales: $10,522,000	2004 Profits: $896,000	Fiscal Year Ends: 12/31
2003 Sales: $9,630,000	2003 Profits: $890,000	Parent Company:

SALARIES/BENEFITS:

Pension Plan: Y	ESOP Stock Plan:	Profit Sharing:	Top Exec. Salary: $1,150,000	Bonus: $1,989,500
Savings Plan: Y	Stock Purch. Plan:		Second Exec. Salary: $551,221	Bonus: $744,700

OTHER THOUGHTS:

Apparent Women Officers or Directors: 6
Hot Spot for Advancement for Women/Minorities: Y

LOCATIONS: ("Y" = Yes)

West:	Southwest:	Midwest:	Southeast:	Northeast:	International:
Y	Y	Y	Y	Y	

FRED'S INC

www.fredsinc.com

Industry Group Code: 452910 Ranks within this company's industry group: Sales: 6 Profits: 6

Management:		Sales/Marketing:		Liberal Arts:		Information Systems:		Professionals:		Technical/Scientific:	
Mgmt. Trainees:	Y	Mktg. Professionals:	Y	Gen. Writing/Editing:	Y	Info. Management:	Y	Finance/Accounting:	Y	Engineers, Elec.:	
Experienced Mgmt.:	Y	Retail Sales:	Y	Technical Writing:		Software Dev.:	Y	Law:	Y	Engineers, Other:	
Int'l Business:		Commercial/Industrial:	Y	Graphic Arts/Photog.:	Y	Hardware Dev.:		HR/Other:	Y	Health/Lab:	
MBA Graduates:	Y	Sales Trainees:	Y	Music:		Systems Integration:		Training:	Y	Scientists/Research:	
		Advertising Pros.:	Y	Broadcasting:		Consulting/Other:		Health Care:		Petroleum/Chemicals:	
				Other:	Y			Consulting:		Math/Other:	

TYPES OF BUSINESS:

Discount Stores
Pharmacies
Photo Processing
General Merchandise

BRANDS/DIVISIONS/AFFILIATES:

Fred's
Fred's Pharmacies

CONTACTS: Note: Officers with more than one job title may be intentionally listed here more than once.

Michael J. Hayes, CEO
Bruce A. Efird, Pres.
Jerry A. Shore, CFO/Exec. VP
James R. Fennema, Exec. VP/Gen. Merch. Mgr.
Charles S. Vail, General Counsel/Corp. Sec./VP-Legal Svcs.
Dennis K. Curtis, Exec. VP-Store Oper.
John A. Casey, Exec. VP-Pharmacy Acquisitions
Rick A. Chambers, Exec. VP-Pharmacy Oper.
Michael J. Hayes, Chmn.

Phone: 901-365-8880	Fax:
Toll-Free:	
Address: 4300 New Getwell Rd., Memphis, TN 38118 US	

GROWTH PLANS/SPECIAL FEATURES:

Fred's, Inc. operates approximately 665 discount general merchandise and pharmacy stores throughout 15 southeastern states. Approximately 65% of Fred's stores are in markets with populations of 15,000 or fewer people. Of these locations, 296 contain full-service pharmacies. The firm also markets goods and services to 24 franchised Fred's stores. Fred's stores feature over 12,000 items, including national brand names, off-brands and Fred's private label. The firm operates distribution centers in Georgia and Tennessee. About half of Fred's stores' merchandise is received through these centers, while the remaining stock is shipped directly from suppliers. The company's strategy for obtaining customers for new pharmacies is through the acquisition of prescription files from independent pharmacies. These acquisitions provide an immediate sales benefit, and in many cases, the independent pharmacist will move to Fred's, thereby providing continuity in the pharmacist-patient relationship. Additionally, the company attempts to meet the general merchandise and pharmacy needs of the towns it serves by offering a variety of merchandise and a more attractive price-to-value relationship than either drug stores or smaller variety/dollar stores. In 2007, Fred's opened 35 stores and closed 20 stores. The majority of the new stores opened were located in Mississippi, Georgia, Texas, South Carolina and North Carolina. The company's new store prototype has 16,000 square feet of space. Opening a new store currently costs between $450,000 and $575,000 for inventory, furniture, fixtures, equipment and leasehold improvements. Also in 2007, the company added 11 new pharmacies and closed 4 pharmacies. Approximately 43% of Fred's stores, as of February 2008, contain a pharmacy and sell prescription drugs. In 2008, the company plans to take a more conservative expansion approach and intends to open approximately 18 stores and 10 to 15 pharmacies. Additionally, the firm plans to increase the number of store closings when compared to historic patterns.

FINANCIALS: Sales and profits are in thousands of dollars—add 000 to get the full amount. 2007 Note: Financial information for 2007 was not available for all companies at press time.

2007 Sales: $1,767,239	2007 Profits: $26,746	U.S. Stock Ticker: FRED	
2006 Sales: $1,589,342	2006 Profits: $26,094	Int'l Ticker: Int'l Exchange:	
2005 Sales: $1,441,781	2005 Profits: $27,952	Employees: 10,370	
2004 Sales: $1,302,700	2004 Profits: $33,700	Fiscal Year Ends: 1/31	
2003 Sales: $1,103,400	2003 Profits: $28,200	Parent Company:	

SALARIES/BENEFITS:

Pension Plan:	ESOP Stock Plan:	Profit Sharing:	Top Exec. Salary: $254,808	Bonus: $50,000
Savings Plan:	Stock Purch. Plan:		Second Exec. Salary: $224,231	Bonus: $75,000

OTHER THOUGHTS:

Apparent Women Officers or Directors:
Hot Spot for Advancement for Women/Minorities:

LOCATIONS: ("Y" = Yes)

West:	Southwest:	Midwest:	Southeast:	Northeast:	International:
	Y	Y	Y	Y	

FRONTIER COMMUNICATIONS CORPORATION
www.frontieronline.com

Industry Group Code: 513300A   **Ranks within this company's industry group:**   Sales: Profits:

Management:	Sales/Marketing:	Liberal Arts:	Information Systems:	Professionals:	Technical/Scientific:
Mgmt. Trainees:	Mktg. Professionals:	Gen. Writing/Editing:	Info. Management:	Finance/Accounting:	Engineers, Elec.:
Experienced Mgmt.:	Retail Sales:	Technical Writing:	Software Dev.:	Law:	Engineers, Other:
Int'l Business:	Commercial/Industrial:	Graphic Arts/Photog.:	Hardware Dev.:	HR/Other:	Health/Lab:
MBA Graduates:	Sales Trainees:	Music:	Systems Integration:	Training:	Scientists/Research:
	Advertising Pros.:	Broadcasting:	Consulting/Other:	Health Care:	Petroleum/Chemicals:
		Other:		Consulting:	Math/Other:

TYPES OF BUSINESS:
Telecommunications
Internet Services
Long-Distance Phone Services
Directory Service
Access Services

BRANDS/DIVISIONS/AFFILIATES:
Frontier Pages
GVN Services
Commonwealth Telephone Enterprises, Inc.
Global Valley Networks

CONTACTS: Note: Officers with more than one job title may be intentionally listed here more than once.
Maggie Wilderotter, CEO
Daniel McCarthy, COO/Exec. VP
Maggie Wilderotter, Pres.
Donald R. Shassian, CFO/Exec. VP
Peter B. Hayes, Exec. VP-Mktg. & Sales
Cecilia K. McKenney, Sr. VP-Human Resources
Hilary E. Glassman, General Counsel/Sr. VP/Sec.
Peter B. Hayes, Exec. VP-Bus. Dev.
Melinda White, Gen. Mgr./Sr. VP-New Bus. Oper.
Cecilia K. McKenney, Sr. VP-Call Center Sales & Svcs.
Maggie Wilderotter, Chmn.

Phone: 203-614-5600	**Fax:** 203-614-4602
Toll-Free:	
Address: 3 High Ridge Pk., Stamford, CT 06905 US	

GROWTH PLANS/SPECIAL FEATURES:

Frontier Communications Corporation, formerly Citizens Communications, provides communication services to homes and business, primarily in rural areas. The firm operates as an incumbent local exchange carrier in 24 states. The company provides access, local, long distance, data and internet, directory, television and wireless services. The firm had 2,955,500 access lines and internet subscribers at the close of 2007. Access services allow other carriers the use of Frontier facilities for long distance voice and data transmissions. Local services include basic telephone wireline services, as well as call forwarding, conference calling, caller identification, voicemail and call waiting. Long distance services use external interexchange carrier facilities. Data and internet services include internet access via high-speed or dial up connections, frame relay, Metro Ethernet and asynchronous transfer mode (ATM) switching services, as well as data transmission services to other carriers and commercial customers with dedicated high-capacity circuits. Directory services include white and yellow page directories of residential and business listings, and the Frontier Pages, an online directory service. Television services are offered in partnership with Echostar's DISH Network, including access to local channels, digital television channels and high-definition programming. Wireless services include wireless data WIFI networks in 13 municipalities, four colleges and universities and over 50 businesses. In March 2007, Frontier Communications acquired Commonwealth Telephone Enterprises, Inc. for approximately $1.1 billion. In October 2007, the company acquired Global Valley Networks, Inc. and GVN Services for $62 million total. In July 2008, the firm changed its name to Frontier Communications Corporation; Frontier was previously the firm's service brand. In August 2008, the firm partnered with Yahoo to create a co-branded personalized home page including search capabilities, with email services being planned.

Frontier employee benefits include medical and vision coverage, flexible spending accounts, life and accident insurance, corporate discounts and tuition reimbursement.

FINANCIALS: Sales and profits are in thousands of dollars—add 000 to get the full amount. 2007 Note: Financial information for 2007 was not available for all companies at press time.

2007 Sales: $2,288,015	2007 Profits: $214,654	**U.S. Stock Ticker: FTR**
2006 Sales: $2,025,367	2006 Profits: $344,555	**Int'l Ticker:** Int'l Exchange:
2005 Sales: $2,017,041	2005 Profits: $202,375	**Employees:** 5,900
2004 Sales: $2,168,422	2004 Profits: $72,150	**Fiscal Year Ends:** 12/31
2003 Sales: $2,424,174	2003 Profits: $187,852	**Parent Company:**

SALARIES/BENEFITS:

Pension Plan:	ESOP Stock Plan:	Profit Sharing:	Top Exec. Salary: $875,000	Bonus: $
Savings Plan:	Stock Purch. Plan:		Second Exec. Salary: $435,834	Bonus: $

OTHER THOUGHTS:
Apparent Women Officers or Directors: 8
Hot Spot for Advancement for Women/Minorities: Y

LOCATIONS: ("Y" = Yes)

West:	Southwest:	Midwest:	Southeast:	Northeast:	International:
Y	Y	Y	Y	Y	

Note: Financial information, benefits and other data can change quickly and may vary from those stated here.

GAMESTOP CORP

www.gamestop.com

Industry Group Code: 451120 **Ranks within this company's industry group:** Sales: 1 Profits: 1

Management:		Sales/Marketing:		Liberal Arts:		Information Systems:		Professionals:		Technical/Scientific:	
Mgmt. Trainees:	Y	Mktg. Professionals:	Y	Gen. Writing/Editing:	Y	Info. Management:	Y	Finance/Accounting:	Y	Engineers, Elec.:	
Experienced Mgmt.:	Y	Retail Sales:	Y	Technical Writing:		Software Dev.:	Y	Law:	Y	Engineers, Other:	
Int'l Business:	Y	Commercial/Industrial:	Y	Graphic Arts/Photog.:	Y	Hardware Dev.:		HR/Other:	Y	Health/Lab:	
MBA Graduates:	Y	Sales Trainees:	Y	Music:		Systems Integration:		Training:	Y	Scientists/Research:	
		Advertising Pros.:	Y	Broadcasting:		Consulting/Other:		Health Care:		Petroleum/Chemicals:	
				Other:	Y			Consulting:		Math/Other:	

TYPES OF BUSINESS:

Video Games-Retail
PC Software Sales
Game Accessories
Online Sales
Magazine Publication

BRANDS/DIVISIONS/AFFILIATES:

EB Games
GameStop.com
ebgames.com
Game Informer Magazine

CONTACTS: *Note: Officers with more than one job title may be intentionally listed here more than once.*

Daniel A. DeMatteo, CEO
J. Paul Raines, COO
Steven R. Morgan, Pres.
David W. Carlson, CFO/Exec. VP
Tony D. Bartel, Exec. VP-Mktg.
Tony D. Bartel, Exec. VP-Merch.
Michael N. Rosen, Sec.
Matt Hodges, Dir. Investor Rel.
Daniel A. DeMatteo, Vice Chmn.
R. Richard Fontaine, Chmn.
Ronald Freeman, Exec. VP-Dist.

Phone: 817-424-2000	Fax: 817-424-2062
Toll-Free: 800-883-8895	
Address: 625 Westport Pkwy., Grapevine, TX 76051 US	

GROWTH PLANS/SPECIAL FEATURES:

GameStop Corp. is one of the world's largest retailers of video games and PC entertainment software. The company operates 5,543 retail stores throughout 50 U.S. states, eleven European countries, Australia and Canada. Approximately 3,800 of the company's stores are located in the U.S., operating primarily under the names GameStop and EB Games. The company opened 586 new stores in 2007. The stores offer both new and used video game hardware, software and accessories, as well as PC entertainment software; they are generally located in power strip centers or high-traffic shopping malls; and average approximately 1,500 square feet. The firm's used video game products provide a unique value proposition to the stores' customers and its purchasing of video game products provides its customers with an opportunity to trade in their used video game products for store credits and apply those credits towards other merchandise, which, in turn, drives more sales. Stores also typically feature several video game sampling areas, which provide our customers the opportunity to play games before purchase, as well as equipment to play video game clips. Additionally, GameStop operates two e-commerce web sites, gamestop.com and ebgames.com, as well as publishing Game Informer, one of the largest multi-platform video game magazines in the U.S., based on its 2.7 million subscribers. Paid Game Informer subscribers receive a GameStop loyalty card, which offers discounts on selected merchandise in the company's stores. In July 2008, GameStop bought the Gamesman, a New Zealand-based independent gaming specialist.

GameStop provides employees flexible spending accounts; 15% discounts at GameStop owned stores and 30% discounts at Barnes & Noble and B. Dalton Bookstores; paid vacation, holidays, sick days, jury duty and bereavement; tuition reimbursement; vision coverage; and dental and preferred provider organization (PPO) medical insurance.

FINANCIALS: Sales and profits are in thousands of dollars—add 000 to get the full amount. 2007 Note: Financial information for 2007 was not available for all companies at press time.

2007 Sales: $5,318,900	2007 Profits: $158,250	**U.S. Stock Ticker:** GME	
2006 Sales: $3,091,783	2006 Profits: $100,784	**Int'l Ticker:** Int'l Exchange:	
2005 Sales: $1,842,806	2005 Profits: $60,926	Employees: 32,000	
2004 Sales: $1,578,838	2004 Profits: $63,467	Fiscal Year Ends: 1/31	
2003 Sales: $1,352,800	2003 Profits: $52,400	Parent Company:	

SALARIES/BENEFITS:

Pension Plan:	ESOP Stock Plan:	Profit Sharing:	Top Exec. Salary: $1,011,539	Bonus: $2,000,000
Savings Plan: Y	Stock Purch. Plan:		Second Exec. Salary: $810,385	Bonus: $1,600,000

OTHER THOUGHTS:

Apparent Women Officers or Directors: 1
Hot Spot for Advancement for Women/Minorities:

LOCATIONS: ("Y" = Yes)

West:	Southwest:	Midwest:	Southeast:	Northeast:	International:
Y	Y	Y	Y	Y	Y

GENENTECH INC

www.gene.com

Industry Group Code: 325412 Ranks within this company's industry group: Sales: 5 Profits: 3

Management:		Sales/Marketing:		Liberal Arts:		Information Systems:		Professionals:		Technical/Scientific:	
Mgmt. Trainees:	Y	Mktg. Professionals:	Y	Gen. Writing/Editing:	Y	Info. Management:	Y	Finance/Accounting:	Y	Engineers, Elec.:	Y
Experienced Mgmt.:	Y	Retail Sales:		Technical Writing:	Y	Software Dev.:	Y	Law:	Y	Engineers, Other:	Y
Int'l Business:	Y	Commercial/Industrial:	Y	Graphic Arts/Photog.:	Y	Hardware Dev.:		HR/Other:	Y	Health/Lab:	Y
MBA Graduates:	Y	Sales Trainees:	Y	Music:		Systems Integration:		Training:	Y	Scientists/Research:	Y
		Advertising Pros.:		Broadcasting:		Consulting/Other:		Health Care:	Y	Petroleum/Chemicals:	
				Other:				Consulting:		Math/Other:	Y

TYPES OF BUSINESS:

Drug Development & Manufacturing
Genetically Engineered Drugs

BRANDS/DIVISIONS/AFFILIATES:

Avastin
TNKase
Herceptin
Rituxan
Activase
Pulmozyme
Nutropin

CONTACTS: *Note: Officers with more than one job title may be intentionally listed here more than once.*

Arthur D. Levinson, CEO
Myrtle S. Potter, COO
Arthur D. Levinson, Pres.
David A. Ebersman, CFO/Exec. VP
Richard H. Scheller, Exec. VP-Research
Susan Desmond-Hellmann, Pres., Prod. Dev.
Stephen G. Juelsgaard, Exec. VP/Corp. Sec.
Ian T. Clark, Exec. VP-Comm. Oper.
Robert E. Andreatta, Chief Acct. Officer/Controller
Stephen G. Juelsgaard, Corp. Sec.
Patrick Y. Yang, Exec. VP-Product Oper.
Stephen G. Juelsgaard, Chief Compliance Officer
Arthur D. Levinson, Chmn.

Phone: 650-225-1000   **Fax:** 650-225-6000
Toll-Free:
Address: 1 DNA Way, South San Francisco, CA 94080 US

GROWTH PLANS/SPECIAL FEATURES:

Genentech, Inc. makes medicines by splicing genes into fast-growing bacteria that then produce therapeutic proteins and combat diseases on a molecular level. Genentech uses cutting-edge technologies such as computer visualization of molecules, micro arrays and sensitive assaying techniques to develop, manufacture and market pharmaceuticals for unmet medical needs. Genentech's research is directed toward the oncology, immunology and vascular biology fields. The company's products consist of a variety of cardio-centric medications, as well as cancer, growth hormone deficiency (GHD) and cystic fibrosis treatments. Biotechnology products offered by Genentech include Herceptin, used to treat metastatic breast cancers; Avastin, used to inhibit angiogenesis of solid-tumor cancers; Nutropin, a growth hormone for the treatment of GHD in children and adults; TNKase, for the treatment of acute myocardial infarction; and Pulmozyme, for the treatment of cystic fibrosis. The company also produces the Rituxan antibody, used for the treatment of patients with non-Hodgkin's lymphoma. Through its long-standing Genentech Access to Care Foundation, Genentech assists those without sufficient health insurance to receive its medicines. In 2007, sales to Genentech's three major distributors represented 86% of its total U.S. net product sales. The firm recently completed the acquisition of Tanox, a firm that focuses on monoclonal antibody technology. Roche Holdings, Ltd. owns 55.8% of Genentech. Roche hopes to acquire all of Genentech's outstanding stock.

For the last ten years, the company has been named to Fortune Magazine's 100 Best Companies to Work For. Every Friday evening, Genentech hosts socials called Ho-Hos, providing free food, beverages and a chance to socialize with co-workers.

FINANCIALS: Sales and profits are in thousands of dollars—add 000 to get the full amount. 2007 Note: Financial information for 2007 was not available for all companies at press time.

2007 Sales: $11,724,000	2007 Profits: $2,769,000	**U.S. Stock Ticker: DNA**
2006 Sales: $9,284,000	2006 Profits: $2,113,000	**Int'l Ticker:** Int'l Exchange:
2005 Sales: $6,633,372	2005 Profits: $1,278,991	Employees: 11,174
2004 Sales: $4,621,157	2004 Profits: $784,816	Fiscal Year Ends: 12/31
2003 Sales: $2,799,400	2003 Profits: $562,527	Parent Company:

SALARIES/BENEFITS:

Pension Plan:	ESOP Stock Plan:	Profit Sharing:	Top Exec. Salary: $995,000	Bonus: $2,725,000
Savings Plan: Y	Stock Purch. Plan: Y		Second Exec. Salary: $625,000	Bonus: $870,000

OTHER THOUGHTS:

Apparent Women Officers or Directors: 2
Hot Spot for Advancement for Women/Minorities: Y

LOCATIONS: ("Y" = Yes)

West:	Southwest:	Midwest:	Southeast:	Northeast:	International:
Y					Y

GENERAL DYNAMICS CORP   www.generaldynamics.com

Industry Group Code: 336410 Ranks within this company's industry group: Sales: 6   Profits: 5

Management:		Sales/Marketing:		Liberal Arts:		Information Systems:		Professionals:		Technical/Scientific:	
Mgmt. Trainees:	Y	Mktg. Professionals:	Y	Gen. Writing/Editing:	Y	Info. Management:	Y	Finance/Accounting:	Y	Engineers, Elec.:	Y
Experienced Mgmt.:	Y	Retail Sales:		Technical Writing:	Y	Software Dev.:	Y	Law:	Y	Engineers, Other:	
Int'l Business:	Y	Commercial/Industrial:	Y	Graphic Arts/Photog.:	Y	Hardware Dev.:	Y	HR/Other:	Y	Health/Lab:	Y
MBA Graduates:	Y	Sales Trainees:		Music:		Systems Integration:	Y	Training:	Y	Scientists/Research:	Y
		Advertising Pros.:		Broadcasting:		Consulting/Other:	Y	Health Care:		Petroleum/Chemicals:	
				Other:				Consulting:	Y	Math/Other:	Y

TYPES OF BUSINESS:

Aerospace Products & Services
Combat Vehicles & Systems
Telecommunications Systems
Naval Vessels & Submarines
Ship Management Services
Information Systems & Technology
Defense Systems & Services
Business Jets

BRANDS/DIVISIONS/AFFILIATES:

Gulfstream Aerospace
TriPoint Global Communications, Inc.
General Dynamics C4 Systems
Spectrum Astro, Inc.
General Dynamics Advanced Information Systems
M1A1 Abrams Tank
Abrams Integrated Management
SNC Technologies, Inc.

CONTACTS: Note: Officers with more than one job title may be intentionally listed here more than once.

Nicholas D. Chabraja, CEO
L. Hugh Redd, CFO/Sr. VP
Raynor B. Reavis, Sr. VP-Mktg. & Sales
Walter M. Oliver, Sr. VP-Human Resources
Tommy R. Augustsson, VP-IT
Gerard J. DeMuro, Exec. VP-Info. Systems & Tech.
Phebe N. Novakovic, Sr. VP-Planning & Dev.
Preston A. Henne, Sr. VP-Eng., Test & Programs
Walter M. Oliver, Sr. VP-Admin.
David A. Savner, General Counsel/Sec./Sr. VP
Phebe N. Novakovic, Sr. VP-Planning & Dev.
Kendell Pease, VP-Gov't Rel. & Comm.
David H. Fogg, Treas./VP
Larry R. Flynn, VP/Pres., Aviation Svcs.
John P. Casey, VP/Pres., Electric Boat Corp.
Lewis F. von Thaer, VP/Pres., Advanced Info. Systems
Charles M. Hall, Exec. VP-Combat Systems
Nicholas D. Chabraja, Chmn.
William O. Schmieder, VP-Int'l

Phone: 703-876-3000	Fax: 703-876-3125
Toll-Free:	
Address: 2941 Fairview Park Dr., Ste. 100, Falls Church, VA 22042-4513 US	

GROWTH PLANS/SPECIAL FEATURES:

General Dynamics Corp. (GDC) is one of the world's largest aerospace and defense contractors. Its customers include the U.S. military, other government organizations, the armed forces of allied nations and a diverse base of corporate and industrial buyers. The firm's operations are divided into four segments: Information systems and technology (IST), marine systems, combat systems and aerospace. The IST group provides defense and commercial customers with infrastructure and systems integration skills required to process, communicate and manage information effectively. The group has market-leading positions in the design, deployment and maintenance of wireline and wireless voice and data networks, telecommunications system security, encryption and fiber optics. The marine systems division provides the U.S. Navy with combat vessels, including nuclear submarines, surface combatants and auxiliary ships. The segment also provides ship management services for the U.S. government and builds commercial ships. The combat systems group provides systems integration, design, development, production and support for armored vehicles, armaments, munitions and components, with product lines including unmanned systems, medium-caliber guns, space propulsion systems, reactive armor and suspensions, engines and transmissions. It is the leading builder of armored vehicles and makes products such as the M1A1 Abrams Tank. The aerospace group designs, develops, manufactures and provides services for technologically advanced business jet aircraft under the Gulfstream name. In early 2008, the firm was awarded roughly $2.5 billion for various government military projects and contracts.

FINANCIALS: Sales and profits are in thousands of dollars—add 000 to get the full amount. 2007 Note: Financial information for 2007 was not available for all companies at press time.

2007 Sales: $27,240,000	2007 Profits: $2,072,000	U.S. Stock Ticker: GD
2006 Sales: $24,063,000	2006 Profits: $1,856,000	Int'l Ticker: Int'l Exchange:
2005 Sales: $20,975,000	2005 Profits: $1,461,000	Employees: 83,500
2004 Sales: $18,868,000	2004 Profits: $1,227,000	Fiscal Year Ends: 12/31
2003 Sales: $16,328,000	2003 Profits: $1,004,000	Parent Company:

SALARIES/BENEFITS:

Pension Plan:	ESOP Stock Plan:	Profit Sharing:	Top Exec. Salary: $1,300,000	Bonus: $3,000,000
Savings Plan:	Stock Purch. Plan:		Second Exec. Salary: $575,000	Bonus: $700,000

OTHER THOUGHTS:

Apparent Women Officers or Directors: 1
Hot Spot for Advancement for Women/Minorities:

LOCATIONS: ("Y" = Yes)

West:	Southwest:	Midwest:	Southeast:	Northeast:	International:
Y	Y	Y	Y	Y	Y

GENERAL ELECTRIC CO (GE)　　　　　　www.ge.com

Industry Group Code: 522220A　Ranks within this company's industry group: Sales: 1　Profits: 1

Management:		Sales/Marketing:		Liberal Arts:		Information Systems:		Professionals:		Technical/Scientific:	
Mgmt. Trainees:	Y	Mktg. Professionals:	Y	Gen. Writing/Editing:	Y	Info. Management:	Y	Finance/Accounting:	Y	Engineers, Elec.:	Y
Experienced Mgmt.:	Y	Retail Sales:		Technical Writing:	Y	Software Dev.:	Y	Law:	Y	Engineers, Other:	
Int'l Business:	Y	Commercial/Industrial:	Y	Graphic Arts/Photog.:	Y	Hardware Dev.:	Y	HR/Other:	Y	Health/Lab:	
MBA Graduates:	Y	Sales Trainees:		Music:		Systems Integration:		Training:	Y	Scientists/Research:	Y
		Advertising Pros.:	Y	Broadcasting:		Consulting/Other:		Health Care:		Petroleum/Chemicals:	
				Other:				Consulting:		Math/Other:	Y

TYPES OF BUSINESS:

Business Leasing & Finance
Energy Systems & Consulting
Insurance & Financial Services
Industrial & Electrical Equipment & Consumer Products
Television & Film Production & Distribution
Real Estate Investments & Finance
Medical Equipment
Transportation, Aircraft Engines, Rail Systems & Truck Fleet Management

BRANDS/DIVISIONS/AFFILIATES:

GE Commercial Finance
GE Infrastructure
GE Healthcare
NBC Universal
GE Money
GE Equipment Services
GE Industrial
GE Aviation

CONTACTS: *Note: Officers with more than one job title may be intentionally listed here more than once.*

Jeffrey R. Immelt, CEO
Keith S. Sherin, CFO
Beth Comstock, Chief Mktg. Officer/Sr. VP
John Lynch, Sr. VP-Corp. Human Resources
Mark M. Little, Sr. VP/Dir.-Global Research
Gary M. Reiner, CIO/Sr. VP
Brackett B. Denniston, III, General Counsel/Sr. VP
Wayne Hewett, VP-Oper.
Pamela Daley, Sr. VP-Corp. Bus. Dev.
Trevor Schauenberg, Corp. Investor Comm.
Kathryn A. Cassidy, Treas./VP
Michael A. Neal, CEO/Pres., GE Commercial Finance
John G. Rice, CEO/Pres., GE Infrastructure
James Campbell, CEO/Pres., GE Industrial
Susan P. Peters, VP-Exec. Dev.
Jeffrey R. Immelt, Chmn.
Ferdinando Beccalli-Falco, CEO/Pres., Int'l
Wayne Hewett, VP-Supply Chain

Phone: 203-373-2211	Fax: 203-373-3131
Toll-Free:	
Address: 3135 Easton Turnpike, Fairfield, CT 06828-0001 US	

GROWTH PLANS/SPECIAL FEATURES:

General Electric Co. (GE) is one of the world's largest and most diversified corporations, with six operating divisions: Infrastructure, commercial finance, GE Money (formerly consumer finance), healthcare, NBC Universal and industrial. GE's infrastructure division, its largest operating segment, produces, sells, finances and services equipment for the air and rail transportation, water treatment and energy generation industries. GE's commercial finance segment offers financial services mainly to manufacturers, distributors and end-users, including loans and leases. GE Money offers credit and deposit products to consumers, retailers, banks and auto dealers in over 50 countries. The healthcare segment develops diagnostic and therapy equipment including MRI and CT scanners, x-ray, nuclear imaging and ultrasound equipment. NBC Universal, the company's network television affiliate, broadcasts to affiliated television stations within the U.S., produces live and recorded television programs, operates television broadcasting stations and produces and distributes films. GE's industrial segment produces and sells products including consumer appliances, industrial equipment and plastics and also provides asset management services for the transportation industry. In 2007, the firm made a number of acquisitions, the most significant of which were Trustreet Properties, Inc.; Diskont und Kredit AG and Disko Leasing GmbH (DISKO) and ASL Auto Service-Leasing GmbH (ASL), the leasing businesses of KG Allgemeine Leasing GmbH & Co.; and Sanyo Electric Credit Co., Ltd. Recent acquisitions include Kelman Limited of Northern Ireland; CitiCapital, Citigroup's North American commercial leasing and commercial equipment finance business; and Bank BPH of Poland.

GE provides its employees with tuition, adoption, parenting and child care assistance; education and career counseling; and legal and financial information services.

FINANCIALS: Sales and profits are in thousands of dollars—add 000 to get the full amount. 2007 Note: Financial information for 2007 was not available for all companies at press time.

2007 Sales: $172,738,000	2007 Profits: $22,208,000	**U.S. Stock Ticker: GE**
2006 Sales: $151,843,000	2006 Profits: $20,742,000	**Int'l Ticker:**　Int'l Exchange:
2005 Sales: $136,580,000	2005 Profits: $16,720,000	Employees: 327,000
2004 Sales: $134,481,000	2004 Profits: $16,285,000	Fiscal Year Ends: 12/31
2003 Sales: $134,187,000	2003 Profits: $15,002,000	Parent Company:

SALARIES/BENEFITS:

Pension Plan:	ESOP Stock Plan:	Profit Sharing:	Top Exec. Salary: $3,300,000	Bonus: $5,000,000
Savings Plan: Y	Stock Purch. Plan:		Second Exec. Salary: $2,500,000	Bonus: $6,900,000

OTHER THOUGHTS:

Apparent Women Officers or Directors: 10
Hot Spot for Advancement for Women/Minorities: Y

LOCATIONS: ("Y" = Yes)

West:	Southwest:	Midwest:	Southeast:	Northeast:	International:
Y	Y	Y	Y	Y	Y

Note: Financial information, benefits and other data can change quickly and may vary from those stated here.

GENERAL MILLS INC
www.generalmills.com

Industry Group Code: 311230 Ranks within this company's industry group: Sales: Profits:

Management:		Sales/Marketing:		Liberal Arts:		Information Systems:		Professionals:		Technical/Scientific:	
Mgmt. Trainees:	Y	Mktg. Professionals:	Y	Gen. Writing/Editing:	Y	Info. Management:	Y	Finance/Accounting:	Y	Engineers, Elec.:	Y
Experienced Mgmt.:	Y	Retail Sales:		Technical Writing:		Software Dev.:		Law:	Y	Engineers, Other:	Y
Int'l Business:	Y	Commercial/Industrial:	Y	Graphic Arts/Photog.:	Y	Hardware Dev.:		HR/Other:	Y	Health/Lab:	Y
MBA Graduates:	Y	Sales Trainees:		Music:		Systems Integration:		Training:	Y	Scientists/Research:	
		Advertising Pros.:	Y	Broadcasting:		Consulting/Other:		Health Care:		Petroleum/Chemicals:	Y
				Other:				Consulting:		Math/Other:	

TYPES OF BUSINESS:
Cereal Manufacturing
Snack Foods
Frozen Foods
Baking Products
Yogurt
Organic Foods
Convenience Meal Products
Canned and Frozen Vegetables

BRANDS/DIVISIONS/AFFILIATES:
Big G Cereals
Cheerios
Betty Crocker
Progresso
Pillsbury
Yoplait
Bisquick
Haagen-Dazs

CONTACTS: Note: Officers with more than one job title may be intentionally listed here more than once.
Kendall J. Powell, CEO
Kendall J. Powell, Pres.
Donal Leo Mulligan, CFO/Exec. VP
Jeffrey J. Rotsch, Exec. VP- Worldwide Sales
Michael A. Peel, Sr. VP-Human Resources
Randy G. Darcy, CTO/Exec. VP-Tech.
Michael A. Peel, Exec. VP-Admin. Svcs.
Roderick A. Palmore, General Counsel/Chief Compliance & Risk Officer
Randy G. Darcy, Exec. VP-Worldwide Oper.
Christina L. Shea, Sr. VP-External Rel./Pres., Community Action
Ian R. Friendly, COO-U.S. Retail/Exec. VP
Peter J. Capell, Pres., Big G Cereal Div.
Gary Chu, Pres., Greater China
Robert F. Waldron, Pres., Yoplait USA/Sr. VP
Kendall J. Powell, Chmn.
Christopher D. O'Leary, COO-Int'l/Exec. VP

Phone: 763-764-7600	Fax: 763-764-7384
Toll-Free:	
Address: One General Mills Blvd., Minneapolis, MN 55426 US	

GROWTH PLANS/SPECIAL FEATURES:
General Mills, Inc. is a leading global producer of packaged consumer foods. The company markets its products in over 100 countries and manufactures its products in 18 countries, according to three divisions: U.S. retail, generating approximately 68% of its net sales; bakeries and food service, generating 15%; and international, generating 17%. The U.S. retail division consists of five segments: Big G Cereals, which controls Cheerios, Chex and Lucky Charms; meals, with products such as Betty Crocker, Hamburger Helper and Progresso; Pillsbury U.S., including frozen dough products and frozen breakfast products; Yoplait, including Yoplait Light, Go-GURT and Yoplait Kids; snacks, which includes Fruit Roll-Ups and Bugles; baking products, including Bisquick baking mix and Warm Delights microwaveable desserts; and small planet foods and other, including Cascadian Farm and Muir Glen. The bakeries and food service segment consists of products marketed to retail and wholesale bakeries; and offered to commercial and noncommercial food service sectors, such as restaurants and school cafeterias, throughout the U.S. and Canada, under the Pillsbury and Gold Medal trademarks. The international segment is made up of retail and food services businesses outside the U.S. and Canada, with major product categories including super-premium ice cream; grain snacks; shelf-stable and frozen vegetables; refrigerated and frozen dough products; and dry dinners. The firm owns a 50% stake in 8th Continent, LLC, a joint venture with DuPont, which develops and markets soy-based products. General Mills also owns 50% of Haagen-Dazs ice cream, as well as 50% interest in Seretram, a joint venture with Co-op de Pau for the production of Green Giant corn in France.

General Mills offers its employees educational assistance; relocation benefits; credit union membership; parenting benefits; on-site services; an employee club; flexible work arrangements; domestic partner benefits; flexible spending accounts; and medical, dental, life, long-term care, legal, auto and homeowners insurance.

FINANCIALS: Sales and profits are in thousands of dollars—add 000 to get the full amount. 2007 Note: Financial information for 2007 was not available for all companies at press time.

2007 Sales: $12,442,000	2007 Profits: $2,058,000	U.S. Stock Ticker: GIS
2006 Sales: $11,712,000	2006 Profits: $1,958,000	Int'l Ticker: Int'l Exchange:
2005 Sales: $11,308,000	2005 Profits: $1,900,000	Employees: 28,500
2004 Sales: $11,070,000	2004 Profits: $1,055,000	Fiscal Year Ends: 5/31
2003 Sales: $10,506,000	2003 Profits: $917,000	Parent Company:

SALARIES/BENEFITS:

Pension Plan:	ESOP Stock Plan:	Profit Sharing:	Top Exec. Salary: $1,241,250	Bonus: $2,513,531
Savings Plan: Y	Stock Purch. Plan: Y		Second Exec. Salary: $700,000	Bonus: $1,323,000

OTHER THOUGHTS:
Apparent Women Officers or Directors: 13
Hot Spot for Advancement for Women/Minorities: Y

LOCATIONS: ("Y" = Yes)

West:	Southwest:	Midwest:	Southeast:	Northeast:	International:
Y	Y	Y	Y	Y	Y

GENESCO INC

www.genesco.com

Industry Group Code: 316213 Ranks within this company's industry group: Sales: 1   Profits: 1

Management:		Sales/Marketing:		Liberal Arts:		Information Systems:		Professionals:		Technical/Scientific:	
Mgmt. Trainees:	Y	Mktg. Professionals:	Y	Gen. Writing/Editing:	Y	Info. Management:	Y	Finance/Accounting:	Y	Engineers, Elec.:	
Experienced Mgmt.:	Y	Retail Sales:	Y	Technical Writing:		Software Dev.:		Law:	Y	Engineers, Other:	
Int'l Business:	Y	Commercial/Industrial:	Y	Graphic Arts/Photog.:	Y	Hardware Dev.:		HR/Other:	Y	Health/Lab:	
MBA Graduates:	Y	Sales Trainees:	Y	Music:		Systems Integration:		Training:	Y	Scientists/Research:	
		Advertising Pros.:	Y	Broadcasting:		Consulting/Other:		Health Care:		Petroleum/Chemicals:	
				Other:	Y			Consulting:		Math/Other:	

TYPES OF BUSINESS:

Men's Shoes, Retail
Retail Stores
Men's Accessories
Wholesale Operations
Hats, Retail
Catalog & Online Operations

BRANDS/DIVISIONS/AFFILIATES:

Johnston & Murphy
Journeys
Underground Station
Journeys Kidz
Hat World Corporation
Hat Zone
Lids
Cap Connection

CONTACTS: *Note: Officers with more than one job title may be intentionally listed here more than once.*

Robert J. Dennis, CEO
Robert J. Dennis, Pres.
James S. Gulmi, CFO/Sr. VP-Finance
John W. Clinard, Sr. VP-Human Resources
John W. Clinard, Sr. VP-Admin.
Roger G. Sisson, General Counsel/Corp. Sec./Sr. VP
Mimi Eckel Vaughn, Sr. VP-Strategy & Bus. Dev.
Claire S. McCall, VP-Investor Rel.
Paul D. Williams, Chief Acct. Officer/VP
Kenneth J. Kocher, Sr. VP/Pres., Hat World
James C. Estepa, Sr. VP/CEO/Pres., Genesco Retail
Jonathan D. Caplan, Sr. VP/CEO-Genesco Branded Group
Hal N. Pennington, Chmn.

Phone: 615-367-7000	**Fax:** 615-367-8579
Toll-Free:	
Address: 1415 Murfreesboro Rd., Nashville, TN 37217 US	

GROWTH PLANS/SPECIAL FEATURES:

Genesco is a leading specialty retailer of footwear, headwear and accessories through 2,175 retail stores in the U.S., Canada and Puerto Rico. The company operates five business segments: Journeys Group, Underground Station Group, Hat World Group, Johnston & Murphy Group and Licensed Brands. The Journey's Group segment operates 967 stores, including Journeys, Journeys Kidz and Shi by Journeys, as well as through a catalog and journeys.com. Journeys stores target customers in the 13-22 year age group through the use of youth-oriented decor and popular music videos. The Underground Station Group segment operates 192 stores, including Underground Station and Jarman. The Hat World Group segment operates 862 stores, including Hat World, Lids, Hat Shack, Hat Zone, Head Quarters, Cap Connection and Lids Kids, as well as through hatworld.com and lidsyco.com. The core adult stores, located in malls, airports, street level stores and factory outlet stores, target customers in the early-teens to mid-20s age group. The 14 Lids Kids stores target toddlers to 10 year olds. The Johnston & Murphy Group segment operates 154 retail and factory stores, as well as through johnstonmurphy.com, selling footwear and accessories for men. Targeting male business and professional customers, retail prices for Johnston & Murphy footwear generally range from $100 to $300. The Licensed Brands segment is comprised primarily of Dockers footwear, sourced and marketed under a license from Levi Strauss & Company. In January 2007, Genesco acquired Hat Shack, Inc. for $16.6 million. In June 2007, Genesco agreed to be acquired by Finish Line, Inc. for $1.5 billion. However, in March 2008, Genesco and Finish Line terminated the agreement.

Genesco offers its employees educational assistance, flexible spending accounts, service awards, adoption assistance, scholarships, dry cleaning service, a hair salon, an employee credit association, child care alternatives, fitness classes, massage therapy and Weight Watchers at Work.

FINANCIALS: Sales and profits are in thousands of dollars—add 000 to get the full amount. 2007 Note: Financial information for 2007 was not available for all companies at press time.

2007 Sales: $1,460,478	2007 Profits: $67,646	**U.S. Stock Ticker:** GCO	
2006 Sales: $1,283,876	2006 Profits: $62,686	**Int'l Ticker:**	**Int'l Exchange:**
2005 Sales: $1,112,681	2005 Profits: $48,249	Employees: 12,750	
2004 Sales: $837,379	2004 Profits: $28,730	Fiscal Year Ends: 1/31	
2003 Sales: $828,300	2003 Profits: $36,200	Parent Company:	

SALARIES/BENEFITS:

Pension Plan:	ESOP Stock Plan:	Profit Sharing:	Top Exec. Salary: $720,000	Bonus: $759,000
Savings Plan: Y	Stock Purch. Plan: Y		Second Exec. Salary: $500,000	Bonus: $462,000

OTHER THOUGHTS:

Apparent Women Officers or Directors: 2
Hot Spot for Advancement for Women/Minorities: Y

LOCATIONS: ("Y" = Yes)

West:	Southwest:	Midwest:	Southeast:	Northeast:	International:
Y	Y	Y	Y	Y	Y

GENWORTH FINANCIAL INC
www.genworth.com

Industry Group Code: 524113 **Ranks within this company's industry group:** Sales: 1 Profits: 1

Management:		Sales/Marketing:		Liberal Arts:		Information Systems:		Professionals:		Technical/Scientific:	
Mgmt. Trainees:	Y	Mktg. Professionals:	Y	Gen. Writing/Editing:	Y	Info. Management:	Y	Finance/Accounting:	Y	Engineers, Elec.:	
Experienced Mgmt.:	Y	Retail Sales:		Technical Writing:	Y	Software Dev.:	Y	Law:	Y	Engineers, Other:	
Int'l Business:		Commercial/Industrial:	Y	Graphic Arts/Photog.:	Y	Hardware Dev.:		HR/Other:	Y	Health/Lab:	
MBA Graduates:	Y	Sales Trainees:		Music:		Systems Integration:		Training:	Y	Scientists/Research:	Y
		Advertising Pros.:	Y	Broadcasting:		Consulting/Other:		Health Care:		Petroleum/Chemicals:	
				Other:				Consulting:		Math/Other:	

TYPES OF BUSINESS:
Life Insurance
Annuities
Group Health, Life, Dental & Disability Insurance
Payment Protection Insurance
Mortgage Insurance
Retirement Income & Investment Products & Services
Long-Term Care Insurance

BRANDS/DIVISIONS/AFFILIATES:
Sun Life Financial, Inc.
Liberty Reverse Mortgage, Inc.

CONTACTS: *Note: Officers with more than one job title may be intentionally listed here more than once.*
Michael D. Fraizer, CEO
Michael D. Fraizer, Pres.
Patrick B. Kelleher, CFO/Sr. VP
Michael S. Laming, Sr. VP-Human Resources
Scott J. McKay, CIO
Leon E. Roday, General Counsel/Sr. VP/Sec.
Scott J. McKay, Sr. VP-Oper. & Quality
Jean S. Peters, Sr. VP-Strategic Analysis
Barbara Faurot, Sr. VP-Comm.
Amy R. Corbin, Controller/VP
Brian L. Hurley, Pres., Int'l Dev. & Australian Oper.
Kevin D. Schneider, Pres., US Mortgage Insurance
William C. Goings, Pres., Life Insurance
Ronald D. Cordes, Pres., Managed Money
Michael D. Fraizer, Chmn.
Robert J. Brannock, Pres., European & Canadian Oper.

Phone: 804-281-6000 **Fax:** 804-662-2414
Toll-Free: 888-436-9678
Address: 6620 W. Broad St., Richmond, VA 23230 US

GROWTH PLANS/SPECIAL FEATURES:
Genworth Financial, Inc. is a financial security company focused on developing solutions that help the investment, protection, homeownership, retirement and independent lifestyle needs of more than 15 million customers with a presence in more than 25 countries. The company operates in three segments: retirement and protection; international; and U.S. mortgage insurance. The retirement and protection segment provides protection, wealth accumulation, retirement income and institutional products, such as: life insurance; long-term care insurance; a linked-benefits product that combines long-term care insurance with universal life insurance; Medicare supplement insurance; wellness and care coordination services for our long-term care policyholders; fixed and variable deferred and immediate individual annuities; group variable annuities offered through retirement plans; a variety of managed account programs, financial planning services and mutual funds; funding agreements; funding agreements backing notes; and guaranteed investment contracts. The international division provides structured, or bulk, mortgage insurance products as well as analytical tools and technology in Canada, Australia, New Zealand, Mexico, Japan and various European countries. This division also provides payment protection in North America and Europe. The U.S. mortgage insurance segment offers flow, or prime-based, individually underwritten residential mortgage loans. Genworth Financial also has corporate and other activities, which consist primarily of unallocated corporate income and expenses, results of a small, non-core business and most interest and other financing expenses. In May 2007, Genworth sold its employee benefits group business to Sun Life Financial, Inc. In October 2007, Genworth's subsidiary Senior Financial, Inc. acquired Liberty Reverse Mortgage, Inc. for $50 million. In May 2008, the firm agreed to acquire CareScout, a U.S. provider of long term care services, for $12.5 million.

The company offers its employees medical, prescription, vision and dental insurance; short- and long-term disability insurance; a 401(k) plan; a retirement plan; life and AD&D insurance; an employee assistance program; and tuition reimbursement.

FINANCIALS: Sales and profits are in thousands of dollars—add 000 to get the full amount. 2007 Note: Financial information for 2007 was not available for all companies at press time.
2007 Sales: $11,125,000	2007 Profits: $1,154,000	**U.S. Stock Ticker:** GNW
2006 Sales: $10,285,000	2006 Profits: $1,283,000	**Int'l Ticker:** Int'l Exchange:
2005 Sales: $10,504,000	2005 Profits: $1,221,000	Employees: 7,200
2004 Sales: $11,057,000	2004 Profits: $1,157,000	Fiscal Year Ends: 12/31
2003 Sales: $11,671,000	2003 Profits: $1,081,000	Parent Company:

SALARIES/BENEFITS:
Pension Plan: Y	ESOP Stock Plan:	Profit Sharing:	Top Exec. Salary: $1,121,403	Bonus: $9,375,000
Savings Plan: Y	Stock Purch. Plan:		Second Exec. Salary: $613,034	Bonus: $5,025,000

OTHER THOUGHTS:
Apparent Women Officers or Directors: 5
Hot Spot for Advancement for Women/Minorities: Y

LOCATIONS: ("Y" = Yes)
West:	Southwest:	Midwest:	Southeast:	Northeast:	International:
Y	Y	Y	Y	Y	Y

Note: Financial information, benefits and other data can change quickly and may vary from those stated here.

GEO GROUP INC
www.wcc-corrections.com

Industry Group Code: 561610 Ranks within this company's industry group: Sales: 2 Profits: 2

Management:		Sales/Marketing:		Liberal Arts:		Information Systems:		Professionals:		Technical/Scientific:	
Mgmt. Trainees:		Mktg. Professionals:		Gen. Writing/Editing:		Info. Management:	Y	Finance/Accounting:	Y	Engineers, Elec.:	
Experienced Mgmt.:	Y	Retail Sales:		Technical Writing:		Software Dev.:		Law:	Y	Engineers, Other:	
Int'l Business:	Y	Commercial/Industrial:	Y	Graphic Arts/Photog.:		Hardware Dev.:		HR/Other:	Y	Health/Lab:	
MBA Graduates:	Y	Sales Trainees:		Music:		Systems Integration:		Training:	Y	Scientists/Research:	
		Advertising Pros.:		Broadcasting:		Consulting/Other:		Health Care:		Petroleum/Chemicals:	
				Other:				Consulting:		Math/Other:	

TYPES OF BUSINESS:
Prison Management
Institutional Facilities Management
Facilities Maintenance
Facilities Design
Support Services

BRANDS/DIVISIONS/AFFILIATES:
GEO Care, Inc.
CentraCore Properties Trust

CONTACTS: Note: Officers with more than one job title may be intentionally listed here more than once.
George C. Zoley, CEO
Wayne H. Calabrese, COO
Wayne H. Calabrese, Pres.
John G. O'Rourke, CFO/Sr. VP
John J. Bulfin, General Counsel/Sr. VP/Corp. Sec.
Jorge A. Dominicis, Sr. VP-Residential Treatment/Pres., Geo Care, Inc.
John M. Hurley, Sr. VP/Pres., US Corrections
Thomas M. Wierdsma, Sr. VP-Project Dev.
George C. Zoley, Chmn.
Mark H. Underwood, Sr. VP/Pres., Int'l Svcs.

Phone: 561-893-0101	Fax: 561-999-7635
Toll-Free: 866-301-4436	
Address: 1 Park Plz., 621 NW 53rd St., Ste. 700, Boca Raton, FL 33487 US	

GROWTH PLANS/SPECIAL FEATURES:
GEO Group, Inc. is a provider of government-outsourced services specializing in the management of correctional, detention and mental health and residential treatment facilities in the U.S., Canada, Australia, South Africa and the U.K. It operates a broad range of correctional and detention facilities including maximum, medium and minimum security prisons; immigration detention centers; minimum security detention centers; and mental health and residential treatment facilities. The company operates in four segments: U.S. corrections; international services; GEO Care; and facility construction and design. The U.S. correction segment primarily encompasses the U.S.-based privatized corrections and detention business. The international services segment primarily consists of privatized corrections and detention operations in South Africa, Australia and the U.K. This division review opportunities to further diversify into related foreign-based governmental-outsourced services on an ongoing basis. The GEO Care segment, which is operated by wholly-owned subsidiary GEO Care, Inc., comprises the privatized mental health and residential treatment services business, all of which is currently conducted in the U.S. The facility construction and design segment primarily consists of contracts with various state, local and federal agencies for the design and construction of facilities for which the firm has management contracts. At its correctional and detention facilities, GEO Group offers services that include a wide array of in-facility rehabilitative and educational programs such as basic education through academic programs designed to improve literacy levels and enhance the opportunity to acquire skills planning programs. The company manages 59 facilities totaling roughly 50,400 beds worldwide and has an additional 6,800 beds under development at 10 facilities, including the expansion of five facilities it currently operates and five new facilities under construction. The firm also has about 730 additional inactive beds available to meet customers' potential future demand for bed space. In early 2007, GEO Group acquired CentraCore Properties Trust.

FINANCIALS: Sales and profits are in thousands of dollars—add 000 to get the full amount. 2007 Note: Financial information for 2007 was not available for all companies at press time.
2007 Sales: $1,024,832	2007 Profits: $41,845	U.S. Stock Ticker: GEO
2006 Sales: $860,882	2006 Profits: $30,031	Int'l Ticker: Int'l Exchange:
2005 Sales: $612,900	2005 Profits: $7,006	Employees: 11,037
2004 Sales: $593,994	2004 Profits: $16,815	Fiscal Year Ends: 12/31
2003 Sales: $549,238	2003 Profits: $40,019	Parent Company:

SALARIES/BENEFITS:
Pension Plan:	ESOP Stock Plan:	Profit Sharing:	Top Exec. Salary: $873,269	Bonus: $1,842,750
Savings Plan:	Stock Purch. Plan:		Second Exec. Salary: $613,654	Bonus: $1,036,152

OTHER THOUGHTS:
Apparent Women Officers or Directors: 1
Hot Spot for Advancement for Women/Minorities:

LOCATIONS: ("Y" = Yes)
West:	Southwest:	Midwest:	Southeast:	Northeast:	International:
Y	Y	Y	Y	Y	Y

Note: Financial information, benefits and other data can change quickly and may vary from those stated here.

GEORGIA GULF CORPORATION

www.ggc.com

Industry Group Code: 325000 Ranks within this company's industry group: Sales: 1 Profits: 3

Management:		Sales/Marketing:		Liberal Arts:		Information Systems:		Professionals:		Technical/Scientific:	
Mgmt. Trainees:		Mktg. Professionals:	Y	Gen. Writing/Editing:		Info. Management:	Y	Finance/Accounting:	Y	Engineers, Elec.:	
Experienced Mgmt.:	Y	Retail Sales:		Technical Writing:	Y	Software Dev.:		Law:	Y	Engineers, Other:	Y
Int'l Business:	Y	Commercial/Industrial:	Y	Graphic Arts/Photog.:		Hardware Dev.:		HR/Other:	Y	Health/Lab:	
MBA Graduates:	Y	Sales Trainees:		Music:		Systems Integration:		Training:	Y	Scientists/Research:	Y
		Advertising Pros.:		Broadcasting:		Consulting/Other:		Health Care:		Petroleum/Chemicals:	Y
				Other:				Consulting:		Math/Other:	

TYPES OF BUSINESS:

Basic Chemicals
Building & Home Improvement Products
Outdoor Building Products

BRANDS/DIVISIONS/AFFILIATES:

Royal Group, Inc.
Colorscapes
Windlok
Royal DuraPlank

CONTACTS: Note: Officers with more than one job title may be intentionally listed here more than once.

Paul D. Carrico, CEO
Paul D. Carrico, Pres.
Gregory C. Thompson, CFO
James Worrell, VP-Human Resources
Joel I. Beerman, General Counsel/VP/Sec.
Mark Buckis, Corp. Controller/VP
Mark J. Seal, VP-Outdoor Building Prod.
William H. Doherty, VP-Custom Products
Art Ramey, Pres., Royal Group Sales & Mktg.
Patrick J. Fleming, Chmn.
Charles Ulik, Pres., Canadian Window & Door Profiles & Mouldings
C. Douglas Shannon, VP-Procurement

Phone: 770-395-4500	Fax: 770-395-4529
Toll-Free:	
Address: 115 Perimeter Center Pl., Ste. 460, Atlanta, GA 30346 US	

GROWTH PLANS/SPECIAL FEATURES:

Georgia Gulf Corporation manufactures and markets two integrated chemical product lines, chlorovinyls and aromatics. The company operates in four segments: Chlorovinyls; window and door profiles and mouldings products; outdoor building products; and aromatics. The chlorovinyls segment sells a chain of products, which includes chlorine, caustic soda, ethylene dichloride (EDC), vinyl chloride monomer (VCM), vinyl resins and compounds. In North America, Georgia Gulf is one of the largest producers of VCM, vinyl resins and vinyl compounds. These chlorovinyls are sold to customers in the electrical, insulation, piping, siding, windows, chemical, pulp, paper and alumina industries. The window and door profiles and mouldings segment consists of extruded vinyl window and door profiles as well as interior and exterior mouldings. The company operates 16 manufacturing facilities located in Canada and the U.S, as well as a number of distribution centers. The outdoor building products segment, operating 12 manufacturing facilities, produces siding; pipe and pipe fittings; and deck, fence and rail outdoor storage buildings. Siding is sold under the brand names Colorscapes, Windlok and Royal DuraPlank. The aromatics segment produces cumene and the co-products phenol and acetone. The company is the second largest worldwide producer of cumene. The firm also markets vinyl-based building and home improvement products under the Royal Group brand names. In 2007, the company announced plans to close one of its Royal Group window and door profile extrusion plant in Winnipeg. In 2008, Georgia Gulf sold its outdoor storage buildings business for $13 million; sold and leased buildings in Ontario for $13.5 million; and proceeded to use the money to pay down debt. Also in 2008, the company closed its polyvinyl chloride (PVC) plant in Oklahoma.

The company offers its employees health and welfare benefits, life insurance, short- and long-term benefits and a 401(k) plan.

FINANCIALS: Sales and profits are in thousands of dollars—add 000 to get the full amount. 2007 Note: Financial information for 2007 was not available for all companies at press time.

2007 Sales: $3,157,270	2007 Profits: $-266,027	U.S. Stock Ticker: GGC
2006 Sales: $2,427,843	2006 Profits: $48,539	Int'l Ticker: Int'l Exchange:
2005 Sales: $2,273,719	2005 Profits: $95,503	Employees: 5,249
2004 Sales: $2,206,239	2004 Profits: $105,892	Fiscal Year Ends: 12/31
2003 Sales: $1,444,483	2003 Profits: $12,495	Parent Company:

SALARIES/BENEFITS:

Pension Plan: Y	ESOP Stock Plan:	Profit Sharing:	Top Exec. Salary: $800,000	Bonus: $
Savings Plan: Y	Stock Purch. Plan:		Second Exec. Salary: $360,000	Bonus: $

OTHER THOUGHTS:

Apparent Women Officers or Directors:
Hot Spot for Advancement for Women/Minorities:

LOCATIONS: ("Y" = Yes)

West:	Southwest:	Midwest:	Southeast:	Northeast:	International:
Y	Y	Y	Y	Y	Y

Note: Financial information, benefits and other data can change quickly and may vary from those stated here.

GLOBAL HYATT CORPORATION

www.hyatt.com

Industry Group Code: 721110 Ranks within this company's industry group: Sales: Profits:

Management:		Sales/Marketing:		Liberal Arts:		Information Systems:		Professionals:		Technical/Scientific:	
Mgmt. Trainees:	Y	Mktg. Professionals:	Y	Gen. Writing/Editing:	Y	Info. Management:	Y	Finance/Accounting:	Y	Engineers, Elec.:	
Experienced Mgmt.:	Y	Retail Sales:		Technical Writing:		Software Dev.:	Y	Law:	Y	Engineers, Other:	
Int'l Business:	Y	Commercial/Industrial:	Y	Graphic Arts/Photog.:	Y	Hardware Dev.:		HR/Other:	Y	Health/Lab:	
MBA Graduates:	Y	Sales Trainees:		Music:		Systems Integration:	Y	Training:	Y	Scientists/Research:	
		Advertising Pros.:	Y	Broadcasting:		Consulting/Other:		Health Care:		Petroleum/Chemicals:	
				Other:	Y			Consulting:		Math/Other:	

TYPES OF BUSINESS:

Hotel Ownership & Management
Timeshares
Golf Courses
Gaming
Retirement Communities
Motels & Inns
Hotel Franchising

BRANDS/DIVISIONS/AFFILIATES:

Hyatt Regency
Grand Hyatt
Hyatt Resorts
Hyatt Summerfield Suites
U.S. Franchise Systems, Inc.
Hyatt Vacation Ownership, Inc.
Hyatt Gold Passport
Andaz

CONTACTS: Note: Officers with more than one job title may be intentionally listed here more than once.

Mark S. Hoplamazian, CEO
Mark S. Hoplamazian, Pres.
Katie Meyer, VP-Corp. Comm.
Steve Sokal, Sr. VP-Global Asset Mgmt.
Steve Haggerty, Exec. VP-Real Estate Dev.
Jill Johnson, VP-Asset Mgmt.
Thomas J. Pritzker, Chmn.

Phone: 312-750-1234	Fax: 312-750-8550
Toll-Free:	
Address: 71 S. Wacker Dr.. 16th Fl., Chicago, IL 60606 US	

GROWTH PLANS/SPECIAL FEATURES:

Global Hyatt Corporation (Hyatt) owns and operates full-service luxury hotels. With its subsidiaries, Hyatt offers approximately 140,000 rooms in over 750 resorts and hotels across 45 countries, and its brands include the following. Its best known brand, Hyatt Regency, caters mainly to corporate travel clients. Grand Hyatt hotels cater to leisure and business travelers and include accommodations for banquets and conferences. Hyatt Resorts often feature professional, PGA golf courses; adventure travel opportunities, such as scuba diving, biking, hot air balloon trips or horseback riding; Hyatt Pure spas; and activities for kids and families. Hyatt Summerfield Suites, an all-suites hotel concept designed to feel more like home, offers 32-inch HDTVs, a full kitchen and complementary shopping service for its outdoor BBQ-pits. Recently introduced Hyatt Place hotels feature high-tech amenities such as 42-inch HDTVs in every room, free Wi-Fi Internet access and a 24-hour, touch-screen room service ordering system. Lastly, Park Hyatt hotels are smaller, full-service luxury hotels that offer unique services including limited time specials and Pamper at the Park, which includes breakfast and spa time. Hyatt is also the owner of U.S. Franchise Systems, Inc., which franchises Hawthorn Suites and Microtel Inns and Suites. Additionally, subsidiary Hyatt Vacation Ownership, Inc. offers vacation ownership and vacation rental opportunities, offering members timeshare or points-based resort vacation opportunities. Hyatt hotel services include Hyatt Gold Passport, a frequent-traveler rewards program; and some properties feature casinos. In February 2007, Hyatt completed the first phase of its $60 million renovation of its Hyatt Regency O'Hare property, one of the world's largest convention hotels. In April 2007, the firm launched its newest brand, Andaz, which has one hotel in London, with three more under development in New York and Texas.

Employees of Hyatt receive complementary hotel rooms; medical, dental, vision and prescription drug coverage; and life insurance.

FINANCIALS: Sales and profits are in thousands of dollars—add 000 to get the full amount. 2007 Note: Financial information for 2007 was not available for all companies at press time.

2007 Sales: $3,750,000	2007 Profits: $	U.S. Stock Ticker: Private
2006 Sales: $3,500,000	2006 Profits: $	Int'l Ticker: Int'l Exchange:
2005 Sales: $7,266,000	2005 Profits: $	Employees:
2004 Sales: $5,500,000	2004 Profits: $	Fiscal Year Ends: 1/31
2003 Sales: $	2003 Profits: $	Parent Company:

SALARIES/BENEFITS:

Pension Plan:	ESOP Stock Plan:	Profit Sharing:	Top Exec. Salary: $	Bonus: $
Savings Plan: Y	Stock Purch. Plan:		Second Exec. Salary: $	Bonus: $

OTHER THOUGHTS:

Apparent Women Officers or Directors: 2
Hot Spot for Advancement for Women/Minorities:

LOCATIONS: ("Y" = Yes)

West:	Southwest:	Midwest:	Southeast:	Northeast:	International:
Y	Y	Y	Y	Y	Y

GLOBAL PAYMENTS INC   www.globalpaymentsinc.com

Industry Group Code: 522320 **Ranks within this company's industry group:** Sales: 6   Profits: 6

Management:		Sales/Marketing:		Liberal Arts:		Information Systems:		Professionals:		Technical/Scientific:	
Mgmt. Trainees:	Y	Mktg. Professionals:	Y	Gen. Writing/Editing:		Info. Management:	Y	Finance/Accounting:	Y	Engineers, Elec.:	Y
Experienced Mgmt.:	Y	Retail Sales:		Technical Writing:		Software Dev.:	Y	Law:	Y	Engineers, Other:	Y
Int'l Business:	Y	Commercial/Industrial:	Y	Graphic Arts/Photog.:		Hardware Dev.:	Y	HR/Other:	Y	Health/Lab:	
MBA Graduates:	Y	Sales Trainees:	Y	Music:		Systems Integration:		Training:	Y	Scientists/Research:	Y
		Advertising Pros.:	Y	Broadcasting:		Consulting/Other:		Health Care:		Petroleum/Chemicals:	
				Other:				Consulting:		Math/Other:	

TYPES OF BUSINESS:

Electronic Payment Processing
Credit & Debit Card Processing
Funds Transfer Services
Check Guarantee Services
Merchant Services

BRANDS/DIVISIONS/AFFILIATES:

Global Payments Europe
DolEx

CONTACTS: Note: Officers with more than one job title may be intentionally listed here more than once.

Paul R. Garcia, CEO
James G. Kelly, COO/Sr. Exec. VP
Paul R. Garcia, Pres.
Joseph C. Hyde, CFO/Exec. VP
Morgan M. (Mac) Schuessler, Exec. VP-Human Resources
Suellyn P. Tornay, General Counsel/Exec. VP
Morgan M. (Mac) Schuessler, Exec. VP-Corp. Comm.
Martin A. Picciano, Chief Acct. Officer/Sr. VP-Acct.
George Zelinski, Pres., North American Money Transfer
Jose Salinas Nilson, Pres., European Money Transfer
Paul R. Garcia, Chmn.
Carl J. Williams, Pres., Worldwide Payment Processing

Phone: 770-829-8236	Fax: 770-829-8267
Toll-Free: 800-560-2960	
Address: 10 Glenlake Pkwy., N. Tower, Atlanta, GA 30328 US	

GROWTH PLANS/SPECIAL FEATURES:

Global Payments, Inc. is a leading payment processing and consumer money transfer company enabling merchants, multinational corporations, financial institutions, consumers, government agencies and other profit and non-profit business enterprises to facilitate payments or further other economic goals. Global Payments markets its products and services throughout the U.S., Canada, Europe and the Asia-Pacific region. It operates in two business segments: merchant services and money transfer. It operates 875 originating retail branch locations in the U.S. and 68 in Europe. Global Payments has settlement arrangements with over 12,000 bank, exchange house and retail locations worldwide. The company's offerings in its merchant services segment provide merchants, independent sales organizations (ISOs) and financial institutions with credit and debit card transaction processing and check-related services. Global Payments also offers sales, installation and servicing of ATM and point of sale terminals and selected card issuing services through its Czech Republic-based Global Payments Europe subsidiary. The company markets its merchant services both directly, using a salaried and commissioned sales force, ISOs and independent sales representatives to sell its products directly to merchants; and indirectly, providing its products and services primarily to financial institutions and a limited number of ISOs on an unbundled basis, which in turn resell its products and services to merchants. Global Payments Europe provides the company's indirect merchant services in Europe. The company's money transfer segment provides consumer money transfer services primarily marketed through its DolEx brand electronic money transfer services targeting first and second generation Latin Americans living in the U.S.

Global Payments offers its employees an educational assistance program, a PC purchase plan, a 529 college savings plan, an employee assistance program, flexible spending accounts and medical, dental, vision, life and disability insurance.

FINANCIALS: Sales and profits are in thousands of dollars—add 000 to get the full amount. 2007 Note: Financial information for 2007 was not available for all companies at press time.

2007 Sales: $1,061,523	2007 Profits: $142,985	U.S. Stock Ticker: GPN
2006 Sales: $908,056	2006 Profits: $125,524	Int'l Ticker: Int'l Exchange:
2005 Sales: $784,331	2005 Profits: $92,896	Employees: 4,680
2004 Sales: $629,320	2004 Profits: $62,443	Fiscal Year Ends: 5/31
2003 Sales: $516,084	2003 Profits: $53,300	Parent Company:

SALARIES/BENEFITS:

Pension Plan:	ESOP Stock Plan:	Profit Sharing:	Top Exec. Salary: $779,077	Bonus: $732,000
Savings Plan: Y	Stock Purch. Plan: Y		Second Exec. Salary: $479,385	Bonus: $351,000

OTHER THOUGHTS:

Apparent Women Officers or Directors: 2
Hot Spot for Advancement for Women/Minorities: Y

LOCATIONS: ("Y" = Yes)

West:	Southwest:	Midwest:	Southeast:	Northeast:	International:
Y	Y	Y	Y	Y	Y

Note: Financial information, benefits and other data can change quickly and may vary from those stated here.

GOOGLE INC

www.google.com

Industry Group Code: 514199B **Ranks within this company's industry group:** Sales: 1　Profits: 1

Management:		Sales/Marketing:		Liberal Arts:		Information Systems:		Professionals:		Technical/Scientific:	
Mgmt. Trainees:	Y	Mktg. Professionals:	Y	Gen. Writing/Editing:	Y	Info. Management:	Y	Finance/Accounting:	Y	Engineers, Elec.:	Y
Experienced Mgmt.:	Y	Retail Sales:		Technical Writing:	Y	Software Dev.:	Y	Law:	Y	Engineers, Other:	
Int'l Business:	Y	Commercial/Industrial:	Y	Graphic Arts/Photog.:	Y	Hardware Dev.:		HR/Other:	Y	Health/Lab:	
MBA Graduates:	Y	Sales Trainees:		Music:		Systems Integration:		Training:	Y	Scientists/Research:	
		Advertising Pros.:	Y	Broadcasting:		Consulting/Other:		Health Care:		Petroleum/Chemicals:	
				Other:				Consulting:		Math/Other:	

TYPES OF BUSINESS:

Search Engine-Internet
Paid Search Listing Advertising Services
News Site Search Service
Catalog Search Service
Shopping Site
Web Log Tool
Search and Advertising on Cellphones

BRANDS/DIVISIONS/AFFILIATES:

Google
Google AdWords
Google AdSense
MySpace
DoubleClick
Adscape Media, Inc.
YouTube
ZAO Begun

CONTACTS: *Note: Officers with more than one job title may be intentionally listed here more than once.*

Eric Schmidt, CEO
Patrick Pichette, CFO/Sr. VP
Omid Kordestani, Sr. VP-Worldwide Sales & Bus. Dev.
Laszlo Bock, VP-People Oper.
Alan Eustace, Sr. VP-Research/Eng.
Ben Fried, CIO
Sergey Brin, Pres., Tech./Co-Founder
Larry Page, Pres., Products/Co-Founder
W.M. Coughran, Jr., Sr. VP-Eng.
David C. Drummond, Chief Legal Officer
David C. Drummond, VP-Corp. Dev.
Vinton G. Cerf., Chief Internet Evangelist/VP
Rachel Whetstone, VP-Global Comm. & Public Affairs
Mark Fuchs, VP-Finance/Chief Acct.
Shona Brown, Sr. VP-Bus. Oper.
Jeff Huber, Sr. VP-Eng.
Jonathan Rosenberg, Sr. VP-Product Management
Penry Price, VP-Advertising Sales, North America
Eric Schmidt, Chmn.
Omid Kordestani, Sr. VP-Global Sales/Bus. Dev.

Phone: 650-623-4000	Fax: 650-253-0001
Toll-Free:	
Address: 1600 Amphitheatre Pkwy., Mountain View, CA 94043 US	

GROWTH PLANS/SPECIAL FEATURES:

Google, Inc. operates Google.com, one of the worlds largest and most used search engines, which indexes the content of over 8 billion Internet pages. While Google charges nothing for its search engine, it charges fees to other sites that use its search technology, and has a lucrative program that enables business clients to bid for ad space. Google provides its services in 116 different languages, with more than 50% of its searches coming from outside the U.S. The company's technology employs a unique, distributed-computing system utilizing thousands of low-end servers rather than a small number of high-powered computers. The company offers Google AdWords, a global advertising program which presents ads to customers precisely when they are looking for what the advertiser has to offer. Google AdSense allows web sites in the Google Network to serve targeted ads from the AdWords advertisers. In March 2008, the firm announced the acquisition of DoubleClick. DoubleClick offers online ad serving and management technology to advertisers, web publishers and ad agencies. In July 2008, the company announced that it has signed an agreement with Rambler Media to acquire ZAO Begun, a Russian context advertising service

Employee benefits include medical, dental and vision insurance; 401(k); 18 weeks maternity leave; flexible spending accounts; college savings plan; adoption assistance; tuition reimbursement; free on-site lunches and dinners; paid vacation that increases with years of service;. Google also provides recreation facilities, financial planning classes and on-site dry cleaning, oil change and car wash facilities.

FINANCIALS: Sales and profits are in thousands of dollars—add 000 to get the full amount. 2007 Note: Financial information for 2007 was not available for all companies at press time.

2007 Sales: $16,593,986	2007 Profits: $4,203,720	**U.S. Stock Ticker: GOOG**
2006 Sales: $10,604,917	2006 Profits: $3,077,446	**Int'l Ticker:**　Int'l Exchange:
2005 Sales: $6,138,560	2005 Profits: $1,465,397	Employees:　16,805
2004 Sales: $3,189,223	2004 Profits: $399,119	Fiscal Year Ends: 12/31
2003 Sales: $1,465,934	2003 Profits: $105,648	Parent Company:

SALARIES/BENEFITS:

Pension Plan: Y	ESOP Stock Plan:	Profit Sharing:	Top Exec. Salary: $250,000	Bonus: $927,000
Savings Plan: Y	Stock Purch. Plan:		Second Exec. Salary: $250,000	Bonus: $764,367

OTHER THOUGHTS:

Apparent Women Officers or Directors: 9
Hot Spot for Advancement for Women/Minorities: Y

LOCATIONS: ("Y" = Yes)

West:	Southwest:	Midwest:	Southeast:	Northeast:	International:
Y	Y			Y	Y

GRANT THORNTON LLP
www.grantthornton.com

Industry Group Code: 541210 Ranks within this company's industry group: Sales: 4 Profits:

Management:		Sales/Marketing:		Liberal Arts:		Information Systems:		Professionals:		Technical/Scientific:	
Mgmt. Trainees:		Mktg. Professionals:	Y	Gen. Writing/Editing:	Y	Info. Management:	Y	Finance/Accounting:	Y	Engineers, Elec.:	
Experienced Mgmt.:	Y	Retail Sales:		Technical Writing:	Y	Software Dev.:		Law:	Y	Engineers, Other:	
Int'l Business:		Commercial/Industrial:	Y	Graphic Arts/Photog.:		Hardware Dev.:		HR/Other:	Y	Health/Lab:	
MBA Graduates:	Y	Sales Trainees:		Music:		Systems Integration:	Y	Training:	Y	Scientists/Research:	
		Advertising Pros.:	Y	Broadcasting:		Consulting/Other:	Y	Health Care:		Petroleum/Chemicals:	
				Other:	Y			Consulting:	Y	Math/Other:	

TYPES OF BUSINESS:
Accounting & Auditing Services
Financial Services
Administration Consulting

BRANDS/DIVISIONS/AFFILIATES:
Grant Thornton International
On The Horizon
Grant Thornton U.S.A.

CONTACTS: *Note: Officers with more than one job title may be intentionally listed here more than once.*
Edward E. Nusbaum, CEO
C. Morgan Kinghorn, COO
William E. Schultz, CFO
David Holyoak, CIO
Trent Gazzaway, Managing Partner-Corp. Gov.
Anne McGeorge, National Managing Partner-Health Care Practice
Lewis W. Crenshaw, Exec. Dir.-Global Public Sector

Phone: 312-856-0200	Fax: 312-602-8099
Toll-Free:	
Address: 175 W. Jackson Blvd., Fl. 20, Chicago, IL 60604 US	

GROWTH PLANS/SPECIAL FEATURES:

Grant Thornton LLP is the U.S. arm of Grant Thornton International, a global accounting, tax and business advisory organization with over 50 offices across the country. The company seeks to become a leading accounting firm in the U.S., as a provider of specialist financial, tax and advisory services, for mid-cap, small-cap and privately held clients. Some of its key audit and assurance services are integrated auditing, benefits management and public finance. The company's investment banking services involve sell side advisory, buy side advisory, management buyouts, restructurings and capital raising. It also offers more general administrative consulting services, such as Sarbanes-Oxley compliance; services for Chief Information Officers and Chief Financial Officers; project management office strategies; and performance improvement. Grant Thornton specializes in the construction, real estate, health care, technology, non-profit and financial services industries. Grant Thornton offers audit and assurance services tailored to particular needs, as well as providing the public with a series of publications, including On the Horizon, which publishes weekly news on developments in the accounting world. With support from Grant Thornton International's investment banking teams in London, Paris, Hamburg and Hong Kong, as well as other offices in the organization, Grant Thornton U.S.A. can assist international clients with cross-border merger and acquisition activities. The company also provides expatriate services, international tax services and transfer pricing. In February 2007, Grant Thornton launched a private equity initiative that will enhance the value of the services that it provides through a point of contact approach. In February 2008, the company unveiled a new brand identity, logo and website. The new brand identity will be adopted by all member firms, domestic and international.

Grant Thornton's employee benefits include medical and dental plans, extended to domestic partners; reimbursement accounts; 401(k); a variety of insurance offerings; employee assistance; elder care; and legal services.

FINANCIALS: Sales and profits are in thousands of dollars—add 000 to get the full amount. 2007 Note: Financial information for 2007 was not available for all companies at press time.

2007 Sales: $1,075,000	2007 Profits: $	U.S. Stock Ticker: Private
2006 Sales: $886,000	2006 Profits: $	Int'l Ticker: Int'l Exchange:
2005 Sales: $795,000	2005 Profits: $	Employees:
2004 Sales: $635,000	2004 Profits: $	Fiscal Year Ends: 7/31
2003 Sales: $485,000	2003 Profits: $	Parent Company:

SALARIES/BENEFITS:

Pension Plan:	ESOP Stock Plan:	Profit Sharing:	Top Exec. Salary: $	Bonus: $
Savings Plan: Y	Stock Purch. Plan:		Second Exec. Salary: $	Bonus: $

OTHER THOUGHTS:
Apparent Women Officers or Directors: 1
Hot Spot for Advancement for Women/Minorities:

LOCATIONS: ("Y" = Yes)

West:	Southwest:	Midwest:	Southeast:	Northeast:	International:
Y	Y	Y	Y	Y	

GTECH HOLDINGS CORP
www.gtech.com

Industry Group Code: 713290 Ranks within this company's industry group: Sales: 1   Profits: 1

Management:		Sales/Marketing:		Liberal Arts:		Information Systems:		Professionals:		Technical/Scientific:	
Mgmt. Trainees:	Y	Mktg. Professionals:	Y	Gen. Writing/Editing:		Info. Management:	Y	Finance/Accounting:	Y	Engineers, Elec.:	Y
Experienced Mgmt.:	Y	Retail Sales:		Technical Writing:	Y	Software Dev.:		Law:	Y	Engineers, Other:	
Int'l Business:	Y	Commercial/Industrial:	Y	Graphic Arts/Photog.:	Y	Hardware Dev.:		HR/Other:	Y	Health/Lab:	
MBA Graduates:	Y	Sales Trainees:		Music:		Systems Integration:		Training:	Y	Scientists/Research:	
		Advertising Pros.:		Broadcasting:		Consulting/Other:		Health Care:		Petroleum/Chemicals:	
				Other:				Consulting:		Math/Other:	Y

TYPES OF BUSINESS:

Lottery Systems
Lottery Technology Services
Online Game Products & Services
Printing

BRANDS/DIVISIONS/AFFILIATES:

Europrint
BillBird
Interlott
Finsoft
Innoka
Veikkaus Oy
Lottomatica S.p.A.
Creative Games International

CONTACTS: *Note: Officers with more than one job title may be intentionally listed here more than once.*

W. Bruce Turner, CEO
Jaymin B. Patel, COO
Jaymin B. Patel, Pres.
Stefano Bortoli, CFO/Sr. VP
Connie Laverty O'Connor, Chief Mktg. Officer/Sr. VP
John L. Pothin, Sr. VP-Human Resources
Charles Cautley, CTO/Sr. VP
Walter G. DeSocio, Chief Admin. Officer/Sr. VP
Michael K. Prescott, General Counsel/Sr. VP/Corp. Sec.
Fabio Celadon, Sr. VP-Strategic Planning
Robert Vincent, VP-Corp. Affairs
Ross Dalton, Sr. VP-Printed Prod. & Licensed Content Markets
Alan Eland, Sr. VP-GTECH Americas
Donald R. Sweitzer, Sr. VP-Global Bus. Dev. & Public Affairs
Gerhard H. Burda, Sr. VP-Gaming Solutions
Donald R. Sweitzer, Chmn.
Declan Harkin, Sr. VP-GTECH Int'l

Phone: 401-392-1000	Fax: 401-392-1234
Toll-Free:	
Address: GTECH Center, 10 Memorial Blvd., Providence, RI 02903 US	

GROWTH PLANS/SPECIAL FEATURES:

GTECH Holdings Corp., a subsidiary of Lottomatica S.p.A., is a global gaming technology and services company. The company's core business is the lottery industry, in which it does business in 45 countries. The company provides integrated online lottery solutions, services and products to governmental lottery authorities and governmental licensees worldwide. GTECH offers its customers a full range of lottery technology services, including the design, assembly, installation, operation, maintenance and marketing of online lottery systems and instant ticket support systems. The firm has introduced several new online products and services, including Aladdin, a credit-card-sized lottery ticket that can be reused up to 500 times; the Extra-Online game, an online lottery game that allows players to purchase an additional game with instant-ticket features; and e-scratch, a web-based interactive suite of scratch and reveal games. The company also owns IGI Europrint, a provider of promotional games, contests and sweepstakes; Leeward Islands Lottery Holding Company, which operates lotteries throughout the Caribbean; BillBird, an electronic bill payment service in Poland; Interlott, a leading ITVM technology company; Leeward Islands Lottery Holding Co., a lottery operator; Finsoft, a provider of real-time transaction and information management systems; Innoka, jointly owned with Veikkaus Oy, the Finish National Lottery and GTECH Printing. GTECH and Medstroms AB acquired roughly 92% of the outstanding share capital and voting rights in Boss Media AB in March 2008. In April 2008, GTECH entered into an agreement to acquire a 90% interest in St Enodoc Holdings Limited and its subsidiaries. In May 2008, the firm acquired the remaining 50% interest in the Atronic group which was owned by Gauselmann Group.

The company offers its employees medical, dental and vision plans; domestic partner benefits; business travel accident insurance; flexible spending accounts; a 401(k) plan; a college savings plan; education assistance; and employee assistance programs.

FINANCIALS: Sales and profits are in thousands of dollars—add 000 to get the full amount. 2007 Note: Financial information for 2007 was not available for all companies at press time.

2007 Sales: $1,206,846	2007 Profits: $	U.S. Stock Ticker: Subsidiary
2006 Sales: $415,699	2006 Profits: $	Int'l Ticker: Int'l Exchange:
2005 Sales: $	2005 Profits: $	Employees: 5,300
2004 Sales: $	2004 Profits: $	Fiscal Year Ends:
2003 Sales: $	2003 Profits: $	Parent Company: LOTTOMATICA SPA

SALARIES/BENEFITS:

Pension Plan:	ESOP Stock Plan:	Profit Sharing:	Top Exec. Salary: $746,154	Bonus: $
Savings Plan: Y	Stock Purch. Plan:		Second Exec. Salary: $488,077	Bonus: $

OTHER THOUGHTS:

Apparent Women Officers or Directors: 1
Hot Spot for Advancement for Women/Minorities:

LOCATIONS: ("Y" = Yes)

West:	Southwest:	Midwest:	Southeast:	Northeast:	International:
Y	Y	Y	Y	Y	Y

Note: Financial information, benefits and other data can change quickly and may vary from those stated here.

GUESS? INC

www.guessinc.com

Industry Group Code: 448000 Ranks within this company's industry group: Sales: 6   Profits: 7

Management:		Sales/Marketing:		Liberal Arts:		Information Systems:		Professionals:		Technical/Scientific:	
Mgmt. Trainees:	Y	Mktg. Professionals:	Y	Gen. Writing/Editing:	Y	Info. Management:	Y	Finance/Accounting:	Y	Engineers, Elec.:	
Experienced Mgmt.:	Y	Retail Sales:	Y	Technical Writing:		Software Dev.:	Y	Law:	Y	Engineers, Other:	
Int'l Business:	Y	Commercial/Industrial:	Y	Graphic Arts/Photog.:	Y	Hardware Dev.:		HR/Other:	Y	Health/Lab:	
MBA Graduates:	Y	Sales Trainees:	Y	Music:		Systems Integration:		Training:	Y	Scientists/Research:	
		Advertising Pros.:	Y	Broadcasting:		Consulting/Other:		Health Care:		Petroleum/Chemicals:	
				Other:	Y			Consulting:		Math/Other:	

TYPES OF BUSINESS:
Casual Clothing Stores
Accessories
Fragrances
Footwear
Online Sales
Jeans

BRANDS/DIVISIONS/AFFILIATES:
Baby GUESS
Guess? Jeans
Triangle Design
Question Mark
Marciano
Brand G
Baby GUESS
Focus Europe, S.r.l.

CONTACTS: *Note: Officers with more than one job title may be intentionally listed here more than once.*
Paul Marciano, CEO
Carlos Alberini, COO
Carlos Alberini, Pres.
Dennis Secor, CFO/Sr. VP
Dennis Secor, Principal Financial & Acct. Officer
Joseph Teklits, Integrated Corp. Rel.
Massimo Macchi, Pres., Guess Europe
Maurice Marciano, Chmn.

Phone: 213-765-3100	Fax:
Toll-Free: 800-224-8377	
Address: 1444 S. Alameda St., Los Angeles, CA 90021 US	

GROWTH PLANS/SPECIAL FEATURES:
Guess?, Inc. designs, markets, distributes and licenses lifestyle collections of contemporary apparel and accessories for men, women and children that reflect the American lifestyle and European fashion sensibilities. The company's apparel is marketed under trademarks including GUESS, GUESS?, GUESS U.S.A., GUESS Jeans, Triangle Design, Question Mark, Brand G, a stylized G, GUESS Kids, Baby GUESS, YES and Marciano. The lines include full collections of denim and cotton clothing, including jeans, pants, overalls, skirts, dresses, shorts, blouses, shirts, jackets and knitwear. The firm also grants licenses to manufacture and distribute a broad range of products that complement its apparel lines, including eyewear, watches, handbags, footwear, infants' and children's apparel, leather apparel, fragrance, jewelry and other fashion accessories. Guess products are sold through three primary distribution channels: its own stores in the U.S. and Canada, a network of wholesale accounts in the U.S. and via the Internet. The company operates 373 stores in U.S. and Canada, consisting of 187 full-price retail stores, 97 factory outlet stores, 38 Marciano stores and 17 Guess Accessories stores; 24 stores in Europe; and three stores in Mexico through a majority owned joint venture. Guess' international licensees and distributors operate 579 Guess stores in about 65 countries outside of North America. The company opened 49 new stores in the U.S. and Canada during 2008.

Guess offers its employees medical, dental and vision insurance; flexible spending accounts; an employee assistance program; life and AD&D insurance; short- and long-term disability; a 401(k) plan; an employee stock purchase plan; a corporate wellness program; access to a credit union; and tuition reimbursement.

FINANCIALS: Sales and profits are in thousands of dollars—add 000 to get the full amount. 2007 Note: Financial information for 2007 was not available for all companies at press time.

2007 Sales: $1,252,664	2007 Profits: $131,172	U.S. Stock Ticker: GES	
2006 Sales: $1,185,184	2006 Profits: $123,168	Int'l Ticker:	Int'l Exchange:
2005 Sales: $936,092	2005 Profits: $58,813	Employees: 8,800	
2004 Sales: $729,262	2004 Profits: $29,566	Fiscal Year Ends: 12/31	
2003 Sales: $636,585	2003 Profits: $7,286	Parent Company:	

SALARIES/BENEFITS:

Pension Plan:	ESOP Stock Plan:	Profit Sharing:	Top Exec. Salary: $1,000,000	Bonus: $4,187,459
Savings Plan: Y	Stock Purch. Plan:		Second Exec. Salary: $900,000	Bonus: $1,440,000

OTHER THOUGHTS:
Apparent Women Officers or Directors: 2
Hot Spot for Advancement for Women/Minorities: Y

LOCATIONS: ("Y" = Yes)

West:	Southwest:	Midwest:	Southeast:	Northeast:	International:
Y	Y	Y	Y	Y	Y

Note: Financial information, benefits and other data can change quickly and may vary from those stated here.

HALLIBURTON COMPANY   www.halliburton.com

Industry Group Code: 213111   Ranks within this company's industry group: Sales: 1   Profits: 3

Management:		Sales/Marketing:		Liberal Arts:		Information Systems:		Professionals:		Technical/Scientific:	
Mgmt. Trainees:	Y	Mktg. Professionals:	Y	Gen. Writing/Editing:		Info. Management:	Y	Finance/Accounting:	Y	Engineers, Elec.:	Y
Experienced Mgmt.:	Y	Retail Sales:		Technical Writing:	Y	Software Dev.:	Y	Law:	Y	Engineers, Other:	
Int'l Business:	Y	Commercial/Industrial:	Y	Graphic Arts/Photog.:	Y	Hardware Dev.:		HR/Other:	Y	Health/Lab:	Y
MBA Graduates:	Y	Sales Trainees:		Music:		Systems Integration:		Training:	Y	Scientists/Research:	Y
		Advertising Pros.:		Broadcasting:		Consulting/Other:		Health Care:		Petroleum/Chemicals:	Y
				Other:				Consulting:		Math/Other:	

TYPES OF BUSINESS:
Oil & Gas Drilling Support Services
Software Information Systems

BRANDS/DIVISIONS/AFFILIATES:
Landmark
Security DBS Drill Bits
Sperry Drilling Services
Easywell
Ultraline Service Corp.
PSL Energy Services, Ltd.
WellDynamics
OOO Burservice

CONTACTS: *Note: Officers with more than one job title may be intentionally listed here more than once.*
David J. Lesar, CEO
Andrew Lane, COO/Exec. VP
David J. Lesar, Pres.
Mark A. McCollum, CFO/Exec. VP
Lawrence Pope, Chief Human Resources Officer
Lawrence Pope, VP-Admin.
Bert Cornelison, General Counsel/Exec. VP
Tim Probert, Exec. VP-Strategy & Corp. Dev.
Christian Garcia, VP-Investor Rel.
Craig Nunez, Treas./Sr. VP
Sherry Williams, Corp. Sec./VP
Christopher (Cris) Gaut, Pres., Halliburton's Drilling & Evaluation Div.
Evelyn Angelle, Corp. Controller/Principal Acct. Officer/VP
David J. Lesar, Chmn.

Phone: 713-759-2605	**Fax:** 713-759-2635
Toll-Free: 888-669-3920	
Address: 5 Houston Center, 1401 McKinney, Ste. 2400, Houston, TX 77010 US	

GROWTH PLANS/SPECIAL FEATURES:
Halliburton Company is a leading provider of products and services to the petroleum and energy industries. The firm is structured into two divisions: Drilling and Evaluation; and Completion and Production. The Drilling and Evaluation division is split into five subdivisions. Baroid Fluid Services provides fluids that support well completion, drilling, solids control and waste management. Landmark offers software and other IT solutions to support and help coordinate various oilfield operations. Security DBS Drill Bits supplies fixed cutter and roller cone drill bits and tools to perform hole enlargement, torque reduction and drag resistance improvement. Sperry Drilling Services offers directional drilling and other services including data logging. Finally, the wireline and perforating subdivision provides measurement and evaluation services. The Completion and Production division provides various testing, measuring and well productivity services. Cementing helps seal well bores, increasing productivity. Stimulation services include acidizing and fracturing, which inject various high-pressure substances into a well, forcing petroleum out. The Easywell subdivision sells a proprietary screen, valve and isolation system. Hydraulic Workover units perform basic well maintenance. The Pipeline & Process Services subdivision provides products that help start, stop and clean wells. Finally, its Sand Control subdivision includes numerous products to aid sandstone wells. The Drilling and Evaluation segment produces approximately 44% of the firm's revenue, Completion and Production, 56%. In 2007, International revenue accounted for 53% while North American revenue represented 47%. In November 2007, Halliburton acquired OOO Burservice, a Russian directional drilling services provider. In July 2008, Halliburton acquired WellDynamics, an intelligent completion technology provider for the oil industry.

FINANCIALS: Sales and profits are in thousands of dollars—add 000 to get the full amount. 2007 Note: Financial information for 2007 was not available for all companies at press time.

2007 Sales: $15,264,000		2007 Profits: $3,499,000	**U.S. Stock Ticker: HAL**
2006 Sales: $12,955,000		2006 Profits: $2,348,000	**Int'l Ticker:** Int'l Exchange:
2005 Sales: $10,100,000		2005 Profits: $2,358,000	Employees: 51,000
2004 Sales: $19,878,000		2004 Profits: $-979,000	Fiscal Year Ends: 12/31
2003 Sales: $16,271,000		2003 Profits: $-820,000	Parent Company:

SALARIES/BENEFITS:

Pension Plan:	ESOP Stock Plan:	Profit Sharing:	Top Exec. Salary: $1,260,000	Bonus: $
Savings Plan: Y	Stock Purch. Plan: Y		Second Exec. Salary: $650,000	Bonus: $

OTHER THOUGHTS:
Apparent Women Officers or Directors: 3
Hot Spot for Advancement for Women/Minorities: Y

LOCATIONS: ("Y" = Yes)

West:	Southwest:	Midwest:	Southeast:	Northeast:	International:
Y	Y		Y		Y

Note: Financial information, benefits and other data can change quickly and may vary from those stated here.

HARRAH'S ENTERTAINMENT INC

www.harrahs.com

Industry Group Code: 721120   Ranks within this company's industry group: Sales: 1   Profits: 3

Management:		Sales/Marketing:		Liberal Arts:		Information Systems:		Professionals:		Technical/Scientific:	
Mgmt. Trainees:	Y	Mktg. Professionals:	Y	Gen. Writing/Editing:	Y	Info. Management:	Y	Finance/Accounting:	Y	Engineers, Elec.:	
Experienced Mgmt.:	Y	Retail Sales:		Technical Writing:		Software Dev.:		Law:	Y	Engineers, Other:	
Int'l Business:	Y	Commercial/Industrial:	Y	Graphic Arts/Photog.:	Y	Hardware Dev.:		HR/Other:	Y	Health/Lab:	
MBA Graduates:	Y	Sales Trainees:		Music:	Y	Systems Integration:		Training:	Y	Scientists/Research:	
		Advertising Pros.:	Y	Broadcasting:		Consulting/Other:		Health Care:		Petroleum/Chemicals:	
				Other:	Y			Consulting:		Math/Other:	

TYPES OF BUSINESS:

Casino Hotels
Dockside & Riverboat Casinos
Racing Venues
Casino Management
Golf Facility

BRANDS/DIVISIONS/AFFILIATES:

Harrah's Operating Company, Inc.
Harrah's
Caesars
Horseshoe
Total Rewards
Caesars Palace Las Vegas
Macau Orient Golf
Apollo Management, L.P.

CONTACTS: Note: Officers with more than one job title may be intentionally listed here more than once.

Gary W. Loveman, CEO
Gary W. Loveman, Pres.
Jonathan S. Halkyard, CFO/Sr. VP/Treas.
David Norton, Chief Mktg. Officer/Sr. VP
Mary Thomas, Sr. VP-Human Resources
Tim Stanley, CIO
Tim Stanley, Sr. VP-Innovation, Gaming & Tech.
Steve Brammell, General Counsel/Sr. VP
Jan Jones, Sr. VP-Comm. & Gov't Rel.
Anthony D. McDuffie, Chief Acct. Officer/Controller/Sr. VP
Tom M. Jenkin, Pres., Western Div.
John Payne, Pres., Central Div.
J. Carlos Tolosa, Pres., Eastern Div.
Charles L. Atwood, Vice Chmn.
Gary W. Loveman, Chmn.

Phone: 702-407-6000	Fax: 702-407-6037
Toll-Free:	
Address: 1 Caesars Palace Dr., Las Vegas, NV 89109 US	

GROWTH PLANS/SPECIAL FEATURES:

Harrah's Entertainment, Inc. is one of the largest gaming companies in the world. It owns or manages 50 casinos, including 35 in the U.S., 10 in the U.K., two in Egypt, and one each in Canada, South Africa and Uruguay. Harrah's also earns fees from managing three casinos for Indian tribes: Harrah's Phoenix Ak-Chin, located near Phoenix, Arizona; Harrah's Rincon Casino and Resort, near San Diego, California; and Harrah's Cherokee Casino and Hotel, in Cherokee, North Carolina. These contracts expire in 2011. Harrah's is developing additional properties in Spain and the Bahamas. The firm offers casino entertainment facilities primarily under the Harrah's, Caesars and Horseshoe brands in the U.S., including land-based casinos; riverboat or dockside casinos; casino clubs; and three racing venues. Besides casinos, the firm's properties generally include hotel and convention space; restaurants; and non-gaming entertainment facilities. Harrah's properties total approximately 3 million square feet of gaming space and 38,000 hotel rooms. For returning customers in the U.S., the firm offers the Total Rewards card plan, allowing holders to earn reward credits for prizes such as vacations, event tickets and cars; Total Rewards currently has over 40 million members. The company owns and operates the World Series of Poker tournament and brand. In July 2007, Harrah's announced plans for a $1.3 billion expansion and renovation effort for Caesars Palace Las Vegas, including adding a 650-room hotel tower. In September 2007, the firm acquired Macau Orient Golf, located on 175 acres near the Lotus Bridge, as well as rights to a land concession contract, for $577.7 million. In January 2008, Harrah's was acquired by Hamlet Holdings LLC, an affiliate of TGP Capital, LP and Apollo Management, L.P., for $29.7 billion dollars, and subsequently taken private.

Employees of Harrah's receive medical, dental and vision plans; educational assistance; and employee assistance programs.

FINANCIALS: Sales and profits are in thousands of dollars—add 000 to get the full amount. 2007 Note: Financial information for 2007 was not available for all companies at press time.

2007 Sales: $10,825,200	2007 Profits: $619,400	**U.S. Stock Ticker: Private**
2006 Sales: $9,673,900	2006 Profits: $535,800	**Int'l Ticker:** Int'l Exchange:
2005 Sales: $7,010,000	2005 Profits: $236,400	Employees: 87,000
2004 Sales: $4,396,800	2004 Profits: $367,709	Fiscal Year Ends: 12/31
2003 Sales: $4,126,200	2003 Profits: $292,700	Parent Company: HAMLET HOLDINGS LLC

SALARIES/BENEFITS:

Pension Plan:	ESOP Stock Plan:	Profit Sharing:	Top Exec. Salary: $2,000,000	Bonus: $2,490,000
Savings Plan: Y	Stock Purch. Plan:		Second Exec. Salary: $1,228,615	Bonus: $1,271,337

OTHER THOUGHTS:

Apparent Women Officers or Directors: 2
Hot Spot for Advancement for Women/Minorities: Y

LOCATIONS: ("Y" = Yes)

West:	Southwest:	Midwest:	Southeast:	Northeast:	International:
Y	Y	Y	Y	Y	Y

HARRIS CORPORATION

www.harris.com

Industry Group Code: 334200 Ranks within this company's industry group: Sales: 2   Profits: 2

Management:		Sales/Marketing:		Liberal Arts:		Information Systems:		Professionals:		Technical/Scientific:	
Mgmt. Trainees:	Y	Mktg. Professionals:	Y	Gen. Writing/Editing:	Y	Info. Management:	Y	Finance/Accounting:	Y	Engineers, Elec.:	Y
Experienced Mgmt.:	Y	Retail Sales:		Technical Writing:	Y	Software Dev.:	Y	Law:	Y	Engineers, Other:	
Int'l Business:	Y	Commercial/Industrial:	Y	Graphic Arts/Photog.:	Y	Hardware Dev.:	Y	HR/Other:	Y	Health/Lab.:	Y
MBA Graduates:	Y	Sales Trainees:		Music:		Systems Integration:	Y	Training:	Y	Scientists/Research:	Y
		Advertising Pros.:	Y	Broadcasting:		Consulting/Other:	Y	Health Care:		Petroleum/Chemicals:	
				Other:				Consulting:		Math/Other:	Y

TYPES OF BUSINESS:

Communications Equipment Manufacturing
Wireless Communications Equipment
Broadcasting Equipment
Microwave Equipment
Aerospace Equipment

BRANDS/DIVISIONS/AFFILIATES:

Orkand Corp.
Encoda Systems Holdings, Inc.
Leitch Technology Corporation
Maritime Communications Services, Inc.
Optimal Solutions, Inc.
Aastra Digital Video
Multimax Incorporated
Zandar Technologies

CONTACTS: *Note: Officers with more than one job title may be intentionally listed here more than once.*

Howard L. Lance, CEO
Robert K. Henry, COO/Exec. VP
Howard L. Lance, Pres.
Gary L. McArthur, CFO/VP
Jeffrey S. Shuman, VP-Human Resources
William H. Miller, Jr., CIO/VP-Info. Svcs.
R. Kent Buchanan, CTO
R. Kent Buchanan, VP-Eng.
Eugene S. Cavallucci, General Counsel/VP
Leon V. Shivamber, VP-Oper.
Ricardo A. Navarro, VP-Corp. Dev.
Pamela Padgett, VP-Corp. Comm.
Pamela Padgett, VP-Investor Rel.
Lewis A. Schwartz, Principal Acct. Officer/VP
Jeremy C. Wensinger, Pres., Gov't Comm. Systems Div.
Daniel R. Pearson, Pres., Defense Comm. & Electronics
Timothy Thorsteinson, Pres., Broadcast Comm. Div.
Peter Challan, VP-Gov't Rel.
Howard L. Lance, Chmn.
Leon V. Shivamber, VP-Supply Chain Mgmt.

Phone: 321-727-9100	Fax: 321-674-4740
Toll-Free: 800-442-7747	
Address: 1025 W. NASA Blvd., Melbourne, FL 32919-0001 US	

GROWTH PLANS/SPECIAL FEATURES:

Harris Corporation, along with its subsidiaries, is an international communications and information technology company that provides sales and services in over 90 countries. Harris operates through fThe divisions: Defense Communications and Electronics, Government Communications Systems, Broadcast Communications and Harris Stratex Networks. The Defense Communications and Electronics segment is a worldwide supplier of secure voice and data radio communications products, systems and networks; conducts advanced research studies; and designs, develops and supplies state-of-the-art communications and information networks and equipment, primarily for the U.S. Department of Defense, other Federal and state agencies, allied government defense and peacekeeping forces, and other aerospace and defense companies. Government Communications Systems segment develops intelligence, surveillance and reconnaissance solutions; designs and supports information systems for image and other data collection, processing, interpretation, storage and retrieval; and offers engineering, operations and support services, primarily for various agencies of the U.S. Government and for other aerospace and defense companies. The Broadcast Communications segment serves the global digital and analog markets, providing video infrastructure and digital media products and solutions; enterprise software systems and solutions; and television and radio transmission equipment and systems. The Harris Stratex Networks segment offers reliable, flexible, scalable and cost-efficient wireless transmission network solutions, including microwave radio systems and network management software, which are backed by comprehensive services and support, primarily to mobile and fixed telephone service providers, private network operators, government agencies, transportation and utility companies, public safety agencies and broadcast system operators. In 2007, the company acquired Multimax Incorporated for approximately $400 million. In 2008, Harris acquired Zandar Technologies, a privately held developer and provider of high-quality multi-image display processors for television broadcast and professional video markets.

FINANCIALS: Sales and profits are in thousands of dollars—add 000 to get the full amount. 2007 Note: Financial information for 2007 was not available for all companies at press time.

2007 Sales: $4,243,000	2007 Profits: $480,400	**U.S. Stock Ticker: HRS**
2006 Sales: $3,474,800	2006 Profits: $237,900	**Int'l Ticker:** Int'l Exchange:
2005 Sales: $3,000,600	2005 Profits: $202,200	Employees: 16,000
2004 Sales: $2,518,600	2004 Profits: $132,800	Fiscal Year Ends: 6/30
2003 Sales: $2,092,700	2003 Profits: $59,500	Parent Company:

SALARIES/BENEFITS:

Pension Plan: Y	ESOP Stock Plan:	Profit Sharing: Y	Top Exec. Salary: $945,673	Bonus: $1,550,000
Savings Plan: Y	Stock Purch. Plan: Y		Second Exec. Salary: $491,346	Bonus: $465,663

OTHER THOUGHTS:

Apparent Women Officers or Directors: 3
Hot Spot for Advancement for Women/Minorities: Y

LOCATIONS: ("Y" = Yes)

West:	Southwest:	Midwest:	Southeast:	Northeast:	International:
		Y	Y	Y	Y

Note: Financial information, benefits and other data can change quickly and may vary from those stated here.

HARTFORD FINANCIAL SERVICES GROUP INC (THE)
www.thehartford.com

Industry Group Code: 524113 Ranks within this company's industry group: Sales: Profits:

Management:		Sales/Marketing:		Liberal Arts:		Information Systems:		Professionals:		Technical/Scientific:	
Mgmt. Trainees:	Y	Mktg. Professionals:	Y	Gen. Writing/Editing:	Y	Info. Management:	Y	Finance/Accounting:	Y	Engineers, Elec.:	
Experienced Mgmt.:	Y	Retail Sales:	Y	Technical Writing:	Y	Software Dev.:	Y	Law:	Y	Engineers, Other:	
Int'l Business:	Y	Commercial/Industrial:	Y	Graphic Arts/Photog.:		Hardware Dev.:		HR/Other:	Y	Health/Lab:	
MBA Graduates:	Y	Sales Trainees:		Music:		Systems Integration:		Training:	Y	Scientists/Research:	Y
		Advertising Pros.:	Y	Broadcasting:		Consulting/Other:		Health Care:	Y	Petroleum/Chemicals:	
				Other:				Consulting:		Math/Other:	Y

TYPES OF BUSINESS:

Life Insurance
Mutual Funds
Property & Casualty Insurance
Group Life & Accident Insurance
Reinsurance
Employee Benefits Administration
Asset Management
Auto Insurance

BRANDS/DIVISIONS/AFFILIATES:

Hartford Fire Insurance Company
Hartford Life Insurance Company
Hartford Life and Accident
Hartford Life Group Insurance Company
Hartford Life and Annuity
Hartford Investment Financial Services, LLC
Hartford International Management Services Company
Hartford Mutual Funds, Inc. (The)

CONTACTS: *Note: Officers with more than one job title may be intentionally listed here more than once.*

Ramani Ayer, CEO
Thomas M. Marra, COO
Thomas M. Marra, Pres.
Lizabeth H. Zlatkus, CFO/Exec. VP
Connie Weaver, Sr. VP-Mktg.
Eileen Whelley, Exec. VP-Human Resources
Alan J. Kreczko, General Counsel/Exec. VP
Connie Weaver, Sr. VP-Comm.
Michael Kalen, Sr. VP-Finance
David M. Znamierowski, Chief Investment Officer
Neal S. Wolin, Pres./COO-Property & Casualty Oper.
Ronald R. Gendreau, Exec. VP-Group Benefits
John C. Walters, Pres./COO-Hartford Life, Inc.
Ramani Ayer, Chmn.
Marc Lieberman, Pres., CEO-Hartford Life, Ltd., Europe

Phone: 860-547-5000	Fax: 860-547-2680

Toll-Free:

Address: 690 Asylum Ave., 1 Hartford Plaza, Hartford, CT 06115-1900 US

GROWTH PLANS/SPECIAL FEATURES:

The Hartford Financial Services Group is a diversified insurance and financial services company that offers insurance and investment products. Through its many subsidiaries, it is among the largest providers of investment products, individual life, group life and group disability insurance products and property and casualty insurance products in the U.S. and Canada. The company also operates in Brazil, Japan, England and Ireland serving millions worldwide through independent agents and brokers, financial institutions and online. Products and services for individuals and families include annuities; mutual funds; college savings plans; and auto, flood, home and life insurance. Business offerings include property and casualty, group benefits, retirement, reinsurance and investment management products and services. Subsidiary Hartford Investment Management Co., offers a range of investment products including multi-sector fixed income, specialty fixed income, cash and enhanced cash and passive investing. Hartford is organized into two major divisions: life and property/casualty. The life division is involved with segments of investment products, individual life, group benefits and corporate-owned life insurance. The property and casualty operations include North American underwriting segments of business insurance, affinity personal lines, personal insurance, specialty commercial and reinsurance. Hartford recently announced its launching of a new target retirement fund, The Hartford Target Retirement Funds, to help baby boomers plan for retirement needs. The Hartford Mutual Funds family now offers 54 retail mutual funds, spanning both equity and fixed income investments; mutual fund assets totaled $48.4 billion in 2007. In December 2007, the firm agreed to acquire Princeton Retirement Group, a defined contribution recordkeeping alliance business. In September 2008, the firm announced a new German branch.

Hartford employees receive a benefits package including adoption and tuition assistance; degree development, on-site fitness center; employee discounts; and health coverage. Qualified employees enjoy the opportunity for additional rewards when Hartford meets or exceeds business objectives.

FINANCIALS: Sales and profits are in thousands of dollars—add 000 to get the full amount. 2007 Note: Financial information for 2007 was not available for all companies at press time.

2007 Sales: $25,916,000	2007 Profits: $2,949,000	**U.S. Stock Ticker: HIG**
2006 Sales: $26,500,000	2006 Profits: $2,745,000	**Int'l Ticker:** Int'l Exchange:
2005 Sales: $27,083,000	2005 Profits: $2,274,000	Employees: 31,000
2004 Sales: $22,693,000	2004 Profits: $2,115,000	Fiscal Year Ends: 12/31
2003 Sales: $18,733,000	2003 Profits: $-91,000	Parent Company:

SALARIES/BENEFITS:

Pension Plan: Y	ESOP Stock Plan:	Profit Sharing:	Top Exec. Salary: $1,150,000	Bonus: $3,650,000
Savings Plan: Y	Stock Purch. Plan: Y		Second Exec. Salary: $990,000	Bonus: $2,316,000

OTHER THOUGHTS:

Apparent Women Officers or Directors: 4
Hot Spot for Advancement for Women/Minorities: Y

LOCATIONS: ("Y" = Yes)

West:	Southwest:	Midwest:	Southeast:	Northeast:	International:
Y	Y	Y	Y	Y	Y

HAWAIIAN ELECTRIC INDUSTRIES INC   www.hei.com

Industry Group Code: 221000A Ranks within this company's industry group: Sales: Profits:

Management:		Sales/Marketing:		Liberal Arts:		Information Systems:		Professionals:		Technical/Scientific:	
Mgmt. Trainees:	Y	Mktg. Professionals:	Y	Gen. Writing/Editing:	Y	Info. Management:	Y	Finance/Accounting:	Y	Engineers, Elec.:	Y
Experienced Mgmt.:	Y	Retail Sales:		Technical Writing:		Software Dev.:		Law:	Y	Engineers, Other:	
Int'l Business:		Commercial/Industrial:	Y	Graphic Arts/Photog.:		Hardware Dev.:		HR/Other:	Y	Health/Lab:	
MBA Graduates:	Y	Sales Trainees:		Music:		Systems Integration:		Training:	Y	Scientists/Research:	
		Advertising Pros.:		Broadcasting:		Consulting/Other:		Health Care:		Petroleum/Chemicals:	
				Other:				Consulting:		Math/Other:	

TYPES OF BUSINESS:

Utilities-Electricity
Savings Bank
Renewable Energy

BRANDS/DIVISIONS/AFFILIATES:

Hawaiian Electric Company
Hawaiian Electric Light Company
Maui Electric Company, Limited
Renewable Hawaii, Inc.
American Savings Bank, F.S.B.
HEI Diversified
Pacific Energy Conservation Services, Inc.
Uluwehiokama Biofuels Corp.

CONTACTS: *Note: Officers with more than one job title may be intentionally listed here more than once.*

Constance H. Lau, CEO
Constance H. Lau, Pres.
Curtis Y. Harada, Acting CFO/VP-Finance/Treas.
Karl E. Stahlkopf, CTO/Sr. VP-Energy Solutions, Hawaiian Electric Co.
Patricia U. Wong, VP-Admin./Corp. Sec.
Chet A. Richardson, General Counsel/VP
Andrew I. T. Chang, VP-External Affairs
Curtis Y. Harada, Controller
T. Michael May, CEO/Pres., Hawaiian Electric Company Inc.
Jay M. Ignacio, Pres., Hawaii Electric Light Company, Inc.
Timothy K. Schools, Pres., American Savings Bank, F.S.B.
Edward L. Reinhardt, Pres., Maui Electric Company, Limited
Jeffrey N. Watanabe, Chmn.

Phone: 808-543-5662	Fax: 808-543-7602
Toll-Free:	
Address: 900 Richards St., Honolulu, HI 96813 US	

GROWTH PLANS/SPECIAL FEATURES:

Hawaiian Electric Industries, Inc. (HEI) is a diversified holding company engaged in independent power and utility services and the operation of a savings bank. HEI's Hawaiian Electric Company (HECO) subsidiary, founded in 1891, is a regulated electric public utility company, along with its subsidiaries Hawaiian Electric Light Company (HELCO) and Maui Electric Company, Limited (MECO). HECO's Renewable Hawaii, Inc. subsidiary invests in renewable energy projects. Additional subsidiaries of HEI include HEI Diversified (HEIDI), a holding company; Pacific Energy Conservation Services, Inc. (PECS), a contract services company; HEI Properties, Inc. (HEIPI); HEI Investments, Inc.; Hawaiian Electric Industries Capital Trusts II and III; and The Old Oahu Tug Service, Inc. (TOOTS). HEIDI's American Savings Bank, F.S.B. subsidiary is a leading financial institution in Hawaii, with more than 60 branch offices offering investment products, financial planning services, insurance, deposit accounts and consumer loans. HECO, HELCO and MELCO are regulated operating electric public utilities engaged in the production, purchase, transmission, distribution and sale of electricity on the islands of Oahu, Maui, Lanai, Molokai and Hawaii. HEI's electric utility operations generate approximately 83% of its revenues. The islands of Oahu, Maui, Lanai, Molokai and Hawaii have a combined population of approximately 1.2 million, or approximately 95% of the Hawaii population, and comprise a service area of 5,766 square miles. The principle communities served include Honolulu on Oahu; Wailuku and Kahului on Maui; and Hilo and Kona on Hawaii. Each island has its own generation and transmission system that is not connected to any other grid, which results in the company maintaining a larger amount of surplus capacity than most utilities. In September 2007, HECO formed a new subsidiary, Uluwehiokama Biofuels Corp., to partially own a biodiesel refining plant which the firm expects to be built on Maui by 2009.

FINANCIALS: Sales and profits are in thousands of dollars—add 000 to get the full amount. 2007 Note: Financial information for 2007 was not available for all companies at press time.

2007 Sales: $2,536,400	2007 Profits: $84,779	**U.S. Stock Ticker:** HE
2006 Sales: $2,460,904	2006 Profits: $108,001	**Int'l Ticker:** Int'l Exchange:
2005 Sales: $2,215,564	2005 Profits: $126,689	Employees: 3,383
2004 Sales: $1,924,057	2004 Profits: $109,652	Fiscal Year Ends: 12/31
2003 Sales: $1,781,316	2003 Profits: $114,178	Parent Company:

SALARIES/BENEFITS:

Pension Plan:	ESOP Stock Plan:	Profit Sharing:	Top Exec. Salary: $680,667	Bonus: $191,449
Savings Plan:	Stock Purch. Plan:		Second Exec. Salary: $571,334	Bonus: $

OTHER THOUGHTS:

Apparent Women Officers or Directors: 8
Hot Spot for Advancement for Women/Minorities: Y

LOCATIONS: ("Y" = Yes)

West:	Southwest:	Midwest:	Southeast:	Northeast:	International:
Y					

HCA INC
www.hcahealthcare.com

Industry Group Code: 622110 Ranks within this company's industry group: Sales: 1 Profits: 1

Management:		Sales/Marketing:		Liberal Arts:		Information Systems:		Professionals:		Technical/Scientific:	
Mgmt. Trainees:	Y	Mktg. Professionals:	Y	Gen. Writing/Editing:	Y	Info. Management:	Y	Finance/Accounting:	Y	Engineers, Elec.:	
Experienced Mgmt.:	Y	Retail Sales:		Technical Writing:	Y	Software Dev.:		Law:	Y	Engineers, Other:	Y
Int'l Business:	Y	Commercial/Industrial:		Graphic Arts/Photog.:	Y	Hardware Dev.:		HR/Other:	Y	Health/Lab:	
MBA Graduates:	Y	Sales Trainees:		Music:		Systems Integration:		Training:	Y	Scientists/Research:	
		Advertising Pros.:	Y	Broadcasting:		Consulting/Other:		Health Care:	Y	Petroleum/Chemicals:	
				Other:				Consulting:		Math/Other:	

TYPES OF BUSINESS:
Hospitals-General
Outpatient Surgery Centers
Sub-Acute Care
Psychiatric Hospitals
Rehabilitation Services
Hospital Management Services

BRANDS/DIVISIONS/AFFILIATES:
Bain Capital LLC
KKR & Co LP (Kohlberg Kravis Roberts & Co)
Merrill Lynch & Co Inc

CONTACTS: Note: Officers with more than one job title may be intentionally listed here more than once.
Jack O. Bovender, Jr., CEO
Richard M. Bracken, COO
Richard M. Bracken, Pres.
R. Milton Johnson, CFO/Exec. VP
John M. Steele, Sr. VP-Human Resources
Noel B. Williams, CIO/Sr. VP
Robert A. Waterman, General Counsel/Sr. VP
V. Carl George, VP-Dev.
David G. Anderson, Sr. VP-Finance/Treas.
Chuck J. Hall, Pres., Eastern Group
Jonathan B. Perlin, Chief Medical Officer/Sr. VP-Quality
Victor L. Campbell, Sr. VP
Rosalyn S. Elton, Sr. VP-Oper. Finance
Jack O. Bovender, Jr., Chmn.

Phone: 615-344-2068 **Fax:**
Toll-Free:
Address: 1 Park Plaza, Nashville, TN 37203 US

GROWTH PLANS/SPECIAL FEATURES:
HCA, Inc., formerly known as HCA Healthcare Co., owns and operates approximately 168 hospitals and approximately 113 outpatient surgery centers in 20 states and the U.K. The company's acute care hospitals provide a full range of services, including internal medicine, general surgery, neurosurgery, orthopedics, obstetrics, cardiac care, diagnostic and emergency services, radiology, respiratory therapy, cardiology and physical therapy. The psychiatric hospitals provide therapeutic programs including child, adolescent and adult psychiatric care and adult and adolescent alcohol and drug abuse treatment and counseling. The outpatient health care facilities operated by HCA include surgery centers, diagnostic and imaging centers, comprehensive outpatient rehabilitation and physical therapy centers. The company's hospitals do not engage in extensive medical research and education programs; however, some facilities are affiliated with medical schools and may participate in the clinical rotation of medical interns and residents. In addition, HCA provides a variety of management services to health care facilities such as patient safety programs; ethics and compliance programs; national supply contracts; equipment purchasing and leasing contracts; and accounting, financial and clinical systems. Other services include governmental reimbursement assistance; construction planning and coordination; information technology systems; legal counsel; human resource services; and internal audit. The firm is owned by a group of private equity companies, including KKR & Co., Merrill Lynch and Bain Capital.

HCA offers its employees a day care flexible spending account; child care center discounts; an adoption assistance program; a ConSern student loan program; laser surgery discounts at LaserVision; a healthcare flexible spending account; and medical, dental and vision coverage.

FINANCIALS: Sales and profits are in thousands of dollars—add 000 to get the full amount. 2007 Note: Financial information for 2007 was not available for all companies at press time.
2007 Sales: $26,900,000	2007 Profits: $	**U.S. Stock Ticker:** Private
2006 Sales: $25,477,000	2006 Profits: $1,036,000	**Int'l Ticker:** Int'l Exchange:
2005 Sales: $24,455,000	2005 Profits: $1,424,000	Employees: 186,000
2004 Sales: $23,502,000	2004 Profits: $1,246,000	Fiscal Year Ends: 12/31
2003 Sales: $21,808,000	2003 Profits: $1,332,000	Parent Company: BAIN CAPITAL LLC

SALARIES/BENEFITS:
Pension Plan: Y ESOP Stock Plan: Profit Sharing: Top Exec. Salary: $1,404,959 Bonus: $
Savings Plan: Y Stock Purch. Plan: Second Exec. Salary: $817,667 Bonus: $

OTHER THOUGHTS:
Apparent Women Officers or Directors: 3
Hot Spot for Advancement for Women/Minorities: Y

LOCATIONS: ("Y" = Yes)
West:	Southwest:	Midwest:	Southeast:	Northeast:	International:
Y	Y	Y	Y	Y	Y

Note: Financial information, benefits and other data can change quickly and may vary from those stated here.

HE BUTT GROCERY COMPANY (HEB)

www.heb.com

Industry Group Code: 445110 Ranks within this company's industry group: Sales: Profits:

Management:		Sales/Marketing:		Liberal Arts:		Information Systems:		Professionals:		Technical/Scientific:	
Mgmt. Trainees:	Y	Mktg. Professionals:	Y	Gen. Writing/Editing:	Y	Info. Management:	Y	Finance/Accounting:	Y	Engineers, Elec.:	
Experienced Mgmt.:	Y	Retail Sales:	Y	Technical Writing:		Software Dev.:	Y	Law:	Y	Engineers, Other:	Y
Int'l Business:	Y	Commercial/Industrial:	Y	Graphic Arts/Photog.:	Y	Hardware Dev.:		HR/Other:	Y	Health/Lab:	
MBA Graduates:	Y	Sales Trainees:	Y	Music:		Systems Integration:		Training:	Y	Scientists/Research:	
		Advertising Pros.:	Y	Broadcasting:		Consulting/Other:		Health Care:	Y	Petroleum/Chemicals:	
				Other:				Consulting:		Math/Other:	

TYPES OF BUSINESS:

Supermarkets
Grocery Stores
Gourmet Food Stores
Dairy Processing
Bakery
Pharmacy Services

BRANDS/DIVISIONS/AFFILIATES:

H-E-B
Central Market
H-E-B plus!
H-E-B Insurance Agency
H-E-B Mobile

CONTACTS: Note: Officers with more than one job title may be intentionally listed here more than once.

Charles C. Butt, CEO
Robert Loeffler, COO
Jack C. Brouillard, CFO
Bob McCullough, VP-Mfg.
Jack C. Brouillard, Chief Admin. Officer
Dya Campos, Dir.-Public Affairs
Kathy Durbin, Dir.-Benefits

Phone: 210-938-8357		**Fax:** 210-938-8169	
Toll-Free: 800-432-3113			
Address: 646 S. Main Ave., San Antonio, TX 78204 US			

GROWTH PLANS/SPECIAL FEATURES:

H.E. Butt Grocery Company (H-E-B) is one of the largest regional food retailers in the southwestern U.S. and Mexico. It operates over 300 grocery stores in 150 communities in Texas and Mexico under H-E-B brand names. The firm owns one of the largest milk plants in Texas, as well as a large bread bakery, a meat plant, a pastry bakery, an ice cream plant, a chip plant and a photo processing lab. The stores carry a wide variety of merchandise, including a line of products under the H-E-B brand name. H-E-B operates the Central Market stores, with single locations in Houston, Dallas, Forth Worth, Plano, San Antonio and Southlake; and two locations in Austin. Central Markets are large gourmet specialty stores featuring vast prepared foods to go areas, eat-in areas, immense wine departments, specialty butcher and fish counters, a European bakery, a deli with meats, a large selection of cheeses from around the globe and a juice and ice cream bar. H-E-B plus! stores offer additional departments including Do-It-Yourself, Bed & Bath, Cook & Grill and Card & Party. H-E-B Insurance Agency offers automobile, life, health, homeowners and renters insurance, and can sign clients up over the phone or through its locations in six Texas cities. H-E-B Mobile offers nation wide cell phone service with free unlimited nights and weekends; and free nation wide long distance, text messaging and data services. To better serve its Mexican markets, the company owns and operates a $30 million retail support center in Monterrey, Mexico. In 2008, the firm opened its fourth H-E-B plus! store in San Antonio at McCreless Market, a redeveloped city landmark.

H-E-B offers its employees a leadership development program, tuition reimbursement, a scholarship program, flexible spending accounts, membership in a federal credit union and use of recreational lodges.

FINANCIALS: Sales and profits are in thousands of dollars—add 000 to get the full amount. 2007 Note: Financial information for 2007 was not available for all companies at press time.

2007 Sales: $13,500,000	2007 Profits: $	**U.S. Stock Ticker: Private**
2006 Sales: $13,500,000	2006 Profits: $	**Int'l Ticker:** Int'l Exchange:
2005 Sales: $11,500,000	2005 Profits: $	Employees: 63,000
2004 Sales: $10,500,000	2004 Profits: $	Fiscal Year Ends: 10/31
2003 Sales: $10,700,000	2003 Profits: $	Parent Company:

SALARIES/BENEFITS:

Pension Plan: Y	ESOP Stock Plan:	Profit Sharing:	Top Exec. Salary: $	Bonus: $
Savings Plan: Y	Stock Purch. Plan:		Second Exec. Salary: $	Bonus: $

OTHER THOUGHTS:

Apparent Women Officers or Directors:
Hot Spot for Advancement for Women/Minorities:

LOCATIONS: ("Y" = Yes)

West:	Southwest:	Midwest:	Southeast:	Northeast:	International:
	Y				Y

Note: Financial information, benefits and other data can change quickly and may vary from those stated here.

HEALTH FITNESS CORP

www.hfit.com

Industry Group Code: 713940 **Ranks within this company's industry group:** Sales: 1 Profits: 1

Management:		Sales/Marketing:		Liberal Arts:		Information Systems:		Professionals:		Technical/Scientific:	
Mgmt. Trainees:	Y	Mktg. Professionals:	Y	Gen. Writing/Editing:	Y	Info. Management:	Y	Finance/Accounting:	Y	Engineers, Elec.:	
Experienced Mgmt.:	Y	Retail Sales:		Technical Writing:		Software Dev.:		Law:	Y	Engineers, Other:	
Int'l Business:	Y	Commercial/Industrial:	Y	Graphic Arts/Photog.:	Y	Hardware Dev.:		HR/Other:	Y	Health/Lab:	
MBA Graduates:	Y	Sales Trainees:	Y	Music:		Systems Integration:		Training:	Y	Scientists/Research:	
		Advertising Pros.:	Y	Broadcasting:		Consulting/Other:		Health Care:		Petroleum/Chemicals:	
				Other:	Y			Consulting:		Math/Other:	

TYPES OF BUSINESS:

Fitness Center Management
Consulting Services
Corporate & Hospital-Based Fitness Centers
Fitness Center Design
Wellness Programs
Health & Fitness Assessment
On-Site Physical Therapy Services

BRANDS/DIVISIONS/AFFILIATES:

HFC Assessment Services
HFC Wellness Programs
HFC Fitness Programs
HFC Corporate Fitness Programs
Science Advisory Board

CONTACTS: Note: Officers with more than one job title may be intentionally listed here more than once.

Greg Lehman, CEO
John Griffin, COO
Greg Lehman, Pres.
Wesley Winnekins, CFO
Debra Marshall, VP-Mktg.
Jeanne Crawford, VP-Human Resources
Jim Reynolds, Chief Medical Officer
John Ellis, CIO
Brian Gagne, National VP-Oper.
Mike Seethaler, National VP-New Bus. Dev.
Wesley Winnekins, Treas.
Scott Kinzer, National VP-Bus. Dev.
Katherine M. Hamlin, VP-Health Mgmt. Acct. Svcs.
David Hurt, VP-Fitness Mgmt. Acct. Svcs.
Mark W. Sheffert, Chmn.

Phone: 952-831-6830	Fax: 952-897-5173
Toll-Free: 800-639-7913	
Address: 1650 W. 82nd St., Ste. 110, Minneapolis, MN 55431 US	

GROWTH PLANS/SPECIAL FEATURES:

Health Fitness Corp. (HFC) and its subsidiaries provide fitness and wellness management services and programs to corporations, hospitals, communities and universities in the U.S. and Canada. The firm also provides injury prevention programs and on-site physical therapy services. Currently, HFC is under contract to manage more than 390 sites, including corporate fitness centers; corporate wellness programs; occupational health programs; hospital-, community- or university-based fitness centers; and corporate sites that do not have full-time staff. The company provides a full range of development, management, marketing and consulting services, including demographic analysis, space planning, interior design, floor plan design, selection and sourcing of fitness equipment, fitness program design and occupational health consulting services. HFC also manages the operations of established fitness centers, including staff selection and implementation of programs. Programs offered include HFC Assessment Services, a full range of tools to assess the health and well-being of individuals, including screenings and education; HFC Wellness Programs, a menu of lifestyle programs addressing the specific needs of a company's workforce, including weight loss and stress management; HFC Fitness Programs, customized exercise-based programs including personal training and specialty group classes; and Corporate Fitness Programs, including fitness needs assessment, facility planning and program design. In 2007, the firm announced the formation of a Science Advisory Board of health industry experts, whose responsibilities will include reviewing the quality of HFC's products and services, delivering guidance of the implementation of products and services and providing peer review to the firm's research programs.

The company offers its employees medical, dental and vision insurance; flexible spending accounts; life and AD&D insurance; an employee assistance program; long-term disability insurance; a 401(k0 plan; and an employee stock purchase plan.

FINANCIALS: Sales and profits are in thousands of dollars—add 000 to get the full amount. 2007 Note: Financial information for 2007 was not available for all companies at press time.

2007 Sales: $69,958	2007 Profits: $ 910	**U.S. Stock Ticker:** HFIT
2006 Sales: $63,578	2006 Profits: $1,352	**Int'l Ticker:** Int'l Exchange:
2005 Sales: $54,942	2005 Profits: $1,204	Employees: 3,809
2004 Sales: $52,455	2004 Profits: $1,588	Fiscal Year Ends: 12/31
2003 Sales: $31,478	2003 Profits: $- 27	Parent Company:

SALARIES/BENEFITS:

Pension Plan:	ESOP Stock Plan:	Profit Sharing:	Top Exec. Salary: $275,000	Bonus: $15,000
Savings Plan: Y	Stock Purch. Plan: Y		Second Exec. Salary: $264,423	Bonus: $66,000

OTHER THOUGHTS:

Apparent Women Officers or Directors: 3
Hot Spot for Advancement for Women/Minorities: Y

LOCATIONS: ("Y" = Yes)

West:	Southwest:	Midwest:	Southeast:	Northeast:	International:
Y	Y	Y	Y	Y	Y

Note: Financial information, benefits and other data can change quickly and may vary from those stated here.

HEALTH MANAGEMENT ASSOCIATES INC   www.hma.com

Industry Group Code: 622110 Ranks within this company's industry group: Sales: 3 Profits: 3

Management:		Sales/Marketing:		Liberal Arts:		Information Systems:		Professionals:		Technical/Scientific:	
Mgmt. Trainees:	Y	Mktg. Professionals:	Y	Gen. Writing/Editing:	Y	Info. Management:	Y	Finance/Accounting:	Y	Engineers, Elec.:	
Experienced Mgmt.:	Y	Retail Sales:		Technical Writing:	Y	Software Dev.:		Law:	Y	Engineers, Other:	Y
Int'l Business:		Commercial/Industrial:		Graphic Arts/Photog.:	Y	Hardware Dev.:		HR/Other:	Y	Health/Lab:	
MBA Graduates:	Y	Sales Trainees:		Music:		Systems Integration:		Training:	Y	Scientists/Research:	
		Advertising Pros.:		Broadcasting:		Consulting/Other:		Health Care:	Y	Petroleum/Chemicals:	
				Other:				Consulting:		Math/Other:	

TYPES OF BUSINESS:
Acute Care Hospitals

BRANDS/DIVISIONS/AFFILIATES:
Brooksville Regional Hospital
River Oaks Health System
Lake Norman Regional Medical Center
Heart of Florida Regional Medical Center

CONTACTS: *Note: Officers with more than one job title may be intentionally listed here more than once.*
Burke W. Whitman, CEO
Kelly E. Curry, COO/Exec. VP
Burke W. Whitman, Pres.
Robert E. Farnham, CFO/Sr. VP
Frederick L. Drow, Sr. VP-Human Resources
Jim L. Jordan, Sr. VP-MIS
Randel J. Holly, Sr., VP-Corp. Eng.
Timothy R. Parry, General Counsel/Sr. VP
Stanley D. McLemore, Sr. VP-Oper.
Peter M. Lawson, Exec. VP-Dev.
Joseph C. Meek, Treas./VP
Kenneth M. Koopman, Sr. VP-Reimbursement
John C. Merriwether, VP-Financial Rel.
Lisa Gore, Sr. VP-Clinical Affairs
William J. Schoen, Chmn.
Johnny A. Owenby, Sr. VP-Support Svcs.

Phone: 239-598-3131	Fax: 239-598-2705
Toll-Free:	
Address: 5811 Pelican Bay Blvd., Ste. 500, Naples, FL 34108 US	

GROWTH PLANS/SPECIAL FEATURES:

Health Management Associates, Inc. (HMA) owns and operates acute care hospitals in non-urban communities. The company operates 59 hospitals, with a total of 8,458 licensed beds. The firm operates facilities in Alabama, Arkansas, Florida, Georgia, Kentucky, Mississippi, Missouri, North Carolina, Oklahoma, Pennsylvania, South Carolina, Tennessee, Texas, Washington and West Virginia. Services provides by the hospitals include general surgery, internal medicine, obstetrics, emergency room care, radiology, oncology, diagnostic care, coronary care and pediatric care. They also provide outpatient services such as one-day surgery, laboratory, x-ray, respiratory therapy, cardiology and physical therapy. In addition, some hospitals provide specialty services in, among other areas, cardiology (e.g., open-heart surgery), neuron-surgery, oncology, radiation therapy, computer-assisted tomography scanning, magnetic resonance imaging, lithotripsy and full-service obstetrics. The facilities benefit from centralized corporate resources such as purchasing; information services; finance and control systems; legal services; facilities planning; physicians recruitment services; administrative personnel management; marketing; and public relations. Some of the company's hospitals provide services to retired and certain other military personnel and their families, pursuant to the Civilian Health and Medical Program of Uniformed Services (CHAMPUS). In 2008, HMA saw expansion at 11 hospitals, including Brooksville Regional Hospital, River Oaks Health System, Lake Norman Regional Medical Center and Heart of Florida Regional Medical Center.

The company offers its employees medical, dental and vision insurance; flexible spending accounts; life insurance; a 401(k) plan; and disability and critical illness insurance.

FINANCIALS: Sales and profits are in thousands of dollars—add 000 to get the full amount. 2007 Note: Financial information for 2007 was not available for all companies at press time.

2007 Sales: $4,392,086	2007 Profits: $119,879	**U.S. Stock Ticker: HMA**
2006 Sales: $4,050,425	2006 Profits: $182,749	**Int'l Ticker:** Int'l Exchange:
2005 Sales: $3,479,568	2005 Profits: $353,077	Employees: 34,500
2004 Sales: $3,092,547	2004 Profits: $325,099	Fiscal Year Ends: 12/31
2003 Sales: $2,560,600	2003 Profits: $283,400	Parent Company:

SALARIES/BENEFITS:

Pension Plan:	ESOP Stock Plan:	Profit Sharing:	Top Exec. Salary: $800,000	Bonus: $
Savings Plan: Y	Stock Purch. Plan:		Second Exec. Salary: $600,000	Bonus: $600,000

OTHER THOUGHTS:

Apparent Women Officers or Directors: 9
Hot Spot for Advancement for Women/Minorities: Y

LOCATIONS: ("Y" = Yes)

West:	Southwest:	Midwest:	Southeast:	Northeast:	International:
Y	Y	Y	Y	Y	

HEALTH NET INC

www.healthnet.com

Industry Group Code: 524114 Ranks within this company's industry group: Sales: Profits:

Management:		Sales/Marketing:		Liberal Arts:		Information Systems:		Professionals:		Technical/Scientific:	
Mgmt. Trainees:		Mktg. Professionals:	Y	Gen. Writing/Editing:		Info. Management:	Y	Finance/Accounting:	Y	Engineers, Elec.:	
Experienced Mgmt.:	Y	Retail Sales:		Technical Writing:		Software Dev.:	Y	Law:	Y	Engineers, Other:	Y
Int'l Business:		Commercial/Industrial:	Y	Graphic Arts/Photog.:		Hardware Dev.:		HR/Other:	Y	Health/Lab:	
MBA Graduates:	Y	Sales Trainees:		Music:		Systems Integration:		Training:	Y	Scientists/Research:	
		Advertising Pros.:	Y	Broadcasting:		Consulting/Other:		Health Care:	Y	Petroleum/Chemicals:	
				Other:				Consulting:		Math/Other:	

TYPES OF BUSINESS:
Insurance-Medical & Health, HMOs & PPOs
Utilization Management
Health Care Services Management
Administrative Services
Health Insurance Underwriting
Life Insurance Underwriting

BRANDS/DIVISIONS/AFFILIATES:
Decision Power
It's Your Life Wellsite
Salud Con Health Net

CONTACTS: *Note: Officers with more than one job title may be intentionally listed here more than once.*
Jay M. Gellert, CEO
James E. Woys, COO
Jay M. Gellert, Pres.
Joseph C. Capezza, CFO
Mark S. El-Tawil, Chief Senior Prod. Officer
Linda V. Tiano, General Counsel/Sr. VP/Sec.
Patricia T. Clarey, Chief Regulatory & External Rel. Officer/Sr. VP
John P. Sivori, Sr. VP/Pres., Health Net Pharmaceutical Svcs.
Paul S. Lambdin, Pres., Health Net of the Northeast, Inc.
Steven Sell, CEO/Pres., MHN
Steven D. Tough, Pres., Health Net Federal Svcs, LLC
Roger F. Greaves, Chmn.

Phone: 818-676-6000	Fax: 818-676-8591
Toll-Free: 800-291-6911	
Address: 21650 Oxnard St., Woodland Hills, CA 91367 US	

GROWTH PLANS/SPECIAL FEATURES:
Health Net, Inc. is an integrated managed care organization that delivers managed health care services through health plans and government sponsored managed care plans. The firm's subsidiaries offer products related to prescription drugs; managed health care product coordination for multi-region employers; and administrative services for medical groups and self-funded benefits programs. HealthNet's managed health care providers include a network of health maintenance organizations (HMOs), insured preferred provider organizations (PPOs) and point-of-service (POS) plans to approximately 6.6 million individuals. These operations extend through group, individual, Medicare, Medicaid, TRICARE and Veterans Affairs programs. HealthNet's HMOs and PPOs contract approximately 71,100 primary care physicians and 203,600 specialist physicians. Health Net's behavioral health subsidiary provides mental health benefits to approximately 7 million individuals. The company owns insurance companies licensed to sell exclusive provider organization (EPO), PPO, POS and indemnity products, as well as auxiliary non-health products such as life and accidental death and dismemberment, dental, vision, behavioral health and disability insurance. In 2007, approximately 53% of the company's commercial members were covered by HMOs; 44% were covered by POS and PPO products; and 3% by EPO and fee-for-service products including consumer-directed health plans. The firm provides the Decision Power series of programs designed to directly involve patients in their health care decisions; the It's Your Life Wellsite, similar to the Decision Power programs, but targeted at Medicare members; the Salud Con Health Net, a project of its Californian branch designed to help uninsured Latino immigrants meet their health care needs; Medicare stores in Phoenix, Arizona and Meriden, Connecticut; and community enrollment and customer service centers in Los Angeles and Modesto, California. In August 2008, the firm disbursed over $5 million in no-interest loans to 12 Central Valley Californian health clinics to keep them open during budget negotiations.

FINANCIALS: Sales and profits are in thousands of dollars—add 000 to get the full amount. 2007 Note: Financial information for 2007 was not available for all companies at press time.

2007 Sales: $14,108,271	2007 Profits: $193,697	U.S. Stock Ticker: HNT
2006 Sales: $12,908,350	2006 Profits: $329,313	Int'l Ticker: Int'l Exchange:
2005 Sales: $11,940,533	2005 Profits: $229,785	Employees: 9,725
2004 Sales: $11,646,393	2004 Profits: $42,604	Fiscal Year Ends: 12/31
2003 Sales: $10,959,000	2003 Profits: $234,000	Parent Company:

SALARIES/BENEFITS:

Pension Plan:	ESOP Stock Plan:	Profit Sharing:	Top Exec. Salary: $1,061,538	Bonus: $1,213,713
Savings Plan: Y	Stock Purch. Plan:		Second Exec. Salary: $545,197	Bonus: $

OTHER THOUGHTS:
Apparent Women Officers or Directors: 5
Hot Spot for Advancement for Women/Minorities: Y

LOCATIONS: ("Y" = Yes)

West:	Southwest:	Midwest:	Southeast:	Northeast:	International:
Y	Y			Y	

Note: Financial information, benefits and other data can change quickly and may vary from those stated here.

HEALTHWAYS INC   www.americanhealthways.com

Industry Group Code: 524298 Ranks within this company's industry group: Sales: 2 Profits: 2

Management:		Sales/Marketing:		Liberal Arts:		Information Systems:		Professionals:		Technical/Scientific:	
Mgmt. Trainees:		Mktg. Professionals:	Y	Gen. Writing/Editing:		Info. Management:	Y	Finance/Accounting:	Y	Engineers, Elec.:	
Experienced Mgmt.:	Y	Retail Sales:		Technical Writing:	Y	Software Dev.:	Y	Law:	Y	Engineers, Other:	
Int'l Business:	Y	Commercial/Industrial:		Graphic Arts/Photog.:		Hardware Dev.:		HR/Other:	Y	Health/Lab:	Y
MBA Graduates:	Y	Sales Trainees:		Music:		Systems Integration:	Y	Training:	Y	Scientists/Research:	
		Advertising Pros.:		Broadcasting:		Consulting/Other:		Health Care:	Y	Petroleum/Chemicals:	
				Other:				Consulting:		Math/Other:	

TYPES OF BUSINESS:

Disease Management Programs
Ambulatory Surgery Centers
Arthritis Care
Osteoporosis Care
Cardiac Disease Management Services
Respiratory Disease Management Services
Online Disease Management
Outsourced Diabetes Treatment Programs

BRANDS/DIVISIONS/AFFILIATES:

CentreVu Customer Care Solution
Cardiac Healthways
Respiratory Healthways
Diabetes Healthways
MyHealthways
Axia Health Management, LLC
Medco Health Solutions

CONTACTS: *Note: Officers with more than one job title may be intentionally listed here more than once.*

Ben R. Leedle, CEO
James E. Pope, COO/Exec. VP
Ben R. Leedle, Pres.
Mary A. Chaput, CFO/Exec. VP
Anne Marie Wilkins, Exec. VP-Mktg. & Strategy
Robert L. Chaput, CIO/Exec. VP
Robert E. Stone, Exec. VP/Chief Strategy Officer
Kriste Goad, Sr. Dir.-Corp. Comm
Alfred Lumsdaine, Chief Acct. Officer/Controller/Sr. VP
Mary D. Hunter, Exec. VP
Dexter W. Shurney, Chief Medical Officer
Thomas G. Cigarran, Chmn.
Matthew E. Kelliher, Exec. VP-Int'l Bus.

Phone: 615-665-1122	Fax: 615-665-7697
Toll-Free: 800-327-3822	
Address: 3841 Green Hills Village Dr., Nashville, TN 37215-6104 US	

GROWTH PLANS/SPECIAL FEATURES:

Healthways, Inc., formerly American Healthways, Inc., provides specialized, comprehensive care enhancement and disease management services to health plans, physicians and hospitals in all 50 states, Washington, D.C., Puerto Rico and Guam. Through its educational programs and life-coaching services, the firm helps customers understand and follow doctors' orders; become aware of and recognize early warning signs associated with a major health episode; and set achievable goals for themselves, such as to exercise more, lose weight, quit smoking or otherwise improve their current health status. The firm also offers specialized support for people with diabetes, coronary artery disease, heart failure, asthma, chronic obstructive pulmonary disease, end-stage renal disease, cancer, chronic kidney disease, acid-related stomach disorders, hepatitis C, inflammatory bowel disease, irritable bowel syndrome, lower-back pain, osteoarthritis, osteoporosis, urinary incontinence and high-risk population management. Healthways also features MyHealthways, a web-based application that allows physicians, patients and care coordinators to actively monitor a chronic disease, receive customized plans of action or identify at-risk individuals through predictive modeling technology. In May 2008, the firm announced plans to partner with Medco Health Solutions, Inc. to open a new health center in San Antonio, Texas that will provide support for patients managing chronic conditions.

Healthways offers its employees a complete benefits package including flexible spending accounts, tuition reimbursement, performance bonuses and a 401(k) savings plan. In April 2008, the firm was featured in Training Magazine's Top 125 list for training and e-learning for the second consecutive year.

FINANCIALS: Sales and profits are in thousands of dollars—add 000 to get the full amount. 2007 Note: Financial information for 2007 was not available for all companies at press time.

2007 Sales: $615,586	2007 Profits: $45,121	**U.S. Stock Ticker: HWAY**
2006 Sales: $412,308	2006 Profits: $37,151	**Int'l Ticker:** Int'l Exchange:
2005 Sales: $312,504	2005 Profits: $33,084	Employees: 3,800
2004 Sales: $245,410	2004 Profits: $26,058	Fiscal Year Ends: 8/31
2003 Sales: $165,500	2003 Profits: $18,500	Parent Company:

SALARIES/BENEFITS:

Pension Plan:	ESOP Stock Plan:	Profit Sharing:	Top Exec. Salary: $660,000	Bonus: $
Savings Plan: Y	Stock Purch. Plan:		Second Exec. Salary: $385,143	Bonus: $

OTHER THOUGHTS:

Apparent Women Officers or Directors: 4
Hot Spot for Advancement for Women/Minorities: Y

LOCATIONS: ("Y" = Yes)

West:	Southwest:	Midwest:	Southeast:	Northeast:	International:
Y	Y	Y	Y	Y	Y

HELMERICH & PAYNE INC

www.hpinc.com

Industry Group Code: 211111 Ranks within this company's industry group: Sales: 8 Profits: 7

Management:		Sales/Marketing:		Liberal Arts:		Information Systems:		Professionals:		Technical/Scientific:	
Mgmt. Trainees:	Y	Mktg. Professionals:	Y	Gen. Writing/Editing:		Info. Management:	Y	Finance/Accounting:	Y	Engineers, Elec.:	Y
Experienced Mgmt.:	Y	Retail Sales:		Technical Writing:	Y	Software Dev.:		Law:	Y	Engineers, Other:	Y
Int'l Business:	Y	Commercial/Industrial:	Y	Graphic Arts/Photog.:		Hardware Dev.:		HR/Other:	Y	Health/Lab:	
MBA Graduates:	Y	Sales Trainees:		Music:		Systems Integration:		Training:	Y	Scientists/Research:	Y
		Advertising Pros.:		Broadcasting:		Consulting/Other:		Health Care:		Petroleum/Chemicals:	Y
				Other:				Consulting:		Math/Other:	

TYPES OF BUSINESS:

Oil & Gas Exploration & Production
Contract Drilling Services
Drilling Technology Development
Commercial Real Estate

BRANDS/DIVISIONS/AFFILIATES:

FlexRigs
FlexRig3
FlexRig4
TerraVici Drilling Solutions

CONTACTS: Note: Officers with more than one job title may be intentionally listed here more than once.

Hans Helmerich, CEO
Hans Helmerich, Pres.
Douglas E. Fears, CFO/VP
M. Alan Orr, Exec. VP-Eng. & Dev., Int'l Drilling Co.
Steven R. Mackey, General Counsel/Exec. VP/Corp. Sec.
W. H. Helmerich, III, Chmn.
John W. Lindsay, Exec. VP-US & Int'l Oper., Int'l Drilling Co.

Phone: 918-742-5531	Fax: 918-742-0237
Toll-Free:	
Address: 1437 S. Boulder Ave., Tulsa, OK 74119 US	

GROWTH PLANS/SPECIAL FEATURES:

Helmerich and Payne, Inc. (HP) operates both on and offshore rigs under contract with oil and gas companies. The firm offers clients drilling rigs, equipment, personnel and camps on a contract basis. These drilling rigs include a number of the newest generation of FlexRigs, which allow a greater depth and flexibility of between 8,000 to 18,000 feet, and provide greater operating efficiency. The company has completed design and manufacturing work on the FlexRig3 and FlexRig4, now available to U.S. and international drilling companies. Drilling rigs consist of engines, drawworks, a mast, pumps, blowout preventers, a drillstring and related equipment. HP has 157 land rigs available for work in the U.S., nine offshore platform rigs in the Gulf of Mexico and 27 international rigs. HP's contract drilling business is composed of three reportable business segments: U.S. land drilling, U.S. offshore platform drilling and international drilling. The firm's U.S. land drilling is conducted primarily in Oklahoma, California, Texas, Wyoming, Colorado, Louisiana, Mississippi, Alabama, Arkansas, New Mexico, and North Dakota. The company's offshore platform operations are conducted in the Gulf of Mexico, California, Trinidad and Equatorial Guinea. It also operates land rigs in seven international locations, including Venezuela, Ecuador, Colombia, Argentina, Bolivia, Tunisia, and Chile. The firm's contract drilling customers include major domestic and international oil companies, such as ExxonMobil or BP. In addition to its oil rig business, HP has real estate operations that are conducted within the metropolitan area of Tulsa, Oklahoma. Its major holding is a shopping center consisting of 15 buildings on about 30 acres. In May 2008, HP acquired TerraVici Drilling Solutions, including their proprietary rotary steerable system that enhances horizontal and directional drilling for $22 million.

HP offers employees benefits such as medical, dental and vision insurance; life insurance; long term disability; and a flexible spending account.

FINANCIALS: Sales and profits are in thousands of dollars—add 000 to get the full amount. 2007 Note: Financial information for 2007 was not available for all companies at press time.

2007 Sales: $1,629,658	2007 Profits: $449,261	U.S. Stock Ticker: HP
2006 Sales: $1,224,813	2006 Profits: $293,858	Int'l Ticker: Int'l Exchange:
2005 Sales: $800,726	2005 Profits: $127,606	Employees: 4,302
2004 Sales: $589,056	2004 Profits: $4,359	Fiscal Year Ends: 9/30
2003 Sales: $504,223	2003 Profits: $17,873	Parent Company:

SALARIES/BENEFITS:

Pension Plan:	ESOP Stock Plan:	Profit Sharing:	Top Exec. Salary: $559,833	Bonus: $789,000
Savings Plan: Y	Stock Purch. Plan:		Second Exec. Salary: $298,056	Bonus: $280,000

OTHER THOUGHTS:

Apparent Women Officers or Directors: 1
Hot Spot for Advancement for Women/Minorities:

LOCATIONS: ("Y" = Yes)

West:	Southwest:	Midwest:	Southeast:	Northeast:	International:
Y	Y	Y	Y		Y

HENRY SCHEIN INC

www.henryschein.com

Industry Group Code: 421450 Ranks within this company's industry group: Sales: 2 Profits: 2

Management:		Sales/Marketing:		Liberal Arts:		Information Systems:		Professionals:		Technical/Scientific:	
Mgmt. Trainees:	Y	Mktg. Professionals:	Y	Gen. Writing/Editing:	Y	Info. Management:	Y	Finance/Accounting:	Y	Engineers, Elec.:	Y
Experienced Mgmt.:	Y	Retail Sales:		Technical Writing:	Y	Software Dev.:	Y	Law:	Y	Engineers, Other:	Y
Int'l Business:	Y	Commercial/Industrial:	Y	Graphic Arts/Photog.:	Y	Hardware Dev.:		HR/Other:	Y	Health/Lab:	
MBA Graduates:	Y	Sales Trainees:		Music:		Systems Integration:		Training:	Y	Scientists/Research:	
		Advertising Pros.:	Y	Broadcasting:		Consulting/Other:		Health Care:	Y	Petroleum/Chemicals:	
				Other:				Consulting:		Math/Other:	

TYPES OF BUSINESS:

Health Care Products Distribution
Dental Supplies Distribution
Veterinary Products Distribution
Electronic Catalogs

BRANDS/DIVISIONS/AFFILIATES:

Aruba
Dentrix
Easy Dental
AVImark
W. & J. Dunlop, Ltd.

CONTACTS: Note: Officers with more than one job title may be intentionally listed here more than once.

Stanley M. Bergman, CEO
James P. Breslawski, COO
James P. Breslawski, Pres.
Steven Paladino, CFO/Exec. VP
James A. Harding, CTO/Sr. VP
Michael Racioppi, Chief Merchandising Officer/Sr. VP
Gerald A. Benjamin, Chief Admin. Officer/Exec. VP
Mark E. Mlotek, Exec. VP-Corp. Bus. Dev.
Leonard A. David, Corp. Sr. VP/Chief Compliance Officer
Stanley Komaroff, Sr. Advisor
Stanley M. Bergman, Chmn.
Michael Zack, Sr. VP/Pres., Int'l Group

Phone: 631-843-5500	Fax: 631-843-5658
Toll-Free:	
Address: 135 Duryea Rd., Melville, NY 11747 US	

GROWTH PLANS/SPECIAL FEATURES:

Henry Schein, Inc. distributes healthcare products and services to office-based healthcare practitioners in North America and Europe. The firm has over 550,000 customers in more than 200 countries, including dental practitioners and dental laboratories; physician practices; and animal health clinics. The company operates in two segments: healthcare distribution and technology. The healthcare distribution segment aggregates the dental, medical (including animal health) and international operating segments. Products distributed include consumable products; small equipment; laboratory products; large dental equipment; branded and generic pharmaceuticals; vaccines; surgical products; diagnostic tests; infection-control products; and vitamins. The technology segment provides software, technology and other value-added services to healthcare practitioners, primarily in the U.S. and Canada. Value-added solutions include practice-management software systems for dental and medical practitioners and animal health clinics. The lead practice-management software solutions include DENTRIX and Easy Dental for dental practices and AVImark for veterinary clinics. The technology group offerings also include financial services and continuing education for practitioners. Henry Schein offers a broad selection of more than 190,000 branded and Henry Schein private-brand products. The firm currently distributes over 34 million pieces of direct marketing material through the Aruba electronic catalog and ordering system. Henry Schein's web site provides an array of value-added features including instant customer registration and improved customer service and supply procurement capabilities. In June 2007, the company agreed to acquire Becker-Parkin Dental Supply Co.'s full-service and special markets business. In August 2007, the firm acquired W. & J. Dunlop, Ltd., a U.K supplier of animal health products and services. In April 2008, the firm acquired Minerva Dental Limited, a U.K. supplier of dental consumables and equipment.

The company offers its employees medical, dental and vision plans; life and AD&D insurance; short- and long-term disability insurance; flexible spending accounts; tuition assistance; a college savings plan; and on-site wellness programs.

FINANCIALS: Sales and profits are in thousands of dollars—add 000 to get the full amount. 2007 Note: Financial information for 2007 was not available for all companies at press time.

2007 Sales: $5,920,190	2007 Profits: $215,173	U.S. Stock Ticker: HSIC
2006 Sales: $5,048,191	2006 Profits: $163,759	Int'l Ticker: Int'l Exchange:
2005 Sales: $4,635,929	2005 Profits: $139,759	Employees: 11,000
2004 Sales: $3,898,485	2004 Profits: $114,274	Fiscal Year Ends: 12/31
2003 Sales: $3,353,805	2003 Profits: $137,501	Parent Company:

SALARIES/BENEFITS:

Pension Plan:	ESOP Stock Plan:	Profit Sharing:	Top Exec. Salary: $1,000,000	Bonus: $1,300,000
Savings Plan: Y	Stock Purch. Plan:		Second Exec. Salary: $513,401	Bonus: $390,000

OTHER THOUGHTS:

Apparent Women Officers or Directors: 3
Hot Spot for Advancement for Women/Minorities: Y

LOCATIONS: ("Y" = Yes)

West:	Southwest:	Midwest:	Southeast:	Northeast:	International:
Y	Y	Y	Y	Y	Y

Note: Financial information, benefits and other data can change quickly and may vary from those stated here.

HERTZ GLOBAL HOLDINGS INC

www.hertz.com

Industry Group Code: 532111 Ranks within this company's industry group: Sales: 2 Profits: 1

Management:		Sales/Marketing:		Liberal Arts:		Information Systems:		Professionals:		Technical/Scientific:	
Mgmt. Trainees:	Y	Mktg. Professionals:	Y	Gen. Writing/Editing:	Y	Info. Management:	Y	Finance/Accounting:	Y	Engineers, Elec.:	
Experienced Mgmt.:	Y	Retail Sales:		Technical Writing:		Software Dev.:	Y	Law:	Y	Engineers, Other:	
Int'l Business:	Y	Commercial/Industrial:	Y	Graphic Arts/Photog.:	Y	Hardware Dev.:		HR/Other:	Y	Health/Lab:	
MBA Graduates:	Y	Sales Trainees:	Y	Music:		Systems Integration:		Training:	Y	Scientists/Research:	
		Advertising Pros.:	Y	Broadcasting:		Consulting/Other:		Health Care:		Petroleum/Chemicals:	
				Other:				Consulting:		Math/Other:	

TYPES OF BUSINESS:

Automobile Rental
Truck Rental
Claims Management
Heavy Equipment Rental
Used Automobile Sales
Leasing
Actuarial Services
Franchising

BRANDS/DIVISIONS/AFFILIATES:

Hertz Local Edition
Hertz Car Sales
Hertz Equipment Rental Corp.
Hertz Rent A Car
Hertz Leasing

CONTACTS: Note: Officers with more than one job title may be intentionally listed here more than once.

Mark Frissora, CEO
Elyse Douglas, CFO/Exec. VP
Brian J. Kennedy, Exec. VP-Mktg. & Sales
LeighAnne Baker, Sr. VP-Chief Human Resources Officer
Joseph F. Eckroth, CIO/Sr. VP
Jeffrey Zimmerman, General Counsel/Sr. VP/Sec.
Jatindar Kapur, Corp. Controller/Sr. VP-Finance
Joseph R. Nothwang, Exec. VP/Pres., Vehicle Renting & Leasing
Gerald A. Plescia, Exec. VP/Pres., Hertz Equipment Rental Corp.
Lois Boyd, Sr VP-Process Improvement & Project Mgmt.
Robert J. Stuart, Sr. VP-Global Sales
Mark Frissora, Chmn.
Michael Taride, Exec. VP/Pres., Hertz Europe Ltd.
John A. Thomas, Exec. VP-Supply Chain Mgmt.

Phone: 201-307-2000	Fax: 201-307-2644
Toll-Free: 800-654-3131	
Address: 225 Brae Blvd., Park Ridge, NJ 07656-0713 US	

GROWTH PLANS/SPECIAL FEATURES:

Hertz Global Holdings, Inc. comprises a family of companies preceded by the name Hertz: Local Edition, which can be found at many airports, specializes in local rentals at affordable rates; Equipment Rental, which rents and sells heavy equipment and tools for construction and industrial applications; Car Sales, which sells one-year-old vehicles from Hertz' rental car fleet; Claim Management, which provides claim management services for liability exposures; Truck & Van Rental, which rents trucks and vans to facilitate customers' moves and large deliveries; and Lease, which offers leasing and fleet management services throughout its franchise network in Europe, the Middle East and Africa. Hertz is best known for its car rental activities, both in the U.S. market and internationally. Hertz and its independent licensees and associates accept reservations for car rentals at approximately 8,000 locations in approximately 145 countries. As of 2007, Hertz had a 28.5% market share at U.S. airport locations, compared to the Avis Budget Group's 30.1%. In March 2008, Hertz acquired Quilovat, a Spanish power generation rental company, to supplement the Equipment Rental's Energy Division. In April 2008, the firm obtained All Reach, LLC, a Connecticut-based aerial lift rental and service company, to service the northeast.

Hertz offers its employees benefits such as U.S. savings bonds, employee discounts and tuition reimbursement.

FINANCIALS: Sales and profits are in thousands of dollars—add 000 to get the full amount. 2007 Note: Financial information for 2007 was not available for all companies at press time.

2007 Sales: $8,685,600	2007 Profits: $264,500	U.S. Stock Ticker: HTZ
2006 Sales: $8,058,400	2006 Profits: $115,900	Int'l Ticker: Int'l Exchange:
2005 Sales: $7,314,700	2005 Profits: $371,300	Employees: 29,350
2004 Sales: $6,676,000	2004 Profits: $365,500	Fiscal Year Ends: 12/31
2003 Sales: $5,207,900	2003 Profits: $158,600	Parent Company:

SALARIES/BENEFITS:

Pension Plan: Y	ESOP Stock Plan:	Profit Sharing:	Top Exec. Salary: $986,539	Bonus: $3,834,000
Savings Plan: Y	Stock Purch. Plan:		Second Exec. Salary: $605,385	Bonus: $1,138,789

OTHER THOUGHTS:

Apparent Women Officers or Directors: 3
Hot Spot for Advancement for Women/Minorities: Y

LOCATIONS: ("Y" = Yes)

West:	Southwest:	Midwest:	Southeast:	Northeast:	International:
Y	Y	Y	Y	Y	Y

Note: Financial information, benefits and other data can change quickly and may vary from those stated here.

HESS CORPORATION

www.hess.com

Industry Group Code: 211111 Ranks within this company's industry group: Sales: Profits:

Management:		Sales/Marketing:		Liberal Arts:	Information Systems:		Professionals:		Technical/Scientific:	
Mgmt. Trainees:	Y	Mktg. Professionals:	Y	Gen. Writing/Editing:	Info. Management:	Y	Finance/Accounting:	Y	Engineers, Elec.:	Y
Experienced Mgmt.:	Y	Retail Sales:		Technical Writing:	Software Dev.:	Y	Law:	Y	Engineers, Other:	
Int'l Business:	Y	Commercial/Industrial:	Y	Graphic Arts/Photog.:	Hardware Dev.:		HR/Other:	Y	Health/Lab:	Y
MBA Graduates:	Y	Sales Trainees:		Music:	Systems Integration:		Training:	Y	Scientists/Research:	Y
		Advertising Pros.:		Broadcasting:	Consulting/Other:		Health Care:		Petroleum/Chemicals:	Y
				Other:			Consulting:		Math/Other:	Y

TYPES OF BUSINESS:

Oil & Gas Exploration & Production
Natural Gas
Refining
Energy Marketing

BRANDS/DIVISIONS/AFFILIATES:

Hovensa

CONTACTS: *Note: Officers with more than one job title may be intentionally listed here more than once.*

John B. Hess, CEO
F. Borden Walker, CFO/Sr. VP
R. J. Lawlor, Exec. VP/Pres., Mktg. & Refining
B. J. Bohling, Sr. VP-Human Resources
P. R. Walton, CIO/VP
S. Heck, Sr. VP-Tech.
S. Heck, Sr. VP-Global Prod.
J. Barclay Collins II, General Counsel/Exec. VP
H. Paver, Sr. VP-Global New Bus. Dev.
John Pepper, VP-Corp. Comm.
Jay R. Wilson, VP-Investor Rel.
J. J. Scelfo, Sr. VP-Finance & Corp. Dev.
John J. O'Connor, Exec. VP/Pres., Worldwide Exploration & Prod.
W. Drennen III, Sr. VP-Global Exploration & New Ventures
J.A. Gartman, Sr. VP-Energy Mktg.
D. Sweet, VP-Terminals & Refining
John B. Hess, Chmn.
D. K. Kirshner, VP-Supply & Trading

Phone: 212-997-8500	Fax: 212-536-8593
Toll-Free:	
Address: 1185 Ave. of the Americas, New York, NY 10036 US	

GROWTH PLANS/SPECIAL FEATURES:

Hess Corporation is a globally integrated energy company that operates in two segments: exploration and production; and marketing and refining. The exploration and production segment explores for, develops, produces, purchases, transports and sells crude oil and natural gas. These exploration and production activities take place in the U.S., the U.K., Norway, Denmark, Equatorial Guinea, Algeria, Malaysia, Thailand, Russia, Gabon, Azerbaijan, Indonesia, Libya, Egypt and other countries. The manufacturing and refining segment manufactures, purchases, transports, trades and markets refined petroleum products, natural gas and electricity. The company also owns 50% of a refinery joint venture with Petroleos de Venezuela in the U.S. Virgin Islands. Hess additionally owns another refining facility, and various terminals and retail gasoline stations, most of which include convenience stores located on the east coast of the U.S. In 2007, the company had 885 million barrels of proven reserves of crude oil and natural gas liquids, and over 2,600 billions of thousands of cubic feet of natural gas. The company markets refined petroleum products in the U.S. to the motoring public; wholesale distributors; industrial and commercial users; other petroleum companies; governmental agencies; and public utilities. The firm operates approximately 1,370 HESS retail facilities from Massachusetts to Florida. In 2007, 19% of the company's total proved reserves were located in the U.S.; 33% were located in Europe; 22% were in Africa; and 26% were in Asia and other regions. Hovensa, the refinery joint venture in the U.S. Virgin Islands, has a daily refining capacity of 7.8 million barrels per day. In June 2008, the company's Glencoe-1 exploration well on Australia's Northwest Shelf discovered natural gas in upper Jurassic sandstones, the first of three such discoveries off the coast of Australia between June and September.

FINANCIALS: Sales and profits are in thousands of dollars—add 000 to get the full amount. 2007 Note: Financial information for 2007 was not available for all companies at press time.

2007 Sales: $31,647,000	2007 Profits: $1,832,000	U.S. Stock Ticker: HES
2006 Sales: $28,067,000	2006 Profits: $1,916,000	Int'l Ticker: Int'l Exchange:
2005 Sales: $22,747,000	2005 Profits: $1,242,000	Employees: 11,610
2004 Sales: $16,733,000	2004 Profits: $977,000	Fiscal Year Ends: 12/31
2003 Sales: $14,311,000	2003 Profits: $643,000	Parent Company:

SALARIES/BENEFITS:

Pension Plan:	ESOP Stock Plan:	Profit Sharing:	Top Exec. Salary: $1,250,000	Bonus: $3,400,000
Savings Plan:	Stock Purch. Plan:		Second Exec. Salary: $1,100,000	Bonus: $2,200,000

OTHER THOUGHTS:

Apparent Women Officers or Directors: 2
Hot Spot for Advancement for Women/Minorities:

LOCATIONS: ("Y" = Yes)

West:	Southwest:	Midwest:	Southeast:	Northeast:	International:
Y	Y	Y	Y	Y	Y

HEWITT ASSOCIATES

www.hewitt.com

Industry Group Code: 541612 Ranks within this company's industry group: Sales: 3   Profits: 2

Management:		Sales/Marketing:		Liberal Arts:		Information Systems:		Professionals:		Technical/Scientific:	
Mgmt. Trainees:	Y	Mktg. Professionals:	Y	Gen. Writing/Editing:	Y	Info. Management:	Y	Finance/Accounting:	Y	Engineers, Elec.:	
Experienced Mgmt.:	Y	Retail Sales:		Technical Writing:	Y	Software Dev.:	Y	Law:	Y	Engineers, Other:	
Int'l Business:	Y	Commercial/Industrial:	Y	Graphic Arts/Photog.:	Y	Hardware Dev.:		HR/Other:	Y	Health/Lab:	
MBA Graduates:	Y	Sales Trainees:		Music:		Systems Integration:	Y	Training:	Y	Scientists/Research:	Y
		Advertising Pros.:	Y	Broadcasting:		Consulting/Other:	Y	Health Care:		Petroleum/Chemicals:	
				Other:				Consulting:	Y	Math/Other:	

TYPES OF BUSINESS:

Human Resources Consulting
Human Resources Outsourcing
Actuarial Services
Payroll & Benefits Consulting

BRANDS/DIVISIONS/AFFILIATES:

HeptaCon
RealLife HR
Global Risk Services
Vista Equity Partners
New Bridge Street Consultants
Csi-The Remuneration Specialists

CONTACTS: *Note: Officers with more than one job title may be intentionally listed here more than once.*

Russell P. Fradin, CEO
Daniel J. Holland, COO
John Park, CFO
Tracy Koegh, Sr. VP-Human Resources
Brad Anderson, CIO
Sanjiv K. Anand, CTO
Steven Kyono, General Counsel/Exec. VP/Corp. Sec.
Matthew Levin, Sr. VP-Corp. Dev. & Strategy
Kristi Savacool, Sr. VP-Global Bus. Svcs. & IT
Monica Burmeister, Global Chief-Consulting Oper.
Julie Gordon, Pres., Client & Market Leadership
Rohail Khan, Dir.-Benefits Outsourcing Oper.
Jay Rising, Pres., HR Outsourcing
Russell P. Fradin, Chmn.
Carlos A. Raposo, Dir.-HR Outsourcing, Latin America

Phone: 847-295-5000	Fax: 847-295-7634
Toll-Free:	
Address: 100 Half Day Rd., Lincolnshire, IL 60069 US	

GROWTH PLANS/SPECIAL FEATURES:

Hewitt Associates, Inc. is a human resources benefits, outsourcing and consulting services provider with offices in 33 countries. The company operates in three segments: Benefits Outsourcing, Human Resource Business Process Outsourcing (HR BPO) and Consulting. The Benefits Outsourcing sector of Hewitt provides integrated, single-system administration with the flexibility of multiple access channels (call centers, interactive voice response and the Internet) for employees to execute transactions and manage benefit programs for both defined contribution, such as a 401(k), and defined benefit (pension) plans, as well as health and welfare programs. The company offers its outsourcing services primarily to large companies with complex benefit programs. In the HR BPO segment, the firm helps more than 300 client companies manage employee data, administer benefits, payroll and other human resources processes, and record and manage transactions across talent management, workforce management and core process management. In the Consulting segment, Hewitt helps more than 3,000 client companies create effective strategies and programs in human resources, retirement plans, compensation, health care, benefits and payroll through its two sectors: benefits consulting and talent and organization consulting. In 2007, the firm acquired HeptaCon, an HR consulting company based in Vienna, and RealLife HR, a leading U.S. provider of benefits management services. The company launched Global Risk Services, a risk management organization for retirement plan sponsors. In January 2008, Hewitt agreed to sell assets related to its Cyborg business, a payroll and HR services organization, to Vista Equity Partners. In March, the company acquired New Bridge Street Consultants, a compensation consultancy in the U.K., and agreed to acquire CSi-The Remuneration Specialists, a compensation consulting company based in Australia.

Hewitt Associates provides its employees with long-term disability insurance, family counseling services, tuition reimbursement, legal assistance, adoption assistance and overnight pet care.

FINANCIALS: Sales and profits are in thousands of dollars—add 000 to get the full amount. 2007 Note: Financial information for 2007 was not available for all companies at press time.

2007 Sales: $2,990,326		2007 Profits: $-175,080		**U.S. Stock Ticker: HEW**	
2006 Sales: $2,857,161		2006 Profits: $-115,938		**Int'l Ticker:** Int'l Exchange:	
2005 Sales: $2,889,650		2005 Profits: $134,732		Employees: 23,000	
2004 Sales: $2,257,400		2004 Profits: $122,844		Fiscal Year Ends: 9/30	
2003 Sales: $2,031,293		2003 Profits: $94,277		Parent Company:	

SALARIES/BENEFITS:

Pension Plan: Y	ESOP Stock Plan:	Profit Sharing: Y	Top Exec. Salary: $882,692	Bonus: $1,539,450
Savings Plan: Y	Stock Purch. Plan:		Second Exec. Salary: $506,667	Bonus: $568,540

OTHER THOUGHTS:

Apparent Women Officers or Directors: 5
Hot Spot for Advancement for Women/Minorities: Y

LOCATIONS: ("Y" = Yes)

West:	Southwest:	Midwest:	Southeast:	Northeast:	International:
Y	Y	Y	Y	Y	Y

HEWLETT-PACKARD CO (HP)

www.hp.com

Industry Group Code: 334111   Ranks within this company's industry group: Sales: 1   Profits: 1

Management:		Sales/Marketing:		Liberal Arts:		Information Systems:		Professionals:		Technical/Scientific:	
Mgmt. Trainees:	Y	Mktg. Professionals:	Y	Gen. Writing/Editing:	Y	Info. Management:	Y	Finance/Accounting:	Y	Engineers, Elec.:	Y
Experienced Mgmt.:	Y	Retail Sales:		Technical Writing:	Y	Software Dev.:	Y	Law:	Y	Engineers, Other:	
Int'l Business:	Y	Commercial/Industrial:	Y	Graphic Arts/Photog.:	Y	Hardware Dev.:	Y	HR/Other:	Y	Health/Lab:	Y
MBA Graduates:	Y	Sales Trainees:	Y	Music:		Systems Integration:	Y	Training:	Y	Scientists/Research:	Y
		Advertising Pros.:	Y	Broadcasting:		Consulting/Other:	Y	Health Care:		Petroleum/Chemicals:	
				Other:	Y			Consulting:	Y	Math/Other:	Y

TYPES OF BUSINESS:

Computer Hardware-PCs
Computer Software
Printers & Supplies
Scanners
Outsourcing
Servers
Consulting

BRANDS/DIVISIONS/AFFILIATES:

StorageWorks
HP Services
Hewlett-Packard Laboratories
Mercury Interactive Corp
Hewlett-Packard Quantum Science Research
Hewlett-Packard Global Soft Limited
Bristol Technologies, Inc.
Neoware, Inc.

CONTACTS: Note: Officers with more than one job title may be intentionally listed here more than once.

Mark Hurd, CEO
Mark Hurd, Pres.
Cathie Lesjak, CFO/Exec. VP
Michael Mendenhall, Chief Mktg. Officer/Sr. VP
Marcela Perez de Alonso, Exec. VP-Human Resources
Prith Banerjee, Sr. VP-Research/Dir.-HP Labs
Randall D. Mott, CIO/Exec. VP
Shane Robison, CTO/Exec. VP
Jon Flaxman, Chief Admin. Officer/Exec. VP
Michael J. Holston, General Counsel/Exec. VP/Sec.
Shane Robison, Chief Strategy Officer
Todd Bradley, Exec. VP-Personal Systems Group
Ann M. Livermore, Exec. VP-Tech. Solutions Group
Vyomesh Joshi, Exec. VP-Imaging & Printing Group
Don Grantham, Sr. VP/Chief Sales Officer
Mark Hurd, Chmn.

Phone: 650-857-1501	Fax: 650-857-5518
Toll-Free:	
Address: 3000 Hanover St., Palo Alto, CA 94304 US	

GROWTH PLANS/SPECIAL FEATURES:

Hewlett-Packard Co. (HP) is a global provider of products, technologies, software and services to customers ranging from individuals to large enterprises, including the public and education sectors. Offerings span personal computing and other access devices; imaging and printing-related products and services; enterprise IT infrastructure; and multi-vendor services. The company operates in seven segments: enterprise storage and servers (ESS); HP services (HPS); HP software; the personal systems group (PSG); the imaging and printing group (IPG); HP financial services (HPFS); and corporate investments. The ESS segment provides a broad portfolio of storage and server solutions such as the HP StorageWorks, whose offerings include entry-level, mid-range and high-end arrays, storage area networks, network attached storage, storage management software and virtualization technologies, as well as tape drives, tape libraries and optical archival storage. The HPS segment provides of portfolio of multi-vendor IT services, including technology services; consulting and integration; and outsourcing services. The HP software segment provides a suite of business technology optimization software solutions, including support, that allow customers to manage and automate their IT infrastructure, operations, applications, IT services and business processes under the OpenView brand. The PSG segment provides PCs, consumer PCs, workstations, handheld computing devices, digital entertainment systems, calculators and related accessories, software and services for the commercial and consumer markets. The IPG segment provides consumer and commercial printer hardware, printing supplies, printing media and scanning devices. The HPFS segment provides a broad range of value-added financial lifecycle management services. The corporate investments segment includes the Hewlett-Packard Laboratories and certain business incubation projects. The division sells certain network infrastructure products, including Ethernet switch products that enhance computing and enterprise solutions under the brand ProCurve Networking. In 2007, HP acquired Bristol Technology, Inc.; SPI Dynamics, Inc.; Opsware, Inc.; and Neoware, Inc. In May 2008, the firm agreed to acquire Electronic Data Systems (EDS) for $13.9 billion.

FINANCIALS: Sales and profits are in thousands of dollars—add 000 to get the full amount. 2007 Note: Financial information for 2007 was not available for all companies at press time.

2007 Sales: $104,286,000	2007 Profits: $7,264,000	U.S. Stock Ticker: HPQ
2006 Sales: $91,658,000	2006 Profits: $6,198,000	Int'l Ticker: Int'l Exchange:
2005 Sales: $86,696,000	2005 Profits: $2,398,000	Employees: 172,000
2004 Sales: $79,905,000	2004 Profits: $3,497,000	Fiscal Year Ends: 10/31
2003 Sales: $73,061,000	2003 Profits: $2,539,000	Parent Company:

SALARIES/BENEFITS:

Pension Plan: Y	ESOP Stock Plan:	Profit Sharing:	Top Exec. Salary: $1,400,000	Bonus: $8,624,000
Savings Plan: Y	Stock Purch. Plan:		Second Exec. Salary: $975,000	Bonus: $4,095,000

OTHER THOUGHTS:

Apparent Women Officers or Directors: 5
Hot Spot for Advancement for Women/Minorities: Y

LOCATIONS: ("Y" = Yes)

West:	Southwest:	Midwest:	Southeast:	Northeast:	International:
Y	Y	Y	Y	Y	Y

HIBBETT SPORTS INC

www.hibbett.com

Industry Group Code: 451110 **Ranks within this company's industry group:** Sales: 3 Profits: 3

Management:		Sales/Marketing:		Liberal Arts:		Information Systems:		Professionals:		Technical/Scientific:	
Mgmt. Trainees:	Y	Mktg. Professionals:	Y	Gen. Writing/Editing:	Y	Info. Management:	Y	Finance/Accounting:	Y	Engineers, Elec.:	
Experienced Mgmt.:	Y	Retail Sales:	Y	Technical Writing:		Software Dev.:	Y	Law:	Y	Engineers, Other:	
Int'l Business:		Commercial/Industrial:	Y	Graphic Arts/Photog.:	Y	Hardware Dev.:		HR/Other:	Y	Health/Lab:	
MBA Graduates:	Y	Sales Trainees:	Y	Music:		Systems Integration:		Training:	Y	Scientists/Research:	
		Advertising Pros.:	Y	Broadcasting:		Consulting/Other:		Health Care:		Petroleum/Chemicals:	
				Other:				Consulting:		Math/Other:	

TYPES OF BUSINESS:

Sporting Goods Stores
Sports Apparel
Athletic Shoes
Training Equipment

BRANDS/DIVISIONS/AFFILIATES:

Hibbett Sports
Sports & Co.
Sports Additions
Hibbett Team Sales, Inc.

CONTACTS: *Note: Officers with more than one job title may be intentionally listed here more than once.*

Michael J. Newsome, CEO
Brian N Priddy, Pres.
Gary A. Smith, CFO/VP
Jeffry O. Rosenthal, VP-Merch.
Cathy E. Pryor, VP-Store Oper.
Michael J. Newsome, Chmn.

Phone: 205-942-4292	Fax: 205-912-7290
Toll-Free:	
Address: 451 Industrial Ln., Birmingham, AL 35211 US	

GROWTH PLANS/SPECIAL FEATURES:

Hibbett Sports, Inc. is an operator of sporting goods stores in small to mid-sized markets predominantly in the Sunbelt, Mid-Atlantic and Midwest. Its stores offer a broad assortment of athletic equipment, footwear and apparel. The company's merchandise assortment features a broad selection of brand name merchandise emphasizing team sports complemented by localized apparel and accessories designed to appeal to a wide range of customers. The firm's primary retail format is Hibbett Sports, a 5,000 square foot store located in enclosed malls or in strip centers that are generally the center of commerce within an area and that are usually anchored by a Wal-Mart store. The Hibbett Sports stores strive to respond quickly to major sporting events of local interests. The Sports Additions stores are small, mall-based stores averaging 2,300 square feet with roughly 90% of merchandise consisting of athletic footwear and the remainder consisting of caps and a limited assortment of apparel. Sports Additions stores offer a broader assortment of athletic footwear, with a greater emphasis on fashion than the athletic footwear assortment offered by Hibbett Sports stores. The Sports & Co. superstores average 25,000 square feet and offer a broader assortment of athletic footwear, apparel and equipment than the Hibbett Sports stores. Hibbett Sports operates over 650 stores in 23 states. Subsidiary Hibbett Team Sales, Inc. supplies customized athletic apparel, equipment and footwear to school, athletic and youth programs primarily in Alabama. It sells its merchandise directly to educational institutions and youth associations.

The company offers its employees health, dental and vision insurance; life and AD&D insurance; short- and long-term disability insurance; a stock purchase plan; a 401(k) plan; employee discounts; and a college savings plan. The Superstars program awards young athletes for sportsmanship and determination with a $1,000 donation to charities in the winners' community.

FINANCIALS: Sales and profits are in thousands of dollars—add 000 to get the full amount. 2007 Note: Financial information for 2007 was not available for all companies at press time.

2007 Sales: $512,094	2007 Profits: $38,073	**U.S. Stock Ticker: HIBB**
2006 Sales: $440,269	2006 Profits: $33,624	**Int'l Ticker:** Int'l Exchange:
2005 Sales: $377,534	2005 Profits: $25,147	Employees: 5,200
2004 Sales: $320,964	2004 Profits: $20,348	Fiscal Year Ends: 1/31
2003 Sales: $279,200	2003 Profits: $14,700	Parent Company:

SALARIES/BENEFITS:

Pension Plan:	ESOP Stock Plan:	Profit Sharing:	Top Exec. Salary: $440,000	Bonus: $360,510
Savings Plan: Y	Stock Purch. Plan: Y		Second Exec. Salary: $308,000	Bonus: $209,468

OTHER THOUGHTS:

Apparent Women Officers or Directors: 1
Hot Spot for Advancement for Women/Minorities:

LOCATIONS: ("Y" = Yes)

West:	Southwest:	Midwest:	Southeast:	Northeast:	International:
	Y	Y	Y	Y	

HILB ROGAL & HOBBS CO

www.hrh.com

Industry Group Code: 524210 **Ranks within this company's industry group:** Sales: 3 Profits: 3

Management:		Sales/Marketing:		Liberal Arts:		Information Systems:		Professionals:		Technical/Scientific:	
Mgmt. Trainees:	Y	Mktg. Professionals:	Y	Gen. Writing/Editing:		Info. Management:	Y	Finance/Accounting:	Y	Engineers, Elec.:	
Experienced Mgmt.:	Y	Retail Sales:		Technical Writing:	Y	Software Dev.:		Law:	Y	Engineers, Other:	
Int'l Business:	Y	Commercial/Industrial:	Y	Graphic Arts/Photog.:		Hardware Dev.:		HR/Other:	Y	Health/Lab:	
MBA Graduates:	Y	Sales Trainees:		Music:		Systems Integration:		Training:	Y	Scientists/Research:	
		Advertising Pros.:	Y	Broadcasting:		Consulting/Other:		Health Care:		Petroleum/Chemicals:	
				Other:				Consulting:		Math/Other:	

TYPES OF BUSINESS:

Insurance Brokerage
Risk Management
Consulting Services
Claims Administration
Employee Benefits

BRANDS/DIVISIONS/AFFILIATES:

Resource Group, L.C. (The)
Brown/Raynor Corporation
Charlton Manley, Inc.
Banc of America Corporate Insurance Agency, L.L.C.
Integrated Group Benefits
Talty Insurance Agency, Inc.
G.A. Pearson and Associates Insurance Brokers, Inc
Willis Group Holdings Ltd.

CONTACTS: *Note: Officers with more than one job title may be intentionally listed here more than once.*

Martin (Mell) Vaughan, III, CEO
F. Michael Crowley, COO
F. Michael Crowley, Pres.
Michael Dinkins, CFO/Exec. VP
Robert S. O'Brien, VP/Nat'l Dir.-Production & Sales Dev.
Joseph Birriel, VP-Human Resources & Corp. Branding
Viren R. Kapadia, CIO/VP-Sourcing
A. Brent King, General Counsel/Sr. VP
Chris Purvis, VP/Dir.-Oper.
Timothy J. Korman, Exec. VP-Mergers & Acquisitions
Elizabeth J. Cougot, Asst. VP-Corp. Comm.
Carolyn Jones, Sr. VP-Investor Rel.
Carolyn Jones, Treas.
Steven C. Deal, VP/Regional Dir.-Mid-Atlantic Region
Frank H. Beard, VP/Nat'l Dir.-Property & Casualty
Walter L. Smith, Sr. VP-Bus. Practices & Quality Assurance/Sec.
John Hamerski, VP/Controller
Martin (Mell) Vaughan, III, Chmn.
Steven P. Hearn, VP/Dir.-Int'l

Phone: 804-747-0200	Fax: 804-747-7307
Toll-Free:	
Address: 4951 Lake Brook Dr., Ste. 500, Glen Allen, VA 23060-9272 US	

GROWTH PLANS/SPECIAL FEATURES:

Hilb, Rogal and Hobbs Co. (HRH) is an U.S insurance and risk management intermediary firms. The company operates over 120 offices in 29 U.S. states and London as well as branch locations in Russia, South Africa and Australia. The firm assists clients in managing their risks in areas such as property and casualty, executive and employee benefits and other areas of specialized exposure. Insurance commissions and fees in lieu of commission account for approximately 94% of HRH's 2007 revenues. The company's offices act as independent agents representing a large number of insurance companies, which gives it access to specialized products and capacity needed by its clients. Offices and regions are staffed to handle the broad variety of insurance needs of clients. HRH also advises clients on risk management and employee benefits, and provides claims administration and loss control consulting services to clients, which accounts for approximately 4% of 2007 revenues. The firm's client base ranges from individuals to large national accounts and is primarily composed of middle-market and major businesses that do not have internal risk management departments. HRH's growth strategy principally involves mergers and acquisitions of independent agencies that operate in small to medium-sized metropolitan areas. Since its establishment, the firm has acquired over 230 independent agencies. In 2007, HRH acquired Brown/Raynor Corporation; Charlton Manley, Inc.; The Resource Group, L.C.; and Banc of America Corporate Insurance Agency, L.L.C. As of September 2008, the firm acquired Integrated Group Benefits; Talty Insurance Agency, Inc.; and G.A. Pearson and Associates Insurance Brokers, Inc. In June 2008, Willis Group Holdings Ltd. agreed to acquire HRH for $1.7 billion; the transaction is expected to close by the end of 2008.

HRH employee benefits include medical, dental, disability, and life insurance; and a 401(k) plan.

FINANCIALS: Sales and profits are in thousands of dollars—add 000 to get the full amount. 2007 Note: Financial information for 2007 was not available for all companies at press time.

2007 Sales: $799,664	2007 Profits: $78,125	**U.S. Stock Ticker: HRH**
2006 Sales: $710,845	2006 Profits: $87,031	**Int'l Ticker:** Int'l Exchange:
2005 Sales: $673,885	2005 Profits: $56,200	Employees: 3,700
2004 Sales: $619,603	2004 Profits: $81,414	Fiscal Year Ends: 12/31
2003 Sales: $563,647	2003 Profits: $74,954	Parent Company:

SALARIES/BENEFITS:

Pension Plan:	ESOP Stock Plan:	Profit Sharing:	Top Exec. Salary: $554,667	Bonus: $482,300
Savings Plan: Y	Stock Purch. Plan:		Second Exec. Salary: $440,000	Bonus: $337,080

OTHER THOUGHTS:

Apparent Women Officers or Directors: 4
Hot Spot for Advancement for Women/Minorities: Y

LOCATIONS: ("Y" = Yes)

West:	Southwest:	Midwest:	Southeast:	Northeast:	International:
Y	Y	Y	Y	Y	Y

Note: Financial information, benefits and other data can change quickly and may vary from those stated here.

HILTON HOTELS CORP

www.hiltonworldwide.com

Industry Group Code: 721110 **Ranks within this company's industry group:** Sales: 2 Profits: 3

Management:		Sales/Marketing:		Liberal Arts:		Information Systems:		Professionals:		Technical/Scientific:	
Mgmt. Trainees:	Y	Mktg. Professionals:	Y	Gen. Writing/Editing:	Y	Info. Management:	Y	Finance/Accounting:	Y	Engineers, Elec.:	
Experienced Mgmt.:	Y	Retail Sales:		Technical Writing:		Software Dev.:		Law:	Y	Engineers, Other:	
Int'l Business:	Y	Commercial/Industrial:	Y	Graphic Arts/Photog.:	Y	Hardware Dev.:		HR/Other:	Y	Health/Lab:	
MBA Graduates:	Y	Sales Trainees:		Music:		Systems Integration:		Training:	Y	Scientists/Research:	
		Advertising Pros.:	Y	Broadcasting:		Consulting/Other:		Health Care:		Petroleum/Chemicals:	
				Other:				Consulting:		Math/Other:	

TYPES OF BUSINESS:

Hotels & Resorts
Timeshare Properties
Conference Centers
Franchising
Management Services
Online Reservations

BRANDS/DIVISIONS/AFFILIATES:

Blackstone Group LP (The)
Hilton Group plc
Hampton Inn
Conrad Hotels and Resorts
Waldorf=Astoria Collection (The)
Embassy Suits
Hilton Garden Vacations Company, LLC
Hhonors

CONTACTS: Note: Officers with more than one job title may be intentionally listed here more than once.

Christopher J. Nassetta, CEO
Christopher J. Nassetta, Pres.
Robert M. La Forgia, CFO/Exec. VP
Kenneth Smith, Pres., Sales & Revenue Mgmt.
Molly McKenzie-Swarts, Exec. VP-Human Resources & Diversity
James Harvey, CIO/Exec. VP-Shared Svcs.
Molly McKenzie-Swarts, Exec. VP-Admin.
Kenneth Smith, Pres., Americas Oper.
Steven Goldman, Pres., Global Dev. & Real Estate
Linda Bain, Sr. VP-Global Comm. & Public Rel.
Atish Shah, VP-Investor Rel.
Thomas L. Keltner, Exec. VP/CEO-Americas & Global Brands
Mark Wang, Pres., Hilton Grand Vacations
Ian R. Carter, Pres., Int'l Oper.

Phone: 310-278-4321	Fax: 310-205-7678
Toll-Free: 800-445-8667	
Address: 9336 Civic Center Dr., Beverly Hills, CA 90210 US	

GROWTH PLANS/SPECIAL FEATURES:

Hilton Hotels Corp. (HHC), founded in 1919, owns, manages and develops hotels, resorts and timeshare properties; and franchises lodging properties. In October 2007, the firm was acquired by an affiliate of The Blackstone Group LP for $26.93 billion and taken private. Having sold numerous properties lately, HHC now consists of over 490,000 rooms in over 2,800 properties across 80 countries. Its hotel brands include Hilton, Hilton Garden Inn, Doubletree, Embassy Suites, Homewood, Hampton Inn, Conrad Hotels and Resorts and The Waldorf=Astoria Collection. HHC recently acquired the lodging assets of Hilton Group plc, known collectively as Hilton International, for approximately $5.71 billion dollars; the international assets of the firm had been spun-off in 1964. Following the acquisition, HHC again owns the worldwide rights to develop and market Hilton and Conrad brands. Although the majority of the company's hotels are located within the U.S., the company also operates luxury lodgings in locations such as Thailand, Ireland, Singapore, Uruguay, Indonesia and Egypt. Hilton Worldwide Resorts offers 56 self-contained resorts in the Middle East, Asia Pacific, Europe, the Americas, the Indian Ocean and the Caribbean. Through Hilton Garden Vacations Company, LLC, the firm also owns and manages 33 vacation timeshare properties. HHonors, the firm's loyalty enrollment program for returning customers, has over 17 million members. The firm is investing in innovative technologies such as check-in kiosks to facilitate an easier and faster check-in process for its customers. HHC, in separate deals with three real estate groups, is developing over 55 properties in Russia, the U.K. and Central America, all planned to be completed by 2012. Over the next decade, the firm will open 300 new hotels in Asia, including properties in India and China. In April 2007, HHC sold its 132 hotel Scandic chain for $1.1 billion to private-equity firm EQT.

Employees of HHC receive health and dependent care spending accounts; employee assistance programs; tuition reimbursements; discounted home and auto insurance options; credit union/banking options; and legal assistance.

FINANCIALS: Sales and profits are in thousands of dollars—add 000 to get the full amount. 2007 Note: Financial information for 2007 was not available for all companies at press time.

2007 Sales: $8,090,000	2007 Profits: $121,000	**U.S. Stock Ticker:** Private
2006 Sales: $7,438,000	2006 Profits: $572,000	**Int'l Ticker:** Int'l Exchange:
2005 Sales: $3,218,000	2005 Profits: $460,000	Employees: 105,000
2004 Sales: $4,146,000	2004 Profits: $238,000	Fiscal Year Ends: 12/31
2003 Sales: $3,853,000	2003 Profits: $164,000	Parent Company: BLACKSTONE GROUP LP (THE)

SALARIES/BENEFITS:

Pension Plan: Y	ESOP Stock Plan:	Profit Sharing:	Top Exec. Salary: $1,000,000	Bonus: $1,977,830
Savings Plan: Y	Stock Purch. Plan:		Second Exec. Salary: $789,438	Bonus: $768,805

OTHER THOUGHTS:

Apparent Women Officers or Directors: 2
Hot Spot for Advancement for Women/Minorities: Y

LOCATIONS: ("Y" = Yes)

West:	Southwest:	Midwest:	Southeast:	Northeast:	International:
Y	Y	Y	Y	Y	Y

HOME DEPOT INC

www.homedepot.com

Industry Group Code: 444110 Ranks within this company's industry group: Sales: 1 Profits: 1

Management:		Sales/Marketing:		Liberal Arts:		Information Systems:		Professionals:		Technical/Scientific:	
Mgmt. Trainees:	Y	Mktg. Professionals:	Y	Gen. Writing/Editing:	Y	Info. Management:	Y	Finance/Accounting:	Y	Engineers, Elec.:	
Experienced Mgmt.:	Y	Retail Sales:	Y	Technical Writing:		Software Dev.:	Y	Law:	Y	Engineers, Other:	
Int'l Business:	Y	Commercial/Industrial:	Y	Graphic Arts/Photog.:	Y	Hardware Dev.:		HR/Other:	Y	Health/Lab:	
MBA Graduates:	Y	Sales Trainees:	Y	Music:		Systems Integration:		Training:	Y	Scientists/Research:	
		Advertising Pros.:	Y	Broadcasting:		Consulting/Other:		Health Care:		Petroleum/Chemicals:	
				Other:	Y			Consulting:		Math/Other:	

TYPES OF BUSINESS:

Home Centers, Retail
Home Improvement Products
Building Materials
Lawn & Garden Products
Online & Catalog Sales
Tool & Truck Rental
Installation & Design Services

BRANDS/DIVISIONS/AFFILIATES:

EXPO Design Centers
Home Way (The)
THD Design Center
Yardbirds

CONTACTS: Note: Officers with more than one job title may be intentionally listed here more than once.

Francis (Frank) Blake, CEO
Joe DeAngelo, COO/Exec. VP
Carol B. Tome, CFO
Frank Bifulco, Sr. VP/Chief Mktg. Officer
Tim Crow, Exec. VP-Human Resources
Matt Carey, CIO/Exec. VP
Craig Menear, Exec. VP-Merch.
Jack A. VanWoerkom, General Counsel/Corp. Sec./Exec. VP
Carol B. Tome, Exec. VP-Corp. Svcs.
Brad Shaw, Sr. VP-Corp Comm. & External Affairs
Dianne Dayhoff, Sr. VP-Investor Rel.
Kelly Barrett, Sr. VP-Enterprise Program Management
Joe McFarland, Pres., Western Div.
Joe Izganics, Pres., Southern Div.
Marvin Ellison, Exec. VP-US Stores
Francis (Frank) Blake, Chmn.
Annette Verschuren, Pres., The Home Depot Canada & Asia
Mark Holifield, Sr. VP-Supply Chain

Phone: 770-433-8211	Fax: 770-384-2356
Toll-Free: 800-533-3199	
Address: 2455 Paces Ferry Rd., Atlanta, GA 30339-4024 US	

GROWTH PLANS/SPECIAL FEATURES:

Home Depot, Inc. is one of the world's largest home improvement retailers. The company operates 2,193 Home Depot stores throughout the U.S., Puerto Rico, the Virgin Islands, Canada, China and Mexico. A typical store encompasses 105,000 square feet of enclosed space, plus 23,000 square feet in the outdoor garden center, and stocks 35,000 to 45,000 items. These stores sell an assortment of building materials, plumbing materials, electrical materials, kitchen products, hardware, seasonal items, paint, flooring and wall coverings. The company also operates 34 full-service interior design and home furnishing stores under the name EXPO Design Centers in 13 states. These focus on interior design products including cabinetry, flooring, appliances, window treatments and lighting fixtures and offer a variety of installation services. Sales per square foot per year average about $380. The company also operates two THD Design Center stores and five Yardbirds stores in California and North Carolina. In August 2007, the company completed the sale of its wholesale construction supply business (HD Supply) to Bain Capital LLC, Carlyle Group LP and Clayton, Dubilier & Rice, Inc. for $8.5 billion. Home Depot retains a 12.5% stake in HD Supply. In 2007, the company closed its 11 Home Depot Landscape Supply stores and two Home Depot Floor stores. The nationwide real estate slowdown of 2007-2008 hurt Home Depot's business. In mid 2008, the firm cancelled plans for about 50 new store openings, and announced that it was closing 15 underperforming stores.

The company offers its employees a 401(k) plan; an employee stock purchase plan; adoption, education and relocation assistance; flexible spending accounts; a legal services plan; auto and homeowners insurance; and veterinary insurance.

FINANCIALS: Sales and profits are in thousands of dollars—add 000 to get the full amount. 2007 Note: Financial information for 2007 was not available for all companies at press time.

2007 Sales: $79,022,000	2007 Profits: $5,761,000	U.S. Stock Ticker: HD
2006 Sales: $77,019,000	2006 Profits: $5,838,000	Int'l Ticker: Int'l Exchange:
2005 Sales: $73,094,000	2005 Profits: $5,001,000	Employees: 345,000
2004 Sales: $64,816,000	2004 Profits: $4,304,000	Fiscal Year Ends: 1/31
2003 Sales: $58,247,000	2003 Profits: $3,664,000	Parent Company:

SALARIES/BENEFITS:

Pension Plan:	ESOP Stock Plan:	Profit Sharing:	Top Exec. Salary: $2,331,538	Bonus: $6,000,000
Savings Plan: Y	Stock Purch. Plan: Y		Second Exec. Salary: $758,384	Bonus: $941,250

OTHER THOUGHTS:

Apparent Women Officers or Directors: 6
Hot Spot for Advancement for Women/Minorities: Y

LOCATIONS: ("Y" = Yes)

West:	Southwest:	Midwest:	Southeast:	Northeast:	International:
Y	Y	Y	Y	Y	Y

Note: Financial information, benefits and other data can change quickly and may vary from those stated here.

HONEYWELL INTERNATIONAL INC   www.honeywell.com

Industry Group Code: 336410   Ranks within this company's industry group: Sales: 4   Profits: 4

Management:		Sales/Marketing:		Liberal Arts:		Information Systems:		Professionals:		Technical/Scientific:	
Mgmt. Trainees:	Y	Mktg. Professionals:	Y	Gen. Writing/Editing:	Y	Info. Management:	Y	Finance/Accounting:	Y	Engineers, Elec.:	
Experienced Mgmt.:	Y	Retail Sales:		Technical Writing:	Y	Software Dev.:	Y	Law:	Y	Engineers, Other:	
Int'l Business:	Y	Commercial/Industrial:	Y	Graphic Arts/Photog.:		Hardware Dev.:	Y	HR/Other:	Y	Health/Lab:	
MBA Graduates:	Y	Sales Trainees:		Music:		Systems Integration:	Y	Training:	Y	Scientists/Research:	
		Advertising Pros.:	Y	Broadcasting:		Consulting/Other:	Y	Health Care:		Petroleum/Chemicals:	
				Other:				Consulting:	Y	Math/Other:	

TYPES OF BUSINESS:
Aerospace & Defense Products
Automation & Control Systems
Turboprop Engines
Performance Polymers
Specialty Chemicals
Nuclear Services
Life Sciences
Nanotechnology & MEMS Research

BRANDS/DIVISIONS/AFFILIATES:
Honeywell Aerospace Solutions
Prestone
FRAM
Enraf Holdings B.V.
Hand Held Products, Inc.
Dimensions International
Maxon Corporation
UOP LLC

CONTACTS: Note: Officers with more than one job title may be intentionally listed here more than once.
David M. Cote, CEO
David J. Anderson, CFO/Sr. VP
Mark James, Sr. VP-Human Resources
Larry E. Kittelberger, Sr. VP-Tech.
Peter M. Kreindler, General Counsel/Sr. VP
Larry E. Kittelberger, Sr. VP-Oper.
Rhonda Germany, VP-Strategy & Bus. Dev.
Mark James, Sr. VP-Comm.
Murray Grainger, VP-Investor Rel.
Rob Gillette, CEO/Pres., Aerospace
Nance K. Dicciani, CEO/Pres., Specialty Materials
Roger Fradin, CEO/Pres., Automation & Control Solutions
David M. Cote, Chmn.
Adriane M. Brown, CEO/Pres., Transportation Systems

Phone: 973-455-2000	Fax: 973-455-4807
Toll-Free: 800-328-5111	
Address: 101 Columbia Rd., Morristown, NJ 07962-1219 US	

GROWTH PLANS/SPECIAL FEATURES:

Honeywell International, Inc. is a leading producer of high-tech control systems, including turboprop engines for airplanes, specialty chemicals for heavy equipment, polymers for electronics, sensing and security technologies for buildings, homes and industry and process technology for refining and petrochemicals. The company is divided into four sectors: Aerospace solutions, automation and control solutions, specialty materials and transportation systems. The aerospace unit is associated with engines, electronic systems, integrated avionics systems and service solutions. It is Honeywell's largest segment, earning 35% of sales. The automation and control solutions division deals with control products such as heating and air conditioning for homes and buildings, water controls and electronic systems for burners, broilers and furnaces, along with security and fire products and services. The specialty materials segment is involved in nylon products and services, fluorocarbons, specialty fibers, nuclear services and customized research chemicals for use in segments such as telecommunications, ballistic protection, pharmaceutical packaging and counterfeit avoidance. The transportation and power systems division includes charge air systems and thermal systems, as well as consumer car care products (under the Prestone, FRAM and Autolite brands). The firm is engaged in manufacturing, sales and research and development mainly in the U.S., Europe, Canada, Asia and Latin America. The firm made a number of acquisitions in 2007, including: Enraf Holding B.V., a division of Delft Industries based in the Netherlands; Hand Held Products, Inc., an Automatic Identification and Data Collection (AIDC) company; and Dimensions International, a company focused on defense logistics. In November 2007, Honeywell agreed to acquire Maxon Corporation, an industrial combustion controls business. In early 2008, the company announced its intention to establish a natural gas processing design center in Malaysia to support the Southeast Asia market.

FINANCIALS: Sales and profits are in thousands of dollars—add 000 to get the full amount. 2007 Note: Financial information for 2007 was not available for all companies at press time.

2007 Sales: $34,589,000	2007 Profits: $2,444,000	U.S. Stock Ticker: HON
2006 Sales: $31,367,000	2006 Profits: $2,083,000	Int'l Ticker: Int'l Exchange:
2005 Sales: $27,652,000	2005 Profits: $1,638,000	Employees: 122,000
2004 Sales: $25,593,000	2004 Profits: $1,246,000	Fiscal Year Ends: 12/31
2003 Sales: $23,103,000	2003 Profits: $1,324,000	Parent Company:

SALARIES/BENEFITS:

Pension Plan: Y	ESOP Stock Plan:	Profit Sharing:	Top Exec. Salary: $1,610,192	Bonus: $11,400,000
Savings Plan: Y	Stock Purch. Plan:		Second Exec. Salary: $753,365	Bonus: $2,950,000

OTHER THOUGHTS:
Apparent Women Officers or Directors: 3
Hot Spot for Advancement for Women/Minorities: Y

LOCATIONS: ("Y" = Yes)

West:	Southwest:	Midwest:	Southeast:	Northeast:	International:
Y	Y	Y	Y	Y	Y

HOT TOPIC INC
www.hottopic.com

Industry Group Code: 448000 Ranks within this company's industry group: Sales: 8   Profits: 9

Management:		Sales/Marketing:		Liberal Arts:		Information Systems:		Professionals:		Technical/Scientific:	
Mgmt. Trainees:	Y	Mktg. Professionals:	Y	Gen. Writing/Editing:	Y	Info. Management:	Y	Finance/Accounting:	Y	Engineers, Elec.:	
Experienced Mgmt.:	Y	Retail Sales:	Y	Technical Writing:		Software Dev.:	Y	Law:	Y	Engineers, Other:	
Int'l Business:	Y	Commercial/Industrial:	Y	Graphic Arts/Photog.:	Y	Hardware Dev.:		HR/Other:	Y	Health/Lab:	
MBA Graduates:	Y	Sales Trainees:	Y	Music:		Systems Integration:		Training:	Y	Scientists/Research:	
		Advertising Pros.:	Y	Broadcasting:		Consulting/Other:		Health Care:		Petroleum/Chemicals:	
				Other:	Y			Consulting:		Math/Other:	

TYPES OF BUSINESS:

Music-Related Apparel Stores
Online Sales
Accessories
Cosmetics
Jewelry

BRANDS/DIVISIONS/AFFILIATES:

Hot Topic
Torrid
HotTopic.com
Torrid.com
Morbid Threads
Morbid Metals
Morbid Makeup
Everything About the Music

CONTACTS: *Note: Officers with more than one job title may be intentionally listed here more than once.*

Elizabeth (Betsy) McLaughlin, CEO
Jerry Cook, COO
James McGinty, CFO
Robin Elledge, Sr. VP-Human Resources
Tom Beauchamp, CIO/Sr. VP
Steffani Stevens, General Counsel/VP
Ed Gusman, VP-Hot Topic Store Oper.
George Wehlitz, VP-Finance
Kelly McGuire Diehl, VP-Employee Rel. & Training
Christopher Daniel, Pres., Torrid
John Neppl, VP-Real Estate & Construction
John Kirkpatrick, Chief Music Officer, Hot Topic
Bruce Quinnell, Chmn.
Bill Bellerose, VP-Dist. & Logistics

Phone: 626-839-4681	**Fax:** 626-839-4686
Toll-Free:	
Address: 18305 E. San Jose Ave., City of Industry, CA 91748 US	

GROWTH PLANS/SPECIAL FEATURES:

Hot Topic, Inc. is a mall-based specialty retailer that operates the Hot Topic and Torrid brand stores. Hot Topic stores targets young men and women primarily between the ages of 12-22, selling a selection of music-inspired apparel and accessories, such as woven and knit tops, skirts, pants, shorts, jackets, shoes, costume jewelry, body jewelry, sunglasses, cosmetics, leather accessories and gift items. Torrid targets plus-size females between the ages of 15-29, selling apparel, lingerie, shoes and accessories designed for various lifestyles. Hot Topic has developed a strategy focused exclusively on offering music-related merchandise in the mall environment. The company tracks alternative and rock music trends by visiting nightclubs, attending concerts and monitoring new music, music videos and radio airplay. The company sells merchandise similar to its two stores through two distinct web sites: HotTopic.com and Torrid.com. Hot Topic produces private-label products including Morbid Threads, a clothing line; Morbid Metals, a body jewelry line; and Morbid Makeup. The firm operates 683 Hot Topic stores throughout the U.S. and Puerto Rico; and 157 Torrid stores in thirty-six states. The company's average store is approximately 1,700 square feet; and sales per square foot averaged $500.

Employees of Hot Topic receive a 40% discount on merchandise, tuition assistance, basic life and accidental death and dismemberment (AD&D) coverage, short term disability coverage and scholarship programs.

FINANCIALS: Sales and profits are in thousands of dollars—add 000 to get the full amount. 2007 Note: Financial information for 2007 was not available for all companies at press time.

2007 Sales: $751,558	2007 Profits: $13,626	**U.S. Stock Ticker: HOTT**
2006 Sales: $725,142	2006 Profits: $22,419	**Int'l Ticker:** Int'l Exchange:
2005 Sales: $656,468	2005 Profits: $39,673	Employees: 9,794
2004 Sales: $572,039	2004 Profits: $48,042	Fiscal Year Ends: 1/31
2003 Sales: $443,300	2003 Profits: $34,600	Parent Company:

SALARIES/BENEFITS:

Pension Plan:	ESOP Stock Plan:	Profit Sharing:	Top Exec. Salary: $700,000	Bonus: $
Savings Plan: Y	Stock Purch. Plan: Y		Second Exec. Salary: $450,000	Bonus: $155,925

OTHER THOUGHTS:

Apparent Women Officers or Directors: 9
Hot Spot for Advancement for Women/Minorities: Y

LOCATIONS: ("Y" = Yes)

West:	Southwest:	Midwest:	Southeast:	Northeast:	International:
Y	Y	Y	Y	Y	Y

HUMANA INC

www.humana.com

Industry Group Code: 524114 Ranks within this company's industry group: Sales: 3 Profits: 3

Management:		Sales/Marketing:		Liberal Arts:		Information Systems:		Professionals:		Technical/Scientific:	
Mgmt. Trainees:	Y	Mktg. Professionals:	Y	Gen. Writing/Editing:	Y	Info. Management:	Y	Finance/Accounting:	Y	Engineers, Elec.:	
Experienced Mgmt.:	Y	Retail Sales:		Technical Writing:	Y	Software Dev.:	Y	Law:	Y	Engineers, Other:	Y
Int'l Business:	Y	Commercial/Industrial:	Y	Graphic Arts/Photog.:	Y	Hardware Dev.:		HR/Other:	Y	Health/Lab:	
MBA Graduates:	Y	Sales Trainees:		Music:		Systems Integration:		Training:	Y	Scientists/Research:	Y
		Advertising Pros.:	Y	Broadcasting:		Consulting/Other:		Health Care:	Y	Petroleum/Chemicals:	
				Other:				Consulting:		Math/Other:	

TYPES OF BUSINESS:

Insurance-Medical & Health, HMOs & PPOs
Insurance-Dental
Employee Benefit Plans
Insurance-Group Life
Wellness Programs

BRANDS/DIVISIONS/AFFILIATES:

Humana Military Healthcare Services, Inc.
Humana Dental
HumanaOne
Humana Ventures
Humana Medicare
CompBenefits Corporation
KMG America Corporation
Medicare Advantage

CONTACTS: Note: Officers with more than one job title may be intentionally listed here more than once.

Michael B. McCallister, CEO
James E. Murray, COO/Sr. VP
Michael B. McCallister, Pres.
James H. Bloem, CFO/Sr. VP/Treas.
Steven O. Moya, Chief Mktg. Officer/Sr. VP
Bonnita C. Hathcock, Chief Human Resources Officer/Sr. VP
Bruce J. Goodman, Chief Svc. & Info. Officer/Sr. VP
Thomas J. Liston, VP-Senior Products
Christopher M. Todoroff, General Counsel/Sr. VP
Thomas J. Liston, Sr. VP-Strategy & Corp. Dev.
Steven E. McCulley, Controller/Principal Acct. Officer/VP
Jonathan T. Lord, Sr. VP/Chief Innovation Officer
Heidi S. Margulis, Sr. VP-Gov't Rel.
Joan O. Lenahan, VP/Corp. Sec.
David A. Jones, Jr., Chmn.

Phone: 502-580-1000	Fax: 502-580-3639
Toll-Free:	
Address: 500 W. Main St., Louisville, KY 40202 US	

GROWTH PLANS/SPECIAL FEATURES:

Humana, Inc. is a leading health benefits company in the U.S., serving approximately 11.5 million members in the U.S. and Puerto Rico. It divides its business between government and commercial operations. Government operations consist of Medicare, military and Medicaid business. Its commercial operations, which are offered to both employer groups and individuals, consist of medical and specialty services. Subsidiary Humana Military Healthcare Services, Inc. provides TRICARE services to 2.8 million military beneficiaries. HumanaDental covers 2.6 million customers, making it one of the largest dental carries in the U.S. HumanaOne offers insurance coverage to individuals. Humana Ventures is a capital investing branch of Humana. Finally, Humana Medicare offers plans for Medicare patients to help them with drug and medical coverage. Humana contracts with approximately 540,000 physicians, 5,300 hospitals, 263,000 other providers and dentists, in one of the largest networks in the U.S. The company also offers a wide variety of services to employers, such as workers' compensation, dental plans, group life plans and an administrative-services-only plan. Humana provides health benefits and related services to companies ranging from fewer than 10 to over 10,000 employees. Many of its products are offered through HMOs (health maintenance organizations), Private Fee-For-Service (PFFS) and preferred provider organizations (PPOs). In October 2007, Humana acquired CompBenefits Corporation, a dental and vision benefits company. In November 2007, the firm acquired KMG America Corporation, a provider of life and health insurance products, for approximately $187.7 million. In May 2008, Humana acquired UnitedHealth Group's Medicare Advantage business for approximately $185 million. In May 2008, the firm acquired OSF HealthPlans, Inc., a managed care company, and agreed to acquire Metcare Health Plans. In August 2008, Humana agreed to acquire Cariten Healthcare.

Humana offers its employees tuition reimbursement, a work-life program, adoption assistance, flexible spending accounts and medical, dental, life and disability insurance.

FINANCIALS: Sales and profits are in thousands of dollars—add 000 to get the full amount. 2007 Note: Financial information for 2007 was not available for all companies at press time.

2007 Sales: $25,289,989	2007 Profits: $833,684	**U.S. Stock Ticker: HUM**
2006 Sales: $21,416,537	2006 Profits: $487,423	**Int'l Ticker:** Int'l Exchange:
2005 Sales: $14,418,127	2005 Profits: $296,730	Employees: 22,300
2004 Sales: $13,104,325	2004 Profits: $269,947	Fiscal Year Ends: 12/31
2003 Sales: $12,226,311	2003 Profits: $228,934	Parent Company:

SALARIES/BENEFITS:

Pension Plan: Y	ESOP Stock Plan:	Profit Sharing:	Top Exec. Salary: $900,000	Bonus: $1,552,419
Savings Plan: Y	Stock Purch. Plan:		Second Exec. Salary: $591,370	Bonus: $849,892

OTHER THOUGHTS:

Apparent Women Officers or Directors: 5
Hot Spot for Advancement for Women/Minorities: Y

LOCATIONS: ("Y" = Yes)

West:	Southwest:	Midwest:	Southeast:	Northeast:	International:
Y	Y	Y	Y	Y	Y

Note: Financial information, benefits and other data can change quickly and may vary from those stated here.

IAC/INTERACTIVECORP

www.iac.com

Industry Group Code: 454110B Ranks within this company's industry group: Sales: 1 Profits: 1

Management:		Sales/Marketing:		Liberal Arts:		Information Systems:		Professionals:		Technical/Scientific:	
Mgmt. Trainees:	Y	Mktg. Professionals:	Y	Gen. Writing/Editing:	Y	Info. Management:	Y	Finance/Accounting:	Y	Engineers, Elec.:	Y
Experienced Mgmt.:	Y	Retail Sales:		Technical Writing:		Software Dev.:	Y	Law:	Y	Engineers, Other:	
Int'l Business:	Y	Commercial/Industrial:		Graphic Arts/Photog.:	Y	Hardware Dev.:		HR/Other:	Y	Health/Lab:	
MBA Graduates:	Y	Sales Trainees:		Music:	Y	Systems Integration:		Training:	Y	Scientists/Research:	
		Advertising Pros.:	Y	Broadcasting:	Y	Consulting/Other:		Health Care:		Petroleum/Chemicals:	
				Other:	Y			Consulting:		Math/Other:	

TYPES OF BUSINESS:

Cable Television Shopping Programs
Entertainment & Event Ticket Sales
Catalog & Online Home Products & Apparel Retailing
e-Commerce, Online Advertising & Search Engines
Online Real Estate Services, Mortgages & Loans
Online Entertainment & Shopping Directories
Online Personals & Dating Services

BRANDS/DIVISIONS/AFFILIATES:

HSN LP (Home Shopping Network)
Cornerstone Brands
Ticketmaster
LendingTree LLC
iNest Realty Inc
IAC Search & Media
Match.com
RealEstate.com

CONTACTS: *Note: Officers with more than one job title may be intentionally listed here more than once.*

Barry Diller, CEO
Thomas J. McInerney, CFO/Exec. VP
Johnny C. Taylor, Jr., Sr. VP-Human Resources
Jason Stewart, Chief Admin. Officer
Greg Blatt, General Counsel/Sec./Exec. VP
Shana Fisher, Sr. VP-Strategy, Mergers & Acquisitions
Jonathan L. Sanchez, Chief Comm. Officer/Sr. VP
Eoin Ryan, VP-Investor Rel.
Joey Levin, Sr. VP-Finance, Mergers & Acquisitions
Victor Kaufman, Vice Chmn.
Joanne Hawkins, Deputy General Counsel/Sr. VP
Michael Jackson, Pres.-Programming
Greg Morrow, VP-Tax
Barry Diller, Chmn.
Jane Thompson, Managing Dir.-Int'l

Phone: 212-314-7300	Fax: 212-314-7309
Toll-Free:	
Address: 555 W. 18th St., New York, NY 10011 US	

GROWTH PLANS/SPECIAL FEATURES:

IAC/InterActiveCorp's operating businesses provide various products and services through four segments: Retailing; Transactions; Media and Advertising; and Membership and Subscriptions. Retailing markets and sells third party and private label merchandise directly to consumers through broadcasts on HSN (formerly Home Shopping Network) television network; catalogs from the Cornerstone Brands portfolio; and websites, primarily hsn.com and shoebuy.com. In 2007, HSN reached 90.6 million households in the U.S. Transactions operates Ticketmaster, a provider of online and offline international ticketing services that sells tickets for the 2008 Beijing Olympic Games and is the Official Resale Ticket Provider for the National Hockey League; LendingTree, which consists of businesses offering online lending products and services; Real Estate, a full service real estate brokerage firm on RealEstate.com; and ServiceMagic, which provides pre-screened, customer-rated home service professional referrals. Media and Advertising consists of IAC Search & Media, formerly Ask Jeeves, Inc., which offers Internet search services through Ask.com; Citysearch, a network of local city guide websites; and Evite, a social planning website. Membership and Subscriptions includes Interval, which provides timeshare exchange, vacation rental and property management services; Match, which offers single adults a forum for meeting each other through various websites; and Entertainment, which consists of Entertainment Publications (EPI), a marketer of coupon book memberships, discounts and merchant promotions serving 155 major markets in North America. In June 2007, the company sold its German TV and Internet retailer, HSE Germany. In November 2007, the company announced that IAC will separate into five publicly traded companies: IAC; HSN; Ticketmaster; Interval International; and LendingTree.

The company provides employees with medical, dental and vision care plans; life insurance; paid vacations; pet insurance; and flexible spending accounts.

FINANCIALS: Sales and profits are in thousands of dollars—add 000 to get the full amount. 2007 Note: Financial information for 2007 was not available for all companies at press time.

2007 Sales: $6,373,410	2007 Profits: $-144,069	**U.S. Stock Ticker: IACI**
2006 Sales: $5,908,902	2006 Profits: $187,065	**Int'l Ticker:** Int'l Exchange:
2005 Sales: $5,024,635	2005 Profits: $869,683	Employees: 21,000
2004 Sales: $3,911,050	2004 Profits: $151,808	Fiscal Year Ends: 12/31
2003 Sales: $6,328,100	2003 Profits: $167,400	Parent Company:

SALARIES/BENEFITS:

Pension Plan:	ESOP Stock Plan:	Profit Sharing:	Top Exec. Salary: $750,000	Bonus: $1,300,000
Savings Plan: Y	Stock Purch. Plan: Y		Second Exec. Salary: $650,000	Bonus: $1,600,000

OTHER THOUGHTS:

Apparent Women Officers or Directors: 7
Hot Spot for Advancement for Women/Minorities: Y

LOCATIONS: ("Y" = Yes)

West:	Southwest:	Midwest:	Southeast:	Northeast:	International:
Y	Y	Y	Y	Y	Y

ICT GROUP INC

www.ictgroup.com

Industry Group Code: 541800 **Ranks within this company's industry group:** Sales: 1 Profits: 1

Management:		Sales/Marketing:		Liberal Arts:	Information Systems:		Professionals:		Technical/Scientific:
Mgmt. Trainees:	Y	Mktg. Professionals:	Y	Gen. Writing/Editing:	Info. Management:	Y	Finance/Accounting:	Y	Engineers, Elec.:
Experienced Mgmt.:	Y	Retail Sales:		Technical Writing:	Software Dev.:	Y	Law:	Y	Engineers, Other:
Int'l Business:	Y	Commercial/Industrial:	Y	Graphic Arts/Photog.:	Hardware Dev.:		HR/Other:	Y	Health/Lab:
MBA Graduates:	Y	Sales Trainees:		Music:	Systems Integration:		Training:	Y	Scientists/Research:
		Advertising Pros.:		Broadcasting:	Consulting/Other:		Health Care:		Petroleum/Chemicals:
				Other:			Consulting:	Y	Math/Other:

TYPES OF BUSINESS:

Customer Relationship Management
Database Marketing
Sales Services
CRM Technologies
Financial Marketing Services
Outsourcing

BRANDS/DIVISIONS/AFFILIATES:

CONTACTS: *Note: Officers with more than one job title may be intentionally listed here more than once.*

John J. Brennan, CEO
Vincent A. Paccapaniccia, CFO/Exec. VP
John D. Campbell, Exec. VP-Global Sales
Gail M. Lebel, Sr. VP-Human Resources
Pamela Goyke, CIO/Sr. VP-Systems & Tech.
Timothy F. Kowalski, Pres./COO-Tech. Svcs.
Jeffrey C. Moore, General Counsel/Sr. VP/Corp. Sec.
Timothy F. Kowalski, Pres./COO-Mktg.
John L. Magee, Pres./COO-North America
Janice A. Jones, Sr. VP-Corp. Svcs.
John J. Brennan, Chmn.
Guy T. Gray, Pres./COO-Int'l

Phone: 267-685-5000	Fax: 267-685-5705
Toll-Free: 800-201-1085	
Address: 100 Brandywine Blvd., Newtown, PA 18940 US	

GROWTH PLANS/SPECIAL FEATURES:

ICT Group, Inc. is a global provider of outsourced customer management and business process outsourcing solutions. Its sales, service, marketing and technology solutions include customer care/retention; technical support and customer acquisition; cross-selling/upselling; as well as market research, database marketing, data capture/collection, e-mail management, collections and other back-office business processing services. The company also offers a suite of customer relationship management (CRM) technologies, which are available on a hosted basis for use by clients at their own in-house facilities, or on a co-sourced basis in conjunction with a fully integrated, web-enabled contact centers. These technologies include automatic call distribution voice processing; interactive voice response and advanced speech recognition; voice over Internet protocol (VoIP); contact management; automated e-mail management and processing, sales force and marketing automation; alert notification; and web self-help for the delivery of consistent quality customer care across multiple channels. The firm's services are provided through contact centers located across the globe. The technology assets may be located at a different physical location or country than the contact center. Accordingly, many of ICT's contact centers are not limited to performing only one service. Rather, they perform a variety of different services for a number of different customers/programs. The company's domestic sales force is organized by specific vertical industries, which enables the sales personnel to develop in-depth industry and product knowledge. Selected industries targeted include financial services and insurance; telecommunications; health care services; and technology and consumer electronics products and services.

FINANCIALS: Sales and profits are in thousands of dollars—add 000 to get the full amount. 2007 Note: Financial information for 2007 was not available for all companies at press time.

		U.S. Stock Ticker: ICTG
2007 Sales: $453,621	2007 Profits: $-11,809	Int'l Ticker: Int'l Exchange:
2006 Sales: $447,912	2006 Profits: $16,811	Employees: 17,500
2005 Sales: $401,300	2005 Profits: $12,200	Fiscal Year Ends: 12/31
2004 Sales: $325,500	2004 Profits: $-2,700	Parent Company:
2003 Sales: $298,142	2003 Profits: $-1,144	

SALARIES/BENEFITS:

Pension Plan:	ESOP Stock Plan:	Profit Sharing: Y	Top Exec. Salary: $674,039	Bonus: $377,982
Savings Plan: Y	Stock Purch. Plan:		Second Exec. Salary: $344,192	Bonus: $167,769

OTHER THOUGHTS:

Apparent Women Officers or Directors: 3
Hot Spot for Advancement for Women/Minorities: Y

LOCATIONS: ("Y" = Yes)

West:	Southwest:	Midwest:	Southeast:	Northeast:	International:
Y	Y	Y	Y	Y	Y

IDEXX LABORATORIES INC

www.idexx.com

Industry Group Code: 325413 Ranks within this company's industry group: Sales: 1   Profits: 1

Management:		Sales/Marketing:		Liberal Arts:		Information Systems:		Professionals:		Technical/Scientific:	
Mgmt. Trainees:	Y	Mktg. Professionals:	Y	Gen. Writing/Editing:		Info. Management:	Y	Finance/Accounting:	Y	Engineers, Elec.:	Y
Experienced Mgmt.:	Y	Retail Sales:		Technical Writing:	Y	Software Dev.:	Y	Law:	Y	Engineers, Other:	Y
Int'l Business:	Y	Commercial/Industrial:	Y	Graphic Arts/Photog.:		Hardware Dev.:	Y	HR/Other:	Y	Health/Lab:	Y
MBA Graduates:	Y	Sales Trainees:		Music:		Systems Integration:		Training:		Scientists/Research:	
		Advertising Pros.:		Broadcasting:		Consulting/Other:		Health Care:	Y	Petroleum/Chemicals:	
				Other:				Consulting:		Math/Other:	

TYPES OF BUSINESS:

Veterinary Laboratory Testing & Consulting
Point-of-Care Diagnostic Products
Veterinary Pharmaceuticals
Information Management Software
Food & Water Testing Products

BRANDS/DIVISIONS/AFFILIATES:

Colilert-18
SNAP
Parallux
Colisure
VetLab
Cardiopet proBNP
Coag Dx

CONTACTS: *Note: Officers with more than one job title may be intentionally listed here more than once.*

Jonathan W. Ayers, CEO
Jonathan W. Ayers, Pres.
Merilee Raines, CFO/VP
William C. Wallen, Sr. VP/Chief Scientific Officer
Conan R. Deady, General Counsel/Sec./VP
Irene C. Kerr, VP-Worldwide Oper.
Merilee Raines, Treas.
James Polewaczyck, VP-Rapid Assay & Digital Radiography
Michael Williams, VP-Instrument Diagnostics
Thomas J. Dupree, VP-Companion Animal Group
S. Sam Fratoni, VP-Computer Systems
Jonathan W. Ayers, Chmn.
Ali Naqui, VP-Intl.

Phone: 207-556-0300	Fax: 207-556-0346
Toll-Free: 800-548-6733	
Address: 1 Idexx Dr., Westbrook, ME 04092-2041 US	

GROWTH PLANS/SPECIAL FEATURES:

IDEXX Laboratories, Inc. develops, manufactures and distributes products and provides services for the veterinary and the food and water testing markets. The company operates in two business segments: The Companion Animal Group, which provides products and services for the veterinary market; water quality products; and the Production Animal Segment, which provides products for production animal health. The company also operated two smaller segments: Dairy, comprising products for dairy quality, and OPTI Medical, comprising products for the human medical diagnostic market. Its primary business focus is on animal health. IDEXX currently markets an integrated and flexible suite of in-house laboratory analyzers for use in veterinary practices, which is referred to as the VetLab suite of analyzers. The suite includes several instrument systems, as well as associated proprietary consumable products such as VetTest, VetLyte, VetStat, LaserCyte and VetAutoread analyzers, the IDEXX SNAP Reader, as well as the Coag Dx Analyzer (released in late 2007), among other offerings. The company is developing and plans to launch a new quantitative immunoassay platform called SNAPshot Dx in 2008. This product will replace the IDEXX SNAP Reader. In addition, it also provides assay kits, software and instrumentation for accurate assessment of infectious disease in production animals, such as cattle, swine and poultry. The company currently offers commercial veterinary laboratory and consulting services in the U.S. through facilities located in Arizona, California, Colorado, Illinois, Maryland, Massachusetts, New Jersey, Oregon and Texas. The water quality segment's products include Colilert-18 and Colisure tests, which simultaneously detect total coliforms and E. coli in water. IDEXX's two principal products for use in testing for antibiotic residue in milk are the SNAP Beta-lactam test and the Parallux system. In July 2008, IDEXX launched its new Cardiopet proBNP test, a minimally invasive blood test that evaluates the cardiovascular status of canine and feline patients.

FINANCIALS: Sales and profits are in thousands of dollars—add 000 to get the full amount. 2007 Note: Financial information for 2007 was not available for all companies at press time.

2007 Sales: $922,555	2007 Profits: $94,014	**U.S. Stock Ticker: IDXX**
2006 Sales: $739,117	2006 Profits: $93,678	**Int'l Ticker:** Int'l Exchange:
2005 Sales: $638,095	2005 Profits: $78,254	Employees: 4,700
2004 Sales: $549,181	2004 Profits: $78,332	Fiscal Year Ends: 12/31
2003 Sales: $475,992	2003 Profits: $57,090	Parent Company:

SALARIES/BENEFITS:

Pension Plan:	ESOP Stock Plan:	Profit Sharing:	Top Exec. Salary: $650,000	Bonus: $650,000
Savings Plan: Y	Stock Purch. Plan: Y		Second Exec. Salary: $365,000	Bonus: $275,000

OTHER THOUGHTS:

Apparent Women Officers or Directors: 2
Hot Spot for Advancement for Women/Minorities: Y

LOCATIONS: ("Y" = Yes)

West:	Southwest:	Midwest:	Southeast:	Northeast:	International:
Y	Y	Y	Y	Y	Y

IGATE CORPORATION

www.igatecorp.com

Industry Group Code: 541512 Ranks within this company's industry group: Sales: 12 Profits: 13

Management:		Sales/Marketing:		Liberal Arts:		Information Systems:		Professionals:		Technical/Scientific:	
Mgmt. Trainees:	Y	Mktg. Professionals:	Y	Gen. Writing/Editing:		Info. Management:	Y	Finance/Accounting:	Y	Engineers, Elec.:	
Experienced Mgmt.:	Y	Retail Sales:		Technical Writing:	Y	Software Dev.:	Y	Law:	Y	Engineers, Other:	
Int'l Business:	Y	Commercial/Industrial:	Y	Graphic Arts/Photog.:	Y	Hardware Dev.:		HR/Other:	Y	Health/Lab:	
MBA Graduates:	Y	Sales Trainees:		Music:		Systems Integration:	Y	Training:	Y	Scientists/Research:	Y
		Advertising Pros.:		Broadcasting:		Consulting/Other:		Health Care:		Petroleum/Chemicals:	
				Other:				Consulting:		Math/Other:	

TYPES OF BUSINESS:

IT Consulting
Data Warehousing
Business Process Outsourcing
Web Integration Services
Software Design Services
Clinical Research

BRANDS/DIVISIONS/AFFILIATES:

iGATE Solutions
IGS
iGATE Global Solutions
iGATE Shared Services
Jobcurry Systems Private Ltd.
iGATE Professional Services
Clinical Research International, Inc.
iGATE Clinical Research International Private Ltd.

CONTACTS: Note: Officers with more than one job title may be intentionally listed here more than once.

Phaneesh Murthy, CEO
Ashok Trivedi, Pres./Co-Chmn.
Ramachandran Natesan, CFO
J. Gordon Garrett, CEO-Interloci Management, Inc.
Michel Berty, Pres., PAC U.S.
Edward Yourdon, Software Eng. Consultant
Steven Shangold, Pres., iGate Mastech, Inc.
Ashok Trivedi, Co-Chmn.

Phone: 412-506-1131	Fax:
Toll-Free:	
Address: 1000 Commerce Dr., Ste. 500, Pittsburgh, PA 15275 US	

GROWTH PLANS/SPECIAL FEATURES:

iGATE Corporation is a global provider of information technology (IT) strategy services to corporations. Together with its offshore subsidiary, iGATE Global Solutions, the company offers a combination of process investment strategies, technology leverage and business process outsourcing. Services offered by the company include consultations, IT services, data analytics, enterprise systems, business process outsourcing (BPO), contact center and infrastructure management services. The company operates in two distinct business segments: iGATE Solutions and iGATE Shared Services. The iGATE Solutions segment offers outsourcing of IT and BPO services using an onsite/offshore delivery model. IT services include software application development services and maintenance; implementation and support of enterprise application; and data management and integration. BPO services include call center services and transaction processing services, the latter of which are designed for mortgage banking, insurance and capital market industries. iGATE Shared Services consists of two segments: Clinical Research International, Inc. and iGATE Clinical Research International Private Ltd. This division is operated in India and offers Phase II - IV clinical trial support services. In 2007, iGATE Global Solutions installed a 100,000 square foot facility in Whitefield, Bangalore, India and also signed a key technology services agreement with Radian group to provide credit solutions to its global financial and capital markets. In December 2007, the company sold Jobcurry Systems Private Ltd., its offshore recruiting and training subsidiary. In early 2008, iGATE acquired all remaining shares of iGATE Global Solutions and delisted its stock on all Indian stock exchanges. In February 2008, the firm announced plans to divest its iGATE Professional Services segment, formerly providing client-managed and supervised IT staffing services. The divestiture may involve the sale of the business or a spin-off to iGATE shareholders.

The company offers its employees educational assistance, relocation assistance and flexible spending accounts.

FINANCIALS: Sales and profits are in thousands of dollars—add 000 to get the full amount. 2007 Note: Financial information for 2007 was not available for all companies at press time.

2007 Sales: $307,258	2007 Profits: $15,585	U.S. Stock Ticker: IGTE
2006 Sales: $283,588	2006 Profits: $8,704	Int'l Ticker: Int'l Exchange:
2005 Sales: $275,992	2005 Profits: $6,969	Employees: 7,140
2004 Sales: $264,585	2004 Profits: $-18,211	Fiscal Year Ends: 12/31
2003 Sales: $240,634	2003 Profits: $-9,020	Parent Company:

SALARIES/BENEFITS:

Pension Plan:	ESOP Stock Plan:	Profit Sharing:	Top Exec. Salary: $450,000	Bonus: $200,000
Savings Plan:	Stock Purch. Plan:		Second Exec. Salary: $300,000	Bonus: $159,000

OTHER THOUGHTS:

Apparent Women Officers or Directors:
Hot Spot for Advancement for Women/Minorities:

LOCATIONS: ("Y" = Yes)

West:	Southwest:	Midwest:	Southeast:	Northeast:	International:
Y	Y			Y	Y

IMS HEALTH INC

www.imshealth.com

Industry Group Code: 541910 Ranks within this company's industry group: Sales: 1 Profits: 1

Management:		Sales/Marketing:		Liberal Arts:		Information Systems:		Professionals:		Technical/Scientific:	
Mgmt. Trainees:		Mktg. Professionals:	Y	Gen. Writing/Editing:	Y	Info. Management:	Y	Finance/Accounting:	Y	Engineers, Elec.:	Y
Experienced Mgmt.:	Y	Retail Sales:		Technical Writing:	Y	Software Dev.:	Y	Law:	Y	Engineers, Other:	
Int'l Business:	Y	Commercial/Industrial:		Graphic Arts/Photog.:	Y	Hardware Dev.:		HR/Other:	Y	Health/Lab:	
MBA Graduates:	Y	Sales Trainees:		Music:		Systems Integration:		Training:	Y	Scientists/Research:	
		Advertising Pros.:	Y	Broadcasting:		Consulting/Other:		Health Care:		Petroleum/Chemicals:	
				Other:				Consulting:		Math/Other:	

TYPES OF BUSINESS:

Market Research - Pharmaceuticals
Pharmaceutical Sales Tracking
Health Care Databases
Software-Sales Management & Market Research
Physician Profiling
Industry Audits
Prescription Tracking Reporting Services

BRANDS/DIVISIONS/AFFILIATES:

MIDAS
Market Research Publications
Pharmaceutical World Review
ValueMedics Research LLC
MIHS Holdings, Inc.
HIS
MedInitiatives

CONTACTS: Note: Officers with more than one job title may be intentionally listed here more than once.

David R. Carlucci, CEO
Giles V. J. Pajot, COO
David R. Carlucci, Pres.
Leslye G. Katz, CFO/Sr. VP
Bruce F. Boggs, Sr. VP-Global Mktg. & External Affairs
Karla L. Packer, Sr. VP-Human Resources
Robert H. Steinfeld, General Counsel/Sr. VP/Corp. Sec.
John R. Walsh, Sr. VP-Strategy & Bus. Dev.
Jeffrey J. Ford, Treas./VP
Murray L. Aitken, Sr. VP-Healthcare Insight
Andrew Howden, Pres., Asia Pacific
Kevin Knightly, Sr. VP-Bus Line Mgmt.
William J. Nelligan, Pres., Americas
David R. Carlucci, Chmn.
Adel Al-Saleh, Pres., EMEA

Phone: 203-845-5200	Fax:
Toll-Free:	
Address: 901 Main Ave., Ste. 612, Norwalk, CT 06851 US	

GROWTH PLANS/SPECIAL FEATURES:

IMS Health, Inc. is a leading global provider of market intelligence to the pharmaceutical and health care industries. IMS offers such products and services as portfolio optimization capabilities; launch and brand management solutions; sales force effectiveness innovations; managed markets and consumer health offerings; and consulting and services solutions that improve ROI and the delivery of quality healthcare worldwide. The company's information products use data secured from a worldwide network of suppliers in over 100 countries. The firm's sales force effectiveness products generated roughly 46% of its worldwide revenue in 2007 and include sales territory reporting services; prescription tracking reporting services; and sales and account management services. Portfolio optimization products generated roughly 29% of IMS's 2007 revenue, and include pharmaceutical, medical, hospital and prescription audits; MIDAS, its online multinational integrated data analysis tool used to assess global pharmaceutical information and trends; other portfolio optimization reports, including personal care reports, reports of bulk chemical shipments and Market Research Publications such as the Pharmaceutical World Review; and consulting and services. Launch, brand management and other offerings comprised roughly 25% of the company's 2007 revenue. Launch and brand management offerings combine information, analytical tools and consulting and services to address client needs relevant to the management of each stage of the lifecycle of their pharmaceutical brands. Additional products offered by IMS include information to quantify the effects of managed markets on the pharmaceutical and healthcare industries and product movement, market share and pricing information for over-the-counter, personal care, patient care and nutritional products. During 2007, IMS acquired ValueMedics Research LLC, a healthcare research and consulting firm, and MIHS Holdings, Inc., which provides healthcare analytics and technology services through its HIS and MedInitiatives subsidiaries. In January 2008, the company announced restructuring plans that include a reduction in its workforce by 10%.

FINANCIALS: Sales and profits are in thousands of dollars—add 000 to get the full amount. 2007 Note: Financial information for 2007 was not available for all companies at press time.

2007 Sales: $2,192,571	2007 Profits: $234,040	U.S. Stock Ticker: RX
2006 Sales: $1,958,588	2006 Profits: $315,511	Int'l Ticker: Int'l Exchange:
2005 Sales: $1,754,791	2005 Profits: $284,091	Employees: 7,950
2004 Sales: $1,569,045	2004 Profits: $285,422	Fiscal Year Ends: 12/31
2003 Sales: $1,381,800	2003 Profits: $639,000	Parent Company:

SALARIES/BENEFITS:

Pension Plan:	ESOP Stock Plan:	Profit Sharing:	Top Exec. Salary: $843,750	Bonus: $680,625
Savings Plan:	Stock Purch. Plan:		Second Exec. Salary: $718,817	Bonus: $431,500

OTHER THOUGHTS:

Apparent Women Officers or Directors: 3
Hot Spot for Advancement for Women/Minorities: Y

LOCATIONS: ("Y" = Yes)

West:	Southwest:	Midwest:	Southeast:	Northeast:	International:
Y				Y	Y

Note: Financial information, benefits and other data can change quickly and may vary from those stated here.

INFOUSA INC
www.infousa.com

Industry Group Code: 511140 **Ranks within this company's industry group:** Sales: 1 Profits: 1

Management:		Sales/Marketing:		Liberal Arts:		Information Systems:		Professionals:		Technical/Scientific:	
Mgmt. Trainees:		Mktg. Professionals:	Y	Gen. Writing/Editing:	Y	Info. Management:	Y	Finance/Accounting:	Y	Engineers, Elec.:	
Experienced Mgmt.:	Y	Retail Sales:		Technical Writing:	Y	Software Dev.:	Y	Law:	Y	Engineers, Other:	
Int'l Business:	Y	Commercial/Industrial:	Y	Graphic Arts/Photog.:	Y	Hardware Dev.:		HR/Other:	Y	Health/Lab:	
MBA Graduates:	Y	Sales Trainees:	Y	Music:		Systems Integration:	Y	Training:	Y	Scientists/Research:	
		Advertising Pros.:	Y	Broadcasting:		Consulting/Other:		Health Care:		Petroleum/Chemicals:	
				Other:				Consulting:		Math/Other:	

TYPES OF BUSINESS:
Online Directories
Sales Leads
Mailing Lists
Direct Marketing
Database Marketing
E-mail Marketing
Market Research Solution

BRANDS/DIVISIONS/AFFILIATES:
Yesmail.com Inc
OneSource Information Services Inc
Walter Karl
MarketZone
Salesgenie.com
Opinion Research Corp
expresscopy.com
NWC Research

CONTACTS: *Note: Officers with more than one job title may be intentionally listed here more than once.*
Vinod Gupta, CEO
Monica Messer, COO
Stormy Dean, CFO
Fred Vakili, Chief Admin. Officer/Exec. VP-Admin.
John Longwell, General Counsel/Corp. Sec.
Edward C. Mallin, Pres., Svcs. Group
Rakesh Gupta, Pres., Enterprise Sales Group
D.J. Thayer, Exec. VP-infoUSA Group
Gerard Miodus, Pres., Opinion Research
Vinod Gupta, Chmn.
Greg Mahnke, Pres., Macro Int'l

Phone: 402-593-4500	**Fax:** 402-593-4671
Toll-Free: 800-321-0869	
Address: 5711 S. 86th Cir., Omaha, NE 68127 US	

GROWTH PLANS/SPECIAL FEATURES:

InfoUSA, Inc. is a provider of sales leads, mailing lists, direct marketing, database marketing, e-mail marketing and market research solutions. It operates in three segments: data, services and research. The data group maintains 12 proprietary databases of U.S. and international businesses and consumers. The division offers business databases, which contain information on about 15 million businesses in the U.S. and Canada; and consumer databases, which contain roughly 200 million individuals and 115 million households. Its flagship offerings are Salesgenie.com, a web-based subscription service that helps sales representatives and business owners find new prospective customers; MarketZone, a customer data solutions combining lead-generation and database marketing functions with data storage, hygiene and updating; and OneSource, a web-based data service with information about the world's largest companies and their executives. The segment also licenses its data to major Internet search providers, including Google, Yahoo! and AOL; and to providers of mapping systems and in-car navigation products. The services group consists of subsidiaries providing customer data management and brokerage services; e-mail marketing services; and catalog marketing services. It is divided into list brokerage and list management, which includes subsidiary Walter Karl, which specializes in e-mail list management and brokerage services for online marketers; catalog vision, a provider of data processing services to the catalog direct marketing industry; Triplex, a provider of data processing services for high-profile political and non-profit organizations; and Yesmail, which specializes in providing e-mail solutions for a wide range of industries. The research group, recently established with the acquisition of Opinion Research Corp., provides customer surveys, opinion polling and other market research services for business, through the Opinion Research division; and for government, through its Macro International division. In 2007, InfoUSA acquired ExpressCopy.com and, through Opinion Research, NWC Research, an Australian company.

FINANCIALS: Sales and profits are in thousands of dollars—add 000 to get the full amount. 2007 Note: Financial information for 2007 was not available for all companies at press time.

2007 Sales: $688,773	2007 Profits: $40,942	**U.S. Stock Ticker:** IUSA
2006 Sales: $434,876	2006 Profits: $33,300	**Int'l Ticker:** Int'l Exchange:
2005 Sales: $383,158	2005 Profits: $31,507	Employees: 4,089
2004 Sales: $344,859	2004 Profits: $17,838	Fiscal Year Ends: 12/31
2003 Sales: $311,345	2003 Profits: $19,695	Parent Company:

SALARIES/BENEFITS:

Pension Plan:	ESOP Stock Plan:	Profit Sharing:	Top Exec. Salary: $836,539	Bonus: $
Savings Plan: Y	Stock Purch. Plan:		Second Exec. Salary: $597,692	Bonus: $300,000

OTHER THOUGHTS:
Apparent Women Officers or Directors:
Hot Spot for Advancement for Women/Minorities:

LOCATIONS: ("Y" = Yes)

West:	Southwest:	Midwest:	Southeast:	Northeast:	International:
		Y			Y

Note: Financial information, benefits and other data can change quickly and may vary from those stated here.

INGRAM MICRO INC

www.ingrammicro.com

Industry Group Code: 421430 Ranks within this company's industry group: Sales: 1 Profits: 1

Management:		Sales/Marketing:		Liberal Arts:		Information Systems:		Professionals:		Technical/Scientific:	
Mgmt. Trainees:	Y	Mktg. Professionals:	Y	Gen. Writing/Editing:		Info. Management:	Y	Finance/Accounting:	Y	Engineers, Elec.:	
Experienced Mgmt.:	Y	Retail Sales:		Technical Writing:	Y	Software Dev.:	Y	Law:	Y	Engineers, Other:	
Int'l Business:	Y	Commercial/Industrial:	Y	Graphic Arts/Photog.:	Y	Hardware Dev.:		HR/Other:	Y	Health/Lab:	
MBA Graduates:	Y	Sales Trainees:		Music:		Systems Integration:		Training:	Y	Scientists/Research:	
		Advertising Pros.:		Broadcasting:		Consulting/Other:		Health Care:		Petroleum/Chemicals:	
				Other:				Consulting:		Math/Other:	

TYPES OF BUSINESS:
Microcomputers, Distribution
Networking Equipment
Software & Accessories Distribution
Supply Chain Management Services
Online Marketing Services

BRANDS/DIVISIONS/AFFILIATES:
Micro Logistics
AVAD
SymTech
Ingram Micro Asia Pacific Pte. Ltd.
Ingram Micro Canada
InGram Micro UK Ltd.
IMOnsite
Ingram Micro Channel Advisor

CONTACTS: *Note: Officers with more than one job title may be intentionally listed here more than once.*
Gregory M. Spierkel, CEO
Alain Monie, COO
Alain Monie, Pres.
William D. Humes, CFO/Exec. VP
Lynn Jolliffe, Sr. VP-Human Resources
Karen Salem, CIO
Larry C. Boyd, General Counsel/Sr. VP
Ria M. Carlson, Corp. VP-Strategy
Ria M. Carlson, Corp. VP-Comm.
James F. Ricketts, Treas./VP
Shailendra Gupta, Exec. VP/Pres., Ingram Micro Asia-Pacific
Keith Bradley, Exec. VP/Pres., Ingram Micro North America
Alain Maquet, Sr. VP/Pres., Ingram Micro Latin America
Kent B. Foster, Chmn.
Jay A. Forbes, Exec. VP/Pres., EMEA

Phone: 714-566-1000	Fax: 714-566-7900
Toll-Free:	
Address: 1600 E. St. Andrew Pl., Santa Ana, CA 92799 US	

GROWTH PLANS/SPECIAL FEATURES:
Ingram Micro is a global distributor of technology products and supply chain management services. The company markets microcomputer hardware, networking equipment and software products to nearly 159,000 resellers in approximately 150 countries. Ingram provides a comprehensive inventory of hundreds of thousands of distinct items from nearly 1,300 suppliers. Networking products include routers, switches, hubs, wireless networks, networking cards, video conferencing, storage area networks and software products such as business application, operating system, entertainment and security software. Systems products include servers, desktops, laptop computers and personal digital assistants. Peripherals include printers, scanners, displays, projectors, monitors, mass storage and tape. In addition, the company offers components, such as processors, motherboards, hard drives and memory; supplies and accessories, including ink and toner supplies, paper, carrying cases and anti-glare screens; and consumer electronic products, such as cell phones, digital cameras, DVD players, game consoles and televisions. Ingram also offers supply chain management services such as sales and marketing, customer care, financial services and logistics to suppliers and resellers. Its Micro Logistics division provides end-to-end order management and fulfillment, retail logistics merchandizing, warehousing and storage, contract manufacturing, distribution center services, product procurement, reverse logistics, transportation management, marketing services and other outsourcing services. Through its web site, Ingram also offers online account management, a vast resource library and advanced marketing tools. Some of the company's supply chain management clients include CompUSA, Intuit, Iomega and Microsoft. In June 2007, the company acquired certain net assets of DBL Distributing, Inc., a distributor of consumer electronics accessories and related products.

Ingram provides its employees with concierge services such as dry cleaning and auto detailing. Other employee benefits include continuing education reimbursement, day care and rideshare programs.

FINANCIALS: Sales and profits are in thousands of dollars—add 000 to get the full amount. 2007 Note: Financial information for 2007 was not available for all companies at press time.

2007 Sales: $35,047,089	2007 Profits: $275,908	**U.S. Stock Ticker: IM**
2006 Sales: $31,357,477	2006 Profits: $265,766	**Int'l Ticker:** Int'l Exchange:
2005 Sales: $28,808,312	2005 Profits: $216,906	Employees: 13,700
2004 Sales: $25,462,071	2004 Profits: $219,901	Fiscal Year Ends: 12/31
2003 Sales: $22,613,000	2003 Profits: $149,200	Parent Company:

SALARIES/BENEFITS:
Pension Plan:	ESOP Stock Plan:	Profit Sharing:	Top Exec. Salary: $617,693	Bonus: $566,688
Savings Plan: Y	Stock Purch. Plan:		Second Exec. Salary: $558,847	Bonus: $484,045

OTHER THOUGHTS:
Apparent Women Officers or Directors: 2
Hot Spot for Advancement for Women/Minorities:

LOCATIONS: ("Y" = Yes)
West:	Southwest:	Midwest:	Southeast:	Northeast:	International:
Y	Y	Y	Y	Y	Y

INTEL CORP

www.intel.com

Industry Group Code: 334413 **Ranks within this company's industry group:** Sales: 1 Profits: 1

Management:		Sales/Marketing:		Liberal Arts:		Information Systems:		Professionals:		Technical/Scientific:	
Mgmt. Trainees:	Y	Mktg. Professionals:	Y	Gen. Writing/Editing:	Y	Info. Management:	Y	Finance/Accounting:	Y	Engineers, Elec.:	Y
Experienced Mgmt.:	Y	Retail Sales:		Technical Writing:	Y	Software Dev.:	Y	Law:	Y	Engineers, Other:	
Int'l Business:	Y	Commercial/Industrial:	Y	Graphic Arts/Photog.:	Y	Hardware Dev.:	Y	HR/Other:	Y	Health/Lab:	Y
MBA Graduates:	Y	Sales Trainees:		Music:		Systems Integration:	Y	Training:	Y	Scientists/Research:	Y
		Advertising Pros.:	Y	Broadcasting:		Consulting/Other:	Y	Health Care:		Petroleum/Chemicals:	
				Other:	Y			Consulting:		Math/Other:	Y

TYPES OF BUSINESS:

Microprocessors
Semiconductors
Circuit Boards
Flash Memory Products
Software Development
Home Network Equipment
Digital Imaging Products
Demodulation & Tuner Applications Products

BRANDS/DIVISIONS/AFFILIATES:

Pentium
Dual Core
Havok
SpectraWatt, Inc.
Dual-Core Intel Itanium
Dual-Core Intel Xeon
Intel Core 2 Quad
SpectraWatt, Inc.

CONTACTS: Note: Officers with more than one job title may be intentionally listed here more than once.

Paul S. Otellini, CEO
Paul S. Otellini, Pres.
Stacy J. Smith, CFO/VP
Sean M. Maloney, Chief Sales & Mktg. Officer
Patricia Murray, Sr. VP/Dir.-Human Resources
Diane M. Bryant, CIO/VP
Justin R. Rattner, CTO/VP/Dir.-Corp. Tech. Group
Robert J. Baker, Sr. VP/Gen. Mgr.-Mfg. & Tech. Group
Andy D. Bryant, Chief Admin. Officer/Exec. VP
D. Bruce Sewell, General Counsel/Sr. VP
Cary I. Klafter, VP-Corp. Affairs
Leslie S. Culbertson, VP/Dir.-Finance
Deborah S. Conrad, VP/Gen. Mgr.-Intel Corp. Mktg. Group
Arvind Sodhani, Exec. VP/Pres., Intel Capital
Cary I. Klafter, VP-Legal Affairs/Dir.-Corp. Legal/Sec.
Ravi Jacob, Treas./VP
Craig R. Barrett, Chmn.

Phone: 408-765-8080	Fax: 408-765-3804
Toll-Free: 800-628-8686	
Address: 2200 Mission College Blvd., Santa Clara, CA 95054 US	

GROWTH PLANS/SPECIAL FEATURES:

Intel Corp. is a major global semiconductor chip maker that develops advanced integrated digital technology platforms and components, primarily integrated circuits, for the computing and communications industries. It operates in five segments: Digital Enterprise, Mobility, NAND Products, Flash Memory and Digital Home. The Digital Enterprise Group's products include microprocessors and related chipsets and motherboards designed for the desktop and enterprise computing market segments; communications infrastructure components such as network processors, communications boards and embedded processors; wired connectivity devices; and products for network and server storage. The Mobility Group's products include microprocessors and related chipsets designed for the notebook market segment and wireless connectivity products. The NAND Products Group produces memory products used in digital audio players, memory cards and solid-state drives. The Flash Memory Group provides NOR flash memory products for a variety of digital devices. The Digital Home Group designs and delivers products and platforms for consumer products such as PCs, digital TVs and networked media devices. In addition, it offers products for demodulation and tuner applications as well as processors and chipsets for embedded consumer electronics designs such as digital televisions, digital video recorders and set-top boxes. In 2007, Intel acquired Havok, Inc., a software and services provider to the game and movie industries; and agreed to sell the telecom-related portion of its optical platform division to EMCORE for $85 million. In 2008, the firm spun off its solar energy technology business into a new company called SpectraWatt, Inc.; sold its RFID business to Impinj, Inc.; and divested itself of its NOR flash memory assets to a new company called Numonyx (in a joint venture with STMicorelectronics).

The company offers its employees medical and dental insurance; a profit sharing plan; and an employee assistance program.

FINANCIALS: Sales and profits are in thousands of dollars—add 000 to get the full amount. 2007 Note: Financial information for 2007 was not available for all companies at press time.

2007 Sales: $38,334,000	2007 Profits: $6,976,000	U.S. Stock Ticker: INTC
2006 Sales: $35,382,000	2006 Profits: $5,044,000	Int'l Ticker: Int'l Exchange:
2005 Sales: $38,826,000	2005 Profits: $8,664,000	Employees: 86,300
2004 Sales: $34,209,000	2004 Profits: $7,516,000	Fiscal Year Ends: 12/31
2003 Sales: $30,141,000	2003 Profits: $5,641,000	Parent Company:

SALARIES/BENEFITS:

Pension Plan: Y	ESOP Stock Plan:	Profit Sharing: Y	Top Exec. Salary: $700,000	Bonus: $1,772,700
Savings Plan: Y	Stock Purch. Plan:		Second Exec. Salary: $463,000	Bonus: $1,110,400

OTHER THOUGHTS:

Apparent Women Officers or Directors: 9
Hot Spot for Advancement for Women/Minorities: Y

LOCATIONS: ("Y" = Yes)

West:	Southwest:	Midwest:	Southeast:	Northeast:	International:
Y	Y	Y	Y	Y	Y

Note: Financial information, benefits and other data can change quickly and may vary from those stated here.

INTERNATIONAL BUSINESS MACHINES CORP (IBM)

www.ibm.com

Industry Group Code: 541512 Ranks within this company's industry group: Sales: 1   Profits: 1

Management:		Sales/Marketing:		Liberal Arts:		Information Systems:		Professionals:		Technical/Scientific:	
Mgmt. Trainees:	Y	Mktg. Professionals:	Y	Gen. Writing/Editing:	Y	Info. Management:	Y	Finance/Accounting:	Y	Engineers, Elec.:	Y
Experienced Mgmt.:	Y	Retail Sales:		Technical Writing:	Y	Software Dev.:	Y	Law:	Y	Engineers, Other:	
Int'l Business:	Y	Commercial/Industrial:	Y	Graphic Arts/Photog.:	Y	Hardware Dev.:	Y	HR/Other:	Y	Health/Lab:	Y
MBA Graduates:	Y	Sales Trainees:	Y	Music:		Systems Integration:	Y	Training:	Y	Scientists/Research:	Y
		Advertising Pros.:	Y	Broadcasting:		Consulting/Other:	Y	Health Care:		Petroleum/Chemicals:	
				Other:	Y			Consulting:	Y	Math/Other:	Y

TYPES OF BUSINESS:

Computer Hardware
Supercomputers
Microelectronic Technology
Software Development
Networking Systems
IT Consulting & Outsourcing
Financial Services

BRANDS/DIVISIONS/AFFILIATES:

Rational Software Corp
Software Inc
Filenet Corp
Global Services
Internet Security Systems Inc
IBM Research
IBM Canada Ltd

CONTACTS: *Note: Officers with more than one job title may be intentionally listed here more than once.*

Samuel J. Palmisano, CEO
Samuel J. Palmisano, Pres.
Mark Loughridge, CFO/Sr. VP
J. Bruce Harreld, Sr. VP-Mktg.
J. Randall MacDonald, Sr. VP-Human Resources
John E. Kelly, III, Sr. VP-IBM Research
Linda S. Sanford, Sr. VP-IT & Enterprise On Demand Transformation
Robert W. Moffat, Jr., Sr. VP-Systems & Tech. Group
Robert C. Weber, General Counsel/Sr. VP-Legal & Regulatory Affairs
J. Bruce Harreld, Sr. VP-Strategy
Jon C. Iwata, Sr. VP-Comm.
Martin Schroeter, Treas.
Rodney C. Adkins, Sr. VP-Dev. & Mfg.-IBM Systems & Tech. Group
Michael E. Daniels, Sr. VP-Global Tech. Svcs.-IBM Global Svcs.
Jesse J. Greene, Jr., VP-Financial Mgmt.
Daniel E. O'Donnell, Corp. Sec./VP
Samuel J. Palmisano, Chmn.
Robert W. Moffat, Jr., Sr. VP-Supply Chain

Phone: 914-499-1900	**Fax:** 866-722-9226
Toll-Free: 800-426-4968	
Address: 1 New Orchard Rd., Armonk, NY 10504 US	

GROWTH PLANS/SPECIAL FEATURES:

International Business Machines Corp. (IBM) is a global producer of computer hardware and software, with one of the largest technology consulting businesses in the world. It operates in five segments: Global technology services; global business services; systems and technology; software; and global financing. The global technology services segment primarily reflects IT infrastructure services and business process services. The division's capabilities include outsourcing services, business transformation services and maintenance. The global business services segment primarily reflects professional services and application outsourcing services. Capabilities include consulting and systems integration; and application management services. The systems and technology division provides IBM's clients with business solutions requiring advanced computing power and storage capabilities. Offerings include services; storage; microelectronics; engineering and technology services; and retail store solutions. The software segment consists primarily of middleware and operating systems software. Middleware software enables clients to integrate systems, processes and applications across a standard software platform. Offerings include information management software; operating systems; and Tivoli software, for infrastructure management, including security and storage management. The global financing division's capabilities include commercial financing, client financing and remarketing. The company has manufacturing locations in Minnesota, New York and California in the U.S.; Mexico; Ireland; Hungary; France; China; and Singapore. In November 2007, the firm agreed to acquire Cognos, an independent analytical software producer, for $4.9 billion.

The company offers its employees medical, dental and vision insurance; sickness and accident income plans; long-term disability and life insurance; travel accident insurance; a 401(k) plan; and an employee stock purchase plan.

FINANCIALS: Sales and profits are in thousands of dollars—add 000 to get the full amount. 2007 Note: Financial information for 2007 was not available for all companies at press time.

2007 Sales: $98,786,000	2007 Profits: $10,418,000	**U.S. Stock Ticker: IBM**
2006 Sales: $91,424,000	2006 Profits: $9,492,000	**Int'l Ticker:** Int'l Exchange:
2005 Sales: $91,134,000	2005 Profits: $7,934,000	Employees: 386,558
2004 Sales: $96,503,000	2004 Profits: $8,430,000	Fiscal Year Ends: 12/31
2003 Sales: $89,131,000	2003 Profits: $7,583,000	Parent Company:

SALARIES/BENEFITS:

Pension Plan:	ESOP Stock Plan:	Profit Sharing:	Top Exec. Salary: $1,800,000	Bonus: $5,800,000
Savings Plan: Y	Stock Purch. Plan: Y		Second Exec. Salary: $775,001	Bonus: $1,265,000

OTHER THOUGHTS:

Apparent Women Officers or Directors: 5
Hot Spot for Advancement for Women/Minorities: Y

LOCATIONS: ("Y" = Yes)

West:	Southwest:	Midwest:	Southeast:	Northeast:	International:
Y	Y	Y	Y	Y	Y

Note: Financial information, benefits and other data can change quickly and may vary from those stated here.

INTIMATE BRANDS INC

www.intimatebrands.com

Industry Group Code: 448120 Ranks within this company's industry group: Sales: 2 Profits:

Management:		Sales/Marketing:		Liberal Arts:		Information Systems:		Professionals:		Technical/Scientific:	
Mgmt. Trainees:	Y	Mktg. Professionals:	Y	Gen. Writing/Editing:	Y	Info. Management:	Y	Finance/Accounting:	Y	Engineers, Elec.:	
Experienced Mgmt.:	Y	Retail Sales:	Y	Technical Writing:		Software Dev.:	Y	Law:	Y	Engineers, Other:	
Int'l Business:	Y	Commercial/Industrial:	Y	Graphic Arts/Photog.:	Y	Hardware Dev.:		HR/Other:	Y	Health/Lab:	
MBA Graduates:	Y	Sales Trainees:	Y	Music:		Systems Integration:		Training:	Y	Scientists/Research:	
		Advertising Pros.:	Y	Broadcasting:		Consulting/Other:		Health Care:		Petroleum/Chemicals:	
				Other:	Y			Consulting:		Math/Other:	

TYPES OF BUSINESS:

Intimate Apparel-Women's, Retail
Cosmetics
Fragrances
Personal Care Products
Online Sales
Catalogs
Candles
Professional Apparel

BRANDS/DIVISIONS/AFFILIATES:

Limited Brands, Inc.
Victoria's Secret
Limited (The)
Bath & Body Works
White Barn Candle Co.
Victoria's Secret Direct
C.O. Bigelow
PINK

CONTACTS: Note: Officers with more than one job title may be intentionally listed here more than once.

Leslie H. Wexner, CEO/Group Pres., Lingerie
Leonard A. Schlesinger, COO/Group Pres., Beauty & Personal Care
Martyn R. Redgrave, CFO
Jane L. Ramsey, Exec. VP-Human Resources
Martyn R. Redgrave, Exec. VP/Chief Admin. Officer
Mark Giresi, Exec. VP-Retail Oper.
V. Ann Hailey, Exec. VP-Corp. Dev.
Jay Margolis, Group Pres., Apparel
Deborah I. Fine, CEO-PINK
Sharen Jester Turney, CEO/Pres., Victoria's Secret Megabrand & Intimates

Phone: 614-415-7000	Fax: 614-415-7278
Toll-Free:	
Address: 3 Limited Pkwy., Columbus, OH 43230 US	

GROWTH PLANS/SPECIAL FEATURES:

Intimate Brands, Inc., a wholly-owned subsidiary of Limited Brands, Inc., purchases, distributes and sells lingerie, personal care products and women's apparel through over 3,500 retail stores, the Internet and direct mail channels. The company operates Victoria's Secret, Express, The Limited, Bath and Body Works, C.O. Bigelow, Henri Bendel and White Barn Candle Co. retail locations. Victoria's Secret is a leading specialty retailer of women's intimate apparel and related products. There are 998 locations that house branded merchandise such as IPEX and PINK. Express is a retail store marketing original designs in work and casual wear to young men and women in 743 stores. The Limited is a retail store dedicated to sophisticated, feminine styles with a total of 292 stores. Bath and Body Works (BB), which also operates White Barn Candle Co., is a retailer of personal and home care products. Through 1,555 stores, BB sells personal care products such as fragrances, body creams, shower washes, cosmetics, hair care products and aromatherapy and spa treatments. The unit sells its products under private labels, such as American Girl and Breathe. White Barn Candle Co. is a retailer of candles and assorted home furnishings through its 100 stores. In addition to its retail stores, which also include C.O. Bigelow and Henri Bendel, Intimate Brands operates Victoria's Secret Direct, which consists of the famous Victoria's Secret Catalog and an e-commerce site, VictoriaSecret.com. The firm's widely distributed catalog offers women's fashion apparel, lingerie, swimwear and footwear through its over 390 million annually distributed copies. Intimate Brands has closed over 200 retail stores since 2005.

The company offers its employees merchandise discounts, education assistance, school loans, adoption assistance, bonus programs and an annual retirement contribution. The Merchant In-Training program is a three month intensive course designed to prepare participants for a career in merchandizing.

FINANCIALS: Sales and profits are in thousands of dollars—add 000 to get the full amount. 2007 Note: Financial information for 2007 was not available for all companies at press time.

2007 Sales: $	2007 Profits: $	U.S. Stock Ticker: **Subsidiary**	
2006 Sales: $6,733,000	2006 Profits: $	**Int'l Ticker:** Int'l Exchange:	
2005 Sales: $6,401,000	2005 Profits: $	Employees: 70,000	
2004 Sales: $5,751,000	2004 Profits: $	Fiscal Year Ends: 1/31	
2003 Sales: $5,367,000	2003 Profits: $	Parent Company: LIMITED BRANDS INC	

SALARIES/BENEFITS:

Pension Plan:	ESOP Stock Plan:	Profit Sharing:	Top Exec. Salary: $1,685,192	Bonus: $758,880
Savings Plan: Y	Stock Purch. Plan:		Second Exec. Salary: $1,105,769	Bonus: $1,380,000

OTHER THOUGHTS:

Apparent Women Officers or Directors: 6
Hot Spot for Advancement for Women/Minorities: Y

LOCATIONS: ("Y" = Yes)

West:	Southwest:	Midwest:	Southeast:	Northeast:	International:
Y	Y	Y	Y	Y	Y

Note: Financial information, benefits and other data can change quickly and may vary from those stated here.

INTUIT INC

www.intuit.com

Industry Group Code: 511201 **Ranks within this company's industry group:** Sales: 2   Profits: 1

Management:		Sales/Marketing:		Liberal Arts:		Information Systems:		Professionals:		Technical/Scientific:	
Mgmt. Trainees:		Mktg. Professionals:	Y	Gen. Writing/Editing:	Y	Info. Management:	Y	Finance/Accounting:	Y	Engineers, Elec.:	
Experienced Mgmt.:	Y	Retail Sales:		Technical Writing:	Y	Software Dev.:	Y	Law:	Y	Engineers, Other:	
Int'l Business:	Y	Commercial/Industrial:	Y	Graphic Arts/Photog.:	Y	Hardware Dev.:		HR/Other:	Y	Health/Lab:	
MBA Graduates:	Y	Sales Trainees:		Music:		Systems Integration:		Training:	Y	Scientists/Research:	
		Advertising Pros.:	Y	Broadcasting:		Consulting/Other:		Health Care:		Petroleum/Chemicals:	
				Other:				Consulting:		Math/Other:	

TYPES OF BUSINESS:

Computer Software-Financial Management
Business Accounting Software
Consumer Finance Software
Tax Preparation Software
Online Financial Services

BRANDS/DIVISIONS/AFFILIATES:

QuickBooks
QuickBooks Payroll
Innovative Merchant Services
Quicken
Quicken.com
Intuit Real Estate Solutions
StepUp Commerce, Inc.
Digital Insight Corp.

CONTACTS: Note: Officers with more than one job title may be intentionally listed here more than once.

Brad D. Smith, CEO
Brad D. Smith, Pres.
Neil Williams, CFO/Sr. VP
Caroline Donahue, VP-Sales
Laura A. Fennell, General Counsel/VP/Corp. Sec.
Alexander Lintner, Sr. VP-Strategy & Corp. Dev.
Jeffrey Hank, Controller/VP
Scott D. Cook, Chmn.-Exec. Committee
Kiran Patel, Gen. Mgr./Sr. VP-Consumer Tax Unit
Peter Karpas, Sr. VP-Quicken Health Group
Sasan Goodarzi, Sr. VP
Bill Campbell, Chmn.

Phone: 650-944-6000	Fax: 650-944-3699
Toll-Free: 800-446-8848	
Address: 2632 Marine Way, Mountain View, CA 94043 US	

GROWTH PLANS/SPECIAL FEATURES:

Intuit, Inc. is a leading provider of software and web-based services designed to provide consumers, small businesses and accounting professionals with financial management and tax solutions. The company has six business segments: QuickBooks, Payroll and Payments, Consumer Tax, Professional Tax, Financial Institutions and Other Businesses. QuickBooks products include QuickBooks Simple Start, which provides accounting functionality suitable for very small, less complex businesses; QuickBooks Pro, which provides accounting functionality suitable for slightly larger businesses, including those with payroll needs; QuickBooks Pro for Mac; QuickBooks Premier; and QuickBooks Enterprise Solutions. The company also offers QuickBooks Online Edition, suitable for multiple users working in various locations. QuickBooks Payroll is a family of products sold on a subscription basis to small businesses that prepare their own payrolls. The Innovative Merchant Services business, part of the company's Payroll and Payments segment, offers credit card, debit card, electronic benefits, check guarantee and gift card processing services as well as web-based transaction processing services for online merchants. The Consumer and Professional Tax segments offer a variety of software and services for customers whose returns have varying levels of complexity and for accountants and tax preparers in public practice who serve multiple clients. The Financial Institutions segment was formed after the acquision of Digital Insight Corp. in February 2007, and primarily consists of outsourced online banking applications and services for banks and credit unions provided by our Digital Insight business. The Other Businesses segment includes the Quicken software, Quicken.com, Intuit Real Estate Solutions and its businesses in Canada and the U.K. In December 2007, Intuit acquired Homestead Technologies, Inc., which provides website and online store services for small businesses, for $170 million. In February 2008, the company acquired Electronic Clearing House, Inc., which provides electronic payment processing solutions, for $131 million.

Intuit's employees enjoy an employee assistance program, tuition assistance, adoption assistance and medical, vision and dental insurance.

FINANCIALS: Sales and profits are in thousands of dollars—add 000 to get the full amount. 2007 Note: Financial information for 2007 was not available for all companies at press time.

2007 Sales: $2,672,947	2007 Profits: $440,003	**U.S. Stock Ticker:** INTU
2006 Sales: $2,293,010	2006 Profits: $416,963	**Int'l Ticker:** **Int'l Exchange:**
2005 Sales: $1,993,102	2005 Profits: $381,627	Employees: 8,200
2004 Sales: $1,867,663	2004 Profits: $317,030	Fiscal Year Ends: 7/31
2003 Sales: $1,581,500	2003 Profits: $343,000	Parent Company:

SALARIES/BENEFITS:

Pension Plan:	ESOP Stock Plan:	Profit Sharing:	Top Exec. Salary: $1,100,000	Bonus: $3,170,000
Savings Plan: Y	Stock Purch. Plan: Y		Second Exec. Salary: $584,134	Bonus: $850,000

OTHER THOUGHTS:

Apparent Women Officers or Directors: 5
Hot Spot for Advancement for Women/Minorities: Y

LOCATIONS: ("Y" = Yes)

West:	Southwest:	Midwest:	Southeast:	Northeast:	International:
Y	Y	Y	Y	Y	Y

Note: Financial information, benefits and other data can change quickly and may vary from those stated here.

INVENTIV HEALTH INC

www.ventiv.com

Industry Group Code: 541613 Ranks within this company's industry group: Sales: 1 Profits: 1

Management:		Sales/Marketing:		Liberal Arts:		Information Systems:		Professionals:		Technical/Scientific:	
Mgmt. Trainees:	Y	Mktg. Professionals:	Y	Gen. Writing/Editing:	Y	Info. Management:	Y	Finance/Accounting:	Y	Engineers, Elec.:	
Experienced Mgmt.:	Y	Retail Sales:		Technical Writing:	Y	Software Dev.:	Y	Law:	Y	Engineers, Other:	Y
Int'l Business:	Y	Commercial/Industrial:	Y	Graphic Arts/Photog.:	Y	Hardware Dev.:		HR/Other:	Y	Health/Lab:	
MBA Graduates:	Y	Sales Trainees:		Music:		Systems Integration:	Y	Training:	Y	Scientists/Research:	Y
		Advertising Pros.:		Broadcasting:		Consulting/Other:		Health Care:	Y	Petroleum/Chemicals:	
				Other:				Consulting:	Y	Math/Other:	

TYPES OF BUSINESS:

Marketing-Life Sciences & Pharmaceuticals
Sales & Marketing Outsourcing
Clinical Staffing
Health Care Communications
Advertising Services
Data Services
Sales Force Deployment
Clinical & Statistical Research

BRANDS/DIVISIONS/AFFILIATES:

inVentiv Commercial Services
inVentiv Communications
inVentiv Clinical Services
Franklin Group (The)
Pharmaceutical Resource Solutions
GSW Worldwide
Stonefly
MedFocus

CONTACTS: Note: Officers with more than one job title may be intentionally listed here more than once.

Eran Broshy, CEO
Terrell Herring, COO
Blane Walter, Pres.
David Bassin, CFO
Terrell Herring, CEO/Pres., iVentiv Commercial
William O'Donnell, COO-inVentiv Communications
Thomas A. Hanley, Jr., CEO/Pres., Smith Hanley Holding Company
Michael Hlinak, Pres., inVentiv Clinical
Daniel M. Snyder, Chmn.

Phone: 732-748-4666	Fax: 732-537-4912
Toll-Free: 800-416-0555	
Address: 200 Cottontail Ln., 8th Fl., Somerset, NJ 08873 US	

GROWTH PLANS/SPECIAL FEATURES:

inVentiv Health, Inc. is a clinical services and marketing services provider for the pharmaceutical and life sciences industry. inVentiv's services include sales and marketing; clinical staffing; planning and analytics; marketing support; professional development and training; and data collection and management. The company is structured into three business units: inVentiv Commercial Services, inVentiv Communications and inVentiv Clinical Services. inVentiv Commercial Services, formerly inVentiv Pharma Services, oversees most of the firm's services such as sales and marketing teams and recruitment of sales representatives in the commercial services area. Additional subsidiaries and acquisitions of this group include the Franklin Group, Pharmaceutical Resource Solutions and Promotech. inVentiv Communications provides advertising, business communications, branding, medical education and contract marketing services via subsidiaries GSW Worldwide, Palio, Navicor, Stonefly and Jeffrey Simbrow and Associates. inVentiv Clinical Services consists of subsidiaries Smith Hanley Associates, Smith Hanley Consulting Group and MedFocus (collectively Smith Hanley), HHI Clinical & Statistical Research Services and Anova Clinical Resources. This segment provides services related to recruitment, clinical staffing and data collection and management. inVentiv's clients include Sanofi-Aventis Group, Bayer Corporation, Bristol-Myers Squibb and Watson Pharmaceuticals, Inc. Daniel M. Snyder, owner of the Washington Redskins football team, retains a significant interest in inVentiv as the company's chairman. Recently, the company acquired the assets of The Maxwell Group (including its MedConference brand of on-demand virtual services) for 8.1 million in cash and stock. In 2007, the firm acquired Ignite (Incendia Health, Inc.), a medical advertising and interactive communications firm, for $20 million in cash and stock. In addition, the company acquired Chamberlain (a public relations firm in the healthcare industry) for $13 million. The new companies are included in the firm's inVentiv Communications segment.

inVentiv has its own training center and offers online courses to enrich its employees' skills and leadership.

FINANCIALS: Sales and profits are in thousands of dollars—add 000 to get the full amount. 2007 Note: Financial information for 2007 was not available for all companies at press time.

2007 Sales: $977,300	2007 Profits: $47,484	**U.S. Stock Ticker: VTIV**
2006 Sales: $766,245	2006 Profits: $51,235	**Int'l Ticker:** Int'l Exchange:
2005 Sales: $556,312	2005 Profits: $43,863	Employees: 5,700
2004 Sales: $352,184	2004 Profits: $31,132	Fiscal Year Ends: 12/31
2003 Sales: $224,453	2003 Profits: $5,776	Parent Company:

SALARIES/BENEFITS:

Pension Plan:	ESOP Stock Plan:	Profit Sharing:	Top Exec. Salary: $560,000	Bonus: $750,000
Savings Plan: Y	Stock Purch. Plan:		Second Exec. Salary: $387,000	Bonus: $

OTHER THOUGHTS:

Apparent Women Officers or Directors:
Hot Spot for Advancement for Women/Minorities:

LOCATIONS: ("Y" = Yes)

West:	Southwest:	Midwest:	Southeast:	Northeast:	International:
Y	Y	Y	Y	Y	

Note: Financial information, benefits and other data can change quickly and may vary from those stated here.

J C PENNEY COMPANY INC   www.jcpenney.com

Industry Group Code: 452110 Ranks within this company's industry group: Sales: 2   Profits: 2

Management:		Sales/Marketing:		Liberal Arts:		Information Systems:		Professionals:		Technical/Scientific:	
Mgmt. Trainees:	Y	Mktg. Professionals:	Y	Gen. Writing/Editing:	Y	Info. Management:	Y	Finance/Accounting:	Y	Engineers, Elec.:	
Experienced Mgmt.:	Y	Retail Sales:	Y	Technical Writing:	Y	Software Dev.:		Law:	Y	Engineers, Other:	
Int'l Business:	Y	Commercial/Industrial:	Y	Graphic Arts/Photog.:	Y	Hardware Dev.:		HR/Other:	Y	Health/Lab:	
MBA Graduates:	Y	Sales Trainees:	Y	Music:		Systems Integration:	Y	Training:	Y	Scientists/Research:	
		Advertising Pros.:	Y	Broadcasting:		Consulting/Other:		Health Care:		Petroleum/Chemicals:	
				Other:	Y			Consulting:		Math/Other:	

TYPES OF BUSINESS:

Department Stores
Online & Catalog Sales
Optometry
Photography Services
Salons
Custom Decorating

BRANDS/DIVISIONS/AFFILIATES:

J.C. Penney Corp., Inc.
jcpenney.com
Leisure Plus
JCPenney Optical Services
JCPenney Portraits
JCPenney Salon
JCPenney Custom Decorating

CONTACTS: Note: Officers with more than one job title may be intentionally listed here more than once.

Myron E. Ullman, III, CEO
Ken C. Hicks, Pres./Chief Merch. Officer
Robert B. Cavanaugh, CFO/Exec. VP
Michael J. Boylson, Chief Mktg. Officer/Exec. VP
Michael T. Theilmann, Chief Human Resources Officer/Exec. VP
Thomas Nealon, CIO/Exec. VP
Peter M. McGrath, Exec. VP/Dir.-Prod. Dev. & Sourcing
Michael T. Theilmann, Chief Admin. Officer
Joanne Bober, General Counsel/Exec. VP/Sec.
Clarence Kelley, Exec. VP/Dir.-Planning & Allocation
Thomas A. Clerkin, Sr. VP/Dir.-Finance-Stores, Catalog & Internet
Michael P. Dastuge, Sr. VP/Dir.-Property Dev.
Elizabeth H. Sweney, Exec. VP/Gen. Merch. Mgr.-Women's Apparel
Steven Lawrence, Exec. VP/Gen. Merch. Mgr.-Men's & Children's
Myron E. Ullman, III, Chmn.
Marie Lacertosa, Sr. VP/Dir.-Supply Chain

Phone: 972-431-1000	Fax: 972-431-1362
Toll-Free:	
Address: 6501 Legacy Dr., Plano, TX 75024 US	

GROWTH PLANS/SPECIAL FEATURES:

J.C. Penney Co., Inc. is a holding company for J.C. Penney Corp., Inc., a department store retailer. J.C. Penney provides merchandise and services through department stores, catalogs and the Internet. The company operates 1,067 JCPenney department stores in 49 U.S. states and Puerto Rico. The firm's major products include family apparel, jewelry, shoes, accessories and home furnishings. The firm operates the nation's largest general catalog businesses, as well as jcpenney.com, one of the largest apparel and home furnishings sites on the Internet. The company's entire product offering of 250,000 items is available online. Local stores receive revenue credit for online and catalog sales made within their regions. The direct and retail segments of J.C. Penney's business are fully integrated, making pickups and returns at retail stores possible for direct sales. Other services offered by the company are JCPenney Optical services, JCPenney Portraits, JCPenney Salon and JCPenney Custom Decorating, all of which departments can be found within JCPenney department stores. Additionally, the firm operates LeisurePlus, a travel and entertainment discount club. In April 2007, the firm announced plans to open 250 new stores over the next five years, but by 2008 had scaled back those plans due to the slowing economy, opening 20 new stores and renovating 10-15 existing store, as opposed to initial plans of 50 new stores and 65 renovations. New stores were opened in Lake Havasu City, Arizona; Council Bluffs, Iowa; Rockwall, Texas; and Panama City Beach, Florida, among others.

The company offers its employees term life insurance; a 401(k) plan; paid time off and holidays; and healthcare benefits, including medical, dental and vision insurance.

FINANCIALS: Sales and profits are in thousands of dollars—add 000 to get the full amount. 2007 Note: Financial information for 2007 was not available for all companies at press time.

2007 Sales: $19,903,000	2007 Profits: $1,153,000	U.S. Stock Ticker: JCP
2006 Sales: $18,781,000	2006 Profits: $1,088,000	Int'l Ticker: Int'l Exchange:
2005 Sales: $18,424,000	2005 Profits: $524,000	Employees: 151,000
2004 Sales: $17,786,000	2004 Profits: $-928,000	Fiscal Year Ends: 1/31
2003 Sales: $32,347,000	2003 Profits: $405,000	Parent Company:

SALARIES/BENEFITS:

Pension Plan:	ESOP Stock Plan:	Profit Sharing:	Top Exec. Salary: $1,500,000	Bonus: $2,673,750
Savings Plan: Y	Stock Purch. Plan:		Second Exec. Salary: $791,250	Bonus: $1,072,932

OTHER THOUGHTS:

Apparent Women Officers or Directors: 4
Hot Spot for Advancement for Women/Minorities: Y

LOCATIONS: ("Y" = Yes)

West:	Southwest:	Midwest:	Southeast:	Northeast:	International:
Y	Y	Y	Y	Y	Y

Note: Financial information, benefits and other data can change quickly and may vary from those stated here.

JABIL CIRCUIT INC

www.jabil.com

Industry Group Code: 334419 Ranks within this company's industry group: Sales: 1 Profits: 1

Management:		Sales/Marketing:		Liberal Arts:		Information Systems:		Professionals:		Technical/Scientific:	
Mgmt. Trainees:	Y	Mktg. Professionals:	Y	Gen. Writing/Editing:		Info. Management:	Y	Finance/Accounting:	Y	Engineers, Elec.:	Y
Experienced Mgmt.:	Y	Retail Sales:		Technical Writing:	Y	Software Dev.:	Y	Law:	Y	Engineers, Other:	Y
Int'l Business:	Y	Commercial/Industrial:	Y	Graphic Arts/Photog.:		Hardware Dev.:	Y	HR/Other:	Y	Health/Lab:	
MBA Graduates:	Y	Sales Trainees:	Y	Music:		Systems Integration:	Y	Training:	Y	Scientists/Research:	
		Advertising Pros.:	Y	Broadcasting:		Consulting/Other:		Health Care:		Petroleum/Chemicals:	
				Other:				Consulting:		Math/Other:	

TYPES OF BUSINESS:
Electronic Manufacturing Services & Solutions
Maintenance & Support Services
Custom Design Services

BRANDS/DIVISIONS/AFFILIATES:
Taiwan Green Point Enterprises Co., Ltd.

CONTACTS: *Note: Officers with more than one job title may be intentionally listed here more than once.*
Timothy L. Main, CEO
Mark T. Mondello, COO
Timothy L. Main, Pres.
Forbes Alexander, CFO
David Couch, CIO
Robert L. Paver, General Counsel/Corp. Sec.
Teck Ping Yuen, Sr. VP-Worldwide Oper.
Donald J. Myers, VP-Corp. Dev.
Beth A. Walters, VP-Comm.
Beth A. Walters, VP-Investor Rel.
Sergio A. Cadavrid, Treas.
John P. Lovato, CEO/Exec. VP-Consumer Div.
William D. Muir, Jr., CEO/Exec. VP-EMS Div.
William E. Peters, Sr. VP-Human Dev.
Meheryar Dastoor, Controller
William D. Morean, Chmn.
Sirjang L. Tandon, CEO-India Bus. Ventures
Jeffrey P. Ameel, VP-Global Supply Chain

Phone: 727-577-9749	Fax: 727-579-8529
Toll-Free:	
Address: 10560 Dr. Martin Luther King Jr. St. N., St. Petersburg, FL 33716 US	

GROWTH PLANS/SPECIAL FEATURES:
Jabil Circuit, Inc. is a provider of worldwide electronic manufacturing services and solutions. It provides electronics and mechanical design, production, product management and after-market services to companies in the aerospace, automotive, computing, consumer, defense, industrial, instrumentation, medical, networking, peripherals, storage and telecommunications industry. The company's business units are capable of providing customers with varying combinations of the following services: Integrated design and engineering; component selection, sourcing and procurement; automate assembly; design and implementation of product testing; parallel global production; enclosure service; systems assembly, direct-order fulfillment and configure-to-order; and after-market services. The firm conducts its operations in facilities located in Austria, Belgium, Brazil, China, England, France, Germany, Hungary, India, Ireland, Italy, Japan, Malaysia, Mexico, the Netherlands, Poland, Scotland, Singapore, Taiwan, Ukraine, Vietnam and the U.S. The largest customers include Cisco Systems, Inc.; EMC Corp.; Hewlett-Packard Co.; International Business Machines Corp. (IBM); Network Appliance; NEC Corp.; Nokia Corp.; Royal Philips Electronics; Tellabs, Inc.; and Valeo S.A. In April 2007, Taiwan Green Point Enterprises Co., Ltd. merged with and into an existing Jabil entity in Taiwan.

FINANCIALS: Sales and profits are in thousands of dollars—add 000 to get the full amount. 2007 Note: Financial information for 2007 was not available for all companies at press time.

		U.S. Stock Ticker: JBL
2007 Sales: $12,290,592	2007 Profits: $73,236	Int'l Ticker: Int'l Exchange:
2006 Sales: $10,265,447	2006 Profits: $164,518	Employees: 61,000
2005 Sales: $7,524,386	2005 Profits: $203,875	Fiscal Year Ends: 8/31
2004 Sales: $6,252,897	2004 Profits: $166,900	Parent Company:
2003 Sales: $3,545,466	2003 Profits: $43,007	

SALARIES/BENEFITS:
Pension Plan:	ESOP Stock Plan:	Profit Sharing:	Top Exec. Salary: $1,000,000	Bonus: $345,488
Savings Plan:	Stock Purch. Plan:		Second Exec. Salary: $600,000	Bonus: $188,448

OTHER THOUGHTS:
Apparent Women Officers or Directors: 2
Hot Spot for Advancement for Women/Minorities: Y

LOCATIONS: ("Y" = Yes)
West:	Southwest:	Midwest:	Southeast:	Northeast:	International:
Y		Y	Y	Y	Y

Note: Financial information, benefits and other data can change quickly and may vary from those stated here.

JACK IN THE BOX INC   www.jackinthebox.com

Industry Group Code: 722110 Ranks within this company's industry group: Sales: Profits:

Management:	Sales/Marketing:	Liberal Arts:	Information Systems:	Professionals:	Technical/Scientific:
Mgmt. Trainees:	Mktg. Professionals:	Gen. Writing/Editing:	Info. Management:	Finance/Accounting:	Engineers, Elec.:
Experienced Mgmt.:	Retail Sales:	Technical Writing:	Software Dev.:	Law:	Engineers, Other:
Int'l Business:	Commercial/Industrial:	Graphic Arts/Photog.:	Hardware Dev.:	HR/Other:	Health/Lab:
MBA Graduates:	Sales Trainees:	Music:	Systems Integration:	Training:	Scientists/Research:
	Advertising Pros.:	Broadcasting:	Consulting/Other:	Health Care:	Petroleum/Chemicals:
		Other:		Consulting:	Math/Other:

TYPES OF BUSINESS:

Fast Food Restaurants
Convenience Stores

BRANDS/DIVISIONS/AFFILIATES:

Jack in the Box
Qdoba Restaurant Corporation
Qdoba Mexican Grill
Jumbo Jack
Jack's Ultimate Salads
Quick Stuff
Breakfast Jack
Jack in the Box Foundation

CONTACTS: Note: Officers with more than one job title may be intentionally listed here more than once.

Linda A. Lang, CEO
Paul L. Schultz, COO
Paul L. Schultz, Pres.
Jerry P. Rebel, CFO/Exec. VP
Terri F. Graham, Chief Mktg. Officer/VP
Carlo E. Cetti, Human Resources/Sr. VP
Stephanie E. Cline, CIO/VP
Lawrence E. Schauf, General Counsel/Exec. VP/Corp. Sec.
Carlo E. Cetti, Sr. VP-Strategic Planning
Paul D. Melancon, VP/Controller
David Kaufhold, VP-Oper., Div. I
Lenny Comma, Regional VP-Quick Stuff Convenience Stores
Debra Jensen, VP-Systems Dev.
David M. Theno, Sr. VP-Logistics & Quality
Linda A. Lang, Chmn.
Carl R. Nank, VP-Supply Chain Svcs.

Phone: 858-571-2121	Fax: 858-571-2101
Toll-Free: 800-955-5225	
Address: 9330 Balboa Ave., San Diego, CA 92123-1516 US	

GROWTH PLANS/SPECIAL FEATURES:

Jack in the Box, Inc. (JB) operates and franchises the Jack in the Box fast food chain and, through its wholly-owned subsidiary Qdoba Restaurant Corporation, the Qdoba Mexican Grill dining chain in 31 states. The Jack in the Box hamburger chain has over 2,000 locations in 17 states, primarily in the Western and Southern U.S. JB is known for being the first fast food chain to introduce drive-through services, breakfast sandwiches and portable salads. The Jack in the Box menu features a variety of hamburgers (Jumbo Jack, Sourdough Jack and Ultimate Cheeseburger), salads (Jack's Ultimate Salads), specialty sandwiches (Ciabatta sandwiches), drinks and side items. Qdoba, which offers Mexican food in a casual dining atmosphere, has 177 locations in 31 states (47 company-operated and 130 franchised). Qdoba's menu features Mexican spices, fresh flavors and customizable menu creations which cater primarily to adult tastes. JB also operates approximately 50 proprietary convenience stores named Quick Stuff, which include fuel stations and are built adjacent to many Jack in the Box Restaurants. In 2006, the company sold 25 company-operated Jack in the Box restaurants in Hawaii to Scanlan Management LLC for $19 million in cash. Additionally, the company recently introduced the first contactless card readers, which allow customers to hold their debit/credit cards in front of a reader instead of swiping them. JB's non-managerial employees enjoy full medical/dental/vision insurance, vacation pay, discounted meals and a family and friends discount card. Managers are entitled to the same benefits, plus a 401(k), tuition reimbursement plan, dependant care and an employee assistance program. JB operates the Jack in the Box Foundation, a nonprofit organization which partners primarily with Big Brothers Big Sisters.

FINANCIALS: Sales and profits are in thousands of dollars—add 000 to get the full amount. 2007 Note: Financial information for 2007 was not available for all companies at press time.

2007 Sales: $2,875,978	2007 Profits: $126,304	U.S. Stock Ticker: JBX
2006 Sales: $2,723,603	2006 Profits: $109,075	Int'l Ticker: Int'l Exchange:
2005 Sales: $2,480,214	2005 Profits: $91,537	Employees: 42,500
2004 Sales: $2,320,465	2004 Profits: $74,684	Fiscal Year Ends: 10/31
2003 Sales: $2,058,290	2003 Profits: $73,618	Parent Company:

SALARIES/BENEFITS:

Pension Plan:	ESOP Stock Plan:	Profit Sharing:	Top Exec. Salary: $700,000	Bonus: $1,050,000
Savings Plan: Y	Stock Purch. Plan:		Second Exec. Salary: $485,000	Bonus: $654,750

OTHER THOUGHTS:

Apparent Women Officers or Directors: 8
Hot Spot for Advancement for Women/Minorities: Y

LOCATIONS: ("Y" = Yes)

West:	Southwest:	Midwest:	Southeast:	Northeast:	International:
Y	Y	Y	Y	Y	

Note: Financial information, benefits and other data can change quickly and may vary from those stated here.

JACOBS ENGINEERING GROUP INC

www.jacobs.com

Industry Group Code: 234000 Ranks within this company's industry group: Sales: 3 Profits: 3

Management:		Sales/Marketing:		Liberal Arts:		Information Systems:		Professionals:		Technical/Scientific:	
Mgmt. Trainees:	Y	Mktg. Professionals:	Y	Gen. Writing/Editing:		Info. Management:	Y	Finance/Accounting:	Y	Engineers, Elec.:	Y
Experienced Mgmt.:	Y	Retail Sales:		Technical Writing:	Y	Software Dev.:	Y	Law:	Y	Engineers, Other:	Y
Int'l Business:	Y	Commercial/Industrial:	Y	Graphic Arts/Photog.:	Y	Hardware Dev.:		HR/Other:	Y	Health/Lab:	
MBA Graduates:	Y	Sales Trainees:		Music:		Systems Integration:	Y	Training:	Y	Scientists/Research:	Y
		Advertising Pros.:		Broadcasting:		Consulting/Other:		Health Care:		Petroleum/Chemicals:	Y
				Other:				Consulting:	Y	Math/Other:	

TYPES OF BUSINESS:

Engineering & Design Services
Facility Management
Construction & Field Services
Technical Consulting Services
Environmental Services

BRANDS/DIVISIONS/AFFILIATES:

Edwards and Kelcey
Carter and Burgess
Neste Jacobs Oy of Kilpilahti
Rintekno

CONTACTS: Note: Officers with more than one job title may be intentionally listed here more than once.

Craig Martin, CEO
Craig Martin, Pres.
John Prosser, CFO/Exec. VP
Robert M. Clement, Sr. VP-Global Sales
Patricia H. Summers, Sr. VP-Human Resources
John W. Prosser Jr., Exec. VP-Admin.
William C. Markley III, Sr. VP/General Counsel/Sec.
Thomas R. Hammond, Exec. VP-Oper.
John W. Prosser Jr., Exec. VP-Finance/Treas.
Thomas R. Hammond, Exec. VP
George A. Kunberger, Exec. VP
Rogers F. Starr, Pres., Jacobs Tech. Inc.
Noel G. Watson, Chmn.

Phone: 626-578-3500	Fax: 626-568-6916
Toll-Free:	
Address: 1111 S. Arroyo Pkwy., Pasadena, CA 91109-7084 US	

GROWTH PLANS/SPECIAL FEATURES:

Jacobs Engineering Group, Inc. offers technical, professional, and construction services to industrial, commercial and governmental clients throughout North America, Europe, Asia, South America, India, the U.K. and Australia. The company's global network includes more than 60 offices in over 15 countries. The company provides project services, which include engineering, design and architecture; process, scientific, and systems consulting services; operations and maintenance services; and construction services, which include direct-hire construction and management services. Services are offered to selected industry groups such as oil and gas exploration, production, and refining; programs for various federal governments; pharmaceuticals and biotechnology; chemicals and polymers; buildings, which includes projects in the fields of health care and education as well as civic, governmental, and other buildings; infrastructure; technology and manufacturing; and pulp and paper, among others. Jacobs also provides pricing studies, project feasibility reports and automation and control system analysis for U.S. government agencies involved in defense and aerospace programs. In addition, the company is one of the leading providers of environmental engineering and consulting services in the U.S. and abroad, including hazardous and nuclear waste management and site cleanup and closure, providing support in such areas as underground storage tank removal, contaminated soil and water remediation, and long-term groundwater monitoring. Jacobs also designs, builds, installs, operates and maintains various types of soil and groundwater cleanup systems. In recent news, Jacobs acquired engineering and design firms Edwards & Kelcey and Carter & Burgess in 2007. In 2008, the company's Neste Jacobs Oy of Kilpilahti subsidiary in Finland acquired Rintekno, an engineering company in Finland.

Company employees receive tuition reimbursement, award and recognition programs, and medical and dental insurance

FINANCIALS: Sales and profits are in thousands of dollars—add 000 to get the full amount. 2007 Note: Financial information for 2007 was not available for all companies at press time.

2007 Sales: $8,473,970	2007 Profits: $287,130	U.S. Stock Ticker: JEC	
2006 Sales: $7,421,270	2006 Profits: $196,883	Int'l Ticker: Int'l Exchange:	
2005 Sales: $5,635,001	2005 Profits: $131,608	Employees: 36,400	
2004 Sales: $4,594,235	2004 Profits: $115,574	Fiscal Year Ends: 9/30	
2003 Sales: $4,615,601	2003 Profits: $128,010	Parent Company:	

SALARIES/BENEFITS:

Pension Plan: Y	ESOP Stock Plan:	Profit Sharing:	Top Exec. Salary: $975,000	Bonus: $1,219,359
Savings Plan: Y	Stock Purch. Plan: Y		Second Exec. Salary: $850,000	Bonus: $1,063,031

OTHER THOUGHTS:

Apparent Women Officers or Directors: 1
Hot Spot for Advancement for Women/Minorities:

LOCATIONS: ("Y" = Yes)

West:	Southwest:	Midwest:	Southeast:	Northeast:	International:
Y	Y	Y	Y	Y	Y

Note: Financial information, benefits and other data can change quickly and may vary from those stated here.

JM SMUCKER CO
www.smucker.com

Industry Group Code: 311000 Ranks within this company's industry group: Sales: 1 Profits: 1

Management:		Sales/Marketing:		Liberal Arts:	Information Systems:		Professionals:		Technical/Scientific:	
Mgmt. Trainees:	Y	Mktg. Professionals:	Y	Gen. Writing/Editing:	Info. Management:	Y	Finance/Accounting:	Y	Engineers, Elec.:	
Experienced Mgmt.:	Y	Retail Sales:		Technical Writing:	Software Dev.:		Law:	Y	Engineers, Other:	Y
Int'l Business:	Y	Commercial/Industrial:	Y	Graphic Arts/Photog.:	Hardware Dev.:		HR/Other:	Y	Health/Lab:	
MBA Graduates:	Y	Sales Trainees:		Music:	Systems Integration:		Training:	Y	Scientists/Research:	
		Advertising Pros.:		Broadcasting:	Consulting/Other:		Health Care:		Petroleum/Chemicals:	
				Other:			Consulting:		Math/Other:	

TYPES OF BUSINESS:
Food Products, Manufacturing
Fruit Spreads
Dessert Toppings
Peanut Butter
Beverages
Shortening and Oils
Baking Mixes
Condiments

BRANDS/DIVISIONS/AFFILIATES:
Smuckers
Jif
Crisco
Uncrustables
Adams
Pillsbury
Eagle Family Foods Holdings, Inc.
Carnation

CONTACTS: *Note: Officers with more than one job title may be intentionally listed here more than once.*
Timothy P. Smucker, Co-CEO
Richard K. Smucker, Pres./Co-CEO
Mark R. Belgya, CFO/Treas./VP
Christopher P. Resweber, VP-Mktg. Svcs.
Andrew G. Platt, CIO/VP-Info. Svcs.
M. Ann Harlan, General Counsel/Corp. Sec./VP
Barry C. Dunaway, VP-Corp. Dev.
John W. Denman, Controller/VP
Vincent C. Byrd, Sr. VP-Consumer Market
Julia L. Sabin, VP/Gen. Mgr.-Smucker Quality Beverages
Donald D. Hurrle, VP-Sales & Grocery Market
Steven Oakland, VP/Gen. Mgr.-Consumer Oils & Baking
Timothy P. Smucker, Chmn.
Mark T. Smucker, VP-Int'l
Dennis J. Armstrong, VP-Logistics & Oper. Support

Phone: 330-682-3000	Fax: 330-684-6410
Toll-Free: 888-550-9555	
Address: 1 Strawberry Ln., Orrville, OH 44667-0280 US	

GROWTH PLANS/SPECIAL FEATURES:
J.M. Smucker Company (Smuckers), established in 1897, manufactures and markets branded food products on a worldwide basis, with the majority of its sales in the U.S. and Canada. Products offered by Smuckers include peanut butter; shortening and oils; flour and baking ingredients; fruit spreads; baking mixes and ready-to-spread frostings; fruit and vegetable juices; beverages; dessert toppings; syrups; frozen sandwiches; pickles and condiments; potato side dishes; and, most recently, canned milk. Products are sold through brokers to food retailers, food wholesalers, club stores, mass merchandisers, discount stores and military commissaries. The company's products are also sold to food service distributors and operators including restaurants, schools and universities; health care operators; and health/natural food stores. The raw fruit materials used by Smuckers in the production of its food products are purchased from independent growers and suppliers. The company's major trademarks include Smuckers, Jif, Crisco, Dutch Girl, White Lily, Hungry Jack, Uncrustables, Adams, Laura Scudder's, Goober, Pet, R. W. Knudsen Family, and Magic Shell. Smuckers also uses the Pillsbury trademark under a royalty-free license. In May 2007, the company acquired Eagle Family Foods Holdings, Inc., a leading producer of sweetened condensed milk in the U.S. and Canada, for $133 million. In October 2007, Smuckers acquired the Canadian Carnation brand canned milk products business from Nestle Canada. In June 2008, the firm agreed to acquire Procter & Gamble's Folgers coffee business for nearly $3 billion.

FINANCIALS: Sales and profits are in thousands of dollars—add 000 to get the full amount. 2007 Note: Financial information for 2007 was not available for all companies at press time.

2007 Sales: $2,148,017	2007 Profits: $157,219	**U.S. Stock Ticker:** SJM
2006 Sales: $2,154,726	2006 Profits: $143,354	**Int'l Ticker:** Int'l Exchange:
2005 Sales: $2,043,877	2005 Profits: $129,073	Employees: 3,025
2004 Sales: $1,417,011	2004 Profits: $111,350	Fiscal Year Ends: 4/30
2003 Sales: $1,311,744	2003 Profits: $96,342	Parent Company:

SALARIES/BENEFITS:
Pension Plan: Y	ESOP Stock Plan:	Profit Sharing:	Top Exec. Salary: $700,000	Bonus: $854,000
Savings Plan: Y	Stock Purch. Plan:		Second Exec. Salary: $700,000	Bonus: $854,000

OTHER THOUGHTS:
Apparent Women Officers or Directors: 7
Hot Spot for Advancement for Women/Minorities: Y

LOCATIONS: ("Y" = Yes)
West:	Southwest:	Midwest:	Southeast:	Northeast:	International:
Y		Y	Y	Y	Y

JOHNSON & JOHNSON

www.jnj.com

Industry Group Code: 325412 Ranks within this company's industry group: Sales: 1 Profits: 1

Management:		Sales/Marketing:		Liberal Arts:		Information Systems:		Professionals:		Technical/Scientific:	
Mgmt. Trainees:	Y	Mktg. Professionals:	Y	Gen. Writing/Editing:	Y	Info. Management:	Y	Finance/Accounting:	Y	Engineers, Elec.:	Y
Experienced Mgmt.:	Y	Retail Sales:		Technical Writing:	Y	Software Dev.:	Y	Law:	Y	Engineers, Other:	Y
Int'l Business:	Y	Commercial/Industrial:	Y	Graphic Arts/Photog.:	Y	Hardware Dev.:		HR/Other:	Y	Health/Lab:	Y
MBA Graduates:	Y	Sales Trainees:	Y	Music:		Systems Integration:		Training:	Y	Scientists/Research:	Y
		Advertising Pros.:	Y	Broadcasting:		Consulting/Other:		Health Care:	Y	Petroleum/Chemicals:	
				Other:				Consulting:		Math/Other:	Y

TYPES OF BUSINESS:

Personal Health Care & Hygiene Products
Sterilization Products
Surgical Products
Pharmaceuticals
Skin Care Products
Baby Care Products
Contact Lenses
Medical Equipment

BRANDS/DIVISIONS/AFFILIATES:

Scios Inc
Centocor Inc
Alza Corp
Depuy Inc
Ethicon Inc
Cordis Corp
LifeScan Inc
Conor Medsystems, Inc.

CONTACTS: Note: Officers with more than one job title may be intentionally listed here more than once.

William C. Weldon, CEO
Dominic J. Caruso, CFO
Kaye I. Foster-Cheek, VP-Human Resources
Russell C. Deyo, General Counsel/VP/Chief Compliance Officer
Nicholas J. Valeriani, VP-Strategy & Growth
Dominic J. Caruso, VP-Finance
Per A. Peterson, Chmn., R&D Pharmaceutical Group
William C. Weldon, Chmn.

Phone: 732-524-0400	Fax: 732-214-0332
Toll-Free:	
Address: 1 Johnson & Johnson Plz., New Brunswick, NJ 08933 US	

GROWTH PLANS/SPECIAL FEATURES:

Johnson & Johnson, founded in 1886, is one of the world's most comprehensive and well-known manufacturers of health care products. The firm owns more than 250 companies in over 90 countries and markets its products in almost every country in the world. Johnson & Johnson's worldwide operations are divided into three segments: consumer, pharmaceutical and medical devices and diagnostics. The company's principal consumer goods are personal care and hygiene products, including nonprescription drugs, adult skin and hair care, baby care, oral care, first aid and sanitary protection products. Major consumer brands include Mylanta, Band-Aid, Tylenol, Aveeno and Monistat. The pharmaceutical segment covers a wide spectrum of health fields, including antifungal, anti-infective, cardiovascular, dermatology, immunology, pain management, psychotropic and women's health. Among its pharmaceutical products are Risperdal, an antipsychotic used to treat schizophrenia, and Remicade for the treatment of Crohn's disease and rheumatoid arthritis. In the medical devices and diagnostics segment, Johnson & Johnson makes a number of products including suture and mechanical wound closure products, surgical instruments, disposable contact lenses, joint replacement products and intravenous catheters. Johnson & Johnson is pursuing nanotechnology applications in the biomedical fields primarily through research and funding agreements with other biotech companies, including Cordis. In early 2007, the firm acquired Conor Medsystems, Inc., a cardiovascular device developer. In late 2007, the company announced that it was in the midst of reorganizing, downsizing from three business segments to two: surgical care and comprehensive care.

Johnson & Johnson offers its employees comprehensive heath and wellness. Some locations offer on-site child care centers and Nurture Space programs through which new mothers get counseling on how to return to work while breastfeeding.

FINANCIALS: Sales and profits are in thousands of dollars—add 000 to get the full amount. 2007 Note: Financial information for 2007 was not available for all companies at press time.

2007 Sales: $61,095,000	2007 Profits: $10,576,000	U.S. Stock Ticker: JNJ
2006 Sales: $53,324,000	2006 Profits: $11,053,000	Int'l Ticker: Int'l Exchange:
2005 Sales: $50,514,000	2005 Profits: $10,060,000	Employees: 119,200
2004 Sales: $47,348,000	2004 Profits: $8,180,000	Fiscal Year Ends: 12/31
2003 Sales: $41,862,000	2003 Profits: $7,197,000	Parent Company:

SALARIES/BENEFITS:

Pension Plan:	ESOP Stock Plan:	Profit Sharing:	Top Exec. Salary: $1,659,231	Bonus: $7,461,440
Savings Plan: Y	Stock Purch. Plan:		Second Exec. Salary: $1,023,846	Bonus: $2,574,880

OTHER THOUGHTS:

Apparent Women Officers or Directors: 6
Hot Spot for Advancement for Women/Minorities: Y

LOCATIONS: ("Y" = Yes)

West:	Southwest:	Midwest:	Southeast:	Northeast:	International:
Y	Y	Y	Y	Y	Y

Note: Financial information, benefits and other data can change quickly and may vary from those stated here.

JOHNSON CONTROLS INC

www.johnsoncontrols.com

Industry Group Code: 336300 Ranks within this company's industry group: Sales: 1 Profits: 1

Management:		Sales/Marketing:		Liberal Arts:		Information Systems:		Professionals:		Technical/Scientific:	
Mgmt. Trainees:	Y	Mktg. Professionals:	Y	Gen. Writing/Editing:	Y	Info. Management:	Y	Finance/Accounting:	Y	Engineers, Elec.:	Y
Experienced Mgmt.:	Y	Retail Sales:		Technical Writing:	Y	Software Dev.:	Y	Law:	Y	Engineers, Other:	
Int'l Business:	Y	Commercial/Industrial:	Y	Graphic Arts/Photog.:	Y	Hardware Dev.:	Y	HR/Other:	Y	Health/Lab:	Y
MBA Graduates:	Y	Sales Trainees:		Music:		Systems Integration:	Y	Training:	Y	Scientists/Research:	Y
		Advertising Pros.:	Y	Broadcasting:		Consulting/Other:	Y	Health Care:		Petroleum/Chemicals:	
				Other:				Consulting:		Math/Other:	Y

TYPES OF BUSINESS:

Automobile Parts & Controls
Automotive Batteries
Plastics
Environmental Services
Energy Management Services
Building Security, Lighting & HVAC Systems
Automotive Interior Components
Facilities Management

BRANDS/DIVISIONS/AFFILIATES:

Matasys Building Management System
Johnson Controls-Saft Advanced Power Solutions
York International
Optima
Varta
The Capital Group
Skymark International, Inc.
Metro Mechanical, Inc.

CONTACTS: Note: Officers with more than one job title may be intentionally listed here more than once.

Stephen A. Roell, CEO
Keith Wandell, COO
Keith Wandell, Pres.
R. Bruce McDonald, CFO/Exec. VP
Susan F. Davis, Exec. VP-Human Resources
Subhash S. Valanju, CIO/VP
Jerome D. Okarma, General Counsel/Sec./VP
Denise Zutz, VP-Strategy
Denise Zutz, VP-Corp. Comm.
Denise Zutz, VP-Investor Rel.
Frank A. Voltolina, Treasurer/VP
Jeffrey G. Augustin, VP-Building Efficiency
Beda Bolzenius, VP-Automotive Experience
Alex A. Molinaroli, Pres., Power Solutions
Charles A. Harvey, VP-Public Affairs & Diversity
Stephen A. Roell, Chmn.
Jeffrey S. Edwards, VP-Automotive Experience, Japan & Asia Pacific

Phone: 414-524-1200	Fax: 414-524-2070
Toll-Free: 800-524-6220	
Address: 5757 N. Green Bay Ave., Milwaukee, WI 53201 US	

GROWTH PLANS/SPECIAL FEATURES:

Johnson Controls, Inc. is a leader in automotive interiors, building controls, facility management and automotive batteries. The firm's automotive interiors segment designs and manufactures complete seat systems, seating components, electronics, instrument panels, overhead, door, cargo management systems and interior trim for manufacturers of cars and light trucks. The automotive segment is also one of the largest replacement and original equipment automotive battery manufacturers in North America, including batteries for hybrid electric vehicles. Johnson's controls segment is a global supplier of systems designed to control heating, ventilating, air conditioning, lighting, security and fire management for buildings. The company manages facilities including over 7,000 school districts and over 2,000 hospitals, as well as factories, airports and government facilities using its patented Matasys Building Management System. Johnson Control's well-known battery brands include Optima, Varta, Heliar (in South America), and LTH (in Mexico). Prominent clients include BMW; DaimlerChrysler; Ford; Toyota; Volkswagen; AutoZone; Interstate Battery System of America; Bank of America; IBM; and Wal-Mart. The U.S. Department of Defense selected Johnson Controls to provide energy management and environmental control systems for the Pentagon, one of the largest such projects in the company's history. The company has a joint venture with Saft SA, a battery company, called Johnson Controls-Saft Advanced Power Solutions. Recent acquisitions include Metro Mechanical, Inc., a mechanical services company; Skymark International, Inc., an indoor packaged HVAC products manufacturer; and The Capital Group, a mechanical services company. The firm recently gained a patent for a wireless communication system that allows hands-free cell phone use in automobiles.

Johnson Controls offers its employees a benefits package that includes health care coverage and tuition reimbursement. Additionally, it operates an educational institute to supplement employees' skills. In 2007, Johnson Controls was ranked among the top 15 of the 40 Best Companies for Diversity by Black Enterprise magazine.

FINANCIALS: Sales and profits are in thousands of dollars—add 000 to get the full amount. 2007 Note: Financial information for 2007 was not available for all companies at press time.

2007 Sales: $34,524,000	2007 Profits: $1,252,000	U.S. Stock Ticker: JCI
2006 Sales: $32,235,000	2006 Profits: $1,028,000	Int'l Ticker: Int'l Exchange:
2005 Sales: $27,479,400	2005 Profits: $909,400	Employees: 140,000
2004 Sales: $26,553,400	2004 Profits: $817,500	Fiscal Year Ends: 9/30
2003 Sales: $22,646,000	2003 Profits: $682,900	Parent Company:

SALARIES/BENEFITS:

Pension Plan: Y	ESOP Stock Plan:	Profit Sharing:	Top Exec. Salary: $1,485,000	Bonus: $8,368,000
Savings Plan: Y	Stock Purch. Plan:		Second Exec. Salary: $975,000	Bonus: $4,104,000

OTHER THOUGHTS:

Apparent Women Officers or Directors: 4
Hot Spot for Advancement for Women/Minorities: Y

LOCATIONS: ("Y" = Yes)

West:	Southwest:	Midwest:	Southeast:	Northeast:	International:
Y	Y	Y	Y	Y	Y

JP MORGAN CHASE & CO INC   www.jpmorganchase.com

Industry Group Code: 522110 Ranks within this company's industry group: Sales: 3   Profits: 3

Management:		Sales/Marketing:		Liberal Arts:		Information Systems:		Professionals:		Technical/Scientific:	
Mgmt. Trainees:	Y	Mktg. Professionals:	Y	Gen. Writing/Editing:	Y	Info. Management:	Y	Finance/Accounting:	Y	Engineers, Elec.:	
Experienced Mgmt.:	Y	Retail Sales:		Technical Writing:		Software Dev.:	Y	Law:	Y	Engineers, Other:	
Int'l Business:	Y	Commercial/Industrial:	Y	Graphic Arts/Photog.:		Hardware Dev.:		HR/Other:	Y	Health/Lab:	
MBA Graduates:	Y	Sales Trainees:		Music:		Systems Integration:		Training:	Y	Scientists/Research:	
		Advertising Pros.:	Y	Broadcasting:		Consulting/Other:		Health Care:		Petroleum/Chemicals:	
				Other:				Consulting:		Math/Other:	

TYPES OF BUSINESS:

Banking
Mortgages
Investment Banking
Stock Brokerage
Credit Cards
Business Finance
Mutual Funds
Annuities

BRANDS/DIVISIONS/AFFILIATES:

JPMorgan Chase Vastera Inc
Bear Stearns Cos Inc (The)
J.P. Morgan Securities
MorganMarkets
JPMorgan Partners
One Equity Partners
Bank of New York
Integrated Investment Services

CONTACTS: *Note: Officers with more than one job title may be intentionally listed here more than once.*

James Dimon, CEO
Michael J. Cavanagh, Dir.-Finance
John F. Bradley, Dir.-Human Resources
Austin A. Adams, Dir.-Tech.
Frank J. Bisignano, Chief Admin. Officer
Stephen M. Cutler, General Counsel/Dir.-Legal & Compliance
Jay Mandelbaum, Dir.-Strategy
Joseph M. Evangelisti, Dir.-Corp. Comm.
Heidi Miller, Treas./Dir.-Securities Svcs.
Barry Zubrow, Chief Risk Officer
Paul T. Bateman, Dir.-Asset Mgmt.
Anthony J. Best, Dir.-Investment Bank
Steven D. Black, Dir.-Investment Bank
James Dimon, Chmn.
Andrew D. Crockett, Dir.-JPMorgan Chase Int'l

Phone: 212-270-6000	Fax: 212-270-2613
Toll-Free: 877-242-7372	
Address: 270 Park Ave., New York, NY 10017-2070 US	

GROWTH PLANS/SPECIAL FEATURES:

J.P. Morgan Chase & Co., Inc. (JPM) is one of the largest banking institutions in the U.S., with operations in more than 50 countries and assets amounting to $1.6 trillion. JPM provides investment banking; financial services; financial transaction processing; asset and wealth management; and private equity services for consumers and businesses. JPM's principal bank subsidiaries are JPMorgan Chase Bank, a national banking association with branches in 17 states; Chase Bank USA, the firm's leading provider of credit cards; and J.P. Morgan Securities, an investment banking firm.   The company is organized into six segments: Investment banking; retail finance; card services; commercial banking; treasury and securities; and asset management. JPM also operates private equity and treasury businesses through its subsidiary, One Equity Partners.   In the investment banking sector, JPM provides strategic advice, capital raising and risk management expertise in areas such as healthcare, technology, energy, real estate and transportation.   JPM also offers global research in areas such as fixed income/rates, credit, foreign exchange, emerging markets, derivatives, structured finance and bond indices.   The firm's research data portal, MorganMarkets, gives information on a range of financial markets by providing reports, commentaries, trading strategies, market data and portfolio management tools. In March 2008, JPM purchased Bear Stearns & Co. for approximately $236 million. The firm plans to merge J.P. Morgan Securities Inc. and Bear Stearns in October 2008.

FINANCIALS: Sales and profits are in thousands of dollars—add 000 to get the full amount. 2007 Note: Financial information for 2007 was not available for all companies at press time.

2007 Sales: $71,372,000	2007 Profits: $15,365,000	**U.S. Stock Ticker: JPM**
2006 Sales: $61,999,000	2006 Profits: $14,444,000	**Int'l Ticker:** Int'l Exchange:
2005 Sales: $54,248,000	2005 Profits: $8,483,000	Employees: 174,360
2004 Sales: $43,097,000	2004 Profits: $4,466,000	Fiscal Year Ends: 12/31
2003 Sales: $33,384,000	2003 Profits: $6,719,000	Parent Company:

SALARIES/BENEFITS:

Pension Plan: Y	ESOP Stock Plan:	Profit Sharing:	Top Exec. Salary: $1,000,000	Bonus: $21,000,000
Savings Plan: Y	Stock Purch. Plan: Y		Second Exec. Salary: $1,000,000	Bonus: $13,000,000

OTHER THOUGHTS:

Apparent Women Officers or Directors: 11
Hot Spot for Advancement for Women/Minorities: Y

LOCATIONS: ("Y" = Yes)

West:	Southwest:	Midwest:	Southeast:	Northeast:	International:
Y	Y	Y	Y	Y	Y

Note: Financial information, benefits and other data can change quickly and may vary from those stated here.

JUNIPER NETWORKS INC

www.juniper.net

Industry Group Code: 334110 Ranks within this company's industry group: Sales: 2 Profits: 2

Management:		Sales/Marketing:		Liberal Arts:		Information Systems:		Professionals:		Technical/Scientific:	
Mgmt. Trainees:		Mktg. Professionals:	Y	Gen. Writing/Editing:		Info. Management:	Y	Finance/Accounting:	Y	Engineers, Elec.:	Y
Experienced Mgmt.:	Y	Retail Sales:		Technical Writing:	Y	Software Dev.:	Y	Law:	Y	Engineers, Other:	Y
Int'l Business:	Y	Commercial/Industrial:	Y	Graphic Arts/Photog.:	Y	Hardware Dev.:	Y	HR/Other:	Y	Health/Lab:	
MBA Graduates:	Y	Sales Trainees:		Music:		Systems Integration:	Y	Training:	Y	Scientists/Research:	Y
		Advertising Pros.:	Y	Broadcasting:		Consulting/Other:		Health Care:		Petroleum/Chemicals:	
				Other:				Consulting:		Math/Other:	Y

TYPES OF BUSINESS:

Networking Equipment
IP Networking Systems
Internet Routers
Network Security Products
Internet Software
Intrusion Prevention
Application Acceleration

BRANDS/DIVISIONS/AFFILIATES:

JUNOS
E-Series
J-Series
M-Series
T-Series
MX-Series
SDX Service Deployment System
SSL VPN

CONTACTS: Note: Officers with more than one job title may be intentionally listed here more than once.

Kevin Johnson, CEO
Stephen Elop, COO
Robyn Denholm, CFO/Exec. VP
Penny Wilson, Chief Mktg. Officer
Steven Rice, Exec. VP-Human Resources
Michele Goins, CIO
Pradeep Sindhu, CTO/Vice Chmn.
Mitchell Gaynor, General Counsel
Eddie Minshull, Exec. VP-Worldwide Field Oper.
Spencer Greene, VP-Corp. Dev.
Kim Perdikou, Exec. VP-Infrastructure Products Group
Kim Perdikou, Gen. Mgr.-Service Provider Bus. Team
Mark Bauhaus, Exec. VP/Gen. Mgr.-Service Layer Tech. Bus. Group
Hitesh Sheth, Exec. VP/Gen. Mgr.-Ethernet Platforms Bus. Group
Scott Kriens, Chmn.
Donna Grothjan, VP-Worldwide Channel Strategy & Oper.

Phone: 408-745-2000	Fax: 408-745-2100
Toll-Free: 888-586-4737	
Address: 1194 N. Mathilda Ave., Sunnyvale, CA 94089-1206 US	

GROWTH PLANS/SPECIAL FEATURES:

Juniper Networks, Inc. is a provider of custom-designed Internet protocol (IP) networking platforms for Internet service providers, enterprises, governments and educational institutions. Operations are organized into three segments: infrastructure, service layer technologies (SLT) and service. The infrastructure segment primarily offers scalable router products used to control and direct network traffic. Product families offered by the firm include the M-Series, T-Series and E-Series. The SLT segment offers services that protect networks as well as maximize existing bandwidth and acceleration of applications across a distributed network. The SLT product families include firewall services, virtual private network (VPN) systems, intrusion detection and prevention (IDP) and application acceleration platforms. The firm outsources manufacturing to companies such as IBM, Toshiba, Celestica and Plexus; these manufacturers create application-specific chips from Juniper's designs. Additionally, the company sells Internet backbone routers, which are offered through a direct sales force to Internet and telecommunication service providers around the world. The firm maintains several strategic alliances with prominent companies including Avaya, Ericsson, Lucent Technologies, Siemens, and more recently, Lockheed Martin, Microsoft and Oracle. Juniper's customers include wireline, wireless and cable ISPs; private enterprises; federal, state and local government agencies; and research and education institutions. The firm maintains international headquarters in the U.K., Hong Kong and Tokyo and sales offices in 39 countries worldwide. The firm added several new national and international clients in 2007 and 2008 including Verizon, GMarket, a leading Korean ecommerce company, Pakistan Private Asset Company; IGDAS, Istanbul's leading gas provider; Mustang Engineering; and T-Mobile, among others. Juniper owns 500 technology patents, either issued or pending, and in 2007, spent more than $500 million on research and development.

FINANCIALS: Sales and profits are in thousands of dollars—add 000 to get the full amount. 2007 Note: Financial information for 2007 was not available for all companies at press time.

2007 Sales: $2,836,100	2007 Profits: $360,800	U.S. Stock Ticker: JNPR
2006 Sales: $2,303,580	2006 Profits: $-1,001,437	Int'l Ticker: Int'l Exchange:
2005 Sales: $2,063,957	2005 Profits: $350,701	Employees: 5,879
2004 Sales: $1,336,019	2004 Profits: $128,228	Fiscal Year Ends: 12/31
2003 Sales: $701,400	2003 Profits: $39,200	Parent Company:

SALARIES/BENEFITS:

Pension Plan:	ESOP Stock Plan:	Profit Sharing:	Top Exec. Salary: $475,000	Bonus: $591,376
Savings Plan: Y	Stock Purch. Plan: Y		Second Exec. Salary: $440,789	Bonus: $631,519

OTHER THOUGHTS:

Apparent Women Officers or Directors: 5
Hot Spot for Advancement for Women/Minorities: Y

LOCATIONS: ("Y" = Yes)

West:	Southwest:	Midwest:	Southeast:	Northeast:	International:
Y	Y	Y	Y	Y	Y

KAISER PERMANENTE

www.kaiserpermanente.org

Industry Group Code: 622110 Ranks within this company's industry group: Sales: Profits:

Management:		Sales/Marketing:		Liberal Arts:		Information Systems:		Professionals:		Technical/Scientific:	
Mgmt. Trainees:		Mktg. Professionals:	Y	Gen. Writing/Editing:	Y	Info. Management:	Y	Finance/Accounting:	Y	Engineers, Elec.:	
Experienced Mgmt.:	Y	Retail Sales:		Technical Writing:		Software Dev.:	Y	Law:	Y	Engineers, Other:	
Int'l Business:		Commercial/Industrial:	Y	Graphic Arts/Photog.:	Y	Hardware Dev.:		HR/Other:	Y	Health/Lab:	
MBA Graduates:	Y	Sales Trainees:	Y	Music:		Systems Integration:	Y	Training:	Y	Scientists/Research:	
		Advertising Pros.:	Y	Broadcasting:		Consulting/Other:		Health Care:	Y	Petroleum/Chemicals:	
				Other:	Y			Consulting:		Math/Other:	

TYPES OF BUSINESS:

Hospitals & Clinics
General & Specialty Hospitals
Outpatient Facilities
HMO
Health Insurance
Integrated Health Care System
Physician Networks

BRANDS/DIVISIONS/AFFILIATES:

Kaiser Foundation Health Plan, Inc.
Kaiser Foundation Hospitals
Permanente Medical Groups
KP HealthConnect
Coalition of Kaiser Permanente Unions (The)
Kaiser Permanente Healthcare Institute
National Labor College

CONTACTS: *Note: Officers with more than one job title may be intentionally listed here more than once.*

George C. Halvorson, CEO
Kathy Lancaster, CFO/Sr. VP
Paul B. Records, Chief Human Resources Officer/Sr. VP
Raymond J. Baxter, Sr. VP-Research
J. Clifford Dodd,
Steven Zatkin, General Counsel/Sr. VP
Arthur M. Southam, Exec. VP-Health Plan Oper.
Jack Cochran, Exec. Dir.-Permanente Federation
Raymond J. Baxter, Sr. VP-Community Benefit & Health Policy
Louise L. Liang, Sr. VP-Quality & Clinical Systems Support
Bernard J. Tyson, Sr. VP-Health Plan & Hospital Oper.
George C. Halvorson, Chmn.

Phone: 510-271-5800	Fax: 510-267-7524
Toll-Free:	
Address: 1 Kaiser Plz., Ste. 2600, Oakland, CA 94612-3673 US	

GROWTH PLANS/SPECIAL FEATURES:

Kaiser Permanente is a non-profit company dedicated to providing integrated health care coverage. The firm operates in Washington, D.C. and nine states: California, Colorado, Georgia, Hawaii, Maryland, Ohio, Oregon, Virginia and Washington. It serves almost 8.7 million members, of which approximately 6.5 million are in California. Kaiser has three main operating divisions: Kaiser Foundation Health Plan, Inc., which contracts with individuals and groups to provide medical coverage; Kaiser Foundation Hospitals and their subsidiaries, operating community hospitals and outpatient facilities in several states; and Permanente Medical Groups, the company's network of physicians providing health care to its members. The company resources include 32 medical centers, including hospitals and outpatient facilities; 421 medical offices; and 14,000 physicians. Kaiser Foundation Hospitals also fund medical and health-related research. The firm, as a participant in the Medicare program, cares for approximately 880,000 Medicare members, making it one of the largest health plans serving the Medicare program. The KP HealthConnect program integrates clinical records with appointments, registration and billing, thereby significantly improving care delivery and patient satisfaction.

The company offers its employees paid time off for vacations, designated holidays, sick leave and what it calls life balance days. Kaiser Permanente's employee health care coverage extends to spouses, domestic partners and unmarried children.

FINANCIALS: Sales and profits are in thousands of dollars—add 000 to get the full amount. 2007 Note: Financial information for 2007 was not available for all companies at press time.

2007 Sales: $37,800,000	2007 Profits: $1,700,000	**U.S. Stock Ticker: Nonprofit**
2006 Sales: $34,600,000	2006 Profits: $	**Int'l Ticker:** Int'l Exchange:
2005 Sales: $31,100,000	2005 Profits: $1,000,000	Employees: 156,000
2004 Sales: $26,600,000	2004 Profits: $1,600,000	Fiscal Year Ends: 12/31
2003 Sales: $25,300,000	2003 Profits: $996,000	Parent Company:

SALARIES/BENEFITS:

Pension Plan: Y	ESOP Stock Plan:	Profit Sharing:	Top Exec. Salary: $	Bonus: $
Savings Plan: Y	Stock Purch. Plan:		Second Exec. Salary: $	Bonus: $

OTHER THOUGHTS:

Apparent Women Officers or Directors: 3
Hot Spot for Advancement for Women/Minorities: Y

LOCATIONS: ("Y" = Yes)

West:	Southwest:	Midwest:	Southeast:	Northeast:	International:
Y		Y	Y	Y	

KEANE INC

www.keane.com

Industry Group Code: 541512　Ranks within this company's industry group:　Sales: 10　Profits: 11

Management:		Sales/Marketing:		Liberal Arts:		Information Systems:		Professionals:		Technical/Scientific:	
Mgmt. Trainees:	Y	Mktg. Professionals:	Y	Gen. Writing/Editing:	Y	Info. Management:	Y	Finance/Accounting:	Y	Engineers, Elec.:	Y
Experienced Mgmt.:	Y	Retail Sales:		Technical Writing:	Y	Software Dev.:	Y	Law:	Y	Engineers, Other:	
Int'l Business:	Y	Commercial/Industrial:	Y	Graphic Arts/Photog.:	Y	Hardware Dev.:		HR/Other:	Y	Health/Lab:	
MBA Graduates:	Y	Sales Trainees:		Music:		Systems Integration:	Y	Training:	Y	Scientists/Research:	Y
		Advertising Pros.:	Y	Broadcasting:		Consulting/Other:	Y	Health Care:		Petroleum/Chemicals:	
				Other:				Consulting:	Y	Math/Other:	Y

TYPES OF BUSINESS:

IT Consulting
Business Management Software
Software Development & Integration
System Design & Implementation
Applications Outsourcing
Health Care Consulting

BRANDS/DIVISIONS/AFFILIATES:

Caritor, Inc.
Adobe Systems Inc
BMC Software Inc
Business Objects SA
Compuware Corp
International Business Machines Corp (IBM)
Microsoft Corp
BestShores

CONTACTS: Note: Officers with more than one job title may be intentionally listed here more than once.

Mani Subramanian, CEO
Jim Puthuff, COO/Exec. VP
Chris Setterington, CFO/Exec. VP
Marv Mouchawar, Exec. VP-Prod. & Corp. Dev.
Sandeep Bhargava, Exec. VP-Bus. Dev. & Industry Solutions
Srikanth Rao, Exec. VP-Quality/Pres., Keane India
Mani Subramanian, Chmn.
Krishna Prabhu, Sr. VP-Global Client Mgmt.
Karen Powell, Sr. VP-Bus. Process Outsourcing & Mgmt. Consulting

Phone: 925-838-8600	Fax: 925-838-7138
Toll-Free:	
Address: 210 Porter Dr., Ste. 315, San Ramon, CA 94583 US	

GROWTH PLANS/SPECIAL FEATURES:

Keane, Inc. is a global services company specializing in enabling the transformation of businesses and IT functions. In June 2007, Keane was acquired by and integrated into Caritor, Inc. for a purchase price of roughly $854 million. The combined company has operations in Australia, Canada, France, India, New Zealand, Switzerland, Singapore, UAE, the U.K. and the U.S., with more than $1 billion in annual revenue. Keane's global delivery approach includes onsite, offsite, nearshore and offshore options. The company has partnerships with Adobe; BMC Software; Business Objects; Cerylion; Compuware; Curam Software; DataCore; Enlighta; ExperSolve; HP Software; IBM; Lombardi Software; Microsoft; Oracle; PlanetSoft; PlanView; SAP; Vertica; and ZC Sterling. Keane provides business services including consulting, process outsourcing, strategy and program and performance management services, and technology services including application, architecture, enterprise application, infrastructure and quality assurance and testing services. The company serves the financial services, insurance, healthcare, manufacturing, public sector, telecom, life sciences, energy and utilities, hospitality; transportation and retail industries. In July 2007, Keane launched a joint-venture named BestShores with ZC Sterling to provide mortgage lenders with business process outsourcing solutions.

Keane offers its employees tuition assistance, an employee assistance program, a 529 College Savings Plan and a variety of healthcare options.

FINANCIALS: Sales and profits are in thousands of dollars—add 000 to get the full amount. 2007 Note: Financial information for 2007 was not available for all companies at press time.

2007 Sales: $1,100,000	2007 Profits: $	U.S. Stock Ticker: Private
2006 Sales: $948,306	2006 Profits: $34,514	Int'l Ticker:　　Int'l Exchange:
2005 Sales: $955,855	2005 Profits: $33,426	Employees: 14,000
2004 Sales: $911,543	2004 Profits: $32,282	Fiscal Year Ends: 12/31
2003 Sales: $804,976	2003 Profits: $29,222	Parent Company:

SALARIES/BENEFITS:

Pension Plan:	ESOP Stock Plan:	Profit Sharing:	Top Exec. Salary: $525,000	Bonus: $309,750
Savings Plan: Y	Stock Purch. Plan:		Second Exec. Salary: $430,000	Bonus: $149,963

OTHER THOUGHTS:

Apparent Women Officers or Directors: 1
Hot Spot for Advancement for Women/Minorities: Y

LOCATIONS: ("Y" = Yes)

West:	Southwest:	Midwest:	Southeast:	Northeast:	International:
Y				Y	Y

KELLOGG CO
www.kelloggs.com

Industry Group Code: 311230 Ranks within this company's industry group: Sales: Profits:

Management:		Sales/Marketing:		Liberal Arts:		Information Systems:		Professionals:		Technical/Scientific:	
Mgmt. Trainees:	Y	Mktg. Professionals:	Y	Gen. Writing/Editing:	Y	Info. Management:	Y	Finance/Accounting:	Y	Engineers, Elec.:	Y
Experienced Mgmt.:	Y	Retail Sales:		Technical Writing:		Software Dev.:		Law:	Y	Engineers, Other:	Y
Int'l Business:	Y	Commercial/Industrial:	Y	Graphic Arts/Photog.:	Y	Hardware Dev.:		HR/Other:	Y	Health/Lab:	
MBA Graduates:	Y	Sales Trainees:		Music:		Systems Integration:		Training:	Y	Scientists/Research:	
		Advertising Pros.:	Y	Broadcasting:		Consulting/Other:		Health Care:		Petroleum/Chemicals:	Y
				Other:				Consulting:		Math/Other:	

TYPES OF BUSINESS:
Cereal Manufacturing
Frozen Foods
Snack Foods
Convenience Foods
Processed Foods

BRANDS/DIVISIONS/AFFILIATES:
Keebler
Pop-Tarts
Nutri-Grain
Eggo
Rice Krispies
Kellogg Snacks Division
Nabisco Fruit Sancks
United Bakers Group

CONTACTS: *Note: Officers with more than one job title may be intentionally listed here more than once.*
A.D. David Mackay, CEO
A.D. David Mackay, Pres.
John A. Bryant, CFO/Exec. VP
Kathleen Wilson-Thompson, Sr. VP-Global Human Resources
Margarget Bath, VP-Research & Quality
Ruth E. Bruch, CIO/Sr. VP
Margarget Bath, VP-Tech.
Gary H. Pilnick, General Counsel/Corp. Sec.
Gary H. Pilnick, Sr. VP-Corp. Dev.
Celeste Clark, SR. VP-Corp. Affairs & Global Nutrition
John A. Bryant, Pres., Kellogg North America
Donna J. Banks, Sr. VP-Global Innovation/Environmental Officer
Juan Pablo Villalobos, Pres., Kellogg Latin America
Jeffrey M. Boromisa, Sr. VP/Pres., Kellogg Asia Pacific
James Jenness, Chmn.
Timothy P. Mobsy, Pres., Kellogg Europe

Phone: 269-961-2000	Fax: 269-961-2871

Toll-Free: 800-962-1413
Address: 1 Kellogg Sq., Battle Creek, MI 49016 US

GROWTH PLANS/SPECIAL FEATURES:

Kellogg Company is one of the world's largest producers of cereal and a major producer of convenience foods, including cookies, crackers, toaster pastries, cereal bars, frozen waffles, meat alternatives, pie crusts and ice cream cones. The firm's products are manufactured in 17 countries and marketed in over 180 countries worldwide. Kellogg's two major divisions are U.S. and international, which is further divided into Europe, Latin America, Canada, Australia and Asia. Kellogg owns a number of familiar cereal trademarks including Apple Jacks, Corn Pops, Kellogg's Corn Flakes, Crispix, Froot Loops, Frosted Mini-Wheats, Rice Krispies and Special K. Other Kellogg trademarks and products include Eggo frozen waffles, Rice Krispies Treats, Nutri-Grain convenience foods, Pop-Tarts toaster pastries, Kashi nutritional foods and Morningstar Farms meat and dairy alternatives. Cookie and cracker trademarks include Cheez-It, E.L. Fudge, Famous Amos, Chips Deluxe, Hydrox, Soft Batch, Town House, Vienna Fingers and Zesta. Kellogg also owns Keebler Foods Company and its line of snack food products. Kellogg's largest customer is Wal-Mart, which accounted for 18% of consolidated net sales in 2006. In 2007, Kellogg started offering a number of new products with a focus on health and wellness. These products include: Smart Start, a cold cereal with ingredients that may help lower blood pressure and cholesterol; Special K Protein Meal and Snack Bars; Special K20 Protein Waters, which each contain five grams of protein and come in three fruit flavors; and Special K Honey Nut Cereal Bars. In January 2008, the company acquired United Bakers Group, a Russian biscuit, cracker and breakfast cereal manufacturer.

The company offers its employees medical and dental insurance; a 401(k) plan; stock purchase plans; a fitness center; tuition reimbursement; employee discounted programs; life and AD&D insurance; life insurance; and long-term care insurance.

FINANCIALS: Sales and profits are in thousands of dollars—add 000 to get the full amount. 2007 Note: Financial information for 2007 was not available for all companies at press time.

2007 Sales: $11,776,000	2007 Profits: $1,103,000	**U.S. Stock Ticker: K**
2006 Sales: $10,906,700	2006 Profits: $1,004,100	**Int'l Ticker:** Int'l Exchange:
2005 Sales: $10,177,200	2005 Profits: $980,400	Employees: 25,600
2004 Sales: $9,613,900	2004 Profits: $890,600	Fiscal Year Ends: 12/31
2003 Sales: $8,811,500	2003 Profits: $787,100	Parent Company:

SALARIES/BENEFITS:

Pension Plan:	ESOP Stock Plan:	Profit Sharing:	Top Exec. Salary: $1,103,720	Bonus: $2,482,900
Savings Plan: Y	Stock Purch. Plan: Y		Second Exec. Salary: $898,743	Bonus: $1,571,400

OTHER THOUGHTS:
Apparent Women Officers or Directors: 7
Hot Spot for Advancement for Women/Minorities: Y

LOCATIONS: ("Y" = Yes)

West:	Southwest:	Midwest:	Southeast:	Northeast:	International:
Y	Y	Y	Y	Y	Y

Note: Financial information, benefits and other data can change quickly and may vary from those stated here.

KELLY SERVICES INC

www.kellyservices.com

Industry Group Code: 561320 Ranks within this company's industry group: Sales: 2 Profits: 3

Management:		Sales/Marketing:		Liberal Arts:		Information Systems:		Professionals:		Technical/Scientific:	
Mgmt. Trainees:	Y	Mktg. Professionals:	Y	Gen. Writing/Editing:	Y	Info. Management:	Y	Finance/Accounting:	Y	Engineers, Elec.:	Y
Experienced Mgmt.:	Y	Retail Sales:		Technical Writing:		Software Dev.:	Y	Law:	Y	Engineers, Other:	Y
Int'l Business:	Y	Commercial/Industrial:	Y	Graphic Arts/Photog.:	Y	Hardware Dev.:		HR/Other:	Y	Health/Lab:	Y
MBA Graduates:	Y	Sales Trainees:	Y	Music:		Systems Integration:	Y	Training:	Y	Scientists/Research:	Y
		Advertising Pros.:	Y	Broadcasting:		Consulting/Other:	Y	Health Care:	Y	Petroleum/Chemicals:	
				Other:	Y			Consulting:	Y	Math/Other:	Y

TYPES OF BUSINESS:

Staffing & Temporary Help
Human Resources Consulting
Outsourcing Solutions
Permanent Hiring Programs
Call Center Services
Benefits & Payroll Outsourcing

BRANDS/DIVISIONS/AFFILIATES:

Kelly Office Services
KellyConnect
KellyDirect
Kelly Scientific Resources
P-Serv
CGR/seven LLC
Tempstaff Kelly
Talents Technology

CONTACTS: *Note: Officers with more than one job title may be intentionally listed here more than once.*

Carl T. Camden, CEO
Carl T. Camden, Pres.
Michael E. Debs, Interim CFO/Sr. VP
Michael S. Webster, Sr. VP-Global Sales, Mktg. & Svc.
Nina M. Ramsey, Sr. VP-Human Resources
Allison M. Everett, Sr. VP-IT
Michael L. Durik, Chief Admin. Officer/Exec. VP
Daniel T. Lis, General Counsel/Corp. Sec.
George S. Corona, Exec. VP-Americas
Rolf E. Kleiner, Sr. VP-Outsourcing & Consulting Group
Michael S. Morrow, Sr. VP-Mktg.
James H. Bradley, Sr. VP-Admin.
Terence E. Adderley, Chmn.
Leif Agneus, Sr. VP/General Mgr.-EMEA

Phone: 248-362-4444	Fax: 248-244-4360
Toll-Free:	
Address: 999 W. Big Beaver Rd., Troy, MI 48084 US	

GROWTH PLANS/SPECIAL FEATURES:

Kelly Services, Inc. is a staffing solutions and services company that offers temporary staffing services, staff leasing, outsourcing and full-time placement, serving customers in 36 countries and territories. It operates in four segments: Americas-commercial; Americas-professional, technical and staffing alternatives (Americas-PTSA); international-commercial; and international-professional, technical and staffing alternatives (international-PTSA). The Americas-commercial segment includes Kelly Office Services, offering trained employees who work in word processing and data entry and as administrative support staff; KellyConnect, providing staff for contact centers, technical support hotlines and telemarketing units; and KellyDirect, a permanent placement service used across all business units. The Americas-PTSA segment includes a number of industry-specific includes a number of industry-specific services including CGR/seven, placing employees in creative services positions; Kelly Financial Resources, serving the needs of corporate finance departments, accounting firms and financial institutions with profession personal; Kelly Law Registry, placing legal professionals including attorneys, paralegals, contract administrators, compliance specialists and legal administrators; and Kelly Scientific Resources, providing entry-level to PhD professionals to a broad spectrum of scientific and clinical research industries. The international-commercial segment provides the full range of commercial staffing services that are offered in the Americas. The international-PTSA segment provides engineering, financial, health care, IT, legal and scientific staffing. Recruitment process outsourcing, consulting, outsourcing and vendor management are also included in this division. The segment places increased emphasis on cross-border recruitment opportunities. In 2007, Kelly Services acquired P-Serv, a firm specializing in temporary staffing, permanent staffing, outsourcing and executive search with operations in China, Hong Kong and Singapore; CGR/seven LLC, a creative services firm in New York; the remaining shares of Tempstaff Kelly, originally a joint venture created with Sony Corp. and Tempstaff; and Talents Technology, a permanence placement and execute search firm with operations in the Czech Republic and Poland.

FINANCIALS: Sales and profits are in thousands of dollars—add 000 to get the full amount. 2007 Note: Financial information for 2007 was not available for all companies at press time.

		U.S. Stock Ticker: KELYA
2007 Sales: $5,667,589	2007 Profits: $61,016	
2006 Sales: $5,546,778	2006 Profits: $63,491	Int'l Ticker: Int'l Exchange:
2005 Sales: $5,186,358	2005 Profits: $39,263	Employees: 750,000
2004 Sales: $4,932,650	2004 Profits: $21,211	Fiscal Year Ends: 12/31
2003 Sales: $4,325,155	2003 Profits: $4,904	Parent Company:

SALARIES/BENEFITS:

Pension Plan:	ESOP Stock Plan:	Profit Sharing:	Top Exec. Salary: $900,000	Bonus: $848,500
Savings Plan:	Stock Purch. Plan:		Second Exec. Salary: $600,000	Bonus: $375,000

OTHER THOUGHTS:

Apparent Women Officers or Directors: 7
Hot Spot for Advancement for Women/Minorities: Y

LOCATIONS: ("Y" = Yes)

West:	Southwest:	Midwest:	Southeast:	Northeast:	International:
Y	Y	Y	Y	Y	Y

Note: Financial information, benefits and other data can change quickly and may vary from those stated here.

KENDLE INTERNATIONAL INC

www.kendle.com

Industry Group Code: 325412 Ranks within this company's industry group: Sales: 9 Profits: 8

Management:		Sales/Marketing:		Liberal Arts:		Information Systems:		Professionals:		Technical/Scientific:	
Mgmt. Trainees:		Mktg. Professionals:	Y	Gen. Writing/Editing:		Info. Management:	Y	Finance/Accounting:	Y	Engineers, Elec.:	Y
Experienced Mgmt.:	Y	Retail Sales:		Technical Writing:	Y	Software Dev.:	Y	Law:	Y	Engineers, Other:	Y
Int'l Business:	Y	Commercial/Industrial:	Y	Graphic Arts/Photog.:		Hardware Dev.:		HR/Other:	Y	Health/Lab:	Y
MBA Graduates:	Y	Sales Trainees:		Music:		Systems Integration:	Y	Training:	Y	Scientists/Research:	Y
		Advertising Pros.:		Broadcasting:		Consulting/Other:	Y	Health Care:	Y	Petroleum/Chemicals:	Y
				Other:				Consulting:		Math/Other:	Y

TYPES OF BUSINESS:

Pharmaceutical Development-Clinical Trials
Statistical Analysis
Technical Writing
Regulatory Assistance
Consulting Services
Clinical Trial Software
Clinical Data Management
e-Learning

BRANDS/DIVISIONS/AFFILIATES:

eKendleCollege
TrialWare
TrialWeb
TrialBase
TrialView
TriaLine

CONTACTS: Note: Officers with more than one job title may be intentionally listed here more than once.

Candace Kendle, CEO
Christopher Bergen, COO
Christopher Bergen, Pres.
Karl Brenkert, III, CFO/Sr. VP
Simon Higginbotham, Chief Mktg. Officer/VP
Karen L. Crone, VP-Global Human Resources
Gary Wedig, CIO/VP
Karl Brenkert, III, Corp. Sec.
Anthony L. Forcellini, VP-Strategic Dev.
Anthony L. Forcellini, Treas.
Martha Feller, Sr. VP-Global Clinical Dev.
Melanie A. Bruno, VP-Global Regulatory Affairs & Quality
Sylva Collins, VP-Global Biometrics
Patricia A. Steigerwald, VP-Global Late Phase
Candace Kendle, Chmn.

Phone: 513-381-5550	Fax: 513-381-5870
Toll-Free: 800-733-1572	
Address: 441 Vine St., Ste. 1200, Cincinnati, OH 45202 US	

GROWTH PLANS/SPECIAL FEATURES:

Kendle International, Inc. is a global clinical research organization that provides a broad range of Phase I-IV global clinical development services to the biopharmaceutical industry. The company augments the research and development activities of biopharmaceutical companies by offering value-added clinical research services and proprietary information technology designed to reduce drug development time and expense. The firm operates in two segments: early stage, which handles all Phase I testing services; and late stage, which handles all Phase II-IV services. Kendle's services include clinical trial management, clinical data management, statistical analysis, technical writing and regulatory consulting and representation. It runs a state-of-the-art clinical pharmacology unit in the Netherlands, where it offers services for drugs undergoing clinical trials. The company's therapeutic expertise covers fields such as cardiovascular, dermatology, hematology, oncology, respiratory and women's health. Through its health care communications division, the firm provides organizational, meeting management and publication services to various professional associations and pharmaceutical companies. The firm's proprietary TrialWare product line includes a database management system, TrialBase; an interactive voice response patient randomization system, TriaLine; a validated medical imaging system, TrialView; a global project management system, TrialWatch; an Internet based collaborative tool, TrialWeb; and a late phase technology system, Trial4. Additionally, the company operates eKendleCollege, an online e-learning division that runs seminars and training programs, focusing on the organization of clinical trials.

The company offers its employees medical, dental and vision insurance; flexible spending accounts; life and AD&D insurance; a 401(k) plan; tuition reimbursement; and a profit sharing plan. The firm also offers opportunities for professional and personal development through eKendle College.

FINANCIALS: Sales and profits are in thousands of dollars—add 000 to get the full amount. 2007 Note: Financial information for 2007 was not available for all companies at press time.

2007 Sales: $568,818	2007 Profits: $18,687	U.S. Stock Ticker: KNDL
2006 Sales: $373,936	2006 Profits: $8,530	Int'l Ticker: Int'l Exchange:
2005 Sales: $250,639	2005 Profits: $10,674	Employees: 3,325
2004 Sales: $215,868	2004 Profits: $3,572	Fiscal Year Ends: 12/31
2003 Sales: $209,657	2003 Profits: $-1,690	Parent Company:

SALARIES/BENEFITS:

Pension Plan:	ESOP Stock Plan:	Profit Sharing: Y	Top Exec. Salary: $383,259	Bonus: $
Savings Plan: Y	Stock Purch. Plan:		Second Exec. Salary: $328,083	Bonus: $

OTHER THOUGHTS:

Apparent Women Officers or Directors: 6
Hot Spot for Advancement for Women/Minorities: Y

LOCATIONS: ("Y" = Yes)

West:	Southwest:	Midwest:	Southeast:	Northeast:	International:
Y		Y		Y	Y

Note: Financial information, benefits and other data can change quickly and may vary from those stated here.

KIMBERLY-CLARK CORP   www.kimberly-clark.com

Industry Group Code: 322000 Ranks within this company's industry group: Sales: 1 Profits: 1

Management:		Sales/Marketing:		Liberal Arts:		Information Systems:		Professionals:		Technical/Scientific:	
Mgmt. Trainees:	Y	Mktg. Professionals:	Y	Gen. Writing/Editing:	Y	Info. Management:	Y	Finance/Accounting:	Y	Engineers, Elec.:	Y
Experienced Mgmt.:	Y	Retail Sales:		Technical Writing:		Software Dev.:		Law:	Y	Engineers, Other:	
Int'l Business:	Y	Commercial/Industrial:	Y	Graphic Arts/Photog.:	Y	Hardware Dev.:		HR/Other:	Y	Health/Lab:	
MBA Graduates:	Y	Sales Trainees:		Music:		Systems Integration:		Training:	Y	Scientists/Research:	
		Advertising Pros.:	Y	Broadcasting:		Consulting/Other:		Health Care:		Petroleum/Chemicals:	
				Other:	Y			Consulting:		Math/Other:	

TYPES OF BUSINESS:

Personal Care Products-Paper
Consumer Tissue Products
Safety Products
Healthcare Products

BRANDS/DIVISIONS/AFFILIATES:

Kleenex
Scott
Huggies
Kotex
Depend
Pull-Ups
Kimberly-Clark of South Africa
P.T. Kimberly-Lever Indonesia

CONTACTS: *Note: Officers with more than one job title may be intentionally listed here more than once.*

Thomas J. Falk, CEO
Thomas J. Falk, Pres.
Mark A. Buthman, CFO/Sr. VP
Anthony J. Palmer, Chief Mktg. Officer/Sr. VP
Lizanne C. Gottung, Sr. VP-Human Resources
Thomas J. Mielke, Sr. VP-Law
Christian Brickman,
Thomas J. Mielke, Chief Compliance Officer & Sr. VP Gov't Affairs
Robert W. Black, Pres., Developing & Emerging Markets
Joanne Bauer, Pres., Healthcare Bus.
Robert. E. Abernathy, Pres., North Atlantic Consumer Prod.
Jan B. Spencer, Pres., Kimberly-Clark Professional
Thomas J. Falk, Chmn.

Phone: 972-281-1200	Fax: 972-281-1490
Toll-Free:	
Address: 351 Phelps Dr., Irving, TX 75038 US	

GROWTH PLANS/SPECIAL FEATURES:

Kimberly-Clark Corp. (KC) is a global health and hygiene company that manufactures and markets a wide range of health and hygiene products around the world. Most of these products are made from natural or synthetic fibers. KC operates in four segments: personal care; consumer tissue; KC professional and other; and healthcare. The personal care segment manufactures and markets disposable diapers, training and youth pants; swim pants; baby wipes; feminine and incontinence care products; and related products. Products in this segment are primarily for household use and are sold under brand names such as Huggies, Pull-Ups, Little Swimmer, GoodNites, Kotex, Lightdays, Depend and Poise. The consumer tissue segment manufactures and markets facial and bathroom tissue; paper towels; napkins; and related products for household use. Products in this division are sold under brands such as Kleenex, Scott, Cottonelle, Viva, Andrex, Scottex, Hakle and Page. The KC professional & other segment manufactures and markets facial and bathroom tissue; paper towels; napkins; wipers; and a range of safety products for the away-from-home marketplace. Brand names in this segment include Kimberly-Clark, Kleenex, Scott, WypAll, Kimtech, Kleenguard and Kimcare. The healthcare segment manufactures and markets surgical gowns; drapes; infection control products; sterilization wrap; disposable face masks and exam gloves; respiratory products; and other disposable medical products. Products in this division are sold under the Kimberly-Clark and Ballard brand names. Sales to Wal-Mart Stores, Inc. accounted for approximately 13% of the company's 2007 revenues. In 2007, Kimberly Clark purchased the remaining 50% stake in its Indonesian subsidiary, P.T. Kimberly-Lever Indonesia. In May 2008, the company purchase the remaining stake in South African subsidiary Kimberly-Clark of South Africa from The Lion Match Company (Proprietary) Limited.

The company offers its employees medical and dental insurance; short- and long-term disability insurance; life insurance; an investment plan; and a retirement contribution plan.

FINANCIALS: Sales and profits are in thousands of dollars—add 000 to get the full amount. 2007 Note: Financial information for 2007 was not available for all companies at press time.

2007 Sales: $18,266,000	2007 Profits: $1,822,900	**U.S. Stock Ticker: KMB**
2006 Sales: $16,746,900	2006 Profits: $1,499,500	**Int'l Ticker:** Int'l Exchange:
2005 Sales: $15,902,600	2005 Profits: $1,568,300	Employees: 53,000
2004 Sales: $15,083,200	2004 Profits: $1,800,200	Fiscal Year Ends: 12/31
2003 Sales: $14,348,000	2003 Profits: $1,694,200	Parent Company:

SALARIES/BENEFITS:

Pension Plan: Y	ESOP Stock Plan:	Profit Sharing:	Top Exec. Salary: $1,175,000	Bonus: $1,367,700
Savings Plan:	Stock Purch. Plan:		Second Exec. Salary: $618,000	Bonus: $476,362

OTHER THOUGHTS:

Apparent Women Officers or Directors: 4
Hot Spot for Advancement for Women/Minorities: Y

LOCATIONS: ("Y" = Yes)

West:	Southwest:	Midwest:	Southeast:	Northeast:	International:
Y	Y	Y	Y	Y	Y

KINDRED HEALTHCARE INC
www.kindredhealthcare.com

Industry Group Code: 623110 Ranks within this company's industry group: Sales: 1 Profits: 2

Management:		Sales/Marketing:		Liberal Arts:		Information Systems:		Professionals:		Technical/Scientific:	
Mgmt. Trainees:	Y	Mktg. Professionals:	Y	Gen. Writing/Editing:		Info. Management:	Y	Finance/Accounting:	Y	Engineers, Elec.:	
Experienced Mgmt.:	Y	Retail Sales:		Technical Writing:		Software Dev.:		Law:	Y	Engineers, Other:	Y
Int'l Business:		Commercial/Industrial:	Y	Graphic Arts/Photog.:		Hardware Dev.:		HR/Other:	Y	Health/Lab:	
MBA Graduates:	Y	Sales Trainees:		Music:		Systems Integration:		Training:	Y	Scientists/Research:	
		Advertising Pros.:		Broadcasting:		Consulting/Other:		Health Care:	Y	Petroleum/Chemicals:	
				Other:				Consulting:		Math/Other:	

TYPES OF BUSINESS:
Hospitals
Nursing Centers
Institutional Pharmacies
Contract Rehabilitation Services

BRANDS/DIVISIONS/AFFILIATES:
Peoplefirst Rehabilitation
AmerisourceBergen Corp.
PharMerica Corp.

CONTACTS: Note: Officers with more than one job title may be intentionally listed here more than once.
Paul J. Diaz, CEO
Frank J. Battafarano, COO
Paul J. Diaz, Pres.
Richard A. Lechleiter, CFO/Exec. VP
Richard E. Chapman, CIO/Exec. VP
Richard E. Chapman, Chief Admin. Officer
M. Suzanne Riedman, General Counsel/Sr. VP
Gregory C. Miller, Sr. VP-Corp. Dev. & Financial Planning
Susan E. Moss, VP-Comm.
Benjamin A. Breier, Exec. VP/Pres., Hospital Division
Lane M. Bowen, Exec. VP/Pres., Health Svcs. Division
William M. Altman, Sr. VP-Strategy & Public Policy
Joseph L. Landenwich, Sr. VP-Corp. Legal Affairs/Corp. Sec.
Edward L. Kuntz, Exec. Chmn.

Phone: 502-596-7300	Fax: 502-596-4170
Toll-Free: 800-545-0749	
Address: 680 S. 4th St., Louisville, KY 40202 US	

GROWTH PLANS/SPECIAL FEATURES:

Kindred Healthcare, Inc. is a healthcare services company that operates hospitals, nursing centers and a contract rehabilitation services business across the U.S. The company runs three operating divisions. The hospital division operates 84 long-term acute care hospitals with 6,567 licensed beds in 24 states. The firm treats medically complex patients, including the critically ill, suffering from multiple organ system failures, most commonly the cardiovascular, pulmonary, gastro-intestinal and cutaneous systems. A number of hospitals in this division offer outpatient services, which may include diagnostic services, rehabilitation therapy, CT scanning, one-day surgery, laboratory and X-ray. More than 62% of patients are over 65 years of age. The health service division operates 228 nursing centers with 29,106 licensed beds in 27 states. Through its nursing centers, Kindred Healthcare provides long-term care services; a full range of pharmacy, medical and clinical services; and routine services, including daily, dietary, social and recreational services. A number of nursing centers offer specialized programs for residents suffering from Alzheimer's disease and other dementias. The contract rehabilitation services business provides rehabilitative services under the name Peoplefirst Rehabilitation primarily in long-term care settings. In addition to standard physical, occupational and speech therapies, the company provides specialized care programs designed to deal with dementia and Alzheimer's disease, wound care, pain management and pulmonary therapies. In July 2007, Kindred Healthcare and AmerisourceBergen Corp. announced the completion of the transaction that combines their respective institutional pharmacy businesses to create PharMerica Corp., a new, independent company. In February 2008, Kindred reopened the relocated and expanded Indianapolis South in Greenwood, Indiana, a 60 bed long term acute care hospital; and opened the new 58 bed long term acute care Northwest Phoenix hospital in Peoria, Arizona.

FINANCIALS: Sales and profits are in thousands of dollars—add 000 to get the full amount. 2007 Note: Financial information for 2007 was not available for all companies at press time.

2007 Sales: $4,220,266	2007 Profits: $-46,870	U.S. Stock Ticker: KND
2006 Sales: $4,266,661	2006 Profits: $78,711	Int'l Ticker: Int'l Exchange:
2005 Sales: $3,852,975	2005 Profits: $144,909	Employees: 55,000
2004 Sales: $3,421,411	2004 Profits: $70,580	Fiscal Year Ends: 12/31
2003 Sales: $3,284,019	2003 Profits: $-75,336	Parent Company:

SALARIES/BENEFITS:

Pension Plan:	ESOP Stock Plan:	Profit Sharing:	Top Exec. Salary: $847,906	Bonus: $1,432,779
Savings Plan:	Stock Purch. Plan:		Second Exec. Salary: $635,928	Bonus: $

OTHER THOUGHTS:
Apparent Women Officers or Directors: 3
Hot Spot for Advancement for Women/Minorities: Y

LOCATIONS: ("Y" = Yes)

West:	Southwest:	Midwest:	Southeast:	Northeast:	International:
Y	Y	Y	Y	Y	

KOCH INDUSTRIES INC

www.kochind.com

Industry Group Code: 324110 Ranks within this company's industry group: Sales: 1   Profits:

Management:		Sales/Marketing:		Liberal Arts:		Information Systems:		Professionals:		Technical/Scientific:	
Mgmt. Trainees:	Y	Mktg. Professionals:	Y	Gen. Writing/Editing:		Info. Management:	Y	Finance/Accounting:	Y	Engineers, Elec.:	Y
Experienced Mgmt.:	Y	Retail Sales:		Technical Writing:	Y	Software Dev.:	Y	Law:	Y	Engineers, Other:	
Int'l Business:	Y	Commercial/Industrial:	Y	Graphic Arts/Photog.:		Hardware Dev.:		HR/Other:	Y	Health/Lab:	
MBA Graduates:	Y	Sales Trainees:		Music:		Systems Integration:		Training:	Y	Scientists/Research:	
		Advertising Pros.:		Broadcasting:		Consulting/Other:		Health Care:		Petroleum/Chemicals:	Y
				Other:				Consulting:		Math/Other:	

TYPES OF BUSINESS:

Petroleum Refining
Chemicals
Textiles
Pipelines
Energy Trading
Chemical Equipment
Asphalt & Paving Supplies
Beef Production

BRANDS/DIVISIONS/AFFILIATES:

Flint Hills Resources
Koch Mineral Services
Matador Cattle Company
Koch Pipeline Company
Koch Chemical Technologies Group
Koch Materials Company
INVISTA
Georgia-Pacific Corp

CONTACTS: Note: Officers with more than one job title may be intentionally listed here more than once.

Charles G. Koch, CEO
David L. (Dave) Robertson, COO
David L. (Dave) Robertson, Pres.
Steve Feilmeier, CFO
Ron Vaupel, VP-Bus. Dev.
David H. Koch, Exec. VP
Charles G. Koch, Chmn.

Phone: 316-828-5500	Fax: 316-828-5739
Toll-Free:	
Address: 4111 E. 37th St. N., Wichita, KS 67220-3203 US	

GROWTH PLANS/SPECIAL FEATURES:

Koch Industries, Inc. is a diversified group of companies engaged in the exploration, production and trade of petroleum, chemicals, asphalt, minerals, fertilizer, natural gas liquids, chemical technology, pipelines, plastics, fibers, textiles and electricity. It also conducts operations in venture capital investments, municipal finance, capital market investments and business development. Subsidiary Flint Hills Resources is engaged in petroleum refining, chemicals and lube oil production, crude oil supply and trading, and wholesale marketing and trading of fuel oil, gasoline, petrochemicals and other products. Subsidiary Koch Mineral Services supplies coal and petroleum coke as well as fertilizer, sulfur, cement and ores internationally. Koch's ranching subsidiary, Matador Cattle Company, produces 5 million pounds of beef a year. Subsidiary Koch Pipeline Company, LP and its affiliates operate a 4,000-mile network of pipelines. Subsidiary Koch Chemical Technologies Group develops, manufactures and sells membrane water filtration systems, high-efficiency waste reduction technologies and other high-technology products. Subsidiary Koch Materials Company develops and markets solutions for road paving and other construction work. Subsidiary INVISTA is a global producer and marketer of premium integrated fibers, resins, polymers and intermediates. Subsidiary Georgia-Pacific manufactures and markets tissue, packaging, paper, building products, related chemicals and fluff, filter and market pulp under such brand names as Quilted Northern, Angel Soft, Brawny and Dixie. In March 2007, Koch Membrane Systems was awarded a multi-million dollar contract to provide a reverse osmosis (RO) system for municipal effluent reuse in Australia. In May 2007, Koch Partners began plans for a 15,000 BPSD gas oil mild hydrocracking unit at Navajo Refining Company's New Mexico refinery. In November 2007, Flint Hills acquired a Port Arthur, Texas manufacturing plant and associated pipelines for $770 million.

Koch offers its employees educational assistance, flexible spending accounts and medical, dental, life, AD&D and disability insurance.

FINANCIALS: Sales and profits are in thousands of dollars—add 000 to get the full amount. 2007 Note: Financial information for 2007 was not available for all companies at press time.

2007 Sales: $98,000,000	2007 Profits: $	**U.S. Stock Ticker: Private**
2006 Sales: $90,000,000	2006 Profits: $	**Int'l Ticker:** Int'l Exchange:
2005 Sales: $80,000,000	2005 Profits: $	Employees: 80,000
2004 Sales: $60,000,000	2004 Profits: $	Fiscal Year Ends: 12/31
2003 Sales: $40,000,000	2003 Profits: $	Parent Company:

SALARIES/BENEFITS:

Pension Plan: Y	ESOP Stock Plan:	Profit Sharing:	Top Exec. Salary: $	Bonus: $
Savings Plan: Y	Stock Purch. Plan:		Second Exec. Salary: $	Bonus: $

OTHER THOUGHTS:

Apparent Women Officers or Directors:
Hot Spot for Advancement for Women/Minorities:

LOCATIONS: ("Y" = Yes)

West:	Southwest:	Midwest:	Southeast:	Northeast:	International:
Y	Y	Y	Y	Y	Y

Note: Financial information, benefits and other data can change quickly and may vary from those stated here.

KOHL'S CORP

www.kohls.com

Industry Group Code: 452910 Ranks within this company's industry group: Sales: 3 Profits: 3

Management:		Sales/Marketing:		Liberal Arts:		Information Systems:		Professionals:		Technical/Scientific:	
Mgmt. Trainees:	Y	Mktg. Professionals:	Y	Gen. Writing/Editing:	Y	Info. Management:	Y	Finance/Accounting:	Y	Engineers, Elec.:	
Experienced Mgmt.:	Y	Retail Sales:	Y	Technical Writing:		Software Dev.:	Y	Law:	Y	Engineers, Other:	
Int'l Business:		Commercial/Industrial:	Y	Graphic Arts/Photog.:	Y	Hardware Dev.:		HR/Other:	Y	Health/Lab:	
MBA Graduates:	Y	Sales Trainees:	Y	Music:		Systems Integration:		Training:	Y	Scientists/Research:	
		Advertising Pros.:	Y	Broadcasting:		Consulting/Other:		Health Care:		Petroleum/Chemicals:	
				Other:	Y			Consulting:		Math/Other:	

TYPES OF BUSINESS:

Discount Department Stores
Online Sales

BRANDS/DIVISIONS/AFFILIATES:

Kohls.com

CONTACTS: Note: Officers with more than one job title may be intentionally listed here more than once.

Kevin Mansell, CEO
Kevin Mansell, Pres.
Wes McDonald, CFO
Tom Kingsbury, Sr. Exec. VP-Mktg.
Tom Kingsbury, Sr. Exec. VP-Info. Svcs.
Donald Brennan, Sr. Exec. VP-Merch.
Richard Schepp, General Counsel/Exec. VP/Sec.
Tom Kingsbury, Sr. Exec. VP-Bus. Dev.
Tom Kingsbury, Sr. Exec. VP-e-Commerce
Vicki Shamion, VP-Public Rel.
John Worthington, Sr. Exec. VP-Store Oper./Store Admin.
John Worthington, Sr. Exec. VP-Merch. Presentation/Loss Prevention
Brian Miller, VP-Corp. Governance
Larry Montgomery, Chmn.

Phone: 262-703-7000	Fax:
Toll-Free:	
Address: N56 W17000 Ridgewood Dr., Menomonee Falls, WI 53051 US	

GROWTH PLANS/SPECIAL FEATURES:

Kohl's Corp. operates family-oriented specialty department stores. The company currently operates 929 stores in 47 states, with three store formats: prototype, small and urban. Kohl's stores offer merchandise that consists of apparel, shoes and accessories for women, children and men; soft home products, such as sheets and pillows; and other home products such as small electrics and luggage. Kohl's offered brands include Dockers, Lee, Levi's, Jockey, Candie's, Nike, Vanity Fair and Chaps. Brands introduced in 2007 include Simply Vera Vera Wang and Food Network. Kohl's operates in a unique niche, positioned between major department stores and true discounters. The company also markets its products online. It opened 112 stores in 2007 and hopes to operate more than 1,200 by the end of 2010. The company has nine distribution centers and a 940,000 square foot fulfillment center for its e-commerce site, kohls.com. In November 2007, the company signed a multi-year licensing agreement with Fila Luxembourg S.a.r.l. making Kohl's the exclusive U.S. retailer of the FILA SPORT collection. In January 2008, Kohl's also signed a licensing agreement with Liz Claiborne, Inc. to become exclusive U.S. retailer for the Dana Buchman brand of merchandise, which includes women's apparel, intimate apparel, accessories, and footwear. In June 2008, Kohl's agreed to become exclusive U.S. retailer for the Hang Ten brand, owned by American Brand Holdings.

The company offers its employees medical, dental and vision insurance; long-term disability and life insurance; a 401(k) plan; an employee stock ownership plan; tuition reimbursement; and merchandise discounts.

FINANCIALS: Sales and profits are in thousands of dollars—add 000 to get the full amount. 2007 Note: Financial information for 2007 was not available for all companies at press time.

2007 Sales: $15,596,910	2007 Profits: $1,108,681	U.S. Stock Ticker: KSS
2006 Sales: $13,402,217	2006 Profits: $841,960	Int'l Ticker: Int'l Exchange:
2005 Sales: $11,700,619	2005 Profits: $730,380	Employees: 125,000
2004 Sales: $10,282,094	2004 Profits: $591,152	Fiscal Year Ends: 1/31
2003 Sales: $9,120,300	2003 Profits: $643,400	Parent Company:

SALARIES/BENEFITS:

Pension Plan:	ESOP Stock Plan: Y	Profit Sharing:	Top Exec. Salary: $1,087,067	Bonus: $1,925,000
Savings Plan: Y	Stock Purch. Plan:		Second Exec. Salary: $946,283	Bonus: $1,674,750

OTHER THOUGHTS:

Apparent Women Officers or Directors: 1
Hot Spot for Advancement for Women/Minorities: Y

LOCATIONS: ("Y" = Yes)

West:	Southwest:	Midwest:	Southeast:	Northeast:	International:
Y	Y	Y	Y	Y	

KPMG LLP

www.us.kpmg.com

Industry Group Code: 541210 Ranks within this company's industry group: Sales: 3 Profits:

Management:		Sales/Marketing:		Liberal Arts:		Information Systems:		Professionals:		Technical/Scientific:	
Mgmt. Trainees:	Y	Mktg. Professionals:	Y	Gen. Writing/Editing:	Y	Info. Management:	Y	Finance/Accounting:	Y	Engineers, Elec.:	
Experienced Mgmt.:	Y	Retail Sales:		Technical Writing:	Y	Software Dev.:	Y	Law:	Y	Engineers, Other:	
Int'l Business:	Y	Commercial/Industrial:	Y	Graphic Arts/Photog.:		Hardware Dev.:		HR/Other:	Y	Health/Lab:	
MBA Graduates:	Y	Sales Trainees:		Music:		Systems Integration:	Y	Training:	Y	Scientists/Research:	Y
		Advertising Pros.:	Y	Broadcasting:		Consulting/Other:	Y	Health Care:		Petroleum/Chemicals:	
				Other:				Consulting:	Y	Math/Other:	Y

TYPES OF BUSINESS:

Accounting Services
Human Resource Advisory Services
Accounting Technology
Publications
Risk Management

BRANDS/DIVISIONS/AFFILIATES:

KPMG International
Audit Committee Institute
KPMG TaxWatch Thought Leadership Series
Japanese Practice
Tax Governance Institute

CONTACTS: *Note: Officers with more than one job title may be intentionally listed here more than once.*

Timothy P. Flynn, CEO
Jack T. Taylor, COO
Jack T. Taylor, Exec. VP-Oper.
Brian Ambrose, Vice Chmn.-Strategy
John B. Veihmeyer, Deputy Chmn.
Mark Barnes, Managing Dir.-Emerging Markets
Timothy P. Flynn, Chmn.
Brian Ambrose, Vice Chmn.-Int'l

Phone: 212-758-9700	Fax: 202-758-9819
Toll-Free:	
Address: 757 3rd Ave., New York, NY 10017 US	

GROWTH PLANS/SPECIAL FEATURES:

KPMG LLP, the U.S. subsidiary of global accounting cooperative KPMG International, is a leading provider of audit, advisory and tax services across the U.S. The firm's audit operations are based on a multidisciplinary approach focused on compliance tools, technological assistance and cultural values central to clients' companies. KPMG founded and maintains the Audit Committee Institute, designed to educate audit committee members about governance, accounting, financial reporting and other audit issues. KPMG's tax services segment provides tax assistance in the areas of economic and valuation services; exempt organizations tax; federal tax; international corporate tax; international executive services; legislative and regulatory services; mergers and acquisitions; state and local tax; and trade and customs. The company also provides tax-related news and trends through its KPMG TaxWatch Thought Leadership Series and tax-related newsletters and publications. The firm's advisory services division assists its clients in achieving strengthened governance, reporting and internal controls; early identification and assessment of risk and control issues that affect performance; improved efficiency and effectiveness of key business processes; and informed responses to existing and proposed regulatory requirements. KPMG serves companies and organizations in such major industry sectors as financial services; industrial markets; consumer markets; information, communications and entertainment; government; and healthcare. The firm also maintains a special focus group that has industry experience with the issues Japanese companies face in the U.S., as well as both Japanese and American business cultures, practices and standards. In 2007, the firm announced the establishment of the Tax Governance Institute, an open forum for government representatives to debate certain aspects of tax oversight and management.

KPMG offers its employees alternative work arrangements; a mortgage assistance program; flexible spending accounts; and medical, dental, vision and disability insurance. The firm was named one of Fortune Magazine's 100 Best Companies to Work For in 2007.

FINANCIALS: Sales and profits are in thousands of dollars—add 000 to get the full amount. 2007 Note: Financial information for 2007 was not available for all companies at press time.

2007 Sales: $	2007 Profits: $	U.S. Stock Ticker: Subsidiary
2006 Sales: $5,000,000	2006 Profits: $	Int'l Ticker: Int'l Exchange:
2005 Sales: $4,700,000	2005 Profits: $	Employees:
2004 Sales: $4,100,000	2004 Profits: $	Fiscal Year Ends: 9/30
2003 Sales: $4,630,000	2003 Profits: $	Parent Company: KPMG INTERNATIONAL

SALARIES/BENEFITS:

Pension Plan: Y	ESOP Stock Plan:	Profit Sharing:	Top Exec. Salary: $	Bonus: $
Savings Plan: Y	Stock Purch. Plan:		Second Exec. Salary: $	Bonus: $

OTHER THOUGHTS:

Apparent Women Officers or Directors:
Hot Spot for Advancement for Women/Minorities:

LOCATIONS: ("Y" = Yes)

West:	Southwest:	Midwest:	Southeast:	Northeast:	International:
Y	Y	Y	Y	Y	

KRAFT FOODS INC   www.kraft.com

Industry Group Code: 311000 Ranks within this company's industry group: Sales: Profits:

Management:		Sales/Marketing:		Liberal Arts:		Information Systems:		Professionals:		Technical/Scientific:	
Mgmt. Trainees:	Y	Mktg. Professionals:	Y	Gen. Writing/Editing:	Y	Info. Management:	Y	Finance/Accounting:	Y	Engineers, Elec.:	Y
Experienced Mgmt.:	Y	Retail Sales:		Technical Writing:		Software Dev.:		Law:	Y	Engineers, Other:	
Int'l Business:	Y	Commercial/Industrial:	Y	Graphic Arts/Photog.:	Y	Hardware Dev.:		HR/Other:	Y	Health/Lab:	Y
MBA Graduates:	Y	Sales Trainees:	Y	Music:		Systems Integration:		Training:	Y	Scientists/Research:	
		Advertising Pros.:	Y	Broadcasting:		Consulting/Other:		Health Care:		Petroleum/Chemicals:	
				Other:				Consulting:		Math/Other:	

TYPES OF BUSINESS:

Food Manufacturing
Snack Foods
Beverages
Prepared Foods
Convenience Meals
Cheese Products
Energy & Nutrition Products
Processed Meats

BRANDS/DIVISIONS/AFFILIATES:

Altria Group Inc
Jacobs
Maxwell House
Philadelphia
Velveeta
Oscar Mayer
Jell-O
Oreo

CONTACTS: Note: Officers with more than one job title may be intentionally listed here more than once.

Irene B. Rosenfeld, CEO
Timothy R. McLevish, CFO/Exec. VP
Mary Beth West, Chief Mktg. Officer/Exec. VP
Karen J. May, Exec. VP-Global Human Resources
Jean E. Spence, Exec. VP-Global Tech. & Quality
Marc S. Firestone, General Counsel/Exec. VP/Corp. Sec.
David Brearton, Exec. VP-Global Bus. Svcs. & Strategy
David Brearton, Sr. VP-Bus. Process Simplification/Controller
Richard G. Searer, Pres., North America Commercial Segment
Irene Rosenfeld, Chmn.
Sanjay Khosla, Pres., Int'l Commercial/Exec. VP
Franz-Josef H. Vogelsang, Exec. VP-Global Supply Chain

Phone: 847-646-2000	Fax: 847-646-6005
Toll-Free:	
Address: 3 Lakes Dr., Northfield, IL 60093 US	

GROWTH PLANS/SPECIAL FEATURES:

Kraft Foods, Inc. is one of the largest food companies in the U.S. In March 2007, Kraft was spun-off from Altria Group, Inc., and in June it completed an initial public offering. The company manufactures and markets packaged food products, consisting principally of snacks, generating roughly 29% of its revenues; beverages, generating roughly 21%; cheese and dairy products, generating roughly 19%; convenient meals, generating roughly 16%; and various packaged grocery products; generating roughly 15%. Kraft has operations in 72 countries and sells its products in more than 155 countries. The company markets many of the world's leading food brands, more than 40 of which are over 100 years old, more than 50 of which have revenues of $100 million and seven of which have revenue of $1 billion. Some of its major brands include Jacobs, Maxwell House, Gevalia, Kool-Aid, Tang, Crystal Light and Country Time beverages; Philadelphia, Velveeta, Cheez Whiz, Deli Deluxe and Knudsen cheese products; DiGiorno, Tombstone, Lunchables, Oscar Mayer, Boca and Stove Top convenient meal products; Jell-O, Cool Whip, Handi-Snacks, Miracle Whip, A.1., Bull's-Eye, Grey Poupon and Shake' N Bake grocery products; and Oreo, Chips Ahoy!, Newtons, Nilla, Nutter Butter, SnackWell's, Ritz, Triscuit, Wheat Thins, Cheese Nips, Teddy Grahams, Planters and Toblerone snacks. These products are generally sold to supermarket chains, wholesalers, club stores, mass merchandisers, distributors, convenience stores, gasoline stations and other retail food outlets. In early 2007, Kraft sold its hot cereal unit to B&G Foods for $200 million, including its Cream of Wheat line of products. In November 2007, the firm agreed to sell its Post cereals business to Ralcorp Holdings, Inc. for $1.6 billion. Also in November, the company acquired the global biscuit business of Groupe Danone.

FINANCIALS: Sales and profits are in thousands of dollars—add 000 to get the full amount. 2007 Note: Financial information for 2007 was not available for all companies at press time.

2007 Sales: $37,241,000	2007 Profits: $2,590,000	**U.S. Stock Ticker: KFT**	
2006 Sales: $34,356,000	2006 Profits: $3,060,000	**Int'l Ticker:** Int'l Exchange:	
2005 Sales: $34,113,000	2005 Profits: $2,632,000	Employees: 98,000	
2004 Sales: $32,168,000	2004 Profits: $2,665,000	Fiscal Year Ends: 12/31	
2003 Sales: $31,010,000	2003 Profits: $3,476,000	Parent Company:	

SALARIES/BENEFITS:

Pension Plan: Y	ESOP Stock Plan:	Profit Sharing:	Top Exec. Salary: $830,769	Bonus: $
Savings Plan:	Stock Purch. Plan:		Second Exec. Salary: $675,000	Bonus: $5,750,000

OTHER THOUGHTS:

Apparent Women Officers or Directors: 8
Hot Spot for Advancement for Women/Minorities: Y

LOCATIONS: ("Y" = Yes)

West:	Southwest:	Midwest:	Southeast:	Northeast:	International:
Y	Y	Y	Y	Y	Y

KROGER CO (THE)   www.kroger.com

Industry Group Code: 445110 Ranks within this company's industry group: Sales: Profits:

Management:		Sales/Marketing:		Liberal Arts:		Information Systems:		Professionals:		Technical/Scientific:	
Mgmt. Trainees:	Y	Mktg. Professionals:	Y	Gen. Writing/Editing:	Y	Info. Management:	Y	Finance/Accounting:	Y	Engineers, Elec.:	
Experienced Mgmt.:	Y	Retail Sales:	Y	Technical Writing:		Software Dev.:		Law:	Y	Engineers, Other:	
Int'l Business:		Commercial/Industrial:		Graphic Arts/Photog.:	Y	Hardware Dev.:		HR/Other:	Y	Health/Lab:	
MBA Graduates:	Y	Sales Trainees:	Y	Music:		Systems Integration:		Training:	Y	Scientists/Research:	
		Advertising Pros.:	Y	Broadcasting:		Consulting/Other:		Health Care:	Y	Petroleum/Chemicals:	
				Other:				Consulting:		Math/Other:	

TYPES OF BUSINESS:
Grocery Stores
Convenience Stores
Jewelry Stores
Pharmacies
Food Processing
Gas Stations
Department Stores

BRANDS/DIVISIONS/AFFILIATES:
Smith's Food & Drug Centers Inc
Fry's
Barclay
QFC
Ralph's
Smith's
King Soopers
Quik Stop

CONTACTS: *Note: Officers with more than one job title may be intentionally listed here more than once.*
David B. Dillon, CEO
Don W. McGeorge, COO
Don W. McGeorge, Pres.
J. Michael Schlotman, CFO/Sr. VP
Christopher T. Hjelm, CIO/Sr. VP
Joseph A. Grieshaber, Jr., VP-Merch. & Procurement
William T. Boehm, Sr. VP/Pres., Mfg.
Paul W. Heldman, General Counsel/Exec. VP/Sec.
Scott M. Henderson, Treas./VP
Donald E. Becker, Exec. VP
Carver L. Johnson, Chief Diversity Officer
R. Pete Williams, Sr. VP
Mike Hoffmann, Dir.-Convenience Stores
David B. Dillon, Chmn.
Kevin M. Dougherty, VP-Logistics

Phone: 513-762-4000	Fax: 513-762-1160
Toll-Free:	
Address: 1014 Vine St., Cincinnati, OH 45202 US	

GROWTH PLANS/SPECIAL FEATURES:

The Kroger Co. is one of the largest supermarket operators in the U.S. The company operates 2,486 supermarkets in 31 states under a variety of names: Kroger, Kroger Marketplace, Ralphs, Fred Meyer, Food 4 Less, King Soopers, Smith's, Smith's Marketplace, Fry's, Fry's Marketplace, Dillons, Dillons Marketplace QFC and City Market. Of these stores, 696 have fuel centers and 1,962 have pharmacies. Kroger's supermarkets operate under one of three store formats: combination food and drug stores; multi-department stores; or price-impact warehouse stores. Kroger stores offer one-stop shopping, including whole health sections, pharmacies, pet centers and world-class perishables, such as fresh seafood and organic produce. Kroger also operates 782 convenience stores under the Quik Stop, Loaf N' Jug, Tom Thumb, Turkey Hill and Kwik Shop names. These stores offer a limited assortment of staple food items and general merchandise, and, in most cases, sell gasoline. The company operates 392 fine jewelry stores under the banners Fred Meyer Jewelers, Littman Jewelers, Barclay Jewelers and Fox's Jewelers. The 42 food processing or manufacturing plants operated by Kroger are primarily bakeries and dairies, which supply approximately 43% of the corporate brand units sold in its retail outlets. These plants consisted of 18 dairies, 11 deli or bakery plants, five grocery product plants, three beverage plants, three meat plants and two cheese plants.

The company offers its employees medical, dental and vision insurance; a 401(k) plan; life and accident insurance; long-term disability, homeowners and auto insurance; a stock purchase plan; and an employee assistance program.

FINANCIALS: Sales and profits are in thousands of dollars—add 000 to get the full amount. 2007 Note: Financial information for 2007 was not available for all companies at press time.

2007 Sales: $66,111,000	2007 Profits: $1,115,000	**U.S. Stock Ticker: KR**
2006 Sales: $60,553,000	2006 Profits: $958,000	**Int'l Ticker:** Int'l Exchange:
2005 Sales: $56,434,000	2005 Profits: $-104,000	Employees: 310,000
2004 Sales: $53,791,000	2004 Profits: $285,000	Fiscal Year Ends: 1/31
2003 Sales: $51,760,000	2003 Profits: $1,205,000	Parent Company:

SALARIES/BENEFITS:

Pension Plan:	ESOP Stock Plan:	Profit Sharing:	Top Exec. Salary: $1,155,991	Bonus: $2,116,770
Savings Plan: Y	Stock Purch. Plan: Y		Second Exec. Salary: $809,969	Bonus: $1,340,621

OTHER THOUGHTS:
Apparent Women Officers or Directors: 4
Hot Spot for Advancement for Women/Minorities: Y

LOCATIONS: ("Y" = Yes)

West:	Southwest:	Midwest:	Southeast:	Northeast:	International:
Y	Y	Y	Y	Y	

Note: Financial information, benefits and other data can change quickly and may vary from those stated here.

L-3 COMMUNICATIONS HOLDINGS INC   www.l-3com.com

Industry Group Code: 334200 Ranks within this company's industry group: Sales: 1 Profits: 1

Management:		Sales/Marketing:		Liberal Arts:		Information Systems:		Professionals:		Technical/Scientific:	
Mgmt. Trainees:	Y	Mktg. Professionals:	Y	Gen. Writing/Editing:		Info. Management:	Y	Finance/Accounting:	Y	Engineers, Elec.:	Y
Experienced Mgmt.:	Y	Retail Sales:		Technical Writing:	Y	Software Dev.:	Y	Law:	Y	Engineers, Other:	
Int'l Business:	Y	Commercial/Industrial:	Y	Graphic Arts/Photog.:		Hardware Dev.:	Y	HR/Other:	Y	Health/Lab:	Y
MBA Graduates:	Y	Sales Trainees:		Music:		Systems Integration:	Y	Training:	Y	Scientists/Research:	Y
		Advertising Pros.:	Y	Broadcasting:		Consulting/Other:	Y	Health Care:		Petroleum/Chemicals:	
				Other:				Consulting:		Math/Other:	Y

TYPES OF BUSINESS:
Electronic Equipment-Specialized Communications
Intelligence, Surveillance & Reconnaissance Systems
Aviation & Aerospace Products
Telemetry Products
Instrumentation Products
Microwave Components
Security Systems
Airport Luggage Screening Systems

BRANDS/DIVISIONS/AFFILIATES:
L-3 Communications Corporation
Vertex Aerospace LLC
TRL Electronics
Crestview Aerospace
L-3 TITAN GROUP
SAM Electronics GmbH
Nova Engineering
SSG Precision Optronics, Inc.

CONTACTS: Note: Officers with more than one job title may be intentionally listed here more than once.
Michael T. Strianese, CEO
Michael T. Strianese, Pres.
Ralph G. D'Ambrosio, CFO
Kenneth W. Manne, VP-Human Resources
Vincent T. Taylor, CIO/VP
A. Michael Andrews, CTO
Sheila M. Sheridan, VP-Admin.
Kathleen E. Karelis, General Counsel/Sr. VP/Sec.
Jimmie V. Adams, Sr. VP-Oper.
Curtis Brunson, Sr. VP-Corp. Strategy & Dev.
Karen C. Tripp, VP-Corp. Comm.
Thomas Ripp, Pres., Security & Detection Systems
Craig P. Coy, COO/Pres., Homeland Security Group
Carl E. Vuono, COO/Pres., Gov't. Svcs. Group
Robert W. Drewes, Sr. VP/COO/Pres., L-3 Integrated Systems Group
Charles F. Wald, VP-Int'l
Ralph Denino, VP-Procurement

Phone: 212-697-1111   **Fax:** 212-867-5249
Toll-Free: 866-463-6555
Address: 600 3rd Ave., 34th Fl., New York, NY 10016 US

GROWTH PLANS/SPECIAL FEATURES:
L-3 Communications Holdings, Inc., which operates solely under its subsidiary L-3 Communications Corp., is a supplier of products used in aerospace and defense platforms. The company operates through four business segments: Command, Control, Communications, Intelligence, Surveillance and Reconnaissance (C3ISR); Government Services; Aircraft Modernization and Maintenance (AM&M); and Specialized Products. The C3ISR segment specializes in signals intelligence and communications intelligence. The businesses in this segment provide equipment for United States and foreign government intelligence and reconnaissance applications. The Government Services division provides: training services; maintenance and logistics support; communications systems support; engineering services; and marksmanship training systems. Through the AM&M segment, the company offers specialized aircraft modernization and logistics support services. The Specialized Products segment provides naval warfare products, security systems, sensors and wireless communication products. L-3's systems and equipment are essential to nearly all major communication, command and control, intelligence-gathering and space systems. The company's customers include the U.S. Department of Defense, U.S. Department of Homeland Security, U.S. government intelligence agencies, Aerospace and defense contractors, Foreign governments and Commercial customers. In 2007, the company acquired Geneva Aerospace, Inc., a provider of unmanned aerial vehicle technology, and Global Communications Solutions, Inc., a provider of portable satellite communications equipment and products.

L-3 Communications offers its employees educational assistance, a 401(k) savings plan and an employee stock purchase plan.

FINANCIALS: Sales and profits are in thousands of dollars—add 000 to get the full amount. 2007 Note: Financial information for 2007 was not available for all companies at press time.
2007 Sales: $13,960,500	2007 Profits: $756,100	**U.S. Stock Ticker:** LLL
2006 Sales: $12,476,900	2006 Profits: $526,100	**Int'l Ticker:** Int'l Exchange:
2005 Sales: $9,444,700	2005 Profits: $508,500	**Employees:** 64,600
2004 Sales: $6,897,000	2004 Profits: $381,900	**Fiscal Year Ends:** 12/31
2003 Sales: $5,061,600	2003 Profits: $277,600	**Parent Company:**

SALARIES/BENEFITS:
| Pension Plan: Y | ESOP Stock Plan: | Profit Sharing: | Top Exec. Salary: $775,192 | Bonus: $1,650,000 |
| Savings Plan: Y | Stock Purch. Plan: Y | | Second Exec. Salary: $461,346 | Bonus: $ |

OTHER THOUGHTS:
Apparent Women Officers or Directors: 4
Hot Spot for Advancement for Women/Minorities: Y

LOCATIONS: ("Y" = Yes)
West:	Southwest:	Midwest:	Southeast:	Northeast:	International:
Y	Y	Y	Y	Y	Y

L-3 TITAN GROUP

www.titan.com

Industry Group Code: 541512 Ranks within this company's industry group: Sales: Profits:

Management:		Sales/Marketing:		Liberal Arts:		Information Systems:		Professionals:		Technical/Scientific:	
Mgmt. Trainees:	Y	Mktg. Professionals:	Y	Gen. Writing/Editing:		Info. Management:	Y	Finance/Accounting:	Y	Engineers, Elec.:	
Experienced Mgmt.:	Y	Retail Sales:		Technical Writing:	Y	Software Dev.:	Y	Law:	Y	Engineers, Other:	
Int'l Business:	Y	Commercial/Industrial:	Y	Graphic Arts/Photog.:	Y	Hardware Dev.:	Y	HR/Other:	Y	Health/Lab:	Y
MBA Graduates:	Y	Sales Trainees:		Music:		Systems Integration:	Y	Training:	Y	Scientists/Research:	Y
		Advertising Pros.:		Broadcasting:		Consulting/Other:		Health Care:		Petroleum/Chemicals:	
				Other:				Consulting:	Y	Math/Other:	

TYPES OF BUSINESS:
Consulting-Government InfoTech
Satellite Communication Systems
Intelligence & Surveillance Systems
Information Technology Systems
Homeland Security Consulting
Aerospace Engineering

BRANDS/DIVISIONS/AFFILIATES:
L-3 Communications Holdings Inc
Center for National Response

CONTACTS: Note: Officers with more than one job title may be intentionally listed here more than once.
A. Anton Frederickson, COO
A. Anton Frederickson, Pres.

Phone: 703-434-4000	Fax: 703-434-5075
Toll-Free:	
Address: 11955 Freedom Dr., Reston, VA 20190 US	

GROWTH PLANS/SPECIAL FEATURES:

L-3 Titan Group, a subsidiary of L-3 Communications, provides information and communications products and services to the Department of Defense, the Department of Homeland Security, intelligence agencies and other government customers. It works on over 2,000 contracts at a time, and more than 8,000 of its personnel have security clearances. It has employees in 46 U.S. states, as well as in 300 locations throughout 24 countries worldwide including Iraq and Afghanistan. Titan focuses on five business areas: Homeland Security and Homeland Defense; Enterprise Information Technology; Command, Control, Communications, Computer, Intelligence, Surveillance and Reconnaissance (C4ISR); Intelligence; and Aerospace. Titan provides the Department of Homeland Security with communication systems, such as APCO 25 compliant radio systems, that support first responders. Other services assist explosives detection, advanced physics research, US-VISIT (United States Visitor and Immigrant Status Indicator Technology Program) border security and U.S. Coast Guard training. The firm also runs the Center for National Response, a training facility that prepares first responders for potential terrorist threats. Titan's Enterprise Information Technology division provides end-to-end IT solutions that connect strategic and tactical levels of a customer's critical enterprise. C4ISR is the cornerstone of Titan's business and involves four distinct activities: gathering military information through intelligence, surveillance and reconnaissance; transmitting the information digitally through high-technology communications systems; processing the digitized information to facilitate command and control decision making; and disseminating commands electronically back to military and intelligence platforms for execution. The firm's Intelligence segment provides services for experts at all levels of security expertise. Finally, Titan's Aerospace division supports military aviation with systems engineering, advance systems design, aircraft modernization, systems integration, avionics technical support and life-cycle support services.

Employees of Titan receive medical, dental and vision coverage; life insurance; educational assistance; flexible spending accounts; and paid time off.

FINANCIALS: Sales and profits are in thousands of dollars—add 000 to get the full amount. 2007 Note: Financial information for 2007 was not available for all companies at press time.

2007 Sales: $	2007 Profits: $	**U.S. Stock Ticker:** Subsidiary
2006 Sales: $	2006 Profits: $	**Int'l Ticker:** Int'l Exchange:
2005 Sales: $2,500,000	2005 Profits: $	Employees:
2004 Sales: $2,046,525	2004 Profits: $-38,397	Fiscal Year Ends: 12/31
2003 Sales: $1,775,007	2003 Profits: $32,097	Parent Company: L-3 COMMUNICATIONS HOLDINGS INC

SALARIES/BENEFITS:

Pension Plan:	ESOP Stock Plan:	Profit Sharing:	Top Exec. Salary: $807,500	Bonus: $
Savings Plan: Y	Stock Purch. Plan: Y		Second Exec. Salary: $342,777	Bonus: $

OTHER THOUGHTS:
Apparent Women Officers or Directors:
Hot Spot for Advancement for Women/Minorities:

LOCATIONS: ("Y" = Yes)

West:	Southwest:	Midwest:	Southeast:	Northeast:	International:
Y	Y	Y	Y	Y	Y

Note: Financial information, benefits and other data can change quickly and may vary from those stated here.

LABORATORY CORP OF AMERICA HOLDINGS

www.labcorp.com

Industry Group Code: 621511 **Ranks within this company's industry group:** Sales: 2 Profits: 2

Management:		Sales/Marketing:		Liberal Arts:		Information Systems:		Professionals:		Technical/Scientific:	
Mgmt. Trainees:	Y	Mktg. Professionals:	Y	Gen. Writing/Editing:	Y	Info. Management:	Y	Finance/Accounting:	Y	Engineers, Elec.:	
Experienced Mgmt.:	Y	Retail Sales:		Technical Writing:	Y	Software Dev.:	Y	Law:	Y	Engineers, Other:	Y
Int'l Business:	Y	Commercial/Industrial:	Y	Graphic Arts/Photog.:	Y	Hardware Dev.:		HR/Other:	Y	Health/Lab:	Y
MBA Graduates:	Y	Sales Trainees:		Music:		Systems Integration:		Training:	Y	Scientists/Research:	Y
		Advertising Pros.:		Broadcasting:		Consulting/Other:		Health Care:	Y	Petroleum/Chemicals:	
				Other:				Consulting:		Math/Other:	

TYPES OF BUSINESS:
Clinical Laboratory Testing
Diagnostics
Urinalyses
Blood Cell Counts
Blood Chemistry Analysis
HIV Tests
Genetic Testing
Specialty & Niche Tests

BRANDS/DIVISIONS/AFFILIATES:
Dianon Systems, Inc.
Esoterix, Inc.
US Pathology Labs, Inc.
Tandem Labs., Inc.

CONTACTS: Note: Officers with more than one job title may be intentionally listed here more than once.
David P. King, CEO
Don Hardison, COO/Exec. VP
David P. King, Pres.
William Hayes, CFO/Exec. VP
Benjamin R. Miller, Exec. VP-Mktg. & Sales
Myla P. Lai-Goldman, Chief Scientific Officer
Andrew S. Walton, CIO
Bradford T. Smith, Chief Legal Officer/Corp. Sec.
Woodrow L. Cook, Exec. VP-Eastern Oper.
Andrew S. Walton, Exec. VP-Strategic Planning
Bradford T. Smith, Exec. VP-Corp. Affairs
Eric Lindblom, Sr. VP-Investor & Media Rel.
William Hayes, Treas.
Myla P. Lai-Goldman, Exec. VP/Medical Dir.
William B. Haas, Exec. VP-Esoteric Bus.
Benjamin R. Miller, Exec. VP-Managed Care
Allen W. Troub, Exec. VP-Western Oper.
Thomas P. Mac Mahon, Chmn.

Phone: 336-584-5171	Fax: 336-436-1205
Toll-Free: 800-334-5261	
Address: 358 S. Main St., Burlington, NC 27215 US	

GROWTH PLANS/SPECIAL FEATURES:

Laboratory Corporation of America Holdings (LabCorp) is one of the top independent clinical laboratory companies in the U.S., offering more than 4,400 health-related laboratory tests to the medical industry. The tests are used primarily in routine screening, patient diagnosis and monitoring and treatment of disease. Its laboratories participated in the development of genomic applications using polymerase chain reaction (PCR) technology and LabCorp was the first commercial laboratory to provide this technology to health care providers. The company operates a nationwide network of 37 primary testing facilities and over 1,700 service centers, consisting of branches, patient service centers and STAT labs, which can perform routine tests quickly and report results to the physician within 24 hours. Some of its labs are operated by subsidiaries Dianon Systems, Inc.; Esoterix, Inc.; and US Pathology Labs, Inc. They are leading providers of anatomic pathology testing services. The most common tests performed by the firm include blood chemistry analysis, urinalyses, blood cell counts, Pap smears, HIV tests, microbiology cultures and substance abuse tests. The company processes an average of approximately 370,000 specimens per day for over 220,000 clients in all 50 states, Washington, D.C., Puerto Rico and Canada. LabCorp also performs specialty and niche testing including infectious disease and allergy testing and a number of genetics testing services and forensic identity tests. The company provides clinical laboratory testing for pharmaceutical companies conducting clinical research trials on new drugs. The expansion of its specialty and niche testing business is currently a primary growth strategy for the company. In early 2008, LabCorp acquired Tandem Labs, Inc., a bioanalytical and inmunoanalytical contract research organization.

LabCorp offers its employees flexible spending accounts, tuition reimbursement, adoption assistance, credit union membership, an employee assistance program and a legal assistance program.

FINANCIALS: Sales and profits are in thousands of dollars—add 000 to get the full amount. 2007 Note: Financial information for 2007 was not available for all companies at press time.

2007 Sales: $4,068,200	2007 Profits: $476,800	**U.S. Stock Ticker: LH**
2006 Sales: $3,590,800	2006 Profits: $431,600	**Int'l Ticker:** Int'l Exchange:
2005 Sales: $3,327,600	2005 Profits: $386,200	Employees: 25,000
2004 Sales: $3,084,800	2004 Profits: $363,000	Fiscal Year Ends: 12/31
2003 Sales: $2,939,400	2003 Profits: $321,000	Parent Company:

SALARIES/BENEFITS:

Pension Plan: Y	ESOP Stock Plan:	Profit Sharing:	Top Exec. Salary: $989,526	Bonus: $2,041,500
Savings Plan: Y	Stock Purch. Plan: Y		Second Exec. Salary: $524,960	Bonus: $850,575

OTHER THOUGHTS:
Apparent Women Officers or Directors: 2
Hot Spot for Advancement for Women/Minorities:

LOCATIONS: ("Y" = Yes)

West:	Southwest:	Midwest:	Southeast:	Northeast:	International:
Y	Y	Y	Y	Y	Y

Note: Financial information, benefits and other data can change quickly and may vary from those stated here.

LANDRY'S RESTAURANTS INC　www.landrysrestaurants.com

Industry Group Code: 722110　Ranks within this company's industry group: Sales: 8　Profits: 9

Management:		Sales/Marketing:		Liberal Arts:		Information Systems:		Professionals:		Technical/Scientific:	
Mgmt. Trainees:	Y	Mktg. Professionals:	Y	Gen. Writing/Editing:	Y	Info. Management:	Y	Finance/Accounting:	Y	Engineers, Elec.:	
Experienced Mgmt.:	Y	Retail Sales:		Technical Writing:		Software Dev.:	Y	Law:	Y	Engineers, Other:	
Int'l Business:		Commercial/Industrial:		Graphic Arts/Photog.:	Y	Hardware Dev.:		HR/Other:	Y	Health/Lab:	
MBA Graduates:	Y	Sales Trainees:		Music:		Systems Integration:		Training:	Y	Scientists/Research:	
		Advertising Pros.:	Y	Broadcasting:		Consulting/Other:		Health Care:		Petroleum/Chemicals:	
				Other:	Y			Consulting:		Math/Other:	

TYPES OF BUSINESS:
Casual Dining Restaurants
Hotel & Casino Resorts
Restaurants

BRANDS/DIVISIONS/AFFILIATES:
Crab House (The)
Landry's Seafood House
Rainforest Cafe
Chart House (The)
Saltgrass Steak House
Golden Nugget Hotels & Casinos
T-Rex Café
Yak & Yeti

CONTACTS: *Note: Officers with more than one job title may be intentionally listed here more than once.*
Tilman J. Fertitta, CEO
Tilman J. Fertitta, Pres.
Richard H. Liem, CFO/Exec. VP
Steven L. Scheinthal, General Counsel/Exec. VP/ Sec.
Jeffrey L. Cantwell, Sr. VP- Dev.
K. Kelly Roberts, Chief Admin. Officer-Hospitality & Gaming Division
Richard E. Ervin, Exec. VP-Restaurant Oper.
Tilman J. Fertitta, Chmn.

Phone: 713-850-1010	Fax: 713-850-7070
Toll-Free: 800-552-6379	
Address: 1510 W. Loop S., Houston, TX 77027 US	

GROWTH PLANS/SPECIAL FEATURES:
Landry's Restaurants, Inc. is a restaurant, hospitality and entertainment company principally engaged in the ownership and operation of casual dining restaurants, primarily under the names of Rainforest Café, Saltgrass Steak House, Landry's Seafood House, The Crab House, Charley's Crab and The Chart House. The firm owns and operates over 179 full-service and certain limited-service restaurants in 28 states. Landry's Restaurants also owns and operates select hospitality businesses including hotel and casino resorts, such as the Golden Nugget Hotels and Casinos in downtown Las Vegas and Laughlin, Nevada. The company operates its restaurants through three divisions: the Landry's Division, its seafood and signature restaurants; Rainforest Café, the rainforest-themed casual dining restaurants; and Saltgrass Steak House, the Texas-Western themed casual dining restaurants. The Landry's division is comprised of Landry's Seafood House, The Crab House, Chart House, C.A. Muer, Grotto, Pesce, Vic & Anthony's Steakhouse, Willie G's Seafood and Steak House, La Griglia and Brenner's Steakhouse. The Rainforest Café restaurants provide casual dining in a rainforest-themed environment, complete with thunderstorms, waterfalls and active wildlife. Each Café consists of a restaurant and a retail village. The Saltgrass Steak House offer casual dining in a Texas-Western theme. Prototype buildings welcome guests into a stone and wood beam ranch house complete with a fireplace and a saloon-style bar. In June 2008, Landry's entered into agreement with Fertitta Holdings, Inc. (the holding company for Landry's) to acquire all of the company's outstanding common stock. Fertitta is a newly formed entity wholly owned by Landry's CEO and founder, Tilman J. Fertitta.

FINANCIALS: Sales and profits are in thousands of dollars—add 000 to get the full amount. 2007 Note: Financial information for 2007 was not available for all companies at press time.

2007 Sales: $1,171,923	2007 Profits: $18,112	U.S. Stock Ticker: LNY
2006 Sales: $1,114,213	2006 Profits: $-21,770	Int'l Ticker:　　Int'l Exchange:
2005 Sales: $897,460	2005 Profits: $44,815	Employees: 20,055
2004 Sales: $804,903	2004 Profits: $66,522	Fiscal Year Ends: 12/31
2003 Sales: $1,105,755	2003 Profits: $44,914	Parent Company:

SALARIES/BENEFITS:
Pension Plan:	ESOP Stock Plan:	Profit Sharing:	Top Exec. Salary: $1,450,000	Bonus: $1,585,000
Savings Plan:	Stock Purch. Plan:		Second Exec. Salary: $350,000	Bonus: $385,000

OTHER THOUGHTS:
Apparent Women Officers or Directors:
Hot Spot for Advancement for Women/Minorities:

LOCATIONS: ("Y" = Yes)
West:	Southwest:	Midwest:	Southeast:	Northeast:	International:
Y	Y	Y	Y	Y	

Note: Financial information, benefits and other data can change quickly and may vary from those stated here.

LAS VEGAS SANDS CORP (THE VENETIAN)
www.lasvegassands.com
Industry Group Code: 721120 Ranks within this company's industry group: Sales: 3   Profits: 4

Management:		Sales/Marketing:		Liberal Arts:		Information Systems:		Professionals:		Technical/Scientific:	
Mgmt. Trainees:	Y	Mktg. Professionals:	Y	Gen. Writing/Editing:	Y	Info. Management:	Y	Finance/Accounting:	Y	Engineers, Elec.:	
Experienced Mgmt.:	Y	Retail Sales:		Technical Writing:		Software Dev.:		Law:	Y	Engineers, Other:	
Int'l Business:	Y	Commercial/Industrial:	Y	Graphic Arts/Photog.:	Y	Hardware Dev.:		HR/Other:	Y	Health/Lab:	
MBA Graduates:	Y	Sales Trainees:		Music:	Y	Systems Integration:		Training:	Y	Scientists/Research:	
		Advertising Pros.:	Y	Broadcasting:		Consulting/Other:		Health Care:		Petroleum/Chemicals:	
				Other:	Y			Consulting:		Math/Other:	

TYPES OF BUSINESS:
Hotel Casinos
Convention & Conference Centers
Shopping Center Development
Casino Property Development

BRANDS/DIVISIONS/AFFILIATES:
Venetian Resort Hotel Casino (The)
Sands Expo and Convention Center (The)
Congress Center (The)
Sands Macao Casino (The)
Palazzo Resort Hotel Casino (The)
Venetian Macao Resort Hotel (The)
Marina Bay Sands
Cotai Strip

CONTACTS: Note: Officers with more than one job title may be intentionally listed here more than once.
Sheldon G. Adelson, CEO
William P. Weidner, COO
William P. Weidner, Pres.
Robert P. Rozek, CFO/Sr. VP
Scott D. Henry, Sr. VP-Finance
Robert G. Goldstein, Sr. VP/Pres., The Venetian & The Palazzo
Bradley H. Stone, Exec. VP
Sheldon G. Adelson, Chmn.
Mark A. Brown, Pres., Sands Macao & The Venetian Macao

Phone: 702-414-1000	Fax: 702-414-4884
Toll-Free:	
Address: 3355 Las Vegas Blvd. S., Las Vegas, NV 89109 US	

GROWTH PLANS/SPECIAL FEATURES:
Las Vegas Sands Corp. (The Venetian) is an international hotel, resort and casino firm. It owns The Venetian Resort Hotel Casino, offering a 120,000-square-foot casino floor with 130 table games and 1,700 slot machines; 4,027 hotel suites; and a 440,000-square-foot enclosed dining, retail and entertainment complex. It connects to the firm's 1.15-million-square-foot convention and trade show facility, The Sands Expo and Convention Center, and to its supplemental upscale business event and conference center The Congress Center. Additionally, the Sands Macao offers 229,000 square feet of gaming space with 630 table games and 1,350 slot machines; a 238-suite hotel tower; and other amenities. In January 2008, The Palazzo Resort Hotel Casino opened adjacent to and directly connected to The Venetian. It features 3,066 suites in a 50-floor tower; 105,000 square feet of gaming space with 130 table games and 1,400 slot machines; one of the Strip's first Lamborghini dealerships; and 400,000 of dining and retail space called The Shoppes at The Palazzo, including 20 Las Vegas-premiering luxury brands and stores; and numerous restaurants, including CarneVino by Mario Batali and Table 10 by Emeril Lagasse. In August 2007, The Venetian Macao Resort Hotel opened in China, featuring a 3,000-suite hotel; a 550,000 square feet casino floor with 870 table games and 3,400 slot machines; 1.2 million square feet of meeting, exhibition and convention space; 1 million square feet of retail and dining space; and the 15,000 seat Venetian Arena. Its two largest projects in development include the $4 billion Marina Bay Sands integrated resort in Singapore and the $12 billion Cotai Strip, a collection of hotel properties, casinos and entertainment venues featuring 19,750 guest rooms; 1.6 million square feet of gaming space with 3,300 table games and 16,470 slot machines; and 3 million square feet of retail space.

FINANCIALS: Sales and profits are in thousands of dollars—add 000 to get the full amount. 2007 Note: Financial information for 2007 was not available for all companies at press time.

		U.S. Stock Ticker: LVS
2007 Sales: $3,104,422	2007 Profits: $116,688	Int'l Ticker: Int'l Exchange:
2006 Sales: $2,340,178	2006 Profits: $442,003	Employees: 28,000
2005 Sales: $1,824,225	2005 Profits: $283,686	Fiscal Year Ends: 12/31
2004 Sales: $1,258,570	2004 Profits: $495,183	Parent Company:
2003 Sales: $641,500	2003 Profits: $37,400	

SALARIES/BENEFITS:
Pension Plan:	ESOP Stock Plan:	Profit Sharing:	Top Exec. Salary: $1,000,000	Bonus: $4,400,000
Savings Plan: Y	Stock Purch. Plan:		Second Exec. Salary: $1,000,000	Bonus: $3,503,200

OTHER THOUGHTS:
Apparent Women Officers or Directors:
Hot Spot for Advancement for Women/Minorities:

LOCATIONS: ("Y" = Yes)
West:	Southwest:	Midwest:	Southeast:	Northeast:	International:
Y				Y	Y

LEVEL 3 COMMUNICATIONS INC   www.level3.com

Industry Group Code: 513390C Ranks within this company's industry group: Sales: 1 Profits: 2

Management:		Sales/Marketing:		Liberal Arts:		Information Systems:		Professionals:		Technical/Scientific:	
Mgmt. Trainees:		Mktg. Professionals:	Y	Gen. Writing/Editing:		Info. Management:	Y	Finance/Accounting:	Y	Engineers, Elec.:	Y
Experienced Mgmt.:	Y	Retail Sales:		Technical Writing:	Y	Software Dev.:	Y	Law:	Y	Engineers, Other:	
Int'l Business:	Y	Commercial/Industrial:	Y	Graphic Arts/Photog.:		Hardware Dev.:	Y	HR/Other:	Y	Health/Lab:	
MBA Graduates:	Y	Sales Trainees:		Music:		Systems Integration:	Y	Training:	Y	Scientists/Research:	
		Advertising Pros.:		Broadcasting:		Consulting/Other:		Health Care:		Petroleum/Chemicals:	
				Other:				Consulting:		Math/Other:	

TYPES OF BUSINESS:
Private Data Networks-Fiber Optic
Broadband Network Services
Managed Modem Access Services

BRANDS/DIVISIONS/AFFILIATES:
Peter Kiewit Sons', Inc. (PKS)
ICG Communications Inc
Softswitch
Broadwing Communications LLC
Telcove Corp

CONTACTS: Note: Officers with more than one job title may be intentionally listed here more than once.
James Q. Crowe, CEO
James Q. Crowe, Pres.
Sunit Patel, CFO/Exec. VP
Sureel Choksi, Chief Mktg. Officer
Meg Porfido, Chief Human Resources Officer
Kevin Hart, CIO
Jack Waters, CTO/Pres., Global Network Svcs.
Thomas C. Stortz, Chief Legal Officer/Exec. VP
Neil Hobbs, Exec. VP-Oper.
Don Gips, Group VP-Corp. Strategy & Dev.
Chris Hardman, VP-Corp. Comm.
Robin Grey, Corp. Treas.
Raoul Abdel, Pres., Bus. Markets
Grant van Rooyen, Pres., Content Markets
Andrew Crouch, Pres., Wholesale Markets
Walter Scott, Jr., Chmn.
James Heard, Pres., European Markets

Phone: 720-888-1000	Fax: 720-888-5085
Toll-Free: 877-253-8353	
Address: 1025 Eldorado Blvd., Broomfield, CO 80021 US	

GROWTH PLANS/SPECIAL FEATURES:
Level 3 Communications, Inc., which operates one of the world's largest Internet backbones, is a leading provider of integrated communications services. The company's main offering is its 48,000 miles of broadband networks in the U.S. and Europe. Using these networks, the firms supplies a portfolio of services including Internet Protocol (IP) services (Internet access, Ethernet and virtual private network, or VPN), broadband transport, colocation services, and patented Softswitch-based managed modem and voice services, which use a distributed computer system to emulate traditional circuit switches. Level 3 divides these services according to customer base into four segments: Wholesale markets group, business markets group, content markets group and the European group. The wholesale group services high bandwidth needs of large communications providers. The business group provides services to enterprises, regional carriers, educational institutions and government agencies. The content group sells services designed for video distribution companies; providers of online gaming and mega-portals; software service providers; social networking providers; and traditional media distribution companies including broadcasters, television networks and sports leagues. Lastly, the European groups supplies communications services in Europe for customers similar to the wholesale and content customers. The firm owns and operates several subsidiaries including Telcove Corp.; Broadwing Corporation, which owns Broadwing Communications, LLC; and ICG Communications, Inc. Originally founded as a part of Peter Kiewit Sons', Inc., a mining, construction and communications company, Level 3 also has holdings in coal mining and other diversified interests. In 2007, the firm purchased assets from AT&T Inc., including the rights to dark fiber connections in 27 buildings and over 450 metro fiber route miles. In 2008, the firm sold its advertising distribution business to DG FastChannel, Inc.

Level 3 offers employees life, medical, dental, and vision insurance; educational assistance; flexible spending accounts; and an employee assistance program.

FINANCIALS: Sales and profits are in thousands of dollars—add 000 to get the full amount. 2007 Note: Financial information for 2007 was not available for all companies at press time.

2007 Sales: $4,269,000	2007 Profits: $-1,114,000	U.S. Stock Ticker: LVLT
2006 Sales: $3,378,000	2006 Profits: $-744,000	Int'l Ticker: Int'l Exchange:
2005 Sales: $1,719,000	2005 Profits: $-638,000	Employees: 6,680
2004 Sales: $1,776,000	2004 Profits: $-458,000	Fiscal Year Ends: 12/31
2003 Sales: $3,947,000	2003 Profits: $-711,000	Parent Company:

SALARIES/BENEFITS:

Pension Plan:	ESOP Stock Plan:	Profit Sharing:	Top Exec. Salary: $790,385	Bonus: $
Savings Plan: Y	Stock Purch. Plan:		Second Exec. Salary: $566,154	Bonus: $

OTHER THOUGHTS:
Apparent Women Officers or Directors: 2
Hot Spot for Advancement for Women/Minorities: Y

LOCATIONS: ("Y" = Yes)

West:	Southwest:	Midwest:	Southeast:	Northeast:	International:
Y	Y		Y	Y	Y

Note: Financial information, benefits and other data can change quickly and may vary from those stated here.

LEXMARK INTERNATIONAL INC

www.lexmark.com

Industry Group Code: 334119 Ranks within this company's industry group: Sales: 1   Profits: 1

Management:		Sales/Marketing:		Liberal Arts:		Information Systems:		Professionals:		Technical/Scientific:	
Mgmt. Trainees:	Y	Mktg. Professionals:	Y	Gen. Writing/Editing:		Info. Management:	Y	Finance/Accounting:	Y	Engineers, Elec.:	Y
Experienced Mgmt.:	Y	Retail Sales:		Technical Writing:	Y	Software Dev.:	Y	Law:	Y	Engineers, Other:	Y
Int'l Business:	Y	Commercial/Industrial:	Y	Graphic Arts/Photog.:	Y	Hardware Dev.:	Y	HR/Other:	Y	Health/Lab:	Y
MBA Graduates:	Y	Sales Trainees:		Music:		Systems Integration:		Training:	Y	Scientists/Research:	Y
		Advertising Pros.:	Y	Broadcasting:		Consulting/Other:		Health Care:		Petroleum/Chemicals:	
				Other:				Consulting:		Math/Other:	

TYPES OF BUSINESS:

Computer Accessories-Printers
Laser & Inkjet Printers
Printer Consumables
Typewriters & Supplies
Connectivity Products
Document Software

BRANDS/DIVISIONS/AFFILIATES:

International Business Machines Corp (IBM)

CONTACTS: *Note: Officers with more than one job title may be intentionally listed here more than once.*

Paul J. Curlander, CEO
John W. Gamble Jr., CFO/Exec. VP
Jeri Isbell, VP-Human Resources
Vincent J. Cole, General Counsel/Sec./VP
Gary D. Stromquist, Corp. Controller/VP
Paul A. Rooke, Exec. VP/Pres., Consumer Printer Div.
Daniel P. Bork, VP-Tax
Martin Canning, VP/Pres., Printing Solutions & Svcs. Div.
Paul J. Curlander, Chmn.
David L. Goodnight, VP-Asia Pacific & Latin America

Phone: 859-232-2000	**Fax:** 859-232-2403
Toll-Free: 800-539-6275	
Address: 740 W. New Circle Rd., Lexington, KY 40550 US	

GROWTH PLANS/SPECIAL FEATURES:

Lexmark International, Inc., a former subsidiary of International Business Machines Corp. (IBM), is a global developer, manufacturer and supplier of laser and inkjet printers and associated consumable supplies for the office and home markets. Its products are sold in over 150 countries across the Americas, Europe, the Middle East, Africa, Asia, the Pacific Rim and the Caribbean. The company's research and development activity for the past several years has focused on laser and inkjet printers, associated supplies and network connectivity products. In addition to its laser and inkjet printers, Lexmark sells dot matrix printers for printing single and multi-part forms by business users, as well as the consumable supplies used by its large installed base of printers. Because consumable supplies must be replaced on average one to three times a year, depending on type of printer and usage, demand for laser and inkjet print cartridges is increasing at a higher rate than their associated printer shipments. Besides its core printer business, the firm manufactures a broad line of other office imaging products, including supplies for IBM-branded printers; after-market supplies for original equipment manufacturer products; and typewriters and typewriter supplies that are sold under the IBM trademark. International sales, including exports from the U.S., accounted for approximately 56% of the firm's revenue.

Employees of Lexmark receive medical, dental and vision benefits, including coverage for a domestic partner or spouse, and children; flexible spending accounts; the Live for Life health and fitness refund program; an employee assistance program; life, business travel, accident long-term disability and long-term care insurance; care services for children with special needs; adoption assistance; training and management development programs; and education assistance. The company's headquarters features an on-site cafeteria as well as onsite banking and medical services, including overseas travel assistance, physical therapy and health screenings.

FINANCIALS: Sales and profits are in thousands of dollars—add 000 to get the full amount. 2007 Note: Financial information for 2007 was not available for all companies at press time.

		U.S. Stock Ticker: LXK
2007 Sales: $4,973,900	2007 Profits: $300,800	**Int'l Ticker:** Int'l Exchange:
2006 Sales: $5,108,100	2006 Profits: $338,400	Employees: 13,800
2005 Sales: $5,221,500	2005 Profits: $356,300	Fiscal Year Ends: 12/31
2004 Sales: $5,313,800	2004 Profits: $568,700	Parent Company:
2003 Sales: $4,754,700	2003 Profits: $439,200	

SALARIES/BENEFITS:

Pension Plan:	ESOP Stock Plan:	Profit Sharing:	Top Exec. Salary: $1,000,000	Bonus: $1,646,820
Savings Plan: Y	Stock Purch. Plan: Y		Second Exec. Salary: $530,000	Bonus: $633,833

OTHER THOUGHTS:

Apparent Women Officers or Directors: 3
Hot Spot for Advancement for Women/Minorities: Y

LOCATIONS: ("Y" = Yes)

West:	Southwest:	Midwest:	Southeast:	Northeast:	International:
Y		Y			Y

LIBERTY GLOBAL INC

www.lgi.com

Industry Group Code: 513220 Ranks within this company's industry group: Sales: 5   Profits: 4

Management:		Sales/Marketing:		Liberal Arts:		Information Systems:		Professionals:		Technical/Scientific:	
Mgmt. Trainees:	Y	Mktg. Professionals:	Y	Gen. Writing/Editing:		Info. Management:	Y	Finance/Accounting:	Y	Engineers, Elec.:	Y
Experienced Mgmt.:	Y	Retail Sales:		Technical Writing:		Software Dev.:	Y	Law:	Y	Engineers, Other:	
Int'l Business:	Y	Commercial/Industrial:	Y	Graphic Arts/Photog.:		Hardware Dev.:		HR/Other:	Y	Health/Lab:	
MBA Graduates:	Y	Sales Trainees:		Music:		Systems Integration:		Training:	Y	Scientists/Research:	
		Advertising Pros.:	Y	Broadcasting:		Consulting/Other:		Health Care:		Petroleum/Chemicals:	
				Other:				Consulting:		Math/Other:	

TYPES OF BUSINESS:
Video, Voice & Broadband Internet Access Services
Telephony Services
VoIP Services
Mobile Telephony Services

BRANDS/DIVISIONS/AFFILIATES:
UPC Holding BV
UPC Broadband Division
Jupiter Telecommunication Co., Ltd. (J:Com)
Austar United Communications Ltd.
VTR Global Com S.A.
Liberty Cablevision of Puerto Rico
Telenet Group Holding NV
Chellomedia BV

CONTACTS: Note: Officers with more than one job title may be intentionally listed here more than once.
Michael T. Fries, CEO
Michael T. Fries, Pres.
Charles H. R. Bracken, Co-CFO/Principal Financial Officer/Sr. VP
Amy M. Blair, Sr. VP-Global Human Resources
Balan Nair, CTO/Sr. VP
Elizabeth M. Markowski, General Counsel/Sec./Sr. VP
Shane O'Neill, Chief Strategy Officer/Sr. VP
Frederick G. (Rick) Westerman, III, Sr. VP-Corp. Comm.
Frederick G. (Rick) Westerman, III, Sr. VP-Investor Rel.
Bernard C. Dvorak, Co-CFO/Principle Acct. Officer/Sr. VP
Mauricio Ramos, Pres., Liberty Global Latin America/CEO-VTR Global
W. Gene Musselman, Pres./COO-UPC Broadband Div.
Shane O'Neill, Pres., Chellomedia BV
Bob Leighton, Sr. VP-Programming
John C. Malone, Chmn.
Miranda Curtis, Pres., Liberty Global Japan

Phone: 303-220-6600	Fax: 303-220-6601
Toll-Free:	
Address: 12300 Liberty Blvd., Englewood, CO 80112 US	

GROWTH PLANS/SPECIAL FEATURES:
Liberty Global, Inc. (LGI) is an international broadband communications provider of video, voice and broadband Internet access services. In select markets, the company also offers telephony, mobile telephony (using third-party networks) and VoIP (Voice over Internet Protocol) services. LGI has roughly 16.1 million customers and 24.5 million service subscribers, including 14.7 million video, 5.6 million broadband and 4.2 million telephone subscribers. It offers broadband services in 15 countries, principally in Europe, Japan and Chile. Through indirect wholly-owned subsidiary UPC Holding BV, the company provides broadband communications services in 10 European countries. The firm refers to these European operations as the UPC Broadband Division. Through its indirect 37.9% controlling interest in Jupiter Telecommunication Co., Ltd. (J:Com), LGI offers broadband communications services in Japan. The firm also offers Direct-to-Home (DTH) satellite services in Australia through 53.4%-owned Austar United Communications Ltd. In the Americas, the firm operates through 80%-owned Chilean subsidiary VTR Global Com S.A., a broadband and cable TV provider; and wholly-owned subsidiary Liberty Cablevision of Puerto Rico. Lastly, through an indirect 51.1% controlling interest in Telenet Group Holding NV, the firm provides broadband services in Belgium. Besides these subsidiaries, LGI's consolidated businesses include broadband communications operations in Puerto Rico and programming businesses in Europe, Japan and Argentina. Most of its consolidated European programming interests are held through Chellomedia BV, which also provides certain digital and interactive services to the firm's broadband operations in that region. Chellomedia also owns various businesses in Europe, including LGI's share in the Telenet Group, which it owns in part through subsidiary Belgian Cable Investors. During 2007, Chellomedia acquired the remaining 10.5% of Belgian Cable Investors that it did not already own, as well as purchasing shares of the Telenet Group, thus raising its ownership in Telenet from 28.8% to 51.1%, for a total consideration of $930.8 million.

FINANCIALS: Sales and profits are in thousands of dollars—add 000 to get the full amount. 2007 Note: Financial information for 2007 was not available for all companies at press time.

2007 Sales: $9,000,000	2007 Profits: $-420,000	**U.S. Stock Ticker: LBTYA**
2006 Sales: $6,487,500	2006 Profits: $706,200	**Int'l Ticker:** Int'l Exchange:
2005 Sales: $5,151,332	2005 Profits: $-80,097	Employees: 20,500
2004 Sales: $2,531,889	2004 Profits: $-21,481	Fiscal Year Ends: 12/31
2003 Sales: $108,390	2003 Profits: $20,889	Parent Company:

SALARIES/BENEFITS:

Pension Plan:	ESOP Stock Plan:	Profit Sharing:	Top Exec. Salary: $920,000	Bonus: $1,600,000
Savings Plan:	Stock Purch. Plan:		Second Exec. Salary: $734,294	Bonus: $1,000,000

OTHER THOUGHTS:
Apparent Women Officers or Directors: 3
Hot Spot for Advancement for Women/Minorities: Y

LOCATIONS: ("Y" = Yes)

West:	Southwest:	Midwest:	Southeast:	Northeast:	International:
Y					Y

Note: Financial information, benefits and other data can change quickly and may vary from those stated here.

LIMITED BRANDS INC
www.limitedbrands.com

Industry Group Code: 448120 Ranks within this company's industry group: Sales: 1 Profits: 1

Management:		Sales/Marketing:		Liberal Arts:		Information Systems:		Professionals:		Technical/Scientific:	
Mgmt. Trainees:	Y	Mktg. Professionals:	Y	Gen. Writing/Editing:	Y	Info. Management:	Y	Finance/Accounting:	Y	Engineers, Elec.:	
Experienced Mgmt.:	Y	Retail Sales:	Y	Technical Writing:		Software Dev.:	Y	Law:	Y	Engineers, Other:	
Int'l Business:	Y	Commercial/Industrial:	Y	Graphic Arts/Photog.:	Y	Hardware Dev.:		HR/Other:	Y	Health/Lab:	
MBA Graduates:	Y	Sales Trainees:	Y	Music:		Systems Integration:		Training:	Y	Scientists/Research:	
		Advertising Pros.:	Y	Broadcasting:		Consulting/Other:		Health Care:		Petroleum/Chemicals:	
				Other:	Y			Consulting:		Math/Other:	

TYPES OF BUSINESS:

Apparel, Retail
Contract Manufacturing
Apparel Importing
Catalog & Online Sales
Lingerie
Cosmetics
Fragrances
Candles

BRANDS/DIVISIONS/AFFILIATES:

Limited, Inc. (The)
Victoria's Secret
Victoria's Secret Beauty
Bath & Body Works
White Barn Candle Company
C.O. Bigelow
Mast Industries
La Senza Corporation

CONTACTS: *Note: Officers with more than one job title may be intentionally listed here more than once.*

Leslie H. Wexner, CEO
Stuart Burgdoerfer, CFO
Jane L. Ramsey, Exec. VP-Human Resources
Martyn R. Redgrave, Chief Admin. Officer/Exec. VP
Tammy Roberts Myers, Assoc. VP-External Comm.
Peter Horvath, Exec. VP-Bus. Integration
Shashi Batra, Pres., Victoria's Secret Beauty
Sharen J. Turney, CEO & Pres., Victoria's Secret Megabrand
Leslie H. Wexner, Chmn.
Martin Waters, Exec. VP-Int'l

Phone: 614-415-7000	Fax: 614-415-7440
Toll-Free:	
Address: 3 Limited Pkwy., Columbus, OH 43216 US	

GROWTH PLANS/SPECIAL FEATURES:

Limited Brands, Inc., formerly The Limited, Inc., is a leading retailer of apparel, lingerie, personal care products, accessories and fragrances. The company operates over 2,660 retail stores, mainly in malls and shopping centers throughout the U.S., through two main business segments: Victoria's Secret and Bath & Body Works. Victoria's Secret and Victoria's Secret Beauty, with aggregate 1,332 stores in the U.S. and Canada, are specialty retailers of women's intimate apparel, beauty products and related accessories. The direct marketing segment is in charge of the famous intimate apparel catalog, which is produced at volumes of approximately 390 million copies annually. Bath & Body Works, with 1,326 stores, features personal care products and also operates White Barn Candle Company and C.O. Bigelow. Apparel retailing for Limited includes a 25% stake in the 260 Limited stores, retailing sophisticated sportswear for modern women and the 658 Express stores selling men's and women's sportswear and accessories. Limited Brands retains full ownership of the two Henri Bendel stores located in New York City and Columbus, Ohio. The firm also owns Mast Industries, a contract manufacturer and apparel importer, which supplies merchandise to Victoria's Secret, Express and Limited Stores. The company runs three e-commerce sites: VictoriasSecret.com, LaSenza.com and bathandbodyworks.com. In July 2007, the firm completed the sale of 75% of Express to affiliates of Golden Gate Capital for $602 million. In July 2007, the firm agreed to transfer 75% of Limited Stores to Sun Capital Partners, Inc., expecting to post a loss of roughly $42 million on the sale.

Limited Brands offers medical, dental and vision insurance; product discounts; tuition assistance; paid time off; and adoption assistance.

FINANCIALS: Sales and profits are in thousands of dollars—add 000 to get the full amount. 2007 Note: Financial information for 2007 was not available for all companies at press time.

2007 Sales: $10,671,000	2007 Profits: $676,000	**U.S. Stock Ticker: LTD**
2006 Sales: $9,699,000	2006 Profits: $683,000	**Int'l Ticker:** Int'l Exchange:
2005 Sales: $9,408,000	2005 Profits: $705,000	Employees: 125,500
2004 Sales: $8,934,000	2004 Profits: $717,000	Fiscal Year Ends: 1/31
2003 Sales: $8,445,000	2003 Profits: $502,000	Parent Company:

SALARIES/BENEFITS:

Pension Plan:	ESOP Stock Plan:	Profit Sharing:	Top Exec. Salary: $1,685,192	Bonus: $758,880
Savings Plan: Y	Stock Purch. Plan: Y		Second Exec. Salary: $1,105,769	Bonus: $1,380,000

OTHER THOUGHTS:

Apparent Women Officers or Directors: 5
Hot Spot for Advancement for Women/Minorities: Y

LOCATIONS: ("Y" = Yes)

West:	Southwest:	Midwest:	Southeast:	Northeast:	International:
Y	Y	Y	Y	Y	Y

Note: Financial information, benefits and other data can change quickly and may vary from those stated here.

LINCARE HOLDINGS INC
www.lincare.com

Industry Group Code: 621610 Ranks within this company's industry group: Sales: 1 Profits: 1

Management:		Sales/Marketing:		Liberal Arts:		Information Systems:		Professionals:		Technical/Scientific:	
Mgmt. Trainees:	Y	Mktg. Professionals:	Y	Gen. Writing/Editing:		Info. Management:	Y	Finance/Accounting:	Y	Engineers, Elec.:	
Experienced Mgmt.:	Y	Retail Sales:		Technical Writing:	Y	Software Dev.:		Law:	Y	Engineers, Other:	
Int'l Business:		Commercial/Industrial:	Y	Graphic Arts/Photog.:		Hardware Dev.:		HR/Other:	Y	Health/Lab:	Y
MBA Graduates:	Y	Sales Trainees:		Music:		Systems Integration:		Training:	Y	Scientists/Research:	
		Advertising Pros.:	Y	Broadcasting:		Consulting/Other:		Health Care:	Y	Petroleum/Chemicals:	Y
				Other:				Consulting:		Math/Other:	

TYPES OF BUSINESS:
Home Health Care-Oxygen & Other Respiratory Therapy Services
Durable Medical Equipment
Home Infusion Therapies

BRANDS/DIVISIONS/AFFILIATES:

CONTACTS: *Note: Officers with more than one job title may be intentionally listed here more than once.*
John P. Byrnes, CEO
Shawn Schabel, COO
Shawn Schabel, Pres.
Paul G. Gabos, CFO
John P. Byrnes, Chmn.

Phone: 727-530-7700	Fax: 727-532-9692
Toll-Free:	
Address: 19387 US 19 N., Clearwater, FL 33764 US	

GROWTH PLANS/SPECIAL FEATURES:
Lincare Holdings, Inc. is a provider of oxygen and other respiratory therapy services to patients in the home. The firm serves roughly 700,000 customers in 47 states through 1,019 operating centers. The company also provides durable medical equipment and home infusion therapies in certain geographic markets. The firm's customers typically suffer from chronic obstructive pulmonary diseases (COPD), such as emphysema, chronic bronchitis or asthma, and require supplemental oxygen or other respiratory therapy services in order to alleviate the symptoms and discomfort of respiratory dysfunction. Lincare's home oxygen equipment comes in two variations. Oxygen concentrators are stationary units that provide a continuous flow of oxygen by filtering ordinary room air and are often supplemented with portable gaseous oxygen cylinders or liquid oxygen systems to meet the ambulatory or emergency needs of the customer. Liquid oxygen systems are thermally insulated containers of liquid oxygen, generally consisting of a stationary unit and a portable unit, which are most commonly used by customers with significant ambulatory requirements. Other respiratory therapy services offered by the company include nebulizers and associated respiratory medications, which provide aerosol therapy for customers suffering from COPD and asthma; non-invasive ventilation, which provides nocturnal ventilatory support for customers with neuromuscular disease and COPD; ventilators, which support respiratory function in severe cases of respiratory failure where the customer can no longer sustain the mechanics of breathing without the assistance of a machine; and continuous positive airway pressure devices, which maintain open airways in customer suffering from obstructive sleep apnea by providing airflow at prescribed pressures during sleep. Home infusion therapy products include parenteral nutrition, intravenous antibiotic therapy, enteral nutrition, chemotherapy, dobutamine infusions, immunoglobulin therapy, continuous pain management and central catheter management.

FINANCIALS: Sales and profits are in thousands of dollars—add 000 to get the full amount. 2007 Note: Financial information for 2007 was not available for all companies at press time.

2007 Sales: $1,595,990	2007 Profits: $226,077	**U.S. Stock Ticker: LNCR**
2006 Sales: $1,409,795	2006 Profits: $212,981	**Int'l Ticker:** Int'l Exchange:
2005 Sales: $1,266,627	2005 Profits: $213,696	Employees: 9,070
2004 Sales: $1,268,531	2004 Profits: $273,428	Fiscal Year Ends: 12/31
2003 Sales: $1,147,356	2003 Profits: $232,111	Parent Company:

SALARIES/BENEFITS:
Pension Plan:	ESOP Stock Plan:	Profit Sharing:	Top Exec. Salary: $840,483	Bonus: $756,435
Savings Plan: Y	Stock Purch. Plan: Y		Second Exec. Salary: $560,602	Bonus: $504,542

OTHER THOUGHTS:
Apparent Women Officers or Directors:
Hot Spot for Advancement for Women/Minorities:

LOCATIONS: ("Y" = Yes)
West:	Southwest:	Midwest:	Southeast:	Northeast:	International:
Y	Y	Y	Y	Y	

LINCOLN NATIONAL CORPORATION

www.lfg.com

Industry Group Code: 524113 Ranks within this company's industry group: Sales: Profits:

Management:		Sales/Marketing:		Liberal Arts:		Information Systems:		Professionals:		Technical/Scientific:	
Mgmt. Trainees:	Y	Mktg. Professionals:	Y	Gen. Writing/Editing:	Y	Info. Management:	Y	Finance/Accounting:	Y	Engineers, Elec.:	
Experienced Mgmt.:	Y	Retail Sales:		Technical Writing:		Software Dev.:	Y	Law:	Y	Engineers, Other:	
Int'l Business:	Y	Commercial/Industrial:	Y	Graphic Arts/Photog.:		Hardware Dev.:		HR/Other:	Y	Health/Lab:	
MBA Graduates:	Y	Sales Trainees:		Music:		Systems Integration:		Training:	Y	Scientists/Research:	Y
		Advertising Pros.:	Y	Broadcasting:		Consulting/Other:		Health Care:	Y	Petroleum/Chemicals:	
				Other:				Consulting:		Math/Other:	Y

TYPES OF BUSINESS:

Life Insurance
Investment Management
Retirement Plans
Mutual Funds
Financial Planning
Annuities

BRANDS/DIVISIONS/AFFILIATES:

Jefferson-Pilot Corp.
Lincoln UK
Lincoln Financial Media
Delaware Management Holdings, Inc.
Lincoln Variable Insurance Product
Jefferson Pilot Variable Fund
Lincoln American Legacy Retirement
Lincoln Director (The)

CONTACTS: *Note: Officers with more than one job title may be intentionally listed here more than once.*

Dennis R. Glass, CEO
Dennis R. Glass, Pres.
Frederick J. Crawford, CFO
Charles C. Cornelio, CIO/Sr. VP-Shared Svcs.
Dennis L. Schoff, General Counsel/Sr. VP
Lisa Marie DeSimone, VP-Corp. Dev.
Robert W. Dineen, Pres., Lincoln Financial Advisors
Patrick P. Coyne, Pres., Delaware Mgmt. Holdings, Inc.
J. Patrick Barrett, Chmn.
Michael Tallett-Williams, Chmn./Managing Dir.-Lincoln UK

Phone: 215-448-1400	Fax: 215-448-3962
Toll-Free: 877-275-5462	
Address: 1500 Market St., Ste. 3900, Philadelphia, PA 19102-2112 US	

GROWTH PLANS/SPECIAL FEATURES:

Lincoln National Corp. is a holding company operating multiple insurance and investment businesses. The operations of the firm's subsidiaries, collectively known as Lincoln Financial Group, are divided into four business segments: Individual Markets, Employer Markets, Investment Management and Lincoln U.K. The Individual Markets business provides its products through Individual Annuities, which provides broker-dealer services and tax-deferred investment growth and lifetime income opportunities through individual fixed annuities, indexed annuities and variable annuities; and Individual Life Insurance, which offers wealth protection and transfer opportunities through universal life, variable universal life, term insurance and linked-benefit product. Lincoln's Employer Markets division offers products focused on retirement income security through its Defined Contribution, Executive Benefits and Group Protection businesses. Some of its primary products cover corporate-owned life insurance, bank-owned life insurance, employer sponsored annuities and mutual fund programs, such as 401(k), 403(b) and 457 plans. These services are offered through the Lincoln American Legacy Retirement, The Lincoln Director, Lincoln Alliance and Multi-Fund products. The Investment Management segment provides mutual funds, investment advisory services and retirement plans to both individual and institutional investors through its subsidiary, Delaware Management Holdings, Inc. The company's Lincoln U.K. segment primarily offers unit-linked life and pension products throughout the U.K. In June 2007, Lincoln announced its intention to sell Lincoln Financial Media. Lincoln divested its television stations, sports programming and certain radio properties to various companies in late 2007 and early 2008. In May 2008, the firm launched its Lincoln 403(b)e SURE Advantage suite to help employers with new 403(b) regulations.

Lincoln employee benefits include medical, dental and vision insurance; domestic partner benefits; on-site fitness centers and massage therapy in certain locations; training programs and its Professional Development Program; tuition reimbursement; disability, life, accidental death and dismemberment insurance; alternative work schedules; adoption assistance; Homework Hotline; counseling services; and matching gifts.

FINANCIALS: Sales and profits are in thousands of dollars—add 000 to get the full amount. 2007 Note: Financial information for 2007 was not available for all companies at press time.

2007 Sales: $10,594,000	2007 Profits: $1,215,000	**U.S. Stock Ticker: LNC**
2006 Sales: $8,962,000	2006 Profits: $1,316,000	**Int'l Ticker:** Int'l Exchange:
2005 Sales: $5,475,000	2005 Profits: $831,055	Employees: 10,744
2004 Sales: $5,351,000	2004 Profits: $707,009	Fiscal Year Ends: 12/31
2003 Sales: $5,283,881	2003 Profits: $511,936	Parent Company:

SALARIES/BENEFITS:

Pension Plan:	ESOP Stock Plan:	Profit Sharing: Y	Top Exec. Salary: $925,000	Bonus: $7,393,423
Savings Plan: Y	Stock Purch. Plan:		Second Exec. Salary: $700,000	Bonus: $2,205,000

OTHER THOUGHTS:

Apparent Women Officers or Directors: 2
Hot Spot for Advancement for Women/Minorities: Y

LOCATIONS: ("Y" = Yes)

West:	Southwest:	Midwest:	Southeast:	Northeast:	International:
Y	Y	Y	Y	Y	Y

Note: Financial information, benefits and other data can change quickly and may vary from those stated here.

LKQ CORP

www.lkqcorp.com

Industry Group Code: 336300 Ranks within this company's industry group: Sales: 4 Profits: 4

Management:		Sales/Marketing:		Liberal Arts:		Information Systems:		Professionals:		Technical/Scientific:	
Mgmt. Trainees:		Mktg. Professionals:	Y	Gen. Writing/Editing:		Info. Management:	Y	Finance/Accounting:	Y	Engineers, Elec.:	
Experienced Mgmt.:	Y	Retail Sales:		Technical Writing:	Y	Software Dev.:		Law:	Y	Engineers, Other:	Y
Int'l Business:		Commercial/Industrial:	Y	Graphic Arts/Photog.:		Hardware Dev.:		HR/Other:	Y	Health/Lab:	
MBA Graduates:	Y	Sales Trainees:		Music:		Systems Integration:		Training:	Y	Scientists/Research:	
		Advertising Pros.:		Broadcasting:		Consulting/Other:		Health Care:		Petroleum/Chemicals:	
				Other:				Consulting:		Math/Other:	

TYPES OF BUSINESS:

Remanufactured OEM Parts
Aftermarket Replacement Parts
Vehicle Salvage
Scrap/Bulk Automotive Parts
Refurbished Aluminum Wheels

BRANDS/DIVISIONS/AFFILIATES:

Transwheel Corporation
Global Automotive Parts
Fit-Rite Body Parts & Affilliates
Pintendre Autos Inc
Keystone Automotive Industries Inc

CONTACTS: *Note: Officers with more than one job title may be intentionally listed here more than once.*

Joseph M. Holsten, CEO
Joseph M. Holsten, Pres.
Mark T. Spears, CFO/Exec. VP
Victor M. Casini, General Counsel/VP/Corp. Sec.
Walter P. Hanley, VP-Dev./Associate General Counsel/Assistant Sec.
Frank P. Erlain, VP-Finance/Controller
Leonard A. Damron, Sr. VP-Southeast Region
H. Bradley Willen, VP-Midwest Region
Steven H. Jones, VP-Central Region & Core Oper.
Robert L. Wagman, VP-Insurance Services & Aftermarket Oper.
Donald F. Flynn, Chmn.

Phone: 312-621-1950	**Fax:** 312-621-1969
Toll-Free: 877-557-2677	
Address: 120 N. LaSalle St., Ste. 3300, Chicago, IL 60602 US	

GROWTH PLANS/SPECIAL FEATURES:

LKQ Corporation is one of the largest providers of recycled OEM (original equipment manufacturer) automotive parts and related services in the U.S. LKQ operates approximately 300 facilities around the world. In the U.S., the company has a network of 70 locations that supply wholesale recycled OEM parts, 55 of which include a combination of processing, sales and redistribution operations, and 15 of which are primarily redistribution facilities. The firm's aftermarket parts business operates from facilities that serve as sales, warehousing or distribution centers, with a total of 191 facilities in the U.S. and Canada. LKQ has 27 locations providing self-service retail recycled vehicle products in Florida, Illinois, Oregon and Tennessee and three locations in Central America. LKQ's aftermarket business operates as Global Automotive Parts. The company refurbishes bumpers and wheels at 64 locations in the U.S. and Canada and one location in northeast Mexico. It also refurbishes head lamps and tail lamps at a facility in Grand Rapids, Michigan. The firm procures salvage vehicles, primarily at auctions, using its local professionals and centralized purchasing systems, and directly from insurance companies, automobile manufacturers and other suppliers. Once LKQ has received the proper title, assuring that the vehicles have not been stolen, it dismantles it for recycled parts. The firm's customers include collision and mechanical repair shops and, indirectly, insurance companies, including extended-warranty companies. LKQ's most popular products include engines, vehicle front-end assemblies, doors, transmissions, trunk lids, bumper assemblies, wheels, head and tail lamp assemblies, mirrors, fenders and axles. In July 2007, the company entered the Canadian market with the acquisition of Pintendre Autos, Inc., a recycled parts business near Quebec City, Canada. In October 2007, LKQ acquired Keystone Automotive Industries, Inc. In August 2008, the firm signed an agreement to acquire Pick-Your-Part Auto Wrecking, an auto recycler with nine recycling locations in California.

FINANCIALS: Sales and profits are in thousands of dollars—add 000 to get the full amount. 2007 Note: Financial information for 2007 was not available for all companies at press time.

2007 Sales: $1,126,825	2007 Profits: $65,901	**U.S. Stock Ticker: LKQX**
2006 Sales: $789,381	2006 Profits: $44,395	**Int'l Ticker:** Int'l Exchange:
2005 Sales: $547,392	2005 Profits: $30,887	Employees: 9,100
2004 Sales: $424,756	2004 Profits: $20,573	Fiscal Year Ends: 12/31
2003 Sales: $327,974	2003 Profits: $14,576	Parent Company:

SALARIES/BENEFITS:

Pension Plan:	ESOP Stock Plan:	Profit Sharing:	Top Exec. Salary: $550,000	Bonus: $1,312,266
Savings Plan: Y	Stock Purch. Plan:		Second Exec. Salary: $370,000	Bonus: $646,406

OTHER THOUGHTS:

Apparent Women Officers or Directors:
Hot Spot for Advancement for Women/Minorities:

LOCATIONS: ("Y" = Yes)

West:	Southwest:	Midwest:	Southeast:	Northeast:	International:
Y	Y	Y	Y	Y	

LOCKHEED MARTIN CORP

www.lockheedmartin.com

Industry Group Code: 336410 Ranks within this company's industry group: Sales: 3 Profits: 2

Management:		Sales/Marketing:		Liberal Arts:		Information Systems:		Professionals:		Technical/Scientific:	
Mgmt. Trainees:	Y	Mktg. Professionals:	Y	Gen. Writing/Editing:	Y	Info. Management:	Y	Finance/Accounting:	Y	Engineers, Elec.:	Y
Experienced Mgmt.:	Y	Retail Sales:		Technical Writing:	Y	Software Dev.:	Y	Law:	Y	Engineers, Other:	Y
Int'l Business:	Y	Commercial/Industrial:	Y	Graphic Arts/Photog.:	Y	Hardware Dev.:	Y	HR/Other:	Y	Health/Lab:	Y
MBA Graduates:	Y	Sales Trainees:		Music:		Systems Integration:	Y	Training:	Y	Scientists/Research:	Y
		Advertising Pros.:		Broadcasting:		Consulting/Other:	Y	Health Care:		Petroleum/Chemicals:	
				Other:				Consulting:	Y	Math/Other:	Y

TYPES OF BUSINESS:

Aerospace & Defense Technology
Military Aircraft
Defense Electronics
Systems Integration & Technology Services
Communications Satellites & Launch Services
Undersea, Shipboard, Land & Airborne Systems & Subsystems

BRANDS/DIVISIONS/AFFILIATES:

Orion
Skunk Works
Management Systens Designers, Inc.
RLM Systems, Ltd.
3Dsolve, Inc.

CONTACTS: Note: Officers with more than one job title may be intentionally listed here more than once.

Robert J. Stevens, CEO
Robert J. Stevens, Pres.
Bruce L. Tanner, CFO/Exec. VP
Linda Gooden, Exec. VP-Info. Systems & Global Svcs.
Ralph D. Heath, Exec. VP-Aeronautics
Christopher E. Kubasik, Exec. VP-Electronic Systems
Joanne M. Maguire, Exec. VP-Space Systems
Robert J. Stevens, Chmn.

Phone: 301-897-6000	Fax: 301-897-6704
Toll-Free:	
Address: 6801 Rockledge Dr., Bethesda, MD 20817 US	

GROWTH PLANS/SPECIAL FEATURES:

Lockheed Martin Corp. specializes in developing and servicing advanced technological systems. It serves domestic and international customers with products and services that have defense, civil and commercial applications, with principal customers being agencies of the U.S. government. The company operates in four segments: aeronautics; electronic systems; information systems & global services (IS&GS); and space systems. The aeronautics segment is engaged in the design, research and development, systems integration, production, sustainment, support and upgrade of advanced military aircraft, air vehicles and related technologies. Major products and programs include design, development, production and sustainment of the F-35 stealth multi-role international coalition fighter; the F-16 international multi-role fighter and U-2 high-altitude reconnaissance aircraft. It also produces major components for Japan's F-2 fighter and is a co-developer of the T-50 advanced jet trainer. The Skunk Works advanced development organization provides system solutions using rapid prototyping and advanced technologies. The electronic systems segment designs, researches, develops, integrates, produces and sustains systems and subsystems for undersea, shipboard, land and airborne applications. Major products include tactical missiles and weapon fire control systems; ground combat vehicle integrations; and surveillance and reconnaissance systems. The IS&GS segment provides federal services, IT solutions and technology expertise across a broad spectrum of applications and customers. It provides full life cycle support and highly specialized talent in the areas of software and systems engineering, including capabilities in space, air and ground systems, and also provides logistics, mission operations support, peacekeeping and nation-building services for a wide variety of U.S. defense and civil government agencies in the U.S. and abroad. The space systems segment designs, researches, develops, engineers and produces satellites, strategic and defensive missile systems and space transportation systems. In 2007, Lockheed acquired Management Systems Designers, Inc.; RLM Systems, Ltd.; and 3Dsolve, Inc.

FINANCIALS: Sales and profits are in thousands of dollars—add 000 to get the full amount. 2007 Note: Financial information for 2007 was not available for all companies at press time.

2007 Sales: $41,862,000	2007 Profits: $3,033,000	U.S. Stock Ticker: LMT
2006 Sales: $39,620,000	2006 Profits: $2,529,000	Int'l Ticker: Int'l Exchange:
2005 Sales: $37,213,000	2005 Profits: $1,825,000	Employees: 140,000
2004 Sales: $35,526,000	2004 Profits: $1,266,000	Fiscal Year Ends: 12/31
2003 Sales: $31,824,000	2003 Profits: $1,053,000	Parent Company:

SALARIES/BENEFITS:

Pension Plan:	ESOP Stock Plan:	Profit Sharing:	Top Exec. Salary: $1,627,500	Bonus: $12,400,000
Savings Plan: Y	Stock Purch. Plan:		Second Exec. Salary: $891,346	Bonus: $2,874,500

OTHER THOUGHTS:

Apparent Women Officers or Directors: 4
Hot Spot for Advancement for Women/Minorities: Y

LOCATIONS: ("Y" = Yes)

West:	Southwest:	Midwest:	Southeast:	Northeast:	International:
Y	Y	Y	Y	Y	Y

Note: Financial information, benefits and other data can change quickly and may vary from those stated here.

LODGIAN INC

www.lodgian.com

Industry Group Code: 721110 Ranks within this company's industry group: Sales: 5 Profits: 5

Management:		Sales/Marketing:		Liberal Arts:		Information Systems:		Professionals:		Technical/Scientific:	
Mgmt. Trainees:	Y	Mktg. Professionals:	Y	Gen. Writing/Editing:		Info. Management:	Y	Finance/Accounting:	Y	Engineers, Elec.:	
Experienced Mgmt.:	Y	Retail Sales:		Technical Writing:		Software Dev.:		Law:	Y	Engineers, Other:	
Int'l Business:	Y	Commercial/Industrial:		Graphic Arts/Photog.:		Hardware Dev.:		HR/Other:	Y	Health/Lab:	
MBA Graduates:	Y	Sales Trainees:		Music:		Systems Integration:	Y	Training:	Y	Scientists/Research:	
		Advertising Pros.:		Broadcasting:		Consulting/Other:		Health Care:		Petroleum/Chemicals:	
				Other:				Consulting:		Math/Other:	

TYPES OF BUSINESS:

Hotels

BRANDS/DIVISIONS/AFFILIATES:

InterContinental Hotels Group plc
Marriott International Inc
Hilton Group plc
Wyndham Worldwide
Crowne Plaza
Holiday Inn
Courtyard by Marriott
Residence Inn by Marriott

CONTACTS: Note: Officers with more than one job title may be intentionally listed here more than once.

Peter T. Cyrus, Interim CEO
Peter T. Cyrus, Interim Pres.
James A. MacLennan, CFO/Exec. VP
Carol L. Mayne, VP-Human Resources
Daniel Webber, Interim VP-IT
Daniel E. (Dan) Ellis, General Counsel/Corp. Sec./Sr. VP
James R. McGrath, VP-Hotel Oper.
Susan King, VP-Franchise Comm.
Deborah N. (Debi) Ethridge, VP-Investor Rel. & Finance
Donna B. Cohen, Controller/VP
Barbra Beaulieu, VP-Internal Audit & Controls
Kevin B. Richards, VP-Asset Mgmt.
Stewart J. Brown, Chmn.

Phone: 404-364-9400	Fax: 404-364-6144
Toll-Free:	
Address: 3445 Peachtree Rd. NE, Ste. 700, Atlanta, GA 30326 US	

GROWTH PLANS/SPECIAL FEATURES:

Lodgian, Inc. is an independent owner and operator of 46 hotels containing 8,432 rooms located in 24 states and Canada. Of its hotels, 35 are held for use and 11 are held for sale. One of the firm's hotels is operated in a joint venture in which a subsidiary serves as the general partner and has a 50% voting interest. Lodgian operates substantially all of its hotels under nationally recognized brands, with 25 operated under franchises obtained from InterContinental Hotels Group, with brands including Crowne Plaza, Holiday Inn, Holiday Inn Select and Holiday Inn Express; 12 operated under franchises from Marriott International, with brands including Marriott, Courtyard by Marriott, Fairfield Inn by Marriott, Residence Inn by Marriott and SpringHill Suites by Marriott; seven operated under other nationally recognized brands, including Hilton and Wyndham; and two non-branded. The company's hotels are primarily full-service properties that offer food and beverage services; meeting and banquet facilities; and compete in the midscale and upscale market segments of the lodging industry. Lodgian operates hotel brands in the Upper Upscale; Upscale; Midscale with Food & Beverage; and Midscale without Food & Beverage segments. Transient revenues, derived from guests staying only for brief periods of time without a long-term contract, generated roughly 71% of the firm's 2007 room revenues, while groups generated 23% and contract revenues (such as contracts with airlines for crew rooms) generated 6%. In June 2007, Lodgian sold 16 hotels to Kronos Hotels & Resorts for $64.9 million. In July 2007, the firm sold two Holiday Inn hotels for an aggregate price of $5.6 million. An additional five hotels are planned to be sold, three of which are currently under contract and two of which are being actively marketed.

Lodgian offers its employees educational assistance, hotel discounts and medical, dental, vision and disability insurance.

FINANCIALS: Sales and profits are in thousands of dollars—add 000 to get the full amount. 2007 Note: Financial information for 2007 was not available for all companies at press time.

2007 Sales: $278,079	2007 Profits: $-8,446	U.S. Stock Ticker: LGN	
2006 Sales: $261,785	2006 Profits: $-15,176	Int'l Ticker:	Int'l Exchange:
2005 Sales: $222,762	2005 Profits: $12,301	Employees: 3,444	
2004 Sales: $217,189	2004 Profits: $-31,834	Fiscal Year Ends: 12/31	
2003 Sales: $301,398	2003 Profits: $-31,677	Parent Company:	

SALARIES/BENEFITS:

Pension Plan:	ESOP Stock Plan:	Profit Sharing:	Top Exec. Salary: $590,164	Bonus: $220,000
Savings Plan: Y	Stock Purch. Plan:		Second Exec. Salary: $300,000	Bonus: $120,000

OTHER THOUGHTS:

Apparent Women Officers or Directors: 5
Hot Spot for Advancement for Women/Minorities: Y

LOCATIONS: ("Y" = Yes)

West:	Southwest:	Midwest:	Southeast:	Northeast:	International:
Y	Y	Y	Y	Y	Y

LOEWS CORPORATION

www.loews.com

Industry Group Code: 524126 **Ranks within this company's industry group:** Sales: Profits:

Management:		Sales/Marketing:		Liberal Arts:		Information Systems:		Professionals:		Technical/Scientific:	
Mgmt. Trainees:	Y	Mktg. Professionals:	Y	Gen. Writing/Editing:	Y	Info. Management:	Y	Finance/Accounting:	Y	Engineers, Elec.:	
Experienced Mgmt.:	Y	Retail Sales:		Technical Writing:		Software Dev.:	Y	Law:	Y	Engineers, Other:	Y
Int'l Business:	Y	Commercial/Industrial:	Y	Graphic Arts/Photog.:		Hardware Dev.:		HR/Other:	Y	Health/Lab:	
MBA Graduates:	Y	Sales Trainees:		Music:		Systems Integration:		Training:	Y	Scientists/Research:	Y
		Advertising Pros.:	Y	Broadcasting:		Consulting/Other:		Health Care:		Petroleum/Chemicals:	
				Other:				Consulting:		Math/Other:	Y

TYPES OF BUSINESS:
Direct Property & Casualty Insurance
Natural Gas Exploration & Production
Offshore Oil & Gas Drilling
Hotel Operation
Drilling Rigs

BRANDS/DIVISIONS/AFFILIATES:
CNA Financial Corp.
Lorillard Inc
Loews Hotels Holding Corporation
Diamond Offshore Drilling, Inc.
Bulova Corp.
Boardwalk Pipeline Partners, LP
HighMount Exploration & Production, LLC

CONTACTS: *Note: Officers with more than one job title may be intentionally listed here more than once.*
James S. Tisch, CEO
James S. Tisch, Pres.
Peter W. Keegan, CFO/Sr. VP
Alan Momeyer, VP-Human Resources
Gary Garson, General Counsel/Sr. VP/Sec.
Jonathan Nathanson, VP-Corp. Dev.
Susan Becker, VP-Tax
Jonathan M. Tisch, Co-Chmn.
Jonathan M. Tisch, CEO/Chmn., Loews Hotels
Mark Schwartz, Controller
Lisa Hess, VP-Chief Investment Officer
Andrew H. Tisch, Co-Chmn.

Phone: 212-521-2000	Fax: 212-521-2525
Toll-Free:	
Address: 667 Madison Ave., New York, NY 10065-8087 US	

GROWTH PLANS/SPECIAL FEATURES:
Loews Corp. is the holding company of CNA Financial Corp.; Boardwalk Pipeline Partners, LP; Diamond Offshore Drilling, Inc.; Loews Hotels Holdings Corp.; and HighMount Exploration & Production, LLC. CNA Financial, a 90% owned subsidiary, is an insurance holding company. CNA's property and casualty insurance operations are conducted by Continental Casualty Co. and its affiliate The Continental Insurance Co. Boardwalk Pipeline, a 70% owned subsidiary, is engaged in the interstate transportation and storage of natural gas. The subsidiary conducts its operations through two subsidiaries: Texas Gas Transmission LLC, which operates roughly 5,850 miles of natural gas pipeline located in Louisiana, Texas, Arkansas, Mississippi, Tennessee, Kentucky, Indiana, Ohio and Illinois; and Gulf South Pipeline, LP, which operates about 7,700 miles of natural gas pipeline located in Texas, Louisiana, Mississippi, Alabama and Florida. Diamond Offshore, a 51% owned subsidiary, owns and operates drilling rigs that are used in the drilling of offshore oil and gas wells on a contract basis for companies that explore and produce hydrocarbons. The subsidiary owns 44 offshore rigs, of which 30 are semi-submersible. Loews Hotels, a wholly-owned subsidiary, operates 18 hotels, including Loews Annapolis; Hard Rock Hotel in Orlando, Florida; The Regency in New York; and Loews Hotel Vogue in Montreal, Canada. HighMount Exploration, a wholly-owned subsidiary, explores and produces natural gas. In July 2007, Loews established subsidiary HighMount Exploration, which acquired natural gas and exploration and production assets from Dominion Resources for $4 billion. In late 2007, the firm announced plans to spin off Lorillard, Inc., its cigarettes producing subsidiary, to holders of its Carolina Group stock and Loews common stock. In January 2008, the company agreed to sell Bulova Corp., its watch and clock distribution subsidiary, to Citizen Watch Company for approximately $250 million.

FINANCIALS: Sales and profits are in thousands of dollars—add 000 to get the full amount. 2007 Note: Financial information for 2007 was not available for all companies at press time.

2007 Sales: $18,380,000	2007 Profits: $2,489,000	**U.S. Stock Ticker: L**	
2006 Sales: $17,702,000	2006 Profits: $2,491,300	**Int'l Ticker:** Int'l Exchange:	
2005 Sales: $16,017,800	2005 Profits: $1,211,600	Employees: 21,600	
2004 Sales: $15,236,900	2004 Profits: $1,215,800	Fiscal Year Ends: 12/31	
2003 Sales: $16,459,700	2003 Profits: $-597,200	Parent Company:	

SALARIES/BENEFITS:

Pension Plan:	ESOP Stock Plan:	Profit Sharing:	Top Exec. Salary: $1,275,000	Bonus: $1,500,000
Savings Plan: Y	Stock Purch. Plan:		Second Exec. Salary: $990,000	Bonus: $1,010,000

OTHER THOUGHTS:
Apparent Women Officers or Directors: 4
Hot Spot for Advancement for Women/Minorities: Y

LOCATIONS: ("Y" = Yes)

West:	Southwest:	Midwest:	Southeast:	Northeast:	International:
Y	Y	Y	Y	Y	Y

Note: Financial information, benefits and other data can change quickly and may vary from those stated here.

LOWE'S COMPANIES INC
www.lowes.com

Industry Group Code: 444110 Ranks within this company's industry group: Sales: 2 Profits: 2

Management:		Sales/Marketing:		Liberal Arts:		Information Systems:		Professionals:		Technical/Scientific:	
Mgmt. Trainees:	Y	Mktg. Professionals:	Y	Gen. Writing/Editing:	Y	Info. Management:	Y	Finance/Accounting:	Y	Engineers, Elec.:	
Experienced Mgmt.:	Y	Retail Sales:	Y	Technical Writing:	Y	Software Dev.:	Y	Law:	Y	Engineers, Other:	
Int'l Business:	Y	Commercial/Industrial:	Y	Graphic Arts/Photog.:	Y	Hardware Dev.:		HR/Other:	Y	Health/Lab:	
MBA Graduates:	Y	Sales Trainees:	Y	Music:		Systems Integration:		Training:	Y	Scientists/Research:	
		Advertising Pros.:	Y	Broadcasting:		Consulting/Other:		Health Care:		Petroleum/Chemicals:	
				Other:				Consulting:		Math/Other:	

TYPES OF BUSINESS:
Home Centers, Retail
Home Improvement Products
Home Installation Services
Special Order Sales

BRANDS/DIVISIONS/AFFILIATES:

CONTACTS:
Note: Officers with more than one job title may be intentionally listed here more than once.
Robert A. Niblock, CEO
Larry D. Stone, COO
Larry D. Stone, Pres.
Robert F. Hull, Jr., CFO/Exec. VP
Robert J. Gfeller, Jr., Sr. VP-Mktg. & Advertising
Maureen K. Ausura, Sr. VP-Human Resources
Steven M. Stone, CIO/Sr. VP
Charles W. (Nick) Canter, Jr., Exec. VP-Merch.
Gaither M. Keener, Jr., General Counsel/Sr. VP/Corp. Sec.
Michael K. Brown, Exec. VP-Store Oper.
Gregory M. Bridgeford, Exec. VP-Bus. Dev.
N. Brian Peace, Sr. VP-Corp. Affairs
Michael V. Hollifield, Chief Acct. Officer/Sr. VP
Theresa A. Anderson, Sr. VP/Gen. Merch. Manager-Home Decor
Scott C. Butterfield, Sr. VP-Research & Strategic Planning
Marshall A. Croom, Sr. VP-Merch. & Store Support
Clinton T. Davis, Sr. VP/Gen. Merch. Manager-Hardlines
Robert A. Niblock, Chmn.
Joseph M. (Mike) Mabry, Jr., Exec. VP-Logistics & Distribution

Phone: 704-758-1000	Fax:
Toll-Free: 800-445-6937	
Address: 1000 Lowe's Blvd., Mooresville, NC 28117 US	

GROWTH PLANS/SPECIAL FEATURES:

Lowe's Companies, Inc., a Fortune 50 company, is one of the largest home improvement retailers in the world. The company owns approximately 1,577 superstores in 50 states and Canada, each carrying approximately 40,000 products. Hundreds of thousands of items are also available through the firm's special order system. Lowe's stores chiefly serve do-it-yourself homeowners and commercial business customers, including contractors, landscapers, electricians, painters and plumbers. Each Lowe's store carries a wide selection of national brand name merchandise such as KitchenAid, Samsung, Whirlpool, Pella, Werner, Kohler, DeWalt, JohnDeere, Troy-Bilt, Jenn-Air and Bosch, as well as exclusive brand names such as Premier Living, Kobalt, Portfolio, Harbor Breeze, Reliabilt, Perfect Flams and Top Choice Lumber. The company's website, Lowes.com, facilitates customers researching, comparing and buying Lowe's products and services. Lowes recently completed the remerchandising of 116 of its earlier format stores to make them more closely resemble its most current store prototypes. The remerchandising efforts focused on moving entire departments, improving adjacencies, replacing or refurbishing the selling centers, adding interior signage and installing self check-out in each of the remerchandised stores. As part of its expansion strategy, Lowe's opened 153 stores in 2007 that included two primary prototypes, a 117,000-square-foot store for large markets and a 94,000-square-foot store to serve smaller markets. In January 2007, the company announced plans to expand into Mexico, expecting to open three to five new stores in Monterrey in fiscal year 2009. For 2008, Lowe's planned to open as many as 120 new stores. However, the slowing of the real estate and construction sector is negatively affecting Lowe's, and stores openings may be delayed as a result.

Lowe's offers its employees merchandise discounts, a pre-paid legal plan, group auto and home insurance, employee assistance, discounted auto purchases, mortgage assistance, flexible spending accounts and relocation assistance.

FINANCIALS:
Sales and profits are in thousands of dollars—add 000 to get the full amount. 2007 Note: Financial information for 2007 was not available for all companies at press time.

2007 Sales: $46,927,000	2007 Profits: $3,105,000	**U.S. Stock Ticker:** LOW
2006 Sales: $43,243,000	2006 Profits: $2,765,000	**Int'l Ticker:** Int'l Exchange:
2005 Sales: $36,464,000	2005 Profits: $2,167,000	Employees: 210,000
2004 Sales: $30,838,000	2004 Profits: $877,000	Fiscal Year Ends: 1/31
2003 Sales: $26,492,000	2003 Profits: $1,471,000	Parent Company:

SALARIES/BENEFITS:

Pension Plan:	ESOP Stock Plan:	Profit Sharing:	Top Exec. Salary: $950,000	Bonus: $1,037,875
Savings Plan: Y	Stock Purch. Plan: Y		Second Exec. Salary: $770,039	Bonus: $491,360

OTHER THOUGHTS:
Apparent Women Officers or Directors: 5
Hot Spot for Advancement for Women/Minorities: Y

LOCATIONS: ("Y" = Yes)

West:	Southwest:	Midwest:	Southeast:	Northeast:	International:
Y	Y	Y	Y	Y	Y

MACY'S INC

www.fds.com

Industry Group Code: 452110 **Ranks within this company's industry group:** Sales: 1   Profits: 1

Management:		Sales/Marketing:		Liberal Arts:		Information Systems:		Professionals:		Technical/Scientific:	
Mgmt. Trainees:	Y	Mktg. Professionals:	Y	Gen. Writing/Editing:	Y	Info. Management:	Y	Finance/Accounting:	Y	Engineers, Elec.:	
Experienced Mgmt.:	Y	Retail Sales:	Y	Technical Writing:		Software Dev.:		Law:	Y	Engineers, Other:	
Int'l Business:	Y	Commercial/Industrial:		Graphic Arts/Photog.:	Y	Hardware Dev.:		HR/Other:	Y	Health/Lab:	
MBA Graduates:	Y	Sales Trainees:	Y	Music:		Systems Integration:		Training:	Y	Scientists/Research:	
		Advertising Pros.:	Y	Broadcasting:		Consulting/Other:		Health Care:		Petroleum/Chemicals:	
				Other:				Consulting:		Math/Other:	

TYPES OF BUSINESS:

Department Stores
Bridal & Formalwear Stores
Direct Marketing
Online Sales
Catalogs
Wedding Planning & Bridal Registries
Credit Services
Furniture Stores

BRANDS/DIVISIONS/AFFILIATES:

Federated Department Stores, Inc.
Macy's
Bloomingdale's
May's Department Stores

CONTACTS: *Note: Officers with more than one job title may be intentionally listed here more than once.*

Terry J. Lundgren, CEO
Terry J. Lundgren, Pres.
Karen M. Hoguet, CFO/Exec. VP
David W. Clark, Sr. VP-Human Resources
Dennis J. Broderick, General Counsel/Sr. VP/Sec.
Amy Hanson, Sr. VP-Property Dev.
James A. Sluzewski, VP-Corp. Comm. & External Affairs
Joel A. Belsky, Controller
William L. Hawthorne, III, Chief Diversity Officer & Legal Affairs
Cynthia Ray Walker, VP-Area Research
Felicia Williams, VP-Internal Audit
Gary J. Nay, VP-Real Estate
Terry J. Lundgren, Chmn.

Phone: 513-579-7000	**Fax:** 513-579-7555
Toll-Free: 800-261-5385	
Address: 7 W. 7th St., Cincinnati, OH 45202 US	

GROWTH PLANS/SPECIAL FEATURES:

Macy's, Inc., formerly Federated Department Stores, Inc., is a U.S. operator of full-line department stores with more than 853 stores in 45 states, Washington, DC, Guam and Puerto Rico. Macy's department stores offer a variety of merchandise, including men's, women's and children's apparel and accessories; cosmetics; home furnishings; and other consumer goods. Through its Bloomingdale's and Macy's stores, the firm conducts direct-to-customer catalog and e-commerce businesses under the names Bloomingdale's By Mail, bloomingdales.com and macys.com. Additionally, the company offers online bridal registry and gift purchase facilities to customers. Macy's Home Store, LLC, a wholly-owned indirect subsidiary of the firm, is responsible for the overall strategy, merchandising and marketing of home-related merchandise categories of all Macy's stores. Feminine accessories, intimate apparel, shoes and cosmetics generated 36% of revenue in 2007, while feminine apparel; men's and children's; and home/miscellaneous generated 27%, 22% and 15%, respectively. By the end of 2006, Macy's re-branded the department stores, as well as the bridal and formalwear stores, that it had acquired from May's Department Stores, including Foley's, Kaufmann's, Hecht's, Marshall Field's, Strawbridge's and Meier & Frank, to either Macy's or Bloomingdale's. In June 2007, the company changed its name to Macy's, Inc.

FINANCIALS: Sales and profits are in thousands of dollars—add 000 to get the full amount. 2007 Note: Financial information for 2007 was not available for all companies at press time.

2007 Sales: $26,970,000		2007 Profits: $995,000		**U.S. Stock Ticker: M**	
2006 Sales: $22,390,000		2006 Profits: $1,406,000		**Int'l Ticker:** Int'l Exchange:	
2005 Sales: $15,776,000		2005 Profits: $689,000		Employees: 188,000	
2004 Sales: $15,412,000		2004 Profits: $693,000		Fiscal Year Ends: 1/31	
2003 Sales: $15,435,000		2003 Profits: $818,000		Parent Company:	

SALARIES/BENEFITS:

Pension Plan:	ESOP Stock Plan:	Profit Sharing:	Top Exec. Salary: $1,383,333	Bonus: $2,704,800
Savings Plan:	Stock Purch. Plan:		Second Exec. Salary: $1,042,500	Bonus: $1,039,300

OTHER THOUGHTS:

Apparent Women Officers or Directors: 8
Hot Spot for Advancement for Women/Minorities: Y

LOCATIONS: ("Y" = Yes)

West:	Southwest:	Midwest:	Southeast:	Northeast:	International:
Y	Y	Y	Y	Y	Y

Note: Financial information, benefits and other data can change quickly and may vary from those stated here.

MANOR CARE INC

www.hcr-manorcare.com

Industry Group Code: 623110 Ranks within this company's industry group: Sales: 2 Profits: 1

Management:		Sales/Marketing:		Liberal Arts:		Information Systems:		Professionals:		Technical/Scientific:	
Mgmt. Trainees:	Y	Mktg. Professionals:	Y	Gen. Writing/Editing:	Y	Info. Management:	Y	Finance/Accounting:	Y	Engineers, Elec.:	
Experienced Mgmt.:	Y	Retail Sales:		Technical Writing:		Software Dev.:		Law:	Y	Engineers, Other:	Y
Int'l Business:	Y	Commercial/Industrial:		Graphic Arts/Photog.:		Hardware Dev.:		HR/Other:	Y	Health/Lab:	
MBA Graduates:	Y	Sales Trainees:		Music:		Systems Integration:		Training:	Y	Scientists/Research:	
		Advertising Pros.:		Broadcasting:		Consulting/Other:		Health Care:	Y	Petroleum/Chemicals:	
				Other:				Consulting:		Math/Other:	

TYPES OF BUSINESS:

Long-Term Health Care/Nursing Homes
Home Health Care
Short-Term Care Facilities
Assisted Living Facilities
Rehabilitation Clinics

BRANDS/DIVISIONS/AFFILIATES:

HCR Manor Care
Springhouse
Heartland
HCR Manor Care Foundation
ManorCare
Arden Courts
ManorCare Health Services

CONTACTS: Note: Officers with more than one job title may be intentionally listed here more than once.

Paul A. Ormond, CEO
Paul A. Ormond, Pres.
Paul A. Ormond, Chmn.

Phone: 419-252-5500	Fax: 419-252-5554
Toll-Free:	
Address: 333 N. Summit St., Toledo, OH 43604-2617 US	

GROWTH PLANS/SPECIAL FEATURES:

Manor Care, Inc. provides a range of health care services, including skilled nursing care, assisted living, post-acute medical and rehabilitation care, hospice care, home health care and rehabilitation therapy. Manor Care operates 278 skilled nursing facilities and 65 assisted living facilities in 30 states, with 62% of its facilities located in Florida, Illinois, Michigan, Ohio and Pennsylvania. These facilities primarily operate under the names Heartland, ManorCare Health Services and Arden Courts. Manor Care's long-term care services consist of skilled nursing centers, assisted living services, post-acute medical and rehabilitation care and Alzheimer's care. The skilled nursing centers use interdisciplinary teams of experienced medical professionals, including registered nurses, licensed practical nurses and certified nursing assistants, to provide services prescribed by physicians. Other services include the design of Quality of Life programs to give the highest practicable level of functional independence to patients, provide physical, speech, respiratory and occupational therapy and provide quality nutrition services, social services, activities and housekeeping and laundry services. Manor Care's assisted living services provide personal care services and assistance with general activities of daily living such as dressing, bathing, meal preparation and medication management. Manor Care provides hospice and home health care through 116 offices in 25 states focusing on the physical, spiritual and psychosocial needs of individuals facing a life-limiting illness. Other health care services include outpatient rehabilitation therapy, which it provides in its 92 outpatient therapy clinics located in Midwestern and Mid-Atlantic states, Texas and Florida as well as through work sites, schools, hospitals and other health care settings. In December 2007, the firm was acquired by private equity firm, the Carlyle Group for roughly $6.3 billion.

Manor's employee benefits include tuition reimbursement, access to a credit union, retirement benefits and medical, dental, prescription drug and vision coverage.

FINANCIALS: Sales and profits are in thousands of dollars—add 000 to get the full amount. 2007 Note: Financial information for 2007 was not available for all companies at press time.

2007 Sales: $	2007 Profits: $	U.S. Stock Ticker: Private
2006 Sales: $3,613,185	2006 Profits: $169,560	Int'l Ticker: Int'l Exchange:
2005 Sales: $3,417,290	2005 Profits: $160,955	Employees: 59,500
2004 Sales: $3,208,867	2004 Profits: $168,222	Fiscal Year Ends: 12/31
2003 Sales: $3,029,441	2003 Profits: $119,007	Parent Company: CARLYLE GROUP (THE)

SALARIES/BENEFITS:

Pension Plan: Y	ESOP Stock Plan:	Profit Sharing:	Top Exec. Salary: $1,000,550	Bonus: $2,864,500
Savings Plan: Y	Stock Purch. Plan:		Second Exec. Salary: $639,015	Bonus: $1,429,000

OTHER THOUGHTS:

Apparent Women Officers or Directors:
Hot Spot for Advancement for Women/Minorities: Y

LOCATIONS: ("Y" = Yes)

West:	Southwest:	Midwest:	Southeast:	Northeast:	International:
Y	Y	Y	Y	Y	

MANPOWER INC
www.manpower.com

Industry Group Code: 561320 Ranks within this company's industry group: Sales: 1 Profits: 1

Management:		Sales/Marketing:		Liberal Arts:		Information Systems:		Professionals:		Technical/Scientific:	
Mgmt. Trainees:	Y	Mktg. Professionals:	Y	Gen. Writing/Editing:	Y	Info. Management:	Y	Finance/Accounting:	Y	Engineers, Elec.:	Y
Experienced Mgmt.:	Y	Retail Sales:		Technical Writing:	Y	Software Dev.:	Y	Law:	Y	Engineers, Other:	Y
Int'l Business:	Y	Commercial/Industrial:	Y	Graphic Arts/Photog.:	Y	Hardware Dev.:		HR/Other:	Y	Health/Lab:	Y
MBA Graduates:	Y	Sales Trainees:	Y	Music:		Systems Integration:	Y	Training:	Y	Scientists/Research:	Y
		Advertising Pros.:	Y	Broadcasting:		Consulting/Other:	Y	Health Care:	Y	Petroleum/Chemicals:	
				Other:				Consulting:		Math/Other:	Y

TYPES OF BUSINESS:

Staffing & Temporary Help
Employee Testing, Training & Development
Internal Audit, Accounting & Tax Services
Organizational Performance Consulting
IT Recruitment & Managed Services
Business Function Outsourcing
Market Research

BRANDS/DIVISIONS/AFFILIATES:

Manpower Professional
Elan
Right Management
Jefferson Wells
Clarendon Parker Middle East FZ LLC
Vitae
CRI, Inc.
Global Learning Center

CONTACTS: Note: Officers with more than one job title may be intentionally listed here more than once.

Jeffrey A. Joerres, CEO
Jeffrey A. Joerres, Pres.
Michael J. Van Handel, CFO/Exec. VP
Emma van Rooyen, VP-Global Mktg.
Mara Swan, Sr. VP-Global Human Resources
Rick Davidson, CIO/Sr. VP
Kenneth C. Hunt, General Counsel/Corp. Sec./Sr. VP
Tammy Johns, Sr. VP-Workforce Strategy
David Arkless, Sr. VP-Global Corp. Affairs
Owen J. Sullivan, Exec. VP/CEO-Right Mgmt. Consultants, Inc.
Francoise Gri, Exec. VP/Managing Dir.-France
Darryl E. Green, Exec. VP/Pres., Asia-Pacific
Jonas Prising, Exec. VP-U.S. & Canadian Oper.
Jeffrey A. Joerres, Chmn.
Barbara J. Beck, Pres., EMEA/Exec. VP

Phone: 414-961-1000	Fax: 414-961-7081
Toll-Free:	
Address: 100 Manpower Pl., Milwaukee, WI 53212 US	

GROWTH PLANS/SPECIAL FEATURES:

Manpower, Inc. is a world leader in the employment services industry, with a global network of roughly 4,500 offices in 80 countries and territories. Manpower offers permanent, temporary and contract recruitment; employee assessment and selection; training; outplacement; outsourcing; consulting; and professional services. The company's recruitment services are offered under the Manpower, Manpower Professional and Elan brands. Under its Right Management brand, Manpower provides transition services and organizational consulting services. The company's transition services range from advising employers on severance packages to assisting displaced employees with resume writing, networking and interviewing skills. Its organizational consulting services use customized tools, interventions and workshops to drive organizational effectiveness, employee engagement and alignment of the workforce. The firm's Jefferson Wells brand is an alternative to public accounting firms and other consulting groups, providing project professionals along four primary solution areas: Internal controls, tax, technology risk management and finance and accounting. During 2007, Manpower found permanent and temporary jobs for nearly 5 million people with its roughly 400,000 clients. Manpower's largest operations are located in Australia, Japan, Mexico, Argentina and Canada, with additional operations located throughout the Americas and Asia. The firm primarily supplies workers to the office (representing 55% of recruitment revenues), industrial (25%) and technical (20%) markets. In January 2008, Right Management opened a new office in Geneva, Switzerland. Manpower acquired Clarendon Parker Middle East FZ LLC, a recruitment provider for the U.A.E., Bahrain, Kuwait, Qatar and Saudi Arabia, in January 2008. In March 2008, Manpower acquired Vitae, a professional placement firm with 10 locations in the Netherlands. Manpower agreed to acquire CRI, Inc., a Los Angeles-based recruitment process outsourcing service provider, in March 2008.

Manpower's Global Learning Center provides Manpower employees with free online access to over 3,600 Direct Training courses, covering subjects in many languages and fields.

FINANCIALS: Sales and profits are in thousands of dollars—add 000 to get the full amount. 2007 Note: Financial information for 2007 was not available for all companies at press time.

2007 Sales: $20,500,300	2007 Profits: $484,700	**U.S. Stock Ticker: MAN**
2006 Sales: $17,562,500	2006 Profits: $398,000	**Int'l Ticker:** Int'l Exchange:
2005 Sales: $15,845,400	2005 Profits: $260,100	Employees: 33,000
2004 Sales: $14,675,000	2004 Profits: $245,700	Fiscal Year Ends: 12/31
2003 Sales: $12,184,500	2003 Profits: $137,700	Parent Company:

SALARIES/BENEFITS:

Pension Plan:	ESOP Stock Plan:	Profit Sharing:	Top Exec. Salary: $1,000,000	Bonus: $2,801,333
Savings Plan: Y	Stock Purch. Plan: Y		Second Exec. Salary: $500,000	Bonus: $932,111

OTHER THOUGHTS:

Apparent Women Officers or Directors: 7
Hot Spot for Advancement for Women/Minorities: Y

LOCATIONS: ("Y" = Yes)

West:	Southwest:	Midwest:	Southeast:	Northeast:	International:
Y	Y	Y	Y	Y	Y

Note: Financial information, benefits and other data can change quickly and may vary from those stated here.

MARATHON OIL CORP

www.marathon.com

Industry Group Code: 211111 Ranks within this company's industry group: Sales: 5 Profits: 4

Management:		Sales/Marketing:		Liberal Arts:		Information Systems:		Professionals:		Technical/Scientific:	
Mgmt. Trainees:	Y	Mktg. Professionals:	Y	Gen. Writing/Editing:		Info. Management:	Y	Finance/Accounting:	Y	Engineers, Elec.:	Y
Experienced Mgmt.:	Y	Retail Sales:		Technical Writing:		Software Dev.:		Law:	Y	Engineers, Other:	
Int'l Business:	Y	Commercial/Industrial:	Y	Graphic Arts/Photog.:		Hardware Dev.:		HR/Other:	Y	Health/Lab:	Y
MBA Graduates:	Y	Sales Trainees:		Music:		Systems Integration:		Training:	Y	Scientists/Research:	
		Advertising Pros.:		Broadcasting:		Consulting/Other:		Health Care:		Petroleum/Chemicals:	Y
				Other:				Consulting:		Math/Other:	

TYPES OF BUSINESS:

Oil & Gas Exploration & Production
Petroleum Marketing, Refining & Transportation
Gas Stations
Energy Marketing

BRANDS/DIVISIONS/AFFILIATES:

Marathon Petroleum Company LLC
Western Oil Sands Inc

CONTACTS: *Note: Officers with more than one job title may be intentionally listed here more than once.*

Clarence P. Cazalot, Jr., CEO
Clarence P. Cazalot, Jr., Pres.
Janet F. Clark, CFO/Exec. VP
Eileen M. Campbell, VP-Human Resources
Thomas K. Sneed, CIO
William F. Schwind, Jr., General Counsel/VP/Sec.
David E. Roberts, Jr, Sr. VP-Bus. Dev.
Howard J. Thill, VP-Public Affairs
Howard J. Thill, VP-Investor Rel.
Paul C. Reinbolt, VP-Finance/Treas.
Steven B. Hinchman, Sr. VP-Worldwide Prod.
Michael K. Stewart, VP-Acct./Controller
Daniel J. Sullenbarger, VP-Corp. Responsibility
Stephen J. Landry, VP-Tax
Thomas J. Usher, Chmn.

Phone: 713-629-6600	Fax: 713-296-2952
Toll-Free:	
Address: 5555 San Felipe St., Houston, TX 77056 US	

GROWTH PLANS/SPECIAL FEATURES:

Marathon Oil Corp. explores for crude oil and natural gas worldwide, operates refineries and maintains U.S. retail gas outlets. It operates in four segments: Exploration and products (E&P); oil sands mining (OSM); refining, marketing and transportation (RM&T); and integrated gas (IG). The E&P segment explores for, produces and markets liquid hydrocarbons and natural gas on a worldwide basis. It conducts its exploration, development and production activities in 11 countries. Principal exploration activities are in the U.S., Angola, Norway and Indonesia. Principal development and production activities are in the U.S., the U.K., Norway, Ireland, Equatorial Guinea and Libya. In 2007, the division's net sales averaged 351,000 barrels of oil equivalent per day. The OSM segment mines, extracts and transports bitumen from oil sands deposits in Alberta, Canada, and upgrades the bitumen to produce and market synthetic crude oil and by-products. The RM&T segment refines, markets and transports crude oil and petroleum products, primarily in the Midwest, upper Great Plain, Gulf Coast and Southeastern regions of the U.S. The IG segments markets and transports products manufactured from natural gas, such as liquefied natural gas and methanol, on a worldwide basis; and is developing other projects to link stranded natural gas resources with demanded areas. In January 2007, through Marathon Petroleum Norge AS and its Volund project partner, Marathon was approved by the Norwegian Ministry of Petroleum and Energy to develop and operate the Volund field with production slated for the second quarter of 2009. The company jointly filed for a 2-year extension of the Kenai Liquefied Natural Gas facility's export license with ConocoPhillips. In October 2007, the company acquired Western Oil Sands, Inc. for roughly $5.8 billion.

The company offers its employees medical and dental coverage; life and disability insurance; Fidelity Investments; tuition reimbursement; and annual cash bonuses and awards for achievement.

FINANCIALS: Sales and profits are in thousands of dollars—add 000 to get the full amount. 2007 Note: Financial information for 2007 was not available for all companies at press time.

2007 Sales: $64,552,000	2007 Profits: $3,956,000	**U.S. Stock Ticker: MRO**
2006 Sales: $64,896,000	2006 Profits: $5,234,000	**Int'l Ticker:** Int'l Exchange:
2005 Sales: $62,986,000	2005 Profits: $3,032,000	Employees: 29,524
2004 Sales: $49,465,000	2004 Profits: $1,261,000	Fiscal Year Ends: 12/31
2003 Sales: $41,234,000	2003 Profits: $1,321,000	Parent Company:

SALARIES/BENEFITS:

Pension Plan: Y	ESOP Stock Plan:	Profit Sharing:	Top Exec. Salary: $1,294,000	Bonus: $6,264,000
Savings Plan: Y	Stock Purch. Plan:		Second Exec. Salary: $706,000	Bonus: $1,745,400

OTHER THOUGHTS:

Apparent Women Officers or Directors: 3
Hot Spot for Advancement for Women/Minorities: Y

LOCATIONS: ("Y" = Yes)

West:	Southwest:	Midwest:	Southeast:	Northeast:	International:
Y	Y	Y	Y	Y	Y

MARRIOTT INTERNATIONAL INC   www.marriott.com

Industry Group Code: 721110   Ranks within this company's industry group: Sales: 1   Profits: 2

Management:		Sales/Marketing:		Liberal Arts:		Information Systems:		Professionals:		Technical/Scientific:	
Mgmt. Trainees:	Y	Mktg. Professionals:	Y	Gen. Writing/Editing:	Y	Info. Management:	Y	Finance/Accounting:	Y	Engineers, Elec.:	
Experienced Mgmt.:	Y	Retail Sales:		Technical Writing:		Software Dev.:		Law:	Y	Engineers, Other:	
Int'l Business:	Y	Commercial/Industrial:	Y	Graphic Arts/Photog.:	Y	Hardware Dev.:		HR/Other:	Y	Health/Lab:	
MBA Graduates:	Y	Sales Trainees:		Music:		Systems Integration:		Training:	Y	Scientists/Research:	
		Advertising Pros.:	Y	Broadcasting:		Consulting/Other:		Health Care:		Petroleum/Chemicals:	
				Other:				Consulting:		Math/Other:	

TYPES OF BUSINESS:
Hotels & Resorts
Hotels and Lodging
Timeshares
Extended Stay Lodging
Resorts
Corporate Apartments
Timeshares
Synthetic Fuel

BRANDS/DIVISIONS/AFFILIATES:
Marriott Hotels and Resorts
Ritz-Carlton (The)
Bulgari Hotel and Resort
Renaissance Hotels, Resorts and Suites
Courtyard Residence Inn
Fairfield Inn
ExecuStay
Synthetic American Fuel Enterprises I, LLC

CONTACTS: *Note: Officers with more than one job title may be intentionally listed here more than once.*
J. W. Marriott, Jr., CEO
William J. Shaw, COO
William J. Shaw, Pres.
Arne M. Sorenson, CFO/Exec. VP
Edward A. Ryan, General Counsel/Exec. VP
Robert J. McCarthy, Exec. VP-North American Lodging Oper.
Arne M. Sorenson, Pres., Continental European Lodging
Simon Cooper, COO/Pres., The Ritz-Carlton Hotel Co., LLC
Stephen P. Weisz, Pres., Marriott Vacation Club International
Robert J. McCarthy, Exec. VP-Global Brand Mgmt.
J. W. Marriott, Jr., Chmn.
Edwin D. Fuller, Pres./Managing Dir.-Marriott Lodging Int'l

Phone: 301-380-3000	Fax: 301-380-3969
Toll-Free: 800-721-7033	
Address: 10400 Fernwood Rd., Bethesda, MD 20817 US	

GROWTH PLANS/SPECIAL FEATURES:
Marriott International, Inc. operates almost 3,000 hotels and related lodging facilities in the U.S. and 67 other countries and territories. Though primarily known for the firm's various hotel brands, Marriot also has operations in time shares. Marriott develops, operates and franchises hotels under 13 brand names, including Marriott Hotels and Resorts; the Ritz-Carlton, featuring luxury hotels and resorts; Bulgari Hotel and Resort; Renaissance Hotels, Resorts and Suites; Courtyard; Residence Inn, the firm's extended-stay brand; Fairfield Inn; SpringHill Suites; and TownePlace Suites. The firm also provides furnished corporate housing units in more than 40 major markets through its ExecuStay brand, as well as operating 15 upscale serviced apartments through Marriott Executive Apartments. The company also develops, sells and operates vacation timesharing resorts in over 45 locations. The resorts are usually adjacent to the firm's hotels, bearing the brand names Marriott Vacation Club International, Horizons by Marriott Vacation Club International, Ritz-Carlton Club and Marriott Grand Residence Club. Additionally, Marriott manages 45 golf courses worldwide. In March 2007, the firm completed a three-year, $187 million renovation, the largest capital investment on any company property, on its Marco Island property. In November 2007, the company discontinued its synthetic fuels operations.

Marriot was named one of the 100 best companies to work for by Fortune and Working Mother in 2007.

FINANCIALS: Sales and profits are in thousands of dollars—add 000 to get the full amount. 2007 Note: Financial information for 2007 was not available for all companies at press time.

		U.S. Stock Ticker: MAR
2007 Sales: $12,990,000	2007 Profits: $696,000	Int'l Ticker: Int'l Exchange:
2006 Sales: $11,995,000	2006 Profits: $608,000	Employees: 151,000
2005 Sales: $11,129,000	2005 Profits: $669,000	Fiscal Year Ends: 12/31
2004 Sales: $10,099,000	2004 Profits: $596,000	Parent Company:
2003 Sales: $9,014,000	2003 Profits: $502,000	

SALARIES/BENEFITS:
Pension Plan:	ESOP Stock Plan:	Profit Sharing:	Top Exec. Salary: $1,175,500	Bonus: $2,166,916
Savings Plan: Y	Stock Purch. Plan:		Second Exec. Salary: $955,000	Bonus: $1,239,018

OTHER THOUGHTS:
Apparent Women Officers or Directors:
Hot Spot for Advancement for Women/Minorities: Y

LOCATIONS: ("Y" = Yes)
West:	Southwest:	Midwest:	Southeast:	Northeast:	International:
Y	Y	Y	Y	Y	Y

MARS INC

www.mars.com

Industry Group Code: 311330 Ranks within this company's industry group: Sales: Profits:

Management:		Sales/Marketing:		Liberal Arts:		Information Systems:		Professionals:		Technical/Scientific:	
Mgmt. Trainees:	Y	Mktg. Professionals:	Y	Gen. Writing/Editing:	Y	Info. Management:	Y	Finance/Accounting:	Y	Engineers, Elec.:	Y
Experienced Mgmt.:	Y	Retail Sales:		Technical Writing:		Software Dev.:		Law:	Y	Engineers, Other:	Y
Int'l Business:	Y	Commercial/Industrial:	Y	Graphic Arts/Photog.:	Y	Hardware Dev.:		HR/Other:	Y	Health/Lab:	Y
MBA Graduates:	Y	Sales Trainees:	Y	Music:		Systems Integration:		Training:	Y	Scientists/Research:	
		Advertising Pros.:	Y	Broadcasting:		Consulting/Other:		Health Care:		Petroleum/Chemicals:	
				Other:				Consulting:		Math/Other:	

TYPES OF BUSINESS:

Chocolate & Confectionery Manufacturing
Snack Foods & Candy Bars
Pet Nutrition
Drink Vending Systems
Prepared Foods
Information Technology Services

BRANDS/DIVISIONS/AFFILIATES:

M&Ms
Snickers
Milky Way
Twix
Sheba
Cesar
Uncle Ben's
Seeds of Change

CONTACTS: Note: Officers with more than one job title may be intentionally listed here more than once.

Paul S. Michaels, Pres.
Harold Schmitz, Chief Science Officer
Alice Nathanson, Dir.-Corp. Comm.
Rodney Snyder, Dir.-R&D Mars Historic Div.
Howard Shapiro, Global Dir.-Plant Science & External Research
John Franklyn Mars, Chmn.

Phone: 703-821-4900	Fax: 908-850-2734
Toll-Free: 800-627-7852	
Address: 6885 Elm St., McLean, VA 22101 US	

GROWTH PLANS/SPECIAL FEATURES:

Mars, Inc., founded in 1911, is family-owned company that operates through five divisions: Snack food, pet care, food and drinks. One of the world's largest family-owned companies, Mars operates over 100 manufacturing facilities and distributes products to over 100 countries. Approximately 50% of the company's sales are in Europe, 40% are in the Americas and 10% are in Australia and Asia. The company makes some of the world's most popular and widely available snacks and confectionery products, including M&Ms, Mars, Snickers, Milky Way, Twix, Skittles, Starburst and Dove candies, as well as Combos snacks and Kudos bars. The firm's pet care products for cats and dogs include such brands as Sheba, Cesar, Whiskas, Pedigree, Royal Canin, My Dog, Kitekat, Buckeye, Frolic, Chappi, Winergy, Trill, Waltham, Aquarian, Rena and Nutro. In the food division, Mars produces rice, entrees, sauces and condiments under brand names including Uncle Ben's, Dolmio, Suzi-Wan, Seeds of Change and Ebly. The firm's beverage segment distributes Mars' KLIX and FLAVIA drink vending machine systems, which are industry leading products that provide in-cup drinks such as fresh ground coffee, leaf tea and hot chocolate. In addition, the company manufactures nutritional foods, snacks and beverages under the Cocoa Via brand. In May 2007, Mars unified its regional corporate brands, including Masterfoods, under a single corporate brand name, Mars. In December 2007, Mars Europe announced that it will no longer advertise to children. Also in December, Mars U.S. and Mars Germany launched websites providing nutritional information on products, as well as material promoting healthy lifestyles. In January 2008, Mars announced its participation in a European Union forum established to reverse obesity trends through voluntary measures. In 2008, the company agreed to a merger with Wm. Wrigley Jr. Company.

FINANCIALS: Sales and profits are in thousands of dollars—add 000 to get the full amount. 2007 Note: Financial information for 2007 was not available for all companies at press time.

2007 Sales: $25,000,000	2007 Profits: $	**U.S. Stock Ticker: Private**
2006 Sales: $21,500,000	2006 Profits: $	**Int'l Ticker:** Int'l Exchange:
2005 Sales: $20,000,000	2005 Profits: $	Employees: 40,500
2004 Sales: $18,000,000	2004 Profits: $	Fiscal Year Ends: 12/31
2003 Sales: $17,000,000	2003 Profits: $	Parent Company:

SALARIES/BENEFITS:

Pension Plan:	ESOP Stock Plan:	Profit Sharing:	Top Exec. Salary: $	Bonus: $
Savings Plan:	Stock Purch. Plan:		Second Exec. Salary: $	Bonus: $

OTHER THOUGHTS:

Apparent Women Officers or Directors:
Hot Spot for Advancement for Women/Minorities:

LOCATIONS: ("Y" = Yes)

West:	Southwest:	Midwest:	Southeast:	Northeast:	International:
Y	Y	Y	Y	Y	Y

MARSH & MCLENNAN COMPANIES INC www.marshmac.com

Industry Group Code: 524210 Ranks within this company's industry group: Sales: Profits:

Management:		Sales/Marketing:		Liberal Arts:		Information Systems:		Professionals:		Technical/Scientific:	
Mgmt. Trainees:	Y	Mktg. Professionals:	Y	Gen. Writing/Editing:	Y	Info. Management:	Y	Finance/Accounting:	Y	Engineers, Elec.:	
Experienced Mgmt.:	Y	Retail Sales:		Technical Writing:	Y	Software Dev.:	Y	Law:	Y	Engineers, Other:	
Int'l Business:	Y	Commercial/Industrial:	Y	Graphic Arts/Photog.:		Hardware Dev.:		HR/Other:	Y	Health/Lab:	
MBA Graduates:	Y	Sales Trainees:		Music:		Systems Integration:		Training:	Y	Scientists/Research:	Y
		Advertising Pros.:	Y	Broadcasting:		Consulting/Other:		Health Care:		Petroleum/Chemicals:	
				Other:				Consulting:	Y	Math/Other:	Y

TYPES OF BUSINESS:
Insurance Brokerage
Consulting Services
Risk Management
Benefits Administration
Human Resources Services

BRANDS/DIVISIONS/AFFILIATES:
Marsh, Inc.
Guy Carpenter & Company, LLC
Marsh & McLennan Risk Capital Holdings
Kroll Inc
Mercer Inc
Oliver Wyman Group
Mercer Specialty Consulting
Putnam LLC

CONTACTS: *Note: Officers with more than one job title may be intentionally listed here more than once.*
Brian Duperreault, CEO
Brian Duperreault, Pres.
Vanessa A. Wittman, CFO/Exec. VP
Peter J. Beshar, General Counsel/Exec. VP
Christine Walton, VP-Public Rel.
M. Michele Burns, Chmn./CEO-Mercer, Inc.
Ben Allen, CEO/Pres., Kroll Inc.
John Drzik, CEO/Pres., Oliver Wyman Group
Daniel S. Glaser, Chmn./CEO-Marsh, Inc.
Stephen R. Hardis, Chmn.
Mathis Cabiallavetta, Chmn.-MCC Int'l

Phone: 212-345-5000	Fax: 212-345-4838
Toll-Free:	
Address: 1166 Ave. of the Americas, New York, NY 10036-2774 US	

GROWTH PLANS/SPECIAL FEATURES:

Marsh and McLennan Companies, Inc. (MMC), an insurance brokerage firm, provides global professional services with transactional capabilities to clients in over 100 countries. The company operates three segments: Risk and Insurance Services; Risk Consulting and Technology; and Consulting. The Risk and Insurance segment, which generated 49% of MMC's operating segments revenue, is primarily composed of two companies and their subsidiaries. Marsh, Inc., operating through 400 offices in 100 countries, provides risk management, insurance broking, consulting and insurance program management services; and Guy Carpenter & Company, LLC provides reinsurance broking, catastrophe and financial modeling services and related advisory functions. This segment also owns investments in private equity funds and other firms through Marsh & McLennan Risk Capital Holdings. Risk Consulting and Technology, which generated 9% of revenues, consists of Kroll, Inc. and its subsidiaries. Besides technology and consulting services, it provides security as well as corporate advisory and restructuring. Its consulting services include finance and risk management. The Consulting segment, which generated 43% of revenue, operates through Mercer, Inc. and its two main subsidiaries: Mercer Human Resource Consulting and Mercer Specialty Consulting. Mercer Human Resource offers consultations covering retirement and investments; health and benefits; talent; and outsourcing. Mercer Specialty offers consultations covering management; organization design and change; and economics. In August 2007, the firm completed the sale of Putnam Investments to Great-West Lifeco, Inc., a unit of Power Financial Corp., for $3.9 billion. Putnam Investments managed over 10 million shareholder accounts and over 300 institutional accounts.

The company provides an employee gifts matching program; and health and welfare benefit programs.

FINANCIALS: Sales and profits are in thousands of dollars—add 000 to get the full amount. 2007 Note: Financial information for 2007 was not available for all companies at press time.

2007 Sales: $11,350,000	2007 Profits: $2,475,000	**U.S. Stock Ticker: MMC**
2006 Sales: $10,547,000	2006 Profits: $990,000	**Int'l Ticker:** Int'l Exchange:
2005 Sales: $11,578,000	2005 Profits: $404,000	Employees: 55,000
2004 Sales: $11,727,000	2004 Profits: $176,000	Fiscal Year Ends: 12/31
2003 Sales: $11,588,000	2003 Profits: $1,540,000	Parent Company:

SALARIES/BENEFITS:

Pension Plan: Y	ESOP Stock Plan:	Profit Sharing:	Top Exec. Salary: $1,000,000	Bonus: $2,650,000
Savings Plan: Y	Stock Purch. Plan: Y		Second Exec. Salary: $1,000,000	Bonus: $2,500,000

OTHER THOUGHTS:
Apparent Women Officers or Directors: 4
Hot Spot for Advancement for Women/Minorities: Y

LOCATIONS: ("Y" = Yes)

West:	Southwest:	Midwest:	Southeast:	Northeast:	International:
Y	Y	Y		Y	Y

MARY KAY INC

www.marykay.com

Industry Group Code: 446191A Ranks within this company's industry group: Sales: Profits:

Management:		Sales/Marketing:		Liberal Arts:		Information Systems:		Professionals:		Technical/Scientific:	
Mgmt. Trainees:	Y	Mktg. Professionals:	Y	Gen. Writing/Editing:	Y	Info. Management:	Y	Finance/Accounting:	Y	Engineers, Elec.:	
Experienced Mgmt.:	Y	Retail Sales:	Y	Technical Writing:		Software Dev.:		Law:	Y	Engineers, Other:	
Int'l Business:	Y	Commercial/Industrial:		Graphic Arts/Photog.:	Y	Hardware Dev.:		HR/Other:	Y	Health/Lab:	
MBA Graduates:	Y	Sales Trainees:	Y	Music:		Systems Integration:		Training:	Y	Scientists/Research:	
		Advertising Pros.:	Y	Broadcasting:		Consulting/Other:		Health Care:		Petroleum/Chemicals:	
				Other:				Consulting:		Math/Other:	

TYPES OF BUSINESS:

Cosmetics & Beauty Supplies, Direct Selling
Online Retail
Fragrances
Over-the-Counter Drugs
Cosmetics & Beauty Supplies, Manufacturing

BRANDS/DIVISIONS/AFFILIATES:

Embrace
TimeWise
Belara
Domain
Velocity
Journey
Angelfire
Elige

CONTACTS: *Note: Officers with more than one job title may be intentionally listed here more than once.*

David B. Holl, CEO
David B. Holl, Pres.
Terry Jacks, VP-R&D
Kregg Jodie, CIO/Exec. VP
Yvette Franco, VP-Brand Dev.
Nathan P. Moore, General Counsel/Sec./Sr. VP
Richard Rogers, Chmn.

Phone: 972-687-6300	**Fax:** 972-687-1611
Toll-Free: 800-627-9529	
Address: 16251 Dallas Pkwy., Dallas, TX 75001 US	

GROWTH PLANS/SPECIAL FEATURES:

Mary Kay, Inc. is one of the largest direct sellers of skin care products in the U.S. Mary Kay Ash, the company's founder, launched the company in 1963 with the help of her son. Mary Kay Ash's vision for the company included a strong commitment to family and allegiance to the golden rule. The company's merchandise includes more than 200 products in four categories: facial skin care, color cosmetics, spa and body care and fragrances. Skin care includes anti-aging creams, cleansers, moisturizers, basic skin care for different skin types, products for specific needs such as acne treatment and oil control, and lip and eye care. Color cosmetics products include lip, eyes, cheeks, nails, foundations and powder color enhancers, as well as travel sets and applicators. The Mary Kay fragrance line has specialty scents for both men and women, including Journey, Belara and Elige for women and Domain and Velocity for men. Mary Kay develops, tests, manufactures and packages the majority of its own products at state-of-the-art plants. Most inventory is manufactured at the Dallas site, where the company headquarters and the Mary Kay Museum are located. An additional plant is located in China. With FDA approval, the company also manufactures and distributes certain products classified as over-the-counter drugs, such as sunscreens and acne treatment products. There are about 1.6 million Mary Kay independent beauty consultants serving customers in 30 markets worldwide. Independent beauty consultants may eventually become independent sales directors and/or independent national sales directors. Since its inception, the family of Mary Kay Ash has owned the majority of the company.

Mary Kay's employees generally work out of their homes and are offered sales incentives such as the use of the company's signature pink Cadillacs.

FINANCIALS: Sales and profits are in thousands of dollars—add 000 to get the full amount. 2007 Note: Financial information for 2007 was not available for all companies at press time.

2007 Sales: $2,400,000	2007 Profits: $	**U.S. Stock Ticker: Private**
2006 Sales: $2,250,000	2006 Profits: $	**Int'l Ticker:** Int'l Exchange:
2005 Sales: $2,200,000	2005 Profits: $	Employees: 3,600
2004 Sales: $1,800,000	2004 Profits: $	Fiscal Year Ends: 12/31
2003 Sales: $1,800,000	2003 Profits: $	Parent Company:

SALARIES/BENEFITS:

Pension Plan:	ESOP Stock Plan:	Profit Sharing:	Top Exec. Salary: $	Bonus: $
Savings Plan:	Stock Purch. Plan:		Second Exec. Salary: $	Bonus: $

OTHER THOUGHTS:

Apparent Women Officers or Directors: 2
Hot Spot for Advancement for Women/Minorities:

LOCATIONS: ("Y" = Yes)

West:	Southwest:	Midwest:	Southeast:	Northeast:	International:
Y	Y	Y	Y	Y	Y

Note: Financial information, benefits and other data can change quickly and may vary from those stated here.

MASSEY ENERGY COMPANY   www.masseyenergyco.com

Industry Group Code: 212110 **Ranks within this company's industry group:** Sales: 3 Profits: 3

Management:		Sales/Marketing:		Liberal Arts:		Information Systems:		Professionals:		Technical/Scientific:	
Mgmt. Trainees:	Y	Mktg. Professionals:	Y	Gen. Writing/Editing:		Info. Management:	Y	Finance/Accounting:	Y	Engineers, Elec.:	Y
Experienced Mgmt.:	Y	Retail Sales:		Technical Writing:		Software Dev.:		Law:	Y	Engineers, Other:	
Int'l Business:		Commercial/Industrial:		Graphic Arts/Photog.:		Hardware Dev.:		HR/Other:	Y	Health/Lab:	Y
MBA Graduates:	Y	Sales Trainees:		Music:		Systems Integration:		Training:	Y	Scientists/Research:	
		Advertising Pros.:		Broadcasting:		Consulting/Other:		Health Care:		Petroleum/Chemicals:	Y
				Other:				Consulting:		Math/Other:	

TYPES OF BUSINESS:

Coal Mining
Natural Gas Gathering
Synthetic Fuel Manufacturing
Rail Cargo Transport

BRANDS/DIVISIONS/AFFILIATES:

CONTACTS: Note: Officers with more than one job title may be intentionally listed here more than once.

Don L. Blankenship, CEO
J. Christopher Adkins, COO/Sr. VP
Don L. Blankenship, Pres.
Eric B. Tolbert, CFO
John M. Poma, VP-Human Resources
Baxter Phillips, Chief Admin. Officer/Exec. VP
M. Shane Harvey, General Counsel
Mark Clemens, Sr. VP-Group Oper.
Michael Bauersachs, VP-Planning
Jeffrey Jarosinski, VP-Finance
Richard R. Grinnan, Corp. Sec./VP
Jeffrey Jarosinski, Chief Compliance Officer
Don L. Blankenship, Chmn.

Phone: 804-788-1800	Fax: 804-788-1870
Toll-Free: 800-766-1320	
Address: 4 N. 4th St., Richmond, VA 23219 US	

GROWTH PLANS/SPECIAL FEATURES:

Massey Energy Company is a leading coal company in the U.S. and is one of the largest in the Central Appalachian region. The company produces, processes and sells bituminous, low-sulfur coal of steam and metallurgical grades, operating 35 underground and 12 surface mine complexes in West Virginia, Kentucky and Virginia. These complexes blend, process and ship coal that is produced the mines to one of the company's 22 resource groups. Any one of these preparation plants can handle the coal production from as many as seven distinct underground or surface mines. The mines have been strategically developed in close proximity to the Massey preparation plants and rail shipping facilities in order to cut down transportation costs. Once prepared, the coal is transported to customers by means of railroad cars, trucks or barges, with rail shipments representing approximately 90% of 2007 coal shipments. Massey's steam coal is primarily purchased by utilities and industrial clients as fuel for power plants, and its metallurgical coal is used primarily to make coke for use in the manufacture of steel. Through its subsidiaries, the company also manages a synthetic fuel manufacturing facility in West Virginia; unloading, storage and conveying facilities; and natural gas gathering operations. Massey owns and operates approximately 188 gas wells, 200 miles of gathering line and various small compression facilities, as well as interests in 30 wells operated by others. In August 2007, the company acquired Belle Coal Company, Inc. and certain assets from Peachtree Ridge Mining Company, Inc., including 15 million tons of leased coal reserves and a deep mine permit in West Virginia. In October 2007, Massey announced plans to expand production at its Central Appalachian coal mining operations over the next two years.

FINANCIALS: Sales and profits are in thousands of dollars—add 000 to get the full amount. 2007 Note: Financial information for 2007 was not available for all companies at press time.

2007 Sales: $2,413,523	2007 Profits: $94,098	U.S. Stock Ticker: MEE
2006 Sales: $2,219,854	2006 Profits: $40,977	Int'l Ticker: Int'l Exchange:
2005 Sales: $1,777,700	2005 Profits: $-101,600	Employees: 5,517
2004 Sales: $1,456,700	2004 Profits: $13,900	Fiscal Year Ends: 12/31
2003 Sales: $1,262,100	2003 Profits: $-40,213	Parent Company:

SALARIES/BENEFITS:

Pension Plan: Y	ESOP Stock Plan:	Profit Sharing:	Top Exec. Salary: $1,000,000	Bonus: $814,054
Savings Plan:	Stock Purch. Plan:		Second Exec. Salary: $550,000	Bonus: $208,417

OTHER THOUGHTS:

Apparent Women Officers or Directors: 3
Hot Spot for Advancement for Women/Minorities: Y

LOCATIONS: ("Y" = Yes)

West:	Southwest:	Midwest:	Southeast:	Northeast:	International:
				Y	

MATTEL INC   www.mattel.com

Industry Group Code: 451120   **Ranks within this company's industry group:** Sales: Profits:

Management:	Sales/Marketing:	Liberal Arts:	Information Systems:	Professionals:	Technical/Scientific:
Mgmt. Trainees:	Mktg. Professionals:	Gen. Writing/Editing:	Info. Management:	Finance/Accounting:	Engineers, Elec.:
Experienced Mgmt.:	Retail Sales:	Technical Writing:	Software Dev.:	Law:	Engineers, Other:
Int'l Business:	Commercial/Industrial:	Graphic Arts/Photog.:	Hardware Dev.:	HR/Other:	Health/Lab:
MBA Graduates:	Sales Trainees:	Music:	Systems Integration:	Training:	Scientists/Research:
	Advertising Pros.:	Broadcasting:	Consulting/Other:	Health Care:	Petroleum/Chemicals:
		Other:		Consulting:	Math/Other:

TYPES OF BUSINESS:

Toy Manufacturing

BRANDS/DIVISIONS/AFFILIATES:

Fisher-Price
American Girl
Barbie
Polly Pocket!
Disney Classics
Hot Wheels
Matchbox
Sesame Street

CONTACTS:
Note: Officers with more than one job title may be intentionally listed here more than once.

Robert A. Eckert, CEO
Kevin M. Farr, CFO
Alan Kaye, Sr. VP-Human Resources
Robert (Bob) Normile, General Counsel/Corp. Sec./Sr. VP
Thomas A. Debrowski, Exec. VP-Worldwide Oper.
Mike Salop, Sr. VP-External Affairs
Neil B. Friedman, Pres., Mattel Brands
Ellen L. Brothers, Pres., American Girl Brands
Geoff Massingberd, Sr. VP-Corp. Responsibility
Robert A. Eckert, Chmn.
Bryan G. Stockton, Pres., Int'l

Phone: 310-252-2000	**Fax:**
Toll-Free:	
Address: 333 Continental Blvd., El Segundo, CA 90245 US	

GROWTH PLANS/SPECIAL FEATURES:

Mattel, Inc., designs, manufactures and markets a variety of toy products worldwide. Mattel's product portfolio of brands and products are grouped into three categories: Mattel Girls & Boys Brands; Fisher-Price Brands; and American Girl Brands. The Mattel Girls & Boys Brands include Barbie fashion dolls and accessories; Polly Pocket!; Pixel Chix; Winx Club; Disney Classics; Hot Wheels; Matchbox and Tyco R/C vehicles and playsets; Batman, CARS, Superman and Radica products; and games and puzzles. Fisher-Price brands include Little People, BabyGear, View-Master, Sesame Street, Dora the Explorer, Go-Diego-Go!, Winnie the Pooh, InteracTV, See 'N Say and Power Wheels. American Girl Brands include Just Like You, the historical collection and Bitty Baby. For 2008, Mattel developed products for entertainment properties such as Warner Bros.' the Dark Knight and Speed Racer and Dreamworks' animated Kung Fu Panda. The Disney Pixar CARS products saw an expansion due to its success. The firm's products in the domestic segment are sold directly to retailers, including discount and free-standing toy stores, chain stores, department stores and other retail outlets. The company's international sales represent approximately 49% of its total sales, of which sales in Europe represent approximately 56%, sales in Latin America represent approximately 28%, sales in Asia Pacific represent approximately 7% and sales in other regions represent approximately 7%. Products marketed internationally are generally the same as those developed and marketed domestically, with the exception of American Girl Brands. During 2007, Wal-Mart, Toys R Us and Target, Mattel's largest customers, accounted for approximately 41% of worldwide net sales.

Mattel offers its employees a retirement plan, a stock purchase plan, an educational assistance program, adoption assistance and medical, prescription and dental insurance.

FINANCIALS:
Sales and profits are in thousands of dollars—add 000 to get the full amount. 2007 Note: Financial information for 2007 was not available for all companies at press time.

2007 Sales: $5,970,090	2007 Profits: $599,993	**U.S. Stock Ticker: MAT**
2006 Sales: $5,650,156	2006 Profits: $592,927	**Int'l Ticker:** Int'l Exchange:
2005 Sales: $5,179,016	2005 Profits: $417,019	Employees:
2004 Sales: $	2004 Profits: $	Fiscal Year Ends:
2003 Sales: $	2003 Profits: $	Parent Company:

SALARIES/BENEFITS:

Pension Plan: Y	ESOP Stock Plan:	Profit Sharing:	Top Exec. Salary: $	Bonus: $
Savings Plan:	Stock Purch. Plan: Y		Second Exec. Salary: $	Bonus: $

OTHER THOUGHTS:

Apparent Women Officers or Directors: 1
Hot Spot for Advancement for Women/Minorities:

LOCATIONS: ("Y" = Yes)

West:	Southwest:	Midwest:	Southeast:	Northeast:	International:
Y	Y	Y	Y	Y	Y

MAXIM INTEGRATED PRODUCTS INC   www.maxim-ic.com

Industry Group Code: 334413 Ranks within this company's industry group: Sales: 7 Profits: 4

Management:		Sales/Marketing:		Liberal Arts:		Information Systems:		Professionals:		Technical/Scientific:	
Mgmt. Trainees:	Y	Mktg. Professionals:	Y	Gen. Writing/Editing:		Info. Management:	Y	Finance/Accounting:	Y	Engineers, Elec.:	Y
Experienced Mgmt.:	Y	Retail Sales:		Technical Writing:	Y	Software Dev.:	Y	Law:	Y	Engineers, Other:	
Int'l Business:	Y	Commercial/Industrial:	Y	Graphic Arts/Photog.:		Hardware Dev.:	Y	HR/Other:	Y	Health/Lab:	Y
MBA Graduates:	Y	Sales Trainees:		Music:		Systems Integration:		Training:	Y	Scientists/Research:	Y
		Advertising Pros.:	Y	Broadcasting:		Consulting/Other:		Health Care:		Petroleum/Chemicals:	
				Other:				Consulting:		Math/Other:	

TYPES OF BUSINESS:

Integrated Circuits-Analog & Mixed Signal
High-Frequency Design Processes
Manufacturing Capabilities
Power Conversion Chips

BRANDS/DIVISIONS/AFFILIATES:

Dallas Semiconductor Corp
RAD Data Communications
Vitesse Semiconductor Corp.

CONTACTS: *Note: Officers with more than one job title may be intentionally listed here more than once.*

Tunc Doluca, CEO
Tunc Doluca, Pres.
Ed Medlin, Sr. Counsel/VP
John F. Gifford, Strategic Advisor
Paresh Maniar, Exec. Dir.-Investor Rel.
Bruce E. Kiddoo, VP-Finance
Vijay Ullal, Group Pres.
Charles (Chuck) Rigg, Sr. VP
Pirooz Parvarandeh, Group Pres.
B. Kipling (Kip) Hagopian, Chmn.

Phone: 408-737-7600	Fax: 408-737-7194
Toll-Free: 800-998-8800	
Address: 120 San Gabriel Dr., Sunnyvale, CA 94086 US	

GROWTH PLANS/SPECIAL FEATURES:

Maxim Integrated Products, Inc. designs, develops, manufactures and markets analog, mixed-signal, high frequency and digital circuits. Its products are primarily created by wholly-owned subsidiary Dallas Semiconductor Corporation, which designs, manufactures and markets mixed-signal semiconductors. Maxim's circuits connect the analog and digital world by detecting, measuring, amplifying and converting real-world signals into the digital signals necessary for computer processing. It produces electronic interface products to interact with people, through audio, video, touchpad, key pad and security devices; the physical world, through motion, time, temperature and humidity sensors; power sources, via conversion, charging, supervision and regulation systems; and other digital systems, including wireless, storage and fiber optic systems. Maxim's products serve the following industries: Automotive, specifically air bags, cruise controls and navigation systems; Communications, including broadband access, cable systems and cordless phones; Consumer, specifically digital cameras, personal digital assistants and DVD players; Data Processing, including printers and storage systems; Industrial Control, concerning robotics; Instrumentation, featuring automatic testing equipment; and Medical, including blood glucose meters and imaging. The company also offers the use of its manufacturing capabilities for custom designs. Some of Maxim's newest products include one of the industry's smallest DC/DC converters; one of the first fully integrated switch-mode/linear LED drivers; bidirectional video filters/buffers for portable consumer devices; high-voltage, low-power linear regulators for automotive and industrial applications; dual-band, dual-mode tuners for Japanese digital broadcasts; a programmable high-brightness LED driver for automotive and other lighting applications; and one of the first chips to convert an all-analog power supply to a fully programmable, digital power-management solution. Maxim and Dallas Semiconductor recently announced that they are working with RAD Data Communications to produce TDM-over-Packet chips. In October 2007, the firm acquired Vitesse Semiconductor Corporation's Storage Products Business, for $63 million.

Employees of Maxim receive medical coverage; life and AD&D insurance; and educational assistance.

FINANCIALS: Sales and profits are in thousands of dollars—add 000 to get the full amount. 2007 Note: Financial information for 2007 was not available for all companies at press time.

2007 Sales: $	2007 Profits: $	**U.S. Stock Ticker: MXIM.PK**
2006 Sales: $1,858,942	2006 Profits: $462,552	**Int'l Ticker:** Int'l Exchange:
2005 Sales: $1,671,713	2005 Profits: $540,837	Employees:
2004 Sales: $1,439,263	2004 Profits: $419,752	Fiscal Year Ends: 8/31
2003 Sales: $1,153,200	2003 Profits: $309,600	Parent Company:

SALARIES/BENEFITS:

Pension Plan:	ESOP Stock Plan:	Profit Sharing:	Top Exec. Salary: $300,000	Bonus: $
Savings Plan: Y	Stock Purch. Plan: Y		Second Exec. Salary: $300,000	Bonus: $

OTHER THOUGHTS:

Apparent Women Officers or Directors:
Hot Spot for Advancement for Women/Minorities:

LOCATIONS: ("Y" = Yes)

West:	Southwest:	Midwest:	Southeast:	Northeast:	International:
Y	Y	Y	Y	Y	Y

Note: Financial information, benefits and other data can change quickly and may vary from those stated here.

MCAFEE INC

www.mcafee.com

Industry Group Code: 511211 Ranks within this company's industry group: Sales: 3   Profits: 3

Management:		Sales/Marketing:		Liberal Arts:		Information Systems:		Professionals:		Technical/Scientific:	
Mgmt. Trainees:	Y	Mktg. Professionals:	Y	Gen. Writing/Editing:	Y	Info. Management:	Y	Finance/Accounting:	Y	Engineers, Elec.:	Y
Experienced Mgmt.:	Y	Retail Sales:		Technical Writing:	Y	Software Dev.:	Y	Law:	Y	Engineers, Other:	
Int'l Business:	Y	Commercial/Industrial:	Y	Graphic Arts/Photog.:		Hardware Dev.:		HR/Other:	Y	Health/Lab:	
MBA Graduates:	Y	Sales Trainees:		Music:		Systems Integration:		Training:	Y	Scientists/Research:	
		Advertising Pros.:	Y	Broadcasting:		Consulting/Other:		Health Care:		Petroleum/Chemicals:	
				Other:				Consulting:	Y	Math/Other:	

TYPES OF BUSINESS:

Software-Security
Virus Protection Software
Network Management Software

BRANDS/DIVISIONS/AFFILIATES:

McAfee Foundstone Professional Services
McAfee System Protection Solutions
McAfee Network Protection Solutions
McAfee Anti-Virus
McAfee Spam Killer
SafeBoot Holding B.V.

CONTACTS: *Note: Officers with more than one job title may be intentionally listed here more than once.*

David DeWalt, CEO
David DeWalt, Pres.
David Milam, Chief Mktg. Officer/Exec. VP
Joseph Gabbert, Exec. VP-Human Resources
Richard J. Decker, CIO
Christopher Bolin, CTO/Exec. VP
Dennis Omanoff, Sr. VP-Worldwide Mfg.
Mark Cochran, General Counsel/Exec. VP
Keith Krzeminski, Chief Acct. Officer/Sr. VP-Finance
Michael DeCesare, Exec. VP-Worldwide Sales
Roger King, Exec. VP-Worldwide Channel Oper.
Takahiro Kato, Pres., Japan
Steve Redman, Pres., Asia Pacific
Charles J. Robel, Chmn.
Mike Dalton, Pres., EMEA

Phone: 408-988-3832	Fax: 408-970-9727
Toll-Free:	
Address: 3965 Freedom Cir., Santa Clara, CA 95054 US	

GROWTH PLANS/SPECIAL FEATURES:

McAfee, Inc. is a developer and supplier of software-based computer security systems that prevent intrusions on networks and protect computer systems from attacks. It allows home users, businesses, government agencies, service providers and partners to block attacks, prevent disruptions and continuously track and improve their security. The company offers two families of products, McAfee System Protection Solutions (SPS) and McAfee Network Protection Solutions (NPS). SPS secures all layers of desktop, server systems and applications. These solutions include McAfee Anti-Virus for desktop vulnerability assessment, McAfee Entercept for preventing system intrusions and McAfee Spam Killer to block unsolicited e-mail. This line of products also includes McAfee VirusScan, McAfee Personal Firewall Plus, McAfee AntiSpyware, McAfee QuickClean and McAfee Internet Security Suite. NPS helps enterprises, small businesses, government agencies, educational organizations and service providers maximize the availability, performance and security of their network infrastructure. Network protection solutions in the portfolio include McAfee IntruShield, which delivers network-based intrusion detection and prevention. The firm's McAfee Foundstone Professional Services division identifies, recommends and implements the right balance of technology, education and training, and process to manage digital risk and leverage security investments for its customers. McAfee conducts its research and development through the Avert Labs organization. In late October 2007, the firm agreed to purchase ScanAlert, Inc., developers of Hacker Safe web site security service, for roughly $51 million. In November 2007, the company acquired SafeBoot Holding B.V. for about $350 million.

FINANCIALS: Sales and profits are in thousands of dollars—add 000 to get the full amount. 2007 Note: Financial information for 2007 was not available for all companies at press time.

2007 Sales: $1,308,220	2007 Profits: $166,980	**U.S. Stock Ticker: MFE**
2006 Sales: $1,142,327	2006 Profits: $137,529	**Int'l Ticker:** Int'l Exchange:
2005 Sales: $987,299	2005 Profits: $138,828	Employees: 4,250
2004 Sales: $910,542	2004 Profits: $225,065	Fiscal Year Ends: 12/31
2003 Sales: $936,336	2003 Profits: $70,242	Parent Company:

SALARIES/BENEFITS:

Pension Plan:	ESOP Stock Plan:	Profit Sharing:	Top Exec. Salary: $835,224	Bonus: $1,000,000
Savings Plan:	Stock Purch. Plan:		Second Exec. Salary: $506,531	Bonus: $420,000

OTHER THOUGHTS:

Apparent Women Officers or Directors:
Hot Spot for Advancement for Women/Minorities: Y

LOCATIONS: ("Y" = Yes)

West:	Southwest:	Midwest:	Southeast:	Northeast:	International:
Y	Y	Y	Y	Y	Y

MCDONALD'S CORP

www.mcdonalds.com

Industry Group Code: 722110 Ranks within this company's industry group: Sales: 1 Profits: 1

Management:		Sales/Marketing:		Liberal Arts:		Information Systems:		Professionals:		Technical/Scientific:	
Mgmt. Trainees:	Y	Mktg. Professionals:	Y	Gen. Writing/Editing:	Y	Info. Management:	Y	Finance/Accounting:	Y	Engineers, Elec.:	
Experienced Mgmt.:	Y	Retail Sales:		Technical Writing:		Software Dev.:	Y	Law:	Y	Engineers, Other:	
Int'l Business:	Y	Commercial/Industrial:	Y	Graphic Arts/Photog.:	Y	Hardware Dev.:		HR/Other:	Y	Health/Lab:	
MBA Graduates:	Y	Sales Trainees:		Music:		Systems Integration:		Training:	Y	Scientists/Research:	
		Advertising Pros.:	Y	Broadcasting:		Consulting/Other:		Health Care:		Petroleum/Chemicals:	
				Other:	Y			Consulting:		Math/Other:	

TYPES OF BUSINESS:

Fast Food Restaurants
Home-Meal Replacement Restaurants
Mexican Restaurants
Franchising

BRANDS/DIVISIONS/AFFILIATES:

Ronald McDonald House
Boston Market
Filet-O-Fish
Quarter Pounder
Big Mac
Chicken McNuggets
Happy Meal

CONTACTS: *Note: Officers with more than one job title may be intentionally listed here more than once.*

Jim Skinner, CEO
Ralph Alvarez, COO
Ralph Alvarez, Pres.
Peter J. Bensen, CFO
Mary Dillon, Global Chief Mktg. Officer/Exec. VP
Richard Floersch, Chief Human Resources Officer/Exec. VP
Gloria Santona, General Counsel/Exec. VP/Corp. Sec.
Jose Armario, Pres., McDonald's Latin America
Don Thompson, Pres., McDonald's USA
Tim Fenton, Pres., Asia, Pacific, Middle East and Africa
Janice L. Fields, Exec. VP/COO-USA
Andrew J. McKenna, Chmn.
Jeff Stratton, Worldwide Chief Restaurant Officer/Corp. Exec. VP

Phone: 630-623-3000	Fax: 630-623-5004
Toll-Free: 800-244-6227	
Address: 2111 McDonald's Dr., Oak Brook, IL 60523 US	

GROWTH PLANS/SPECIAL FEATURES:

McDonald's Corp. operates more than 31,375 fast-food restaurants in over 118 countries serving approximately 48 million customers per day. McDonald's has expanded primarily based on its successful franchising model, whereby independent businessmen and women provide capital by initially investing in equipment, signs, seating and decor of their restaurants and personally operating them. The company shares the investment by owning or leasing the land and buildings. Approximately 70% of McDonald's worldwide restaurants are franchises, the rest being operated directly by the company or under joint-venture agreements. The McDonald's menu includes items such as hamburgers, cheeseburgers, fish and chicken sandwiches, chicken nuggets, french fries, salads, milkshakes, desserts and soft drinks. McDonald's restaurants are also open during breakfast hours and offer egg sandwiches, hotcakes, biscuit and bagel sandwiches and muffins. As part of a multi-year beverage business strategy designed to take advantage of the significant and growing beverage category, the company will begin introducing hot specialty coffee offerings on a market-by-market basis, all of which will serve as a platform for the anticipated future introduction of smoothies, frappes and other beverage options. McDonald's also owns a minority ownership interest in U.K.-based Pret A Manger. In 2007, the company sold its interest in Boston Market, a limited-service restaurant serving chicken, meatloaf and a variety of side dishes, for approximately $250 million.

The firm offers its employees medical, dental and vision insurance; short- and long-term disability; profit sharing and savings plans; adoption assistance; vacation and holiday pay; and a child care discount. McDonald's U.S. employees at corporate division and region offices may receive benefits including a bonus program, educational assistance, credit union membership and sabbaticals of eight weeks every 10 years. Hamburger University is McDonald's worldwide management training center located in Illinois.

FINANCIALS: Sales and profits are in thousands of dollars—add 000 to get the full amount. 2007 Note: Financial information for 2007 was not available for all companies at press time.

2007 Sales: $22,786,600	2007 Profits: $2,395,100	**U.S. Stock Ticker: MCD**
2006 Sales: $20,895,200	2006 Profits: $3,544,200	**Int'l Ticker:** Int'l Exchange:
2005 Sales: $19,832,500	2005 Profits: $2,602,200	Employees: 465,000
2004 Sales: $19,064,700	2004 Profits: $2,278,500	Fiscal Year Ends: 12/31
2003 Sales: $17,140,000	2003 Profits: $1,471,000	Parent Company:

SALARIES/BENEFITS:

Pension Plan:	ESOP Stock Plan:	Profit Sharing: Y	Top Exec. Salary: $1,177,692	Bonus: $8,833,195
Savings Plan: Y	Stock Purch. Plan:		Second Exec. Salary: $962,500	Bonus: $5,243,438

OTHER THOUGHTS:

Apparent Women Officers or Directors: 4
Hot Spot for Advancement for Women/Minorities: Y

LOCATIONS: ("Y" = Yes)

West:	Southwest:	Midwest:	Southeast:	Northeast:	International:
Y	Y	Y	Y	Y	Y

MCKESSON CORPORATION

www.mckesson.com

Industry Group Code: 422210 Ranks within this company's industry group: Sales: 1 Profits: 2

Management:		Sales/Marketing:		Liberal Arts:		Information Systems:		Professionals:		Technical/Scientific:	
Mgmt. Trainees:	Y	Mktg. Professionals:	Y	Gen. Writing/Editing:	Y	Info. Management:	Y	Finance/Accounting:	Y	Engineers, Elec.:	
Experienced Mgmt.:	Y	Retail Sales:		Technical Writing:	Y	Software Dev.:	Y	Law:	Y	Engineers, Other:	
Int'l Business:	Y	Commercial/Industrial:	Y	Graphic Arts/Photog.:	Y	Hardware Dev.:		HR/Other:	Y	Health/Lab:	
MBA Graduates:	Y	Sales Trainees:	Y	Music:		Systems Integration:		Training:	Y	Scientists/Research:	
		Advertising Pros.:	Y	Broadcasting:		Consulting/Other:		Health Care:	Y	Petroleum/Chemicals:	
				Other:				Consulting:		Math/Other:	

TYPES OF BUSINESS:

Pharmaceutical Solutions
Medical-Surgical Solutions
Provider Technologies

BRANDS/DIVISIONS/AFFILIATES:

McKesson U.S. Pharmaceutical
McKesson Canada
McKesson Health Solutions
McKesson Pharmacy Systems
InterQual
ZEE Medical
Per-Se Technologies Inc
Oncology Technology Network

CONTACTS: Note: Officers with more than one job title may be intentionally listed here more than once.

John H. Hammergren, CEO
John H. Hammergren, Pres.
Jeffrey C. Campbell, CFO/Exec. VP
Paul E. Kirincic, Exec. VP-Human Resources
Randall N. Spratt, CIO/Exec. VP
Laureen E. Seeger, General Counsel/Exec. VP/Sec.
Marc E. Owen, Exec. VP-Corp. Strategy & Bus. Dev.
Nigel A. Rees, Controller
Paul C. Julian, Exec. VP/ Pres., McKesson Distribution Solutions
Pamela Pure, Exec. VP/Pres., McKesson Technology Solutions
John H. Hammergren, Chmn.

Phone: 415-983-8300	**Fax:** 415-983-7160
Toll-Free:	
Address: 1 Post St., San Francisco, CA 94104 US	

GROWTH PLANS/SPECIAL FEATURES:

McKesson Corp. provides supply, information and care management products and services to the healthcare industry. The company operates in two segments, McKesson distribution solutions and McKesson technology solutions. The McKesson distribution solutions segment distributes ethical and proprietary drugs, medical-surgical supplies and equipment, and health and beauty care products throughout North America. This segment also provides specialty pharmaceutical solutions for biotech and pharmaceutical manufacturers, sells pharmacy software and provides consulting, outsourcing and other services. This segment includes a 49% interest in Nadro, S.A. de C.V., the leading pharmaceutical distributor in Mexico and a 39% interest in Parata Systems, LLC, which sells automated pharmacy and supply management systems and services to retail and institutional outpatient pharmacies. The McKesson technology solutions segment delivers enterprise-wide clinical, patient care, financial, supply chain, and strategic management software solutions, pharmacy automation for hospitals, as well as connectivity, outsourcing and other services. The firm's payor group of businesses, which includes InterQual, clinical auditing and compliance and medical management software businesses and care management programs, are also included in this segment. This segment's customers include hospitals, physicians, homecare providers, retail pharmacies and payors from North America, the U. K., other European countries and Asia Pacific. During 2007, McKesson acquired Per-Se, RelayHealth Corporation and Sterling Medical Services. In April 2008, the firm acquired Rosebud Solutions, LLC which is a provider of software solutions. In May 2008, the firm acquired McQueary Brothers Drug Company, Inc. In July 2008, it acquired EN-Chart Scanning Program, LLC, a provider of computer-assisted facility coding and compliance solutions for emergency department visits. During the third quarter of 2008, McKesson acquired Oncology Therapeutics Network, a U.S. distributor of specialty pharmaceuticals.

The company offers its employees medical, dental and vision insurance; life and AD&D insurance; flexible spending accounts; a 401(k) plan; an employee stock purchase plan; and an employee assistance program.

FINANCIALS: Sales and profits are in thousands of dollars—add 000 to get the full amount. 2007 Note: Financial information for 2007 was not available for all companies at press time.

2007 Sales: $92,977,000	2007 Profits: $913,000	**U.S. Stock Ticker: MCK**
2006 Sales: $86,983,000	2006 Profits: $751,000	**Int'l Ticker:** Int'l Exchange:
2005 Sales: $79,096,000	2005 Profits: $-157,000	Employees: 31,800
2004 Sales: $69,210,000	2004 Profits: $646,500	Fiscal Year Ends: 3/31
2003 Sales: $57,120,800	2003 Profits: $555,400	Parent Company:

SALARIES/BENEFITS:

Pension Plan:	ESOP Stock Plan:	Profit Sharing:	Top Exec. Salary: $1,366,716	Bonus: $10,981,932
Savings Plan: Y	Stock Purch. Plan: Y		Second Exec. Salary: $830,829	Bonus: $4,450,000

OTHER THOUGHTS:

Apparent Women Officers or Directors: 5
Hot Spot for Advancement for Women/Minorities: Y

LOCATIONS: ("Y" = Yes)

West:	Southwest:	Midwest:	Southeast:	Northeast:	International:
Y	Y	Y	Y	Y	Y

Note: Financial information, benefits and other data can change quickly and may vary from those stated here.

MCKINSEY & COMPANY INC

www.mckinsey.com

Industry Group Code: 541611 Ranks within this company's industry group: Sales: 2   Profits:

Management:		Sales/Marketing:		Liberal Arts:		Information Systems:		Professionals:		Technical/Scientific:	
Mgmt. Trainees:	Y	Mktg. Professionals:	Y	Gen. Writing/Editing:	Y	Info. Management:	Y	Finance/Accounting:	Y	Engineers, Elec.:	
Experienced Mgmt.:	Y	Retail Sales:		Technical Writing:	Y	Software Dev.:	Y	Law:	Y	Engineers, Other:	
Int'l Business:	Y	Commercial/Industrial:	Y	Graphic Arts/Photog.:	Y	Hardware Dev.:		HR/Other:	Y	Health/Lab:	
MBA Graduates:	Y	Sales Trainees:		Music:		Systems Integration:	Y	Training:	Y	Scientists/Research:	Y
		Advertising Pros.:	Y	Broadcasting:		Consulting/Other:	Y	Health Care:		Petroleum/Chemicals:	
				Other:				Consulting:	Y	Math/Other:	Y

TYPES OF BUSINESS:

Management Consulting
Strategic & Logistics Consulting
Industry-Specific Consulting
Business Research
Business Publications

BRANDS/DIVISIONS/AFFILIATES:

McKinsey & Co.
McKinsey Global Institute
McKinsey Quarterly (The)

CONTACTS: *Note: Officers with more than one job title may be intentionally listed here more than once.*

Ian Davis, Managing Dir.
Bill Bradley, Advisor-Non-profit

Phone: 212-446-7000	Fax: 212-446-8575
Toll-Free:	
Address: 55 E. 52nd St., 21st Fl., New York, NY 10022 US	

GROWTH PLANS/SPECIAL FEATURES:

McKinsey & Company, Inc. is a privately held international business consulting firm that was established in 1926. Headquartered in New York, the firm maintains 90 offices in 51 countries, as well as a cross-functional global business technology office. The firm provides consulting services for companies seeking functional assistance or market insights. Through a variety of leadership and financial consulting services, McKinsey helps clients sustain growth and maximize revenue. McKinsey serves companies within a wide range of industries including banking, insurance, telecom, information services, media/entertainment, industrial, health care, public sector and retail/consumer. The company helps clients achieve functional efficiency with consulting services such as outsourcing, information technology (IT) services, financial strategy, operations strategy, organization and leadership. McKinsey's consultants publish a variety of books and articles with topics ranging from company productivity and structural engineering to accentuating the positive. The firm also publishes The McKinsey Quarterly, a business journal expounding the company's current views about business strategy, finance and management. Through the McKinsey Global Institute (MGI), the company conducts business research and develops points of view relating to the economic issues faced by businesses and governments. In 2007, the firm added Usha International, a home appliances and electrical equipment manufacturer, to its portfolio of clients.

FINANCIALS: Sales and profits are in thousands of dollars—add 000 to get the full amount. 2007 Note: Financial information for 2007 was not available for all companies at press time.

2007 Sales: $4,500,000	2007 Profits: $	**U.S. Stock Ticker: Private**
2006 Sales: $4,200,000	2006 Profits: $	**Int'l Ticker:** Int'l Exchange:
2005 Sales: $3,900,000	2005 Profits: $	Employees: 14,100
2004 Sales: $3,700,000	2004 Profits: $	Fiscal Year Ends: 12/31
2003 Sales: $3,400,000	2003 Profits: $	Parent Company:

SALARIES/BENEFITS:

Pension Plan:	ESOP Stock Plan:	Profit Sharing:	Top Exec. Salary: $	Bonus: $
Savings Plan:	Stock Purch. Plan:		Second Exec. Salary: $	Bonus: $

OTHER THOUGHTS:

Apparent Women Officers or Directors: 1
Hot Spot for Advancement for Women/Minorities: Y

LOCATIONS: ("Y" = Yes)

West:	Southwest:	Midwest:	Southeast:	Northeast:	International:
Y	Y	Y	Y	Y	Y

MEDCO HEALTH SOLUTIONS

www.medco.com

Industry Group Code: 522320A **Ranks within this company's industry group:** Sales: 1 Profits: 2

Management:		Sales/Marketing:		Liberal Arts:		Information Systems:		Professionals:		Technical/Scientific:	
Mgmt. Trainees:	Y	Mktg. Professionals:	Y	Gen. Writing/Editing:	Y	Info. Management:	Y	Finance/Accounting:	Y	Engineers, Elec.:	
Experienced Mgmt.:	Y	Retail Sales:		Technical Writing:	Y	Software Dev.:	Y	Law:	Y	Engineers, Other:	Y
Int'l Business:		Commercial/Industrial:	Y	Graphic Arts/Photog.:		Hardware Dev.:		HR/Other:	Y	Health/Lab:	
MBA Graduates:	Y	Sales Trainees:		Music:		Systems Integration:		Training:	Y	Scientists/Research:	
		Advertising Pros.:	Y	Broadcasting:		Consulting/Other:		Health Care:	Y	Petroleum/Chemicals:	
				Other:				Consulting:		Math/Other:	

TYPES OF BUSINESS:
Pharmacy Benefits Management
Payment & Transaction Processing
Online Services

BRANDS/DIVISIONS/AFFILIATES:
Medicare Part D Prescription Drug Program
Accredo Health Group Inc
Medco Therapeutic Resource Centers
Optimal Health
RationalMed
Physician Service Center
PolyMedica Corporation
Europa Apotheek Venlo

CONTACTS: Note: Officers with more than one job title may be intentionally listed here more than once.
David B. Snow, Jr., CEO
Kenneth O. Klepper, COO
Kenneth O. Klepper, Pres.
Richard J. Rubino, CFO/Sr. VP-Finance
Jack A. Smith, Chief Mktg. Officer/Sr. VP
Karin Princivalle, Sr. VP-Human Resources
Robert S. Epstein, Chief Medical Officer/Sr. VP-Medical & Analytical
John P. Driscoll, Sr. VP-Prod. Dev.
Thomas M. Moriarty, General Counsel/Corp. Sec./Sr. VP-Pharmaceutical
John P. Driscoll, Sr. VP-Bus. Dev.
Gabriel R. Cappucci, Chief Acct. Officer/Sr. VP/Controller
Timothy C. Wentworth, CEO/Pres., Accredo Health Group, Inc.
Bryan D. Birch, Group Pres., Employer Accounts
Brian T. Griffin, Group Pres., Health Plans
Glenn C. Taylor, Group Pres., Key Accounts
David B. Snow, Jr., Chmn.

Phone: 201-269-3400	Fax: 201-269-1109
Toll-Free:	
Address: 100 Parsons Pond Dr., Franklin Lakes, NJ 07417-2603 US	

GROWTH PLANS/SPECIAL FEATURES:
Medco Health Solutions, Inc. is a leading national pharmacy benefit manager. Its prescription drug benefit programs are designed to drive down the cost of pharmacy healthcare for private and public employers, health plans, labor unions, government agencies of all sizes and individuals served by the Medicare Part D Prescription Drug Program. Medco collaborates with retail pharmacies, physicians, the Centers for Medicare & Medicaid Services for Medicare and state Medicaid agencies. It provides its services through a national network of retail pharmacies, its mail-order pharmacies and its Specialty Pharmacy segment, Accredo Health Group. In 2007, Medco introduced Medco Therapeutic Resource Centers, staffed with hundreds of pharmacists trained and certified in specific complex and chronic conditions and associated medications. The company's services include benefit plan design services, which take into account formulary, pharmacy management, mail-order initiatives, specialty pharmacy, drug coverage, cost-share options and generic drug utilization initiatives; clinical management services, including utilization management and its RationalMed patient safety program and Optimal Health support solution; pharmacy management services, such as its mail-order service, specialty pharmacy management, retail pharmacy networks, call center pharmacies and reimbursement services; physician services, such as its Physician Service Center, designed to motivate physicians to prescribe more cost-effective medications; and web-based services for members, clients and pharmacists. In October 2007, Medco acquired PolyMedica Corporation, which provides blood glucose testing supplies, for $1.5 billion. In November 2007, it acquired Critical Care Systems for $218 million. In March 2008, Medco broke ground on its $140 million automated pharmacy in Indiana, which will be the world's largest automated pharmacy and will house a research center for personalized medicine. In April 2008, Medco acquired a majority interest in Europa Apotheek Venlo, a provider of clinical health care and mail-order pharmacy services in Germany, for approximately $120 million.

Medco offers its employees flexible working arrangements.

FINANCIALS: Sales and profits are in thousands of dollars—add 000 to get the full amount. 2007 Note: Financial information for 2007 was not available for all companies at press time.

2007 Sales: $44,506,200	2007 Profits: $912,000	U.S. Stock Ticker: MHS
2006 Sales: $42,543,700	2006 Profits: $630,200	Int'l Ticker: Int'l Exchange:
2005 Sales: $37,870,900	2005 Profits: $602,000	Employees: 19,900
2004 Sales: $35,351,900	2004 Profits: $481,600	Fiscal Year Ends: 12/31
2003 Sales: $34,264,500	2003 Profits: $425,800	Parent Company:

SALARIES/BENEFITS:
Pension Plan:	ESOP Stock Plan:	Profit Sharing:	Top Exec. Salary: $1,273,204	Bonus: $2,600,000
Savings Plan:	Stock Purch. Plan:		Second Exec. Salary: $738,368	Bonus: $1,100,000

OTHER THOUGHTS:
Apparent Women Officers or Directors: 3
Hot Spot for Advancement for Women/Minorities: Y

LOCATIONS: ("Y" = Yes)
West:	Southwest:	Midwest:	Southeast:	Northeast:	International:
Y	Y	Y	Y	Y	

Note: Financial information, benefits and other data can change quickly and may vary from those stated here.

MEDTRONIC INC

www.medtronic.com

Industry Group Code: 339113 Ranks within this company's industry group: Sales: 2 Profits: 2

Management:		Sales/Marketing:		Liberal Arts:		Information Systems:		Professionals:		Technical/Scientific:	
Mgmt. Trainees:	Y	Mktg. Professionals:	Y	Gen. Writing/Editing:	Y	Info. Management:	Y	Finance/Accounting:	Y	Engineers, Elec.:	Y
Experienced Mgmt.:	Y	Retail Sales:		Technical Writing:	Y	Software Dev.:	Y	Law:	Y	Engineers, Other:	Y
Int'l Business:	Y	Commercial/Industrial:	Y	Graphic Arts/Photog.:	Y	Hardware Dev.:	Y	HR/Other:	Y	Health/Lab:	Y
MBA Graduates:	Y	Sales Trainees:	Y	Music:		Systems Integration:		Training:	Y	Scientists/Research:	Y
		Advertising Pros.:	Y	Broadcasting:		Consulting/Other:		Health Care:	Y	Petroleum/Chemicals:	
				Other:				Consulting:		Math/Other:	Y

TYPES OF BUSINESS:

Equipment-Defibrillators & Pacing Products
Neurological Devices
Diabetes Management Devices
Ear, Nose & Throat Surgical Equipment
Pain Management Devices
Catheters & Stents
Cardiac Surgery Equipment

BRANDS/DIVISIONS/AFFILIATES:

Medtronic ENT
Medtronic Xomed
Kyphon, Inc.
Breakaway Imaging LLC
LifeScan, Inc.
INFUSE Bone Graft
Continuous Glucose Monitoring

CONTACTS: *Note: Officers with more than one job title may be intentionally listed here more than once.*

Bill Hawkins, CEO
Bill Hawkins, Pres.
Gary Ellis, CFO/Sr. VP
Stephen N. Oesterle, Sr. VP-Medicine & Tech.
Terrance Carlson, General Counsel/Corp. Sec./Sr. VP
H. James Dallas, Sr. VP-Quality & Oper.
Dan Lemaitre, Sr. VP-Corp Strategy & Dev.
Susan Alpert, Chief Regulatory Officer/Sr. VP
Oern R. Stuge, Sr. VP/Pres., Europe, Canada, Latin America
Scott Ward, Sr. VP/Pres., Cardiovascular
Stephen Mahle, Exec. VP-Healthcare Policy & Regulatory
Arthur D. Collins, Jr., Chmn.
Jean-Luc Butel, Sr. VP/Pres., Medtronic Int'l

Phone: 763-514-4000	Fax: 763-514-4879
Toll-Free:	
Address: 710 Medtronic Pkwy., Minneapolis, MN 55432 US	

GROWTH PLANS/SPECIAL FEATURES:

Medtronic, Inc. is a global leader in medical technology, whose professed mission is alleviating pain, restoring health and extending life for millions of people around the world. The firm operates in eight business sectors: cardiac rhythm disease management; cardiac surgery; neurological; spinal and navigation; ear, nose and throat (ENT) surgery; vascular; physio-control; and diabetes. Medtronic is one of the world's largest suppliers of medical devices for cardiac rhythm management, including pacemakers and implantable cardiac defibrillators. The Cardiac Surgery division specializes in revascularization, heart valve repair and replacement, surgical ablation and blood management, offering cardiac surgeons a broad range of products for the operating room. The Navigation and Spinal division offers spinal products and image-guided surgery systems that facilitate surgical planning. The ENT surgery unit operates under the name Xomed Surgical Products, Inc. and is a leading manufacturer ENT surgical products. The Neurological division develops, manufactures, and markets devices for the treatment of neurological, urological, and gastrointestinal disorders. The Vascular Therapy division offers minimally invasive products and therapies to treat coronary artery disease, aortic and thoracic aneurysms, and peripheral vascular disease. The Diabetes unit provides glucose monitors, insulin pumps and other products, as well as informational resources available on the firm's web site. In 2007, the FDA approved the firm's Continuous Glucose Monitoring devices for children and teenagers. The FDA also approved Medtronic's INFUSE Bone Graft treatment for certain oral maxillofacial and dental regenerative bone grafting procedures. The company formed an alliance with LifeScan, Inc. to distribute and co-market blood glucose meters for diabetes patients. In April 2007, Medtronic acquired the O-arm Imaging System assets of Breakaway Imaging LLC, and in November the firm completed its acquisition of Kyphon, Inc. for roughly $4.2 billion.

FINANCIALS: Sales and profits are in thousands of dollars—add 000 to get the full amount. 2007 Note: Financial information for 2007 was not available for all companies at press time.

2007 Sales: $12,299,000	2007 Profits: $2,802,000	**U.S. Stock Ticker: MDT**
2006 Sales: $11,292,000	2006 Profits: $2,546,700	**Int'l Ticker:** **Int'l Exchange:**
2005 Sales: $10,054,600	2005 Profits: $1,803,900	Employees: 37,800
2004 Sales: $9,087,200	2004 Profits: $1,959,300	Fiscal Year Ends: 4/30
2003 Sales: $7,665,200	2003 Profits: $1,599,800	Parent Company:

SALARIES/BENEFITS:

Pension Plan:	ESOP Stock Plan:	Profit Sharing:	Top Exec. Salary: $1,275,000	Bonus: $1,020,000
Savings Plan: Y	Stock Purch. Plan: Y		Second Exec. Salary: $775,000	Bonus: $490,963

OTHER THOUGHTS:

Apparent Women Officers or Directors: 2
Hot Spot for Advancement for Women/Minorities: Y

LOCATIONS: ("Y" = Yes)

West:	Southwest:	Midwest:	Southeast:	Northeast:	International:
Y	Y	Y	Y	Y	Y

Note: Financial information, benefits and other data can change quickly and may vary from those stated here.

MEIJER INC

www.meijer.com

Industry Group Code: 445110 Ranks within this company's industry group: Sales: Profits:

Management:		Sales/Marketing:		Liberal Arts:	Information Systems:		Professionals:		Technical/Scientific:	
Mgmt. Trainees:	Y	Mktg. Professionals:	Y	Gen. Writing/Editing:	Info. Management:	Y	Finance/Accounting:	Y	Engineers, Elec.:	
Experienced Mgmt.:	Y	Retail Sales:	Y	Technical Writing:	Software Dev.:		Law:	Y	Engineers, Other:	
Int'l Business:		Commercial/Industrial:		Graphic Arts/Photog.:	Hardware Dev.:		HR/Other:	Y	Health/Lab:	
MBA Graduates:	Y	Sales Trainees:	Y	Music:	Systems Integration:		Training:	Y	Scientists/Research:	
		Advertising Pros.:	Y	Broadcasting:	Consulting/Other:		Health Care:		Petroleum/Chemicals:	
				Other:			Consulting:		Math/Other:	

TYPES OF BUSINESS:
Grocery Stores
General Merchandise
Hardware
Photo Services
Pharmacies
In-Store Restaurants
Gasoline, Retail
Home Decor

BRANDS/DIVISIONS/AFFILIATES:

CONTACTS: Note: Officers with more than one job title may be intentionally listed here more than once.
Hendrik G. Meijer, CEO
Mark Murray, Pres.
Bob Mooney, VP-Mfg.
Stacie Behler, VP-Corp. Comm. & Public Rel.
Doug Meijer, Co-Chmn.
Fred Meijer, Chmn. Emeritus
Hendrik G. Meijer, Co-Chmn.
Bob Mooney, VP-Distribution Oper.

Phone: 616-453-6711 Fax: 616-791-2572
Toll-Free: 877-363-4537
Address: 2929 Walker Ave. N.W., Grand Rapids, MI 49544 US

GROWTH PLANS/SPECIAL FEATURES:
Meijer, Inc. is a leading grocery retailer in the Midwest, with 182 superstores throughout Illinois, Indiana, Kentucky, Michigan and Ohio. The firm's combination grocery and general merchandise stores range in size from 200,000 to 250,000 square feet, which is about four times the size of typical grocery stores. Each Meijer store carries about 120,000 brand-name and private-label products, including bulk foods, fresh produce, frozen items, seafood and meat products. Most stores feature nearly 40 departments, such as electronics, hardware, toys, garden, entertainment, jewelry, photo, banking, pharmacy, books, apparel, automotive and furniture. In addition, some stores offer a discount gas station. The superstores also offer several in-store restaurants, including delis and cafes. Meijer stores are open 24-hours-a-day and close only on Christmas. In addition to its retail stores, the firm operates a web site that features a baby club, wine guides, contests, advertisements, pharmaceutical help and gardening tips. The company recently launched a branded prepaid wireless phone and phone card program, in conjunction with Fusion Mobile. In September 2008, the company announced the construction of a new bakery facility at its Middlebury, Indiana food-service plant.

The company offers extensive benefits to both full- and part-time employees, including casual dress, competitive pay, flexible hours and health plans. Benefits vary with position.

FINANCIALS: Sales and profits are in thousands of dollars—add 000 to get the full amount. 2007 Note: Financial information for 2007 was not available for all companies at press time.
2007 Sales: $13,900,000 2007 Profits: $ U.S. Stock Ticker: Private
2006 Sales: $12,500,000 2006 Profits: $ Int'l Ticker: Int'l Exchange:
2005 Sales: $ 2005 Profits: $ Employees: 65,000
2004 Sales: $11,900,000 2004 Profits: $ Fiscal Year Ends: 1/31
2003 Sales: $10,900,000 2003 Profits: $ Parent Company:

SALARIES/BENEFITS:
Pension Plan: ESOP Stock Plan: Profit Sharing: Top Exec. Salary: $ Bonus: $
Savings Plan: Y Stock Purch. Plan: Second Exec. Salary: $ Bonus: $

OTHER THOUGHTS:
Apparent Women Officers or Directors:
Hot Spot for Advancement for Women/Minorities:

LOCATIONS: ("Y" = Yes)
West:	Southwest:	Midwest:	Southeast:	Northeast:	International:
		Y			

MEN'S WEARHOUSE INC (THE) www.menswearhouse.com

Industry Group Code: 448110 Ranks within this company's industry group: Sales: 1 Profits: 1

Management:		Sales/Marketing:		Liberal Arts:		Information Systems:		Professionals:		Technical/Scientific:	
Mgmt. Trainees:	Y	Mktg. Professionals:	Y	Gen. Writing/Editing:	Y	Info. Management:	Y	Finance/Accounting:	Y	Engineers, Elec.:	
Experienced Mgmt.:	Y	Retail Sales:	Y	Technical Writing:		Software Dev.:	Y	Law:	Y	Engineers, Other:	
Int'l Business:	Y	Commercial/Industrial:	Y	Graphic Arts/Photog.:	Y	Hardware Dev.:		HR/Other:	Y	Health/Lab:	
MBA Graduates:	Y	Sales Trainees:	Y	Music:		Systems Integration:		Training:	Y	Scientists/Research:	
		Advertising Pros.:	Y	Broadcasting:		Consulting/Other:		Health Care:		Petroleum/Chemicals:	
				Other:	Y			Consulting:		Math/Other:	

TYPES OF BUSINESS:

Men's Apparel, Retail
Men's Suits
Shoes & Accessories
Business Casual Wear
Sportswear
Shoes & Accessories
Ladies' Career Apparel

BRANDS/DIVISIONS/AFFILIATES:

K&G
Moores Clothing for Men
MW Tux
Perfect Fit
After Hours Formalwear

CONTACTS: Note: Officers with more than one job title may be intentionally listed here more than once.

George A. Zimmer, CEO
Douglas S. Ewert, COO
Douglas S. Ewert, Pres.
Neill P. Davis, CFO/Exec. VP
Charles Bresler, Exec. VP-Mktg.
Charles Bresler, Exec. VP-Human Resources
Neill P. Davis, Treas./Principal Financial Officer
David H. Edwab, Vice Chmn.
George A. Zimmer, Chmn.

Phone: 713-592-7200	Fax: 713-657-0872
Toll-Free:	
Address: 5803 Glenmont Dr., Houston, TX 77081 US	

GROWTH PLANS/SPECIAL FEATURES:

The Men's Wearhouse, Inc. is a leading specialty retailer of men's suits and provider of tuxedo rental products in the U.S. and Canada. The company's U.S. operations include more than 668 stores in 46 states and Washington, D.C., primarily operating under the brand names of Men's Wearhouse and K&G. In Canada, operations include 116 retail apparel stores in ten provinces operating under the brand name of Moores Clothing for Men. Its tuxedo rental stores are operated under the brand name of MW Tux in 35 states. Men's Wearhouse apparel stores target middle and upper-middle income men and offer designer, brand name and private label merchandise at discounted prices through 563 locations. Merchandise offered includes suits, sport coats, slacks, formalwear, business casual, sportswear, outerwear, dress shirts, shoes and accessories. Most of these stores also offer tuxedo rental products in a section branded as MW Tux. The Men's Wearhouse's 105 K&G branded stores target more price sensitive customers and include ladies' career apparel at 89 locations. Under the Moores brand, the company targets middle and upper-middle income men in Canada. During 2007, 54.1% of The Men's Wearhouse's clothing product sales were attributable to tailored clothing and 45.9% were attributable to casual attire, sportswear, shoes, shirts, ties, outerwear and other clothing product revenues. The firm offers a private label credit card as well as a Perfect Fit loyalty program to its customers. In April 2007, The Men's Wearhouse acquired After Hours Formalwear, a chain of 507 men's formalwear stores, for roughly $100 million. In July 2008, the company closed its manufacturing facility in Montreal, Quebec.

The Men's Wearhouse offers its employees a tuition reimbursement program, a sabbatical leave program, a wellness program, merchandise discounts and medical, dental, life and disability insurance.

FINANCIALS: Sales and profits are in thousands of dollars—add 000 to get the full amount. 2007 Note: Financial information for 2007 was not available for all companies at press time.

2007 Sales: $1,882,064	2007 Profits: $148,575	U.S. Stock Ticker: MW
2006 Sales: $1,724,898	2006 Profits: $103,903	Int'l Ticker: Int'l Exchange:
2005 Sales: $1,546,679	2005 Profits: $71,356	Employees: 14,900
2004 Sales: $1,392,680	2004 Profits: $50,026	Fiscal Year Ends: 2/1
2003 Sales: $1,295,000	2003 Profits: $42,400	Parent Company:

SALARIES/BENEFITS:

Pension Plan:	ESOP Stock Plan: Y	Profit Sharing:	Top Exec. Salary: $428,077	Bonus: $134,000
Savings Plan: Y	Stock Purch. Plan: Y		Second Exec. Salary: $428,077	Bonus: $134,000

OTHER THOUGHTS:

Apparent Women Officers or Directors:
Hot Spot for Advancement for Women/Minorities:

LOCATIONS: ("Y" = Yes)

West:	Southwest:	Midwest:	Southeast:	Northeast:	International:
Y	Y	Y	Y	Y	Y

MERCER INC

www.mercer.com

Industry Group Code: 541612 Ranks within this company's industry group: Sales: 2 Profits:

Management:		Sales/Marketing:		Liberal Arts:		Information Systems:		Professionals:		Technical/Scientific:	
Mgmt. Trainees:		Mktg. Professionals:	Y	Gen. Writing/Editing:	Y	Info. Management:	Y	Finance/Accounting:	Y	Engineers, Elec.:	
Experienced Mgmt.:	Y	Retail Sales:		Technical Writing:		Software Dev.:		Law:	Y	Engineers, Other:	
Int'l Business:	Y	Commercial/Industrial:	Y	Graphic Arts/Photog.:		Hardware Dev.:		HR/Other:	Y	Health/Lab:	
MBA Graduates:	Y	Sales Trainees:		Music:		Systems Integration:	Y	Training:	Y	Scientists/Research:	
		Advertising Pros.:	Y	Broadcasting:		Consulting/Other:	Y	Health Care:		Petroleum/Chemicals:	
				Other:	Y			Consulting:	Y	Math/Other:	

TYPES OF BUSINESS:

Consulting-Human Resources
Employee Benefits Consulting
Compensation Consulting
Investment Consulting
Outsourced Human Resources Services (BPO)
Employee Benefits Administration
Retirement Plan Administration
Absence Management

BRANDS/DIVISIONS/AFFILIATES:

Mercer HR
Mercer Investment Consulting
Mercer Retirement
Mercer Global Investments
Mercer Human Capital
Mercer HR Services
Marsh & McLennan Companies, Inc.
Höfer Vorsorge-Management

CONTACTS: *Note: Officers with more than one job title may be intentionally listed here more than once.*

M. Michele Burns, CEO
Tom Elliott, COO
Pat Milligan, Head-Sales & Mktg.
Steve Mele, Chief Human Resources Officer
Larry Woerner, Chief Admin. Officer
David Goldenberg, General Counsel
Terry Thompson, Head-Corp. Strategy
Terry Thompson, Head-Finance
Patricia Milligan, Leader-Global Market Dev.
Phil de Cristo, Pres., Investment Mgmt.
Jeff Miller, Pres., Outsourcing
Pat Milligan, Chief Markets Officer/Head-Global Client Mgmt.
M. Michele Burns, Chmn.

Phone: 212-345-7000	Fax: 212-345-7414
Toll-Free:	
Address: 1166 Ave. of the Americas, New York, NY 10036 US	

GROWTH PLANS/SPECIAL FEATURES:

Mercer, Inc. (Mercer HR) is a global provider of a broad range of human resource advice and solutions. Mercer HR also provides related financial advice, products and services in the retirement, health and benefits areas. The firm has four lines of business: Retirement & Investments; Health & Benefits; Talent; and Outsourcing. The Retirement & Investments segment is divided into three units: Mercer Retirement, Mercer Investment Consulting and Mercer Global Investments. Mercer Retirement offers consulting services in defined benefit and defined contribution plans, executive retirement plans, retiree medical benefits and the retiree benefits aspects of mergers and acquisitions. Mercer Investment Consulting offers customized guidance at each stage of an investment decision, risk management and investment monitoring process. Mercer Global Investments provides global, multi-manager investment solutions to institutional investors (primarily retirement plan sponsors and trustees) and individual investors (in Australia and prospectively in other countries), primarily for investment of their retirement plan assets. The Health & Benefits segment offers advice and solutions related to a broad spectrum of health and welfare related issues including health care strategy, health care funding, pharmacy, disease management and absentee management. The Talent segment works through subsidiary Mercer Human Capital to design, analyze and align clients' compensation and performance management systems, including both executive compensation and broad-based employee compensation programs. It also provides data, software and compensation administration services to help companies manage and operate their compensation and total rewards programs. The Outsourcing segment, through subsidiary Mercer HR Services, provides outsourced human resources administration, technology and business process solutions globally. The majority of Mercer HR's clients are Fortune 1000 and FTSE 100 companies. Mercer HR has offices in 41 countries around the globe, and the firm is a subsidiary of Marsh & McLennan Companies, Inc.

FINANCIALS: Sales and profits are in thousands of dollars—add 000 to get the full amount. 2007 Note: Financial information for 2007 was not available for all companies at press time.

2007 Sales: $3,368,000	2007 Profits: $	**U.S. Stock Ticker: Subsidiary**
2006 Sales: $3,021,000	2006 Profits: $	**Int'l Ticker:** Int'l Exchange:
2005 Sales: $2,794,000	2005 Profits: $	Employees: 16,500
2004 Sales: $	2004 Profits: $	Fiscal Year Ends: 12/31
2003 Sales: $	2003 Profits: $	Parent Company: MARSH & MCLENNAN COMPANIES INC

SALARIES/BENEFITS:

Pension Plan:	ESOP Stock Plan:	Profit Sharing:	Top Exec. Salary: $	Bonus: $
Savings Plan:	Stock Purch. Plan:		Second Exec. Salary: $	Bonus: $

OTHER THOUGHTS:

Apparent Women Officers or Directors: 2
Hot Spot for Advancement for Women/Minorities: Y

LOCATIONS: ("Y" = Yes)

West:	Southwest:	Midwest:	Southeast:	Northeast:	International:
Y	Y	Y	Y	Y	Y

Note: Financial information, benefits and other data can change quickly and may vary from those stated here.

MERCK & CO INC

www.merck.com

Industry Group Code: 325412 **Ranks within this company's industry group:** Sales: Profits:

Management:		Sales/Marketing:		Liberal Arts:		Information Systems:		Professionals:		Technical/Scientific:	
Mgmt. Trainees:	Y	Mktg. Professionals:	Y	Gen. Writing/Editing:	Y	Info. Management:	Y	Finance/Accounting:	Y	Engineers, Elec.:	Y
Experienced Mgmt.:	Y	Retail Sales:		Technical Writing:	Y	Software Dev.:	Y	Law:	Y	Engineers, Other:	Y
Int'l Business:	Y	Commercial/Industrial:	Y	Graphic Arts/Photog.:	Y	Hardware Dev.:		HR/Other:	Y	Health/Lab:	Y
MBA Graduates:	Y	Sales Trainees:	Y	Music:		Systems Integration:		Training:	Y	Scientists/Research:	Y
		Advertising Pros.:	Y	Broadcasting:		Consulting/Other:		Health Care:	Y	Petroleum/Chemicals:	
				Other:				Consulting:		Math/Other:	Y

TYPES OF BUSINESS:

Pharmaceuticals Development & Manufacturing
Cholesterol Drugs
Hypertension Drugs
Heart Failure Drugs
Allergy & Asthma Drugs
Animal Health Products
Vaccines
Preventative Drugs

BRANDS/DIVISIONS/AFFILIATES:

Merck Institute for Science Education
Sirna Therapeutics, Inc.
Singulair
Propecia
Cozaar
Fosamax
Gardasil
EMEND

CONTACTS: *Note: Officers with more than one job title may be intentionally listed here more than once.*

Richard Clark, CEO
Richard Clark, Pres.
Peter Kellogg, CFO/Exec. VP
Mirian Graddick-Weir, Sr. VP-Human Resources
Peter Kim, Pres., Research Laboratories
Chris Scalet, CIO
Willie Deese, Pres., Mfg. Div.
Bruce N. Kuhlik, General Counsel/Exec. VP
David W. Anstice, Exec. VP-Strategy Initiatives
Peter Kellogg, Exec. VP-Investor Rel.
Judy Lewent, Chief-Finance
Kenneth C. Frazier, Pres., Global Human Health
Richard T. Clark, Chmn.
Chris Scalet, Sr. VP-Global Svcs.

Phone: 908-423-1000	Fax: 908-735-1253
Toll-Free:	
Address: 1 Merck Dr., Whitehouse Station, NJ 08889-0100 US	

GROWTH PLANS/SPECIAL FEATURES:

Merck & Co., Inc. is a leading research-driven pharmaceutical company that manufactures a broad range of products sold in approximately 150 countries. These products include therapeutic and preventative drugs generally sold by prescription and medications used to control and alleviate disease. As one of the world's largest pharmaceutical companies, Merck's line of big selling medicines include Gardasil, a vaccine for HPV which causes cervical cancer and warts; Fosamax a drug for the prevention of osteoporosis; and Zocor for cholesterol. The company also manufactures Propecia, a popular treatment for male pattern baldness, and Singulair, a seasonal allergy and asthma medicine, both of which are offered in tablet form. In addition to medicines, the company manufactures vaccines such as Rotateq, designed to prevent gastroenteritis in infants and children; and Gardasil, a new product designed to reduce the probabilities of cancer. Drugs approved by the FDA in 2007 include: EMEND, a drug that prevents chemotherapy-induced nausea and ISENTRESS (raltegravir) tablets, which treats patients with the HIV-1 infection. Additionally, the FDA is currently reviewing approval applications for CORDAPTIVE , a drug designed to reduce flushing often associated with niacin treatment and loratadine/montelukast, a treatment of allergic rhinitis symptoms. In 2007, Merck acquired NovaCardia, Inc., a privately held clinical-stage pharmaceutical company focused on cardiovascular disease, for $366.4 million.

Merck offers its employees on-site fitness facilities, day care and summer camp programs, tuition reimbursement and financial planning assistance.

FINANCIALS: Sales and profits are in thousands of dollars—add 000 to get the full amount. 2007 Note: Financial information for 2007 was not available for all companies at press time.

2007 Sales: $24,197,700	2007 Profits: $3,275,400	**U.S. Stock Ticker: MRK**
2006 Sales: $22,636,000	2006 Profits: $4,433,800	**Int'l Ticker:** Int'l Exchange:
2005 Sales: $22,011,900	2005 Profits: $4,631,300	Employees: 59,800
2004 Sales: $22,938,600	2004 Profits: $5,813,400	Fiscal Year Ends: 12/31
2003 Sales: $22,485,900	2003 Profits: $6,830,900	Parent Company:

SALARIES/BENEFITS:

Pension Plan: Y	ESOP Stock Plan:	Profit Sharing:	Top Exec. Salary: $1,616,670	Bonus: $4,311,059
Savings Plan: Y	Stock Purch. Plan:		Second Exec. Salary: $922,560	Bonus: $1,395,554

OTHER THOUGHTS:

Apparent Women Officers or Directors: 2
Hot Spot for Advancement for Women/Minorities: Y

LOCATIONS: ("Y" = Yes)

West:	Southwest:	Midwest:	Southeast:	Northeast:	International:
Y	Y	Y	Y	Y	Y

Note: Financial information, benefits and other data can change quickly and may vary from those stated here.

METLIFE INC

www.metlife.com

Industry Group Code: 524113 Ranks within this company's industry group: Sales: 1 Profits: 1

Management:		Sales/Marketing:		Liberal Arts:		Information Systems:		Professionals:		Technical/Scientific:	
Mgmt. Trainees:	Y	Mktg. Professionals:	Y	Gen. Writing/Editing:	Y	Info. Management:	Y	Finance/Accounting:	Y	Engineers, Elec.:	
Experienced Mgmt.:	Y	Retail Sales:	Y	Technical Writing:	Y	Software Dev.:	Y	Law:	Y	Engineers, Other:	
Int'l Business:	Y	Commercial/Industrial:	Y	Graphic Arts/Photog.:	Y	Hardware Dev.:		HR/Other:	Y	Health/Lab:	
MBA Graduates:	Y	Sales Trainees:	Y	Music:		Systems Integration:		Training:	Y	Scientists/Research:	Y
		Advertising Pros.:	Y	Broadcasting:		Consulting/Other:		Health Care:	Y	Petroleum/Chemicals:	
				Other:				Consulting:		Math/Other:	Y

TYPES OF BUSINESS:

Insurance
Banking
Investment Products
Mutual Funds
Life Insurance
Property & Casualty Insurance
Auto Insurance
Reinsurance

BRANDS/DIVISIONS/AFFILIATES:

MetLife Bank
Reinsurance Group of America, Inc.

CONTACTS: Note: Officers with more than one job title may be intentionally listed here more than once.

C. Robert Henrikson, CEO
C. Robert Henrikson, Pres.
William J. Wheeler, CFO/Exec. VP
Maria R. Morris, Technology & Operations
Exec. VP-Tech. & Oper.
Ruth A. Fattori, Chief Admin. Officer/Sr. Exec. VP
James L. Lipscomb, General Counsel/Exec. VP
Steven A. Kandarian, Chief Investment Officer/Exec. VP
Lisa M. Weber, Pres., Individual Bus.
William J. Mullaney, Pres., Institutional Bus.
C. Robert Henrikson, Chmn.
William J. Toppeta, Pres., Int'l

Phone: 212-578-2211	Fax: 212-578-3320
Toll-Free: 800-638-5433	
Address: 200 Park Ave., New York, NY 10166 US	

GROWTH PLANS/SPECIAL FEATURES:

MetLife, Inc. is a provider of insurance and other financial services with operations throughout the U.S. and regions of Latin America, Europe and Asia Pacific. Through its domestic and international subsidiaries and affiliates, the company offers life insurance; annuities; automobile and homeowners insurance; retail banking; and other financial services to individuals, as well as group insurance, reinsurance and retirement & savings products and services to corporations and other institutions. The firm operates in five segments. The institutional segment offers group insurance, retirement and savings products and services to corporations and other institutions. The individual segment offers asset protection and accumulation products, primarily life and disability insurance. The auto and home group operates through the Metropolitan Property and Casualty Insurance Company subsidiary and offers personal lines property and casualty insurance including renters', homeowners', car and recreational vehicle insurance. The international segment provides accident and health insurance; credit insurance; annuities; and savings and retirement products to customers within the Latin America, Europe and Asia Pacific regions. The reinsurance segment includes Reinsurance Group of America, Inc. and MetLife's ancillary life reinsurance business. Corporate and other segment contains the excess capital not allocated to the business segments; various start-up entities, including MetLife Bank; National Association, and run-off entities and interest expense related to the majority of the company's outstanding debt and expenses associated with certain legal proceedings and income tax audit issues. In June 2008, MetLife announced its intent to split-off substantially all of its 52% interest in RGA. Also in 2008, MetLife Bank N.A. entered an agreement to acquire First Tennessee Bank N.A., a subsidiary of First Horizon National Corp. Metlife will not be assuming any subprime mortgages in the First Horizon acquisition. MetLife Bank also acquired EverBank Reverse Mortgage LLC in May 2008.

FINANCIALS: Sales and profits are in thousands of dollars—add 000 to get the full amount. 2007 Note: Financial information for 2007 was not available for all companies at press time.

2007 Sales: $53,070,000	2007 Profits: $4,317,000	**U.S. Stock Ticker: MET**
2006 Sales: $48,254,000	2006 Profits: $6,293,000	**Int'l Ticker:** Int'l Exchange:
2005 Sales: $44,683,000	2005 Profits: $4,714,000	Employees: 47,000
2004 Sales: $38,712,000	2004 Profits: $2,758,000	Fiscal Year Ends: 12/31
2003 Sales: $35,190,000	2003 Profits: $2,217,000	Parent Company:

SALARIES/BENEFITS:

Pension Plan: Y	ESOP Stock Plan:	Profit Sharing:	Top Exec. Salary: $950,000	Bonus: $4,000,000
Savings Plan:	Stock Purch. Plan:		Second Exec. Salary: $583,334	Bonus: $1,300,000

OTHER THOUGHTS:

Apparent Women Officers or Directors: 5
Hot Spot for Advancement for Women/Minorities: Y

LOCATIONS: ("Y" = Yes)

West:	Southwest:	Midwest:	Southeast:	Northeast:	International:
Y	Y	Y	Y	Y	Y

Note: Financial information, benefits and other data can change quickly and may vary from those stated here.

MGM MIRAGE   www.mgmmirage.com

Industry Group Code: 721120 Ranks within this company's industry group: Sales: 2 Profits: 1

Management:		Sales/Marketing:		Liberal Arts:		Information Systems:		Professionals:		Technical/Scientific:	
Mgmt. Trainees:	Y	Mktg. Professionals:	Y	Gen. Writing/Editing:	Y	Info. Management:	Y	Finance/Accounting:	Y	Engineers, Elec.:	
Experienced Mgmt.:	Y	Retail Sales:		Technical Writing:		Software Dev.:		Law:	Y	Engineers, Other:	
Int'l Business:	Y	Commercial/Industrial:	Y	Graphic Arts/Photog.:	Y	Hardware Dev.:		HR/Other:	Y	Health/Lab:	
MBA Graduates:	Y	Sales Trainees:		Music:	Y	Systems Integration:		Training:	Y	Scientists/Research:	
		Advertising Pros.:	Y	Broadcasting:		Consulting/Other:		Health Care:		Petroleum/Chemicals:	
				Other:	Y			Consulting:		Math/Other:	

TYPES OF BUSINESS:

Casino Hotels & Resorts
Golf Courses

BRANDS/DIVISIONS/AFFILIATES:

Bellagio
MGM Grand Las Vegas
Mandalay Bay
Mirage (The)
Luxor
Excalibur
Treasure Island
MGM Grand Macau

CONTACTS: *Note: Officers with more than one job title may be intentionally listed here more than once.*

J. Terrence Lanni, CEO
James Murren, COO
James Murren, Pres.
Daniel J. D'Arrigo, CFO/Exec. VP
Richard Vosburgh, Sr. VP-Human Resources
Thomas R. Peck, Jr., CIO/Sr. VP
Robert Baldwin, Chief Design & Construction Officer
Aldo Manzini, Chief Admin. Officer/Exec. VP
Gary N. Jacobs, General Counsel/Sec./Exec. VP
Cathy Santoro, Treas.
Randy Morton, Pres./COO-Bellagio
Bill Hornbuckle, Pres./COO-Mandalay Bay & MGM Grand Atlantic City
Robert Baldwin, Pres./CEO-CityCenter
Lorenzo Creighton, Pres./COO-MGM Grand Detroit
J. Terrence Lanni, Chmn.
Pansy Ho Chiu-king, Managing Dir.-MGM Grand Macau
Teresa Reynolds, Chief Procurement Officer

Phone: 702-693-7120	Fax: 702-693-8626
Toll-Free:	
Address: 3600 Las Vegas Blvd. S., Las Vegas, NV 89109 US	

GROWTH PLANS/SPECIAL FEATURES:

MGM Mirage (MGM) operates 16 wholly-owned casino resorts in Nevada, Mississippi and Michigan; and four 50%-owned casino resorts in Nevada, Macau, New Jersey and Illinois. Its casinos on the Las Vegas Strip include Bellagio, MGM Grand Las Vegas, Mandalay Bay, The Mirage, Luxor, Treasure Island, New York-New York, Excalibur, Monte Carlo and Circus Circus Las Vegas. Combined, they feature 37,696 guestrooms, nearly 1.2 million square feet of gaming space, 19,335 slot machines and 994 gaming tables. Its other Nevada properties, including Circus Circus Reno, Silver Legacy (50% owned), Gold Strike (in Jean, NV) and Railroad Pass, offer 4,212 guestrooms, 207,000 square feet of gaming space, 3,477 slot machines and 127 gaming tables. Finally, its other operations include MGM Grand Detroit, Beau Rivage and Gold Strike (in Tunica, MI), all wholly-owned; and MGM Grand Macau, Borgata and Grand Victoria, all 50%-owned. These facilities offer 5,666 guestrooms, 663,000 square feet of gaming space, 13,874 slot machines and 835 gaming tables. MGM's casinos often feature restaurants, bars, spas, salons, retail space, nightclubs and lounges. It also owns and operates three championship golf courses: Shadow Creek, Fallen Oak and Primm Valley Golf Club. Over half of MGM's revenue is generated by non-gaming activities. Following its November 2007 joint venture agreement with Dubai World, MGM now owns 50% of the $8.7 billion Project CityCenter, still under development, located between Bellagio and Monte Carlo. It will feature a 4,000-room casino resort; two 400-room non-casino hotels; 425,000 square feet of retail, restaurant and entertainment space; and 2.3 million square feet of residential space for 2,700 luxury condominiums. In April 2007, MGM sold three casinos (Whiskey Pete's, Buffalo Bill's and Primm Valley Resorts) to Herbst Gaming, Inc. for $398 million. In June 2007, it sold two hotel-casinos in Laughlin, NV (Colorado Belle and Edgewater) to a group led by Anthony Marnell III for $199 million.

FINANCIALS: Sales and profits are in thousands of dollars—add 000 to get the full amount. 2007 Note: Financial information for 2007 was not available for all companies at press time.

2007 Sales: $7,691,637	2007 Profits: $1,584,419	**U.S. Stock Ticker: MGM**
2006 Sales: $7,175,956	2006 Profits: $648,264	**Int'l Ticker:** Int'l Exchange:
2005 Sales: $6,128,843	2005 Profits: $443,256	Employees: 67,400
2004 Sales: $4,001,804	2004 Profits: $412,332	Fiscal Year Ends: 12/31
2003 Sales: $3,908,800	2003 Profits: $243,700	Parent Company:

SALARIES/BENEFITS:

Pension Plan:	ESOP Stock Plan:	Profit Sharing:	Top Exec. Salary: $2,000,000	Bonus: $6,567,893
Savings Plan: Y	Stock Purch. Plan:		Second Exec. Salary: $1,500,000	Bonus: $4,896,493

OTHER THOUGHTS:

Apparent Women Officers or Directors: 4
Hot Spot for Advancement for Women/Minorities: Y

LOCATIONS: ("Y" = Yes)

West:	Southwest:	Midwest:	Southeast:	Northeast:	International:
Y		Y	Y	Y	Y

Note: Financial information, benefits and other data can change quickly and may vary from those stated here.

MICROCHIP TECHNOLOGY INC

www.microchip.com

Industry Group Code: 334413 Ranks within this company's industry group: Sales: 8 Profits: 7

Management:		Sales/Marketing:		Liberal Arts:		Information Systems:		Professionals:		Technical/Scientific:	
Mgmt. Trainees:	Y	Mktg. Professionals:	Y	Gen. Writing/Editing:		Info. Management:	Y	Finance/Accounting:	Y	Engineers, Elec.:	Y
Experienced Mgmt.:	Y	Retail Sales:		Technical Writing:	Y	Software Dev.:	Y	Law:	Y	Engineers, Other:	
Int'l Business:	Y	Commercial/Industrial:	Y	Graphic Arts/Photog.:		Hardware Dev.:	Y	HR/Other:	Y	Health/Lab:	Y
MBA Graduates:	Y	Sales Trainees:		Music:		Systems Integration:		Training:	Y	Scientists/Research:	Y
		Advertising Pros.:	Y	Broadcasting:		Consulting/Other:		Health Care:		Petroleum/Chemicals:	
				Other:				Consulting:		Math/Other:	

TYPES OF BUSINESS:

Semiconductors-Specialized
Microcontrollers
Battery Management & Interface Devices
Development Tools
Memory Products

BRANDS/DIVISIONS/AFFILIATES:

PIC
dsPIC
Digital Signal Controllers
EEPROM
EPROM Memory
Flash

CONTACTS: Note: Officers with more than one job title may be intentionally listed here more than once.

Steve Sanghi, CEO
Steve Sanghi, Pres.
Gordon W. Parnell, CFO/VP
Robert H. Owen, VP-Information Svcs.
Kenneth N. Pye, VP-Worldwide Applications Eng.
J. Eric Bjornholt, Sec.
Paul R. Breault, VP-Greater China Sales
Randall L. Drwinga, VP-Memory Prod. Div.
Dan L. Termer, VP-Vertical Markets Group
William Yang, VP-Pacific Rim Finance
Steve Sanghi, Chmn.
Gary P. Marsh, VP-European Sales

Phone: 480-792-7200	Fax: 480-899-9210
Toll-Free:	
Address: 2355 W. Chandler Blvd., Chandler, AZ 85224 US	

GROWTH PLANS/SPECIAL FEATURES:

Microchip Technology, Inc. develops and manufactures specialized semiconductor products used for a wide variety of embedded control applications. In addition, the company offers a broad spectrum of high-performance linear, mixed-signal, power management, thermal management, battery management and interface devices. The firm focuses on embedded control solutions, including microcontrollers; development tools; analog and interface products; and memory products. Microchip offers a broad family of microcontroller products featuring the proprietary architecture PIC. They feature a variety of memory technology configurations, low voltage and power, small footprint and ease of use. With over 400 microcontrollers in its portfolio, the company targets the 8-bit and 16-bit microcontroller markets. Additionally, the scalable product architecture allows it to target both the entry-level of the 32-bit microcontroller markets, as well as the 4-bit microcontroller marketplace. In addition, the firm is able to incorporate non-volatile memory, such as Flash, EEPROM and EPROM Memory, into the microcontroller and offers reprogrammable microcontroller products. The development tools enable system designers to program a PIC microcontroller and dsPIC Digital Signal Controllers for specific applications. Microchip's family of development tools operate in the standard Windows environment on standard PC hardware. These tools range from entry-level systems, which include an assembler and programmer or in-circuit debugging hardware, to fully configured systems that provide in-circuit emulation hardware. Analog and interface products consist of several families with over 500 power management, linear, mixed-signal, thermal management and interface products. Memory products consists primarily of serial electrically erasable programmable read only memory, referred to as Serial EEPROMs. Serial EEPROM products are used for non-volatile program and data storage systems where such data must be either modified frequently or retained for long periods.

FINANCIALS: Sales and profits are in thousands of dollars—add 000 to get the full amount. 2007 Note: Financial information for 2007 was not available for all companies at press time.

2007 Sales: $1,039,671	2007 Profits: $357,029	**U.S. Stock Ticker:** MCHP
2006 Sales: $927,893	2006 Profits: $242,369	**Int'l Ticker:** Int'l Exchange:
2005 Sales: $846,936	2005 Profits: $213,785	Employees: 4,582
2004 Sales: $699,260	2004 Profits: $137,262	Fiscal Year Ends: 3/31
2003 Sales: $651,500	2003 Profits: $88,300	Parent Company:

SALARIES/BENEFITS:

Pension Plan:	ESOP Stock Plan:	Profit Sharing: Y	Top Exec. Salary: $515,010	Bonus: $1,195,743
Savings Plan: Y	Stock Purch. Plan: Y		Second Exec. Salary: $241,808	Bonus: $139,264

OTHER THOUGHTS:

Apparent Women Officers or Directors:
Hot Spot for Advancement for Women/Minorities:

LOCATIONS: ("Y" = Yes)

West:	Southwest:	Midwest:	Southeast:	Northeast:	International:
Y	Y	Y	Y	Y	Y

MICRON TECHNOLOGY INC

www.micron.com

Industry Group Code: 334413 Ranks within this company's industry group: Sales: 4 Profits: 5

Management:		Sales/Marketing:		Liberal Arts:		Information Systems:		Professionals:		Technical/Scientific:	
Mgmt. Trainees:		Mktg. Professionals:	Y	Gen. Writing/Editing:		Info. Management:	Y	Finance/Accounting:	Y	Engineers, Elec.:	Y
Experienced Mgmt.:	Y	Retail Sales:		Technical Writing:	Y	Software Dev.:	Y	Law:	Y	Engineers, Other:	Y
Int'l Business:	Y	Commercial/Industrial:	Y	Graphic Arts/Photog.:	Y	Hardware Dev.:	Y	HR/Other:	Y	Health/Lab:	
MBA Graduates:	Y	Sales Trainees:		Music:		Systems Integration:	Y	Training:	Y	Scientists/Research:	Y
		Advertising Pros.:		Broadcasting:		Consulting/Other:		Health Care:		Petroleum/Chemicals:	
				Other:				Consulting:		Math/Other:	Y

TYPES OF BUSINESS:

Components-Semiconductor Memory
PCs & Peripherals
Flash Memory Devices
CMOS Image Sensors

BRANDS/DIVISIONS/AFFILIATES:

IM Flash Technologies, LLC
Intel Corp
Avago Technologies Ltd.

CONTACTS: Note: Officers with more than one job title may be intentionally listed here more than once.

Steven R. Appleton, CEO
D. Mark Durcan, COO
D. Mark Durcan, Pres.
Ronald C. Foster, CFO/VP-Finance
Michael W. Sadler, VP-Worldwide Sales
Pat Otte, VP-Human Resources
James E. Mahoney, VP-Info. Sys.
Brian J. Shields, VP-Worldwide Wafer Fabrication
Roderic W. Lewis, General Counsel/Corp. Sec./VP-Legal Affairs
Jay L. Hawkins, VP-Oper.
Kipp A. Bedard, VP-Investor Rel.
Norman L. Schlachter, Treas.
Mark Adams, VP-Digital Media
Brian M. Shirley, VP-Memory
Dean A. Klein, VP-Memory System Dev.
Frankie F. Roohparvar, VP-NAND Dev.
Steven R. Appleton, Chmn.
Steve Thorsen, VP-Procurement

Phone: 208-368-4000	Fax: 208-368-4435
Toll-Free:	
Address: 8000 S. Federal Way, Boise, ID 83716-9632 US	

GROWTH PLANS/SPECIAL FEATURES:

Micron Technology, Inc. and its subsidiaries design, develop, manufacture and market semiconductor memory products and personal computer systems. Its products are used in a range of electronic devices, including personal computers, workstations, servers, cell phones, digital cameras and other consumer and industrial products. The products are sold to computing and consumer, networking, telecommunications and imaging markets. Micron has two segments: Memory, producing dynamic random access memory (DRAM), accounting for 65% of 2007 sales, and NAND flash memory, 23% of sales; and Imaging, producing complementary metal-oxide semiconductor (CMOS) image sensors, 12%. DRAMs are high-density, low-cost-per-bit RAM storage units. Micron offers double data rate (DDR) and DDR2 DRAM, primarily used for the main system memory in computers; and synchronous DRAM (SDRAM), used in networking devices, servers, consumer electronics, communications equipment, computer peripherals and as memory upgrades to older computers. NAND products are re-writable, non-volatile semiconductor devices, meaning they retain memory after power has been shut off. It is used in mobile devices such as digital cameras, MP3 players, USB Flash Drives and cellular phones. IM Flash Technologies, LLC, a joint venture with Intel Corp., produces Micron's NAND products. CMOS image sensors are semiconductor devices that capture and process images into pictures or video for consumer and industrial applications. They are used in digital cameras, automotive systems and other emerging applications. The firm has manufacturing facilities located in the U.S., Italy, Japan, Puerto Rico and Singapore. Recently, Micron acquired Avago Technologies Ltd., an image-sensor business, for $53 million. During 2007, the company began sampling a 1 gigabyte (Gb) DDR3 device, introduced an 8 Gb Multi-Cell Level (MCL) NAND device and began sampling a 16 Gb MCL NAND device.

Micron's employees receive medical, dental, vision, life, AD&D, disability and business travel accident insurance; and paid time off.

FINANCIALS: Sales and profits are in thousands of dollars—add 000 to get the full amount. 2007 Note: Financial information for 2007 was not available for all companies at press time.

2007 Sales: $5,688,000	2007 Profits: $-320,000	U.S. Stock Ticker: MU
2006 Sales: $5,272,000	2006 Profits: $408,000	Int'l Ticker: Int'l Exchange:
2005 Sales: $4,880,200	2005 Profits: $188,000	Employees: 23,500
2004 Sales: $4,404,200	2004 Profits: $157,200	Fiscal Year Ends: 8/31
2003 Sales: $3,901,300	2003 Profits: $-1,273,200	Parent Company:

SALARIES/BENEFITS:

Pension Plan:	ESOP Stock Plan:	Profit Sharing:	Top Exec. Salary: $948,169	Bonus: $
Savings Plan: Y	Stock Purch. Plan: Y		Second Exec. Salary: $515,115	Bonus: $203,850

OTHER THOUGHTS:

Apparent Women Officers or Directors: 1
Hot Spot for Advancement for Women/Minorities: Y

LOCATIONS: ("Y" = Yes)

West:	Southwest:	Midwest:	Southeast:	Northeast:	International:
Y	Y	Y	Y	Y	Y

Note: Financial information, benefits and other data can change quickly and may vary from those stated here.

MICROSOFT CORP

www.microsoft.com

Industry Group Code: 511204 Ranks within this company's industry group: Sales: 1   Profits: 1

Management:		Sales/Marketing:		Liberal Arts:		Information Systems:		Professionals:		Technical/Scientific:	
Mgmt. Trainees:	Y	Mktg. Professionals:	Y	Gen. Writing/Editing:	Y	Info. Management:	Y	Finance/Accounting:	Y	Engineers, Elec.:	Y
Experienced Mgmt.:	Y	Retail Sales:		Technical Writing:	Y	Software Dev.:	Y	Law:	Y	Engineers, Other:	
Int'l Business:	Y	Commercial/Industrial:	Y	Graphic Arts/Photog.:	Y	Hardware Dev.:	Y	HR/Other:	Y	Health/Lab:	
MBA Graduates:	Y	Sales Trainees:		Music:	Y	Systems Integration:	Y	Training:	Y	Scientists/Research:	Y
		Advertising Pros.:	Y	Broadcasting:		Consulting/Other:	Y	Health Care:		Petroleum/Chemicals:	
				Other:	Y			Consulting:		Math/Other:	Y

TYPES OF BUSINESS:

Computer Software
Personal Communications Services
Video Games Systems
Mobile Communications
Voice-Enabled Mobile Search
Internet Search Engine
E-Mail Services
Instant Messaging

BRANDS/DIVISIONS/AFFILIATES:

Windows
Windows Vista
MSN
Xbox 360
Windows Live
Microsoft Dynamics
Microsroft Office
aQuantive Inc

CONTACTS: *Note: Officers with more than one job title may be intentionally listed here more than once.*

Steve Ballmer, CEO
Kevin Turner, COO
Jeff Raikes, Pres.
Christopher Liddell, CFO
Mich Mathews, Sr. VP-Central Mktg. Group
Lisa Brummel, Sr. VP-Human Resources
Rick Rashid, Sr. VP-Research
David Vaskevitch, CTO/Sr. VP
Brad Smith, General Counsel/Sr. VP-Legal & Corp. Affairs/Sec.
Robert (Robbie) Bach, Pres., Entertainment & Devices Div.
Stephen Elop, Pres., Microsoft Bus. Div.
Ray Ozzie, Chief Software Architect
Bill Gates, Chmn.
Jean-Philippe Courtois, Pres., Microsoft Int'l

Phone: 425-882-8080	Fax: 545-936-7329
Toll-Free: 800-642-7676	
Address: 1 Microsoft Way, Redmond, WA 98052-6399 US	

GROWTH PLANS/SPECIAL FEATURES:

Microsoft Corp. develops, manufactures and supports software for businesses, government and consumers. Microsoft operates in five segments. The client segment produces technical architecture, engineering and product delivery of the Windows product family. Vista, the latest generation of Windows operating system, includes advances in security, digital media, user interfaces, and other areas that enhance the user and developer experience. The server and tools segment develops and markets Windows server products and operating systems; builds standalone and software development lifecycle tools for software architects, developers, testers and project managers; and provides consulting and product support services. The online services business segment provides personal services including MSN Search; Windows Live; Windows Live Hotmail and others. The business division offers the Microsoft Dynamics business solutions and the Microsoft Office system. The entertainment and devices division is responsible for developing, producing and marketing the Xbox video game system, including consoles and accessories, third-party games, games published under the Microsoft brand and Xbox Live operations, as well as research, sales and support of those products. The Xbox is a major generator of the company's revenue at present time, with over 10 million consoles sold in the U.S. and 19 million worldwide. In 2007, Microsoft acquired Fast Search & Transfer, a leading provider of enterprise search solutions; Danger, Inc., which will become a part of the new Premium Mobile Experiences (PMX) team within the Mobile Communications Business of the Entertainment and Devices Division at Microsoft; Rapt, Inc., a leading provider of advertising yield management solutions for digital media publishers; and, for roughly $6 billion, aQuantive, Inc., which acquisition will help Microsoft deliver on its previously outlined goal to provide the advertising industry with a world-class advertising platform across devices and media that will create the best experiences for users, advertisers and publishers.

FINANCIALS: Sales and profits are in thousands of dollars—add 000 to get the full amount. 2007 Note: Financial information for 2007 was not available for all companies at press time.

2007 Sales: $51,122,000	2007 Profits: $14,065,000	**U.S. Stock Ticker: MSFT**
2006 Sales: $44,282,000	2006 Profits: $12,599,000	**Int'l Ticker:** Int'l Exchange:
2005 Sales: $39,788,000	2005 Profits: $12,254,000	Employees: 79,000
2004 Sales: $36,835,000	2004 Profits: $8,168,000	Fiscal Year Ends: 6/30
2003 Sales: $32,187,000	2003 Profits: $9,993,000	Parent Company:

SALARIES/BENEFITS:

Pension Plan:	ESOP Stock Plan:	Profit Sharing:	Top Exec. Salary: $620,000	Bonus: $650,000
Savings Plan: Y	Stock Purch. Plan: Y		Second Exec. Salary: $600,000	Bonus: $600,000

OTHER THOUGHTS:

Apparent Women Officers or Directors: 1
Hot Spot for Advancement for Women/Minorities: Y

LOCATIONS: ("Y" = Yes)

West:	Southwest:	Midwest:	Southeast:	Northeast:	International:
Y	Y	Y	Y	Y	Y

MILLIPORE CORP

www.millipore.com

Industry Group Code: 334500 Ranks within this company's industry group: Sales: 4   Profits: 4

Management:		Sales/Marketing:		Liberal Arts:		Information Systems:		Professionals:		Technical/Scientific:	
Mgmt. Trainees:		Mktg. Professionals:	Y	Gen. Writing/Editing:		Info. Management:	Y	Finance/Accounting:	Y	Engineers, Elec.:	Y
Experienced Mgmt.:	Y	Retail Sales:		Technical Writing:	Y	Software Dev.:	Y	Law:	Y	Engineers, Other:	Y
Int'l Business:	Y	Commercial/Industrial:	Y	Graphic Arts/Photog.:	Y	Hardware Dev.:	Y	HR/Other:	Y	Health/Lab:	Y
MBA Graduates:	Y	Sales Trainees:		Music:		Systems Integration:	Y	Training:	Y	Scientists/Research:	Y
		Advertising Pros.:		Broadcasting:		Consulting/Other:		Health Care:		Petroleum/Chemicals:	
				Other:				Consulting:		Math/Other:	

TYPES OF BUSINESS:

Biotechnology Instruments
Fluid Analysis, Identification & Purification Equipment
Chromatography Technologies

BRANDS/DIVISIONS/AFFILIATES:

Direct-Q 3
Lynx S2S
MicroSafe, B.V.
Newport Bio Systems
Serologicals Corporation
MilliPROBE

CONTACTS: Note: Officers with more than one job title may be intentionally listed here more than once.

Martin D. Madaus, CEO
Martin D. Madaus, Pres.
Charles Wagner, CFO/VP
Bruce Bonnevier, VP-Worldwide Human Resources
Dennis W. Harris, Chief Scientific Officer/VP
Peter C. Kershaw, VP-Worldwide Mfg. Oper.
Jeffrey Rudin, General Counsel/VP/Corp. Sec.
Wei Zhang, VP-Strategic & Corp. Dev.
Karen Marinella Hall, Dir.-Corp. Comm.
Joshua S. Young, Dir.-Investor Rel.
Jon DiVincenzo, VP/Pres., Bioscience Div.
Gregory J. Sam, VP-Quality
Jean-Paul Mangeolle, VP/Pres., Bioprocess Div.
Martin D. Madaus, Chmn.
Geoffrey F. Ide, VP-Millipore Int'l
Peter C. Kershaw, VP-Global Supply Chain

Phone: 978-715-4321	Fax: 800-645-5439
Toll-Free: 800-645-5476	
Address: 290 Concord Rd., Billerica, MA 01821 US	

GROWTH PLANS/SPECIAL FEATURES:

Millipore Corp. is a multinational bioscience company that provides technologies, tools and services for research, development and production. The company's products and services are based on technologies such as filtration, chromatography, cell culture supplements, antibodies and cell lines. The firm's products are offered through its two segments, the Bioscience division and the Bioprocess division. Millipore's Bioscience division, which accounted for 43% of 2007 revenue, is organized around four specific market segments: Biotools for the separation, isolation and purification of biological samples; research reagents such as antibodies, dyes and biochemical reagents; drug discovery reagent for the analysis of drug candidates; and laboratory water purification systems that remove contaminants for critical laboratory analysis. The Bioprocess division, which accounted for 57% of 2007 revenue, provides bio-products and technologies for the manufacturing of biologic drugs in mammalian cell cultures; filtration, purification and chromatography technologies to clarify, concentrate, purify and remove viruses; process monitoring tools for the sampling and testing of drugs and intermediate products and advanced manufacturing systems for use in sterile biomanufacturing environments. The firm operates 10 manufacturing sites in Massachusetts, New Hampshire, Missouri, Illinois, California, France and the U.K., and a total of 47 offices worldwide. In 2008, the firm entered into a license agreement with Bayer HeathCare AG. In January 2008, Millipore and Gen-Probe created the MilliPROBE system for real time tests of contaminants in manufacturing.

Millipore offers employees flexible spending accounts, tuition reimbursement, employee assistance programs and adoption assistance.

FINANCIALS: Sales and profits are in thousands of dollars—add 000 to get the full amount. 2007 Note: Financial information for 2007 was not available for all companies at press time.

2007 Sales: $1,531,555	2007 Profits: $136,472	U.S. Stock Ticker: MIL	
2006 Sales: $1,255,371	2006 Profits: $96,984	Int'l Ticker: Int'l Exchange:	
2005 Sales: $991,031	2005 Profits: $80,168	Employees: 6,000	
2004 Sales: $883,263	2004 Profits: $105,556	Fiscal Year Ends: 12/31	
2003 Sales: $799,622	2003 Profits: $100,796	Parent Company:	

SALARIES/BENEFITS:

Pension Plan:	ESOP Stock Plan:	Profit Sharing:	Top Exec. Salary: $742,307	Bonus: $488,000
Savings Plan: Y	Stock Purch. Plan:		Second Exec. Salary: $339,612	Bonus: $132,002

OTHER THOUGHTS:

Apparent Women Officers or Directors: 3
Hot Spot for Advancement for Women/Minorities: Y

LOCATIONS: ("Y" = Yes)

West:	Southwest:	Midwest:	Southeast:	Northeast:	International:
Y	Y	Y	Y	Y	Y

Note: Financial information, benefits and other data can change quickly and may vary from those stated here.

MOLEX INC

www.molex.com

Industry Group Code: 334119 Ranks within this company's industry group: Sales: 2   Profits: 2

Management:		Sales/Marketing:		Liberal Arts:		Information Systems:		Professionals:		Technical/Scientific:	
Mgmt. Trainees:		Mktg. Professionals:	Y	Gen. Writing/Editing:		Info. Management:	Y	Finance/Accounting:	Y	Engineers, Elec.:	Y
Experienced Mgmt.:	Y	Retail Sales:		Technical Writing:	Y	Software Dev.:	Y	Law:	Y	Engineers, Other:	
Int'l Business:	Y	Commercial/Industrial:	Y	Graphic Arts/Photog.:		Hardware Dev.:	Y	HR/Other:	Y	Health/Lab:	
MBA Graduates:	Y	Sales Trainees:		Music:		Systems Integration:	Y	Training:	Y	Scientists/Research:	
		Advertising Pros.:		Broadcasting:		Consulting/Other:		Health Care:		Petroleum/Chemicals:	
				Other:				Consulting:		Math/Other:	

TYPES OF BUSINESS:

Electronic Components
Transportation Products
Commercial Products
Micro Products
Automation & Electrical Products
Integrated Products
Global Sales & Marketing Organization

BRANDS/DIVISIONS/AFFILIATES:

Woodhead
Brad

CONTACTS: Note: Officers with more than one job title may be intentionally listed here more than once.

Martin P. Slark, CEO
Liam G. McCarthy, COO
Liam G. McCarthy, Pres.
David D. Johnson, CFO/Exec. VP
Graham C. Brock, Exec. VP/Pres., Global Sales & Mktg. Div.
David D. Johnson, Treas.
James E. Fleischhacker, Exec. VP/Pres., Global Transportation Prod. Div.
John H. Krehbiel, Co-Chmn.
David B. Root, Exec. VP/Pres., Global Commercial Prod. Div.
Katsumi Hirokawa, Exec. VP/Pres., Global Micro Prod. Div.
Frederick A. Krehbiel, Co-Chmn.

Phone: 630-969-4550	Fax: 630-968-8356
Toll-Free: 800-786-6539	
Address: 2222 Wellington Ct., Lisle, IL 60532 US	

GROWTH PLANS/SPECIAL FEATURES:

Molex, Inc. is a manufacturer of electronic components. It designs, manufactures and sells more than 100,000 products, including terminals, connectors, planar cables, cable assemblies, interconnection systems, backplanes, integrated products and mechanical and electronic switches. The company also provides manufacturing services to integrate specific components into a customer's product. The firm is organized into six divisions: transportation products; commercial products; micro products; automation and electrical products; integrated products; and global sales and marketing organization. The transportation products segment specializes in interconnection for cockpit, engine and infotainment functions in automobiles and other transportation equipment. The commercial products segment specializes in high-speed, high-signal-integrity, high-signal interconnect applications. The micro products segment focuses on portable digital product applications. The automation and electrical products segment focuses on harsh-environment technology for factory automation, temporary lighting, power and ergonomic products in construction, industrial and other applications. The integrated products segment produces higher-level assemblies using Molex interconnect technologies, usually in fiber optic, printed circuit board, flex circuit and other applications. The global sales and marketing organization segment comprises regional sales and industry marketing support teams, which provide customers with access to the Molex products. Molex operates 59 manufacturing facilities in 19 countries including France, Germany, Ireland, Italy, Poland, Japan, Brazil, China, India and Thailand. Major customers include AT&T; AMD; Canon; Cisco; IBM; Lucent; Motorola; Sony; Toshiba; and Xerox.

FINANCIALS: Sales and profits are in thousands of dollars—add 000 to get the full amount. 2007 Note: Financial information for 2007 was not available for all companies at press time.

2007 Sales: $3,265,874	2007 Profits: $240,768	U.S. Stock Ticker: MOLX
2006 Sales: $2,861,289	2006 Profits: $236,091	Int'l Ticker: Int'l Exchange:
2005 Sales: $2,554,458	2005 Profits: $150,116	Employees: 33,200
2004 Sales: $2,246,700	2004 Profits: $176,000	Fiscal Year Ends: 6/30
2003 Sales: $1,843,098	2003 Profits: $84,918	Parent Company:

SALARIES/BENEFITS:

Pension Plan:	ESOP Stock Plan:	Profit Sharing:	Top Exec. Salary: $833,333	Bonus: $
Savings Plan:	Stock Purch. Plan:		Second Exec. Salary: $564,635	Bonus: $

OTHER THOUGHTS:

Apparent Women Officers or Directors:
Hot Spot for Advancement for Women/Minorities:

LOCATIONS: ("Y" = Yes)

West:	Southwest:	Midwest:	Southeast:	Northeast:	International:
Y		Y	Y	Y	Y

MONRO MUFFLER BRAKE INC

www.monro.com

Industry Group Code: 811100 Ranks within this company's industry group: Sales: 1   Profits: 1

Management:		Sales/Marketing:		Liberal Arts:		Information Systems:		Professionals:		Technical/Scientific:	
Mgmt. Trainees:	Y	Mktg. Professionals:	Y	Gen. Writing/Editing:		Info. Management:	Y	Finance/Accounting:	Y	Engineers, Elec.:	
Experienced Mgmt.:	Y	Retail Sales:		Technical Writing:		Software Dev.:	Y	Law:	Y	Engineers, Other:	
Int'l Business:		Commercial/Industrial:		Graphic Arts/Photog.:		Hardware Dev.:		HR/Other:	Y	Health/Lab:	
MBA Graduates:	Y	Sales Trainees:		Music:		Systems Integration:		Training:	Y	Scientists/Research:	
		Advertising Pros.:	Y	Broadcasting:		Consulting/Other:		Health Care:		Petroleum/Chemicals:	
				Other:				Consulting:		Math/Other:	

TYPES OF BUSINESS:

Automotive Repair & Maintenance
Under-Car Repair Services
Inspection Services
Tires

BRANDS/DIVISIONS/AFFILIATES:

Monro Muffler Brake & Service
Mr. Tire
Tread Quarters Discount Tire
Monro Service Corporation

CONTACTS: Note: Officers with more than one job title may be intentionally listed here more than once.

Robert G. Gross, CEO
John W. Van Heel, Pres.
Catherine D'Amico, CFO
John W. Van Heel, Sec.
Catherine D'Amico, Exec. VP-Finance/Treas.
Joseph Tomarchio, Jr., Exec. VP-Store Oper.
Christopher R. Hoornbeck, Div. VP-Western Oper.
Craig L. Hoyle, Div. VP-Southern Oper.
Robert G. Gross, Chmn.

Phone: 585-647-6400	Fax: 585-647-0945
Toll-Free:	
Address: 200 Holleder Pkwy., Rochester, NY 14615 US	

GROWTH PLANS/SPECIAL FEATURES:

Monro Muffler Brake, Inc., based in Rochester, New York, oversees a chain of 720 company-operated stores and 14 dealer-operated stores providing automotive under-car repair services in the U.S. These stores are located in Connecticut, Delaware, Indiana, Maryland, Massachusetts, New Hampshire, New Jersey, New York, North Carolina, Ohio, Pennsylvania, Rhode Island, South Carolina, Vermont, Virginia, Maine and West Virginia. The stores operate under the names Monro Muffler Brake and Service, Tread Quarters Discount Tire and Mr. Tire. Monro provides a broad range of services on passenger cars, light trucks and vans, including mufflers and exhaust systems, brakes, steering, drive train, suspension and wheel alignment. Other products and services include tires, scheduled maintenance and state inspections. The company specializes in the repair and replacement of parts that must be periodically replaced due to normal wear and tear. Typically, the firm does not perform under-the-hood repair, except for oil change services, heating and cooling system flush and fill services and some minor tune-ups. Monro operates one subsidiary, Monro Service Corporation, which provides purchasing, distribution, merchandising, advertising, accounting and other store support functions. In 2008, the firm serviced 3.4 million vehicles with sales as follows: 23% brakes, 8% exhaust, 14% steering, 24% tires and 31% maintenance.

Monro provides employees with benefits including medical and dental coverage; disability and life insurance; tool insurance; employee parts and labor discounts; an employee assistance program; and recreational discounts.

FINANCIALS: Sales and profits are in thousands of dollars—add 000 to get the full amount. 2007 Note: Financial information for 2007 was not available for all companies at press time.

2007 Sales: $417,226		2007 Profits: $21,921		U.S. Stock Ticker: MNRO	
2006 Sales: $368,727		2006 Profits: $22,666		Int'l Ticker: Int'l Exchange:	
2005 Sales: $337,409		2005 Profits: $19,669		Employees: 4,066	
2004 Sales: $279,457		2004 Profits: $17,005		Fiscal Year Ends: 3/31	
2003 Sales: $258,026		2003 Profits: $13,728		Parent Company:	

SALARIES/BENEFITS:

Pension Plan:	ESOP Stock Plan:	Profit Sharing:	Top Exec. Salary: $769,125	Bonus: $150,000
Savings Plan: Y	Stock Purch. Plan: Y		Second Exec. Salary: $360,000	Bonus: $

OTHER THOUGHTS:

Apparent Women Officers or Directors: 2
Hot Spot for Advancement for Women/Minorities: Y

LOCATIONS: ("Y" = Yes)

West:	Southwest:	Midwest:	Southeast:	Northeast:	International:
		Y		Y	

MURPHY OIL CORPORATION   www.murphyoilcorp.com

Industry Group Code: 211111   Ranks within this company's industry group: Sales: Profits:

Management:		Sales/Marketing:		Liberal Arts:		Information Systems:		Professionals:		Technical/Scientific:	
Mgmt. Trainees:	Y	Mktg. Professionals:		Gen. Writing/Editing:		Info. Management:	Y	Finance/Accounting:	Y	Engineers, Elec.:	Y
Experienced Mgmt.:	Y	Retail Sales:		Technical Writing:		Software Dev.:		Law:	Y	Engineers, Other:	
Int'l Business:	Y	Commercial/Industrial:	Y	Graphic Arts/Photog.:		Hardware Dev.:		HR/Other:	Y	Health/Lab:	Y
MBA Graduates:	Y	Sales Trainees:		Music:		Systems Integration:		Training:	Y	Scientists/Research:	
		Advertising Pros.:		Broadcasting:		Consulting/Other:		Health Care:		Petroleum/Chemicals:	Y
				Other:				Consulting:		Math/Other:	

TYPES OF BUSINESS:
Oil & Gas Exploration & Production
Refining
Pipelines
Retail Gas Stations
Wholesale Marketing
Synthetic Crude

BRANDS/DIVISIONS/AFFILIATES:
Syncrude Canada, Ltd.
Murco Petroleum, Ltd.
Murphy Oil USA, Inc.
SPUR
Murphy USA
Murphy Canada
Murphy Oil Company, Ltd.
Bear Ridge Resources, Ltd.

CONTACTS: Note: Officers with more than one job title may be intentionally listed here more than once.
David M. Wood, CEO
David M. Wood, Pres.
Kevin G. Fitzgerald, CFO/Sr. VP
Harvey Doerr, Exec. VP-Mktg.
Steven A. Cosse, General Counsel/Exec. VP
David M. Wood, Exec. VP-Exploration & Production Oper.
Harvey Doerr, Exec. VP-Strategic Planning
John W. Eckart, Controller/VP
Bill H. Stobaugh, Sr. VP
Harvey Doerr, Exec. VP-Refining
Mindy K. West, Treasurer/VP
William Nolan, Chmn.

Phone: 870-862-6411   Fax: 870-864-6373
Toll-Free:
Address: 200 Peach St., El Dorado, AR 71730 US

GROWTH PLANS/SPECIAL FEATURES:
Murphy Oil Corporation, through its subsidiaries, is a global oil and gas exploration and production company with refining and marketing operations in North America and the U.K. The company's U.S. exploration and production activities are located primarily in the Gulf of Mexico, onshore Louisiana and Alaska. The company operates 13 of these fields itself, while 15 are operated by others. Murphy's Canadian assets include interests in the Hibernia and Terra Nova properties offshore Newfoundland and in Syncrude Canada, Ltd., which produces synthetic crude from bitumen oil sands. The company's crude oil, condensate and natural gas liquids production averages 87,000 barrels per day from its facilities in the U.S., Canada, Malaysia, Ecuador, the Republic of Congo and the North Sea. Murphy conducts its refining and marketing operations through Murphy Oil USA, Inc. and the U.K. subsidiary Murco Petroleum, Ltd. These companies refine crude oil and feedstock into petroleum products such as gasoline and distillates; buy and sell crude oil and refined products; and transport and market petroleum products. Murphy owns interests in three refineries in Louisiana, Wisconsin and Wales. These refineries have a production capacity of 192,400 barrels per day. The company's petroleum products are marketed under the brands SPUR and Murphy USA, with most locations in the parking areas of Wal-Mart stores. The company also has an agreement to market products through Murphy Canada stations at Canadian Wal-Mart stores. Murphy also owns interests in a number of pipelines in North America and the U.K. In August 2007, Murco Petroleum, Ltd. acquired the Milford Haven, Wales refinery from TOTAL. In January 2008, the firm's Canadian subsidiary Murphy Oil Company Ltd. acquired three land parcels in British Columbia.

FINANCIALS: Sales and profits are in thousands of dollars—add 000 to get the full amount. 2007 Note: Financial information for 2007 was not available for all companies at press time.
2007 Sales: $18,423,771   2007 Profits: $766,529
2006 Sales: $14,279,325   2006 Profits: $638,279
2005 Sales: $11,680,079   2005 Profits: $846,452
2004 Sales: $8,299,147   2004 Profits: $701,315
2003 Sales: $5,094,518   2003 Profits: $294,197

U.S. Stock Ticker: MUR
Int'l Ticker: Int'l Exchange:
Employees: 6,248
Fiscal Year Ends: 12/31
Parent Company:

SALARIES/BENEFITS:
Pension Plan: Y   ESOP Stock Plan: Profit Sharing: Top Exec. Salary: $1,064,167   Bonus: $1,500,000
Savings Plan: Stock Purch. Plan: Y   Second Exec. Salary: $496,667   Bonus: $600,000

OTHER THOUGHTS:
Apparent Women Officers or Directors: 1
Hot Spot for Advancement for Women/Minorities:

LOCATIONS: ("Y" = Yes)
West:	Southwest:	Midwest:	Southeast:	Northeast:	International:
Y	Y	Y	Y	Y	Y

NATIONAL OILWELL VARCO INC

www.natoil.com

Industry Group Code: 213111 Ranks within this company's industry group: Sales: 5   Profits: 8

Management:		Sales/Marketing:		Liberal Arts:		Information Systems:		Professionals:		Technical/Scientific:	
Mgmt. Trainees:		Mktg. Professionals:	Y	Gen. Writing/Editing:		Info. Management:	Y	Finance/Accounting:	Y	Engineers, Elec.:	Y
Experienced Mgmt.:	Y	Retail Sales:		Technical Writing:	Y	Software Dev.:	Y	Law:	Y	Engineers, Other:	Y
Int'l Business:	Y	Commercial/Industrial:	Y	Graphic Arts/Photog.:		Hardware Dev.:		HR/Other:	Y	Health/Lab:	
MBA Graduates:	Y	Sales Trainees:		Music:		Systems Integration:		Training:	Y	Scientists/Research:	
		Advertising Pros.:		Broadcasting:		Consulting/Other:		Health Care:		Petroleum/Chemicals:	Y
				Other:				Consulting:		Math/Other:	

TYPES OF BUSINESS:

Oil & Gas Drilling Equipment & Systems
Distribution & Logistics Services
Waste Management Services

BRANDS/DIVISIONS/AFFILIATES:

National-Oilwell, Inc.
Varco International, Inc.
Grant Prideco Inc
Marlex Energy Services Company
Grammaloy Holdings, L.P.
NQL Energy Services, Inc.

CONTACTS: Note: Officers with more than one job title may be intentionally listed here more than once.

Merrill (Pete) Miller, Jr., CEO
Merrill (Pete) Miller, Jr., Pres.
Clay C. Williams, CFO/Sr. VP
Kenneth Nibling, VP-Human Resources
Dwight W. Rettig, General Counsel/Sec./VP
Robert Blanchard, Chief Acct. Officer/Corp. Controller/VP
Mark Reese, Pres., Rig Tech.
Jeremy Thigpen, Pres., Downhole & Pumping Solutions
Haynes B. Smith, III, Pres., Svcs.
Merrill (Pete) Miller, Jr., Chmn.

Phone: 713-375-3700	Fax:
Toll-Free: 888-262-8645	
Address: 7909 Parkwood Circle Dr., Houston, TX 77036 US	

GROWTH PLANS/SPECIAL FEATURES:

National Oilwell Varco, Inc., formed when National-Oilwell, Inc. acquired Varco International, Inc., designs, manufactures and sells comprehensive systems, components and products used in oil and gas drilling and production, as well as distributing products and providing services to the exploration and production segment of the oil and gas industry, with operations in over 700 locations across six continents. The firm's rig technology segment offers a variety of products that automates well construction such as drilling rigs, derricks, pressure pumping units, wired winches and cranes. It also provides spare parts and other services. Its operations extend to Canada, Norway, the U.K., China and Belarus. The petroleum services and supplies segment manufactures, rents and sells transfer pumps, drilling motors, rig instrumentation systems and other equipment. Its services include inspection and internal coating services for drillpipe, linepipe, tubing and pipelines. Its operations extend to Canada, the U.K., China, Kazakhstan and Mexico. The company's distribution services segment provides maintenance, repair, operating supplies and spare parts to drill site and production locations throughout North America, Mexico, the Middle East, Europe, Southeast Asia and South America. With its information technology platforms and processes, this segment can provide complete procurement, inventory management and logistics services to its customers. It operates a network of over 180 locations worldwide, although approximately 77% of its 2007 revenue came from the U.S. and Canada. In February 2008, the firm, in partnership with Fabtech International Limited, created a joint venture for the provision of rig up and structural refurbishment services for the Middle East and North African land rig markets. In April 2008, the company finalized its acquisition of Grant Prideco, Inc.

FINANCIALS: Sales and profits are in thousands of dollars—add 000 to get the full amount. 2007 Note: Financial information for 2007 was not available for all companies at press time.

2007 Sales: $9,789,000	2007 Profits: $1,337,100	U.S. Stock Ticker: NOV
2006 Sales: $7,025,800	2006 Profits: $684,000	Int'l Ticker: Int'l Exchange:
2005 Sales: $4,644,500	2005 Profits: $286,900	Employees: 26,861
2004 Sales: $2,318,100	2004 Profits: $115,200	Fiscal Year Ends: 12/31
2003 Sales: $2,004,920	2003 Profits: $79,700	Parent Company:

SALARIES/BENEFITS:

Pension Plan:	ESOP Stock Plan:	Profit Sharing:	Top Exec. Salary: $800,000	Bonus: $1,600,000
Savings Plan: Y	Stock Purch. Plan:		Second Exec. Salary: $474,800	Bonus: $800,000

OTHER THOUGHTS:

Apparent Women Officers or Directors:
Hot Spot for Advancement for Women/Minorities:

LOCATIONS: ("Y" = Yes)

West:	Southwest:	Midwest:	Southeast:	Northeast:	International:
	Y				Y

NEIMAN MARCUS GROUP INC (THE) www.neimanmarcus.com

Industry Group Code: 452110 Ranks within this company's industry group: Sales: 4 Profits: 4

Management:		Sales/Marketing:		Liberal Arts:		Information Systems:		Professionals:		Technical/Scientific:	
Mgmt. Trainees:	Y	Mktg. Professionals:	Y	Gen. Writing/Editing:	Y	Info. Management:	Y	Finance/Accounting:	Y	Engineers, Elec.:	
Experienced Mgmt.:	Y	Retail Sales:	Y	Technical Writing:		Software Dev.:		Law:	Y	Engineers, Other:	
Int'l Business:		Commercial/Industrial:		Graphic Arts/Photog.:	Y	Hardware Dev.:		HR/Other:	Y	Health/Lab:	
MBA Graduates:	Y	Sales Trainees:	Y	Music:		Systems Integration:		Training:	Y	Scientists/Research:	
		Advertising Pros.:	Y	Broadcasting:		Consulting/Other:		Health Care:		Petroleum/Chemicals:	
				Other:				Consulting:		Math/Other:	

TYPES OF BUSINESS:

Upscale Department Stores
Online & Catalog Sales
Corporate Gifts
Fine Jewelry
Fine Apparel
Cosmetics
Housewares & Linens

BRANDS/DIVISIONS/AFFILIATES:

InCircle
Horchow
Bergdorf Goodman, Inc.
Cusp
Last-Call
Warburg Pincus LLC
TPG (Texas Pacific Group)
Neiman Marcus Christmas Book

CONTACTS: *Note: Officers with more than one job title may be intentionally listed here more than once.*

Burton M. Tansky, CEO
Burton M. Tansky, Pres.
James E. Skinner, CFO/Exec. VP
Steven Dennis, Sr. VP-Mktg.
Marita O'Dea, Chief Human Resources Officer/Sr. VP
Phillip L. Maxwell, CIO/Sr. VP
Nelson Bangs, General Counsel/Sr. VP
Steven Dennis, Sr. VP-Strategy & Bus. Dev.
Ginger Reeder, Corp. Comm. Contact
Karen W. Katz, CEO/Pres., Neiman Marcus Stores
James Gold, CEO/Pres., Bergdorf Goodman
Brendan Hoffman, CEO/Pres., Neiman Marcus Direct
Wayne Hussey, Sr. VP-Properties & Store Dev.
Richard A. Smith, Chmn.

Phone: 214-741-6911	Fax: 214-573-5320
Toll-Free: 888-888-4757	
Address: 1 Marcus Sq., 1618 Main St., Dallas, TX 75201 US	

GROWTH PLANS/SPECIAL FEATURES:

The Neiman Marcus Group, Inc. specializes in high-end retail sales and focuses on a largely affluent customer base. The company's 39 Neiman Marcus and two Bergdorf Goodman stores showcase global designer brands such as Prada, Armani, Chanel and Gucci. These stores average an eye-popping $611 per square foot in annual sales, about double the figure for a typical department store. In addition to apparel, the firm offers distinctive and unusual upscale merchandise such as fine jewelry, chocolates, perfumes and accessories. Neiman Marcus is well-known for its emphasis on maintaining its customer base through personal contact, including invitations to events, thank-you notes, birthday greetings and personal correspondence alerting customers that new merchandise has arrived. The firm's highly successful rewards program, InCircle helps drive sales. To qualify, customers must spend at least $5,000 yearly. Over 100,000 customers are members, each spending an average $11,000 yearly. Additionally, Neiman Marcus Direct offers a mix of apparel and home furnishings online and through catalogs, including Horchow and the world-famous Neiman Marcus Christmas Book, complementary to its store merchandise. The firm operates two Bergdorf Goodman stores in New York City and 21 Last-Call clearance centers that sell marked down goods. The company is owned by an investor group led by TPG (Texas Pacific Group) and Warburg Pincus LLC. Neiman Marcus is planning to gradually expand its 39 stores to 44 by 2010. The company also operates a new concept called Cusp. These smaller stores in Virginia, Illinois and California are designed to appeal to fashion-forward women aged 21 to 45.

Neiman Marcus offers its employees a range of benefits including credit union membership, educational assistance, an employee assistance program, prenatal programs, domestic partner benefits, Dell personal computer discounts, paid counseling, adoption benefits, scholarships for children, discounts on merchandise, a matching gift program and financial planning seminars.

FINANCIALS: Sales and profits are in thousands of dollars—add 000 to get the full amount. 2007 Note: Financial information for 2007 was not available for all companies at press time.

2007 Sales: $4,419,700	2007 Profits: $111,900	**U.S. Stock Ticker: Private**
2006 Sales: $4,105,596	2006 Profits: $56,609	**Int'l Ticker:** Int'l Exchange:
2005 Sales: $3,774,798	2005 Profits: $248,800	Employees:
2004 Sales: $3,545,600	2004 Profits: $204,832	Fiscal Year Ends: 7/31
2003 Sales: $3,098,100	2003 Profits: $109,300	Parent Company:

SALARIES/BENEFITS:

Pension Plan: Y	ESOP Stock Plan:	Profit Sharing:	Top Exec. Salary: $	Bonus: $1,574,219
Savings Plan: Y	Stock Purch. Plan:		Second Exec. Salary: $650,000	Bonus: $650,000

OTHER THOUGHTS:

Apparent Women Officers or Directors: 3
Hot Spot for Advancement for Women/Minorities: Y

LOCATIONS: ("Y" = Yes)

West:	Southwest:	Midwest:	Southeast:	Northeast:	International:
Y	Y	Y	Y	Y	

NETWORK APPLIANCE INC

www.netapp.com

Industry Group Code: 334112 Ranks within this company's industry group: Sales: 3   Profits: 3

Management:		Sales/Marketing:		Liberal Arts:		Information Systems:		Professionals:		Technical/Scientific:	
Mgmt. Trainees:		Mktg. Professionals:		Gen. Writing/Editing:		Info. Management:	Y	Finance/Accounting:	Y	Engineers, Elec.:	Y
Experienced Mgmt.:	Y	Retail Sales:		Technical Writing:	Y	Software Dev.:	Y	Law:	Y	Engineers, Other:	
Int'l Business:	Y	Commercial/Industrial:	Y	Graphic Arts/Photog.:		Hardware Dev.:	Y	HR/Other:	Y	Health/Lab:	
MBA Graduates:	Y	Sales Trainees:		Music:		Systems Integration:		Training:	Y	Scientists/Research:	
		Advertising Pros.:		Broadcasting:		Consulting/Other:		Health Care:		Petroleum/Chemicals:	
				Other:				Consulting:		Math/Other:	

TYPES OF BUSINESS:

Data Management Solutions
Storage Solutions
Data Protection Software Products
Data Protection Platform Products
Storage Security Products
Data Retention & Archive Software Products
Storage Management & Application Software
Management Tools

BRANDS/DIVISIONS/AFFILIATES:

Data ONTAP
NetApp
NetCache
NetStore
NearStore
Data ONTAP
FlexVol
Onaro Inc

CONTACTS: *Note: Officers with more than one job title may be intentionally listed here more than once.*

Daniel Warmenhoven, CEO
Thomas F. Mendoza, Pres.
Steve Gomo, CFO
Jay Kidd, Chief Mktg. Officer
Gwen McDonald, Sr. VP-Human Resources
Steve Kleiman, Chief Scientist/Sr. VP
Marina Levinson, CIO/Sr. VP
Mark Jon Bluth, Sr. VP-Oper.
James Lau, Chief Strategy Officer/Exec. VP
Steve Gomo, Exec. VP-Finance
Ed Deenihan, Exec. VP-NetApp Global Svcs.
Tom Georgens, Exec. VP-Prod. Oper.
Rob Salmon, Exec. VP-Field Oper.
D. Patrick Linehan, Sr. VP-Worldwide Sales
Don Valentine, Chmn.

Phone: 408-822-6000	Fax: 408-822-4501
Toll-Free:	
Address: 495 E. Java Dr., Sunnyvale, CA 94089 US	

GROWTH PLANS/SPECIAL FEATURES:

Network Appliance, Inc. (NetApp) is a provider of data management solutions. The NetApp enterprise-class storage solutions are interoperable across all platforms. The storage solutions are all based on Data ONTAP, an optimized, scalable and flexible operating system that supports any mix of SAN, NAS and IP SAN environments concurrently. Data ONTAP software integrated seamlessly into UNIX, Windows and web environments. The Data ONTAP operating system provides the foundation to build storage infrastructure and an enterprise-wide data fabric for business applications. It includes the patented NetApp WAFL (Write Anywhere File Layout) file management system and the RADI-DP (RAID Double Parity), a double-parity software RAID architecture. It supports all of the major industry-standard protocols' storage, as well as a suite of data management, data replication and data protection software products. The operating system also includes FlexVol, which creates volume that can be expanded or contracted while reducing the need for spare capacity; FlexShare, which enables the consolidation and prioritization of disparate workloads; and FilerView, a web-based element manager. The firm offers a variety of management tools, including the FlexClone technology, which enables data cloning or the instant replication of data volumes and data sets; FlexCache technology, which allows the creation of read-writeable replicas of volumes by creating caching volumes on multiple storage controllers; and MultiStore software, which allows for the creation of separate logical partitions in storage systems and network storage resources. Additionally, NetApp offers data protection software products; data protection platform products; storage security products; data retention and archive software products; and storage management and application software. In January 2008, NetApp agreed to acquire Onaro, Inc.

The company offers its employees medical, dental and vision insurance; an employee assistance program; life and AD&D insurance; a 401(k) plan; an employee stock purchase plan; and educational assistance.

FINANCIALS: Sales and profits are in thousands of dollars—add 000 to get the full amount. 2007 Note: Financial information for 2007 was not available for all companies at press time.

2007 Sales: $2,804,282	2007 Profits: $297,735	**U.S. Stock Ticker: NTAP**
2006 Sales: $2,066,456	2006 Profits: $266,452	**Int'l Ticker:** Int'l Exchange:
2005 Sales: $1,598,131	2005 Profits: $225,754	Employees: 6,635
2004 Sales: $1,170,310	2004 Profits: $152,087	Fiscal Year Ends: 4/30
2003 Sales: $892,068	2003 Profits: $76,472	Parent Company:

SALARIES/BENEFITS:

Pension Plan:	ESOP Stock Plan:	Profit Sharing:	Top Exec. Salary: $709,615	Bonus: $986,365
Savings Plan: Y	Stock Purch. Plan: Y		Second Exec. Salary: $440,385	Bonus: $520,314

OTHER THOUGHTS:

Apparent Women Officers or Directors: 3
Hot Spot for Advancement for Women/Minorities: Y

LOCATIONS: ("Y" = Yes)

West:	Southwest:	Midwest:	Southeast:	Northeast:	International:
Y				Y	Y

NEWS CORP

www.newscorp.com

Industry Group Code: 513120 Ranks within this company's industry group: Sales: Profits:

Management:		Sales/Marketing:		Liberal Arts:		Information Systems:		Professionals:		Technical/Scientific:	
Mgmt. Trainees:	Y	Mktg. Professionals:	Y	Gen. Writing/Editing:	Y	Info. Management:	Y	Finance/Accounting:	Y	Engineers, Elec.:	Y
Experienced Mgmt.:	Y	Retail Sales:		Technical Writing:		Software Dev.:	Y	Law:	Y	Engineers, Other:	
Int'l Business:	Y	Commercial/Industrial:	Y	Graphic Arts/Photog.:	Y	Hardware Dev.:		HR/Other:	Y	Health/Lab:	
MBA Graduates:	Y	Sales Trainees:		Music:	Y	Systems Integration:		Training:	Y	Scientists/Research:	
		Advertising Pros.:	Y	Broadcasting:	Y	Consulting/Other:		Health Care:		Petroleum/Chemicals:	
				Other:	Y			Consulting:		Math/Other:	

TYPES OF BUSINESS:

Television Broadcasting & Distribution
Film & Television Production
Newspaper Publishing
Online Media
Advertising Services
Magazine & Book Publishing
Satellite Television

BRANDS/DIVISIONS/AFFILIATES:

MySpace
Intermix Media
Fox Entertainment Group Inc
Fox Broadcasting Company
HarperCollins Publishers Inc
Fox Sports Net Inc
IGN Entertainment
Dow Jones & Co Inc

CONTACTS: Note: Officers with more than one job title may be intentionally listed here more than once.

K. Rupert Murdoch, CEO
Peter Chernin, COO
Peter Chernin, Pres.
David F. DeVoe, CFO/Sr. Exec. VP
Gary Ginsberg, Exec. VP-Global Mktg.
Beryl Cook, Chief Human Resources Officer
Lawrence A. Jacobs, General Counsel/Sr. Exec. VP
Gary Ginsberg, Exec. VP-Corp. Affairs
Anthea Disney, Exec. VP-Content
Michael Regan, Exec. VP-Gov't Affairs
Genie Gavenchak, Chief Compliance & Ethics Officer/Sr. VP
Mark Williams, CFO-Europe & Asia
K. Rupert Murdoch, Chmn.
James Murdoch, Chmn./CEO-Europe & Asia

Phone: 212-852-7000	Fax: 212-852-7147
Toll-Free:	
Address: 1211 Ave. of the Americas, 8th Fl., New York, NY 10036 US	

GROWTH PLANS/SPECIAL FEATURES:

News Corp. is an entertainment company with operations in eight industry segments: filmed entertainment; television; cable network programming; direct broadcast satellite television; magazines and inserts; newspapers; book publishing; and other. The filmed entertainment segment produces and acquires live-action and animated motion pictures for distribution and licensing in all formats in entertainment media; and the production and licensing of television programming worldwide. Subsidiaries include Fox Filmed Entertainment and Twentieth Century Fox Television. The television segment operates broadcast television stations; broadcasts network programming in the U.S.; and develops, produces and broadcasts television programming in Asia. The cable networking programming division produces and licenses news, sports, general entertainment and movie programming for distribution to distributors worldwide. The direct broadcast satellite television segment operates through SKY Italia, which currently distributes over 100 channels of basic and premium programming services via satellite and broadband to subscribers in Italy. The magazines and inserts group is engaged in marketing operations, primarily the publication of free standing inserts and the provision of in-store marketing products and services; and magazine publishing, such as The Weekly Standard. The newspapers segment publishes newspapers and magazines in the U.K., Ireland, Australia and the U.S., including The Sun, News of the World and the New York Post. The book publishing division operates through HarperCollins Publishers, which primarily publishes fiction and non-fiction for the general consumer. The other segment includes News' Internet businesses, including Myspace.com; interests in various companies; and other operations. In December 2007, News acquired Dow Jones & Co., Inc. for roughly $5 billion. In February 2008, Liberty Media Corp. completed a significant asset swap with News. Under the agreement, Liberty received News' 41% stake in DIRECTV, $625 million in cash and three regional sports networks. News received Liberty's $10.1 billion stake in News itself. This gives Liberty controlling interest in DIRECTV.

FINANCIALS: Sales and profits are in thousands of dollars—add 000 to get the full amount. 2007 Note: Financial information for 2007 was not available for all companies at press time.

2007 Sales: $28,655,000	2007 Profits: $3,426,000	U.S. Stock Ticker: NWS	
2006 Sales: $25,327,000	2006 Profits: $2,314,000	Int'l Ticker: Int'l Exchange:	
2005 Sales: $23,859,000	2005 Profits: $2,128,000	Employees: 44,000	
2004 Sales: $20,959,000	2004 Profits: $1,647,000	Fiscal Year Ends: 6/30	
2003 Sales: $17,474,000	2003 Profits: $1,046,000	Parent Company:	

SALARIES/BENEFITS:

Pension Plan:	ESOP Stock Plan:	Profit Sharing:	Top Exec. Salary: $8,100,000	Bonus: $15,795,000
Savings Plan: Y	Stock Purch. Plan:		Second Exec. Salary: $8,100,000	Bonus: $10,397,500

OTHER THOUGHTS:

Apparent Women Officers or Directors: 3
Hot Spot for Advancement for Women/Minorities: Y

LOCATIONS: ("Y" = Yes)

West:	Southwest:	Midwest:	Southeast:	Northeast:	International:
Y	Y	Y	Y	Y	Y

NII HOLDINGS INC

www.nii.com

Industry Group Code: 513322 **Ranks within this company's industry group:** Sales: 5 Profits: 3

Management:		Sales/Marketing:		Liberal Arts:	Information Systems:		Professionals:		Technical/Scientific:	
Mgmt. Trainees:	Y	Mktg. Professionals:	Y	Gen. Writing/Editing:	Info. Management:	Y	Finance/Accounting:	Y	Engineers, Elec.:	Y
Experienced Mgmt.:	Y	Retail Sales:		Technical Writing:	Software Dev.:	Y	Law:	Y	Engineers, Other:	
Int'l Business:	Y	Commercial/Industrial:		Graphic Arts/Photog.:	Hardware Dev.:		HR/Other:	Y	Health/Lab:	
MBA Graduates:	Y	Sales Trainees:		Music:	Systems Integration:		Training:	Y	Scientists/Research:	
		Advertising Pros.:	Y	Broadcasting:	Consulting/Other:		Health Care:		Petroleum/Chemicals:	
				Other:			Consulting:		Math/Other:	

TYPES OF BUSINESS:
Cell Phone Service

BRANDS/DIVISIONS/AFFILIATES:
Motorola Inc
iDEN
Nextel Direct Connect
International Direct Connect
Nextel Online
Nextel Worldwide
Sprint Nextel Corp
TELUS Corporation

CONTACTS: *Note: Officers with more than one job title may be intentionally listed here more than once.*
Steven P. Dussek, CEO
Lodewijk (Lo) van Gemert, COO
Lodewijk (Lo) van Gemert, Pres.
Gokul V. Hemmady, CFO/VP
Gregory J. (Greg) Santoro, Chief Mktg. Officer
Alan Strauss, CTO/VP
Gary Begeman, General Counsel/VP
John M. McMahon, VP-Bus. Oper.
Gregory J. (Greg) Santoro, Chief Strategy Officer
Daniel E. Freiman, Controller/VP
Miguel E. Rivera, Pres., Nextel Peru
Sergio Borges Chaia, CEO/Pres., Nextel Brazil
Ruben Butvilofsky, Pres., Nextel Argentina
Jose Felipe, Pres., Mercosur
Steven M. Shindler, Chmn.
Peter A. Foyo, Pres., Nextel Mexico

Phone: 703-390-5100	Fax: 703-547-5269
Toll-Free:	
Address: 1875 Explorer St., Ste. 1000, Reston, VA 20190 US	

GROWTH PLANS/SPECIAL FEATURES:
NII Holdings, Inc. provides digital wireless communication services through operating companies located in selected Latin American markets, including major business centers and related transportation corridors in Mexico, Brazil, Argentina and Peru. NII additionally offers its digital services on a limited basis in Santiago, Chile. The company uses a transmission technology developed by Motorola called integrated digital enhanced network, or iDEN, to provide its digital mobile services on 800 MHz spectrum holdings in all of its markets. This technology, which is currently the only digital technology available that can be used on non-contiguous spectrum frequencies, allows NII to use its spectrum efficiently and to offer multiple wireless services integrated into a variety of handset devices. Services offered by NII include mobile telephone, Nextel Direct Connect, International Direct Connect, Nextel Online and Nextel Worldwide services. The company's mobile telephone service includes such features as speakerphone, conference calling, voice mail, call forwarding and additional line service. Nextel Direct Connect is a long-range walkie-talkie service enabling users to set up a conference more quickly than would be possible with a traditional mobile telephone call. International Direct Connect allows subscribers to communicate instantly across national borders with other subscribers in Mexico, Brazil, Argentina, Peru and Chile; any Sprint Nextel Corporation subscriber in the U.S. using a compatible handset; and, with the exception of Chilean subscribers, any TELUS subscriber in Canada using a compatible handset. Nextel Online provides mobile Internet services; text messaging services; email services, including Blackberry services; location-based services, including those using global positioning system (GPS) technologies; digital media services; and advanced Java enabled business applications. Nextel Worldwide provides international roaming capabilities. NII's operating companies have roughly 4.7 million digital handsets in commercial service. During 2007, the company added 885 transmitter and receiver sites to its networks, focused primarily on Mexico and Brazil.

FINANCIALS: Sales and profits are in thousands of dollars—add 000 to get the full amount. 2007 Note: Financial information for 2007 was not available for all companies at press time.

2007 Sales: $3,296,295	2007 Profits: $378,418	U.S. Stock Ticker: NIHD
2006 Sales: $2,371,340	2006 Profits: $294,490	Int'l Ticker: Int'l Exchange:
2005 Sales: $1,745,839	2005 Profits: $174,781	Employees: 9,873
2004 Sales: $1,279,908	2004 Profits: $57,289	Fiscal Year Ends: 12/31
2003 Sales: $938,687	2003 Profits: $172,960	Parent Company:

SALARIES/BENEFITS:
Pension Plan:	ESOP Stock Plan:	Profit Sharing:	Top Exec. Salary: $711,250	Bonus: $599,040
Savings Plan:	Stock Purch. Plan:		Second Exec. Salary: $426,899	Bonus: $269,594

OTHER THOUGHTS:
Apparent Women Officers or Directors: 2
Hot Spot for Advancement for Women/Minorities:

LOCATIONS: ("Y" = Yes)
West:	Southwest:	Midwest:	Southeast:	Northeast:	International:
				Y	Y

Note: Financial information, benefits and other data can change quickly and may vary from those stated here.

NIKE INC

www.nike.com

Industry Group Code: 316219 **Ranks within this company's industry group:** Sales: 1 Profits: 1

Management:		Sales/Marketing:		Liberal Arts:		Information Systems:		Professionals:		Technical/Scientific:	
Mgmt. Trainees:	Y	Mktg. Professionals:	Y	Gen. Writing/Editing:	Y	Info. Management:	Y	Finance/Accounting:	Y	Engineers, Elec.:	
Experienced Mgmt.:	Y	Retail Sales:	Y	Technical Writing:		Software Dev.:		Law:	Y	Engineers, Other:	
Int'l Business:	Y	Commercial/Industrial:	Y	Graphic Arts/Photog.:	Y	Hardware Dev.:		HR/Other:	Y	Health/Lab:	
MBA Graduates:	Y	Sales Trainees:	Y	Music:		Systems Integration:		Training:	Y	Scientists/Research:	
		Advertising Pros.:	Y	Broadcasting:		Consulting/Other:		Health Care:		Petroleum/Chemicals:	
				Other:	Y			Consulting:		Math/Other:	

TYPES OF BUSINESS:

Athletic Shoes/Apparel Manufacturing
Athletic Equipment
Sports Accessories
Retail Stores
Sports Apparel
Plastic Products
Hockey Products
Swimwear

BRANDS/DIVISIONS/AFFILIATES:

Cole Haan Holdings, Inc.
Nike Bayer Hockey Corp.
Nike Bauer Hockey U.S.A., Inc
Converse Inc
Hurley International, LLC
Chuck Taylor
Bragano
All Star

CONTACTS: Note: Officers with more than one job title may be intentionally listed here more than once.

Mark G. Parker, CEO
Mark G. Parker, Pres.
Donald Blair, CFO/VP
Joaquin Hidalgo, VP-Global Mktg.
David Ayre, VP-Global Human Resources
Roland Paanakker, CIO/VP
Hans van Alebeek, VP-Nike Global Oper. & Tech.
Ron McCray, Chief Admin. Officer/VP
James C. Carter, General Counsel/VP/Chief Legal Officer
Gary M. DeStefano, VP/Pres., Global Oper.
Andy Campion, VP-Corp. Planning
Nigel Powell, VP-Global Comm.
Pamela Catlett, VP-Investor Rel.
Charlie Denson, Pres., Nike Brand
Mary Kate Buckley, VP-EMEA Apparel
Thomas E. Clarke, Pres., New Bus. Ventures
John F. Coburn III, Corp. Sec.
Philip H. Knight, Chmn.
Jim Allaker, VP/Gen. Mgr.-UK & Ireland
Nick Athanasakos, VP-Global Supply Chain

Phone: 503-671-6453	Fax: 503-671-6300
Toll-Free: 800-344-6453	
Address: 1 Bowerman Dr., Beaverton, OR 97005 US	

GROWTH PLANS/SPECIAL FEATURES:

Nike, Inc. designs, develops and markets footwear, apparel, equipment and accessory products. It is one of the largest sellers of athletic footwear and athletic apparel in the world. The company's athletic footwear products are designed primarily for specific athletic use, although a large percentage of the products are worn for casual or leisure purposes. Running, training, basketball, soccer, sport-inspired urban shoes and children's shoes are the firm's top-selling product categories. Nike also markets shoes designed for tennis, golf, baseball, football, lacrosse, walking, outdoor activities, skateboarding, bicycling, volleyball, wrestling, cheerleading, aquatic activities and other athletic and recreational uses. The company also sells sports apparel and accessories; athletic bags and accessory items; a line of performance equipment including bags, socks, sport balls, eyewear, timepieces, electronic devices, bats, gloves and protective equipment; swimwear, cycling apparel, children's clothing, school supplies, electronic devices, eyewear, golf accessories and belts; and a line of dress and casual footwear, apparel and accessories for men and women under the brand names Cole Haan, G. Series, and Bragano, through wholly-owned subsidiary Cole Haan Holdings, Inc. Subsidiary Nike IHM, Inc. manufactures various plastic products. Subsdiary Converse, Inc. designs and distributes athletic and casual footwear, apparel and accessories under brands such as Converse, Chuck Taylor, All Star and One Star. Subsidiary Hurley International, LLC designs and distributes action sports apparel for surfing, skateboarding and snowboarding. Nike Bauer Hockey Corp. and Nike Bauer Hockey U.S.A., Inc. manufacture and distribute hockey equipment, apparel and accessories. Nike sells its products to retail accounts, through Nike-owned retail stores and through a mix of independent distributors and licensees, in over 180 countries.

The company offers its employees medical, dental and vision insurance; life and AD&D insurance; short- and long-term disability insurance; tuition assistance; employee discounts; and an employee assistance plan.

FINANCIALS: Sales and profits are in thousands of dollars—add 000 to get the full amount. 2007 Note: Financial information for 2007 was not available for all companies at press time.

2007 Sales: $16,325,900	2007 Profits: $1,491,500	**U.S. Stock Ticker:** NKE
2006 Sales: $14,954,900	2006 Profits: $1,392,000	**Int'l Ticker:** Int'l Exchange:
2005 Sales: $13,739,700	2005 Profits: $1,211,600	Employees: 30,200
2004 Sales: $12,253,100	2004 Profits: $945,600	Fiscal Year Ends: 5/31
2003 Sales: $10,697,000	2003 Profits: $474,000	Parent Company:

SALARIES/BENEFITS:

Pension Plan:	ESOP Stock Plan:	Profit Sharing: Y	Top Exec. Salary: $1,250,000	Bonus: $2,147,537
Savings Plan: Y	Stock Purch. Plan: Y		Second Exec. Salary: $1,150,000	Bonus: $1,868,030

OTHER THOUGHTS:

Apparent Women Officers or Directors: 14
Hot Spot for Advancement for Women/Minorities: Y

LOCATIONS: ("Y" = Yes)

West:	Southwest:	Midwest:	Southeast:	Northeast:	International:
Y	Y	Y	Y	Y	Y

Note: Financial information, benefits and other data can change quickly and may vary from those stated here.

NOBLE CORPORATION

www.noblecorp.com

Industry Group Code: 213111   Ranks within this company's industry group: Sales: 11   Profits: 6

Management:		Sales/Marketing:		Liberal Arts:	Information Systems:		Professionals:		Technical/Scientific:	
Mgmt. Trainees:	Y	Mktg. Professionals:	Y	Gen. Writing/Editing:	Info. Management:	Y	Finance/Accounting:	Y	Engineers, Elec.:	Y
Experienced Mgmt.:	Y	Retail Sales:		Technical Writing:	Software Dev.:	Y	Law:	Y	Engineers, Other:	Y
Int'l Business:	Y	Commercial/Industrial:	Y	Graphic Arts/Photog.:	Hardware Dev.:		HR/Other:	Y	Health/Lab:	
MBA Graduates:	Y	Sales Trainees:		Music:	Systems Integration:		Training:	Y	Scientists/Research:	Y
		Advertising Pros.:		Broadcasting:	Consulting/Other:		Health Care:		Petroleum/Chemicals:	Y
				Other:			Consulting:		Math/Other:	

TYPES OF BUSINESS:

Oil & Gas Services
Drilling Services
Well Site Services
Project Management Services
Engineering Services

BRANDS/DIVISIONS/AFFILIATES:

Triton Engineering Services
Noble Engineering & Development (NED)
Maurer Technology, Inc.
Noble Downhole Technology
Well Director Rotary Steerable System
Noble Category 5
Noble Amos Runner

CONTACTS: *Note: Officers with more than one job title may be intentionally listed here more than once.*

David W. Williams, CEO
David W. Williams, Pres.
Thomas L. Mitchell, CFO/Sr. VP
Robert D. Campbell, General Counsel/Sr. VP
Lee M. Ahlstrom, VP-Planning
Lee M. Ahlstrom, VP-Investor Rel.
Thomas L. Mitchell, Controller/Treas.
Julie J. Robertson, Exec. VP/Corp. Sec.
Ross W. Gallup, VP-Tax, Noble Drilling Svcs., Inc.
David W. Williams, Chmn.

Phone: 281-276-6100	**Fax:** 281-491-2092

Toll-Free:

Address: 13135 S. Dairy Ashford Rd., Ste. 800, Sugar Land, TX 77478 US

GROWTH PLANS/SPECIAL FEATURES:

Noble Corporation provides diversified services for the oil and gas industry. The company performs drilling services on a contract basis through its fleet of 62 mobile offshore drilling units located in key markets worldwide. The fleet includes 43 jackup drilling rigs, 13 semi-submersible rigs, three dynamically positioned drillships and three submersible drilling platforms. Approximately 85% of Noble's fleet is currently deployed in international markets including the North Sea, Mexico, Brazil, West Africa, the Middle East and India; and offshore drilling accounted for approximately 93% of the company's 2006 operating revenue. Unlike other firms in the industry, Noble only buys specially contracted rigs, and not those built on speculation. In addition to contract drilling services, the company provides well site and project management services, as well as engineering services through subsidiary Triton Engineering Services Company. The company's Noble Engineering and Development and Maurer Technology, Inc., subsidiaries focus on the design and development of drilling products as well as drilling-related technical solutions and applications that allow for more cost-effective deepwater drilling. The company's Noble Downhole Technology subsidiary provides the Well Director Rotary Steerable System to the oil and gas industry worldwide. In January 2008, the company sold its North Sea labor contract drilling services business to Seawell Holding UK Limited for approximately $35 million.

FINANCIALS: Sales and profits are in thousands of dollars—add 000 to get the full amount. 2007 Note: Financial information for 2007 was not available for all companies at press time.

2007 Sales: $2,995,311	2007 Profits: $1,206,011	**U.S. Stock Ticker: NE**
2006 Sales: $2,100,239	2006 Profits: $731,866	**Int'l Ticker:** Int'l Exchange:
2005 Sales: $1,382,137	2005 Profits: $296,696	Employees: 6,000
2004 Sales: $1,066,231	2004 Profits: $146,086	Fiscal Year Ends: 12/31
2003 Sales: $987,380	2003 Profits: $166,416	Parent Company:

SALARIES/BENEFITS:

Pension Plan: Y	ESOP Stock Plan:	Profit Sharing:	Top Exec. Salary: $946,735	Bonus: $1,780,000
Savings Plan: Y	Stock Purch. Plan:		Second Exec. Salary: $604,367	Bonus: $1,270,000

OTHER THOUGHTS:

Apparent Women Officers or Directors: 1
Hot Spot for Advancement for Women/Minorities: Y

LOCATIONS: ("Y" = Yes)

West:	Southwest:	Midwest:	Southeast:	Northeast:	International:
	Y		Y		Y

Note: Financial information, benefits and other data can change quickly and may vary from those stated here.

NORDSTROM INC

www.nordstrom.com

Industry Group Code: 452110 Ranks within this company's industry group: Sales: 3 Profits: 3

Management:		Sales/Marketing:		Liberal Arts:		Information Systems:		Professionals:		Technical/Scientific:	
Mgmt. Trainees:	Y	Mktg. Professionals:	Y	Gen. Writing/Editing:	Y	Info. Management:	Y	Finance/Accounting:	Y	Engineers, Elec.:	
Experienced Mgmt.:	Y	Retail Sales:	Y	Technical Writing:		Software Dev.:	Y	Law:	Y	Engineers, Other:	
Int'l Business:	Y	Commercial/Industrial:	Y	Graphic Arts/Photog.:	Y	Hardware Dev.:		HR/Other:	Y	Health/Lab:	
MBA Graduates:	Y	Sales Trainees:	Y	Music:		Systems Integration:		Training:	Y	Scientists/Research:	
		Advertising Pros.:	Y	Broadcasting:		Consulting/Other:		Health Care:		Petroleum/Chemicals:	
				Other:	Y			Consulting:		Math/Other:	

TYPES OF BUSINESS:

Department Stores
Outlet Stores
Online Retailing
Catalog Sales
Financial Services
Federal Savings Bank

BRANDS/DIVISIONS/AFFILIATES:

Nordstrom Bank
Nordstrom Rack
Facconable
Last Chance
Brass Plum
Rubbish
Classiques Entier
Halogen

CONTACTS: *Note: Officers with more than one job title may be intentionally listed here more than once.*

Blake W. Nordstrom, Pres.
Michael G. Koppel, CFO/Exec. VP
Linda Toschi Finn, Exec. VP-Mktg.
Delena M. Sunday, Exec. VP-Human Resources & Diversity Affairs
Peter E. Nordstrom, Pres., Merch.
Daniel F. Little, Chief Admin. Officer/Exec. VP
Lisa G. Iglesias, General Counsel/Corp. Sec./Exec. VP
Paul Favaro, Exec. VP-Strategy & Dev.
James A. Howell, VP-Fin.
Laurie M. Black, Exec. VP/Gen. Merch. Manager, Cosmetic Div.
Erik B. Nordstrom, Pres., Stores
Jeffrey S. Kalinski, Exec. VP-Designer Merch.
James R. O'Neal, Pres./Exec. VP- Nordstrom Product Group
Bruce A. Nordstrom, Chmn.

Phone: 206-628-2111	Fax: 206-628-1795
Toll-Free: 888-282-6060	
Address: 1617 6th Ave., Ste. 500, Seattle, WA 98101 US	

GROWTH PLANS/SPECIAL FEATURES:

Nordstrom, Inc., founded in 1901, is one of the nation's largest upscale fashion apparel and shoe retailers, with 157 U.S. stores in 28 states that sell a wide selection of apparel, shoes and accessories for women, men and children. Nordstrom is comprised of four segments: Retail Stores, Direct, Credit, and Other. Retail Stores derive its revenues from the sale of designer, luxury and high end apparel, shoes, cosmetics and accessories. The company operates 103 full-line stores, 50 Nordstrom Rack stores, two Last Chance clearance stores and two Jeffrey boutiques. The Nordstrom Rack stores serve as outlets for clearance merchandise from the full-line stores and purchase merchandise directly from manufacturers. In 2007, the firm opened three full-line stores, one Rack store, and increased its ownership in two Jeffrey boutiques. The company is scheduled to open six more full-line stores, relocate one full-line store and open three Rack stores in 2008. In 2009, Nordstrom is scheduled to open five full-line stores, relocate one full-line store and open two Rack stores. The Direct segment generates revenues from the sale of designer, luxury and high end apparel, shoes, cosmetics and accessories by serving customers on the internet at www.nordstrom.com and through catalogs. The Credit segment generates income through finance charges and fees on Nordstrom credit cards. The final, Other segment includes the company's product development team, called Nordstrom Product Group, which designs and coordinates the production of private label merchandise sold in its Retail Stores and Direct. In July 2007, Nordstrom announced it agreed to sell Facconable, a wholly owned subsidiary, to M1 Group for $210 Million.

Nordstrom offers employees medical, dental and vision insurance; 401(k) and profit sharing; adoption assistance; dependent care, health care and commuter spending accounts; employee stock purchase plan; a Nordstrom Bank account; and Nordstrom Federal Credit Union membership.

FINANCIALS: Sales and profits are in thousands of dollars—add 000 to get the full amount. 2007 Note: Financial information for 2007 was not available for all companies at press time.

2007 Sales: $8,560,698	2007 Profits: $667,999	**U.S. Stock Ticker: JWN**
2006 Sales: $7,722,860	2006 Profits: $551,339	**Int'l Ticker:** Int'l Exchange:
2005 Sales: $7,131,400	2005 Profits: $393,500	Employees: 52,900
2004 Sales: $6,491,673	2004 Profits: $242,841	Fiscal Year Ends: 1/31
2003 Sales: $5,975,100	2003 Profits: $90,200	Parent Company:

SALARIES/BENEFITS:

Pension Plan:	ESOP Stock Plan:	Profit Sharing: Y	Top Exec. Salary: $711,302	Bonus: $1,645,506
Savings Plan: Y	Stock Purch. Plan:		Second Exec. Salary: $490,932	Bonus: $1,460,843

OTHER THOUGHTS:

Apparent Women Officers or Directors: 5
Hot Spot for Advancement for Women/Minorities: Y

LOCATIONS: ("Y" = Yes)

West:	Southwest:	Midwest:	Southeast:	Northeast:	International:
Y	Y	Y	Y	Y	Y

Note: Financial information, benefits and other data can change quickly and may vary from those stated here.

NORFOLK SOUTHERN CORP

www.nscorp.com

Industry Group Code: 482110 Ranks within this company's industry group: Sales: 4   Profits: 3

Management:		Sales/Marketing:		Liberal Arts:		Information Systems:		Professionals:		Technical/Scientific:	
Mgmt. Trainees:	Y	Mktg. Professionals:	Y	Gen. Writing/Editing:	Y	Info. Management:	Y	Finance/Accounting:	Y	Engineers, Elec.:	Y
Experienced Mgmt.:	Y	Retail Sales:		Technical Writing:	Y	Software Dev.:	Y	Law:	Y	Engineers, Other:	Y
Int'l Business:	Y	Commercial/Industrial:		Graphic Arts/Photog.:		Hardware Dev.:		HR/Other:	Y	Health/Lab:	
MBA Graduates:	Y	Sales Trainees:		Music:		Systems Integration:		Training:	Y	Scientists/Research:	
		Advertising Pros.:		Broadcasting:		Consulting/Other:		Health Care:		Petroleum/Chemicals:	
				Other:				Consulting:		Math/Other:	

TYPES OF BUSINESS:

Railroad Transportation
Cargo Services
Logistics Services
Commercial Real Estate Development
Natural Resources Acquisition Leasing & Management

BRANDS/DIVISIONS/AFFILIATES:

Norfolk Southern Railway Co.
CSX Corp
Conrail, Inc.
Consolidated Rail Corp.
Triple Crown Services Co.
RoadRailer
Watco Companies

CONTACTS: *Note: Officers with more than one job title may be intentionally listed here more than once.*

Charles W. Moorman, CEO
Stephen Tobias, COO
Charles W. Moorman, Pres.
James A. Squires, CFO
Donald W. Seale, Chief Mktg. Officer/Exec. VP
Cindy Earhart, VP-Human Resources
Debbie Butler, CIO
Timothy Drake, VP-Eng.
John P. Rathbone, Exec. VP-Admin.
James A. Hixon, Exec. VP-Law
Mark D. Manion, Exec. VP-Oper.
Debbie Butler, Exec. VP-Planning
James Hixon, Exec. VP-Corp. Rel.
James A. Squires, Exec. VP-Finance
Robert Martinez, VP-Bus. Dev.
Danny Smith, Sr. VP-Energy & Properties
Terry Evans, VP-Oper. Planning & Budget
John Friedmann, VP-Strategic Planning
Charles W. Moorman, Chmn.

Phone: 757-629-2861	Fax:
Toll-Free:	
Address: 3 Commercial Pl., Norfolk, VA 23510 US	

GROWTH PLANS/SPECIAL FEATURES:

Norfolk Southern Corp., based in Norfolk, Virginia, controls a major freight railroad through Norfolk Southern Railway Co. Norfolk Southern Railway Co. is principally engaged in the rail transportation of raw materials, intermediate products and finished goods in the Southeast, East and Midwest and, via interchange with rail carriers, the rest of the U.S.. Norfolk Southern also transports overseas freight through several Atlantic and Gulf Coast ports. The company's general merchandise traffic is composed of five major commodity groupings: automotive; chemicals; metals and construction; agriculture, consumer products and government; and paper, clay and forest products. Coal, coke and iron ore comprise the company's largest commodity group as measured by revenues, about 25%. Total coal handled through all system ports in 2007 was 186 million tons. The firm also provides logistics services and offers an intermodal network in the eastern U.S. Norfolk Southern operates about 21,000 route miles in 22 eastern states and Washington, D.C. The lines reach many individual industries, electric generating facilities, mines, distribution centers, transload facilities and other businesses located in smaller communities in its service area. Through a limited liability company, the firm and CSX Corp. jointly own Conrail, Inc., whose primary subsidiary is Consolidated Rail Corp. The Triple Crown Services Co. subsidiary offers door-to-door intermodal service using RoadRailer equipment and domestic containers. The company's noncarrier subsidiaries engage principally in the acquisition, leasing and management of coal, oil, gas and minerals; the development of commercial real estate; telecommunications; and the leasing or sale of rail property and equipment. In 2007, Norfolk agreed to form a joint venture with Watco Companies for freight rail service in Michigan and Indiana.

The company offers its employees medical, dental and vision coverage; a 401(k) plan; railroad retirement, which includes an additional benefit based on railroad earnings; education assistance; and on-site child care.

FINANCIALS: Sales and profits are in thousands of dollars—add 000 to get the full amount. 2007 Note: Financial information for 2007 was not available for all companies at press time.

2007 Sales: $9,432,000	2007 Profits: $1,464,000	**U.S. Stock Ticker: NSC**	
2006 Sales: $9,407,000	2006 Profits: $1,481,000	**Int'l Ticker:** Int'l Exchange:	
2005 Sales: $8,527,000	2005 Profits: $1,281,000	Employees: 30,541	
2004 Sales: $7,312,000	2004 Profits: $923,000	Fiscal Year Ends: 12/31	
2003 Sales: $6,468,000	2003 Profits: $535,000	Parent Company:	

SALARIES/BENEFITS:

Pension Plan:	ESOP Stock Plan:	Profit Sharing:	Top Exec. Salary: $750,000	Bonus: $1,312,500
Savings Plan: Y	Stock Purch. Plan:		Second Exec. Salary: $600,000	Bonus: $810,000

OTHER THOUGHTS:

Apparent Women Officers or Directors: 2
Hot Spot for Advancement for Women/Minorities: Y

LOCATIONS: ("Y" = Yes)

West:	Southwest:	Midwest:	Southeast:	Northeast:	International:
	Y	Y	Y	Y	Y

NORTHROP GRUMMAN CORP www.northropgrumman.com

Industry Group Code: 336410 Ranks within this company's industry group: Sales: 5 Profits: 6

Management:		Sales/Marketing:		Liberal Arts:		Information Systems:		Professionals:		Technical/Scientific:	
Mgmt. Trainees:	Y	Mktg. Professionals:	Y	Gen. Writing/Editing:	Y	Info. Management:	Y	Finance/Accounting:	Y	Engineers, Elec.:	Y
Experienced Mgmt.:	Y	Retail Sales:		Technical Writing:	Y	Software Dev.:	Y	Law:	Y	Engineers, Other:	
Int'l Business:	Y	Commercial/Industrial:	Y	Graphic Arts/Photog.:	Y	Hardware Dev.:	Y	HR/Other:	Y	Health/Lab:	Y
MBA Graduates:	Y	Sales Trainees:		Music:		Systems Integration:	Y	Training:	Y	Scientists/Research:	Y
		Advertising Pros.:		Broadcasting:		Consulting/Other:	Y	Health Care:		Petroleum/Chemicals:	
				Other:				Consulting:	Y	Math/Other:	Y

TYPES OF BUSINESS:

Aerospace & Defense Technology
Shipbuilding & Engineering
Aircraft Manufacturing
Electronic Systems & Components
Hardware & Software Manufacturing
Design & Engineering Services
IT Systems & Services
Nuclear-Powered Aircraft Carriers & Submarines

BRANDS/DIVISIONS/AFFILIATES:

F/A-18
F-35
B-2
Multi-Platform Radar Technology Insertion Program
Global Hawk
James Webb Space Telescope
Airborne Laser
EA-6B

CONTACTS: Note: Officers with more than one job title may be intentionally listed here more than once.

Ronald D. Sugar, CEO
Wesley G. Bush, COO
Wesley G. Bush, Pres.
James F. Palmer, CFO/Corp. VP
Ian V. Ziskin, Chief Human Resources Officer/Corp. VP
Linda A. Mills, Corp. VP/Pres., IT
Ian V. Ziskin, Chief Admin. Officer
W. Burks Terry, General Counsel/Corp. VP
Rosanne O'Brien, Corp. VP-Comm.
Kenneth N. Heintz, Chief Acct. Officer/Controller/Corp. VP
Robert W. Helm, Corp. VP-Gov't Rel.
James F. Pitts, Corp. VP/Pres., Electronic Systems
Alexis Livanos, Corp. VP/Pres., Space Tech.
Mike Petters, Corp. VP/Pres., Shipbuilding
Ronald D. Sugar, Chmn.

Phone: 310-553-6262	Fax: 310-553-2076
Toll-Free:	
Address: 1840 Century Park E., Los Angeles, CA 90067-2199 US	

GROWTH PLANS/SPECIAL FEATURES:

Northrop Grumman Corp. is a global aerospace and defense technology company. 90% of its revenue comes from the U.S. Government. It has four primary businesses: Information and Services (I&S), Aerospace, Electronics and Ships. I&S encompasses three divisions: Mission Systems, Information Technology (IT) and Technical Services. Mission Systems offers land forces and global combat support, satellite ground stations and signals intelligence. The IT division offers data analysis; document management; data center, IT security, storage and help desk management; R&D and test centers; and education and training commands. Technical Services offers base support, including civil engineering, and support functions, including space launch services, combat vehicle maintenance and protective and emergency services. It also covers training and simulation services. The Aerospace business encompasses Space Technology and Integrated Systems. The Space Technology division's major projects include the James Webb Space Telescope; Space Tracking and Surveillance System; and the Airborne Laser. In 2008, the missile systems business (offering fire control systems, simulation and warfighter operations) was transferred from Mission Systems to Space Technology. Integrated Systems has two business areas. Integrated Systems Western Region is working on the F/A-18, F-35 and B-2 manned aircraft programs; the Multi-Platform Radar Technology Insertion Program (MP-RTIP); and the Global Hawk and Fire Scout unmanned vehicle programs. Integrated Systems Eastern Region produced the E-2C Hawkeye command plane; and developed the EA-6B (Prowler) offensive tactical radar jamming aircraft. The Electronics business offers missile tracking and warning systems; fire control radars; advanced simulation systems; infrared detection and countermeasures systems; night vision goggles; laser designators; Chemical, Biological, Radiological, Nuclear and Explosive (CBRNE) material detection and alert systems; U.S. Postal Service bio-detection systems; and power generation systems for aircraft carriers. Finally, the Ships business designs, builds, maintains and refuels nuclear-powered aircraft carriers; and designs and constructs amphibious assault ships, Aegis guided missile destroyers, nuclear-powered submarines and oil tankers.

FINANCIALS: Sales and profits are in thousands of dollars—add 000 to get the full amount. 2007 Note: Financial information for 2007 was not available for all companies at press time.

2007 Sales: $32,018,000	2007 Profits: $1,790,000	U.S. Stock Ticker: NOC
2006 Sales: $30,113,000	2006 Profits: $1,542,000	Int'l Ticker: Int'l Exchange:
2005 Sales: $29,978,000	2005 Profits: $1,400,000	Employees: 122,600
2004 Sales: $29,000,000	2004 Profits: $1,080,000	Fiscal Year Ends: 12/31
2003 Sales: $26,206,000	2003 Profits: $866,000	Parent Company:

SALARIES/BENEFITS:

Pension Plan: Y	ESOP Stock Plan:	Profit Sharing:	Top Exec. Salary: $1,414,128	Bonus: $3,500,000
Savings Plan: Y	Stock Purch. Plan:		Second Exec. Salary: $667,307	Bonus: $730,000

OTHER THOUGHTS:

Apparent Women Officers or Directors: 3
Hot Spot for Advancement for Women/Minorities: Y

LOCATIONS: ("Y" = Yes)

West:	Southwest:	Midwest:	Southeast:	Northeast:	International:
Y	Y	Y	Y	Y	Y

Note: Financial information, benefits and other data can change quickly and may vary from those stated here.

OCCIDENTAL PETROLEUM CORP

www.oxy.com

Industry Group Code: 211111 Ranks within this company's industry group: Sales: 6 Profits: 5

Management:		Sales/Marketing:		Liberal Arts:	Information Systems:		Professionals:		Technical/Scientific:	
Mgmt. Trainees:	Y	Mktg. Professionals:	Y	Gen. Writing/Editing:	Info. Management:	Y	Finance/Accounting:	Y	Engineers, Elec.:	Y
Experienced Mgmt.:	Y	Retail Sales:		Technical Writing:	Software Dev.:	Y	Law:	Y	Engineers, Other:	
Int'l Business:	Y	Commercial/Industrial:	Y	Graphic Arts/Photog.:	Hardware Dev.:		HR/Other:	Y	Health/Lab:	Y
MBA Graduates:	Y	Sales Trainees:		Music:	Systems Integration:		Training:	Y	Scientists/Research:	
		Advertising Pros.:		Broadcasting:	Consulting/Other:		Health Care:		Petroleum/Chemicals:	Y
				Other:			Consulting:		Math/Other:	

TYPES OF BUSINESS:

Oil & Natural Gas Exploration & Production
Basic Chemicals
Vinyls

BRANDS/DIVISIONS/AFFILIATES:

OxyChem

CONTACTS: *Note: Officers with more than one job title may be intentionally listed here more than once.*

Ray R. Irani, CEO
Stephen I. Chazen, Pres.
Stephen I. Chazen, CFO
Martin Cozyn, Exec. VP-Human Resources
Donald L. Moore, Jr., CIO/VP
Donald P. de Brier, General Counsel/Exec. VP/Sec.
Richard S. Kline, VP-Comm. & Public Affairs
Christopher G. Stavros, VP-Investor Rel.
James M. Lienert, Exec. VP-Finance & Planning
B. Chuck Anderson, Pres., OxyChem
James R. Havert, VP/Treas.
William E. Albrecht, Pres., Oxy Oil & Gas
Gary L. Daugherty, VP-Internal Audit
Ray R. Irani, Chmn.
R. Casey Olson, Exec. VP/Pres., Oil & Gas Eastern Hemisphere

Phone: 310-208-8800	**Fax:** 310-443-6690
Toll-Free:	
Address: 10889 Wilshire Blvd., Los Angeles, CA 90024-4201 US	

GROWTH PLANS/SPECIAL FEATURES:

Occidental Petroleum Corp. (OPC) explores for, develops, produces and markets crude oil and natural gas. The company also manufactures and markets basic chemicals, vinyls and specialty chemicals. The firm operates in two segments: Oil and gas; and chemical. It has proven reserves of oil amounting to 4,452 million barrels and of natural gas amounting to 7,686 billion cubic feet, including the reserves of its consolidated subsidiaries. OPC's primary domestic oil and gas operations, responsible for 63% of production, are in California; the Hugoton field in Kansas and Oklahoma; and the Permian field in west Texas and New Mexico. International operations are principally located in Colombia, Argentina, Oman, Qatar, Libya and Yemen, with exploration interests in other countries. The firm's chemicals business, run by OxyChem, owns and operates 23 chemical manufacturing plants in the U.S. and three internationally. The segment produces chlorine; caustic soda; potassium chemicals for use in glass, fertilizer, cleaning products and rubber; and other chemicals including chlorinated isocyanurates, resorcinol and sodium silicates for use in pool sanitation, home soaps and detergents. The company is also a leading producer of vinyls for piping, medical, building and automotive products, focusing on polyvinyl chloride (PVC) resins and vinyl chloride monomers (VCM). OxyChem is the only producer of mercury-free caustic potash. In April 2007, OPC announced that it would acquire BP's West Texas pipeline system and that BP would acquire all of OPC's remaining interests in Pakistan. In December 2007, the firm acquired 50% of Plains Exploration & Production's oil and gas interests in the Permian and Piceance Basins. In 2008, the company entered a joint investment agreement with Abu Dhabi's International Petroleum Investment Company to make hydrocarbon investments.

OPC offers employees medical and dental insurance, matches contributions to a personal savings account, provides educational assistance and has employee retirement accounts.

FINANCIALS: Sales and profits are in thousands of dollars—add 000 to get the full amount. 2007 Note: Financial information for 2007 was not available for all companies at press time.

2007 Sales: $18,784,000	2007 Profits: $5,400,000	**U.S. Stock Ticker: OXY**
2006 Sales: $17,175,000	2006 Profits: $4,191,000	**Int'l Ticker:** Int'l Exchange:
2005 Sales: $15,208,000	2005 Profits: $5,281,000	Employees: 9,700
2004 Sales: $11,368,000	2004 Profits: $2,568,000	Fiscal Year Ends: 12/31
2003 Sales: $9,447,000	2003 Profits: $1,527,000	Parent Company:

SALARIES/BENEFITS:

Pension Plan: Y	ESOP Stock Plan:	Profit Sharing:	Top Exec. Salary: $1,300,000	Bonus: $4,290,000
Savings Plan: Y	Stock Purch. Plan:		Second Exec. Salary: $720,000	Bonus: $1,584,000

OTHER THOUGHTS:

Apparent Women Officers or Directors: 1
Hot Spot for Advancement for Women/Minorities:

LOCATIONS: ("Y" = Yes)

West:	Southwest:	Midwest:	Southeast:	Northeast:	International:
Y	Y	Y	Y	Y	Y

Note: Financial information, benefits and other data can change quickly and may vary from those stated here.

OCEANEERING INTERNATIONAL INC   www.oceaneering.com

Industry Group Code: 213111 Ranks within this company's industry group: Sales: 13   Profits: 13

Management:		Sales/Marketing:		Liberal Arts:	Information Systems:		Professionals:		Technical/Scientific:	
Mgmt. Trainees:	Y	Mktg. Professionals:	Y	Gen. Writing/Editing:	Info. Management:	Y	Finance/Accounting:	Y	Engineers, Elec.:	Y
Experienced Mgmt.:	Y	Retail Sales:		Technical Writing:	Software Dev.:	Y	Law:	Y	Engineers, Other:	Y
Int'l Business:	Y	Commercial/Industrial:	Y	Graphic Arts/Photog.:	Hardware Dev.:		HR/Other:	Y	Health/Lab:	Y
MBA Graduates:	Y	Sales Trainees:		Music:	Systems Integration:		Training:	Y	Scientists/Research:	Y
		Advertising Pros.:		Broadcasting:	Consulting/Other:		Health Care:		Petroleum/Chemicals:	Y
				Other:			Consulting:		Math/Other:	Y

TYPES OF BUSINESS:
Oil & Gas Drilling Support Services
Subsea Construction
Engineered Services & Hardware
Maintenance & Repair Services
Production Systems
Remotely Operated Vehicles
Robotic Systems

BRANDS/DIVISIONS/AFFILIATES:
Oceaneering Intervention Engineering
Grayloc Products
Oceaneering Multiflex
Oceaneering Rotator
Advanced Technologies
Ifokus Engineering AS

CONTACTS: Note: Officers with more than one job title may be intentionally listed here more than once.
T. Jay Collins, CEO
T. Jay Collins, Pres.
Marvin J. Migura, CFO/Sr. VP
Janet G. Charles, VP-Human Resources
Gregg K. Farris, VP-IT
F. Richard Frisbie, Sr. VP-Deepwater Tech.
George R. Haubenreich, Jr., General Counsel/Sr. VP/Sec.
Stephen E. Bradshaw, VP-Bus. Dev.
Jack Jurkoshek, Dir.-Investor Rel.
W. Cardon Gerner, VP/Chief Acct. Officer
M. Kevin McEvoy, Exec. VP
John R. Huff, Chmn.

Phone: 713-329-4500	Fax: 713-329-4951
Toll-Free:	
Address: 11911 FM 529, Houston, TX 77041 US	

GROWTH PLANS/SPECIAL FEATURES:
Oceaneering International, Inc. primarily provides oilfield products and services worldwide to the oil and gas industry. The oil and gas business of the company has five segments: Remotely Operated Vehicles (ROVs), Subsea Products, Subsea Projects, Inspection and Mobile Offshore Production Systems (MOPS). The company uses submersible ROVs to support drilling and construction; pipeline inspection; and subsea production facility operation and maintenance. It designs and builds ROVs, having constructed over 150 to date; and it owns a total of 186, one of the largest ROV fleets worldwide. The firm is an industry leader in providing ROV services on deepwater wells, a highly technically demanding operation. Its Subsea Products segment manufactures typically built-to-order items including hydraulic hoses, ROV tooling, control valves, production control equipment and pipeline repair systems. These products are manufactured mainly by the Oceaneering Intervention Engineering, Grayloc Products, Oceaneering Multiflex and Oceaneering Rotator divisions. The Subsea Projects segment primarily operates in the Gulf of Mexico (GOM), offering subsea installation, inspection, maintenance and repair services. The Inspection segment provides nondestructive testing and inspection services, including to the power generation, engineering and petrochemical industries; and it also publishes The Inspection Standard newsletter twice a year, informing customers of technical developments. Finally, the MOPS segment owns three MOPS oil processing rigs currently in place offshore West Africa, Indonesia and Western Australia; and also provides engineering services. The company's non-oilfield business is accomplished by its Advanced Technologies unit, which manufactures remotely operated diving vessels used extensively by the U.S. Navy, as well as life-support and robotic systems for use in government space programs. In July 2007, Oceaneering acquired Ifokus Engineering AS, a Norwegian manufacturer of subsea products, for approximately $20 million. In May 2007, it obtained contracts from BP Americas Production Company to assist in decommissioning its GOM platforms in preparation for hurricane season.

FINANCIALS: Sales and profits are in thousands of dollars—add 000 to get the full amount. 2007 Note: Financial information for 2007 was not available for all companies at press time.

2007 Sales: $1,743,080	2007 Profits: $180,374	U.S. Stock Ticker: OII
2006 Sales: $1,280,198	2006 Profits: $124,494	Int'l Ticker: Int'l Exchange:
2005 Sales: $998,543	2005 Profits: $62,680	Employees: 6,500
2004 Sales: $780,181	2004 Profits: $40,300	Fiscal Year Ends: 3/31
2003 Sales: $639,249	2003 Profits: $29,301	Parent Company:

SALARIES/BENEFITS:
Pension Plan: Y	ESOP Stock Plan:	Profit Sharing:	Top Exec. Salary: $800,000	Bonus: $1,000,000
Savings Plan: Y	Stock Purch. Plan:		Second Exec. Salary: $457,000	Bonus: $469,000

OTHER THOUGHTS:
Apparent Women Officers or Directors:
Hot Spot for Advancement for Women/Minorities:

LOCATIONS: ("Y" = Yes)
West:	Southwest:	Midwest:	Southeast:	Northeast:	International:
Y	Y		Y	Y	Y

Note: Financial information, benefits and other data can change quickly and may vary from those stated here.

ODYSSEY HEALTHCARE INC

www.odsyhealth.com

Industry Group Code: 621610 **Ranks within this company's industry group:** Sales: 4   Profits: 4

Management:		Sales/Marketing:		Liberal Arts:		Information Systems:		Professionals:		Technical/Scientific:	
Mgmt. Trainees:	Y	Mktg. Professionals:	Y	Gen. Writing/Editing:		Info. Management:	Y	Finance/Accounting:	Y	Engineers, Elec.:	
Experienced Mgmt.:	Y	Retail Sales:		Technical Writing:		Software Dev.:		Law:	Y	Engineers, Other:	Y
Int'l Business:		Commercial/Industrial:		Graphic Arts/Photog.:		Hardware Dev.:		HR/Other:	Y	Health/Lab:	
MBA Graduates:	Y	Sales Trainees:		Music:		Systems Integration:		Training:	Y	Scientists/Research:	
		Advertising Pros.:		Broadcasting:		Consulting/Other:		Health Care:	Y	Petroleum/Chemicals:	
				Other:				Consulting:		Math/Other:	

TYPES OF BUSINESS:

Hospice Care Services
Medical Supplies & Equipment

BRANDS/DIVISIONS/AFFILIATES:

CONTACTS: Note: Officers with more than one job title may be intentionally listed here more than once.

Robert A. Lefton, CEO
Craig P. Goguen, COO/Sr. VP
Robert A. Lefton, Pres.
R. Dirk Allison, CFO/Sr. VP
Frank W. Anastasio, Sr. VP-Sales & Mktg.
Brenda A. Belger, Sr. VP-Human Resources
W. Bradley Bickham, General Counsel/Sr. VP/Corp. Sec.
R. Dirk Allison, Treas./Asst. Sec.
Kathleen A. Ventre, Dir.-Clinical & Regulatory Affairs
Richard R. Burnham, Chmn.

Phone: 214-922-9711	Fax: 214-922-9752
Toll-Free: 888-922-9711	
Address: 717 N. Harwood St., Ste. 1500, Dallas, TX 75201 US	

GROWTH PLANS/SPECIAL FEATURES:

Odyssey HealthCare, Inc. is a leading provider of hospice care in the U.S., with 110 Medicare-certified hospice programs in 30 states and over 12,000 patients. Odyssey assigns each of its hospice patients to an interdisciplinary team, comprised of a physician, a patient care manager, one or more registered nurses, one or more certified home health aides, a medical social worker, a chaplain, a homemaker and one or more specially trained volunteers. The team assesses the clinical, psychosocial and spiritual needs of the patient and his or her family; develops a plan of care; and delivers, monitors and coordinates that plan of care with the goal of providing appropriate care for the patient and his or her family. Services provided by the company include nursing care; medical social services, physician services, dietary, spiritual and other patient counseling; general inpatient care; medical supplies and equipment; drugs for pain control and symptom management; home health aide services; homemaker services; physical, occupational and speech therapy; respite inpatient care; and family bereavement counseling. Services provided under the Medicare program represented approximately 92.4% of Odyssey's net patient service revenue for 2007. Approximately 97.2% of Odyssey's total days of care during 2007 were comprised of routine home care; 0.9% were comprised of continuous home care; 1.7% were comprised of general inpatient care; and 0.2% were comprised of respite inpatient care. In March 2008, Odyssey acquired VistaCare, Inc. for approximately $148 million.

Odyssey offers its employees tuition reimbursement; employee recognition programs; an employee referral bonus; flexible spending accounts; and medical, dental, vision, life, AD&D and disability insurance.

FINANCIALS: Sales and profits are in thousands of dollars—add 000 to get the full amount. 2007 Note: Financial information for 2007 was not available for all companies at press time.

2007 Sales: $404,872	2007 Profits: $12,111	**U.S. Stock Ticker:** ODSY	
2006 Sales: $384,981	2006 Profits: $19,729	**Int'l Ticker:** Int'l Exchange:	
2005 Sales: $378,073	2005 Profits: $18,556	**Employees:** 4,185	
2004 Sales: $340,180	2004 Profits: $34,996	**Fiscal Year Ends:** 12/31	
2003 Sales: $274,309	2003 Profits: $31,207	**Parent Company:**	

SALARIES/BENEFITS:

Pension Plan:	ESOP Stock Plan:	Profit Sharing:	Top Exec. Salary: $525,000	Bonus: $
Savings Plan: Y	Stock Purch. Plan: Y		Second Exec. Salary: $335,000	Bonus: $

OTHER THOUGHTS:

Apparent Women Officers or Directors: 2
Hot Spot for Advancement for Women/Minorities: Y

LOCATIONS: ("Y" = Yes)

West:	Southwest:	Midwest:	Southeast:	Northeast:	International:
Y	Y	Y	Y	Y	

Note: Financial information, benefits and other data can change quickly and may vary from those stated here.

OFFICE DEPOT INC　　　　www.officedepot.com

Industry Group Code: 453210　**Ranks within this company's industry group:** Sales: 2　Profits: 2

Management:		Sales/Marketing:		Liberal Arts:		Information Systems:		Professionals:		Technical/Scientific:	
Mgmt. Trainees:	Y	Mktg. Professionals:	Y	Gen. Writing/Editing:	Y	Info. Management:	Y	Finance/Accounting:	Y	Engineers, Elec.:	
Experienced Mgmt.:	Y	Retail Sales:	Y	Technical Writing:		Software Dev.:	Y	Law:	Y	Engineers, Other:	
Int'l Business:	Y	Commercial/Industrial:	Y	Graphic Arts/Photog.:	Y	Hardware Dev.:		HR/Other:	Y	Health/Lab:	
MBA Graduates:	Y	Sales Trainees:	Y	Music:		Systems Integration:	Y	Training:	Y	Scientists/Research:	
		Advertising Pros.:	Y	Broadcasting:		Consulting/Other:		Health Care:		Petroleum/Chemicals:	
				Other:	Y			Consulting:		Math/Other:	

TYPES OF BUSINESS:

Office Supplies, Retail
Contract Stationery
Online Retailing
Copy Services
Office Design Services
Office Furnishings
Direct Marketing

BRANDS/DIVISIONS/AFFILIATES:

Niceday
Foray
Ativa
Break Escapes
Worklife
Christopher Lowell

CONTACTS: *Note: Officers with more than one job title may be intentionally listed here more than once.*

Steve Odland, CEO
Mike Newman, CFO/Exec. VP
Daisy Vanderlinde, Exec. VP-Human Resources
Monica Luechtefeld, Exec. VP-IT
Elisa D. Garcia C., General Counsel/Corp. Sec./Exec. VP
Carl (Chuck) Rubin, Pres., North American Retail
Steven M. Schmidt, Pres., North American Bus. Solutions Div.
David Fannin, Exec. VP
Steve Odland, Chmn.
Charles E. Brown, Pres., Int'l Bus.
Monica Luechtefeld, Exec. VP-Supply Chain

Phone: 561-266-4800	**Fax:** 800-685-5010
Toll-Free: 800-463-3768	
Address: 2200 Old Germantown Rd., Delray Beach, FL 33445 US	

GROWTH PLANS/SPECIAL FEATURES:

Office Depot, Inc. is one of the largest retail office products businesses in the world by sales volume, with nearly 1,600 stores in 43 countries. Office Depot operates through three business segments: North American Retail Division, North American Business Solutions Division and International Division. The North American Retail Division sells an assortment of merchandise, including general office supplies, computer supplies, business machines and office furniture from national brands to its own private brands, which include Office Depot, Niceday, Foray, Ativa, Break Escapes, Worklife and Christopher Lowell. Most stores also contain a design, print and ship center offering graphic design, printing, reproduction, mailing, shipping and other services. Office Depot's North American Business Solutions Division provides office supply products and services directly to businesses through its delivery operations in the U.S. and Canada. The division sells branded and private brand products and services by means of a dedicated sales force, through catalogs and electronically through its Internet sites. The firm's International Division sells office products and services through direct mail catalogs, contract sales forces, Internet sites and retail stores, using a mix of company-owned operations; joint ventures; licensing and franchise agreements; alliances; and other arrangements. In March 2008, Office Depot was listed for the seventh consecutive year by the WBENC (Women's Business Enterprise National Council) as one of America's Top Corporations for Women's Business Enterprises and was also recognized by the National Association for Female Executives as a Top Company for Female Professionals for the fourth consecutive year. The firm had originally planned to open 150 new stores during 2008, but scaled that back to 75 new stores due to the slowing economy.

Office Depot offers its employees tuition reimbursement, employee discounts, an employee assistance program and matching gifts programs.

FINANCIALS: Sales and profits are in thousands of dollars—add 000 to get the full amount. 2007 Note: Financial information for 2007 was not available for all companies at press time.

2007 Sales: $15,527,537	2007 Profits: $395,615	**U.S. Stock Ticker:** ODP
2006 Sales: $15,010,781	2006 Profits: $503,471	**Int'l Ticker:**　**Int'l Exchange:**
2005 Sales: $14,278,944	2005 Profits: $273,792	Employees: 52,000
2004 Sales: $13,564,699	2004 Profits: $335,504	Fiscal Year Ends: 12/31
2003 Sales: $12,358,566	2003 Profits: $276,295	Parent Company:

SALARIES/BENEFITS:

Pension Plan:	ESOP Stock Plan:	Profit Sharing:	Top Exec. Salary: $1,000,000	Bonus: $2,220,840
Savings Plan: Y	Stock Purch. Plan: Y		Second Exec. Salary: $615,000	Bonus: $616,821

OTHER THOUGHTS:

Apparent Women Officers or Directors: 3
Hot Spot for Advancement for Women/Minorities: Y

LOCATIONS: ("Y" = Yes)

West:	Southwest:	Midwest:	Southeast:	Northeast:	International:
Y	Y	Y	Y	Y	Y

OIL STATES INTERNATIONAL INC
www.oilstatesintl.com

Industry Group Code: 213111 **Ranks within this company's industry group:** Sales: Profits:

Management:		Sales/Marketing:		Liberal Arts:		Information Systems:		Professionals:		Technical/Scientific:	
Mgmt. Trainees:	Y	Mktg. Professionals:	Y	Gen. Writing/Editing:		Info. Management:	Y	Finance/Accounting:	Y	Engineers, Elec.:	Y
Experienced Mgmt.:	Y	Retail Sales:		Technical Writing:		Software Dev.:	Y	Law:	Y	Engineers, Other:	
Int'l Business:	Y	Commercial/Industrial:	Y	Graphic Arts/Photog.:		Hardware Dev.:		HR/Other:	Y	Health/Lab:	
MBA Graduates:	Y	Sales Trainees:		Music:		Systems Integration:		Training:	Y	Scientists/Research:	
		Advertising Pros.:		Broadcasting:		Consulting/Other:		Health Care:		Petroleum/Chemicals:	Y
				Other:				Consulting:		Math/Other:	

TYPES OF BUSINESS:
Oil & Gas Drilling Support Services
Offshore Products
Well Site Services
Tubular Services
Drilling Services
Catering & Logistics Services
Construction Services
Equipment Rental

BRANDS/DIVISIONS/AFFILIATES:
Sooner, Inc.
HWC Energy Services, Inc.
PTI Group, Inc.
Phillips Casing & Tubing
Boots & Coots International Well Control, Inc.

CONTACTS: Note: Officers with more than one job title may be intentionally listed here more than once.
Cindy B. Taylor, CEO
Cindy B. Taylor, Pres.
Bradley J. Dodson, CFO/Treas./VP
Robert W. Hampton, Corp. Sec.
Christopher E. Cragg, Sr. VP-Oper.
Robert W. Hampton, Sr. VP-Acct.
Ron R. Green, CEO/Pres., PTI Group Inc.
Howard Hughes, VP-Offshore Products/Pres., Oil States Industries
Stephen A. Wells, Chmn.

Phone: 713-652-0582	Fax: 713-652-0499

Toll-Free:

Address: 3 Allen Ctr., 333 Clay St., Ste. 4620, Houston, TX 77002 US

GROWTH PLANS/SPECIAL FEATURES:
Oil States International, Inc. is a leading provider of specialty products and services to oil and gas drilling and production companies throughout the world. Areas of operation include the Gulf of Mexico, West Africa, the North Sea, Canada, South America and Southeast Asia as well as onshore U.S. It operates in three principal business segments. Its offshore products segment designs and manufactures products for the offshore energy industry, such as flexible bearings and connector products; subsea pipeline products; marine winches, mooring and lifting systems and rig equipment; and blowout prevention stack assembly, integration, testing and repair services. Oil States' tubular services segment offers tubular services and casing, premium tubing and line pipe, which are purchased from manufacturers and sold to oil and gas companies and drilling contractors. It has also developed an e-commerce portal for pricing, ordering and tracking tubular products, operating under Sooner, Inc. The firm's well site services segment provides worker services, drilling services, rental equipment, remote site accommodations, catering and logistics services and modular building construction services. Subsidiary HWC Energy Services, Inc. provides worldwide well control services, drilling services and rental equipment to the oil and gas industry; while subsidiary PTI Group, Inc. is a supplier of integrated housing, food, site management and logistics support services to remote sites. In August 2007, the company acquired the business of Schooner Petroleum Services, Inc., a provider of rental tools and services in Texas, Louisiana, Wyoming and Arkansas, for approximately $66.4 million. In February 2008, Oil States acquired an accommodations lodge in the oil sands area of Alberta, Canada for roughly $6.1 million and a waterfront facility on the ship channel in Houston, Texas for $22.5 million.

Employees of the firm receive medical, dental and vision plans; life and AD&D insurance; and a 529 college savings plan.

FINANCIALS: Sales and profits are in thousands of dollars—add 000 to get the full amount. 2007 Note: Financial information for 2007 was not available for all companies at press time.

2007 Sales: $2,088,235	2007 Profits: $203,372	**U.S. Stock Ticker:** OIS
2006 Sales: $1,923,357	2006 Profits: $197,634	**Int'l Ticker:** Int'l Exchange:
2005 Sales: $1,531,636	2005 Profits: $121,813	Employees: 5,236
2004 Sales: $971,012	2004 Profits: $59,362	Fiscal Year Ends: 12/31
2003 Sales: $723,681	2003 Profits: $44,432	Parent Company:

SALARIES/BENEFITS:
Pension Plan:	ESOP Stock Plan:	Profit Sharing:	Top Exec. Salary: $372,269	Bonus: $409,496
Savings Plan: Y	Stock Purch. Plan:		Second Exec. Salary: $351,500	Bonus: $351,500

OTHER THOUGHTS:
Apparent Women Officers or Directors: 1
Hot Spot for Advancement for Women/Minorities: Y

LOCATIONS: ("Y" = Yes)
West:	Southwest:	Midwest:	Southeast:	Northeast:	International:
	Y	Y	Y		Y

Note: Financial information, benefits and other data can change quickly and may vary from those stated here.

OLD DOMINION FREIGHT LINE INC

www.odfl.com

Industry Group Code: 484122 Ranks within this company's industry group: Sales: 2   Profits: 1

Management:		Sales/Marketing:		Liberal Arts:		Information Systems:		Professionals:		Technical/Scientific:	
Mgmt. Trainees:		Mktg. Professionals:		Gen. Writing/Editing:		Info. Management:	Y	Finance/Accounting:	Y	Engineers, Elec.:	
Experienced Mgmt.:	Y	Retail Sales:		Technical Writing:		Software Dev.:	Y	Law:	Y	Engineers, Other:	
Int'l Business:		Commercial/Industrial:	Y	Graphic Arts/Photog.:		Hardware Dev.:		HR/Other:	Y	Health/Lab:	
MBA Graduates:	Y	Sales Trainees:		Music:		Systems Integration:		Training:	Y	Scientists/Research:	
		Advertising Pros.:		Broadcasting:		Consulting/Other:		Health Care:		Petroleum/Chemicals:	
				Other:				Consulting:		Math/Other:	

TYPES OF BUSINESS:

Trucking
LTL Trucking
Freight Logistics

BRANDS/DIVISIONS/AFFILIATES:

OD Domestic
OD Expedited
OD Global
OD Technology

CONTACTS: *Note: Officers with more than one job title may be intentionally listed here more than once.*

David S. Congdon, CEO
John B. Yowell, COO/Exec. VP
David S. Congdon, Pres.
J. Wes Frye, CFO
Joel B. McCarty, Jr., General Counsel/Sr. VP/Corp. Sec.
J. Wes Frye, Sr. VP-Finance/Treas.
Earl E. Congdon, Chmn.

Phone: 336-889-5000	Fax: 336-822-5229
Toll-Free: 800-432-6335	
Address: 500 Old Dominion Way, Thomasville, NC 27360 US	

GROWTH PLANS/SPECIAL FEATURES:

Old Dominion Freight Line, Inc. is a less-than-truckload multi-regional motor carrier providing one- to five-day service among five regions in the U.S., and next-day and second-day service within these regions. It offers an expanding array of products and services through four branded product groups: OD-Domestic, OD-Expedited, OD-Global and OD-Technology. The company provides full-state coverage to 37 of the 47 states that it serves directly. Through marketing and carrier relationships, the firm also provides service to and from the remaining states, as well as international services around the globe. Old Dominion conducts operations though more than 180 service center locations, of which it owns over 85 and leases over 90. The company operates major breakbulk facilities in Atlanta, GA; Rialto, CA; Indianapolis, IN; Greensboro, NC; Harrisburg, PA; Memphis and Morristown, TN; and Dallas, TX. Additionally, the company uses some smaller service centers for limited breakbulk activity in order to serve next-day markets. The service centers are strategically located in five regions of the country to help minimize freight handling costs. Each of the firm's service centers is responsible of the pickup and delivery of freight for its service area. All inbound freight received by the service center in the evening or during the night is scheduled for local delivery the next business day, unless a customer requests a different delivery schedule. Old Dominion's linehaul dispatchers control the movement of freight among service centers through integrated freight movement systems. The company uses 28-foot trailers exclusively in its linehaul operations, which permits it to transport freight directly from its point of origin to destination. Additionally, the firm operates over 4,600 tractors. These are generally used in linehaul operations for roughly three to five years and are then transferred to pickup and delivery operations for the remainder of the assets' useful lives.

FINANCIALS: Sales and profits are in thousands of dollars—add 000 to get the full amount. 2007 Note: Financial information for 2007 was not available for all companies at press time.

2007 Sales: $1,401,542	2007 Profits: $71,832	**U.S. Stock Ticker: ODFL**
2006 Sales: $1,279,431	2006 Profits: $72,569	**Int'l Ticker:** Int'l Exchange:
2005 Sales: $1,061,403	2005 Profits: $53,475	Employees: 10,762
2004 Sales: $824,051	2004 Profits: $38,992	Fiscal Year Ends: 12/31
2003 Sales: $667,531	2003 Profits: $27,600	Parent Company:

SALARIES/BENEFITS:

Pension Plan:	ESOP Stock Plan:	Profit Sharing:	Top Exec. Salary: $439,740	Bonus: $2,258,402
Savings Plan:	Stock Purch. Plan:		Second Exec. Salary: $309,740	Bonus: $475,453

OTHER THOUGHTS:

Apparent Women Officers or Directors:
Hot Spot for Advancement for Women/Minorities:

LOCATIONS: ("Y" = Yes)

West:	Southwest:	Midwest:	Southeast:	Northeast:	International:
Y	Y	Y	Y	Y	

OMNICARE INC
www.omnicare.com

Industry Group Code: 446110A **Ranks within this company's industry group:** Sales: 1 Profits: 1

Management:		Sales/Marketing:		Liberal Arts:		Information Systems:		Professionals:		Technical/Scientific:	
Mgmt. Trainees:	Y	Mktg. Professionals:	Y	Gen. Writing/Editing:	Y	Info. Management:	Y	Finance/Accounting:	Y	Engineers, Elec.:	
Experienced Mgmt.:	Y	Retail Sales:		Technical Writing:	Y	Software Dev.:	Y	Law:	Y	Engineers, Other:	Y
Int'l Business:	Y	Commercial/Industrial:	Y	Graphic Arts/Photog.:		Hardware Dev.:		HR/Other:	Y	Health/Lab:	
MBA Graduates:	Y	Sales Trainees:	Y	Music:		Systems Integration:		Training:	Y	Scientists/Research:	
		Advertising Pros.:	Y	Broadcasting:		Consulting/Other:		Health Care:	Y	Petroleum/Chemicals:	
				Other:				Consulting:		Math/Other:	

TYPES OF BUSINESS:

Specialty Pharmacies
Infusion Therapy
Consulting Services
Pharmaceutical Research
Medical Records Services
Billing Services
Pharmaceutical Distribution
Software Information Systems

BRANDS/DIVISIONS/AFFILIATES:

Omnicare Clinical Research
Advanced Care Scripts Inc.

CONTACTS: Note: Officers with more than one job title may be intentionally listed here more than once.

Joel F. Gemunder, CEO
Patrick E. Keefe, COO/Exec. VP
Joel F. Gemunder, Pres.
David W. Froesel, Jr., CFO/Sr. VP
Stephen S. Brown, Sr. VP/CIO
Mark G. Kobasuk, General Counsel/VP
Robert E. Dries, VP & Group Exec.-Oper. Finance Group
Tracy Finn, VP-Strategic Planning & Dev.
Paul W. Baldwin, VP-Public Affairs
Bradley S. Abbott, Controller/VP/Group Exec.-Corp. Financial Svcs.
Cheryl D. Hodges, Sr. VP/Corp. Sec.
Donald E. Amorosi, VP-Trade Rel.
Dale B. Evans, VP/CEO-Omnicare Clinical Research
W. Gary Erwin, Pres., Omnicare Senior Health Outcomes
John T. Crotty, Chmn.
Daniel J. Maloney, VP-Purchasing

Phone: 859-392-3300	Fax:
Toll-Free:	
Address: 100 E. RiverCenter Blvd., Ste. 1600, Covington, KY 41011 US	

GROWTH PLANS/SPECIAL FEATURES:

Omnicare, Inc. is a provider of geriatric pharmaceuticals and related geriatric pharmacy services to long-term care institutions such as skilled nursing facilities, assisted living facilities and retirement centers, as well as hospitals and other institutional health care facilities. The firm's main business segment, pharmacy services, provides pharmaceutical distribution, related pharmacy consulting, data management services and medical supplies to long-term care facilities. Services include purchasing, repackaging and dispensing pharmaceuticals, computerized medical record keeping and third-party billing for residents in the institutions. Omnicare also provides consultant pharmacist services, including evaluating monthly patient drug therapy, monitoring the drug distribution system within the nursing facility, assisting in compliance with state and federal regulations and providing proprietary clinical and health management programs. In addition, Omnicare's pharmacy services segment provides ancillary services, such as providing medications and nutrition for intravenous administration , or infusion therapy services, and furnishing respiratory therapy services, medical supplies and equipment, clinical care planning, financial software information systems, pharmaceutical informatics services, mail order pharmacy and other pharmacy distribution and patient assistance services for specialty pharmaceuticals. Another business segment, contract research organization services (CRO) is a leading international provider of comprehensive product development and research services to client companies in the pharmaceutical, biotechnology, medical device and diagnostics industries. Subsidiary Omnicare Clinical Research has expertise in various fields including cardiovascular, anti-infectives, oncology, central nervous system and geriatrics areas. During 2007, the pharmacy services segment accounted for 97% of total net sales while CRO services accounted for 3%. In July 2008, Omnicare purchased Advanced Care Scripts Inc., a specialty pharmacy that dispenses oral and injectable medications. In August 2008, Omnicare acquired four pharmacy outlets in Edinburgh, Scotland.

FINANCIALS: Sales and profits are in thousands of dollars—add 000 to get the full amount. 2007 Note: Financial information for 2007 was not available for all companies at press time.

2007 Sales: $6,220,010	2007 Profits: $114,056	**U.S. Stock Ticker:** OCR
2006 Sales: $6,492,993	2006 Profits: $183,572	**Int'l Ticker:** Int'l Exchange:
2005 Sales: $5,292,782	2005 Profits: $226,491	Employees: 17,100
2004 Sales: $4,119,891	2004 Profits: $236,011	Fiscal Year Ends: 12/31
2003 Sales: $3,499,174	2003 Profits: $194,368	Parent Company:

SALARIES/BENEFITS:

Pension Plan: Y	ESOP Stock Plan:	Profit Sharing:	Top Exec. Salary: $1,600,000	Bonus: $
Savings Plan: Y	Stock Purch. Plan:		Second Exec. Salary: $472,000	Bonus: $

OTHER THOUGHTS:

Apparent Women Officers or Directors: 5
Hot Spot for Advancement for Women/Minorities: Y

LOCATIONS: ("Y" = Yes)

West:	Southwest:	Midwest:	Southeast:	Northeast:	International:
Y	Y	Y	Y	Y	Y

Note: Financial information, benefits and other data can change quickly and may vary from those stated here.

OMNICOM GROUP INC

www.omnicomgroup.com

Industry Group Code: 541810 Ranks within this company's industry group: Sales: 1 Profits: 1

Management:		Sales/Marketing:		Liberal Arts:		Information Systems:		Professionals:		Technical/Scientific:	
Mgmt. Trainees:	Y	Mktg. Professionals:	Y	Gen. Writing/Editing:		Info. Management:	Y	Finance/Accounting:	Y	Engineers, Elec.:	
Experienced Mgmt.:	Y	Retail Sales:		Technical Writing:		Software Dev.:	Y	Law:	Y	Engineers, Other:	
Int'l Business:	Y	Commercial/Industrial:	Y	Graphic Arts/Photog.:	Y	Hardware Dev.:		HR/Other:	Y	Health/Lab:	
MBA Graduates:	Y	Sales Trainees:		Music:		Systems Integration:		Training:	Y	Scientists/Research:	
		Advertising Pros.:	Y	Broadcasting:		Consulting/Other:		Health Care:		Petroleum/Chemicals:	
				Other:				Consulting:	Y	Math/Other:	

TYPES OF BUSINESS:

Advertising Services
Public Relations
Market Research
Marketing & Brand Consulting
Interactive & Search Engine Marketing
Media Planning & Buying
Health Care Communications
Printing

BRANDS/DIVISIONS/AFFILIATES:

BBDO Worldwide Network
DDB Worldwide
TBWA Worldwide
Arnell Group
Goodby, Silverstein & Partners
OMD Worldwide
Ketchum
Porter Novelli

CONTACTS: *Note: Officers with more than one job title may be intentionally listed here more than once.*

John D. Wren, CEO
John D. Wren, Pres.
Randall J. Weisenburger, CFO/Exec. VP
Michael J. O'Brien, General Counsel/Sr. VP/Corp. Sec.
Philip J. Angelastro, Sr. VP-Finance/Controller
Asit Mehra, Exec. VP
Bruce Redditt, Exec. VP
Janet Riccio, Exec. VP
Cynder Niemela, Sr. VP/Chief Talent Officer-Creative Channel Svcs.
Bruce Crawford, Chmn.
Michael Birkin, Chmn./CEO-Asia Pacific

Phone: 212-415-3600	Fax: 212-415-3530
Toll-Free:	
Address: 437 Madison Ave., New York, NY 10022 US	

GROWTH PLANS/SPECIAL FEATURES:

Omnicom Group, Inc. is a holding company that, through its subsidiaries, is one of the largest advertising, marketing and corporate communications companies in the world. The firm owns more than 160 subsidiary agencies that operate in all major markets worldwide. Its agencies provide an extensive range of services, mainly focusing on four fundamental disciplines, including traditional media advertising, customer relationship management, public relations and specialty communications. The company's holdings are managed by the Diversified Agency Services (DAS) division. Omnicom's traditional media advertising is based in three areas: Global advertising brands, such as BBDO Worldwide, DDB Worldwide and TBWA Worldwide; national advertising agencies, including Arnell Group, Element 79 Partners, GSD&M, Martin/Williams, Merkley + Partners, Zimmerman Advertising and Goodby, Silverstein & Parners; and media services, which has two dull service media companies, OMD Worldwide and PHD Network, and several media specialist companies. Customer relationship management includes three of the top 10 promotional marketing agencies, and the segment focuses on marketing for sports and events, promotions, non-profit organizations and events, the entertainment industry, as well as field marketing and branding, consultants and design. Within the public relations segment, Omnicom's Diversified Agency Services includes Fleishman-Hillard, Ketchum and Porter Novelli, all of which are within the top seven public relationship firms in the world. The company also has a number of specialist agencies within the division. Specialty communications contains healthcare communications companies, as well as recruitment communications, multicultural marketing and financial and corporate advertising. Other group activities of note include experiential marketing, instore design, mobile marketing, package design, custom printing, reputation consulting and search engine marketing.

FINANCIALS: Sales and profits are in thousands of dollars—add 000 to get the full amount. 2007 Note: Financial information for 2007 was not available for all companies at press time.

2007 Sales: $12,700,000	2007 Profits: $975,700	**U.S. Stock Ticker: OMC**
2006 Sales: $11,376,900	2006 Profits: $864,000	**Int'l Ticker:** Int'l Exchange:
2005 Sales: $10,481,100	2005 Profits: $790,700	Employees: 66,000
2004 Sales: $9,747,200	2004 Profits: $723,500	Fiscal Year Ends: 12/31
2003 Sales: $8,621,404	2003 Profits: $675,883	Parent Company:

SALARIES/BENEFITS:

Pension Plan:	ESOP Stock Plan:	Profit Sharing:	Top Exec. Salary: $1,000,000	Bonus: $7,000,000
Savings Plan:	Stock Purch. Plan:		Second Exec. Salary: $975,000	Bonus: $5,580,884

OTHER THOUGHTS:

Apparent Women Officers or Directors: 3
Hot Spot for Advancement for Women/Minorities: Y

LOCATIONS: ("Y" = Yes)

West:	Southwest:	Midwest:	Southeast:	Northeast:	International:
Y	Y	Y	Y	Y	Y

Note: Financial information, benefits and other data can change quickly and may vary from those stated here.

ONEOK INC

www.oneok.com

Industry Group Code: 221000B **Ranks within this company's industry group:** Sales: 1 Profits: 1

Management:		Sales/Marketing:		Liberal Arts:		Information Systems:		Professionals:		Technical/Scientific:	
Mgmt. Trainees:	Y	Mktg. Professionals:	Y	Gen. Writing/Editing:		Info. Management:	Y	Finance/Accounting:	Y	Engineers, Elec.:	Y
Experienced Mgmt.:	Y	Retail Sales:		Technical Writing:		Software Dev.:		Law:	Y	Engineers, Other:	Y
Int'l Business:		Commercial/Industrial:		Graphic Arts/Photog.:		Hardware Dev.:		HR/Other:	Y	Health/Lab:	
MBA Graduates:	Y	Sales Trainees:		Music:		Systems Integration:		Training:	Y	Scientists/Research:	
		Advertising Pros.:		Broadcasting:		Consulting/Other:		Health Care:		Petroleum/Chemicals:	Y
				Other:				Consulting:		Math/Other:	

TYPES OF BUSINESS:

Utilities-Natural Gas
Wholesale Gas Marketing & Trading
Oil & Natural Gas Production
Gas Transportation & Storage
Natural Gas Liquids

BRANDS/DIVISIONS/AFFILIATES:

ONEOK Partners, L.P.

CONTACTS: Note: Officers with more than one job title may be intentionally listed here more than once.

John W. Gibson, CEO
James C. Kneale, COO
James C. Kneale, Pres.
Curtis L. Dinan, CFO/Sr. VP/Treas.
Steve Guy, Sr. VP-Tech. Svcs.
Daniel Walker, VP-Eng.
David Roth, Sr. VP-Admin. Svcs.
John R. Barker, General Counsel/Sr. VP
Daniel Walker, VP-Oper.
Dan Harrison, VP-Public Affairs
Dan Harrison, VP-Investor Rel.
Caron A. Lawhorn, Chief Acct. Officer
Pierce Norton, Exec. VP-Natural Gas
Terry Spencer, Exec. VP-Natural Gas Liquids
Eric Grimshaw, VP/Corp. Sec.
Samuel Combs, III, Pres., ONEOK Distribution Companies
David L. Kyle, Chmn.

Phone: 918-588-7000	Fax: 918-588-7273
Toll-Free:	
Address: 100 W. 5th St., P.O. Box 871, Tulsa, OK 74103 US	

GROWTH PLANS/SPECIAL FEATURES:

ONEOK, Inc. purchases, transports, stores and distributes natural gas in the south central areas of the U.S. The firm's largest distribution markets are Oklahoma City and Tulsa, Oklahoma; Kansas City, Wichita and Topeka, Kansas; and Austin and El Paso, Texas. Its energy services operation is engaged in wholesale and retail natural gas and trading activities and provides services to customers in the U.S. and Canada. ONEOK is the sole general partner and owns 45.7% of ONEOK Partners, L.P., which is engaged in gathering, processing, storing and transporting natural gas in the U.S. and owns natural gas liquids systems that connect much of the natural gas and NGL supply in the mid-continent and Gulf Coast regions with market centers in Conway, Kansas; Mont Belvieu, Texas; and Chicago, Illinois. ONEOK's distribution segment provides natural gas distribution services to over two million customers in Oklahoma, Kansas and Texas through Oklahoma Natural Gas, Kansas Gas Service and Texas Gas Service, respectively. It serves residential, commercial, industrial and transportation customers in all three states. In addition, the firm's distribution companies in Oklahoma and Kansas serve wholesale customers and in Texas its distribution companies serve public authority customers, such as cities, governmental agencies and schools. ONEOK's energy services segment delivers physical natural gas products and risk management services through its network of contracted transportation and storage capacity and natural gas supply. These services include meeting its customers' baseload, swing and peaking natural gas commodity requirements on a year-round basis. In July 2007, ONEOK announced its acquisition of an interstate NGL and refined petroleum products pipeline system from Kinder Morgan Energy Partners, L.P. for approximately $300 million.

FINANCIALS: Sales and profits are in thousands of dollars—add 000 to get the full amount. 2007 Note: Financial information for 2007 was not available for all companies at press time.

2007 Sales: $13,488,027	2007 Profits: $304,921	**U.S. Stock Ticker: OKE**	
2006 Sales: $11,913,529	2006 Profits: $306,312	**Int'l Ticker:** Int'l Exchange:	
2005 Sales: $12,676,230	2005 Profits: $546,545	Employees: 4,536	
2004 Sales: $5,785,528	2004 Profits: $242,178	Fiscal Year Ends: 12/31	
2003 Sales: $2,870,466	2003 Profits: $112,488	Parent Company:	

SALARIES/BENEFITS:

Pension Plan:	ESOP Stock Plan:	Profit Sharing:	Top Exec. Salary: $850,000	Bonus: $1,912,500
Savings Plan:	Stock Purch. Plan:		Second Exec. Salary: $435,000	Bonus: $655,000

OTHER THOUGHTS:

Apparent Women Officers or Directors: 4
Hot Spot for Advancement for Women/Minorities: Y

LOCATIONS: ("Y" = Yes)

West:	Southwest:	Midwest:	Southeast:	Northeast:	International:
	Y	Y			

Note: Financial information, benefits and other data can change quickly and may vary from those stated here.

ORACLE CORP

www.oracle.com

Industry Group Code: 511207 Ranks within this company's industry group: Sales: 1   Profits: 1

Management:		Sales/Marketing:		Liberal Arts:		Information Systems:		Professionals:		Technical/Scientific:	
Mgmt. Trainees:	Y	Mktg. Professionals:	Y	Gen. Writing/Editing:	Y	Info. Management:	Y	Finance/Accounting:	Y	Engineers, Elec.:	Y
Experienced Mgmt.:	Y	Retail Sales:		Technical Writing:	Y	Software Dev.:	Y	Law:	Y	Engineers, Other:	
Int'l Business:	Y	Commercial/Industrial:	Y	Graphic Arts/Photog.:	Y	Hardware Dev.:		HR/Other:	Y	Health/Lab:	
MBA Graduates:	Y	Sales Trainees:		Music:		Systems Integration:		Training:	Y	Scientists/Research:	Y
		Advertising Pros.:	Y	Broadcasting:		Consulting/Other:		Health Care:		Petroleum/Chemicals:	
				Other:				Consulting:		Math/Other:	

TYPES OF BUSINESS:

Computer Software-Database Management
e-Business Applications Software
Internet-Based Software
Consulting Services
Human Resources Management Software
CRM Software
Middleware

BRANDS/DIVISIONS/AFFILIATES:

BEA Systems Inc
Bridgestream Inc
Agile Software Corp
Portal Software Inc
Sunopsis
SPL World Group
MetaSolv Software
Stellant, Inc.

CONTACTS: *Note: Officers with more than one job title may be intentionally listed here more than once.*

Larry Ellison, CEO
Charles Phillips, Co-Pres.
Safra Catz, CFO/Co-Pres.
Judith Sim, Sr. VP/Chief Mktg. Officer
Dorian Daley, General Counsel/Sr. VP/Sec.
Keith G. Block, Exec. VP-North America
Mary Ann Davidson, Chief Security Officer
Luiz Meisler, Sr. VP-Latin America
Charles Rozwat, Exec. VP-Oracle Server Technologies
Jeffrey O. Henley, Chmn.
Masaaki Shintaku, Pres./CEO-Japan

Phone: 650-506-7000	Fax: 650-506-7200
Toll-Free: 800-672-2531	
Address: 500 Oracle Pkwy., Redwood Shores, CA 94065 US	

GROWTH PLANS/SPECIAL FEATURES:

Oracle Corporation is one of the largest enterprise software companies in the world. The firm markets its software directly to corporations rather than dealing in the consumer market. Oracle's products can be categorized into two broad areas: software (representing 79% of revenue) and services. The company's core software business segment is based upon its prepackaged enterprise data management software and Internet applications including Oracle Database, Oracle Fusion Middleware, Oracle Enterprise Manager, Oracle Collaboration Suite, Oracle Developer Suite and Oracle E-Business Suite. Oracle's services business is comprised of Oracle Consulting and Oracle On Demand. Oracle Consulting specializes in the design, implementation, deployment, upgrade and migration of its database technology and applications software. Oracle On Demand offers distributed application services including E-Business Suite On Demand, Technology On Demand and Collaboration Suite On Demand. In early 2007, the firm unveiled Oracle Retail Promotion Planning and Optimization, a data mining application for retail analysis, forecasting and planning. In addition, the company launched Oracle SQL Developer, an upgrade to Oracle's free database development and debugging application, as well as Oracle Management Pack for Linux. In March 2007, Oracle agreed to acquire Hyperion Solutions Corp. for roughly $3.3 billion. In April 2007, the firm released Oracle Manufacturing Execution System for Discrete Manufacturing (Oracle MES for Discrete Manufacturing), a new application that lets manufacturers set up Oracle Applications on the shop floor. In September 2007, the company acquired enterprise software manufacturer Bridgestream, Inc. Oracle's acquisition strategy continued in December 2007 with the purchase of software vendor Moniforce and the $8.3 billion deal for enterprise infrastructure software firm BEA Systems, Inc. in early 2008.

FINANCIALS: Sales and profits are in thousands of dollars—add 000 to get the full amount. 2007 Note: Financial information for 2007 was not available for all companies at press time.

2007 Sales: $17,996,000	2007 Profits: $4,274,000	U.S. Stock Ticker: ORCL
2006 Sales: $14,380,000	2006 Profits: $3,381,000	Int'l Ticker: Int'l Exchange:
2005 Sales: $11,799,000	2005 Profits: $2,886,000	Employees: 74,674
2004 Sales: $10,156,000	2004 Profits: $2,681,000	Fiscal Year Ends: 5/31
2003 Sales: $9,475,000	2003 Profits: $2,307,000	Parent Company:

SALARIES/BENEFITS:

Pension Plan: Y	ESOP Stock Plan:	Profit Sharing:	Top Exec. Salary: $1,000,000	Bonus: $8,369,000
Savings Plan: Y	Stock Purch. Plan:		Second Exec. Salary: $800,000	Bonus: $4,882,000

OTHER THOUGHTS:

Apparent Women Officers or Directors: 4
Hot Spot for Advancement for Women/Minorities: Y

LOCATIONS: ("Y" = Yes)

West:	Southwest:	Midwest:	Southeast:	Northeast:	International:
Y	Y	Y	Y	Y	Y

O'REILLY AUTOMOTIVE INC

www.oreillyauto.com

Industry Group Code: 441310 **Ranks within this company's industry group:** Sales: 3 Profits: 3

Management:		Sales/Marketing:		Liberal Arts:		Information Systems:		Professionals:		Technical/Scientific:	
Mgmt. Trainees:	Y	Mktg. Professionals:	Y	Gen. Writing/Editing:	Y	Info. Management:	Y	Finance/Accounting:	Y	Engineers, Elec.:	
Experienced Mgmt.:	Y	Retail Sales:	Y	Technical Writing:		Software Dev.:		Law:	Y	Engineers, Other:	
Int'l Business:		Commercial/Industrial:	Y	Graphic Arts/Photog.:	Y	Hardware Dev.:		HR/Other:	Y	Health/Lab:	
MBA Graduates:	Y	Sales Trainees:	Y	Music:		Systems Integration:		Training:	Y	Scientists/Research:	
		Advertising Pros.:	Y	Broadcasting:		Consulting/Other:		Health Care:		Petroleum/Chemicals:	
				Other:				Consulting:		Math/Other:	

TYPES OF BUSINESS:

Auto Parts, Retail
Tools
Auto Accessories

BRANDS/DIVISIONS/AFFILIATES:

O'Reilly Auto Parts
SuperStart
BrakeBest
Ultima
Master-Pro
Omnispark
Ozark Automotive Distributors, Inc.

CONTACTS: Note: Officers with more than one job title may be intentionally listed here more than once.

Greg L. Henslee, CEO/Co-Pres.
Ted F. Wise, COO
Ted F. Wise, Co-Pres.
Tom McFall, CFO/Exec. VP-Finance
Tony Bartholomew, VP-Sales
Phillip Thompson, VP-Human Resources
Mike Williams, VP-Advanced Tech.
Steve Jasinski, VP-Info. Systems
Mike Swearengin, Sr. VP-Merch.
Phyllis Evans, VP-Store Admin.
Tricia Headley, Corp. Sec./VP
Jeff Shaw, Sr. VP-Store Sales & Oper.
Tom McFall, Exec. VP-Finance
Doug Ruble, VP-Advertising & Mktg.
Alan Fears, VP-Store Acquisitions & Expansion
Greg Johnson, Sr. VP-Dist. Oper.
Barry Sabor, VP-Loss Prevention
David E. O'Reilly, Chmn.
Randy Johnson, VP-Store Inventories

Phone: 417-862-2674	Fax: 417-863-2242
Toll-Free:	
Address: 233 S. Patterson Ave., Springfield, MO 65802 US	

GROWTH PLANS/SPECIAL FEATURES:

O'Reilly Automotive, Inc., founded in 1957, is one of the largest specialty retailers of automotive aftermarket parts, tools, supplies, equipment and accessories in the U.S., selling products to both do-it-yourself customers and professional installers. This dual-market strategy allows the firm to target a larger customer base, operate profitably in large and small markets and provide superior customer service to do-it-yourself (DIY) customers. The company operates 1,830 stores in 26 states across the U.S. Stores carry an extensive product line consisting of new and remanufactured automotive hard parts such as chassis parts and engine parts; maintenance items, such as oil, antifreeze, fluids, engine additives and appearance products; accessories, such as floor mats and seat covers; and a complete line of auto body paint and related materials, automotive tools and professional service equipment. Store merchandise generally consists of nationally recognized, well-advertised, name-brand products such as AC Delco, Moog, Wagner, Gates Rubber, Federal Mogul, Monroe, Prestone, Quaker State, Pennzoil, Castrol, Valvoline, STP, BWD, Cardone, Wix, Armor All and Turtle Wax. In addition to name-brand products, stores carry a wide variety of high-quality private-label products under the O'Reilly Auto Parts, SuperStart, BrakeBest, Ultima, Master-Pro and Omnispark name-brands. In 2007, O'Reilly derived approximately 52% of sale from DIY customers and 48% from professional installer customers. O'Reilly operates 14 distribution centers, each equipped with highly automated conveyor systems that expedite the movement of its products to loading areas for shipment to individual stores on a nightly basis. In April 2008, the firm agreed to acquire CSK Auto Corporation for approximately $1 billion.

O'Reilly offers its employees a benefits package that includes medical, dental, vision and pharmacy insurance, purchase discounts, a credit union membership and an employee assistance program.

FINANCIALS: Sales and profits are in thousands of dollars—add 000 to get the full amount. 2007 Note: Financial information for 2007 was not available for all companies at press time.

2007 Sales: $2,522,319	2007 Profits: $193,988	**U.S. Stock Ticker:** ORLY
2006 Sales: $2,283,222	2006 Profits: $178,085	**Int'l Ticker:** Int'l Exchange:
2005 Sales: $2,045,318	2005 Profits: $164,266	Employees: 21,920
2004 Sales: $1,721,241	2004 Profits: $139,566	Fiscal Year Ends: 12/31
2003 Sales: $1,511,816	2003 Profits: $100,087	Parent Company:

SALARIES/BENEFITS:

Pension Plan:	ESOP Stock Plan:	Profit Sharing: Y	Top Exec. Salary: $649,120	Bonus: $381,875
Savings Plan: Y	Stock Purch. Plan: Y		Second Exec. Salary: $525,579	Bonus: $249,100

OTHER THOUGHTS:

Apparent Women Officers or Directors: 3
Hot Spot for Advancement for Women/Minorities: Y

LOCATIONS: ("Y" = Yes)

West:	Southwest:	Midwest:	Southeast:	Northeast:	International:
Y	Y	Y	Y	Y	

OSHKOSH CORPORATION   www.oshkoshcorporation.com

Industry Group Code: 336120 Ranks within this company's industry group: Sales: 1 Profits: 1

Management:		Sales/Marketing:		Liberal Arts:		Information Systems:		Professionals:		Technical/Scientific:	
Mgmt. Trainees:	Y	Mktg. Professionals:	Y	Gen. Writing/Editing:		Info. Management:	Y	Finance/Accounting:	Y	Engineers, Elec.:	Y
Experienced Mgmt.:	Y	Retail Sales:		Technical Writing:	Y	Software Dev.:		Law:	Y	Engineers, Other:	Y
Int'l Business:	Y	Commercial/Industrial:	Y	Graphic Arts/Photog.:	Y	Hardware Dev.:		HR/Other:	Y	Health/Lab:	
MBA Graduates:	Y	Sales Trainees:		Music:		Systems Integration:		Training:	Y	Scientists/Research:	
		Advertising Pros.:		Broadcasting:		Consulting/Other:		Health Care:		Petroleum/Chemicals:	
				Other:				Consulting:		Math/Other:	

TYPES OF BUSINESS:
Fire & Emergency Vehicles
Military Trucks
Truck Bodies
Specialty Trucks
Cement Mixers
Refuse Trucks

BRANDS/DIVISIONS/AFFILIATES:
Oshkosh
Pierce
McNeilus
Medtec
Geesink
Norba
Jerr-Dan
Oshkosh Truck Corporation

CONTACTS: Note: Officers with more than one job title may be intentionally listed here more than once.
Robert G. Bohn, CEO
Charles L. Szews, COO/Pres.
David M. Sagehorn, CFO/Exec. VP
Ann Stawski, VP-Mktg. Comm.
Michael K. Rohrkaste, VP-Human Resources
Michael Guzowski, VP-IT
Donald H. Verhoff, Exec. VP-Tech.
Wayne P. MacDonald, Sr. VP-Eng., Access Equipment Div.
Matthew J. Zolnowski, Chief Admin. Officer/Exec. VP
Bryan J. Blankfield, General Counsel/Exec. VP/Sec.
Joseph (Jay) H. Kimmitt, Exec. VP-Gov't Oper.
Michael K. Rohrkaste, VP-Bus. Dev.
Joseph (Jay) H. Kimmitt, Exec. VP-Industry Rel.
Patrick N. Davidson, VP-Investor Rel.
Thomas J. Polnaszek, Sr. VP-Finance/Controller
Michael J. Wuest, Exec. VP/Pres., Commercial
Kirsten Skyba, VP-Global Mktg., JLG Industries, Inc.
W. John Stoddart, Exec. VP/Pres., Defense
Robert G. Bohn, Chmn.
Desmond Soh, Pres., Asian Oper.
Gregory L. Fredericksen, Chief Procurement Officer/Sr. VP

Phone: 920-235-9150	Fax:
Toll-Free:	
Address: 2307 Oregon St., Oshkosh, WI 54902 US	

GROWTH PLANS/SPECIAL FEATURES:
Oshkosh Corporation is a leading designer, manufacturer and marketer of a broad range of specialty vehicles and vehicle bodies. The company operates in four segments: Access equipment, defense, fire and emergency and commercial. The access equipment segment manufactures aerial work platforms and telehandlers used in a wide variety of construction, industrial, institutional and general maintenance applications to position workers and materials at elevated heights. Access equipment customers include equipment rental companies, construction contractors, manufacturing companies, home improvement centers and the U.S. military. The defense segment supplies severe-duty, heavy-payload tactical trucks to the U.S. Department of Defense (DoD). The fire and emergency segment manufactures commercial and custom firefighting vehicles and equipment, aircraft rescue and firefighting (ARFF) vehicles, snow removal vehicles, ambulances, wreckers, carriers and other emergency vehicles primarily sold to fire departments, airports, other governmental units and towing companies in the U.S. and abroad. It also sells mobile medical trailers sold to hospitals and third party medical service providers in the U.S. and Europe and broadcast vehicles sold to broadcasters and TV stations in North America and abroad. The commercial segment manufactures rear- and front-discharge concrete mixers, refuse collection vehicles, mobile and stationary compactors and waste transfer units, portable and stationary concrete batch plants and vehicle components. The company's brands include Oshkosh, Pierce, McNeilus, Medtec, Jerr-Dan, BAI, London, Geesink, Norba, Frontline and CON-E-CO. In February 2008, the company changed its name from Oshkosh Truck Corporation to Oshkosh Corporation. In March 2008, Oshkosh opened its third office in China.

FINANCIALS: Sales and profits are in thousands of dollars—add 000 to get the full amount. 2007 Note: Financial information for 2007 was not available for all companies at press time.

2007 Sales: $6,307,300	2007 Profits: $268,100	U.S. Stock Ticker: OSK
2006 Sales: $3,427,388	2006 Profits: $205,529	Int'l Ticker: Int'l Exchange:
2005 Sales: $2,959,900	2005 Profits: $160,205	Employees: 14,200
2004 Sales: $2,262,305	2004 Profits: $112,806	Fiscal Year Ends: 9/30
2003 Sales: $1,926,000	2003 Profits: $75,600	Parent Company:

SALARIES/BENEFITS:

Pension Plan: Y	ESOP Stock Plan:	Profit Sharing:	Top Exec. Salary: $1,070,000	Bonus: $1,526,034
Savings Plan: Y	Stock Purch. Plan: Y		Second Exec. Salary: $518,950	Bonus: $444,117

OTHER THOUGHTS:
Apparent Women Officers or Directors: 4
Hot Spot for Advancement for Women/Minorities: Y

LOCATIONS: ("Y" = Yes)

West:	Southwest:	Midwest:	Southeast:	Northeast:	International:
Y		Y	Y	Y	Y

Note: Financial information, benefits and other data can change quickly and may vary from those stated here.

OSI RESTAURANT PARTNERS INC
www.osirestaurantpartners.com
Industry Group Code: 722110 Ranks within this company's industry group: Sales: 5 Profits: 5

Management:		Sales/Marketing:		Liberal Arts:		Information Systems:		Professionals:		Technical/Scientific:	
Mgmt. Trainees:	Y	Mktg. Professionals:	Y	Gen. Writing/Editing:		Info. Management:	Y	Finance/Accounting:	Y	Engineers, Elec.:	
Experienced Mgmt.:	Y	Retail Sales:		Technical Writing:		Software Dev.:	Y	Law:	Y	Engineers, Other:	
Int'l Business:	Y	Commercial/Industrial:		Graphic Arts/Photog.:		Hardware Dev.:		HR/Other:	Y	Health/Lab:	
MBA Graduates:	Y	Sales Trainees:		Music:		Systems Integration:		Training:	Y	Scientists/Research:	
		Advertising Pros.:	Y	Broadcasting:		Consulting/Other:		Health Care:		Petroleum/Chemicals:	
				Other:	Y			Consulting:		Math/Other:	

TYPES OF BUSINESS:
Restaurants
Catering
Event Hosting

BRANDS/DIVISIONS/AFFILIATES:
Bain Capital LLC
Carrabba's Italian Grill
Fleming's Prime Steakhouse
Cheeseburger in Paradise
Roy's
Lee Roy Selmon's
Bonefish Grill
Blue Coral Seafood & Spirits

CONTACTS: Note: Officers with more than one job title may be intentionally listed here more than once.
A. William Allen, III, CEO
Paul E. Avery, COO
Dirk A. Montgomery, CFO/Sr. VP
Lindon Richardson, Sr. VP-Equipment & Design
Steven C. Stanley, Sr. VP-Construction
Joseph J. Kadow, Chief Corp. & Legal Affairs Officer/Exec. VP/Sec.
Richard L. Renninger, Chief Dev. Officer
Lisa Hathcoat, Mgr.-Investor Rel.
Jeff Smith, Pres., Outback Steakhouse
Steven T. Shlemon, Pres., Carrabba's Italian Grill
John W. Cooper, Pres., Bonefish Grill
C.H. (Skip) Fox, Pres., Blue Coral Seafood & Spirits
Chris T. Sullivan, Chmn.
Michael W. Coble, Pres., Outback Int'l
Irene Wenzel, Sr. VP-Purchasing

Phone: 813-282-1225	Fax:
Toll-Free:	
Address: 2202 N. Westshore Blvd., 5th Fl., Tampa, FL 33607 US	

GROWTH PLANS/SPECIAL FEATURES:
OSI Restaurant Partners, Inc. (OSI), formerly Outback Steakhouse, Inc., owns and operates over 1,400 casual dining restaurants under the names Outback Steakhouse, Carrabba's Italian Grill, Fleming's Prime Steakhouse, Bonefish Grill, Roy's, Lee Roy Selmon's, Cheeseburger in Paradise and Blue Coral Seafood and Spirits. The corporation owns and operates the majority of its restaurants. Outback Steakhouse restaurants have an Australian-styled atmosphere that emphasizes quality food in large portions. Carrabba's restaurants have a small, focused menu and a casual, traditional Italian atmosphere. Bonefish Grill is a mid-scale seafood restaurant emphasizing hand-cut fish prepared over a wood-burning grill with original sauces. Fleming's has an upscale contemporary menu, exhibition-style kitchen and an extensive wine list. Cheeseburger in Paradise has Key West style architecture, a Tiki bar and its famous gourmet cheeseburger. Roy's also features an exhibition kitchen and serves primarily Hawaiian-influenced cuisine. Lee Roy Selmon's provides Southern comfort cooking and warm hospitality. Blue Coral Seafood features a modern take on fresh seafood and includes an extensive vodka bar. In all of the restaurants, kitchens are uncommonly large and designed for rapid production of a wide variety of food. Servers never cover more than three tables at once, and most restaurants are only open for dinner. In June 2007, OSI was acquired by an investor group including Bain Capital LLC and Catterton Partners.

OSI offers its employees a 401(k) plan; adoption assistance; a flexible spending account; an employee assistance program; and medical, dental and prescription coverage.

FINANCIALS: Sales and profits are in thousands of dollars—add 000 to get the full amount. 2007 Note: Financial information for 2007 was not available for all companies at press time.

2007 Sales: $	2007 Profits: $	**U.S. Stock Ticker: Private**
2006 Sales: $3,940,959	2006 Profits: $100,160	**Int'l Ticker:** Int'l Exchange:
2005 Sales: $3,612,717	2005 Profits: $146,746	Employees: 116,000
2004 Sales: $3,215,989	2004 Profits: $151,571	Fiscal Year Ends: 12/31
2003 Sales: $2,665,777	2003 Profits: $167,255	Parent Company: BAIN CAPITAL LLC

SALARIES/BENEFITS:
Pension Plan:	ESOP Stock Plan:	Profit Sharing:	Top Exec. Salary: $787,500	Bonus: $59,063
Savings Plan: Y	Stock Purch. Plan:		Second Exec. Salary: $661,500	Bonus: $297,675

OTHER THOUGHTS:
Apparent Women Officers or Directors: 4
Hot Spot for Advancement for Women/Minorities: Y

LOCATIONS: ("Y" = Yes)
West:	Southwest:	Midwest:	Southeast:	Northeast:	International:
Y	Y	Y	Y	Y	Y

Note: Financial information, benefits and other data can change quickly and may vary from those stated here.

OWENS & MINOR INC

www.owens-minor.com

Industry Group Code: 421450 Ranks within this company's industry group: Sales: 1 Profits: 3

Management:		Sales/Marketing:		Liberal Arts:		Information Systems:		Professionals:		Technical/Scientific:	
Mgmt. Trainees:	Y	Mktg. Professionals:	Y	Gen. Writing/Editing:	Y	Info. Management:	Y	Finance/Accounting:	Y	Engineers, Elec.:	
Experienced Mgmt.:	Y	Retail Sales:		Technical Writing:	Y	Software Dev.:	Y	Law:	Y	Engineers, Other:	Y
Int'l Business:		Commercial/Industrial:	Y	Graphic Arts/Photog.:	Y	Hardware Dev.:		HR/Other:	Y	Health/Lab:	
MBA Graduates:	Y	Sales Trainees:	Y	Music:		Systems Integration:		Training:	Y	Scientists/Research:	
		Advertising Pros.:	Y	Broadcasting:		Consulting/Other:		Health Care:	Y	Petroleum/Chemicals:	
				Other:				Consulting:		Math/Other:	

TYPES OF BUSINESS:
Distribution-Medical & Surgical Equipment
Supply Chain Management

BRANDS/DIVISIONS/AFFILIATES:
Pandac
CostTrack
WISDOM
OM DIRECT
SurgiTrack

CONTACTS: Note: Officers with more than one job title may be intentionally listed here more than once.
Craig R. Smith, CEO
Craig R. Smith, Pres.
James L. Bierman, CFO
W. Marshall Simpson, Sr. VP-Sales & Mktg.
Erika T. Davis, Sr. VP-Human Resources
Richard W. Mears, CIO/Sr. VP
Charles C. Colpo, Exec. VP-Admin.
Grace R. den Hartog, General Counsel/Sr. VP/Corp. Sec.
Mark A. Van Sumeren, Sr. VP-Bus. Dev.
Hugh F. Gouldthorpe, VP-Comm. & Quality
Richard F. Bozard, Treas./VP
Olwen B. Cape, VP/Controller
Scott W. Perkins, VP-West
G. Gilmer Minor, III, Chmn.
E. V. Clarke, Exec. VP-Dist.

Phone: 804-723-7000	Fax: 804-723-7100
Toll-Free:	
Address: 9120 Lockwood Blvd., Mechanicsville, VA 23116 US	

GROWTH PLANS/SPECIAL FEATURES:
Owens & Minor, Inc. (OMI) is a distributor of medical and surgical supplies to the acute-care market, a healthcare supply-chain management company and a national direct-to-consumer supplier of testing and monitoring supplies for diabetics. In its acute-care supply distribution, the company distributes 180,000 finished medical and surgical products produced by over 1,200 suppliers to about 4,000 healthcare provider customers from 50 distribution centers nationwide. The firm's primary distribution customers are acute-care hospitals and integrated healthcare networks, which account for more than 90% of the company's revenue. Other customers include the federal government, for which OMI serves as a vendor for medical and surgical supply distribution services for the U.S. Department of Defense. On a more limited basis, the company serves alternate care providers including clinics, home healthcare organizations, nursing homes, physicians' offices, rehabilitation facilities and surgery centers. The firm typically provides its distribution services under contractual arrangements with terms ranging from three to five years. Most of OMI's sales consist of consumable goods such as disposable gloves; dressings; endoscopic products; intravenous products; needles and syringes; sterile procedure trays; surgical products and gowns; urological products; and wound closure products. CostTrack separates product and process costs to clearly reflect the cost of individual distribution activities. Pandac and SurgiTrack are both programs that help with operating room equipment management. Online services and order forms are available through OM DIRECT and WISDOM. In September 2006, OMI acquired McKesson Corp.'s acute-care medical supply assets for $170 million.

OMI offers its employees educational assistance, incentive pay, flexible benefit plans and medical, dental, vision, life and disability insurance.

FINANCIALS: Sales and profits are in thousands of dollars—add 000 to get the full amount. 2007 Note: Financial information for 2007 was not available for all companies at press time.
2007 Sales: $6,800,466   2007 Profits: $72,710   U.S. Stock Ticker: OMI
2006 Sales: $5,533,736   2006 Profits: $48,752   Int'l Ticker: Int'l Exchange:
2005 Sales: $4,822,414   2005 Profits: $64,420   Employees: 4,600
2004 Sales: $4,525,105   2004 Profits: $60,500   Fiscal Year Ends: 12/31
2003 Sales: $4,244,067   2003 Profits: $53,641   Parent Company:

SALARIES/BENEFITS:
Pension Plan: ESOP Stock Plan: Profit Sharing: Top Exec. Salary: $717,307   Bonus: $
Savings Plan: Y   Stock Purch. Plan: Y   Second Exec. Salary: $415,768   Bonus: $

OTHER THOUGHTS:
Apparent Women Officers or Directors: 3
Hot Spot for Advancement for Women/Minorities: Y

LOCATIONS: ("Y" = Yes)
West:	Southwest:	Midwest:	Southeast:	Northeast:	International:
Y	Y	Y	Y	Y	

Note: Financial information, benefits and other data can change quickly and may vary from those stated here.

PACIFIC SUNWEAR OF CALIFORNIA INC   www.pacsun.com

Industry Group Code: 448000 Ranks within this company's industry group: Sales: 5 Profits: 6

Management:		Sales/Marketing:		Liberal Arts:		Information Systems:		Professionals:		Technical/Scientific:	
Mgmt. Trainees:	Y	Mktg. Professionals:	Y	Gen. Writing/Editing:	Y	Info. Management:	Y	Finance/Accounting:	Y	Engineers, Elec.:	
Experienced Mgmt.:	Y	Retail Sales:	Y	Technical Writing:		Software Dev.:	Y	Law:	Y	Engineers, Other:	
Int'l Business:	Y	Commercial/Industrial:	Y	Graphic Arts/Photog.:	Y	Hardware Dev.:		HR/Other:	Y	Health/Lab:	
MBA Graduates:	Y	Sales Trainees:	Y	Music:		Systems Integration:		Training:	Y	Scientists/Research:	
		Advertising Pros.:	Y	Broadcasting:		Consulting/Other:		Health Care:		Petroleum/Chemicals:	
				Other:	Y			Consulting:		Math/Other:	

TYPES OF BUSINESS:

Casual Apparel, Retail
Teen & Young Adult Apparel
Accessories
Footwear
Online Sales

BRANDS/DIVISIONS/AFFILIATES:

PacSun
PacSun Outlet
pacsun.com

CONTACTS: Note: Officers with more than one job title may be intentionally listed here more than once.

Sally Frame Kasaks, CEO
Michael L. Henry, CFO/Sr. VP
Caroline Kenyon, Sr. VP-Human Resources
Jon Brewer, VP-Prod. Dev.
Whitney Walker, VP-Bus. Strategy
Gar Jackson, VP-Investor Rel.
Thomas Kennedy, Div. Pres., PacSun
Reenie Benziger, Exec. VP-Merch., PacSun
Charlie Mescher, Sr. VP-Gen. Merch. Mgr. PacSun Young Men's
Linda Eddy, VP-Real Estate
Sally Frame Kasaks, Chmn.

Phone: 714-414-4000	Fax: 714-414-4251
Toll-Free: 800-444-6770	
Address: 3450 E. Miraloma Ave., Anaheim, CA 92806 US	

GROWTH PLANS/SPECIAL FEATURES:

Pacific Sunwear of California, Inc. is a leading specialty retailer of everyday casual apparel, accessories and footwear designed to meet the lifestyle needs of active teens and young adults. The company operates two nationwide primarily mall-based chains of retail stores under the names PacSun and PacSun Outlet with approximately 938 stores in 50 states and Puerto Rico. PacSun's typical customers are young people ages 12-22 who prefer a casual, fun look. Much of the fashion influence at the 815 PacSun stores comes from surfing, skateboarding and snowboarding, as well as from brand names associated with these sports. A typical Pacific Sunwear store offers accessories such as sunglasses and hats, footwear and casual apparel such as shorts, jeans, swimwear and shirts under brand names including Roxy, Quiksilver, Billabong, O'Neill, Etnies and newer brands like Volcom, Fox Racing and Paul Frank. The company also offers merchandise under its private labels Bullhead, Breakdown, Good Vibes and Tilt. In addition to its retail operations, Pacific Sunwear operates the e-commerce site pacsun.com. In October 2007, Pacific Sunwear announced it would close its nine One Thousand Step Stores. In January 2008, the firm announced that it would close its 150 d.e.m.o.'s stores. These stores featured casual apparel and related accessories influenced by hip-hop music, music personalities and mainstream sports personalities, targeted at customers aged 16-24.

FINANCIALS: Sales and profits are in thousands of dollars—add 000 to get the full amount. 2007 Note: Financial information for 2007 was not available for all companies at press time.

2007 Sales: $1,447,204	2007 Profits: $39,621	U.S. Stock Ticker: PSUN
2006 Sales: $1,391,500	2006 Profits: $126,200	Int'l Ticker: Int'l Exchange:
2005 Sales: $1,229,762	2005 Profits: $106,900	Employees: 17,000
2004 Sales: $1,040,294	2004 Profits: $80,213	Fiscal Year Ends: 1/31
2003 Sales: $846,400	2003 Profits: $49,700	Parent Company:

SALARIES/BENEFITS:

Pension Plan:	ESOP Stock Plan:	Profit Sharing:	Top Exec. Salary: $712,308	Bonus: $
Savings Plan:	Stock Purch. Plan:		Second Exec. Salary: $595,192	Bonus: $60,000

OTHER THOUGHTS:

Apparent Women Officers or Directors: 6
Hot Spot for Advancement for Women/Minorities: Y

LOCATIONS: ("Y" = Yes)

West:	Southwest:	Midwest:	Southeast:	Northeast:	International:
Y	Y	Y	Y	Y	Y

PANTRY INC (THE)

www.thepantry.com

Industry Group Code: 445120 Ranks within this company's industry group: Sales: 1 Profits: 1

Management:		Sales/Marketing:		Liberal Arts:		Information Systems:		Professionals:		Technical/Scientific:	
Mgmt. Trainees:	Y	Mktg. Professionals:	Y	Gen. Writing/Editing:		Info. Management:	Y	Finance/Accounting:	Y	Engineers, Elec.:	
Experienced Mgmt.:	Y	Retail Sales:	Y	Technical Writing:		Software Dev.:		Law:	Y	Engineers, Other:	
Int'l Business:		Commercial/Industrial:	Y	Graphic Arts/Photog.:		Hardware Dev.:		HR/Other:	Y	Health/Lab:	
MBA Graduates:	Y	Sales Trainees:	Y	Music:		Systems Integration:		Training:	Y	Scientists/Research:	
		Advertising Pros.:	Y	Broadcasting:		Consulting/Other:		Health Care:		Petroleum/Chemicals:	
				Other:				Consulting:		Math/Other:	

TYPES OF BUSINESS:

Convenience Stores
Gas Stations
Fast Food

BRANDS/DIVISIONS/AFFILIATES:

Kangaroo Express
McLane Company

CONTACTS: *Note: Officers with more than one job title may be intentionally listed here more than once.*

Peter J. Sodini, CEO
Peter J. Sodini, Pres.
Frank G. Paci, CFO
Melissa H. Anderson, Sr. VP-Human Resources
Steven J. Ferreira, Sr. VP-Admin.
Frank G. Paci, Sec.
Brad Williams, VP-Oper.
Frank G. Paci, Sr. VP-Finance
Keith S. Bell, Sr. VP-Fuels
Peter J. Sodini, Chmn.

Phone: 919-774-6700	Fax: 919-775-5428
Toll-Free:	
Address: 1801 Douglas Dr., P.O. Box 1410, Sanford, NC 27330 US	

GROWTH PLANS/SPECIAL FEATURES:

The Pantry, Inc. is a leading operator of convenience stores in the Southeast U.S., operating 1,644 convenience stores under a variety of brand names including its primary operating banner, Kangaroo Express. The company operates 234 quick service restaurants within 222 of its locations, of which 142 offer products from nationally branded food franchises including Subway, Quiznos, Hardee's, Krystal, Church's, Dairy Queen and Bojangles. In addition, The Pantry offers a variety of proprietary food service programs in 92 of its quick service restaurants featuring breakfast biscuits, fried chicken, a deli and other hot food offerings. Its stores offer merchandise, gasoline and ancillary products and services. The biggest selling items have historically been tobacco products, which accounted for approximately 31% of 2007 merchandise sales; packaged beverages, 17.5%; and beer and wine, 15.6%. Merchandise sales in 2007 generated approximately 23% of The Pantry's total revenues. Its services revenue is derived from sales of lottery tickets, prepaid products, money orders, public telephones, ATMs and amusement and video gaming service offerings. The Pantry purchases over 50% of its merchandise, including most tobacco and grocery items, from McLane Company, Inc., a subsidiary of Berkshire Hathaway, Inc. The company purchases gasoline from major oil companies and independent refiners and offers a mix of branded and private brand gasoline at its locations based on an evaluation of local market conditions. Approximately 67% of the firm's locations that sell gasoline are branded under the BP, CITGO, Chevron or ExxonMobil brand names. Gasoline revenues generated approximately 77% of The Pantry's total revenues in 2007. Approximately 32% of the firm's stores are strategically located in coastal or resort areas, while roughly 25% are situated along major interstates and highways. In 2007, The Pantry acquired 126 convenience stores.

FINANCIALS: Sales and profits are in thousands of dollars—add 000 to get the full amount. 2007 Note: Financial information for 2007 was not available for all companies at press time.

2007 Sales: $6,911,163	2007 Profits: $26,732	**U.S. Stock Ticker: PTRY**
2006 Sales: $5,961,700	2006 Profits: $89,200	**Int'l Ticker:** Int'l Exchange:
2005 Sales: $4,429,200	2005 Profits: $57,800	Employees: 11,248
2004 Sales: $3,493,100	2004 Profits: $17,600	Fiscal Year Ends: 9/30
2003 Sales: $2,776,361	2003 Profits: $11,504	Parent Company:

SALARIES/BENEFITS:

Pension Plan:	ESOP Stock Plan:	Profit Sharing:	Top Exec. Salary: $719,923	Bonus: $1,092,000
Savings Plan:	Stock Purch. Plan:		Second Exec. Salary: $308,538	Bonus: $312,000

OTHER THOUGHTS:

Apparent Women Officers or Directors: 2
Hot Spot for Advancement for Women/Minorities:

LOCATIONS: ("Y" = Yes)

West:	Southwest:	Midwest:	Southeast:	Northeast:	International:
		Y	Y	Y	

PARAMETRIC TECHNOLOGY CORP

www.ptc.com

Industry Group Code: 511215 Ranks within this company's industry group: Sales: 2 Profits: 1

Management:		Sales/Marketing:		Liberal Arts:		Information Systems:		Professionals:		Technical/Scientific:	
Mgmt. Trainees:		Mktg. Professionals:	Y	Gen. Writing/Editing:		Info. Management:	Y	Finance/Accounting:	Y	Engineers, Elec.:	Y
Experienced Mgmt.:	Y	Retail Sales:		Technical Writing:	Y	Software Dev.:	Y	Law:	Y	Engineers, Other:	
Int'l Business:	Y	Commercial/Industrial:	Y	Graphic Arts/Photog.:		Hardware Dev.:		HR/Other:	Y	Health/Lab:	
MBA Graduates:	Y	Sales Trainees:		Music:		Systems Integration:	Y	Training:	Y	Scientists/Research:	
		Advertising Pros.:		Broadcasting:		Consulting/Other:		Health Care:		Petroleum/Chemicals:	
				Other:				Consulting:		Math/Other:	

TYPES OF BUSINESS:

Computer Software-Engineering & Manufacturing
Engineering Consulting Services
Enterprise Publishing Software
Product Data Management

BRANDS/DIVISIONS/AFFILIATES:

Pro/ENGINEER
Arbortext, Inc.
Arbortext Advanced Print Publisher
Mathsoft Engineering & Education, Inc.
Mathcad
ITEDO Software LLC
CoCreate Software GmbH
OneSpace

CONTACTS: *Note: Officers with more than one job title may be intentionally listed here more than once.*

C. Richard Harrison, CEO
C. Richard Harrison, Pres.
Neil F. Moses, CFO/Exec. VP
Paul J. Cunningham, Exec. VP-Worldwide Sales & Dist.
Steve Horan, CIO/Corp. VP
James E. Heppelmann, Chief Prod. Officer/Exec. VP-Software Solutions
Aaron C. von Staats, General Counsel/Sr. VP
Barry F. Cohen, Exec. VP-Strategic Svcs. & Partners
Meredith Mendola, VP-Corp. Comm.
Anthony DiBona, Exec. VP-Global Maintenance Support
Noel G. Posternak, Chmn.

Phone: 781-370-5000	Fax: 781-370-6000
Toll-Free: 877-275-4782	
Address: 140 Kendrick St., Needham, MA 02494 US	

GROWTH PLANS/SPECIAL FEATURES:

Parametric Technology Corp. (PTC) develops markets and supports product lifecycle management (PLM) and enterprise content management (ECM) software that helps manufacturers improve the competitiveness of their products and product development processes. PTC offers product data management, dynamic publishing solutions, supplier management, digital mockup, enterprise application integration, project management, after-market service, customer needs management and manufacturing planning. Parametric's leading product family, Pro/ENGINEER, is a 3D modeling software used by large enterprises including NASA. The Pro/ENGINEER family includes Pro/ENGINEER CAD, CAM and CAE. The firm's Windchill Software enables users to enhance their businesses via the Internet through digital mock-up collaboration, internal library design, product data management tools and cross-application integration. PTC recently acquired Arbortext, Inc., a leader in the dynamic enterprise publishing market, and subsequently released Arbortext Advanced Print Publisher 9.0, designed assist in the production of technical documentation; financial reports; scientific, technical and medical journals; legislation and amendments; marketing brochures; telephone directories; and product catalogs. PTC also recently acquired Mathsoft Engineering & Education, Inc., which creates Mathcad software essential to the PLM process, for $64.4 million; and ITEDO Software GmbH and ITEDO Software LLC, designers of software which creates technical illustrations, for approximately $17 million in cash. PTC has partnered with many companies in recent years, including Autodesk, Inc., to expand its manufacturing capabilities; International Business Machines Corp. (IBM), to integrate with the IBM Rational Software Development platform and focus on the PLM market in China; and IHS, Inc., to deliver electronic components content to users of PTC Windchill. In December 2007, the firm acquired CoCreate Software GmbH, a product development solutions provider and developer of the OneSpace line of drawing and modeling software, for $250 million.

Parametric provides its employees with tuition reimbursement; paid time off; medical, dental and vision plans; life insurance; and short- and long-term disability coverage.

FINANCIALS: Sales and profits are in thousands of dollars—add 000 to get the full amount. 2007 Note: Financial information for 2007 was not available for all companies at press time.

2007 Sales: $941,279	2007 Profits: $143,656	**U.S. Stock Ticker: PMTC**
2006 Sales: $847,983	2006 Profits: $56,804	**Int'l Ticker:** Int'l Exchange:
2005 Sales: $707,975	2005 Profits: $73,187	Employees: 4,449
2004 Sales: $660,029	2004 Profits: $34,813	Fiscal Year Ends: 9/30
2003 Sales: $671,940	2003 Profits: $-98,280	Parent Company:

SALARIES/BENEFITS:

Pension Plan:	ESOP Stock Plan:	Profit Sharing:	Top Exec. Salary: $520,000	Bonus: $1,050,254
Savings Plan: Y	Stock Purch. Plan:		Second Exec. Salary: $487,000	Bonus: $450,096

OTHER THOUGHTS:

Apparent Women Officers or Directors:
Hot Spot for Advancement for Women/Minorities:

LOCATIONS: ("Y" = Yes)

West:	Southwest:	Midwest:	Southeast:	Northeast:	International:
Y	Y	Y	Y	Y	Y

Note: Financial information, benefits and other data can change quickly and may vary from those stated here.

PAREXEL INTERNATIONAL CORP   www.parexel.com

Industry Group Code: 541710 Ranks within this company's industry group: Sales: 4   Profits: 3

Management:		Sales/Marketing:		Liberal Arts:		Information Systems:		Professionals:		Technical/Scientific:	
Mgmt. Trainees:	Y	Mktg. Professionals:	Y	Gen. Writing/Editing:	Y	Info. Management:	Y	Finance/Accounting:	Y	Engineers, Elec.:	Y
Experienced Mgmt.:	Y	Retail Sales:		Technical Writing:	Y	Software Dev.:	Y	Law:	Y	Engineers, Other:	
Int'l Business:	Y	Commercial/Industrial:	Y	Graphic Arts/Photog.:		Hardware Dev.:		HR/Other:	Y	Health/Lab:	Y
MBA Graduates:	Y	Sales Trainees:		Music:		Systems Integration:	Y	Training:	Y	Scientists/Research:	Y
		Advertising Pros.:		Broadcasting:		Consulting/Other:	Y	Health Care:	Y	Petroleum/Chemicals:	
				Other:				Consulting:	Y	Math/Other:	Y

TYPES OF BUSINESS:

Clinical Trial & Data Management
Biostatistical Analysis & Reporting
Medical Communications Services
Clinical Pharmacology Services
Educational & Training Services
Web-Based Solutions
Medical Software Solutions
Consulting Services

BRANDS/DIVISIONS/AFFILIATES:

Clinical Research Services
PAREXEL Consulting & Medical Communications Svcs.
Perceptive Informatics, Inc.
Barnett Educational Services
PAREXEL International Synchron Private Limited
California Clinical Trials Medical Group, Inc.
Behavioral and Medical Research, LLC
PAREXEL APEX International

CONTACTS: *Note: Officers with more than one job title may be intentionally listed here more than once.*

Josef H. von Rickenbach, CEO
Mark A. Goldberg, COO
James F. Winschel, Jr., CFO/Sr. VP
Ulf Schneider, Chief Admin. Officer/Sr. VP
Douglas A. Batt, General Counsel/Corp. Sec./Sr. VP
Jennifer Baird, Dir.-Public Rel.
Mark A. Goldberg, Pres., Perceptive Informatics, Inc./Pres., CRS
Kurt A. Brykman, Pres., PAREXEL Consulting & Medical Comm. Svcs.
Todd A. Joron, Corp. VP/General Mgr.-Perceptive Informatics, Inc.
Josef H. von Rickenbach, Chmn.

Phone: 781-487-9900	Fax: 781-768-5512
Toll-Free:	
Address: 200 West St., Waltham, MA 02451-1163 US	

GROWTH PLANS/SPECIAL FEATURES:

PAREXEL International is a biopharmaceutical services company serving the pharmaceutical, biotechnology and medical device industries worldwide. Operating in 64 locations throughout 51 countries, PAREXEL has three business segments: Clinical Research Services (CRS); PAREXEL Consulting and Medical Communications Services (PCMS); and Perceptive Informatics, Inc. PAREXEL's core business, CRS, provides clinical trials management; biostatistical analysis and reporting; data management; patient recruiting; clinical pharmacology; and related medical advisory and investigator site services. PCMS provides technical expertise and advice for drug development and regulatory affairs; offers product launch support, including market development, product development and targeted communications services; registration and commercialization; and provides policy consulting and strategic reimbursement services. Additionally, PCMS division Barnett Educational Services offers educational and training services ranging from webcast seminars to on-site training. Lastly, Perceptive provides information technology designed to improve clients' product development processes, including medical imaging services, interactive voice response systems, clinical trials management systems, web-based portals, systems integration and patient diary applications. In recent years, the firm and Synchron Research Services Private Ltd. created joint venture PAREXEL International Synchron Private Limited, located in Bangalore, India, to conduct clinical trial business operations; and it acquired a minority equity interest in Synchron's clinical pharmacology business of in Ahmedabad, India. PAREXEL also recently acquired California Clinical Trials Medical Group, Inc. and Behavioral and Medical Research, LLC for $66.5 million; and opened an office in Mexico City to provide clinical research and consulting services. In September 2007, subsidiary PAREXEL (Taiwan), Inc. acquired Apex International Clinical Research Co., Ltd., now called PAREXEL APEX International, for $50.9 million. Apex operates mainly in the Asia-Pacific region.

Employees of PAREXEL receive health, dental, life and disability insurance; paid time off; and numerous career development opportunities, including leadership development programs and personalized learning plans.

FINANCIALS: Sales and profits are in thousands of dollars—add 000 to get the full amount. 2007 Note: Financial information for 2007 was not available for all companies at press time.

2007 Sales: $741,955	2007 Profits: $37,289	U.S. Stock Ticker: PRXL
2006 Sales: $614,947	2006 Profits: $23,544	Int'l Ticker: Int'l Exchange:
2005 Sales: $544,726	2005 Profits: $-35,177	Employees: 6,485
2004 Sales: $540,983	2004 Profits: $13,791	Fiscal Year Ends: 6/30
2003 Sales: $615,838	2003 Profits: $10,662	Parent Company:

SALARIES/BENEFITS:

Pension Plan:	ESOP Stock Plan:	Profit Sharing:	Top Exec. Salary: $500,000	Bonus: $409,072
Savings Plan: Y	Stock Purch. Plan:		Second Exec. Salary: $361,233	Bonus: $126,541

OTHER THOUGHTS:

Apparent Women Officers or Directors: 1
Hot Spot for Advancement for Women/Minorities: Y

LOCATIONS: ("Y" = Yes)

West:	Southwest:	Midwest:	Southeast:	Northeast:	International:
Y				Y	Y

PARSONS BRINCKERHOFF INC

www.pbworld.com

Industry Group Code: 234000 Ranks within this company's industry group: Sales: 7 Profits:

Management:		Sales/Marketing:		Liberal Arts:		Information Systems:		Professionals:		Technical/Scientific:	
Mgmt. Trainees:		Mktg. Professionals:	Y	Gen. Writing/Editing:		Info. Management:	Y	Finance/Accounting:	Y	Engineers, Elec.:	Y
Experienced Mgmt.:	Y	Retail Sales:		Technical Writing:	Y	Software Dev.:	Y	Law:	Y	Engineers, Other:	Y
Int'l Business:	Y	Commercial/Industrial:	Y	Graphic Arts/Photog.:	Y	Hardware Dev.:		HR/Other:	Y	Health/Lab:	
MBA Graduates:	Y	Sales Trainees:		Music:		Systems Integration:	Y	Training:	Y	Scientists/Research:	
		Advertising Pros.:		Broadcasting:		Consulting/Other:	Y	Health Care:		Petroleum/Chemicals:	
				Other:				Consulting:	Y	Math/Other:	

TYPES OF BUSINESS:

Engineering Services
Planning, Design & Construction
Civic Construction Projects
Commercial Construction
Transportation Consulting
Program Management Services
Telecommunications & Environmental Projects

BRANDS/DIVISIONS/AFFILIATES:

PB Facilities, Inc.
PB Aviation, Inc.
PB Farradyne, Inc.
PB Buildings, Inc.
PB Constructors, Inc.
PB Telecommunications, Inc.
Parsons Brinckerhoff Power, Inc.
PB Research Library

CONTACTS: Note: Officers with more than one job title may be intentionally listed here more than once.

Thomas J. O'Neill, CEO
Richard A. Schrader, CFO/Exec. VP
John J. Ryan, Exec. VP/Dir.-Human Resources
Hugh Inglis, Sr. VP-Alltech
Gay Knipper, Dir.-National Program Management, PB Americas
Paul Skoutelas, Market Leader-Transit, PB Americas
Patrick Lun, Deputy COO-PB Int'l
Thomas J. O'Neill, Chmn.

Phone: 212-465-5000	Fax: 212-465-5096
Toll-Free:	
Address: 1 Penn Plaza, New York, NY 10119 US	

GROWTH PLANS/SPECIAL FEATURES:

Parsons Brinckerhoff, Inc. provides engineering, consulting, and management services to local governments and the transportation, energy, and commercial market sectors. The company also offers construction services, program and project management, and facilities management. Parsons Brinckerhoff has taken on projects for clients such as Bangkok Mass Transit System Corporation and the City of Austin, Texas; and its signature works include the design of New York City's first subway and the reconfiguration of the Fort Washington Way interstate connector in Cincinnati. In recent years, the company worked with the Delhi Metro Rail Corporation to build a mass transit system designed as an urban transport system to move over 3 million passengers a day. Other relevant projects have included contracts to build an oil and gas fired power station in Kuwait; to design a website and communications plan for lower Manhattan, known as lowermanhatten.info; and to design and engineer the Greater Cairo Metro system. Potential clients can view the company's work through the PB Research Library, a body that showcases and publishes the details of important projects. The firm is organized into three divisions: Americas, International and Facilities. The company is employee-owned with roughly 200 offices worldwide. In March 2008, the firm was awarded the contract for Section One of the New Jersey Turnpike Interchange 6-9 Widening Program in Burlington County, New Jersey.

FINANCIALS: Sales and profits are in thousands of dollars—add 000 to get the full amount. 2007 Note: Financial information for 2007 was not available for all companies at press time.

2007 Sales: $	2007 Profits: $	U.S. Stock Ticker: Private	
2006 Sales: $1,689,964	2006 Profits: $46,386	Int'l Ticker: Int'l Exchange:	
2005 Sales: $1,447,756	2005 Profits: $27,160	Employees: 10,080	
2004 Sales: $1,389,400	2004 Profits: $18,400	Fiscal Year Ends: 10/31	
2003 Sales: $1,370,000	2003 Profits: $	Parent Company:	

SALARIES/BENEFITS:

Pension Plan:	ESOP Stock Plan:	Profit Sharing:	Top Exec. Salary: $	Bonus: $
Savings Plan:	Stock Purch. Plan:		Second Exec. Salary: $	Bonus: $

OTHER THOUGHTS:

Apparent Women Officers or Directors: 4
Hot Spot for Advancement for Women/Minorities: Y

LOCATIONS: ("Y" = Yes)

West:	Southwest:	Midwest:	Southeast:	Northeast:	International:
Y	Y	Y	Y	Y	Y

PATTERSON COMPANIES INC www.pattersoncompanies.com

Industry Group Code: 421450 Ranks within this company's industry group: Sales: 3 Profits: 1

Management:		Sales/Marketing:		Liberal Arts:		Information Systems:		Professionals:		Technical/Scientific:	
Mgmt. Trainees:	Y	Mktg. Professionals:	Y	Gen. Writing/Editing:	Y	Info. Management:	Y	Finance/Accounting:	Y	Engineers, Elec.:	
Experienced Mgmt.:	Y	Retail Sales:		Technical Writing:	Y	Software Dev.:	Y	Law:	Y	Engineers, Other:	Y
Int'l Business:	Y	Commercial/Industrial:	Y	Graphic Arts/Photog.:	Y	Hardware Dev.:		HR/Other:	Y	Health/Lab:	
MBA Graduates:	Y	Sales Trainees:	Y	Music:		Systems Integration:		Training:	Y	Scientists/Research:	
		Advertising Pros.:	Y	Broadcasting:		Consulting/Other:		Health Care:	Y	Petroleum/Chemicals:	
				Other:				Consulting:		Math/Other:	

TYPES OF BUSINESS:

Dental Products & Related Services
Veterinary Products
Non-Wheelchair Assistive Products

BRANDS/DIVISIONS/AFFILIATES:

Patterson Dental Co.
Accu-Bite Dental Products, LLC
Webster Management LP
Patterson Medical Holdings, Inc.
Dale Surgical Professional Supply, Inc.
Metri Medical, Inc.
Sammons Preston Rolyan
Homecraft

CONTACTS: Note: Officers with more than one job title may be intentionally listed here more than once.

James W. Wiltz, CEO
James W. Wiltz, Pres.
R. Stephen Armstrong, CFO/Exec. VP
Jerome E. Thygesen, VP-Human Resources
Lynn E. Askew, VP-IT
Matthew L. Levitt, General Counsel/Sec.
Dan Peckskamp, VP-Oper.
R. Stephen Armstrong, Treas.
George L. Henriques, Pres., Webster Veterinary Supply, Inc.
David P. Sproat, Pres., Patterson Medical
Scott P. Anderson, Pres., Patterson Dental
Peter L. Frechette, Chmn.

Phone: 651-686-1600	Fax: 651-686-9331
Toll-Free: 800-328-5536	
Address: 1031 Mendota Heights Rd., St. Paul, MN 55120 US	

GROWTH PLANS/SPECIAL FEATURES:

Patterson Companies, Inc., formerly Patterson Dental Co., is a value-added products distributor in the dental; companion pet and equine veterinary; and rehabilitation and non-wheelchair assistive products markets. The company operates in three segments: dental supply, veterinary supply and rehabilitation supply. The dental supply segment, Patterson Dental, is one of the two largest distributors of dental products in North America. The division provides consumable products, including x-ray film, restorative materials, hand instruments and sterilization products; basic and advanced technology dental equipment; practice management and clinical software; patient education systems; and office forms and stationery. Patterson Dental also offers related services including dental equipment installation; maintenance and repair; dental office design; and equipment financing. The veterinary supply segment, Webster Veterinary, provides products for the diagnosis, treatment and/or prevention of diseases in companion pets and equine animals. Webster's more than 11,000 products are sold by about 175 field sales representatives. The segment also has an agency commission business with several pharmaceutical manufacturers. The rehabilitation supply segment, Patterson Medical, formerly AbilityOne Corp., distributes rehabilitation medical supplies and non-wheelchair assistive products. Patterson Medical operates as Sammons Preston Rolyan in North America and Homecraft in international markets. Subsidiaries include Patterson Dental Holdings, Inc.; Direct Dental Supply Co.; Webster Management LP; Patterson Medical Holdings, Inc.; Accu-Bite Dental Products, LLC; Williamston Industrial Center, LLC; Strategic Dental Marketing, Inc.; AbilityOne, Ltd.; Metro Medical, Inc.; and Dale Surgical Professional Supply, Inc. In November 2008, Patterson acquired Advanced Practice Systems, also known as PTOS Software, a designer and marketer of physical therapist management software. In April 2008, the firm acquired Leventhal & Sons, Inc., a regional dental distributor.

The company offers its employees medical, dental and vision insurance; short- and long-term disability insurance; life and personal accident insurance; education assistance; and an employee assistance program.

FINANCIALS: Sales and profits are in thousands of dollars—add 000 to get the full amount. 2007 Note: Financial information for 2007 was not available for all companies at press time.

2007 Sales: $2,798,398	2007 Profits: $208,336	U.S. Stock Ticker: PDCO
2006 Sales: $2,615,123	2006 Profits: $198,425	Int'l Ticker: Int'l Exchange:
2005 Sales: $2,421,457	2005 Profits: $183,698	Employees: 6,580
2004 Sales: $1,969,349	2004 Profits: $149,465	Fiscal Year Ends: 4/30
2003 Sales: $1,657,000	2003 Profits: $119,700	Parent Company:

SALARIES/BENEFITS:

Pension Plan:	ESOP Stock Plan: Y	Profit Sharing:	Top Exec. Salary: $557,338	Bonus: $250,250
Savings Plan: Y	Stock Purch. Plan: Y		Second Exec. Salary: $300,000	Bonus: $171,500

OTHER THOUGHTS:

Apparent Women Officers or Directors: 2
Hot Spot for Advancement for Women/Minorities:

LOCATIONS: ("Y" = Yes)

West:	Southwest:	Midwest:	Southeast:	Northeast:	International:
Y	Y	Y	Y	Y	Y

Note: Financial information, benefits and other data can change quickly and may vary from those stated here.

PATTERSON-UTI ENERGY INC   www.patenergy.com

Industry Group Code: 213111   Ranks within this company's industry group: Sales: 9   Profits: 9

Management:		Sales/Marketing:		Liberal Arts:	Information Systems:		Professionals:		Technical/Scientific:	
Mgmt. Trainees:	Y	Mktg. Professionals:	Y	Gen. Writing/Editing:	Info. Management:	Y	Finance/Accounting:	Y	Engineers, Elec.:	Y
Experienced Mgmt.:	Y	Retail Sales:		Technical Writing:	Software Dev.:		Law:	Y	Engineers, Other:	
Int'l Business:	Y	Commercial/Industrial:	Y	Graphic Arts/Photog.:	Hardware Dev.:		HR/Other:	Y	Health/Lab:	Y
MBA Graduates:	Y	Sales Trainees:		Music:	Systems Integration:		Training:	Y	Scientists/Research:	
		Advertising Pros.:		Broadcasting:	Consulting/Other:		Health Care:		Petroleum/Chemicals:	Y
				Other:			Consulting:		Math/Other:	

TYPES OF BUSINESS:

Oil & Gas Services
Onshore Contract Drilling Services
Drilling & Completion Fluid Services
Pressure Pumping Services
Oil & Gas Production

BRANDS/DIVISIONS/AFFILIATES:

TMBR/Sharp Drilling, Inc.

CONTACTS: *Note: Officers with more than one job title may be intentionally listed here more than once.*

Douglas J. Wall, CEO
Douglas J. Wall, Pres.
John E. Vollmer, III, CFO/Treas.
William L. Moll Jr., General Counsel/Sec.
John E. Vollmer, III, Sr. VP-Corp. Dev.
Greg Pipkin, Chief Acct. Officer
Kenneth N. Berns, Sr. VP
Mark S. Siegel, Chmn.

Phone: 281-765-7100	Fax: 281-765-7175
Toll-Free:	
Address: 450 Gears Rd., Ste. 500, Houston, TX 77067 US	

GROWTH PLANS/SPECIAL FEATURES:

Patterson-UTI Energy, Inc. serves land-based oil and natural gas exploration and production companies. The company operates in Texas, New Mexico, Oklahoma, Arkansas, Louisiana, Mississippi, Colorado, Utah, Wyoming, Montana, North Dakota, South Dakota, Pennsylvania and Western Canada through four business segments: contract drilling; pressure pumping; drilling and completion fluids; and oil and natural gas. The firm operates 350 currently marketable contract drilling rigs, with a maximum drilling depth capacity ranging from 5,000 to 30,000 feet; of these rigs, 281 are mechanical and 69 silicon-controlled rectifier (SCR) electric. Patterson-UTI dug 4,237 wells in 2007, each dug on average in 21 days. It operates 336 trucks and 439 trailers used to transport and support its rigs. Pressure pumping services includes stimulation, which enhances well flow by pumping corrosive acid, nitrogen gas or highly pressurized fracturing fluid into a well; and cementing, which involves inserting a substance between a wellbore and its casing to add support. It operates approximately 344 trucks and three trailers to transport and handle stimulation and cementing materials. Patterson-UTI's drilling fluids cool and lubricate the bit during drilling operations, contain formation pressures to prevent blowout, and remove rock cuttings from the hole; and completion fluids are used to accurately manipulate well pressures as well as meeting other requirements. It owns and operates 20 trucks and 92 trailers and leases another 34 trucks to transport drilling and completion fluids; and owns two mills used to process barite, a material used in drilling fluids. The oil and gas segment operates in Texas, New Mexico, Utah and Mississippi as a working interest owner. Contract drilling provided 82% of the company's 2007 revenue; pressure pumping, 10%; drilling and completion fluids, 6%; and oil and natural gas, 2%. In November 2007, the firm sold the exploration and production portions of the oil and gas segment.

FINANCIALS: Sales and profits are in thousands of dollars—add 000 to get the full amount. 2007 Note: Financial information for 2007 was not available for all companies at press time.

2007 Sales: $2,114,194	2007 Profits: $438,639	U.S. Stock Ticker: PTEN
2006 Sales: $2,546,586	2006 Profits: $673,254	Int'l Ticker: Int'l Exchange:
2005 Sales: $1,740,455	2005 Profits: $372,740	Employees: 9,000
2004 Sales: $1,000,769	2004 Profits: $94,346	Fiscal Year Ends: 12/31
2003 Sales: $776,170	2003 Profits: $43,187	Parent Company:

SALARIES/BENEFITS:

Pension Plan:	ESOP Stock Plan:	Profit Sharing:	Top Exec. Salary: $450,000	Bonus: $2,750,000
Savings Plan: Y	Stock Purch. Plan:		Second Exec. Salary: $350,000	Bonus: $2,750,000

OTHER THOUGHTS:

Apparent Women Officers or Directors:
Hot Spot for Advancement for Women/Minorities:

LOCATIONS: ("Y" = Yes)

West:	Southwest:	Midwest:	Southeast:	Northeast:	International:
Y	Y	Y	Y	Y	Y

PAXAR CORP

www.paxar.com

Industry Group Code: 334119 Ranks within this company's industry group: Sales: 3 Profits: 3

Management:		Sales/Marketing:		Liberal Arts:		Information Systems:		Professionals:		Technical/Scientific:	
Mgmt. Trainees:	Y	Mktg. Professionals:	Y	Gen. Writing/Editing:		Info. Management:	Y	Finance/Accounting:	Y	Engineers, Elec.:	Y
Experienced Mgmt.:	Y	Retail Sales:		Technical Writing:		Software Dev.:		Law:	Y	Engineers, Other:	
Int'l Business:	Y	Commercial/Industrial:	Y	Graphic Arts/Photog.:	Y	Hardware Dev.:		HR/Other:	Y	Health/Lab:	
MBA Graduates:	Y	Sales Trainees:		Music:		Systems Integration:		Training:	Y	Scientists/Research:	
		Advertising Pros.:	Y	Broadcasting:		Consulting/Other:		Health Care:		Petroleum/Chemicals:	
				Other:				Consulting:		Math/Other:	

TYPES OF BUSINESS:

Tags & Labels
Manufacturing-Printers & Supplies
Logistics Systems
RFID Systems
Inventory Systems
Retail Information Services

BRANDS/DIVISIONS/AFFILIATES:

Avery Dennison Corp
Monarch

CONTACTS: Note: Officers with more than one job title may be intentionally listed here more than once.

Dean A. Scarborough, CEO
Dean A. Scarborough, Pres.
Anthony S. Colatrella, CFO/VP
Terry L. Hemmelgarn, Group VP-Retail Info. Ser.
Robert Cornick, VP-Printer Systems Division

Phone:	Fax: 914-696-4128
Toll-Free: 800-337-2927	
Address: 105 Corporate Park Dr., White Plains, NY 10604 US	

GROWTH PLANS/SPECIAL FEATURES:

Paxar Corporation, a subsidiary of Avery Dennison Corp., designs, manufactures and distributes a wide variety of tags and labels, including labels with bar codes, as well as printers and the associated supplies, for retailers and apparel manufacturers. The company's services are targeted toward customers who prefer the flexibility of creating labels and tags on an as-needed basis in their facilities. Paxar's activities and services include graphic design, coating, laminating, weaving, design of mechanical and electronic printers and systems integration. It manufactures the printers, paper and fabric substrates, as well as the inks for in-plant tag and label-printing systems. The corporation manufactures electronic bar code systems, RFID (radio frequency identification) systems and hand-held mechanical labelers for use in retail stores and distribution centers, as well as for remote tracking applications. Paxar has lately been investing in RFID technology, introducing a tabletop printer/encoder designed to write RFID chips and adding manufacturing equipment in its plants to process smart tags at high speeds. Paxar markets its bar code and RFID products under the Monarch brand name. The firm also designs integrated systems for large in-store and warehouse applications, such as inventory control and distribution management. The company provides service for its printers and mechanical labelers at customer locations worldwide and in its own facilities at multiple locations. In June 2007, Avery Dennison Corp. acquired Paxar for approximately $1.3 billion.

FINANCIALS: Sales and profits are in thousands of dollars—add 000 to get the full amount. 2007 Note: Financial information for 2007 was not available for all companies at press time.

2007 Sales: $	2007 Profits: $	U.S. Stock Ticker: Subsidiary
2006 Sales: $880,800	2006 Profits: $56,800	Int'l Ticker: Int'l Exchange:
2005 Sales: $809,100	2005 Profits: $23,000	Employees: 12,100
2004 Sales: $804,400	2004 Profits: $47,400	Fiscal Year Ends: 12/31
2003 Sales: $712,000	2003 Profits: $14,600	Parent Company: AVERY DENNISON CORP

SALARIES/BENEFITS:

Pension Plan:	ESOP Stock Plan:	Profit Sharing:	Top Exec. Salary: $636,000	Bonus: $590,213
Savings Plan:	Stock Purch. Plan:		Second Exec. Salary: $610,000	Bonus: $906,360

OTHER THOUGHTS:

Apparent Women Officers or Directors:
Hot Spot for Advancement for Women/Minorities:

LOCATIONS: ("Y" = Yes)

West:	Southwest:	Midwest:	Southeast:	Northeast:	International:
Y	Y	Y	Y	Y	Y

Note: Financial information, benefits and other data can change quickly and may vary from those stated here.

PAYCHEX INC

www.paychex.com

Industry Group Code: 514210 Ranks within this company's industry group: Sales: 2   Profits: 2

Management:		Sales/Marketing:		Liberal Arts:		Information Systems:		Professionals:		Technical/Scientific:	
Mgmt. Trainees:	Y	Mktg. Professionals:	Y	Gen. Writing/Editing:		Info. Management:	Y	Finance/Accounting:	Y	Engineers, Elec.:	
Experienced Mgmt.:	Y	Retail Sales:		Technical Writing:		Software Dev.:	Y	Law:	Y	Engineers, Other:	
Int'l Business:	Y	Commercial/Industrial:	Y	Graphic Arts/Photog.:		Hardware Dev.:		HR/Other:	Y	Health/Lab:	
MBA Graduates:	Y	Sales Trainees:		Music:		Systems Integration:		Training:	Y	Scientists/Research:	
		Advertising Pros.:	Y	Broadcasting:		Consulting/Other:		Health Care:		Petroleum/Chemicals:	
				Other:				Consulting:		Math/Other:	

TYPES OF BUSINESS:

Payroll Processing Services
Payroll & Tax Preparation
Internal Accounting Records
Human Resources Outsourcing
Employee Benefits Outsourcing
Regulatory Compliance
Workers' Compensation Insurance
Online Payroll Services

BRANDS/DIVISIONS/AFFILIATES:

Core Payroll
Major Market Services
Paychex Online
Paychex Online Reports
General Ledger Services
Hawthorne Benefit Technologies, Inc.
BeneTrac
Paychex FSA Debit Card

CONTACTS: Note: Officers with more than one job title may be intentionally listed here more than once.

Jonathan J. Judge, CEO
Jonathan J. Judge, Pres.
John M. Morphy, CFO/Sr. VP/Corp. Sec.
Walter Turek, Sr. VP-Sales & Mktg.
Daniel A. Canzano, VP-IT
Stephanie Schaeffer, Chief Legal Officer/VP
Martin Mucci, Sr. VP-Oper.
William G. Kuchta, VP-Organizational Dev.
Laura S. Lynch, Dir.-Corp. Comm.
Terri Allen, Dir.-Investor Rel.
Melinda A. Janik, VP-Finance
Martin Stowe, VP-Human Resources Svcs.
Kevin N. Hill, VP-Insurance Oper.
Leonard E. Redon, VP-Western Oper.
Lynn J. Miley, VP-Eastern Oper.
B. Thomas Golisano, Chmn.

Phone: 585-385-6666	Fax: 585-383-3428
Toll-Free: 800-322-7292	
Address: 911 Panorama Trail S., Rochester, NY 14625-2396 US	

GROWTH PLANS/SPECIAL FEATURES:

Paychex, Inc. offers payroll and human resource outsourcing services to small- and medium-sized businesses. It serves approximately 561,000 clients through more than 100 offices in the U.S. and serves 900 customers in Germany through offices in Hamburg, Berlin, Munich and Dusseldorf. Paychex mainly targets businesses with fewer than 100 employees, with 81% of its customers employing 19 people or less. The company offers services covering payroll processing; employee benefits administration; time and attendance solutions; workers' compensation insurance; and other human resource services and products. Payroll processing is the backbone of the Paychex product portfolio. Its Core Payroll services include calculating, preparing and delivering employee payroll checks; producing internal accounting records and management reports; and preparing federal, state and local payroll tax returns. Another product is Major Market Services, which primarily targets companies that have outgrown the Core Payroll service or have more complex needs.   Payroll services also include Paychex Online, a secure Internet site with a suite of interactive, always-available self-service products and services, offering employees current and historical time sheets through Paychex Online Reports; and downloadable payroll information through General Ledger Services. In September 2007, Paychex acquired Hawthorne Benefit Technologies, Inc. (now called Paychex Benefit Technologies, Inc.), including BeneTrac, its online benefits management and administration system. In January 2008, the firm launched a debit card that client's employees can use to draw directly from their Flexible Spending Account (FSA) funds. Using the Paychex FSA Debit Card thus allows employees to avoid having pay fees out of pocket, submit a claim and wait for reimbursement. Paychex offers the card to its clients free of charge.

Employees of Paychex receive medical, vision and dental coverage; life insurance; business travel accident insurance; short- and long-term disability coverage; child care and employee assistance programs; tuition reimbursement; and travel and relocation assistance.

FINANCIALS: Sales and profits are in thousands of dollars—add 000 to get the full amount. 2007 Note: Financial information for 2007 was not available for all companies at press time.

2007 Sales: $1,886,964	2007 Profits: $515,447	U.S. Stock Ticker: PAYX
2006 Sales: $1,674,596	2006 Profits: $464,914	Int'l Ticker: Int'l Exchange:
2005 Sales: $1,445,143	2005 Profits: $368,849	Employees: 11,700
2004 Sales: $1,240,093	2004 Profits: $302,950	Fiscal Year Ends: 5/31
2003 Sales: $1,046,000	2003 Profits: $293,500	Parent Company:

SALARIES/BENEFITS:

Pension Plan:	ESOP Stock Plan:	Profit Sharing:	Top Exec. Salary: $868,144	Bonus: $1,030,979
Savings Plan: Y	Stock Purch. Plan: Y		Second Exec. Salary: $397,426	Bonus: $257,390

OTHER THOUGHTS:

Apparent Women Officers or Directors: 6
Hot Spot for Advancement for Women/Minorities: Y

LOCATIONS: ("Y" = Yes)

West:	Southwest:	Midwest:	Southeast:	Northeast:	International:
Y	Y	Y	Y	Y	Y

Note: Financial information, benefits and other data can change quickly and may vary from those stated here.

PEABODY ENERGY CORP   www.peabodyenergy.com

Industry Group Code: 212110 Ranks within this company's industry group: Sales: 1   Profits: 1

Management:		Sales/Marketing:		Liberal Arts:		Information Systems:		Professionals:		Technical/Scientific:	
Mgmt. Trainees:	Y	Mktg. Professionals:	Y	Gen. Writing/Editing:		Info. Management:	Y	Finance/Accounting:	Y	Engineers, Elec.:	Y
Experienced Mgmt.:	Y	Retail Sales:		Technical Writing:		Software Dev.:		Law:	Y	Engineers, Other:	Y
Int'l Business:	Y	Commercial/Industrial:		Graphic Arts/Photog.:		Hardware Dev.:		HR/Other:	Y	Health/Lab:	
MBA Graduates:	Y	Sales Trainees:		Music:		Systems Integration:		Training:	Y	Scientists/Research:	
		Advertising Pros.:		Broadcasting:		Consulting/Other:		Health Care:		Petroleum/Chemicals:	Y
				Other:				Consulting:		Math/Other:	

TYPES OF BUSINESS:

Coal Production
Energy Trading & Marketing
Transportation Services
Coalbed Methane Production

BRANDS/DIVISIONS/AFFILIATES:

Excel Coal Ltd.
COALSALES LLC

CONTACTS: Note: Officers with more than one job title may be intentionally listed here more than once.

Gregory H. Boyce, CEO
Eric Ford, COO/Exec. VP
Gregory H. Boyce, Pres.
Michael C. Crews, CFO/Exec. VP
Richard M. Whiting, Chief Mktg. Officer/Exec. VP
Sharon D. Fiehler, Exec. VP-Human Resources
Sharon D. Fiehler, Exec. VP-Admin.
Alexander C. Scoch, Chief Legal Officer/Exec. VP
Kemal Williamson, Group Vice President of Operations
Richard A. Navarre, Exec. VP-Corp. Dev.
John C. Hull, Dir. Sales-COALSALES
Rick Bowen, Pres., Generation & Btu Conversion
Roger B. Walcott, Jr., Exec. VP-Strategy & Bus. Svcs.
Rob Hammond, COO-Australia Oper.
Gregory H. Boyce, Chmn.
L. Cartan Sumner, Jr., VP-Intl. Gov't Rel.
Christopher J. Hagedorn, VP-Supply Chain Management

Phone: 314-342-3400	Fax: 314-342-7799
Toll-Free:	
Address: 701 Market St., St. Louis, MO 63101 US	

GROWTH PLANS/SPECIAL FEATURES:

Peabody Energy Corp. is a private-sector coal company with operations worldwide. The firm sells approximately 237 million tons of coal annually to a clientele of nearly 340 electricity generating and industrial plants in 19 countries. It shipped 192.3 million tons from 20 U.S. mining operations and 21.4 million tons from 11 Australia operations in 2007. The company has approximately 9.3 billion tons of proven and probable coal reserves. The mining operations consist of three principal operating segments, western U.S. mining, eastern U.S. mining, and australian mining. In addition to mining operations, the firm markets, brokers and trades coal through a trading and brokerage operations segment. The firm's total tons traded were 166.5 million for the year ended December 31, 2007. In response to growing international markets, Peabody established an international trading group in 2006 and added a trading operations office in Europe in early 2007. It also has a business development, sales and marketing office in Beijing, China. Other energy-related commercial activities include the development of mine-mouth coal-fueled generating plants, the management of vast coal reserve and real estate holdings, and Btu conversion technologies, which are designed to convert coal to natural gas and transportation fuels. In July 2008, Peabody Energy announced that it has reached an agreement to acquire 15 percent of the Millennium Mine in Queensland, Australia, and intends to acquire the remaining 0.5 percent ownership in the near future. The company currently owns 84.5 percent of the operation, and intends to purchase the remaining equity interest following regulatory approvals. July 2008, the firm also announced it has completed the $50-plus million expansion of its Wambo Coal Preparation Facility, the final phase in a multi-year build out of Peabody's Wambo complex. The plant serves the North Wambo underground and Wambo open-cut mines in New South Wales, Australia.

FINANCIALS: Sales and profits are in thousands of dollars—add 000 to get the full amount. 2007 Note: Financial information for 2007 was not available for all companies at press time.

2007 Sales: $4,574,712	2007 Profits: $264,285	U.S. Stock Ticker: BTU
2006 Sales: $4,108,396	2006 Profits: $600,697	Int'l Ticker: Int'l Exchange:
2005 Sales: $4,644,453	2005 Profits: $422,653	Employees: 9,200
2004 Sales: $3,631,582	2004 Profits: $175,387	Fiscal Year Ends: 12/31
2003 Sales: $2,815,296	2003 Profits: $31,348	Parent Company:

SALARIES/BENEFITS:

Pension Plan:	ESOP Stock Plan:	Profit Sharing:	Top Exec. Salary: $887,500	Bonus: $1,329,620
Savings Plan:	Stock Purch. Plan:		Second Exec. Salary: $612,500	Bonus: $850,000

OTHER THOUGHTS:

Apparent Women Officers or Directors: 2
Hot Spot for Advancement for Women/Minorities:

LOCATIONS: ("Y" = Yes)

West:	Southwest:	Midwest:	Southeast:	Northeast:	International:
Y		Y			Y

Note: Financial information, benefits and other data can change quickly and may vary from those stated here.

PEPSI BOTTLING GROUP INC

www.pbg.com

Industry Group Code: 312111 Ranks within this company's industry group: Sales: Profits:

Management:		Sales/Marketing:		Liberal Arts:		Information Systems:		Professionals:		Technical/Scientific:	
Mgmt. Trainees:	Y	Mktg. Professionals:	Y	Gen. Writing/Editing:		Info. Management:	Y	Finance/Accounting:	Y	Engineers, Elec.:	Y
Experienced Mgmt.:	Y	Retail Sales:		Technical Writing:		Software Dev.:		Law:	Y	Engineers, Other:	
Int'l Business:	Y	Commercial/Industrial:	Y	Graphic Arts/Photog.:		Hardware Dev.:		HR/Other:	Y	Health/Lab:	
MBA Graduates:	Y	Sales Trainees:	Y	Music:		Systems Integration:		Training:	Y	Scientists/Research:	
		Advertising Pros.:	Y	Broadcasting:		Consulting/Other:		Health Care:		Petroleum/Chemicals:	
				Other:				Consulting:		Math/Other:	

TYPES OF BUSINESS:

Beverages-Soft Drinks Manufacturing
Bottled Water
Iced Tea

BRANDS/DIVISIONS/AFFILIATES:

Mirinda
Pepsi-Cola
Aquafina
Lipton
Mountain Dew
Sobe
Electropura
Garci Crespo

CONTACTS: Note: Officers with more than one job title may be intentionally listed here more than once.

Eric J. Foss, CEO
Eric J. Foss, Pres.
Alfred H. Drewes, CFO/Sr. VP
Brent J. Franks, Sr. VP-Global Sales/Chief Customer Officer
John L. Berisford, Sr. VP-Human Resources
Neal A. Bronzo, CIO/Sr. VP
Steven M. Rapp, General Counsel/Sr. VP/Corp. Sec.
Victor L. Crawford, Sr. VP-Worldwide Oper.
Kathleen M. Dwyer, VP-Strategy
Thomas M. Lardieri, Controller/VP
Pablo Lagos, Pres./Gen. Mgr.-PBG Mexico
Robert C. King, Pres., PBG North America
Barry H. Beracha, Chmn.
Yiannis Petrides, Pres., PBG Europe

Phone: 914-767-6000	Fax: 914-767-7761
Toll-Free:	
Address: 1 Pepsi Way, Somers, NY 10589 US	

GROWTH PLANS/SPECIAL FEATURES:

The Pepsi Bottling Group, Inc. (PBG), a 38% subsidiary of PepsiCo, Inc., is one of the world's largest manufacturers and distributors of Pepsi-Cola beverages, with the exclusive right to manufacture, sell and distribute Pepsi-Cola beverages in all or a portion of 41 states, Washington, D.C., nine Canadian provinces, Spain, Greece, Russia, Turkey and Mexico, including the carbonated and non-carbonated beverages Pepsi-Cola, Diet Pepsi, Mountain Dew, Sierra Mist, Lipton tea products, Sobe, Dole and Aquafina bottled water. In certain regions, PBG owns the rights to manufacture, sell and distribute the soft drink products of other companies, such as Starbucks Frappuccino, Dr Pepper and 7UP. In addition, PBG manufactures, sells and distributes beverages under its own trademarks, including Electropura and Garci Crespo. PBG's sales represent over half of all Pepsi-Cola beverages sold in the U.S. and Canada. Its three largest U.S. brands in terms of volume are Pepsi-Cola, Diet Pepsi and Mountain Dew. Worldwide, the company operates 95 plants and 515 distribution centers. In early 2007, the firm announced plans to acquire the distribution and bottling rights for certain Cadbury Schweppes brands in Northern California. In late 2007, PBG agreed to acquire Pepsi-Cola Batavia Bottling Corp., a family owned and operated business in New York.

The company offers its employees a 401(k) plan; medical, dental and vision insurance; life and accident insurance; short- and long-term disability insurance; same sex domestic partner coverage; a stock purchase program; and tuition reimbursement.

FINANCIALS: Sales and profits are in thousands of dollars—add 000 to get the full amount. 2007 Note: Financial information for 2007 was not available for all companies at press time.

2007 Sales: $13,591,000	2007 Profits: $532,000	U.S. Stock Ticker: PBG
2006 Sales: $12,730,000	2006 Profits: $522,000	Int'l Ticker: Int'l Exchange:
2005 Sales: $11,885,000	2005 Profits: $466,000	Employees: 66,900
2004 Sales: $10,906,000	2004 Profits: $457,000	Fiscal Year Ends: 12/31
2003 Sales: $10,265,000	2003 Profits: $416,000	Parent Company:

SALARIES/BENEFITS:

Pension Plan:	ESOP Stock Plan:	Profit Sharing:	Top Exec. Salary: $1,025,000	Bonus: $5,000,000
Savings Plan: Y	Stock Purch. Plan: Y		Second Exec. Salary: $754,500	Bonus: $1,289,000

OTHER THOUGHTS:

Apparent Women Officers or Directors: 5
Hot Spot for Advancement for Women/Minorities: Y

LOCATIONS: ("Y" = Yes)

West:	Southwest:	Midwest:	Southeast:	Northeast:	International:
Y	Y	Y	Y	Y	Y

Note: Financial information, benefits and other data can change quickly and may vary from those stated here.

PEPSICO INC   www.pepsico.com

Industry Group Code: 312111 Ranks within this company's industry group: Sales: 1   Profits: 1

Management:		Sales/Marketing:		Liberal Arts:		Information Systems:		Professionals:		Technical/Scientific:	
Mgmt. Trainees:	Y	Mktg. Professionals:	Y	Gen. Writing/Editing:	Y	Info. Management:	Y	Finance/Accounting:	Y	Engineers, Elec.:	Y
Experienced Mgmt.:	Y	Retail Sales:		Technical Writing:		Software Dev.:	Y	Law:	Y	Engineers, Other:	
Int'l Business:	Y	Commercial/Industrial:	Y	Graphic Arts/Photog.:	Y	Hardware Dev.:		HR/Other:	Y	Health/Lab:	Y
MBA Graduates:	Y	Sales Trainees:	Y	Music:		Systems Integration:		Training:	Y	Scientists/Research:	Y
		Advertising Pros.:	Y	Broadcasting:		Consulting/Other:		Health Care:		Petroleum/Chemicals:	
				Other:	Y			Consulting:		Math/Other:	

TYPES OF BUSINESS:

Soft Drink Manufacturing
Snack Food Manufacturing
Juice & Sports Drink Manufacturing
Cereal Manufacturing
Rice & Pasta Product Manufacturing
Oatmeal Product Manufacturing
Bottled Water Production
Cereal Bar Manufacturing

BRANDS/DIVISIONS/AFFILIATES:

Frito-Lay Inc
Pepsi
Doritos
Quaker Foods And Beverages
Tropicana Products Inc
Gatorade
PepsiAmericas Inc
Sandora, LLC

CONTACTS: Note: Officers with more than one job title may be intentionally listed here more than once.

Indra K. Nooyi, CEO
Cynthia M. Trudell, Chief Personnel Officer/Sr. VP
Mehmood Khan, Chief Scientific Officer
Larry D. Thompson, General Counsel/Sec.
Larry D. Thompson, Sr. VP-Gov't Affairs
Lionel L. Nowell III, Treas./Sr. VP
Ronald C. Parker, Chief Diversity & Inclusion Officer
Peter A. Bridgman, Controller/Sr. VP
Julie Hamp, Sr. VP-PepsiCo Comm.
Sarah McGill, Sr. VP-Tax
Indra K. Nooyi, Chmn.
Michael D. White, CEO-PepsiCO Int'l
Mitch Adamek, Chief Procurement Officer/Sr. VP

Phone: 914-253-2000	Fax: 914-253-2070
Toll-Free:	
Address: 700 Anderson Hill Rd., Purchase, NY 10577 US	

GROWTH PLANS/SPECIAL FEATURES:

PepsiCo, Inc. is a global snack and beverage company that sells a variety of salty, convenient, sweet and grain-based snacks; carbonated and non-carbonated beverages; and foods. The company operates in three segments: PepsiCo Americas food, PepsiCo Americas beverages; and PepsiCo International. The PepsiCo Americas food segment is comprised of Frito-Lay North America; Quaker; and all Latin American food and snack businesses, including the Sabritas and Gamesa businesses in Mexico. Frito-Lay manufactures, markets, sells and distributes branded snacks, which include Lay's potato chips, Doritos tortilla chips, Tostitos tortilla chips, Cheetos cheese flavored snacks, Fritos corn chips, branded dips, Ruffles potato chips, Quaker Chewy granola bars, SunChips multigrain snacks, Rold Gold pretzels, Santitas tortilla chips, Frito-Lay nuts, Grandma's cookies, Munchies snack mix, Lay's Stax potato crisps, Quaker Quakes corn and rice snacks, Miss Vickie's potato chips, branded crackers, Quaker snack mix, Smartfood popcorn, Chester's fries, Stacy's pita chips and Quaker Fruit & Oatmeal bars. Quaker manufactures, markets and sells cereals, pasta and other branded products such as Quaker oatmeal, Aunt Jemima mixes and syrups, Cap'n Crunch cereal, Quaker grits, Life cereal, Rice-A-Roni, Pasta Roni and Near East side dishes. The PepsiCo Americas beverages segment encompasses Pepsi-Cola North America, Gatorade, Tropicana and all Latin American beverage businesses. The division manufactures, markets and sells beverage concentrates, fountain syrups and finished goods, under brands including Pepsi, Mountain Dew, Gatorade, Tropicana, Pure Premium, Lipton, Sierra Mist, Propel, Dole and SoBe. It also sells tea, coffee and water products through joint ventures with Unilever and Starbucks. In addition, the segment licenses the Aquafina water brand to its bottlers and markets this brand. The PepsiCo International segment is comprised of all PepsiCo businesses in the U.K., Europe, Asia, Middle East and Africa. In 2007, PepsiCo and PepsiAmericas, Inc. jointly acquired Sandora, LLC, a Ukrainian juice company.

FINANCIALS: Sales and profits are in thousands of dollars—add 000 to get the full amount. 2007 Note: Financial information for 2007 was not available for all companies at press time.

2007 Sales: $39,474,000	2007 Profits: $5,658,000	**U.S. Stock Ticker: PEP**
2006 Sales: $35,137,000	2006 Profits: $5,642,000	**Int'l Ticker:** Int'l Exchange:
2005 Sales: $32,562,000	2005 Profits: $4,078,000	Employees: 168,000
2004 Sales: $29,261,000	2004 Profits: $4,212,000	Fiscal Year Ends: 12/31
2003 Sales: $26,971,000	2003 Profits: $3,568,000	Parent Company:

SALARIES/BENEFITS:

Pension Plan:	ESOP Stock Plan:	Profit Sharing:	Top Exec. Salary: $1,000,000	Bonus: $5,000,000
Savings Plan:	Stock Purch. Plan:		Second Exec. Salary: $964,413	Bonus: $3,000,000

OTHER THOUGHTS:

Apparent Women Officers or Directors: 5
Hot Spot for Advancement for Women/Minorities: Y

LOCATIONS: ("Y" = Yes)

West:	Southwest:	Midwest:	Southeast:	Northeast:	International:
Y	Y	Y	Y	Y	Y

Note: Financial information, benefits and other data can change quickly and may vary from those stated here.

PEROT SYSTEMS CORP

www.perotsystems.com

Industry Group Code: 541512 Ranks within this company's industry group: Sales: 5 Profits: 7

Management:		Sales/Marketing:		Liberal Arts:		Information Systems:		Professionals:		Technical/Scientific:	
Mgmt. Trainees:	Y	Mktg. Professionals:	Y	Gen. Writing/Editing:	Y	Info. Management:	Y	Finance/Accounting:	Y	Engineers, Elec.:	Y
Experienced Mgmt.:	Y	Retail Sales:		Technical Writing:	Y	Software Dev.:	Y	Law:	Y	Engineers, Other:	
Int'l Business:	Y	Commercial/Industrial:	Y	Graphic Arts/Photog.:	Y	Hardware Dev.:	Y	HR/Other:	Y	Health/Lab:	
MBA Graduates:	Y	Sales Trainees:		Music:		Systems Integration:	Y	Training:	Y	Scientists/Research:	
		Advertising Pros.:	Y	Broadcasting:		Consulting/Other:	Y	Health Care:		Petroleum/Chemicals:	
				Other:				Consulting:	Y	Math/Other:	

TYPES OF BUSINESS:

IT Consulting
Business Process Outsourcing
Management Consulting
Government Services
Infrastructure Services
Systems & Software Development

BRANDS/DIVISIONS/AFFILIATES:

QSS Group, Inc.
JJWild, Inc.

CONTACTS: Note: Officers with more than one job title may be intentionally listed here more than once.

Peter Altabef, CEO
Russell Freeman, COO
Peter Altabef, Pres.
John Harper, CFO
Jeff Renzi, Exec. VP-Mktg. & Sales
Darcy Anderson, Chief People Officer/VP-Corp. Support
Del Williams, General Counsel/VP/Corp. Sec
John King, VP
James Champy, Chmn.-Consulting
Scott Barnes, VP-Infrastructure Solutions
Atul Vohra, Chief Mktg. Officer
Ross Perot, Jr., Chmn.

Phone: 972-577-0000	Fax:
Toll-Free: 888-317-3768	
Address: 2300 W. Plano Pkwy., Plano, TX 75075 US	

GROWTH PLANS/SPECIAL FEATURES:

Perot Systems Corp. is a worldwide provider of information technology (IT) services and business solutions to a broad range of customers. The firm offers integrated solutions designed around specific business objectives, with services including technology outsourcing, business process outsourcing, development and integration of systems and applications, and business and technology consulting services. Services are divided into four primary segments: infrastructure services, applications services, business process services and consulting services. The infrastructure services segment forms multi-year contracts through which it assumes operational responsibility for various aspects of customers' businesses. Perot Systems can take charge of a company's data center management, web hosting and Internet access, desktop solutions, messaging services, network management, program management and security. The applications services segment includes the development and continued maintenance of packaged or custom application software. The division also provides application systems migration and testing. The business process services segment includes services such as claims processing, life insurance policy administration, call center management, payment and settlement management, security and services to improve the collection of receivables. This group also provides engineering support and other technical and administrative services to the U.S. government. Consulting services include strategy, enterprise and technology consulting, research and software implementation. The firm's clients include government agencies, healthcare providers, the construction and manufacturing industries and financial services companies. In June 2007, Perot Systems acquired QSS Group, Inc., a federal government IT services company. In September 2007, the company purchased JJWild, Inc., a preferred provider of integrated healthcare delivery solutions.

FINANCIALS: Sales and profits are in thousands of dollars—add 000 to get the full amount. 2007 Note: Financial information for 2007 was not available for all companies at press time.

2007 Sales: $2,612,000	2007 Profits: $115,000	U.S. Stock Ticker: PER
2006 Sales: $2,298,000	2006 Profits: $81,000	Int'l Ticker: Int'l Exchange:
2005 Sales: $1,998,286	2005 Profits: $111,120	Employees: 21,200
2004 Sales: $1,773,452	2004 Profits: $94,347	Fiscal Year Ends: 12/31
2003 Sales: $1,460,751	2003 Profits: $2,506	Parent Company:

SALARIES/BENEFITS:

Pension Plan:	ESOP Stock Plan:	Profit Sharing:	Top Exec. Salary: $592,505	Bonus: $905,000
Savings Plan:	Stock Purch. Plan:		Second Exec. Salary: $577,904	Bonus: $301,000

OTHER THOUGHTS:

Apparent Women Officers or Directors:
Hot Spot for Advancement for Women/Minorities:

LOCATIONS: ("Y" = Yes)

West:	Southwest:	Midwest:	Southeast:	Northeast:	International:
Y	Y	Y	Y	Y	Y

PERRIGO CO

www.perrigo.com

Industry Group Code: 325416 **Ranks within this company's industry group:** Sales: 2   Profits: 1

Management:		Sales/Marketing:		Liberal Arts:		Information Systems:		Professionals:		Technical/Scientific:	
Mgmt. Trainees:	Y	Mktg. Professionals:	Y	Gen. Writing/Editing:		Info. Management:	Y	Finance/Accounting:	Y	Engineers, Elec.:	Y
Experienced Mgmt.:	Y	Retail Sales:		Technical Writing:	Y	Software Dev.:	Y	Law:	Y	Engineers, Other:	Y
Int'l Business:	Y	Commercial/Industrial:	Y	Graphic Arts/Photog.:		Hardware Dev.:		HR/Other:	Y	Health/Lab:	Y
MBA Graduates:	Y	Sales Trainees:	Y	Music:		Systems Integration:		Training:	Y	Scientists/Research:	Y
		Advertising Pros.:	Y	Broadcasting:		Consulting/Other:		Health Care:	Y	Petroleum/Chemicals:	
				Other:				Consulting:		Math/Other:	Y

TYPES OF BUSINESS:

Generic Prescription Drugs
Over-the-Counter Pharmaceuticals
Nutritional Products
Active Pharmaceutical Ingredients
Consumer Products

BRANDS/DIVISIONS/AFFILIATES:

Careline
Neca
Natural Formula
Perrigo New York, Inc.
Perrigo Israel Pharmaceuticals, Ltd.
Quimica Y Famarcia S.A. de C.V.
Wrafton Laboratories, Ltd.
Galpharm Healthcare, Ltd.

CONTACTS: Note: Officers with more than one job title may be intentionally listed here more than once.

Joseph C. Papa, CEO
Joseph C. Papa, Pres.
Judy L. Brown, CFO/Exec. VP
Michael Stewart, Sr. VP-Global Human Resources
Thomas M. Farrington, CIO
Todd W. Kingma, General Counsel/Exec. VP/Sec.
John T. Hendrickson, Exec. VP-Global Oper.
Jeffrey R. Needham, Sr. VP-Global Bus. Dev.
David T. Gibbons, Chmn.
Refael Lebel, Exec VP/Gen. Mgr.-Perrigo Israel
John T. Hendrickson, Exec. VP-Supply Chain

Phone: 269-673-8451	Fax: 269-673-7534
Toll-Free:	
Address: 515 Eastern Ave., Allegan, MI 49010 US	

GROWTH PLANS/SPECIAL FEATURES:

Perrigo Co. is a global healthcare supplier and one of the world's largest manufacturers of over-the-counter pharmaceutical and nutritional products for the store brand market. The company also develops and manufactures generic prescription drugs, active pharmaceutical ingredients (API) and consumer products. The firm operates through three segments: consumer healthcare, prescription pharmaceuticals and API. The consumer healthcare segment makes a broad line of products including analgesics, cough/cold/allergy/sinus, gastrointestinal, smoking cessation, first aid, vitamin and nutritional supplement products. The pharmaceuticals segment's primary activity is the development, manufacture and sale of generic prescription drug products, generally for the U.S. market. The company currently markets roughly 230 generic prescription products to approximately 110 customers. The API segment develops, manufactures and markets API for the drug industry and branded pharmaceutical companies. In addition, Perrigo's operations also include the Israel consumer products segment, which consist of cosmetics, toiletries and detergents generally sold under brands such as Careline, Neca and Natural Formula; and the Israel pharmaceutical and diagnostic products segment, which includes the marketing and manufacturing of branded prescription drugs under long-term exclusive licenses and the importation of pharmaceutical, diagnostics and other medical products into Israel based on exclusive agreement with the manufacturers. Perrigo operates through several wholly-owned subsidiaries. In the U.S., these subsidiaries consist primarily of L. Perrigo Co.; Perrigo Co. of South Carolina; and Perrigo New York, Inc. Outside the U.S., the subsidiaries consist primarily of Perrigo Israel Pharmaceuticals, Ltd.; Chemagis, Ltd.; Quimica Y Farmacia S.A. de C.V.; Wrafton Laboratories, Ltd.; and Perrigo U.K., Ltd. In January 2008, the firm acquired Galpharm Healthcare, Ltd. for $86 million in cash. Galpharm is a supplier of over-the-counter store brand pharmaceutical products sold in the U.K.

FINANCIALS: Sales and profits are in thousands of dollars—add 000 to get the full amount. 2007 Note: Financial information for 2007 was not available for all companies at press time.

2007 Sales: $1,447,428	2007 Profits: $73,797	**U.S. Stock Ticker:** PRGO
2006 Sales: $1,366,821	2006 Profits: $71,400	**Int'l Ticker:** Int'l Exchange:
2005 Sales: $1,024,098	2005 Profits: $-325,983	Employees: 6,200
2004 Sales: $898,204	2004 Profits: $80,567	Fiscal Year Ends: 6/30
2003 Sales: $826,000	2003 Profits: $54,000	Parent Company:

SALARIES/BENEFITS:

Pension Plan:	ESOP Stock Plan:	Profit Sharing:	Top Exec. Salary: $581,250	Bonus: $244,126
Savings Plan:	Stock Purch. Plan:		Second Exec. Salary: $509,295	Bonus: $341,228

OTHER THOUGHTS:

Apparent Women Officers or Directors: 2
Hot Spot for Advancement for Women/Minorities:

LOCATIONS: ("Y" = Yes)

West:	Southwest:	Midwest:	Southeast:	Northeast:	International:
				Y	Y

PETCO ANIMAL SUPPLIES INC

www.petco.com

Industry Group Code: 453910 Ranks within this company's industry group: Sales: 2   Profits: 2

Management:		Sales/Marketing:		Liberal Arts:		Information Systems:		Professionals:		Technical/Scientific:	
Mgmt. Trainees:	Y	Mktg. Professionals:	Y	Gen. Writing/Editing:	Y	Info. Management:	Y	Finance/Accounting:	Y	Engineers, Elec.:	
Experienced Mgmt.:	Y	Retail Sales:	Y	Technical Writing:		Software Dev.:	Y	Law:	Y	Engineers, Other:	
Int'l Business:		Commercial/Industrial:	Y	Graphic Arts/Photog.:	Y	Hardware Dev.:		HR/Other:	Y	Health/Lab:	
MBA Graduates:	Y	Sales Trainees:	Y	Music:		Systems Integration:		Training:	Y	Scientists/Research:	
		Advertising Pros.:	Y	Broadcasting:		Consulting/Other:		Health Care:		Petroleum/Chemicals:	
				Other:				Consulting:		Math/Other:	

TYPES OF BUSINESS:

Pets & Pet Supplies, Retail
Online Sales
Pet Grooming
Veterinary Services
Obedience Training
Pet Photography

BRANDS/DIVISIONS/AFFILIATES:

Petco Foundation (The)
P.A.L.S.
Think Adoption First
Leonard Green & Partners LP
TPG (Texas Pacific Group)

CONTACTS: Note: Officers with more than one job title may be intentionally listed here more than once.

James M. Myers, CEO
Bruce C. Hall, COO
Bruce C. Hall, Pres.
Michael E. Foss, CFO/Exec. VP
Janet D. Mitchell, Sr. VP-Human Resources
Frederick W. Major, Sr. VP-Info. Systems
David Bolen, Chief Merch. Officer/Exec. VP
Janet D. Mitchell, Sr. VP-Admin.
William M. Woodard, Sr. VP-Bus. Dev.
Brian K. Devine, Chmn.
Razia Richter, Sr. VP-Supply Chain

Phone: 858-453-7845	Fax: 858-784-3489
Toll-Free: 888-824-7257	
Address: 9125 Rehco Rd., San Diego, CA 92121 US	

GROWTH PLANS/SPECIAL FEATURES:

Petco Animal Supplies, Inc. is a leading specialty retailer of premium pet food, supplies and services. The company currently operates over 850 stores and 11 distribution centers in 49 states and Washington, D.C. Petco's superstores carry more than 10,000 competitively priced products, including premium pet food and treats; small animals, such as fish, birds, reptiles and related supplies; collars and leashes; grooming products; toys; pet carriers; cat furniture; dog houses; vitamins; and veterinary supplies. Most stores also provide a variety of pet services, including professional grooming, veterinary clinics, vaccinations, obedience training and pet photography. Several services are performed in glass-walled stations in order to increase customer awareness and confidence in the services. In light of overpopulation problems, Petco chooses not to sell dogs and cats, though it does support adoption programs such as Petfinder.com through in-store Think Adoption First kiosks in many stores. Petco also operates the P.A.L.S. (Petco Animal Lovers Save) customer loyalty program. P.A.L.S. members receive special benefits and savings through the use of the P.A.L.S. card, which allows Petco to target customers and track shopping habits. In addition to its retail stores, the company operates an e-commerce site, which offers Petco merchandise, pet tips, a community forum, online specials and information about the Petco Foundation, an animal welfare and rights group. The company is owned by Leonard Green & Partners LP and TPG (Texas Pacific Group), two private equity investment firms.

Petco offers its employees health insurance plans, discounted pet insurance, a 401(k) retirement savings plan and merchandise discounts. The company also offers a Management Achievement Program and training programs related to specific types of animals.

FINANCIALS: Sales and profits are in thousands of dollars—add 000 to get the full amount. 2007 Note: Financial information for 2007 was not available for all companies at press time.

2007 Sales: $	2007 Profits: $	U.S. Stock Ticker: Private
2006 Sales: $1,996,089	2006 Profits: $75,170	Int'l Ticker: Int'l Exchange:
2005 Sales: $1,812,145	2005 Profits: $82,373	Employees: 17,900
2004 Sales: $1,654,138	2004 Profits: $64,713	Fiscal Year Ends: 1/31
2003 Sales: $1,476,600	2003 Profits: $32,100	Parent Company: TPG (TEXAS PACIFIC GROUP)

SALARIES/BENEFITS:

Pension Plan:	ESOP Stock Plan:	Profit Sharing:	Top Exec. Salary: $855,000	Bonus: $
Savings Plan: Y	Stock Purch. Plan:		Second Exec. Salary: $625,000	Bonus: $

OTHER THOUGHTS:

Apparent Women Officers or Directors: 2
Hot Spot for Advancement for Women/Minorities: Y

LOCATIONS: ("Y" = Yes)

West:	Southwest:	Midwest:	Southeast:	Northeast:	International:
Y	Y	Y	Y	Y	

PETSMART INC

www.petsmart.com

Industry Group Code: 453910 Ranks within this company's industry group: Sales: 1 Profits: 1

Management:		Sales/Marketing:		Liberal Arts:		Information Systems:		Professionals:		Technical/Scientific:	
Mgmt. Trainees:	Y	Mktg. Professionals:	Y	Gen. Writing/Editing:	Y	Info. Management:	Y	Finance/Accounting:	Y	Engineers, Elec.:	
Experienced Mgmt.:	Y	Retail Sales:	Y	Technical Writing:		Software Dev.:	Y	Law:	Y	Engineers, Other:	
Int'l Business:	Y	Commercial/Industrial:		Graphic Arts/Photog.:	Y	Hardware Dev.:		HR/Other:	Y	Health/Lab:	Y
MBA Graduates:	Y	Sales Trainees:	Y	Music:		Systems Integration:	Y	Training:	Y	Scientists/Research:	
		Advertising Pros.:	Y	Broadcasting:		Consulting/Other:		Health Care:	Y	Petroleum/Chemicals:	
				Other:	Y			Consulting:		Math/Other:	

TYPES OF BUSINESS:

Pets & Pet Supplies, Retail
Online & Catalog Sales
Pet Training
In-Store Adoption Centers
Veterinary Services
Pet Boarding
Pet Grooming

BRANDS/DIVISIONS/AFFILIATES:

Medical Management International, Inc.
Banfield, The Pet Hospital
PetsHotels
PetPerks
PetSmart.com
petsmartbebettertogether.com

CONTACTS: Note: Officers with more than one job title may be intentionally listed here more than once.

Philip L. Francis, CEO
Robert F. Moran, COO
Robert F. Moran, Pres.
Lawrence (Chip) Molloy, CFO/Sr. VP
Mary Miller, Chief Mktg. Officer/Sr. VP
Francesca Spinelli, Sr. VP-People
Donald Beaver, CIO/Sr. VP
Kenneth T. Hall, Sr. VP-Merch.
Scott A. Crozier, General Counsel/Sr. VP/Chief Compliance Officer
David K. Lenhardt, Sr. VP-Svcs. & Store Oper.
Jaye Perricone, Sr. VP-Real Estate
Philip L. Francis, Chmn.
Joseph O'Leary, Sr. VP-Supply Chain

Phone: 623-580-6100	Fax: 623-580-6183
Toll-Free: 800-738-1385	
Address: 19601 N. 27th Ave., Phoenix, AZ 85027 US	

GROWTH PLANS/SPECIAL FEATURES:

PetSmart, Inc. is a leading operator of superstores specializing in pet food, supplies and services. The company operates more than 1,043 stores in the U.S. and Canada offering an assortment of pet products and pet services. PetSmart stores also offer value-added pet services, including grooming, training, boarding and day camp, and the firm operates full-service veterinary hospitals in 685 of its stores. Medical Management International, Inc., an operator of veterinary hospitals, operates 673 of PetSmart's hospitals under the name of Banfield, The Pet Hospital. The remaining hospitals are located in Canada and operated by other third parties. PetSmart offers pet boarding at 97 of its stores through its PetSmart PetsHotels. The company opened or acquired 100 new stores during 2007. Its stores range in size from 19,000 to 27,000 square feet and carry more than 10,500 distinct items, including nationally recognized brand names and a selection of proprietary or private label brands. PetSmart stores sell supplies for dogs, cats, fresh-water tropical fish, birds and other small pets, such as hamsters, gerbils and guinea pigs. Sales of pet food, treats, litter and supplies and pet sales generate approximately 90% of PetSmart's net sales. The firm also actively supports pet adoption through its in-store adoption centers. The firm offers a PetPerks loyalty program and sells its products online through PetSmart.com. In 2007, PetSmart completed the exit of its equine product line including the sale of StateLineTack.com and its equine catalog.

PetSmart offers its employees education assistance, a nurse hotline, store discounts, an employee assistance program, adoption assistance, flexible spending accounts, pet insurance, domestic partner benefits, credit union membership and medical, dental, vision, prescription, life, AD&D and disability insurance.

FINANCIALS: Sales and profits are in thousands of dollars—add 000 to get the full amount. 2007 Note: Financial information for 2007 was not available for all companies at press time.

2007 Sales: $4,233,857	2007 Profits: $185,069	U.S. Stock Ticker: PETM
2006 Sales: $3,760,499	2006 Profits: $182,490	Int'l Ticker: Int'l Exchange:
2005 Sales: $3,363,452	2005 Profits: $171,228	Employees: 34,600
2004 Sales: $2,996,051	2004 Profits: $139,549	Fiscal Year Ends: 1/29
2003 Sales: $2,695,200	2003 Profits: $88,900	Parent Company:

SALARIES/BENEFITS:

Pension Plan:	ESOP Stock Plan:	Profit Sharing:	Top Exec. Salary: $905,769	Bonus: $783,490
Savings Plan: Y	Stock Purch. Plan: Y		Second Exec. Salary: $693,077	Bonus: $449,634

OTHER THOUGHTS:

Apparent Women Officers or Directors: 5
Hot Spot for Advancement for Women/Minorities: Y

LOCATIONS: ("Y" = Yes)

West:	Southwest:	Midwest:	Southeast:	Northeast:	International:
Y	Y	Y	Y	Y	Y

PFIZER INC
www.pfizer.com

Industry Group Code: 325412 Ranks within this company's industry group: Sales: Profits:

Management:		Sales/Marketing:		Liberal Arts:		Information Systems:		Professionals:		Technical/Scientific:	
Mgmt. Trainees:	Y	Mktg. Professionals:	Y	Gen. Writing/Editing:	Y	Info. Management:	Y	Finance/Accounting:	Y	Engineers, Elec.:	Y
Experienced Mgmt.:	Y	Retail Sales:		Technical Writing:	Y	Software Dev.:	Y	Law:	Y	Engineers, Other:	Y
Int'l Business:	Y	Commercial/Industrial:	Y	Graphic Arts/Photog.:	Y	Hardware Dev.:		HR/Other:	Y	Health/Lab:	Y
MBA Graduates:	Y	Sales Trainees:	Y	Music:		Systems Integration:		Training:	Y	Scientists/Research:	Y
		Advertising Pros.:	Y	Broadcasting:		Consulting/Other:		Health Care:	Y	Petroleum/Chemicals:	
				Other:				Consulting:		Math/Other:	Y

TYPES OF BUSINESS:
Pharmaceutical Drugs
Prescription Pharmaceuticals
Veterinary Pharmaceuticals
Gelatin Capsules Manufacturing
Contract Manufacturing
Bulk Pharmaceutical Chemicals

BRANDS/DIVISIONS/AFFILIATES:
Norvasc
Viagra
Zoloft
Revolution/Stronghold
Draxxin
Lipitor
Excede
Rimadyl

CONTACTS: *Note: Officers with more than one job title may be intentionally listed here more than once.*
Jeffrey B. Kindler, CEO
Frank D'Amelio, CFO
Mary McLeod, Sr. VP-Worldwide Human Resources
Martin Mackay, Pres., Pfizer Global R&D
Natale Ricciardi, Pres./Team Leader-Pfizer Global Mfg.
Allen Waxman, General Counsel
Sally Susman, Chief Comm. Officer/Sr. VP
Joe Feckzo, Chief Medical Officer
Corey Goodman, Pres., Biotherapeutics & Bioinnovation Center
Ian Read, Pres., Worldwide Pharmaceutical Oper.
Rich Bagger, Sr. VP-Worldwide Public Affairs & Policy
Jeffrey B. Kindler, Chmn.

Phone: 212-733-2323	Fax:
Toll-Free:	
Address: 235 E. 42nd St., New York, NY 10017 US	

GROWTH PLANS/SPECIAL FEATURES:
Pfizer, Inc. is a research-based, global pharmaceutical company. It discovers, develops, manufactures and markets prescription medicines for humans and animals. The company operates in two segments: pharmaceutical and animal health. The pharmaceutical business is one of the largest in the world. With medicines across 11 therapeutic areas, it helps to treat and prevent many of the most common conditions. The segment's products are in cardiovascular and metabolic diseases; central nervous system disorders; arthritis and pain; infectious and respiratory diseases; urology; oncology; ophthalmology; and endocrine disorders. Major pharmaceutical products include Lipitor, for the treatment of LDL-cholesterol levels in the blood; Norvasc, for treating hypertension; Zoloft, for the treatment of major depressive disorder, panic disorder, obsessive-compulsive disorder, post-traumatic stress disorder, premenstrual dysphoric disorder and social anxiety disorder; and Viagra, a treatment for erectile dysfunction. The animal health segment discovers, develops and sells products for the prevention and treatment of diseases in livestock and companion animals. Among the products it markets are parasiticides, anti-inflammatories, antibiotics, vaccines, atiemetics and anti-obesity agents. Products include Revolution/Stronghold, a parasiticide for dogs and cats; Rimadyl, an arthritis pain medication; and Draxxin, an antibiotic used to treat infections in dairy cows, beef cattle and swine. Pfizer also operates several other businesses, including the manufacture of gelatin capsules, contract manufacturing and bulk pharmaceutical chemicals. In early 2007, Pfizer announced it would eliminate 10,000 positions (10% of its workforce) over the next two years. Additionally, the firm plans to close up to five of its research laboratories. In early 2008, the company agreed to acquire Encysive Pharmaceuticals, Inc. and Serenex, Inc.

The firm offers its employees medical, dental and vision insurance; short- and long-term disability insurance; a savings and a retirement plan; life and business travel accident insurance; and tuition reimbursement.

FINANCIALS: Sales and profits are in thousands of dollars—add 000 to get the full amount. 2007 Note: Financial information for 2007 was not available for all companies at press time.

2007 Sales: $48,418,000	2007 Profits: $8,144,000	U.S. Stock Ticker: PFE
2006 Sales: $48,371,000	2006 Profits: $19,337,000	Int'l Ticker: Int'l Exchange:
2005 Sales: $47,405,000	2005 Profits: $8,085,000	Employees: 86,600
2004 Sales: $48,988,000	2004 Profits: $11,361,000	Fiscal Year Ends: 12/31
2003 Sales: $45,188,000	2003 Profits: $3,910,000	Parent Company:

SALARIES/BENEFITS:
Pension Plan: Y	ESOP Stock Plan:	Profit Sharing:	Top Exec. Salary: $2,270,500	Bonus: $
Savings Plan: Y	Stock Purch. Plan:		Second Exec. Salary: $1,220,300	Bonus: $1,383,000

OTHER THOUGHTS:
Apparent Women Officers or Directors: 4
Hot Spot for Advancement for Women/Minorities: Y

LOCATIONS: ("Y" = Yes)
West:	Southwest:	Midwest:	Southeast:	Northeast:	International:
Y	Y	Y	Y	Y	Y

PG&E CORPORATION

www.pgecorp.com

Industry Group Code: 221000 Ranks within this company's industry group: Sales: Profits:

Management:		Sales/Marketing:		Liberal Arts:		Information Systems:		Professionals:		Technical/Scientific:	
Mgmt. Trainees:	Y	Mktg. Professionals:	Y	Gen. Writing/Editing:	Y	Info. Management:	Y	Finance/Accounting:	Y	Engineers, Elec.:	Y
Experienced Mgmt.:	Y	Retail Sales:		Technical Writing:		Software Dev.:	Y	Law:	Y	Engineers, Other:	
Int'l Business:	Y	Commercial/Industrial:	Y	Graphic Arts/Photog.:		Hardware Dev.:		HR/Other:	Y	Health/Lab:	
MBA Graduates:	Y	Sales Trainees:		Music:		Systems Integration:		Training:	Y	Scientists/Research:	
		Advertising Pros.:	Y	Broadcasting:		Consulting/Other:		Health Care:		Petroleum/Chemicals:	
				Other:				Consulting:		Math/Other:	

TYPES OF BUSINESS:

Utilities-Electricity & Natural Gas
Energy Trading
Electricity Generation
Pipelines
Hydroelectric & Nuclear Generation
Natural Gas

BRANDS/DIVISIONS/AFFILIATES:

Pacific Gas and Electric Co.
Elm Power Corp.
PG&E Strategic Capital, Inc.

CONTACTS: Note: Officers with more than one job title may be intentionally listed here more than once.

Peter A. Darbee, CEO
Peter A. Darbee, Pres.
Christopher P. Johns, CFO/Sr. VP
John R. Simon, Sr. VP-Human Resources
Pat Lawicki, CIO/Sr. VP
Edward A. Salas, Sr. VP-Eng.
Hyun Park, General Counsel/Sr. VP
Edward A. Salas, Sr. VP-Oper.
Rand L. Rosenberg, Sr. VP-Corp. Strategy & Dev.
Nancy E. McFadden, Sr. VP-Public Affairs
Gabriel B. Togneri, VP-Investor Rel.
Christopher P. Johns, Treas.
Kent M. Harvey, Sr. VP-Chief Risk & Audit Officer
Greg S. Pruett, Sr. VP-Corp. Rel.
Linda Y.H. Cheng, VP-Corp. Governance/Corp. Sec.
Steven L. Kline, VP-Corp. Environmental & Federal Affairs
Peter A. Darbee, Chmn.

Phone: 415-267-7000	Fax: 415-267-7268
Toll-Free: 1-800-743-5000	
Address: 1 Market, Spear Tower, Ste. 2400, San Francisco, CA 94105 US	

GROWTH PLANS/SPECIAL FEATURES:

PG&E Corp. is a holding company that markets energy services and products in northern and central California through subsidiary Pacific Gas and Electric Co. The subsidiary is one of the largest electric and natural gas utilities in the U.S., serving roughly 5.1 million electric and 4.3 million natural gas customers. With over 140,684 circuit miles of distribution lines, the company's electricity distribution network extends through most of northern and central California. Additionally, the firm is interconnected with electric power systems in the Western Electricity Coordinating Council, which includes 14 western states, Alberta and British Columbia, Canada and parts of Mexico. Pacific owns and operates power plants producing nearly half of the power it sells, including 110 hydroelectric, two nuclear and four fossil fuel facilities. The company's hydroelectric generation system covers 16 counties in northern and central California. It includes 99 reservoirs, 56 diversions, 170 dams, 184 miles of canals, 44 miles of flumes, 135 miles of tunnels, 19 miles of pipe and 5 miles of natural waterways. The company's natural gas operations consist of an integrated transportation, storage and distribution system throughout 39 counties, including most of northern and central California. This system consists of 41,805 miles of distribution pipelines; over 6,300 miles of backbone and local transmission pipelines; and three storage facilities. Through interconnections with various interstate pipelines, the company receives gas from every major natural gas basin in western North America, including basins in Canada and the southwestern U.S. In December 2007, the company entered into a letter of intent to acquire a 25.5% interest in El Paso's Ruby Pipeline project.

The company offers employees medical, dental and vision insurance; supplemental life insurance; health care and dependent care reimbursement accounts; 401(k); adoption reimbursement; and tuition refund opportunities.

FINANCIALS: Sales and profits are in thousands of dollars—add 000 to get the full amount. 2007 Note: Financial information for 2007 was not available for all companies at press time.

2007 Sales: $13,237,000	2007 Profits: $1,006,000	U.S. Stock Ticker: PCG
2006 Sales: $12,539,000	2006 Profits: $2,108,000	Int'l Ticker: Int'l Exchange:
2005 Sales: $11,703,000	2005 Profits: $1,970,000	Employees: 20,200
2004 Sales: $11,080,000	2004 Profits: $7,118,000	Fiscal Year Ends: 12/31
2003 Sales: $10,435,000	2003 Profits: $420,000	Parent Company:

SALARIES/BENEFITS:

Pension Plan: Y	ESOP Stock Plan:	Profit Sharing:	Top Exec. Salary: $975,000	Bonus: $1,485,900
Savings Plan: Y	Stock Purch. Plan:		Second Exec. Salary: $615,000	Bonus: $702,945

OTHER THOUGHTS:

Apparent Women Officers or Directors: 7
Hot Spot for Advancement for Women/Minorities: Y

LOCATIONS: ("Y" = Yes)

West:	Southwest:	Midwest:	Southeast:	Northeast:	International:
Y					

PHARMACEUTICAL PRODUCT DEVELOPMENT INC
www.ppdi.com

Industry Group Code: 541710 Ranks within this company's industry group: Sales: 3 Profits: 1

Management:		Sales/Marketing:		Liberal Arts:		Information Systems:		Professionals:		Technical/Scientific:	
Mgmt. Trainees:	Y	Mktg. Professionals:	Y	Gen. Writing/Editing:		Info. Management:	Y	Finance/Accounting:	Y	Engineers, Elec.:	Y
Experienced Mgmt.:	Y	Retail Sales:		Technical Writing:	Y	Software Dev.:	Y	Law:	Y	Engineers, Other:	Y
Int'l Business:	Y	Commercial/Industrial:	Y	Graphic Arts/Photog.:	Y	Hardware Dev.:		HR/Other:	Y	Health/Lab:	Y
MBA Graduates:	Y	Sales Trainees:		Music:		Systems Integration:	Y	Training:	Y	Scientists/Research:	Y
		Advertising Pros.:		Broadcasting:		Consulting/Other:	Y	Health Care:	Y	Petroleum/Chemicals:	
				Other:				Consulting:	Y	Math/Other:	Y

TYPES OF BUSINESS:
Contract Research
Drug Discovery & Development Services
Clinical Data Consulting Services
Medical Marketing & Information Support Services
Drug Development Software
Medical Device Development

BRANDS/DIVISIONS/AFFILIATES:
PPD Discovery
PPD Development
CSS Informatics
PPD Medical Communications
PPD Virtual
Nimbus Partners
Peking Union Lawke Biomedical Development, Ltd.
InnoPharm, Ltd.

CONTACTS: Note: Officers with more than one job title may be intentionally listed here more than once.
Fred N. Eshelman, CEO
William Sharbaugh, COO
Daniel Darazsdi, CFO
Susan Atkinson, Sr. VP-Data Mgmt. & Global Biostatistics
Paul S. Covington, Exec. VP-Dev.
Judd Hartman, General Counsel/Corp. Sec.
William Richardson, Sr. VP-Global Bus. Dev.
Sue Ann Pentecost, Mgr.-Corp. Comm.
Craig Eastwood, Dir.-Investor Rel.
Simon Britton, VP-Asia
Louise Caudle, Dir.-Corp. Comm.
Philip Mathew, Dir.-Strategic Dev.
Paul Colvin, Sr. VP-North America
Ernest Mario, Chmn.
Sebastian Pacios, Sr. VP-EMEA

Phone: 910-251-0081	Fax: 910-762-5820
Toll-Free:	
Address: 929 N. Front St., Wilmington, NC 28401 US	

GROWTH PLANS/SPECIAL FEATURES:
Pharmaceutical Product Development, Inc. (PPD) provides drug discovery and development services to pharmaceutical and biotechnology companies as well as academic and government organizations. PPD's services are primarily divided into two company segments: PPD Discovery and PPD Development. Through the combined services of these segments, PPD helps pharmaceutical companies through all stages of clinical testing. The stages of testing can be specifically divided into preclinical, phase I, phase II-IIIb and post-approval. In the preclinical stages of drug testing, PPD provides information concerning the pharmaceutical composition of a new drug, its safety, its formulaic design and how it will be administered to children and adults. During phase I of testing, PPD conducts healthy volunteer clinics, provides data management services and guides companies/laboratories through regulatory affairs. In phase II and III tests, PPD oversees the later stages of product development and government approval, providing project management and clinical monitoring. In the post-approval stage of a drug's development, PPD provides technology and marketing services aimed to maximize the new drug's lifecycle. PPD has experience conducting research and drug development in the areas of antiviral studies, cardiovascular diseases, critical care studies, endocrine/metabolic studies, vaccine development, hematology/oncology studies, immunology studies and ophthalmology studies. The firm conducts regional, national and global studies and research projects through offices in 30 countries worldwide. In early 2008, PPD signed an agreement to acquire InnoPharm, Ltd., an independent contract research company based in Russia. The firm's data management consulting division, CSS Informatics, entered an agreement with Nimbus Partners. The division will use Nimbus' Control 2007 software to expand its client services. In 2007, PPD opened a new facility in Lanarkshire, Scotland, and expanded its central lab services into China through an agreement with Peking Union Lawke Biomedical Development, Ltd. The firm also opened offices in Greece, Australia, Denmark, Peru and Portugal.

FINANCIALS: Sales and profits are in thousands of dollars—add 000 to get the full amount. 2007 Note: Financial information for 2007 was not available for all companies at press time.

2007 Sales: $1,414,465	2007 Profits: $163,401	U.S. Stock Ticker: PPDI
2006 Sales: $1,247,682	2006 Profits: $156,652	Int'l Ticker: Int'l Exchange:
2005 Sales: $1,037,090	2005 Profits: $119,897	Employees: 10,200
2004 Sales: $841,256	2004 Profits: $91,684	Fiscal Year Ends: 12/31
2003 Sales: $726,983	2003 Profits: $46,310	Parent Company:

SALARIES/BENEFITS:

Pension Plan:	ESOP Stock Plan:	Profit Sharing:	Top Exec. Salary: $689,167	Bonus: $250,000
Savings Plan: Y	Stock Purch. Plan:		Second Exec. Salary: $357,253	Bonus: $100,000

OTHER THOUGHTS:
Apparent Women Officers or Directors: 3
Hot Spot for Advancement for Women/Minorities: Y

LOCATIONS: ("Y" = Yes)

West:	Southwest:	Midwest:	Southeast:	Northeast:	International:
Y	Y	Y	Y	Y	Y

PITNEY BOWES INC

www.pb.com

Industry Group Code: 333313 Ranks within this company's industry group: Sales: 1 Profits: 1

Management:		Sales/Marketing:		Liberal Arts:		Information Systems:		Professionals:		Technical/Scientific:	
Mgmt. Trainees:	Y	Mktg. Professionals:	Y	Gen. Writing/Editing:	Y	Info. Management:	Y	Finance/Accounting:	Y	Engineers, Elec.:	Y
Experienced Mgmt.:	Y	Retail Sales:		Technical Writing:	Y	Software Dev.:	Y	Law:	Y	Engineers, Other:	Y
Int'l Business:	Y	Commercial/Industrial:	Y	Graphic Arts/Photog.:	Y	Hardware Dev.:	Y	HR/Other:	Y	Health/Lab:	
MBA Graduates:	Y	Sales Trainees:	Y	Music:		Systems Integration:		Training:	Y	Scientists/Research:	
		Advertising Pros.:	Y	Broadcasting:		Consulting/Other:		Health Care:		Petroleum/Chemicals:	
				Other:				Consulting:		Math/Other:	

TYPES OF BUSINESS:

Business Machines-Mail and Messaging
Business Equipment
Outsourced Services

BRANDS/DIVISIONS/AFFILIATES:

Global Business Services
MapInfo Corp.
Global Mailstream Solutions
Pitney Bowes Legal Solutions
Axciom France
Encom Holdings Pty Ltd.
Asterion SAS
Group 1 Software, Inc.

CONTACTS: Note: Officers with more than one job title may be intentionally listed here more than once.

Murray D. Martin, CEO
Murray D. Martin, Pres.
Bruce P. Nolop, CFO/Exec. VP
Mark Cattini, Pres., Pitney Bowes Mktg. Svcs.
Johnna G. Torsone, Chief Human Resources Officer/Sr. VP
Gregory E. Buoncontri, CIO/Sr. VP
Joseph E. Wall, CTO/Sr. VP
Amy C. Corn, Sec./VP
Juanita T. James, Chief Comm. Officer/VP
Charles F. McBride, VP-Investor Rel.
Steven J. Green, Chief Acct. Officer/VP-Finance
Leslie Abi-Karam, Exec. VP/Pres., Document Messaging Tech.
Elise R. DeBois, Exec. VP/Pres., Global Financial Svcs.
Amy C. Corn, VP-Chief Governance Officer
Helen Shan, VP/Treas.
Michael J. Critelli, Exec. Chmn.
Patrick Keddy, Exec. VP/Pres., Mailstream Int'l
Neil Metviner, Exec. VP/Pres., Global Small Bus. & Supplies

Phone: 203-356-5000	Fax: 203-351-6858
Toll-Free: 800-672-6937	
Address: 1 Elmcroft Rd., Stamford, CT 06926-0700 US	

GROWTH PLANS/SPECIAL FEATURES:

Pitney Bowes, Inc. is a global provider of informed mail and messaging management for corporations and businesses of all sizes. The company has recently revised its business segments into three units: the Global Mailstream Solutions Segment, Global Business Services Segment and the Capital Services Segment. The Global Mailstream Solutions Segment includes the sales, rental and financing of production mail and inserting equipment, mail finishing, mail creation and shipping equipment, related supplies and maintenance services, mailing and customer communication software, postal payment solutions and small business solutions. The Global Business Services Segment includes advanced mailing, secure mail services, reprographic, document management and other value-added services in the Global Management Services segment, as well as presort mail services, international outbound mail services and direct mail marketing services in its Mail Services segment. In April 2007, the firm completed the acquisition of MapInfo Corp., a location intelligence company. Pitney Bowes acquired two other location intelligence software companies, Encom Holdings Pty Ltd. and Acxiom France, as well as Asterion SAS, a provider of transactional print and document process services. The firm also acquired Digital Cement Inc., a professional services firm that assists companies in maintaining and growing customer relationships. In November 2007, the firm announced that it would cut roughly 1,500 jobs as part of a cost-cutting plan, and that an additional 170 jobs would be moved to the Pitney Bowes Software facility in Troy, New York.

Pitney Bowes offers employees a health and wellness program, disability and life insurance, and tuition reimbursement.

FINANCIALS: Sales and profits are in thousands of dollars—add 000 to get the full amount. 2007 Note: Financial information for 2007 was not available for all companies at press time.

2007 Sales: $6,129,795	2007 Profits: $366,781	U.S. Stock Ticker: PBI
2006 Sales: $5,730,018	2006 Profits: $105,347	Int'l Ticker: Int'l Exchange:
2005 Sales: $5,366,936	2005 Profits: $508,611	Employees: 26,267
2004 Sales: $4,832,304	2004 Profits: $461,996	Fiscal Year Ends: 12/31
2003 Sales: $4,576,853	2003 Profits: $498,117	Parent Company:

SALARIES/BENEFITS:

Pension Plan:	ESOP Stock Plan:	Profit Sharing:	Top Exec. Salary: $1,032,500	Bonus: $4,714,044
Savings Plan: Y	Stock Purch. Plan:		Second Exec. Salary: $741,667	Bonus: $2,152,500

OTHER THOUGHTS:

Apparent Women Officers or Directors: 8
Hot Spot for Advancement for Women/Minorities: Y

LOCATIONS: ("Y" = Yes)

West:	Southwest:	Midwest:	Southeast:	Northeast:	International:
Y	Y	Y	Y	Y	Y

Note: Financial information, benefits and other data can change quickly and may vary from those stated here.

PLANTRONICS INC
www.plantronics.com

Industry Group Code: 334200 Ranks within this company's industry group: Sales: 3 Profits: 3

Management:		Sales/Marketing:		Liberal Arts:		Information Systems:		Professionals:		Technical/Scientific:	
Mgmt. Trainees:	Y	Mktg. Professionals:	Y	Gen. Writing/Editing:		Info. Management:	Y	Finance/Accounting:	Y	Engineers, Elec.:	Y
Experienced Mgmt.:	Y	Retail Sales:		Technical Writing:	Y	Software Dev.:	Y	Law:	Y	Engineers, Other:	
Int'l Business:	Y	Commercial/Industrial:	Y	Graphic Arts/Photog.:	Y	Hardware Dev.:	Y	HR/Other:	Y	Health/Lab:	Y
MBA Graduates:	Y	Sales Trainees:		Music:		Systems Integration:		Training:	Y	Scientists/Research:	Y
		Advertising Pros.:	Y	Broadcasting:		Consulting/Other:		Health Care:		Petroleum/Chemicals:	
				Other:				Consulting:		Math/Other:	Y

TYPES OF BUSINESS:
Communications Headsets
Communications Accessories
Specialty Telephone Products
Wireless Headsets

BRANDS/DIVISIONS/AFFILIATES:
Clarity
Volume Logic
Altec Lansing

CONTACTS: Note: Officers with more than one job title may be intentionally listed here more than once.
Ken Kannappan, CEO
Ken Kannappan, Pres.
Barbara Scherer, CFO/Sr. VP
Clay Hausmann, VP-Corp. Mktg.
Owen Brown, CTO/VP
Jim Sotelo, VP-Prod. Dev. & Tech.
Barbara Scherer, Sr. VP-Admin.
Larry Wuerz, Sr. VP-Worldwide Oper.
Barry Margerum, VP-Strategy & Bus. Dev.
Jennifer Shanks, Dir.-Public Rel.
Barbara Scherer, Sr. VP-Finance
Donald Houston, Sr. VP-Sales
Renee Niemi, VP/General Mgr.-Mobile & Entertainment
Joyce Shimizu, VP/General Mgr.-Home & Home Office
Carsten Trads, Pres., Clarity Div.
Marvin Tseu, Chmn.
Philip Vanhoutte, Managing Dir.-EMEA

Phone: 831-426-5858	Fax: 831-426-6098
Toll-Free: 800-544-4660	
Address: 345 Encinal St., Santa Cruz, CA 95060 US	

GROWTH PLANS/SPECIAL FEATURES:
Plantronics, Inc. is a worldwide designer, manufacturer and marketer of lightweight communications headsets, telephone headset systems and accessories for the business and consumer markets under the Plantronics brand. The company is organized in two segments: The audio entertainment group (AEG) and the audio communications group (ACG). The AEG segment, the firm's core business, designs, manufactures, markets and sells headsets for business and consumer applications and other specialty products. The segment also designs, manufactures, sells and markets audio solutions and related technologies. Plantronics manufactures and markets computer and home entertainment sound systems; docking audio products; and a line of headsets and headphones for personal digital media under Altec Landing brand. In addition, the company manufactures and markets under the Clarity brand specialty telephone products, such as telephones for the hearing impaired and other related products for people with special communicated needs. The firm also provides audio enhancement solutions to consumers, audio professionals and businesses under the Volume Logic brand. The company ships a broad range of communications products to over 70 countries through a worldwide network of distributors, retailers, wireless carriers, original equipment manufacturers (OEMs) and telephony service providers. The firm has well-developed distribution channels in North America, Europe, Australia and New Zeeland. In 2007, the company announced a reorganization of its Asia-Pacific operations that include the close of a manufacturing facility in Dongguan, China and a corporate office in Hong Kong. Additionally, it plans two consolidations which include the joining of its procurement, research and development activities for AEG within a new Shenzhen, China site, and its selling, general and administrative functions of AEG with ACG throughout the region.

Plantronics offers its employees medical, dental and vision insurance; a 401(k) plan; life insurance; an employee stock purchase plan; an employee assistance plan; and access to a credit union.

FINANCIALS: Sales and profits are in thousands of dollars—add 000 to get the full amount. 2007 Note: Financial information for 2007 was not available for all companies at press time.

2007 Sales: $800,154	2007 Profits: $50,143	U.S. Stock Ticker: PLT
2006 Sales: $750,394	2006 Profits: $81,150	Int'l Ticker: Int'l Exchange:
2005 Sales: $559,995	2005 Profits: $97,520	Employees: 6,000
2004 Sales: $417,000	2004 Profits: $62,300	Fiscal Year Ends: 3/31
2003 Sales: $337,508	2003 Profits: $41,476	Parent Company:

SALARIES/BENEFITS:

Pension Plan:	ESOP Stock Plan:	Profit Sharing:	Top Exec. Salary: $550,001	Bonus: $147,013
Savings Plan: Y	Stock Purch. Plan: Y		Second Exec. Salary: $305,332	Bonus: $121,758

OTHER THOUGHTS:
Apparent Women Officers or Directors: 5
Hot Spot for Advancement for Women/Minorities: Y

LOCATIONS: ("Y" = Yes)

West:	Southwest:	Midwest:	Southeast:	Northeast:	International:
Y					Y

PLEXUS CORP

www.plexus.com

Industry Group Code: 334419 Ranks within this company's industry group: Sales: 3   Profits: 3

Management:		Sales/Marketing:		Liberal Arts:		Information Systems:		Professionals:		Technical/Scientific:	
Mgmt. Trainees:	Y	Mktg. Professionals:	Y	Gen. Writing/Editing:		Info. Management:	Y	Finance/Accounting:	Y	Engineers, Elec.:	Y
Experienced Mgmt.:	Y	Retail Sales:		Technical Writing:	Y	Software Dev.:	Y	Law:	Y	Engineers, Other:	Y
Int'l Business:	Y	Commercial/Industrial:	Y	Graphic Arts/Photog.:		Hardware Dev.:	Y	HR/Other:	Y	Health/Lab:	
MBA Graduates:	Y	Sales Trainees:		Music:		Systems Integration:	Y	Training:	Y	Scientists/Research:	
		Advertising Pros.:	Y	Broadcasting:		Consulting/Other:		Health Care:		Petroleum/Chemicals:	
				Other:				Consulting:		Math/Other:	

TYPES OF BUSINESS:

Contract Manufacturing-Diversified Electronics
Hardware & Software Design
Printed Circuit Board Design
Prototyping Services
Material Procurement & Management

BRANDS/DIVISIONS/AFFILIATES:

CONTACTS: *Note: Officers with more than one job title may be intentionally listed here more than once.*

Dean Foate, CEO
Paul Ehlers, COO/Exec. VP
Dean Foate, Pres.
Ginger M. Jones, CFO/VP
Kristian Talvitie, VP-Mktg. & Branding
David Rust, VP-Human Resources
Tom Czajkowski, CIO/VP
Bob Kronser, CTO/Exec. VP
Angelo Ninivaggi, General Counsel/Sec.
Bob Kronser, Chief Strategy Officer
Kristian Talvitie, VP-Corp. Comm.
George Setton, Corp. Treas./Chief Treasury Officer
David A. Clark, VP-Materials, Plexus Electronic Assembly
Michael Verstegen, VP/Pres., Tech. Group
Simon J. Painter, Corp. Controller/Chief Acct. Officer
Y. J. Lim, Pres., Asia-Pacific
John L. Nussbaum, Chmn.
Michael Verstegen, Sr. VP-Global Market Dev.
David A. Clark, VP-Supply Chain

Phone: 920-722-3451	Fax: 920-751-5395
Toll-Free:	
Address: 55 Jewelers Park Dr., Neenah, WI 54957-0156 US	

GROWTH PLANS/SPECIAL FEATURES:

Plexus Corp. is a leading global provider of electronics manufacturing services.   The company's customers may outsource all stages of the product realization process, including development and design, materials procurement and management, prototyping and new product introduction, testing, manufacturing configuration, logistics and repair. Increasingly, the company is providing its customers with fulfillment and logistics services including Direct Order Fulfilment, Build to Order and Configure to Order.   Plexus offers a complete menu of engineering services, including digital and analog design, mechanical and industrial design, embedded software design, printed circuit board design, test equipment and software development, product verification and new product introduction services.   Throughout the production process, Plexus offers logistics services such as materials procurement, inventory management, packaging and distribution. Plexus serves companies from industries including wireline/networking, 38% net sales; medical, 26%; industrial/commercial, 18%; defense/security/aerospace, 9%; and wireless infrastructure, 9%. Plexus has no proprietary products, although its product realization services have created complex, high-tech products for large original equipment manfacturers and start-ups. The firm's customer service is provided to over 120 customers in North America, Europe and Asia.   The company's 10 largest customers accounted for roughly 59% of net sales. Of these, Juniper Networks, Inc. and General Electric Corp. (GE) respectively accounted for 19% and 12%. At the beginning of 2007, Plexus had 18 active facilities in 14 locations in Malaysia, Mexico, China, the U.K. and the U.S. Facilities representing approximately 70% of net sales run on a common enterprise resource planning platform.

Plexus offers its employees an interest-free computer loan program, medical and dental insurance, a 401(k) plan, flexible spending accounts, tuition reimbursement and an employee assistance program.

FINANCIALS: Sales and profits are in thousands of dollars—add 000 to get the full amount. 2007 Note: Financial information for 2007 was not available for all companies at press time.

2007 Sales: $1,546,264	2007 Profits: $65,718	U.S. Stock Ticker: PLXS
2006 Sales: $1,460,557	2006 Profits: $100,025	Int'l Ticker: Int'l Exchange:
2005 Sales: $1,228,882	2005 Profits: $-12,417	Employees: 7,500
2004 Sales: $1,040,858	2004 Profits: $-31,580	Fiscal Year Ends: 9/30
2003 Sales: $807,837	2003 Profits: $-67,978	Parent Company:

SALARIES/BENEFITS:

Pension Plan:	ESOP Stock Plan:	Profit Sharing:	Top Exec. Salary: $528,846	Bonus: $835,218
Savings Plan: Y	Stock Purch. Plan: Y		Second Exec. Salary: $310,577	Bonus: $305,816

OTHER THOUGHTS:

Apparent Women Officers or Directors: 1
Hot Spot for Advancement for Women/Minorities:

LOCATIONS: ("Y" = Yes)

West:	Southwest:	Midwest:	Southeast:	Northeast:	International:
Y		Y	Y	Y	Y

POLO RALPH LAUREN CORP
www.polo.com

Industry Group Code: 315000 Ranks within this company's industry group: Sales: 1   Profits: 1

Management:		Sales/Marketing:		Liberal Arts:		Information Systems:		Professionals:		Technical/Scientific:	
Mgmt. Trainees:	Y	Mktg. Professionals:	Y	Gen. Writing/Editing:	Y	Info. Management:	Y	Finance/Accounting:	Y	Engineers, Elec.:	
Experienced Mgmt.:	Y	Retail Sales:	Y	Technical Writing:		Software Dev.:		Law:	Y	Engineers, Other:	
Int'l Business:	Y	Commercial/Industrial:	Y	Graphic Arts/Photog.:	Y	Hardware Dev.:		HR/Other:	Y	Health/Lab:	
MBA Graduates:	Y	Sales Trainees:	Y	Music:		Systems Integration:		Training:	Y	Scientists/Research:	
		Advertising Pros.:	Y	Broadcasting:		Consulting/Other:		Health Care:		Petroleum/Chemicals:	
				Other:	Y			Consulting:		Math/Other:	

TYPES OF BUSINESS:
Men's & Women's Branded Fashions
Apparel Design & Marketing
Accessories
Fragrances
Home Furnishings
Cosmetics
Retail Stores

BRANDS/DIVISIONS/AFFILIATES:
Polo
Ralph Lauren
Club Monaco
American Living
Chaps
Caban
Rugby
Polo.com

CONTACTS: *Note: Officers with more than one job title may be intentionally listed here more than once.*
Ralph Lauren, CEO
Roger N. Farah, COO
Roger N. Farah, Pres.
Tracy Travis, CFO/Sr. VP-Finance
Mitchell A. Kosh, Sr. VP-Human Resources
Ryan Lally, Dir.-Corp. Comm.
Jackwyn L. Nemerov, Exec. VP
Wayne Meichner, COO/Pres.-Polo Retail Group
Susie Coulter, Pres., Polo Ralph Lauren Retail Stores
Ralph Lauren, Chmn.

Phone: 212-318-7000	Fax: 212-888-5780
Toll-Free: 800-377-7656	
Address: 650 Madison Ave., New York, NY 10022 US	

GROWTH PLANS/SPECIAL FEATURES:
Polo Ralph Lauren Corporation (Polo) is a leader in the design, marketing and distribution of premium lifestyle products. Over the past 30 years, the firm has expanded its line of clothing, accessories, fragrances and home furnishings into worldwide markets. Polo licenses the manufacturing of its products to companies worldwide. Capitalizing on the creative force of its founder, Ralph Lauren, the firm's various brand names have become recognizable cultural symbols across the globe. The firm offers four categories of lifestyle products: Apparel products (including extensive collections of men's, women's and children's clothing); home products (including bedding and bath products, furniture, fabric, wallpaper, paints, tabletop and giftware); accessories (including footwear, eyewear, jewelry, leather goods, handbags and luggage); and fragrance products (consisting of fragrances and skin care products and sold under the Glamorous, Romance, Polo, Lauren, Safari, Blue Label, Black Label, and Polo Sport brands, among others). The company markets its products through department, specialty, golf and Polo Ralph Lauren stores, as well as via the Internet and mail order catalogs. It currently operates 147 full price stores including Ralph Lauren, Caban and Rugby stores; and 10,600 shop-within-shops. The company formed Ralph Lauren Media in a joint venture with NBC in order to reach consumers through various media outlets, including the Internet, television, cable and print. Its first initiative was the creation of Polo.com, a web site that brings products and information to consumers in an online magazine format.

FINANCIALS: Sales and profits are in thousands of dollars—add 000 to get the full amount. 2007 Note: Financial information for 2007 was not available for all companies at press time.

			U.S. Stock Ticker: RL	
2007 Sales: $4,295,400	2007 Profits: $400,900		Int'l Ticker: Int'l Exchange:	
2006 Sales: $3,746,300	2006 Profits: $308,000		Employees: 14,000	
2005 Sales: $3,305,415	2005 Profits: $190,425		Fiscal Year Ends: 3/28	
2004 Sales: $2,380,844	2004 Profits: $170,954		Parent Company:	
2003 Sales: $2,439,300	2003 Profits: $174,200			

SALARIES/BENEFITS:
Pension Plan:	ESOP Stock Plan:	Profit Sharing:	Top Exec. Salary: $1,000,000	Bonus: $16,500,000
Savings Plan:	Stock Purch. Plan:		Second Exec. Salary: $900,000	Bonus: $2,970,000

OTHER THOUGHTS:
Apparent Women Officers or Directors: 2
Hot Spot for Advancement for Women/Minorities: Y

LOCATIONS: ("Y" = Yes)
West:	Southwest:	Midwest:	Southeast:	Northeast:	International:
Y	Y	Y	Y	Y	Y

PRAXAIR INC

www.praxair.com

Industry Group Code: 325120 **Ranks within this company's industry group:** Sales: 2   Profits: 1

Management:		Sales/Marketing:		Liberal Arts:		Information Systems:		Professionals:		Technical/Scientific:	
Mgmt. Trainees:	Y	Mktg. Professionals:	Y	Gen. Writing/Editing:		Info. Management:	Y	Finance/Accounting:	Y	Engineers, Elec.:	Y
Experienced Mgmt.:	Y	Retail Sales:		Technical Writing:	Y	Software Dev.:		Law:	Y	Engineers, Other:	
Int'l Business:	Y	Commercial/Industrial:	Y	Graphic Arts/Photog.:		Hardware Dev.:		HR/Other:	Y	Health/Lab:	Y
MBA Graduates:	Y	Sales Trainees:		Music:		Systems Integration:		Training:	Y	Scientists/Research:	Y
		Advertising Pros.:	Y	Broadcasting:		Consulting/Other:		Health Care:		Petroleum/Chemicals:	Y
				Other:				Consulting:		Math/Other:	

TYPES OF BUSINESS:

Industrial Gases
Atmospheric & Process Gases
Coatings & Powders
On-Site Production Plants
Distribution

BRANDS/DIVISIONS/AFFILIATES:

Praxair Distribution, Inc.
Wilson Welding & Medical Gases
Praair Surface Technologies, Inc.

CONTACTS: *Note: Officers with more than one job title may be intentionally listed here more than once.*

Stephen F. Angel, CEO
Stephen F. Angel, Pres.
James S. Sawyer, CFO/Exec. VP
Sunil Mattoo, VP-Mktg.
Sally A. Savoia, VP-Human Resources
Melissa Buckwalter, CIO/VP-Financial Svcs.
Steven L. Lerner, CTO/Sr. VP
James T. Breedlove, General Counsel/Sr. VP/Sec.
Richard P. Kenny, VP-Global Oper.
Sunil Mattoo, VP-Strategic Planning
Nigel D. Muir, VP-Comm. & Public Rel.
Elizabeth T. Hirsch, Dir.-Investor Rel.
Patrick M. Clark, Controller/VP
Ricardo S. Malfitano, Exec. VP
Michael J. Allan, VP/Treas.
Domingos Bulus, Pres., Praxair South America
Murray G. Covello, Pres., Praxair Asia
Stephen F. Angel, Chmn.
Eduardo Menezes, Pres., Europe

Phone: 716-879-4077	Fax: 716-879-2040
Toll-Free: 800-772-9247	
Address: 39 Old Ridgebury Rd., Danbury, CT 06810 US	

GROWTH PLANS/SPECIAL FEATURES:

Praxair, Inc. is an industrial gas supplier in North and South America, Asia and Europe. Praxair's primary products are atmospheric gases, which include oxygen, nitrogen, argon and rare gases, and process gases, which include carbon dioxide, helium, hydrogen, electronic gases, specialty gases and acetylene. Praxair serves industries such as aerospace, food and beverages, healthcare, semiconductors, chemicals and refining, as well as other areas of general industry. The company also designs, engineers, and builds equipment that produces industrial gases for internal use and external sale. In 2007, 94% of sales were generated in four regional segments (North America, Europe, South America and Asia) primarily from the sale of industrial gases with the balance generated from the surface technologies segment. Atmospheric gases are the highest volume products produced by Praxair. Using air as its raw material, Praxair produces oxygen, nitrogen and argon through several air separation processes of which cryogenic air separation is the most prevalent. Process gases, including carbon dioxide, hydrogen, carbon monoxide, helium and acetylene are produced by methods other than air separation. Praxair uses three distribution methods for industrial gases: On-site or tonnage; merchant liquid; and packaged or cylinder gases. Through its subsidiary Praxair Surface Technologies, the company supplies wear-resistant and high-temperature corrosion-resistant metallic and ceramic coatings and powders to the aircraft, printing, textile, plastics, primary metals and petrochemical industries. It also manufactures a complete line of electric arc, plasma and high-velocity oxygen fuel spray equipment, as well as arc and flame wire equipment used for the application of wear resistant coatings. In March 2008, Beijing Praxair Inc., an affiliate of Praxair China, signed an oxygen supply contract with Beijing Drainage Group Co., Ltd to be the exclusive supplier of oxygen to three wastewater treatment plants in Beijing for the 2008 Beijing Olympic Games.

FINANCIALS: Sales and profits are in thousands of dollars—add 000 to get the full amount. 2007 Note: Financial information for 2007 was not available for all companies at press time.

2007 Sales: $9,402,000	2007 Profits: $1,177,000	**U.S. Stock Ticker:** PX
2006 Sales: $8,324,000	2006 Profits: $988,000	**Int'l Ticker:** Int'l Exchange:
2005 Sales: $7,656,000	2005 Profits: $726,000	Employees: 27,992
2004 Sales: $6,594,000	2004 Profits: $697,000	Fiscal Year Ends: 12/31
2003 Sales: $5,613,000	2003 Profits: $585,000	Parent Company:

SALARIES/BENEFITS:

Pension Plan:	ESOP Stock Plan:	Profit Sharing:	Top Exec. Salary: $1,000,000	Bonus: $2,800,000
Savings Plan:	Stock Purch. Plan:		Second Exec. Salary: $550,000	Bonus: $1,029,600

OTHER THOUGHTS:

Apparent Women Officers or Directors: 2
Hot Spot for Advancement for Women/Minorities: Y

LOCATIONS: ("Y" = Yes)

West:	Southwest:	Midwest:	Southeast:	Northeast:	International:
				Y	Y

PRICEWATERHOUSECOOPERS   www.pwcglobal.com

Industry Group Code: 541210 Ranks within this company's industry group: Sales: 1 Profits:

Management:		Sales/Marketing:		Liberal Arts:		Information Systems:		Professionals:		Technical/Scientific:	
Mgmt. Trainees:	Y	Mktg. Professionals:	Y	Gen. Writing/Editing:	Y	Info. Management:	Y	Finance/Accounting:	Y	Engineers, Elec.:	
Experienced Mgmt.:	Y	Retail Sales:		Technical Writing:	Y	Software Dev.:	Y	Law:	Y	Engineers, Other:	
Int'l Business:	Y	Commercial/Industrial:	Y	Graphic Arts/Photog.:	Y	Hardware Dev.:		HR/Other:	Y	Health/Lab:	
MBA Graduates:	Y	Sales Trainees:		Music:		Systems Integration:	Y	Training:	Y	Scientists/Research:	Y
		Advertising Pros.:	Y	Broadcasting:		Consulting/Other:	Y	Health Care:		Petroleum/Chemicals:	
				Other:				Consulting:	Y	Math/Other:	Y

TYPES OF BUSINESS:
Accounting Services
Business Advisory
Corporate Finance Services
Employee Benefits Services
Tax Services
Business Publications

BRANDS/DIVISIONS/AFFILIATES:
PricewaterhouseCoopers, LLP
XPRL
Global VATOnline
Global Best Practices
CFOdirect Network
Comperio

CONTACTS: *Note: Officers with more than one job title may be intentionally listed here more than once.*
Samuel DiPiazza, Jr., CEO
Richard Baird, Global Human Capital Leader
Javier H. Rubinstein, General Counsel
Paul Boorman, Global Managing Partner-Oper. & Markets
Mike Kubena, CEO-PwC Central & Eastern Europe
Robert Ward, VP-Global Assurance
Gene Donnelly, Global Managing Partner-Advisory & Tax
Alec Jones, VP-Global Industries
Gautam Banerjee, Exec. Chmn./Sr. Partner-Singapore
Chris Clark, Sr. Partner/CEO-PricewaterhouseCoopers Canada LLP

Phone: 646-471-4000	Fax: 646-471-4444
Toll-Free:	
Address: 300 Madison Ave., Fl. 24, New York, NY 10017 US	

GROWTH PLANS/SPECIAL FEATURES:
PricewaterhouseCoopers (PwC) is a global accounting firm with offices in 148 countries. Locations of PwC offices include Africa, the Americas, Asia/Asia Pacific, Europe and the Middle East. PwC provides accounting and advisory services to a large number of mid-sized and small companies and caters to about 80% of Fortune magazine's Global 500 companies in 29 different industries, which includes aerospace and defense; banking and capital markets; forest, paper and packaging; government/public services; health care; and telecommunications. The firm provides industry-focused services for public and private clients primarily in six areas: audit and assurance; crisis management; human resources; performance improvement; tax; and transactions. Audit and assurance provides financial statement audits, regulatory and Sarbanes-Oxley compliance and financial accounting while the crisis management sector offers business recovery services with dispute analysis and investigations. Human resource services include employee communications, international assignment solutions and retirement benefits services. The performance improvement sector provides financial, IT, government and risk and compliance services and tax services for business compliance, mergers and acquisitions and global tax structuring. Lastly, transactions services are offered for accounting valuations and modeling and business planning. PwC also produces a number of publications that provide authoritative information on better business practices and emerging issues facing management and breaking trends in the business world. Online services offered by the company include CFOdirect Network, Comperio, Global Best Practices, Global VATOnline and XBRL. In 2007, Ambit RSM, a well established financial firm in India, merged its tax practice into PricewaterhouseCoopers'. Operating under the PricewaterhouseCoopers brand, the affiliate now encompasses approximately 4,000 people across different offices in India.

The company offers employees mortgage and insurance plans and additional benefits for child care and working mothers. Additionally, the company organizes an annual International Leadership Summit, which is a five-day program of business case studies for top international students.

FINANCIALS: Sales and profits are in thousands of dollars—add 000 to get the full amount. 2007 Note: Financial information for 2007 was not available for all companies at press time.
2007 Sales: $25,150,000	2007 Profits: $	U.S. Stock Ticker: Private
2006 Sales: $22,000,000	2006 Profits: $	Int'l Ticker: Int'l Exchange:
2005 Sales: $20,300,000	2005 Profits: $	Employees: 146,700
2004 Sales: $16,283,000	2004 Profits: $	Fiscal Year Ends: 6/30
2003 Sales: $14,683,000	2003 Profits: $	Parent Company:

SALARIES/BENEFITS:
Pension Plan: Y	ESOP Stock Plan:	Profit Sharing:	Top Exec. Salary: $	Bonus: $
Savings Plan: Y	Stock Purch. Plan:		Second Exec. Salary: $	Bonus: $

OTHER THOUGHTS:
Apparent Women Officers or Directors: 1
Hot Spot for Advancement for Women/Minorities:

LOCATIONS: ("Y" = Yes)
West:	Southwest:	Midwest:	Southeast:	Northeast:	International:
Y	Y	Y	Y	Y	Y

PRIDE INTERNATIONAL INC   www.prideinternational.com

Industry Group Code: 213111 Ranks within this company's industry group: Sales: 10   Profits: 11

Management:		Sales/Marketing:		Liberal Arts:		Information Systems:		Professionals:		Technical/Scientific:	
Mgmt. Trainees:	Y	Mktg. Professionals:		Gen. Writing/Editing:		Info. Management:	Y	Finance/Accounting:	Y	Engineers, Elec.:	Y
Experienced Mgmt.:	Y	Retail Sales:		Technical Writing:		Software Dev.:		Law:	Y	Engineers, Other:	Y
Int'l Business:	Y	Commercial/Industrial:	Y	Graphic Arts/Photog.:		Hardware Dev.:		HR/Other:	Y	Health/Lab:	
MBA Graduates:	Y	Sales Trainees:		Music:		Systems Integration:		Training:	Y	Scientists/Research:	
		Advertising Pros.:		Broadcasting:		Consulting/Other:		Health Care:		Petroleum/Chemicals:	Y
				Other:				Consulting:		Math/Other:	

TYPES OF BUSINESS:
Contract Drilling Services
Oil Rig Management Services

BRANDS/DIVISIONS/AFFILIATES:
GP Investments, Ltd.
Ferncliff TIH AS
Blake International LLC

CONTACTS: Note: Officers with more than one job title may be intentionally listed here more than once.
Louis A. Raspino, CEO
Rodney W. Eads, COO/Exec. VP
Louis A. Raspino, Pres.
Brian C. Voegele, CFO/Sr. VP
Kevin C. Robert, VP-Mktg.
Lonnie D. Bane, Sr. VP-Human Resources
Jenny M. Rub, CIO/VP
Imran (Ron) Toufeeq, Sr. VP-Eng. & Asset Mgmt.
Lonnie D. Bane, Sr. VP-Admin.
W. Gregory Looser, General Counsel/Corp. Sec
Kevin C. Robert, Sr. VP-Bus. Dev.
Jeffrey L. Chastain, VP-Comm.
Jeffrey L. Chastain, VP-Investor Rel.
Steven D. Oldham, Treas./VP
David E. Bruce, VP-Regional Oper.
Leonard Travis, VP/Chief Acct. Officer
Robert Warren, VP-Industry & Gov't Affairs
Brady Long, Chief Compliance Officer/Deputy General Counsel
David A. B. Brown, Chmn.

Phone: 713-789-1400   Fax: 713-789-1430
Toll-Free:
Address: 5847 San Felipe St., Ste. 3300, Houston, TX 77057 US

GROWTH PLANS/SPECIAL FEATURES:
Pride International, Inc. is a leading international provider of offshore contract drilling and related services to oil and natural gas companies worldwide, operating in approximately 15 countries and marine provinces. Pride owns a fleet of 46 rigs, consisting of two deepwater drillships, 13 semisubmersible rigs and 28 jackup rigs, as well as three ultra-deepwater drillships under construction in Korea. Pride's operations are conducted in many of the most active oil and natural gas basins of the world, including South America, the Gulf of Mexico, the Mediterranean Sea, West Africa, the Middle East and Asia Pacific. Pride's customers consist of large multinational oil and natural gas companies, government-owned oil and natural gas companies and independent oil and natural gas producers. The company also provides rig management services, such as technical drilling assistance, personnel, repair and maintenance services and drilling operation management services for a variety of rigs. The company also has management contracts for two deepwater TLP rigs, two deepwater spar rigs and one semisubmersible rig. In July 2007, Pride acquired an ultra-deepwater drillship, currently under construction, from Lexton, Inc. for approximately $675 million. In August 2007, Pride agreed to sell its Latin America Land and E&P Services segments to GP Investments Ltd. for $1 billion. Also in August 2007, the company agreed to sell its fleet of three self-erecting, tender-assist rigs to Ferncliff TIH AS for $213 million and acquired the remaining 9% of its Angolan joint venture. In May 2008, Pride completed the sale of its platform rig fleet Blake International LLC for $66 million.

Employees receive a full benefits package that includes medical, vision and dental insurance, a flexible spending account and an employee assistance program.

FINANCIALS: Sales and profits are in thousands of dollars—add 000 to get the full amount. 2007 Note: Financial information for 2007 was not available for all companies at press time.

2007 Sales: $2,043,800	2007 Profits: $784,300	U.S. Stock Ticker: PDE
2006 Sales: $2,495,400	2006 Profits: $295,300	Int'l Ticker: Int'l Exchange:
2005 Sales: $2,033,300	2005 Profits: $128,300	Employees: 14,300
2004 Sales: $1,712,200	2004 Profits: $27,600	Fiscal Year Ends: 12/31
2003 Sales: $1,689,720	2003 Profits: $-16,000	Parent Company:

SALARIES/BENEFITS:
Pension Plan:	ESOP Stock Plan:	Profit Sharing:	Top Exec. Salary: $800,000	Bonus: $600,000
Savings Plan: Y	Stock Purch. Plan: Y		Second Exec. Salary: $475,000	Bonus: $118,750

OTHER THOUGHTS:
Apparent Women Officers or Directors:
Hot Spot for Advancement for Women/Minorities:

LOCATIONS: ("Y" = Yes)
West:	Southwest:	Midwest:	Southeast:	Northeast:	International:
	Y		Y		Y

Note: Financial information, benefits and other data can change quickly and may vary from those stated here.

PRINCIPAL FINANCIAL GROUP (THE)   www.principal.com

Industry Group Code: 524113 Ranks within this company's industry group: Sales: Profits:

Management:		Sales/Marketing:		Liberal Arts:		Information Systems:		Professionals:		Technical/Scientific:	
Mgmt. Trainees:	Y	Mktg. Professionals:	Y	Gen. Writing/Editing:	Y	Info. Management:	Y	Finance/Accounting:	Y	Engineers, Elec.:	
Experienced Mgmt.:	Y	Retail Sales:		Technical Writing:	Y	Software Dev.:	Y	Law:	Y	Engineers, Other:	
Int'l Business:	Y	Commercial/Industrial:	Y	Graphic Arts/Photog.:		Hardware Dev.:		HR/Other:	Y	Health/Lab:	
MBA Graduates:	Y	Sales Trainees:	Y	Music:		Systems Integration:		Training:	Y	Scientists/Research:	Y
		Advertising Pros.:	Y	Broadcasting:		Consulting/Other:		Health Care:	Y	Petroleum/Chemicals:	
				Other:				Consulting:		Math/Other:	Y

TYPES OF BUSINESS:
Asset Management
Life Insurance
Health Insurance
Annuities
Disability Insurance
Investment Services
Specialty Benefits Insurance

BRANDS/DIVISIONS/AFFILIATES:
Principal Life Insurance Co.
Principal Financial Services, Inc.
Principal International, Inc.

CONTACTS: Note: Officers with more than one job title may be intentionally listed here more than once.
Larry D. Zimpleman, CEO
Larry D. Zimpleman, Pres.
Terry Lillis, CFO/Sr. VP
Michael T. Daley, Exec. VP-Mktg.
James D. DeVries, Sr. VP-Human Resources
Gary P. Scholten, CIO/Sr. VP
Karen E. Shaff, General Counsel/Exec. VP
Norman Sorensen, Exec. VP-Bus. Dev. & Strategy
Mary A. O'Keefe, Sr. VP-Corp. Rel.
Greg Elming, Controller/Sr. VP
James P. McCaughan, Pres., Global Asset Mgmt.
Julia M. Lawler, Sr. VP/Chief Investment Officer
John E. Aschenbrenner, Pres., Insurance & Financial Svcs.
Ellen Z. Lamale, Sr. VP/Chief Actuary
J. Barry Griswell, Chmn.
Michael T. Daley, Exec. VP-Dist.

Phone: 515-247-5111	Fax: 515-246-5475
Toll-Free: 800-986-3343	
Address: 711 High St., Des Moines, IA 50392-0001 US	

GROWTH PLANS/SPECIAL FEATURES:

The Principal Financial Group is a leading provider of retirement savings, investment and insurance products and services. It holds a total of $311.1 billion in assets, which it manages for approximately 19 million customers throughout the world. The company is organized into four primary business segments: U.S. asset management; global asset management; international asset management and accumulation; and life and health insurance. Its flagship unit is Principal Life Insurance Co., which provides life, health, dental and disability insurance. The firm's U.S. and international operations concentrate on asset accumulation and management, additionally offering individual and group life insurance; group health insurance; and individual and group disability insurance. Principal Financial Group focuses primarily on small and medium sized businesses, which it defines as companies with less than 1,000 employees. The U.S. asset management segment consists of asset management operations, which provide retirement savings and related investment products and services to businesses, their employees and other individuals. The global asset management segment consists of Principal Global Investors and its affiliates, which focus on providing a range of asset management services covering a broad range of asset classes, investment styles and portfolio structures to Principle Financial Group's other segments and third-party institutional clients. The international asset management and accumulation division consists of Principal International, which has operations in Chile, Mexico, Hong Kong, Brazil, India, China and Malaysia. The life and health insurance segment offers individual life and disability insurance as well as group health insurance, group dental, group vision, group life and group long-term and short-term disability insurance in the U.S. In December 2007, the company acquired Retirement Consulting Actuaries, Inc.

Principal offers its employees a range of benefits, including a pension plan, 401(k) with company match, and life and health insurance.

FINANCIALS: Sales and profits are in thousands of dollars—add 000 to get the full amount. 2007 Note: Financial information for 2007 was not available for all companies at press time.

2007 Sales: $10,906,500	2007 Profits: $860,300	U.S. Stock Ticker: PFG
2006 Sales: $9,873,100	2006 Profits: $1,064,300	Int'l Ticker: Int'l Exchange:
2005 Sales: $9,041,700	2005 Profits: $919,000	Employees: 14,507
2004 Sales: $8,320,900	2004 Profits: $825,600	Fiscal Year Ends: 12/31
2003 Sales: $9,404,200	2003 Profits: $746,300	Parent Company:

SALARIES/BENEFITS:

Pension Plan: Y	ESOP Stock Plan: Y	Profit Sharing:	Top Exec. Salary: $1,000,000	Bonus: $2,500,000
Savings Plan: Y	Stock Purch. Plan: Y		Second Exec. Salary: $582,904	Bonus: $1,092,945

OTHER THOUGHTS:
Apparent Women Officers or Directors: 13
Hot Spot for Advancement for Women/Minorities: Y

LOCATIONS: ("Y" = Yes)

West:	Southwest:	Midwest:	Southeast:	Northeast:	International:
Y	Y	Y	Y	Y	Y

PROCTER & GAMBLE CO

www.pg.com

Industry Group Code: 325600 Ranks within this company's industry group: Sales: 1   Profits: 1

Management:		Sales/Marketing:		Liberal Arts:		Information Systems:		Professionals:		Technical/Scientific:	
Mgmt. Trainees:	Y	Mktg. Professionals:	Y	Gen. Writing/Editing:		Info. Management:	Y	Finance/Accounting:	Y	Engineers, Elec.:	Y
Experienced Mgmt.:	Y	Retail Sales:		Technical Writing:	Y	Software Dev.:		Law:	Y	Engineers, Other:	
Int'l Business:	Y	Commercial/Industrial:	Y	Graphic Arts/Photog.:		Hardware Dev.:		HR/Other:	Y	Health/Lab:	Y
MBA Graduates:	Y	Sales Trainees:		Music:		Systems Integration:		Training:	Y	Scientists/Research:	Y
		Advertising Pros.:	Y	Broadcasting:		Consulting/Other:		Health Care:		Petroleum/Chemicals:	
				Other:	Y			Consulting:		Math/Other:	

TYPES OF BUSINESS:

Household Products Manufacturing
Pharmaceuticals
Foods & Beverages
Beauty Products

BRANDS/DIVISIONS/AFFILIATES:

Cover Girl
Crest
Tide
Pringles
Gillette
Clairol
Wella
HDS Cosmetics Lab, Inc.

CONTACTS: *Note: Officers with more than one job title may be intentionally listed here more than once.*

Alan G. Lafley, CEO
Robert A. McDonald, COO
Clayton C. Daley, Jr., CFO
Marc Pritchard, Global Mktg. Officer
Moheet Nagrath, Global Human Resources Officer
Filippo Passerini, CIO/Pres., Global Bus. Svcs.
G. Gilbert Cloyd, CTO
Steven W. Jemison, Chief Legal Officer/Sec.
Werner Geissler, Vice Chair-Global Oper.
Jon Moeller, Treas./VP
Susan E. Arnold, Pres., Global Bus. Units
Mark S. Bertolami, Pres., Duracell
Gina Drosos, Pres., Global Personal Beauty
Valarie L. Sheppard, Comptroller/VP
Alan G. Lafley, Chmn.
Giovanni Ciserani, Pres., Western Europe

Phone: 513-983-1100	Fax: 513-983-9369
Toll-Free:	
Address: 1 Procter & Gamble Plz., Cincinnati, OH 45202 US	

GROWTH PLANS/SPECIAL FEATURES:

The Procter & Gamble Co. develops and manufactures a wide range of household goods, including fabric and home care, baby care, feminine care, tissue and towel, beauty care, health care and food and beverage products. Its operations are divided in three segments: beauty, including beauty and grooming products; health and well being, encompassing health care products, snacks, coffee and pet care products; and household care, which includes fabric care, home care, baby care and family care. Laundry products generated roughly 16% of net sales in 2007. The company markets almost 300 brands to more than 5 billion consumers in over 180 countries. These brands include Tide, Crest, Pantene, Tampax, Pringles, Pampers, Folgers, Jif, Cover Girl, Gillette, Downy, Dawn, Bounty, Charmin and Iams pet food. The firm's products are primarily distributed through food, drug and mass merchandise retail outlets, with Wal-Mart providing a large percentage of sales. In the U.S., Procter & Gamble operates 33 manufacturing facilities in 21 states. Moreover, it owns and operates 91 facilities in 42 other countries, including Canada, Japan and Western European countries. The company has continued to experience increased earnings and revenue, nearly doubling its revenues since 2000, with major acquisitions such as Clairol, Wella and Gillette. In early 2007, Procter & Gamble acquired HDS Cosmetics Lab, Inc., which manufactures and markets Doctor's Dermatologic Formula skin care, from private equity firm North Castle Partners. In June 2008, the firm agreed to sell its Folgers Coffee unit to JM Smucker Co. for nearly $3 billion.

FINANCIALS: Sales and profits are in thousands of dollars—add 000 to get the full amount. 2007 Note: Financial information for 2007 was not available for all companies at press time.

2007 Sales: $76,476,000	2007 Profits: $10,340,000	**U.S. Stock Ticker: PG**
2006 Sales: $68,222,000	2006 Profits: $8,684,000	**Int'l Ticker:** Int'l Exchange:
2005 Sales: $56,741,000	2005 Profits: $6,923,000	Employees: 138,000
2004 Sales: $51,407,000	2004 Profits: $6,156,000	Fiscal Year Ends: 6/30
2003 Sales: $43,377,000	2003 Profits: $5,186,000	Parent Company:

SALARIES/BENEFITS:

Pension Plan:	ESOP Stock Plan:	Profit Sharing:	Top Exec. Salary: $1,700,000	Bonus: $6,101,000
Savings Plan:	Stock Purch. Plan:		Second Exec. Salary: $910,000	Bonus: $1,760,000

OTHER THOUGHTS:

Apparent Women Officers or Directors: 12
Hot Spot for Advancement for Women/Minorities: Y

LOCATIONS: ("Y" = Yes)

West:	Southwest:	Midwest:	Southeast:	Northeast:	International:
Y	Y	Y	Y	Y	Y

PROGRESSIVE CORPORATION (THE) www.progressive.com

Industry Group Code: 524126 Ranks within this company's industry group: Sales: 1 Profits: 2

Management:		Sales/Marketing:		Liberal Arts:		Information Systems:		Professionals:		Technical/Scientific:	
Mgmt. Trainees:	Y	Mktg. Professionals:	Y	Gen. Writing/Editing:	Y	Info. Management:	Y	Finance/Accounting:	Y	Engineers, Elec.:	
Experienced Mgmt.:	Y	Retail Sales:		Technical Writing:	Y	Software Dev.:	Y	Law:	Y	Engineers, Other:	
Int'l Business:	Y	Commercial/Industrial:		Graphic Arts/Photog.:	Y	Hardware Dev.:		HR/Other:	Y	Health/Lab:	
MBA Graduates:	Y	Sales Trainees:	Y	Music:		Systems Integration:		Training:	Y	Scientists/Research:	Y
		Advertising Pros.:	Y	Broadcasting:		Consulting/Other:		Health Care:		Petroleum/Chemicals:	
				Other:				Consulting:		Math/Other:	Y

TYPES OF BUSINESS:
Insurance, Direct Property & Casualty
Automobile Insurance
Specialty Insurance

BRANDS/DIVISIONS/AFFILIATES:
www.progressiveresponds.com

CONTACTS: *Note: Officers with more than one job title may be intentionally listed here more than once.*
Glenn M. Renwick, CEO
Glenn M. Renwick, Pres.
Brian C. Domeck, CFO/VP
Larry Bloomenkranz, Chief Mktg. Officer
Valerie Krasowski, Chief Human Resources Officer
Raymond M. Voelker, CIO
Charles (Chuck) Jarret, Chief Legal Officer/Corp. Sec.
Jeffery W. Basch, Chief Acct. Officer/VP
John P. Sauerland, Pres., Personal Lines Group
John Barbagallo, Pres., Commercial Lines Group
William (Bill) Cody, Chief Investment Officer
Susan Griffith, Pres., Claims Group
Peter B. Lewis, Chmn.

Phone: 440-461-5000	**Fax:** 440-603-4420
Toll-Free: 800-776-4737	
Address: 6300 Wilson Mills Rd., Mayfield Village, OH 44143 US	

GROWTH PLANS/SPECIAL FEATURES:
The Progressive Corporation, together with its 65 subsidiaries, is one of the largest auto insurers in the U.S. Progressive is divided into three business areas: personal lines, commercial auto and claims. The firm's personal lines segment writes insurance for private passenger automobiles and recreational and other vehicles, including motorcycles, all-terrain vehicles, boats and recreational vehicles. The personal lines business accounted for 87% of total net premiums written in 2007. The commercial auto business writes primary liability and physical damage insurance for automobiles and trucks owned by small businesses and represented 13% of Progressive's total net premiums written in 2007. The company's claims business area is organized into six geographical regions, with a general manager responsible for each region. The firm manages its claims handling on a companywide basis through approximately 475 claims offices located throughout the U.S. The company has 54 centers, in 41 metropolitan areas across the country, that provide concierge-level claims service. These facilities are designed to provide end-to-end resolution for auto physical damage losses. Customers can choose to bring their vehicles to one of these sites, where they can pick up a rental vehicle. Progressive's representatives will then write the estimate, select a qualified repair shop, arrange the repair and inspect the vehicle once the repairs are complete. The company plans to construct five new centers in 2008 and 2009. Progressive recently launched a new catastrophe web site (www.progressiveresponds.com) to provide consumers with information about how to stay safe and protect their vehicles and boats before, during and after a catastrophic event. In September 2007, Progressive started offering pet injury coverage at no extra cost for customers with collision coverage. In November 2007, Progressive began providing golf cart insurance for electric and gas vehicles.

FINANCIALS: Sales and profits are in thousands of dollars—add 000 to get the full amount. 2007 Note: Financial information for 2007 was not available for all companies at press time.

2007 Sales: $14,686,800	2007 Profits: $1,182,500	**U.S. Stock Ticker: PGR**
2006 Sales: $14,786,400	2006 Profits: $1,647,500	**Int'l Ticker:** Int'l Exchange:
2005 Sales: $14,303,400	2005 Profits: $1,393,900	Employees: 26,851
2004 Sales: $13,782,100	2004 Profits: $1,648,700	Fiscal Year Ends: 12/31
2003 Sales: $11,892,000	2003 Profits: $1,255,400	Parent Company:

SALARIES/BENEFITS:
Pension Plan: Y	ESOP Stock Plan:	Profit Sharing:	Top Exec. Salary: $750,000	Bonus: $832,500
Savings Plan: Y	Stock Purch. Plan:		Second Exec. Salary: $438,270	Bonus: $324,319

OTHER THOUGHTS:
Apparent Women Officers or Directors: 5
Hot Spot for Advancement for Women/Minorities: Y

LOCATIONS: ("Y" = Yes)
West:	Southwest:	Midwest:	Southeast:	Northeast:	International:
Y	Y	Y	Y	Y	

Note: Financial information, benefits and other data can change quickly and may vary from those stated here.

PRUDENTIAL FINANCIAL INC

www.prudential.com

Industry Group Code: 524113 Ranks within this company's industry group: Sales: Profits:

Management:		Sales/Marketing:		Liberal Arts:		Information Systems:		Professionals:		Technical/Scientific:	
Mgmt. Trainees:	Y	Mktg. Professionals:	Y	Gen. Writing/Editing:	Y	Info. Management:	Y	Finance/Accounting:	Y	Engineers, Elec.:	
Experienced Mgmt.:	Y	Retail Sales:	Y	Technical Writing:	Y	Software Dev.:	Y	Law:	Y	Engineers, Other:	
Int'l Business:	Y	Commercial/Industrial:	Y	Graphic Arts/Photog.:		Hardware Dev.:		HR/Other:	Y	Health/Lab:	
MBA Graduates:	Y	Sales Trainees:	Y	Music:		Systems Integration:		Training:	Y	Scientists/Research:	Y
		Advertising Pros.:	Y	Broadcasting:		Consulting/Other:		Health Care:	Y	Petroleum/Chemicals:	
				Other:				Consulting:		Math/Other:	Y

TYPES OF BUSINESS:

Insurance-Life
Property & Casualty Insurance
Asset Management, Pension & Benefit Plans
Mutual Funds
Brokerage Services
Credit Card Services
Trust Services

BRANDS/DIVISIONS/AFFILIATES:

Prudential Insurance Company of America (The)
Prudential Relocation
Prudential Real Estate Affiliates, Inc.
Prudential Equity Group
Prudential Bank
Prudential Retirement Insurance and Annuity Co.
Wachovia Securities, LLC

CONTACTS: *Note: Officers with more than one job title may be intentionally listed here more than once.*

John Strangfeld, CEO
Arthur F. Ryan, Pres.
Richard J. Carbone, CFO/Sr. VP
Sharon C. Taylor, Sr. VP-Human Resources
Robert C. Golden, Exec. VP-Systems
Susan L. Blount, General Counsel/Sr. VP
Robert C. Golden, Exec. VP-Oper.
Sharon C. Taylor, Sr. VP-Community Resources
Bernard Jacob, Sr. VP/Treas.
Bernard B. Winograd, Exec. VP/COO-U.S. Businesses
Stephen Pelletier, Pres., Prudential Annuities
Arthur F. Ryan, Chmn.
Edward P. Baird, Exec. VP/COO-Int'l Businesses

Phone: 973-802-6000	Fax: 973-367-4479
Toll-Free: 800-346-3778	
Address: 751 Broad St., Newark, NJ 07102 US	

GROWTH PLANS/SPECIAL FEATURES:

Prudential Financial, Inc. is one of the largest financial services groups in the U.S. It provides a range of products in three divisions: insurance; investments; and international insurance and investments. The insurance division operates through the Prudential Insurance Company of America, its major subsidiary, which is one of the largest life insurance companies in the country. Prudential Insurance has two segments: individual life and annuities, which offers individual variable life, term life, universal life and other non-participating life insurance services, as well as variable and fixed annuity products which are distributed to the U.S. retail market through proprietary and third-party distribution channels; and group insurance, which distributes a range of group life insurance, long-term and short-term group disability insurance, long-term care and corporate and trust owned life insurance to institutional clients for use in conjunction with benefit plans. The company's investments division has three segments: asset management, financial advisory and retirement. The financial advisory segment consists of the firm's joint venture, Wachovia Securities, LLC, which is one of the nation's largest retail financial advisory organizations. The international division provides the same services as the other two divisions to international clients in 30 countries, primarily Japan. All of the company's operations are divided into either Financial Services Businesses, which are publicly traded on the New York Stock Exchange, or Closed Block Businesses, which represent a former operating division and are not traded in any exchange. The company has approximately $638 billion in assets under management. In June 2007, Prudential launched Prudential Bank as a part of Prudential Financial Group, operating in its 18 re-branded offices throughout Mexico. Also in June 2007, the company discontinued its institutional equity research, sales and trading firm, Prudential Equity Group. In October 2007, Wachovia completed the acquisition of A.G. Edwards, Inc.

FINANCIALS: Sales and profits are in thousands of dollars—add 000 to get the full amount. 2007 Note: Financial information for 2007 was not available for all companies at press time.

2007 Sales: $34,401,000	2007 Profits: $3,704,000	U.S. Stock Ticker: PRU
2006 Sales: $32,268,000	2006 Profits: $3,428,000	Int'l Ticker: Int'l Exchange:
2005 Sales: $31,599,000	2005 Profits: $3,540,000	Employees: 39,814
2004 Sales: $28,096,000	2004 Profits: $2,256,000	Fiscal Year Ends: 12/31
2003 Sales: $27,907,000	2003 Profits: $1,264,000	Parent Company:

SALARIES/BENEFITS:

Pension Plan: Y	ESOP Stock Plan:	Profit Sharing:	Top Exec. Salary: $1,000,000	Bonus: $6,300,000
Savings Plan: Y	Stock Purch. Plan:		Second Exec. Salary: $600,000	Bonus: $3,800,000

OTHER THOUGHTS:

Apparent Women Officers or Directors: 4
Hot Spot for Advancement for Women/Minorities: Y

LOCATIONS: ("Y" = Yes)

West:	Southwest:	Midwest:	Southeast:	Northeast:	International:
Y	Y	Y	Y	Y	Y

PSYCHIATRIC SOLUTIONS INC
www.psysolutions.com

Industry Group Code: 622210 Ranks within this company's industry group: Sales: 2 Profits: 1

Management:		Sales/Marketing:		Liberal Arts:		Information Systems:		Professionals:		Technical/Scientific:	
Mgmt. Trainees:	Y	Mktg. Professionals:	Y	Gen. Writing/Editing:		Info. Management:	Y	Finance/Accounting:	Y	Engineers, Elec.:	
Experienced Mgmt.:	Y	Retail Sales:		Technical Writing:	Y	Software Dev.:		Law:	Y	Engineers, Other:	Y
Int'l Business:		Commercial/Industrial:		Graphic Arts/Photog.:		Hardware Dev.:		HR/Other:	Y	Health/Lab:	
MBA Graduates:	Y	Sales Trainees:		Music:		Systems Integration:		Training:	Y	Scientists/Research:	
		Advertising Pros.:		Broadcasting:		Consulting/Other:		Health Care:	Y	Petroleum/Chemicals:	
				Other:				Consulting:		Math/Other:	

TYPES OF BUSINESS:
Clinics-Psychiatric
Contract Management Services
Employee Assistance Program Administration

BRANDS/DIVISIONS/AFFILIATES:
Horizon Health Corp.

CONTACTS: Note: Officers with more than one job title may be intentionally listed here more than once.
Joey A. Jacobs, CEO
Terrance R. (Terry) Bridges, COO
Joey A. Jacobs, Pres.
Brent Turner, Exec. VP-Admin.
Christopher L. (Chris) Howard, General Counsel/Sec./Exec. VP
Steven T. Davidson, Chief Dev. Officer
Brent Turner, Exec. VP-Finance
Jack E. Polson, Chief Acct. Officer/Exec. VP
Joey A. Jacobs, Chmn.

Phone: 615-312-5700	Fax: 615-312-5711
Toll-Free:	
Address: 6640 Carothers Pkwy., Ste. 500, Franklin, TN 37067 US	

GROWTH PLANS/SPECIAL FEATURES:
Psychiatric Solutions, Inc. (PSI) is a leading provider of inpatient behavioral health care services in the U.S. It operates 90 inpatient behavioral health care facilities with over 10,000 beds in 31 states, the U.S. Virgin Islands and Puerto Rico. These facilities offer a wide range of inpatient services for children, adolescents and adults through a combination of acute inpatient behavioral facilities and residential treatment centers (RTCs). Acute inpatient behavioral facilities provide intensive psychiatric care: 24-hour skilled nursing observation; daily interventions and oversight by a psychiatrist; and intensive, coordinated treatment by a physician-led team of mental health professionals. RTCs provide longer term treatment programs primarily for children and adolescents with long-standing chronic behavioral health problems. RTCs offer physician-led multi-disciplinary treatments that address the patient's medical, psychiatric, social and academic needs. Both of these facilities work closely with others, including psychiatrists; non-psychiatric physicians; emergency rooms; counselors, therapists and social workers; school systems; insurance companies; employee assistance programs (EAPs); and law enforcement and community agencies that interact with individuals who require mental illness or substance abuse treatment. Many of PSI's facilities have mobile assessment teams who travel to prospective clients, assess their condition and determine if they meet established criteria for inpatient care. Those clients not meeting the criteria may qualify for outpatient care or a less intensive level of care provided by the facility. Besides its facilities, PSI also offers behavioral health care services, primarily contract management, comprising the development, organization and management of behavioral health care programs within hospitals; and EAPs, involving contracting with employers to assist employees and their dependents with behavioral and other problems. The inpatient behavioral health care facilities accounted for 91.6% of 2007 revenue; behavioral health care services, the remaining 8.4%. In May 2007, PSI acquired behavioral health care services provider Horizon Health Corp. for $426.7 million.

FINANCIALS: Sales and profits are in thousands of dollars—add 000 to get the full amount. 2007 Note: Financial information for 2007 was not available for all companies at press time.

2007 Sales: $1,481,952	2007 Profits: $76,208	U.S. Stock Ticker: PSYS
2006 Sales: $1,022,428	2006 Profits: $60,632	Int'l Ticker: Int'l Exchange:
2005 Sales: $715,324	2005 Profits: $27,154	Employees: 18,700
2004 Sales: $470,969	2004 Profits: $16,801	Fiscal Year Ends: 12/31
2003 Sales: $293,665	2003 Profits: $5,216	Parent Company:

SALARIES/BENEFITS:
Pension Plan:	ESOP Stock Plan:	Profit Sharing:	Top Exec. Salary: $890,865	Bonus: $1,204,200
Savings Plan:	Stock Purch. Plan:		Second Exec. Salary: $340,625	Bonus: $230,344

OTHER THOUGHTS:
Apparent Women Officers or Directors: 1
Hot Spot for Advancement for Women/Minorities:

LOCATIONS: ("Y" = Yes)
West:	Southwest:	Midwest:	Southeast:	Northeast:	International:
Y	Y	Y	Y	Y	

PUBLIC STORAGE INC

www.publicstorage.com

Industry Group Code: 525930 Ranks within this company's industry group: Sales: 1 Profits: 1

Management:		Sales/Marketing:	Liberal Arts:	Information Systems:		Professionals:		Technical/Scientific:	
Mgmt. Trainees:	Y	Mktg. Professionals:	Gen. Writing/Editing:	Info. Management:	Y	Finance/Accounting:	Y	Engineers, Elec.:	
Experienced Mgmt.:	Y	Retail Sales:	Technical Writing:	Software Dev.:		Law:	Y	Engineers, Other:	
Int'l Business:		Commercial/Industrial:	Graphic Arts/Photog.:	Hardware Dev.:		HR/Other:	Y	Health/Lab:	
MBA Graduates:	Y	Sales Trainees:	Music:	Systems Integration:		Training:		Scientists/Research:	
		Advertising Pros.:	Broadcasting:	Consulting/Other:		Health Care:		Petroleum/Chemicals:	
			Other:			Consulting:		Math/Other:	

TYPES OF BUSINESS:

Real Estate Investment Trust
Self-Storage Facilities
Commercial Properties
Transportation Services
Online Storage Reservations

BRANDS/DIVISIONS/AFFILIATES:

PS Business Parks, Inc.
Carson Storage Partners, Ltd.
Del Amo Storage Partners, Ltd.
Connecticut Storage Fund
PS Partners, Ltd.
Van Nuys Storage Partners, Ltd.
Secure Mini-Storage
Shurgard Storage Centers, Inc.

CONTACTS: Note: Officers with more than one job title may be intentionally listed here more than once.

Ronald L. Havner, Jr., CEO
Ronald L. Havner, Jr., Pres.
John Reyes, CFO/Sr. VP
Candace N. Krol, Sr. VP-Human Resources
John S. Baumann, Chief Legal Officer/Sr. VP
John E. Graul, Pres., Self-Storage Oper.
David F. Doll, Pres., Real Estate Div.
B. Wayne Hughes, Chmn.

Phone: 818-244-8080	Fax: 818-553-2376
Toll-Free:	
Address: 701 Western Ave., Ste. 200, Glendale, CA 91201 US	

GROWTH PLANS/SPECIAL FEATURES:

Public Storage, Inc. is a fully integrated, self-administered and self-managed equity real estate investment trust (REIT) that acquires, develops, owns and operates self-storage facilities. It is one of the largest owners and operators of self-storage space in the U.S., with direct and indirect equity investments in over 2,100 self-storage facilities containing approximately 92 million square feet of net rentable space in 37 states, with 800,000 self-service storage spaces in 80 U.S. cities. The company's growth strategy consists of improving the operating performance of its existing traditional self-storage properties; acquiring interests in properties that are owned or operated by others; expanding and repackaging existing real estate facilities; developing properties in selected markets; and participating in the growth of commercial facilities owned primarily by PS Business Parks, Inc. (a publicly traded REIT in which Public Storage holds a 44% interest). Public Storage also controls or has a minority interest in many subsidiary companies, which include Carson Storage Partners, Ltd.; Connecticut Storage Fund; Del Amo Storage Partners, Ltd.; PS Partners, Ltd.; Secure Mini-Storage; and Van Nuys Storage Partners, Ltd.

FINANCIALS: Sales and profits are in thousands of dollars—add 000 to get the full amount. 2007 Note: Financial information for 2007 was not available for all companies at press time.

2007 Sales: $1,816,371	2007 Profits: $457,527	U.S. Stock Ticker: PSA
2006 Sales: $1,381,011	2006 Profits: $314,026	Int'l Ticker: Int'l Exchange:
2005 Sales: $1,059,838	2005 Profits: $456,393	Employees: 5,700
2004 Sales: $958,157	2004 Profits: $366,213	Fiscal Year Ends: 12/31
2003 Sales: $893,956	2003 Profits: $336,653	Parent Company:

SALARIES/BENEFITS:

Pension Plan:	ESOP Stock Plan:	Profit Sharing:	Top Exec. Salary: $550,000	Bonus: $650,000
Savings Plan: Y	Stock Purch. Plan:		Second Exec. Salary: $392,700	Bonus: $275,000

OTHER THOUGHTS:

Apparent Women Officers or Directors: 1
Hot Spot for Advancement for Women/Minorities:

LOCATIONS: ("Y" = Yes)

West:	Southwest:	Midwest:	Southeast:	Northeast:	International:
Y	Y	Y	Y	Y	

PUBLIX SUPER MARKETS INC

www.publix.com

Industry Group Code: 445110 **Ranks within this company's industry group:** Sales: Profits:

Management:		Sales/Marketing:		Liberal Arts:		Information Systems:		Professionals:		Technical/Scientific:	
Mgmt. Trainees:	Y	Mktg. Professionals:	Y	Gen. Writing/Editing:	Y	Info. Management:	Y	Finance/Accounting:	Y	Engineers, Elec.:	
Experienced Mgmt.:	Y	Retail Sales:	Y	Technical Writing:		Software Dev.:		Law:	Y	Engineers, Other:	
Int'l Business:		Commercial/Industrial:		Graphic Arts/Photog.:	Y	Hardware Dev.:		HR/Other:	Y	Health/Lab:	
MBA Graduates:	Y	Sales Trainees:	Y	Music:		Systems Integration:		Training:	Y	Scientists/Research:	
		Advertising Pros.:	Y	Broadcasting:		Consulting/Other:		Health Care:	Y	Petroleum/Chemicals:	
				Other:				Consulting:		Math/Other:	

TYPES OF BUSINESS:

Grocery Stores
Dairy, Deli & Bakery Products

BRANDS/DIVISIONS/AFFILIATES:

CONTACTS: Note: Officers with more than one job title may be intentionally listed here more than once.

William E. Crenshaw, CEO
Randall T. Jones, Sr., Pres.
David P. Phillips, CFO/Treas.
John Hrabusa, Sr. VP-Human Resources
Laurie S. Zeitlin, CIO/Sr. VP
Mike Smith, VP-Mfg.
John A. Attaway, Jr., General Counsel/Sec./Sr. VP
Sandra J. Woods, VP/Controller
Robert H. Moore, VP
David E. Bridges, VP
G. Gino DiGrazia, VP/Controller
Howard M. Jenkins, Chmn.

Phone: 863-688-1188	Fax: 863-284-5532
Toll-Free: 800-242-1227	
Address: 3300 Publix Corporate Pkwy., Lakeland, FL 33811 US	

GROWTH PLANS/SPECIAL FEATURES:

Publix Super Markets, Inc. is a leading operator of supermarkets, with 926 locations in Alabama, Florida, Georgia, South Carolina and Tennessee. The firm's supermarkets sell groceries, dairy products, produce, deli foods, bakery items, meat, seafood, housewares and health and beauty care merchandise. Many stores also feature pharmacies, floral departments, photo labs and in-store banking areas. Publix's lines of merchandise include a variety of nationally advertised and private label brands, as well as some unbranded merchandise, such as produce, meat and seafood. In addition to its retail operations, Publix manufactures dairy, bakery and deli products through manufacturing facilities located in Jacksonville, Lakeland and Deerfield Beach, Florida and Lawrenceville and Atlanta, Georgia. The firm is one of the largest employee-owned grocery stores in the U.S. In September 2007, the company opened a new Publix GreenWise Market in Lakeland, Florida. This 39,000 square foot facility is focused on all-natural and organic products, combined with conventional products. In July 2008, Pbluix agreed to acquire 49 Florida stores from Albertson's LLC.

Employee benefits include an employee stock ownership plan; health, dental and vision insurance; employee assistance program; tuition reimbursement; and 401(k) savings plan.

FINANCIALS: Sales and profits are in thousands of dollars—add 000 to get the full amount. 2007 Note: Financial information for 2007 was not available for all companies at press time.

		U.S. Stock Ticker: PUSH
2007 Sales: $23,016,568	2007 Profits: $1,183,925	Int'l Ticker: Int'l Exchange:
2006 Sales: $21,654,774	2006 Profits: $1,097,209	Employees: 140,000
2005 Sales: $20,589,130	2005 Profits: $989,156	Fiscal Year Ends: 12/31
2004 Sales: $18,554,486	2004 Profits: $819,383	Parent Company:
2003 Sales: $16,760,749	2003 Profits: $660,933	

SALARIES/BENEFITS:

Pension Plan:	ESOP Stock Plan: Y	Profit Sharing: Y	Top Exec. Salary: $735,900	Bonus: $151,767
Savings Plan: Y	Stock Purch. Plan:		Second Exec. Salary: $590,155	Bonus: $121,709

OTHER THOUGHTS:

Apparent Women Officers or Directors: 8
Hot Spot for Advancement for Women/Minorities: Y

LOCATIONS: ("Y" = Yes)

West:	Southwest:	Midwest:	Southeast:	Northeast:	International:
			Y		

Note: Financial information, benefits and other data can change quickly and may vary from those stated here.

QUALCOMM INC

www.qualcomm.com

Industry Group Code: 334413 Ranks within this company's industry group: Sales: 2 Profits: 2

Management:		Sales/Marketing:		Liberal Arts:		Information Systems:		Professionals:		Technical/Scientific:	
Mgmt. Trainees:	Y	Mktg. Professionals:	Y	Gen. Writing/Editing:		Info. Management:	Y	Finance/Accounting:	Y	Engineers, Elec.:	Y
Experienced Mgmt.:	Y	Retail Sales:		Technical Writing:	Y	Software Dev.:	Y	Law:	Y	Engineers, Other:	
Int'l Business:	Y	Commercial/Industrial:	Y	Graphic Arts/Photog.:		Hardware Dev.:	Y	HR/Other:	Y	Health/Lab:	Y
MBA Graduates:	Y	Sales Trainees:		Music:		Systems Integration:		Training:	Y	Scientists/Research:	Y
		Advertising Pros.:	Y	Broadcasting:	Y	Consulting/Other:		Health Care:		Petroleum/Chemicals:	
				Other:				Consulting:		Math/Other:	

TYPES OF BUSINESS:

Telecommunications Equipment
Digital Wireless Communications Products
Integrated Circuits
Mobile Communications Systems
Wireless Software & Services
E-Mail Software
Code Division Multiple Access

BRANDS/DIVISIONS/AFFILIATES:

MediaFLO USA, Inc.
Qualcomm Flarion Technologies, Inc.
Qualcomm MEMS Technologies, Inc.
Firethorn Holdings, LLC
SoftMax, Inc.

CONTACTS: Note: Officers with more than one job title may be intentionally listed here more than once.

Paul E. Jacobs, CEO
Steven R. Altman, Pres.
William E. Keitel, CFO/Exec. VP
Jeffrey A. Jacobs, Chief Mktg. Officer/Exec. VP
Daniel L. Sullivan, Exec. VP-Human Resources
Norm Fjeldheim, CIO/Sr. VP
Roberto Padovani, CTO/Exec. VP
Donald J. Rosenberg, General Counsel/Exec. VP/Corp. Sec.
William Bold, Sr. VP-Gov't Affairs
William F. Davidson, Jr., Sr. VP-Investor Rel. & Global Mktg.
Jing Wang, Exec. VP-Asia Pacific, Middle East & Africa
Len. J. Lauer, Exec. VP
Marvin Blecker, Exec. VP/Pres., Qualcomm Tech. Licensing
Irwin M. Jacobs, Chmn.
Margaret L. Johnson, Exec. VP-Americas & India

Phone: 858-587-1121	Fax: 858-658-2100
Toll-Free:	
Address: 5775 Morehouse Dr., San Diego, CA 92121 US	

GROWTH PLANS/SPECIAL FEATURES:

Qualcomm, Inc. provides digital wireless communications products, technologies and services. It designs application-specific integrated circuits based on Code Division Multiple Access (CDMA) technology and licenses its technology to domestic and international telecommunications equipment suppliers. CDMA technology is an industry standard for all forms of digital wireless communications networks. The company also produces the e-mail software Eudora and sells Binary Runtime Environment for Wireless (BREW) software to network operators, handset manufacturers and application developers. BREW is an open-standard platform that can interface with many different wireless applications. The firm's wireless business services, which consist of satellite and terrestrial-based two-way data messaging and position reporting, serve transportation companies, private and construction equipment fleets and U.S. government agencies through its government technologies division. Subsidiary Qualcomm MEMS Technologies develops improved graphical systems for handheld devices. Subsidiary MediaFLO USA, Inc. began offering services over a nationwide multicast network based on the MediaFLO Media Distribution System (MDS) and Forward Link Only (FLO) technology in 2007. This network is utilized as a shared resource for wireless operators and their partners. Subsidiary Qualcomm Flarion Technologies is a developer and provider of FLASH-OFDM (Orthogonal Frequency Division Multiplexing Access). In 2007, the firm announced partnerships with a variety of media networks including NBC, CBS, FOX and MTV to offer mobile entertainment services. The company is sampling its Universal Broadcast Modem (UBM) chip, which supports Digital Video Broadcasting Handheld (DVB-H) and Terrestrial (ISDB-T) in a single chip. It also unveiled the uiOne Handset Development Kit (HDK) version 2.0, which supports seamless integration of third-party application engines. In late 2007, Qualcomm acquired Firethorn Holdings, LLC, a mobile banking enabler; and SoftMax, Inc., which focuses on noise reduction for mobile devices.

The company offers its employees medical, dental and vision insurance; a 401(k) plan; an employee stock purchase plan; and tuition reimbursement.

FINANCIALS: Sales and profits are in thousands of dollars—add 000 to get the full amount. 2007 Note: Financial information for 2007 was not available for all companies at press time.

2007 Sales: $8,871,000	2007 Profits: $3,303,000	**U.S. Stock Ticker: QCOM**
2006 Sales: $7,526,000	2006 Profits: $2,470,000	**Int'l Ticker:** Int'l Exchange:
2005 Sales: $5,673,000	2005 Profits: $2,143,000	Employees: 12,800
2004 Sales: $4,880,000	2004 Profits: $1,720,000	Fiscal Year Ends: 9/30
2003 Sales: $3,970,636	2003 Profits: $827,441	Parent Company:

SALARIES/BENEFITS:

Pension Plan:	ESOP Stock Plan:	Profit Sharing:	Top Exec. Salary: $1,063,467	Bonus: $1,013,200
Savings Plan: Y	Stock Purch. Plan: Y		Second Exec. Salary: $862,813	Bonus: $765,100

OTHER THOUGHTS:

Apparent Women Officers or Directors: 6
Hot Spot for Advancement for Women/Minorities: Y

LOCATIONS: ("Y" = Yes)

West:	Southwest:	Midwest:	Southeast:	Northeast:	International:
Y	Y	Y	Y	Y	Y

Note: Financial information, benefits and other data can change quickly and may vary from those stated here.

QUEST DIAGNOSTICS INC

www.questdiagnostics.com

Industry Group Code: 621511 Ranks within this company's industry group: Sales: 1 Profits: 1

Management:		Sales/Marketing:		Liberal Arts:		Information Systems:		Professionals:		Technical/Scientific:	
Mgmt. Trainees:	Y	Mktg. Professionals:	Y	Gen. Writing/Editing:		Info. Management:	Y	Finance/Accounting:	Y	Engineers, Elec.:	
Experienced Mgmt.:	Y	Retail Sales:		Technical Writing:	Y	Software Dev.:	Y	Law:	Y	Engineers, Other:	Y
Int'l Business:	Y	Commercial/Industrial:	Y	Graphic Arts/Photog.:	Y	Hardware Dev.:		HR/Other:	Y	Health/Lab:	Y
MBA Graduates:	Y	Sales Trainees:		Music:		Systems Integration:		Training:	Y	Scientists/Research:	Y
		Advertising Pros.:		Broadcasting:		Consulting/Other:		Health Care:	Y	Petroleum/Chemicals:	
				Other:				Consulting:		Math/Other:	

TYPES OF BUSINESS:

Services-Testing & Diagnostics
Clinical Laboratory Testing
Clinical Trials Testing
Esoteric Testing Laboratories

BRANDS/DIVISIONS/AFFILIATES:

Cardio CRP
HEPTIMAX
Focus Diagnostics, Inc.
CF Complete
CellSearch
Bio-Intact PTH
Leumeta
LabOne

CONTACTS: *Note: Officers with more than one job title may be intentionally listed here more than once.*

Surya N. Mohapatra, CEO
Surya N. Mohapatra, Pres.
Robert A. Hagemann, CFO/Sr. VP
Michael E. Prevoznik, General Counsel/VP-Legal & Compliance
Wayne R. Simmons, VP-Oper.
Laura Park, VP-Investor Rel. & Comm.
Joan E. Miller, Sr. VP-Pathology & Hospital Svcs.
Surya N. Mohapatra, Chmn.

Phone: 973-520-2700	Fax:
Toll-Free: 800-222-0446	
Address: 3 Giralda Farms, Madison, NJ 07940 US	

GROWTH PLANS/SPECIAL FEATURES:

Quest Diagnostics, Inc. is a U.S. clinical laboratory testing company, offering diagnostic testing and related services to the health care industry. The firm's operations consist of routine, esoteric and clinical trials testing. Quest operates through its national network of 2,100 patient service centers, principal laboratories in more than 30 major metropolitan areas, approximately 150 rapid-response laboratories, 40 outpatient anatomic pathology centers, hospital-based laboratories and esoteric testing laboratories on both coasts. Routine tests measure various important bodily health parameters. Tests in this category include blood cholesterol level tests, complete blood cell counts, pap smears, HIV-related tests, urinalyses, pregnancy and prenatal tests, and substance-abuse tests. Esoteric tests require more sophisticated technology and highly skilled personnel. The firm's tests in this field include Cardio CRP and HEPTIMAX. Quest's two esoteric testing laboratories, comprising the Nichols Institute, are among the leading esoteric clinical testing laboratories in the world. Esoteric tests involve endocrinology, genetics, immunology, microbiology, oncology, serology and special chemistry. Clinical trial testing primarily involves assessing the safety and efficacy of new drugs to meet FDA requirements, with services including Bio-Intact PTH. In recent news, Quest received FDA clearance to market its Plexus HerpeSelect 1 and 2 IgG test kit. Additionally, the company acquired diagnostic testing company AmeriPath, Inc. for approximately $2 billion. In July 2007, Quest introduced a new diagnostic testing technique to help physicians diagnose genetic metabolic disorders such as phenylketonuria (PKU) and homocystinuria. Late in 2007, Quest entered a non-exclusive license agreement for heteroduplex tracking technology, essential to Pathway Diagnostics' SensiTrop HIV co-receptor tropism test. In May 2008, the firm worked with Google to develop Google Heath, a product allowing patients to store medical and health information online.

Quest offers employees educational assistance, adoption assistance, free lab testing, annual development training and credit union access.

FINANCIALS: Sales and profits are in thousands of dollars—add 000 to get the full amount. 2007 Note: Financial information for 2007 was not available for all companies at press time.

2007 Sales: $6,704,907	2007 Profits: $339,939	**U.S. Stock Ticker: DGX**
2006 Sales: $6,268,659	2006 Profits: $586,421	**Int'l Ticker:** Int'l Exchange:
2005 Sales: $5,456,726	2005 Profits: $546,277	Employees: 43,500
2004 Sales: $5,066,986	2004 Profits: $499,195	Fiscal Year Ends: 12/31
2003 Sales: $4,737,958	2003 Profits: $436,717	Parent Company:

SALARIES/BENEFITS:

Pension Plan:	ESOP Stock Plan:	Profit Sharing: Y	Top Exec. Salary: $1,094,610	Bonus: $1,669,007
Savings Plan: Y	Stock Purch. Plan: Y		Second Exec. Salary: $495,419	Bonus: $453,234

OTHER THOUGHTS:

Apparent Women Officers or Directors: 4
Hot Spot for Advancement for Women/Minorities: Y

LOCATIONS: ("Y" = Yes)

West:	Southwest:	Midwest:	Southeast:	Northeast:	International:
Y	Y	Y	Y	Y	Y

Note: Financial information, benefits and other data can change quickly and may vary from those stated here.

QUIKSILVER INC

www.quiksilverinc.com

Industry Group Code: 315000A Ranks within this company's industry group: Sales: 1   Profits: 1

Management:		Sales/Marketing:		Liberal Arts:		Information Systems:		Professionals:		Technical/Scientific:	
Mgmt. Trainees:	Y	Mktg. Professionals:	Y	Gen. Writing/Editing:	Y	Info. Management:	Y	Finance/Accounting:	Y	Engineers, Elec.:	
Experienced Mgmt.:	Y	Retail Sales:	Y	Technical Writing:		Software Dev.:	Y	Law:	Y	Engineers, Other:	
Int'l Business:	Y	Commercial/Industrial:	Y	Graphic Arts/Photog.:	Y	Hardware Dev.:		HR/Other:	Y	Health/Lab:	
MBA Graduates:	Y	Sales Trainees:	Y	Music:		Systems Integration:		Training:	Y	Scientists/Research:	
		Advertising Pros.:	Y	Broadcasting:		Consulting/Other:		Health Care:		Petroleum/Chemicals:	
				Other:	Y			Consulting:		Math/Other:	

TYPES OF BUSINESS:

Sports Apparel & Equipment
Snow & Surf Apparel & Equipment
Accessories
Swimwear
Retail Stores

BRANDS/DIVISIONS/AFFILIATES:

Boardriders Club
Roxy
Rossignol
DC
Roxy Girl
Dynastar
Lange
Kerma

CONTACTS: *Note: Officers with more than one job title may be intentionally listed here more than once.*

Robert B. McKnight, Jr., CEO
David H. Morgan, COO/Exec. VP
Bernard Mariette, Pres.
Joseph Scirocco, CFO/Exec. VP
Charles S. Exon, General Counsel/Corp. Sec.
Charles S. Exon, Exec. VP-Bus. & Legal Affairs
Robert B. McKnight, Jr., Chmn.

Phone: 714-889-2200	Fax: 714-889-3700
Toll-Free:	
Address: 15202 Graham St., Huntington Beach, CA 92649 US	

GROWTH PLANS/SPECIAL FEATURES:

Quiksilver, Inc. is a globally diversified company that designs, produces, retails and distributes branded apparel, wintersports equipment, footwear, accessories and related products. It operates in three segments: the Americas, which includes the U.S. and Canada; Europe, which includes primarily countries located in Western Europe; and Asia/Pacific, which includes Australia, Japan, New Zealand and Indonesia. The company's brands are focused on different sports within the outdoor market. Quiksilver and Roxy are rooted in the sport of surfing and are leading brands representing the boardriding lifestyle, which includes not only surfing, but also skateboarding and snowboarding. Quiksilver has grown to include shirts, walkshorts, t-shirts, pants, jackets, fleece, pants, snowboardwear, footwear, hats, backpacks, wetsuits, watches, eyewear and other accessories. In addition, the brand has expanded its target market to include boys, toddlers and infants. The Roxy brand includes sportswear, footwear, backpacks, snowboardwear, swimwear, backpacks, snowboard boots, skis, fragrance, beauty care, bedroom furnishings and other accessories for young women. The brand now contains the Teenie Wahine and Roxy Girl brands for girls and infants. DC's reputation is based on its technical shoes made for skateboarding. The firm also developed a portfolio of other brands also inspired by surfing, skateboarding and snowboarding. The wintersports brands include Rossignol, Dynastar, Look, Lange and Kerma, which are focused on equipment for alpine skiing but have extended into areas of wintersports, including snowboarding, freestyle skiing, Nordic skiing and technical outwear. Quiksilver's products are sold in over 90 countries in a wide range of distribution channels, including surf shops, ski shops, snowboard shops, the proprietary Boardriders Club shops, other specialty stores and select department stores. In December 2007, the company successfully completed the selling of its golf equipment operations for $132.5 million. In 2008, the firm launched a new retro styled line targeting women in their 20s.

FINANCIALS: Sales and profits are in thousands of dollars—add 000 to get the full amount. 2007 Note: Financial information for 2007 was not available for all companies at press time.

2007 Sales: $2,426,035	2007 Profits: $-121,119	U.S. Stock Ticker: ZQK
2006 Sales: $2,200,234	2006 Profits: $93,016	Int'l Ticker: Int'l Exchange:
2005 Sales: $1,780,869	2005 Profits: $107,120	Employees: 9,600
2004 Sales: $1,266,939	2004 Profits: $81,369	Fiscal Year Ends: 10/31
2003 Sales: $975,005	2003 Profits: $58,516	Parent Company:

SALARIES/BENEFITS:

Pension Plan:	ESOP Stock Plan:	Profit Sharing:	Top Exec. Salary: $950,000	Bonus: $650,000
Savings Plan: Y	Stock Purch. Plan:		Second Exec. Salary: $800,000	Bonus: $650,000

OTHER THOUGHTS:

Apparent Women Officers or Directors:
Hot Spot for Advancement for Women/Minorities:

LOCATIONS: ("Y" = Yes)

West:	Southwest:	Midwest:	Southeast:	Northeast:	International:
Y					Y

R R DONNELLEY & SONS CO

www.rrdonelley.com

Industry Group Code: 323000 Ranks within this company's industry group: Sales: 2 Profits: 2

Management:		Sales/Marketing:		Liberal Arts:		Information Systems:		Professionals:		Technical/Scientific:	
Mgmt. Trainees:	Y	Mktg. Professionals:	Y	Gen. Writing/Editing:	Y	Info. Management:	Y	Finance/Accounting:	Y	Engineers, Elec.:	Y
Experienced Mgmt.:	Y	Retail Sales:		Technical Writing:		Software Dev.:		Law:	Y	Engineers, Other:	
Int'l Business:	Y	Commercial/Industrial:	Y	Graphic Arts/Photog.:	Y	Hardware Dev.:		HR/Other:	Y	Health/Lab:	
MBA Graduates:	Y	Sales Trainees:		Music:		Systems Integration:		Training:	Y	Scientists/Research:	
		Advertising Pros.:		Broadcasting:		Consulting/Other:		Health Care:		Petroleum/Chemicals:	
				Other:				Consulting:		Math/Other:	

TYPES OF BUSINESS:

Commercial Printing
Distributors-Books, Magazines, Catalogs & Direct Mail
Digital Content Management
Creative Services
Logistics Services

BRANDS/DIVISIONS/AFFILIATES:

RR Donnelley Global Document Solutions
Office Tiger
Banta Corporation
Perry-Judd's Holdings, Inc.
Von Hoffmann
Cardinal Brands, Inc.
Pro Line Printing, Inc.

CONTACTS: Note: Officers with more than one job title may be intentionally listed here more than once.

Thomas J. Quinlan III, CEO
John Paloian, COO
Thomas J. Quinlan III, Pres.
George Zengo, CFO
Andrew B. Panega, Sr. VP-Human Resources
Kenneth E. O'Brien, CIO
Suzanne S. Bettman, General Counsel/Corp. Sec/Chief Compliance Officer
Thomas J. Quinlan III, Exec. VP-Oper.
Andrew Coxhead, Controller/Chief Acct. Officer/Sr. VP
Stephen M. Wolf, Chmn.

Phone: 312-326-8000	Fax:
Toll-Free:	
Address: 111 S. Wacker Dr., Chicago, IL 60606 US	

GROWTH PLANS/SPECIAL FEATURES:

R. R. Donnelley & Sons Co. provides print and related services, including business process outsourcing, to customers in the publishing, healthcare, advertising, retail, technology, financial services and other industries. R. R. Donnelley operates through Global Print Solutions and Global Services. Global Print Solutions provides print services to consumer magazine and catalog publishers; retailers; yellow and white pages directory publishers; and religious, educational and specialty book publishers. The segment also consolidates and delivers company-printed products, as well as products printed by third parties; offers content creation, database management, printing, personalization, finishing and distribution services; and provides short-run commercial print services. Global Services provides digital solutions for conventional and digital photography; creative, color matching, page production and content management services; and information management, content assembly and print services for such products as annual reports, marketing brochures and marketing inserts. Within the Global Services segment, RR Donnelley Global Document Solutions provides business outsourcing services, transactional print and mail services, data and print management and document production, primarily in the U.K. Office Tiger provides integrated process outsourcing and transaction processing services throughout North America, Europe, India, the Philippines and Sri Lanka. In 2007, R. R. Donnelley completed the purchase of Banta Corporation, Perry-Judd's Holdings, Inc., Von Hoffmann and Cardinal Brands, Inc. In June 2007, the company unified its services under the R. R. Donnelley brand, including its Office Tiger brand. In December 2007, the firm opened a new outsourcing facility in India. In March 2008, the firm acquired Pro Line Printing, Inc.

R. R. Donnelley offers its employees a dependent care plan, a pension plan, a 401(k) plan, an employee stock purchase plan, an employee assistance program, an adoption assistance program, a health care flexible spending account and medical, dental and vision coverage programs.

FINANCIALS: Sales and profits are in thousands of dollars—add 000 to get the full amount. 2007 Note: Financial information for 2007 was not available for all companies at press time.

2007 Sales: $11,587,100	2007 Profits: $-48,900	U.S. Stock Ticker: RRD
2006 Sales: $9,316,600	2006 Profits: $400,600	Int'l Ticker: Int'l Exchange:
2005 Sales: $8,430,200	2005 Profits: $137,100	Employees: 53,000
2004 Sales: $7,156,400	2004 Profits: $178,300	Fiscal Year Ends: 12/31
2003 Sales: $4,787,162	2003 Profits: $176,509	Parent Company:

SALARIES/BENEFITS:

Pension Plan: Y	ESOP Stock Plan:	Profit Sharing:	Top Exec. Salary: $1,000,000	Bonus: $4,250,000
Savings Plan: Y	Stock Purch. Plan: Y		Second Exec. Salary: $500,000	Bonus: $1,000,000

OTHER THOUGHTS:

Apparent Women Officers or Directors: 1
Hot Spot for Advancement for Women/Minorities: Y

LOCATIONS: ("Y" = Yes)

West:	Southwest:	Midwest:	Southeast:	Northeast:	International:
Y	Y	Y	Y	Y	Y

Note: Financial information, benefits and other data can change quickly and may vary from those stated here.

RAYTHEON CO

www.raytheon.com

Industry Group Code: 336410 Ranks within this company's industry group: Sales: 7 Profits: 7

Management:		Sales/Marketing:		Liberal Arts:		Information Systems:		Professionals:		Technical/Scientific:	
Mgmt. Trainees:	Y	Mktg. Professionals:	Y	Gen. Writing/Editing:		Info. Management:	Y	Finance/Accounting:	Y	Engineers, Elec.:	Y
Experienced Mgmt.:	Y	Retail Sales:		Technical Writing:	Y	Software Dev.:	Y	Law:	Y	Engineers, Other:	Y
Int'l Business:	Y	Commercial/Industrial:	Y	Graphic Arts/Photog.:	Y	Hardware Dev.:	Y	HR/Other:	Y	Health/Lab:	Y
MBA Graduates:	Y	Sales Trainees:		Music:		Systems Integration:	Y	Training:	Y	Scientists/Research:	Y
		Advertising Pros.:	Y	Broadcasting:		Consulting/Other:	Y	Health Care:		Petroleum/Chemicals:	Y
				Other:				Consulting:		Math/Other:	Y

TYPES OF BUSINESS:

Aerospace & Defense Technology
Commercial Electronics
Technical Services
Communications & Information Systems
Sensors & Surveillance Equipment
Missile Systems
Space Exploration Devices
Software Engineering

BRANDS/DIVISIONS/AFFILIATES:

Patriot Air & Missile Defense System
Flight Options LLC
Raytheon Aircraft Company

CONTACTS: *Note: Officers with more than one job title may be intentionally listed here more than once.*

William H. Swanson, CEO
David C. Wajsgras, CFO
Keith J. Peden, Sr. VP-Human Resources
Rebecca Rhoads, CIO/VP
Taylor W. Lawrence, VP-Tech. & Mission Assurance
Taylor W. Lawrence, VP-Eng.
Jay B. Stephens, General Counsel/Sec./Sr. VP
William J. Lynn, VP-Gov't Oper. & Strategy
Thomas M. Culligan, Exec. VP-Bus. Dev.
Pamela A. Wickham, VP-Corp. Affairs & Comm.
Michael J. Wood, Chief Acct. Officer/VP
Jon C. Jones, VP/Pres., Space & Airborne Systems
Louise L. Francesconi, VP/Pres., Missile Systems
Colin Schottlaender, VP/Pres., Network Centric Systems
Daniel L. Smith, VP/Pres., Integrated Defense Systems
William H. Swanson, Chmn.
Thomas M. Culligan, CEO-Raytheon Int'l, Inc.
John D. Harris, II, VP-Contracts & Supply Chain

Phone: 781-522-3000	Fax: 781-522-3001
Toll-Free:	
Address: 870 Winter St., Waltham, MA 02451 US	

GROWTH PLANS/SPECIAL FEATURES:

Raytheon Co. offers defense and government electronics; aerospace systems; IT equipment; and technical services. It operates six business segments. The Integrated Defense Systems segment provides integrated space, air, surface and subsurface solutions; and homeland security products. It offers advanced radar and sonar systems; surveillance equipment; sensors; air and missile defense systems, including the Patriot Air & Missile Defense System; technical services; and other defense equipment. The Intelligence and Information Systems segment offers commercial and government customers weather and environmental management; geospatial intelligence; signal and image processing; and ground engineering support. The Missile Systems segment offers a variety of missiles, including one anti-satellite system, as well as smart projectiles, missile defense guns and even a microwave-based anti-missile system. The Network Centric Systems segment develops and produces mission solutions for networking and communications; command and control; battlefield awareness; and transportation management. The Space and Airborne Systems segment provides electro-optic/infrared sensors, airborne radars, high-energy lasers, precision guidance systems and space-qualified systems for civil and military applications. Lastly, the Technical Services segment provides technical, scientific and professional services for defense, federal and commercial customers worldwide. The U.S. Government accounted for 86% of Raytheon's 2007 sales. Customers include all branches of the U.S. armed forces, the National Guard, the Department of Homeland Security, the F.A.A., the Japanese Defense Agency and the Royal Saudi Air Defense Forces. In March 2007, the firm sold Raytheon Aircraft Company to Canadian-based Onex Partners and Hawker Beechcraft Corporation for almost $3.32 billion. In November 2007, it sold Flight Options LLC to H.I.G. Capital for an undisclosed amount. As a result these two sales, Raytheon has basically exited the commercial aircraft market.

Raytheon employees receive dental, prescription drug and vision care coverage; short- and long-term disability options; life and AD&D insurance; paid time off; adoption assistance; educational assistance; and investment services.

FINANCIALS: Sales and profits are in thousands of dollars—add 000 to get the full amount. 2007 Note: Financial information for 2007 was not available for all companies at press time.

2007 Sales: $21,301,000	2007 Profits: $2,578,000	**U.S. Stock Ticker: RTN**
2006 Sales: $19,707,000	2006 Profits: $1,283,000	**Int'l Ticker:** Int'l Exchange:
2005 Sales: $18,491,000	2005 Profits: $871,000	Employees: 72,100
2004 Sales: $17,825,000	2004 Profits: $417,000	Fiscal Year Ends: 12/31
2003 Sales: $18,109,000	2003 Profits: $365,000	Parent Company:

SALARIES/BENEFITS:

Pension Plan:	ESOP Stock Plan:	Profit Sharing:	Top Exec. Salary: $1,200,014	Bonus: $2,800,000
Savings Plan: Y	Stock Purch. Plan:		Second Exec. Salary: $603,067	Bonus: $730,000

OTHER THOUGHTS:

Apparent Women Officers or Directors: 3
Hot Spot for Advancement for Women/Minorities: Y

LOCATIONS: ("Y" = Yes)

West:	Southwest:	Midwest:	Southeast:	Northeast:	International:
Y	Y	Y	Y	Y	Y

Note: Financial information, benefits and other data can change quickly and may vary from those stated here.

REGIS CORPORATION

www.regiscorp.com

Industry Group Code: 812110 Ranks within this company's industry group: Sales: 1 Profits: 1

Management:		Sales/Marketing:		Liberal Arts:	Information Systems:		Professionals:		Technical/Scientific:	
Mgmt. Trainees:	Y	Mktg. Professionals:	Y	Gen. Writing/Editing:	Info. Management:	Y	Finance/Accounting:	Y	Engineers, Elec.:	
Experienced Mgmt.:	Y	Retail Sales:		Technical Writing:	Software Dev.:		Law:	Y	Engineers, Other:	
Int'l Business:	Y	Commercial/Industrial:		Graphic Arts/Photog.:	Hardware Dev.:		HR/Other:	Y	Health/Lab:	
MBA Graduates:	Y	Sales Trainees:		Music:	Systems Integration:		Training:	Y	Scientists/Research:	
		Advertising Pros.:	Y	Broadcasting:	Consulting/Other:		Health Care:		Petroleum/Chemicals:	
				Other:			Consulting:		Math/Other:	

TYPES OF BUSINESS:

Hair Salons
Hair Care Products
Beauty Schools
Hair Restoration Services

BRANDS/DIVISIONS/AFFILIATES:

Regis Salons
MasterCuts
Trade Secret
SmartStyle
SuperCuts
Cameron Capital Investments Inc
Provalliance
Hair Club for Men & Women

CONTACTS: Note: Officers with more than one job title may be intentionally listed here more than once.

Paul D. Finkelstein, CEO
Kris Bergly, COO/Exec. VP
Paul D. Finkelstein, Pres.
Randy L. Pearce, CFO/Sr. Exec. VP
Gordon Nelson, Exec. VP-Mktg., Fashion & Education
Randy L. Pearce, Chief Admin. Officer
Eric A. Bakken, General Counsel/Sr. VP
Bruce Johnson, Exec. VP-Real Estate & Construction
Mark Kartarik, Exec. VP/Pres., Franchise Division
Norma Knudsen, Exec. VP-Merchandising/COO-Trade Secret Division
C. John Briggs, Sr. VP/Pres., SmartStyle Family Hair Salons
Paul D. Finkelstein, Chmn.
Andy Cohen, Pres., Int'l Div.

Phone: 952-947-7777	Fax: 952-947-7600
Toll-Free:	
Address: 7201 Metro Blvd., Edina, MN 55439 US	

GROWTH PLANS/SPECIAL FEATURES:

Regis Corporation is a global owner, operator, franchiser and consolidator of hair and retail product salons. The company owns, franchises or holds ownership interests in over 13,550 worldwide locations. The company's locations consist of 10,745 company-owned and franchise salons, 92 hair restoration centers and 2,714 locations in which the company maintains an ownership interest of less than 100%. The company is organized to manage its operations based on significant lines of business, salons and hair restoration centers. Salon operations are managed based on geographical location, North America and International. The company's North American salon operations are comprised of 8,110 company-owned salons and 2,163 franchise salons. The company's international operations are comprised of 472 company-owned salons. The company's worldwide salon locations operate primarily under the trade names of Regis Salons, MasterCuts, Trade Secret, SmartStyle, Supercuts, Cost Cutters and Sassoon. In August 2007, the company contributed 51 of its wholly-owned accredited cosmetology schools to Empire Education Group, Inc (EEG) in exchange for a 49% equity interest in EEG. In January 2008, the company's effective ownership interest increased to 55.1% related to the buyout of EEG's equity interest shareholder. In January 2008, the company merged its continental European franchise salon operations with the operations of the Franck Provost Salon Group in exchange for a 30% equity interest in the newly formed Provalliance entity. The merger with the operations of the Franck Provost Salon Group, which are also located in continental Europe, created Europe's largest salon operator with approximately 2,300 company-owned and franchise salons as of June 2008. In February 2008, the company acquired the capital stock of Cameron Capital I, Inc., a wholly-owned subsidiary of Cameron Capital Investments, Inc. (CCI). CCI owns and operates PureBeauty and BeautyFirst salons and is now accounted for as a wholly-owned subsidiary of the company.

FINANCIALS: Sales and profits are in thousands of dollars—add 000 to get the full amount. 2007 Note: Financial information for 2007 was not available for all companies at press time.

2007 Sales: $2,626,588	2007 Profits: $83,170	U.S. Stock Ticker: RGS
2006 Sales: $2,430,864	2006 Profits: $109,578	Int'l Ticker: Int'l Exchange:
2005 Sales: $2,194,294	2005 Profits: $64,631	Employees: 59,000
2004 Sales: $1,923,143	2004 Profits: $105,478	Fiscal Year Ends: 6/30
2003 Sales: $1,684,500	2003 Profits: $86,700	Parent Company:

SALARIES/BENEFITS:

Pension Plan:	ESOP Stock Plan:	Profit Sharing:	Top Exec. Salary: $888,890	Bonus: $342,600
Savings Plan: Y	Stock Purch. Plan: Y		Second Exec. Salary: $743,310	Bonus: $

OTHER THOUGHTS:

Apparent Women Officers or Directors: 5
Hot Spot for Advancement for Women/Minorities: Y

LOCATIONS: ("Y" = Yes)

West:	Southwest:	Midwest:	Southeast:	Northeast:	International:
Y	Y	Y	Y	Y	Y

RELIANT ENERGY INC

www.reliant.com

Industry Group Code: 221000 Ranks within this company's industry group: Sales: Profits:

Management:		Sales/Marketing:		Liberal Arts:		Information Systems:		Professionals:		Technical/Scientific:	
Mgmt. Trainees:	Y	Mktg. Professionals:	Y	Gen. Writing/Editing:	Y	Info. Management:	Y	Finance/Accounting:	Y	Engineers, Elec.:	Y
Experienced Mgmt.:	Y	Retail Sales:		Technical Writing:		Software Dev.:	Y	Law:	Y	Engineers, Other:	
Int'l Business:		Commercial/Industrial:	Y	Graphic Arts/Photog.:		Hardware Dev.:		HR/Other:	Y	Health/Lab:	
MBA Graduates:	Y	Sales Trainees:		Music:		Systems Integration:		Training:	Y	Scientists/Research:	
		Advertising Pros.:	Y	Broadcasting:		Consulting/Other:		Health Care:		Petroleum/Chemicals:	
				Other:				Consulting:		Math/Other:	

TYPES OF BUSINESS:

Utilities-Electricity
Power Generation
Wholesale Energy Trading & Marketing
Landfill Gas Generation

BRANDS/DIVISIONS/AFFILIATES:

Reliant Resources, Inc.
Liberty Electric PA, LLC
Reliant Energy Solutions East, LLC
Smart Energy

CONTACTS: *Note: Officers with more than one job title may be intentionally listed here more than once.*

Mark Jacobs, CEO
Brian Landrum, COO/Exec. VP
Mark Jacobs, Pres.
Rick J. Dobson, CFO/Exec. VP
David Roylance, Sr. VP-Commercial & Industrial Mktg. & Sales
Karen D. Taylor, Sr. VP-Human Resources/Chief Diversity Officer
Michael L. Jines, Sr. VP/General Counsel/Sec.
David Brast, Sr. VP-Commercial Oper. & Organization
James A. Ajello, Sr. VP-Bus. Dev.
Thomas C. Livengood, Controller/Sr. VP
Suzanne L. Kupiec, Sr. VP-Risk & Structuring
Jason Few, Sr. VP-Smart Energy
Dave Freysinger, Sr. VP-Generation Oper.
Charles Griffey, Sr. VP-Regulatory Affairs
Joel V. Staff, Chmn.

Phone: 713-497-3000	Fax: 713-488-5925
Toll-Free: 866-872-6656	
Address: 1000 Main St., Houston, TX 77002 US	

GROWTH PLANS/SPECIAL FEATURES:

Reliant Energy, Inc., formerly Reliant Resources, Inc., is an electricity and energy services provider. The company's retail energy segment provides electricity and related services to 1.8 million residential, commercial, industrial and institutional customers in Texas. It also acquires and manages the electric energy, capacity and ancillary services associated with supplying these retail customers. Power is purchased from third parties and sold at unregulated or price-to-beat prices. Reliant's wholesale energy segment provides competitive energy generation and procures natural gas, coal, fuel oil, natural gas transportation and storage capacity and other energy-related commodities. It owns interest in or leases operating 38 electric power generation facilities with an aggregate net generating capacity of approximately 16,337 megawatts (MW). These are located in Pennsylvania, New Jersey, Illinois, Ohio, Texas, Mississippi, Florida, California and Nevada, and run on coal, gas and oil power, with one that runs on landfill gas. Recently, the firm sold its two remaining hydroelectric generating stations to Brascan Corp. for $42 million. This was followed by the sale of Reliant's Ceredo natural-gas fired plant to Appalachian Power Company for $100 million and the sale of its three New York City plants to Madison Dearborn Partners and U.S. Power Generating Company for $975 million. In 2007, Reliant announced its intention to enter the Delaware market via subsidiary Reliant Energy Solutions East, LLC. Also in 2007, the firm introduced Smart Energy products and services to its Texas markets; these products to help reduce consumption during peak usage periods, such as meters that raise or lower thermostat settings a few degrees in peak hot and cold temperatures. In February 2008, the firm agreed to sell its Channelview Cogeneration Plant. In April 2008, the company entered the New York electricity market. Also in April 2008, Reliant agreed to sell its Bighorn Generating Station.

FINANCIALS: Sales and profits are in thousands of dollars—add 000 to get the full amount. 2007 Note: Financial information for 2007 was not available for all companies at press time.

2007 Sales: $11,209,000	2007 Profits: $365,000	U.S. Stock Ticker: RRI
2006 Sales: $10,877,000	2006 Profits: $-328,000	Int'l Ticker: Int'l Exchange:
2005 Sales: $9,711,995	2005 Profits: $-330,556	Employees: 3,675
2004 Sales: $8,098,222	2004 Profits: $-29,370	Fiscal Year Ends: 12/31
2003 Sales: $11,000,319	2003 Profits: $-1,342,117	Parent Company:

SALARIES/BENEFITS:

Pension Plan:	ESOP Stock Plan:	Profit Sharing: Y	Top Exec. Salary: $1,000,000	Bonus: $993,800
Savings Plan: Y	Stock Purch. Plan: Y		Second Exec. Salary: $575,000	Bonus: $577,185

OTHER THOUGHTS:

Apparent Women Officers or Directors: 3
Hot Spot for Advancement for Women/Minorities: Y

LOCATIONS: ("Y" = Yes)

West:	Southwest:	Midwest:	Southeast:	Northeast:	International:
Y	Y	Y	Y	Y	

Note: Financial information, benefits and other data can change quickly and may vary from those stated here.

RENT-A-CENTER INC

www.rentacenter.com

Industry Group Code: 532200 **Ranks within this company's industry group:** Sales: 1 Profits: 1

Management:		Sales/Marketing:		Liberal Arts:		Information Systems:		Professionals:		Technical/Scientific:	
Mgmt. Trainees:	Y	Mktg. Professionals:	Y	Gen. Writing/Editing:		Info. Management:	Y	Finance/Accounting:	Y	Engineers, Elec.:	
Experienced Mgmt.:	Y	Retail Sales:	Y	Technical Writing:		Software Dev.:	Y	Law:	Y	Engineers, Other:	
Int'l Business:	Y	Commercial/Industrial:	Y	Graphic Arts/Photog.:	Y	Hardware Dev.:		HR/Other:	Y	Health/Lab:	
MBA Graduates:	Y	Sales Trainees:	Y	Music:		Systems Integration:		Training:	Y	Scientists/Research:	
		Advertising Pros.:	Y	Broadcasting:		Consulting/Other:		Health Care:		Petroleum/Chemicals:	
				Other:				Consulting:		Math/Other:	

TYPES OF BUSINESS:
Assorted Merchandise, Rental

BRANDS/DIVISIONS/AFFILIATES:
Get It Now
Rent-A-Centre
ColorTyme, Inc.
Cash AdvantEdge

CONTACTS: *Note: Officers with more than one job title may be intentionally listed here more than once.*
Mark E. Speese, CEO
Mitchell E. Fadel, COO
Mitchell E. Fadel, Pres.
Robert D. Davis, CFO
Ann. L. Davids, Chief Mktg. Officer/Sr. VP-Mktg.
Melvin D. McCall, Sr. VP-Human Resources
Tony F. Fuller, CIO/Sr. VP-IT
Robert W. Rapp, CTO/VP-IT
Dan Glasky, VP-Merch.
Christopher A. Korst, General Counsel/Corp. Sec./Exec. VP
Christopher A. Korst, Exec. VP-Oper.
Daniel R. Eichelberger, VP-Bus. Dev.
August E. Whitcomb, VP-Public Affairs
David E. Carpenter, VP-Investor Rel.
Robert D. Davis, Exec. VP-Finance/Treas.
Robert F. Bloom, Pres./CEO-ColorTyme, Inc.
William S. Short, Exec. VP-Oper.
David E. West, Exec. VP-Oper. Svcs.
Kent W. Brown, VP-Dev.
Mark E. Speese, Chmn.

Phone: 972-801-1100	Fax: 972-943-0113
Toll-Free: 800-275-2996	
Address: 5501 Headquarters Dr., Plano, TX 75024 US	

GROWTH PLANS/SPECIAL FEATURES:
Rent-A-Center, Inc. operates rent-to-own stores in the U.S., with approximately 3,081 stores in 50 states, Canada and Puerto Rico, including 24 Get It Now stores and eight Rent-A-Centre stores in Canada. ColorTyme, Inc., a subsidiary of the company, franchises rent-to-own stores, with approximately 227 stores in 33 states under the ColorTyme and Rent-A-Center brand names. The stores provide home electronics, appliances, computers, furniture and assorted accessories including brands such as Sony, Philips and Hitachi home electronics; Whirlpool appliances; Dell, Toshiba and Hewlett-Packard computers; and Ashley, England, Berkshire and Standard furniture. Rent-a-Center offers additional services such as free repair, pick-up and delivery. The company provides rental purchase agreements that allow the customer to obtain ownership of merchandise at the conclusion of a set rental period. Rent-A-Center also offers such financial services as short term and unsecured loans; debit cards; check cashing; and money transfer in 276 of its store locations in 15 states under the trade name Cash AdvantEdge.

FINANCIALS: Sales and profits are in thousands of dollars—add 000 to get the full amount. 2007 Note: Financial information for 2007 was not available for all companies at press time.

2007 Sales: $2,906,121	2007 Profits: $76,268	U.S. Stock Ticker: RCII
2006 Sales: $2,433,908	2006 Profits: $103,092	Int'l Ticker: Int'l Exchange:
2005 Sales: $2,339,107	2005 Profits: $135,738	Employees: 19,740
2004 Sales: $2,313,255	2004 Profits: $155,855	Fiscal Year Ends: 12/31
2003 Sales: $2,228,150	2003 Profits: $181,496	Parent Company:

SALARIES/BENEFITS:

Pension Plan:	ESOP Stock Plan:	Profit Sharing:	Top Exec. Salary: $740,000	Bonus: $532,800
Savings Plan: Y	Stock Purch. Plan: Y		Second Exec. Salary: $510,000	Bonus: $298,350

OTHER THOUGHTS:
Apparent Women Officers or Directors: 4
Hot Spot for Advancement for Women/Minorities: Y

LOCATIONS: ("Y" = Yes)

West:	Southwest:	Midwest:	Southeast:	Northeast:	International:
Y	Y	Y	Y	Y	Y

Note: Financial information, benefits and other data can change quickly and may vary from those stated here.

RES CARE INC

www.rescare.com

Industry Group Code: 622210 Ranks within this company's industry group: Sales: 1   Profits: 2

Management:		Sales/Marketing:		Liberal Arts:		Information Systems:		Professionals:		Technical/Scientific:	
Mgmt. Trainees:	Y	Mktg. Professionals:	Y	Gen. Writing/Editing:		Info. Management:	Y	Finance/Accounting:	Y	Engineers, Elec.:	
Experienced Mgmt.:	Y	Retail Sales:		Technical Writing:	Y	Software Dev.:		Law:	Y	Engineers, Other:	Y
Int'l Business:	Y	Commercial/Industrial:		Graphic Arts/Photog.:		Hardware Dev.:		HR/Other:	Y	Health/Lab:	
MBA Graduates:	Y	Sales Trainees:		Music:		Systems Integration:		Training:	Y	Scientists/Research:	
		Advertising Pros.:		Broadcasting:		Consulting/Other:		Health Care:	Y	Petroleum/Chemicals:	
				Other:				Consulting:		Math/Other:	

TYPES OF BUSINESS:

Community Services
Job Corps Training Services
Employment Training Services

BRANDS/DIVISIONS/AFFILIATES:

Armstrong Unicare
Armstrong Uniserve
Workforce Services Group
Select Health Care Services
Caregivers Home Health, Inc.

CONTACTS: *Note: Officers with more than one job title may be intentionally listed here more than once.*

Ralph G. Gronefeld, Jr., CEO
Ralph G. Gronefeld, Jr., Pres.
David W. Miles, CFO
Nina P. Seigle, Chief People Officer
George Watts, CIO
David S. Waskey, General Counsel/Chief Compliance Officer
Richard Tinsley, Chief Dev. Officer
Nel Taylor, Chief Comm. Officer
Derwin A. Wallace, Dir.-Investor Rel.
Vincent Doran, Pres., Employment & Training Svcs. Group
Paul G. Dunn, Pres., Arbor E&T
Kelley Abell, Consultant-Gov. Rel.
Michael J. Reibel, Sr. VP-Support Svcs.
Ronald G. Geary, Chmn.

Phone: 502-394-2100	Fax: 502-394-2206
Toll-Free: 800-866-0860	
Address: 9901 Linn Station Rd., Louisville, KY 40223-3808 US	

GROWTH PLANS/SPECIAL FEATURES:

Res-Care, Inc. provides residential, therapeutic, job training and educational supports to adults and youths with intellectual, cognitive and other developmental disabilities; youths who have special educational or support needs, are from disadvantaged backgrounds or have severe emotional disorders; and adults who experience barriers to employment. The firm also offers, through drop-in or live-in services, personal care, meal preparation, housekeeping and transportation to the elderly in their own homes. In addition, Res-Care provides services to welfare recipients, young people and people who have been laid off or have special barriers to employment, to transition into the workforce and become productive employees. The company operates in three segments: community services, job corps training services and employment training services. Through the community services segment, the firm offers programs in 32 states for individual with developmental disabilities designed to encourage greater independence and the development or maintenance of daily living skills. The job corps training services segment operates 17 job corps centers that provide for the educational and vocational skills training, healthcare, employment counseling and other support necessary to enable disadvantaged youths to become responsible working adults. The employment training services segment operate 240 career centers, which offer job training and placement programs that assist welfare recipients and disadvantaged job seekers in finding employment and improving their careers prospects. The company provides services in 37 states, Washington, D.C., Puerto Rico, Canada, the U.K., the Netherlands, Germany, Haiti, Bahrain and the United Arab Emirates. In May 2008, the firm acquired Select Health Care Services, a home health care agency in Texas, providing companion care; skilled nursing; and physical, occupational and speech therapy. In July 2008, Res-Care acquired Caregivers Home Health, Inc., a home and personal care provider for seniors.

FINANCIALS: Sales and profits are in thousands of dollars—add 000 to get the full amount. 2007 Note: Financial information for 2007 was not available for all companies at press time.

2007 Sales: $1,433,298	2007 Profits: $43,891	**U.S. Stock Ticker:** RSCR
2006 Sales: $1,302,118	2006 Profits: $36,696	**Int'l Ticker:** Int'l Exchange:
2005 Sales: $1,046,556	2005 Profits: $21,222	Employees: 37,000
2004 Sales: $966,185	2004 Profits: $21,507	Fiscal Year Ends: 12/31
2003 Sales: $961,333	2003 Profits: $13,387	Parent Company:

SALARIES/BENEFITS:

Pension Plan:	ESOP Stock Plan:	Profit Sharing:	Top Exec. Salary: $379,796	Bonus: $370,000
Savings Plan: Y	Stock Purch. Plan: Y		Second Exec. Salary: $309,994	Bonus: $155,000

OTHER THOUGHTS:

Apparent Women Officers or Directors: 4
Hot Spot for Advancement for Women/Minorities: Y

LOCATIONS: ("Y" = Yes)

West:	Southwest:	Midwest:	Southeast:	Northeast:	International:
Y	Y	Y	Y	Y	Y

RESPIRONICS INC

www.respironics.com

Industry Group Code: 339113 Ranks within this company's industry group: Sales: 15 Profits: 13

Management:		Sales/Marketing:		Liberal Arts:		Information Systems:		Professionals:		Technical/Scientific:	
Mgmt. Trainees:	Y	Mktg. Professionals:	Y	Gen. Writing/Editing:		Info. Management:	Y	Finance/Accounting:	Y	Engineers, Elec.:	Y
Experienced Mgmt.:	Y	Retail Sales:		Technical Writing:	Y	Software Dev.:	Y	Law:	Y	Engineers, Other:	Y
Int'l Business:	Y	Commercial/Industrial:		Graphic Arts/Photog.:	Y	Hardware Dev.:		HR/Other:	Y	Health/Lab:	Y
MBA Graduates:	Y	Sales Trainees:		Music:		Systems Integration:		Training:	Y	Scientists/Research:	Y
		Advertising Pros.:	Y	Broadcasting:		Consulting/Other:		Health Care:	Y	Petroleum/Chemicals:	
				Other:				Consulting:		Math/Other:	Y

TYPES OF BUSINESS:
Equipment/Supplies-Respiratory Devices

BRANDS/DIVISIONS/AFFILIATES:
Sleep Well Ventures
Children's Medical Ventures
OxyTec Medical Corporation
OxyTec 900
Royal Philips Electronics NV

CONTACTS: *Note: Officers with more than one job title may be intentionally listed here more than once.*
John L. Miclot, CEO
Craig B. Reynolds, COO/Exec. VP
John L. Miclot, Pres.
Daniel J. Bevevino, CFO/VP
David P. White, Chief Medical Officer
Steven Fulton, General Counsel/VP
Susan A. Lloyd, VP-Respiratory Drug Delivery Div.
Derek Smith, Pres., Hospital Group
Donald Spence, Pres., Sleep & Home Respiratory Group
Gerald E. McGinnis, Chmn.
Geoffrey C. Waters, Pres., Int'l Div.

Phone: 724-387-5200	Fax:
Toll-Free: 800-345-6443	
Address: 1010 Murry Ridge Ln., Murrysville, PA 15668-8525 US	

GROWTH PLANS/SPECIAL FEATURES:

Respironics, Inc. is a leading developer, manufacturer and marketer of medical devices that are used for the treatment of patients suffering from sleep and respiratory disorders. The company's products comprise the following two categories: Sleep and Home Respiratory Products, which include sleep disordered breathing products, home respiratory care products and Sleep Well Ventures products; and Hospital Products, which include critical care products, respiratory drug delivery products and Children's Medical Ventures products. Sleep disordered breathing products include devices and accessories used in the home for the treatment of Obstructive Sleep Apnea (OSA); patient interface products, including nasal pillows and full face masks; and products that are used to diagnose sleep disorders in sleep labs and for patient testing in the home. Home respiratory care products include noninvasive ventilation products that provide positive airway pressure by mask to supplement the patient's own breathing; portable life support ventilators used in the home on patients requiring continuous support; stationary and portable oxygen delivery products; and oximetry products. Sleep Well Ventures' products target undiagnosed and untreated sleep and sleep-related movement disorders such as insomnia, circadian rhythm disorders and restless leg syndrome. Critical care products include noninvasive ventilators, patient masks, accessories, patient monitoring technologies and spontaneous breathing trial products. Respiratory drug delivery products include methods of delivering drugs via the respiratory pathway to help treat chronic obstructive pulmonary disease, asthma, pulmonary arterial hypertension and cystic fibrosis. Children's Medical Ventures provide developmentally supportive products for premature and ill infants in the hospital or home, including apnea monitors and diagnostic and treatment tools for jaundice. In 2008, the company was acquired by Royal Phillips Electronics.

Respironics offers its employees wellness programs, fitness centers, flex time, service awards, recognition programs, patent awards, educational assistance and credit union membership.

FINANCIALS: Sales and profits are in thousands of dollars—add 000 to get the full amount. 2007 Note: Financial information for 2007 was not available for all companies at press time.

2007 Sales: $1,195,035	2007 Profits: $122,285	**U.S. Stock Ticker:** Subsidiary
2006 Sales: $1,046,141	2006 Profits: $99,893	**Int'l Ticker:** Int'l Exchange:
2005 Sales: $911,500	2005 Profits: $84,400	Employees: 4,900
2004 Sales: $759,550	2004 Profits: $65,020	Fiscal Year Ends: 6/30
2003 Sales: $629,800	2003 Profits: $46,600	Parent Company: ROYAL PHILIPS ELECTRONICS NV

SALARIES/BENEFITS:

Pension Plan:	ESOP Stock Plan:	Profit Sharing: Y	Top Exec. Salary: $634,616	Bonus: $490,000
Savings Plan: Y	Stock Purch. Plan: Y		Second Exec. Salary: $500,225	Bonus: $312,096

OTHER THOUGHTS:
Apparent Women Officers or Directors: 1
Hot Spot for Advancement for Women/Minorities:

LOCATIONS: ("Y" = Yes)

West:	Southwest:	Midwest:	Southeast:	Northeast:	International:
Y	Y		Y	Y	Y

Note: Financial information, benefits and other data can change quickly and may vary from those stated here.

RITE AID CORPORATION

www.riteaid.com

Industry Group Code: 446110 **Ranks within this company's industry group:** Sales: Profits:

Management:	Sales/Marketing:	Liberal Arts:	Information Systems:	Professionals:	Technical/Scientific:
Mgmt. Trainees:	Mktg. Professionals:	Gen. Writing/Editing:	Info. Management:	Finance/Accounting:	Engineers, Elec.:
Experienced Mgmt.:	Retail Sales:	Technical Writing:	Software Dev.:	Law:	Engineers, Other:
Int'l Business:	Commercial/Industrial:	Graphic Arts/Photog.:	Hardware Dev.:	HR/Other:	Health/Lab:
MBA Graduates:	Sales Trainees:	Music:	Systems Integration:	Training:	Scientists/Research:
	Advertising Pros.:	Broadcasting:	Consulting/Other:	Health Care:	Petroleum/Chemicals:
		Other:		Consulting:	Math/Other:

TYPES OF BUSINESS:

Drug Stores
Pharmacy Benefits Management

BRANDS/DIVISIONS/AFFILIATES:

FLAVORx
Rite Aid Health Solutions
Brooks Eckerd
Saint Alphonsus Express Care
MedStar PromptCare
c.booth derma
Pure Spring
MultiCare Express Clinics

CONTACTS: *Note: Officers with more than one job title may be intentionally listed here more than once.*

Mary Sammons, CEO
Robert J. Easley, COO
Mary Sammons, Pres.
Kevin Twomey, CFO/Exec. VP
Mark Panzer, Chief Mktg. Officer/Sr. Exec. VP
Steve Parsons, Sr. VP-Human Resources
Don P. Davis, CIO/Sr. VP
Pierre Legault, Chief Admin. Officer
Robert Sari, General Counsel/Exec. VP
Christopher Hall, Sr. VP-Strategic Bus. Dev.
Karen Rugen, Sr. VP-Corp. Comm.
Doug Donley, Chief Acct. Officer/Sr. VP
Mark de Bruin, Exec. VP-Pharmacy
Brian Fiala, Exec. VP-Store Oper.
Tony Bellezza, Sr. VP/Chief Compliance Officer
John Learish, Sr. VP-Mktg.
Mary Sammons, Chmn.
Wilson A. Lester, Jr., Sr. VP-Supply Chain

Phone: 717-761-2633	Fax: 717-975-5871
Toll-Free: 800-748-3243	
Address: 30 Hunter Ln., Camp Hill, PA 17011 US	

GROWTH PLANS/SPECIAL FEATURES:

Rite Aid Corp. operates over 5,000 drug stores in 31 states and Washington, D.C. Rite Aid stores sell prescription drugs, which accounted for about 66.7% of revenue in fiscal year 2008, and other merchandise such as non-prescription medications; health and beauty aids; personal care items; cosmetics; household items; beverages; convenience foods; greeting cards; and seasonal merchandise. Rite Aid offers over 26,300 products, approximately 3,000 of which are under the Rite Aid private brand. Approximately 56% of Rite Aid's stores are freestanding; 47% include a drive-through pharmacy; 62% include one-hour photo shops; and 29% include a GNC store-within-Rite Aid-store. The company's Rite Aid Health Solutions segment provides pharmacy benefit management services to employers, health plans and insurance companies. In June 2007, the company acquired 1,854 Brooks and Eckerd Stores and six distribution centers from The Jean Coutu Group, Inc. In October 2007, Rite Aid opened two Saint Alphonsus Express Care in-store clinics in Idaho. A third opened in April 2008. As of March 2008, The Jean Coutu Group owns 28.6% of Rite Aid common stock. In April 2008, the firm announced plans for four MedStar PromptCare in-store health clinics in Baltimore and Washington, D.C. Also in April, the firm announced the new c.booth derma skin care line and new Rite Aid's Pure Spring bath and body products, as well as new natural organic sections in many nationwide stores. Rite Aid agreed in April to purchase certain assets of 12 Pharm retail stores from Spartan Stores, Inc. In May 2008, the company partnered with MultiCare Health System to open two in-store MultiCare Express Clinics in Washington. Rite Aid and Fujifilm announced new expanded, state-of-the-art services beginning in summer 2008.

The company offers its employees health, dental and vision insurance; life and AD&D insurance; and an employee assistance program.

FINANCIALS: Sales and profits are in thousands of dollars—add 000 to get the full amount. 2007 Note: Financial information for 2007 was not available for all companies at press time.

2007 Sales: $17,507,719	2007 Profits: $26,826	**U.S. Stock Ticker:** RAD
2006 Sales: $17,270,968	2006 Profits: $1,273,006	**Int'l Ticker:** Int'l Exchange:
2005 Sales: $16,816,439	2005 Profits: $302,478	Employees: 69,700
2004 Sales: $16,600,449	2004 Profits: $83,311	Fiscal Year Ends: 2/28
2003 Sales: $15,800,900	2003 Profits: $-112,100	Parent Company:

SALARIES/BENEFITS:

Pension Plan:	ESOP Stock Plan:	Profit Sharing:	Top Exec. Salary: $1,000,000	Bonus: $1,543,631
Savings Plan: Y	Stock Purch. Plan: Y		Second Exec. Salary: $775,000	Bonus: $877,297

OTHER THOUGHTS:

Apparent Women Officers or Directors: 4
Hot Spot for Advancement for Women/Minorities: Y

LOCATIONS: ("Y" = Yes)

West:	Southwest:	Midwest:	Southeast:	Northeast:	International:
Y	Y	Y	Y	Y	

RITZ-CARLTON HOTEL COMPANY LLC (THE)
www.ritzcarlton.com

Industry Group Code: 721110 Ranks within this company's industry group: Sales: Profits:

Management:		Sales/Marketing:		Liberal Arts:		Information Systems:		Professionals:		Technical/Scientific:	
Mgmt. Trainees:	Y	Mktg. Professionals:	Y	Gen. Writing/Editing:	Y	Info. Management:	Y	Finance/Accounting:	Y	Engineers, Elec.:	
Experienced Mgmt.:	Y	Retail Sales:		Technical Writing:		Software Dev.:		Law:	Y	Engineers, Other:	
Int'l Business:	Y	Commercial/Industrial:	Y	Graphic Arts/Photog.:	Y	Hardware Dev.:		HR/Other:	Y	Health/Lab:	
MBA Graduates:	Y	Sales Trainees:		Music:		Systems Integration:		Training:	Y	Scientists/Research:	
		Advertising Pros.:	Y	Broadcasting:		Consulting/Other:		Health Care:		Petroleum/Chemicals:	
				Other:				Consulting:		Math/Other:	

TYPES OF BUSINESS:
Hotels, Luxury
Condominiums
Golf Courses
Spas
Time Share Units

BRANDS/DIVISIONS/AFFILIATES:
Marriott International Inc
Ritz-Carlton Club
Taj Boston
Six Senses
La Prairie
2SPA

CONTACTS: Note: Officers with more than one job title may be intentionally listed here more than once.
Simon F. Cooper, COO
Simon F. Cooper, Pres.
Jim Connelly, CFO
Herve Humler, Pres., Int'l

Phone: 301-547-4700	Fax: 301-547-4723
Toll-Free:	
Address: 4445 Willard Ave., Ste. 800, Chevy Chase, MD 20815 US	

GROWTH PLANS/SPECIAL FEATURES:

The Ritz-Carlton Hotel Co., LLC, a subsidiary of Marriott International, Inc., is one of the world's best-known luxury hotel chains, operating 70 hotels in 23 countries. In an attempt to cater to an upscale clientele base, full-service luxury spas are offered at most of the company's resorts, and plans have been made for additional spas at new or existing hotel locations. Some spas at Ritz-Carlton hotels operate under the brand names Six Senses, La Prairie and 2SPA. Additionally, Ritz-Carlton markets its 15 luxury golf courses (many designed by leading names in the golf world such as Greg Norman and Jack Nicklaus) and fitness facilities to both local residents and visitors. The Ritz-Carlton Club is the firm's time share ownership unit, offering a flexible alternative to a second home. This concept features luxury condominiums located at Ritz-Carlton's hotels and resorts worldwide, with features such as marble foyers, walk-in closets, daily housekeeping services, 24-hour room service and access to fitness facilities and spa services. Membership is currently available in locations such as Aspen, St. Thomas, Bachelor Gulch and Jupiter, Florida. The firm plans to expand hotel operations to such locations as Toronto, Canada and Rose Island, Bahamas. In 2007, the firm opened resorts in Tokyo, Japan; Bali; and Doha, Qatar. Indian-based chain Taj Hotels took over Ritz-Carlton operations at the Ritz-Carlton Boston, renaming the hotel Taj Boston.

The company offers its employees benefits that include medical, dental and vision insurance; short- and long-term disability insurance; life and AD&D insurance; flexible spending accounts; a 401(k) plan; an employee stock purchase plan; domestic partner benefits; educational assistance; employee discounts; and an employee assistance program. It also sponsors a leadership training center, the Ritz-Carlton Leadership Center, that has benefited managers from diverse industries such as financial, hospitality and automotive.

FINANCIALS: Sales and profits are in thousands of dollars—add 000 to get the full amount. 2007 Note: Financial information for 2007 was not available for all companies at press time.

2007 Sales: $1,576,000	2007 Profits: $72,000	U.S. Stock Ticker: Subsidiary
2006 Sales: $1,423,000	2006 Profits: $	Int'l Ticker: Int'l Exchange:
2005 Sales: $	2005 Profits: $	Employees:
2004 Sales: $	2004 Profits: $	Fiscal Year Ends: 12/31
2003 Sales: $	2003 Profits: $	Parent Company: MARRIOTT INTERNATIONAL INC

SALARIES/BENEFITS:

Pension Plan:	ESOP Stock Plan:	Profit Sharing:	Top Exec. Salary: $	Bonus: $
Savings Plan: Y	Stock Purch. Plan: Y		Second Exec. Salary: $	Bonus: $

OTHER THOUGHTS:
Apparent Women Officers or Directors: 1
Hot Spot for Advancement for Women/Minorities:

LOCATIONS: ("Y" = Yes)

West:	Southwest:	Midwest:	Southeast:	Northeast:	International:
Y	Y	Y	Y	Y	Y

ROBERT HALF INTERNATIONAL INC

www.rhi.com

Industry Group Code: 561320 Ranks within this company's industry group: Sales: 3 Profits: 2

Management:		Sales/Marketing:		Liberal Arts:		Information Systems:		Professionals:		Technical/Scientific:	
Mgmt. Trainees:		Mktg. Professionals:	Y	Gen. Writing/Editing:	Y	Info. Management:	Y	Finance/Accounting:	Y	Engineers, Elec.:	
Experienced Mgmt.:	Y	Retail Sales:		Technical Writing:		Software Dev.:		Law:	Y	Engineers, Other:	
Int'l Business:	Y	Commercial/Industrial:	Y	Graphic Arts/Photog.:		Hardware Dev.:		HR/Other:	Y	Health/Lab:	
MBA Graduates:	Y	Sales Trainees:		Music:		Systems Integration:	Y	Training:	Y	Scientists/Research:	
		Advertising Pros.:	Y	Broadcasting:		Consulting/Other:		Health Care:		Petroleum/Chemicals:	
				Other:	Y			Consulting:	Y	Math/Other:	

TYPES OF BUSINESS:

Staffing
Risk Consulting
Internal Audit Services
Litigation Consulting & Forensic Accounting

BRANDS/DIVISIONS/AFFILIATES:

Accountemps
Robert Half Finance & Accounting
Robert Half Management Resources
Robert Half Technology
OfficeTeam
Robert Half Legal
Creative Group (The)
Protiviti, Inc.

CONTACTS: *Note: Officers with more than one job title may be intentionally listed here more than once.*

Harold M. Messmer, Jr., CEO
M. Keith Waddell, Pres./Vice Chmn.
M. Keith Waddell, CFO
Elena West, Sr. VP-Mktg.
Michael C. Buckley, Chief Admin. Officer/Treas./Exec. VP
Steven Karel, General Counsel/Sr. VP/Corp. Sec.
Robert W. Glass, Exec. VP-Corp. Dev.
Reesa M. Staten, VP-Corp. Comm.
Paula Streit, Sr. VP-Operational Finance & Acct.
Paul F. Gentzkow, COO/Pres., Staffing Svcs.
Evelyn Crane-Oliver, VP/Associate General Counsel
Harold M. Messmer, Jr., Chmn.

Phone: 650-234-6000	Fax: 650-234-6999
Toll-Free:	
Address: 2884 Sand Hill Rd., Ste. 200, Menlo Park, CA 94025 US	

GROWTH PLANS/SPECIAL FEATURES:

Robert Half International, Inc. (RHI) is a global staffing firm that provides professional staffing and risk consulting services. RHI operates through more than 360 company operated or owned locations in 19 countries around the world, including Europe, Asia, Australia and New Zealand. The company provides temporary, project and full-time workers to firms in areas such as accounting, finance, administrative and legal support, information technology, advertising and marketing. RHI consists of seven staffing divisions: Accountemps for the staffing of accounting and finance professionals; Robert Half Finance and Accounting and Robert Half Management Resources for senior-level accounting and financing professionals; OfficeTeam, a division for highly skilled temporary administrative support; Robert Half Technology for information technology professionals; Robert Half Legal, a staffing sector for attorneys, paralegals and legal support personnel; and the Creative Group for advertising, marketing and web design professionals. The company's wholly-owned subsidiary, Protiviti, Inc., provides internal audit and risk consulting services by aiding clients in identifying, measuring and managing operational and technology-related risks in areas such as the media, hospitality, communications, energy, financial services, real estate, healthcare, government, education, non-profit, manufacturing, distribution and technology industries. Business risk consultations involve areas such as anti-money laundering, capital projects and construction, energy commodity risks, fraud investigation and forensic accounting. Technology risk consultations provide solutions for security and privacy, continuity, change management, IT assets and application effectiveness. In April 2007, RHI acquired Penta Advisory Services, a provider of restructuring, bankruptcy-related litigation and tax services. Penta was acquired through Protiviti, which integrated Penta into its event response practice.

FINANCIALS: Sales and profits are in thousands of dollars—add 000 to get the full amount. 2007 Note: Financial information for 2007 was not available for all companies at press time.

2007 Sales: $4,645,666	2007 Profits: $296,212	U.S. Stock Ticker: RHI
2006 Sales: $4,013,546	2006 Profits: $283,178	Int'l Ticker: Int'l Exchange:
2005 Sales: $3,338,439	2005 Profits: $237,870	Employees: 15,300
2004 Sales: $2,675,696	2004 Profits: $140,604	Fiscal Year Ends: 12/31
2003 Sales: $1,974,991	2003 Profits: $6,390	Parent Company:

SALARIES/BENEFITS:

Pension Plan:	ESOP Stock Plan:	Profit Sharing:	Top Exec. Salary: $525,000	Bonus: $6,339,334
Savings Plan: Y	Stock Purch. Plan:		Second Exec. Salary: $265,000	Bonus: $3,173,586

OTHER THOUGHTS:

Apparent Women Officers or Directors: 4
Hot Spot for Advancement for Women/Minorities: Y

LOCATIONS: ("Y" = Yes)

West:	Southwest:	Midwest:	Southeast:	Northeast:	International:
Y	Y	Y	Y	Y	Y

ROSS STORES INC

www.rossstores.com

Industry Group Code: 448000 Ranks within this company's industry group: Sales: 2 Profits: 4

Management:		Sales/Marketing:		Liberal Arts:		Information Systems:		Professionals:		Technical/Scientific:	
Mgmt. Trainees:	Y	Mktg. Professionals:	Y	Gen. Writing/Editing:	Y	Info. Management:	Y	Finance/Accounting:	Y	Engineers, Elec.:	
Experienced Mgmt.:	Y	Retail Sales:	Y	Technical Writing:		Software Dev.:	Y	Law:	Y	Engineers, Other:	
Int'l Business:	Y	Commercial/Industrial:	Y	Graphic Arts/Photog.:	Y	Hardware Dev.:		HR/Other:	Y	Health/Lab:	
MBA Graduates:	Y	Sales Trainees:	Y	Music:		Systems Integration:		Training:	Y	Scientists/Research:	
		Advertising Pros.:	Y	Broadcasting:		Consulting/Other:		Health Care:		Petroleum/Chemicals:	
				Other:	Y			Consulting:		Math/Other:	

TYPES OF BUSINESS:

Discount Apparel Stores
Home Furnishings

BRANDS/DIVISIONS/AFFILIATES:

dd's DISCOUNTS
Ross Dress for Less

CONTACTS: Note: Officers with more than one job title may be intentionally listed here more than once.

Michael A. Balmuth, CEO
Gary Cribb, COO/Exec. VP
Michael Balmuth, Pres.
John G. Call, CFO/Sr. VP/Corp. Sec.
D. Jane Marvin, Sr. VP-Human Resources
Michael K. Kobayashi, CIO/Sr. VP
Lisa Panattoni, Exec. VP-Merch.
Michael B. O'Sullivan, Chief Admin. Officer/Exec. VP
Mark LeHocky, General Counsel/Sr. VP
Ken Caruana, Sr. VP-Strategy, Mktg-Store Planning & Allocation
Douglas Baker, Sr. VP/Gen. Merch. Mgr., dd's DISCOUNTS
Art Roth, Sr. VP-Merch. Control
Barbara Rentler, Exec. VP-Merch.
James S. Fassio, Exe. VP-Property Dev., Construction & Store Design
Norman A. Ferber, Chmn.
Michael K. Kobayashi, Sr. VP-Supply Chain

Phone: 925-965-4400	Fax: 925-965-4388
Toll-Free:	
Address: 4440 Rosewood Dr., Pleasanton, CA 94588-3050 US	

GROWTH PLANS/SPECIAL FEATURES:

Ross Stores, Inc. operates two chains of off-price retail apparel and home accessories stores in 27 states and Guam, including 890 Ross Dress for Less locations and 52 dd's DISCOUNTS locations in California. Most of the stores are located in predominantly community and neighborhood strip shopping centers in heavily populated urban and suburban areas. The company's chains target value-conscious women and men age 18-54. With customers primarily from middle-income households, Ross offers first-quality, in-season, name-brand and designer apparel, accessories, footwear and home merchandise at savings of 20% to 60% off department and specialty store regular prices, while dd's DISCOUNTS, targeting customers from lower-income households, offers similar merchandise, but at savings of up to 70% off department and specialty store prices. The company's stores are supplied by four distribution processing facilities. Ross has combined a network of approximately 6,400 vendors and manufacturers, purchasing the vast majority of its merchandise directly from the manufacturer. By purchasing later in the merchandise buying cycle than department and specialty stores, Ross is able to take advantage of imbalances between retailers' demand for products and manufacturers' supply of those products. In addition, the company typically does not require that manufacturers provide promotional and markdown allowances, return privileges, split shipments, drop shipments to stores or delayed deliveries of merchandise, further enabling the company to provide significant discounts on in-season merchandise.

Ross offers its employees a merchandise discount, accidental death and dismemberment insurance, long term disability, sick pay, health care spending account, a commuter reimbursement account and a dependent day care spending account.

FINANCIALS: Sales and profits are in thousands of dollars—add 000 to get the full amount. 2007 Note: Financial information for 2007 was not available for all companies at press time.

2007 Sales: $5,570,210	2007 Profits: $241,634	U.S. Stock Ticker: ROST
2006 Sales: $4,944,179	2006 Profits: $199,632	Int'l Ticker: Int'l Exchange:
2005 Sales: $4,239,990	2005 Profits: $169,902	Employees: 35,800
2004 Sales: $3,920,583	2004 Profits: $228,102	Fiscal Year Ends: 1/31
2003 Sales: $3,531,300	2003 Profits: $201,200	Parent Company:

SALARIES/BENEFITS:

Pension Plan:	ESOP Stock Plan:	Profit Sharing:	Top Exec. Salary: $993,791	Bonus: $1,099,848
Savings Plan: Y	Stock Purch. Plan: Y		Second Exec. Salary: $612,613	Bonus: $588,181

OTHER THOUGHTS:

Apparent Women Officers or Directors: 7
Hot Spot for Advancement for Women/Minorities: Y

LOCATIONS: ("Y" = Yes)

West:	Southwest:	Midwest:	Southeast:	Northeast:	International:
Y	Y		Y	Y	Y

Note: Financial information, benefits and other data can change quickly and may vary from those stated here.

ROYAL CARIBBEAN CRUISES   www.royalcaribbean.com

Industry Group Code: 483112   Ranks within this company's industry group: Sales: 2   Profits: 2

Management:		Sales/Marketing:		Liberal Arts:		Information Systems:		Professionals:		Technical/Scientific:	
Mgmt. Trainees:	Y	Mktg. Professionals:	Y	Gen. Writing/Editing:	Y	Info. Management:	Y	Finance/Accounting:	Y	Engineers, Elec.:	Y
Experienced Mgmt.:	Y	Retail Sales:		Technical Writing:		Software Dev.:	Y	Law:	Y	Engineers, Other:	Y
Int'l Business:	Y	Commercial/Industrial:	Y	Graphic Arts/Photog.:	Y	Hardware Dev.:		HR/Other:	Y	Health/Lab:	
MBA Graduates:	Y	Sales Trainees:		Music:	Y	Systems Integration:		Training:	Y	Scientists/Research:	
		Advertising Pros.:	Y	Broadcasting:		Consulting/Other:		Health Care:	Y	Petroleum/Chemicals:	
				Other:	Y			Consulting:		Math/Other:	

TYPES OF BUSINESS:

Cruise Line
Rail Tours
Online Travel Services
Academic Tours

BRANDS/DIVISIONS/AFFILIATES:

Royal Caribbean International
Celebrity Cruises
Royal Celebrity Tours
Pullmantur
Azamara
Freedom of the Seas
Scholar Ship (The)
Liberty of the Seas

CONTACTS: Note: Officers with more than one job title may be intentionally listed here more than once.

Richard D. Fain, CEO
Adam M. Goldstein, Pres.
Brian Rice, CFO/Exec. VP
Alice Norsworthy, Sr. VP-Mktg.
Mike Sutten, CIO
William Wright, Sr. VP-Marine Oper.
Dan Hanrahan, Pres., Celebrity Cruises
Harri Kulovaara, Exec. VP-Maritime
Lisa Bauer, Sr. VP-Hotel Oper.
Susan Hooper, Managing Dir./Sr. VP-EMEA
Richard D. Fain, Chmn.
Adam Goldstein, Pres., Royal Caribbean Int'l

Phone: 305-539-6000	Fax: 305-374-7354
Toll-Free:	
Address: 1050 Caribbean Way, Miami, FL 33132-2096 US	

GROWTH PLANS/SPECIAL FEATURES:

Royal Caribbean Cruises, Ltd. is a global cruise vacation company serving the contemporary, premium and deluxe cruise markets, which also includes the budget and luxury segments. The firm operates 35 ships in the cruise vacation industry with approximately 71,200 berths. It owns Royal Caribbean International, Celebrity Cruises, Pullmantur Cruises, Azamara Cruises, and CDF Croisieres de France, and has a 50% investment in a joint venture with TUI Travel PLC, which operates Island Cruises. The company's worldwide destinations include Alaska, Australia/New Zealand, the Bahamas, Canada/New England, the Caribbean, Europe, Asia, Hawaii, Mexico, the U.S. Pacific Northwest, the Panama Canal and South America. The ships operate worldwide with a selection of itineraries that call on approximately 380 destinations. Its ships offer a wide range of activities, services and amenities, including swimming pools, sun decks, salons, gyms, spas, ice skating rinks, rock climbing walls, casinos, lounges, bars, on-board entertainment, retail shopping and movie theaters. The Celebrity Cruises brand targets the higher-end segment of the industry with superior service and facilities and cruises to unusual destinations such as the Arctic, Antarctic and the Galapagos. Subsidiary Royal Celebrity Tours operates land-tour vacations in several locations, including Alaska, using the world's largest glass-domed train cars; Canada, alongside Rocky Mountaineer Railtours; and Europe. Royal Caribbean will launch a new ship, Oasis of the Seas, in December 2009, projected to be the world's largest cruise ship. Her sister ship will follow in 2010.

The firm offers special rates for employees, their families and relatives. For sea-based employees, Royal Caribbean operates on a 14-weeks-on, 14-weeks-off plan.

FINANCIALS: Sales and profits are in thousands of dollars—add 000 to get the full amount. 2007 Note: Financial information for 2007 was not available for all companies at press time.

2007 Sales: $6,149,139	2007 Profits: $603,405	U.S. Stock Ticker: RCL
2006 Sales: $5,229,584	2006 Profits: $633,922	Int'l Ticker: Int'l Exchange:
2005 Sales: $4,903,174	2005 Profits: $715,956	Employees: 5,068
2004 Sales: $4,555,375	2004 Profits: $474,691	Fiscal Year Ends: 12/31
2003 Sales: $3,784,249	2003 Profits: $280,664	Parent Company:

SALARIES/BENEFITS:

Pension Plan: Y	ESOP Stock Plan:	Profit Sharing:	Top Exec. Salary: $1,001,923	Bonus: $2,990,625
Savings Plan:	Stock Purch. Plan: Y		Second Exec. Salary: $644,231	Bonus: $1,179,393

OTHER THOUGHTS:

Apparent Women Officers or Directors: 4
Hot Spot for Advancement for Women/Minorities: Y

LOCATIONS: ("Y" = Yes)

West:	Southwest:	Midwest:	Southeast:	Northeast:	International:
Y		Y	Y		Y

RUSSELL CORP

www.russellcorp.com

Industry Group Code: 315000A Ranks within this company's industry group: Sales: Profits:

Management:		Sales/Marketing:		Liberal Arts:		Information Systems:		Professionals:		Technical/Scientific:	
Mgmt. Trainees:	Y	Mktg. Professionals:	Y	Gen. Writing/Editing:		Info. Management:	Y	Finance/Accounting:	Y	Engineers, Elec.:	
Experienced Mgmt.:	Y	Retail Sales:		Technical Writing:		Software Dev.:		Law:	Y	Engineers, Other:	
Int'l Business:	Y	Commercial/Industrial:	Y	Graphic Arts/Photog.:		Hardware Dev.:		HR/Other:	Y	Health/Lab:	
MBA Graduates:	Y	Sales Trainees:		Music:		Systems Integration:		Training:	Y	Scientists/Research:	
		Advertising Pros.:	Y	Broadcasting:		Consulting/Other:		Health Care:		Petroleum/Chemicals:	
				Other:	Y			Consulting:		Math/Other:	

TYPES OF BUSINESS:

Athletic Apparel & Equipment
Athletic Uniforms

BRANDS/DIVISIONS/AFFILIATES:

Spalding
Russell Athletic
Mossy Oak Apparel
JERZEES
Moving Comfort
Russell Artwear
Brooks Sports
Berkshire Hathaway

CONTACTS: *Note: Officers with more than one job title may be intentionally listed here more than once.*

John B. Holland, CEO
Robert D. Koney, Jr., CFO
Edsel W. Flowers, Sr. VP-Human Resources
Robert P. Keefe, CIO
Floyd G. Hoffman, General Counsel/Corp. Sec.
Floyd G. Hoffman, Sr. VP-Corp. Dev.
Nancy N. Young, VP-Comm.
Victoria W. Beck, VP/Corp. Controller
Scott H. Creelman, VP/CEO-Spalding
James Weber, VP/CEO-Brooks Sports
John B. Holland, Chmn.

Phone: 678-742-8000	**Fax:** 678-742-8300

Toll-Free:

Address: 3330 Cumberland Blvd., Ste. 800, Atlanta, GA 30339 US

GROWTH PLANS/SPECIAL FEATURES:

Russell Corp., a Berkshire Hathaway company, is a leading branded athletic, active wear and outdoor gear company that markets athletic uniforms, apparel, footwear, sporting goods, athletic equipment and accessories for a wide variety of sports, outdoor and fitness activities. The firm's well-known brands include Russell Athletic, JERZEES, Brooks Sports, Mossy Oak, Cross Creek, Moving Comfort, Discus, Bike, Spalding, Dudley, Huffy and Sherrin. The company markets and manufactures a variety of apparel products, including fleece, t-shirts, casual shirts, jackets, athletic shorts, socks and camouflage attire for men, women, boys and girls. Russell is also a leading supplier of uniforms and related apparel to college, high school and other organized sports teams. The company is the largest provider of basketball equipment in the world, due in part to its eight-year global partnership with the National Basketball Association. Russell markets its products in the U.S., Canada and approximately 100 additional countries through mass merchandisers, sporting goods dealers, department and sports specialty stores, college stores, online retailers, mail-order houses, art wear distributors, screen printers and embroiderers. The company's largest customer is Wal-Mart, making up approximately 20% of annual sales. Early in 2008, Russell Corp. obtained a patent for a basketball hoop ratchet elevator system that allows players to adjust the height of the net and backboard without the use of tools.

FINANCIALS: Sales and profits are in thousands of dollars—add 000 to get the full amount. 2007 Note: Financial information for 2007 was not available for all companies at press time.

2007 Sales: $561,800	2007 Profits: $	**U.S. Stock Ticker:** Subsidiary
2006 Sales: $	2006 Profits: $	**Int'l Ticker:** **Int'l Exchange:**
2005 Sales: $1,434,605	2005 Profits: $34,430	Employees: 14,400
2004 Sales: $1,298,252	2004 Profits: $47,936	Fiscal Year Ends: 12/31
2003 Sales: $1,186,263	2003 Profits: $43,039	Parent Company: BERKSHIRE HATHAWAY INC

SALARIES/BENEFITS:

Pension Plan: Y	ESOP Stock Plan:	Profit Sharing:	Top Exec. Salary: $845,600	Bonus: $
Savings Plan: Y	Stock Purch. Plan:		Second Exec. Salary: $343,834	Bonus: $71,099

OTHER THOUGHTS:

Apparent Women Officers or Directors: 1
Hot Spot for Advancement for Women/Minorities:

LOCATIONS: ("Y" = Yes)

West:	Southwest:	Midwest:	Southeast:	Northeast:	International:
Y		Y	Y	Y	Y

RYDER SYSTEM INC

www.ryder.com

Industry Group Code: 532120 Ranks within this company's industry group: Sales: 1 Profits: 1

Management:		Sales/Marketing:		Liberal Arts:	Information Systems:		Professionals:		Technical/Scientific:
Mgmt. Trainees:	Y	Mktg. Professionals:	Y	Gen. Writing/Editing:	Info. Management:	Y	Finance/Accounting:	Y	Engineers, Elec.:
Experienced Mgmt.:	Y	Retail Sales:		Technical Writing:	Software Dev.:	Y	Law:	Y	Engineers, Other:
Int'l Business:	Y	Commercial/Industrial:	Y	Graphic Arts/Photog.:	Hardware Dev.:		HR/Other:	Y	Health/Lab:
MBA Graduates:	Y	Sales Trainees:		Music:	Systems Integration:		Training:	Y	Scientists/Research:
		Advertising Pros.:		Broadcasting:	Consulting/Other:		Health Care:		Petroleum/Chemicals:
				Other:			Consulting:		Math/Other:

TYPES OF BUSINESS:

Truck Rental & Leasing
Trucking
Logistics & Consulting Services
Supply Chain Management
Dedicated Fleet Services
Fleet Management Services

BRANDS/DIVISIONS/AFFILIATES:

Pollock NationaLease

CONTACTS: Note: Officers with more than one job title may be intentionally listed here more than once.

Gregory T. Swienton, CEO
Robert E. Sanchez, CFO/Exec. VP
Gregory F. Greene, Chief Human Resources Officer/Exec. VP
Robert D. Fatovic, Chief Legal Officer/Exec. VP/Corp. Sec.
Lisa Brumfield, Dir.-Corp. Comm.
Robert Brunn, VP-Investor Rel. & Public Affairs
David Bruce, VP-Corp. Comm.
Anthony G. Tegnelia, Pres., U.S. Fleet Mgmt. Solutions
Thomas S. Renehan, Exec. VP-Sales & Mktg., U.S. Fleet Mgmt. Solutions
Gregory T. Swienton, Chmn.
David P. Bouchard, Managing Dir.-Int'l

Phone: 305-500-3726	Fax: 305-500-3203
Toll-Free:	
Address: 11690 N.W. 105th St., Miami, FL 33178 US	

GROWTH PLANS/SPECIAL FEATURES:

Ryder System, Inc. is a global provider of transportation and supply chain management solutions. It operates in three segments: Fleet management solutions, supply chain solutions and dedicated contract carriage. The fleet management solutions segment provides full service leasing, contract maintenance, contract-related maintenance and commercial renal of trucks, tractors and trailers to customers principally in the U.S., Canada and the U.K. The division also offers transaction fleet solutions, including commercial truck rental, maintenance services and value-added fleet support services such as insurance, vehicle administration and fuel services. In addition, it provides customers with access to a large selection of used trucks, tractors and trailers through the used vehicle sales program. The supply chain solutions segment provides supply chain solutions including distribution and transportation services throughout North America and in Latin America, Europe and Asia. The division's product offerings are organized into three categories: Professional services, distribution operations and transportation solutions. Additionally, the firm offers customers a variety of information technology solutions, or e-fulfillment. The dedicated contract carriage segment combines equipment, maintenance and administrative services with additional services such as driver hiring and training, routing and scheduling, fleet sizing, safety, regulatory compliance, risk management, technology and communication systems support, including on-board computers and other technical support. In October 2007, Ryder System acquired Pollock NationaLease, a Canadian private commercial truck leasing and rental company. In January 2008, the company acquired full service truck leasing, commercial truck rental and contract maintenance businesses of Lily Transportation Corp.

FINANCIALS: Sales and profits are in thousands of dollars—add 000 to get the full amount. 2007 Note: Financial information for 2007 was not available for all companies at press time.

		U.S. Stock Ticker: R
2007 Sales: $6,565,995	2007 Profits: $253,861	Int'l Ticker: Int'l Exchange:
2006 Sales: $6,306,643	2006 Profits: $248,959	Employees: 28,800
2005 Sales: $5,740,847	2005 Profits: $226,929	Fiscal Year Ends: 12/31
2004 Sales: $5,150,278	2004 Profits: $215,609	Parent Company:
2003 Sales: $4,802,294	2003 Profits: $131,436	

SALARIES/BENEFITS:

Pension Plan:	ESOP Stock Plan:	Profit Sharing:	Top Exec. Salary: $843,750	Bonus: $1,744,716
Savings Plan:	Stock Purch. Plan:		Second Exec. Salary: $490,250	Bonus: $624,088

OTHER THOUGHTS:

Apparent Women Officers or Directors: 4
Hot Spot for Advancement for Women/Minorities: Y

LOCATIONS: ("Y" = Yes)

West:	Southwest:	Midwest:	Southeast:	Northeast:	International:
			Y		Y

SABRE HOLDINGS CORP

www.sabre.com

Industry Group Code: 561500A **Ranks within this company's industry group:** Sales: 1 Profits: 1

Management:		Sales/Marketing:		Liberal Arts:		Information Systems:		Professionals:		Technical/Scientific:	
Mgmt. Trainees:		Mktg. Professionals:	Y	Gen. Writing/Editing:	Y	Info. Management:	Y	Finance/Accounting:	Y	Engineers, Elec.:	Y
Experienced Mgmt.:	Y	Retail Sales:		Technical Writing:	Y	Software Dev.:	Y	Law:	Y	Engineers, Other:	
Int'l Business:	Y	Commercial/Industrial:		Graphic Arts/Photog.:		Hardware Dev.:		HR/Other:	Y	Health/Lab:	
MBA Graduates:	Y	Sales Trainees:		Music:		Systems Integration:	Y	Training:	Y	Scientists/Research:	
		Advertising Pros.:		Broadcasting:		Consulting/Other:		Health Care:		Petroleum/Chemicals:	
				Other:				Consulting:		Math/Other:	

TYPES OF BUSINESS:

Online Travel Reservations
Travel Marketing Solutions
Distribution & Technology Solutions
Consulting Services

BRANDS/DIVISIONS/AFFILIATES:

Silver Lake Partners
Texas Pacific Group
Sabre Travel Network
Travelocity.com LP
LastMinute.com
Sabre Airline Solutions
getthere.com
E-site Marketing

CONTACTS: Note: Officers with more than one job title may be intentionally listed here more than once.

Sam Gilliland, CEO
Jeffery Jackson, CFO/Exec. VP
David Schwarte, General Counsel/Exec. VP
Thomas Klein, Exec. VP/Pres., Sabre Travel Network
Thomas Klein, Exec. VP/Pres., Sabre Airline Solutions
Michelle Peluso, Exec. VP/Pres./CEO-Travelocity

Phone: 682-605-1000	Fax: 682-605-8267
Toll-Free:	
Address: 3150 Sabre Dr., Southlake, TX 76092 US	

GROWTH PLANS/SPECIAL FEATURES:

Sabre Holdings Corp., an entity owned by private equity giants Silver Lake Partners and Texas Pacific Group, is a provider of travel commerce. It offers a broad portfolio of travel marketing, distribution and technology solutions. The company operates in three segments: Travelocity, Sabre Travel Network and Sabre Airline Solutions. The Travelocity segment markets and distributes travel-related products and services directly to individuals, including leisure travelers and business travelers, through the travelocity.com, lastminute.com and zuji.com web sites and contact centers. Travelers can access offerings, pricing and information about airlines, hotels, car rental companies, cruise lines, vacation and last-minute travel packages and other travel-related services. It also provides content and functionality to, and markets and sells products and services through private-label web sites for, suppliers, distribution partners and travel agencies. The Travelocity Business online corporate travel agency provides business travelers the offerings of the GetThere products. The Sabre Travel Network segment markets and distributes travel-related products and services for the travel supplier participants through the online and offline travel agency and corporate channels. Users of the Sabre system can access information about, book reservations for and purchase a variety of travel offerings, including airline trips, hotel stays, car rentals, cruises and tour packages. The division provides travel agencies with office automation tools and enables them to provide services via the Internet. In addition, Sabre Travel provides marketing information to suppliers and reservation management and technology services to hotel properties. The Sabre Airline Solutions segment provides passenger management solutions; software products and related services; and consulting services, which range from one time to extended engagements. It offers airline reservations, inventory and check-in hosting solutions. In 2007, the firm was acquired by private equity firms Silver Lake Partners and Texas Pacific Group for roughly $5 billion. In June 2007, Sabre Holdings purchased E-site Marketing.

FINANCIALS: Sales and profits are in thousands of dollars—add 000 to get the full amount. 2007 Note: Financial information for 2007 was not available for all companies at press time.

2007 Sales: $	2007 Profits: $	U.S. Stock Ticker: Private
2006 Sales: $2,823,797	2006 Profits: $155,638	Int'l Ticker: Int'l Exchange:
2005 Sales: $2,521,255	2005 Profits: $172,152	Employees: 9,000
2004 Sales: $2,130,971	2004 Profits: $190,419	Fiscal Year Ends: 12/31
2003 Sales: $2,000,869	2003 Profits: $83,301	Parent Company: SILVER LAKE PARTNERS

SALARIES/BENEFITS:

Pension Plan:	ESOP Stock Plan:	Profit Sharing:	Top Exec. Salary: $739,500	Bonus: $540,000
Savings Plan: Y	Stock Purch. Plan:		Second Exec. Salary: $424,000	Bonus: $585,000

OTHER THOUGHTS:

Apparent Women Officers or Directors: 1
Hot Spot for Advancement for Women/Minorities: Y

LOCATIONS: ("Y" = Yes)

West:	Southwest:	Midwest:	Southeast:	Northeast:	International:
Y	Y		Y	Y	Y

SAFECO CORP

www.safeco.com

Industry Group Code: 524126 Ranks within this company's industry group: Sales: Profits:

Management:		Sales/Marketing:		Liberal Arts:		Information Systems:		Professionals:		Technical/Scientific:	
Mgmt. Trainees:	Y	Mktg. Professionals:	Y	Gen. Writing/Editing:		Info. Management:	Y	Finance/Accounting:	Y	Engineers, Elec.:	
Experienced Mgmt.:	Y	Retail Sales:		Technical Writing:		Software Dev.:	Y	Law:	Y	Engineers, Other:	
Int'l Business:	Y	Commercial/Industrial:	Y	Graphic Arts/Photog.:		Hardware Dev.:		HR/Other:	Y	Health/Lab:	
MBA Graduates:	Y	Sales Trainees:		Music:		Systems Integration:		Training:	Y	Scientists/Research:	
		Advertising Pros.:	Y	Broadcasting:		Consulting/Other:		Health Care:		Petroleum/Chemicals:	
				Other:				Consulting:		Math/Other:	

TYPES OF BUSINESS:

Direct Property & Casualty Insurance
Business Insurance
Workers' Compensation
Surety Bonds
Personal Insurance
Specialty Insurance

BRANDS/DIVISIONS/AFFILIATES:

CONTACTS: *Note: Officers with more than one job title may be intentionally listed here more than once.*

Paula Rosput Reynolds, CEO
Paula R. Reynolds, Pres.
Ross Kari, CFO/Exec. VP
Rauline Ochs, Exec. VP-Sales & Mktg.
William Jenks, CIO
Arthur Chong, Chief Legal Officer/Exec. VP
Allie Mysliwy, Chief Bus. Officer/Exec. VP
David M. Monfried, VP-Corp. Comm.
Neal Fuller, Investor Rel.
Mike Hughes, Exec. VP-Insurance Oper.
R. Eric Martinez, Jr., Exec. VP-Claims, Customer Care & Procurement
Kim Garland, Pres., Open Seas Insurance
Joseph W. Brown, Chmn.

Phone: 206-545-5000	Fax: 206-545-5995
Toll-Free:	
Address: Safeco Plz., 1001 Fourth Avenue,, Seattle, WA 98154 US	

GROWTH PLANS/SPECIAL FEATURES:

Safeco Corp. is a provider of property and casualty insurance to homeowners, drivers and small- and mid-sized businesses.   The company operates in four segments, personal insurance, business insurance, surety and other. The personal insurance segment, which was responsible for about 66% of total revenue in 2007, offers auto, homeowners and other property and specialty insurance products for individuals.   Specialty insurance includes umbrella, motorcycle, recreational vehicle and boat owners' insurance coverage for individuals. The business insurance segment, which generated roughly 28% of net sales in 2007, provides business-owner policies, commercial auto, commercial multi-peril, workers' compensation, commercial property and general liability policies for small- and mid-sized businesses. The surety segment offers bonds that provide payment and performance guarantees primarily for construction businesses and corporations. The P&C other segment includes run-off assumed reinsurance, large commercial and business accounts and commercial specialty programs in run-off, and other business and programs the firm has exited. In 2008, the firm agreed to be acquired by Liberty Mutual for $6.2 billion. The transaction is expected to close by the end of third quarter 2008

The company offers its employees medical, dental and vision insurance; life and travel accident insurance; short- and long-term disability insurance; flexible spending accounts; a 401(k) plan; a profit sharing plan; tuition assistance and an employee discount program.

FINANCIALS: Sales and profits are in thousands of dollars—add 000 to get the full amount. 2007 Note: Financial information for 2007 was not available for all companies at press time.

2007 Sales: $6,208,800	2007 Profits: $707,800	U.S. Stock Ticker: SAF
2006 Sales: $6,289,900	2006 Profits: $880,000	Int'l Ticker: Int'l Exchange:
2005 Sales: $6,350,900	2005 Profits: $691,100	Employees: 7,208
2004 Sales: $6,195,400	2004 Profits: $562,400	Fiscal Year Ends: 12/31
2003 Sales: $7,358,100	2003 Profits: $339,200	Parent Company:

SALARIES/BENEFITS:

Pension Plan:	ESOP Stock Plan:	Profit Sharing: Y	Top Exec. Salary: $925,000	Bonus: $1,998,000
Savings Plan: Y	Stock Purch. Plan:		Second Exec. Salary: $400,000	Bonus: $796,000

OTHER THOUGHTS:

Apparent Women Officers or Directors: 3
Hot Spot for Advancement for Women/Minorities: Y

LOCATIONS: ("Y" = Yes)

West:	Southwest:	Midwest:	Southeast:	Northeast:	International:
Y	Y	Y	Y	Y	

SAFEWAY INC

www.safeway.com

Industry Group Code: 445110 Ranks within this company's industry group: Sales: Profits:

Management:		Sales/Marketing:		Liberal Arts:		Information Systems:		Professionals:		Technical/Scientific:	
Mgmt. Trainees:	Y	Mktg. Professionals:	Y	Gen. Writing/Editing:	Y	Info. Management:	Y	Finance/Accounting:	Y	Engineers, Elec.:	
Experienced Mgmt.:	Y	Retail Sales:	Y	Technical Writing:		Software Dev.:	Y	Law:	Y	Engineers, Other:	
Int'l Business:	Y	Commercial/Industrial:		Graphic Arts/Photog.:	Y	Hardware Dev.:		HR/Other:	Y	Health/Lab:	
MBA Graduates:	Y	Sales Trainees:		Music:		Systems Integration:		Training:	Y	Scientists/Research:	
		Advertising Pros.:	Y	Broadcasting:		Consulting/Other:		Health Care:	Y	Petroleum/Chemicals:	
				Other:				Consulting:		Math/Other:	

TYPES OF BUSINESS:
Grocery Stores
Food Processing & Packaging
Online Grocery Sales & Home Delivery
Pharmacies
Gift Cards & Payment Processing Technology

BRANDS/DIVISIONS/AFFILIATES:
Carr-Gottstein Foods Co
Randall's Food Markets Inc
Vons Companies Inc (The)
Canada Safeway Limited
GroceryWorks
Safeway SELECT
Casa Ley, S.A. de C.V.
Blackhawk Network

CONTACTS: Note: Officers with more than one job title may be intentionally listed here more than once.
Steven A. Burd, CEO
Steven A. Burd, Pres.
Robert L. Edwards, CFO/Exec. VP
Diane M. Deitz, Chief Mktg. Officer
Russell M. Jackson, Sr. VP-Human Resources
David T. Ching, CIO/Sr. VP
Donald P. Wright, Sr. VP-Real Estate & Eng.
Larree M. Renda, Chief Strategist & Admin. Officer/Exec. VP
Robert A. Gordon, General Counsel/Sr. VP
Bruce L. Everette, Exec. VP-Retail Oper.
David R. Stern, Sr. VP-Bus. Dev. & Planning
Melissa C. Plaisance, Sr. VP-Finance & Investor Rel.
David F. Bond, Sr. VP-Finance & Control
Kelly Griffith, Pres., Perishables
Kenneth M. Shachmut, Sr. VP-Reengineering & Mktg. Analysis
Steven A. Burd, Chmn.
Jerry Tidwell, Sr. VP-Supply Oper.

Phone: 925-467-3000	Fax: 925-467-3321
Toll-Free: 877-723-3929	
Address: 5918 Stoneridge Mall Rd., Pleasanton, CA 94588 US	

GROWTH PLANS/SPECIAL FEATURES:
Safeway, Inc., originally incorporated as SSI Holdings Corporations and then Safeway Stores, is one of the largest food retailers in North America, operating 1,740 stores located principally in California, Oregon, Washington, Alaska, Colorado, Arizona, Texas, the Chicago metropolitan area and the Mid-Atlantic region. The company's Canadian retail operations are located principally in British Columbia, Alberta and Saskatchewan. These stores operate regionally under the names Safeway, Carrs, Genuardi's, Pavilions, Tom Thumb, Dominick's, Randall's and Vons, which each offer a wide selection of both food and general merchandise and feature a variety of special departments such as bakery, delicatessen, pharmacy and floral departments. In addition, the company offers online grocery shopping and home delivery through its wholly-owned subsidiary, GroceryWorks. Safeway has developed a line of more than 1,250 Safeway SELECT brand products, ranging from packaged foods to laundry detergent, and offers an additional 2,500 corporate-brand products under the Safeway and subsidiary labels. Throughout 2007, the company expanded its O Organics line of certified organic foods and beverages to almost 300 exclusive products. Safeway operates 32 processing plants and 17 distribution/warehousing centers in the U.S. and Canada. Safeway also owns a 49% interest in Casa Ley, S.A. de C.V., which operates over 135 general merchandise and food stores in Mexico. The company also manages its Blackhawk Network subsidiary, which is one of the largest providers of third-party prepaid gift cards in the country with a gift card offering of more than 100 brands from retailers such as Barnes & Noble Booksellers, Best Buy, Pizza Hut and Starbucks Coffee. In September 2007, Safeway began a new environmental project designed to transition over 23 of its California-based stores to solar power as part of a renewable energy initiative.

FINANCIALS: Sales and profits are in thousands of dollars—add 000 to get the full amount. 2007 Note: Financial information for 2007 was not available for all companies at press time.

2007 Sales: $42,286,000	2007 Profits: $888,400	**U.S. Stock Ticker: SWY**	
2006 Sales: $40,185,000	2006 Profits: $870,600	**Int'l Ticker:** Int'l Exchange:	
2005 Sales: $38,416,000	2005 Profits: $561,100	Employees: 207,000	
2004 Sales: $35,822,900	2004 Profits: $560,200	Fiscal Year Ends: 12/31	
2003 Sales: $35,552,700	2003 Profits: $-169,800	Parent Company:	

SALARIES/BENEFITS:

Pension Plan: Y	ESOP Stock Plan:	Profit Sharing:	Top Exec. Salary: $1,332,250	Bonus: $2,639,825
Savings Plan: Y	Stock Purch. Plan: Y		Second Exec. Salary: $691,425	Bonus: $854,739

OTHER THOUGHTS:
Apparent Women Officers or Directors: 2
Hot Spot for Advancement for Women/Minorities: Y

LOCATIONS: ("Y" = Yes)

West:	Southwest:	Midwest:	Southeast:	Northeast:	International:
Y	Y	Y		Y	Y

Note: Financial information, benefits and other data can change quickly and may vary from those stated here.

SAIC INC

www.saic.com

Industry Group Code: 541512 Ranks within this company's industry group: Sales: 3 Profits: 3

Management:		Sales/Marketing:		Liberal Arts:		Information Systems:		Professionals:		Technical/Scientific:	
Mgmt. Trainees:	Y	Mktg. Professionals:	Y	Gen. Writing/Editing:		Info. Management:	Y	Finance/Accounting:	Y	Engineers, Elec.:	Y
Experienced Mgmt.:	Y	Retail Sales:		Technical Writing:	Y	Software Dev.:	Y	Law:	Y	Engineers, Other:	
Int'l Business:	Y	Commercial/Industrial:	Y	Graphic Arts/Photog.:	Y	Hardware Dev.:		HR/Other:	Y	Health/Lab:	
MBA Graduates:	Y	Sales Trainees:		Music:		Systems Integration:	Y	Training:	Y	Scientists/Research:	Y
		Advertising Pros.:		Broadcasting:		Consulting/Other:		Health Care:		Petroleum/Chemicals:	
				Other:				Consulting:	Y	Math/Other:	

TYPES OF BUSINESS:

Systems Integration Services
Consulting Services
Research & Development
Software Development
Venture Capital
Engineering

BRANDS/DIVISIONS/AFFILIATES:

Science Applications International Corporation
Defense Transformation
Intelligence
Homeland Security and Defense
Benham Investment Holdings, LLC
Scicom Technologies Private Limited
AMSEC, LLC
ANXeBusiness Corp.

CONTACTS: Note: Officers with more than one job title may be intentionally listed here more than once.

Kenneth C. Dahlberg, CEO
Lawrence B. Prior, III, COO
Mark W. Sopp, CFO/Exec. VP
Brian F. Keenan, Exec. VP-Human Resources
Charles F. Koontz, Pres., IT & Network Solutions Group
Amy E. Alving, CTO
Joseph W. Craver, III, Pres., Prod. Solutions
Douglas E. Scott, General Counsel/Exec. VP/Corp. Sec.
Greg Henson, Sr. VP-Bus. Dev.
Arnold L. Punaro, Exec. VP-Comm., Gov't. Affairs & Support Oper.
Donald H. Foley, Exec. VP-Special Projects
Larry J. Peck, Exec. VP-Homeland Security
Joesph P. Walkush, Exec. VP-Strategic Projects
Deborah H. Alderson, Pres., Defense Solutions Group
Kenneth C. Dahlberg, Chmn.
Joseph W. Craver, III, Pres., Logistics & Infrastructure

Phone: 858-826-6000	Fax: 858-826-6800
Toll-Free: 800-430-7629	
Address: 10260 Campus Point Dr., San Diego, CA 92121 US	

GROWTH PLANS/SPECIAL FEATURES:

SAIC, Inc., formerly Science Applications International Corporation, provides scientific, engineering, systems integration and technical services for all branches of the U.S. military, agencies of the U.S. Department of Defense (DoD), the intelligence community, the U.S. Department of Homeland Security (DHS) and other U.S. government civil agencies, as well as to customers in selected commercial markets. The company completed a reorganization merger in late 2006, changing its name to SAIC. SAIC offers products and solutions in three segments: government, commercial and corporate. Government offers services such as Defense Transformation; Intelligence; Homeland Security and Defense; Logistics and Products Support; Systems Engineering and Integration; and Research and Development to a wide array of national, state and local governments. The commercial segment provides technology-driven consulting, systems integration and outsourcing services and solutions in selected commercial markets such as oil and gas exploration, utilities and pharmaceuticals, in the U.S. and abroad. Revenue from the government segment accounts for approximately 93% of the company's total consolidated revenue, while the commercial segment generates approximately 7% of its total revenue. SAIC owns 55% of AMSEC, LLC, a joint venture that provides maintenance engineering and technical support services to the U.S. Navy and marine industry customers. In August 2007, SAIC acquired Benham Investment Holdings, LLC, an engineering and life-cycle technology implementation firm that serves Fortune 500 commercial and federal government subsidiaries. In September 2007, the company acquired Scicom Technologies Private Limited, a provider of onsite and offshore hydrocarbon exploration product development services and technology consulting in the science and engineering sector.

SAIC offers its workers an employee assistance program, flexible spending accounts, comprehensive leave and education assistance.

FINANCIALS: Sales and profits are in thousands of dollars—add 000 to get the full amount. 2007 Note: Financial information for 2007 was not available for all companies at press time.

2007 Sales: $8,294,000	2007 Profits: $391,000	U.S. Stock Ticker: SAI	
2006 Sales: $7,775,000	2006 Profits: $927,000	Int'l Ticker:	Int'l Exchange:
2005 Sales: $7,172,000	2005 Profits: $409,000	Employees: 44,100	
2004 Sales: $6,720,000	2004 Profits: $351,000	Fiscal Year Ends: 1/31	
2003 Sales: $5,902,700	2003 Profits: $246,300	Parent Company:	

SALARIES/BENEFITS:

Pension Plan:	ESOP Stock Plan:	Profit Sharing:	Top Exec. Salary: $1,000,000	Bonus: $1,325,000
Savings Plan: Y	Stock Purch. Plan: Y		Second Exec. Salary: $467,308	Bonus: $415,000

OTHER THOUGHTS:

Apparent Women Officers or Directors: 4
Hot Spot for Advancement for Women/Minorities: Y

LOCATIONS: ("Y" = Yes)

West:	Southwest:	Midwest:	Southeast:	Northeast:	International:
Y	Y	Y	Y	Y	Y

SAM'S CLUB

www.samsclub.com

Industry Group Code: 452910A Ranks within this company's industry group: Sales: 2 Profits:

Management:		Sales/Marketing:		Liberal Arts:		Information Systems:		Professionals:		Technical/Scientific:	
Mgmt. Trainees:	Y	Mktg. Professionals:	Y	Gen. Writing/Editing:	Y	Info. Management:	Y	Finance/Accounting:	Y	Engineers, Elec.:	
Experienced Mgmt.:	Y	Retail Sales:	Y	Technical Writing:		Software Dev.:	Y	Law:	Y	Engineers, Other:	
Int'l Business:	Y	Commercial/Industrial:		Graphic Arts/Photog.:	Y	Hardware Dev.:		HR/Other:	Y	Health/Lab:	
MBA Graduates:	Y	Sales Trainees:	Y	Music:		Systems Integration:	Y	Training:	Y	Scientists/Research:	
		Advertising Pros.:	Y	Broadcasting:		Consulting/Other:		Health Care:		Petroleum/Chemicals:	
				Other:	Y			Consulting:		Math/Other:	

TYPES OF BUSINESS:

Warehouse Clubs, Retail

BRANDS/DIVISIONS/AFFILIATES:

Wal-Mart Stores, Inc.
Member's Mark
Bakers & Chefs
Business Membership
Advantage Membership
Plus Membership Card
Sam's Café

CONTACTS: *Note: Officers with more than one job title may be intentionally listed here more than once.*

C. Douglas McMillon, CEO
C. Douglas McMillon, Pres.
Liz Kirkwood, CFO
Mark D. Goodman, Exec. VP-Mktg. & Membership
Sharon Orlopp, Sr. VP-Sam's Club People Div.
Greg Spragg, Exec. VP-Merch.
Whitney Head, General Counsel
Greg Johnston, Exec. VP-Oper.
Cindy Davis, Exec. VP-E-Commerce
Liz Kirkwood, Sr. VP-Finance

Phone: 479-277-7000	Fax:
Toll-Free: 800-331-0085	
Address: 608 SW 8th St., Bentonville, AR 72712-6097 US	

GROWTH PLANS/SPECIAL FEATURES:

Sam's Club, a subsidiary of Wal-Mart Stores, Inc., is one of the nation's largest members-only warehouse clubs, with more than 47 million U.S. members and 594 stores in the U.S. and over 100 international locations in Brazil, Canada, China, Mexico and Puerto Rico. Sam's offers discounted prices on more than 4,000 items, including appliances and electronics, office supplies, fresh food, clothing, optical and pharmacy services, home furnishings, books, batteries and auto supplies. It also sells selected private-label items under the Member's Mark, Bakers & Chefs and Sam's Club brands. Most locations also offer photo processing, pharmaceuticals, optical departments, gasoline stations and fresh departments, including bakery, meat, produce, floral and Sam's Cafe. Sam's Club requires a customer to become a member, providing two options: Business Membership or Advantage Membership. Both member groups pay an annual fee. Business members include anyone who holds a valid city/state business or tax permit or anyone who holds a professional license. Everyone else can purchase an Advantage Membership. In addition, Sam's offers a PLUS Membership Card, which offers extra benefits on either level. In addition to merchandise discounts, Sam's offers its members discounted services that include various types of insurance, a travel club, an auto purchase program, discount credit card processing, software training, mail-order pharmacy services, Internet access and long-distance services. Store sizes for Sam's Club generally range between 72,000 and 190,000 square feet and are designed to resemble a warehouse, with merchandise displayed on shipping pallets or in large freezer/cooler units. In 2008, Sam's Club opens its first business center format at its Dunvale Road store in Houston, Texas to serve food service industry professionals, convenience store owners, vending operators, office administrators, florists, hotel/motel operators and more.

Sam's Club offers its employees medical, dental and life insurance; merchandise discounts; education assistance; GED reimbursement; and scholarships.

FINANCIALS: Sales and profits are in thousands of dollars—add 000 to get the full amount. 2007 Note: Financial information for 2007 was not available for all companies at press time.

2007 Sales: $41,582,000	2007 Profits: $1,480,000	U.S. Stock Ticker: Subsidiary
2006 Sales: $39,798,000	2006 Profits: $	Int'l Ticker: Int'l Exchange:
2005 Sales: $37,100,000	2005 Profits: $1,280,000	Employees:
2004 Sales: $34,537,000	2004 Profits: $1,126,000	Fiscal Year Ends: 1/31
2003 Sales: $31,702,000	2003 Profits: $1,023,000	Parent Company: WAL-MART STORES INC

SALARIES/BENEFITS:

Pension Plan:	ESOP Stock Plan: Y	Profit Sharing:	Top Exec. Salary: $	Bonus: $
Savings Plan: Y	Stock Purch. Plan:		Second Exec. Salary: $	Bonus: $

OTHER THOUGHTS:

Apparent Women Officers or Directors: 2
Hot Spot for Advancement for Women/Minorities:

LOCATIONS: ("Y" = Yes)

West:	Southwest:	Midwest:	Southeast:	Northeast:	International:
Y	Y	Y	Y	Y	Y

Note: Financial information, benefits and other data can change quickly and may vary from those stated here.

SARA LEE CORP

www.saralee.com

Industry Group Code: 311800 Ranks within this company's industry group: Sales: Profits:

Management:		Sales/Marketing:		Liberal Arts:		Information Systems:		Professionals:		Technical/Scientific:	
Mgmt. Trainees:	Y	Mktg. Professionals:	Y	Gen. Writing/Editing:	Y	Info. Management:	Y	Finance/Accounting:	Y	Engineers, Elec.:	Y
Experienced Mgmt.:	Y	Retail Sales:		Technical Writing:		Software Dev.:		Law:	Y	Engineers, Other:	Y
Int'l Business:	Y	Commercial/Industrial:	Y	Graphic Arts/Photog.:	Y	Hardware Dev.:		HR/Other:	Y	Health/Lab:	Y
MBA Graduates:	Y	Sales Trainees:		Music:		Systems Integration:		Training:	Y	Scientists/Research:	
		Advertising Pros.:	Y	Broadcasting:		Consulting/Other:		Health Care:		Petroleum/Chemicals:	Y
				Other:				Consulting:		Math/Other:	

TYPES OF BUSINESS:

Food & Beverage, Manufacturing
Household Products
Bakery Products
Processed Meats
Coffee & Tea
Foodservice Distribution
Apparel

BRANDS/DIVISIONS/AFFILIATES:

Ball Park
Hillshire Farm
Jimmy Dean
State Fair
Maison du Cafe
Superior
Douwe Egberts
Kiwi

CONTACTS: *Note: Officers with more than one job title may be intentionally listed here more than once.*

Brenda C. Barnes, CEO
Christopher J. Fraleigh, COO/Exec. VP
L. M. de Kool, CFO/Exec. VP
Christopher J. Fraleigh, Chief Customer & Mktg. Officer
Stephen J. Cerrone, Exec. VP-Human Resources
Heidi Kleinbach-Sauter, Sr. VP-R&D
George Chappelle, CIO/Sr. VP
L. M. de Kool, Chief Admin. Officer/Exec. VP
Roderick A. Palmore, General Counsel/Exec. VP/Corp. Sec.
B. Thomas Hansson, Sr. VP-Strategic Planning & Corp. Dev.
Mike Cummins, Dir.-Corp. Comm.
Shalabh Gupta, Treas.
Frank van Oers, Sr. VP/CEO-Coffee & Tea, Sara Lee Int'l
Randy White, Sr. VP-Corp. Affairs
Christopher J. Fraleigh, CEO-Sara Lee Food & Beverage
James W. Nolan, Sr. VP/CEO-Sara Lee Foodservice
Brenda C. Barnes, Chmn.
Vincent Janssen, Exec. VP/CEO-Household & Body, Sara Lee Int'l
Garry Berryman, Chief Procurement Officer

Phone: 630-598-6000	Fax: 630-598-8482
Toll-Free:	
Address: 3500 Lacey Rd., Downers Grove, IL 60515-5424 US	

GROWTH PLANS/SPECIAL FEATURES:

Sara Lee Corp. manufactures and markets brand-name food products worldwide. The company is divided into six operating segments: North American retail meats, North American retail bakery, foodservice, international beverage, international bakery and household and body care. These in turn are organized into: international, food and beverage, and foodservice. The Sara Lee Food and Beverage subsidiary manufactures packaged meat products under the names Ball Park, Best's Kosher, Hillshire Farm and Jimmy Dean, and the Sara Lee Bakery Group produces specialty breads, fresh and frozen pies, pound cakes, cheesecakes and Danishes in North America. Sara Lee Foodservice oversees the bakery, coffee and meats foodservice business in North America. Sara Lee International manages the firm's worldwide coffee and tea operations (including the Superior tea and Maison du Cafe brands), its household products segment and the direct-selling operations, which distributes a range of products including cosmetics, jewelry, nutritional supplements and household products, such as Endust furniture cleaner, Kiwi shoe care products and Ambi Pure air fresheners, through a network of independent sales representatives. Sara Lee's apparel business, Hanesbrands, Inc., includes well known brands such as Hanes, Playtex, Barely There, Wonder Bra and Champion. Roughly 43% of sales are derived outside of North America. As part of a five-year transformation plan, started in 2005, the company plans to drive growth in key categories via its strongest brands, including Ambi Pur, Ball Park, Douwe Egberts, Hillshire Farm, Jimmy Dean, Kiwi, Sanex, Senseo and Sara Lee. In early 2007, the company finalized plans for a new multi-million dollar research and development center to be called The Kitchens of Sara Lee and completed in early 2009. The firm also recently completed the consolidation of its North American headquarters to one location in the Chicago area.

FINANCIALS: Sales and profits are in thousands of dollars—add 000 to get the full amount. 2007 Note: Financial information for 2007 was not available for all companies at press time.

2007 Sales: $12,278,000	2007 Profits: $504,000	**U.S. Stock Ticker:** SLE
2006 Sales: $11,460,000	2006 Profits: $555,000	**Int'l Ticker:** Int'l Exchange:
2005 Sales: $11,346,000	2005 Profits: $719,000	Employees: 52,000
2004 Sales: $15,892,000	2004 Profits: $1,272,000	Fiscal Year Ends: 7/1
2003 Sales: $18,291,000	2003 Profits: $1,221,000	Parent Company:

SALARIES/BENEFITS:

Pension Plan: Y	ESOP Stock Plan:	Profit Sharing:	Top Exec. Salary: $1,000,000	Bonus: $1,761,610
Savings Plan:	Stock Purch. Plan:		Second Exec. Salary: $780,000	Bonus: $1,086,629

OTHER THOUGHTS:

Apparent Women Officers or Directors: 4
Hot Spot for Advancement for Women/Minorities: Y

LOCATIONS: ("Y" = Yes)

West:	Southwest:	Midwest:	Southeast:	Northeast:	International:
Y	Y	Y	Y	Y	Y

SAS INSTITUTE INC

www.sas.com

Industry Group Code: 511207 Ranks within this company's industry group: Sales: 2 Profits:

Management:		Sales/Marketing:		Liberal Arts:		Information Systems:		Professionals:		Technical/Scientific:	
Mgmt. Trainees:	Y	Mktg. Professionals:	Y	Gen. Writing/Editing:	Y	Info. Management:	Y	Finance/Accounting:	Y	Engineers, Elec.:	Y
Experienced Mgmt.:	Y	Retail Sales:		Technical Writing:	Y	Software Dev.:	Y	Law:	Y	Engineers, Other:	
Int'l Business:	Y	Commercial/Industrial:		Graphic Arts/Photog.:	Y	Hardware Dev.:		HR/Other:	Y	Health/Lab:	
MBA Graduates:	Y	Sales Trainees:		Music:		Systems Integration:	Y	Training:	Y	Scientists/Research:	Y
		Advertising Pros.:	Y	Broadcasting:		Consulting/Other:	Y	Health Care:		Petroleum/Chemicals:	
				Other:				Consulting:	Y	Math/Other:	Y

TYPES OF BUSINESS:

Software-Statistical Analysis
Business Intelligence Software
Data Warehousing
Online Bookstore

BRANDS/DIVISIONS/AFFILIATES:

SAS9
SAS Enterprise BI Server
DataFlux
SAS Revenue Optimization
SAS Promotion Optimization
SAS Enterprise Intelligence Platform

CONTACTS: *Note: Officers with more than one job title may be intentionally listed here more than once.*

James Goodnight, CEO
James Goodnight, Pres.
Don Parker, CFO/VP
Jim Davis, Chief Mktg. Officer/Sr. VP
Jeff Chambers, VP-Human Resources
Amitava Ghosh, VP-R&D
Suzanne Gordon, CIO/VP-IT
Keith Collins, CTO/Sr. VP
Alexi Sarnevitz, Sr. Dir.-Global Retail Strategy
John Sall, Exec. VP
James Goodnight, Chmn.
Mikael Hagstrom, Exec. VP-EMEA & Asia Pacific

Phone: 919-677-8000	Fax: 919-677-4444
Toll-Free: 800-727-0025	
Address: 100 SAS Campus Dr., Cary, NC 27513-2414 US	

GROWTH PLANS/SPECIAL FEATURES:

SAS Institute, Inc., one of the world's largest privately held software specialty companies, is a provider of statistical analysis software. The company's products are essentially designed to extract, manage and analyze large volumes of data, often assisting in financial reporting and credit analysis. Individual contracts can be tailored to specific global and local industries, such as banking, manufacturing and government. SAS's top products are SAS9 and SAS Enterprise BI Server. The SAS9 platform is centered on providing extensive data management and analytics integration. It also features predictive applications, a highly adaptable interface and unique grid computing capabilities. SAS Enterprise BI Server is an enhanced reporting and analysis system for the organization and reporting of business intelligence. SAS also provides data warehousing services for large amounts of data, as well as consulting, training and technical support through its SAS Services unit. The company's DataFlux subsidiary helps it deliver quality capabilities in SAS Data Integration solutions. In addition, the firm operates an online bookstore offering a library of SAS-produced books, documentation and training materials. SAS serves more than 43,000 business, government and university sites in 108 different countries, including 96 of the top 100 companies on the Fortune Global 500 list. Some of the firm's more prominent clients are Hewlett Packard; Brooks Brothers; the U.S. Department of Defense; Staples, Subway; and Allstate Financial.

The SAS headquarters features on-site childcare centers, an eldercare information and referral program, an employee health care center, wellness programs and a 58,000 square foot recreation and fitness center. The firm has been listed in Fortune's Top 100 Companies to Work For in America for 10 consecutive years.

FINANCIALS: Sales and profits are in thousands of dollars—add 000 to get the full amount. 2007 Note: Financial information for 2007 was not available for all companies at press time.

		U.S. Stock Ticker: Private
2007 Sales: $2,150,000	2007 Profits: $	Int'l Ticker: Int'l Exchange:
2006 Sales: $1,900,000	2006 Profits: $	Employees: 10,094
2005 Sales: $1,680,000	2005 Profits: $	Fiscal Year Ends: 12/31
2004 Sales: $1,530,000	2004 Profits: $	Parent Company:
2003 Sales: $1,180,000	2003 Profits: $	

SALARIES/BENEFITS:

Pension Plan:	ESOP Stock Plan:	Profit Sharing: Y	Top Exec. Salary: $	Bonus: $
Savings Plan: Y	Stock Purch. Plan:		Second Exec. Salary: $	Bonus: $

OTHER THOUGHTS:

Apparent Women Officers or Directors: 2
Hot Spot for Advancement for Women/Minorities: Y

LOCATIONS: ("Y" = Yes)

West:	Southwest:	Midwest:	Southeast:	Northeast:	International:
Y	Y	Y	Y	Y	Y

SCANA CORPORATION

www.scana.com

Industry Group Code: 221000   Ranks within this company's industry group: Sales: 5   Profits: 5

Management:		Sales/Marketing:		Liberal Arts:		Information Systems:		Professionals:		Technical/Scientific:	
Mgmt. Trainees:	Y	Mktg. Professionals:	Y	Gen. Writing/Editing:	Y	Info. Management:	Y	Finance/Accounting:	Y	Engineers, Elec.:	Y
Experienced Mgmt.:	Y	Retail Sales:		Technical Writing:	Y	Software Dev.:		Law:	Y	Engineers, Other:	Y
Int'l Business:		Commercial/Industrial:	Y	Graphic Arts/Photog.:	Y	Hardware Dev.:		HR/Other:	Y	Health/Lab:	
MBA Graduates:	Y	Sales Trainees:		Music:		Systems Integration:		Training:	Y	Scientists/Research:	
		Advertising Pros.:	Y	Broadcasting:		Consulting/Other:		Health Care:		Petroleum/Chemicals:	
				Other:				Consulting:		Math/Other:	

TYPES OF BUSINESS:

Electricity & Natural Gas
Telecommunications Services
Ethernet Services & Data Center Facilities
Communications Towers Management
Management & Maintenance Services
Service Contracts
Risk Management Services

BRANDS/DIVISIONS/AFFILIATES:

South Carolina Electric & Gas Co.
South Carolina Generating Co., Inc.
South Carolina Fuel Co., Inc.
Public Service Co. of North Carolina, Inc.
Carolina Gas Transmission Corp.
SCANA Communications, Inc.
SCANA Energy Marketing, Inc.
ServiceCare, Inc.

CONTACTS: *Note: Officers with more than one job title may be intentionally listed here more than once.*

William B. Timmerman, CEO
William B. Timmerman, Pres.
Jimmy Addison, CFO/Sr. VP
Joseph C. Bouknight, Sr. VP-Human Resources
Francis P. Mood, Jr., General Counsel/Sr. VP/Assistant Sec.
Mark R. Cannon, Treas./Risk Mgmt. Officer
Kevin B. Marsh, Pres./COO-South Carolina Electric & Gas Co.
Sarena D. Burch, Sr. VP-Fuel Procurement & Asset Mgmt.
Paul V. Fant, Pres./COO-Carolina Gas Transmission
Charles McFadden, Sr. VP-Gov't Affairs & Economic Dev.
William B. Timmerman, Chmn.

Phone: 803-217-9000	**Fax:** 803-217-8119
Toll-Free: 800-763-5891	
Address: 1426 Main St., Columbia, SC 29218 US	

GROWTH PLANS/SPECIAL FEATURES:

SCANA Corp. is an energy-based holding company that operates through wholly-owned subsidiaries. South Carolina Electric & Gas Company (SCE&G) generates and sells electricity to retail and wholesale customers, and purchases, sells and transports natural gas to retail customers. South Carolina Generating Company, Inc. owns and operates Williams Station and sells electricity solely to SCE&G. South Carolina Fuel Company, Inc. owns and provides financing for SCE&G's nuclear fuel, fossil fuel and emission allowances. Public Service Company of North Carolina, Inc. purchases, sells and transports natural gas to retail customers. Carolina Gas Transmission Corp. (CGTC) transports natural gas in southeastern Georgia and South Carolina. SCANA Communications, Inc. (SCI) provides fiber optic communications, ethernet services and data center facilities through a 500-mile fiber optic telecommunications network. SCI also builds, manages and leases communications towers in South Carolina, North Carolina and Georgia. SCANA Energy Marketing, Inc. (SEMI) markets natural gas, primarily in the southeast, and provides energy-related risk management services. Through its SCANA Energy division, SEMI markets natural gas in Georgia's retail natural gas market. ServiceCare, Inc. provides service contracts on home appliances and heating and air conditioning units. SCANA Services, Inc. provides administrative, management and other services to the subsidiaries and business units within SCANA. These are the firm's 10 primary subsidiaries, in addition to which the firm also owns three smaller energy-related companies. All together, SCANA's electric service area extends into 24 counties covering roughly 16,000 square miles and serving 639,300 customers. The company's natural gas operations own liquefied natural gas liquefaction and storage facilities and transports natural gas to over one million customers. In 2008, SCE&G and Santee Cooper, a state-owned electric and water utility in South Carolina, joined together to construct two nuclear electric-generating units.

The company offers its employees medical, dental and vision insurance; a retirement plan; and a 401(k) plan.

FINANCIALS: Sales and profits are in thousands of dollars—add 000 to get the full amount. 2007 Note: Financial information for 2007 was not available for all companies at press time.

2007 Sales: $4,621,000	2007 Profits: $320,000	**U.S. Stock Ticker:** SCG
2006 Sales: $4,563,000	2006 Profits: $310,000	**Int'l Ticker:** Int'l Exchange:
2005 Sales: $4,777,000	2005 Profits: $320,000	Employees: 5,683
2004 Sales: $3,885,000	2004 Profits: $257,000	Fiscal Year Ends: 12/31
2003 Sales: $3,416,000	2003 Profits: $282,000	Parent Company:

SALARIES/BENEFITS:

Pension Plan: Y	ESOP Stock Plan:	Profit Sharing:	Top Exec. Salary: $1,043,408	Bonus: $622,846
Savings Plan: Y	Stock Purch. Plan:		Second Exec. Salary: $548,115	Bonus: $250,250

OTHER THOUGHTS:

Apparent Women Officers or Directors: 4
Hot Spot for Advancement for Women/Minorities: Y

LOCATIONS: ("Y" = Yes)

West:	Southwest:	Midwest:	Southeast:	Northeast:	International:
			Y	Y	

SCHERING-PLOUGH CORP
www.schering-plough.com

Industry Group Code: 325412 Ranks within this company's industry group: Sales: 4 Profits: 5

Management:		Sales/Marketing:		Liberal Arts:		Information Systems:		Professionals:		Technical/Scientific:	
Mgmt. Trainees:		Mktg. Professionals:	Y	Gen. Writing/Editing:		Info. Management:	Y	Finance/Accounting:	Y	Engineers, Elec.:	Y
Experienced Mgmt.:	Y	Retail Sales:		Technical Writing:	Y	Software Dev.:	Y	Law:	Y	Engineers, Other:	Y
Int'l Business:	Y	Commercial/Industrial:	Y	Graphic Arts/Photog.:	Y	Hardware Dev.:		HR/Other:	Y	Health/Lab:	Y
MBA Graduates:	Y	Sales Trainees:	Y	Music:		Systems Integration:	Y	Training:	Y	Scientists/Research:	Y
		Advertising Pros.:	Y	Broadcasting:		Consulting/Other:		Health Care:	Y	Petroleum/Chemicals:	Y
				Other:				Consulting:		Math/Other:	Y

TYPES OF BUSINESS:

Drugs-Diversified
Anti-Infective & Anti-Cancer Drugs
Dermatologicals
Cardiovascular Drugs
Animal Health Products
Over-the-Counter Drugs
Foot & Sun Care Products

BRANDS/DIVISIONS/AFFILIATES:

Schering-Plough Research Institute
Collateral Therapeutics
Dr. Scholl's
Coppertone
Nuflor
Livial
Nobilon
Organon Biosciences N.V.

CONTACTS: Note: Officers with more than one job title may be intentionally listed here more than once.

Fred Hassan, CEO
Robert J. Bertolini, CFO/Exec. VP
C. Ron Cheeley, Sr. VP-Global Human Resources
Thomas P. Koestler, Exec. VP/Pres., Schering-Plough Research Institute
Thomas Sabatino, Jr., General Counsel/Exec. VP
Richard S. Bowles III, Sr. VP-Global Quality Oper.
Carrie S. Cox, Exec. VP/Pres., Global Pharmaceuticals
Lori Queisser, Sr. VP-Global Compliance & Bus. Practices
Brent Saunders, Sr. VP/Pres., Consumer Health Care
Fred Hassan, Chmn.
Ian McInnes, Sr. VP/Pres., Global Supply Chain

Phone: 908-298-4000	Fax: 908-298-7653
Toll-Free:	
Address: 2000 Galloping Hill Rd., Kenilworth, NJ 07033 US	

GROWTH PLANS/SPECIAL FEATURES:

Schering-Plough Corp. is a science-centered global heath care company. It applies its research and development platform to human prescription, animal health and consumer products. The company operates in three segments: Human prescription pharmaceuticals, animal health and consumer health care. The human prescription pharmaceuticals segment discovers, develops, manufactures and markets human pharmaceutical products. Within the segment, the firm has a broad range of research projects and marketed products in six therapeutic areas: Cardiovascular, central nervous system, immunology and infectious disease, oncology, respiratory and women's health. The division also includes Nobilon, a human vaccine development unit and Diosynth, a third-party manufacturing unit. Marketed products include Vytorin, a cholesterol-lowering tablet; Remeron, an antidepressant; Livial, a menopausal therapy; and Temodar/Temodal capsules for certain types of brain tumors including newly diagnosed glioblastoma multiforme. The animal health segment discovers, develops, manufactures and markets animal health products including vaccines. Principal marketed products in this segment include Nuflor bovine and swine antibiotics; Bovilis/Vista vaccine lines for infectious diseases in cattle; Nobilis/Innovax vaccine lines for poultry; Zubrin, an anti-inflammatory/analgesic for dogs; and Slice parasiticide for sea lice in salmon. The consumer health care segment develops, manufactures and markets over-the-counter, foot care and sun care products. Principal products in this division include Claritin non-sedating antihistamines; Dr. Scholl's foot care products; Lotrimin topical antifungal products; and Coppertone sun care lotions, sprays, dry oils, lip protection products and sunless tanning products. In late 2007, Schering-Plough acquired Organon BioSciences N.V.

FINANCIALS: Sales and profits are in thousands of dollars—add 000 to get the full amount. 2007 Note: Financial information for 2007 was not available for all companies at press time.

2007 Sales: $12,690,000	2007 Profits: $-1,473,000	U.S. Stock Ticker: SGP
2006 Sales: $10,594,000	2006 Profits: $1,143,000	Int'l Ticker: Int'l Exchange:
2005 Sales: $9,508,000	2005 Profits: $269,000	Employees: 55,000
2004 Sales: $8,272,000	2004 Profits: $-947,000	Fiscal Year Ends: 12/31
2003 Sales: $8,334,000	2003 Profits: $-92,000	Parent Company:

SALARIES/BENEFITS:

Pension Plan:	ESOP Stock Plan:	Profit Sharing:	Top Exec. Salary: $1,646,250	Bonus: $12,771,698
Savings Plan:	Stock Purch. Plan:		Second Exec. Salary: $987,500	Bonus: $4,894,543

OTHER THOUGHTS:

Apparent Women Officers or Directors: 4
Hot Spot for Advancement for Women/Minorities: Y

LOCATIONS: ("Y" = Yes)

West:	Southwest:	Midwest:	Southeast:	Northeast:	International:
Y	Y	Y	Y	Y	Y

SCHLUMBERGER LIMITED

www.slb.com

Industry Group Code: 213111 Ranks within this company's industry group: Sales: 2 Profits: 1

Management:		Sales/Marketing:		Liberal Arts:		Information Systems:		Professionals:		Technical/Scientific:	
Mgmt. Trainees:		Mktg. Professionals:	Y	Gen. Writing/Editing:		Info. Management:	Y	Finance/Accounting:	Y	Engineers, Elec.:	Y
Experienced Mgmt.:	Y	Retail Sales:		Technical Writing:	Y	Software Dev.:	Y	Law:	Y	Engineers, Other:	
Int'l Business:	Y	Commercial/Industrial:	Y	Graphic Arts/Photog.:	Y	Hardware Dev.:		HR/Other:	Y	Health/Lab:	Y
MBA Graduates:	Y	Sales Trainees:		Music:		Systems Integration:		Training:	Y	Scientists/Research:	Y
		Advertising Pros.:		Broadcasting:		Consulting/Other:		Health Care:		Petroleum/Chemicals:	Y
				Other:				Consulting:		Math/Other:	Y

TYPES OF BUSINESS:

Oil & Gas Drilling Support Services
Seismic Services
Reservoir Imaging
Data & IT Consulting Services
Outsourcing
Stimulation Services

BRANDS/DIVISIONS/AFFILIATES:

Schlumberger Oilfield Services
WesternGeco
Smith International
M-I Drilling Fluids
Insensys Oil & Gas, Ltd.
InnerLogix
TerraTek, Inc.
Reslink

CONTACTS: *Note: Officers with more than one job title may be intentionally listed here more than once.*

Andrew Gould, CEO
Simon Ayat, CFO/Exec. VP
Olivier Le Peuch, Pres., Information Solutions
Ashok Belani, CTO
Mark Corrigan, VP-Oper.
Malcolm Theobald, VP-Investor Rel.
Chakib Sbiti, Exec. VP/Dir.-Oilfield Svcs.
Antonio Campo, Pres., Latin America
Dalton Boutte, Pres., WesternGeco
Zaki Selim, Pres., Middle East & Asia
Andrew Gould, Chmn.
Satish Pai, Pres., Europe & Africa

Phone: 713-513-2000	Fax: 281-285-8548
Toll-Free:	
Address: 5599 San Felipe St., Fl. 17, Houston, TX 77056 US	

GROWTH PLANS/SPECIAL FEATURES:

Schlumberger, Ltd. (SLB) is a leading oil field service company offering technology, project management and information solutions for customers in the international oil and gas industry. Schlumberger operates in 80 countries throughout North America, Latin America, Europe, Africa, the Middle East and Asia in 27 oilfield service GeoMarket regions and 23 research and engineering facilities. The SLB Oilfield Services segment is divided into ten technology-based service lines, which include wireline, drilling and measurements, well testing, well service, completions, artificial lift, data and consulting services and SLB information solutions. The overall purpose of the Oilfield Services sector is to provide proper exploration with production services and technologies throughout the entire life cycle of a reservoir. Another SLB service is its Integrated Project Management (IPM) line, which provides consulting, project management and engineering services for well construction using SLB technology. The company owns 40% of M-I Drilling Fluids along with Smith International, which offers drilling and completion fluids to stabilize rock and minimize formation damage. In addition, the firm owns a majority stake in Framo Engineering, a Norwegian-based company that provides multiphase booster pumps, flow metering equipment and swivel stack systems. Another subsidiary of SLB, WesternGeco, offers worldwide marine and seismic reservoir imaging, data processing centers and a multiclient seismic library for monitoring and development services. Additional services include 3-D, time-lapse and multicomponent surveys for delineating prospects and reservoir management. In late 2007, SLB acquired Reslink, a Norwegian company that offers engineering applications for zonal isolation and intelligent well completions, InnerLogix, a data quality management company and TerraTek, Inc., a geomechanics company in Salt Lake City. SLB also completed the relocation of its corporate office from New York to Houston, Texas and expanded its Singapore Artificial Lift center.

Schlumberger offers its employees adoption assistance, tuition reimbursement and credit union services.

FINANCIALS: Sales and profits are in thousands of dollars—add 000 to get the full amount. 2007 Note: Financial information for 2007 was not available for all companies at press time.

2007 Sales: $23,777,000	2007 Profits: $5,177,000	U.S. Stock Ticker: SLB
2006 Sales: $19,230,000	2006 Profits: $3,710,000	Int'l Ticker: Int'l Exchange:
2005 Sales: $14,309,000	2005 Profits: $2,207,000	Employees: 80,000
2004 Sales: $11,480,200	2004 Profits: $1,223,900	Fiscal Year Ends: 12/31
2003 Sales: $13,892,604	2003 Profits: $383,002	Parent Company:

SALARIES/BENEFITS:

Pension Plan: Y	ESOP Stock Plan:	Profit Sharing:	Top Exec. Salary: $2,500,000	Bonus: $3,750,000
Savings Plan: Y	Stock Purch. Plan: Y		Second Exec. Salary: $964,516	Bonus: $1,401,907

OTHER THOUGHTS:

Apparent Women Officers or Directors:
Hot Spot for Advancement for Women/Minorities:

LOCATIONS: ("Y" = Yes)

West:	Southwest:	Midwest:	Southeast:	Northeast:	International:
Y	Y	Y		Y	Y

SCIENTIFIC GAMES CORPORATION www.scientificgames.com

Industry Group Code: 713290 Ranks within this company's industry group: Sales: 2 Profits: 2

Management:		Sales/Marketing:		Liberal Arts:		Information Systems:		Professionals:		Technical/Scientific:	
Mgmt. Trainees:	Y	Mktg. Professionals:	Y	Gen. Writing/Editing:		Info. Management:	Y	Finance/Accounting:	Y	Engineers, Elec.:	Y
Experienced Mgmt.:	Y	Retail Sales:		Technical Writing:		Software Dev.:	Y	Law:	Y	Engineers, Other:	Y
Int'l Business:	Y	Commercial/Industrial:	Y	Graphic Arts/Photog.:	Y	Hardware Dev.:	Y	HR/Other:	Y	Health/Lab:	
MBA Graduates:	Y	Sales Trainees:		Music:		Systems Integration:		Training:	Y	Scientists/Research:	
		Advertising Pros.:	Y	Broadcasting:		Consulting/Other:		Health Care:		Petroleum/Chemicals:	
				Other:				Consulting:		Math/Other:	

TYPES OF BUSINESS:

Gambling Equipment-Computer-Based Lottery Systems
Pari-Mutuel Wagering Systems
Satellite Broadcasting Services
Telecommunications Products
Off-Track Betting Facilities Management
Lottery Services
Race Simulcasting
Prepaid Phone Cards

BRANDS/DIVISIONS/AFFILIATES:

The Global Draw Limited
Scientific Games Racing LLC
Games Media Limited
Games Media Ltd.
Guard Libang
Inspur

CONTACTS: *Note: Officers with more than one job title may be intentionally listed here more than once.*

A. Lorne Weil, CEO
Michael R. Chambrello, COO
Michael R. Chambrello, Pres.
DeWayne E. Laird, CFO/VP
Brooks Pierce, VP-Corp. Mktg.
Sally L. Conkright, Chief Human Resource Officer/VP-Admin.
Steven W. Beason, CTO/VP/Pres., Lottery Systems Group
Sally L. Conkright, VP-Admin.
Ira H. Raphaelson, General Counsel/Corp. Sec./VP
David Pye, VP-Corp. Dev.
Lisa D. Lettieri, Dir.-Corp. Comm.
Stephen L. Gibbs, Chief Acct. Officer/VP
Robert C. Becker, VP/Treas.
Larry A. Potts, VP/Chief Compliance Officer/Corp. Dir.-Security
William J. Huntley, VP/Pres., Racing & Sports
Steven M. Saferin, VP/Pres., Properties
A. Lorne Weil, Chmn.
Yan Xuan, Pres., Greater China/Sr. VP-Scientific Games Int'l

Phone: 212-754-2233	Fax: 212-754-2372
Toll-Free: 800-367-9345	
Address: 750 Lexington Ave., New York, NY 10022 US	

GROWTH PLANS/SPECIAL FEATURES:

Scientific Games Corp. is a leading supplier of technology-based products, systems and services to gaming markets worldwide, including 40 of the 42 U.S. jurisdictions that currently sell lottery tickets and over 50 countries. Scientific Games operates in three business segments: Printed Products Group, Lottery Systems Group and Diversified Gaming Group. The Printed Products Group is composed of its instant lottery ticket business and its prepaid phone card business, providing lotteries with some of the world's most popular entertainment brands, including Major League Baseball, NASCAR, National Basketball Association, Wheel-of-Fortune, Monopoly, World Poker Tour and The World Series of Poker. The Lottery Systems Group provides sophisticated, customized computer software, equipment and data communication services to government-sponsored and privately-operated lotteries in the U.S. and internationally. This business includes the provision of transaction processing software for the accounting and validation of both instant and online lottery games, point-of-sale terminals, central site computers, communications technology and ongoing support and maintenance for these products. The Diversified Gaming Group provides services and systems to private and public operators in the wide area gaming markets and in the pari-mutuel wagering industry, with products including fixed odds betting terminals; video lottery terminals; monitor games; wagering systems for the pari-mutuel racing industry; sports betting systems and services; and Amusement With Prize and Skill With Prize terminals. Business units within the Diversified Gaming Group include The Global Draw Limited, Scientific Games Racing LLC and Games Media Limited. In September 2007, Scientific Games closed its San Antonio plant, affecting 350 jobs in the San Antonio metro area. In November 2007, Scientific Games acquired 50% interest in Guard Libang, a provider of instant lottery ticket services in China.

Scientific Games offers its employees tuition reimbursement, flexible spending accounts, service awards, free parking and credit union membership.

FINANCIALS: Sales and profits are in thousands of dollars—add 000 to get the full amount. 2007 Note: Financial information for 2007 was not available for all companies at press time.

2007 Sales: $1,046,704	2007 Profits: $65,367	U.S. Stock Ticker: SGMS
2006 Sales: $897,230	2006 Profits: $66,761	Int'l Ticker: Int'l Exchange:
2005 Sales: $781,683	2005 Profits: $75,319	Employees: 5,500
2004 Sales: $725,495	2004 Profits: $65,742	Fiscal Year Ends: 12/31
2003 Sales: $560,900	2003 Profits: $52,100	Parent Company:

SALARIES/BENEFITS:

Pension Plan:	ESOP Stock Plan:	Profit Sharing:	Top Exec. Salary: $870,000	Bonus: $
Savings Plan: Y	Stock Purch. Plan: Y		Second Exec. Salary: $616,270	Bonus: $

OTHER THOUGHTS:

Apparent Women Officers or Directors: 1
Hot Spot for Advancement for Women/Minorities: Y

LOCATIONS: ("Y" = Yes)

West:	Southwest:	Midwest:	Southeast:	Northeast:	International:
Y	Y	Y	Y	Y	Y

SCOTTS MIRACLE GROW CO

www.scotts.com

Industry Group Code: 115112   Ranks within this company's industry group: Sales: 1   Profits: 1

Management:		Sales/Marketing:		Liberal Arts:		Information Systems:		Professionals:		Technical/Scientific:	
Mgmt. Trainees:	Y	Mktg. Professionals:	Y	Gen. Writing/Editing:	Y	Info. Management:	Y	Finance/Accounting:	Y	Engineers, Elec.:	Y
Experienced Mgmt.:	Y	Retail Sales:	Y	Technical Writing:	Y	Software Dev.:		Law:	Y	Engineers, Other:	
Int'l Business:	Y	Commercial/Industrial:	Y	Graphic Arts/Photog.:		Hardware Dev.:		HR/Other:	Y	Health/Lab:	Y
MBA Graduates:	Y	Sales Trainees:	Y	Music:		Systems Integration:		Training:	Y	Scientists/Research:	
		Advertising Pros.:	Y	Broadcasting:		Consulting/Other:		Health Care:		Petroleum/Chemicals:	
				Other:				Consulting:		Math/Other:	

TYPES OF BUSINESS:

Horticulture & Turf Products Manufacturer
Fertilizers
Herbicides
Plant Foods
Lawn Services
Outdoor & Garden Products
Plants & Seeds
Mowers & Tractors

BRANDS/DIVISIONS/AFFILIATES:

Turf Builder
Miracle-Gro
Osmocote
Ortho
Weedol
EverGreen
Scotts LawnService
Smith & Hawken

CONTACTS: *Note: Officers with more than one job title may be intentionally listed here more than once.*

James Hagedorn, CEO
James Hagedorn, Pres.
Dave Evans, CFO/Exec. VP
Claude Lopez, Chief Mktg. Officer
Denise S. Stump, Exec. VP-Global Human Resources
Mike Lukemire, Sr. VP-Global Tech.
Vincent Brockman, General Counsel/Exec. VP/Corp. Sec.
Mike Lukemire, Sr. VP-Oper.
Barry Sanders, Exec. VP-North America Consumer Bus.
Richard Shank, Chief Environmental Officer
Michel Gasnier, Sr. VP/CFO-Int'l Oper.
James Hagedorn, Chmn.
Claude Lopez, Exec. VP-Int'l

Phone: 614-719-5500	**Fax:** 614-719-5750
Toll-Free: 888-270-3714	
Address: 14111 Scottslawn Rd., Marysville, OH 43041 US	

GROWTH PLANS/SPECIAL FEATURES:

The Scotts Miracle-Gro Company (SMG) is a marketer of do-it-yourself lawn, garden and home protection products in North America and Europe. Its products include consumer fertilizers, plant foods, soils and mulches, pest controls, grass seed and bird food. The company's principal brands in North America are Scotts, Miracle-Gro, and Ortho. International consumer brands include Miracle-Gro, Evergreen, Fertiligene, Celaflor, KB, Substral, Levington and Weedol. SMG operates through the following business segments: North America; Scotts LawnService; International; and Corporate & Other. The North America segment sells products in the following categories: Lawns, including lawn fertilizer, crabgrass control, weed control or pest control; Gardens, which offers a complete line of plant foods marketed under the Miracle-Gro brand name; Growing Media, which includes potting mix, garden soils, topsoil and manures; Grass Seed products for both the consumer and the professional user; and Controls, which includes a broad line of weed control, indoor and outdoor pest control and plant disease control products. The Scotts LawnService segment provides residential lawn care, lawn aeration, tree and shrub care and external pest control services in the U.S. The International segment sells consumer lawn and garden products in more than 25 countries outside of North America. The Corporate and Other segment includes the Smith & Hawken brand of lifestyle products such as high-end outdoor furniture, pottery, garden tools, gardening containers and live goods. In April 2008, SMG launched a $30 million campaign to educate homeowners about water conservation and the environmental benefits of healthy turf, as well as introduced Scotts Turf Builder Water smart, a fertilizer product meant to conserve water.

Scotts Miracle-Gro offers its employee benefits that include medical and prescription drugs plan; dental and vision insurance; fitness club reimbursement; and a 401(k) plan.

FINANCIALS: Sales and profits are in thousands of dollars—add 000 to get the full amount. 2007 Note: Financial information for 2007 was not available for all companies at press time.

2007 Sales: $2,871,800	2007 Profits: $113,400	**U.S. Stock Ticker:** SMG
2006 Sales: $2,697,100	2006 Profits: $132,700	**Int'l Ticker:** Int'l Exchange:
2005 Sales: $2,369,300	2005 Profits: $100,600	Employees: 5,081
2004 Sales: $2,106,500	2004 Profits: $100,900	Fiscal Year Ends: 9/30
2003 Sales: $1,941,600	2003 Profits: $103,800	Parent Company:

SALARIES/BENEFITS:

Pension Plan: Y	ESOP Stock Plan:	Profit Sharing:	Top Exec. Salary: $600,000	Bonus: $30,926
Savings Plan: Y	Stock Purch. Plan: Y		Second Exec. Salary: $400,000	Bonus: $19,257

OTHER THOUGHTS:

Apparent Women Officers or Directors: 1
Hot Spot for Advancement for Women/Minorities:

LOCATIONS: ("Y" = Yes)

West:	Southwest:	Midwest:	Southeast:	Northeast:	International:
Y	Y	Y	Y	Y	Y

SEACOR HOLDINGS INC

www.seacorholdings.com

Industry Group Code: 483111 Ranks within this company's industry group: Sales: 1 Profits: 1

Management:		Sales/Marketing:		Liberal Arts:		Information Systems:		Professionals:		Technical/Scientific:	
Mgmt. Trainees:	Y	Mktg. Professionals:	Y	Gen. Writing/Editing:	Y	Info. Management:	Y	Finance/Accounting:	Y	Engineers, Elec.:	Y
Experienced Mgmt.:	Y	Retail Sales:		Technical Writing:		Software Dev.:	Y	Law:	Y	Engineers, Other:	Y
Int'l Business:	Y	Commercial/Industrial:		Graphic Arts/Photog.:		Hardware Dev.:		HR/Other:	Y	Health/Lab:	
MBA Graduates:	Y	Sales Trainees:		Music:		Systems Integration:		Training:	Y	Scientists/Research:	
		Advertising Pros.:		Broadcasting:		Consulting/Other:		Health Care:		Petroleum/Chemicals:	Y
				Other:				Consulting:		Math/Other:	

TYPES OF BUSINESS:

Offshore Oil Platform Logistics
Inland Shipping
Aviation Services
Environmental Services
Maritime Communications
Helicopter Services

BRANDS/DIVISIONS/AFFILIATES:

SEACOR SMIT, Inc.
EraMed LLC
National Response Corp.
SCF Marine Inc.
O'Brien's Group, Inc. (The)
Era Aviation Inc.

CONTACTS: Note: Officers with more than one job title may be intentionally listed here more than once.

Charles Fabrikant, CEO
Charles Fabrikant, Pres.
Richard Ryan, CFO/Sr. VP
Alice Gran, Sr. VP/General Counsel/Corp. Sec.
Dick Fagerstal, Sr. VP-Corp. Dev./Treas.
Molly Hottinger, VP-Corp. Comm.
Molly Hottinger, VP-Investor Rel.
Matthew Cenac, VP/Chief Acct. Officer
John Gellert, Sr. VP-Offshore Marine Svcs.
James Cowderoy, Sr. VP
Randall Blank, Sr. VP/Pres./CEO-Environmental Svcs.
Charles Fabrikant, Chmn.

Phone: 954-523-2200	Fax: 954-524-9185
Toll-Free:	
Address: 2200 Eller Dr., Ft. Lauderdale, FL 33316 US	

GROWTH PLANS/SPECIAL FEATURES:

SEACOR Holdings, Inc. is in the business of owning, operating, investing in, marketing and remarketing equipment primarily in the offshore oil and gas and inland transportation industries, as well as providing oil spill response and environmental remediation services. The company's operations are divided into six business segments. The firm's principal business segment, offshore marine services, the firm's principal business, operates a diversified fleet of offshore support vessels primarily servicing offshore oil and gas exploration, development and production facilities worldwide. The marine transportation services segment operates a fleet of 10 U.S.-flag tankers providing marine transportation services for petroleum products, petrochemicals and chemicals moving in the U.S. domestic or coastwise trade. The inland river services division, trading under the name SCF Marine, Inc., operates a fleet of 1,139 dry cargo barges, which carry ore, grain, coal, aggregate, steel, scrap and fertilizers on the U.S rivers and their tributaries and the Gulf Intracoastal Waterways. The aviation services segment, or Tex-Air Helicopters, Inc., operates 46 helicopters primarily servicing the offshore oil and gas markets in Texas and Louisiana and Era Aviation, Inc., which operates 81 helicopters and an airline with 16 fixed wing aircraft. The firm's harbor and offshore towing services subsidiary, Seabulk Towing, is one of the leading tugboat operators in the United States. Finally, the environmental services group, which is comprised of various subsidiaries including National Response Corporation, The O'Brien's Group, Inc. and others, provides emergency preparedness services and response services such as management of industrial fires, hazardous materials releases and oil spills.

FINANCIALS: Sales and profits are in thousands of dollars—add 000 to get the full amount. 2007 Note: Financial information for 2007 was not available for all companies at press time.

2007 Sales: $1,359,230	2007 Profits: $241,648	U.S. Stock Ticker: CKH
2006 Sales: $1,323,445	2006 Profits: $234,394	Int'l Ticker: Int'l Exchange:
2005 Sales: $972,004	2005 Profits: $170,709	Employees: 4,994
2004 Sales: $491,860	2004 Profits: $19,889	Fiscal Year Ends: 12/31
2003 Sales: $406,209	2003 Profits: $11,954	Parent Company:

SALARIES/BENEFITS:

Pension Plan:	ESOP Stock Plan:	Profit Sharing:	Top Exec. Salary: $600,000	Bonus: $2,000,000
Savings Plan:	Stock Purch. Plan:		Second Exec. Salary: $335,000	Bonus: $1,550,000

OTHER THOUGHTS:

Apparent Women Officers or Directors: 3
Hot Spot for Advancement for Women/Minorities: Y

LOCATIONS: ("Y" = Yes)

West:	Southwest:	Midwest:	Southeast:	Northeast:	International:
Y	Y	Y	Y	Y	Y

SELECT MEDICAL CORPORATION www.selectmedicalcorp.com

Industry Group Code: 622110 Ranks within this company's industry group: Sales: 5 Profits: 4

Management:		Sales/Marketing:		Liberal Arts:		Information Systems:		Professionals:		Technical/Scientific:	
Mgmt. Trainees:	Y	Mktg. Professionals:	Y	Gen. Writing/Editing:		Info. Management:	Y	Finance/Accounting:	Y	Engineers, Elec.:	
Experienced Mgmt.:	Y	Retail Sales:		Technical Writing:	Y	Software Dev.:		Law:	Y	Engineers, Other:	
Int'l Business:	Y	Commercial/Industrial:		Graphic Arts/Photog.:		Hardware Dev.:		HR/Other:	Y	Health/Lab:	Y
MBA Graduates:	Y	Sales Trainees:		Music:		Systems Integration:		Training:	Y	Scientists/Research:	
		Advertising Pros.:		Broadcasting:		Consulting/Other:		Health Care:	Y	Petroleum/Chemicals:	
				Other:				Consulting:		Math/Other:	

TYPES OF BUSINESS:
Specialty Acute Care Hospitals
Long-Term Acute Care
Outpatient Rehabilitation Clinics
Contract Therapy Services
Medical Equipment Distribution

BRANDS/DIVISIONS/AFFILIATES:
EGL Acquisition Corp.
Welsh, Carson, Anderson & Stowe
HealthSouth
Nexus Health Systems, Inc.
CORA Health Services, Inc

CONTACTS: *Note: Officers with more than one job title may be intentionally listed here more than once.*
Robert A. Ortenzio, CEO
Patricia A. Rice, COO
Patricia A. Rice, Pres.
Martin F. Jackson, CFO/Exec. VP
S. Frank Fritsch, Exec. VP-Human Resources
James J. Talalai, CIO/Exec. VP
Michael E. Tarvin, Chief Legal Officer/Exec. VP/Corp. Sec.
David W. Cross, Chief Dev. Officer/Exec. VP
Scott A. Ramberger, Controller/Chief Acct. Officer/Sr. VP
Robert G. Breighner, Jr., VP-Compliance & Audit Svcs.
Robert G. Breighner, Jr., Corp. Compliance Officer
Rocco A. Ortenzio, Exec. Chmn.

Phone: 717-972-1100	Fax: 717-972-1042
Toll-Free:	
Address: 4716 Old Gettysburg Rd., Mechanicsburg, PA 17055 US	

GROWTH PLANS/SPECIAL FEATURES:
Select Medical Corporation operates specialty acute care hospitals for long-term stay patients in the U.S. The firm also operates outpatient rehabilitation clinics in the U.S., as well as a provider of contract therapy services. Select operates four acute medical rehabilitation hospitals, 970 outpatient rehabilitation clinics and 92 long-term acute care hospitals in 37 states and Washington D.C. The company also provides medical rehabilitation services on a contract basis at nursing homes, hospitals, assisted living and senior care centers, schools and worksites. The firm's business is divided between specialty hospitals and outpatient rehabilitation. The company's hospitals treat patients with serious, often complex medical conditions, such as respiratory failure, neuromuscular disorders, cardiac disorders, non-healing wounds, renal disorders and cancer. Patients are admitted to the hospitals from general acute care facilities, as general hospitals are not the optimum setting for patients requiring longer stays and higher levels of clinical attention than typical acute care patients. Most of Select's specialty hospitals are located in leased space within a host general hospital. Select's outpatient rehabilitation segment is designed to help patients minimize physical and cognitive impairments and maximize functional ability. Therapies taking place at its clinics include physical, occupational and speech rehabilitation programs. In addition to rehabilitation services, the firm also distributes home medical equipment, orthotics, prosthetics, oxygen and ventilator systems, infusion/intravenous and certain non-healthcare services. In January 2007, Select agreed to acquire the outpatient rehabilitation division of HealthSouth for approximately $245 million and in March 2007 it agreed to acquire all of the assets of Nexus Health Systems, Inc. for $49 million. In October 2007, the firm agreed to acquire CORA Health Services, Inc. for $46 million.

Select employee benefits include health, dental, vision and prescription insurance; life insurance; short and long-term disability coverage; continuing education; and tuition reimbursement.

FINANCIALS: Sales and profits are in thousands of dollars—add 000 to get the full amount. 2007 Note: Financial information for 2007 was not available for all companies at press time.

2007 Sales: $1,991,666	2007 Profits: $35,430	**U.S. Stock Ticker:** Private	
2006 Sales: $1,851,498	2006 Profits: $94,879	**Int'l Ticker:**	Int'l Exchange:
2005 Sales: $1,580,706	2005 Profits: $85,575	Employees: 18,200	
2004 Sales: $1,601,524	2004 Profits: $118,184	Fiscal Year Ends: 12/31	
2003 Sales: $1,341,657	2003 Profits: $74,471	Parent Company:	

SALARIES/BENEFITS:

Pension Plan:	ESOP Stock Plan:	Profit Sharing:	Top Exec. Salary: $824,000	Bonus: $640,000
Savings Plan: Y	Stock Purch. Plan:		Second Exec. Salary: $824,000	Bonus: $1,648,000

OTHER THOUGHTS:
Apparent Women Officers or Directors: 1
Hot Spot for Advancement for Women/Minorities:

LOCATIONS: ("Y" = Yes)

West:	Southwest:	Midwest:	Southeast:	Northeast:	International:
Y	Y	Y	Y	Y	Y

Note: Financial information, benefits and other data can change quickly and may vary from those stated here.

SEMPRA ENERGY

www.sempra.com

Industry Group Code: 221000 Ranks within this company's industry group: Sales: 3 Profits: 2

Management:		Sales/Marketing:		Liberal Arts:		Information Systems:		Professionals:		Technical/Scientific:	
Mgmt. Trainees:	Y	Mktg. Professionals:	Y	Gen. Writing/Editing:		Info. Management:	Y	Finance/Accounting:	Y	Engineers, Elec.:	Y
Experienced Mgmt.:	Y	Retail Sales:	Y	Technical Writing:	Y	Software Dev.:		Law:	Y	Engineers, Other:	Y
Int'l Business:	Y	Commercial/Industrial:	Y	Graphic Arts/Photog.:		Hardware Dev.:		HR/Other:	Y	Health/Lab:	
MBA Graduates:	Y	Sales Trainees:	Y	Music:		Systems Integration:		Training:	Y	Scientists/Research:	Y
		Advertising Pros.:		Broadcasting:		Consulting/Other:		Health Care:		Petroleum/Chemicals:	Y
				Other:				Consulting:		Math/Other:	

TYPES OF BUSINESS:

Utilities-Electricity & Natural Gas
Energy Management
Energy Marketing
Power Generation-Natural Gas Plants
LNG Pipelines, Storage & Terminals
Financial Management

BRANDS/DIVISIONS/AFFILIATES:

Southern California Gas Company
San Diego Gas & Electric
Sempra Generation
Sempra Commodities
Sempra Pipeline & Storage
Sempra LNG
Sempra Financial

CONTACTS: Note: Officers with more than one job title may be intentionally listed here more than once.

Donald E. Felsinger, CEO
Neal E. Schmale, COO
Neal E. Schmale, Pres.
Mark A. Snell, CFO/Exec. VP
G. Joyce Rowland, Sr. VP-Human Resources
Javade Chaudhri, General Counsel/Exec. VP
Edwin A. Guiles, Exec. VP-Corp. Dev.
Steven D. Davis, VP-Comm. & Community Partnerships
Jeff Martin, VP-Investor Rel.
Joseph A. Householder, Controller/Chief Acct. Officer/Sr. VP
Jessie J. Knight, Jr., Exec. VP-External Affairs
Amy Chiu, VP-Audit Svcs.
Randall B. Peterson, VP/Chief Compliance Officer
Monica Haas, VP-Corp. Planning
Donald E. Felsinger, Chmn.
Mike Morgan, VP-Int'l Affairs

Phone: 619-696-2000	Fax: 619-696-2374
Toll-Free: 877-736-7721	
Address: 101 Ash St., San Diego, CA 92101 US	

GROWTH PLANS/SPECIAL FEATURES:

Sempra Energy is a provider of energy-related products and services mainly to California and abroad. The company operates through two main branches, Sempra Utilities and Sempra Global. Sempra Utilities includes the Southern California Gas Co., a natural gas distribution utility that supplies natural gas to 20 million customers in a 20,000-square-mile service territory that extends from central California to the Mexican border. The other segment of Sempra Utilities is San Diego Gas and Electric, a regulated distribution utility that provides electric and natural gas services to 3.4 million customers across 4,100 square miles from Orange County to the Mexican Border. The Sempra Global subsidiaries handle financial, international, facilities development, business outsourcing and energy trading businesses and include Sempra Generation, Sempra Commodities, Sempra Pipeline and Storage and Sempra LNG. Sempra Generation delivers electricity to the market and operates a fleet of natural gas power plants that produce 2,600 megawatts of electricity. Sempra Commodities is a trading company that markets and trades physical and financial commodity products, through negotiating contracts on natural gas, electricity, petroleum products, base materials and other commodities. Sempra Pipeline and Storage acquires, builds and operates natural gas pipelines and storage facilities in Mexico and the United States. Sempra Energy LNG Corp. is developing liquefied natural gas receipt terminals in North America, recently in partnership with Mexico's state-owned electric utility company. In February 2008, San Diego Gas and Electric added 40 geothermal megawatts from Esmerelda Truckhaven. In April 2008, Sempra formed a joint venture, RBS Sempra Commodities, with the Royal Bank of Scotland. In May 2008, the company's new LNG terminal in Baja California became operational. In July 2008, the firm agreed to acquire EnergySouth, Inc. for $510 million.

Sempra offers its employees tuition reimbursement, a health club membership subsidy, volunteer/giving incentive programs and a mass-transit/parking subsidy.

FINANCIALS: Sales and profits are in thousands of dollars—add 000 to get the full amount. 2007 Note: Financial information for 2007 was not available for all companies at press time.

2007 Sales: $11,438,000	2007 Profits: $1,099,000	U.S. Stock Ticker: SRE
2006 Sales: $11,761,000	2006 Profits: $1,406,000	Int'l Ticker: Int'l Exchange:
2005 Sales: $11,512,000	2005 Profits: $920,000	Employees: 14,061
2004 Sales: $9,234,000	2004 Profits: $895,000	Fiscal Year Ends: 12/31
2003 Sales: $7,891,000	2003 Profits: $649,000	Parent Company:

SALARIES/BENEFITS:

Pension Plan: Y	ESOP Stock Plan:	Profit Sharing:	Top Exec. Salary: $943,320	Bonus: $1,900,000
Savings Plan: Y	Stock Purch. Plan:		Second Exec. Salary: $745,039	Bonus: $1,200,000

OTHER THOUGHTS:

Apparent Women Officers or Directors: 5
Hot Spot for Advancement for Women/Minorities: Y

LOCATIONS: ("Y" = Yes)

West:	Southwest:	Midwest:	Southeast:	Northeast:	International:
Y	Y	Y	Y	Y	Y

SENSIENT TECHNOLOGIES CORPORATION   www.sensient-tech.com

Industry Group Code: 325000 **Ranks within this company's industry group:** Sales: 3   Profits: 2

Management:		Sales/Marketing:		Liberal Arts:	Information Systems:		Professionals:		Technical/Scientific:	
Mgmt. Trainees:	Y	Mktg. Professionals:	Y	Gen. Writing/Editing:	Info. Management:	Y	Finance/Accounting:	Y	Engineers, Elec.:	
Experienced Mgmt.:	Y	Retail Sales:		Technical Writing:	Software Dev.:		Law:	Y	Engineers, Other:	
Int'l Business:	Y	Commercial/Industrial:	Y	Graphic Arts/Photog.:	Hardware Dev.:		HR/Other:	Y	Health/Lab:	Y
MBA Graduates:	Y	Sales Trainees:		Music:	Systems Integration:		Training:	Y	Scientists/Research:	Y
		Advertising Pros.:		Broadcasting:	Consulting/Other:		Health Care:		Petroleum/Chemicals:	
				Other:			Consulting:		Math/Other:	

TYPES OF BUSINESS:

Flavor, Fragrance & Color Chemicals
Inks & Pigments
Pharmaceutical & Cosmetic Ingredients
Specialty Chemicals
Dehydrated Vegetables

BRANDS/DIVISIONS/AFFILIATES:

Sensient Food Colors
Sensient Pharmaceutical Technologies
Sensient Imaging Technologies
Sensient Dehydrated Flavors Company
Sensient Flavors, Inc.

CONTACTS: Note: Officers with more than one job title may be intentionally listed here more than once.

Kenneth P. Manning, CEO
Robert J. Edmonds, COO
Robert J. Edmonds, Pres.
Richard (Dick) Hobbs, CFO/VP
Douglas S. Pepper, VP-Admin.
John L. Hammond, General Counsel/Sec./VP
Stephen J. Rolfs, Chief Acct. Officer/Controller/VP
Peter Bradley, Pres., Color Group
Neil G. Cracknell, Pres., Flavors & Fragrances Group
John F. Collopy, VP/Treas.
Kenneth P. Manning, Chmn.

Phone: 414-271-6755	Fax: 414-347-3785
Toll-Free: 800-558-9892	
Address: 777 E. Wisconsin Ave., Milwaukee, WI 53202-5304 US	

GROWTH PLANS/SPECIAL FEATURES:

Sensient Technologies Corporation, incorporated in 1882, manufactures and markets fragrances, flavors and colors worldwide. Its operations include producing specialty food and beverage systems; cosmetic and pharmaceutical ingredient systems; and inkjet and specialty inks and colors. The company's customers include major international manufacturers representing some of the world's best-known brands. Sensient is composed of two segments: Flavors & Fragrances, which generated 64.6% of 2007 revenue; and Color, 31.2%. The remaining 4.2% came from corporate and other activities, including the Asia Pacific Group, which is not a segment. The Flavors & Fragrances group manufactures and markets flavor and fragrance systems for food, beverage, household and personal care products. Dehydrated flavors generated 27% of this segment's 2007 revenue; dairy flavors, 20%; savory flavors, 18%; beverage flavors, 10%; confectionary & bakery flavors, 5%; all other flavors, 10%; and all fragrances combined, 10%. Group subsidiaries include Sensient Dehydrated Flavors Company and Sensient Flavors, Inc. The Color group manufactures and markets natural and synthetic colors, including those for textiles and papers. Food and beverage colors generated 60% of this segment's 2007 revenue; cosmetics, 20%; inkjet & specialty inks and colors, 9%; pharmaceuticals, 4%; and other technical colors, 7%. Trade names within the group include Sensient Food Colors, Sensient Pharmaceutical Technologies and Sensient Imaging Technologies. Headquartered in Australia, the Asia Pacific Group markets the full line of products for Pacific Rim countries, as well as specialty products designed to appeal to local preferences. It maintains manufacturing facilities in Australia, New Zealand and the Philippines. In all, Sensient has 70 offices located across 30 countries, and 59.8% of its revenue is generated outside the U.S.

FINANCIALS: Sales and profits are in thousands of dollars—add 000 to get the full amount. 2007 Note: Financial information for 2007 was not available for all companies at press time.

2007 Sales: $1,212,561	2007 Profits: $111,243	**U.S. Stock Ticker: SXT**
2006 Sales: $1,124,896	2006 Profits: $93,529	**Int'l Ticker:** Int'l Exchange:
2005 Sales: $1,023,930	2005 Profits: $44,195	Employees: 3,623
2004 Sales: $1,047,133	2004 Profits: $73,918	Fiscal Year Ends: 12/31
2003 Sales: $987,408	2003 Profits: $81,432	Parent Company:

SALARIES/BENEFITS:

Pension Plan:	ESOP Stock Plan:	Profit Sharing:	Top Exec. Salary: $845,500	Bonus: $1,437,350
Savings Plan:	Stock Purch. Plan:		Second Exec. Salary: $411,500	Bonus: $534,950

OTHER THOUGHTS:

Apparent Women Officers or Directors:
Hot Spot for Advancement for Women/Minorities:

LOCATIONS: ("Y" = Yes)

West:	Southwest:	Midwest:	Southeast:	Northeast:	International:
Y		Y		Y	Y

SHAW GROUP INC (THE)

www.shawgrp.com

Industry Group Code: 234000 Ranks within this company's industry group: Sales: 4 Profits: 5

Management:		Sales/Marketing:		Liberal Arts:		Information Systems:		Professionals:		Technical/Scientific:	
Mgmt. Trainees:	Y	Mktg. Professionals:	Y	Gen. Writing/Editing:		Info. Management:	Y	Finance/Accounting:	Y	Engineers, Elec.:	Y
Experienced Mgmt.:	Y	Retail Sales:		Technical Writing:	Y	Software Dev.:		Law:	Y	Engineers, Other:	
Int'l Business:	Y	Commercial/Industrial:	Y	Graphic Arts/Photog.:	Y	Hardware Dev.:		HR/Other:	Y	Health/Lab:	
MBA Graduates:	Y	Sales Trainees:		Music:		Systems Integration:		Training:	Y	Scientists/Research:	
		Advertising Pros.:		Broadcasting:		Consulting/Other:		Health Care:		Petroleum/Chemicals:	
				Other:				Consulting:		Math/Other:	

TYPES OF BUSINESS:

Pipe Manufacturing
Construction & Engineering
Consulting Services
Environmental Services
Facilities Management
Power Plant Construction

BRANDS/DIVISIONS/AFFILIATES:

Westinghouse
Ezeflow, Inc.

CONTACTS: Note: Officers with more than one job title may be intentionally listed here more than once.

James M. Bernhard, Jr., CEO
James M. Bernhard, Jr., Pres.
Brian K. Ferraioli, CFO/Exec. VP
David L. Chapman Sr., Pres., Fabrication & Mfg. Group
Dirk J. Wild, Sr. VP-Admin.
Cliff S. Rankin, General Counsel/Corp. Sec.
Gary P. Graphia, Exec. VP-Corp. Dev. & Strategy
Michael J. Kershaw, Controller/Sr. VP
Richard F. Gill, Exec. VP/Chmn./Pres., Power Group
Lou Pucher, Pres., Energy & Chemicals Group
Ronald W. Oakley, Pres., Environmental & Infrastructure Group
David P. Barry, Pres., Nuclear Div.-Power Group
James M. Bernhard, Jr., Chmn.

Phone: 225-932-2500	Fax: 225-987-3328
Toll-Free:	
Address: 4171 Essen Ln., Baton Rouge, LA 70809 US	

GROWTH PLANS/SPECIAL FEATURES:

The Shaw Group, Inc. is a diverse engineering, technology, construction, fabrication, environmental and industrial services organizations. It provides services to a diverse customer base that includes multinational oil companies and industrial corporations, regulated utilities, independent and merchant power producers, government agencies and other equipment manufacturers. The company operates in six segments: fossil & nuclear (F&N); energy & chemicals (E&C); environmental & infrastructure (E&I); maintenance; fabrication & manufacturing (F&M); and investment in Westinghouse. The F&N segment provides a range of project-related services, primarily to the global fossil and nuclear power generation industries. The E&C division's offerings include design, engineering, construction, procurement, technology and consulting services, primarily to the oil and gas, refinery, petrochemical and chemical industries. The E&I segment designs and executes remediation solutions involving contaminants in soil, air and water. It also provides project and facilities management and other related services for non-environmental construction, watershed restoration, emergency response services, outsourcing of privatization markets, program management, operations and maintenance solutions to support and enhance domestic and global land, water and air transportation systems. The maintenance segment performs routine and outage/turnaround maintenance including restorative, repair, renovation, modification, predictive and preventive maintenance services. The F&M segment supplies fabricated piping systems. Westinghouse serves the nuclear electric power industry by supplying advanced nuclear plant designs, licensing, engineering services, equipment, fuel and a wide range of other products and services to the owners and operators of nuclear power plants. In early 2007, the firm announced that the Shaw/Westinghouse Consortium completed an agreement with China's State Nuclear Power Technology Company, whereby the consortium will build four nuclear power plants in China by 2013. In mid-2007, Shaw acquired Ezeflow, Inc., a manufacturer of pipe fittings.

The company offers its employees medical, dental and vision insurance; a 401(k) plan; life and AD&D insurance; short- and long-term disability; and tuition reimbursement.

FINANCIALS: Sales and profits are in thousands of dollars—add 000 to get the full amount. 2007 Note: Financial information for 2007 was not available for all companies at press time.

2007 Sales: $5,723,712	2007 Profits: $-19,000	U.S. Stock Ticker: SGR
2006 Sales: $4,775,649	2006 Profits: $50,226	Int'l Ticker: Int'l Exchange:
2005 Sales: $3,267,702	2005 Profits: $15,671	Employees: 27,000
2004 Sales: $3,014,709	2004 Profits: $-33,075	Fiscal Year Ends: 8/31
2003 Sales: $3,306,800	2003 Profits: $20,900	Parent Company:

SALARIES/BENEFITS:

Pension Plan:	ESOP Stock Plan:	Profit Sharing:	Top Exec. Salary: $1,579,400	Bonus: $2,112,000
Savings Plan: Y	Stock Purch. Plan:		Second Exec. Salary: $619,629	Bonus: $100,000

OTHER THOUGHTS:

Apparent Women Officers or Directors:
Hot Spot for Advancement for Women/Minorities:

LOCATIONS: ("Y" = Yes)

West:	Southwest:	Midwest:	Southeast:	Northeast:	International:
Y	Y	Y	Y	Y	Y

Note: Financial information, benefits and other data can change quickly and may vary from those stated here.

SHELL OIL CO

www.shelloil.com

Industry Group Code: 211111 Ranks within this company's industry group: Sales: 4   Profits:

Management:		Sales/Marketing:		Liberal Arts:		Information Systems:		Professionals:		Technical/Scientific:	
Mgmt. Trainees:		Mktg. Professionals:	Y	Gen. Writing/Editing:	Y	Info. Management:	Y	Finance/Accounting:	Y	Engineers, Elec.:	Y
Experienced Mgmt.:	Y	Retail Sales:		Technical Writing:	Y	Software Dev.:	Y	Law:	Y	Engineers, Other:	Y
Int'l Business:	Y	Commercial/Industrial:	Y	Graphic Arts/Photog.:	Y	Hardware Dev.:		HR/Other:	Y	Health/Lab:	
MBA Graduates:	Y	Sales Trainees:		Music:		Systems Integration:	Y	Training:	Y	Scientists/Research:	Y
		Advertising Pros.:	Y	Broadcasting:		Consulting/Other:	Y	Health Care:		Petroleum/Chemicals:	Y
				Other:				Consulting:		Math/Other:	Y

TYPES OF BUSINESS:

Oil & Gas Exploration & Production
Chemicals
Power Generation
Nanocomposites
Nanocatalysts
Refineries
Pipelines & Shipping
Hydrogen Storage Technology

BRANDS/DIVISIONS/AFFILIATES:

Shell Oil Products US
Shell Chemicals Limited
Shell Gas and Power
Shell Exploration and Production
Royal Dutch Shell (Shell Group)
Motiva Enterprises LLC
Tesoro Corp
Luminant

CONTACTS: Note: Officers with more than one job title may be intentionally listed here more than once.

Marvin E. Odum, Pres.
William C. (Bill) Lowrey, General Counsel/Corp. Sec./Sr. VP
Curtis R. Frasier, Exec. VP-Americas Shell Gas & Power
Mark Hanafin, CEO-Shell Trading Gas & Power Houston
Stacy Methvin, CEO/Pres., Shell Chemical LP
Marvin E. Odum, Exec. VP-Americas Shell Exploration & Production
Mark Hanafin, Global VP-Shell Trading Gas & Power

Phone: 713-241-6161	Fax: 713-241-4044
Toll-Free:	
Address: 1 Shell Plaza, 910 Louisiana St., Houston, TX 77002 US	

GROWTH PLANS/SPECIAL FEATURES:

Shell Oil Company, an affiliate of the Shell Group, is a chemical, oil and natural gas producer in the U.S., with operations in all 50 states. Shell Oil has a number of division and operations, including Shell Oil Products U.S., Motiva Enterprises, Shell Chemicals, Shell Gas and Power, Shell Exploration and Production (SEPCo) and others. These companies discover, develop, manufacture, transport and market crude oil, natural gas and chemical products. Specifically, Shell Oil Products has four refineries which produce a total of 753,000 barrels of oil per day. Shell Oil Products also maintains 50% ownership of Motiva Enterprises LLC, with whom the firm refines and ships gasoline to more than 7,300 gas stations in the eastern and southern U.S., along with about 3,500 Texaco stations. Shell Chemicals is involved in manufacturing chemicals, including ethylene and propylene, for use in cars, computers, packaging and paints. SEPCo explores and develops natural gas in the U.S, with interests in five states and the Gulf of Mexico. Shell Oil's Gas and Power business is involved in power generation, gas pipeline transmission, receiving terminals, liquefied natural gas, shipping and coal gasification. Newer divisions of Shell Oil include Shell Hydrogen and Shell Renewables, the latter of which invests heavily in wind and solar power research. In May 2007, the company sold its Los Angeles Refinery, Wilmington Products Terminal and roughly 250 retail sites and supply agreements in and around Los Angeles and San Diego to Tesoro Corporation. In July 2007, Shell Oil announced a joint development agreement with Luminant for a 3,000 megawatt wind project in the Texas Panhandle. In September 2007, Shell Oil began construction on a capacity expansion project at its joint venture refinery in Port Arthur, Texas to make it the largest in the U.S., with a 600,000 barrel-per-day capacity.

FINANCIALS: Sales and profits are in thousands of dollars—add 000 to get the full amount. 2007 Note: Financial information for 2007 was not available for all companies at press time.

2007 Sales: $87,548,000	2007 Profits: $	**U.S. Stock Ticker:** Subsidiary
2006 Sales: $80,974,000	2006 Profits: $	**Int'l Ticker:** Int'l Exchange:
2005 Sales: $70,000,000	2005 Profits: $	Employees: 24,008
2004 Sales: $60,000,000	2004 Profits: $	Fiscal Year Ends: 12/31
2003 Sales: $41,468,000	2003 Profits: $3,421,000	Parent Company: ROYAL DUTCH SHELL (SHELL GROUP)

SALARIES/BENEFITS:

Pension Plan:	ESOP Stock Plan:	Profit Sharing:	Top Exec. Salary: $	Bonus: $
Savings Plan: Y	Stock Purch. Plan:		Second Exec. Salary: $	Bonus: $

OTHER THOUGHTS:

Apparent Women Officers or Directors: 1
Hot Spot for Advancement for Women/Minorities: Y

LOCATIONS: ("Y" = Yes)

West:	Southwest:	Midwest:	Southeast:	Northeast:	International:
Y	Y	Y	Y	Y	Y

SHERWIN WILLIAMS COMPANY (THE)
www.sherwin-williams.com

Industry Group Code: 444120   Ranks within this company's industry group: Sales: 1   Profits: 1

Management:		Sales/Marketing:		Liberal Arts:		Information Systems:		Professionals:		Technical/Scientific:	
Mgmt. Trainees:	Y	Mktg. Professionals:	Y	Gen. Writing/Editing:	Y	Info. Management:	Y	Finance/Accounting:	Y	Engineers, Elec.:	
Experienced Mgmt.:	Y	Retail Sales:	Y	Technical Writing:	Y	Software Dev.:	Y	Law:	Y	Engineers, Other:	
Int'l Business:	Y	Commercial/Industrial:	Y	Graphic Arts/Photog.:	Y	Hardware Dev.:		HR/Other:	Y	Health/Lab:	
MBA Graduates:	Y	Sales Trainees:	Y	Music:		Systems Integration:		Training:	Y	Scientists/Research:	Y
		Advertising Pros.:	Y	Broadcasting:		Consulting/Other:		Health Care:		Petroleum/Chemicals:	Y
				Other:				Consulting:		Math/Other:	

TYPES OF BUSINESS:
Paints & Coatings Manufacturing
Retail Paint Stores
Wallcoverings
Automotive Finishing Products
Design Consulting

BRANDS/DIVISIONS/AFFILIATES:
Duron Inc
Martin-Senour
Dutch Boy
Thompson's
Becker Powder Coatings, Inc
Flex Recubrimientos, Acabados Automotrices
Nitco Paints
Columbia Paint & Coatings Co.

CONTACTS: *Note: Officers with more than one job title may be intentionally listed here more than once.*
Christopher M. Connor, CEO
John G. Morikis, COO
John G. Morikis, Pres.
Sean P. Hennessy, CFO/Sr. VP-Finance
Thomas E. Hopkins, Sr. VP-Human Resources
Richard M. Weaver, VP-Admin.
Louis E. Stellato, General Counsel/Corp. Sec./VP
Timothy A. Knight, Sr. VP-Corp. Planning & Dev.
Robert J. Wells, VP-Corp. Comm. & Public Affairs
Cynthia D. Brogran, Treas./VP
Thomas W. Seitz, Sr. VP-Strategic Excellence Initiatives
Steven J. Oberfeld, Pres., Paint Stores Group
George E. Heath, Pres./Gen. Mgr.-Chemical Coatings Div. Global
Thomas C. Hablitzel, Pres./Gen. Mgr.-Automotive Div. Global
Christopher M. Connor, Chmn.
Alexander Zalesky, Pres./Gen. Mgr.-Int'l Div. Global Group

Phone: 216-566-2200	Fax:
Toll-Free:	
Address: 101 Prospect Ave. N.W., Cleveland, OH 44115-1075 US	

GROWTH PLANS/SPECIAL FEATURES:
The Sherwin-Williams Company is one of the largest international manufacturers, distributors and retailers of paint and related products to professional, industrial, commercial and retail customers. The company operates in three segments: Paint stores group, consumer group and global group. The paint stores group consists of seven manufacturing/distribution facilities and 3,325 company-operated stores, which sell Sherwin-Williams brand architectural paint and coating and other associated products and brands. Several subsidiaries operate under this division, including Duron, Inc., a Maryland paint producer. In the last year, this segment opened over 100 new stores. It has operations in the U.S., Canada, Puerto Rico, Jamaica and the Virgin Islands. This division also sells industrial products, marine products, and finishes for original equipment manufacturers. The consumer group produces and distributes paint, coatings and related products to third-party customers and to the paint stores group (which represented 56% of the consumer group's sales in 2007). The global group, through 519 branches, manufactures, licenses, distributes and sells paints and coatings, industrial and marine products, automotive finishes, refinish products and OEM coatings. In all three segments, the company's varnish, applicators, paint, finishes and coatings are marketed under various name brands, including several private labels such as Sherwin-Williams, Pratt and Lambert, Martin-Senour, Dutch Boy, Thompson's, Minwax and Krylon. Additionally, the firm sells wallpaper and flooring such as Shaw carpet. In 2007, Sherwin-Williams acquired the Indian company Nitco Paints; M.A. Bruder & Sons Incorporated paint company; and Columbia Paint & Coatings Co., which became a subsidiary. In 2008, the firm acquired the assets of Mexican company Flex Recubrimientos, Acabados Automotrices; agreed to acquire the liquid coatings subsidiaries of Inchem Holdings; and acquired Becker Powder Coatings, Inc. in North America.

Sherwin-Williams offers employees health care plans; disability and life insurance; and tuition assistance.

FINANCIALS: Sales and profits are in thousands of dollars—add 000 to get the full amount. 2007 Note: Financial information for 2007 was not available for all companies at press time.

2007 Sales: $8,005,000	2007 Profits: $616,000	**U.S. Stock Ticker: SHW**
2006 Sales: $7,810,000	2006 Profits: $576,000	**Int'l Ticker:** Int'l Exchange:
2005 Sales: $7,191,000	2005 Profits: $463,000	Employees: 31,572
2004 Sales: $6,113,789	2004 Profits: $393,254	Fiscal Year Ends: 12/31
2003 Sales: $5,407,764	2003 Profits: $332,058	Parent Company:

SALARIES/BENEFITS:
Pension Plan: Y	ESOP Stock Plan:	Profit Sharing:	Top Exec. Salary: $1,161,047	Bonus: $1,544,000
Savings Plan: Y	Stock Purch. Plan: Y		Second Exec. Salary: $663,481	Bonus: $697,000

OTHER THOUGHTS:
Apparent Women Officers or Directors: 3
Hot Spot for Advancement for Women/Minorities: Y

LOCATIONS: ("Y" = Yes)
West:	Southwest:	Midwest:	Southeast:	Northeast:	International:
Y	Y	Y	Y	Y	Y

SIGMA-ALDRICH CORP

www.sigmaaldrich.com

Industry Group Code: 325000 Ranks within this company's industry group: Sales: 2 Profits: 1

Management:		Sales/Marketing:		Liberal Arts:		Information Systems:		Professionals:		Technical/Scientific:	
Mgmt. Trainees:	Y	Mktg. Professionals:	Y	Gen. Writing/Editing:		Info. Management:	Y	Finance/Accounting:	Y	Engineers, Elec.:	Y
Experienced Mgmt.:	Y	Retail Sales:		Technical Writing:		Software Dev.:		Law:	Y	Engineers, Other:	
Int'l Business:	Y	Commercial/Industrial:	Y	Graphic Arts/Photog.:		Hardware Dev.:		HR/Other:	Y	Health/Lab:	Y
MBA Graduates:	Y	Sales Trainees:		Music:		Systems Integration:		Training:	Y	Scientists/Research:	Y
		Advertising Pros.:	Y	Broadcasting:		Consulting/Other:		Health Care:		Petroleum/Chemicals:	
				Other:				Consulting:		Math/Other:	

TYPES OF BUSINESS:

Chemicals Manufacturing
Biotechnology Equipment
Pharmaceutical Ingredients
Fine Chemicals
Chromatography Products

BRANDS/DIVISIONS/AFFILIATES:

Research Essentials
Research Specialties
Research Biotech
SAFC
Molecular Medicine BioServices, Inc.
Epichem Group, Ltd.

CONTACTS: Note: Officers with more than one job title may be intentionally listed here more than once.

Jai Nagarkatti, CEO
Jai Nagarkatti, Pres.
Mike Hogan, CFO
Gerrit van den Dool, VP-Sales
Doug Rau, VP-Human Resources
Carl Turza, CIO
Michael R. Hogan, Chief Admin. Officer
Richard A. Keffer, General Counsel/VP/Sec.
Karen Miller, Controller
Giles Cottier, Pres., Research Essentials
Dave Julien, Pres., Research Specialties
Franklin D. Wicks, Pres., SAFC
David Smoller, Pres., Research Biotech
David R. Harvey, Chmn.

Phone: 314-771-5765	Fax: 314-771-5757
Toll-Free: 800-521-8956	
Address: 3050 Spruce St., St. Louis, MO 63103 US	

GROWTH PLANS/SPECIAL FEATURES:

Sigma-Aldrich Corp. is a life science and technology company that develops, manufactures, purchases and distributes a broad range of biochemicals and organic chemicals. The company offers roughly 100,000 chemicals (including 46,000 chemicals manufactured in-house) and 30,000 equipment products used for scientific and genomic research; biotechnology; pharmaceutical development; disease diagnosis; and pharmaceutical and high technology manufacturing. Sigma-Aldrich is structured into four units: Research essentials, research specialties, research biotech and SAFC, a fine chemicals unit. The research essentials unit sells biological buffers; cell culture reagents; biochemicals; chemicals; solvents; and other reagents and kits. The research specialties unit provides organic chemicals, biochemicals, analytical reagents, chromatography consumables, reference materials and high-purity products. The research biotech unit supplies immunochemical, molecular biology, cell signaling and neuroscience biochemicals and kits used in biotechnology, genomic, proteomic and other life science research applications. Lastly, the SAFC unit offers large-scale organic chemicals and biochemicals used in development and production by pharmaceutical, biotechnology, industrial and diagnostic companies. In 2007, the research essentials unit accounted for 19% of sales; the research specialties unit for 37%; the research biotech unit for 15%; and the SAFC unit for 29%. The company operates in 36 countries, selling its products in nearly 160 countries and servicing over 1 million customers. Customers include commercial laboratories; pharmaceutical and industrial companies; universities; diagnostics, chemical and biotechnology companies and hospitals; non-profit organizations; and governmental institutions. In 2007, Sigma-Aldrich acquired two new businesses: Epichem Group, Ltd., a U.K.-based company, for roughly $60 million, and Molecular Medicine BioServices, Inc., a California based biopharmaceutical company. Also in 2007, the firm announced plans to build a new active pharmaceutical ingredients suite at its St. Louis manufacturing facility and announced its intent to build a new manufacturing hub in China. In 2008, the company opened a $9 million cleanroom in Wisconsin.

FINANCIALS: Sales and profits are in thousands of dollars—add 000 to get the full amount. 2007 Note: Financial information for 2007 was not available for all companies at press time.

2007 Sales: $2,038,700	2007 Profits: $311,100	U.S. Stock Ticker: SIAL
2006 Sales: $1,797,500	2006 Profits: $276,800	Int'l Ticker: Int'l Exchange:
2005 Sales: $1,666,500	2005 Profits: $258,300	Employees: 7,299
2004 Sales: $1,409,200	2004 Profits: $232,900	Fiscal Year Ends: 12/31
2003 Sales: $1,298,146	2003 Profits: $193,102	Parent Company:

SALARIES/BENEFITS:

Pension Plan: Y	ESOP Stock Plan:	Profit Sharing:	Top Exec. Salary: $660,000	Bonus: $439,105
Savings Plan: Y	Stock Purch. Plan:		Second Exec. Salary: $430,000	Bonus: $213,495

OTHER THOUGHTS:

Apparent Women Officers or Directors: 2
Hot Spot for Advancement for Women/Minorities:

LOCATIONS: ("Y" = Yes)

West:	Southwest:	Midwest:	Southeast:	Northeast:	International:
Y	Y	Y	Y	Y	Y

Note: Financial information, benefits and other data can change quickly and may vary from those stated here.

SISTERS OF MERCY HEALTH SYSTEMS

www.mercy.net

Industry Group Code: 622110 Ranks within this company's industry group: Sales: 4 Profits: 5

Management:		Sales/Marketing:		Liberal Arts:		Information Systems:		Professionals:		Technical/Scientific:	
Mgmt. Trainees:		Mktg. Professionals:		Gen. Writing/Editing:	Y	Info. Management:	Y	Finance/Accounting:	Y	Engineers, Elec.:	
Experienced Mgmt.:	Y	Retail Sales:		Technical Writing:		Software Dev.:		Law:	Y	Engineers, Other:	
Int'l Business:	Y	Commercial/Industrial:		Graphic Arts/Photog.:		Hardware Dev.:		HR/Other:	Y	Health/Lab:	
MBA Graduates:	Y	Sales Trainees:		Music:		Systems Integration:		Training:	Y	Scientists/Research:	
		Advertising Pros.:		Broadcasting:		Consulting/Other:		Health Care:	Y	Petroleum/Chemicals:	
				Other:				Consulting:		Math/Other:	

TYPES OF BUSINESS:

Hospitals-General
Outpatient Care
Health Classes
Long-Term Care
Community Service & Outreach

BRANDS/DIVISIONS/AFFILIATES:

Mercy Health Plans
Sisters of Mercy-St. Louis Regional Community
Mercy Ministries of Laredo

CONTACTS: *Note: Officers with more than one job title may be intentionally listed here more than once.*

John Sullivan, CEO
John Sullivan, Pres.
James R. Jaacks, CFO/Sr. VP
Anthony Kinslow, VP-Human Resources
Mike McCurry, CIO/VP
Philip Wheeler, General Counsel/VP
Vance Moore, VP-Resource Optimization/Pres., ROi
Myra K. Aubuchon, Sr. VP
Jolene Goedken, VP-Medical Svcs.
Glenn Mitchell, VP-Clinical Safety
Joseph M. Sullivan, Chmn.

Phone: 314-579-6100	**Fax:** 314-628-3723
Toll-Free:	
Address: 14528 S. Outer Forty, Ste. 100, Chesterfield, MO 63017 US	

GROWTH PLANS/SPECIAL FEATURES:

Sisters of Mercy Health Systems (Mercy), established in 1986, is one of the largest Catholic health care systems in the U.S. It operates outpatient clinics, physician practices, hospitals, health plants, human services and community outreach programs in seven states: Arkansas, Louisiana, Kansas, Mississippi, Missouri, Oklahoma and Texas. The organization's members include a heart hospital, outpatient care facilities, skilled nursing services providers, long-term residential care facilities, stand-alone clinics and over 4,000 licensed beds in 18 acute care hospitals. It runs Mercy Health Plans, an HMO and third-party administrator in communities served by Mercy. The group also operates an active advocacy program for issues of social justice, especially in the field of health care, providing participants with updates on issues of concern and the means of contacting elected officials. Mercy offers a variety of free or inexpensive classes at its hospitals, including a healing-through-the-arts program, babysitter skills, massage classes, infant care and CPR/first aid classes, as well as substance abuse and terminal illness support groups. It is sponsored by the Sisters of Mercy-St. Louis Regional Community. With outreach programs in Louisiana, Texas, Mississippi and Belize, Mercy allocates money for subsidized care, community outreach ministries and charity care. It operates Mercy Ministries of Laredo, an outpatient program that provides culturally sensitive services from 14 sites in the Laredo, Texas, area. Services include women's and children's health, health education, a diabetes center, a domestic violence shelter, and medication assistance and nutritional assistance programs. In April 2008, the company broke ground on a new data center in Washington, Missouri, scheduled to open in 2010.

Mercy offers education assistance for certified nurse assistants to obtain full nursing degrees.

FINANCIALS: Sales and profits are in thousands of dollars—add 000 to get the full amount. 2007 Note: Financial information for 2007 was not available for all companies at press time.

2007 Sales: $3,653,898	2007 Profits: $67,667	**U.S. Stock Ticker: Nonprofit**
2006 Sales: $3,574,416	2006 Profits: $45,708	**Int'l Ticker:** Int'l Exchange:
2005 Sales: $3,246,696	2005 Profits: $55,460	Employees: 29,500
2004 Sales: $3,012,669	2004 Profits: $97,731	Fiscal Year Ends: 6/30
2003 Sales: $2,721,900	2003 Profits: $	Parent Company:

SALARIES/BENEFITS:

Pension Plan:	ESOP Stock Plan:	Profit Sharing:	Top Exec. Salary: $	Bonus: $
Savings Plan:	Stock Purch. Plan:		Second Exec. Salary: $	Bonus: $

OTHER THOUGHTS:

Apparent Women Officers or Directors: 4
Hot Spot for Advancement for Women/Minorities: Y

LOCATIONS: ("Y" = Yes)

West:	Southwest:	Midwest:	Southeast:	Northeast:	International:
	Y	Y	Y		Y

Note: Financial information, benefits and other data can change quickly and may vary from those stated here.

SMITH INTERNATIONAL INC

www.smith.com

Industry Group Code: 213111 Ranks within this company's industry group: Sales: 4   Profits: 10

Management:		Sales/Marketing:		Liberal Arts:		Information Systems:		Professionals:		Technical/Scientific:	
Mgmt. Trainees:	Y	Mktg. Professionals:	Y	Gen. Writing/Editing:		Info. Management:	Y	Finance/Accounting:	Y	Engineers, Elec.:	Y
Experienced Mgmt.:	Y	Retail Sales:		Technical Writing:		Software Dev.:		Law:	Y	Engineers, Other:	Y
Int'l Business:	Y	Commercial/Industrial:	Y	Graphic Arts/Photog.:		Hardware Dev.:		HR/Other:	Y	Health/Lab:	
MBA Graduates:	Y	Sales Trainees:		Music:		Systems Integration:		Training:	Y	Scientists/Research:	
		Advertising Pros.:		Broadcasting:		Consulting/Other:		Health Care:		Petroleum/Chemicals:	Y
				Other:				Consulting:		Math/Other:	

TYPES OF BUSINESS:

Oil & Gas Drilling Support Services
Waste Management Services
Drilling Equipment
Supply Chain Services

BRANDS/DIVISIONS/AFFILIATES:

M-I SWACO
Smith Technologies
Smith Services
Wilson
Smith Borehole Enlargement
Integra Group
W-H Energy Services, Inc.

CONTACTS: *Note: Officers with more than one job title may be intentionally listed here more than once.*

Douglas L. Rock, CEO
Douglas L. Rock, COO
Douglas L. Rock, Pres.
Margaret K. Dorman, CFO/Sr. VP/Treas.
Malcolm W. Anderson, Sr. VP-Human Resources
Richard E. Chandler, Jr., General Counsel/Sr. VP/Corp. Sec.
Peter J. Pintar, VP-Corp. Strategy & Bus. Dev.
Geraldine Wilde, VP-Taxes/Asst. Treas.
Bryan L. Dudman, Exec. VP/Pres., Smith Drilling & Evaluation
Donald McKenzie, CEO/Pres., M-I SWACO
John J. Kennedy, Pres./CEO-Wilson
Michael D. Pearce, Exec. VP/Pres., Smith Technologies
Douglas L. Rock, Chmn.

Phone: 281-443-3370	Fax: 281-233-5199
Toll-Free: 800-877-6484	
Address: P.O. Box 60068, Houston, TX 77205-0068 US	

GROWTH PLANS/SPECIAL FEATURES:

Smith International, Inc. is a leading worldwide supplier of premium products and services to the oil and gas exploration and production industry. The company operates through two segments: oilfield and distribution. The company's oil field products and services segment consists of M-I SWACO, Smith Technologies and Smith Services. M-I SWACO, a 60% owned joint-venture, provides drilling and completion fluid systems, solids-control and separation equipment, engineering and technical services, waste management and oil field production chemicals. Key products include the MUD D-GASSER and SUPER CHOKE pressure controllers. Smith Technologies designs, manufactures and sells three-cone and diamond drill bits, turbines and borehole enlargement tools. Smith Services manufactures and markets products and services for drilling, workover, well completion and well re-entry operations. It sells and rents impact drilling tools such as Hydra-Jar and Accelerator, as well as selling drill collars, subs, stabilizers, kellys and the Hevi-Wate DrillPipe. Smith Services also provides complete fishing, remedial and thru-tubing services. Smith International's distribution segment consists of the Wilson supply chain management company. The company markets pipe, valves and fittings as well as mill, safety and other maintenance products to energy and industrial markets. In February 2007, Smith Services and Smith Technologies combined both company's wellbore enlargement products, including Smith Services' wellbore enlargement technologies and drilling products from Smith Technologies, into a single operating group that will be called Smith Borehole Enlargement. In March 2008, Smith agreed to form a 50/50 joint venture with Integra Group to supply technologically-advanced downhole oilfield service and engineering solutions to Russia and other countries. In June 2008, the company announced that it had agreed to acquire W-H Energy Services, Inc., an oilfield service company that offers directional drilling services.

Smith International offers its employees educational assistance, scholarships for dependents, an employee assistance program and in-house training programs.

FINANCIALS: Sales and profits are in thousands of dollars—add 000 to get the full amount. 2007 Note: Financial information for 2007 was not available for all companies at press time.

2007 Sales: $8,764,330	2007 Profits: $647,051	**U.S. Stock Ticker: SII**
2006 Sales: $7,333,559	2006 Profits: $502,006	**Int'l Ticker:** Int'l Exchange:
2005 Sales: $5,579,003	2005 Profits: $302,305	Employees: 17,377
2004 Sales: $4,419,015	2004 Profits: $182,451	Fiscal Year Ends: 12/31
2003 Sales: $3,594,828	2003 Profits: $123,480	Parent Company:

SALARIES/BENEFITS:

Pension Plan:	ESOP Stock Plan:	Profit Sharing:	Top Exec. Salary: $1,100,000	Bonus: $2,200,000
Savings Plan: Y	Stock Purch. Plan:		Second Exec. Salary: $525,000	Bonus: $840,000

OTHER THOUGHTS:

Apparent Women Officers or Directors: 2
Hot Spot for Advancement for Women/Minorities:

LOCATIONS: ("Y" = Yes)

West:	Southwest:	Midwest:	Southeast:	Northeast:	International:
Y	Y	Y	Y	Y	Y

SMITHFIELD FOODS INC
www.smithfieldfoods.com

Industry Group Code: 112000 Ranks within this company's industry group: Sales: Profits:

Management:		Sales/Marketing:		Liberal Arts:	Information Systems:		Professionals:		Technical/Scientific:	
Mgmt. Trainees:	Y	Mktg. Professionals:	Y	Gen. Writing/Editing:	Info. Management:	Y	Finance/Accounting:	Y	Engineers, Elec.:	
Experienced Mgmt.:	Y	Retail Sales:		Technical Writing:	Software Dev.:		Law:	Y	Engineers, Other:	
Int'l Business:	Y	Commercial/Industrial:	Y	Graphic Arts/Photog.:	Hardware Dev.:		HR/Other:	Y	Health/Lab:	
MBA Graduates:	Y	Sales Trainees:		Music:	Systems Integration:		Training:	Y	Scientists/Research:	
		Advertising Pros.:	Y	Broadcasting:	Consulting/Other:		Health Care:		Petroleum/Chemicals:	
				Other:			Consulting:		Math/Other:	

TYPES OF BUSINESS:
Meat Processing, Pork
Hog Production
Beef Production
Turkey Production and Processing

BRANDS/DIVISIONS/AFFILIATES:
Premium Standard Firms Inc
Smithfield Beef Group
Butterball LLC

CONTACTS: Note: Officers with more than one job title may be intentionally listed here more than once.
C. Larry Pope, CEO
C. Larry Pope, Pres.
Carey J. Dubois, CFO/VP
James D. Schloss, VP-Mktg. & Sales
Mansour T. Zadeh, CIO
Michael H. Cole, Chief Legal Officer/VP/Sec.
Henry L. Morris, VP-Oper.
Jerry Hostetter, VP-Corp. Comm.
Jerry Hostetter, VP-Investor Rel.
Kenneth M. Sullivan, Chief Acct. Officer/VP
Bart Ellis, VP-Oper. Analysis
Dhamu Thamodaran, VP-Price-Risk Mgmt.
Jeffrey A. Deel, Controller/VP
Joseph W. Luter, III, Chmn.
Jeffrey M. Luckman, VP-Livestock Procurement

Phone: 757-365-3000	Fax: 757-365-3017
Toll-Free: 888-366-6767	
Address: 200 Commerce St., Smithfield, VA 23430 US	

GROWTH PLANS/SPECIAL FEATURES:
Smithfield Foods, Inc. is a hog producer and pork and beef processor. It operates in six segments: pork, beef, international, hog production, other and corporate. The pork segment produces a wide variety of fresh pork and packaged meats products in the U.S. and markets them nationwide and to numerous foreign markets, including Japan, Mexico, Canada and Australia. The division currently operates over 40 processing plants. The beef segment is composed mainly of two U.S. beef processing subsidiaries, the cattle feeding operations and interests in cattle feeding. The division produces mainly boxed beef and ground beef (both chub and case-ready) and markets these products in large portions in the U.S. The international segment includes the company's international meat processing operations that produce a wide variety of fresh and packaged meats products. The firm has interests and controlling interests in Western Europe, Mexico, Romania, Poland and China. The hog producing segment operates numerous hog production facilities with roughly 888,000 sows producing about 13.9 million market hogs annually. In addition, through its joint ventures, the division has about 114,000 sows producing around 1.5 million market hogs annually. The segment also owns certain genetic lines of specialized breeding stock that are marketed using the name Smithfield Premium Genetics. The other segment is comprised of the turnkey production and hatchery operations; and the 40% interests in Butterball, LLC. The corporate segment is comprised of firm operations not related to the other segments. In May 2007, Smithfield Foods acquired Premium Standard Farms, Inc., a leading pork producer, for $800 million, including the assumption of $125 million in debt.

The company offers its employees medical, vision and dental insurance; life and disability insurance; a 401(k) plan; a retirement plan; and education assistance.

FINANCIALS: Sales and profits are in thousands of dollars—add 000 to get the full amount. 2007 Note: Financial information for 2007 was not available for all companies at press time.

2007 Sales: $11,911,100	2007 Profits: $166,800	U.S. Stock Ticker: SFD
2006 Sales: $11,403,600	2006 Profits: $172,700	Int'l Ticker: Int'l Exchange:
2005 Sales: $11,248,400	2005 Profits: $296,200	Employees: 53,100
2004 Sales: $9,178,200	2004 Profits: $227,100	Fiscal Year Ends: 4/30
2003 Sales: $7,904,500	2003 Profits: $26,300	Parent Company:

SALARIES/BENEFITS:
Pension Plan: Y	ESOP Stock Plan:	Profit Sharing:	Top Exec. Salary: $992,667	Bonus: $2,750,000
Savings Plan: Y	Stock Purch. Plan:		Second Exec. Salary: $766,667	Bonus: $2,383,263

OTHER THOUGHTS:
Apparent Women Officers or Directors: 1
Hot Spot for Advancement for Women/Minorities:

LOCATIONS: ("Y" = Yes)
West:	Southwest:	Midwest:	Southeast:	Northeast:	International:
	Y	Y	Y	Y	Y

Note: Financial information, benefits and other data can change quickly and may vary from those stated here.

SOUTHERN COMPANY (THE)   www.southerncompany.com

Industry Group Code: 221000A   Ranks within this company's industry group: Sales: 2   Profits: 1

Management:		Sales/Marketing:		Liberal Arts:		Information Systems:		Professionals:		Technical/Scientific:	
Mgmt. Trainees:	Y	Mktg. Professionals:	Y	Gen. Writing/Editing:	Y	Info. Management:	Y	Finance/Accounting:	Y	Engineers, Elec.:	Y
Experienced Mgmt.:	Y	Retail Sales:		Technical Writing:	Y	Software Dev.:	Y	Law:	Y	Engineers, Other:	Y
Int'l Business:		Commercial/Industrial:	Y	Graphic Arts/Photog.:	Y	Hardware Dev.:		HR/Other:	Y	Health/Lab:	
MBA Graduates:	Y	Sales Trainees:		Music:		Systems Integration:		Training:	Y	Scientists/Research:	
		Advertising Pros.:	Y	Broadcasting:		Consulting/Other:		Health Care:		Petroleum/Chemicals:	
				Other:				Consulting:		Math/Other:	

TYPES OF BUSINESS:

Utilities-Electricity & Natural Gas
Wireless Communications Services
Fiber Optic Solutions
Nuclear Power Operating Services
Consulting Services

BRANDS/DIVISIONS/AFFILIATES:

Alabama Power Company
Georgia Power Company
Mississippi Power Company
Gulf Power Company
Southern Power
SEGCO
Southern Nuclear
SouthernLINC Wireless

CONTACTS: *Note: Officers with more than one job title may be intentionally listed here more than once.*

David M. Ratcliffe, CEO
Thomas A. Fanning, COO/Exec. VP
David M. Ratcliffe, Pres.
W. Paul Bowers, CFO/Exec. VP
Becky Blalock, CIO/Sr. VP
G. Edison Holland, Jr., General Counsel/Exec. VP/Corp. Sec.
Kimberly S. Greene, Sr. VP-Finance
J. Barnie Beasley Jr., Chmn./CEO/Pres., Southern Nuclear
Michael D. Garrett, Exec. VP/CEO/Pres., Georgia Power
C. Alan Martin, Exec. VP/CEO/Pres., Alabama Power
Susan N. Story, CEO/Pres., Gulf Power
David M. Ratcliffe, Chmn.

Phone: 404-506-5000	Fax: 404-506-0455
Toll-Free:	
Address: 30 Ivan Allen Jr. Blvd. N.W., Atlanta, GA 30308 US	

GROWTH PLANS/SPECIAL FEATURES:

The Southern Company, through its subsidiaries, is a producer and distributor of electricity in the U.S. Its four main subsidiaries (Alabama Power Company, Georgia Power Company, Mississippi Power Company and Gulf Power Company) have a combined service territory of 120,000 square miles. It also owns Southern Power, which constructs, acquires and manages power generation assets as well as selling electricity wholesale. Southern Power currently owns almost 5,400 megawatts of generating capacity, through a total of six power plants, and serves 75 utilities, electric cooperatives and municipalities across six states. Alabama Power and Georgia Power each own 50% of SEGCO, which operates a power generation plant and 230,000 miles of transmission lines in Alabama, supplying electricity to both Alabama and Georgia. Combined, the company's utility subsidiaries have a generating capacity of nearly 42,000 megawatts and serve more than 4.3 million residential, commercial and industrial electricity customers in the southeastern U.S. through approximately 27,000 miles of transmission lines. The firm also owns Southern Nuclear, which operates the company's three nuclear power plants; SouthernLINC Wireless, which provides communications services to approximately 300,000 subscribers; and Southern Telecom, which is a wholesaler of fiber optics.

The Southern Company offers its employees tuition reimbursement, credit union membership, a U.S. savings bond program, financial planning services, an employee assistance program, flexible spending accounts and medical, prescription, business travel, disability and life insurance.

FINANCIALS: Sales and profits are in thousands of dollars—add 000 to get the full amount. 2007 Note: Financial information for 2007 was not available for all companies at press time.

2007 Sales: $15,353,000	2007 Profits: $1,734,000	U.S. Stock Ticker: SO
2006 Sales: $14,356,000	2006 Profits: $1,573,000	Int'l Ticker: Int'l Exchange:
2005 Sales: $13,554,000	2005 Profits: $1,591,000	Employees: 26,091
2004 Sales: $11,729,000	2004 Profits: $1,532,000	Fiscal Year Ends: 12/31
2003 Sales: $11,018,000	2003 Profits: $1,474,000	Parent Company:

SALARIES/BENEFITS:

Pension Plan: Y	ESOP Stock Plan:	Profit Sharing:	Top Exec. Salary: $1,028,471	Bonus: $2,563,680
Savings Plan: Y	Stock Purch. Plan:		Second Exec. Salary: $609,407	Bonus: $900,736

OTHER THOUGHTS:

Apparent Women Officers or Directors: 2
Hot Spot for Advancement for Women/Minorities: Y

LOCATIONS: ("Y" = Yes)

West:	Southwest:	Midwest:	Southeast:	Northeast:	International:
			Y		

SOUTHWEST AIRLINES CO

www.southwest.com

Industry Group Code: 481000 Ranks within this company's industry group: Sales: 3 Profits: 1

Management:		Sales/Marketing:		Liberal Arts:		Information Systems:		Professionals:		Technical/Scientific:	
Mgmt. Trainees:		Mktg. Professionals:	Y	Gen. Writing/Editing:	Y	Info. Management:	Y	Finance/Accounting:	Y	Engineers, Elec.:	Y
Experienced Mgmt.:	Y	Retail Sales:		Technical Writing:	Y	Software Dev.:	Y	Law:	Y	Engineers, Other:	
Int'l Business:		Commercial/Industrial:		Graphic Arts/Photog.:	Y	Hardware Dev.:		HR/Other:	Y	Health/Lab:	
MBA Graduates:	Y	Sales Trainees:		Music:		Systems Integration:		Training:	Y	Scientists/Research:	Y
		Advertising Pros.:	Y	Broadcasting:		Consulting/Other:		Health Care:	Y	Petroleum/Chemicals:	
				Other:				Consulting:		Math/Other:	

TYPES OF BUSINESS:
Airline-Domestic
Air Freight

BRANDS/DIVISIONS/AFFILIATES:

CONTACTS: *Note: Officers with more than one job title may be intentionally listed here more than once.*
Gary Kelly, CEO
Michael G. Van De Ven, COO/Exec. VP
Gary Kelly, Pres.
Laura H. Wright, CFO
Kevin M. Krone, VP- Mktg., Sales & Dist.
Jeff Lamb, Sr. VP-People
Darren Dayley, VP-Tech.
Jim Sokol, VP-Eng. & Maintenance
Jeff Lamb, Chief Admin. Officer
Deborah Ackerman, General Counsel/VP
Gregory N. Crum, VP-Oper.
Robert E. Jordan, Exec. VP-Strategy, Procurement & Tech.
Ginger C. Hardage, Sr. VP-Corp. Comm.
Laura H. Wright, Sr. VP-Finance
Ellen Torbert, VP-Reservations
Ron Ricks, Exec. VP-Corp. Svcs./Sec.
Barry Brown, VP-Safety & Security
Linda B. Rutherford, VP-Public Relations & Community Affairs
Gary Kelly, Chmn.
Ray Sears, VP-Purchasing

Phone: 214-792-4000	Fax: 214-792-5015
Toll-Free: 800-435-9792	
Address: 2702 Love Field Dr., Dallas, TX 75235 US	

GROWTH PLANS/SPECIAL FEATURES:
Southwest Airlines Co. is a low-fare domestic airline that provides short haul, high-frequency airline services. Southwest is one of the four largest carriers in the U.S. based on number of domestic passengers. The firm operates 520 Boeing 737 planes, serving 64 cities in 32 states throughout the U.S. The firm serves 411 nonstop city pairs, and operates over 3,200 flights daily. Its busiest routes include those to Las Vegas, Phoenix, Baltimore, Houston, Chicago and Dallas. Using only one type of airplane simplifies the company's scheduling, maintenance, flight operations and training activities. Southwest also utilizes a very simple fare structure that features unlimited, low-cost coach fares. The firm employs a point-to-point route system which provides for more direct nonstop flights that minimize connections, delays and total trip time. Southwest primarily flies to downtown airports. The airline flies its planes an average of seven flights totaling 12 hours daily. The company made a profit for 30 straight years. In 2007, the firm made a number of new additions to its routes, including several new nonstop flights. Additionally, it recommenced service to San Francisco International Airport. By the first half of 2008, Southwest will implement an upgraded gate design at each of its 62 airports to complement its numerical-style boarding procedure introduced in November 2007. The upgrades will include television monitors, family-friendly seating areas and kid-friendly programming.

Southwest's employees and family members have flight discounts.

FINANCIALS: Sales and profits are in thousands of dollars—add 000 to get the full amount. 2007 Note: Financial information for 2007 was not available for all companies at press time.

2007 Sales: $9,860,000	2007 Profits: $645,000	U.S. Stock Ticker: LUV
2006 Sales: $9,086,000	2006 Profits: $499,000	Int'l Ticker: Int'l Exchange:
2005 Sales: $7,584,000	2005 Profits: $484,000	Employees: 41,000
2004 Sales: $6,530,000	2004 Profits: $215,000	Fiscal Year Ends: 12/31
2003 Sales: $5,937,000	2003 Profits: $442,000	Parent Company:

SALARIES/BENEFITS:
Pension Plan:	ESOP Stock Plan:	Profit Sharing: Y	Top Exec. Salary: $450,000	Bonus: $332,000
Savings Plan: Y	Stock Purch. Plan: Y		Second Exec. Salary: $362,487	Bonus: $483,000

OTHER THOUGHTS:
Apparent Women Officers or Directors: 11
Hot Spot for Advancement for Women/Minorities: Y

LOCATIONS: ("Y" = Yes)
West:	Southwest:	Midwest:	Southeast:	Northeast:	International:
	Y	Y		Y	

SRA INTERNATIONAL INC

www.sra.com

Industry Group Code: 541512 Ranks within this company's industry group: Sales: 8 Profits: 8

Management:		Sales/Marketing:		Liberal Arts:		Information Systems:		Professionals:		Technical/Scientific:	
Mgmt. Trainees:		Mktg. Professionals:	Y	Gen. Writing/Editing:	Y	Info. Management:	Y	Finance/Accounting:	Y	Engineers, Elec.:	
Experienced Mgmt.:	Y	Retail Sales:		Technical Writing:	Y	Software Dev.:	Y	Law:	Y	Engineers, Other:	
Int'l Business:		Commercial/Industrial:	Y	Graphic Arts/Photog.:		Hardware Dev.:		HR/Other:	Y	Health/Lab:	
MBA Graduates:	Y	Sales Trainees:		Music:		Systems Integration:	Y	Training:	Y	Scientists/Research:	
		Advertising Pros.:	Y	Broadcasting:		Consulting/Other:	Y	Health Care:		Petroleum/Chemicals:	
				Other:	Y			Consulting:	Y	Math/Other:	Y

TYPES OF BUSINESS:

Technology Consulting
Strategic Consulting
Systems Design
Systems Integration
Managed Services
Outsourcing

BRANDS/DIVISIONS/AFFILIATES:

RABA Technologies, LLC
NetOwl
ORIONMagic

CONTACTS: Note: Officers with more than one job title may be intentionally listed here more than once.

Stanton D. Sloane, CEO
Stanton D. Sloane, Pres.
Stephen C. Hughes, CFO
Michael M. Fox, Sr. VP-Mktg. & Sales
Mary E. Good, Sr. VP-Human Resources
Scott W. Bennett, Dir.-R&D/VP/Chief Technologist
Frank Kist, CIO/VP
Kevin W. Layton, Sr. VP-Tech. Oper.
Anne M. Donohue, Chief Legal Officer
Stephen C. Hughes, Exec. VP-Oper.
Barry S. Landew, Exec. VP-Strategic Dev.
Sheila Blackwell, VP-Comm. & Public Affairs
David Keefer, VP-Investor Rel.
Timothy J. Atkin, Sr. VP-Global Health Sector
Patrick Burke, Sr. VP-National Security Sector
Max N. Hall, Sr. VP-Civil Sector
Melissa A. Burgum, Controller
Ernst Volgenau, Chmn.

Phone: 703-803-1500	Fax: 703-803-1509
Toll-Free:	
Address: 4300 Fair Lakes Ct., Fairfax, VA 22033 US	

GROWTH PLANS/SPECIAL FEATURES:

SRA International, Inc. provides technology and strategic consulting services and solutions to a broad range of clients involved in national security; civil government; and health care and public health. Its largest market is national security, in which the firm services the Department of Defense, the National Guard, the Department of Homeland Security, the CIA and FBI and various other federal agencies with homeland security missions. The company's services across all sectors include strategic consulting; systems design, development and integration; outsourcing and managed services; contingency and disaster response planning; information assurance; business intelligence; privacy protection; enterprise architecture; infrastructure management; and wireless integration. Currently, SRA serves over 275 government clients on over 900 active engagements. Business from the U.S. federal government made up over 59% of SRA's total revenue in 2006; civil government made up 32%; health care and public health 8%; and commercial enterprises made up a scant .6%. The firm uses proprietary NetOwl text mining software tools and ORIONMagic knowledge management software to improve a client's method of managing, exploiting and analyzing large amounts of data.

FINANCIALS: Sales and profits are in thousands of dollars—add 000 to get the full amount. 2007 Note: Financial information for 2007 was not available for all companies at press time.

2007 Sales: $1,268,872	2007 Profits: $63,430	U.S. Stock Ticker: SRX
2006 Sales: $1,179,267	2006 Profits: $62,520	Int'l Ticker: Int'l Exchange:
2005 Sales: $881,770	2005 Profits: $57,723	Employees: 5,200
2004 Sales: $615,802	2004 Profits: $38,937	Fiscal Year Ends: 6/30
2003 Sales: $450,375	2003 Profits: $29,660	Parent Company:

SALARIES/BENEFITS:

Pension Plan:	ESOP Stock Plan:	Profit Sharing:	Top Exec. Salary: $435,000	Bonus: $354,123
Savings Plan:	Stock Purch. Plan:		Second Exec. Salary: $290,000	Bonus: $234,080

OTHER THOUGHTS:

Apparent Women Officers or Directors: 14
Hot Spot for Advancement for Women/Minorities: Y

LOCATIONS: ("Y" = Yes)

West:	Southwest:	Midwest:	Southeast:	Northeast:	International:
Y	Y	Y	Y	Y	

ST JUDE MEDICAL INC
www.sjm.com

Industry Group Code: 339113 Ranks within this company's industry group: Sales: 7 Profits: 6

Management:		Sales/Marketing:		Liberal Arts:		Information Systems:		Professionals:		Technical/Scientific:	
Mgmt. Trainees:	Y	Mktg. Professionals:	Y	Gen. Writing/Editing:	Y	Info. Management:	Y	Finance/Accounting:	Y	Engineers, Elec.:	Y
Experienced Mgmt.:	Y	Retail Sales:		Technical Writing:	Y	Software Dev.:	Y	Law:	Y	Engineers, Other:	Y
Int'l Business:	Y	Commercial/Industrial:	Y	Graphic Arts/Photog.:	Y	Hardware Dev.:	Y	HR/Other:	Y	Health/Lab:	Y
MBA Graduates:	Y	Sales Trainees:	Y	Music:		Systems Integration:		Training:	Y	Scientists/Research:	Y
		Advertising Pros.:	Y	Broadcasting:		Consulting/Other:		Health Care:	Y	Petroleum/Chemicals:	
				Other:				Consulting:		Math/Other:	Y

TYPES OF BUSINESS:
Cardiovascular Medical Devices
Cardiac Rhythm Management Devices
Cardiac Surgery Devices
Cardiology Devices
Atrial Fibrillation Devices

BRANDS/DIVISIONS/AFFILIATES:
Atlas II ICD
Atlas II HF CRT-D
Eon
TigerWire
Reflexion Spiral X
EP MedSystems, Inc.

CONTACTS: *Note: Officers with more than one job title may be intentionally listed here more than once.*
Daniel J. Starks, CEO
Daniel J. Starks, Pres.
John C. Heinmiller, CFO/Exec. VP
Paul Bae, VP-Human Resources
Thomas R. Northenscold, CIO/VP-IT
Thomas R. Northenscold, VP-Admin.
Pamela S. Krop, General Counsel/VP/Sec.
Angela D. Craig, VP-Corp. Rel.
Mark D. Carlson, Chief Medical Officer/Sr. VP-Clinical Affairs
Christopher G. Chavez, Pres., Neuromodulation Division
Eric S. Fain, Pres., Cardiac Rhythm Mgmt. Division
Frank J. Callaghan, Pres., Cardiovascular Division
Daniel J. Starks, Chmn.
Denis M. Gestin, Pres., Int'l Div.

Phone: 651-483-2000 **Fax:** 651-482-8318
Toll-Free: 800-328-9634
Address: 1 Lillehei Plaza, St. Paul, MN 55117 US

GROWTH PLANS/SPECIAL FEATURES:

St. Jude Medical, Inc. develops, manufactures and distributes cardiovascular medical devices for global cardiac rhythm management, cardiac surgery, cardiology and atrial fibrillation therapy and implantable neuromodulation devices for the management of chronic pain. The company operates in four segments: cardiac rhythm management, whose products include tachycardia implantable cardioverter defibrillator systems and bradycardia pacemaker systems; cardiovascular, whose products include vascular closure devices, heart valves and valve repair products; advanced neuromodulation systems, whose products include neurostimulation devices; and atrial fibrillation, whose products include electrophysiology introducers and catheters, advanced cardiac mapping and navigation systems and ablation systems. St. Jude's Neuromodulation Division focuses its efforts on the related therapy areas. Neuromodulation is the delivery of very small, precise doses of electric current or drugs directly to nerve sites and is aimed at treating patients suffering from chronic pain or other disabling nervous system disorders. The firm markets and sells its products through a direct sales force and independent distributors. The principal geographic markets for its products are the U.S., Europe, Japan and the Asia-Pacific region. St. Jude also sells products in Canada and Latin America. The cardiac rhythm management products generated 62.7% of revenue in 2007. In recent news, St. Jude received clearance in the U.S., Canada and Europe on a large variety of products, including the Eon neurostimulator line to treat chronic pain. In 2008, the firm launched its TigerWire steerable guidewire and Reflexion Spiral X variable radius mapping catheter in the U.S. In July 2008, the company acquired EP MedSystems, Inc., which develops, manufactures and markets products for cardiac rhythm management.

The company offers its employees medical, dental and vision insurance; flexible spending accounts; access to a credit union; disability insurance; life insurance; a physical fitness program; a matching gift program; and tuition reimbursement.

FINANCIALS: Sales and profits are in thousands of dollars—add 000 to get the full amount. 2007 Note: Financial information for 2007 was not available for all companies at press time.

2007 Sales: $3,779,277	2007 Profits: $559,038	**U.S. Stock Ticker: STJ**
2006 Sales: $3,302,447	2006 Profits: $548,251	**Int'l Ticker:** Int'l Exchange:
2005 Sales: $2,915,280	2005 Profits: $393,490	Employees: 11,000
2004 Sales: $2,294,173	2004 Profits: $409,934	Fiscal Year Ends: 12/31
2003 Sales: $1,932,500	2003 Profits: $339,400	Parent Company:

SALARIES/BENEFITS:
Pension Plan:	ESOP Stock Plan:	Profit Sharing: Y	Top Exec. Salary: $975,000	Bonus: $1,009,125
Savings Plan: Y	Stock Purch. Plan: Y		Second Exec. Salary: $580,000	Bonus: $500,250

OTHER THOUGHTS:
Apparent Women Officers or Directors: 5
Hot Spot for Advancement for Women/Minorities: Y

LOCATIONS: ("Y" = Yes)
West:	Southwest:	Midwest:	Southeast:	Northeast:	International:
Y	Y	Y	Y	Y	Y

STAPLES INC

www.staples.com

Industry Group Code: 453210 **Ranks within this company's industry group:** Sales: 1 Profits: 1

Management:		Sales/Marketing:		Liberal Arts:		Information Systems:		Professionals:		Technical/Scientific:	
Mgmt. Trainees:	Y	Mktg. Professionals:	Y	Gen. Writing/Editing:	Y	Info. Management:	Y	Finance/Accounting:	Y	Engineers, Elec.:	
Experienced Mgmt.:	Y	Retail Sales:	Y	Technical Writing:		Software Dev.:	Y	Law:	Y	Engineers, Other:	
Int'l Business:	Y	Commercial/Industrial:	Y	Graphic Arts/Photog.:	Y	Hardware Dev.:		HR/Other:	Y	Health/Lab:	
MBA Graduates:	Y	Sales Trainees:	Y	Music:		Systems Integration:		Training:	Y	Scientists/Research:	
		Advertising Pros.:	Y	Broadcasting:		Consulting/Other:		Health Care:		Petroleum/Chemicals:	
				Other:	Y			Consulting:		Math/Other:	

TYPES OF BUSINESS:

Office Supplies, Retail
Contract Stationery Services
Online & Catalog Sales
Catalogs
Office Furniture

BRANDS/DIVISIONS/AFFILIATES:

Quill Corp.
Staples Business Delivery
Staples National Advantage
Staples Business Advantage

CONTACTS: *Note: Officers with more than one job title may be intentionally listed here more than once.*

Ronald L. Sargent, CEO
Michael Miles, COO
Michael Miles, Pres.
John J. Mahoney, CFO
Jevin Eagle, Head-Merch.
Kristin A. Campbell, General Counsel/Sr. VP/Sec.
Christine T. Komola, Corp. Controller/Sr. VP
Joseph G. Doody, Pres., North American Delivery
Demos Parneros, Pres., US Retail
Michael Patriarca, Sr. VP-Quill
Ronald L. Sargent, Chmn.

Phone: 508-253-5000	Fax: 508-253-8989
Toll-Free: 800-378-2753	
Address: 500 Staples Dr., Framingham, MA 01702 US	

GROWTH PLANS/SPECIAL FEATURES:

The firm markets products through three sales channels designed to be convenient to the needs of its customers, retail stores, catalog, and internet. The North American retail segment, consisting of 1,738 stores throughout the United States and Canada at the end of fiscal 2007, generates the majority of the firm's sales and profits. The North American retail stores are located in 47 states, the District of Columbia, 10 Canadian provinces and 2 Canadian territories in both major metropolitan markets and smaller markets. A typical Staples superstore carries over 1,000 Staples-brand and 7,000 brand-name products, including ink and toner; paper; small business machines; computers; and peripherals, as well as a copy center and a business technology center. The North American delivery segment is, in turn, comprised of three business units: Staples business delivery, Quill Corp. and the contract business. The Staples business delivery segment operations consist of the combined direct mail catalog and Internet sales both in the U.S. and Canada, and it is tailored primarily to the needs of small and medium-sized businesses. Quill Corp., a direct mail catalog and Internet distributor, serves the business products needs of more than 1 million small- medium-sized businesses in the U.S. Staples National Advantage and Staples Business Advantage, the firm's contract stationery operations, focus primarily on serving medium to large businesses. The international operations division handles all retail stores, catalog and Internet businesses operating in 19 countries in Europe, South America and Asia. In July 2008, Staples and its wholly owned subsidiary, Staples Acquisition B.V. completed the acquisition of Corporate Express N.V. In August 2008, the firm had a 58.79% interest in Corporate Express Australia Limited.

The company offers its employees medical, dental and vision insurance; life and disability insurance; a 401(k) plan; an employee stock purchase plan; domestic partner benefits; homeowners, auto, legal and pet insurance; tuition reimbursement; shopping discounts; and training opportunities at Staples University.

FINANCIALS: Sales and profits are in thousands of dollars—add 000 to get the full amount. 2007 Note: Financial information for 2007 was not available for all companies at press time.

2007 Sales: $18,160,789	2007 Profits: $973,677	**U.S. Stock Ticker:** SPLS
2006 Sales: $16,078,852	2006 Profits: $834,409	**Int'l Ticker:** Int'l Exchange:
2005 Sales: $14,448,378	2005 Profits: $708,388	Employees: 73,646
2004 Sales: $13,181,222	2004 Profits: $490,211	Fiscal Year Ends: 1/31
2003 Sales: $11,596,100	2003 Profits: $446,100	Parent Company:

SALARIES/BENEFITS:

Pension Plan:	ESOP Stock Plan:	Profit Sharing:	Top Exec. Salary: $1,070,192	Bonus: $1,523,018
Savings Plan: Y	Stock Purch. Plan: Y		Second Exec. Salary: $650,529	Bonus: $554,596

OTHER THOUGHTS:

Apparent Women Officers or Directors: 3
Hot Spot for Advancement for Women/Minorities: Y

LOCATIONS: ("Y" = Yes)

West:	Southwest:	Midwest:	Southeast:	Northeast:	International:
Y	Y	Y	Y	Y	Y

STARTEK INC

www.startek.com

Industry Group Code: 561300   Ranks within this company's industry group: Sales: 1   Profits: 1

Management:		Sales/Marketing:		Liberal Arts:		Information Systems:		Professionals:		Technical/Scientific:	
Mgmt. Trainees:	Y	Mktg. Professionals:	Y	Gen. Writing/Editing:		Info. Management:	Y	Finance/Accounting:	Y	Engineers, Elec.:	
Experienced Mgmt.:	Y	Retail Sales:		Technical Writing:	Y	Software Dev.:	Y	Law:	Y	Engineers, Other:	
Int'l Business:	Y	Commercial/Industrial:	Y	Graphic Arts/Photog.:	Y	Hardware Dev.:		HR/Other:	Y	Health/Lab:	
MBA Graduates:	Y	Sales Trainees:		Music:		Systems Integration:		Training:	Y	Scientists/Research:	
		Advertising Pros.:		Broadcasting:		Consulting/Other:		Health Care:		Petroleum/Chemicals:	
				Other:				Consulting:		Math/Other:	

TYPES OF BUSINESS:

Outsourcing-Supply Chain Management
Business Process Management
Telecommunications Services
Internet Domain Name Licensing

BRANDS/DIVISIONS/AFFILIATES:

StarTek Connect

CONTACTS: *Note: Officers with more than one job title may be intentionally listed here more than once.*

Larry Jones, CEO
Patrick Hayes, COO
Larry Jones, Pres.
David Durham, CFO
Mary Beth Loesch, Sr. VP-Mktg.
Susan Morse, Sr. VP-Human Resources
Doug Pontious, CIO
Michael Clayton, General Counsel/Corp. Sec.
Mary Beth Loesch, Sr. VP-Bus. Dev.
David Durham, Treas.
Michael Griffith, Sr. VP- Sales
Julie Pierce, Dir.-SEC Reporting
A. Emmet Stephenson, Jr., Chmn.

Phone: 303-262-4500	Fax: 303-388-9970
Toll-Free:	
Address: 44 Cook St., Ste. 400, Denver, CO 80206 US	

GROWTH PLANS/SPECIAL FEATURES:

Startek, Inc. provides business process management services to the communications industry through its provision management, customer care, receivables management, wireless telephone activations and high-end technical support and wireline telephone number portability services. The company provides these services through 21 operational facilities across the U.S. and Canada. The firm's business process optimization services include large scale project implementation, distributed resource planning and extended training and quality assurance, which ultimately lowers operational costs, improves quality and adds value to client companies. Current technologies of the company include data center configuration; disaster recovery; call recording and monitoring; CRM/order entry solutions; and reporting and tracking solutions. In addition, Startek offers a communications package that provides software, infrastructure and service through Telephony via TDM (Time Division Multiplexing), Telephony via VoIP (Voice Over Internet Protocol), Unified e-Mail, IVR (Interactive Voice Response), CTI (Computer Telephony Integration) and StarTek Connect, which allows end-to-end integrated, real time reporting. In 2008, the company announced plans to open a new customer care center in Jonesboro, Arkansas. The 55,000 square foot facility will provide in-bound customer care services for an existing Fortune 1000 telecom client, and at capacity, will employ more than 500 people.

The firm offers its employees life insurance, flexible vacation time, bereavement leave and military leave.

FINANCIALS: Sales and profits are in thousands of dollars—add 000 to get the full amount. 2007 Note: Financial information for 2007 was not available for all companies at press time.

2007 Sales: $245,304	2007 Profits: $-2,831	U.S. Stock Ticker: SRT
2006 Sales: $237,612	2006 Profits: $5,764	Int'l Ticker: Int'l Exchange:
2005 Sales: $216,371	2005 Profits: $12,860	Employees: 8,200
2004 Sales: $221,906	2004 Profits: $20,976	Fiscal Year Ends: 12/31
2003 Sales: $225,408	2003 Profits: $22,198	Parent Company:

SALARIES/BENEFITS:

Pension Plan:	ESOP Stock Plan:	Profit Sharing:	Top Exec. Salary: $484,996	Bonus: $
Savings Plan:	Stock Purch. Plan:		Second Exec. Salary: $443,365	Bonus: $225,000

OTHER THOUGHTS:

Apparent Women Officers or Directors: 3
Hot Spot for Advancement for Women/Minorities: Y

LOCATIONS: ("Y" = Yes)

West:	Southwest:	Midwest:	Southeast:	Northeast:	International:
Y	Y	Y	Y	Y	Y

STARWOOD HOTELS & RESORTS WORLDWIDE INC
www.starwoodhotels.com

Industry Group Code: 721110 Ranks within this company's industry group: Sales: 3 Profits: 1

Management:		Sales/Marketing:		Liberal Arts:		Information Systems:		Professionals:		Technical/Scientific:	
Mgmt. Trainees:	Y	Mktg. Professionals:	Y	Gen. Writing/Editing:	Y	Info. Management:	Y	Finance/Accounting:	Y	Engineers, Elec.:	
Experienced Mgmt.:	Y	Retail Sales:		Technical Writing:		Software Dev.:		Law:	Y	Engineers, Other:	
Int'l Business:	Y	Commercial/Industrial:	Y	Graphic Arts/Photog.:	Y	Hardware Dev.:		HR/Other:	Y	Health/Lab:	
MBA Graduates:	Y	Sales Trainees:		Music:		Systems Integration:		Training:	Y	Scientists/Research:	
		Advertising Pros.:	Y	Broadcasting:		Consulting/Other:		Health Care:		Petroleum/Chemicals:	
				Other:				Consulting:		Math/Other:	

TYPES OF BUSINESS:
Hotels & Resorts
Financial Services
Hotel Management & Franchising
Spa Services
Online Auction Web Site
Preferred Guest Club

BRANDS/DIVISIONS/AFFILIATES:
Sheraton
W
Four Points
Westin
Le Meridien
St. Regis
Luxury Collection
Aloft

CONTACTS: Note: Officers with more than one job title may be intentionally listed here more than once.
Frits van Paasschen, CEO
Frits van Paasschen, Pres.
Vasant M. Prabhu, CFO/Exec. VP
Christie Hicks, Sr. VP-Global Sales
Jeffrey M. (Jeff) Cava, Chief Human Resources Officer/Exec. VP
Phil McAveety, Chief Brand Officer
Kenneth S. Siegel, Chief Admin. Officer
Kenneth S. Siegel, General Counsel
Alan Schnaid, Controller/Sr. VP
Raymond L. Gellein, Jr., Pres., Global Dev. Group
Lynne Hicks, Sr. VP-Owner Rel. & Franchise
Helen Horsham-Bertels, Sr. VP-Global Customer Service
Osvaldo V. Librizzi, Pres., Latin America
Bruce W. Duncan, Chmn.
Roeland Vos, Pres., EMEA Division

Phone: 914-640-8100	Fax: 914-640-8310
Toll-Free:	
Address: 1111 Westchester Ave., White Plains, NY 10604 US	

GROWTH PLANS/SPECIAL FEATURES:

Starwood Hotels & Resorts Worldwide, Inc. manages the global operation of hotels and resorts, primarily in the luxury and upscale segments of the industry. It owns, leases, manages or franchises nearly 900 hotels containing about 275,000 rooms in roughly 100 countries. The company's brand names include Sheraton, Westin, St. Regis, The Luxury Collection, W, Aloft, Le Meridien, Four Points and Element. The firm's earnings are derived mainly from its hotel and leisure operations; the receipt of franchise fees; and the development, ownership and operation of vacation ownership resorts. Additionally, Starwood provides financing to customers who purchase interests in resorts. The firm's frequent guest loyalty program, Starwood Preferred Guest, boasts over 27 million members and is unique in the hotel industry for its lack of capacity controls and blackout dates. Starwood's property portfolio includes The Phoenician in Scottsdale, Arizona; the Hotel Gritti Palace in Venice, Italy; the St. Regis in Beijing, China; and the Westin Palace in Madrid, Spain. The company's growth strategy includes reducing investments in owned real estate and focusing on the management and franchise business. The firm is also incorporating signature experiences in all upscale properties with the addition of Bliss Spas, Remede Spas and gourmet restaurants. From 2008 through 2012, Starwood plans the construction of 600 new hotels, at least half of which will be in countries such as China, India and Qatar. The firm also plans to open 500 Aloft hotels in North America through 2013, which combine the hip design of the W brand with the limited service model offered by Marriott Courtyard.

The company offers its employees medical, dental and vision insurance; a 401(k) plan; life and disability insurance; an employee stock purchase plan; an employee assistance program; and domestic partner benefits.

FINANCIALS: Sales and profits are in thousands of dollars—add 000 to get the full amount. 2007 Note: Financial information for 2007 was not available for all companies at press time.

2007 Sales: $6,153,000	2007 Profits: $542,000	**U.S. Stock Ticker: HOT**
2006 Sales: $5,979,000	2006 Profits: $1,043,000	**Int'l Ticker:** Int'l Exchange:
2005 Sales: $5,977,000	2005 Profits: $422,000	Employees: 155,000
2004 Sales: $5,368,000	2004 Profits: $395,000	Fiscal Year Ends: 12/31
2003 Sales: $4,075,500	2003 Profits: $268,300	Parent Company:

SALARIES/BENEFITS:
Pension Plan:	ESOP Stock Plan:	Profit Sharing:	Top Exec. Salary: $794,657	Bonus: $1,495,053
Savings Plan: Y	Stock Purch. Plan: Y		Second Exec. Salary: $721,000	Bonus: $639,082

OTHER THOUGHTS:
Apparent Women Officers or Directors: 6
Hot Spot for Advancement for Women/Minorities: Y

LOCATIONS: ("Y" = Yes)
West:	Southwest:	Midwest:	Southeast:	Northeast:	International:
Y	Y	Y	Y	Y	Y

STERIS CORP

www.steris.com

Industry Group Code: 339113 Ranks within this company's industry group: Sales: 14 Profits: 14

Management:		Sales/Marketing:		Liberal Arts:		Information Systems:		Professionals:		Technical/Scientific:	
Mgmt. Trainees:	Y	Mktg. Professionals:	Y	Gen. Writing/Editing:		Info. Management:	Y	Finance/Accounting:	Y	Engineers, Elec.:	Y
Experienced Mgmt.:	Y	Retail Sales:		Technical Writing:	Y	Software Dev.:	Y	Law:	Y	Engineers, Other:	Y
Int'l Business:	Y	Commercial/Industrial:	Y	Graphic Arts/Photog.:	Y	Hardware Dev.:		HR/Other:	Y	Health/Lab:	
MBA Graduates:	Y	Sales Trainees:		Music:		Systems Integration:		Training:	Y	Scientists/Research:	
		Advertising Pros.:		Broadcasting:		Consulting/Other:		Health Care:	Y	Petroleum/Chemicals:	
				Other:				Consulting:		Math/Other:	

TYPES OF BUSINESS:

Healthcare Products & Related Services
Life Sciences Products
Sterilization Services

BRANDS/DIVISIONS/AFFILIATES:

STERIS Isomedix Services
STERIS SYSTEM 1
Finn-Aqua
Amsco
Reliance
Basil
Detach
Lyovac

CONTACTS: Note: Officers with more than one job title may be intentionally listed here more than once.

Walter M. Rosebrough Jr., CEO
Walter M. Rosebrough Jr., Pres.
Michael J. Tokich, CFO/Sr. VP
Peter A. Burke, CTO/Sr. VP
Gerard J. Reis, Sr. VP/Group Pres., Admin. & Gov't
Mark D. McGinley, General Counsel/Sr. VP/Sec.
Timothy L. Chapman, Sr. VP-Bus. Strategy
Stephen Norton, Dir.-Corp. Comm.
William L. Aamoth, Corp. Treas.
Timothy L. Chapman, Sr. VP/Group Pres., Healthcare
Robert E. Moss, Sr. VP/Pres., Steris Isomedix Svcs.
John N. Voyzey, VP/Gen. Mgr.-Life Sciences
John P. Wareham, Chmn.

Phone: 440-354-2600	Fax: 440-392-8972
Toll-Free: 800-548-4873	
Address: 5960 Heisley Rd., Mentor, OH 44060 US	

GROWTH PLANS/SPECIAL FEATURES:

Steris Corp. provides infection prevention and surgical products and services, focused primarily on the healthcare, pharmaceutical and research markets. The company offers capital products such as sterilizers and surgical tables; consumable products such as detergents and skin care products; and services, including equipment installation and maintenance, as well as the bulk sterilization of single-use medical devices. The firm operates in four segments: healthcare; life sciences; STERIS Isomedix Services; and corporate and other. The healthcare segment, which accounted for about 70.1% of 2008 fiscal year revenues, manufactures and sells capital equipment and accessories used in surgical and critical environments; emergency departments; gastrointestinal and sterile processing environments; and in infection control processes. This segment also provides various equipment maintenance programs and repair services to support effective operation of health care equipment. The health care segment includes products such as the company's STERIS SYSTEM 1, a complete system for sterile processing at or near the site of patient care. The life sciences segment, responsible for roughly 18.1% of 2008 revenue, provides decontamination and sterilization technologies, products and services to pharmaceutical manufacturers and research facilities. Systems and products offered include brand names such as Finn-Aqua and Amsco sterilizers; Reliance washers; Vaporized Hydrogen Peroxide (VHP) bio-decontamination systems; and consumable products for contamination prevention, surface cleaning and sterility assurance. STERIS Isomedix Services, which contributed about 11.1% of 2008 revenue, performs sterilization services on a contract basis through 21 facilities in North America, where the company sterilizes medical devices and other products in bulk prior to their delivery to the end user. The corporate and other segment houses the defense and industrial segment, after fiscal 2008 reorganizations, and contributed 0.7% of 2008 revenue. In fiscal 2008, the firm transferred Pennsylvanian manufacturing operations to Mexico; the company also plans to close two sales offices and reduce workforce.

FINANCIALS: Sales and profits are in thousands of dollars—add 000 to get the full amount. 2007 Note: Financial information for 2007 was not available for all companies at press time.

2007 Sales: $1,197,407	2007 Profits: $82,155	**U.S. Stock Ticker: STE**	
2006 Sales: $1,160,285	2006 Profits: $70,289	**Int'l Ticker:** Int'l Exchange:	
2005 Sales: $1,081,674	2005 Profits: $85,980	Employees: 5,100	
2004 Sales: $1,031,908	2004 Profits: $94,243	Fiscal Year Ends: 3/31	
2003 Sales: $972,100	2003 Profits: $79,400	Parent Company:	

SALARIES/BENEFITS:

Pension Plan:	ESOP Stock Plan:	Profit Sharing:	Top Exec. Salary: $722,843	Bonus: $443,586
Savings Plan: Y	Stock Purch. Plan:		Second Exec. Salary: $308,449	Bonus: $107,500

OTHER THOUGHTS:

Apparent Women Officers or Directors:
Hot Spot for Advancement for Women/Minorities:

LOCATIONS: ("Y" = Yes)

West:	Southwest:	Midwest:	Southeast:	Northeast:	International:
Y	Y	Y	Y	Y	Y

STRYKER CORP

www.stryker.com

Industry Group Code: 339113 Ranks within this company's industry group: Sales: 5 Profits: 4

Management:		Sales/Marketing:		Liberal Arts:		Information Systems:		Professionals:		Technical/Scientific:	
Mgmt. Trainees:	Y	Mktg. Professionals:	Y	Gen. Writing/Editing:	Y	Info. Management:	Y	Finance/Accounting:	Y	Engineers, Elec.:	Y
Experienced Mgmt.:	Y	Retail Sales:		Technical Writing:	Y	Software Dev.:	Y	Law:	Y	Engineers, Other:	Y
Int'l Business:	Y	Commercial/Industrial:	Y	Graphic Arts/Photog.:	Y	Hardware Dev.:	Y	HR/Other:	Y	Health/Lab:	Y
MBA Graduates:	Y	Sales Trainees:		Music:		Systems Integration:		Training:	Y	Scientists/Research:	Y
		Advertising Pros.:	Y	Broadcasting:		Consulting/Other:		Health Care:	Y	Petroleum/Chemicals:	
				Other:				Consulting:		Math/Other:	Y

TYPES OF BUSINESS:

Equipment-Orthopedic Implants
Powered Surgical Instruments
Endoscopic Systems
Patient Care & Handling Equipment
Outpatient Physical Therapy Services
Imaging Software

BRANDS/DIVISIONS/AFFILIATES:

Stryker Orthopaedics
Stryker Osteosynthesis
Stryker Spine
Stryker Biotech
Stryker Instruments
Stryker Endoscopy
Stryker Medical
Sightline Technologies

CONTACTS: *Note: Officers with more than one job title may be intentionally listed here more than once.*

Stephen P. MacMillan, CEO
Stephen P. MacMillan, Pres.
Dean H. Bergy, CFO/VP
Michael W. Rude, VP-Human Resources
Thomas R. Winkel, VP/Sec.
Curtis E. Hall, General Counsel/VP
Bryant S. Zanko, VP-Corp. Bus. Dev.
J. Patrick Anderson, VP-Corp. Affairs
Katherine A. Owen, VP-Investor Rel. & Strategy
Jeanne M. Blondia, Treas./VP
James E. Kemler, VP/Group Pres., Biotech, Osteosynthesis & Dev.
Stephen Si Johnson, VP/Group Pres., MedSurg Equipment
Edward B. Lipes, Exec. VP
Bronwen R. Taylor, VP-Internal Audit & Compliance
John W. Brown, Chmn.
Andrew G. Fox-Smith, Pres., Intl.

Phone: 269-385-2600	**Fax:** 269-385-1062
Toll-Free:	
Address: 2825 Airview Blvd., Kalamazoo, MI 49002 US	

GROWTH PLANS/SPECIAL FEATURES:

Stryker Corp. develops, manufactures and markets specialty surgical and medical products for the global market. These products include orthopedic implants, patient care and handling equipment, powered surgical instruments and endoscopic systems. Founded in 1941, the firm's products are produced by two segments: Orthopaedic Implants, which generated approximately 60% of Stryker's 2007 sales; and MedSurg equipment, the remaining 40%. The Orthopaedic Implant segment's products include reconstructive implants for knee, hip, elbow, shoulder and other joint surgeries; nailing, plating and external fixation systems to mend trauma injuries; spine implants; micro implants for craniomaxillofacial and hand surgery; bone cement; and OP-1, a natural protein that induces bone formation. These products are designed and manufactured by subsidiaries Stryker Orthopaedics, Stryker Osteosynthesis, Stryker Spine and Stryker Biotech. Stryker MedSurg Equipment provides powered surgical instruments, surgical navigation systems, hospital beds and stretchers, endoscopic products, emergency medical equipment and medical video imaging equipment. These devices are produced by Stryker Instruments, Stryker Endoscopy, Stryker Medical and Sightline Technologies Ltd., a recently acquired Israeli company that develops flexible endoscopes. Stryker maintains administrative, sales, warehousing and distribution sites in 41 countries in Europe, Asia, Africa and the Americas; and exports products to numerous international destinations. Geographically, domestic regions generated 64% of the 2007 sales; international regions, the remaining 36%. In June 2007, Physiotherapy Associates was sold for $150 million to Water Street Healthcare Partners. Physiotherapy Associates provided outpatient physical therapy services in the U.S., principally physical, occupational and speech therapy services.

Employees of Stryker receive benefits including medical, dental, vision, prescription, disability and life insurance; flexible spending accounts; an employee assistance program; onsite fitness centers and cafeterias; tuition reimbursement; adoption assistance; and paid vacations, holidays and maternity leave.

FINANCIALS: Sales and profits are in thousands of dollars—add 000 to get the full amount. 2007 Note: Financial information for 2007 was not available for all companies at press time.

2007 Sales: $6,000,500	2007 Profits: $1,017,400	**U.S. Stock Ticker:** SYK
2006 Sales: $5,147,200	2006 Profits: $777,700	**Int'l Ticker:** Int'l Exchange:
2005 Sales: $4,871,500	2005 Profits: $643,600	Employees: 18,806
2004 Sales: $4,262,300	2004 Profits: $440,000	Fiscal Year Ends: 12/31
2003 Sales: $3,625,300	2003 Profits: $453,500	Parent Company:

SALARIES/BENEFITS:

Pension Plan:	ESOP Stock Plan:	Profit Sharing:	Top Exec. Salary: $900,000	Bonus: $877,500
Savings Plan: Y	Stock Purch. Plan: Y		Second Exec. Salary: $781,045	Bonus: $161,052

OTHER THOUGHTS:

Apparent Women Officers or Directors: 5
Hot Spot for Advancement for Women/Minorities: Y

LOCATIONS: ("Y" = Yes)

West:	Southwest:	Midwest:	Southeast:	Northeast:	International:
Y	Y	Y	Y	Y	Y

Note: Financial information, benefits and other data can change quickly and may vary from those stated here.

SUN HEALTHCARE GROUP

www.sunh.com

Industry Group Code: 623110 Ranks within this company's industry group: Sales: 3 Profits: 3

Management:		Sales/Marketing:		Liberal Arts:		Information Systems:		Professionals:		Technical/Scientific:	
Mgmt. Trainees:		Mktg. Professionals:		Gen. Writing/Editing:	Y	Info. Management:	Y	Finance/Accounting:	Y	Engineers, Elec.:	
Experienced Mgmt.:	Y	Retail Sales:		Technical Writing:		Software Dev.:	Y	Law:	Y	Engineers, Other:	
Int'l Business:		Commercial/Industrial:		Graphic Arts/Photog.:		Hardware Dev.:		HR/Other:	Y	Health/Lab:	
MBA Graduates:	Y	Sales Trainees:		Music:		Systems Integration:		Training:	Y	Scientists/Research:	
		Advertising Pros.:		Broadcasting:		Consulting/Other:		Health Care:	Y	Petroleum/Chemicals:	
				Other:				Consulting:		Math/Other:	

TYPES OF BUSINESS:

Long-Term Care
Sub-Acute Care
Assisted Living Services
Temporary Medical Staffing
Mobile Radiology
Medical Laboratory Services
Home Health Care Services
Physical Therapy

BRANDS/DIVISIONS/AFFILIATES:

SunDance Rehabilitation Corp.
CareerStaff Unlimited, Inc.
SunPlus Home Health Services
Harborside Healthcare Corporation
Twilight Wish Foundation

CONTACTS: *Note: Officers with more than one job title may be intentionally listed here more than once.*

Richard K. Matros, CEO
L. Bryan Shaul, CFO/Exec. VP
Heidi J. Fisher, Sr. VP-Human Resources
Michael Newman, General Counsel/Exec. VP
Deborah Haugh, Sr. VP-Bus. Dev.
Jeffrey M. Kreger, VP-Corp. Controller
Michael Montevideo, VP/Treas.
Chauncey J. Hunker, Sr. VP/Corp. Compliance Officer/Chief Risk Officer
Sue Gwyn, Pres., SunDance Rehabilitation Corp.
Richard Peranton, Pres., CareerStaff Unlimited
Richard K. Matros, Chmn.

Phone: 949-255-7100	Fax:
Toll-Free: 800-729-6600	
Address: 18831 Von Karman, Ste. 400, Irvine, CA 92612 US	

GROWTH PLANS/SPECIAL FEATURES:

Sun Healthcare Group, Inc., through its subsidiaries, is a nationwide provider of long-term, sub-acute and related specialty healthcare services primarily to the senior population in the U.S. The firm operates in three principal business segments: inpatient services, rehabilitation therapy services and medical staffing services. Its core business is providing inpatient services, primarily through 190 skilled nursing facilities, 15 assisted and independent living facilities and eight mental health facilities with 24,002 licensed beds located in 25 states. These facilities provide inpatient skilled nursing and custodial services including daily nursing, therapeutic rehabilitation, social services, housekeeping, dietary and administrative services for individuals requiring certain assistance for activities in daily living. Specialized care is available for patients with Alzheimer's disease. The firm's rehabilitation services are provided at over 416 facilities in 33 states through SunDance Rehabilitation Corporation. These services include speech pathology, physical therapy and occupational therapy. Sun Healthcare's medical staffing services, through CareerStaff Unlimited, Inc., provides licensed therapists skilled in physical, occupational and speech therapy; nurses; pharmacists, pharmacist technicians and medical imaging technicians; physicians; and related medical personnel. CareerStaff customers include hospitals, skilled nursing facilities, schools and prisons. In April 2007, Sun Healthcare completed the acquisition of Harborside Healthcare Corporation, a private healthcare company based in Boston, Massachusetts operating 73 skilled nursing facilities, one assisted living facility and one independent living facility, for $349.4 million. In February 2008, the firm announced a partnership with the Twilight Wish Foundation, a non-profit organization which helps seniors realize some of their wishes; the partnership is expected to effect over 200 locations.

FINANCIALS: Sales and profits are in thousands of dollars—add 000 to get the full amount. 2007 Note: Financial information for 2007 was not available for all companies at press time.

2007 Sales: $1,587,307	2007 Profits: $57,510	U.S. Stock Ticker: SUNH
2006 Sales: $1,004,897	2006 Profits: $27,118	Int'l Ticker: Int'l Exchange:
2005 Sales: $765,782	2005 Profits: $24,761	Employees: 19,350
2004 Sales: $700,863	2004 Profits: $-18,627	Fiscal Year Ends: 12/31
2003 Sales: $834,043	2003 Profits: $ 354	Parent Company:

SALARIES/BENEFITS:

Pension Plan:	ESOP Stock Plan:	Profit Sharing:	Top Exec. Salary: $757,692	Bonus: $1,034,375
Savings Plan: Y	Stock Purch. Plan:		Second Exec. Salary: $446,373	Bonus: $500,625

OTHER THOUGHTS:

Apparent Women Officers or Directors: 4
Hot Spot for Advancement for Women/Minorities: Y

LOCATIONS: ("Y" = Yes)

West:	Southwest:	Midwest:	Southeast:	Northeast:	International:
Y	Y	Y	Y	Y	

Note: Financial information, benefits and other data can change quickly and may vary from those stated here.

SUN MICROSYSTEMS INC

www.sun.com

Industry Group Code: 334111 Ranks within this company's industry group: Sales: 3   Profits: 4

Management:		Sales/Marketing:		Liberal Arts:		Information Systems:		Professionals:		Technical/Scientific:	
Mgmt. Trainees:	Y	Mktg. Professionals:	Y	Gen. Writing/Editing:	Y	Info. Management:	Y	Finance/Accounting:	Y	Engineers, Elec.:	Y
Experienced Mgmt.:	Y	Retail Sales:		Technical Writing:	Y	Software Dev.:	Y	Law:	Y	Engineers, Other:	Y
Int'l Business:	Y	Commercial/Industrial:	Y	Graphic Arts/Photog.:		Hardware Dev.:	Y	HR/Other:	Y	Health/Lab:	Y
MBA Graduates:	Y	Sales Trainees:		Music:		Systems Integration:	Y	Training:	Y	Scientists/Research:	Y
		Advertising Pros.:	Y	Broadcasting:		Consulting/Other:	Y	Health Care:		Petroleum/Chemicals:	
				Other:				Consulting:	Y	Math/Other:	Y

TYPES OF BUSINESS:

Computer Hardware
UNIX-Based Workstation Computers
Multiprocessing Servers
Operating System Software
Systems Integration
Office Application Software
Network Products
Consulting Services

BRANDS/DIVISIONS/AFFILIATES:

NetBeans IDE
UltraSPARC
Sun Fire
Solaris OS
Java
StorEdge
SunSpectrum
Tarantella Inc

CONTACTS: Note: Officers with more than one job title may be intentionally listed here more than once.

Jonathan I. Schwartz, CEO
Jonathan I. Schwartz, Pres.
Michael E. Lehman, CFO/Exec. VP-Corp. Resources
Anil Gadre, Chief Mktg. Officer/Exec. VP
William N. MacGowan, Chief Human Resources Officer/Exec. VP
Greg Papadopoulos, Exec. VP-R&D
Robert Worrall, CIO
Greg Papadopoulos, CTO
Michael A. Dillon, General Counsel/Exec. VP
Brian Sutphin, Exec. VP-Corp. Dev. & Alliances
Ingrid Van Den Hoogen, Sr. VP-Brand, Global Comm. & Integrated Mktg.
David W. Yen, Ph.D., Exec. VP-Microelectronics
Bill Vass, COO/Pres., Sun Microsystems Federal
Rich Green, Exec. VP-Software
Scott G. McNealy, Chmn.
Eugene McCabe, Exec. VP-Worldwide Oper.

Phone: 650-960-1300	Fax: 408-276-3804
Toll-Free: 800-786-0404	
Address: 4150 Network Cir., Santa Clara, CA 95054 US	

GROWTH PLANS/SPECIAL FEATURES:

Sun Microsystems, Inc. (Sun) is a worldwide provider of scalable computer systems, networks, storage systems, software, microprocessors and support services. The company has two segments: products and services. The products segment encompasses computer systems and data management products. Sun's services segment consists maintenance contracts and client solutions; and educational services, which consist of technical consulting to help customers plan, implement, and manage distributed network computing environments and developing integrated learning solutions for enterprises, IT organizations and individual IT professionals. Sun's desktops and workstations, including the Sun Ultra series, facilitate a wide range of activities such as software development, mechanical design, financial analysis and education. Sun's proprietary microprocessor, the 64-bit UltraSPARC, powers most Sun platforms, including the Sun Fire series. The software segment of the computer systems group consists of Solaris OS and Java, Sun's universal software platform. Solaris OS is a secure operating system for Sun platforms. Sun's storage systems segment includes the StorEdge system and StorEdge software, offering multi-level storage solutions. SunSpectrum support service products allow customers to customize their services, choosing among four levels of support that range from mission-critical to self-support. The company employs independent distributors in over 100 countries; its channel partners account for 65% of revenues. In 2007, the company announced plans to acquire Vaau, a provider of Enterprise Role Management (ERM) and identity compliance solutions. Sun also recently announced a broad strategic partnership with Intel Corporation based on Intel's endorsement of the Solaris Operating System and Sun's commitment to deliver a comprehensive family of enterprise and telecommunications servers and workstations based on Intel's Xeon processor. Late in 2007, Sun partnered with Dell in a multi-year original equipment manufacturer agreement to combine Sun's Solaris Operating System (OS) and support services with Dell's PowerEdge servers.

Sun offers employees fitness centers, adoption assistance and discounted computer equipment.

FINANCIALS: Sales and profits are in thousands of dollars—add 000 to get the full amount. 2007 Note: Financial information for 2007 was not available for all companies at press time.

2007 Sales: $13,873,000	2007 Profits: $473,000	U.S. Stock Ticker: SUNW
2006 Sales: $13,068,000	2006 Profits: $-864,000	Int'l Ticker: Int'l Exchange:
2005 Sales: $11,070,000	2005 Profits: $-107,000	Employees: 34,200
2004 Sales: $11,185,000	2004 Profits: $-388,000	Fiscal Year Ends: 6/30
2003 Sales: $11,434,000	2003 Profits: $-3,429,000	Parent Company:

SALARIES/BENEFITS:

Pension Plan: Y	ESOP Stock Plan:	Profit Sharing:	Top Exec. Salary: $980,769	Bonus: $2,507,000
Savings Plan: Y	Stock Purch. Plan: Y		Second Exec. Salary: $748,449	Bonus: $938,180

OTHER THOUGHTS:

Apparent Women Officers or Directors: 1
Hot Spot for Advancement for Women/Minorities: Y

LOCATIONS: ("Y" = Yes)

West:	Southwest:	Midwest:	Southeast:	Northeast:	International:
Y	Y	Y	. Y	Y	Y

Note: Financial information, benefits and other data can change quickly and may vary from those stated here.

SUNGARD DATA SYSTEMS INC
www.sungard.com

Industry Group Code: 511201 Ranks within this company's industry group: Sales: 1 Profits: 2

Management:		Sales/Marketing:		Liberal Arts:		Information Systems:		Professionals:		Technical/Scientific:	
Mgmt. Trainees:	Y	Mktg. Professionals:	Y	Gen. Writing/Editing:	Y	Info. Management:	Y	Finance/Accounting:	Y	Engineers, Elec.:	Y
Experienced Mgmt.:	Y	Retail Sales:		Technical Writing:	Y	Software Dev.:	Y	Law:	Y	Engineers, Other:	
Int'l Business:	Y	Commercial/Industrial:	Y	Graphic Arts/Photog.:	Y	Hardware Dev.:		HR/Other:	Y	Health/Lab:	
MBA Graduates:	Y	Sales Trainees:		Music:		Systems Integration:	Y	Training:	Y	Scientists/Research:	Y
		Advertising Pros.:	Y	Broadcasting:		Consulting/Other:	Y	Health Care:		Petroleum/Chemicals:	
				Other:				Consulting:		Math/Other:	Y

TYPES OF BUSINESS:
Outsourced Information Processing & Services
Workflow Management Systems
Data Protection
Financial Services Software
Education Software
Administrative Software

BRANDS/DIVISIONS/AFFILIATES:

CONTACTS: Note: Officers with more than one job title may be intentionally listed here more than once.
Cristobal Conde, CEO
Cristobal Conde, Pres.
Michale J. Ruane, CFO
Brian Robins, Sr. VP-Mktg./Chief Mktg. Officer
Kathleen Asser Weslock, Chief Human Resources Officer/Sr. VP
Victoria E. Silbey, General Counsel/VP-Legal
Richard C. Tarbox, Sr. VP-Corp. Dev.
Gil Santos, CEO-Public Sector
Michale J. Ruane, Sr. VP-Finance
Jim Ashton, Div. CEO-Financial Systems
Harold Finders, Div. CEO-Financial Systems
Eric Berg, Group CEO-Availability Svcs.
Ron Lang, CEO-Enterprise Solutions
James L. Mann, Chmn.

Phone: 484-582-2000 **Fax:** 610-225-1120
Toll-Free: 800-825-2518
Address: 680 E. Swedesford Rd., Wayne, PA 19087-1586 US

GROWTH PLANS/SPECIAL FEATURES:
SunGard Data Systems, Inc. is a leading global provider of integrated software and information technology services for financial services companies, higher education and the public sector. The firm serves more than 25,000 clients in over 50 countries. SunGard is organized into four business segments: Financial Systems, Higher Education, Public Sector and Availability Services. SunGard Financial Systems serves financial services companies specializing in alternative investments; banking; benefit administration; brokerage and clearance; capital markets and investment banking; energy trading and risk management; institutional asset management; insurance; trading; treasury management; and wealth management. The Higher Education segment provides specialized enterprise resource planning and administrative software to higher education institutions. SunGard Public Sector serves school districts, nonprofit organizations and local, state and federal government agencies, with solutions for accounting; human resources; payroll; utility billing; land management; public safety and criminal justice; and grant and project management. The Availability Services segment provides solutions to information-dependent companies across virtually all industries protecting against breaches of security; network or hardware failures; data loss; power failure; and extreme events, such as natural disaster and terrorism. In January 2007, SunGard completed the acquisition of XRT's high-end treasury product lines, Globe$ and TWS. In February 2007, it acquired Maxim Insurance Software Corporation and Aceva Technologies. In April 2007, SunGard acquired Energy Softworx and Finetix LLC. In June 2007, SunGard acquired Aspiren, and in July it acquired GTI Consultants. In August 2007, the company acquired VeriCenter, Inc., a leading managed services, application hosting and IT infrastructure outsourcing company. In October 2007, the firm acquired The ASTEC Group, a specialist research consultancy. In November 2007, SunGard acquired DSPA Software, Inc., a supplier of sales compensation and distribution management software.

FINANCIALS: Sales and profits are in thousands of dollars—add 000 to get the full amount. 2007 Note: Financial information for 2007 was not available for all companies at press time.

2007 Sales: $4,901,000	2007 Profits: $-60,000	**U.S. Stock Ticker: Private**
2006 Sales: $4,323,000	2006 Profits: $-118,000	**Int'l Ticker:** Int'l Exchange:
2005 Sales: $4,002,000	2005 Profits: $117,000	Employees: 16,600
2004 Sales: $3,555,900	2004 Profits: $453,600	Fiscal Year Ends: 12/31
2003 Sales: $2,955,252	2003 Profits: $370,310	Parent Company:

SALARIES/BENEFITS:
Pension Plan:	ESOP Stock Plan:	Profit Sharing:	Top Exec. Salary: $874,000	Bonus: $1,517,972
Savings Plan:	Stock Purch. Plan:		Second Exec. Salary: $557,000	Bonus: $850,423

OTHER THOUGHTS:
Apparent Women Officers or Directors: 2
Hot Spot for Advancement for Women/Minorities:

LOCATIONS: ("Y" = Yes)
West:	Southwest:	Midwest:	Southeast:	Northeast:	International:
Y	Y	Y	Y	Y	Y

SUNOCO INC

www.sunocoinc.com

Industry Group Code: 324110A Ranks within this company's industry group: Sales: 2   Profits: 2

Management:		Sales/Marketing:		Liberal Arts:		Information Systems:		Professionals:		Technical/Scientific:	
Mgmt. Trainees:	Y	Mktg. Professionals:	Y	Gen. Writing/Editing:		Info. Management:	Y	Finance/Accounting:	Y	Engineers, Elec.:	Y
Experienced Mgmt.:	Y	Retail Sales:		Technical Writing:	Y	Software Dev.:		Law:	Y	Engineers, Other:	
Int'l Business:	Y	Commercial/Industrial:	Y	Graphic Arts/Photog.:		Hardware Dev.:		HR/Other:	Y	Health/Lab:	Y
MBA Graduates:	Y	Sales Trainees:		Music:		Systems Integration:		Training:	Y	Scientists/Research:	Y
		Advertising Pros.:		Broadcasting:		Consulting/Other:		Health Care:		Petroleum/Chemicals:	
				Other:				Consulting:		Math/Other:	

TYPES OF BUSINESS:

Petroleum Refiner & Chemicals Manufacturer
Petrochemicals & Lubricants
Coke Manufacturing

BRANDS/DIVISIONS/AFFILIATES:

SunCoke Energy, Inc.
Sunoco Logistic Partners L.P.
Gateway Energy and Coke Company
Sunoco Chemicals

CONTACTS: *Note: Officers with more than one job title may be intentionally listed here more than once.*

Lynn Elsenhans, CEO
John G. Drosdick, Pres.
Thomas W. Hofmann, CFO/Sr. VP
Robert W. Owens, Sr. VP-Mktg.
Rolf D. Naku, Sr. VP-Human Resources
Charles K. Valutas, Chief Admin. Officer/Sr. VP
Michael S. Kuritzkes, General Counsel/Sr. VP
Terence P. Delaney, VP-Planning
Rolf D. Naku, Sr. VP-Public Affairs
Terence P. Delaney, VP-Investor Rel.
Joseph P. Krott, Comptroller
Michael J. Thomson, Sr. VP/Pres., SunCoke Energy, Inc.
Vincent J. Kelley, Sr. VP-Refining
Ann C. Mule, Chief Governance Officer/Corp. Sec.
Bruce G. Fischer, Sr. VP-Sunoco Chemicals
John G. Drosdick, Chmn.
Michael J. Hennigan, Sr. VP-Supply, Sales, Trading & Transportation

Phone: 215-977-3000	**Fax:** 215-977-3409
Toll-Free: 800-786-6261	
Address: 1735 Market St., Ste. LL, Philadelphia, PA 19103-7583 US	

GROWTH PLANS/SPECIAL FEATURES:

Sunoco, Inc. is a petroleum refiner and chemicals manufacturer with interests in logistics and cokemaking. Sunoco operates in five segments: Refining and supply, retail marketing, chemicals, logistics and coke. Additionally, the firm has a holding company and a professional services group. The holding company is a non-operating parent company and the professional services group consists of a number of staff functions including finance, risk management, human resources, information systems and engineering services. The refining and supply business, with operations in the Northeast and Midwest, manufactures petroleum products, including gasoline, middle distillates and residual fuel oil; commodity petrochemicals including olefins and their derivatives; and aromatics and their derivates. Sunoco has a refining capacity of roughly 910,000 barrels per day. The retail marketing business consists of the retail sale of gasoline and middle distillates and the operation of convenience stores in 27 states. The chemicals segment, operating through Sunoco Chemicals, manufactures, distributes and markets commodity and intermediate petrochemicals. The logistics division, including Sunoco Logistic Partners L.P., operates refined product and crude oil pipelines and terminals and conducts crude oil acquisition and marketing activities primarily in the Northeast, Midwest and South Central regions of the U.S. The coke segment operates metallurgical coke plants and metallurgical coal mines, through SunCoke Energy, Inc. Sunoco also owns and operates facilities in Pennsylvania and Ohio, which produce phenol and acetone; and in Texas and West Virginia, which produce polypropylene. The firm operates five refineries and markets gasoline, middle distillates and other convenience store merchandise through 4,684 retail outlets. In 2008, Gateway Energy and Coke Company, a subsidiary of SunCoke, announced plans to build a heat recovery coke facility in Illinois.

The company offers employees a 401(k) plan; medical and dental insurance; an employee assistance program; flexible spending accounts; short- and long-term disability insurance; and an educational assistance plan.

FINANCIALS: Sales and profits are in thousands of dollars—add 000 to get the full amount. 2007 Note: Financial information for 2007 was not available for all companies at press time.

2007 Sales: $44,470,000	2007 Profits: $891,000	**U.S. Stock Ticker:** SUN
2006 Sales: $38,636,000	2006 Profits: $979,000	**Int'l Ticker:** Int'l Exchange:
2005 Sales: $33,754,000	2005 Profits: $974,000	Employees: 14,200
2004 Sales: $25,468,000	2004 Profits: $605,000	Fiscal Year Ends: 12/31
2003 Sales: $17,969,000	2003 Profits: $312,000	Parent Company:

SALARIES/BENEFITS:

Pension Plan:	ESOP Stock Plan:	Profit Sharing:	Top Exec. Salary: $1,200,000	Bonus: $1,826,496
Savings Plan: Y	Stock Purch. Plan:		Second Exec. Salary: $525,000	Bonus: $466,137

OTHER THOUGHTS:

Apparent Women Officers or Directors: 3
Hot Spot for Advancement for Women/Minorities: Y

LOCATIONS: ("Y" = Yes)

West:	Southwest:	Midwest:	Southeast:	Northeast:	International:
Y	Y	Y	Y	Y	Y

Note: Financial information, benefits and other data can change quickly and may vary from those stated here.

SUNRISE SENIOR LIVING
www.sunriseseniorliving.com

Industry Group Code: 623110   Ranks within this company's industry group: Sales: Profits:

Management:		Sales/Marketing:		Liberal Arts:		Information Systems:		Professionals:		Technical/Scientific:	
Mgmt. Trainees:	Y	Mktg. Professionals:	Y	Gen. Writing/Editing:	Y	Info. Management:	Y	Finance/Accounting:	Y	Engineers, Elec.:	
Experienced Mgmt.:	Y	Retail Sales:		Technical Writing:	Y	Software Dev.:		Law:	Y	Engineers, Other:	Y
Int'l Business:	Y	Commercial/Industrial:		Graphic Arts/Photog.:		Hardware Dev.:		HR/Other:	Y	Health/Lab:	
MBA Graduates:	Y	Sales Trainees:		Music:		Systems Integration:		Training:	Y	Scientists/Research:	
		Advertising Pros.:		Broadcasting:		Consulting/Other:		Health Care:	Y	Petroleum/Chemicals:	
				Other:				Consulting:		Math/Other:	

TYPES OF BUSINESS:

Long-Term Health Care
Assisted Living Centers
Independent Living Centers
Nursing Homes

BRANDS/DIVISIONS/AFFILIATES:

Sunrise Assisted Living
Aston Gardens
Trinity Hospice, Inc.

CONTACTS: Note: Officers with more than one job title may be intentionally listed here more than once.

Paul J. Klaassen, CEO
Tiffany L. Tomasso, COO
Richard J. Nadeau, CFO
Jeffery M. Jasnoff, Sr. VP-Human Resources
Mark S. Ordan, Chief Admin. Officer
John F. Gaul, General Counsel
Mark S. Ordan, Chief Investment Officer
Julie A. Pangelinan, Chief Acct. Officer
Teresa M. Klaassen, Chief Cultural Officer/Exec. VP
Michael B. Lanahan, Chmn.-Greystone Div.
Lynn Krominga, Chmn.

Phone: 703-273-7500	Fax: 703-744-1601
Toll-Free: 888-434-4648	
Address: 7902 Westpark Dr., McLean, VA 22102 US	

GROWTH PLANS/SPECIAL FEATURES:

Sunrise Senior Living, formerly Sunrise Assisted Living, Inc., operates more than 439 senior living communities in the U.S., the U.K., Germany and Canada, with a resident capacity of approximately 54,000; and it has 44 more communities under construction. The firm offers services tailored to its individual resident needs, typically in apartment-like assisted living environments. Upon move-in, Sunrise assists the resident in developing an individualized service plan, including selection of resident accommodations and the appropriate level of care. The services provided range from basic care, consisting of assistance with activities of daily living; to reminiscence care, which consists of programs and services to help cognitively impaired residents, including residents with Alzheimer's disease. The firm targets sites for development located in major metropolitan areas and their surrounding suburban communities, considering factors such as population, age demographics and estimated level of market demand. The company often revitalizes existing senior living centers and operates the home for a third-party owner. It owns or has interest in 261 of the properties where it maintains services. In August 2007, the company changed its meal options, no longer using trans fat oils in its food, as well as offering Davidson's Safest Choice Pasteurized Shell Eggs, allowing the company to offer poached and sunny side up eggs that are safe for adults over the age of 50 to eat without risk of salmonella and other food borne illnesses. In November 2007, the firm opened its first community specifically designed for early, mid and late stages of memory loss illness, such as Alzheimer's, in Illinois. In 2008, the firm opened facilities in Nevada, Utah and Quebec.

Sunrise offers employees flexible spending accounts; a scholarship program; tuition assistance; a meal discount program; a dental and vision care plan; life insurance; and scholarship program.

FINANCIALS: Sales and profits are in thousands of dollars—add 000 to get the full amount. 2007 Note: Financial information for 2007 was not available for all companies at press time.

2007 Sales: $1,652,550	2007 Profits: $-70,275	U.S. Stock Ticker: SRZ
2006 Sales: $1,651,081	2006 Profits: $15,284	Int'l Ticker: Int'l Exchange:
2005 Sales: $1,509,438	2005 Profits: $87,089	Employees: 39,000
2004 Sales: $1,446,471	2004 Profits: $50,687	Fiscal Year Ends: 12/31
2003 Sales: $1,188,300	2003 Profits: $62,200	Parent Company:

SALARIES/BENEFITS:

Pension Plan:	ESOP Stock Plan:	Profit Sharing:	Top Exec. Salary: $463,742	Bonus: $
Savings Plan: Y	Stock Purch. Plan: Y		Second Exec. Salary: $360,688	Bonus: $446,000

OTHER THOUGHTS:

Apparent Women Officers or Directors: 3
Hot Spot for Advancement for Women/Minorities: Y

LOCATIONS: ("Y" = Yes)

West:	Southwest:	Midwest:	Southeast:	Northeast:	International:
Y	Y	Y	Y	Y	Y

Note: Financial information, benefits and other data can change quickly and may vary from those stated here.

SUPERVALU INC

www.supervalu.com

Industry Group Code: 445110 Ranks within this company's industry group: Sales: Profits:

Management:		Sales/Marketing:		Liberal Arts:		Information Systems:		Professionals:		Technical/Scientific:	
Mgmt. Trainees:	Y	Mktg. Professionals:	Y	Gen. Writing/Editing:	Y	Info. Management:	Y	Finance/Accounting:	Y	Engineers, Elec.:	
Experienced Mgmt.:	Y	Retail Sales:	Y	Technical Writing:		Software Dev.:		Law:	Y	Engineers, Other:	
Int'l Business:		Commercial/Industrial:		Graphic Arts/Photog.:	Y	Hardware Dev.:		HR/Other:	Y	Health/Lab:	
MBA Graduates:	Y	Sales Trainees:	Y	Music:		Systems Integration:		Training:	Y	Scientists/Research:	
		Advertising Pros.:	Y	Broadcasting:		Consulting/Other:		Health Care:	Y	Petroleum/Chemicals:	
				Other:				Consulting:		Math/Other:	

TYPES OF BUSINESS:

Grocery Stores
Food Distribution & Logistics
Natural & Organic Foods

BRANDS/DIVISIONS/AFFILIATES:

Albertsons
Save-A-Lot
Shaw's Supermarkets
Jewel-Osco
Acme Markets
Sunflower Market
Club Foods
Farm Fresh

CONTACTS: *Note: Officers with more than one job title may be intentionally listed here more than once.*

Jeffrey Noddle, CEO
Michael L. Jackson, COO
Michael L. Jackson, Pres.
Pamela K. Knous, CFO/Exec. VP
Duncan Mac Naughton, Exec. VP-Mktg.
Dave Pylipow, Sr. VP-Human Resources
Duncan Mac Naughton, Exec. VP-Merch.
David Boehnen, Exec. VP-Legal, Real Estate & Gov't Affairs
David Boehnen, Exec. VP-Corp. Dev.
Pete Van Helden, Sr. VP/Pres., Retail West
Kevin Tripp, Exec. VP/Pres., Retail Midwest
Jeffrey Noddle, Chmn.
Janel Haugarth, Exec VP/Pres./COO-Supply Chain Svcs.

Phone: 952-828-4000	Fax: 952-828-8998
Toll-Free:	
Address: 11840 Valley View Rd., Eden Prairie, MN 55344 US	

GROWTH PLANS/SPECIAL FEATURES:

Supervalu, Inc. is a supermarket retailer and food distributor. Supervalu conducts its retail operations under three retail food store formats: combination stores, food stores and limited assortment food stores. The company operates approximately 2,468 stores under the following banners: Albertson's, Save-A-Lot, Shaw's Supermarkets, Jewel-Osco, Acme Markets, Shoppers Food & Pharmacy, Club Foods, Farm Fresh, Lucky, Shop 'n Save, Scott's, Star Markets, Bristol Farms, bigg's, Hornbacher's and Sunflower Market. Supervalu's roughly 900 combination stores combine a grocery and a drug store under one roof, most often including a complete grocery offering, prescription drugs and expanded sections of cosmetics and general merchandise, in addition to specialty departments such as service seafood and meat, bakery, service delicatessen, liquor, floral and in-store banks. Typical combination stores carry about 50,000 items and average approximately 60,000 square feet. Supervalu's food stores focus primarily on food departments and include many of the same product and service offerings as combination stores, but on a more limited basis and without a pharmacy. Typical food stores carry about 40,000 items and average approximately 40,000 square feet. Supervalu operates 865 limited assortment stores, including 328 under the Save-A-Lot banner and four under the Sunflower Market banner. The company licenses 858 Save-A-Lot stores to independent operators.   Supervalu also operates approximately 130 fuel centers. Save-A-Lot stores are typically 15,000 square feet in size, stocking approximately 1,400 high volume food items generally in a single size for each product sold, as well as a limited offering of general merchandise items. At a Save-A-Lot store, the majority of the food products offered for sale are custom branded products. In 2008, the company's pharmacies deployed a pharmacy management system, ARx, that features technologies such as prescription label imaging and thermal printing.

FINANCIALS: Sales and profits are in thousands of dollars—add 000 to get the full amount. 2007 Note: Financial information for 2007 was not available for all companies at press time.

2007 Sales: $37,406,000	2007 Profits: $452,000	**U.S. Stock Ticker:** SVU	
2006 Sales: $19,863,599	2006 Profits: $206,169	**Int'l Ticker:** Int'l Exchange:	
2005 Sales: $19,543,240	2005 Profits: $385,823	Employees: 191,400	
2004 Sales: $20,209,700	2004 Profits: $280,100	Fiscal Year Ends: 2/28	
2003 Sales: $19,160,400	2003 Profits: $257,000	Parent Company:	

SALARIES/BENEFITS:

Pension Plan:	ESOP Stock Plan:	Profit Sharing:	Top Exec. Salary: $1,100,000	Bonus: $1,489,125
Savings Plan: Y	Stock Purch. Plan:		Second Exec. Salary: $630,962	Bonus: $537,625

OTHER THOUGHTS:

Apparent Women Officers or Directors: 5
Hot Spot for Advancement for Women/Minorities: Y

LOCATIONS: ("Y" = Yes)

West:	Southwest:	Midwest:	Southeast:	Northeast:	International:
Y	Y	Y	Y	Y	

Note: Financial information, benefits and other data can change quickly and may vary from those stated here.

SYKES ENTERPRISES INC

www.sykes.com

Industry Group Code: 561422 Ranks within this company's industry group: Sales: 3 Profits: 3

Management:		Sales/Marketing:		Liberal Arts:		Information Systems:		Professionals:		Technical/Scientific:	
Mgmt. Trainees:	Y	Mktg. Professionals:	Y	Gen. Writing/Editing:		Info. Management:	Y	Finance/Accounting:	Y	Engineers, Elec.:	
Experienced Mgmt.:	Y	Retail Sales:		Technical Writing:		Software Dev.:	Y	Law:	Y	Engineers, Other:	
Int'l Business:	Y	Commercial/Industrial:	Y	Graphic Arts/Photog.:		Hardware Dev.:		HR/Other:	Y	Health/Lab:	
MBA Graduates:	Y	Sales Trainees:		Music:		Systems Integration:	Y	Training:	Y	Scientists/Research:	
		Advertising Pros.:		Broadcasting:		Consulting/Other:		Health Care:		Petroleum/Chemicals:	
				Other:				Consulting:	Y	Math/Other:	

TYPES OF BUSINESS:

Consulting-Technical Support
Outsourcing Services
Staffing Services

BRANDS/DIVISIONS/AFFILIATES:

Contact Center Services
TeleHealth Services

CONTACTS: *Note: Officers with more than one job title may be intentionally listed here more than once.*

Charles E. Sykes, CEO
Charles E. Sykes, Pres.
W. Michael Kipphut, CFO/Sr. VP
Lawrence R. Zingale, Sr. VP-Global Sales & Client Mgmt.
Jenna R. Nelson, Sr. VP-Human Resources
David L. Pearson, CIO/Sr. VP
James T. Holder, General Counsel/Sr. VP/Corp. Sec.
James C. Hobby, Sr. VP-Global Oper.
Daniel L.Hernandez, Sr. VP-Global Strategy
William N. Rocktoff, Controller/VP
David P. Reule, Pres., Sykes Realty, Inc.
Paul L. Whiting, Chmn.

Phone: 813-274-1000	Fax: 813-273-0148
Toll-Free:	
Address: 400 N. Ashley Dr., Tampa, FL 33602 US	

GROWTH PLANS/SPECIAL FEATURES:

Sykes Enterprises, Inc. provides outsourced customer contact management solutions and services in the business process outsourcing arena. Clients range from Fortune 100 companies to medium-sized businesses and public institutions in the communications, consumer technology, financial services, healthcare, transportation and leisure industries. The company operates within the U.S., Canada, Latin America, India, the Asia Pacific Rim, Europe, the Middle East and Africa. Sykes provides support via phone, e-mail, web and chat interfaces through global network customer support centers, which provide support capabilities in more than 30 languages. The company offers services in three areas: Outsourced customer contact management services, fulfillment services and enterprise support services. Outsourced customer care management services operate in 18 countries in 42 contact management centers and provides customer care by processing product information requests, activating customer accounts, resolving complaints, warranty management, billing inquiries, technical support, communications services, communications equipment, Internet access technology and portal usage. This sector also offers support in acquisitions, which are primarily focused on inbound up-selling/cross-selling of each client's products and services. The fulfillment services segment is integrated with customer care and technical support services and involves multilingual sales order processing via the Internet and phone; payment processing; inventory control; product delivery; and product returns handling. The enterprise support segment offers services in technical staffing and solutions for outsourced corporate health desks. The company's Contact Center Services division handles customer service, billing and complex technical support problems of companies in such industries as broadband, wireless, managed telecom services, consumer electronics, high-tech, card services and retail banking. Its TeleHealth Services division develops programs including chronic care, symptom management, health information services, wellness and prevention services and behavioral health services.

FINANCIALS: Sales and profits are in thousands of dollars—add 000 to get the full amount. 2007 Note: Financial information for 2007 was not available for all companies at press time.

2007 Sales: $710,120	2007 Profits: $39,859	**U.S. Stock Ticker:** SYKE
2006 Sales: $574,223	2006 Profits: $42,323	**Int'l Ticker:** Int'l Exchange:
2005 Sales: $494,918	2005 Profits: $23,408	Employees: 29,560
2004 Sales: $466,713	2004 Profits: $10,814	Fiscal Year Ends: 12/31
2003 Sales: $480,359	2003 Profits: $9,305	Parent Company:

SALARIES/BENEFITS:

Pension Plan:	ESOP Stock Plan:	Profit Sharing:	Top Exec. Salary: $518,990	Bonus: $590,103
Savings Plan: Y	Stock Purch. Plan:		Second Exec. Salary: $368,500	Bonus: $348,902

OTHER THOUGHTS:

Apparent Women Officers or Directors: 2
Hot Spot for Advancement for Women/Minorities: Y

LOCATIONS: ("Y" = Yes)

West:	Southwest:	Midwest:	Southeast:	Northeast:	International:
Y	Y	Y	Y	Y	Y

SYMANTEC CORP

www.symantec.com

Industry Group Code: 511211 Ranks within this company's industry group: Sales: 1 Profits: 2

Management:		Sales/Marketing:		Liberal Arts:		Information Systems:		Professionals:		Technical/Scientific:	
Mgmt. Trainees:	Y	Mktg. Professionals:	Y	Gen. Writing/Editing:	Y	Info. Management:	Y	Finance/Accounting:	Y	Engineers, Elec.:	Y
Experienced Mgmt.:	Y	Retail Sales:		Technical Writing:	Y	Software Dev.:	Y	Law:	Y	Engineers, Other:	
Int'l Business:	Y	Commercial/Industrial:	Y	Graphic Arts/Photog.:	Y	Hardware Dev.:		HR/Other:	Y	Health/Lab:	
MBA Graduates:	Y	Sales Trainees:		Music:		Systems Integration:	Y	Training:	Y	Scientists/Research:	Y
		Advertising Pros.:	Y	Broadcasting:		Consulting/Other:	Y	Health Care:		Petroleum/Chemicals:	
				Other:				Consulting:	Y	Math/Other:	Y

TYPES OF BUSINESS:

Software-Security
Remote Management Products
IT Consulting Services

BRANDS/DIVISIONS/AFFILIATES:

Norton
LiveUpdate
Norton AntiVirus
Norton Internet Security
Altiris Inc
Vontu, Inc.

CONTACTS: *Note: Officers with more than one job title may be intentionally listed here more than once.*

John W. Thompson, CEO
Enrique T. Salem, COO
James Beer, CFO/Exec. VP
Enrique Salem, Pres., Worldwide Sales & Mktg.
Rebecca Ranninger, Chief Human Resources Officer/Exec. VP
David Thompson, CIO/Exec. VP
Mark Bregman, CTO/Exec. VP
Art Courville, Exec. VP-Legal Affairs/Sec.
Helyn Corcos, VP-Investor Rel.
Greg Butterfield, Pres., Altiris Bus. Unit
Janice Chaffin, Pres., Consumer Bus. Unit
Greg Hughes, Pres., Global Svcs.
Tom Kendra, Pres., Security & Data Mgmt.
John W. Thompson, Chmn.
John Brigden, Sr. VP-EMEA

Phone: 408-517-8000	Fax: 408-517-8186
Toll-Free:	
Address: 20330 Stevens Creek Blvd., Cupertino, CA 95014 US	

GROWTH PLANS/SPECIAL FEATURES:

Symantec Corp. provides a range of software, appliances and services designed to secure and manage information technology (IT) infrastructure. The company is a provider of virus protection, risk management, Internet content, e-mail filtering, remote management and mobile code detection technologies. Symantec operates in five operating segments: consumer products; security and data management; data center management; services; and other. The consumer products segment delivers Internet security, PC tuneup and backup products. The Norton brand of consumer security software products provides protection for Windows and Macintosh platforms. Primary consumer products include Norton Antivirus, which safeguards against viruses, spyware and other security risks; and Norton Internet Security, which helps defend home and home office users by blocking online identity theft, detecting and eliminating spyware, removing viruses and worms and protecting against hackers from entering a user's system. The security and data management segment provides solutions for compliance and security management, endpoint security, messaging management and data protection management software solutions that allow customers to secure, provision, backup and remotely access laptops, PCs, mobile devices and servers. The data center management segment provides storage and server management; data protection; and application performance management solutions across heterogeneous storage and server platforms. The services segment consists of consultants with technical knowledge, business expertise and global insight across multi-vendor environments who assist organizations in managing IT risk on an ongoing basis. It provides maintenance and technical support, consulting, education and business critical services. The other segment includes sunset products and products nearing the end of their life cycle; general and administrative expenses; amortization of acquired product rights; charges; and certain indirect costs. In 2007, Symantec acquired Altiris, Inc. and Vontu, Inc.

The company offers employees medical, dental and vision insurance; a 401(k) plan; stock options; life and dismemberment insurance; tuition reimbursement; and an employee assistance program.

FINANCIALS: Sales and profits are in thousands of dollars—add 000 to get the full amount. 2007 Note: Financial information for 2007 was not available for all companies at press time.

2007 Sales: $5,199,370	2007 Profits: $404,380	**U.S. Stock Ticker: SYMC**
2006 Sales: $4,143,392	2006 Profits: $156,852	**Int'l Ticker:** Int'l Exchange:
2005 Sales: $2,582,849	2005 Profits: $536,159	Employees: 17,500
2004 Sales: $1,870,129	2004 Profits: $370,619	Fiscal Year Ends: 3/31
2003 Sales: $1,406,946	2003 Profits: $248,438	Parent Company:

SALARIES/BENEFITS:

Pension Plan:	ESOP Stock Plan:	Profit Sharing:	Top Exec. Salary: $800,000	Bonus: $350,000
Savings Plan: Y	Stock Purch. Plan: Y		Second Exec. Salary: $650,000	Bonus: $760,000

OTHER THOUGHTS:

Apparent Women Officers or Directors: 2
Hot Spot for Advancement for Women/Minorities: Y

LOCATIONS: ("Y" = Yes)

West:	Southwest:	Midwest:	Southeast:	Northeast:	International:
Y	Y	Y	Y	Y	Y

Note: Financial information, benefits and other data can change quickly and may vary from those stated here.

SYNOPSYS INC
www.synopsys.com

Industry Group Code: 511215 Ranks within this company's industry group: Sales: 1 Profits: 2

Management:		Sales/Marketing:		Liberal Arts:		Information Systems:		Professionals:		Technical/Scientific:	
Mgmt. Trainees:		Mktg. Professionals:		Gen. Writing/Editing:		Info. Management:	Y	Finance/Accounting:	Y	Engineers, Elec.:	Y
Experienced Mgmt.:	Y	Retail Sales:		Technical Writing:	Y	Software Dev.:	Y	Law:	Y	Engineers, Other:	
Int'l Business:	Y	Commercial/Industrial:	Y	Graphic Arts/Photog.:		Hardware Dev.:		HR/Other:	Y	Health/Lab:	
MBA Graduates:	Y	Sales Trainees:		Music:		Systems Integration:	Y	Training:	Y	Scientists/Research:	
		Advertising Pros.:		Broadcasting:		Consulting/Other:		Health Care:		Petroleum/Chemicals:	
				Other:				Consulting:		Math/Other:	

TYPES OF BUSINESS:
Computer Software-Electronic Design Automation
Consulting & Support Services

BRANDS/DIVISIONS/AFFILIATES:
Galaxy Design Platform
Discovery Verification Platform
ArchPro Design Automation, Inc.
Sandwork Design
MOSAID Technologies Incorporated

CONTACTS: *Note: Officers with more than one job title may be intentionally listed here more than once.*
Aart de Geus, CEO
Chi-Foon Chan, COO
Chi-Foon Chan, Pres.
Brian Beattie, CFO
John Chilton, Sr. VP-Mktg.
Jan Collinson, Sr. VP-Human Resources & Facilities
Raul Camposano, CTO/Sr. VP/Gen. Mgr.
Brian Cabrera, General Counsel/VP/Corp. Sec.
John Chilton, Sr. VP-Strategic Dev.
Deirdre Hanford, Sr. VP-Global Tech. Svcs.
Antun Domic, Sr. VP/Gen. Mgr.-Implementation Group
Manoj Gandhi, Sr. VP/Gen. Mgr.-Verification Group
Wolfgang Fichtner, Sr. VP/Gen. Mgr.-Silicon Engineering Group
Aart de Geus, Chmn.
Joe Logan, Sr. VP-Worldwide Sales

Phone: 650-584-5000	Fax:
Toll-Free: 800-541-7737	
Address: 700 E. Middlefield Rd., Mountain View, CA 94043 US	

GROWTH PLANS/SPECIAL FEATURES:
Synopsys, Inc. is a leading supplier of electronic design automation (EDA) software for semiconductor design. Its products are used by designers of integrated circuits (ICs), including system-on-a-chip ICs, and of electronic products, such as computers, cell phones and Internet routers, that use ICs to automate significant portions of their chip design process. The firm's products offer customers the opportunity to design ICs that are optimized for speed, area, power consumption and production cost, while reducing overall design time. The firm's products and services fall into six divisions: Implementation; Verification; Silicon Engineering; Analog/Mixed-Signal; Systems and IP; and Global Technical Services. Products come in five common groupings. The Galaxy Design Platform, which provides customers with many diverse common design requirements in a single application, and the Discovery Verification Platform, which combines simulation and verification products and design-for-verification methodologies to provide a consistent control environment, are generally sold together as Core EDA. Other product groupings include the Intellectual Property and Systems-Level Solutions grouping, which includes a library of standardized designs; Design for Manufacturing, including computer aided design (CAD) products, among others; and Professional Services, which includes consulting and design services. In addition, Synopsys provides consulting services to assist customers with their IC designs, as well as training and support services. The firm has licensed products to most of the world's leading semiconductor, computer, communications and electronics companies. In 2007, Synopsis acquired Sandwork Design, a leading provider of analog and mixed-signal (AMS) verification and debugging programs. The firm also acquired ArchPro Design Automation, Inc., which designs technology to assist in managing power for multi-voltage designs, and the semiconductor intellectual property (IP) assets of MOSAID Technologies, Inc., a developer of semiconductor IP.

Employees at Synopsys are offered an employee assistance program, as well as education assistance, adoption benefits, shopping discounts, referral bonuses and telecommuting options.

FINANCIALS: Sales and profits are in thousands of dollars—add 000 to get the full amount. 2007 Note: Financial information for 2007 was not available for all companies at press time.

2007 Sales: $1,212,469	2007 Profits: $130,491	**U.S. Stock Ticker:** SNPS
2006 Sales: $1,095,560	2006 Profits: $24,742	**Int'l Ticker:** Int'l Exchange:
2005 Sales: $991,931	2005 Profits: $-17,114	Employees: 5,196
2004 Sales: $1,092,104	2004 Profits: $74,337	Fiscal Year Ends: 10/31
2003 Sales: $1,176,983	2003 Profits: $149,724	Parent Company:

SALARIES/BENEFITS:

Pension Plan:	ESOP Stock Plan:	Profit Sharing:	Top Exec. Salary: $450,000	Bonus: $1,257,100
Savings Plan: Y	Stock Purch. Plan: Y		Second Exec. Salary: $420,000	Bonus: $1,100,000

OTHER THOUGHTS:
Apparent Women Officers or Directors: 3
Hot Spot for Advancement for Women/Minorities: Y

LOCATIONS: ("Y" = Yes)

West:	Southwest:	Midwest:	Southeast:	Northeast:	International:
Y	Y	Y	Y	Y	Y

SYNTEL INC

www.syntelinc.com

Industry Group Code: 541512 **Ranks within this company's industry group:** Sales: 13   Profits: 9

Management:		Sales/Marketing:		Liberal Arts:		Information Systems:		Professionals:		Technical/Scientific:	
Mgmt. Trainees:	Y	Mktg. Professionals:	Y	Gen. Writing/Editing:		Info. Management:	Y	Finance/Accounting:	Y	Engineers, Elec.:	Y
Experienced Mgmt.:	Y	Retail Sales:		Technical Writing:	Y	Software Dev.:	Y	Law:	Y	Engineers, Other:	
Int'l Business:	Y	Commercial/Industrial:	Y	Graphic Arts/Photog.:	Y	Hardware Dev.:		HR/Other:	Y	Health/Lab:	
MBA Graduates:	Y	Sales Trainees:		Music:		Systems Integration:	Y	Training:	Y	Scientists/Research:	
		Advertising Pros.:		Broadcasting:		Consulting/Other:		Health Care:		Petroleum/Chemicals:	
				Other:				Consulting:	Y	Math/Other:	

TYPES OF BUSINESS:
IT Consulting
Outsourcing Services
e-Business Solutions
Application Development & Management

BRANDS/DIVISIONS/AFFILIATES:
TeamSourcing
Identeon

CONTACTS: *Note: Officers with more than one job title may be intentionally listed here more than once.*
Bharat Desai, CEO
Keshav Murugesh, COO
Keshav Murugesh, Pres.
Arvind Godbole, CFO
Jonathan James, Chief Mktg. Officer
Srikanth Karra, VP-Global Human Resources
Daniel Moore, Chief Admin. Officer
Daniel Moore, General Counsel
R. Ramdas, Sr. VP-Finance & Corp. Svcs.
Neerja Sethi, VP-Corp. Affairs
Arvind Godbole, Chief Info. Security Officer
Anil Jain, Sr. VP-Insurance Verital
Lakshmanan Chidambaram, VP-Sales
Bharat Desai, Chmn.

Phone: 248-619-2800	Fax: 248-619-2888
Toll-Free:	
Address: 525 E. Big Beaver Rd., 3rd. Fl., Troy, MI 48083 US	

GROWTH PLANS/SPECIAL FEATURES:
Syntel, Inc. delivers flexible, custom information technology (IT) and business process outsourcing (BPO) services to its Global 2000 companies and government entities. Service offerings are grouped into four segments: Applications Outsourcing, which outsources services for ongoing management, development and maintenance of business applications; e-Business, which focuses on Internet services, customer relationship management and data warehousing; KPO, which focuses on transaction processing, loan servicing, retirement processing and collections; and TeamSourcing, which consists of professional IT consulting service and responsiveness. The Applications outsourcing division assumes responsibility for and manages application support for clients; this division contributes 72% of consolidated revenues. The e-business unit provides customized technology services in web solutions (including architecture, web-enablement of legacy applications and portal development), customer relationship management services and maintains alliances with major IT application software infrastructure providers (such as IBM, Oracle and AB Initio); this division accounts for 14% of revenues. The BPO division focuses on the financial services, health care and insurance sectors and operates through the use of Identeon, which assists in strategic assessments of business processes; it accounts for 8% of revenue. Finally, TeamSourcing provides professional IT consulting services including systems specification, design, development, implementation and maintenance of applications involving diverse computer hardware, software and networking technologies; it accounts for 6% of total revenues. The Services Procurement Optimization program tackles procurement challenges by focusing on reducing overall spend while improving business efficiency through process optimization. Syntel's focus and priorities are on the benefits new delivery models unique to each business' need.

FINANCIALS: Sales and profits are in thousands of dollars—add 000 to get the full amount. 2007 Note: Financial information for 2007 was not available for all companies at press time.

2007 Sales: $337,673	2007 Profits: $62,860	**U.S. Stock Ticker: SYNT**
2006 Sales: $270,229	2006 Profits: $50,916	**Int'l Ticker:** Int'l Exchange:
2005 Sales: $226,189	2005 Profits: $30,321	Employees: 11,709
2004 Sales: $186,573	2004 Profits: $40,974	Fiscal Year Ends: 12/31
2003 Sales: $179,500	2003 Profits: $40,300	Parent Company:

SALARIES/BENEFITS:

Pension Plan:	ESOP Stock Plan:	Profit Sharing:	Top Exec. Salary: $300,000	Bonus: $
Savings Plan: Y	Stock Purch. Plan: Y		Second Exec. Salary: $204,326	Bonus: $100,000

OTHER THOUGHTS:
Apparent Women Officers or Directors:
Hot Spot for Advancement for Women/Minorities:

LOCATIONS: ("Y" = Yes)

West:	Southwest:	Midwest:	Southeast:	Northeast:	International:
Y	Y	Y		Y	Y

SYSCO CORP

www.sysco.com

Industry Group Code: 422410 Ranks within this company's industry group: Sales: 1 Profits: 1

Management:		Sales/Marketing:		Liberal Arts:		Information Systems:		Professionals:		Technical/Scientific:	
Mgmt. Trainees:	Y	Mktg. Professionals:	Y	Gen. Writing/Editing:	Y	Info. Management:	Y	Finance/Accounting:	Y	Engineers, Elec.:	
Experienced Mgmt.:	Y	Retail Sales:		Technical Writing:		Software Dev.:	Y	Law:	Y	Engineers, Other:	
Int'l Business:	Y	Commercial/Industrial:	Y	Graphic Arts/Photog.:	Y	Hardware Dev.:		HR/Other:	Y	Health/Lab:	
MBA Graduates:	Y	Sales Trainees:	Y	Music:		Systems Integration:		Training:	Y	Scientists/Research:	
		Advertising Pros.:	Y	Broadcasting:		Consulting/Other:		Health Care:		Petroleum/Chemicals:	
				Other:				Consulting:		Math/Other:	

TYPES OF BUSINESS:

Food-Wholesale Distribution
Restaurant Supplies Distribution
Medical & Surgical Supplies Distribution
Cleaning Supplies Distribution

BRANDS/DIVISIONS/AFFILIATES:

SYGMA Network
Baugh Supply Chain Cooperative
Bunn Capitol

CONTACTS: *Note: Officers with more than one job title may be intentionally listed here more than once.*

Richard J. Schnieders, CEO
Kenneth F. Spitler, COO/Pres.
William J. DeLaney, III, CFO/Exec. VP
James D. Hope, Sr. VP-Sales & Mktg
Thomas P. Randt, VP-Employee Rel.
Lucas Wagenaar, VP-IT
Twila M. Day, CIO/VP
Kenneth J. Carrig, Chief Admin. Officer/Exec. VP
Michael C. Nichols, General Counsel/Sr. VP/Corp. Sec.
James E. Lankford, Sr. VP-Foodservice Oper. (South Region)
Robert J. Davis, Sr. VP-Market Development
Mark A. Palmer, VP-Corp. Comm.
Neil A. Russell, VP-Investor Rel.
Kirk G. Drummond, Sr. VP-Finance/Treasurer
William B. Day, Sr. VP-Supply Chain
James M. Danahy, Sr. VP-Foodservice Oper. (Northeast Region)
Albert L. Gaylor, VP-Industry Rel. & Diversity
William B. Day, Sr. VP-Supply Chain
Richard J. Schnieders, Chmn.
Lesley J. Woodard, CEO/Pres., SYSCO Food Services of Quebec
Larry G. Pulliam, Exec. VP-Global Sourcing & Supply Chain

Phone: 281-584-1390	Fax: 281-584-2721
Toll-Free:	
Address: 1390 Enclave Pkwy., Houston, TX 77077-2099 US	

GROWTH PLANS/SPECIAL FEATURES:

SYSCO Corp., through its subsidiaries, is one of the largest distributors of food and food-related products to the foodservice industry in North America. The firm provides products and services to more than 400,000 customers, including restaurants, healthcare and educational facilities and lodging establishments. Restaurants accounted for 63% of the company's sales in 2007. Hospitals and nursing homes accounted for 10%; school and colleges accounted for 5%; hotels and motels accounted for 6%; and 16% fell into the other category. SYSCO distributes a wide variety of frozen foods, fresh meats, imported foods, fresh produce and nonfood items, including tableware, restaurant and kitchen equipment and supplies, medical and surgical supplies and cleaning supplies. Subsidiary SYGMA Network specializes in serving chain restaurants, especially Wendy's International, which accounts for 5% of SYSCO's sales and 39% of SYGMA's sales. Subsidiary Baugh Supply Chain Cooperative covers the purchasing and marketing of SYSCO-brand merchandise, as well as private-label and national-brand merchandise. The firm operates 180 distribution facilities throughout the U.S. and Canada, with a fleet of approximately 9,100 delivery trucks; approximately 87% of these vehicles are owned. SYSCO has recently begun to transform its supply chain management with plans to launch up to seven redistribution centers, the first of which was completed in Fort Royal, Virginia. This system will reduce the size of the firm's fleet of delivery trucks and their loading and unloading times. The company's primary focus is on growing and optimizing the core foodservice distribution business in North America, however it will also continue to explore and identify opportunities to grow its global capabilities and stay abreast of international acquisition opportunities.

SYSCO offers its employees annual performance incentives; employee assistance program; tuition assistance; a retirement plan; stock purchase plan; matching charity gifts; 401(k); performance incentives; and product discounts.

FINANCIALS: Sales and profits are in thousands of dollars—add 000 to get the full amount. 2007 Note: Financial information for 2007 was not available for all companies at press time.

2007 Sales: $35,042,075	2007 Profits: $1,001,076	**U.S. Stock Ticker:** SYY
2006 Sales: $32,628,438	2006 Profits: $855,325	**Int'l Ticker:** Int'l Exchange:
2005 Sales: $30,281,914	2005 Profits: $961,457	Employees: 50,900
2004 Sales: $29,335,403	2004 Profits: $907,214	Fiscal Year Ends: 6/30
2003 Sales: $26,140,337	2003 Profits: $778,288	Parent Company:

SALARIES/BENEFITS:

Pension Plan: Y	ESOP Stock Plan:	Profit Sharing:	Top Exec. Salary: $1,062,500	Bonus: $
Savings Plan: Y	Stock Purch. Plan: Y		Second Exec. Salary: $580,000	Bonus: $

OTHER THOUGHTS:

Apparent Women Officers or Directors: 10
Hot Spot for Advancement for Women/Minorities: Y

LOCATIONS: ("Y" = Yes)

West:	Southwest:	Midwest:	Southeast:	Northeast:	International:
Y	Y	Y	Y	Y	Y

TALBOTS INC (THE)

www.thetalbotsinc.com

Industry Group Code: 448120 Ranks within this company's industry group: Sales: 6 Profits: 5

Management:		Sales/Marketing:		Liberal Arts:		Information Systems:		Professionals:		Technical/Scientific:	
Mgmt. Trainees:	Y	Mktg. Professionals:	Y	Gen. Writing/Editing:	Y	Info. Management:	Y	Finance/Accounting:	Y	Engineers, Elec.:	
Experienced Mgmt.:	Y	Retail Sales:	Y	Technical Writing:		Software Dev.:	Y	Law:	Y	Engineers, Other:	
Int'l Business:	Y	Commercial/Industrial:	Y	Graphic Arts/Photog.:	Y	Hardware Dev.:		HR/Other:	Y	Health/Lab:	
MBA Graduates:	Y	Sales Trainees:	Y	Music:		Systems Integration:		Training:	Y	Scientists/Research:	
		Advertising Pros.:	Y	Broadcasting:		Consulting/Other:		Health Care:		Petroleum/Chemicals:	
				Other:	Y			Consulting:		Math/Other:	

TYPES OF BUSINESS:

Women's Apparel, Retail
Children's Apparel
Footwear
Accessories
Online & Catalog Sales
Men's Apparel

BRANDS/DIVISIONS/AFFILIATES:

J. Jill Group, Inc. (The)
Talbots Woman
Talbots Outlet
Talbots Petite
Talbots Misses
Talbots Accessories & Shoes
Talbots Mens
AEON

CONTACTS: Note: Officers with more than one job title may be intentionally listed here more than once.

Trudy F. Sullivan, CEO
Philip H. Kowalczyk, COO
Trudy F. Sullivan, Pres.
Edward L. Larsen, CFO
John Fiske III, Sr. VP-Human Resources
Randy Richardon, Sr. VP-Info. Svcs.
John Fiske, III, Exec. VP-Admin.
Richard T. O'Connell, Jr., Corp. Sec./Exec. VP-Legal & Real Estate
Betsy Thompson, Dir.-Corp. Comm. & Public Rel.
Julie Lorigan, Sr. VP-Investor Rel.
Edward L. Larsen, Sr. VP-Finance/Treas.
Michele M. Mandell, Exec. VP-Retail Talbots Brand
Paula Bennett, Pres., J. Jill Brand
Bruce Lee Prescott, Sr. VP-Direct Mktg, Talbots Brand & Customer Svcs.
Michael Smaldone, Chief Creative Officer
Tom Kajita, Chmn.
Gregory Poole, Exec. VP-Supply Chain Officer

Phone: 781-749-7600	**Fax:** 781-741-4369
Toll-Free: 800-825-2687	
Address: One Talbots Dr., Hingham, MA 02043-1586 US	

GROWTH PLANS/SPECIAL FEATURES:

Talbots, Inc. is a leading international specialty retailer and cataloger of women's, children's, and men's apparel, accessories and shoes. The company currently operates 1,421 stores in 47 states, Washington, D.C., Canada and the U.K. Talbots brand stores include 541 Misses stores; 298 Petites stores; 37 Accessories & Shoes stores; 63 Kids stores; 142 Woman stores; 12 Men's stores; two Collection stores; and 24 Outlet stores. In addition to its single-concept stores, the company operates superstores, which combine three or more concepts into one store, as well as a new basic men's wear line. The company is a limited-promotion retailer, with six sale events annually. Talbots stores and catalogs offer a collection of classic sportswear, casual wear, dresses, coats, sweaters, accessories and shoes, consisting primarily of Talbots' own private-label merchandise in misses, woman and petite sizes. Talbots Kids stores, some of which contain Talbots Babies departments, offer an assortment of clothing and accessories for infants, toddlers, boys and girls. Talbots circulated approximately 126 million catalogs worldwide in 2007. Of these catalogs, 48 million were under the Talbots brand and 78 million under the J. Jill brand. In addition to retail operations and catalogs, Talbots operates an e-commerce site, Talbots.com. About 19% of total revenues are generated by catalogs and the web site. As of September 2008, Talbots has closed its 78 Talbots Kids and Talbots Mens stores. In addition, the firm plans to close 20 underperforming Talbots and J. Jill brand stores, including all three stores in the U.K. in 2008. In July 2008, Talbots announced it would reduce its corporate staff by 9%. In 2008, the company put expansion on hold.

The company offers its employees an associate merchandise discount; health and dental insurance; paid time off, life and disability insurance and tuition assistance.

FINANCIALS: Sales and profits are in thousands of dollars—add 000 to get the full amount. 2007 Note: Financial information for 2007 was not available for all companies at press time.

2007 Sales: $2,231,033	2007 Profits: $31,576	**U.S. Stock Ticker: TLB**	
2006 Sales: $1,808,606	2006 Profits: $93,151	**Int'l Ticker:**	Int'l Exchange:
2005 Sales: $1,697,843	2005 Profits: $95,366	Employees: 16,102	
2004 Sales: $1,624,339	2004 Profits: $104,683	Fiscal Year Ends: 1/31	
2003 Sales: $1,595,300	2003 Profits: $120,800	Parent Company:	

SALARIES/BENEFITS:

Pension Plan:	ESOP Stock Plan:	Profit Sharing:	Top Exec. Salary: $1,197,792	Bonus: $359,300
Savings Plan: Y	Stock Purch. Plan:		Second Exec. Salary: $596,334	Bonus: $176,600

OTHER THOUGHTS:

Apparent Women Officers or Directors: 6
Hot Spot for Advancement for Women/Minorities: Y

LOCATIONS: ("Y" = Yes)

West:	Southwest:	Midwest:	Southeast:	Northeast:	International:
Y	Y	Y	Y	Y	Y

TARGET CORPORATION
www.target.com

Industry Group Code: 452910   Ranks within this company's industry group: Sales: 2   Profits: 2

Management:		Sales/Marketing:		Liberal Arts:		Information Systems:		Professionals:		Technical/Scientific:	
Mgmt. Trainees:	Y	Mktg. Professionals:	Y	Gen. Writing/Editing:	Y	Info. Management:	Y	Finance/Accounting:	Y	Engineers, Elec.:	
Experienced Mgmt.:	Y	Retail Sales:	Y	Technical Writing:		Software Dev.:	Y	Law:	Y	Engineers, Other:	
Int'l Business:	Y	Commercial/Industrial:	Y	Graphic Arts/Photog.:	Y	Hardware Dev.:		HR/Other:	Y	Health/Lab:	
MBA Graduates:	Y	Sales Trainees:	Y	Music:		Systems Integration:		Training:	Y	Scientists/Research:	
		Advertising Pros.:	Y	Broadcasting:		Consulting/Other:		Health Care:		Petroleum/Chemicals:	
				Other:	Y			Consulting:		Math/Other:	

TYPES OF BUSINESS:

Discount Department Stores
Online Sales
Catalog Sales
Groceries
Credit Cards

BRANDS/DIVISIONS/AFFILIATES:

SuperTarget
target.com
Market Pantry
Archer Farms
Merona
Xhilaration
Choxie
Target Card

CONTACTS: *Note: Officers with more than one job title may be intentionally listed here more than once.*

Gregg W. Steinhafel, CEO
Gregg W. Steinhafel, Pres.
Douglas A. Scovanner, CFO/Exec. VP
Michael R. Francis, Exec. VP-Mktg.
Jodeen A. Kozlak, Exec. VP-Human Resources
Janet M. Schalk, Sr. VP-Tech. Svcs.
Beth M. Jacob, CIO/Sr. VP-Tech. Svcs.
Kathryn A. Tesija, Exec. VP-Merch.
Timothy R. Baer, General Counsel/Corp. Sec./Exec. VP
Ellen Tansey, Exec. VP-Target Sourcing Svcs., Global Oper.
John D. Griffith, Exec. VP-Property Dev.
Steve Eastman, Pres., Target.com
Susan D. Kahn, VP-Comm.
Susan D. Kahn, VP-Investor Rel.
Jane P. Windmeier, Sr. VP-Finance
Troy H. Risch, Exec. VP-Stores
Terrence J. Scully, Pres., Target Financial Svcs.
Stacia J. Anderson, Pres., Target Sourcing Svcs.
Carmela Batacchi, Sr. VP-Target Sourcing Svcs., Regions II & III
Robert J. Ulrich, Chmn.
Mitchell L. Stover, Sr. VP-Dist.

Phone: 612-304-6073	Fax: 612-696-3731
Toll-Free:	
Address: 1000 Nicollet Mall, Minneapolis, MN 55403 US	

GROWTH PLANS/SPECIAL FEATURES:

Target Corporation operates large-format general merchandise and food discount stores in the U.S., which include Target and SuperTarget stores. The company operates 1,500 stores in 47 states, as well as 26 regional distribution centers in 19 states. Target also owns 231 SuperTarget stores, which combine grocery and general merchandise in a superstore format. SuperTarget stores feature coffee bars, bakeries, banking areas, pharmacies and photo services. The company also has operations in India, with its third facility under construction and a fourth planned for 2009. Target store merchandise includes men's, women's and children's apparel, housewares, electronics, CDs and DVDs, toys, sporting goods, books and personal care items. The median age of Target customers is 42, and the median household income is approximately $58,000; about 33% have children at home and 51% have completed college. Target successfully positions itself as more upscale than most other discount retailers by offering exclusively branded products from designers such as Michael Graves, Todd Oldham and Isaac Mizrahi. In addition, Target sells merchandise under its own private-label brands including, Market Pantry, Archer Farms, Merona, Xhilaration, Choxie, Trutech and Target Limited Edition. The company's branded proprietary credit card products (REDcard) are an integral component of its retail business. Target also sells merchandise via its e-commerce site, Target.com, the sales from which are growing at a much more rapid annual pace than the company's other sales. Sales per square foot per year average about $310.

Target offers it employees dental coverage, prescription drug coverage, educational loans, tuition reimbursement, home loans, home buyer's assistance, adoption assistance, a legal services plan, child care assistance, fitness center discounts, a Sprint PCS discount, a Dell computer system discount, tax preparation assistance, a credit union membership and Target purchase discounts.

FINANCIALS: Sales and profits are in thousands of dollars—add 000 to get the full amount. 2007 Note: Financial information for 2007 was not available for all companies at press time.

2007 Sales: $63,367,000	2007 Profits: $2,849,000	**U.S. Stock Ticker: TGT**
2006 Sales: $59,490,000	2006 Profits: $2,787,000	**Int'l Ticker:** Int'l Exchange:
2005 Sales: $52,620,000	2005 Profits: $2,408,000	Employees: 366,000
2004 Sales: $48,163,000	2004 Profits: $1,841,000	Fiscal Year Ends: 1/31
2003 Sales: $43,917,000	2003 Profits: $1,654,000	Parent Company:

SALARIES/BENEFITS:

Pension Plan:	ESOP Stock Plan:	Profit Sharing:	Top Exec. Salary: $1,659,616	Bonus: $6,128,960
Savings Plan: Y	Stock Purch. Plan: Y		Second Exec. Salary: $1,130,000	Bonus: $1,043,608

OTHER THOUGHTS:

Apparent Women Officers or Directors: 15
Hot Spot for Advancement for Women/Minorities: Y

LOCATIONS: ("Y" = Yes)

West:	Southwest:	Midwest:	Southeast:	Northeast:	International:
Y	Y	Y	Y	Y	Y

Note: Financial information, benefits and other data can change quickly and may vary from those stated here.

TBC CORPORATION

www.tbccorp.com

Industry Group Code: 441300 Ranks within this company's industry group: Sales: Profits:

Management:		Sales/Marketing:		Liberal Arts:		Information Systems:		Professionals:		Technical/Scientific:	
Mgmt. Trainees:	Y	Mktg. Professionals:	Y	Gen. Writing/Editing:	Y	Info. Management:	Y	Finance/Accounting:	Y	Engineers, Elec.:	
Experienced Mgmt.:	Y	Retail Sales:	Y	Technical Writing:		Software Dev.:	Y	Law:	Y	Engineers, Other:	
Int'l Business:	Y	Commercial/Industrial:	Y	Graphic Arts/Photog.:	Y	Hardware Dev.:		HR/Other:	Y	Health/Lab:	
MBA Graduates:	Y	Sales Trainees:	Y	Music:		Systems Integration:		Training:	Y	Scientists/Research:	
		Advertising Pros.:	Y	Broadcasting:		Consulting/Other:		Health Care:		Petroleum/Chemicals:	
				Other:				Consulting:		Math/Other:	

TYPES OF BUSINESS:

Tire Stores
Wholesale Tire Distribution

BRANDS/DIVISIONS/AFFILIATES:

Big O Tires, Inc.
Tire Kingdom, Inc.
Cordovan
Multi-Mile
Sigma
National Tire & Battery
Carroll Tire Company
Vanderbilt Tires

CONTACTS: Note: Officers with more than one job title may be intentionally listed here more than once.

Lawrence C. Day, CEO
Lawrence C. Day, Pres.
Orland M. Wolford, Pres./CEO-Tire Kingdom
John B. Adams, Pres./CEO-Big O Tires, Inc.
Kenneth P. Dick, Pres./CEO-TBC Wholesale Div.
J. Glen Gravatt, Exec. VP-Purchasing

Phone: 561-227-0955	Fax:
Toll-Free:	
Address: 7111 Fairway Dr., Ste. 201, Palm Beach Gardens, FL 33418 US	

GROWTH PLANS/SPECIAL FEATURES:

TBC Corporation markets and distributes replacement automobile tires, through wholesale and retail operations. The wholesale segment of TBC's business markets and distributes its proprietary brands of tires, as well as other tires and related products, through a network of distributors covering the U.S., Canada and Mexico. The company also markets directly to independent tire dealers in the Eastern and Southeastern United States through its Carroll Tire wholesale distribution centers. Tires marketed under the company's proprietary brand trademarks are produced under contract with leading manufacturers, and include the Cordovan, Multi-Mile, Sigma, Vanderbilt and Big O brands of tires. The firm also distributes tires under other brands for automobile, truck, sport utility vehicle, farm, industrial, recreational and other applications. The retail segment of the company's business consists of both the franchised retail tire business conducted by the company's Big O Tires, Inc. subsidiary, as well as the retail tire stores operated by subsidiary Tire Kingdom, Inc. TBC also operates the National Tire and Battery chain, which it acquired from Sears Roebuck and Co. In addition to retail tire sales, TBC stores provide full service tire replacement including balancing, wheel alignment, extended service programs and warranties, as well as additional services such as brake repairs, suspension system replacement and oil changes. The firm owns and operates over 1,100 retail locations, predominantly located in the eastern two-thirds of the U.S., and 32 warehouse locations. TBC is owned by the Sumitomo Corporation, one of Japan's largest integrated trading and investment business organizations.

FINANCIALS: Sales and profits are in thousands of dollars—add 000 to get the full amount. 2007 Note: Financial information for 2007 was not available for all companies at press time.

2007 Sales: $1,779,400	2007 Profits: $	**U.S. Stock Ticker: Subsidiary**
2006 Sales: $	2006 Profits: $	**Int'l Ticker:** Int'l Exchange:
2005 Sales: $	2005 Profits: $	Employees: 9,400
2004 Sales: $1,855,418	2004 Profits: $37,598	Fiscal Year Ends: 12/31
2003 Sales: $1,318,500	2003 Profits: $33,400	Parent Company: SUMITOMO CORPORATION

SALARIES/BENEFITS:

Pension Plan:	ESOP Stock Plan:	Profit Sharing:	Top Exec. Salary: $607,889	Bonus: $290,024
Savings Plan:	Stock Purch. Plan:		Second Exec. Salary: $331,923	Bonus: $110,000

OTHER THOUGHTS:

Apparent Women Officers or Directors:
Hot Spot for Advancement for Women/Minorities:

LOCATIONS: ("Y" = Yes)

West:	Southwest:	Midwest:	Southeast:	Northeast:	International:
Y	Y		Y		Y

TECH DATA CORP

www.techdata.com

Industry Group Code: 421430 Ranks within this company's industry group: Sales: 2 Profits: 2

Management:		Sales/Marketing:		Liberal Arts:		Information Systems:		Professionals:		Technical/Scientific:	
Mgmt. Trainees:	Y	Mktg. Professionals:	Y	Gen. Writing/Editing:		Info. Management:	Y	Finance/Accounting:	Y	Engineers, Elec.:	
Experienced Mgmt.:	Y	Retail Sales:		Technical Writing:	Y	Software Dev.:	Y	Law:	Y	Engineers, Other:	
Int'l Business:	Y	Commercial/Industrial:	Y	Graphic Arts/Photog.:	Y	Hardware Dev.:		HR/Other:	Y	Health/Lab:	
MBA Graduates:	Y	Sales Trainees:		Music:		Systems Integration:		Training:	Y	Scientists/Research:	
		Advertising Pros.:		Broadcasting:		Consulting/Other:		Health Care:		Petroleum/Chemicals:	
				Other:				Consulting:		Math/Other:	

TYPES OF BUSINESS:
Computer & Software Products, Distribution
Training
Assembly Services

BRANDS/DIVISIONS/AFFILIATES:
Tech Data Germany AG
Globelle Corp.

CONTACTS: *Note: Officers with more than one job title may be intentionally listed here more than once.*
Robert M. Dutkowsky, CEO
Jeffery P. Howells, CFO/Exec. VP
Joseph A. Osbourn, Worldwide CIO/Exec. VP
David R. Vetter, General Counsel/Sr. VP/Sec.
Charles V. Dannewitz, Treas./Sr. VP-Taxes
Kenneth Lamneck, Pres., Americas
Joseph B. Trepani, Controller/Sr. VP
Steven A. Raymund, Chmn.
Nestor Cano, Pres., Europe
William K. Todd, Jr., Sr. VP-Logistics & Integration Svcs.

Phone: 727-539-7429	Fax: 727-538-7803
Toll-Free: 800-237-8931	
Address: 5350 Tech Data Dr., Clearwater, FL 33760 US	

GROWTH PLANS/SPECIAL FEATURES:

Tech Data Corp. is a worldwide distributor of information technology (IT) products, logistics management and other value-added services. It sells more than 100,000 products from peripheral, system and networking manufacturers and software publishers such as Acer, Adobe, American Power, Apple, Asus Computer, Autodesk, Canon, Cisco Systems, Epson, Fujitsu-Siemens, Hewlett-Packard, IBM, Kingston, Lexmark, Lenovo, Microsoft, Nortel Networks, Samsung, Sony, Symantec, Toshiba, Viewsonic and Xerox. Products are generally shipped from regionally located logistics centers the same day the orders are received. Products are typically purchased directly from the manufacturer or software publisher on a non-exclusive basis. The company's vendor agreements do not restrict it from selling similar products manufactured by competitors, nor do they require it to sell a specified quantity of product. The firm also provides extensive pre- and post-sale training, service and support, as well as configuration and assembly services and e-commerce tools. Tech Data provides products and services to the online reseller channel and does business with thousands of resellers via its web site. The firm's entire electronic catalog is available online, and its electronic software distribution initiative allows resellers and vendors to easily access software titles directly from a secure location on the web site. The company serves more than 90,000 customers, including resellers, direct marketers, retailers and corporate resellers in more than 100 countries in North America, the Caribbean, Latin America, Europe, the Middle East and Africa. It owns Tech Data Germany AG, a European distributor, and Globelle Corp., a Canadian information technology firm.

The company offers its employees medical, dental and life insurance; short- and long-term disability insurance; tuition reimbursement; a 401(k) plan; and an employee stock purchase program.

FINANCIALS: Sales and profits are in thousands of dollars—add 000 to get the full amount. 2007 Note: Financial information for 2007 was not available for all companies at press time.

2007 Sales: $21,440,445	2007 Profits: $-96,981	U.S. Stock Ticker: TECD	
2006 Sales: $20,482,851	2006 Profits: $26,586	Int'l Ticker: Int'l Exchange:	
2005 Sales: $19,730,917	2005 Profits: $162,460	Employees: 8,000	
2004 Sales: $17,358,525	2004 Profits: $104,147	Fiscal Year Ends: 1/31	
2003 Sales: $15,738,945	2003 Profits: $-199,800	Parent Company:	

SALARIES/BENEFITS:

Pension Plan:	ESOP Stock Plan:	Profit Sharing:	Top Exec. Salary: $1,000,000	Bonus: $935,000
Savings Plan: Y	Stock Purch. Plan: Y		Second Exec. Salary: $650,000	Bonus: $243,800

OTHER THOUGHTS:
Apparent Women Officers or Directors: 1
Hot Spot for Advancement for Women/Minorities:

LOCATIONS: ("Y" = Yes)

West:	Southwest:	Midwest:	Southeast:	Northeast:	International:
Y	Y	Y	Y	Y	Y

TEKTRONIX INC

www.tek.com

Industry Group Code: 334500 Ranks within this company's industry group: Sales: 5   Profits: 5

Management:		Sales/Marketing:		Liberal Arts:		Information Systems:		Professionals:		Technical/Scientific:	
Mgmt. Trainees:		Mktg. Professionals:		Gen. Writing/Editing:		Info. Management:	Y	Finance/Accounting:	Y	Engineers, Elec.:	Y
Experienced Mgmt.:	Y	Retail Sales:		Technical Writing:	Y	Software Dev.:	Y	Law:	Y	Engineers, Other:	Y
Int'l Business:	Y	Commercial/Industrial:	Y	Graphic Arts/Photog.:		Hardware Dev.:	Y	HR/Other:	Y	Health/Lab:	
MBA Graduates:	Y	Sales Trainees:		Music:		Systems Integration:	Y	Training:	Y	Scientists/Research:	
		Advertising Pros.:		Broadcasting:		Consulting/Other:		Health Care:		Petroleum/Chemicals:	
				Other:				Consulting:		Math/Other:	

TYPES OF BUSINESS:

Test & Measurement Equipment
Support Services
Oscilloscopes
Logic analyzers
Video test equipment
Communications test equipment

BRANDS/DIVISIONS/AFFILIATES:

MAXTEK
TEKTRONIX
Danaher Corp

CONTACTS: Note: Officers with more than one job title may be intentionally listed here more than once.

Jim Lico, Pres.
Gary Grossman, Sr. Mgr.-Press Rel.
Neil Huddlestone, Pres., Tektronix China
Arif Kareem, VP-Video Products
Fuki Yoneyama, Pres., Japan Region/ VP-Japan Sales

Phone: 503-627-1000	Fax:
Toll-Free: 800-835-9433	
Address: 14200 SW Karl Braun Dr., Beaverton, OR 97077 US	

GROWTH PLANS/SPECIAL FEATURES:

Tektronix, Inc. develops, manufactures and markets test, measurement and monitoring products to a wide variety of customers in the computing, communications semiconductors, education, computer, military/aerospace, research and consumer electronics industries. The company is organized under two business platforms, instruments and communications. The instruments sector provides general purpose testing products and video test, measurement and monitoring products, which includes oscilloscopes, logic analyzers, signal sources and spectrum analyzers. Additional video products include waveform monitors, video signal generators, compressed digital video test products and other test and measurement for video equipment manufacturers, content developers and traditional television broadcasters. The general testing products are designed to capture, display and analyze streams of electrical data, while video products ensure the delivery of the best possible video experience to the viewer. Tektronix's communications sector offers telecommunications network management and network diagnostics products. Network management products consist of network monitoring systems that actively test networks and provide troubleshooting, provisioning and automated service quality monitoring. The firm's products are sold under the TEKTRONIX and MAXTEK brand names. In 2007, Tektronix was bought by Danaher Corporation and because its subsidiary. Danaher Corporation is a designer and manufacturer of a variety of professional, medical, industrial and consumer products.

Tektronix offers employees medical coverage, educational reimbursement and a 401(k) savings plan.

FINANCIALS: Sales and profits are in thousands of dollars—add 000 to get the full amount. 2007 Note: Financial information for 2007 was not available for all companies at press time.

2007 Sales: $1,105,172	2007 Profits: $90,408	**U.S. Stock Ticker: Subsidiary**
2006 Sales: $1,039,870	2006 Profits: $92,355	**Int'l Ticker:** Int'l Exchange:
2005 Sales: $1,034,654	2005 Profits: $81,596	Employees: 4,541
2004 Sales: $920,620	2004 Profits: $116,095	Fiscal Year Ends:
2003 Sales: $103,819	2003 Profits: $25,329	Parent Company: DANAHER CORP

SALARIES/BENEFITS:

Pension Plan:	ESOP Stock Plan:	Profit Sharing:	Top Exec. Salary: $648,077	Bonus: $472,900
Savings Plan:	Stock Purch. Plan:		Second Exec. Salary: $349,231	Bonus: $165,600

OTHER THOUGHTS:

Apparent Women Officers or Directors:
Hot Spot for Advancement for Women/Minorities:

LOCATIONS: ("Y" = Yes)

West:	Southwest:	Midwest:	Southeast:	Northeast:	International:
Y	Y			Y	Y

TELEDYNE TECHNOLOGIES INCORPORATED

www.teledyne.com

Industry Group Code: 336410 Ranks within this company's industry group: Sales: 8 Profits: 8

Management:		Sales/Marketing:		Liberal Arts:		Information Systems:		Professionals:		Technical/Scientific:	
Mgmt. Trainees:		Mktg. Professionals:		Gen. Writing/Editing:		Info. Management:	Y	Finance/Accounting:	Y	Engineers, Elec.:	Y
Experienced Mgmt.:	Y	Retail Sales:		Technical Writing:		Software Dev.:	Y	Law:		Engineers, Other:	Y
Int'l Business:		Commercial/Industrial:		Graphic Arts/Photog.:		Hardware Dev.:	Y	HR/Other:		Health/Lab:	Y
MBA Graduates:	Y	Sales Trainees:		Music:		Systems Integration:		Training:	Y	Scientists/Research:	Y
		Advertising Pros.:		Broadcasting:		Consulting/Other:		Health Care:		Petroleum/Chemicals:	Y
				Other:				Consulting:		Math/Other:	Y

TYPES OF BUSINESS:

Electronics & Communications Products
Systems Engineering Solutions
Aerospace Engines & Components
Energy Systems

BRANDS/DIVISIONS/AFFILIATES:

Teledyne Isco Inc
Teledyne Brown Engineering
Teledyne Tekmar Co
Teledyne Solutions Inc
Teledyne Energy Systems Inc
Teledyne Cougar Inc
Teledyne Titan
Tindall Technologies Inc

CONTACTS: Note: Officers with more than one job title may be intentionally listed here more than once.

Robert Mehrabian, CEO
Robert Mehrabian, Pres.
Dale A. Schnittjer, CFO/Sr. VP
Robyn E. McGowan, VP-Human Resources
Robert W. Steenberge, CTO/VP
Robyn E. McGowan, VP-Admin.
John T. Kuelbs, General Counsel/Exec. VP/Sec.
Jason VanWees, VP-Corp. Dev.
Jason VanWees, VP-Investor Rel.
Susan L. Main, Controller/VP
Ivars R. Blukis, Chief Bus. Risk Assurance Officer
Aldo Pichelli, COO/Sr. VP-Electronics & Comm. Segment
Bryan R. Lewis, Pres., Teledyne Continental Motors
Rex Geveden, Pres., Teledyne Brown Eng.
Robert Mehrabian, Chmn.

Phone: 805-373-4545	Fax: 805-373-4775
Toll-Free:	
Address: 1049 Camino Dos Rios, Thousand Oaks, CA 91360 US	

GROWTH PLANS/SPECIAL FEATURES:

Teledyne Technologies, Inc. provides electronic components, instruments and communications products including defense electronics, monitoring and control instrumentation for marine, environmental and industrial applications; data acquisition and communications equipment for airlines and business aircraft and components; and subsystems for wireless and satellite communications. The company also provides systems engineering and information technology services for defense, space and environmental applications, and manufactures general aviation engines and components, supply energy generation, energy storage and small propulsion products. The firm operates in four segments, electronics and communications, responsible for 66% of revenue in 2007; engineered systems, which accounted for 19% of revenue in 2007; aerospace engines and components, which generated 11% of revenue; and energy and power systems, 4%. Subsidiaries include Teledyne Isco, Inc., a producer of water quality monitoring products such as wastewater samplers and open channel flow meters; Teledyne Brown Engineering, a full-service missile defense contractor; Teledyne Solutions, Inc., a missile defense systems engineering contractor for the U.S. Army; Teledyne Energy Systems, Inc., a provider of Teledyne Titan hydrogen gas generators and thermoelectric and fuel cell-based power sources; and Teledyne Tekmar Co., a manufacturer of instruments that automate the preparation and concentrations of drinking water and wastewater. Teledyne Technologies operates the Rapid Response System, a mobile chemical waste treatment system used to process chemical agents. Customers include government agencies; aerospace prime contractors; major industrial, communications and aviation companies. In 2007, the firm acquired Storm Products Co and the assets of Impulse Enterprise. In February 2008, it acquired assets of Judson Technologies, LLC, which manufactures infrared detectors. In January 2008, the firm acquired S G Brown Limited and its wholly-owned subsidiary TSS (International) Limited, which is headquartered in Watford, U. K. In July 2008, it acquired assets of Webb Research Corp. In August 2008, it acquired Filtronic PLC in the U.K.

FINANCIALS: Sales and profits are in thousands of dollars—add 000 to get the full amount. 2007 Note: Financial information for 2007 was not available for all companies at press time.

		U.S. Stock Ticker: TDY
2007 Sales: $1,622,300	2007 Profits: $98,500	
2006 Sales: $1,433,200	2006 Profits: $80,300	Int'l Ticker: Int'l Exchange:
2005 Sales: $1,206,500	2005 Profits: $64,200	Employees: 7,700
2004 Sales: $1,016,600	2004 Profits: $41,700	Fiscal Year Ends: 12/31
2003 Sales: $840,700	2003 Profits: $29,700	Parent Company:

SALARIES/BENEFITS:

Pension Plan:	ESOP Stock Plan:	Profit Sharing:	Top Exec. Salary: $718,271	Bonus: $1,200,000
Savings Plan:	Stock Purch. Plan:		Second Exec. Salary: $375,796	Bonus: $398,288

OTHER THOUGHTS:

Apparent Women Officers or Directors: 3
Hot Spot for Advancement for Women/Minorities: Y

LOCATIONS: ("Y" = Yes)

West:	Southwest:	Midwest:	Southeast:	Northeast:	International:
Y	Y	Y	Y	Y	Y

Note: Financial information, benefits and other data can change quickly and may vary from those stated here.

TELEPHONE AND DATA SYSTEMS INC (TDS) www.teldta.com

Industry Group Code: 513300A Ranks within this company's industry group: Sales: 2   Profits: 4

Management:		Sales/Marketing:		Liberal Arts:		Information Systems:		Professionals:		Technical/Scientific:	
Mgmt. Trainees:	Y	Mktg. Professionals:	Y	Gen. Writing/Editing:	Y	Info. Management:	Y	Finance/Accounting:	Y	Engineers, Elec.:	Y
Experienced Mgmt.:	Y	Retail Sales:		Technical Writing:	Y	Software Dev.:	Y	Law:	Y	Engineers, Other:	
Int'l Business:		Commercial/Industrial:	Y	Graphic Arts/Photog.:	Y	Hardware Dev.:		HR/Other:	Y	Health/Lab:	
MBA Graduates:	Y	Sales Trainees:		Music:		Systems Integration:		Training:	Y	Scientists/Research:	
		Advertising Pros.:	Y	Broadcasting:		Consulting/Other:		Health Care:		Petroleum/Chemicals:	
				Other:				Consulting:		Math/Other:	

TYPES OF BUSINESS:

Local Telephone Service
Cellular Telephone Services
Internet Access
Printing Services
Long-Distance Telephone Service
Data Networks

BRANDS/DIVISIONS/AFFILIATES:

US Cellular
TDS Telecom
TDS Metrocom
Suttle Straus, Inc.

CONTACTS: *Note: Officers with more than one job title may be intentionally listed here more than once.*

LeRoy T. Carlson, Jr., CEO
LeRoy T. Carlson, Jr., Pres.
Kenneth R. Meyers, CFO/Exec. VP
C. Theodore Herbert, VP-Human Resources
Kurt Thaus, CIO/Sr. VP
Joseph R. Hanley, VP-Tech. Planning & Svcs.
Kevin C. Gallagher, VP/Corp. Sec.
Scott H. Williamson, Sr. VP-Corp. Dev. & Acquisitions
Mark A. Steinkrauss, VP-Corp. Rel.
Douglas A. Shuma, Sr. VP/Corp. Controller
John E. Rooney, CEO/Pres., U.S. Cellular Corp.
David A. Wittwer, CEO/Pres., TDS Telecommunications Corp.
Peter L. Sereda, VP/Treas.
James Twesme, VP-Corp. Finance
Walter C. D. Carlson, Chmn.

Phone: 312-630-1900	Fax: 312-630-1908
Toll-Free:	
Address: 30 N. LaSalle St., Ste. 4000, Chicago, IL 60602 US	

GROWTH PLANS/SPECIAL FEATURES:

Telephone and Data Systems, Inc. (TDS), a Fortune 500 company, is a diversified telecommunications service company with wireless telephone and wireline telephone operations. It has approximately 7.3 million customers in 36 states. TDS has four subsidiary companies through which it operates: U.S. Cellular (USM), which generates the majority of revenues; TDS Telecommunications Corporation (TDS Telecom); TDS Metrocom; and Suttle-Strauss. The firm owns approximately 82% of USM, which is the nation's sixth-largest wireless telecommunications provider, with more than 6.1 million customers in five major regions of the U.S. TDS conducts substantially all its wireless operations through USM. TDS conducts its wireline telephone operations through wholly-owned subsidiary TDS Telecom. This branch offers local, long-distance, broadband and entertainment solutions. TDS Telecom serves rural and suburban communities in 30 states through its incumbent local exchange carrier (ILEC) business and its competitive local exchange carrier (CLEC) business, which operates under the brand TDS Metrocom. TDS Metrocom provides telecommunications services in a five-state footprint in the Midwest. Majority-owned subsidiary (80%) Suttle-Straus is a full-service printing and communications company that offers customers a wide range of services.

TDS offers its employees a comprehensive benefits package, including medical, dental, disability, vision and term life insurance plans; pension and 401(k) contributions; domestic partner coverage; a flexible spending account; career planning, education and training opportunities; and education reimbursement. The company also offers discounts for personal computers, new cars, fitness centers and Sam's Club memberships.

FINANCIALS: Sales and profits are in thousands of dollars—add 000 to get the full amount. 2007 Note: Financial information for 2007 was not available for all companies at press time.

2007 Sales: $4,829,000	2007 Profits: $386,100	**U.S. Stock Ticker: TDS**
2006 Sales: $4,364,500	2006 Profits: $161,800	**Int'l Ticker:** Int'l Exchange:
2005 Sales: $3,953,000	2005 Profits: $647,700	**Employees:** 7,837
2004 Sales: $3,720,400	2004 Profits: $49,000	**Fiscal Year Ends:** 12/31
2003 Sales: $3,417,900	2003 Profits: $61,500	**Parent Company:**

SALARIES/BENEFITS:

Pension Plan: Y	ESOP Stock Plan:	Profit Sharing:	Top Exec. Salary: $1,193,000	Bonus: $800,000
Savings Plan: Y	Stock Purch. Plan: Y		Second Exec. Salary: $790,000	Bonus: $525,000

OTHER THOUGHTS:

Apparent Women Officers or Directors:
Hot Spot for Advancement for Women/Minorities:

LOCATIONS: ("Y" = Yes)

West:	Southwest:	Midwest:	Southeast:	Northeast:	International:
Y	Y	Y	Y	Y	

TELETECH HOLDINGS INC

www.teletech.com

Industry Group Code: 561422 **Ranks within this company's industry group:** Sales: 2 Profits: 2

Management:		Sales/Marketing:		Liberal Arts:		Information Systems:		Professionals:		Technical/Scientific:	
Mgmt. Trainees:	Y	Mktg. Professionals:	Y	Gen. Writing/Editing:	Y	Info. Management:	Y	Finance/Accounting:	Y	Engineers, Elec.:	
Experienced Mgmt.:	Y	Retail Sales:		Technical Writing:		Software Dev.:	Y	Law:	Y	Engineers, Other:	
Int'l Business:	Y	Commercial/Industrial:	Y	Graphic Arts/Photog.:		Hardware Dev.:		HR/Other:	Y	Health/Lab:	
MBA Graduates:	Y	Sales Trainees:		Music:		Systems Integration:	Y	Training:	Y	Scientists/Research:	
		Advertising Pros.:	Y	Broadcasting:		Consulting/Other:		Health Care:		Petroleum/Chemicals:	
				Other:				Consulting:		Math/Other:	

TYPES OF BUSINESS:

Call Centers
Database & Direct Marketing Services
Outsourced Customer Service
Customer Retention Services
Consulting

BRANDS/DIVISIONS/AFFILIATES:

Percepta
Ford Motor Co.
Aspen Marketing Services, Inc.

CONTACTS: *Note: Officers with more than one job title may be intentionally listed here more than once.*

Kenneth Tuchman, CEO
John Troka, Jr., Interim CFO
John Simon, Exec. VP-Global Human Capital
Carol Kline, CIO/Exec. VP
Alan Schuzman, Exec. VP/General Counsel/Corp. Sec.
K.C. Higgins, Media Rel.
Jennifer Martin, Dir.-Investor Rel.
Karen Breen, VP-Investor Rel./Treas.
Brian Delaney, Exec. VP-Global Svcs. Delivery
James Barlett, Vice Chmn.
Judi Hand, Pres./General Mgr.-Direct Alliance Corp.
Kenneth Tuchman, Chmn.

Phone: 303-397-8100	Fax: 303-397-8671
Toll-Free: 800-835-3832	
Address: 9197 S. Peoria St., Englewood, CO 80112-5833 US	

GROWTH PLANS/SPECIAL FEATURES:

TeleTech Holdings, Inc. provides outsourced customer management services to a significant number of Global 1000 companies. The firm focuses on large global corporations in the automotive, communications and media, financial services, government, health care, logistics, retail, technology and travel industries. TeleTech has 88 office locations in 17 countries, and about 60% of the firm's revenue is generated outside the U.S. With service offered in 150 languages, TeleTech's customer management services business provides outsourced customer support and marketing services via call centers throughout the world. This business is divided into North American customer care, serving the U.S. and Canada, and international customer care. The customer management services business manages telephone, e-mail, automated/interactive voice response and web-based customer interactions. Services include customer acquisition, provisioning, support, development and other customer-related programs. This section represents approximately 89% of total revenue. Also within this segment is subsidiary Percepta, a joint venture with Ford Motor Company, which provides customer management services to Ford customers. TeleTech's database marketing and consulting business provides outsourced database management, direct marketing and related customer retention services for automotive dealerships and manufacturers in North America. In 2007, the firm sold its subsidiary Newgen Results Corp., its database marketing and consulting business, to Aspen Marketing Services, Inc. (Aspen), in conjunction with which it entered a multi-year software use agreement with Aspen. Also in 2007, TeleTech opened its first delivery center in San Jose, Costa Rica, to better serve global clients seeking multiple levels of support.

TeleTech offers its employees benefits including a dependent care reimbursement plan, tuition reimbursement and medical, dental and vision insurance.

FINANCIALS: Sales and profits are in thousands of dollars—add 000 to get the full amount. 2007 Note: Financial information for 2007 was not available for all companies at press time.

2007 Sales: $1,369,632	2007 Profits: $53,103	U.S. Stock Ticker: TTEC
2006 Sales: $1,210,753	2006 Profits: $50,981	Int'l Ticker: Int'l Exchange:
2005 Sales: $1,085,903	2005 Profits: $26,286	Employees: 53,000
2004 Sales: $1,052,690	2004 Profits: $24,003	Fiscal Year Ends: 12/31
2003 Sales: $992,340	2003 Profits: $-41,206	Parent Company:

SALARIES/BENEFITS:

Pension Plan:	ESOP Stock Plan:	Profit Sharing:	Top Exec. Salary: $350,000	Bonus: $
Savings Plan: Y	Stock Purch. Plan:		Second Exec. Salary: $275,000	Bonus: $550,000

OTHER THOUGHTS:

Apparent Women Officers or Directors: 4
Hot Spot for Advancement for Women/Minorities: Y

LOCATIONS: ("Y" = Yes)

West:	Southwest:	Midwest:	Southeast:	Northeast:	International:
Y	Y	Y	Y	Y	Y

Note: Financial information, benefits and other data can change quickly and may vary from those stated here.

TESORO CORP

www.tsocorp.com

Industry Group Code: 324110A Ranks within this company's industry group: Sales: Profits:

Management:		Sales/Marketing:		Liberal Arts:		Information Systems:		Professionals:		Technical/Scientific:	
Mgmt. Trainees:		Mktg. Professionals:		Gen. Writing/Editing:		Info. Management:	Y	Finance/Accounting:	Y	Engineers, Elec.:	Y
Experienced Mgmt.:	Y	Retail Sales:		Technical Writing:		Software Dev.:		Law:	Y	Engineers, Other:	
Int'l Business:		Commercial/Industrial:	Y	Graphic Arts/Photog.:		Hardware Dev.:		HR/Other:	Y	Health/Lab:	
MBA Graduates:	Y	Sales Trainees:		Music:		Systems Integration:		Training:	Y	Scientists/Research:	
		Advertising Pros.:		Broadcasting:		Consulting/Other:		Health Care:		Petroleum/Chemicals:	Y
				Other:				Consulting:		Math/Other:	

TYPES OF BUSINESS:

Petroleum Refining
Gas Stations
Aviation & Heavy Fuels

BRANDS/DIVISIONS/AFFILIATES:

Mirastar

CONTACTS: *Note: Officers with more than one job title may be intentionally listed here more than once.*

Bruce A. Smith, CEO
Everett Lewis, COO/Exec. VP
Bruce A. Smith, Pres.
Otto C. Schwethelm, CFO/Sr. VP
Otto C. Schwethelm, Sr. VP-IT
Gregory A. Wright, Chief Admin. Officer/Exec. VP
Charles S. Parrish, General Counsel/Sr. VP/Sec.
William J. Finnerty, Exec. VP-Strategy & Corp. Dev.
Sarah S. Simpson, VP-Corp. Comm.
Otto C. Schwethelm, Sr. VP-Investor Rel.
Otto C. Schwethelm, Treas.
C.A. Flagg, Sr. VP-System Optimization
Arlen Glenewinkel, Jr., Controller/VP
Dan Porter, Sr. VP-Refining
Susan A. Lerette, Sr. VP-Admin.
Bruce A. Smith, Chmn.
Joseph G. McCoy, Sr. VP-Supply & Training

Phone: 210-828-8484	Fax: 210-283-2045
Toll-Free: 800-837-6768	
Address: 300 Concord Plaza Dr., San Antonio, TX 78216 US	

GROWTH PLANS/SPECIAL FEATURES:

Tesoro Corporation, formerly known as Tesoro Petroleum Corp., is one of the largest independent petroleum refiners in the U.S. The company operates in two segments: refining, and marketing and distribution. Through the refining segment, the firm owns and operates six petroleum refineries located in California, Alaska, Washington, Hawaii, North Dakota and Utah and sells refined products to a wide variety of customers in the western and mid-continental U.S. Tesoro's refineries produce a high proportion of its refined product sales volumes, and the company purchases the remainder from its other refiners and suppliers. The firm's six refineries have a combined crude oil capacity of 530,000 barrels per day. Tesoro operates some of the largest refineries in Hawaii, Utah, northern California and Alaska, in addition to the only refinery in North Dakota. Through the marketing and distribution segment, the company sells refined products including gasoline and gasoline blendstocks, jet fuel, diesel fuel, heavy fuel oils and residual products in both the bulk and wholesale markets. The majority of its wholesale volumes are sold in 10 states to independent unbranded distributors that sell refined products through the firm's owned and third-party terminals. Tesoro's bulk volumes are primarily sold to independent and other oil companies; electric power producers; railroads; airlines; and marine and industrial end-users, which are distributed by pipelines, ships, railcars and trucks. In addition, the company sells refined products that it manufactures, purchases or receives on exchange from third parties. Tesoro's retail marketing operations include about 460 branded retail locations in the western U.S., Alaska and Hawaii, including Mirastar-brand stations at Wal-Mart locations in the western U.S. In August 2008, Tesoro closed 42 of its 74 Mirastar fueling stations at Wal-Mart locations.

Most Tesoro employees are eligible for dental and vision care benefits, accidental death insurance, short term disability, educational assistance and paid holidays.

FINANCIALS: Sales and profits are in thousands of dollars—add 000 to get the full amount. 2007 Note: Financial information for 2007 was not available for all companies at press time.

2007 Sales: $21,915,000	2007 Profits: $566,000	**U.S. Stock Ticker:** TSO
2006 Sales: $18,104,000	2006 Profits: $801,000	**Int'l Ticker:** Int'l Exchange:
2005 Sales: $16,581,000	2005 Profits: $507,000	**Employees:** 3,928
2004 Sales: $12,262,200	2004 Profits: $327,900	**Fiscal Year Ends:** 12/31
2003 Sales: $8,845,700	2003 Profits: $76,100	**Parent Company:**

SALARIES/BENEFITS:

Pension Plan:	ESOP Stock Plan:	Profit Sharing:	Top Exec. Salary: $1,180,822	Bonus: $2,190,000
Savings Plan: Y	Stock Purch. Plan:		Second Exec. Salary: $659,890	Bonus: $1,136,211

OTHER THOUGHTS:

Apparent Women Officers or Directors: 2
Hot Spot for Advancement for Women/Minorities: Y

LOCATIONS: ("Y" = Yes)

West:	Southwest:	Midwest:	Southeast:	Northeast:	International:
Y	Y	Y			Y

TIFFANY & CO

www.tiffany.com

Industry Group Code: 448310 Ranks within this company's industry group: Sales: 1 Profits: 1

Management:		Sales/Marketing:		Liberal Arts:		Information Systems:		Professionals:		Technical/Scientific:	
Mgmt. Trainees:	Y	Mktg. Professionals:	Y	Gen. Writing/Editing:	Y	Info. Management:	Y	Finance/Accounting:	Y	Engineers, Elec.:	
Experienced Mgmt.:	Y	Retail Sales:	Y	Technical Writing:		Software Dev.:	Y	Law:	Y	Engineers, Other:	
Int'l Business:	Y	Commercial/Industrial:	Y	Graphic Arts/Photog.:	Y	Hardware Dev.:		HR/Other:	Y	Health/Lab:	
MBA Graduates:	Y	Sales Trainees:	Y	Music:		Systems Integration:		Training:	Y	Scientists/Research:	
		Advertising Pros.:	Y	Broadcasting:		Consulting/Other:		Health Care:		Petroleum/Chemicals:	
				Other:	Y			Consulting:		Math/Other:	

TYPES OF BUSINESS:

Jewelry & Other Luxury Items, Retail
Catalog & Online Sales
Jewelry
Fragrance
Timepieces
Stationery
Home Décor

BRANDS/DIVISIONS/AFFILIATES:

Tiffany and Company
Tiffany & Co. Japan, Inc.
Mitsukoshi Ltd.
Iridesse, Inc.
Little Switzerland
NXP Corporation

CONTACTS: *Note: Officers with more than one job title may be intentionally listed here more than once.*

Michael J. Kowalski, CEO
James E. Quinn, Pres.
James N. Fernandez, CFO/Exec. VP
Caroline D. Naggiar, Chief Mkt. Officer
Victoria Berger-Gross, Sr. VP-Human Resources
Robert W. Davidson, CIO
Philip C. Alberta, VP-IT Bus. & Tech. Mgmt.
Pamela H. Cloud, Sr. VP-Merch.
Patrick B. Dorsey, General Counsel/Sec./Sr. VP
John S. Petterson, Sr. VP-Oper.
Patrick F. McGuiness, Sr. VP-Finance
Beth O. Canavan, Exec. VP
Jon M. King, Exec. VP
Michael J. Kowalski, Chmn.

Phone: 212-755-8000	Fax: 212-230-6633
Toll-Free:	
Address: 727 Fifth Ave., New York, NY 10022 US	

GROWTH PLANS/SPECIAL FEATURES:

Tiffany & Co. is a holding company that operates through its principle subsidiary, Tiffany and Company, founded in 1837, a retail firm mainly selling jewelry, but also selling timepieces, sterling silver goods, china, crystal, stationery, fragrances and personal accessories. Its products are sold through U.S. and international Tiffany & Co. stores; as well as through direct marketing, including business-to-business, mail-order, Internet and wholesale sales. The firm operates approximately 69 branch stores in the U.S.; 10 stores divided between Canada, Central and South America; 53 stores in Japan; 34 in other Asia-Pacific regions; and 17 Europe. In fiscal 2007, 86% of net sales were attributed to Tiffany & CO. jewelry, the remaining 15% of sales came from all other brand products. Tiffany & Co. Japan, Inc. has a partnership with Mitsukoshi Ltd., operating 15 Mitsukoshi department stores and other retail locations in Japan. Tiffany's flagship New York City store's retail business accounted for approximately 10% of the company's total net sales in 2007. The typical store has traditionally measured less than 10,000 square feet; however the company has switched to a smaller store format and plans to begin opening 5-7 new 5,000 square-foot Tiffany & Co. branch stores each year. In 2007, the company opened seven new stores in various parts of the U.S., including Texas, Nevada, Massachusetts, New York, New Jersey, Rhode Island and California. In December 2007, Tiffany & CO. entered into an alliance with The Swatch Group LTD. The collaboration will place Tiffany brand watches within the collection of watch brands manufactured and distributed by the Swatch Group. Currently, the firm is contemplating opening six new stores in the U.S. in 2008 and eight to 12 stores in 2009.

FINANCIALS: Sales and profits are in thousands of dollars—add 000 to get the full amount. 2007 Note: Financial information for 2007 was not available for all companies at press time.

2007 Sales: $2,560,734	2007 Profits: $253,927	U.S. Stock Ticker: TIF
2006 Sales: $2,312,792	2006 Profits: $254,655	Int'l Ticker: Int'l Exchange:
2005 Sales: $2,204,831	2005 Profits: $304,299	Employees: 8,100
2004 Sales: $2,000,045	2004 Profits: $215,517	Fiscal Year Ends: 1/31
2003 Sales: $1,706,600	2003 Profits: $189,900	Parent Company:

SALARIES/BENEFITS:

Pension Plan:	ESOP Stock Plan:	Profit Sharing:	Top Exec. Salary: $972,382	Bonus: $1,123,541
Savings Plan:	Stock Purch. Plan:		Second Exec. Salary: $738,013	Bonus: $628,334

OTHER THOUGHTS:

Apparent Women Officers or Directors: 4
Hot Spot for Advancement for Women/Minorities: Y

LOCATIONS: ("Y" = Yes)

West:	Southwest:	Midwest:	Southeast:	Northeast:	International:
				Y	

Note: Financial information, benefits and other data can change quickly and may vary from those stated here.

TIME WARNER INC

www.timewarner.com

Industry Group Code: 513220 Ranks within this company's industry group: Sales: 1 Profits: 1

Management:		Sales/Marketing:		Liberal Arts:		Information Systems:		Professionals:		Technical/Scientific:	
Mgmt. Trainees:	Y	Mktg. Professionals:	Y	Gen. Writing/Editing:	Y	Info. Management:	Y	Finance/Accounting:	Y	Engineers, Elec.:	Y
Experienced Mgmt.:	Y	Retail Sales:		Technical Writing:		Software Dev.:	Y	Law:	Y	Engineers, Other:	
Int'l Business:	Y	Commercial/Industrial:	Y	Graphic Arts/Photog.:	Y	Hardware Dev.:		HR/Other:	Y	Health/Lab:	
MBA Graduates:	Y	Sales Trainees:		Music:	Y	Systems Integration:		Training:	Y	Scientists/Research:	
		Advertising Pros.:	Y	Broadcasting:	Y	Consulting/Other:		Health Care:		Petroleum/Chemicals:	
				Other:	Y			Consulting:		Math/Other:	

TYPES OF BUSINESS:

Cable TV Networks
Television Production
Cable TV Service
Magazine Publishing
Entertainment Investments
Film Production

BRANDS/DIVISIONS/AFFILIATES:

AOL LLC
Time Warner Cable Inc
Warner Bros Entertainment Inc
Time Inc
New Line Cinema
Turner Broadcasting System
Sports Illustrated
Goowy Media, Inc.

CONTACTS: Note: Officers with more than one job title may be intentionally listed here more than once.

Jeffrey Bewkes, CEO
Jeffrey Bewkes, Pres.
John Martin, CFO/Exec. VP
Patricia Fili-Krushel, Exec. VP-Admin.
Paul Cappuccio, General Counsel/Exec. VP
Edward Adler, Exec. VP-Corp. Comm.
James Burtson, Sr. VP-Investor Rel.
Carol Melton, Exec. VP-Global Public Policy
Olaf Olafsson, Exec. VP
Richard Parsons, Chmn.

Phone: 212-484-8000	Fax:
Toll-Free:	
Address: 1 Time Warner Ctr., New York, NY 10019 US	

GROWTH PLANS/SPECIAL FEATURES:

Time Warner, Inc. is a global media and entertainment company. The firm operates in five segments: AOL, cable, filmed entertainment, networks and publishing. The company's AOL segment is an advertising supported global web services business. The cable business, Time Warner Cable, Inc. (TWC) and its subsidiaries together form one of the largest cable operators in the U.S. This segment offers high speed data services and digital voice services to residential and business customers. The filmed entertainment segment, operated principally through subsidiary Warner Bros. Entertainment Group, produces and distributes theatrical motion pictures, television shows, animation and other programming, distributes home video product, and licenses rights to the company's feature films, television programming and characters. The networks segment consists principally of domestic and international basic cable networks and pay television programming services. This division includes basic cable networks owned by subsidiary Turner Broadcasting System, Inc. (TBS) and pay television programming, such as the HBO and Cinemax channels, operated by Home Box Office, Inc. Time Warner's publishing business publishes 145 magazines worldwide, including Sports Illustrated, offers direct book marketing and publishes a collection of niche books. In December 2007, AOL acquired Quigo, a site and content-targeted advertising company. In February 2008, AOL acquired Goowy Media, Inc., a widget technology company, and Buy.at, an affiliate network that offers a platform for e-commerce marketing programs to advertisers and publishers.

FINANCIALS: Sales and profits are in thousands of dollars—add 000 to get the full amount. 2007 Note: Financial information for 2007 was not available for all companies at press time.

2007 Sales: $46,482,000	2007 Profits: $4,387,000	**U.S. Stock Ticker:** TWX
2006 Sales: $43,690,000	2006 Profits: $6,552,000	**Int'l Ticker:** Int'l Exchange:
2005 Sales: $42,401,000	2005 Profits: $2,671,000	Employees: 86,400
2004 Sales: $40,993,000	2004 Profits: $3,108,000	Fiscal Year Ends: 12/31
2003 Sales: $39,565,000	2003 Profits: $2,639,000	Parent Company:

SALARIES/BENEFITS:

Pension Plan:	ESOP Stock Plan:	Profit Sharing:	Top Exec. Salary: $1,500,000	Bonus: $8,500,000
Savings Plan:	Stock Purch. Plan:		Second Exec. Salary: $1,250,000	Bonus: $7,500,000

OTHER THOUGHTS:

Apparent Women Officers or Directors: 4
Hot Spot for Advancement for Women/Minorities: Y

LOCATIONS: ("Y" = Yes)

West:	Southwest:	Midwest:	Southeast:	Northeast:	International:
Y	Y	Y	Y	Y	Y

Note: Financial information, benefits and other data can change quickly and may vary from those stated here.

TJX COMPANIES INC (THE)

www.tjx.com

Industry Group Code: 448000 Ranks within this company's industry group: Sales: 1 Profits: 1

Management:		Sales/Marketing:		Liberal Arts:		Information Systems:		Professionals:		Technical/Scientific:	
Mgmt. Trainees:	Y	Mktg. Professionals:	Y	Gen. Writing/Editing:	Y	Info. Management:	Y	Finance/Accounting:	Y	Engineers, Elec.:	
Experienced Mgmt.:	Y	Retail Sales:	Y	Technical Writing:		Software Dev.:		Law:	Y	Engineers, Other:	
Int'l Business:	Y	Commercial/Industrial:	Y	Graphic Arts/Photog.:	Y	Hardware Dev.:		HR/Other:	Y	Health/Lab:	
MBA Graduates:	Y	Sales Trainees:	Y	Music:		Systems Integration:		Training:	Y	Scientists/Research:	
		Advertising Pros.:	Y	Broadcasting:		Consulting/Other:		Health Care:		Petroleum/Chemicals:	
				Other:	Y			Consulting:		Math/Other:	

TYPES OF BUSINESS:

Discount Apparel Stores
Domestics
Footwear
Jewelry
Home Furnishings
Accessories

BRANDS/DIVISIONS/AFFILIATES:

T.J. Maxx
Marshalls
HomeGoods
A.J. Wright
Winners
T.K. Maxx
HomeSense
Bob's Stores

CONTACTS: Note: Officers with more than one job title may be intentionally listed here more than once.

Carol Meyrowitz, CEO
Carol Meyrowitz, Pres.
Nirmal K. Tripathy, CFO/Exec. VP
John Gilbert, Chief Mktg. Officer/Exec. VP
Jeffrey G. Naylor, Chief Admin. Officer
Jeffrey G. Naylor, Chief Bus. Dev. Officer
Ernie Herman, Sr. Exec. VP/Pres., The Marmaxx Group
Arnold S. Barron, Sr. Exec. VP/Group Pres.
Donald G. Campbell, Vice Chmn.
Jerome R. Rossi, Sr. Exec. VP/Group Pres.
Bernard Cammarata, Chmn.
Paul Sweetenham, Sr. Exec. VP/Group Pres., Europe

Phone: 508-390-1000	Fax: 508-390-2828
Toll-Free:	
Address: 770 Cochituate Rd., Framingham, MA 01701 US	

GROWTH PLANS/SPECIAL FEATURES:

The TJX Companies, Inc. is a low-price apparel and home fashions retailer, operating over 2,500 stores through eight businesses including T.J. Maxx, Marshalls, HomeGoods, A.J. Wrights and Bob's Stores in the U.S.; Winners and HomeSense in Canada; and T.K. Maxx in Europe. TJX's 847 T.J. Maxx stores and 762 Marshalls stores offer brand-name family apparel, giftware, domestics and accessories in 42 states across the U.S. and 14 in Puerto Rico. The chains are similar, although Marshalls features a full-line shoe department and a larger men's department while T.J. Maxx now carries an extended line of jewelry and accessories. TJX also operates 191 HomeGoods stores, which sell low-priced home fashions. The chain offers a broad array of giftware, accent furniture, lamps, rugs, accessories and seasonal merchandise. The company also combines HomeGoods stores with a T.J. Maxx or a Marshalls store under the names T.J. Maxx 'N More and Marshalls Mega-Store. TJX's 129 A.J. Wright stores, catering to moderate-income customers, provide low-price family apparel and home fashions. TJX also operates the 191 store Winners chain, patterned after T.J. Maxx, in Canada. The firm's 221 T.K. Maxx stores in Europe resemble its domestic stores, although with a slight name change. TJX also operates a - store chain in Canada, 71 HomeSense, patterned after its American HomeGoods stores. The store sells much of its merchandise off-price, which means that the company purchases its inventory on an opportunistic basis, doing business with over 10,000 vendors worldwide. The 34 Bob's Stores were sold to private equity firms Versa Capital Management and Crystal Capital in August 2008.

The company offers its employees medical, dental, vision, disability and life insurance; a 401(k) plan; a profit sharing plan; auto and home insurance; a college savings program; store discounts; a mortgage discount program; a tuition assistance program; and long term care insurance. Corporate employees have access to basketball courts, fitness classes and indoor golf driving ranges.

FINANCIALS: Sales and profits are in thousands of dollars—add 000 to get the full amount. 2007 Note: Financial information for 2007 was not available for all companies at press time.

2007 Sales: $17,404,637	2007 Profits: $776,756	**U.S. Stock Ticker: TJX**
2006 Sales: $15,955,943	2006 Profits: $689,834	**Int'l Ticker:** Int'l Exchange:
2005 Sales: $14,860,746	2005 Profits: $610,217	Employees: 125,000
2004 Sales: $13,327,938	2004 Profits: $609,412	Fiscal Year Ends: 1/31
2003 Sales: $11,981,200	2003 Profits: $578,400	Parent Company:

SALARIES/BENEFITS:

Pension Plan:	ESOP Stock Plan:	Profit Sharing:	Top Exec. Salary: $1,076,731	Bonus: $2,017,580
Savings Plan: Y	Stock Purch. Plan:		Second Exec. Salary: $911,539	Bonus: $

OTHER THOUGHTS:

Apparent Women Officers or Directors: 3
Hot Spot for Advancement for Women/Minorities: Y

LOCATIONS: ("Y" = Yes)

West:	Southwest:	Midwest:	Southeast:	Northeast:	International:
Y	Y	Y	Y	Y	Y

Note: Financial information, benefits and other data can change quickly and may vary from those stated here.

T-MOBILE USA

www.t-mobile.com

Industry Group Code: 513322 Ranks within this company's industry group: Sales: 3   Profits: 1

Management:		Sales/Marketing:		Liberal Arts:		Information Systems:		Professionals:		Technical/Scientific:	
Mgmt. Trainees:	Y	Mktg. Professionals:	Y	Gen. Writing/Editing:	Y	Info. Management:	Y	Finance/Accounting:	Y	Engineers, Elec.:	Y
Experienced Mgmt.:	Y	Retail Sales:	Y	Technical Writing:		Software Dev.:	Y	Law:	Y	Engineers, Other:	
Int'l Business:	Y	Commercial/Industrial:	Y	Graphic Arts/Photog.:	Y	Hardware Dev.:		HR/Other:	Y	Health/Lab:	
MBA Graduates:	Y	Sales Trainees:		Music:		Systems Integration:		Training:	Y	Scientists/Research:	
		Advertising Pros.:	Y	Broadcasting:		Consulting/Other:		Health Care:		Petroleum/Chemicals:	
				Other:				Consulting:		Math/Other:	

TYPES OF BUSINESS:

PCS Cellular Telephone Service
Wireless Internet Services

BRANDS/DIVISIONS/AFFILIATES:

Deutsche Telekom AG
T-Mobile International AG
T-Mobile HotSpot
SunCom Wireless Holdings, Inc.

CONTACTS: Note: Officers with more than one job title may be intentionally listed here more than once.

Robert P. Dotson, CEO
Robert P. Dotson, Pres.
Brian W. Kirkpatrick, CFO/Exec. VP
Mike Buttler, Chief Mktg. Officer
Manuel Sousa, Chief People Officer/Sr. VP
Rob Strickland, CIO/Sr. VP
Cole Brodman, CTO
Cole Brodman, Sr. VP-Product & Systems Dev.
Neville Ray, Sr. VP-Eng. Oper.
Dave Miller, General Counsel/Sr. VP
Susan Nokes, Chief Customs & Oper. Officer
John W. Stanton, Chmn.

Phone: 425-378-4000	Fax: 425-378-4040
Toll-Free: 800-318-9270	
Address: 12920 S.E. 38th St., Bellevue, WA 98006 US	

GROWTH PLANS/SPECIAL FEATURES:

T-Mobile USA (T-Mobile) is a national provider of wireless voice, messaging and data services in the U.S. The company is the U.S. operating entity of T-Mobile International AG & Co., the mobile communications subsidiary of Deutsche Telekom AG & Co. K.G. T-Mobile uses GSM (global system for mobile communications) technology and is a member of the North American GSM Alliance, a group of U.S. and Canadian digital wireless carriers that helps provide seamless GSM wireless communications for its members in North America and internationally. The firm has international roaming agreements with 192 of the major GSM operators worldwide, providing service to 30.8 million customers in the U.S. who are also able to connect to the GSM network of its parent company when in Europe. The company offers wireless Internet service to phones through its T-Mobile Internet program and high-speed wireless access through its T-Mobile HotSpot service. HotSpot locations can be found at airports, airline clubs and lounges of American Airlines, Delta Air Lines and United Airlines; Borders Books and Music; Kinko's; and Starbucks coffeehouses. With more than 4,700 locations, the T-Mobile HotSpot network is the largest public Wi-Fi network in the U.S. In February 2008, the firm strengthened its footprint in Puerto Rico and the Carolinas with the acquisition of SunCom Wireless Holdings, Inc. for $1.6 billion, plus $800 million in debt. In mid-2008, the firm reached the 30 million customer mark.

T-Mobile offers its employees an educational assistance program.

FINANCIALS: Sales and profits are in thousands of dollars—add 000 to get the full amount. 2007 Note: Financial information for 2007 was not available for all companies at press time.

2007 Sales: $19,288,000	2007 Profits: $5,350,000	U.S. Stock Ticker: Subsidiary
2006 Sales: $17,138,000	2006 Profits: $4,712,000	Int'l Ticker: Int'l Exchange:
2005 Sales: $14,806,000	2005 Profits: $	Employees: 36,000
2004 Sales: $11,679,000	2004 Profits: $	Fiscal Year Ends: 12/31
2003 Sales: $8,358,100	2003 Profits: $	Parent Company: DEUTSCHE TELEKOM AG

SALARIES/BENEFITS:

Pension Plan:	ESOP Stock Plan:	Profit Sharing:	Top Exec. Salary: $	Bonus: $1,000,000
Savings Plan: Y	Stock Purch. Plan: Y		Second Exec. Salary: $232,210	Bonus: $232,210

OTHER THOUGHTS:

Apparent Women Officers or Directors: 1
Hot Spot for Advancement for Women/Minorities:

LOCATIONS: ("Y" = Yes)

West:	Southwest:	Midwest:	Southeast:	Northeast:	International:
Y	Y	Y	Y	Y	

TOTAL SYSTEM SERVICES INC (TSYS)   www.tsys.com

Industry Group Code: 522320 Ranks within this company's industry group: Sales: 5 Profits: 3

Management:		Sales/Marketing:		Liberal Arts:		Information Systems:		Professionals:		Technical/Scientific:	
Mgmt. Trainees:	Y	Mktg. Professionals:	Y	Gen. Writing/Editing:		Info. Management:	Y	Finance/Accounting:	Y	Engineers, Elec.:	
Experienced Mgmt.:	Y	Retail Sales:		Technical Writing:		Software Dev.:	Y	Law:	Y	Engineers, Other:	
Int'l Business:	Y	Commercial/Industrial:	Y	Graphic Arts/Photog.:		Hardware Dev.:		HR/Other:	Y	Health/Lab:	
MBA Graduates:	Y	Sales Trainees:		Music:		Systems Integration:		Training:	Y	Scientists/Research:	
		Advertising Pros.:	Y	Broadcasting:		Consulting/Other:		Health Care:		Petroleum/Chemicals:	
				Other:				Consulting:		Math/Other:	

TYPES OF BUSINESS:

Credit Card Processing
Risk Management Tools
Direct Mail Services
Fraud Detection
Printing Services
Debt Collection Services
Reward Programs
Staffing Services

BRANDS/DIVISIONS/AFFILIATES:

Synovus Financial Corp.
Columbus Depot Equipment Company
Columbus Productions
TSYS Canada, Inc.
TSYS Total Debt Management, Inc.
TSYS Technology Center, Inc.
Total System Services de Mexico
UnionPay Data Co., Ltd.

CONTACTS: *Note: Officers with more than one job title may be intentionally listed here more than once.*

Philip W. Tomlinson, CEO
M. Troy Woods, COO
M. Troy Woods, Pres.
James B. Lipham, CFO/Sr. Exec. VP
Gaylon M. Jowers, Jr., Exec. VP-Sales
Kenneth L. Tye, CIO/Sr. Exec. VP
Stephen W. Humber, CTO/Exec. VP
Connie C. Dudley, Exec. VP-Prod. & Client Dev.
Ryland L. Harrelson, Exec. VP-Admin. Svcs.
Gaylon M. Jowers, Jr., Exec. VP-Strategy & Emerging Markets
Dorenda K. Weaver, Chief Acct. Officer/Controller/Exec. VP
William A. Pruett, Chief Customer Officer/Sr. Exec. VP
Colleen W. Kynard, Exec. VP-Customer Care
Philip W. Tomlinson, Chmn.

Phone: 706-649-2310	**Fax:** 706-644-8065
Toll-Free:	
Address: 1600 1st Ave., Columbus, GA 31901 US	

GROWTH PLANS/SPECIAL FEATURES:

Total System Services (TSYS) is one of the world's largest electronic payment processors of consumer credit, debit, commercial, stored-value, chip and retail cards. Its majority owner, Synovus Financial Corp., has an 81% stake in the firm. TSYS serves institutions throughout the U.S., Canada, Mexico, Honduras, the Caribbean and Europe. The company also offers value-added products and services, including risk management tools and techniques like credit evaluation, fraud detection and prevention and behavior analysis tools, as well as revenue enhancement tools, such as loyalty programs and bonus rewards. The firm's subsidiaries include Columbus Depot Equipment Company, which sells and leases computer-related equipment; Columbus Productions, which provides full-service commercial printing and related services; TSYS Acquiring Solutions, a supplier of acquiring solutions, related systems and integrated support services; TSYS Canada, Inc., which provides programming support and assistance with conversion of card portfolios to TS2; and TSYS Total Debt Management, Inc., which provides debt collection and bankruptcy management services. TSYS Technology Center, Inc. provides flexible staffing solutions to help TSYS address its implementation and development pipeline of clients and prospective clients. The company also owns an equity interest in a joint venture company called Total System Services de Mexico, as well as a 45% interest in China UnionPay Data Co., Ltd.

The company offers its employees medical, dental and vision insurance; flexible spending accounts; a 401(k) plan; a profit sharing plan; an employee stock purchase plan; long-term disability insurance; and a scholarship program for employees' children.

FINANCIALS: Sales and profits are in thousands of dollars—add 000 to get the full amount. 2007 Note: Financial information for 2007 was not available for all companies at press time.

2007 Sales: $1,805,836	2007 Profits: $237,443	**U.S. Stock Ticker: TSS**
2006 Sales: $1,787,171	2006 Profits: $249,163	**Int'l Ticker:** **Int'l Exchange:**
2005 Sales: $1,602,931	2005 Profits: $194,520	Employees: 6,799
2004 Sales: $1,187,008	2004 Profits: $150,558	Fiscal Year Ends: 12/31
2003 Sales: $1,053,500	2003 Profits: $141,000	Parent Company:

SALARIES/BENEFITS:

Pension Plan: Y	ESOP Stock Plan:	Profit Sharing: Y	Top Exec. Salary: $711,833	Bonus: $960,930
Savings Plan: Y	Stock Purch. Plan: Y		Second Exec. Salary: $500,000	Bonus: $675,000

OTHER THOUGHTS:

Apparent Women Officers or Directors: 3
Hot Spot for Advancement for Women/Minorities: Y

LOCATIONS: ("Y" = Yes)

West:	Southwest:	Midwest:	Southeast:	Northeast:	International:
Y	Y	Y	Y	Y	Y

TOWERS PERRIN
www.towersperrin.com

Industry Group Code: 541612 Ranks within this company's industry group: Sales: 1 Profits:

Management:		Sales/Marketing:		Liberal Arts:		Information Systems:		Professionals:		Technical/Scientific:	
Mgmt. Trainees:		Mktg. Professionals:		Gen. Writing/Editing:	Y	Info. Management:	Y	Finance/Accounting:	Y	Engineers, Elec.:	
Experienced Mgmt.:	Y	Retail Sales:		Technical Writing:		Software Dev.:		Law:	Y	Engineers, Other:	
Int'l Business:	Y	Commercial/Industrial:	Y	Graphic Arts/Photog.:		Hardware Dev.:		HR/Other:	Y	Health/Lab:	
MBA Graduates:	Y	Sales Trainees:		Music:		Systems Integration:		Training:	Y	Scientists/Research:	
		Advertising Pros.:		Broadcasting:		Consulting/Other:		Health Care:	Y	Petroleum/Chemicals:	
				Other:				Consulting:	Y	Math/Other:	

TYPES OF BUSINESS:
Human Resources Consulting
Benefit Plan & Compensation Consulting
Actuarial & Management Consulting
Reinsurance Consulting
Human Resources Outsourcing
Human Resources Consulting

BRANDS/DIVISIONS/AFFILIATES:
Tillinghast
Towers Perrin Reinsurance
ExcellerateHRO

CONTACTS: *Note: Officers with more than one job title may be intentionally listed here more than once.*
Mark Mactas, CEO
Bob Hogan, CFO
Tony Candito, Chief Admin. Officer
Kevin Young, General Counsel/Sec.
Tricia Guinn, Managing Dir.-Risk & Financial Svcs.
James K. Foreman, Managing Dir.-Human Capital Group
Don Lowman, Managing Dir.-Human Capital Group
Mark Mactas, Chmn.

Phone: 203-326-5400 **Fax:** 203-326-5499
Toll-Free:
Address: 1 Stamford Plaza, 263 Tresser Blvd., Stamford, CT 06901-3226 US

GROWTH PLANS/SPECIAL FEATURES:
Towers Perrin is an international provider of human resources, benefit plan and compensation consultation, operating out of more than 90 offices in 26 countries. The firm has worked with three-quarters of the world's 500 largest companies and three-quarters of the Fortune 1000 U.S. companies. Towers Perrin's services include third-party administration for retirement, health and welfare plans and compensation administration; human resources consulting, including communication training; employee hiring research; and rewards and performance management. The company is divided into three sections: HR services, reinsurance and the subsidiary Tillinghast. The HR services business provides international human resources consulting and related services. Services include assistance with employee benefits, compensation, and communication and change management. Towers Perrin's reinsurance business provides intermediary services and consulting expertise for reinsurance through a blend of risk transfer vehicles. The firm helps with reinsurance strategy and program review; claims management and program administration; catastrophe exposure management; contract negotiation and placement; and market security issues. Tillinghast provides global actuarial and management consulting to insurance and financial services companies and advises other organizations on risk financing and self-insurance including mergers, acquisitions and restructuring; financial and regulatory reporting; risk, capital and value management; products, markets and distribution; and financial modeling software solutions. In January 2008, the firm launched a new reinsurance business in France, expanding its European market.

FINANCIALS: Sales and profits are in thousands of dollars—add 000 to get the full amount. 2007 Note: Financial information for 2007 was not available for all companies at press time.
2007 Sales: $ 2007 Profits: $
2006 Sales: $2,200,000   2006 Profits: $
2005 Sales: $2,000,000   2005 Profits: $
2004 Sales: $1,700,000   2004 Profits: $
2003 Sales: $1,500,000   2003 Profits: $

U.S. Stock Ticker: Private
Int'l Ticker: **Int'l Exchange:**
Employees:
Fiscal Year Ends: 12/31
Parent Company:

SALARIES/BENEFITS:
Pension Plan: Y   ESOP Stock Plan: Profit Sharing: Top Exec. Salary: $ Bonus: $
Savings Plan: Stock Purch. Plan: Second Exec. Salary: $ Bonus: $

OTHER THOUGHTS:
Apparent Women Officers or Directors: 1
Hot Spot for Advancement for Women/Minorities:

LOCATIONS: ("Y" = Yes)
West:	Southwest:	Midwest:	Southeast:	Northeast:	International:
Y	Y	Y	Y	Y	Y

TRANSOCEAN INC
www.deepwater.com

Industry Group Code: 211111 Ranks within this company's industry group: Sales: 7   Profits: 6

Management:		Sales/Marketing:		Liberal Arts:		Information Systems:		Professionals:		Technical/Scientific:	
Mgmt. Trainees:	Y	Mktg. Professionals:	Y	Gen. Writing/Editing:		Info. Management:	Y	Finance/Accounting:	Y	Engineers, Elec.:	Y
Experienced Mgmt.:	Y	Retail Sales:		Technical Writing:		Software Dev.:		Law:	Y	Engineers, Other:	Y
Int'l Business:	Y	Commercial/Industrial:	Y	Graphic Arts/Photog.:		Hardware Dev.:		HR/Other:	Y	Health/Lab:	Y
MBA Graduates:	Y	Sales Trainees:		Music:		Systems Integration:		Training:	Y	Scientists/Research:	
		Advertising Pros.:		Broadcasting:		Consulting/Other:		Health Care:		Petroleum/Chemicals:	Y
				Other:				Consulting:		Math/Other:	

TYPES OF BUSINESS:
Oil & Gas Exploration & Production
Mobile Offshore Production Units
Inland Drilling
Offshore Drilling & Production
Dual-Activity Drilling
High-Specification Drillships

BRANDS/DIVISIONS/AFFILIATES:

CONTACTS: Note: Officers with more than one job title may be intentionally listed here more than once.
Robert L. Long, CEO
Steven L. Newman, COO
Steven L. Newman, Pres.
Gregory L. Cauthen, CFO/Sr. VP
Terry B. Bonno, Sr. VP-Mktg.
Sherry Richard, Sr. VP-Human Resources
John L. Truschinger, CIO/VP
Eric B. Brown, General Counsel/Corp. Sec./Sr. VP
Simon Crowe, Sr. VP-Planning & Strategy
Gregory S. Panagos, VP-Comm.
Gregory S. Panagos, VP-Investor Rel.
John H. Briscoe, Controller/VP
Adrian P. Rose, VP-Quality, Health, Safety & Environment
Arnaud A.Y. Bobillier, Exec. VP-Assets
Ricardo H. Rosa, VP-Europe & Africa Unit
Rob Saltiel, Exec. VP-Performance
Robert E. Rose, Chmn.
Deepak C. Munganahalli, VP-Asia & Pacific Unit
Michael R. Hoke, VP-Global Supply Chain

Phone: 713-232-7500	Fax: 713-232-7027
Toll-Free:	
Address: 4 Greenway Plz., Houston, TX 77046 US	

GROWTH PLANS/SPECIAL FEATURES:

Transocean, Inc., together with its subsidiaries, is a leading international provider of deepwater and harsh environment contract drilling services for oil and gas wells. The company owned, partially owned or operated 139 mobile offshore and barge drilling units, consisting of 39 high-specification floaters, 29 midwater floaters, 10 high specification jackups, 57 standard jackups, and four other rigs. These units operate all over the world, with 21 units in Asia Pacific, 12 units in India, 16 units in the U.S. Gulf of Mexico, 19 units in the United Kingdom's North Sea, 13 units in Nigeria, 18 units in Southwest Asia, eight units in Brazil, five units in Norway, five units in Angola, five units in other West African countries, three units in the Caspian Sea, three units in Trinidad, two units in Australia, two units in the Mediterranean and one unit in Canada. Transocean obtains most of its contracts through competitive bidding against other contractors. Drilling contracts generally provide for payment on a dayrate basis, with higher rates while the drilling unit is operating and lower rates for periods of mobilization or when drilling operations are interrupted or restricted by equipment breakdowns, adverse environmental conditions or other conditions beyond its control. Major customers include Chevron, accounting for 12% of the company's revenues; BP, 10%; and Shell, 11%. The company's drilling equipment is suitable for both exploration and development drilling and is normally engaged in both types of activity. In July 2007, the firm merged with GlobalSantaFe Corp. in a deal that created a company with a combined market capitalization of $53 billion. The new company retained the Transocean name and ticker.

FINANCIALS: Sales and profits are in thousands of dollars—add 000 to get the full amount. 2007 Note: Financial information for 2007 was not available for all companies at press time.

2007 Sales: $6,377,000	2007 Profits: $3,131,000	U.S. Stock Ticker: RIG
2006 Sales: $3,882,000	2006 Profits: $1,385,000	Int'l Ticker: Int'l Exchange:
2005 Sales: $2,891,700	2005 Profits: $715,600	Employees: 12,500
2004 Sales: $2,613,900	2004 Profits: $152,200	Fiscal Year Ends: 12/31
2003 Sales: $2,434,300	2003 Profits: $19,200	Parent Company:

SALARIES/BENEFITS:

Pension Plan: Y	ESOP Stock Plan:	Profit Sharing:	Top Exec. Salary: $795,833	Bonus: $634,494
Savings Plan:	Stock Purch. Plan:		Second Exec. Salary: $471,667	Bonus: $313,372

OTHER THOUGHTS:
Apparent Women Officers or Directors: 2
Hot Spot for Advancement for Women/Minorities:

LOCATIONS: ("Y" = Yes)

West:	Southwest:	Midwest:	Southeast:	Northeast:	International:
	Y				Y

Note: Financial information, benefits and other data can change quickly and may vary from those stated here.

TRAVELERS COMPANIES INC (THE)   www.travelers.com

Industry Group Code: 524126 Ranks within this company's industry group: Sales: Profits:

Management:		Sales/Marketing:		Liberal Arts:		Information Systems:		Professionals:		Technical/Scientific:	
Mgmt. Trainees:	Y	Mktg. Professionals:	Y	Gen. Writing/Editing:		Info. Management:	Y	Finance/Accounting:	Y	Engineers, Elec.:	
Experienced Mgmt.:	Y	Retail Sales:		Technical Writing:		Software Dev.:	Y	Law:	Y	Engineers, Other:	Y
Int'l Business:	Y	Commercial/Industrial:	Y	Graphic Arts/Photog.:		Hardware Dev.:		HR/Other:	Y	Health/Lab:	
MBA Graduates:	Y	Sales Trainees:		Music:		Systems Integration:		Training:	Y	Scientists/Research:	Y
		Advertising Pros.:	Y	Broadcasting:		Consulting/Other:		Health Care:		Petroleum/Chemicals:	
				Other:				Consulting:		Math/Other:	Y

TYPES OF BUSINESS:
Direct Property & Casualty Insurance
Reinsurance
Automobile & Homeowners' Insurance
General Liability & Commercial Multi-Peril Insurance
Marine Insurance
Risk Management Services

BRANDS/DIVISIONS/AFFILIATES:
St. Paul Companies Inc
Mendota Insurance Co
Afianzadora Insurgentes S.A. de C.V.

CONTACTS: *Note: Officers with more than one job title may be intentionally listed here more than once.*
Jay S. Fishman, CEO
Brian W. MacLean, COO/Exec. VP
Brian W. MacLean, Pres.
Jay Benet, CFO
Kathleen Bolduc, Chief Marketing Officer
John Clifford, Exec. VP-Human Resources
William Bloom, CIO/Exec. VP-Insurance Oper.
Andy F. Bessette, Chief Admin. Officer/Exec. VP
Kenneth F. Spence III, General Counsel/Exec. VP
Samuel Liss, Exec. VP-Strategic Dev.
Maria Olivo, Exec. VP-Corp. Comm.
Gabriella Nawi, Sr. VP-Investor Rel.
William H. Heyman, Chief Investment Officer
John J. Albano, Exec. VP-Bus. Insurance
Alan D. Schnitzer, Chief Legal Officer
Joan Kois Woodward, Exec. VP-Public Policy
Jay S. Fishman, Chmn.

Phone: 651-310-7911	Fax: 651-310-3386
Toll-Free: 800-328-2189	
Address: 385 Washington St., St. Paul, MN 55102 US	

GROWTH PLANS/SPECIAL FEATURES:

The Travelers Companies, Inc., formerly St. Paul Travelers Companies, Inc., is a holding company principally engaged in providing commercial and personal property and casualty insurance products and services to businesses, government units, associations and individuals. The company operates in three segments, business insurance; financial, professional and international insurance; and personal insurance. The business insurance segment offers a broad array of property and casualty insurance and insurance-related services primarily in the U.S. The division is organized in six groups, select accounts, commercial accounts, national accounts, industry-focused underwriting, target risk underwriting and specialized distribution. The groups provide a wide array of insurance coverage, including commercial multi-peril, property, general liability, commercial auto, workers' compensation and marine. The financial, professional and international insurance segment includes surety and financial liability coverages, which require a primarily credit-based underwriting process, as well as property and casualty products that are primarily marketed on an international basis. The division includes the bond and financial products, which provides bond and insurance products and risk management services, and International and Lloyd's, which includes coverages marketed to and underwritten for several customer groups within the U.K., Canada and Ireland. The personal insurance segment writes virtually all types of property and casualty insurance covering personal risks. The primary coverages in this segment are automobile and homeowners insurance. Travelers reinsures a portion of the risks it underwrites. In April 2007, the firm sold Mendota Insurance Co., its non-standard automobile insurance unit, to a subsidiary of Kingsway Financial Services, Inc.; and its Mexican surety company, Afianzadora Insurgentes, S.A. de C.V. to Estrainver S.A. de C.V.

The company offers its employees medical, dental, vision and prescription drug insurance; life insurance; short- and long-term disability insurance; educational assistance; an employee assistance program; a pension plan; and a 401(k) plan.

FINANCIALS: Sales and profits are in thousands of dollars—add 000 to get the full amount. 2007 Note: Financial information for 2007 was not available for all companies at press time.

2007 Sales: $26,017,000	2007 Profits: $4,601,000	**U.S. Stock Ticker:** TRV
2006 Sales: $25,090,000	2006 Profits: $4,208,000	**Int'l Ticker:** Int'l Exchange:
2005 Sales: $24,365,000	2005 Profits: $1,622,000	Employees: 32,800
2004 Sales: $22,544,000	2004 Profits: $955,000	Fiscal Year Ends: 12/31
2003 Sales: $8,854,000	2003 Profits: $661,000	Parent Company:

SALARIES/BENEFITS:

Pension Plan: Y	ESOP Stock Plan:	Profit Sharing:	Top Exec. Salary: $1,000,000	Bonus: $6,500,000
Savings Plan: Y	Stock Purch. Plan:		Second Exec. Salary: $700,000	Bonus: $3,000,000

OTHER THOUGHTS:
Apparent Women Officers or Directors: 7
Hot Spot for Advancement for Women/Minorities: Y

LOCATIONS: ("Y" = Yes)

West:	Southwest:	Midwest:	Southeast:	Northeast:	International:
Y	Y	Y	Y	Y	Y

TW TELECOM INC

www.twtelecom.com

Industry Group Code: 513390C Ranks within this company's industry group: Sales: 2 Profits: 1

Management:		Sales/Marketing:		Liberal Arts:		Information Systems:		Professionals:		Technical/Scientific:	
Mgmt. Trainees:		Mktg. Professionals:	Y	Gen. Writing/Editing:	Y	Info. Management:	Y	Finance/Accounting:	Y	Engineers, Elec.:	Y
Experienced Mgmt.:	Y	Retail Sales:		Technical Writing:	Y	Software Dev.:	Y	Law:	Y	Engineers, Other:	
Int'l Business:		Commercial/Industrial:	Y	Graphic Arts/Photog.:	Y	Hardware Dev.:		HR/Other:	Y	Health/Lab:	
MBA Graduates:	Y	Sales Trainees:		Music:		Systems Integration:	Y	Training:	Y	Scientists/Research:	
		Advertising Pros.:	Y	Broadcasting:		Consulting/Other:		Health Care:		Petroleum/Chemicals:	
				Other:				Consulting:		Math/Other:	

TYPES OF BUSINESS:

Voice & Data Networking Solutions
Ethernet Services
Internet Access

BRANDS/DIVISIONS/AFFILIATES:

Xspedius Communications LLC

CONTACTS: Note: Officers with more than one job title may be intentionally listed here more than once.

Larissa Herda, CEO
John Blount, COO
Larissa Herda, Pres.
Mark A. Peters, CFO/Exec. VP
Graham Taylor, Sr. VP-Mktg. & Sales
Steve Hardardt, Sr. VP-Human Resources
Harold W. Teets, Sr. VP-IT
Paul B. Jones, General Counsel
Michael A. Rouleau, Sr. VP-Bus. Dev. & Strategy
Mark Willency, Sr. VP-Corp. Oper.
Carole Curtin, Sr. Dir.-Investor Rel.
Jill R. Stuart, Sr. VP-Finance & Acct./Chief Acct. Officer
Robert W. Gaskins, Sr. VP-Corp. Dev. & Strategy
Larissa Herda, Chmn.

Phone: 303-566-1000	**Fax:** 303-566-1011
Toll-Free:	
Address: 10475 Park Meadows Dr., Littleton, CO 80124 US	

GROWTH PLANS/SPECIAL FEATURES:

TW Telecom (TW), formerly known as Time Warner Telecom, Inc., is a provider of managed voice and data networking solutions to a broad range of business customers and organizations throughout the U.S. The company provides data, Internet access and local and long distance voice services and operates in 75 metropolitan areas in 30 states and D.C. over its 25,753 route-miles network of fiber-optic cable, directly connecting 8,355 building served directly by its facilities. The firm's customers are principally long-distance carriers, Internet service providers, incumbent local exchange carriers, competitive local exchange carriers, wireless communications companies, governmental entities and telecommunications-intensive enterprise organizations in the health care, finance, higher education, manufacturing and hospitality industries. The company's Xspedius subsidiary, a facilities-based provider of integrated communications services, provides services such as Ethernet; local and long distance voice; and data and Internet access services. AT&T Inc. accounted for 8% of total revenue in 2007. In 2007, the company greatly expanded its Voice over Internet Protocol (VoIP) network, allowing customers access to its carrier grade system. In July 2008, the firm changed its name to TW Telecom.

The company offers its employees medical, vision and dental insurance; life and disability insurance; flexible spending accounts; a 401(k) plan; an employee assistance program; and a stock option plan.

FINANCIALS: Sales and profits are in thousands of dollars—add 000 to get the full amount. 2007 Note: Financial information for 2007 was not available for all companies at press time.

2007 Sales: $1,083,679	2007 Profits: $-40,269	**U.S. Stock Ticker:** TWTC
2006 Sales: $812,375	2006 Profits: $-98,819	**Int'l Ticker:** Int'l Exchange:
2005 Sales: $708,727	2005 Profits: $-108,064	Employees: 2,859
2004 Sales: $653,087	2004 Profits: $-133,037	Fiscal Year Ends: 12/31
2003 Sales: $669,591	2003 Profits: $-89,336	Parent Company:

SALARIES/BENEFITS:

Pension Plan:	ESOP Stock Plan:	Profit Sharing:	Top Exec. Salary: $800,000	Bonus: $
Savings Plan: Y	Stock Purch. Plan: Y		Second Exec. Salary: $476,000	Bonus: $

OTHER THOUGHTS:

Apparent Women Officers or Directors: 3
Hot Spot for Advancement for Women/Minorities: Y

LOCATIONS: ("Y" = Yes)

West:	Southwest:	Midwest:	Southeast:	Northeast:	International:
Y	Y	Y	Y	Y	

TWEEN BRANDS INC

www.tweenbrands.com

Industry Group Code: 448130 Ranks within this company's industry group: Sales: 1 Profits: 1

Management:		Sales/Marketing:		Liberal Arts:		Information Systems:		Professionals:		Technical/Scientific:	
Mgmt. Trainees:	Y	Mktg. Professionals:		Gen. Writing/Editing:	Y	Info. Management:	Y	Finance/Accounting:	Y	Engineers, Elec.:	
Experienced Mgmt.:	Y	Retail Sales:	Y	Technical Writing:		Software Dev.:		Law:	Y	Engineers, Other:	
Int'l Business:	Y	Commercial/Industrial:		Graphic Arts/Photog.:	Y	Hardware Dev.:		HR/Other:	Y	Health/Lab:	
MBA Graduates:	Y	Sales Trainees:	Y	Music:		Systems Integration:		Training:	Y	Scientists/Research:	
		Advertising Pros.:	Y	Broadcasting:		Consulting/Other:		Health Care:		Petroleum/Chemicals:	
				Other:				Consulting:		Math/Other:	

TYPES OF BUSINESS:

Apparel-Children's, Retail
Footwear
Sportswear
Jewelry
Accessories
Online & Catalog Sales

BRANDS/DIVISIONS/AFFILIATES:

Too, Inc.
Limited Too
Justice
It's a Girls World
Family Invest AB

CONTACTS: *Note: Officers with more than one job title may be intentionally listed here more than once.*

Michael W. Rayden, CEO
Rolando de Aguiar, CFO/Exec. VP
Michael Keane, Sr. VP-Human Resources
Karen S. Etzkorn, CIO/Sr. VP
Gregory J. Henchel, General Counsel/Sr. VP/Sec.
Alan J. Hochman, Sr. VP-Real Estate & Store Planning
Julie Sloat, VP-Investor Relations
Kurt E. Gatterdam, Treas./VP
Scott M. Bracale, Pres., Tween Brands Agency
Michael W. Rayden, Chmn.
Ronnie Robinson, Exec. VP-Supply Chain

Phone: 614-775-3500	Fax:
Toll-Free:	
Address: 8323 Walton Pkwy., New Albany, OH 43054-9522 US	

GROWTH PLANS/SPECIAL FEATURES:

Tween Brands, Inc., formerly Too, Inc. is a retail clothing and accessories retailer that primarily works through two subsidiaries, Limited Too and Justice which target girls aged 7-14 years old, also known as tweens. Originally established as a subsidiary of Limited Brands, Inc., formerly The Limited, Inc., the firm became an independent company after a stock spin-off in 1999. It currently owns and operates 582 Limited Too and 260 Justice stores in 37 states and Puerto Rico. Limited Too sells apparel, underwear, sleepwear, swimwear, lifestyle and personal care products; and it also sells non-apparel merchandise, such as candy, electronic toys and games. Justice operates primarily in non-mall locations, such as power centers which attract customer's intent on apparel shopping; and sells less expensive apparel, sportswear and accessory items. Tween Brands clothing and other products are developed internally, with manufacturing mainly sourced to factories in the Pacific Rim. The company has two direct sourcing offices located in Hong Kong and South Korea, which were established in 2002 and 2006, respectively. Direct sourcing purchases represented 25% of its total purchases in fiscal 2007. In addition to the company's direct sourcing offices, it makes use a variety of external sourcing arrangements. Ultimately, the firm expects direct sourcing to account for approximately 45% of its total merchandise purchases. Tween stores feature furniture, fixtures, lighting and music to create a shopping experience matching the energetic lifestyle of young girls. To keep the store atmosphere fresh, the firm continually reassess the layout of its stores. To this end, roughly 49% of its stores are less than three years old. In 2007, the company entered into a new partnership with Family Invest AB, to operate Limited Too stores in Scandinavia beginning in fiscal 2008. Currently the firm has one store open and operating under this agreement.

FINANCIALS: Sales and profits are in thousands of dollars—add 000 to get the full amount. 2007 Note: Financial information for 2007 was not available for all companies at press time.

2007 Sales: $883,683	2007 Profits: $64,821	**U.S. Stock Ticker:** TWB
2006 Sales: $757,936	2006 Profits: $54,451	**Int'l Ticker:** Int'l Exchange:
2005 Sales: $675,834	2005 Profits: $41,589	Employees: 12,400
2004 Sales: $598,681	2004 Profits: $22,551	Fiscal Year Ends: 1/31
2003 Sales: $647,455	2003 Profits: $47,338	Parent Company:

SALARIES/BENEFITS:

Pension Plan:	ESOP Stock Plan:	Profit Sharing:	Top Exec. Salary: $1,050,000	Bonus: $1,423,800
Savings Plan:	Stock Purch. Plan:		Second Exec. Salary: $516,538	Bonus: $440,700

OTHER THOUGHTS:

Apparent Women Officers or Directors: 2
Hot Spot for Advancement for Women/Minorities: Y

LOCATIONS: ("Y" = Yes)

West:	Southwest:	Midwest:	Southeast:	Northeast:	International:
Y	Y	Y	Y	Y	Y

TYSON FOODS INC

www.tyson.com

Industry Group Code: 112300 Ranks within this company's industry group: Sales: Profits:

Management:		Sales/Marketing:		Liberal Arts:		Information Systems:		Professionals:		Technical/Scientific:	
Mgmt. Trainees:	Y	Mktg. Professionals:	Y	Gen. Writing/Editing:		Info. Management:	Y	Finance/Accounting:	Y	Engineers, Elec.:	
Experienced Mgmt.:	Y	Retail Sales:		Technical Writing:		Software Dev.:		Law:	Y	Engineers, Other:	
Int'l Business:	Y	Commercial/Industrial:	Y	Graphic Arts/Photog.:	Y	Hardware Dev.:		HR/Other:	Y	Health/Lab:	
MBA Graduates:	Y	Sales Trainees:		Music:		Systems Integration:		Training:	Y	Scientists/Research:	
		Advertising Pros.:	Y	Broadcasting:		Consulting/Other:		Health Care:		Petroleum/Chemicals:	
				Other:				Consulting:		Math/Other:	

TYPES OF BUSINESS:

Poultry Processing
Beef & Pork Products
Ethnic Foods
Soups & Sauces
Frozen & Refrigerated Food

BRANDS/DIVISIONS/AFFILIATES:

Cobb

CONTACTS: *Note: Officers with more than one job title may be intentionally listed here more than once.*

Richard L. Bond, CEO
Richard L. Bond, Pres.
Wade D. Miquelon, CFO/Exec. VP
Kenneth J. Kimbro, Sr. VP-Human Resources
Howell P. Carper, Sr. VP-R&D
Gary Cooper, CIO/Sr. VP
J. Alberto Gonzalez-Pita, General Counsel/Exec. VP
Ruth Ann Wisener, VP-Investor Rel.
Craig J. Hart, Chief Acct. Officer/Controller/Sr. VP
Karen Gilbert, Sr. VP-Ethics, Compliance & Internal Audit
R. Read Hudson, Corp. Sec./VP
Dennis Leatherby, Sr. VP-Finance/Treas.
Scott McNair, VP-Consumer Prod.
John Tyson, Chmn.
Mike Baker, Sr. VP-Int'l & Cobb-Vantress Oper.
Donnie Smith, VP-Logistics & Oper. Svcs.

Phone: 479-290-4000	Fax: 501-290-4061
Toll-Free:	
Address: 2210 W. Oaklawn Dr., Springdale, AR 72762 US	

GROWTH PLANS/SPECIAL FEATURES:

Tyson Foods, Inc. is a processor and marketer of chicken, beef and pork products. It produces a wide range of fresh, value-added, frozen and refrigerated food products. The company operates in four segments: chicken, beef, pork and prepared foods. The chicken operations include breeding and raising chickens, as well as processing live chickens into fresh, frozen and value-added chicken products. The beef operations include processing live cattle and fabrication of dressed beef carcasses into primal and sub-primal meat cuts and case-ready products. This segment also includes sales from allied products such as hides and variety meats. The pork operations include processing live market hogs and fabricating pork carcasses into primal and sub-primal cuts and case-ready products. This segment also includes the live swine group and related allied product processing activities. The prepared food operations manufacture and market frozen food products. Products include pepperoni, bacon, beef and pork pizza toppings, pizza crusts, flour and corn tortilla products, appetizers, prepared meals, ethnic foods, soups, sauces, side dishes, meat dishes and processed meats. Products are marketed domestically to food retailers, foodservices distributors, restaurant operators and noncommercial foodservice establishments such as schools, hotel chains, health care facilities, the military and other food processors, as well as to international markets. The firm also has international operations, including a Mexican poultry production subsidiary; a Canadian subsidiary, which has a cattle feeding facility, beef carcass production, a boxed beef processing facility, a farming operation and a fertilizer operation; a chicken breeding stock subsidiary, Cobb, with business interests in Latin America, India, Europe and the Philippines; and a majority interest in a chicken further processing and beef processing facilities in China.

FINANCIALS: Sales and profits are in thousands of dollars—add 000 to get the full amount. 2007 Note: Financial information for 2007 was not available for all companies at press time.

2007 Sales: $26,900,000	2007 Profits: $268,000	U.S. Stock Ticker: TSN
2006 Sales: $25,559,000	2006 Profits: $-196,000	Int'l Ticker: Int'l Exchange:
2005 Sales: $26,014,000	2005 Profits: $372,000	Employees: 104,000
2004 Sales: $26,441,000	2004 Profits: $403,000	Fiscal Year Ends: 9/30
2003 Sales: $24,549,000	2003 Profits: $337,000	Parent Company:

SALARIES/BENEFITS:

Pension Plan:	ESOP Stock Plan:	Profit Sharing:	Top Exec. Salary: $1,198,462	Bonus: $1,743,320
Savings Plan: Y	Stock Purch. Plan: Y		Second Exec. Salary: $1,170,000	Bonus: $

OTHER THOUGHTS:

Apparent Women Officers or Directors: 4
Hot Spot for Advancement for Women/Minorities: Y

LOCATIONS: ("Y" = Yes)

West:	Southwest:	Midwest:	Southeast:	Northeast:	International:
Y	Y	Y	Y	Y	Y

Note: Financial information, benefits and other data can change quickly and may vary from those stated here.

UNION PACIFIC CORP

www.up.com

Industry Group Code: 482110 Ranks within this company's industry group: Sales: 1 Profits: 2

Management:		Sales/Marketing:		Liberal Arts:		Information Systems:		Professionals:		Technical/Scientific:	
Mgmt. Trainees:		Mktg. Professionals:		Gen. Writing/Editing:		Info. Management:	Y	Finance/Accounting:	Y	Engineers, Elec.:	Y
Experienced Mgmt.:	Y	Retail Sales:		Technical Writing:		Software Dev.:	Y	Law:	Y	Engineers, Other:	Y
Int'l Business:		Commercial/Industrial:	Y	Graphic Arts/Photog.:		Hardware Dev.:		HR/Other:	Y	Health/Lab:	
MBA Graduates:	Y	Sales Trainees:		Music:		Systems Integration:	Y	Training:	Y	Scientists/Research:	
		Advertising Pros.:		Broadcasting:		Consulting/Other:		Health Care:		Petroleum/Chemicals:	
				Other:				Consulting:		Math/Other:	

TYPES OF BUSINESS:
Railroad

BRANDS/DIVISIONS/AFFILIATES:
Union Pacific Railroad Company

CONTACTS: *Note: Officers with more than one job title may be intentionally listed here more than once.*
James R. Young, CEO
James R. Young, Pres.
Robert M. Knight, Jr., CFO/Exec. VP
John J. Koraleski, Exec. VP-Sales & Mktg.
Barbara W. Schaefer, Sr. VP-Human Resources
Lynden Tennison, CIO/Sr. VP
J. Michael Hemmer, General Counsel/Sr. VP-Law
Dennis J. Duffy, Exec. VP-Oper.
Charles R. Eisele, Sr. VP-Strategic Planning
Robert W. Turner, Sr. VP-Corp. Rel.
Mary S. Jones, Treas./VP
Barbara W. Schaefer, Corp. Sec.
John J. Marchant, VP-Labor Rel.
Richard R. McClish, VP-Continuous Improvement
Mike Rock, VP-External Rel.
James R. Young, Chmn.

Phone: 402-544-5000	Fax: 402-501-2133
Toll-Free: 888-870-8777	
Address: 1400 Douglas St., Omaha, NE 68179 US	

GROWTH PLANS/SPECIAL FEATURES:

Union Pacific Corp. operates primarily as a rail transportation provider through Union Pacific Railroad Company, which is one of the largest railroads in North America, covering 23 states across the western two-thirds of the U.S. Union Pacific Railroad is a Class I railroad with approximately 32,339 route miles linking Pacific Coast and Gulf Coast ports with the Midwest and Eastern U.S. gateways and providing several north/south corridors to key Mexican gateways. The firm handles freight in six commodity groups: agriculture, including grains, food products, beverages and sweeteners; automotive, as the largest automotive carrier west of the Mississippi River; chemicals, including liquid and dry chemicals, plastics and liquid petroleum products; energy, including coal transportation; industrial products, such as stone, cement, lumber, paper and government and consumer goods; and intermodal. In January 2007, Union Pacific put into service the first of 60 environmentally friendly next-generation locomotives for service in the Los Angeles Basin rail yards, in which the company recently invested over $38 million in improvements and upgrades. In February 2008, the firm announced a plan to invest $3.1 billion in capital projects during 2008. Proposed projects include strengthening track infrastructure; increasing terminal capacity; upgrading the locomotive and freight car fleet; and upgrading information technology systems.

Union Pacific offers its employees comprehensive health and dental coverage, flexible spending accounts, life and accident insurance, long-term disability, educational assistance and a relocation program, among other benefits.

FINANCIALS: Sales and profits are in thousands of dollars—add 000 to get the full amount. 2007 Note: Financial information for 2007 was not available for all companies at press time.

2007 Sales: $16,283,000	2007 Profits: $1,855,000	**U.S. Stock Ticker:** UNP
2006 Sales: $15,578,000	2006 Profits: $1,606,000	**Int'l Ticker:** Int'l Exchange:
2005 Sales: $13,578,000	2005 Profits: $1,026,000	Employees: 50,739
2004 Sales: $12,215,000	2004 Profits: $604,000	Fiscal Year Ends: 12/31
2003 Sales: $11,551,000	2003 Profits: $1,585,000	Parent Company:

SALARIES/BENEFITS:

Pension Plan: Y	ESOP Stock Plan:	Profit Sharing:	Top Exec. Salary: $1,450,000	Bonus: $2,500,000
Savings Plan: Y	Stock Purch. Plan:		Second Exec. Salary: $1,000,000	Bonus: $2,250,000

OTHER THOUGHTS:
Apparent Women Officers or Directors: 2
Hot Spot for Advancement for Women/Minorities: Y

LOCATIONS: ("Y" = Yes)

West:	Southwest:	Midwest:	Southeast:	Northeast:	International:
Y	Y	Y	Y		

UNITED NATURAL FOODS INC
www.unfi.com

Industry Group Code: 422410 **Ranks within this company's industry group:** Sales: 2 Profits: 2

Management:		Sales/Marketing:		Liberal Arts:		Information Systems:		Professionals:		Technical/Scientific:	
Mgmt. Trainees:		Mktg. Professionals:	Y	Gen. Writing/Editing:	Y	Info. Management:	Y	Finance/Accounting:	Y	Engineers, Elec.:	
Experienced Mgmt.:	Y	Retail Sales:		Technical Writing:		Software Dev.:	Y	Law:	Y	Engineers, Other:	
Int'l Business:		Commercial/Industrial:	Y	Graphic Arts/Photog.:	Y	Hardware Dev.:		HR/Other:	Y	Health/Lab:	
MBA Graduates:	Y	Sales Trainees:		Music:		Systems Integration:		Training:	Y	Scientists/Research:	
		Advertising Pros.:		Broadcasting:		Consulting/Other:		Health Care:		Petroleum/Chemicals:	
				Other:				Consulting:		Math/Other:	

TYPES OF BUSINESS:
Food Distribution
Natural & Organic Foods Distribution
Nutritional Supplements Distribution
Personal Care Products Distribution
Retail Stores

BRANDS/DIVISIONS/AFFILIATES:
Natural Retail Group
Hershey Import Co.
Albert's Organics
Blooming Prairie Cooperative Warehouse
Grateful Harvest
Woodstock Farms
Select Nutrition Distributors, Inc.
Roots & Fruits Cooperative Produce

CONTACTS: *Note: Officers with more than one job title may be intentionally listed here more than once.*
Michael S. Funk, CEO
Michael S. Funk, Pres.
Mark E. Shamber, CFO/VP
Daniel V. Atwood, Chief Mktg. Officer/Pres., United Natural Brands
Carl F. Koch III, VP-Human Resources
John Stern, CIO
Mark E. Shamber, Treas.
Michael D. Beaudry, Pres., Eastern Region
Thomas A. Dziki, VP-Sustainable Dev.
Randle E. Lindberg, Pres., Western Region
Casey Van Rysdam, Pres., Specialty Foods
Thomas Simone, Chmn.

Phone: 860-779-2800	Fax:
Toll-Free: 800-877-8898	
Address: 260 Lake Rd., Dayville, CT 06241 US	

GROWTH PLANS/SPECIAL FEATURES:

United Natural Foods, Inc. (UNFI) is a national distributor of natural and organic foods and related products. The company carries more than 40,000 natural and organic products, consisting of national bran, regional brand, private label and master distribution products, in six product categories: grocery and general merchandise, produce, perishables and frozen foods, nutritional supplements, bulk and food service products. The firm serves more than 17,000 customers, including independently owned natural products retailers, supernatural chains, which are comprised of large chains of natural foods supermarkets, and conventional supermarkets located across the U.S. Other distribution channels include food service, international and buying clubs. The company has been the primary distributor to the largest natural foods chain in the United States, Whole Foods Market, Inc., for more than 10 years. The company's operations are comprised of three principal divisions: wholesale, which includes its distribution business; retail, which consists of UNFI's 12 retail stores; and manufacturing, which is comprised of its subsidiary, Hershey Imports Co. and its branded product lines. Other subsidiaries include Albert's Organics, Boulder Fruit Express, Inc., Blooming Prairie Cooperative Warehouse, Mountain People's Warehouse and Rainbow Natural Foods. UNFI has a number of company-owned brands including Woodstock Farms, Grateful Harvest, Natural Sea, Old Wessex, Organic Baby and others.

UNFI offers employees medical and dental insurance for full- and part-time regular employees, profit sharing, 401(k), paid holidays and vacations, paid sick leave, life insurance, long-term disability insurance, an employee assistance program which provides free counseling and other assistance for employees and a tuition assistance program.

FINANCIALS: Sales and profits are in thousands of dollars—add 000 to get the full amount. 2007 Note: Financial information for 2007 was not available for all companies at press time.

2007 Sales: $2,754,280	2007 Profits: $50,153	**U.S. Stock Ticker: UNFI**
2006 Sales: $2,433,594	2006 Profits: $43,277	**Int'l Ticker:** Int'l Exchange:
2005 Sales: $2,059,568	2005 Profits: $41,572	Employees: 4,800
2004 Sales: $1,669,952	2004 Profits: $31,986	Fiscal Year Ends: 8/02
2003 Sales: $1,379,900	2003 Profits: $20,200	Parent Company:

SALARIES/BENEFITS:

Pension Plan:	ESOP Stock Plan:	Profit Sharing: Y	Top Exec. Salary: $511,564	Bonus: $
Savings Plan: Y	Stock Purch. Plan:		Second Exec. Salary: $376,923	Bonus: $700,000

OTHER THOUGHTS:
Apparent Women Officers or Directors:
Hot Spot for Advancement for Women/Minorities:

LOCATIONS: ("Y" = Yes)

West:	Southwest:	Midwest:	Southeast:	Northeast:	International:
Y		Y	Y	Y	

UNITED PARCEL SERVICE INC (UPS)   www.ups.com

Industry Group Code: 492110 Ranks within this company's industry group: Sales: 1 Profits: 1

Management:		Sales/Marketing:		Liberal Arts:		Information Systems:		Professionals:		Technical/Scientific:	
Mgmt. Trainees:	Y	Mktg. Professionals:	Y	Gen. Writing/Editing:	Y	Info. Management:	Y	Finance/Accounting:	Y	Engineers, Elec.:	Y
Experienced Mgmt.:	Y	Retail Sales:		Technical Writing:	Y	Software Dev.:	Y	Law:	Y	Engineers, Other:	
Int'l Business:	Y	Commercial/Industrial:	Y	Graphic Arts/Photog.:	Y	Hardware Dev.:		HR/Other:	Y	Health/Lab:	
MBA Graduates:	Y	Sales Trainees:		Music:		Systems Integration:		Training:	Y	Scientists/Research:	Y
		Advertising Pros.:	Y	Broadcasting:		Consulting/Other:		Health Care:		Petroleum/Chemicals:	
				Other:				Consulting:	Y	Math/Other:	Y

TYPES OF BUSINESS:

Express Delivery Service
Logistics Services
Supply Chain Services
International Products & Services
Ground & Air Delivery Services
Visibility & Technology Services

BRANDS/DIVISIONS/AFFILIATES:

UPS Freight
UPS Supply Chain Solutions
UPS WorldShip
Quantum View
UPS Next Day Air
UPS Hundredweight Services
Flex Global View
UPS Billing Analysis Tool

CONTACTS: *Note: Officers with more than one job title may be intentionally listed here more than once.*

D. Scott Davis, CEO
David Abney, COO
Kurt Kuehn, CFO
Alan Gershenhorn, Sr. VP-Worldwide Sales & Mktg.
Allen E. Hill, Sr. VP-Human Resources
David Barnes, CIO/Sr. VP
Bob Stoffel, Sr. VP-Eng.
Teri P. McClure, General Counsel/Sr. VP-Legal/Corp. Sec.
Bob Stoffel, Sr. VP-Strategy
Christine M. Owens, Sr. VP-Comm. & Brand Mgmt.
John McDevitt, Sr. VP-Global Transportation Svcs.
David Abney, Pres., UPS Airlines
Jim Winestock, Sr. VP-US Oper.
D. Scott Davis, Chmn.
Daniel J. Brutto, Pres., UPS Int'l
Bob Stoffel, Sr. VP-Supply Chain

Phone: 404-828-6000	Fax: 404-828-6562
Toll-Free: 800-874-5877	
Address: 55 Glenlake Pkwy., NE, Atlanta, GA 30328 US	

GROWTH PLANS/SPECIAL FEATURES:

United Parcel Service, Inc. (UPS) is a package delivery company and a global provider of supply chain management. It delivers packages each business day for 1.8 million shipping customers to 6.1 million consignees in over 200 countries. The company delivers an average of 15.8 million pieces per day worldwide. In addition, the supply chain solutions capabilities are available in over 175 countries. The firm is also a major provider of less-than-truckload transportation services. Offerings include domestic and international package products and services; supply chain and freight services; and visibility and technology solutions. The domestic package products and services business delivers packages traveling by ground or air transportation. In addition to the standard ground delivery products, UPS Hundredweight Services offers guaranteed, time-definite service to customers sending multiple packages shipments. UPS Next Day Air offers guaranteed next business day delivery by 10:30 am to 75% of the U.S. population and delivery by noon to areas covering an additional 15% of the population. International services include guaranteed early morning, morning and noon delivery to major cities around the world, as well as scheduled day-definite air and ground services. Supply chain and freight services comprise the freight forwarding and logistics business and encompass more than 60 services. Visibility and technology products provide solutions that support automated shipping and tracking, including UPS WorldShip, that helps streamline shipping activities by processing shipments, printing address labels, tracking packages and providing management reports, all from a computer; and Quantum View, a suite of visibility services that provides detailed, timely information about the status of UPS outbound and inbound shipments.

The company offers its employees medical, dental and vision insurance; life and business travel accident insurance; cancer insurance; a 401(k) plan; a defined benefit pension plan; an employee stock purchase plan; and education assistance.

FINANCIALS: Sales and profits are in thousands of dollars—add 000 to get the full amount. 2007 Note: Financial information for 2007 was not available for all companies at press time.

2007 Sales: $49,700,000	2007 Profits: $447,000	**U.S. Stock Ticker: UPS**
2006 Sales: $47,547,000	2006 Profits: $4,202,000	**Int'l Ticker:** Int'l Exchange:
2005 Sales: $42,581,000	2005 Profits: $3,870,000	Employees: 428,000
2004 Sales: $36,582,000	2004 Profits: $3,333,000	Fiscal Year Ends: 12/31
2003 Sales: $33,485,000	2003 Profits: $2,898,000	Parent Company:

SALARIES/BENEFITS:

Pension Plan: Y	ESOP Stock Plan:	Profit Sharing:	Top Exec. Salary: $988,000	Bonus: $215,800
Savings Plan: Y	Stock Purch. Plan: Y		Second Exec. Salary: $538,000	Bonus: $117,260

OTHER THOUGHTS:

Apparent Women Officers or Directors: 4
Hot Spot for Advancement for Women/Minorities: Y

LOCATIONS: ("Y" = Yes)

West:	Southwest:	Midwest:	Southeast:	Northeast:	International:
Y	Y	Y	Y	Y	Y

UNITED STATES CELLULAR CORP   www.uscellular.com

Industry Group Code: 513322 Ranks within this company's industry group: Sales: 4   Profits: 4

Management:		Sales/Marketing:		Liberal Arts:		Information Systems:		Professionals:		Technical/Scientific:	
Mgmt. Trainees:	Y	Mktg. Professionals:	Y	Gen. Writing/Editing:	Y	Info. Management:	Y	Finance/Accounting:	Y	Engineers, Elec.:	Y
Experienced Mgmt.:	Y	Retail Sales:	Y	Technical Writing:		Software Dev.:	Y	Law:	Y	Engineers, Other:	
Int'l Business:		Commercial/Industrial:	Y	Graphic Arts/Photog.:	Y	Hardware Dev.:		HR/Other:	Y	Health/Lab:	
MBA Graduates:	Y	Sales Trainees:	Y	Music:		Systems Integration:		Training:	Y	Scientists/Research:	
		Advertising Pros.:	Y	Broadcasting:		Consulting/Other:		Health Care:		Petroleum/Chemicals:	
				Other:				Consulting:		Math/Other:	

TYPES OF BUSINESS:

Cellular Telephone Service
PCS Service

BRANDS/DIVISIONS/AFFILIATES:

Telephone and Data Systems Inc
easyedge
Qualcomm Inc
Smartphone
Windows Mobile
Motorola Q
BlackBerry 8830
My Contacts Backup

CONTACTS: Note: Officers with more than one job title may be intentionally listed here more than once.

John E. Rooney, CEO
Jay M. Ellison, COO/Exec. VP
John E. Rooney, Pres.
Steven T. (Steve) Campbell, CFO/Exec. VP-Finance/Treas.
Alan D. Ferber, VP-Sales Oper./Chief Mktg. Officer
Jeffrey J. (Jeff) Childs, Chief Human Resources Officer/Sr. VP
John M. Cregier, VP-IT Delivery
Michael S. (Mike) Irizarry, CTO/Exec. VP
John C. Gockley, VP-Legal & Regulatory Affairs
Kevin R. Lowell, VP-National Network Oper.
Karen C. Ehlers, VP-Public Affairs & Comm.
Thomas S. (Tom) Weber, VP-Financial Strategy
Rochelle J. (Shelley) Boersma, VP-Midwest Oper.
Thomas P. (Tom) Catani, VP-East Oper.
Nick B. Wright, VP-West Oper.
George W. Irving, VP-Bus. Support Svcs.
LeRoy T. Carlson, Jr., Chmn.

Phone: 773-399-8900	Fax: 773-399-7054
Toll-Free: 888-944-9400	
Address: 8410 W. Bryn Mawr Ave., Ste. 700, Chicago, IL 60631 US	

GROWTH PLANS/SPECIAL FEATURES:

United States Cellular Corporation (U.S. Cellular), a majority-owned subsidiary of Telephone and Data Systems, Inc., is a leading wireless service provider in the U.S., serving roughly 6.1 million customers in 26 states. The company owns interests in 218 consolidated wireless markets that cover portions of 34 states and a total population of roughly 82.4 million. U.S. Cellular operates approximately 6,400 cell sites and over 400 retail stores. The company's ownership interests in wireless licenses include both consolidated and investment interests in cellular licenses covering metropolitan statistical areas and rural service areas; digital PCS (personal communication service) licenses; advanced wireless service licenses; and 700 megahertz (MHz) licenses. It manages the operations of all but two of the licenses in which it owns a controlling interest. U.S. Cellular offers a range of wireless handset devices, laptop cards and such accessories as carrying cases, hands-free devices, batteries and battery chargers. The company's easyedge brand of enhanced data services uses a binary runtime environment for wireless (BREW) technology, licensed from Qualcomm, and adds limited computer-like functionality to handsets, enabling applications to be downloaded over-the-air directly to the customer's wireless device. These enhanced data services include downloading news, weather, sports information, games, ringtones and other services. During 2007, U.S. Cellular expanded its Smartphone category with the addition of its first Windows Mobile handset device, the Motorola Q, and with the launch of a multimedia Blackberry device, the BlackBerry 8830 Smartphone. In May 2007, the company announced the introduction of My Contacts Backup, a data backup application available through easyedge. My Contacts Backup is powered by Asurion, a provider of enhanced services to the wireless industry.

U.S. Cellular offers its employees an associate scholar program; a PC purchase program; flexible hours; adoption assistance; a flexible spending account; and medical, dental, vision, life and disability insurance.

FINANCIALS: Sales and profits are in thousands of dollars—add 000 to get the full amount. 2007 Note: Financial information for 2007 was not available for all companies at press time.

2007 Sales: $3,946,264	2007 Profits: $314,734	U.S. Stock Ticker: USM
2006 Sales: $3,473,155	2006 Profits: $179,490	Int'l Ticker: Int'l Exchange:
2005 Sales: $3,030,765	2005 Profits: $154,951	Employees: 7,837
2004 Sales: $2,808,201	2004 Profits: $109,516	Fiscal Year Ends: 12/31
2003 Sales: $2,582,783	2003 Profits: $42,660	Parent Company: TELEPHONE AND DATA SYSTEMS INC

SALARIES/BENEFITS:

Pension Plan: Y	ESOP Stock Plan:	Profit Sharing:	Top Exec. Salary: $790,000	Bonus: $525,000
Savings Plan: Y	Stock Purch. Plan: Y		Second Exec. Salary: $502,920	Bonus: $336,414

OTHER THOUGHTS:

Apparent Women Officers or Directors: 3
Hot Spot for Advancement for Women/Minorities: Y

LOCATIONS: ("Y" = Yes)

West:	Southwest:	Midwest:	Southeast:	Northeast:	International:
Y	Y	Y	Y	Y	

Note: Financial information, benefits and other data can change quickly and may vary from those stated here.

UNITED TECHNOLOGIES CORPORATION

www.utc.com

Industry Group Code: 336410 Ranks within this company's industry group: Sales: 2 Profits: 1

Management:		Sales/Marketing:		Liberal Arts:		Information Systems:		Professionals:		Technical/Scientific:	
Mgmt. Trainees:	Y	Mktg. Professionals:	Y	Gen. Writing/Editing:	Y	Info. Management:	Y	Finance/Accounting:	Y	Engineers, Elec.:	Y
Experienced Mgmt.:	Y	Retail Sales:		Technical Writing:	Y	Software Dev.:	Y	Law:	Y	Engineers, Other:	
Int'l Business:	Y	Commercial/Industrial:	Y	Graphic Arts/Photog.:	Y	Hardware Dev.:	Y	HR/Other:	Y	Health/Lab:	Y
MBA Graduates:	Y	Sales Trainees:		Music:		Systems Integration:	Y	Training:	Y	Scientists/Research:	Y
		Advertising Pros.:		Broadcasting:		Consulting/Other:	Y	Health Care:		Petroleum/Chemicals:	
				Other:				Consulting:	Y	Math/Other:	Y

TYPES OF BUSINESS:

Aerospace Technology
Elevator & Escalator Systems
HVAC Systems
Fuel Cells & Power Generation
Industrial Systems
Aircraft Parts & Maintenance
Flight Systems
Security Products & Services

BRANDS/DIVISIONS/AFFILIATES:

Otis Elevator Company
Carrier Corp.
Sikorsky
Pratt & Whitney
Hamilton Sundstrand
UTC Fire and Security
UTC Power

CONTACTS: Note: Officers with more than one job title may be intentionally listed here more than once.

Louis Chenevert, CEO
Louis Chenevert, Pres.
William L. Bucknall, Jr., Sr. VP-Human Resources & Organization
J. Michael McQuade, Sr. VP-Science
John Doucette, CIO/VP
J. Michael McQuade, Sr. VP-Tech.
William H. Trachsel, General Counsel/Sr. VP
Jothi Purushotaman, VP-Oper.
Michael A. Monts, VP-Bus. Practices
Nancy T. Lintner, VP-Comm.
Gregory J. Hayes, VP-Finance & Acct.
Ari Bousbib, Pres., Otis Elevator
Geraud Darnis, Pres., Carrier Corp.
Steven N. Finger, Pres., Pratt & Whitney
Jan van Dokkum, Pres., UTC Power
George David, Chmn.
Alison Kaufman, Sr. VP-Int'l & Gov't Affairs

Phone: 860-728-7000	Fax: 860-728-7979
Toll-Free:	
Address: 1 Financial Plz., Hartford, CT 06101 US	

GROWTH PLANS/SPECIAL FEATURES:

United Technologies Corporation (UTC) owns six operating companies and a research facility, all involved in the technology research, development and production sector. Its main companies consist of Otis Elevator Company; Carrier Corp.; Pratt & Whitney; Sikorsky; Hamilton Sundstrand; and UTC Fire and Security. Otis is one of the world's largest elevator and escalator manufacturing, installation, modernization and maintenance companies. Carrier manufactures commercial and residential heating, ventilation and air conditioning (HVAC) systems and equipment. It also produces, sells, services and provides components for commercial and transport refrigeration equipment. Pratt & Whitney produces and services commercial, general aviation and military aircraft engines. It also handles rocket engine production for commercial and government space applications. Sikorsky is a world leader in helicopters manufacturing and design, whose customers include the U.S. military and 40 other countries. Hamilton Sundstrand serves commercial, military, regional and corporate aviation, as well as space and undersea applications. Its products, found in 90% of the world's aircraft, include power generation management and distribution systems; auxiliary power units; and flight, propeller, engine, environmental control and fire protection and detection systems. Lastly, UTC Fire and Security operates in the electronic security industry, manufacturing intruder alarms, video surveillance systems and other products; and the fire safety industry, manufacturing fixed suppression systems, fire extinguishers and other products. In addition to the above companies, it owns UTC Power, with products including fuel cells, waste-power recycling, heat-to-energy solutions and mobile power plants. UTC's research and development unit strengthens its position in its various markets and provides contract work for government and other customers.

Employees of UTC receive health and life insurance; vision care discounts; adoption assistance; a matching gift program; employee assistance; and tuition reimbursement. UTC also offers fitness centers at some of its facilities.

FINANCIALS: Sales and profits are in thousands of dollars—add 000 to get the full amount. 2007 Note: Financial information for 2007 was not available for all companies at press time.

2007 Sales: $54,759,000	2007 Profits: $4,224,000	**U.S. Stock Ticker: UTX**
2006 Sales: $47,829,000	2006 Profits: $3,732,000	**Int'l Ticker:** Int'l Exchange:
2005 Sales: $42,725,000	2005 Profits: $3,069,000	Employees: 225,600
2004 Sales: $37,445,000	2004 Profits: $2,788,000	Fiscal Year Ends: 12/31
2003 Sales: $31,034,000	2003 Profits: $2,361,000	Parent Company:

SALARIES/BENEFITS:

Pension Plan: Y	ESOP Stock Plan:	Profit Sharing:	Top Exec. Salary: $1,791,667	Bonus: $6,834,287
Savings Plan: Y	Stock Purch. Plan:		Second Exec. Salary: $808,333	Bonus: $2,052,894

OTHER THOUGHTS:

Apparent Women Officers or Directors: 2
Hot Spot for Advancement for Women/Minorities:

LOCATIONS: ("Y" = Yes)

West:	Southwest:	Midwest:	Southeast:	Northeast:	International:
Y	Y	Y	Y	Y	Y

UNITEDHEALTH GROUP INC   www.unitedhealthgroup.com

Industry Group Code: 524114 Ranks within this company's industry group: Sales: 1 Profits: 1

Management:		Sales/Marketing:		Liberal Arts:		Information Systems:		Professionals:		Technical/Scientific:	
Mgmt. Trainees:	Y	Mktg. Professionals:	Y	Gen. Writing/Editing:	Y	Info. Management:	Y	Finance/Accounting:	Y	Engineers, Elec.:	
Experienced Mgmt.:	Y	Retail Sales:		Technical Writing:		Software Dev.:	Y	Law:	Y	Engineers, Other:	Y
Int'l Business:		Commercial/Industrial:	Y	Graphic Arts/Photog.:	Y	Hardware Dev.:		HR/Other:	Y	Health/Lab:	
MBA Graduates:	Y	Sales Trainees:		Music:		Systems Integration:		Training:	Y	Scientists/Research:	Y
		Advertising Pros.:	Y	Broadcasting:		Consulting/Other:		Health Care:	Y	Petroleum/Chemicals:	
				Other:				Consulting:		Math/Other:	

TYPES OF BUSINESS:
Medical Insurance
Wellness Plans
Dental & Vision Insurance

BRANDS/DIVISIONS/AFFILIATES:
Sierra Health Services0 Inc
Uniprise Incorporated
Golden Rule Insurance Company
Ingenix
Definity Health
Mid Atlantic Medical Services Inc
Pacificare Health Systems Inc
Dental Benefits Providers

CONTACTS: *Note: Officers with more than one job title may be intentionally listed here more than once.*
Stephen J. Hemsley, CEO
Stephen J. Hemsley, Pres.
G. Mike Mikan, CFO/Exec. VP
Lori Sweere, Exec. VP-Human Capital
Thomas L. Strickland, Chief Legal Officer/Exec. VP
Peter Gill, VP-Corp. Dev.
Don Nathan, Chief Comm. Officer/Sr. VP
Eric S. Rangen, Chief Acct. Officer/Sr. VP
Anthony Welters, Exec. VP/Head-Public & Social Markets Group
David S. Wichmann, Exec. VP/Pres., Individual & Employer Market Group
Reed V. Tuckson, Exec. VP/Chief-Medical Affairs
Jeannine M. Rivet, Exec. VP
Richard T. Burke, Chmn.

Phone: 952-936-1300	Fax: 952-936-7430
Toll-Free: 800-328-5979	
Address: 9900 Bren Rd. E., Minnetonka, MN 55343 US	

GROWTH PLANS/SPECIAL FEATURES:
UnitedHealth Group, Inc. is a diversified health and well-being company, serving about 70 million Americans. The company provides individuals with access to healthcare services and resources through more than 560,000 physicians and other care providers and 4,800 hospitals across the U.S. The company has four operating segments: Health Care Services; OptumHealth; Ingenix; and Prescription Solutions (formerly included in Ovations). The Health Care Services segment, which includes UnitedHealthcare (comprising UnitedHealthcare National Accounts, formerly Uniprise) and Public and Senior Markets Group (Ovations and AmeriChoice), provides consumer-oriented health benefit plans and services for public sector and small and mid-sized private sector employers health care and well-being services nationwide to large national employers, individual consumers and other health care organizations, for individuals age 50 and older. The OptumHealth segment is engaged in care solutions, behavioral solutions, specialty benefits and financial services in fields such as dental, vision, life, disability and stop-loss coverage. The Ingenix segment offers database and data management services; software products; publications; consulting services; outsourced services; and pharmaceutical development and consulting services nationwide and internationally. Ingenix's customers include more than 5,000 hospitals; 240,000 physicians; 1,500 payers and intermediaries; more than 245 Fortune 500 companies; and more than 250 life sciences companies. The Prescription Solutions segment offers a comprehensive suite of integrated pharmacy benefit management (PBM) services to approximately 10.3 million people, through approximately 64,000 retail network pharmacies and two mail service facilities. In February 2008, UnitedHealth acquired Sierra Health Services, Inc. for $2.6 billion. In May 2008, the company acquired Unison Health Plans (Unison) for approximately $930 million. Unison provides government-sponsored health plan coverage to people in Pennsylvania, Ohio, Tennessee, Delaware, South Carolina and Washington, D.C.

The company offers its employees medical, vision and dental insurance; flexible spending accounts; life and AD&D insurance; and tuition reimbursement.

FINANCIALS: Sales and profits are in thousands of dollars—add 000 to get the full amount. 2007 Note: Financial information for 2007 was not available for all companies at press time.

2007 Sales: $75,431,000	2007 Profits: $4,654,000	**U.S. Stock Ticker: UNH**	
2006 Sales: $71,542,000	2006 Profits: $4,159,000	**Int'l Ticker:**	Int'l Exchange:
2005 Sales: $46,425,000	2005 Profits: $3,083,000	Employees: 58,000	
2004 Sales: $38,217,000	2004 Profits: $2,411,000	Fiscal Year Ends: 12/31	
2003 Sales: $28,823,000	2003 Profits: $1,825,000	Parent Company:	

SALARIES/BENEFITS:

Pension Plan:	ESOP Stock Plan:	Profit Sharing:	Top Exec. Salary: $2,146,923	Bonus: $
Savings Plan: Y	Stock Purch. Plan: Y		Second Exec. Salary: $1,019,615	Bonus: $2,875,000

OTHER THOUGHTS:
Apparent Women Officers or Directors: 3
Hot Spot for Advancement for Women/Minorities: Y

LOCATIONS: ("Y" = Yes)

West:	Southwest:	Midwest:	Southeast:	Northeast:	International:
Y	Y	Y	Y	Y	

Note: Financial information, benefits and other data can change quickly and may vary from those stated here.

UNIVISION COMMUNICATIONS INC   www.univision.com

Industry Group Code: 513120 Ranks within this company's industry group: Sales: 1   Profits: 1

Management:		Sales/Marketing:		Liberal Arts:		Information Systems:		Professionals:		Technical/Scientific:	
Mgmt. Trainees:	Y	Mktg. Professionals:	Y	Gen. Writing/Editing:	Y	Info. Management:	Y	Finance/Accounting:	Y	Engineers, Elec.:	Y
Experienced Mgmt.:	Y	Retail Sales:		Technical Writing:	Y	Software Dev.:	Y	Law:	Y	Engineers, Other:	
Int'l Business:	Y	Commercial/Industrial:	Y	Graphic Arts/Photog.:	Y	Hardware Dev.:		HR/Other:	Y	Health/Lab:	
MBA Graduates:	Y	Sales Trainees:		Music:	Y	Systems Integration:		Training:	Y	Scientists/Research:	
		Advertising Pros.:	Y	Broadcasting:	Y	Consulting/Other:		Health Care:		Petroleum/Chemicals:	
				Other:	Y			Consulting:		Math/Other:	

TYPES OF BUSINESS:
Spanish Television Broadcasting
Cable Television Programming
Online Portal
Radio Broadcasting

BRANDS/DIVISIONS/AFFILIATES:
Univision Television Group
Galavision
TeleFutura
Univision Online, Inc.
Univision Radio, Inc.
Broadcasting Media Partners, Inc.

CONTACTS: *Note: Officers with more than one job title may be intentionally listed here more than once.*
Joe Uva, CEO
Ray Rodriguez, COO
Ray Rodriguez, Pres.
Andrew W. Hobson, CFO/Sr. Exec. VP
C. Douglas Kranwinkle, General Counsel/Exec. VP
Andrew W. Hobson, Chief Strategic Officer
Haim Saban, Chmn.

Phone: 212-455-5200	Fax:
Toll-Free:	
Address: 605 3rd Ave., 12th Fl., New York, NY 10158 US	

GROWTH PLANS/SPECIAL FEATURES:
Univision Communications, Inc. is the leading Spanish-language media company in the U.S. The company currently operates in three business segments: television, which is the company's principle business segment, representing 77% of Univision's net revenue, consists of the Univision and TeleFutura national broadcast networks, and the Galavisión cable television network; radio, which is operated through Univision Radio, Inc. and consists of 21% of the firm's net revenue, owns 69 radio stations in 16 of the top 25 U.S. Hispanic markets, in addition to four stations in Puerto Rico; and Internet, which is run through Univision Online, Inc. and consists of univision.com, a web portal with an annual average of 3 billion hits. Each of these three segments represents the largest Spanish-language media application in their respective fields within the U.S. Following the completion of the,. The firm is able to reach 99% of all U.S. Hispanic households via its nationwide Univision broadcast and cable channels. TeleFutura is the company's 24-hour Spanish-language broadcast television network, reaching 87% of U.S. Hispanic households. The company's Galavision network is the leading Spanish-language cable television network, with more than 5.9 million Hispanic cable subscribers. Broadcast is supported by the Univision Television Group, which owns and operates 20 full-power and 10 low-power Univision Network stations, and one full-power UPN station. In March 2007, Broadcasting Media Partners, Inc., a consortium of private-equity investors, acquired Univision and all of its subsidiaries. In February 2008, the company sold its music and recording business subsidiaries, including the Univision, Fonovisa, Disa and La Calle labels, to Universal Music Group for approximately $153 million. In May 2008, the company unveiled a new video on demand component of its Internet division, offering more than 1,000 hours of sports, news, movies and entertainment from all of the company's cable stations.

FINANCIALS: Sales and profits are in thousands of dollars—add 000 to get the full amount. 2007 Note: Financial information for 2007 was not available for all companies at press time.

2007 Sales: $2,196,000	2007 Profits: $-314,900	**U.S. Stock Ticker: Subsidiary**
2006 Sales: $2,166,652	2006 Profits: $349,174	Int'l Ticker: Int'l Exchange:
2005 Sales: $1,952,531	2005 Profits: $187,179	Employees: 4,233
2004 Sales: $1,786,935	2004 Profits: $255,883	Fiscal Year Ends: 12/31
2003 Sales: $1,311,015	2003 Profits: $155,427	Parent Company: BROADCASTING MEDIA PARTNERS, INC

SALARIES/BENEFITS:
Pension Plan:	ESOP Stock Plan:	Profit Sharing:	Top Exec. Salary: $800,000	Bonus: $1,000,000
Savings Plan:	Stock Purch. Plan:		Second Exec. Salary: $750,000	Bonus: $1,000,000

OTHER THOUGHTS:
Apparent Women Officers or Directors:
Hot Spot for Advancement for Women/Minorities:

LOCATIONS: ("Y" = Yes)
West:	Southwest:	Midwest:	Southeast:	Northeast:	International:
Y	Y	Y	Y	Y	Y

UPS SUPPLY CHAIN SOLUTIONS
www.ups-scs.com

Industry Group Code: 488510 Ranks within this company's industry group: Sales: Profits:

Management:		Sales/Marketing:		Liberal Arts:		Information Systems:		Professionals:		Technical/Scientific:	
Mgmt. Trainees:	Y	Mktg. Professionals:		Gen. Writing/Editing:	Y	Info. Management:	Y	Finance/Accounting:	Y	Engineers, Elec.:	
Experienced Mgmt.:	Y	Retail Sales:		Technical Writing:	Y	Software Dev.:	Y	Law:	Y	Engineers, Other:	
Int'l Business:	Y	Commercial/Industrial:	Y	Graphic Arts/Photog.:		Hardware Dev.:		HR/Other:	Y	Health/Lab:	
MBA Graduates:	Y	Sales Trainees:		Music:		Systems Integration:	Y	Training:	Y	Scientists/Research:	
		Advertising Pros.:	Y	Broadcasting:		Consulting/Other:		Health Care:		Petroleum/Chemicals:	
				Other:				Consulting:	Y	Math/Other:	

TYPES OF BUSINESS:
Logistics Services
Courier Services
Trade Management
Customs Brokerage
Supply Chain Design Services
Service Parts Logistics

BRANDS/DIVISIONS/AFFILIATES:
United Parcel Service Inc (UPS)
UPS Trade Direct

CONTACTS: Note: Officers with more than one job title may be intentionally listed here more than once.
John Sutthoff, VP-Mktg.
Laurie Johnson, VP-Tech.
Robert E. (Bob) Stoffel, Sr. VP-UPS Eng.
Robert E. (Bob) Stoffel, Sr. VP-Strategy
John Sutthoff, VP-Strategy & Supply Chain
Robert E. (Bob) Stoffel, Sr. VP-Supply Chain

Phone: 913-693-6151	Fax: 913-469-8824
Toll-Free: 800-742-5727	
Address: 12380 Morris Rd., Alpharetta, GA 30005 US	

GROWTH PLANS/SPECIAL FEATURES:

UPS Supply Chain Solutions, a subsidiary of United Parcel Service, Inc. (UPS), provides transportation and freight services (via ground, sea, air and rail), logistics services, international trade management, consulting services and industry solutions to customers worldwide. In addition, the company provides specialty services such as service parts logistics, technical repair and configuration, multi-modal transportation network management, supply chain design and planning, returns management and urgent parts delivery. The firm is currently one of the largest logistics providers in the world, relying on the extensive UPS transportation network to suit the needs of its customers. Its UPS Trade Direct service, for example, bypasses distribution centers, providing freight consolidation and delivery to multiple addresses. UPS picks up and consolidates shipments, transports the shipments to their destination, clears them through customs, deconsolidates the shipment into individual shipments, then drops them into the UPS package network and ships directly to the customer. The company's distribution services network combines a shared IT platform with a network of multi-client distribution centers located strategically across the U.S. The firm's consulting services allow small and large companies, organizations and governments to align their supply chain processes with their business strategies. Additionally, the company provides industry-specific services for a number of markets, including automotive and industrial manufacturing; consumer goods; healthcare; retail; and government. UPS Supply Chain Solutions has over 930 facilities at its disposal, ranging from regional logistics and technology centers to small strategic stocking locations and critical parts depots, refrigerated facilities and bonded distribution centers in more than 120 countries.

UPS Supply Chain offers its employees medical, dental, vision, prescription, life and disability insurance. Additional employee benefits offered include tuition assistance programs, flexible spending accounts, adoption assistance, a dependent scholarship program, an employee assistance program, an employee mortgage program, an employee discount program and a work/life assistance program.

FINANCIALS: Sales and profits are in thousands of dollars—add 000 to get the full amount. 2007 Note: Financial information for 2007 was not available for all companies at press time.

2007 Sales: $	2007 Profits: $	U.S. Stock Ticker: Subsidiary
2006 Sales: $	2006 Profits: $	Int'l Ticker: Int'l Exchange:
2005 Sales: $4,737,000	2005 Profits: $	Employees:
2004 Sales: $2,346,000	2004 Profits: $	Fiscal Year Ends: 12/31
2003 Sales: $2,126,000	2003 Profits: $	Parent Company: UNITED PARCEL SERVICE INC (UPS)

SALARIES/BENEFITS:
Pension Plan: Y	ESOP Stock Plan:	Profit Sharing:	Top Exec. Salary: $	Bonus: $
Savings Plan: Y	Stock Purch. Plan: Y		Second Exec. Salary: $	Bonus: $

OTHER THOUGHTS:
Apparent Women Officers or Directors: 1
Hot Spot for Advancement for Women/Minorities:

LOCATIONS: ("Y" = Yes)
West:	Southwest:	Midwest:	Southeast:	Northeast:	International:
Y	Y	Y	Y	Y	Y

Note: Financial information, benefits and other data can change quickly and may vary from those stated here.

URBAN OUTFITTERS INC

www.urbanoutfittersinc.com

Industry Group Code: 448000 Ranks within this company's industry group: Sales: 7 Profits: 5

Management:		Sales/Marketing:		Liberal Arts:		Information Systems:		Professionals:		Technical/Scientific:	
Mgmt. Trainees:	Y	Mktg. Professionals:	Y	Gen. Writing/Editing:	Y	Info. Management:	Y	Finance/Accounting:	Y	Engineers, Elec.:	
Experienced Mgmt.:	Y	Retail Sales:	Y	Technical Writing:		Software Dev.:	Y	Law:	Y	Engineers, Other:	
Int'l Business:	Y	Commercial/Industrial:	Y	Graphic Arts/Photog.:	Y	Hardware Dev.:		HR/Other:	Y	Health/Lab:	
MBA Graduates:	Y	Sales Trainees:	Y	Music:		Systems Integration:		Training:	Y	Scientists/Research:	
		Advertising Pros.:	Y	Broadcasting:		Consulting/Other:		Health Care:		Petroleum/Chemicals:	
				Other:	Y			Consulting:		Math/Other:	

TYPES OF BUSINESS:

Casual Apparel Stores
Household & Gift Merchandise
Accessories
Wholesale Distribution
Online Sales
Footwear
Catalog Sales

BRANDS/DIVISIONS/AFFILIATES:

Urban Outfitters
Anthropologie
Free People

CONTACTS: Note: Officers with more than one job title may be intentionally listed here more than once.

Glen T. Senk, CEO
Richard A. Hayne, Pres.
John E. Kyees, CFO
Freeman M. Zausner, Chief Admin. Officer
Glen A. Bodzy, General Counsel/Corp. Sec.
Robert Ross, Controller
Glen T. Senk, Pres., Anthropologie, Inc.
Tedford G. Marlow, Pres., Urban Retail
Richard A. Hayne, Chmn.

Phone: 215-454-5500	Fax: 215-454-5163
Toll-Free:	
Address: 5000 S. Broad St., Philadelphia, PA 19112-1495 US	

GROWTH PLANS/SPECIAL FEATURES:

Urban Outfitters, Inc. is a clothing and accessories company that operates specialty retail stores under the Urban Outfitters, Anthropologie and Free People brands, as well as a wholesale division under the Free People brand. Urban Outfitters targets young adults aged 18-30 through its upscale, style-conscious merchandise mix and store environment. The company manages and owns 125 Urban Outfitters stores throughout the U.S., Canada and Europe. Its stores are located in major metropolitan areas, near large universities or in other youth-saturated markets. A typical store has over 30,000 to 35,000 stock keeping units (SKUs), including women's and men's fashion apparel, footwear, accessories, apartment wares and gifts. In 2008, Urban Outfitters circulated approximately 13 million catalogs in an effort to expand its distribution channels and increase brand awareness. Anthropologie targets upscale female customers from 30-45 years old. The more than 108 Anthropologie stores are all located near affluent suburban or urban locations, offering women's casual apparel, accessories, home furnishings, gifts and decorative items. Stores average 8,000 square feet and carry 20,000 to 25,000 SKUs. During 2008, Anthropologie circulated 22 million catalogs. Free People, the firm's wholesale division, designs, develops and markets young women's casual apparel through 15 stores in the U.S. Its products, including tops, bottoms, sweaters and dresses, are sold worldwide through approximately 1,500 department and specialty stores, such as Bloomingdale's, Nordstrom and Urban Outfitters, using a shop-within-shops sales model. In 2008, the company circulated approximately 5 million catalogs. About 14% of total revenues are created via mailings and the web site.

Urban Outfitters offers employees wellness programs, financial planning and protection, product discounts, bonuses and associate referral rewards.

FINANCIALS: Sales and profits are in thousands of dollars—add 000 to get the full amount. 2007 Note: Financial information for 2007 was not available for all companies at press time.

2007 Sales: $1,224,717	2007 Profits: $116,206	U.S. Stock Ticker: URBN
2006 Sales: $1,092,107	2006 Profits: $130,796	Int'l Ticker: Int'l Exchange:
2005 Sales: $827,750	2005 Profits: $90,489	Employees: 8,400
2004 Sales: $548,361	2004 Profits: $48,376	Fiscal Year Ends: 1/31
2003 Sales: $422,800	2003 Profits: $27,400	Parent Company:

SALARIES/BENEFITS:

Pension Plan:	ESOP Stock Plan:	Profit Sharing:	Top Exec. Salary: $577,218	Bonus: $55,000
Savings Plan: Y	Stock Purch. Plan:		Second Exec. Salary: $436,676	Bonus: $55,000

OTHER THOUGHTS:

Apparent Women Officers or Directors:
Hot Spot for Advancement for Women/Minorities:

LOCATIONS: ("Y" = Yes)

West:	Southwest:	Midwest:	Southeast:	Northeast:	International:
Y	Y	Y	Y	Y	Y

URS CORPORATION

www.urscorp.com

Industry Group Code: 541330 Ranks within this company's industry group: Sales: 1 Profits: 1

Management:		Sales/Marketing:		Liberal Arts:		Information Systems:		Professionals:		Technical/Scientific:	
Mgmt. Trainees:	Y	Mktg. Professionals:	Y	Gen. Writing/Editing:		Info. Management:	Y	Finance/Accounting:	Y	Engineers, Elec.:	Y
Experienced Mgmt.:	Y	Retail Sales:		Technical Writing:	Y	Software Dev.:	Y	Law:	Y	Engineers, Other:	Y
Int'l Business:	Y	Commercial/Industrial:	Y	Graphic Arts/Photog.:	Y	Hardware Dev.:		HR/Other:	Y	Health/Lab:	
MBA Graduates:	Y	Sales Trainees:		Music:		Systems Integration:		Training:	Y	Scientists/Research:	Y
		Advertising Pros.:		Broadcasting:		Consulting/Other:		Health Care:		Petroleum/Chemicals:	
				Other:				Consulting:	Y	Math/Other:	Y

TYPES OF BUSINESS:

Engineering Design Services
Systems Engineering & Technical Assistance
Operations & Maintenance Services

BRANDS/DIVISIONS/AFFILIATES:

EG&G Division
URS Division
Washington Division
LopezGarcia Group, Inc.
Washington Group International

CONTACTS: *Note: Officers with more than one job title may be intentionally listed here more than once.*

Martin M. Koffel, CEO
Martin M. Koffel, Pres.
H. Thomas Hicks, CFO/VP-Finance
Joseph Masters, General Counsel/Sec.
Thomas W. Bishop, VP-Strategy/Sr. VP-Construction Svcs.
Susan B. Kilgannon, VP-Comm.
Reed N. Brimhall, VP/Controller/Chief Acct. Officer
Thomas H. Zarges, Pres., Washington Div.
Gary V. Jandegian, VP/Pres., URS Div.
Randall A. Wotring, VP/Pres., EG&G Div.
Martin M. Koffel, Chmn.

Phone: 415-774-2700	Fax: 415-398-1905
Toll-Free:	
Address: 600 Montgomery St., Fl. 26, San Francisco, CA 94111 US	

GROWTH PLANS/SPECIAL FEATURES:

URS Corp. is an engineering design services worldwide firm and a U.S. federal government contractor for systems engineering and technical assistance and operations and maintenance services. The company focuses primarily on providing fee-based professional and technical services in the engineering and construction services and defense markets, although it performs some limited construction work. The firm operates in two divisions: URS division and the EG&G division. The URS division provides professional planning and design; program management; construction management; and operations and maintenance services to various government agencies and departments in the U.S. and internationally, as well as to private industry clients. The EG&G division provides planning; systems engineering and technical assistance; operations and maintenance; and program management services to various U.S. federal government agencies, primarily the Departments of Defense and Homeland Security. URS focuses its services on eight key markets: transportation; environmental; facilities; industrial infrastructure and process; water/wastewater; homeland security; defense systems; and installations and logistics. The company has a network of offices and job sites across the U.S. and in more than 30 foreign countries in the Americas, Europe, the Middle East and Asia-Pacific. The federal government accounted for 41% of the company's revenues in 2007, while state and local governments, private industry and international clients accounted for 21%, 27% and 11%, respectively. In November 2007, the company acquired rival Washington Group International, Inc. for about $3.1 billion. These assets became the Washington Division of URS, a third operating division. In August 2008, the firm acquired LopezGarcia Group, Inc. as well as most of the assets of Tryck Nyman Hayes, Inc.

The company offers its employees health and dental insurance; a 401(k) plan; an employee stock purchase plan; short- and long-term insurance; life and accident insurance; an employee assistance program; flexible spending accounts; and group legal services.

FINANCIALS: Sales and profits are in thousands of dollars—add 000 to get the full amount. 2007 Note: Financial information for 2007 was not available for all companies at press time.

2007 Sales: $5,383,007	2007 Profits: $132,243	U.S. Stock Ticker: URS
2006 Sales: $4,222,869	2006 Profits: $113,012	Int'l Ticker: Int'l Exchange:
2005 Sales: $3,890,282	2005 Profits: $82,475	Employees: 56,000
2004 Sales: $3,381,963	2004 Profits: $61,704	Fiscal Year Ends: 12/31
2003 Sales: $3,186,714	2003 Profits: $58,104	Parent Company:

SALARIES/BENEFITS:

Pension Plan:	ESOP Stock Plan:	Profit Sharing:	Top Exec. Salary: $950,019	Bonus: $1,451,145
Savings Plan: Y	Stock Purch. Plan: Y		Second Exec. Salary: $500,513	Bonus: $372,218

OTHER THOUGHTS:

Apparent Women Officers or Directors: 1
Hot Spot for Advancement for Women/Minorities: Y

LOCATIONS: ("Y" = Yes)

West:	Southwest:	Midwest:	Southeast:	Northeast:	International:
Y	Y	Y	Y	Y	Y

Note: Financial information, benefits and other data can change quickly and may vary from those stated here.

USAA
www.usaa.com

Industry Group Code: 524126 Ranks within this company's industry group: Sales: 2   Profits: 1

Management:		Sales/Marketing:		Liberal Arts:		Information Systems:		Professionals:		Technical/Scientific:	
Mgmt. Trainees:	Y	Mktg. Professionals:	Y	Gen. Writing/Editing:	Y	Info. Management:	Y	Finance/Accounting:	Y	Engineers, Elec.:	
Experienced Mgmt.:	Y	Retail Sales:		Technical Writing:	Y	Software Dev.:	Y	Law:	Y	Engineers, Other:	
Int'l Business:	Y	Commercial/Industrial:		Graphic Arts/Photog.:	Y	Hardware Dev.:		HR/Other:	Y	Health/Lab:	
MBA Graduates:	Y	Sales Trainees:	Y	Music:		Systems Integration:		Training:	Y	Scientists/Research:	Y
		Advertising Pros.:	Y	Broadcasting:		Consulting/Other:		Health Care:	Y	Petroleum/Chemicals:	
				Other:				Consulting:		Math/Other:	Y

TYPES OF BUSINESS:

Insurance, Direct Property & Casualty
Banking
Life Insurance
Real Estate Development
Discount Brokerage
Investment Management
Mutual Funds

BRANDS/DIVISIONS/AFFILIATES:

USAA Alliance Services
USAA Investment Management Company
USAA Educational Foundation

CONTACTS: *Note: Officers with more than one job title may be intentionally listed here more than once.*

Josue Robles, Jr., CEO
Robert T. Handren, COO
Kristi A. Matus, CFO
Elizabeth D. Conklyn, Exec. VP-People Svcs.
Steven A. Bennett, General Counsel/Corp. Sec/Exec. VP
Wayne Peacock, Exec. VP-Enterprise Bus. Oper.
Wendi E. Strong, Exec. VP-Corp. Comm.
F. David Bohne, Pres., USAA Fed. Savings Bank
Stuart Parker, Pres., USAA Property & Casualty Insurance Group
Christopher W. claus, Pres., USAA Financial Svcs. Group
John H. Moellering, Chmn.

Phone: 210-498-2211	Fax: 210-498-9940
Toll-Free: 800-531-8722	
Address: 9800 Fredericksburg Rd., San Antonio, TX 78288 US	

GROWTH PLANS/SPECIAL FEATURES:

USAA is a mutual insurance company that exclusively serves U.S. military personnel and their families which currently number 6.4 million members. The firm owns and manages over $81 billion in assets from offices in Texas, Arizona, Virginia, Colorado, Florida and California, in addition to international offices in London, England and Frankfurt, Germany. The company offers automobile, homeowner's and renter's insurance and automobile, mortgage and home equity loans. USAA also manages checking accounts, savings accounts, credit cards and personal loans for its military customers. The firm's USAA Investment Management Company provides a full line of mutual funds and brokerage services. Subsidiary USAA Alliance Services has formed a series of partnerships to provide members with discounts home security, travel services and insurance, floral services, car rentals and diamond and fine jewelry. The firm's USAA Educational Foundation division is a nonprofit entity that provides consumer education to the general public. Educational topics include personal finance, safety and quality of life. Members of USAA are able to access their accounts and conduct investing, banking and insurance business online. In 2008, USAA expanded its membership eligibility to include: military retirees, regardless of when they retired; military personnel who were honorably discharged on or after Jan. 1, 1996; and widows or widowers of military personnel killed in action while eligible. After they join, spouses and children of the above may also be eligible for membership.

USAA employee benefits include educational assistance, flextime, flexible spending accounts, business casual dress, wellness benefits and blood pressure screenings. Company employees who are called to active military duty receive their accustomed pay for four weeks, and pay differential for up to two years after deployment. USAA employees are eligible to receive benefits, holiday bonuses and corporate performance bonuses during the time they are deployed. Women account for 62% of USAA's employees.

FINANCIALS: Sales and profits are in thousands of dollars—add 000 to get the full amount. 2007 Note: Financial information for 2007 was not available for all companies at press time.

2007 Sales: $14,417,900	2007 Profits: $1,855,500	**U.S. Stock Ticker: Mutual Company**
2006 Sales: $13,416,000	2006 Profits: $2,330,000	**Int'l Ticker:** Int'l Exchange:
2005 Sales: $11,980,000	2005 Profits: $1,388,000	Employees: 22,000
2004 Sales: $11,273,000	2004 Profits: $1,597,000	Fiscal Year Ends: 12/31
2003 Sales: $10,593,000	2003 Profits: $1,501,000	Parent Company:

SALARIES/BENEFITS:

Pension Plan: Y	ESOP Stock Plan:	Profit Sharing:	Top Exec. Salary: $	Bonus: $
Savings Plan: Y	Stock Purch. Plan:		Second Exec. Salary: $	Bonus: $

OTHER THOUGHTS:

Apparent Women Officers or Directors: 6
Hot Spot for Advancement for Women/Minorities: Y

LOCATIONS: ("Y" = Yes)

West:	Southwest:	Midwest:	Southeast:	Northeast:	International:
Y	Y		Y	Y	Y

VALERO ENERGY CORP

www.valero.com

Industry Group Code: 324110A Ranks within this company's industry group: Sales: Profits:

Management:	Sales/Marketing:	Liberal Arts:	Information Systems:	Professionals:	Technical/Scientific:
Mgmt. Trainees:	Mktg. Professionals:	Gen. Writing/Editing:	Info. Management:	Finance/Accounting:	Engineers, Elec.:
Experienced Mgmt.:	Retail Sales:	Technical Writing:	Software Dev.:	Law:	Engineers, Other:
Int'l Business:	Commercial/Industrial:	Graphic Arts/Photog.:	Hardware Dev.:	HR/Other:	Health/Lab:
MBA Graduates:	Sales Trainees:	Music:	Systems Integration:	Training:	Scientists/Research:
	Advertising Pros.:	Broadcasting:	Consulting/Other:	Health Care:	Petroleum/Chemicals:
		Other:		Consulting:	Math/Other:

TYPES OF BUSINESS:

Petroleum Refineries & Retail Marketing
Convenience Stores
Home Heating Fuels
Wholesale Fuel Marketing
Asphalt
Marine Transportation

BRANDS/DIVISIONS/AFFILIATES:

Valero Refining & Marketing Company
Corner Store
Stop N Go
Diamond Shamrock
Road Runner

CONTACTS: *Note: Officers with more than one job title may be intentionally listed here more than once.*

William R. Klesse, CEO
Richard J. Marcogliese, COO/Exec. VP
William R. Klesse, Pres.
Michael S. Ciskowski, CFO/Exec. VP
Joseph W. Gorder, Exec. VP-Mktg. & Supply
Mike Crownover, Sr. VP-Human Resources
Hal Zesch, CIO/Sr. VP
Kim Bowers, General Counsel/Sr. VP
S. Eugene Edwards, Exec. VP-Corp. Dev. & Strategic Planning
Eric Fisher, VP-Investor & Corp. Comm.
Donna Titzman, Treas./VP
Gary Arthur, Jr., Sr. VP-Retail Mktg.
Jay D. Browning, Sec./Sr. VP-Corp. Law
Clay Killinger, Sr. VP/Controller
Steve Gilbert, Asst. Sec./Disclosure & Compliance Officer
William R. Klesse, Chmn.

Phone: 210-345-2000	Fax: 210-345-2646
Toll-Free: 800-531-7911	
Address: 1 Valero Way, San Antonio, TX 78249-1616 US	

GROWTH PLANS/SPECIAL FEATURES:

Valero Energy Corporation, formerly Valero Refining & Marketing Company, is a refiner and retailer of gasoline and other oil related products. Valero owns and operates 17 refineries located in the U.S., Canada and Aruba that produce conventional gasolines, distillates, jet fuel, asphalt, petrochemicals, lubricants and other refined products as well as a slate of premium products including diesel fuel, low-sulfur and ultra-low-sulfur diesel fuel, and oxygenates (liquid hydrocarbon compounds containing oxygen). The firm markets branded and unbranded refined products on a wholesale basis in the U.S. and Canada through an extensive bulk and rack marketing network. Valero also sells refined products through a network of about 5,800 retail and wholesale branded outlets in the U.S., Canada and Aruba. The company's business is organized into two reportable segments: refining and retail. The refining segment includes refining operations, wholesale marketing, product supply and distribution and transportation operations. The segment has a total throughput capacity of approximately 3.1 million barrels per day. Valero's retail segment sells transportation fuels at retail stores and unattended, self-service cardlocks; convenience store merchandise in retail stores; and home heating oil to residential customers. The segment is separated into two groups: Retail-U.S., which owns or leases 953 stores under the names Corner Store and Stop N Go and sells transportation fuel under the Valero and Diamond Shamrock brands; and Retail-Canada, which owns or leases 432 retail stores, distributes gasoline to 488 dealers and jobbers and sells transportation fuels under the Ultramar brand through a network of 920 outlets. In 2007, Valero sold its Lima, Ohio refinery to Husky Energy, Inc. for $1.9 billion. Also in 2007, the firm unveiled a new 5,500 Road Runner retail store concept in San Antonio, Texas that devotes more space to prepared foods and meals to go.

FINANCIALS: Sales and profits are in thousands of dollars—add 000 to get the full amount. 2007 Note: Financial information for 2007 was not available for all companies at press time.

2007 Sales: $95,327,000	2007 Profits: $5,234,000	U.S. Stock Ticker: VLO
2006 Sales: $87,640,000	2006 Profits: $5,463,000	Int'l Ticker: Int'l Exchange:
2005 Sales: $80,616,000	2005 Profits: $3,590,000	Employees: 22,000
2004 Sales: $54,589,000	2004 Profits: $	Fiscal Year Ends: 12/31
2003 Sales: $37,951,000	2003 Profits: $	Parent Company:

SALARIES/BENEFITS:

Pension Plan:	ESOP Stock Plan:	Profit Sharing:	Top Exec. Salary: $900,000	Bonus: $1,305,000
Savings Plan:	Stock Purch. Plan:		Second Exec. Salary: $707,000	Bonus: $820,000

OTHER THOUGHTS:

Apparent Women Officers or Directors: 2
Hot Spot for Advancement for Women/Minorities:

LOCATIONS: ("Y" = Yes)

West:	Southwest:	Midwest:	Southeast:	Northeast:	International:
Y	Y	Y	Y	Y	Y

VALSPAR CORPORATION (THE)   www.valspar.com

Industry Group Code: 325510 Ranks within this company's industry group: Sales: 1   Profits: 1

Management:		Sales/Marketing:		Liberal Arts:		Information Systems:		Professionals:		Technical/Scientific:	
Mgmt. Trainees:		Mktg. Professionals:	Y	Gen. Writing/Editing:		Info. Management:	Y	Finance/Accounting:	Y	Engineers, Elec.:	
Experienced Mgmt.:	Y	Retail Sales:		Technical Writing:	Y	Software Dev.:		Law:	Y	Engineers, Other:	Y
Int'l Business:	Y	Commercial/Industrial:	Y	Graphic Arts/Photog.:	Y	Hardware Dev.:		HR/Other:	Y	Health/Lab:	
MBA Graduates:	Y	Sales Trainees:		Music:		Systems Integration:		Training:	Y	Scientists/Research:	Y
		Advertising Pros.:	Y	Broadcasting:		Consulting/Other:		Health Care:		Petroleum/Chemicals:	Y
				Other:				Consulting:		Math/Other:	

TYPES OF BUSINESS:

Coatings & Paints
Packaging Products
Specialty Polymers
General Industrial, Coil & Wood Products
Colorants & Gelcoats
Furniture Protection Plans

BRANDS/DIVISIONS/AFFILIATES:

Valspar Refinish
De Beer
House of Kolor
Teknos Nova Coil TNC Oy
Tekno S.A.
Huarun Paints
H.B. Fuller

CONTACTS: Note: Officers with more than one job title may be intentionally listed here more than once.

William L. Mansfield, CEO
Gary E. Hendrickson, COO
Gary E. Hendrickson, Pres.
Lori A. Walker, CFO/Sr. VP
Anthony L. Blaine, Sr. VP-Human Resources
Rolf Engh, General Counsel/Exec. VP/Sec.
Tyler N. Treat, Contact-Investor Rel.
Paul C. Reyelts, Exec. VP-Finance
Steven L. Erdahl, Exec. VP
Tracy C. Jokinen, VP/Controller
Tyler N. Treat, VP/Treas.
William L. Mansfield, Chmn.

Phone: 612-332-7371	Fax: 612-375-7723
Toll-Free:	
Address: 1101 3rd St. S., Minneapolis, MN 55415-1211 US	

GROWTH PLANS/SPECIAL FEATURES:

The Valspar Corporation is a provider of paints, coatings and related products. The company operates in two segments, coatings and paints. The coatings segment includes a range of decorative and protective coatings for metal, wood, plastic and glass, primarily for sale to original equipment manufacturers (OEMs). Products within this segment include fillers, primers, varnishes, inks, sprays, stains and other coatings used by customers in manufacturing industries such as building products, appliances, automotive parts, furniture and metal fabrication. This segment includes the firm's packaging product line and three industrial product lines: General industrial, coil and wood coatings. The packaging product line includes coatings for the interior and exterior of metal packaging containers, principally food containers and beverage cans. The firm also produces coatings for aerosol and paint cans; bottle crowns for glass; plastic packaging; and bottle closures. The coil coatings unit includes the firm's Finland subsidiary Teknos Nova Coil TNC Oy and the Brazilian joint venture, Tekno S.A.; the wood coatings unit includes an 80% interest in Huarun Paints; and the industrial coatings unit includes H.B. Fuller, an English powder coatings business. The paints segment offers interior and exterior paints; stains; primers; varnishes; high performance floor paints; and specialty decorative products for sale through merchants such as Lowe's. This segment also markets automotive refinish paints under brand names Valspar Refinish, De Beer and House of Kolor. In addition to the product lines offered through its two segments, Valspar makes and sells specialty polymers, colorants, gelcoats and furniture protection plans. The company's gelcoats and related products are sold to boat manufacturers, shower and tub manufacturers and others.

Valspar offers employees medical, dental and life insurance; education assistance; disability insurance; and an employee assistance program.

FINANCIALS: Sales and profits are in thousands of dollars—add 000 to get the full amount. 2007 Note: Financial information for 2007 was not available for all companies at press time.

2007 Sales: $3,249,287	2007 Profits: $172,115	U.S. Stock Ticker: VAL	
2006 Sales: $2,978,062	2006 Profits: $175,252	Int'l Ticker:	Int'l Exchange:
2005 Sales: $2,713,950	2005 Profits: $147,618	Employees: 10,000	
2004 Sales: $2,440,692	2004 Profits: $142,836	Fiscal Year Ends: 10/31	
2003 Sales: $2,247,926	2003 Profits: $112,514	Parent Company:	

SALARIES/BENEFITS:

Pension Plan:	ESOP Stock Plan: Y	Profit Sharing:	Top Exec. Salary: $850,000	Bonus: $736,350
Savings Plan:	Stock Purch. Plan:		Second Exec. Salary: $531,000	Bonus: $415,907

OTHER THOUGHTS:

Apparent Women Officers or Directors: 5
Hot Spot for Advancement for Women/Minorities: Y

LOCATIONS: ("Y" = Yes)

West:	Southwest:	Midwest:	Southeast:	Northeast:	International:
Y	Y	Y	Y	Y	Y

Note: Financial information, benefits and other data can change quickly and may vary from those stated here.

VARIAN MEDICAL SYSTEMS INC

www.varian.com

Industry Group Code: 339113 Ranks within this company's industry group: Sales: 11 Profits: 8

Management:		Sales/Marketing:		Liberal Arts:		Information Systems:		Professionals:		Technical/Scientific:	
Mgmt. Trainees:		Mktg. Professionals:	Y	Gen. Writing/Editing:	Y	Info. Management:	Y	Finance/Accounting:	Y	Engineers, Elec.:	Y
Experienced Mgmt.:	Y	Retail Sales:		Technical Writing:	Y	Software Dev.:	Y	Law:	Y	Engineers, Other:	Y
Int'l Business:		Commercial/Industrial:	Y	Graphic Arts/Photog.:	Y	Hardware Dev.:	Y	HR/Other:	Y	Health/Lab:	Y
MBA Graduates:	Y	Sales Trainees:		Music:		Systems Integration:		Training:	Y	Scientists/Research:	Y
		Advertising Pros.:	Y	Broadcasting:		Consulting/Other:		Health Care:	Y	Petroleum/Chemicals:	
				Other:				Consulting:		Math/Other:	Y

TYPES OF BUSINESS:

Oncology Systems
X-Ray Equipment
Software Systems
Security & Inspection Products

BRANDS/DIVISIONS/AFFILIATES:

Clinac
Ginzton Technology Center
PortalVision
Millennium
RapidArc

CONTACTS: Note: Officers with more than one job title may be intentionally listed here more than once.

Timothy E. Guertin, CEO
Timothy E. Guertin, Pres.
Elisha W. Finney, CFO/Sr. VP
Wendy S. Reitherman, VP-Human Resources
Jessia Denocour, CIO/VP
John W. Kuo, General Counsel/VP/Corp. Sec.
J. A. Thorson, VP-Bus. Dev.
Spencer R. Sias, VP-Corp. Comm.
Spencer R. Sias, VP-Investor Rel.
Franco N. Palomba, VP-Finance
Tai-Yun Chen, Controller/VP
Robert H. Kluge, VP/Pres., X-Ray Prod.
Dow R. Wilson, Exec. VP/Pres., Oncology Systems
George A. Zdasiuk, VP/CTO-Ginzton Tech. Center
Richard M. Levy, Chmn.

Phone: 650-493-4000	Fax: 650-842-5196
Toll-Free:	
Address: 3100 Hansen Way, Palo Alto, CA 94304 US	

GROWTH PLANS/SPECIAL FEATURES:

Varian Medical Systems, Inc. designs, manufactures, sells and services advanced equipment and software products for treating cancer and other conditions with radiotherapy, proton therapy, radiosurgery and brachytherapy. The firm operates in three segments: oncology systems, X-ray products and other. The oncology systems segment provides software and hardware for treating cancer with radiation, including linear accelerators; treatment simulation and verification products; information management and treatment planning software; advanced brachytherapy products and software; and other accessory products and services. The Clinac series of medical linear accelerators treats cancer by producing electrons and x-rays in shaped beams that target tumors and other abnormalities in a patient. The Millennium series of multi-leaf collimators are used with a linear accelerator to define the size, shape and intensity of the radiation beams generated by the linear accelerator. PortalVision, an electronic portal-imaging product, verifies a patient's treatment position, a critical component for accurate delivery of radiotherapy treatment. The X-ray products segment manufactures and sells X-ray imaging components and subsystems, namely X-ray tubes for use in a range of applications including computed tomography, or CT, scanning; radioscopic/fluoroscopic imaging; mammography; special procedures and flat panel detectors for digital X-ray image capture, which is an alternative to image intensifier tubes for fluoroscopy and X-ray film for radiography. The other segment includes the security and inspection products business, which provides Linatron X-ray accelerators to OEMs; and technologies developed by the Ginzton Technology Center, including digital X-ray imaging technology; volumetric and functional imaging; improved X-ray sources; and technology for security and cargo screening applications. In January 2008, the firm received FDA 510(k) clearance for its RapidArc radiotherapy technology, which delivers image-guided, intensity-modulated radiation therapy (IMRT) two to eight times faster than conventional IMRT.

FINANCIALS: Sales and profits are in thousands of dollars—add 000 to get the full amount. 2007 Note: Financial information for 2007 was not available for all companies at press time.

2007 Sales: $1,776,600	2007 Profits: $239,500	U.S. Stock Ticker: VAR			
2006 Sales: $1,597,800	2006 Profits: $245,100	Int'l Ticker: Int'l Exchange:			
2005 Sales: $1,382,600	2005 Profits: $206,600	Employees: 3,900			
2004 Sales: $1,235,523	2004 Profits: $167,700	Fiscal Year Ends: 9/30			
2003 Sales: $1,041,600	2003 Profits: $130,900	Parent Company:			

SALARIES/BENEFITS:

Pension Plan:	ESOP Stock Plan:	Profit Sharing:	Top Exec. Salary: $681,766	Bonus: $319,801
Savings Plan:	Stock Purch. Plan:		Second Exec. Salary: $629,359	Bonus: $561,076

OTHER THOUGHTS:

Apparent Women Officers or Directors: 4
Hot Spot for Advancement for Women/Minorities: Y

LOCATIONS: ("Y" = Yes)

West:	Southwest:	Midwest:	Southeast:	Northeast:	International:
Y				Y	Y

VCA ANTECH INC

www.vcaantech.com

Industry Group Code: 541940 Ranks within this company's industry group: Sales: 1   Profits: 1

Management:		Sales/Marketing:		Liberal Arts:	Information Systems:		Professionals:		Technical/Scientific:	
Mgmt. Trainees:	Y	Mktg. Professionals:	Y	Gen. Writing/Editing:	Info. Management:	Y	Finance/Accounting:	Y	Engineers, Elec.:	
Experienced Mgmt.:	Y	Retail Sales:		Technical Writing:	Software Dev.:	Y	Law:	Y	Engineers, Other:	Y
Int'l Business:		Commercial/Industrial:		Graphic Arts/Photog.:	Hardware Dev.:		HR/Other:	Y	Health/Lab:	
MBA Graduates:	Y	Sales Trainees:		Music:	Systems Integration:		Training:	Y	Scientists/Research:	
		Advertising Pros.:		Broadcasting:	Consulting/Other:		Health Care:	Y	Petroleum/Chemicals:	
				Other:			Consulting:		Math/Other:	

TYPES OF BUSINESS:

Animal Health Care Services
Veterinary Diagnostic Laboratories
Full-Service Animal Hospitals
Veterinary Equipment
Ultrasound Imaging

BRANDS/DIVISIONS/AFFILIATES:

Antech Diagnostics
Zoasis.com
VCA Animal Hospitals
Sound Technologies, Inc.
Healthy Pet Corp.

CONTACTS: *Note: Officers with more than one job title may be intentionally listed here more than once.*

Robert (Bob) Antin, CEO
Arthur J. Antin, COO/Sr. VP
Robert (Bob) Antin, Pres.
Tomas W. Fuller, CFO
Tomas W. Fuller, Corp. Sec./VP
Neil Tauber, Sr. VP-Dev.
Dawn R. Olsen, Principal Acct. Officer/Controller/VP
Robert (Bob) Antin, Chmn.

Phone: 310-571-6500	Fax: 310-571-6700
Toll-Free: 800-966-1822	
Address: 12401 W. Olympic Blvd., Los Angeles, CA 90064-1022 US	

GROWTH PLANS/SPECIAL FEATURES:

VCA Antech, Inc. (VCA) provides animal health care services and operates one of the largest networks of veterinary diagnostic laboratories and freestanding, full-service animal hospitals in the U.S.   The firm's veterinary diagnostic laboratories, run by the Antech Diagnostics division, provides 300 different testing services as well as consulting services to veterinarians, who use these services in the detection, diagnosis, evaluation, monitoring, treatment and prevention of diseases and other conditions. The division operates 36 laboratories. Services rendered in major metropolitan areas accounted for 70% of laboratory revenue for 2007. The laboratories provide testing daily to over 17,000 animal hospitals and zoos in all 50 states, as well as government agencies, and it offers clients access to results online through zoasis.com. The VCA Animal Hospitals division operates 465 animal hospitals in 39 states, offering a full range of general medical and surgical services for animals, as well as specialized treatments including advanced diagnostic services, internal medicine, oncology, ophthalmology, dermatology and cardiology. The division, which has most of its hospitals located in California, Florida and Illinois, is supported by 1,800 veterinarians. VCA animal hospitals typically have three to five full-time veterinarians on staff, and are open 10-15 hours per day, six or seven days a week. Subsidiary Sound Technologies, Inc., the company's medical technology segment, sells medical imaging, primarily ultrasound and digital radiography, equipment and related software and services.

FINANCIALS: Sales and profits are in thousands of dollars—add 000 to get the full amount. 2007 Note: Financial information for 2007 was not available for all companies at press time.

2007 Sales: $1,156,145	2007 Profits: $121,012	U.S. Stock Ticker: WOOF
2006 Sales: $983,313	2006 Profits: $105,529	Int'l Ticker: Int'l Exchange:
2005 Sales: $839,666	2005 Profits: $67,816	Employees: 8,000
2004 Sales: $674,089	2004 Profits: $63,572	Fiscal Year Ends: 12/31
2003 Sales: $544,665	2003 Profits: $43,423	Parent Company:

SALARIES/BENEFITS:

Pension Plan:	ESOP Stock Plan:	Profit Sharing:	Top Exec. Salary: $683,617	Bonus: $825,000
Savings Plan: Y	Stock Purch. Plan:		Second Exec. Salary: $508,846	Bonus: $472,500

OTHER THOUGHTS:

Apparent Women Officers or Directors: 1
Hot Spot for Advancement for Women/Minorities:

LOCATIONS: ("Y" = Yes)

West:	Southwest:	Midwest:	Southeast:	Northeast:	International:
Y	Y	Y	Y	Y	

VERISIGN INC

www.verisign.com

Industry Group Code: 511211 Ranks within this company's industry group: Sales: 2 Profits: 1

Management:		Sales/Marketing:		Liberal Arts:		Information Systems:		Professionals:		Technical/Scientific:	
Mgmt. Trainees:		Mktg. Professionals:		Gen. Writing/Editing:	Y	Info. Management:	Y	Finance/Accounting:	Y	Engineers, Elec.:	Y
Experienced Mgmt.:	Y	Retail Sales:		Technical Writing:	Y	Software Dev.:	Y	Law:	Y	Engineers, Other:	
Int'l Business:	Y	Commercial/Industrial:	Y	Graphic Arts/Photog.:		Hardware Dev.:		HR/Other:	Y	Health/Lab:	
MBA Graduates:	Y	Sales Trainees:		Music:		Systems Integration:	Y	Training:	Y	Scientists/Research:	
		Advertising Pros.:	Y	Broadcasting:		Consulting/Other:		Health Care:		Petroleum/Chemicals:	
				Other:				Consulting:		Math/Other:	

TYPES OF BUSINESS:

Software-Security
Telecommunications Services
Network & e-Mail Security
Managed Security Services
Digital Brand Management
Wireless Content Services
Wireless & Wireline Billing Services
Domain Name Registration

BRANDS/DIVISIONS/AFFILIATES:

SSL

CONTACTS: *Note: Officers with more than one job title may be intentionally listed here more than once.*

William Roper Jr., CEO
William Roper Jr., Pres.
Albert E. Clement, CFO/Sr. VP
John M. Donovan, Exec. VP-Sales
Anne-Marie Law, Sr. VP-Global Human Resources
Kenneth J. Silva, CTO/Sr. VP
John M. Donovan, Exec. VP-Prod. Dev. & Customer Care
Grant L. Clark, Chief Admin. Officer/Sr. VP
Richard H. Goshorn, General Counsel/Sr. VP/Corp. Sec.
John M. Donovan, Exec. VP-Oper.
Kevin A. Werner, Sr. VP-Corp. Dev. & Strategy
Russell S. Lewis, Sr. VP-Strategic Dev.
D. James Bidzos, Chmn.
Teruhide Hashimoto, Pres./CEO-VeriSign Japan

Phone: 650-961-7500	Fax: 650-961-7300
Toll-Free:	
Address: 487 E. Middlefield Rd., Mountain View, CA 94043 US	

GROWTH PLANS/SPECIAL FEATURES:

VeriSign, Inc. operates infrastructure services that enable and protect billions of interactions every day across the world's voice, video and data networks. It offers a variety of Internet and communications-related service that are marketed through web site sales, direct field sales, channel sales, telesales and member organizations in its global affiliate network. The company operates in two segments: the Internet services group and the communications services group. The Internet services group consists of the information and security services business; and the Naming services business. The information and security services business provides products and services that protect online and network interactions, enabling companies to manage reputational, operational and compliance risks. Offerings include SSL certificate services, which enable enterprises and Internet merchants to implements and operate secure networks and web sites that utilize SSL protocol; identity and authentication services, which include the Managed PKI service, the Unified Authentication services and the VeriSign Identity Protection service; managed security services, which enable enterprises to monitor and manage their network security infrastructure; and real-time publisher services, which allow organizations to obtain access to and organize large amounts of constantly updated content and distribute it to enterprises, web-portal developers, application developers and consumers. The Naming services business is the authoritative directory provider of all .com, .net, .cc and .tv domain names. The communications services group provides communications services such as connectivity and interoperability services and intelligent database services; commerce services such as billing and operations support system services, and mobile commerce services; and content services, such as digital content and messaging services. VeriSign is currently undergoing restructuring, which will result in the divestiture of non-core businesses such as communications, billing and commerce, content delivery, messaging and enterprise security services.

The company offers its employees benefits that include tuition reimbursement; health, welfare and financial plans; and health club reimbursement.

FINANCIALS: Sales and profits are in thousands of dollars—add 000 to get the full amount. 2007 Note: Financial information for 2007 was not available for all companies at press time.

2007 Sales: $1,496,000	2007 Profits: $-145,000	U.S. Stock Ticker: VRSN
2006 Sales: $1,575,249	2006 Profits: $379,015	Int'l Ticker: Int'l Exchange:
2005 Sales: $1,612,574	2005 Profits: $428,978	Employees: 4,251
2004 Sales: $1,120,595	2004 Profits: $152,820	Fiscal Year Ends: 12/31
2003 Sales: $1,054,780	2003 Profits: $-249,846	Parent Company:

SALARIES/BENEFITS:

Pension Plan:	ESOP Stock Plan:	Profit Sharing:	Top Exec. Salary: $932,130	Bonus: $
Savings Plan:	Stock Purch. Plan:		Second Exec. Salary: $417,000	Bonus: $

OTHER THOUGHTS:

Apparent Women Officers or Directors: 2
Hot Spot for Advancement for Women/Minorities: Y

LOCATIONS: ("Y" = Yes)

West:	Southwest:	Midwest:	Southeast:	Northeast:	International:
Y	Y	Y	Y	Y	Y

Note: Financial information, benefits and other data can change quickly and may vary from those stated here.

VERIZON COMMUNICATIONS

www.verizon.com

Industry Group Code: 513300A Ranks within this company's industry group: Sales: 1   Profits: 2

Management:		Sales/Marketing:		Liberal Arts:		Information Systems:		Professionals:		Technical/Scientific:	
Mgmt. Trainees:	Y	Mktg. Professionals:	Y	Gen. Writing/Editing:	Y	Info. Management:	Y	Finance/Accounting:	Y	Engineers, Elec.:	Y
Experienced Mgmt.:	Y	Retail Sales:	Y	Technical Writing:	Y	Software Dev.:	Y	Law:	Y	Engineers, Other:	
Int'l Business:	Y	Commercial/Industrial:	Y	Graphic Arts/Photog.:	Y	Hardware Dev.:		HR/Other:	Y	Health/Lab:	
MBA Graduates:	Y	Sales Trainees:	Y	Music:		Systems Integration:		Training:	Y	Scientists/Research:	
		Advertising Pros.:	Y	Broadcasting:		Consulting/Other:		Health Care:		Petroleum/Chemicals:	
				Other:				Consulting:		Math/Other:	

TYPES OF BUSINESS:

Local Telephone Service
Telecommunications Services
Wireless Services
Long-Distance Services
High-Speed Internet Access
Video-on-Demand Services
e-Commerce & Online Services

BRANDS/DIVISIONS/AFFILIATES:

Verizon Wireless
Verizon Business
Verizon Telecom

CONTACTS: *Note: Officers with more than one job title may be intentionally listed here more than once.*

Ivan G. Seidenberg, CEO
Dennis F. Strigl, COO
Dennis F. Strigl, Pres.
Doreen A. Toben, CFO/Exec. VP
John G. Stratton, Chief Mktg. Officer/Exec. VP
Marc C. Reed, Exec. VP-Human Resources
Shaygan Kheradpir, CIO/Exec. VP
Richard J. Lynch, CTO/Exec. VP
William P. Barr, General Counsel/Exec. VP
John W. Diercksen, Exec. VP-Strategy, Dev. & Planning
Thomas J. Tauke, Exec. VP-Public Affairs, Policy & Comm.
Ronald H. Lataille, Sr. VP-Investor Rel.
Catherine T. Webster, Treas./Sr. VP
Lowell C. McAdam, Pres./CEO-Verizon Wireless
John F. Killian, Pres., Verizon Bus.
Marianne Drost, Corp. Sec.
Thomas A. Bartlett, Controller/Sr. VP
Ivan G. Seidenberg, Chmn.

Phone: 212-395-1000	Fax: 212-571-1897
Toll-Free: 800-621-9900	
Address: 140 West St., New York, NY 10007 US	

GROWTH PLANS/SPECIAL FEATURES:

Verizon Communications, Inc. and its subsidiaries form one of the world's largest providers of communications services, including wireline, wireless and Internet services. It operates in two segments: Wireline and domestic wireless. The wireline segment comprises two units: Verizon Telecom and Verizon Business. Verizon Telecom provides voice, video and data services to residential and small business customers in 28 states and Washington, D.C. It is organized in three marketing units: Mass markets, offering services to residential and small businesses; wholesale, offerings long distance and local exchange network facilities for resale to interexchange carriers, competitive local exchange carriers, wireless carriers and Internet identification; and other, whose offerings include operator services, public telephone and dial around services. Verizon Business provides voice, data, Internet communications, next-generation Internet protocol (IP) networking and IT products and service to medium and large businesses and government customers, both domestically and internationally. It is organized in three units: Enterprise business; wholesale; and international and other. The domestic wireless segment's products and services include wireless voice, data products and other value added services and equipment sales across the U.S. The division includes Verizon Wireless, in which Verizon holds a 55% controlling interest, with Vodafone controlling the rest. The firm has over 41 million access line and 8.2 million broadband connections, as well as about 66 million customers. Global operations encompass over 30 countries in the Americas, Europe and Asia Pacific. In June 2008, the firm agreed to acquire Alltel Corp. for $5.9 billion and $22.2 billion in debt acquisition.

FINANCIALS: Sales and profits are in thousands of dollars—add 000 to get the full amount. 2007 Note: Financial information for 2007 was not available for all companies at press time.

2007 Sales: $93,469,000	2007 Profits: $5,521,000	**U.S. Stock Ticker:** VZ
2006 Sales: $88,182,000	2006 Profits: $6,197,000	**Int'l Ticker:** Int'l Exchange:
2005 Sales: $69,518,000	2005 Profits: $7,397,000	Employees: 235,000
2004 Sales: $65,751,000	2004 Profits: $7,831,000	Fiscal Year Ends: 12/31
2003 Sales: $67,752,000	2003 Profits: $3,077,000	Parent Company:

SALARIES/BENEFITS:

Pension Plan:	ESOP Stock Plan:	Profit Sharing:	Top Exec. Salary: $2,100,000	Bonus: $4,200,000
Savings Plan: Y	Stock Purch. Plan:		Second Exec. Salary: $1,250,000	Bonus: $2,000,000

OTHER THOUGHTS:

Apparent Women Officers or Directors: 7
Hot Spot for Advancement for Women/Minorities: Y

LOCATIONS: ("Y" = Yes)

West:	Southwest:	Midwest:	Southeast:	Northeast:	International:
Y	Y	Y	Y	Y	Y

Note: Financial information, benefits and other data can change quickly and may vary from those stated here.

VIACOM INC

www.viacom.com

Industry Group Code: 513210 Ranks within this company's industry group: Sales: Profits:

Management:		Sales/Marketing:		Liberal Arts:		Information Systems:		Professionals:		Technical/Scientific:	
Mgmt. Trainees:	Y	Mktg. Professionals:	Y	Gen. Writing/Editing:	Y	Info. Management:	Y	Finance/Accounting:	Y	Engineers, Elec.:	Y
Experienced Mgmt.:	Y	Retail Sales:		Technical Writing:		Software Dev.:	Y	Law:	Y	Engineers, Other:	
Int'l Business:	Y	Commercial/Industrial:	Y	Graphic Arts/Photog.:	Y	Hardware Dev.:		HR/Other:	Y	Health/Lab:	
MBA Graduates:	Y	Sales Trainees:		Music:	Y	Systems Integration:		Training:	Y	Scientists/Research:	
		Advertising Pros.:	Y	Broadcasting:	Y	Consulting/Other:		Health Care:		Petroleum/Chemicals:	
				Other:	Y			Consulting:		Math/Other:	

TYPES OF BUSINESS:

Cable TV Networks
Television Production/Syndication
Film Production
Online Media
Video Distribution
Video Games

BRANDS/DIVISIONS/AFFILIATES:

National Amusement, Inc.
MTV Networks
Nickelodeon
Comedy Central
CMT: Country Music Television
Paramount Pictures Corp
United Paramount Network (UPN)
DreamWorks SKG

CONTACTS: Note: Officers with more than one job title may be intentionally listed here more than once.

Philippe Dauman, CEO
Philippe P. Dauman, Pres.
Thomas E. Dooley, CFO
JoAnne A. Griffith, Exec. VP-Human Resources
Thomas E. Dooley, Chief Admin. Officer/Sr. Exec. VP
Michael D. Fricklas, General Counsel/Sec./Exec. VP
Wade Davis, Sr. VP-Strategy, Mergers & Acquisitions
Carl D. Folta, Exec. VP-Corp. Comm.
James Bombassei, Sr. VP-Investor Rel.
Jacques Tortoroli, Chief Acct. Officer/Corp. Controller/Sr. VP
Brad Grey, Chmn./CEO-Paramount Motion Picture Group
Debra Lee, CEO/Pres., BET Networks
Judy McGrath, Chmn./CEO-MTV Networks
DeDe Lea, Exec. VP-Gov't Affairs
Sumner M. Redstone, Exec. Chmn.

Phone: 212-258-6000	Fax: 212-258-6464
Toll-Free: 800-516-4399	
Address: 1515 Broadway, New York, NY 10036 US	

GROWTH PLANS/SPECIAL FEATURES:

Viacom, Inc., spun off from now CBS Corp. (formerly Viacom, Inc.), is an international media conglomerate. National Amusement, Inc., owned by the Redstone family, owns 73% of Viacom. Viacom is composed of two segments: Media Networks (formerly Cable Networks) and Filmed Entertainment. Media Networks, operating more than 135 television networks, consist of BET Network, which consists of BET, BETJ, BET Gospel and BET Hip Hop, and the MTV Network. MTV owns the cable television program services MTV: Music Television, VH1, CMT: Country Music Television, Logo, Nickelodeon, Nick at Nite, Comedy Central, Spike TV, TV Land and others, and the digital properties MTV.com, URGE, Comedycentral.com, VSPOT, TurboNick, NeoPets, Xfire and iFilm. Media Networks offers its television content via 171 web sites, with plans to offer content to mobile phones. The Filmed Entertainment segment consists of Paramount Pictures Corp. Paramount produces, finances and distributes feature motion pictures; and has a film library of over 3,500 movies and programs. Online gaming communication and community platform include Xfire, Inc.; Atom Entertainment, Inc., an online game, short film and animation destination; and Harmonix Music Systems, Inc., popular videogame title Guitar Hero developer. Viacom also owns DreamWorks, which produces movies and television programming and markets these properties for home entertainment. Other Paramount companies include Paramount Vantage, Paramount Classics, MTV Films and Nickelodeon Movies. In August 2007, Viacom sold its music publishing business, Famous Music Publishing, to Sony/ATV Music Publishing for around $370 million. Also in August 2007, MTV Networks and RealNetworks, Inc. created Rhapsody America, a venture offering a single, integrated digital music experience that consumers can access through their personal computer (PC), portable music device or mobile phone.

FINANCIALS: Sales and profits are in thousands of dollars—add 000 to get the full amount. 2007 Note: Financial information for 2007 was not available for all companies at press time.

2007 Sales: $13,423,100	2007 Profits: $1,838,100	U.S. Stock Ticker: VIA
2006 Sales: $11,361,100	2006 Profits: $1,592,100	Int'l Ticker: Int'l Exchange:
2005 Sales: $9,609,600	2005 Profits: $1,256,900	Employees: 10,800
2004 Sales: $8,132,200	2004 Profits: $293,700	Fiscal Year Ends: 12/31
2003 Sales: $7,304,400	2003 Profits: $338,500	Parent Company:

SALARIES/BENEFITS:

Pension Plan: Y	ESOP Stock Plan:	Profit Sharing:	Top Exec. Salary: $4,101,954	Bonus: $
Savings Plan: Y	Stock Purch. Plan:		Second Exec. Salary: $3,050,000	Bonus: $5,500,000

OTHER THOUGHTS:

Apparent Women Officers or Directors: 6
Hot Spot for Advancement for Women/Minorities: Y

LOCATIONS: ("Y" = Yes)

West:	Southwest:	Midwest:	Southeast:	Northeast:	International:
Y		Y		Y	Y

Note: Financial information, benefits and other data can change quickly and may vary from those stated here.

VOLT INFORMATION SCIENCES INC

www.volt.com

Industry Group Code: 561320 Ranks within this company's industry group: Sales: 4 Profits: 4

Management:		Sales/Marketing:		Liberal Arts:		Information Systems:		Professionals:		Technical/Scientific:	
Mgmt. Trainees:	Y	Mktg. Professionals:	Y	Gen. Writing/Editing:	Y	Info. Management:	Y	Finance/Accounting:	Y	Engineers, Elec.:	Y
Experienced Mgmt.:	Y	Retail Sales:		Technical Writing:	Y	Software Dev.:	Y	Law:	Y	Engineers, Other:	Y
Int'l Business:	Y	Commercial/Industrial:	Y	Graphic Arts/Photog.:	Y	Hardware Dev.:		HR/Other:	Y	Health/Lab:	Y
MBA Graduates:	Y	Sales Trainees:		Music:		Systems Integration:	Y	Training:	Y	Scientists/Research:	Y
		Advertising Pros.:	Y	Broadcasting:		Consulting/Other:	Y	Health Care:	Y	Petroleum/Chemicals:	
				Other:				Consulting:		Math/Other:	Y

TYPES OF BUSINESS:

Temporary Staffing Services
Telecommunications Services
Information Services
Directory Publishing
Computer Systems

BRANDS/DIVISIONS/AFFILIATES:

Volt Human Resources
Volt Services Group
Volt Europe
VoltDelta
LSSi Data

CONTACTS: Note: Officers with more than one job title may be intentionally listed here more than once.

Steven A. Shaw, CEO
Steven A. Shaw, COO
Steven A. Shaw, Pres.
Jack Eagan, CFO/Sr. VP
Louise Ross, VP-Human Resources
Howard B. Weinreich, General Counsel/Sr. VP
Ludwig M. Guarino, Treas./Sr. VP
Jerome Shaw, Sec./Exec. VP
Thomas Daley, Sr. VP
Daniel G. Hallihan, VP-Acct. Oper.
Ronald Kochman, VP

Phone: 212-704-2400	Fax: 212-704-2417
Toll-Free:	
Address: 560 Lexington Ave., 15th Fl., New York, NY 10022 US	

GROWTH PLANS/SPECIAL FEATURES:

Volt Information Sciences, Inc. provides staffing services, telecommunications services and computer systems to businesses in the U.S., Canada, the U.K. and the Asia-Pacific region. Volt Services Group, Volt Europe and Volt Human Resources provide employee staffing and professional services through over 300 branches and on-site client offices. The company's staffing services include managed staffing, temporary personnel employment and direct hire placement; information technology solutions such as consulting, project management and software and web development; and e-procurement solutions. The firm's telecommunications services segment provides design, engineering, installation, maintenance and removal of telecommunications equipment for outside plant and central offices of cable companies and government entities. In addition, it provides turnkey services such as engineering services, feasibility studies, right-of-way acquisition, network design and detailed engineering services for wireless telecommunications providers and wireless infrastructure suppliers. The computer systems segment provides information and other operator services, and also designs, develops, sells, leases and maintains computer-based directory assistance outsourcing to wireline and wireless telecommunications companies. This segment operates under the brand name VoltDelta. In September 2007, the company completed the purchase of LSSi Corp., and merged it with a subsidiary of VoltDelta to become LSSi Data. In September 2008, the firm sold its directory systems and its directory publishing operations to Yellow Pages Group.

Volt employee benefits include health, dental and vision coverage, life insurance, disability plans, flexible spending accounts, training programs, referral bonuses and reward programs.

FINANCIALS: Sales and profits are in thousands of dollars—add 000 to get the full amount. 2007 Note: Financial information for 2007 was not available for all companies at press time.

2007 Sales: $2,353,082	2007 Profits: $39,332	U.S. Stock Ticker: VOL
2006 Sales: $2,338,453	2006 Profits: $30,650	Int'l Ticker: Int'l Exchange:
2005 Sales: $2,177,619	2005 Profits: $17,040	Employees: 46,000
2004 Sales: $1,924,777	2004 Profits: $33,716	Fiscal Year Ends: 10/31
2003 Sales: $1,609,857	2003 Profits: $4,761	Parent Company:

SALARIES/BENEFITS:

Pension Plan:	ESOP Stock Plan:	Profit Sharing:	Top Exec. Salary: $498,462	Bonus: $100,000
Savings Plan: Y	Stock Purch. Plan:		Second Exec. Salary: $400,192	Bonus: $100,000

OTHER THOUGHTS:

Apparent Women Officers or Directors: 3
Hot Spot for Advancement for Women/Minorities: Y

LOCATIONS: ("Y" = Yes)

West:	Southwest:	Midwest:	Southeast:	Northeast:	International:
Y				Y	Y

W R BERKLEY CORPORATION

www.wrberkley.com

Industry Group Code: 524126 Ranks within this company's industry group: Sales: 3   Profits: 3

Management:		Sales/Marketing:		Liberal Arts:		Information Systems:		Professionals:		Technical/Scientific:	
Mgmt. Trainees:	Y	Mktg. Professionals:	Y	Gen. Writing/Editing:		Info. Management:	Y	Finance/Accounting:	Y	Engineers, Elec.:	
Experienced Mgmt.:	Y	Retail Sales:		Technical Writing:	Y	Software Dev.:	Y	Law:	Y	Engineers, Other:	
Int'l Business:	Y	Commercial/Industrial:	Y	Graphic Arts/Photog.:		Hardware Dev.:		HR/Other:	Y	Health/Lab:	
MBA Graduates:	Y	Sales Trainees:		Music:		Systems Integration:		Training:	Y	Scientists/Research:	Y
		Advertising Pros.:	Y	Broadcasting:		Consulting/Other:		Health Care:		Petroleum/Chemicals:	
				Other:				Consulting:		Math/Other:	Y

TYPES OF BUSINESS:

Insurance, Direct Property & Casualty
Reinsurance
Regional Insurance
Specialty Insurance
Risk Management
Liability Insurance

BRANDS/DIVISIONS/AFFILIATES:

Admiral Insurance Company
Berkley Specialty Underwriting Managers LLC
Select Specialty Managers LLC
CGH Insurance Group
American Mining Insurance Company
Berkley Asset Protection Underwriters LLC
FinSecure LLC

CONTACTS: Note: Officers with more than one job title may be intentionally listed here more than once.

William R. Berkley, CEO
Eugene G. Ballard, CFO/Sr. VP
Joseph Pennachio, VP-Human Resources
Kevin Ebers, Sr. VP-IT
Ira S. Lederman, General Counsel/Sr. VP/Corp. Sec.
Eugene G. Ballard, Treas.
W. Robert Berkley, Jr., Exec. VP
Robert W. Gosselink, Sr. VP-Insurance Risk Mgmt.
Paul J. Hancock, Sr. VP/Chief Corp. Actuary
Robert P. Cole, Sr. VP-Regional Oper.
William R. Berkley, Chmn.
Steven W. Taylor, Sr. VP-Int'l Oper.
Robert C. Hewitt, Sr. VP-Excess & Surplus Lines

Phone: 203-629-3000	Fax: 203-629-3073
Toll-Free:	
Address: 475 Steamboat Rd., Greenwich, CT 06830 US	

GROWTH PLANS/SPECIAL FEATURES:

W. R. Berkley Corporation is one of the largest insurance holding companies in the U.S., operating in five segments of the property casualty insurance business: regional property/casualty insurance; reinsurance; specialty lines of insurance; international operations; and alternative markets, including management of alternative insurance market mechanisms and workers' compensation services. Berkley's subsidiaries operate throughout the U.S. and its international operations are conducted in Europe, South America, Australia and Asia. The specialty insurance unit's services include general, professional, product, excess and umbrella liability, workers' compensation and property coverages, as well as aviation, commercial transportation and program business. Admiral Insurance Company, the largest of Berkley's specialty insurance subsidiaries, provides a diversified portfolio of specialty insurance products in four primary business lines: general liability, professional liability; commercial excess and umbrella liability; and commercial property. The company's alternative market operations specialize in developing and administering self-insurance programs and other alternative risk transfer mechanisms, as well as offering insurance products. The segment's primary line of business is workers' compensation, though it also offers hospital professional liability and medical stop loss insurance. Berkley's regional subsidiaries provide commercial lines coverage for small and mid-sized business firms and governmental entities in 48 states. Berkley Specialty Underwriting Managers LLC offers specialty insurance products on behalf of various insurance subsidiaries. The company's operations include 33 total business units. In May 2007, Berkley launched Select Specialty Managers LLC to offer specialty casualty insurance products to the excess and surplus lines marketplace. In September 2007, the company acquired CGH Insurance Group, the owner of American Mining Insurance Company. In 2008, the company formed Berkley Asset Protection Underwriters LLC, offering coverage for fine arts, jewelers block and fidelity and crime; and FinSecure LLC, offering integrated property and liability insurance for financial institutions and financial services companies.

FINANCIALS: Sales and profits are in thousands of dollars—add 000 to get the full amount. 2007 Note: Financial information for 2007 was not available for all companies at press time.

2007 Sales: $4,575,989	2007 Profits: $743,646	U.S. Stock Ticker: WRB
2006 Sales: $4,818,993	2006 Profits: $699,518	Int'l Ticker: Int'l Exchange:
2005 Sales: $4,996,839	2005 Profits: $544,892	Employees: 5,429
2004 Sales: $4,512,235	2004 Profits: $438,105	Fiscal Year Ends: 12/31
2003 Sales: $3,630,108	2003 Profits: $337,220	Parent Company:

SALARIES/BENEFITS:

Pension Plan:	ESOP Stock Plan:	Profit Sharing:	Top Exec. Salary: $1,000,000	Bonus: $14,931,200
Savings Plan:	Stock Purch. Plan:		Second Exec. Salary: $650,000	Bonus: $2,388,800

OTHER THOUGHTS:

Apparent Women Officers or Directors: 5
Hot Spot for Advancement for Women/Minorities: Y

LOCATIONS: ("Y" = Yes)

West:	Southwest:	Midwest:	Southeast:	Northeast:	International:
Y	Y	Y	Y	Y	Y

Note: Financial information, benefits and other data can change quickly and may vary from those stated here.

WALGREEN CO

www.walgreens.com

Industry Group Code: 446110 **Ranks within this company's industry group:** Sales: 1 Profits: 1

Management:		Sales/Marketing:		Liberal Arts:		Information Systems:		Professionals:		Technical/Scientific:	
Mgmt. Trainees:	Y	Mktg. Professionals:	Y	Gen. Writing/Editing:	Y	Info. Management:	Y	Finance/Accounting:	Y	Engineers, Elec.:	
Experienced Mgmt.:	Y	Retail Sales:	Y	Technical Writing:		Software Dev.:	Y	Law:	Y	Engineers, Other:	Y
Int'l Business:	Y	Commercial/Industrial:	Y	Graphic Arts/Photog.:	Y	Hardware Dev.:		HR/Other:	Y	Health/Lab:	
MBA Graduates:	Y	Sales Trainees:	Y	Music:		Systems Integration:		Training:	Y	Scientists/Research:	
		Advertising Pros.:	Y	Broadcasting:		Consulting/Other:		Health Care:	Y	Petroleum/Chemicals:	
				Other:				Consulting:		Math/Other:	

TYPES OF BUSINESS:

Drug Stores
Mail-Order Pharmacy Services
Pharmacy Benefit Management
Health Care Center Management
Online Pharmacy Services
Photo Printing Services
Specialty Pharmacy Services
Home Infusion Services

BRANDS/DIVISIONS/AFFILIATES:

Whole Health Management
I-trax, Inc.
WHP Health Initiatives, Inc.
Walgreen's Health Services
Walgreen Advance Care, Inc.
Option Care, Inc.
Medmark Specialty Pharmacy
Take Care Health Systems LLC

CONTACTS: *Note: Officers with more than one job title may be intentionally listed here more than once.*

Jeffrey A. Rein, CEO
Gregory D. Wasson, COO
Gregory D. Wasson, Pres.
Wade D. Miquelon, CFO/Sr. VP
George J. Riedl, Exec. VP-Mktg.
Kenneth R. Weigand, Sr. VP-Human Resources
Dana I. Green, General Counsel/Sr. VP/Corp. Sec.
Mark A. Wagner, Exec. VP-Store Oper.
Sona Chawla, Sr. VP-E-commerce
Stanley B. Blaylock, Sr. VP-Walgreens/Pres., Walgreens Health Services
Donald C. Huonker, Sr. VP-Health Care Innovation
Kevin P. Walgreen, Sr. VP-Store Oper.
R. Bruce Bryant, Sr. VP-Store Oper.
Jeffrey A. Rein, Chmn.
J. Randolph Lewis, Sr. VP-Dist. & Logistics

Phone: 847-940-2500	Fax: 847-914-2804
Toll-Free:	
Address: 200 Wilmot Rd., Deerfield, IL 60015 US	

GROWTH PLANS/SPECIAL FEATURES:

Walgreen Co. operates the largest chain of U.S. drug stores based on sales. The company has 5,461 drugstores in 45 U.S. states and Puerto Rico, 12 full-service distribution centers and three prescription mail service facilities. Walgreen currently opens approximately 450 new stores per year and expects to increase its total store count to 7,000 by 2010. The company's pharmacy business fills 529 million prescriptions annually. To coordinate its operations, the firm uses Intercom Plus, a proprietary computer system for filling prescriptions, linking all stores into a single network. Walgreen operates several health care-related businesses, such as WHP Health Initiatives, Inc., a pharmacy benefits management company; Walgreens Health Services, a managed care business; and Walgreens Advance Care, Inc., a retailer of health care maintenance services. A large percentage of the company's stores have drive-through pharmacies, and most stores offer one-hour photo processing, in addition to cosmetics, toiletries, liquor, beverages and tobacco. The firm also accepts prescription refill orders online through its web site. Prescription sales account for approximately 64.3% of total sales and continue to increase each year. Part of the firm's strategy is to build large, free-standing retail buildings on prominent, high traffic corners. A new growth strategy is Walgreen's plan to provide health clinics within the premises of major employers. In May 2008, the company acquired I-trax, Inc. and Whole Health Management, two leaders in this field. It then established a new division where it combined these businesses with its Take Care Health unit. The firm has recently announced plans to slow its rapid growth, forecasting an 8% increase in stores in fiscal 2009, followed by a 6% increase in fiscal 2010 and a 5% increase in fiscal 2011. In July 2008, Walgreens acquired CuraScript Infusion Pharmacy Inc.

FINANCIALS: Sales and profits are in thousands of dollars—add 000 to get the full amount. 2007 Note: Financial information for 2007 was not available for all companies at press time.

2007 Sales: $53,762,000	2007 Profits: $2,041,300	U.S. Stock Ticker: WAG	
2006 Sales: $47,409,000	2006 Profits: $1,750,600	Int'l Ticker: Int'l Exchange:	
2005 Sales: $42,201,600	2005 Profits: $1,559,500	Employees: 195,000	
2004 Sales: $37,508,200	2004 Profits: $1,360,200	Fiscal Year Ends: 8/31	
2003 Sales: $32,505,400	2003 Profits: $1,175,700	Parent Company:	

SALARIES/BENEFITS:

Pension Plan:	ESOP Stock Plan:	Profit Sharing:	Top Exec. Salary: $1,516,667	Bonus: $884,286
Savings Plan: Y	Stock Purch. Plan: Y		Second Exec. Salary: $883,333	Bonus: $500,005

OTHER THOUGHTS:

Apparent Women Officers or Directors: 2
Hot Spot for Advancement for Women/Minorities:

LOCATIONS: ("Y" = Yes)

West:	Southwest:	Midwest:	Southeast:	Northeast:	International:
Y	Y	Y	Y	Y	Y

WAL-MART STORES INC   www.walmartstores.com

Industry Group Code: 452910 Ranks within this company's industry group: Sales: 1 Profits: 1

Management:		Sales/Marketing:		Liberal Arts:		Information Systems:		Professionals:		Technical/Scientific:	
Mgmt. Trainees:	Y	Mktg. Professionals:	Y	Gen. Writing/Editing:	Y	Info. Management:	Y	Finance/Accounting:	Y	Engineers, Elec.:	
Experienced Mgmt.:	Y	Retail Sales:	Y	Technical Writing:		Software Dev.:	Y	Law:	Y	Engineers, Other:	
Int'l Business:	Y	Commercial/Industrial:	Y	Graphic Arts/Photog.:	Y	Hardware Dev.:		HR/Other:	Y	Health/Lab:	
MBA Graduates:	Y	Sales Trainees:	Y	Music:		Systems Integration:		Training:	Y	Scientists/Research:	
		Advertising Pros.:	Y	Broadcasting:	Y	Consulting/Other:		Health Care:		Petroleum/Chemicals:	
				Other:	Y			Consulting:		Math/Other:	

TYPES OF BUSINESS:

Discount Department Stores
Supermarkets
Warehouse Membership Clubs
Online Sales
Pharmacies
Auto Repair Centers
Vision Centers

BRANDS/DIVISIONS/AFFILIATES:

SAM'S CLUB
Wal-Mart Supercenter
Neighborhood Market

CONTACTS: *Note: Officers with more than one job title may be intentionally listed here more than once.*

H. Lee Scott, Jr., CEO/Pres.
William Simon, COO/Exec. VP, Wal-Mart Stores Div.
Thomas M. Schoewe, CFO/Exec. VP
Stephen Quinn, Chief Mktg. Officer/Exec. VP, Wal-Mart Stores Div.
Patricia Curran, Exec. VP-People
Rollin L. Ford, CIO/Exec. VP
John E. Fleming, Chief Merch. Officer/Exec. VP
Thomas A. Mars, General Counsel/Exec. VP
Gregory L. Johnston, Exec. VP-Oper., Sam's Club
John T. Westling, Exec. VP-Replenishment, Pricing & Planning
Raul Vazquez, Pres./CEO-Walmart.com
Leslie A. Dach, Exec. VP-Corp. Affairs & Gov't Rel.
Carol Schumacher, VP-Investor Rel.
Charles M. Holley, Jr., Exec. VP-Finance/Treas.
Eduardo Castro-Wright, CEO/Pres., Wal-Mart Stores USA
C. Douglas McMillon, Exec. VP/CEO/Pres., Sam's Club
Craig R. Herkert, Exec. VP/Pres./CEO-Americas, Int'l
Thomas D. Hyde, Corp. Sec./Exec. VP
S. Robson Walton, Chmn.
Michael T. Duke, Vice Chmn.-Wal-Mart Stores, Inc. Int'l
Johnnie C. Dobbs, Exec. VP-Logistics & Supply Chain

Phone: 479-273-4000	Fax: 479-273-4053
Toll-Free: 800-925-6278	
Address: 702 S.W. 8th St., Bentonville, AR 72716 US	

GROWTH PLANS/SPECIAL FEATURES:

Wal-Mart Stores, Inc., the world's largest retailer, operates through a massive base of Wal-Mart stores, Wal-Mart Supercenters, Sam's Clubs, Neighborhood Markets and walmart.com. The company operates in three business segments: Wal-Mart Stores, representing 64% of net sales for 2008; Sam's Club, generating 11.8% for 2008; and International, accounting for 24.2% of net sales during 2008. The company serves over 200 million customers annually through 7,390 stores and offices, with 2,900 of its stores located internationally. Wal-Mart offers a wide variety of discount merchandise in 36 departments, including family apparel, electronics, toys, lawn and garden and automotive. Additionally, most stores contain a pharmacy, snack bar, vision center, tire and lube center and photo-processing department. The average Wal-Mart customer is 42 to 46 years old, with a household income of $30,000 to $35,000 and an average purchase of $30. Wal-Mart Supercenters, located in 45 states, are larger stores that combine a full-line supermarket with a discount department store. Sam's Club is a members-only warehouse club that sells merchandise at warehouse prices to consumers and small businesses. Club membership exceeds 46 million. The International segment consists of wholly-owned subsidiaries operating in Argentina, Brazil, Canada, Puerto Rico and the U.K.; majority-owned subsidiaries operating in Central America, Japan and Mexico; joint ventures in India and China; and minority-owned subsidiaries in China. From 2008 through 2010, Wal-Mart will open about 170 new Supercenters yearly in the U.S. The company has recently opened health clinics in several locations. In December 2007, Wal-Mart's ownership of The Seiyu, Ltd., a leading Japanese retailer, rose from 50.9% to 95.1%. In June 2008, Wal-Mart agreed to sell Gazeley Limited Group to Economic Zones World.

Wal-Mart is the largest corporate employer of African-Americans and Hispanics in the U.S. It is also the nation's largest non-government employer.

FINANCIALS: Sales and profits are in thousands of dollars—add 000 to get the full amount. 2007 Note: Financial information for 2007 was not available for all companies at press time.

2007 Sales: $344,992,000	2007 Profits: $11,284,000	U.S. Stock Ticker: WMT
2006 Sales: $308,945,000	2006 Profits: $11,231,000	Int'l Ticker: Int'l Exchange:
2005 Sales: $281,488,000	2005 Profits: $10,267,000	Employees: 1,900,000
2004 Sales: $256,329,000	2004 Profits: $9,054,000	Fiscal Year Ends: 1/31
2003 Sales: $244,524,000	2003 Profits: $8,039,000	Parent Company:

SALARIES/BENEFITS:

Pension Plan:	ESOP Stock Plan:	Profit Sharing: Y	Top Exec. Salary: $1,300,000	Bonus: $4,285,840
Savings Plan: Y	Stock Purch. Plan: Y		Second Exec. Salary: $1,000,000	Bonus: $2,435,700

OTHER THOUGHTS:

Apparent Women Officers or Directors: 7
Hot Spot for Advancement for Women/Minorities: Y

LOCATIONS: ("Y" = Yes)

West:	Southwest:	Midwest:	Southeast:	Northeast:	International:
Y	Y	Y	Y	Y	Y

Note: Financial information, benefits and other data can change quickly and may vary from those stated here.

WALT DISNEY COMPANY (THE)

disney.go.com

Industry Group Code: 513210 Ranks within this company's industry group: Sales: 1 Profits: 1

Management:		Sales/Marketing:		Liberal Arts:		Information Systems:		Professionals:		Technical/Scientific:	
Mgmt. Trainees:	Y	Mktg. Professionals:	Y	Gen. Writing/Editing:	Y	Info. Management:	Y	Finance/Accounting:	Y	Engineers, Elec.:	Y
Experienced Mgmt.:	Y	Retail Sales:		Technical Writing:		Software Dev.:	Y	Law:	Y	Engineers, Other:	
Int'l Business:	Y	Commercial/Industrial:		Graphic Arts/Photog.:	Y	Hardware Dev.:		HR/Other:	Y	Health/Lab:	
MBA Graduates:	Y	Sales Trainees:		Music:		Systems Integration:		Training:	Y	Scientists/Research:	
		Advertising Pros.:	Y	Broadcasting:		Consulting/Other:		Health Care:		Petroleum/Chemicals:	
				Other:				Consulting:		Math/Other:	

TYPES OF BUSINESS:

Cable TV Networks, Broadcasting & Entertainment
Filmed Entertainment
Merchandising
Television Networks
Music & Book Publishing
Online Entertainment Programs
Theme Parks, Resorts & Cruise Lines

BRANDS/DIVISIONS/AFFILIATES:

Walt Disney Parks & Resorts
Pixar Animation Studios Inc
ABC Inc
Walt Disney Studios (The)
Miramax Film Corp
ESPN Inc
Walt Disney Pictures
Disney En Familia

CONTACTS: Note: Officers with more than one job title may be intentionally listed here more than once.

Robert A. Iger, CEO
Robert A. Iger, Pres.
Thomas O. Staggs, CFO/Sr. Exec. VP
Dennis W. Shuler, Chief Human Resources Officer/Exec. VP
Kevin Mayer, Exec. VP-Tech. Group
Alan Braverman, General Counsel/Sr. Exec. VP/Corp. Sec.
Kevin Mayer, Exec. VP-Corp. Strategy & Bus. Dev.
Zenia Mucha, Exec. VP-Corp. Comm.
Christine M. McCarthy, Exec. VP-Corp. Finance & Real Estate/Treas.
Ronald L. Iden, Sr. VP-Security
Preston Padden, Exec. VP-Gov't Rel.
Brent Woodford, Sr. VP-Planning & Control
Richard Cook, Chmn.-The Walt Disney Studios
John E. Pepper, Jr., Chmn.
Andy Bird, Chmn.-Walt Disney Int'l

Phone: 818-560-1000	Fax: 818-560-1930
Toll-Free:	
Address: 500 S. Buena Vista St., Burbank, CA 91521 US	

GROWTH PLANS/SPECIAL FEATURES:

The Walt Disney Company is an international entertainment company operating in four major business segments: media networks; studio entertainment; consumer products; and parks and resorts. The media networks segment contributes 43% of revenue. The segment is comprised of domestic broadcast television networks, domestic television stations, cable/satellite networks and international broadcast operations, television production and distribution, domestic broadcast radio networks and stations, as well as Internet and mobile operations. The company also owns and operates cable networks, including ESPN, ABC Family, the History Channel, the Biography Channel, Lifetime Television, E! Entertainment Television, Style and A&E. The studio entertainment segment produces and acquires live action and animated motion pictures, direct-to-video programming, musical recordings and live stage plays. The consumer products segment designs, promotes and sells merchandise based on the firm's intellectual property. The parks and resorts segment manages the operations of the Walt Disney World Resort and the Disney Cruise Line in Florida, the Disneyland resort in California and ESPN Zone facilities in several states, as well as managing the Disneyland Resort Paris and Hong Kong Disneyland (in which the company has a 51% and a 43% interest, respectively) and licenses the Tokyo Disney Resort in Japan. The Walt Disney World Resort includes the Magic Kingdom, Epcot, Disney-MGM Studios and Disney's Animal Kingdom; hotels; vacation ownership units; a retail, dining and entertainment complex; a sports complex; conference centers; campgrounds; golf courses; water parks and other recreational facilities. Currently Disney operates 8 ESPN Zones, located in California, Georgia, Maryland, Illinois, Colorado, Nevada, New York and Washington, D.C. In 2008, Disney launched Disney En Familia, a Spanish magazine for parents.

Disney employees receive theme park passports, educational reimbursement, credit union membership, a personal assistant network and on-site child care services. In addition, the company holds employee and cast member contests.

FINANCIALS: Sales and profits are in thousands of dollars—add 000 to get the full amount. 2007 Note: Financial information for 2007 was not available for all companies at press time.

2007 Sales: $35,510,000	2007 Profits: $4,687,000	U.S. Stock Ticker: DIS
2006 Sales: $33,747,000	2006 Profits: $3,374,000	Int'l Ticker: Int'l Exchange:
2005 Sales: $31,374,000	2005 Profits: $2,533,000	Employees: 137,000
2004 Sales: $30,752,000	2004 Profits: $2,345,000	Fiscal Year Ends: 9/30
2003 Sales: $27,061,000	2003 Profits: $1,267,000	Parent Company:

SALARIES/BENEFITS:

Pension Plan: Y	ESOP Stock Plan:	Profit Sharing:	Top Exec. Salary: $2,000,000	Bonus: $13,670,686
Savings Plan: Y	Stock Purch. Plan:		Second Exec. Salary: $1,106,250	Bonus: $4,450,000

OTHER THOUGHTS:

Apparent Women Officers or Directors: 4
Hot Spot for Advancement for Women/Minorities: Y

LOCATIONS: ("Y" = Yes)

West:	Southwest:	Midwest:	Southeast:	Northeast:	International:
Y	Y	Y	Y	Y	Y

WASTE MANAGEMENT INC

www.wm.com

Industry Group Code: 562000 Ranks within this company's industry group: Sales: 1 Profits: 1

Management:		Sales/Marketing:		Liberal Arts:		Information Systems:		Professionals:		Technical/Scientific:	
Mgmt. Trainees:	Y	Mktg. Professionals:	Y	Gen. Writing/Editing:		Info. Management:	Y	Finance/Accounting:	Y	Engineers, Elec.:	Y
Experienced Mgmt.:	Y	Retail Sales:		Technical Writing:	Y	Software Dev.:	Y	Law:	Y	Engineers, Other:	Y
Int'l Business:		Commercial/Industrial:	Y	Graphic Arts/Photog.:	Y	Hardware Dev.:		HR/Other:	Y	Health/Lab:	Y
MBA Graduates:	Y	Sales Trainees:		Music:		Systems Integration:		Training:	Y	Scientists/Research:	Y
		Advertising Pros.:		Broadcasting:		Consulting/Other:		Health Care:		Petroleum/Chemicals:	
				Other:				Consulting:		Math/Other:	

TYPES OF BUSINESS:
Waste Disposal
Recycling Services
Landfill Operation
Hazardous Waste Management
Transfer Stations
Recycled Commodity Trading
Medical Waste Disposal
Waste Methane Generation

BRANDS/DIVISIONS/AFFILIATES:
Recycle America Alliance
TOSS
Bio-In-A-Box
BioSite
Wheelbrator
Think Green
Republic Services Inc

CONTACTS: Note: Officers with more than one job title may be intentionally listed here more than once.
David P. Steiner, CEO
Lawrence O'Donnell, III, COO
Lawrence O'Donnell, III, Pres.
Robert G. Simpson, CFO/Sr. VP
David Aardsma, Sr. VP-Mktg. & Sales
Michael (Jay) Romans, Sr. VP-People
Lynn M. Caddell, CIO/Sr. VP
Rick L. Wittenbraker, General Counsel/Chief Compliance Officer/Sr. VP
Barry H. Caldwell, Sr. VP-Gov't Affairs & Corp. Comm.
Cherie C. Rice, VP-Finance/Treas.
Patrick J. DeRueda, Pres., Waste Management Recycle America
Mark A. Weidman, Pres., Wheelabrator Technologies Inc.
Carlton Yearwood, VP-Bus. Ethics/Chief Diversity Officer
John (Jack) Pope, Chmn.

Phone: 713-512-6200	Fax: 713-512-6299
Toll-Free:	
Address: 1001 Fannin St., Ste. 4000, Houston, TX 77002 US	

GROWTH PLANS/SPECIAL FEATURES:
Waste Management, Inc. provides comprehensive waste management services to municipal, commercial, industrial and residential customers throughout North America. The company utilizes a number of transfer stations when it is not economical to transport solid waste generated from urban markets directly to landfills. Within these transfer stations, waste is consolidated, compacted and loaded onto long-haul trailers for transport to landfills. Waste Management is the nation's largest collector of recyclables from businesses and households, collecting recyclable materials through subsidiary Recycle America Alliance and depositing them at over a hundred local materials recovery facilities. The company also has a pulp and paper trading group that reduces paper's overall long-term commodity price exposure. The firm operates about 277 solid waste landfills and five secure hazardous waste landfills. Waste Management's hazardous waste management services include geosynthetic manufacturing, radioactive waste services and landfill liner installation. The company has developed TOSS, Bio-In-A-Box and BioSite, bioremediation systems for materials contaminated with petrochemicals, pesticides, explosives or hazardous organics. Through the subsidiary Wheelbrator, the company operates 16 waste-to-energy facilities, which produce electricity through burning solid waste at high temperatures. Additionally, Waste Management promotes environmental initiatives such as Keep America Beautiful, Habitat for Humanity, Red Cross/FEMA, Wildlife Habitat Council, as well as Waste Management's own Think Green. In 2008, the company entered into a definitive merger agreement with Republic Services, Inc.

Waste Management offers its employees family assistance, a prescription drug plan, dental plan, flexible spending accounts, education savings accounts, scholarship programs, discounted banking services and tuition reimbursement.

FINANCIALS: Sales and profits are in thousands of dollars—add 000 to get the full amount. 2007 Note: Financial information for 2007 was not available for all companies at press time.

2007 Sales: $13,310,000	2007 Profits: $1,163,000	U.S. Stock Ticker: WMI
2006 Sales: $13,363,000	2006 Profits: $1,149,000	Int'l Ticker: Int'l Exchange:
2005 Sales: $13,074,000	2005 Profits: $1,182,000	Employees: 48,000
2004 Sales: $12,516,000	2004 Profits: $939,000	Fiscal Year Ends: 12/31
2003 Sales: $11,574,000	2003 Profits: $630,000	Parent Company:

SALARIES/BENEFITS:

Pension Plan:	ESOP Stock Plan:	Profit Sharing:	Top Exec. Salary: $904,808	Bonus: $1,758,270
Savings Plan: Y	Stock Purch. Plan: Y		Second Exec. Salary: $686,094	Bonus: $1,158,117

OTHER THOUGHTS:
Apparent Women Officers or Directors: 2
Hot Spot for Advancement for Women/Minorities:

LOCATIONS: ("Y" = Yes)

West:	Southwest:	Midwest:	Southeast:	Northeast:	International:
Y	Y	Y	Y	Y	

Note: Financial information, benefits and other data can change quickly and may vary from those stated here.

WATERS CORP

www.waters.com

Industry Group Code: 339113 Ranks within this company's industry group: Sales: 12 Profits: 9

Management:		Sales/Marketing:		Liberal Arts:		Information Systems:		Professionals:		Technical/Scientific:	
Mgmt. Trainees:	Y	Mktg. Professionals:	Y	Gen. Writing/Editing:		Info. Management:	Y	Finance/Accounting:	Y	Engineers, Elec.:	Y
Experienced Mgmt.:	Y	Retail Sales:		Technical Writing:	Y	Software Dev.:	Y	Law:	Y	Engineers, Other:	Y
Int'l Business:	Y	Commercial/Industrial:	Y	Graphic Arts/Photog.:	Y	Hardware Dev.:	Y	HR/Other:	Y	Health/Lab:	Y
MBA Graduates:	Y	Sales Trainees:		Music:		Systems Integration:		Training:	Y	Scientists/Research:	Y
		Advertising Pros.:		Broadcasting:		Consulting/Other:		Health Care:		Petroleum/Chemicals:	Y
				Other:				Consulting:		Math/Other:	Y

TYPES OF BUSINESS:

Equipment-Liquid Chromatography Instruments
Mass Spectrometry Systems
Thermal Analyzers
Rheometry Equipment
Software Development
Food Safety Technology

BRANDS/DIVISIONS/AFFILIATES:

Waters Division
Alliance 2795
TA Instruments, Inc.
BiopharmaLynx TM
MassLynx MS
MassTrak Immunosuppressant Kit

CONTACTS: Note: Officers with more than one job title may be intentionally listed here more than once.

Douglas A. Berthiaume, CEO
Douglas A. Berthiaume, Pres.
John Ornell, CFO
Elizabeth B. Rae, VP-Human Resources
John Ornell, VP-Admin.
Mark T. Beaudouin, General Counsel/Sec./VP
John Ornell, VP-Finance
Arthur G. Caputo, Exec. VP/Pres., Waters Div.
Terrence P. Kelly, Pres., TA Instruments, Inc.
Douglas A. Berthiaume, Chmn.

Phone: 508-478-2000	Fax: 508-872-1990
Toll-Free: 800-252-4752	
Address: 34 Maple St., Milford, MA 01757 US	

GROWTH PLANS/SPECIAL FEATURES:

Waters Corporation designs, manufactures and markets analytical instruments in two segments: the Waters division and TA Instruments, Inc. The Waters division offers high-performance liquid chromatography (HPLC) and mass spectrometry instrument systems and associated service and support products, including chromatography columns and laboratory informatics software. HPLC equipment detects, identifies, monitors and measures the chemical, physical and biological composition of materials and purifies compounds. Waters' liquid chromatography instruments allow for different degrees of automation from component-configured systems to its fully automated proprietary Alliance 2795 systems. Mass spectrometry (MS) is an analytical technique that identifies unknown compounds and quantifies known materials. These instruments are used primarily in conjunction with the firm's HPLC products and are used by a wide array of industries, particularly by the life sciences, pharmaceutical, biomedical, clinical and environmental market segments. Through its TA Instruments, Inc. division, the company designs, manufactures, services and sells thermal analysis instruments, which measure the physical characteristics of materials as a function of temperature. In addition to thermal analyzers, TA Instruments produces rheometry instruments, which complement thermal analyzers by characterizing materials' viscosities and fluid behavior. TA Instruments is also a developer and supplier of software-based products that interface with the company's instruments. The thermal analytic and rheometry instruments are used by material testing laboratories for the development and production of materials used in such industries as plastics, automotive, electronics and chemicals. In June 2007, Waters introduced the BiopharmaLynx TM software, an application manager for its MassLynx MS software that automates data processing and protein analysis. In July 2007, it introduced the MassTrak Immunosuppressant Kit, the first commercially available monitor of tacrolimus, an immunosuppressant, in liver and kidney transplant patients. In August 2007, the company purchased Calorimetry Sciences Corporation, a manufacturer of high-performance calorimeters in Utah. In July 2008, the firm acquired VTI Corporation.

FINANCIALS: Sales and profits are in thousands of dollars—add 000 to get the full amount. 2007 Note: Financial information for 2007 was not available for all companies at press time.

2007 Sales: $1,072,864	2007 Profits: $268,072	U.S. Stock Ticker: WAT
2006 Sales: $922,532	2006 Profits: $222,200	Int'l Ticker: Int'l Exchange:
2005 Sales: $1,158,236	2005 Profits: $201,975	Employees: 4,700
2004 Sales: $1,104,536	2004 Profits: $224,053	Fiscal Year Ends: 12/31
2003 Sales: $958,205	2003 Profits: $170,891	Parent Company:

SALARIES/BENEFITS:

Pension Plan: Y	ESOP Stock Plan:	Profit Sharing:	Top Exec. Salary: $650,000	Bonus: $1,625,000
Savings Plan:	Stock Purch. Plan: Y		Second Exec. Salary: $375,000	Bonus: $787,500

OTHER THOUGHTS:

Apparent Women Officers or Directors: 3
Hot Spot for Advancement for Women/Minorities: Y

LOCATIONS: ("Y" = Yes)

West:	Southwest:	Midwest:	Southeast:	Northeast:	International:
Y				Y	Y

WATSON PHARMACEUTICALS INC
www.watson.com

Industry Group Code: 325416 Ranks within this company's industry group: Sales: 1 Profits: 2

Management:		Sales/Marketing:		Liberal Arts:		Information Systems:		Professionals:		Technical/Scientific:	
Mgmt. Trainees:	Y	Mktg. Professionals:	Y	Gen. Writing/Editing:	Y	Info. Management:	Y	Finance/Accounting:	Y	Engineers, Elec.:	Y
Experienced Mgmt.:	Y	Retail Sales:		Technical Writing:	Y	Software Dev.:	Y	Law:	Y	Engineers, Other:	Y
Int'l Business:	Y	Commercial/Industrial:	Y	Graphic Arts/Photog.:	Y	Hardware Dev.:		HR/Other:	Y	Health/Lab:	Y
MBA Graduates:	Y	Sales Trainees:	Y	Music:		Systems Integration:		Training:	Y	Scientists/Research:	Y
		Advertising Pros.:		Broadcasting:		Consulting/Other:		Health Care:	Y	Petroleum/Chemicals:	
				Other:				Consulting:		Math/Other:	Y

TYPES OF BUSINESS:

Generic Pharmaceuticals
Branded Drugs
Urology Drugs
Anti-Hypertensive Drugs
Psychiatric Drugs
Pain Management Drugs
Dermatology Drugs
Nephrology Drugs

BRANDS/DIVISIONS/AFFILIATES:

Watson Laboratories
Watson Pharma
Rugby
Ferrlecit
Trelstar Depot
Oxytrol
Anda
Tilia Fe

CONTACTS: *Note: Officers with more than one job title may be intentionally listed here more than once.*

Paul M. Bisaro, CEO
Paul M. Bisaro, Pres.
Mark Durand, CFO
Clare Carmichael, Sr. VP-Human Resources
Charles D. Ebert, Sr. VP-R&D
Thomas R. Giordano, CIO/Sr. VP
David A. Buchen, General Counsel/Sr. VP/Sec.
Edward F. Heimers, Jr., Exec. VP/Pres., Brand Division
David C. Hsia, Sr. VP-Scientific Affairs
Gordon Munro, Sr. VP-Quality Assurance
Thomas R. Russillo, Exec. VP/Pres., U.S. Generics Division
Allen Chao, Chmn.

Phone: 951-493-5300	Fax: 973-355-8301
Toll-Free:	
Address: 311 Bonnie Cir., Corona, CA 92880 US	

GROWTH PLANS/SPECIAL FEATURES:

Watson Pharmaceuticals, Inc. manufactures and distributes over 27 branded and over 150 generic pharmaceutical products. The company offers generic versions of popular brand-name pharmaceuticals including Zyban, Wellbutrin, Lorcet, Vicodin, Percocet, Ocycontin, Nicorette, Lortab, Triphasil and Demulen. The firm markets its generic products through a network of 25 sales and marketing professionals under the Watson Laboratories and Watson Pharma labels. Over-the-counter products are sold under the Rugby label or private label. Generic products accounted for roughly 60% of net revenues in 2007. Watson Pharmaceuticals' brand business segment develops, manufactures, markets, sells and distributes products primarily through two sales and marketing groups: Specialty groups and nephrology. The specialty products include urology, anti-hypertensive, psychiatry, pain management and dermatology products and a genital warts treatment. Brand names include Trelstar Depot and Trelstar LA, treatments for advanced prostate cancer; Androderm, a male hormone replacement therapy; Oxytrol, an overactive bladder treatment; and Ferrlecit, an iron replacement therapy for patients with iron deficiency anemia. The company markets its brand products through 330 sales professionals. Brand products accounted for roughly 17% of total revenue in 2007. The company's distribution business subsidiaries include Anda, Anda Pharmaceuticals and Valmed. Watson sold its 50% interest in the Somerset Pharmaceuticals, Inc., a research and development joint venture, to Mylan Inc., a generic and specialty pharmaceutical company. The company also received final approval from the U.S. Food and Drug Administration (FDA) for its Abbreviated New Drug Application (ANDA) for Omeprazole Delayed-Release Capsules USP, a short-term treatment for active duodenal ulcers. Watson recently launched several new drugs, including Tilia Fe, the generic version of Warner Chilcott's oral contraceptive Estrostep Fe.

The company offers employees medical, dental and vision insurance; a 401(k) plan; life and AD&D insurance; domestic partner coverage; business travel accident insurance; short- and long-term disability; pet insurance; and tuition reimbursement.

FINANCIALS: Sales and profits are in thousands of dollars—add 000 to get the full amount. 2007 Note: Financial information for 2007 was not available for all companies at press time.

2007 Sales: $2,496,651	2007 Profits: $141,030	**U.S. Stock Ticker: WPI**
2006 Sales: $1,979,244	2006 Profits: $-445,005	**Int'l Ticker:** Int'l Exchange:
2005 Sales: $1,646,203	2005 Profits: $138,557	Employees: 5,640
2004 Sales: $1,640,551	2004 Profits: $150,018	Fiscal Year Ends: 12/31
2003 Sales: $1,457,722	2003 Profits: $202,864	Parent Company:

SALARIES/BENEFITS:

Pension Plan:	ESOP Stock Plan:	Profit Sharing:	Top Exec. Salary: $1,052,940	Bonus: $1,200,000
Savings Plan: Y	Stock Purch. Plan:		Second Exec. Salary: $744,719	Bonus: $560,116

OTHER THOUGHTS:

Apparent Women Officers or Directors: 2
Hot Spot for Advancement for Women/Minorities: Y

LOCATIONS: ("Y" = Yes)

West:	Southwest:	Midwest:	Southeast:	Northeast:	International:
Y		Y	Y	Y	Y

Note: Financial information, benefits and other data can change quickly and may vary from those stated here.

WATSON WYATT WORLDWIDE INC   www.watsonwyatt.com

Industry Group Code: 541612 Ranks within this company's industry group: Sales: 4 Profits: 1

Management:		Sales/Marketing:		Liberal Arts:		Information Systems:		Professionals:		Technical/Scientific:	
Mgmt. Trainees:		Mktg. Professionals:	Y	Gen. Writing/Editing:	Y	Info. Management:	Y	Finance/Accounting:	Y	Engineers, Elec.:	
Experienced Mgmt.:	Y	Retail Sales:		Technical Writing:		Software Dev.:		Law:	Y	Engineers, Other:	
Int'l Business:	Y	Commercial/Industrial:	Y	Graphic Arts/Photog.:		Hardware Dev.:		HR/Other:	Y	Health/Lab:	
MBA Graduates:	Y	Sales Trainees:		Music:		Systems Integration:	Y	Training:	Y	Scientists/Research:	
		Advertising Pros.:	Y	Broadcasting:		Consulting/Other:	Y	Health Care:		Petroleum/Chemicals:	
				Other:	Y			Consulting:	Y	Math/Other:	

TYPES OF BUSINESS:

Human Resources Consulting
Compensation Consulting
Benefit Plan Consulting
Technology Services

BRANDS/DIVISIONS/AFFILIATES:

Watson Wyatt & Company Holdings
Watson Wyatt Brans & Co.

CONTACTS: *Note: Officers with more than one job title may be intentionally listed here more than once.*

John J. Haley, CEO
John J. Haley, Pres.
Roger Millay, CFO/VP
Robert J. McKee, VP/Global Dir.-Mktg.
Stephen E. Mele, Chief Human Resources Officer/VP
Jeffrey J. Held, CIO/VP
Walter W. Bardenwerper, General Counsel/VP/Corp. Sec.
David M. E. Dow, VP/Global Practice Dir.-Tech, & Admin. Solutions
Roger C. Urwin, Practice Dir.-Investment Consulting
Gene H. Wickes, VP/Dir.-Global Benefits Practice
Philip G. H. Brook, VP/Global Practice Dir.-Insurance & Financial Svcs
John J. Haley, Chmn.
Chandrasekhar Ramamurthy, Regional Manager-Europe/VP

Phone: 703-258-8000	Fax: 703-258-7495
Toll-Free:	
Address: 901 N. Glebe Rd., Arlington, VA 22203 US	

GROWTH PLANS/SPECIAL FEATURES:

Watson Wyatt Worldwide, Inc. (WW), formerly Watson Wyatt & Company Holdings, is a global consulting firm focused on providing human capital and financial management consulting services. WW helps its clients enhance their business performance by improving their ability to attract, retain and motivate qualified employees. The company operates through roughly 96 offices in 30 countries, and divides its operations into five groups: Benefits; technology and administration; human capital; investment consulting; and insurance and financial services. WW's benefits group, which generates over 50% of its revenues, provides benefit program design and management; funding and risk management strategies; expatriate and international human resource strategies; strategic workforce planning; and compliance and governance. Services of the technology and administration solutions group include web-based applications and outsourcing solutions for health, welfare, pension and compensation administration; call center strategy, design and tools; strategic human resources technology; service delivery consulting; targeted online compensation and benefits statements; content management; and call center case management solutions. WW's human capital group offers advice concerning compensation plans, including broad-based and executive compensation, stock and other long-term incentive programs; strategies to align workforce performance with business objectives; organization effectiveness consulting, including talent management; strategies for attracting, retaining and motivating employees; and data services. The investment consulting group provides investment consulting services to pension plans and other institutional funds; input on governance and regulatory issues; analysis of asset allocation and investment strategies; investment structure analysis; selection and evaluation of managers; and performance monitoring. WW's insurance and financial services group provides independent actuarial and strategic advice; assessment and advice regarding financial condition and risk management; and financial modeling software tools for product design, pricing, planning, projections, reporting, valuations and risk management. In 2007, the company acquired Watson Wyatt Brans & Co., its long-time alliance partner in the Netherlands.

FINANCIALS: Sales and profits are in thousands of dollars—add 000 to get the full amount. 2007 Note: Financial information for 2007 was not available for all companies at press time.

2007 Sales: $1,486,523	2007 Profits: $116,275	**U.S. Stock Ticker: WW**
2006 Sales: $1,271,811	2006 Profits: $87,191	**Int'l Ticker:** Int'l Exchange:
2005 Sales: $737,421	2005 Profits: $52,162	Employees: 6,600
2004 Sales: $702,005	2004 Profits: $50,593	Fiscal Year Ends: 6/30
2003 Sales: $709,616	2003 Profits: $57,166	Parent Company:

SALARIES/BENEFITS:

Pension Plan: Y	ESOP Stock Plan:	Profit Sharing:	Top Exec. Salary: $826,250	Bonus: $876,750
Savings Plan: Y	Stock Purch. Plan: Y		Second Exec. Salary: $531,250	Bonus: $335,000

OTHER THOUGHTS:

Apparent Women Officers or Directors: 1
Hot Spot for Advancement for Women/Minorities:

LOCATIONS: ("Y" = Yes)

West:	Southwest:	Midwest:	Southeast:	Northeast:	International:
Y	Y	Y	Y	Y	Y

WEATHERFORD INTERNATIONAL LTD www.weatherford.com

Industry Group Code: 213111 Ranks within this company's industry group: Sales: 6 Profits: 4

Management:		Sales/Marketing:		Liberal Arts:	Information Systems:		Professionals:		Technical/Scientific:	
Mgmt. Trainees:	Y	Mktg. Professionals:	Y	Gen. Writing/Editing:	Info. Management:	Y	Finance/Accounting:	Y	Engineers, Elec.:	Y
Experienced Mgmt.:	Y	Retail Sales:		Technical Writing:	Software Dev.:		Law:	Y	Engineers, Other:	Y
Int'l Business:	Y	Commercial/Industrial:	Y	Graphic Arts/Photog.:	Hardware Dev.:		HR/Other:	Y	Health/Lab:	Y
MBA Graduates:	Y	Sales Trainees:		Music:	Systems Integration:		Training:	Y	Scientists/Research:	
		Advertising Pros.:		Broadcasting:	Consulting/Other:		Health Care:		Petroleum/Chemicals:	Y
				Other:			Consulting:		Math/Other:	

TYPES OF BUSINESS:

Oil & Gas Drilling Support Services
Artificial Lift Systems
Completion Systems
Research & Development

BRANDS/DIVISIONS/AFFILIATES:

Precision Energy Services
Precision International Contract Drilling
International Logging, Inc.

CONTACTS: *Note: Officers with more than one job title may be intentionally listed here more than once.*

Bernard J. Duroc-Danner, CEO
E. Lee Colley III, COO/Sr. VP
Bernard J. Duroc-Danner, Pres.
Andrew P. Becnel, CFO/Sr. VP
Stuart E. Ferguson, CTO
M. David Colley, VP-Global Mfg.
Burt M. Martin, Gen. Counsel/Sr. VP
Keith R. Morley, Sr. VP-Well Construction & Oper.
Keith R. Morley, Chief Safety Officer
Stuart E. Ferguson, Sr. VP-Reservoir & Production
Bernard J. Duroc-Danner, Chmn.

Phone: 713-693-4000	Fax:
Toll-Free:	
Address: 515 Post Oak Blvd., Ste. 600, Houston, TX 77027 US	

GROWTH PLANS/SPECIAL FEATURES:

Weatherford International, Inc. provides equipment and services for the drilling, evaluation, completion, production and intervention of oil and natural gas wells. The firm conducts operations throughout the U.S. and in over 100 countries around the world, with more than 800 service, sales and manufacturing locations. Its drilling and intervention service activities provide drilling systems, well installation services, cementing products and underbalanced drilling. The completion system activities offer proprietary and patented technologies that minimize formation damage and maximize production. The firm's artificial lift system activities provide all forms of artificial lift primarily used for the production of oil. This operation also provides production optimization services and automation and monitoring of well head production. Weatherford's strategy includes creating, through research and development efforts and acquisitions, industry-changing products and services that allow it to capitalize on industry trends, such as the maturation of the world's major hydrocarbon reserves and the growth of deepwater activity. In recent years, the company has shifted much of its business overseas. In 2007, the firm's consolidated revenues by product line were as follows: artificial lift systems (18%); well construction (16%); drilling services (15%); drilling tools (12%); completion systems (10%); wireline (8%); re-entry and fishing (8%); stimulation and chemicals (6%); integrated drilling (5%); and pipeline & specialty services (2%). In 2007, the company approved a plan to sell its oil and gas development and production business. A portion of this business was sold in late 2007. The sale of the remaining portion of this business is expected to be completed in 2008. In August 2008, the firm acquired International Logging, Inc. a provider of surface logging and formation evaluation and drilling related services at the well site.

FINANCIALS: Sales and profits are in thousands of dollars—add 000 to get the full amount. 2007 Note: Financial information for 2007 was not available for all companies at press time.

2007 Sales: $7,832,062	2007 Profits: $1,070,606	U.S. Stock Ticker: WFT
2006 Sales: $6,578,928	2006 Profits: $896,369	Int'l Ticker: Int'l Exchange:
2005 Sales: $4,333,227	2005 Profits: $467,420	Employees: 33,000
2004 Sales: $3,131,774	2004 Profits: $330,146	Fiscal Year Ends: 12/31
2003 Sales: $2,591,408	2003 Profits: $143,352	Parent Company:

SALARIES/BENEFITS:

Pension Plan:	ESOP Stock Plan:	Profit Sharing:	Top Exec. Salary: $1,372,604	Bonus: $
Savings Plan:	Stock Purch. Plan:		Second Exec. Salary: $449,339	Bonus: $

OTHER THOUGHTS:

Apparent Women Officers or Directors:
Hot Spot for Advancement for Women/Minorities:

LOCATIONS: ("Y" = Yes)

West:	Southwest:	Midwest:	Southeast:	Northeast:	International:
Y	Y	Y	Y	Y	Y

WEIGHT WATCHERS INTERNATIONAL INC

www.weightwatchers.com

Industry Group Code: 446190 **Ranks within this company's industry group:** Sales: 1 Profits: 1

Management:		Sales/Marketing:		Liberal Arts:		Information Systems:		Professionals:		Technical/Scientific:	
Mgmt. Trainees:	Y	Mktg. Professionals:	Y	Gen. Writing/Editing:	Y	Info. Management:	Y	Finance/Accounting:	Y	Engineers, Elec.:	
Experienced Mgmt.:	Y	Retail Sales:	Y	Technical Writing:		Software Dev.:		Law:	Y	Engineers, Other:	Y
Int'l Business:	Y	Commercial/Industrial:	Y	Graphic Arts/Photog.:	Y	Hardware Dev.:		HR/Other:	Y	Health/Lab:	
MBA Graduates:	Y	Sales Trainees:	Y	Music:		Systems Integration:		Training:	Y	Scientists/Research:	
		Advertising Pros.:	Y	Broadcasting:		Consulting/Other:		Health Care:	Y	Petroleum/Chemicals:	
				Other:	Y			Consulting:		Math/Other:	

TYPES OF BUSINESS:

Weight Management Programs
Franchising
Branded Diet Products

BRANDS/DIVISIONS/AFFILIATES:

Weight Watchers Corporate Solutions
Weight Watchers eTools
Weight Watchers Online
FlexPoints

CONTACTS: *Note: Officers with more than one job title may be intentionally listed here more than once.*

David P. Kirchhoff, CEO
David P. Kirchhoff, Pres.
Ann M. Sardini, CFO/VP
Jeffrey A. Fiarman, General Counsel/Exec. VP/Sec.
Raymond Debbane, Chmn.

Phone: 212-589-2700	Fax: 212-589-2601
Toll-Free:	
Address: 11 Madison Ave., 17th Fl., New York, NY 10010 US	

GROWTH PLANS/SPECIAL FEATURES:

Weight Watchers International, Inc. is a global provider of weight management services, with a presence in 28 countries around the world. The company hosts weekly meetings that promote weight loss through diet, exercise, behavior modification and group support. Each week, over 1.5 million people attend approximately 50,000 Weight Watchers meetings around the world, which are run by roughly 15,000 classroom leaders. Weight Watchers uses a combination of company-owned operations and franchised operations. The firm also offers Weight Watchers Corporate Solutions, a line of weight loss products that can be customized to suit the employees in any company. This at-work program addresses the weight-loss needs of working people by holding classes at their place of employment. The company's web site offers Internet subscription weight management products to consumers and maintains an interactive presence for the Weight Watchers brand. Customers can subscribe to Weight Watchers Online, which provides interactive and personalized resources that allow users to follow its weight management plans via the Internet; and Weight Watchers eTools, the Internet weight management companion for Weight Watchers meetings members who want to interactively manage the day-to-day aspects of their weight management plans on the Internet. As of late 2007, the web site had approximately 584,000 active subscribers. The company offers these two products in the U.S., the U.K., Canada, Germany, Australia and New Zealand. FlexPoints is the firm's proprietary system for tracking and maintaining food amounts. For self-help dieters, Weight Watchers also offers an at-home kit, which is a complete mail-order system including the full set of program materials used in meetings.

FINANCIALS: Sales and profits are in thousands of dollars—add 000 to get the full amount. 2007 Note: Financial information for 2007 was not available for all companies at press time.

2007 Sales: $1,467,167	2007 Profits: $201,180	**U.S. Stock Ticker: WTW**
2006 Sales: $1,233,300	2006 Profits: $209,800	**Int'l Ticker:** Int'l Exchange:
2005 Sales: $1,151,300	2005 Profits: $174,400	Employees: 47,000
2004 Sales: $1,024,900	2004 Profits: $183,100	Fiscal Year Ends: 12/31
2003 Sales: $943,932	2003 Profits: $143,941	Parent Company:

SALARIES/BENEFITS:

Pension Plan:	ESOP Stock Plan:	Profit Sharing:	Top Exec. Salary: $742,156	Bonus: $464,775
Savings Plan:	Stock Purch. Plan:		Second Exec. Salary: $356,924	Bonus: $205,855

OTHER THOUGHTS:

Apparent Women Officers or Directors: 3
Hot Spot for Advancement for Women/Minorities: Y

LOCATIONS: ("Y" = Yes)

West:	Southwest:	Midwest:	Southeast:	Northeast:	International:
Y	Y	Y	Y	Y	Y

WELLPOINT INC
www.wellpoint.com

Industry Group Code: 524114 **Ranks within this company's industry group:** Sales: 2 Profits: 2

Management:		Sales/Marketing:		Liberal Arts:		Information Systems:		Professionals:		Technical/Scientific:	
Mgmt. Trainees:	Y	Mktg. Professionals:	Y	Gen. Writing/Editing:	Y	Info. Management:	Y	Finance/Accounting:	Y	Engineers, Elec.:	
Experienced Mgmt.:	Y	Retail Sales:		Technical Writing:	Y	Software Dev.:	Y	Law:	Y	Engineers, Other:	Y
Int'l Business:		Commercial/Industrial:	Y	Graphic Arts/Photog.:	Y	Hardware Dev.:		HR/Other:	Y	Health/Lab:	
MBA Graduates:	Y	Sales Trainees:		Music:		Systems Integration:		Training:	Y	Scientists/Research:	Y
		Advertising Pros.:	Y	Broadcasting:		Consulting/Other:		Health Care:	Y	Petroleum/Chemicals:	
				Other:				Consulting:		Math/Other:	

TYPES OF BUSINESS:
Health Insurance
Workers' Compensation Plans
Point-of-Service Plans
Dental Plans
Pharmaceutical Plans
Managed Care Services
Actuarial Services

BRANDS/DIVISIONS/AFFILIATES:
WellPoint Behavioral Health
Unicare
BLUE CROSS OF CALIFORNIA
BLUE CROSS AND BLUE SHIELD OF GEORGIA INC
WellPoint Dental Services
HealthLink, Inc.
WellPoint Pharmacy Management
American Imaging Management

CONTACTS: *Note: Officers with more than one job title may be intentionally listed here more than once.*
Angela F. Braly, CEO
Angela F. Braly, Pres.
Wayne S. DeVeydt, CFO/Exec. VP
Randy L. Brown, Exec. VP/Chief Human Resources Officer
Lori Beer, CIO/Exec. VP
John Cannon III, General Counsel/Exec. VP
Brad M. Fluegel, Exec. VP-Chief Strategy Officer
Martin Miller, Sr. VP/Chief Acct. Officer
Mark L. Boxer, Pres./CEO-Oper., Tech. & Gov't Svcs. Bus. Unit
Dijuana Lewi, Pres./CEO-Wellpoint Comprehensive Health Solutions
Randall J. Lewis, Exec. VP-Internal Audit & Chief Compliance Officer
Samuel R. Nussbaum, Exec. VP/Chief Medical Officer
Larry C. Glasscock, Chmn.

Phone: 317-532-6000	Fax: 317-488-6028
Toll-Free:	
Address: 120 Monument Cir., Indianapolis, IN 46204 US	

GROWTH PLANS/SPECIAL FEATURES:

WellPoint, Inc. is a health benefits company, serving more than 34 million medical members. The company is an independent licensee of the Blue Cross and Blue Shield Association, an association of independent health benefit plans, and also serves customers as Unicare. The firm offers network-based managed care plans to the large and small employer, individual, Medicaid and senior markets. The managed care plans include preferred provider organizations, health maintenance organizations, point-of-service plans, traditional indemnity plans and other hybrid plans including consumer-driven health plans, hospital only and limited benefit products. In addition, WellPoint provides managed care services to self-funded customers, including claims processing, underwriting, stop loss insurance, actuarial services, provider network access, medical cost management and other administrative services. The company also provides specialty and other products and services including life and disability insurance benefits; pharmacy benefit management; specialty pharmacy; dental; vision; behavioral health benefit services; long-term care insurance; and flexible spending accounts. The firm markets its products through a network of independent agents and brokers and through its in-house sales force. Subsidiaries include Blue Cross of California and Blue Cross Blue Shield of Georgia, as well as non-Blue Cross subsidiaries such as Healthlink, PrecisionRx, WellPoint Behavioral Health, WellPoint Dental Services and WellPoint Workers' Compensation Managed Care Services. Subsidiary WellPoint Pharmacy Management markets clinical management programs, drug formulary management, benefit design consultation, pharmacy network management, local network contract development, manufacturer discount programs and prescription drug databases. In June 2008, the company launched the Maternity Depression Program, aimed at providing new mothers with depression screenings, education and support in order to help them receive behavioral health treatment post-pregnancy.

WellPoint offers employees tuition assistance; a 401(k) plan; an employee stock purchase plan; retiree medical spending accounts; life insurance; long-term disability insurance; and financial education.

FINANCIALS: Sales and profits are in thousands of dollars—add 000 to get the full amount. 2007 Note: Financial information for 2007 was not available for all companies at press time.

2007 Sales: $61,134,300	2007 Profits: $3,345,400	**U.S. Stock Ticker:** WLP
2006 Sales: $57,038,800	2006 Profits: $3,094,900	**Int'l Ticker:** Int'l Exchange:
2005 Sales: $44,541,300	2005 Profits: $2,463,800	Employees: 42,000
2004 Sales: $20,707,900	2004 Profits: $960,100	Fiscal Year Ends: 12/31
2003 Sales: $20,101,500	2003 Profits: $935,200	Parent Company:

SALARIES/BENEFITS:

Pension Plan:	ESOP Stock Plan:	Profit Sharing:	Top Exec. Salary: $1,290,385	Bonus: $2,013,206
Savings Plan: Y	Stock Purch. Plan: Y		Second Exec. Salary: $703,295	Bonus: $666,190

OTHER THOUGHTS:
Apparent Women Officers or Directors: 4
Hot Spot for Advancement for Women/Minorities: Y

LOCATIONS: ("Y" = Yes)

West:	Southwest:	Midwest:	Southeast:	Northeast:	International:
Y	Y	Y	Y	Y	

Note: Financial information, benefits and other data can change quickly and may vary from those stated here.

WENDYS INTERNATIONAL INC

www.wendys.com

Industry Group Code: 722110 Ranks within this company's industry group: Sales: 6   Profits: 6

Management:		Sales/Marketing:		Liberal Arts:		Information Systems:		Professionals:		Technical/Scientific:	
Mgmt. Trainees:	Y	Mktg. Professionals:	Y	Gen. Writing/Editing:	Y	Info. Management:	Y	Finance/Accounting:	Y	Engineers, Elec.:	
Experienced Mgmt.:	Y	Retail Sales:		Technical Writing:		Software Dev.:	Y	Law:	Y	Engineers, Other:	
Int'l Business:	Y	Commercial/Industrial:	Y	Graphic Arts/Photog.:	Y	Hardware Dev.:		HR/Other:	Y	Health/Lab:	
MBA Graduates:	Y	Sales Trainees:		Music:		Systems Integration:		Training:	Y	Scientists/Research:	
		Advertising Pros.:	Y	Broadcasting:		Consulting/Other:		Health Care:		Petroleum/Chemicals:	
				Other:	Y			Consulting:		Math/Other:	

TYPES OF BUSINESS:

Fast Food Restaurants
Casual Dining Restaurants
Franchising

BRANDS/DIVISIONS/AFFILIATES:

Wendy's
Pasta Pomodoro
New Bakery Co., Inc. (The)
Frosty
Vanilla Frosty
Twisted Frosty
Cafe Express
Baconator

CONTACTS: *Note: Officers with more than one job title may be intentionally listed here more than once.*

Kerrii B. Anderson, CEO
David J. Near, COO
Kerrii B. Anderson, Pres.
Joseph J. Fitzsimmons, CFO/Exec. VP
Paul Kershisnik, Sr. VP-Interim Chief Mktg. Officer
Karen F. Ickes, Interim Sr. VP-Corp. Human Resources
Lori D. Estrada, Sr. VP-R&D
Robert M. Whittington, CIO/Sr. VP
Leon M. McCorkle, Jr., General Counsel/Exec. VP/Sec.
Edward K. Choe, Exec. VP-Restaurant Svcs.
Michael C. Watson, Sr. VP-Oper. Admin. & Strategic Planning
John D. Barker, Sr. VP-Corp. Affairs
John D. Barker, Sr. VP-Investor Rel.
Brendan P. Foley, Jr., Gen. Controller/Sr. VP
Everett E. Gallagher, Jr, Sr. VP-Enterprise Tax & Risk Mgmt.
Neil Lester, Sr. VP-Canada
Tom Spero, Sr. VP-Northern Region
Bob Holtcamp, Sr. VP-Brand Management
James V. Pickett, Chmn.
James C. Hartenstein, Sr. VP-Int'l
Tad G. Wampfler, Sr. VP-Supply Chain & Bakery

Phone: 614-764-3100	Fax: 614-764-3330
Toll-Free:	
Address: One Dave Thomas Blvd., Dublin, OH 43017 US	

GROWTH PLANS/SPECIAL FEATURES:

Wendy's International, Inc. operates, develops and franchises a chain of quick-service restaurants. There are 6,645 Wendy's restaurants in operation across the U.S. and in 19 international markets. Only 1,414 are operated by the company, while 5,231 are operated by franchisees. Each Wendy's restaurant offers a standard menu featuring hamburgers and chicken breast sandwiches, prepared to order with the customer's choice of condiments, as well as chicken nuggets, chili, baked potatoes, french-fries, salads, desserts, soft drinks and children's meals. Wendy's also owns approximately 29% of Pasta Pomodoro, which offers Italian food through its 49 restaurants in California and Arizona. Company subsidiary The New Bakery Co., Inc., supplies buns for 637 Wendy's operated by the company and 2,366 restaurants operated by franchisees, and some third parties. A few of the company's latest additions to the menu include the new Vanilla Frosty, the first companion to the company's trademark combination of a chocolate milk shake and soft-serve ice cream , and the Twisted Frosty, featuring toppings mixed into the shake. About 600 million Frosties are sold annually. In October 2007, Wendy's International and Berjaya Corporation Berhad agreed to build Wendy's restaurants in Malaysia. In April 2008, Wendy's International and Triarc Companies Inc., the franchisor of Arby's restaurants, signed a merger agreement that will bring them together for a total of 10,000 restaurants and estimated annual sales of $12.5 billion. The respective restaurant systems will continue operating as autonomous brands.

FINANCIALS: Sales and profits are in thousands of dollars—add 000 to get the full amount. 2007 Note: Financial information for 2007 was not available for all companies at press time.

2007 Sales: $2,450,244	2007 Profits: $87,896	U.S. Stock Ticker: WEN
2006 Sales: $2,439,277	2006 Profits: $94,312	Int'l Ticker: Int'l Exchange:
2005 Sales: $2,455,418	2005 Profits: $224,067	Employees: 46,000
2004 Sales: $3,635,438	2004 Profits: $52,035	Fiscal Year Ends: 12/31
2003 Sales: $3,148,912	2003 Profits: $235,999	Parent Company:

SALARIES/BENEFITS:

Pension Plan:	ESOP Stock Plan:	Profit Sharing:	Top Exec. Salary: $620,058	Bonus: $1,998,750
Savings Plan:	Stock Purch. Plan:		Second Exec. Salary: $404,842	Bonus: $1,440,000

OTHER THOUGHTS:

Apparent Women Officers or Directors: 5
Hot Spot for Advancement for Women/Minorities: Y

LOCATIONS: ("Y" = Yes)

West:	Southwest:	Midwest:	Southeast:	Northeast:	International:
Y	Y	Y	Y	Y	Y

WEST CORPORATION

www.west.com

Industry Group Code: 561422 Ranks within this company's industry group: Sales: 1 Profits: 1

Management:		Sales/Marketing:		Liberal Arts:		Information Systems:		Professionals:		Technical/Scientific:	
Mgmt. Trainees:	Y	Mktg. Professionals:	Y	Gen. Writing/Editing:		Info. Management:	Y	Finance/Accounting:	Y	Engineers, Elec.:	
Experienced Mgmt.:	Y	Retail Sales:		Technical Writing:		Software Dev.:	Y	Law:	Y	Engineers, Other:	
Int'l Business:	Y	Commercial/Industrial:	Y	Graphic Arts/Photog.:		Hardware Dev.:		HR/Other:	Y	Health/Lab:	
MBA Graduates:	Y	Sales Trainees:		Music:		Systems Integration:		Training:	Y	Scientists/Research:	
		Advertising Pros.:		Broadcasting:		Consulting/Other:		Health Care:		Petroleum/Chemicals:	
				Other:				Consulting:	Y	Math/Other:	

TYPES OF BUSINESS:

Call Centers
Voice Transaction Services
Business Process Outsourcing
Conferencing Communications
Receivables Management

BRANDS/DIVISIONS/AFFILIATES:

West Interactive Corp.
West Telemarketing Corp.
InterCall, Inc.
West Asset Management
IntelliCast
Omnium Worldwide, Inc.
Intrado, Inc.
West Business Services Corp.

CONTACTS: *Note: Officers with more than one job title may be intentionally listed here more than once.*

Thomas B. Barker, CEO
Nancee S. Berger, COO
Nancee S. Berger, Pres.
Paul M. Mendlik, CFO
Mike Sturgeon, Exec. VP-Sales & Mktg.
Mark Lavin, Chief Admin. Officer/Exec. VP
Dave Mussman, General Counsel/Sec./Exec. VP
Dave Treinen, Exec. VP-Corp. Dev. & Planning.
Steven M. Stangl, Pres., West Comm. Svcs.
Paul M. Mendlik, Treas./Exec. VP-Finance
Skip Hanson, Pres., West Telemarketing Corp.
George Heinrichs, Pres., Intrado, Inc.
Pam Mortenson, Exec. VP- West Interactive Corp.
John Sanley, Pres., West Business Services Corp.
Thomas B. Barker, Chmn.

Phone: 402-963-1200	Fax: 402-963-1602
Toll-Free: 800-232-0900	
Address: 11808 Miracle Hills Dr., Omaha, NE 68154 US	

GROWTH PLANS/SPECIAL FEATURES:

West Corporation, based in Nebraska, provides business process outsourcing services to many of the world's largest companies, organizations and government agencies. The firm provides a broad portfolio of voice transaction services, delivered through three segments: Communication services, conferencing services and receivables management. Communication services include both agent and automated services. Agent services provide clients with a range of customer-initiated (inbound) and West-initiated (outbound) transactions, including large-volume transaction processes such as order processing, customer acquisition, customer retention and customer care. The firm's automated services operate over 137,000 interactive voice response ports, with services including automated credit card activation, prepaid calling services, automated product information requests, answers to frequently-asked-questions and call routing and transfer services. West's conferencing services include an integrated suite of audio, video and web conferencing services, including reservationless, operator-assisted conferencing, operating through facilities in the U.S., U.K., Canada, Singapore, Australia, Hong Kong, Japan and New Zealand. The company's receivables management operations include first-party collections, contingent/third-party collections, governmental collections, commercial collections and purchasing. The company additionally collects charged-off consumer and commercial debt. In 2007, West's operations managed and processed more than 11.5 billion telephony minutes, more than 32 million conference calls and more than 200 million 9-1-1 calls. Additionally, the firm completed its acquisition of Omnium Worldwide, Inc., a provider of revenue cycle management solutions. West also recently launched IntelliCast, a multi-channel, automated notification solution that allows employers to communicate information to their customers, employees and partners through automated voice, email, fax and text messaging. In 2008, the company announced plans to purchase Genesys, a global multimedia collaboration service provider, with plans to combine it with InterCall, Inc., a conferencing services provider and West subsidiary.

West employees are offered comprehensive medical benefits, a college savings plan and the West Scholarship Program.

FINANCIALS: Sales and profits are in thousands of dollars—add 000 to get the full amount. 2007 Note: Financial information for 2007 was not available for all companies at press time.

2007 Sales: $2,099,492	2007 Profits: $5,382	**U.S. Stock Ticker: WSTC**
2006 Sales: $1,856,038	2006 Profits: $68,763	**Int'l Ticker:** Int'l Exchange:
2005 Sales: $1,523,923	2005 Profits: $150,349	Employees: 42,000
2004 Sales: $1,217,383	2004 Profits: $113,171	Fiscal Year Ends: 12/31
2003 Sales: $988,341	2003 Profits: $87,876	Parent Company:

SALARIES/BENEFITS:

Pension Plan:	ESOP Stock Plan:	Profit Sharing:	Top Exec. Salary: $850,000	Bonus: $1,977,848
Savings Plan: Y	Stock Purch. Plan:		Second Exec. Salary: $550,000	Bonus: $1,316,717

OTHER THOUGHTS:

Apparent Women Officers or Directors: 2
Hot Spot for Advancement for Women/Minorities: Y

LOCATIONS: ("Y" = Yes)

West:	Southwest:	Midwest:	Southeast:	Northeast:	International:
Y	Y	Y	Y	Y	Y

Note: Financial information, benefits and other data can change quickly and may vary from those stated here.

WEST PHARMACEUTICAL SERVICES INC
www.westpharma.com
Industry Group Code: 322210   Ranks within this company's industry group: Sales: 1   Profits: 1

Management:		Sales/Marketing:		Liberal Arts:		Information Systems:		Professionals:		Technical/Scientific:	
Mgmt. Trainees:		Mktg. Professionals:	Y	Gen. Writing/Editing:		Info. Management:	Y	Finance/Accounting:	Y	Engineers, Elec.:	Y
Experienced Mgmt.:	Y	Retail Sales:		Technical Writing:	Y	Software Dev.:	Y	Law:	Y	Engineers, Other:	Y
Int'l Business:	Y	Commercial/Industrial:	Y	Graphic Arts/Photog.:	Y	Hardware Dev.:	Y	HR/Other:	Y	Health/Lab:	Y
MBA Graduates:	Y	Sales Trainees:		Music:		Systems Integration:	Y	Training:	Y	Scientists/Research:	Y
		Advertising Pros.:		Broadcasting:		Consulting/Other:		Health Care:	Y	Petroleum/Chemicals:	Y
				Other:				Consulting:		Math/Other:	

TYPES OF BUSINESS:
Injectable Drug Delivery Systems Components
Plastic Packaging Systems Components
Elastomer & Metal Components

BRANDS/DIVISIONS/AFFILIATES:
Medimop Medical Projects, Ltd.
The Tech Group
West Analytical Services
Flip-Off
Mixject
Mix2Vial

CONTACTS:
Note: Officers with more than one job title may be intentionally listed here more than once.
Donald E. Morel, Jr., CEO
Steven A. Ellers, COO
Steven A. Ellers, Pres.
William J. Federici, CFO/VP
Richard D. Luzzi, VP-Human Resources
John R. Gailey, III, General Counsel/VP/Sec.
Michael A. Anderson, Treas./VP
Robert S. Hargesheimer, Pres., Tech Group
Donald A. McMillan, Pres., North America-Pharmaceutical Systems Div.
Joseph E. Abbott, VP/Corp. Controller
Donald E. Morel, Jr., Chmn.
Robert J. Keating, Pres., Europe & Asia Pacific-Pharmaceutical Div.

Phone: 610-594-2900	Fax: 610-594-3000
Toll-Free:	
Address: 101 Gordon Dr., Lionville, PA 19341 US	

GROWTH PLANS/SPECIAL FEATURES:
West Pharmaceutical Services, Inc. manufactures components and systems for injectable drug delivery and plastic packaging and markets delivery system components for the healthcare, personal care and consumer products industries. The company's products include stoppers and seals for vials; components used in syringes; intravenous delivery systems; and blood collection systems. The firm operates in two segments: Pharmaceutical systems and The Tech Group. The pharmaceutical systems segment designs, manufactures and sells pharmaceutical packaging components and a variety of plastic, elastomer and metal components used in parenteral drug delivery for the branded pharmaceutical, generic and biopharmaceutical markets. Products include elastomeric stoppers and discs; secondary closures for pharmaceutical vials, called Flip-Off aluminum seals; elastomeric syringe plungers, components for blood collection systems, flashback bulbs and sleeve stoppers; elastomer and co-molded elastomer/plastic components for infusion sets; dropper bulbs for dispensing systems such as eye, ear and nasal drops; needle shields and tip caps; and sterile devices including Mixject and Mix2Vial. Operating under this segment, Medimop Medical Projects, Ltd. provides transfer, mixing and administration systems for injectable pharmaceuticals. The firm also offers contract analytical laboratory services with support from West Analytical Services. The Tech Group, a West Pharmaceutical company, serves the drug delivery, consumer and healthcare markets with custom injection molding products and services. It designs and manufactures unique components for surgical, ophthalmic, diagnostic and drug delivery systems such as contact lens storage kits, pill dispensers and disposable blood collection systems and components. West Pharmaceutical also offers pharmaceutical systems and tech services to international customers. Sales outside of the U.S. account for roughly 51% of net sales.

The company offers employees medical, life, dental and disability insurance; a 401(k) plan; a retirement plan; an employee stock purchase plan; an employee assistance program; an education assistance program; and flexible spending accounts.

FINANCIALS:
Sales and profits are in thousands of dollars—add 000 to get the full amount. 2007 Note: Financial information for 2007 was not available for all companies at press time.

2007 Sales: $1,020,100	2007 Profits: $70,700	**U.S. Stock Ticker: WST**
2006 Sales: $913,300	2006 Profits: $67,100	**Int'l Ticker:** Int'l Exchange:
2005 Sales: $699,700	2005 Profits: $45,600	Employees: 6,478
2004 Sales: $541,600	2004 Profits: $19,400	Fiscal Year Ends: 12/31
2003 Sales: $490,700	2003 Profits: $31,900	Parent Company:

SALARIES/BENEFITS:
Pension Plan: Y	ESOP Stock Plan:	Profit Sharing:	Top Exec. Salary: $778,382	Bonus: $676,005
Savings Plan: Y	Stock Purch. Plan:		Second Exec. Salary: $446,843	Bonus: $288,466

OTHER THOUGHTS:
Apparent Women Officers or Directors: 2
Hot Spot for Advancement for Women/Minorities:

LOCATIONS: ("Y" = Yes)
West:	Southwest:	Midwest:	Southeast:	Northeast:	International:
	Y	Y	Y	Y	Y

WESTERN DIGITAL CORP
www.wdc.com

Industry Group Code: 334112 Ranks within this company's industry group: Sales: 2 Profits: 2

Management:		Sales/Marketing:		Liberal Arts:		Information Systems:		Professionals:		Technical/Scientific:	
Mgmt. Trainees:		Mktg. Professionals:	Y	Gen. Writing/Editing:		Info. Management:	Y	Finance/Accounting:	Y	Engineers, Elec.:	Y
Experienced Mgmt.:	Y	Retail Sales:		Technical Writing:	Y	Software Dev.:	Y	Law:	Y	Engineers, Other:	
Int'l Business:	Y	Commercial/Industrial:	Y	Graphic Arts/Photog.:	Y	Hardware Dev.:	Y	HR/Other:	Y	Health/Lab:	Y
MBA Graduates:	Y	Sales Trainees:		Music:		Systems Integration:		Training:	Y	Scientists/Research:	Y
		Advertising Pros.:		Broadcasting:		Consulting/Other:		Health Care:		Petroleum/Chemicals:	
				Other:				Consulting:		Math/Other:	Y

TYPES OF BUSINESS:
Data Storage Hardware
Hard Drives

BRANDS/DIVISIONS/AFFILIATES:
Read-Rite Corp.
WD Raptor X
FireWire
Media Center
Caviar
Scorpio
Raptor
Komag Inc

CONTACTS: Note: Officers with more than one job title may be intentionally listed here more than once.
John F. Coyne, CEO
John F. Coyne, Pres.
Timothy M. Leyden, CFO/Exec. VP
Hossein M. Moghadam, CTO/Sr. VP
Raymond M. Bukaty, Sr. VP-Admin.
Raymond M. Bukaty, General Counsel/Corp. Sec.
Thomas E. Pardun, Chmn.

Phone: 949-672-7000	Fax: 949-672-5408
Toll-Free:	
Address: 20511 Lake Forest Dr., Lake Forest, CA 92630-7741 US	

GROWTH PLANS/SPECIAL FEATURES:

Western Digital Corporation is a leader in the data storage industry through hard drive manufacturing for desktop and notebook computers, mobile and hand-held devices, corporate networks and home entertainment applications. In addition, the company's hard disk drives are used in external hard disk drive products that feature high-speed buses such as 1394/FireWire/iLink, Universal Serial Bus (USB) and Ethernet. A range of hard drives are available including Caviar drives available in both EIDE and Serial ATA for desktop computers; high performance, low power consumption Scorpio drives for notebook computing; Raptor drives, the world's only 10,000 RPM Serial ATA hard drive used for enterprise storage; and drives for consumer electronics and home use. The company's hard drives include 3.5-inch and 2.5-inch form factor drives with capacities ranging from 40 gigabytes to 1 terabyte; rotation speeds of 5,400, 7,200 and 10,000 revolutions per minute; and the Enhanced Integrated Drive Electronics (EIDE) interfaces in both external and internal models. Recently introduced hard drives include the 320 GB capacity WD Passport Portable Drive, WD RE2 (RAID Edition) 750 GB hard drive and the 3.5-inch WD AV hard drive family. Late in 2007, the firm announced its hard drive density achievement of 520 Gb/in2, the hard drive industry's highest demonstrated density using continuous media. Currently the company's manufacturing is done in Malaysia and Thailand, while design is performed in its California offices. In September 2007, the firm's wholly-owned subsidiary, State M Corporation, completed the acquisition of Komag, Inc., a manufacturer of data-recording rotating disks.

Western Digital employees receive full partner health care benefits, health care, dependent care and educational reimbursements and an employee assistance program.

FINANCIALS: Sales and profits are in thousands of dollars—add 000 to get the full amount. 2007 Note: Financial information for 2007 was not available for all companies at press time.

2007 Sales: $5,468,000	2007 Profits: $564,000	U.S. Stock Ticker: WDC
2006 Sales: $4,341,300	2006 Profits: $395,900	Int'l Ticker: Int'l Exchange:
2005 Sales: $3,638,800	2005 Profits: $198,400	Employees: 29,572
2004 Sales: $2,046,700	2004 Profits: $151,300	Fiscal Year Ends: 6/30
2003 Sales: $2,718,517	2003 Profits: $199,874	Parent Company:

SALARIES/BENEFITS:
Pension Plan:	ESOP Stock Plan:	Profit Sharing: Y	Top Exec. Salary: $800,000	Bonus: $1,000,000
Savings Plan: Y	Stock Purch. Plan:		Second Exec. Salary: $724,423	Bonus: $2,663,500

OTHER THOUGHTS:
Apparent Women Officers or Directors:
Hot Spot for Advancement for Women/Minorities:

LOCATIONS: ("Y" = Yes)
West:	Southwest:	Midwest:	Southeast:	Northeast:	International:
Y					Y

Note: Financial information, benefits and other data can change quickly and may vary from those stated here.

WESTERN UNION COMPANY (THE)   www.westernunion.com

Industry Group Code: 522320   Ranks within this company's industry group: Sales: Profits:

Management:	Sales/Marketing:	Liberal Arts:	Information Systems:	Professionals:	Technical/Scientific:
Mgmt. Trainees:	Mktg. Professionals:	Gen. Writing/Editing:	Info. Management:	Finance/Accounting:	Engineers, Elec.:
Experienced Mgmt.:	Retail Sales:	Technical Writing:	Software Dev.:	Law:	Engineers, Other:
Int'l Business:	Commercial/Industrial:	Graphic Arts/Photog.:	Hardware Dev.:	HR/Other:	Health/Lab:
MBA Graduates:	Sales Trainees:	Music:	Systems Integration:	Training:	Scientists/Research:
	Advertising Pros.:	Broadcasting:	Consulting/Other:	Health Care:	Petroleum/Chemicals:
		Other:		Consulting:	Math/Other:

TYPES OF BUSINESS:

Money Transfers
Money Orders
Bill Payment Services

BRANDS/DIVISIONS/AFFILIATES:

Orlandi Valuta
Vigo
Pago Facil
Servicio Electronico De Pago S.A.
Transfer Express de Panama

CONTACTS: *Note: Officers with more than one job title may be intentionally listed here more than once.*

Christina A. Gold, CEO
Christina A. Gold, Pres.
Scott T. Scheirman, CFO/Exec. VP
Gail Galuppo, Chief Mktg. Officer/Exec. VP
Grover Wray, Exec. VP-Human Resources
Robin Heller, Exec. VP-IT
David Schlapbach, General Counsel/Exec. VP/Sec.
Robin Heller, Exec. VP-Oper.
David Barnes, Exec. VP-U.S., Canada & Strategic Dev.
Anne McCarthy, Exec. VP-Corp. Affairs
Stewart A. Stockdare, Exec. VP/Pres., US & Canada
Liz Alicea-Velez, Exec. VP-Latin America & Caribbean
Ian Marsh, Exec. VP/Managing Dir.-Asia Pacific Region
Guy A. Battista, Exec. VP/Pres., Western Union Financial Svc., Inc.
Hikmet Ersek, Exec. VP/Managing Dir.-EMEA & South Asia

Phone: 720-332-1000	Fax: 720-332-4753
Toll-Free: 866-405-5012	
Address: 12500 E. Belford Ave., Englewood, CO 80112 US	

GROWTH PLANS/SPECIAL FEATURES:

Western Union Co. (The) is a provider of global money transfers, offering ways for customers to send money, pay bills and purchase money orders around the globe. The company operates in two segments, consumer-to-consumer and consumer-to-business. The consumer-to-consumer segment provides money transfer services between consumers, primarily through a global network of third-party agents using multi-currency, real-time money transfer processing systems. The consumer-to-business segment focuses on payments to billers through the firm's networks of third-party agents and various electronic channels. The company offers its services under the Western Union, Orlandi Valuta, Vigo and Pago Facil brands through a network of about 335,000 agent locations in more than 200 countries and territories. About 80% of its agent locations are outside the U.S. The company's revenue is derived primarily from fees that customers pay to transfer money, as well as from foreign currency exchange rate discrepancies. Western Union agents include large networks such as post offices, banks and retailers. The firm has agreements with postal organizations in postal organizations in Argentina, Australia, China, France, Germany, India, New Zealand, Russia, Spain and elsewhere. Western Union's services are offered through banks such as Agricultural Bank of China, BNP Paribas, Credit Lyonnais, Millennium BCP and the State Bank of India. National and international retailers in the network include Kroger and Publix in the United States and Elektra and Travelex internationally. Many agents have multiple locations. In August 2008, the firm acquired Transfer Express de Panama, which will directly operate its own 15 locations and manage relationships with sub-Agents who represent nearly 100 sites throughout Panama.

FINANCIALS: Sales and profits are in thousands of dollars—add 000 to get the full amount. 2007 Note: Financial information for 2007 was not available for all companies at press time.

2007 Sales: $4,900,200	2007 Profits: $857,300	U.S. Stock Ticker: WU
2006 Sales: $4,470,200	2006 Profits: $914,000	Int'l Ticker: Int'l Exchange:
2005 Sales: $3,987,900	2005 Profits: $927,400	Employees: 4,900
2004 Sales: $3,547,600	2004 Profits: $751,600	Fiscal Year Ends: 12/31
2003 Sales: $3,120,800	2003 Profits: $638,700	Parent Company:

SALARIES/BENEFITS:

Pension Plan:	ESOP Stock Plan:	Profit Sharing:	Top Exec. Salary: $714,600	Bonus: $1,550,000
Savings Plan:	Stock Purch. Plan:		Second Exec. Salary: $532,100	Bonus: $1,025,000

OTHER THOUGHTS:

Apparent Women Officers or Directors: 7
Hot Spot for Advancement for Women/Minorities: Y

LOCATIONS: ("Y" = Yes)

West:	Southwest:	Midwest:	Southeast:	Northeast:	International:
Y	Y	Y	Y	Y	Y

WHOLE FOODS MARKET INC   www.wholefoodsmarket.com

Industry Group Code: 445110 Ranks within this company's industry group: Sales: 1   Profits: 1

Management:		Sales/Marketing:		Liberal Arts:		Information Systems:		Professionals:		Technical/Scientific:	
Mgmt. Trainees:	Y	Mktg. Professionals:	Y	Gen. Writing/Editing:	Y	Info. Management:	Y	Finance/Accounting:	Y	Engineers, Elec.:	
Experienced Mgmt.:	Y	Retail Sales:	Y	Technical Writing:		Software Dev.:	Y	Law:	Y	Engineers, Other:	
Int'l Business:	Y	Commercial/Industrial:	Y	Graphic Arts/Photog.:	Y	Hardware Dev.:		HR/Other:	Y	Health/Lab:	
MBA Graduates:	Y	Sales Trainees:	Y	Music:		Systems Integration:		Training:	Y	Scientists/Research:	
		Advertising Pros.:	Y	Broadcasting:		Consulting/Other:		Health Care:		Petroleum/Chemicals:	
				Other:				Consulting:		Math/Other:	

TYPES OF BUSINESS:

Natural Foods Grocery Stores
Nutritional Supplements
Seafood Processing
Coffee Roasting

BRANDS/DIVISIONS/AFFILIATES:

365 Organic Everyday Value
365 Everyday Value
Whole Kitchen
Whole Pantry
Allegro Coffee Company
Pigeon Cove
Select Fish
Wild Oats Markets Inc

CONTACTS: Note: Officers with more than one job title may be intentionally listed here more than once.

John Mackey, CEO
Walter Robb, Co-COO/Co-Pres.
A. C. Gallo, Co-Pres./Co-COO
Glenda Chamberlain, CFO/Exec. VP
Mike Clifford, CIO/VP
Roberta Lang, General Counsel
Jim Sud, Exec. VP-Growth & Bus. Dev.
Margaret Wittenberg, Global VP-Public Affairs & Quality Standards
Cindy McCann, Global VP-Investor Rel.
Sam Ferguson, Global VP-Acct./Controller
Paula Labian, Global VP-Team Member Service.
Bruce Silverman, Global VP-Private Label
Lee Matecko, Global VP-Construction & Store Dev.
Brian O'Connell, Global VP-Oper. Finance
John Mackey, Chmn.
Lee Valkenaar, Exec. VP-Global Support
Bart Beilman, Global VP-Distribution

Phone: 512-477-4455	Fax: 512-482-7000
Toll-Free:	
Address: 550 Bowie St., Austin, TX 78703-4644 US	

GROWTH PLANS/SPECIAL FEATURES:

Whole Foods Market, Inc. owns and operates a chain of natural organic food supermarkets in the U.S. and internationally. The firm's stores generally feature foods made from natural ingredients and free of chemical additives. The company's merchandise line of over 1,500 items includes organically grown and high-grade commercial produce; grocery products; environmentally safe household items; hormone- and antibiotic- free meats; bulk foods; fresh bakery goods; soups, salads, entrees and sandwiches; vitamins; cosmetics; and miscellaneous items. Merchandise is also sold under four private-label brands: 365 Everyday Value, 365 Organic Everyday Value and Whole Kitchen and Whole Pantry, which are chef quality, all natural foods. The company owns about 276 store locations in 37 states and Washington, D.C., as well as seven stores in Canada and six stores in the U.K. Its stores are supplemented by regional distribution centers, bakeries, commissary kitchens, seafood-processing facilities, produce procurement centers and a coffee roasting operation. The company operates a web site that offers features such as online recipes, health information and environmental issue information. The firm's subsidiaries include Allegro Coffee Company; Pigeon Cove, a seafood processing facility; Select Fish, a West Coast seafood processing facility; and Produce Field Inspection Office. In August 2007, Whole Foods acquired Wild Oats Markets, Inc. for $565 million. Wild Oats owned 109 North American stores that operate under the names Wild Oats, Henry's Farmers Market, Sun Harvest and Capers Community Market.

Whole Foods has been named one of the 100 Best Companies to Work For in America by Fortune Magazine for 11 consecutive years. Employees vote on their benefit package every three years, and all employees are eligible to receive stock options. Employees are offered medical, dental and vision insurance; a personal wellness account; health and dependent care reimbursement accounts; 401(k); merchandise discount; gainsharing; team member stock purchase plan and stock option plan; and team member emergency funds.

FINANCIALS: Sales and profits are in thousands of dollars—add 000 to get the full amount. 2007 Note: Financial information for 2007 was not available for all companies at press time.

2007 Sales: $6,591,773	2007 Profits: $182,740	**U.S. Stock Ticker: WFMI**
2006 Sales: $5,607,376	2006 Profits: $203,828	**Int'l Ticker:** Int'l Exchange:
2005 Sales: $4,701,289	2005 Profits: $136,351	Employees: 39,500
2004 Sales: $3,864,950	2004 Profits: $137,113	Fiscal Year Ends: 9/30
2003 Sales: $3,148,593	2003 Profits: $103,687	Parent Company:

SALARIES/BENEFITS:

Pension Plan: Y	ESOP Stock Plan:	Profit Sharing: Y	Top Exec. Salary: $371,600	Bonus: $583,798
Savings Plan: Y	Stock Purch. Plan: Y		Second Exec. Salary: $333,600	Bonus: $684,961

OTHER THOUGHTS:

Apparent Women Officers or Directors: 8
Hot Spot for Advancement for Women/Minorities: Y

LOCATIONS: ("Y" = Yes)

West:	Southwest:	Midwest:	Southeast:	Northeast:	International:
Y	Y	Y	Y	Y	

WILLIAMS COMPANIES INC (THE)

www.williams.com

Industry Group Code: 211111   Ranks within this company's industry group: Sales: Profits:

Management:		Sales/Marketing:		Liberal Arts:		Information Systems:		Professionals:		Technical/Scientific:	
Mgmt. Trainees:		Mktg. Professionals:	Y	Gen. Writing/Editing:		Info. Management:	Y	Finance/Accounting:	Y	Engineers, Elec.:	Y
Experienced Mgmt.:	Y	Retail Sales:		Technical Writing:		Software Dev.:		Law:	Y	Engineers, Other:	
Int'l Business:	Y	Commercial/Industrial:	Y	Graphic Arts/Photog.:		Hardware Dev.:		HR/Other:	Y	Health/Lab:	
MBA Graduates:	Y	Sales Trainees:		Music:		Systems Integration:		Training:	Y	Scientists/Research:	
		Advertising Pros.:		Broadcasting:		Consulting/Other:		Health Care:		Petroleum/Chemicals:	Y
				Other:				Consulting:		Math/Other:	

TYPES OF BUSINESS:

Gas Exploration & Production
Natural Gas Transportation
Pipelines
Wholesale Power

BRANDS/DIVISIONS/AFFILIATES:

Williams Production Co., LLC
Williams Production RMT Co.
Williams Gas Pipeline Co., LLC
Williams Field Services Group, LLC
Williams NAtural Gas Liquids, Inc.
Williams Partners L.P.
Williams Power Co., Inc.
Transco

CONTACTS: *Note: Officers with more than one job title may be intentionally listed here more than once.*

Steven J. Malcomb, CEO
Steven J. Malcomb, Pres.
Don R. Chappel, CFO/Sr. VP
Robyn L. Ewing, Chief Admin. Officer
James J. Bender, General Counsel/Sr. VP
Robyn L. Ewing, Sr. VP-Strategic Srvcs. & Administration
Alan Armstrong, Pres., Midstream Gathering & Processing
Ralph A. Hill, Pres., Exploration & Prod.
Bill Hobbs, Pres., Power
Phillip D. Wright, Pres., Gas Pipeline
Steven J. Malcolm, Chmn.

Phone: 918-573-2000	Fax:
Toll-Free: 800-945-5426	
Address: 1 Williams Ctr., Tulsa, OK 74172 US	

GROWTH PLANS/SPECIAL FEATURES:

The Williams Companies, Inc. finds, produces, gathers, processes and transports natural gas. The firm also manages a wholesale power business. Company operations are concentrated in the Pacific Northwest, Rocky Mountains, Gulf Coast, and the Eastern Seaboard. The company operates in five segments: exploration and production; gas pipeline; midstream gas and liquids; gas marketing services; and other. The exploration and production segment produces, develops and manages natural gas reserves primarily located in the Rocky Mountain and mid-continent regions of the U.S. The gas pipeline segment includes natural gas pipelines and pipeline joint venture investments organized under subsidiary Williams Gas Pipeline Co., LLC. The midstream and gas liquids segment includes our natural gas gathering, treating and processing business and is comprised of several subsidiaries including Williams Field Services Group LLC, Williams Natural Gas Liquids, Inc. and Williams Partners L.P. The gas marketing services segment manages the firm's natural gas commodity risk through purchases, sales and other related transactions, under its wholly owned subsidiary Williams Gas Marketing, Inc. The other segment primarily consists of corporate operations. The division includes the company's interest in Longhorn Partners Pipeline, L.P. Williams operates 14,600 miles of interstate natural gas pipeline and has five interstate natural gas pipelines, including the Transco system, which runs from Texas to New York. The company owns holdings in four production basins: the Piceance Basin in Colorado, the San Juan Basin in New Mexico, the Powder River Basin in Wyoming and the Arkoma Basin in Arkansas and Oklahoma.

The company offers its employees medical and dental insurance; a 401(k) plan; pension benefits; life and disability insurance; flexible spending accounts; an employee assistance program; and access to a credit union.

FINANCIALS: Sales and profits are in thousands of dollars—add 000 to get the full amount. 2007 Note: Financial information for 2007 was not available for all companies at press time.

2007 Sales: $105,558,000	2007 Profits: $990,000	U.S. Stock Ticker: WMB
2006 Sales: $9,376,000	2006 Profits: $309,000	Int'l Ticker: Int'l Exchange:
2005 Sales: $12,583,600	2005 Profits: $317,400	Employees: 3,913
2004 Sales: $12,461,300	2004 Profits: $93,200	Fiscal Year Ends: 12/31
2003 Sales: $16,834,100	2003 Profits: $-492,200	Parent Company:

SALARIES/BENEFITS:

Pension Plan: Y	ESOP Stock Plan:	Profit Sharing:	Top Exec. Salary: $1,040,385	Bonus: $2,309,630
Savings Plan: Y	Stock Purch. Plan:		Second Exec. Salary: $545,192	Bonus: $892,956

OTHER THOUGHTS:

Apparent Women Officers or Directors: 1
Hot Spot for Advancement for Women/Minorities: Y

LOCATIONS: ("Y" = Yes)

West:	Southwest:	Midwest:	Southeast:	Northeast:	International:
Y	Y	Y	Y	Y	Y

WILLIAMS SONOMA INC www.williams-sonomainc.com

Industry Group Code: 442299 Ranks within this company's industry group: Sales: 2 Profits: 2

Management:		Sales/Marketing:		Liberal Arts:		Information Systems:		Professionals:		Technical/Scientific:	
Mgmt. Trainees:	Y	Mktg. Professionals:	Y	Gen. Writing/Editing:	Y	Info. Management:	Y	Finance/Accounting:	Y	Engineers, Elec.:	
Experienced Mgmt.:	Y	Retail Sales:	Y	Technical Writing:		Software Dev.:	Y	Law:	Y	Engineers, Other:	
Int'l Business:	Y	Commercial/Industrial:	Y	Graphic Arts/Photog.:	Y	Hardware Dev.:		HR/Other:	Y	Health/Lab:	
MBA Graduates:	Y	Sales Trainees:	Y	Music:		Systems Integration:		Training:	Y	Scientists/Research:	
		Advertising Pros.:	Y	Broadcasting:		Consulting/Other:		Health Care:		Petroleum/Chemicals:	
				Other:	Y			Consulting:		Math/Other:	

TYPES OF BUSINESS:

Housewares, Retail
Garden Supplies & Accessories
Home Furnishings & Accessories
Specialty Foods
Online & Catalog Sales
Outlet Stores

BRANDS/DIVISIONS/AFFILIATES:

Pottery Barn
Pottery Barn Kids
Grande Cuisine
Design Studio
Hold Everything
Williams-Sonoma Home
West Elm
PBteen

CONTACTS: *Note: Officers with more than one job title may be intentionally listed here more than once.*

W. Howard Lester, CEO
Sharon L. McCollam, COO/Exec. VP
Laura J. Alber, Pres.
Sharon L. McCollam, CFO
Patrick J. Connolly, Chief Mktg. Officer/Exec. VP
W. Howard Lester, Chmn.

Phone: 415-421-7900	Fax: 415-616-8359
Toll-Free:	
Address: 3250 Van Ness Ave., San Francisco, CA 94109 US	

GROWTH PLANS/SPECIAL FEATURES:

Williams-Sonoma, Inc. is a national specialty retailer of high-quality cooking and serving equipment, home furnishings and home and garden accessories, which it markets through 600 retail stores spread across 44 states Washington D.C. and Canada, seven direct-mail catalogs and six e-commerce sites. The company offers home merchandise through five retail store concepts, none of which the company franchises: Williams-Sonoma, Pottery Barn, Pottery Barn Kids, West Elm and Williams-Sonoma Home. Williams-Sonoma stores offer culinary and serving equipment, including cookware, cookbooks, cutlery, informal dinnerware, glassware and table linens. In addition, the stores carry a variety of quality food, including a line of Williams-Sonoma food products. The firm also operates a larger version of its Williams-Sonoma stores called Grande Cuisine. These stores, typically 30% larger than Williams-Sonoma stores, feature tasting bars and kitchen demonstrations. The company also owns and operates 16 Williams-Sonoma outlet stores. Pottery Barn features casual home furnishings, flatware and table accessories. The firm also operates a large-format version of these stores under the name Design Studio. Design Studio stores offer more departments, as well as worktables where customers can plan room arrangements. Pottery Barn Kids features child-sized versions of much of the merchandise offered at Pottery Barn. In addition to its retail stores, Williams-Sonoma owns seven catalogs, including Williams-Sonoma, Pottery Barn, Pottery Barn Kids, Pottery Barn Bed and Bath, PBteen, West Elm and Williams-Sonoma Home. The company's PBteen catalog focuses on the teenage market in home retail. In 2007, retail sales accounted for 57.8% of net revenues while direct-to-customer sales represented 42.2%.

The company's employee benefits package includes merchandise discounts; health and dependent care tax-free spending accounts; short and long-term disability programs; medical, family and bereavement leave; tuition reimbursement; and same-sex domestic partner benefits.

FINANCIALS: Sales and profits are in thousands of dollars—add 000 to get the full amount. 2007 Note: Financial information for 2007 was not available for all companies at press time.

2007 Sales: $3,727,513	2007 Profits: $208,868	U.S. Stock Ticker: WSM
2006 Sales: $3,538,947	2006 Profits: $214,866	Int'l Ticker: Int'l Exchange:
2005 Sales: $3,136,900	2005 Profits: $191,200	Employees: 37,200
2004 Sales: $2,754,368	2004 Profits: $157,211	Fiscal Year Ends: 1/28
2003 Sales: $2,360,800	2003 Profits: $124,400	Parent Company:

SALARIES/BENEFITS:

Pension Plan:	ESOP Stock Plan: Y	Profit Sharing: Y	Top Exec. Salary: $975,000	Bonus: $
Savings Plan: Y	Stock Purch. Plan:		Second Exec. Salary: $700,770	Bonus: $

OTHER THOUGHTS:

Apparent Women Officers or Directors: 2
Hot Spot for Advancement for Women/Minorities: Y

LOCATIONS: ("Y" = Yes)

West:	Southwest:	Midwest:	Southeast:	Northeast:	International:
Y	Y	Y	Y	Y	Y

Note: Financial information, benefits and other data can change quickly and may vary from those stated here.

WM WRIGLEY JR COMPANY
www.wrigley.com

Industry Group Code: 311300   Ranks within this company's industry group: Sales: 1   Profits: 1

Management:		Sales/Marketing:		Liberal Arts:		Information Systems:		Professionals:		Technical/Scientific:	
Mgmt. Trainees:	Y	Mktg. Professionals:	Y	Gen. Writing/Editing:	Y	Info. Management:	Y	Finance/Accounting:	Y	Engineers, Elec.:	Y
Experienced Mgmt.:	Y	Retail Sales:		Technical Writing:		Software Dev.:	Y	Law:	Y	Engineers, Other:	
Int'l Business:	Y	Commercial/Industrial:	Y	Graphic Arts/Photog.:	Y	Hardware Dev.:		HR/Other:	Y	Health/Lab:	Y
MBA Graduates:	Y	Sales Trainees:	Y	Music:		Systems Integration:		Training:	Y	Scientists/Research:	
		Advertising Pros.:	Y	Broadcasting:		Consulting/Other:		Health Care:		Petroleum/Chemicals:	
				Other:				Consulting:		Math/Other:	

TYPES OF BUSINESS:
Chewing Gum Manufacturing
Candy & Confections
Breath Mints
Packaging Materials
Flavorings

BRANDS/DIVISIONS/AFFILIATES:
Wrigley's Spearmint
Doublemint
Juicy Fruit
Life Savers
Big Red
Altoids
L.A. Dreyfus Company
Northwestern Flavors, LLC

CONTACTS: *Note: Officers with more than one job title may be intentionally listed here more than once.*
William D. Perez, CEO
William D. Perez, Pres.
Reuben Gamoran, CFO/Sr. VP
Martin Schlatter, Chief Mktg. Officer/VP
Tawfik Sharkasi, VP/Chief Science & Technology Officer
Dushan Petrovich, Chief Admin. Officer/Sr. VP
Howard Malovany, General Counsel/Sr. VP/Sec.
Susan Henderson, VP-Corp. Comm.
Shaun Mara, Controller/VP
Patrick D. Mitchell, Chief Procurement Officer/VP
Rob Peterson, Chief Innovation Officer
Carol Knight, VP-Scientific & Regulatory Affairs
Mary Kay Haben, Group VP/Managing Dir.-North America
William Wrigley, Jr., Chmn.
Michael Wong, VP/Managing Dir.-Asia/Pacific

Phone: 312-644-2121	Fax: 312-644-0097
Toll-Free:	
Address: 410 N. Michigan Ave., Chicago, IL 60611 US	

GROWTH PLANS/SPECIAL FEATURES:

Wm. Wrigley Jr. Company, founded as a partnership in 1891, is the world's largest gum maker and has products distributed in over 180 countries and territories. The firm manufactures and markets its chewing gum products in the U.S. and around the world. In addition to selling gum, the company is also focusing on sales of non-gum items, including mints, breath strips and candies, both through internal brand development and acquisitions. Its brands include Juicy Fruit, Wrigley's Spearmint, Doublemint, Winterfresh, Big Red, Eclipse, Orbit, Freedent, Big League Chew, Hubba Bubba, Life Savers and Altoids. The firm also has two associated companies, L. A. Dreyfus Company, which manufactures chewing gum base for Wrigley and associated companies, and Northwestern Flavors, LLC, a manufacturer of flavorings and rectified mint oil for the firm's production facilities. The company markets its products through distributors, wholesalers, corporate chains and cooperative buying groups that distribute the products through retail outlets. Additional direct customers are vending distributors, concessionaires and other established customers purchasing in wholesale quantities. In April 2008, the company agreed to a merger with confectionary manufacturer Mars, Inc. Wrigley will become a private company and subsidiary of Mars, Inc.

Wrigley offers employees health care benefits, dental benefits, a retirement plan, an employee assistance program, flexible spending plans, educational assistance, matching charitable grants and transit vouchers. The firm also funds the Wrigley Scholarship Program for children of full-time employees.

FINANCIALS: Sales and profits are in thousands of dollars—add 000 to get the full amount. 2007 Note: Financial information for 2007 was not available for all companies at press time.

2007 Sales: $5,389,100	2007 Profits: $632,005	U.S. Stock Ticker: WWY
2006 Sales: $4,683,437	2006 Profits: $529,377	Int'l Ticker: Int'l Exchange:
2005 Sales: $4,159,306	2005 Profits: $517,252	Employees: 15,800
2004 Sales: $3,648,600	2004 Profits: $493,000	Fiscal Year Ends: 12/31
2003 Sales: $3,069,088	2003 Profits: $445,894	Parent Company:

SALARIES/BENEFITS:

Pension Plan: Y	ESOP Stock Plan:	Profit Sharing:	Top Exec. Salary: $1,412,500	Bonus: $2,171,013
Savings Plan: Y	Stock Purch. Plan:		Second Exec. Salary: $610,833	Bonus: $603,503

OTHER THOUGHTS:
Apparent Women Officers or Directors: 4
Hot Spot for Advancement for Women/Minorities: Y

LOCATIONS: ("Y" = Yes)

West:	Southwest:	Midwest:	Southeast:	Northeast:	International:
		Y	Y	Y	Y

WW GRAINGER INC
www.grainger.com

Industry Group Code: 421800 Ranks within this company's industry group: Sales: 1 Profits: 1

Management:		Sales/Marketing:		Liberal Arts:		Information Systems:		Professionals:		Technical/Scientific:	
Mgmt. Trainees:	Y	Mktg. Professionals:	Y	Gen. Writing/Editing:	Y	Info. Management:	Y	Finance/Accounting:	Y	Engineers, Elec.:	Y
Experienced Mgmt.:	Y	Retail Sales:	Y	Technical Writing:	Y	Software Dev.:	Y	Law:	Y	Engineers, Other:	
Int'l Business:	Y	Commercial/Industrial:	Y	Graphic Arts/Photog.:	Y	Hardware Dev.:		HR/Other:	Y	Health/Lab:	
MBA Graduates:	Y	Sales Trainees:	Y	Music:		Systems Integration:		Training:	Y	Scientists/Research:	
		Advertising Pros.:	Y	Broadcasting:		Consulting/Other:		Health Care:	Y	Petroleum/Chemicals:	
				Other:				Consulting:		Math/Other:	

TYPES OF BUSINESS:
Industrial Equipment & Products-Wholesale
Maintenance & Repair Products
Online Sales
Safety Products
Logistics Services
Outsourcing

BRANDS/DIVISIONS/AFFILIATES:
Acklands-Grainger, Inc.
Lab Safety Supply, Inc.
Grainger Industrial Supply
Grainger, S.A. de C.V.
Grainger Caribe, Inc.
Grainger China LLC
DAYTON
SPEEDAIRE

CONTACTS: Note: Officers with more than one job title may be intentionally listed here more than once.
James T. Ryan, CEO
James T. Ryan, COO
James T. Ryan, Pres.
Ronald L. Jadin, CFO
John L. Howard, General Counsel/Sr. VP
Nancy A. Hobor, Sr. VP-Comm. & Investor Rel.
Gregory S. Irving, Principal Acct. Officer/VP/Controller
Timothy M. Ferrarell, Sr. VP-Enterprise Processes & Systems
Y.C. Chen, Pres., Industrial Supply.
Richard L. Keyser, Chmn.

Phone: 847-535-1000 **Fax:**
Toll-Free:
Address: 100 Grainger Pkwy., Lake Forest, IL 60045-5201 US

GROWTH PLANS/SPECIAL FEATURES:
W. W. Grainger, Inc. (Grainger) offers maintenance, repair and operating (MRO) products, services and information products to approximately 1.8 million businesses and institutions. The company is divided into three segments: Grainger Branch-based, Acklands-Grainger Branch-based (Acklands-Grainger) and Lab Safety Supply, Inc. (Lab Safety). The Grainger Branch-based businesses serve the MRO needs of North American businesses through 434 locations in all 50 states, catalogs and the Internet. This segment includes Grainger Industrial Supply; Grainger, S.A. de C.V. (Mexico); Grainger Caribe, Inc. (Puerto Rico); and Grainger China LLC (China). Grainger Industrial Supply serves outsourcing customers on-site business process reengineering, inventory and tool crib management, purchasing management and information management. Acklands-Grainger is Canada's leading broad-line distributor of industrial, automotive fleet and safety supplies. It serves customers through 153 branches and five distribution centers across Canada. Lab Safety is a direct marketer of safety and other industrial products to U.S. and Canadian businesses, primarily reaching its customers through the distribution of multiple branded catalogs and other marketing materials distributed throughout the year to targeted markets. Lab Safety provides access to approximately 163,000 products through its targeted catalogs and distributes its products from two distribution centers. The company's registered trademarks include DAYTON, SPEEDAIRE, AIR HANDLER, DEM-KOTE, WESTWARD, CONDOR and LUMAPRO. In June 2008, Acklands-Grainger acquired Excel Industriel, a distributor of MRO supplies. In July 2008, Lab Safety acquired Highsmith, Inc., a library equipment, furniture and supplies marketer. Also in July, Grainger announced a 49.9% stake in Asia Pacific Brands India Ltd., an Indian industrial and electrical wholesale distributor.

Employee benefits at Grainger include an employee assistance program, adoption benefits, an educational assistance program, a dependent care assistance plan and a 3-for-1 matching charitable gifts program. The company works with INROADS, a nationwide program, to hire and retain minority employees.

FINANCIALS: Sales and profits are in thousands of dollars—add 000 to get the full amount. 2007 Note: Financial information for 2007 was not available for all companies at press time.

2007 Sales: $6,418,014	2007 Profits: $420,120	**U.S. Stock Ticker:** GWW	
2006 Sales: $5,883,654	2006 Profits: $383,399	**Int'l Ticker:** Int'l Exchange:	
2005 Sales: $5,526,636	2005 Profits: $346,324	Employees: 17,074	
2004 Sales: $5,049,800	2004 Profits: $286,900	Fiscal Year Ends: 12/31	
2003 Sales: $4,667,014	2003 Profits: $226,971	Parent Company:	

SALARIES/BENEFITS:
Pension Plan: Y	ESOP Stock Plan:	Profit Sharing: Y	Top Exec. Salary: $1,075,000	Bonus: $1,149,500
Savings Plan:	Stock Purch. Plan:		Second Exec. Salary: $566,680	Bonus: $436,980

OTHER THOUGHTS:
Apparent Women Officers or Directors: 2
Hot Spot for Advancement for Women/Minorities: Y

LOCATIONS: ("Y" = Yes)
West:	Southwest:	Midwest:	Southeast:	Northeast:	International:
Y	Y	Y	Y	Y	Y

Note: Financial information, benefits and other data can change quickly and may vary from those stated here.

WYETH

www.wyeth.com

Industry Group Code: 325412 Ranks within this company's industry group: Sales: Profits:

Management:		Sales/Marketing:		Liberal Arts:		Information Systems:		Professionals:		Technical/Scientific:	
Mgmt. Trainees:	Y	Mktg. Professionals:	Y	Gen. Writing/Editing:	Y	Info. Management:	Y	Finance/Accounting:	Y	Engineers, Elec.:	Y
Experienced Mgmt.:	Y	Retail Sales:		Technical Writing:	Y	Software Dev.:	Y	Law:	Y	Engineers, Other:	Y
Int'l Business:	Y	Commercial/Industrial:	Y	Graphic Arts/Photog.:	Y	Hardware Dev.:		HR/Other:	Y	Health/Lab:	Y
MBA Graduates:	Y	Sales Trainees:	Y	Music:		Systems Integration:		Training:	Y	Scientists/Research:	Y
		Advertising Pros.:	Y	Broadcasting:		Consulting/Other:		Health Care:	Y	Petroleum/Chemicals:	
				Other:				Consulting:		Math/Other:	Y

TYPES OF BUSINESS:

Drugs-Diversified
Wholesale Pharmaceuticals
Animal Health Care Products
Biologicals
Vaccines
Over-the-Counter Drugs
Women's Health Care Products
Nutritional Supplements

BRANDS/DIVISIONS/AFFILIATES:

Chap Stick
Premarin
Dimetapp
Advil
Robitussin
Preparation H
Centrum
Wyeth K.K.

CONTACTS: *Note: Officers with more than one job title may be intentionally listed here more than once.*

Bernard Poussot, CEO
Bernard Poussot, Pres.
Greg Norden, CFO/Sr. VP
Denise Peppard, Sr. VP-Human Resources
Jeffrey Keisling, CIO/VP-Corp. Info. Svcs.
Lawrence Stein, General Counsel/Sr. VP
Thomas Hofstaetter, Sr. VP-Corp. Bus. Dev.
Marilyn Rhudy, Sr. VP-Public Affairs
Justin Victoria, VP-Investor Rel.
Mary K. Wold, Sr. VP-Finance
James Pohlman, VP-Corp. Strategic Initiatives
Joseph M. Mahady, Sr. VP/Pres., Pharmaceuticals
Rene R. Lewin, Sr. VP-Human Resources
Andrew F. Davidson, VP-Internal Audit
Robert Essner, Chmn.

Phone: 973-660-5000	Fax: 973-660-7026
Toll-Free:	
Address: 5 Giralda Farms, Madison, NJ 07940-0874 US	

GROWTH PLANS/SPECIAL FEATURES:

Wyeth is a global leader in pharmaceuticals, consumer health care products and animal health care products. The firm discovers, develops, manufactures, distributes and sells a diversified line of products arising from three divisions: pharmaceuticals, consumer health care and animal care. The pharmaceuticals segment is itself divided into women's health care, neuroscience, vaccines and infectious disease, musculoskeletal, internal medicine, hemophilia and immunology and oncology. The division sells branded and generic pharmaceuticals, biological and nutraceutical products as well as animal biological products and pharmaceuticals. Its branded products include Premarin, Prempro, Premphase, Triphasil, Ativan, Effexor, Altace, Inderal, Zoton, Protonix and Enbrel. The consumer health care segment's products include analgesics, cough/cold/allergy remedies, nutritional supplements, lip balm and hemorrhoidal, antacid, asthma and other relief items sold over-the-counter. The segment's well-known over-the-counter products include Advil, cold medicines Robitussin and Dimetapp and nutritional supplement Centrum, as well as Chap Stick, Caltrate, Preparation H and Solgar. The company's animal health care products include vaccines, pharmaceuticals, endectocides (dewormers that control both internal and external parasites) and growth implants under the brand names LymeVax, Duramune and Fel-O-Vax. In March 2008, the firm announced plans to invest $280 million to build a state-of-the-art nutritional manufacturing facility in Suzhou Industrial Park, Jiangsu Province, China. The new facility will primarily produce infant formula milk powder and other nutritional products.

FINANCIALS: Sales and profits are in thousands of dollars—add 000 to get the full amount. 2007 Note: Financial information for 2007 was not available for all companies at press time.

2007 Sales: $22,399,798	2007 Profits: $4,615,960	**U.S. Stock Ticker: WYE**
2006 Sales: $20,350,655	2006 Profits: $4,196,706	**Int'l Ticker:** Int'l Exchange:
2005 Sales: $18,755,790	2005 Profits: $3,656,298	Employees: 50,527
2004 Sales: $17,358,028	2004 Profits: $1,233,997	Fiscal Year Ends: 12/31
2003 Sales: $15,850,600	2003 Profits: $2,051,600	Parent Company:

SALARIES/BENEFITS:

Pension Plan: Y	ESOP Stock Plan:	Profit Sharing:	Top Exec. Salary: $1,728,500	Bonus: $3,200,000
Savings Plan: Y	Stock Purch. Plan:		Second Exec. Salary: $1,050,400	Bonus: $2,000,000

OTHER THOUGHTS:

Apparent Women Officers or Directors: 6
Hot Spot for Advancement for Women/Minorities: Y

LOCATIONS: ("Y" = Yes)

West:	Southwest:	Midwest:	Southeast:	Northeast:	International:
Y	Y	Y	Y	Y	Y

WYNDHAM WORLDWIDE   www.wyndhamworldwide.com

Industry Group Code: 721110 Ranks within this company's industry group: Sales: 4   Profits: 4

Management:		Sales/Marketing:		Liberal Arts:		Information Systems:		Professionals:		Technical/Scientific:	
Mgmt. Trainees:	Y	Mktg. Professionals:	Y	Gen. Writing/Editing:	Y	Info. Management:	Y	Finance/Accounting:	Y	Engineers, Elec.:	
Experienced Mgmt.:	Y	Retail Sales:		Technical Writing:		Software Dev.:		Law:	Y	Engineers, Other:	
Int'l Business:	Y	Commercial/Industrial:	Y	Graphic Arts/Photog.:	Y	Hardware Dev.:		HR/Other:	Y	Health/Lab:	
MBA Graduates:	Y	Sales Trainees:	Y	Music:		Systems Integration:		Training:	Y	Scientists/Research:	
		Advertising Pros.:	Y	Broadcasting:		Consulting/Other:		Health Care:		Petroleum/Chemicals:	
				Other:				Consulting:		Math/Other:	

TYPES OF BUSINESS:

Hotels, Motels & Resorts
Property Management
Hotel Development
Vacation Property Exchange and Rental
Timeshare Resorts
Franchising
Vacation Ownership

BRANDS/DIVISIONS/AFFILIATES:

Wyndham Hotels
Wingate Inns
Ramada
Days Inn
Super 8
Howard Johnson
AmeriHost
Trendwest

CONTACTS: Note: Officers with more than one job title may be intentionally listed here more than once.

Stephen P. Holmes, CEO
Virginia M. Wilson, CFO/Exec. VP
Betsy O'Rourke, Sr. VP-Mktg.
Mary R. Falvey, Exec. VP/Chief Human Resources Officer
Scott G. McLester, General Counsel/Exec. VP
Betsy O'Rourke, Sr. VP-Comm.
Nicola Rossi, Sr. VP/Chief Acct. Officer
Franz S. Hanning, Pres./CEO-Wyndham Vacation Ownership
Steven A. Rudnitsky, Pres./CEO-Wyndham Hotel Group
Geoff Ballotti, Pres./CEO-Group RCI
Tom Anderson, Exec. VP/Chief Real Estate Dev. Officer
Stephen P. Holmes, Chmn.

Phone: 973-428-9700	Fax:
Toll-Free:	
Address: 7 Sylvan Way, Parsippany, NJ 07054 US	

GROWTH PLANS/SPECIAL FEATURES:

Wyndham Worldwide (WW) is a hospitality company offering individual consumers and business customers an array of hospitality products and services as well as various accommodation alternatives and price ranges through its portfolio of world-renowned brands. The company encompasses nearly 6,500 hotels representing approximately 550,000 rooms on six continents. Wyndham Hotel Group offers the TripRewards loyalty program. Group RCI, the firm's vacation exchange business, offers its 3.6 million members access for specified periods to 67,000 vacation properties in 100 countries around the world. WW also offers Wyndham Vacation Ownership, which includes marketing and sales of vacation ownership interests, consumer financing in conjunction with the purchase of vacation ownership interests, property management services to property owners' associations and development and acquisition of vacation ownership resorts. Wyndham Vacation has approximately 145 vacation ownership resorts in U.S., Canada, Mexico, the Caribbean and the South Pacific representing over 800,000 owners of vacation ownership interests. WW's extensive portfolio of brands includes AmeriHost Inn; Baymont Inn & Suites; Days Inn; Howard Johnson; Ramada; Super 8; Travelodge; Wingate Inn; Wyndham Hotels and Resorts; Wyndham Vacation Resorts; Chez Nous; Cuendet; Novasol; RCI; Ski Life; Dansk Familiefierie; French Life; Country Cottages; Country Holidays; and Country Manors. The firm also holds 30% interest in CHI Limited; this joint venture provides management services to luxury and upscale hotels in Europe, the Middle East and Africa. The firm provided management services to 14 hotels, as of 2007, many of which were re-branded as a Wyndham brand in early 2008. In 2007, WW unveiled The Blue Harmony Spa and Fitness Experience for its Wyndham hotels and timeshare resorts. In July 2008, the company acquired the Microtel Inns & Suites and Hawthorn Suites brands.

FINANCIALS: Sales and profits are in thousands of dollars—add 000 to get the full amount. 2007 Note: Financial information for 2007 was not available for all companies at press time.

2007 Sales: $4,360,000	2007 Profits: $403,000	U.S. Stock Ticker: WYN
2006 Sales: $3,842,000	2006 Profits: $287,000	Int'l Ticker: Int'l Exchange:
2005 Sales: $3,471,000	2005 Profits: $431,000	Employees: 33,200
2004 Sales: $3,014,000	2004 Profits: $349,000	Fiscal Year Ends: 12/31
2003 Sales: $2,652,000	2003 Profits: $	Parent Company:

SALARIES/BENEFITS:

Pension Plan:	ESOP Stock Plan:	Profit Sharing:	Top Exec. Salary: $1,013,848	Bonus: $2,212,435
Savings Plan: Y	Stock Purch. Plan:		Second Exec. Salary: $561,821	Bonus: $795,300

OTHER THOUGHTS:

Apparent Women Officers or Directors: 4
Hot Spot for Advancement for Women/Minorities: Y

LOCATIONS: ("Y" = Yes)

West:	Southwest:	Midwest:	Southeast:	Northeast:	International:
Y	Y	Y	Y	Y	Y

Note: Financial information, benefits and other data can change quickly and may vary from those stated here.

WYNN RESORTS LIMITED

www.wynnresorts.com

Industry Group Code: 721120 Ranks within this company's industry group: Sales: 4 Profits: 2

Management:		Sales/Marketing:		Liberal Arts:		Information Systems:		Professionals:		Technical/Scientific:	
Mgmt. Trainees:	Y	Mktg. Professionals:	Y	Gen. Writing/Editing:	Y	Info. Management:	Y	Finance/Accounting:	Y	Engineers, Elec.:	
Experienced Mgmt.:	Y	Retail Sales:		Technical Writing:		Software Dev.:		Law:	Y	Engineers, Other:	
Int'l Business:	Y	Commercial/Industrial:	Y	Graphic Arts/Photog.:	Y	Hardware Dev.:		HR/Other:	Y	Health/Lab:	
MBA Graduates:	Y	Sales Trainees:		Music:	Y	Systems Integration:		Training:	Y	Scientists/Research:	
		Advertising Pros.:	Y	Broadcasting:		Consulting/Other:		Health Care:		Petroleum/Chemicals:	
				Other:	Y			Consulting:		Math/Other:	

TYPES OF BUSINESS:

Hotel Casinos

BRANDS/DIVISIONS/AFFILIATES:

Wynn Las Vegas, LLC
Wynn Resorts (Macau), S.A.
Encore Suites at Wynn Las Vegas
Wynn Diamond Suites at Wynn Macau

CONTACTS: *Note: Officers with more than one job title may be intentionally listed here more than once.*

Stephen A. Wynn, CEO
Marc D. Schorr, COO
Matt Maddox, CFO/Exec. VP
Linda Chen, Pres., Wynn Int'l Mktg., Ltd.
John Strzemp, Chief Admin. Officer/Exec. VP
Kim Sinatra, General Counsel/Sec./Sr. VP
Matt Maddox, Treas.
Andrew Pascal, COO/Pres., Wynn Las Vegas, LLC
David R. Sisk, Exec. VP/CFO-Wynn Las Vegas, LLC
Scott Peterson, CFO-Wynn Resorts (Macau), S.A.
Kazuo Okada, Vice Chmn.
Stephen A. Wynn, Chmn.
Ian M. Coughlan, Pres., Wynn Resorts (Macau), S.A.

Phone: 702-770-7555	Fax: 702-697-5009
Toll-Free:	
Address: 3131 Las Vegas Blvd. S., Las Vegas, NV 89109 US	

GROWTH PLANS/SPECIAL FEATURES:

Wynn Resorts Limited is a leading developer, owner and operator of destination casino resorts. It owns and operates two destination casino resorts: The Wynn Las Vegas on the Strip in Las Vegas, NV and the Wynn Macau in the Macau Special Administrative Region of China. The firm is currently constructing Encore Suites at Wynn Las Vegas and Wynn Diamond Suites at Wynn Macau. Wynn Las Vegas offers 2,716 rooms and suites distributed between its 45-story tower, 36 fairway villas and six private-entry villas for its premium guests. The approximately 111,000-square-foot casino features 140 table games, a baccarat salon, private VIP gaming rooms, a poker room, 1,970 slot machines and a race and sports book. The resort's 22 food and beverage outlets feature six fine dining restaurants, including three that have been awarded Michelin stars. Other amenities include a nightclub; a spa and salon; a Ferrari and Maserati automobile dealership; wedding chapels; an 18-hole golf course; approximately 223,000 square feet of meeting space; and an approximately 74,000-square-foot retail promenade featuring boutiques from Chanel, Dior, Graff, Manolo Blahnik, Oscar de la Renta, Cartier and Louis Vuitton. Wynn Las Vegas also has two showrooms, The Le Reve Theater and The Broadway Theater. During 2007, Wynn Las Vegas experienced an overall 96% average occupancy and $300 average daily room rate, compared to the overall 90.4% average occupancy and $132 average daily room rate of the Las Vegas Strip. The recently opened Wynn Macau features approximately 600 hotel rooms and suites; 380 table games and 1,270 slot machines in 205,000 square feet of casino gaming space; five restaurants; 46,000 square feet of retail space featuring boutiques from Prada, Ferrari, Giorgio Armani and Tiffany; a spa and salon; entertainment lounges; and meeting facilities.

Wynn Resorts offers its employees financial assistance with continuing education, an employee assistance program, annual social events and athletic team sponsorship.

FINANCIALS: Sales and profits are in thousands of dollars—add 000 to get the full amount. 2007 Note: Financial information for 2007 was not available for all companies at press time.

2007 Sales: $2,687,519	2007 Profits: $258,148	**U.S. Stock Ticker: WYNN**
2006 Sales: $1,432,257	2006 Profits: $628,728	**Int'l Ticker:** Int'l Exchange:
2005 Sales: $721,981	2005 Profits: $-90,836	Employees: 16,500
2004 Sales: $ 195	2004 Profits: $-204,171	Fiscal Year Ends: 12/31
2003 Sales: $1,018	2003 Profits: $-40,099	Parent Company:

SALARIES/BENEFITS:

Pension Plan:	ESOP Stock Plan:	Profit Sharing:	Top Exec. Salary: $3,173,077	Bonus: $7,500,000
Savings Plan: Y	Stock Purch. Plan:		Second Exec. Salary: $1,750,000	Bonus: $3,500,000

OTHER THOUGHTS:

Apparent Women Officers or Directors: 3
Hot Spot for Advancement for Women/Minorities: Y

LOCATIONS: ("Y" = Yes)

West:	Southwest:	Midwest:	Southeast:	Northeast:	International:
Y					Y

XEROX CORP

www.xerox.com

Industry Group Code: 333313 **Ranks within this company's industry group:** Sales: Profits:

Management:	Sales/Marketing:	Liberal Arts:	Information Systems:	Professionals:	Technical/Scientific:
Mgmt. Trainees:	Mktg. Professionals:	Gen. Writing/Editing:	Info. Management:	Finance/Accounting:	Engineers, Elec.:
Experienced Mgmt.:	Retail Sales:	Technical Writing:	Software Dev.:	Law:	Engineers, Other:
Int'l Business:	Commercial/Industrial:	Graphic Arts/Photog.:	Hardware Dev.:	HR/Other:	Health/Lab:
MBA Graduates:	Sales Trainees:	Music:	Systems Integration:	Training:	Scientists/Research:
	Advertising Pros.:	Broadcasting:	Consulting/Other:	Health Care:	Petroleum/Chemicals:
		Other:		Consulting:	Math/Other:

TYPES OF BUSINESS:

Business Machines-Copiers, Printers & Scanners
Office Consumables
Software
Fax Machines

BRANDS/DIVISIONS/AFFILIATES:

Fuji Xerox
DocuColor
CopyCentre
Xerox Canada Inc
Palo Alto Research Center
Global Imaging Systems, Inc.
Advectis, Inc.
Image Quest, Inc.

CONTACTS: Note: Officers with more than one job title may be intentionally listed here more than once.

Anne M. Mulcahy, CEO
Ursula M. Burns, Pres.
Lawrence A. Zimmerman, CFO/Exec. VP
Michael C. Mac Donald, Sr. VP/Pres., Mktg. Oper.
Patricia M. Nazemetz, Chief Human Resources & Ethics Officer/VP
John McDermott, CIO/VP
Sophie V. Vandebroek, CTO/VP/Pres., Xerox Innovation Group
Anthony M. Federico, Chief Engineer
Don Liu, General Counsel/Sr. VP/Sec.
Eric Armour, VP-Strategy
James H. Lesko, VP-Investor Rel.
Gary R. Kabureck, Chief Acct. Officer/VP
James A. Firestone, Exec. VP/Pres., Xerox North America
Leslie F. Varon, Controller/VP
Richard F. Cerrone, VP-Mktg. Integration & Strategy
Rhonda L. Seegal, Treas./VP
Anne M. Mulcahy, Chmn.
Armando Zagalo de Lima, Sr. VP/Pres., Xerox Europe

Phone: 203-968-3000	Fax: 203-968-3944
Toll-Free:	
Address: 45 Glober Ave., P.O. Box 4505, Norwalk, CT 06856 US	

GROWTH PLANS/SPECIAL FEATURES:

Xerox Corp. is a technology and services enterprise operating in the global document market. It operates in four segments: production, office, developing markets operations (DMO) and other. The production segment provides high-end digital monochrome and color systems designed for customers in the graphic communications industry and for large enterprises. These products enable digital on-demand printing, digital full-color printing and enterprise printing. The division offers a complete family of monochrome production systems from 65-180 pages per minute (ppm) and color production systems from 40-110 ppm. Additionally, it offers a variety of pre-press and post-press options, as well as workflow software. The Freeflow digital workflow collection allows customers to improve everything from content creation and management to production and fulfillment. The office segment systems and services, which include monochrome devices at speeds up to 90 ppm and color devices up to 50 ppm, include the family of CopyCentre, WorkCentre and WorkCentre Pro digital multifunction systems; DocuColor printer/copiers; color laser, LED (light emitting diode), solid ink and monochrome laser desktop printers; digital copiers; and light-lens copiers and facsimile products. The DMO segment includes the marketing, sales and servicing of Xerox products, supplies and services in Latin America, Brazil, the Middle East, India, Eurasia and Central-Eastern Europe and Africa. The other segment primarily includes revenue from paper sales, value-added services and wide-format systems. Fuji Xerox, an unconsolidated entity of which Xerox owns 25%, develops, manufactures and distributes document management system, supplies and services. In 2007, Xerox acquired Global Imaging Systems, Inc. for $1.46 billion; and Advectis, Inc. for $32 million. In November 2007, Global Imaging Systems acquired Image Quest, Inc.

The company offers its employees medical, dental and vision insurance; life and accident insurance; a 401(k) plan; an employee assistance program; tuition reimbursement; and access to a credit union.

FINANCIALS: Sales and profits are in thousands of dollars—add 000 to get the full amount. 2007 Note: Financial information for 2007 was not available for all companies at press time.

2007 Sales: $17,228,000	2007 Profits: $1,135,000	U.S. Stock Ticker: XRX
2006 Sales: $15,895,000	2006 Profits: $1,210,000	Int'l Ticker: Int'l Exchange:
2005 Sales: $15,701,000	2005 Profits: $978,000	Employees: 57,400
2004 Sales: $15,722,000	2004 Profits: $859,000	Fiscal Year Ends: 12/31
2003 Sales: $15,701,000	2003 Profits: $360,000	Parent Company:

SALARIES/BENEFITS:

Pension Plan:	ESOP Stock Plan:	Profit Sharing:	Top Exec. Salary: $1,320,000	Bonus: $2,178,000
Savings Plan: Y	Stock Purch. Plan:		Second Exec. Salary: $685,559	Bonus: $531,754

OTHER THOUGHTS:

Apparent Women Officers or Directors: 9
Hot Spot for Advancement for Women/Minorities: Y

LOCATIONS: ("Y" = Yes)

West:	Southwest:	Midwest:	Southeast:	Northeast:	International:
Y	Y	Y	Y	Y	Y

YAHOO! INC

www.yahoo.com

Industry Group Code: 514199B Ranks within this company's industry group: Sales: 2 Profits: 2

Management:		Sales/Marketing:		Liberal Arts:		Information Systems:		Professionals:		Technical/Scientific:	
Mgmt. Trainees:	Y	Mktg. Professionals:	Y	Gen. Writing/Editing:	Y	Info. Management:	Y	Finance/Accounting:	Y	Engineers, Elec.:	Y
Experienced Mgmt.:	Y	Retail Sales:		Technical Writing:	Y	Software Dev.:	Y	Law:	Y	Engineers, Other:	
Int'l Business:	Y	Commercial/Industrial:	Y	Graphic Arts/Photog.:	Y	Hardware Dev.:		HR/Other:	Y	Health/Lab:	
MBA Graduates:	Y	Sales Trainees:		Music:		Systems Integration:		Training:	Y	Scientists/Research:	
		Advertising Pros.:	Y	Broadcasting:		Consulting/Other:		Health Care:		Petroleum/Chemicals:	
				Other:	Y			Consulting:		Math/Other:	

TYPES OF BUSINESS:

Online Portal-Search Engine
Broadcast Media
Job Placement Services
Paid Positioning Services
Advertising Services
Online Business & Consumer Information
Search Technology Licensing
E-Commerce

BRANDS/DIVISIONS/AFFILIATES:

Yahoo.com
Yahoo! Mail
Yahoo! Messenger
Yahoo! Shopping
Gmarket Inc.
HotJobs.com, Ltd.
BlueLithium
Right Media, Inc.

CONTACTS: *Note: Officers with more than one job title may be intentionally listed here more than once.*

Jerry Yang, CEO
Susan Decker, Pres.
Blake Jorgensen, CFO/Exec. VP
David Windley, Chief Human Resources Officer
Usama Fayyad, Exec. VP-Research & Strategic Data Solutions
Usama Fayyad, Chief Data Officer
Aristotle Balogh, Exec. VP-Networks Div.
Qi Lu, Exec. VP-Search & Advertising Tech. Group
Michael Callahan, General Counsel/Sec./Exec. VP
Jill Nash, Chief Comm. Officer
Michael Murray, Chief Acct. Officer
David Filo, Chief Yahoo
Marco Boerries, Exec. VP-Connected Life Div.
Ash Patel, Exec. VP-Audience Prod. Div.
Hilary Schneider, Exec. VP-Yahoo U.S.
Carl Icahn, Chmn.

Phone: 408-349-3300	Fax: 408-349-3301
Toll-Free:	
Address: 701 First Ave., Sunnyvale, CA 94089 US	

GROWTH PLANS/SPECIAL FEATURES:

Yahoo!, Inc. is a provider of online products and services to consumers and businesses worldwide. The company has two main business segments: The Audience Group; and the Advertiser & Publisher Group; both of which will be supported by the Technology Group. The Audience Group focuses on growing and developing the typically free Yahoo! Tools used by everyday consumers, such as Yahoo! Mail, Yahoo! Messenger, Yahoo! Calendar, Yahoo! Chat, Yahoo! Greetings, Yahoo! Clubs and Yahoo! Photos. Commerce services include Yahoo! Shopping, Yahoo! Auctions, Yahoo! Finance and Yahoo! Travel. The Advertisers & Publishers Group was created by combining Yahoo!'s marketing solutions, sales teams and distribution partners to streamline the firm's advertising and marketing offerings. The Technology Group engineers and provides upkeep for the advertising and Internet platforms. Yahoo! is present in 20 markets in Europe, Latin America, the Asia Pacific and Canada; and is available in twenty languages. The company has entered into relationships with business partners that offer content, technology and distribution capabilities, which permit the company to bring Yahoo!-branded, targeted media products to the market more quickly. Yahoo! owns a 10% stake in Gmarket Inc., an e-commerce marketplace provider in Korea. The company also operates HotJobs.com, Ltd., a leading Internet job placement and recruiting company. In September 2007, Yahoo acquired Zimbra, Inc., an e-mail and collaboration software provider for approximately $350 million. In February 2008, Yahoo! acquired Maven Networks Inc., an online video platform provider. In April 2008, Yahoo! entered into an agreement to acquire Index Tools, a provider of Web analytics software for online marketing.

Yahoo! offers employees discount movie passes; basic life insurance and accidental death and dismemberment insurance, short and long term disability, commuter subsidies; a game room; health club membership and massages; on-site dental care, car washes and haircuts; and tuition reimbursement.

FINANCIALS: Sales and profits are in thousands of dollars—add 000 to get the full amount. 2007 Note: Financial information for 2007 was not available for all companies at press time.

2007 Sales: $6,969,274	2007 Profits: $660,000	**U.S. Stock Ticker:** YHOO
2006 Sales: $6,425,679	2006 Profits: $751,391	**Int'l Ticker:** Int'l Exchange:
2005 Sales: $5,257,668	2005 Profits: $1,896,230	Employees: 11,400
2004 Sales: $3,575,000	2004 Profits: $839,553	Fiscal Year Ends: 12/31
2003 Sales: $1,625,097	2003 Profits: $237,879	Parent Company:

SALARIES/BENEFITS:

Pension Plan:	ESOP Stock Plan:	Profit Sharing:	Top Exec. Salary: $500,000	Bonus: $900,000
Savings Plan: Y	Stock Purch. Plan: Y		Second Exec. Salary: $500,000	Bonus: $850,000

OTHER THOUGHTS:

Apparent Women Officers or Directors: 3
Hot Spot for Advancement for Women/Minorities: Y

LOCATIONS: ("Y" = Yes)

West:	Southwest:	Midwest:	Southeast:	Northeast:	International:
Y	Y	Y	Y	Y	Y

YUM! BRANDS INC

www.yum.com

Industry Group Code: 722110 Ranks within this company's industry group: Sales: 2 Profits: 2

Management:		Sales/Marketing:		Liberal Arts:		Information Systems:		Professionals:		Technical/Scientific:	
Mgmt. Trainees:	Y	Mktg. Professionals:	Y	Gen. Writing/Editing:	Y	Info. Management:	Y	Finance/Accounting:	Y	Engineers, Elec.:	
Experienced Mgmt.:	Y	Retail Sales:		Technical Writing:		Software Dev.:	Y	Law:	Y	Engineers, Other:	
Int'l Business:	Y	Commercial/Industrial:	Y	Graphic Arts/Photog.:	Y	Hardware Dev.:		HR/Other:	Y	Health/Lab:	
MBA Graduates:	Y	Sales Trainees:		Music:		Systems Integration:		Training:	Y	Scientists/Research:	
		Advertising Pros.:	Y	Broadcasting:		Consulting/Other:		Health Care:		Petroleum/Chemicals:	
				Other:	Y			Consulting:		Math/Other:	

TYPES OF BUSINESS:

Fast Food Restaurants

BRANDS/DIVISIONS/AFFILIATES:

Pizza Hut
KFC
Taco Bell
Long John Silver's
A&W All-American Food
Yum! Restaurants International
Yum! China

CONTACTS: *Note: Officers with more than one job title may be intentionally listed here more than once.*

David C. Novak, CEO
Emil J. Brolick, COO
David C. Novak, Pres.
Richard T. Carucci, CFO
Anne P. Byerlein, Chief People Officer
Christian L. Campbell, General Counsel/Sr. VP/Sec.
Roger Eaton, Chief Dev. Officer
Jonathan D. Blum, Sr. VP-Public Affairs
Timothy P. Jerzyk, Sr. VP-Investor Rel./Treas.
Ted F. Knopf, Sr. VP-Finance/Corp. Controller
Scott O. Bergren, Pres./Chief Concept Officer-Pizza Hut
Roger Eaton, Pres., KFC
Greg Creed, Pres./Chief Concept Officer-Taco Bell
Sam Su, Pres., Yum! China Div.
David C. Novak, Chmn.
Graham D. Allan, Pres., Yum Restaurants Int'l

Phone: 502-874-8300	Fax: 502-874-8790
Toll-Free:	
Address: 1441 Gardiner Ln., Louisville, KY 40213 US	

GROWTH PLANS/SPECIAL FEATURES:

Yum! Brands, Inc. is a fast-food restaurant company with over 34,000 restaurants in more than 100 countries and territories. The firm is divided into five operating companies, organized around the five restaurant chains of KFC, Pizza Hut, Taco Bell, A&W and Long John Silver's. Through these concepts, the company develops, operates, franchises and licenses a system of restaurants that operate, package and sell a menu of competitively priced food items. The restaurants are operated by the company, independent third-party franchisees, or by affiliates in which it owns a non-controlling equity interest. In all five chains, customers are offered dine in, carry out and, in some locations, drive-through options. Yum!'s International Division comprises more than 11,000 restaurants, primarily KFCs and Pizza Huts, operating in over 100 countries. The China Division has more than 3,000 system restaurants, predominantly KFCs and in 2007 it reported $2.1 billion in revenue. Mainland China is the company's biggest market for new company restaurant development. KFC, Pizza Hut, Taco Bell and Long John Silver's are the global leaders, respectively, in the chicken, pizza, Mexican-style and seafood fast-food segments. The company is actively pursuing multi-branding, primarily in the U.S., where two or more of its restaurants are operated as a single unit. At the end of 2007, there were 3,989 multibranded units in the worldwide system, of which 3,699 were in the U.S. In August 2008, Yum! Brand Incorporated's Brazilian Pizza Hut franchise, Internacional Restaurantes do Brasil (IRB) sold 60% of its shares to Brazil Fast Food Corp.

Yum! offers its employees medical, dental, vision and hearing coverage; a management incentive plan; health care and dependent care flexible spending accounts; adoption assistance; life and disability insurance, an employee assistance program; a group legal plan; tuition reimbursement; employee discount programs; and a credit union.

FINANCIALS: Sales and profits are in thousands of dollars—add 000 to get the full amount. 2007 Note: Financial information for 2007 was not available for all companies at press time.

2007 Sales: $10,416,000	2007 Profits: $909,000	U.S. Stock Ticker: YUM	
2006 Sales: $9,561,000	2006 Profits: $824,000	Int'l Ticker:	Int'l Exchange:
2005 Sales: $9,349,000	2005 Profits: $762,000	Employees: 280,000	
2004 Sales: $9,011,000	2004 Profits: $740,000	Fiscal Year Ends: 12/31	
2003 Sales: $8,380,000	2003 Profits: $617,000	Parent Company:	

SALARIES/BENEFITS:

Pension Plan:	ESOP Stock Plan:	Profit Sharing:	Top Exec. Salary: $1,215,000	Bonus: $3,347,680
Savings Plan: Y	Stock Purch. Plan: Y		Second Exec. Salary: $629,577	Bonus: $723,233

OTHER THOUGHTS:

Apparent Women Officers or Directors: 3
Hot Spot for Advancement for Women/Minorities: Y

LOCATIONS: ("Y" = Yes)

West:	Southwest:	Midwest:	Southeast:	Northeast:	International:
Y	Y	Y	Y	Y	Y

ZIMMER HOLDINGS INC

www.zimmer.com

Industry Group Code: 339113 Ranks within this company's industry group: Sales: 6   Profits: 3

Management:		Sales/Marketing:		Liberal Arts:		Information Systems:		Professionals:		Technical/Scientific:	
Mgmt. Trainees:	Y	Mktg. Professionals:	Y	Gen. Writing/Editing:	Y	Info. Management:	Y	Finance/Accounting:	Y	Engineers, Elec.:	Y
Experienced Mgmt.:	Y	Retail Sales:		Technical Writing:	Y	Software Dev.:	Y	Law:	Y	Engineers, Other:	Y
Int'l Business:	Y	Commercial/Industrial:	Y	Graphic Arts/Photog.:	Y	Hardware Dev.:		HR/Other:	Y	Health/Lab:	Y
MBA Graduates:	Y	Sales Trainees:	Y	Music:		Systems Integration:		Training:	Y	Scientists/Research:	
		Advertising Pros.:	Y	Broadcasting:		Consulting/Other:		Health Care:	Y	Petroleum/Chemicals:	
				Other:				Consulting:		Math/Other:	

TYPES OF BUSINESS:

Orthopedic Supplies
Surgical Supplies & Systems
Joint Implants
Knee & Hip Replacement Systems
Fracture Management Products

BRANDS/DIVISIONS/AFFILIATES:

NexGen
VerSys
M/DN Intermedullary Fixation
Pulsavac Plus Wound Debridement System
A.T.S. Tourniquet System
Endius, Inc.
ORTHOsoft, Inc.
NexGen LPS-Flex Mobile Knee

CONTACTS: Note: Officers with more than one job title may be intentionally listed here more than once.

David C. Dvorak, CEO
David C. Dvorak, Pres.
James T. Crines, CFO/Exec. VP
David Weidenbenner, Sr. VP-Global Mktg.
Renee Rogers, VP-Global Human Resources
Cheryl R. Blanchard, Sr. VP-R&D/Chief Scientific Officer
Chad F. Phipps, General Counsel/Sr. VP/Sec.
Richard C. Stair, Sr. VP-Global Oper.
Paul G. Blair, VP-Investor Rel.
Derek Davis, VP-Finance/Corp. Controller/Chief Acct. Officer
Mark Throdahl, Group Pres., Global Bus.
Jon E. Kramer, Pres., US Sales
Laura C. O'Donnell, Chief Compliance Officer
Stephen H. L. Ooi, Pres., Asia Pacific
John McGoldrick, Chmn.
Bruno A. Melzi, Chmn.-Europe, Africa & Middle East
Richard C. Stair, Sr. VP-Logistics

Phone: 574-267-6131	Fax:
Toll-Free:	
Address: 345 E. Main St., Warsaw, IN 46580 US	

GROWTH PLANS/SPECIAL FEATURES:

Zimmer Holdings, Inc. designs, develops, manufactures and markets reconstructive orthopedic implants, including joint and dental; spinal implants; trauma products; and related orthopedic surgical products. The company also provides hospital-focused consulting services to help member institutions design, implement and manage orthopedic programs. Through its subsidiaries, the firm has operations in more than 25 countries and markets products in over 100 countries. Zimmer's main products are hip and knee replacements, trauma products and various orthopedic surgical products. The NexGen line consists of knee replacement system surgery products for stabilization and revision procedures. The VerSys hip system is a family of hip products that offer design-specific options for varying patient needs. Trauma products are used primarily to reattach or stabilize damaged bone or tissue to support the body's natural healing process. The M/DN Intramedullary Fixation, Sirus Intramedullary Nail System, and I.T.S.T. Intertrochanteric/Subtrochanteric Fixation System are all used for the internal fixation of long bone fractures through a minimally invasive approach. The company's surgical products include the Pulsavac Plus LP Wound Debridement System and the A.T.S. Tourniquet System. Dental products include reconstructive implants, dental restorative products and regenerative products, used for soft tissue and bone rehabilitation The firm's primary customers include musculoskeletal surgeons, neurosurgeons, oral surgeons, dentists, hospitals, distributors, healthcare dealers and healthcare purchasing organizations or buying groups. In April 2007, Zimmer acquired Endius, Inc., a developer and manufacturer of minimally invasive spine surgery products. In November 2007, the firm acquired ORTHOsoft, Inc., a computer navigation provider for orthopedic surgery. In December 2007, the company announced that its NexGen LPS-Flex Mobile Knee, featuring mobile bearing design, had received FDA approval.

Zimmer offers its employees medical, dental and vision insurance; flexible spending accounts; life and AD&D insurance; disability income protection plans; an employee stock purchase program; and tuition reimbursement.

FINANCIALS: Sales and profits are in thousands of dollars—add 000 to get the full amount. 2007 Note: Financial information for 2007 was not available for all companies at press time.

2007 Sales: $3,897,500	2007 Profits: $773,200	**U.S. Stock Ticker: ZMH**
2006 Sales: $3,495,400	2006 Profits: $834,500	**Int'l Ticker:** Int'l Exchange:
2005 Sales: $3,286,100	2005 Profits: $732,500	Employees: 6,900
2004 Sales: $2,980,900	2004 Profits: $541,800	Fiscal Year Ends: 12/31
2003 Sales: $1,901,000	2003 Profits: $346,300	Parent Company:

SALARIES/BENEFITS:

Pension Plan:	ESOP Stock Plan: Y	Profit Sharing:	Top Exec. Salary: $750,000	Bonus: $1,140,416
Savings Plan: Y	Stock Purch. Plan:		Second Exec. Salary: $510,000	Bonus: $464,730

OTHER THOUGHTS:

Apparent Women Officers or Directors: 3
Hot Spot for Advancement for Women/Minorities: Y

LOCATIONS: ("Y" = Yes)

West:	Southwest:	Midwest:	Southeast:	Northeast:	International:
Y	Y	Y	Y	Y	Y

ADDITIONAL INDEXES

CONTENTS:

Index of Firms Noted as "Hot Spots for Advancement" for Women/Minorities   624

Index by Subsidiaries, Brand Names and Selected Affiliations   627

INDEX OF FIRMS NOTED AS HOT SPOTS FOR ADVANCEMENT FOR WOMEN & MINORITIES

3M COMPANY
7-ELEVEN INC
ABBOTT LABORATORIES
ABERCROMBIE & FITCH CO
ABM INDUSTRIES INC
ACCENTURE LTD
ACXIOM CORP
ADC TELECOMMUNICATIONS INC
ADESA INC
ADOBE SYSTEMS INC
ADVANCE AUTO PARTS INC
AECOM TECHNOLOGY CORPORATION
AEROPOSTALE INC
AES CORPORATION (THE)
AETNA INC
AFFILIATED COMPUTER SERVICES INC
AFLAC INC
AGILENT TECHNOLOGIES INC
AIR PRODUCTS & CHEMICALS INC
ALBERTO-CULVER COMPANY
ALLERGAN INC
ALLSTATE CORPORATION (THE)
ALTRIA GROUP INC
AMAZON.COM INC
AMEDISYS INC
AMERICAN EAGLE OUTFITTERS INC
AMERICAN ELECTRIC POWER COMPANY INC (AEP)
AMERICAN EXPRESS CO
AMGEN INC
ANALOG DEVICES INC
ANNTAYLOR STORES CORP
APACHE CORP
APOLLO GROUP INC
ARCHER DANIELS MIDLAND CO
ARROW ELECTRONICS INC
ARTHUR J GALLAGHER & CO
AT&T INC
AUTOMATIC DATA PROCESSING INC
AVERY DENNISON CORP
AVIS BUDGET GROUP INC
AVON PRODUCTS INC
AXA FINANCIAL INC
BAKER HUGHES INC
BANK OF AMERICA CORP
BARNES & NOBLE INC
BASS PRO SHOPS INC
BAXTER INTERNATIONAL INC
BEBE STORES INC
BECHTEL GROUP INC
BECKMAN COULTER INC
BED BATH & BEYOND INC
BERKSHIRE HATHAWAY INC
BEST BUY CO INC
BIO RAD LABORATORIES INC
BJ'S WHOLESALE CLUB INC

BLACK & DECKER CORP
BOEING COMPANY (THE)
BOOZ ALLEN HAMILTON
BOSTON SCIENTIFIC CORP
BRINKER INTERNATIONAL INC
BRISTOL MYERS SQUIBB CO
BROWN & BROWN INC
BUCKLE INC (THE)
BUILD-A-BEAR WORKSHOP INC
BURGER KING HOLDINGS INC
BURLINGTON NORTHERN SANTA FE CORP
CACI INTERNATIONAL INC
CARDINAL HEALTH INC
CARGILL INC
CARMAX GROUP
CARNIVAL CORPORATION
CATERPILLAR INC
CATERPILLAR LOGISTICS
CATHOLIC HEALTH INITIATIVES
CDW CORPORATION
CELLCO PARTNERSHIP (VERIZON WIRELESS)
CH ROBINSON WORLDWIDE INC
CH2M HILL COMPANIES LTD
CHARLOTTE RUSSE HOLDING
CHARMING SHOPPES INC
CHEMED CORPORATION
CHESAPEAKE ENERGY CORP
CHICO'S FAS INC
CHRISTOPHER & BANKS CORP
CHUBB CORPORATION (THE)
CIBER INC
CISCO SYSTEMS INC
CLEAR CHANNEL COMMUNICATIONS INC
CLUBCORP INC
COACH INC
COCA COLA COMPANY (THE)
COCA COLA ENTERPRISES INC
COLDWATER CREEK INC
COLGATE PALMOLIVE CO
COMCAST CORP
CONAGRA FOODS INC
CONOCOPHILLIPS COMPANY
CONSOL ENERGY INC
CONSOLIDATED EDISON INC
COST PLUS INC
COVANCE INC
COX COMMUNICATIONS INC
CR BARD INC
CSX CORP
CUMMINS INC
CVS CAREMARK CORPORATION
DARDEN RESTAURANTS INC
DAVITA INC
DEAN FOODS CO
DEERE & CO
DELOITTE & TOUCHE USA LLP
DELOITTE CONSULTING LLP
DENNY'S CORPORATION
DEVON ENERGY CORPORATION
DEVRY INC
DICK'S SPORTING GOODS INC
DIEBOLD INC

DINEEQUITY INC
DOLLAR GENERAL CORPORATION
DOLLAR THRIFTY AUTOMOTIVE GROUP INC
DRESS BARN INC (THE)
DTE ENERGY COMPANY
DUKE ENERGY CORP
E I DU PONT DE NEMOURS & CO (DUPONT)
EBAY INC
EDISON INTERNATIONAL
ELECTRONIC ARTS INC
ELI LILLY & COMPANY
EMBARQ CORP
EMC CORP
ENTERGY CORP
ENTERPRISE RENT-A-CAR
ERNST & YOUNG LLP
ESTEE LAUDER COMPANIES INC (THE)
EXELON CORPORATION
EXPEDITORS INTERNATIONAL OF WASHINGTON INC
EXPERIAN AMERICAS
EXXON MOBIL CORPORATION (EXXONMOBIL)
FAMILY DOLLAR STORES INC
FEDEX CORPORATION
FIRST ADVANTAGE CORPORATION
FIRST DATA CORP
FIRSTENERGY CORP
FISERV INC
FLUOR CORP
FOREST LABORATORIES INC
FORTUNE BRANDS INC
FOSSIL INC
FOSTER WHEELER LTD
FPL GROUP INC
FRONTIER COMMUNICATIONS CORPORATION
GENENTECH INC
GENERAL ELECTRIC CO (GE)
GENERAL MILLS INC
GENESCO INC
GENWORTH FINANCIAL INC
GLOBAL PAYMENTS INC
GOOGLE INC
GUESS? INC
HALLIBURTON COMPANY
HARRAH'S ENTERTAINMENT INC
HARRIS CORPORATION
HARTFORD FINANCIAL SERVICES GROUP INC (THE)
HAWAIIAN ELECTRIC INDUSTRIES INC
HCA INC
HEALTH FITNESS CORP
HEALTH MANAGEMENT ASSOCIATES INC
HEALTH NET INC
HEALTHWAYS INC
HENRY SCHEIN INC
HERTZ GLOBAL HOLDINGS INC
HEWITT ASSOCIATES
HEWLETT-PACKARD CO (HP)

HILB ROGAL & HOBBS CO
HILTON HOTELS CORP
HOME DEPOT INC
HONEYWELL INTERNATIONAL INC
HOT TOPIC INC
HUMANA INC
IAC/INTERACTIVECORP
ICT GROUP INC
IDEXX LABORATORIES INC
IMS HEALTH INC
INTEL CORP
INTERNATIONAL BUSINESS
MACHINES CORP (IBM)
INTIMATE BRANDS INC
INTUIT INC
J C PENNEY COMPANY INC
JABIL CIRCUIT INC
JACK IN THE BOX INC
JM SMUCKER CO
JOHNSON & JOHNSON
JOHNSON CONTROLS INC
JP MORGAN CHASE & CO INC
JUNIPER NETWORKS INC
KAISER PERMANENTE
KEANE INC
KELLOGG CO
KELLY SERVICES INC
KENDLE INTERNATIONAL INC
KIMBERLY-CLARK CORP
KINDRED HEALTHCARE INC
KOHL'S CORP
KRAFT FOODS INC
KROGER CO (THE)
L-3 COMMUNICATIONS HOLDINGS
INC
LEVEL 3 COMMUNICATIONS INC
LEXMARK INTERNATIONAL INC
LIBERTY GLOBAL INC
LIMITED BRANDS INC
LINCOLN NATIONAL CORPORATION
LOCKHEED MARTIN CORP
LODGIAN INC
LOEWS CORPORATION
LOWE'S COMPANIES INC
MACY'S INC
MANOR CARE INC
MANPOWER INC
MARATHON OIL CORP
MARRIOTT INTERNATIONAL INC
MARSH & MCLENNAN COMPANIES
INC
MASSEY ENERGY COMPANY
MCAFEE INC
MCDONALD'S CORP
MCKESSON CORPORATION
MCKINSEY & COMPANY INC
MEDCO HEALTH SOLUTIONS
MEDTRONIC INC
MERCER INC
MERCK & CO INC
METLIFE INC
MGM MIRAGE
MICRON TECHNOLOGY INC
MICROSOFT CORP
MILLIPORE CORP

MONRO MUFFLER BRAKE INC
NEIMAN MARCUS GROUP INC (THE)
NETWORK APPLIANCE INC
NEWS CORP
NIKE INC
NOBLE CORPORATION
NORDSTROM INC
NORFOLK SOUTHERN CORP
NORTHROP GRUMMAN CORP
ODYSSEY HEALTHCARE INC
OFFICE DEPOT INC
OIL STATES INTERNATIONAL INC
OMNICARE INC
OMNICOM GROUP INC
ONEOK INC
ORACLE CORP
O'REILLY AUTOMOTIVE INC
OSHKOSH CORPORATION
OSI RESTAURANT PARTNERS INC
OWENS & MINOR INC
PACIFIC SUNWEAR OF CALIFORNIA
INC
PAREXEL INTERNATIONAL CORP
PARSONS BRINCKERHOFF INC
PAYCHEX INC
PEPSI BOTTLING GROUP INC
PEPSICO INC
PETCO ANIMAL SUPPLIES INC
PETSMART INC
PFIZER INC
PG&E CORPORATION
PHARMACEUTICAL PRODUCT
DEVELOPMENT INC
PITNEY BOWES INC
PLANTRONICS INC
POLO RALPH LAUREN CORP
PRAXAIR INC
PRINCIPAL FINANCIAL GROUP (THE)
PROCTER & GAMBLE CO
PROGRESSIVE CORPORATION (THE)
PRUDENTIAL FINANCIAL INC
PUBLIX SUPER MARKETS INC
QUALCOMM INC
QUEST DIAGNOSTICS INC
R R DONNELLEY & SONS CO
RAYTHEON CO
REGIS CORPORATION
RELIANT ENERGY INC
RENT-A-CENTER INC
RES CARE INC
RITE AID CORPORATION
ROBERT HALF INTERNATIONAL INC
ROSS STORES INC
ROYAL CARIBBEAN CRUISES
RYDER SYSTEM INC
SABRE HOLDINGS CORP
SAFECO CORP
SAFEWAY INC
SAIC INC
SARA LEE CORP
SAS INSTITUTE INC
SCANA CORPORATION
SCHERING-PLOUGH CORP
SCIENTIFIC GAMES CORPORATION
SEACOR HOLDINGS INC

SEMPRA ENERGY
SHELL OIL CO
SHERWIN WILLIAMS COMPANY
(THE)
SISTERS OF MERCY HEALTH
SYSTEMS
SOUTHERN COMPANY (THE)
SOUTHWEST AIRLINES CO
SRA INTERNATIONAL INC
ST JUDE MEDICAL INC
STAPLES INC
STARTEK INC
STARWOOD HOTELS & RESORTS
WORLDWIDE INC
STRYKER CORP
SUN HEALTHCARE GROUP
SUN MICROSYSTEMS INC
SUNOCO INC
SUNRISE SENIOR LIVING
SUPERVALU INC
SYKES ENTERPRISES INC
SYMANTEC CORP
SYNOPSYS INC
SYSCO CORP
TALBOTS INC (THE)
TARGET CORPORATION
TELEDYNE TECHNOLOGIES
INCORPORATED
TELETECH HOLDINGS INC
TESORO CORP
TIFFANY & CO
TIME WARNER INC
TJX COMPANIES INC (THE)
TOTAL SYSTEM SERVICES INC
(TSYS)
TRAVELERS COMPANIES INC (THE)
TW TELECOM INC
TWEEN BRANDS INC
TYSON FOODS INC
UNION PACIFIC CORP
UNITED PARCEL SERVICE INC (UPS)
UNITED STATES CELLULAR CORP
UNITEDHEALTH GROUP INC
URS CORPORATION
USAA
VALSPAR CORPORATION (THE)
VARIAN MEDICAL SYSTEMS INC
VERISIGN INC
VERIZON COMMUNICATIONS
VIACOM INC
VOLT INFORMATION SCIENCES INC
W R BERKLEY CORPORATION
WAL-MART STORES INC
WALT DISNEY COMPANY (THE)
WATERS CORP
WATSON PHARMACEUTICALS INC
WEIGHT WATCHERS
INTERNATIONAL INC
WELLPOINT INC
WENDYS INTERNATIONAL INC
WEST CORPORATION
WESTERN UNION COMPANY (THE)
WHOLE FOODS MARKET INC
WILLIAMS COMPANIES INC (THE)
WILLIAMS SONOMA INC

WM WRIGLEY JR COMPANY
WW GRAINGER INC
WYETH
WYNDHAM WORLDWIDE
WYNN RESORTS LIMITED
XEROX CORP
YAHOO! INC
YUM! BRANDS INC
ZIMMER HOLDINGS INC

INDEX OF SUBSIDIARIES, BRAND NAMES AND AFFILIATIONS

Brand or subsidiary, followed by the name of the related corporation

2SPA; **RITZ-CARLTON HOTEL COMPANY LLC (THE)**
365 Everyday Value; **WHOLE FOODS MARKET INC**
365 Organic Everyday Value; **WHOLE FOODS MARKET INC**
3Dsolve, Inc.; **LOCKHEED MARTIN CORP**
3M eStore; **3M COMPANY**
5 A Day for Better Health; **DOLE FOOD COMPANY INC**
76; **CONOCOPHILLIPS COMPANY**
77kids; **AMERICAN EAGLE OUTFITTERS INC**
787 Dreamliner; **BOEING COMPANY (THE)**
A&F Film; **ABERCROMBIE & FITCH CO**
A&W All-American Food; **YUM! BRANDS INC**
A.J. Wright; **TJX COMPANIES INC (THE)**
A.T.S. Tourniquet System; **ZIMMER HOLDINGS INC**
A9.com, Inc.; **AMAZON.COM INC**
Aastra Digital Video; **HARRIS CORPORATION**
Abacus; **FOSSIL INC**
ABC Inc; **WALT DISNEY COMPANY (THE)**
ABeBooks; **AMAZON.COM INC**
Abercrombie & Fitch; **ABERCROMBIE & FITCH CO**
Abercrombie.com; **ABERCROMBIE & FITCH CO**
AbercrombieKids.com; **ABERCROMBIE & FITCH CO**
ABM Engineering Services; **ABM INDUSTRIES INC**
ABM Janitorial Services; **ABM INDUSTRIES INC**
ABM Security Services; **ABM INDUSTRIES INC**
Abrams Integrated Management; **GENERAL DYNAMICS CORP**
Accountemps; **ROBERT HALF INTERNATIONAL INC**
Accredo Health Group Inc; **MEDCO HEALTH SOLUTIONS**
Accu-Bite Dental Products, LLC; **PATTERSON COMPANIES INC**
ACCU-SORT; **DANAHER CORP**
Accuspray Application Technologies; **3M COMPANY**

Acklands-Grainger, Inc.; **WW GRAINGER INC**
Acme Markets; **SUPERVALU INC**
Acorn; **CHRISTOPHER & BANKS CORP**
Actiq; **CEPHALON INC**
Activase; **GENENTECH INC**
Acushnet Co.; **FORTUNE BRANDS INC**
Acxiom Access-X Express; **ACXIOM CORP**
Acxiom Digital; **ACXIOM CORP**
Acxiom Information Security Services; **ACXIOM CORP**
Adams; **JM SMUCKER CO**
ADC Krone; **ADC TELECOMMUNICATIONS INC**
ADESA LiveBlock; **ADESA INC**
ADESA Market Guide; **ADESA INC**
ADESA Notify Me; **ADESA INC**
ADESA Run Lists; **ADESA INC**
ADESA Virtual Inventory; **ADESA INC**
ADM Cocoa; **ARCHER DANIELS MIDLAND CO**
ADM Milling Co.; **ARCHER DANIELS MIDLAND CO**
Admiral Insurance Company; **W R BERKLEY CORPORATION**
Adobe Acrobat; **ADOBE SYSTEMS INC**
Adobe Creative Suite; **ADOBE SYSTEMS INC**
Adobe Flash Player; **ADOBE SYSTEMS INC**
Adobe Photoshop; **ADOBE SYSTEMS INC**
Adobe Reader LE; **ADOBE SYSTEMS INC**
Adobe Systems Inc; **KEANE INC**
ADP TotalSource; **AUTOMATIC DATA PROCESSING INC**
Adscape Media, Inc.; **GOOGLE INC**
Advance Discount Auto Parts; **ADVANCE AUTO PARTS INC**
Advanced Bionics Corp.; **BOSTON SCIENTIFIC CORP**
Advanced Care Scripts Inc.; **OMNICARE INC**
Advanced Select; **EXPERIAN AMERICAS**
Advanced Stent Technologies; **BOSTON SCIENTIFIC CORP**
Advanced Technologies; **OCEANEERING INTERNATIONAL INC**
Advantage Membership; **SAM'S CLUB**
ADVATE; **BAXTER INTERNATIONAL INC**
Advectis, Inc.; **XEROX CORP**
Advil; **WYETH**
AE; **AMERICAN EAGLE OUTFITTERS INC**
ae.com; **AMERICAN EAGLE OUTFITTERS INC**
Aearo Technologies Inc; **3M COMPANY**
AECOM Austin; **AECOM TECHNOLOGY CORPORATION**

AEON; **TALBOTS INC (THE)**
AEP Ohio; **AMERICAN ELECTRIC POWER COMPANY INC (AEP)**
AEP Texas; **AMERICAN ELECTRIC POWER COMPANY INC (AEP)**
aerie by American Eagle; **AMERICAN EAGLE OUTFITTERS INC**
aerie.com; **AMERICAN EAGLE OUTFITTERS INC**
Aeropostale West, Inc.; **AEROPOSTALE INC**
aeropostale.com; **AEROPOSTALE INC**
AES Eletropaulo; **AES CORPORATION (THE)**
AES SONEL; **AES CORPORATION (THE)**
Aetna Global Benefits; **AETNA INC**
Aexa.com; **AMAZON.COM INC**
Afianzadora Insurgentes S.A. de C.V.; **TRAVELERS COMPANIES INC (THE)**
AFLAC Japan; **AFLAC INC**
AFLAC U.S.; **AFLAC INC**
Afren plc; **DEVON ENERGY CORPORATION**
After Hours Formalwear; **MEN'S WEARHOUSE INC (THE)**
Agile Software Corp; **ORACLE CORP**
Agilent Technologies Laboratories; **AGILENT TECHNOLOGIES INC**
Agilysys Keylink Systems Group; **ARROW ELECTRONICS INC**
Agroindustrial Santa Juliana; **BUNGE LTD**
AGS; **AECOM TECHNOLOGY CORPORATION**
AH-64D Apache; **BOEING COMPANY (THE)**
AIB Merchant Services; **FIRST DATA CORP**
Air Force One; **BOEING COMPANY (THE)**
Air Products Asia; **AIR PRODUCTS & CHEMICALS INC**
Air Products Europe; **AIR PRODUCTS & CHEMICALS INC**
Air Products Japan; **AIR PRODUCTS & CHEMICALS INC**
Airborne Laser; **NORTHROP GRUMMAN CORP**
Aircast, Inc.; **DJO INC**
AirForce; **BROADCOM CORP**
Ajax; **COLGATE PALMOLIVE CO**
Alabama Power Company; **SOUTHERN COMPANY (THE)**
Alamo Rental; **ENTERPRISE RENT-A-CAR**
Alantos; **AMGEN INC**
Alaris; **CARDINAL HEALTH INC**
Alberto VO5; **ALBERTO-CULVER COMPANY**
Albert's Organics; **UNITED NATURAL FOODS INC**
Albertsons; **SUPERVALU INC**
Alegant Health; **CATHOLIC HEALTH INITIATIVES**

INDEX OF SUBSIDIARIES, BRAND NAMES AND AFFILIATIONS, CONT.

Alexia Foods, Inc.; **CONAGRA FOODS INC**

All Star; **NIKE INC**

ALLDATA; **AUTOZONE INC**

Allegro Coffee Company; **WHOLE FOODS MARKET INC**

Alliance 2795; **WATERS CORP**

AllianceBernstein LP; **AXA FINANCIAL INC**

Allstate; **ALLSTATE CORPORATION (THE)**

Allstate Insurance Co.; **ALLSTATE CORPORATION (THE)**

Allstate Life Insurance Co.; **ALLSTATE CORPORATION (THE)**

Allstate Motor Club, Inc.; **ALLSTATE CORPORATION (THE)**

Aloft; **STARWOOD HOTELS & RESORTS WORLDWIDE INC**

Alpha Ceramics Inc; **CTS CORP**

Altec Lansing; **PLANTRONICS INC**

Alternative Technology, Inc.; **ARROW ELECTRONICS INC**

Altiris Inc; **SYMANTEC CORP**

Altius Health Plans; **COVENTRY HEALTH CARE INC**

Altoids; **WM WRIGLEY JR COMPANY**

Altria Group Inc; **KRAFT FOODS INC**

Alza Corp; **JOHNSON & JOHNSON**

Amazon Marketplace; **AMAZON.COM INC**

AMD Athlon 64; **ADVANCED MICRO DEVICES INC (AMD)**

AMD Athlon 64 FX; **ADVANCED MICRO DEVICES INC (AMD)**

AMD Athlon XP; **ADVANCED MICRO DEVICES INC (AMD)**

AMD Duron; **ADVANCED MICRO DEVICES INC (AMD)**

AMD Opteron; **ADVANCED MICRO DEVICES INC (AMD)**

AMD Sempron; **ADVANCED MICRO DEVICES INC (AMD)**

American Building Maintenance; **ABM INDUSTRIES INC**

American Express Business Travel; **AMERICAN EXPRESS CO**

American Express Publishing Corporation; **AMERICAN EXPRESS CO**

American Express Travel Related Services Company; **AMERICAN EXPRESS CO**

American Family Life Assurance Company of Columbus; **AFLAC INC**

American Girl; **MATTEL INC**

American Health Packaging; **AMERISOURCEBERGEN CORP**

American Imaging Management; **WELLPOINT INC**

American Living; **POLO RALPH LAUREN CORP**

American Mining Insurance Company; **W R BERKLEY CORPORATION**

American Rod & Gun; **BASS PRO SHOPS INC**

American Savings Bank, F.S.B.; **HAWAIIAN ELECTRIC INDUSTRIES INC**

American Transmission Systems, Inc.; **FIRSTENERGY CORP**

AmeriHost; **WYNDHAM WORLDWIDE**

Ameriprise Financial, Inc.; **AMERICAN EXPRESS CO**

AmerisourceBergen Corp.; **KINDRED HEALTHCARE INC**

AmerisourceBergen Drug Corp.; **AMERISOURCEBERGEN CORP**

AmerisourceBergen Packaging Group; **AMERISOURCEBERGEN CORP**

AmerisourceBergen Specialty Group; **AMERISOURCEBERGEN CORP**

AMRIX; **CEPHALON INC**

Amsbra, Ltd.; **BUILD-A-BEAR WORKSHOP INC**

Amsco; **STERIS CORP**

AMSEC, LLC; **SAIC INC**

Amtech Lighting Services; **ABM INDUSTRIES INC**

Anadarko Algeria Company LLC; **ANADARKO PETROLEUM CORPORATION**

Anadarko Energy Services Company; **ANADARKO PETROLEUM CORPORATION**

Anadarko Land Corp.; **ANADARKO PETROLEUM CORPORATION**

Anda; **WATSON PHARMACEUTICALS INC**

Andaz; **GLOBAL HYATT CORPORATION**

Anderson Packaging; **AMERISOURCEBERGEN CORP**

Anew; **AVON PRODUCTS INC**

Angelfire; **MARY KAY INC**

Ann Taylor; **ANNTAYLOR STORES CORP**

Ann Taylor Factory Store; **ANNTAYLOR STORES CORP**

Ann Taylor LOFT; **ANNTAYLOR STORES CORP**

Antech Diagnostics; **VCA ANTECH INC**

Anthropologie; **URBAN OUTFITTERS INC**

ANXeBusiness Corp.; **SAIC INC**

AOL LLC; **TIME WARNER INC**

Apache Canada Ltd.; **APACHE CORP**

Apache Energy Ltd.; **APACHE CORP**

Apache North America, Inc.; **APACHE CORP**

Apache Overseas, Inc.; **APACHE CORP**

Apollo Management, L.P.; **HARRAH'S ENTERTAINMENT INC**

Appalachian Power; **AMERICAN ELECTRIC POWER COMPANY INC (AEP)**

Apple Computer Inc; **APPLE INC**

Applebee's International Inc; **DINEEQUITY INC**

Applied Molecular Evolution Inc; **ELI LILLY & COMPANY**

Aquafina; **PEPSI BOTTLING GROUP INC**

aQuantive Inc; **MICROSOFT CORP**

ARAMARK Uniform Services; **ARAMARK CORPORATION**

Aramis; **ESTEE LAUDER COMPANIES INC (THE)**

Aranesp; **AMGEN INC**

Arbor Place at Silverlake; **EMERITUS CORP**

Arbortext Advanced Print Publisher; **PARAMETRIC TECHNOLOGY CORP**

Arbortext, Inc.; **PARAMETRIC TECHNOLOGY CORP**

Archer Farms; **TARGET CORPORATION**

ArchPro Design Automation, Inc.; **SYNOPSYS INC**

Arden Courts; **MANOR CARE INC**

Aristokraft; **FORTUNE BRANDS INC**

Armstrong Unicare; **RES CARE INC**

Armstrong Uniserve; **RES CARE INC**

Arnell Group; **OMNICOM GROUP INC**

Aromax; **CHEVRON PHILLIPS CHEMICAL COMPANY LLC**

Arrow ECS; **ARROW ELECTRONICS INC**

Arrow Hose & Tubing, Inc.; **EATON CORP**

ArrowDevTools.com; **ARROW ELECTRONICS INC**

Artesyn Technologies; **EMERSON ELECTRIC CO**

Arthur J. Gallagher (UK), Ltd.; **ARTHUR J GALLAGHER & CO**

Aruba; **HENRY SCHEIN INC**

Aspen Marketing Services, Inc.; **TELETECH HOLDINGS INC**

Asterion SAS; **PITNEY BOWES INC**

Aston Gardens; **SUNRISE SENIOR LIVING**

Athena Innovative Solutions, Inc.; **CACI INTERNATIONAL INC**

Ativa; **OFFICE DEPOT INC**

Atlas II HF CRT-D; **ST JUDE MEDICAL INC**

Atlas II ICD; **ST JUDE MEDICAL INC**

Atrium; **DRESS BARN INC (THE)**

Attiki Gas Supply S.A.; **DUKE ENERGY CORP**

Audit Committee Institute; **KPMG LLP**

Austar United Communications Ltd.; **LIBERTY GLOBAL INC**

Autozone.com; **AUTOZONE INC**

AVAD; **INGRAM MICRO INC**

Avago Technologies Ltd.; **MICRON TECHNOLOGY INC**

INDEX OF SUBSIDIARIES, BRAND NAMES AND AFFILIATIONS, CONT.

Avastin; **GENENTECH INC**

Aveda; **ESTEE LAUDER COMPANIES INC (THE)**

Avery; **AVERY DENNISON CORP**

Avery Dennison Corp; **PAXAR CORP**

Avidyn Inc; **FISERV INC**

AVImark; **HENRY SCHEIN INC**

Avis; **AVIS BUDGET GROUP INC**

Avon Color; **AVON PRODUCTS INC**

Avon Fragrance; **AVON PRODUCTS INC**

Avon Skin-So-Soft; **AVON PRODUCTS INC**

AXA Advisors LLC; **AXA FINANCIAL INC**

AXA Distributors; **AXA FINANCIAL INC**

AXA Equitable Life Insurance Company; **AXA FINANCIAL INC**

AXA Group; **AXA FINANCIAL INC**

Axciom France; **PITNEY BOWES INC**

Axia Health Management, LLC; **HEALTHWAYS INC**

Azamara; **ROYAL CARIBBEAN CRUISES**

B. Dalton Bookseller; **BARNES & NOBLE INC**

B-2; **NORTHROP GRUMMAN CORP**

Babco Electric Group; **EATON CORP**

Baby GUESS; **GUESS? INC**

Baby GUESS; **GUESS? INC**

Baconator; **WENDYS INTERNATIONAL INC**

Bahama Breeze; **DARDEN RESTAURANTS INC**

Bain Capital LLC; **HCA INC**

Bain Capital LLC; **OSI RESTAURANT PARTNERS INC**

Bain Capital LLC; **CLEAR CHANNEL COMMUNICATIONS INC**

Baker Atlas; **BAKER HUGHES INC**

Baker Hughes Drilling Fluids; **BAKER HUGHES INC**

Baker Hughes INTEQ; **BAKER HUGHES INC**

Baker Oil Tools; **BAKER HUGHES INC**

Baker Petrolite; **BAKER HUGHES INC**

Bakers & Chefs; **SAM'S CLUB**

Ball Park; **SARA LEE CORP**

Banc of America Corporate Insurance Agency, L.L.C.; **HILB ROGAL & HOBBS CO**

BancIntelligence.com, Inc.; **FISERV INC**

Banfield, The Pet Hospital; **PETSMART INC**

Bank of New York; **JP MORGAN CHASE & CO INC**

Banta Corporation; **R R DONNELLEY & SONS CO**

Barbie; **MATTEL INC**

Barclay; **KROGER CO (THE)**

Bard Medical Systems; **CR BARD INC**

Bard Peripheral Vascular-Biopsy; **CR BARD INC**

Bard Peripheral Vascular-Interventional; **CR BARD INC**

Bargain Cave; **CABELA'S INC**

Barnes & Noble Bookseller; **BARNES & NOBLE INC**

Barnes & Noble Classics; **BARNES & NOBLE COLLEGE BOOKSTORES**

Barnes & Noble College Marketing Network; **BARNES & NOBLE COLLEGE BOOKSTORES**

Barnes & Noble Inc; **BARNES & NOBLE COLLEGE BOOKSTORES**

BarnesandNoble.com Inc; **BARNES & NOBLE INC**

Barnett Banks, Inc.; **BANK OF AMERICA CORP**

Barnett Educational Services; **PAREXEL INTERNATIONAL CORP**

Barnett Shale; **DEVON ENERGY CORPORATION**

Basil; **STERIS CORP**

Bath & Body Works; **INTIMATE BRANDS INC**

Bath & Body Works; **LIMITED BRANDS INC**

Baugh Supply Chain Cooperative; **SYSCO CORP**

BBDO Worldwide Network; **OMNICOM GROUP INC**

BDO Business Resource Network; **BDO SEIDMAN LLP**

BDO Consulting Services; **BDO SEIDMAN LLP**

BDO International; **BDO SEIDMAN LLP**

BDO Seidman Alliance; **BDO SEIDMAN LLP**

BEA Systems Inc; **ORACLE CORP**

Beam Global Spirits & Wine, Inc.; **FORTUNE BRANDS INC**

Bear Bunk Trunk; **BUILD-A-BEAR WORKSHOP INC**

Bear Factory Limited (The); **BUILD-A-BEAR WORKSHOP INC**

Bear Ridge Resources, Ltd.; **MURPHY OIL CORPORATION**

Bear Stearns Cos Inc (The); **JP MORGAN CHASE & CO INC**

bebe; **BEBE STORES INC**

bebe Outlet; **BEBE STORES INC**

BEBE SPORT; **BEBE STORES INC**

bebe.com; **BEBE STORES INC**

Bechtel Power Corp.; **BECHTEL GROUP INC**

Bechtel Systems & Infrastructure, Inc.; **BECHTEL GROUP INC**

Becker Powder Coatings, Inc; **SHERWIN WILLIAMS COMPANY (THE)**

Becker Professional Review; **DEVRY INC**

Becton Dickinson Biosciences; **BECTON DICKINSON & CO**

Becton Dickinson Diagnostics; **BECTON DICKINSON & CO**

Becton Dickinson Medical; **BECTON DICKINSON & CO**

Bed Bath & Beyond Superstores; **BED BATH & BEYOND INC**

Behavioral and Medical Research, LLC; **PAREXEL INTERNATIONAL CORP**

Belara; **MARY KAY INC**

Bellagio; **MGM MIRAGE**

BellSouth; **AT&T INC**

BenefitPort Northwest; **ARTHUR J GALLAGHER & CO**

BeneTrac; **PAYCHEX INC**

Benham Investment Holdings, LLC; **SAIC INC**

Benicar; **FOREST LABORATORIES INC**

Benjamin Moore & Co; **BERKSHIRE HATHAWAY INC**

Berbee Information Networks Corp; **CDW CORPORATION**

Bergdorf Goodman, Inc.; **NEIMAN MARCUS GROUP INC (THE)**

Berkeley Data Systems; **EMC CORP**

Berkley & Jensen; **BJ'S WHOLESALE CLUB INC**

Berkley Asset Protection Underwriters LLC; **W R BERKLEY CORPORATION**

Berkley Specialty Underwriting Managers LLC; **W R BERKLEY CORPORATION**

Berkshire Hathaway; **RUSSELL CORP**

BestShores; **KEANE INC**

Betty Crocker; **GENERAL MILLS INC**

Beverage Partners Worldwide; **COCA COLA COMPANY (THE)**

Beyond Color; **AVON PRODUCTS INC**

Big Bite; **7-ELEVEN INC**

Big Cedar Lodge; **BASS PRO SHOPS INC**

Big G Cereals; **GENERAL MILLS INC**

Big Gulp; **7-ELEVEN INC**

Big Mac; **MCDONALD'S CORP**

Big O Tires, Inc.; **TBC CORPORATION**

Big Red; **WM WRIGLEY JR COMPANY**

Big Tic; **FOSSIL INC**

BillBird; **GTECH HOLDINGS CORP**

Bio-In-A-Box; **WASTE MANAGEMENT INC**

Bio-Intact PTH; **QUEST DIAGNOSTICS INC**

BioLife Plasma Services; **BAXTER INTERNATIONAL INC**

BiopharmaLynx TM; **WATERS CORP**

BioPlex 2200; **BIO RAD LABORATORIES INC**

BioScience; **BAXTER INTERNATIONAL INC**

BioSite; **WASTE MANAGEMENT INC**

BioWare Corp.; **ELECTRONIC ARTS INC**

INDEX OF SUBSIDIARIES, BRAND NAMES AND AFFILIATIONS, CONT.

Bisquick; **GENERAL MILLS INC**
BK Fish Filet; **BURGER KING HOLDINGS INC**
BK Veggie Burger; **BURGER KING HOLDINGS INC**
Black River Asset Management; **CARGILL INC**
BlackBerry 8830; **UNITED STATES CELLULAR CORP**
Blackhawk Network; **SAFEWAY INC**
Blackstone Group LP (The); **HILTON HOTELS CORP**
Bladerunner; **BROADCOM CORP**
Blake International LLC; **PRIDE INTERNATIONAL INC**
Bloomberg Electronic Trading Systems; **BLOOMBERG LP**
Bloomberg Magazine; **BLOOMBERG LP**
Bloomberg News; **BLOOMBERG LP**
Bloomberg Professional; **BLOOMBERG LP**
Bloomberg Roadshows; **BLOOMBERG LP**
Bloomberg Television; **BLOOMBERG LP**
Bloomberg Terminals; **BLOOMBERG LP**
Bloomberg Tradebook; **BLOOMBERG LP**
Blooming Prairie Cooperative Warehouse; **UNITED NATURAL FOODS INC**
Bloomingdale's; **MACY'S INC**
Blount; **CATERPILLAR INC**
blu chic; **CHARLOTTE RUSSE HOLDING**
Blue Coral Seafood & Spirits; **OSI RESTAURANT PARTNERS INC**
BLUE CROSS AND BLUE SHIELD OF GEORGIA INC; **WELLPOINT INC**
BLUE CROSS OF CALIFORNIA; **WELLPOINT INC**
BlueLithium; **YAHOO! INC**
BMC Software Inc; **KEANE INC**
BNSF Logistics; **BURLINGTON NORTHERN SANTA FE CORP**
Boardriders Club; **QUIKSILVER INC**
Boardwalk Pipeline Partners, LP; **LOEWS CORPORATION**
Bobbie Brown; **ESTEE LAUDER COMPANIES INC (THE)**
Bob's Stores; **TJX COMPANIES INC (THE)**
Boeing Business Jets; **BOEING COMPANY (THE)**
Boeing Capital; **BOEING COMPANY (THE)**
Bondo; **3M COMPANY**
Bonefish Grill; **OSI RESTAURANT PARTNERS INC**
Boots & Coots International Well Control, Inc.; **OIL STATES INTERNATIONAL INC**
Boston College Club; **CLUBCORP INC**

Boston Market; **MCDONALD'S CORP**
Botox; **ALLERGAN INC**
Bowers & Associates; **AFFILIATED COMPUTER SERVICES INC**
Brad; **MOLEX INC**
Bragano; **NIKE INC**
BrakeBest; **O'REILLY AUTOMOTIVE INC**
Brand G; **GUESS? INC**
Brass Plum; **NORDSTROM INC**
Braun Consulting, Inc.; **FAIR ISAAC CORPORATION**
Braun's; **CHRISTOPHER & BANKS CORP**
Break Escapes; **OFFICE DEPOT INC**
Breakaway Imaging LLC; **MEDTRONIC INC**
Breakfast Jack; **JACK IN THE BOX INC**
Brecon Pharmaceutical, Ltd.; **AMERISOURCEBERGEN CORP**
Bridgestream Inc; **ORACLE CORP**
Brink's Home Security, Inc.; **BRINKS COMPANY (THE)**
Brink's, Inc.; **BRINKS COMPANY (THE)**
Broadcasting Media Partners, Inc.; **UNIVISION COMMUNICATIONS INC**
Broadridge Financial Solutions, Inc.; **AUTOMATIC DATA PROCESSING INC**
Broadwing Communications LLC; **LEVEL 3 COMMUNICATIONS INC**
Brooks Eckerd; **RITE AID CORPORATION**
Brooks Sports; **RUSSELL CORP**
Brooksville Regional Hospital; **HEALTH MANAGEMENT ASSOCIATES INC**
Brown/Raynor Corporation; **HILB ROGAL & HOBBS CO**
BSNF Railway Company; **BURLINGTON NORTHERN SANTA FE CORP**
Buckle; **BUCKLE INC (THE)**
Buckle [The]; **BUCKLE INC (THE)**
Buckle Screenprinting; **BUCKLE INC (THE)**
buckle.com; **BUCKLE INC (THE)**
Budget; **AVIS BUDGET GROUP INC**
Budget Truck; **AVIS BUDGET GROUP INC**
Bufferin; **BRISTOL MYERS SQUIBB CO**
BuildaBearville.com; **BUILD-A-BEAR WORKSHOP INC**
Bulgari Hotel and Resort; **MARRIOTT INTERNATIONAL INC**
Bulova Corp.; **LOEWS CORPORATION**
Bunn Capitol; **SYSCO CORP**
Business Membership; **SAM'S CLUB**
Business Objects SA; **KEANE INC**
Butterball LLC; **SMITHFIELD FOODS INC**

buybuy BABY; **BED BATH & BEYOND INC**
c.booth derma; **RITE AID CORPORATION**
C.J. Banks; **CHRISTOPHER & BANKS CORP**
C.O. Bigelow; **LIMITED BRANDS INC**
C.O. Bigelow; **INTIMATE BRANDS INC**
Caban; **POLO RALPH LAUREN CORP**
Cabela's Club; **CABELA'S INC**
CACI Limited; **CACI INTERNATIONAL INC**
Cacique; **CHARMING SHOPPES INC**
Caesars; **HARRAH'S ENTERTAINMENT INC**
Caesars Palace Las Vegas; **HARRAH'S ENTERTAINMENT INC**
Cafe Express; **WENDYS INTERNATIONAL INC**
Cafe Select; **7-ELEVEN INC**
California Clinical Trials Medical Group, Inc.; **PAREXEL INTERNATIONAL CORP**
Caltex; **CHEVRON CORPORATION**
Cameron Capital Investments Inc; **REGIS CORPORATION**
Cameron Compression; **CAMERON INTERNATIONAL CORPORATION**
Cameron Offshore Systems; **CAMERON INTERNATIONAL CORPORATION**
Cameron Valves & Measurement; **CAMERON INTERNATIONAL CORPORATION**
Canada Dry; **COCA COLA COMPANY (THE)**
Canada Safeway Limited; **SAFEWAY INC**
Cap Connection; **GENESCO INC**
Captiva; **EMC CORP**
Captive Management Initiatives; **CATHOLIC HEALTH INITIATIVES**
Cardiac Healthways; **HEALTHWAYS INC**
Cardinal Brands, Inc.; **R R DONNELLEY & SONS CO**
Cardio CRP; **QUEST DIAGNOSTICS INC**
Cardiopet proBNP; **IDEXX LABORATORIES INC**
CareerStaff Unlimited, Inc.; **SUN HEALTHCARE GROUP**
CareFusion; **CARDINAL HEALTH INC**
Caregivers Home Health, Inc.; **RES CARE INC**
Careline; **PERRIGO CO**
Carelink Health Plans; **COVENTRY HEALTH CARE INC**
Caremark Pharmacy Services; **CVS CAREMARK CORPORATION**
Caremark Rx., Inc.; **CVS CAREMARK CORPORATION**

Carey International; **AVIS BUDGET GROUP INC**
Cargill AgHorizons U.S.; **CARGILL INC**
Cargill Animal Nutrition; **CARGILL INC**
Caritor, Inc.; **KEANE INC**
Carlyle Group (The); **MANOR CARE INC**
CarMax Foundation; **CARMAX GROUP**
Carnation; **JM SMUCKER CO**
Carnival Cruise Lines; **CARNIVAL CORPORATION**
Carolina Gas Transmission Corp.; **SCANA CORPORATION**
Carrabba's Italian Grill; **OSI RESTAURANT PARTNERS INC**
Carr-Gottstein Foods Co; **SAFEWAY INC**
Carrier Corp.; **UNITED TECHNOLOGIES CORPORATION**
Carroll Tire Company; **TBC CORPORATION**
Carson Storage Partners, Ltd.; **PUBLIC STORAGE INC**
Carter and Burgess; **JACOBS ENGINEERING GROUP INC**
Casa Ley, S.A. de C.V.; **SAFEWAY INC**
Cash AdvantEdge; **RENT-A-CENTER INC**
Cash America Payday Advance; **CASH AMERICA INTERNATIONAL INC**
Cash Net Holdings, LLC; **CASH AMERICA INTERNATIONAL INC**
Cashland Financial Services, Inc.; **CASH AMERICA INTERNATIONAL INC**
CashNet USA; **CASH AMERICA INTERNATIONAL INC**
Catalytica Energy Systems, Inc.; **EATON CORP**
Caterpillar Inc; **CATERPILLAR LOGISTICS**
Caterpillar Remanufacturing Services; **CATERPILLAR INC**
Catherine's Plus Sizes; **CHARMING SHOPPES INC**
Caviar; **WESTERN DIGITAL CORP**
CC Media Holdings; **CLEAR CHANNEL COMMUNICATIONS INC**
CCMP Capital Advisors; **ARAMARK CORPORATION**
CDW Canada Inc; **CDW CORPORATION**
CDW Government Inc; **CDW CORPORATION**
Cederroth International; **ALBERTO-CULVER COMPANY**
Celebrity Cruises; **ROYAL CARIBBEAN CRUISES**
Celera; **EMC CORP**
CellSearch; **QUEST DIAGNOSTICS INC**
Center for Esoteric Testing (The); **LABORATORY CORP OF AMERICA HOLDINGS**

Center for Molecular Biology and Pathology (The); **LABORATORY CORP OF AMERICA HOLDINGS**
Center for National Response; **L-3 TITAN GROUP**
Centia Group Limited; **ARROW ELECTRONICS INC**
Centocor Inc; **JOHNSON & JOHNSON**
CentraCore Properties Trust; **GEO GROUP INC**
Central Market; **HE BUTT GROCERY COMPANY (HEB)**
CentreVu Customer Care Solution; **HEALTHWAYS INC**
Centrilift; **BAKER HUGHES INC**
Centrum; **WYETH**
Centura Health; **CATHOLIC HEALTH INITIATIVES**
Century Man Communication; **ADC TELECOMMUNICATIONS INC**
Cerestar Sweeteners Europe; **CARGILL INC**
Cerexa, Inc.; **FOREST LABORATORIES INC**
Cerveillance Scope; **COOPER COMPANIES INC**
Cesar; **MARS INC**
CF Complete; **QUEST DIAGNOSTICS INC**
CFOdirect Network; **PRICEWATERHOUSECOOPERS**
CGH Insurance Group; **W R BERKLEY CORPORATION**
CGR/seven LLC; **KELLY SERVICES INC**
CH2M HILL Canada, Ltd.; **CH2M HILL COMPANIES LTD**
CH2M-IDC China; **CH2M HILL COMPANIES LTD**
Chamberlain College of Nursing; **DEVRY INC**
Chap Stick; **WYETH**
Chaps; **POLO RALPH LAUREN CORP**
Charlotte Russe; **CHARLOTTE RUSSE HOLDING**
Charlton Manley, Inc.; **HILB ROGAL & HOBBS CO**
Chart House (The); **LANDRY'S RESTAURANTS INC**
Check Giant, LLC (The); **CASH AMERICA INTERNATIONAL INC**
CheckFree Corp.; **FISERV INC**
Cheerios; **GENERAL MILLS INC**
Cheeseburger in Paradise; **OSI RESTAURANT PARTNERS INC**
CheetahMail; **EXPERIAN AMERICAS**
Chef Boyardee; **CONAGRA FOODS INC**
Chellomedia BV; **LIBERTY GLOBAL INC**
ChemTreat, Inc.; **DANAHER CORP**
Chemtura Corporation; **E I DU PONT DE NEMOURS & CO (DUPONT)**

Chevron Phillips Chemical Company LLC; **CONOCOPHILLIPS COMPANY**
Chevron Technology Ventures; **CHEVRON CORPORATION**
Chicken McNuggets; **MCDONALD'S CORP**
Chick's Sporting Goods; **DICK'S SPORTING GOODS INC**
Chico's; **CHICO'S FAS INC**
Chico's Outlet; **CHICO'S FAS INC**
Children's Medical Ventures; **RESPIRONICS INC**
Chili's Grill and Bar; **BRINKER INTERNATIONAL INC**
China Construction Bank; **BANK OF AMERICA CORP**
ChloraPrep; **CARDINAL HEALTH INC**
Choxie; **TARGET CORPORATION**
CHREX; **CH ROBINSON WORLDWIDE INC**
Christmas Tree Shops; **BED BATH & BEYOND INC**
Christopher Lowell; **OFFICE DEPOT INC**
Chubb Commercial Insurance; **CHUBB CORPORATION (THE)**
Chubb Custom Insurance Company; **CHUBB CORPORATION (THE)**
Chubb Personal Insurance; **CHUBB CORPORATION (THE)**
Chubb Specialty Insurance; **CHUBB CORPORATION (THE)**
Chuck Taylor; **NIKE INC**
CIBER Europe; **CIBER INC**
Cingular Wireless; **AT&T INC**
Citizen's Gas Fuel Corp.; **DTE ENERGY COMPANY**
Clairol; **PROCTER & GAMBLE CO**
Clarendon Parker Middle East FZ LLC; **MANPOWER INC**
CLARiiON; **EMC CORP**
Clarity; **PLANTRONICS INC**
Classiques Entier; **NORDSTROM INC**
Clayton Homes Inc; **BERKSHIRE HATHAWAY INC**
Clear Channel Independent; **CLEAR CHANNEL COMMUNICATIONS INC**
Cleveland Electric Illuminating Co. (The); **FIRSTENERGY CORP**
Clinac; **VARIAN MEDICAL SYSTEMS INC**
Clinical Research International, Inc.; **IGATE CORPORATION**
Clinical Research Services; **PAREXEL INTERNATIONAL CORP**
Clinique; **ESTEE LAUDER COMPANIES INC (THE)**
Club Foods; **SUPERVALU INC**
Club Monaco; **POLO RALPH LAUREN CORP**
clubbebe; **BEBE STORES INC**

INDEX OF SUBSIDIARIES, BRAND NAMES AND AFFILIATIONS, CONT.

CMT: Country Music Television; **VIACOM INC**

CNA Financial Corp.; **LOEWS CORPORATION**

CNX Gas Corporation; **CONSOL ENERGY INC**

CNX Land Resources Inc; **CONSOL ENERGY INC**

Coach Japan, Inc.; **COACH INC**

Coach Legacy; **COACH INC**

Coach.com; **COACH INC**

Coag Dx; **IDEXX LABORATORIES INC**

Coalition of Kaiser Permanente Unions (The); **KAISER PERMANENTE COALSALES LLC; PEABODY ENERGY CORP**

Coban; **ELI LILLY & COMPANY**

Cobb; **TYSON FOODS INC**

Coca Cola Co; **COCA COLA ENTERPRISES INC**

CoCreate Software GmbH; **PARAMETRIC TECHNOLOGY CORP**

Cognio, Inc.; **CISCO SYSTEMS INC**

Coldwatercreek.com; **COLDWATER CREEK INC**

Cole Haan Holdings, Inc.; **NIKE INC**

Colilert-18; **IDEXX LABORATORIES INC**

Colisure; **IDEXX LABORATORIES INC**

Collateral Therapeutics; **SCHERING-PLOUGH CORP**

Colleague CX; **BAXTER INTERNATIONAL INC**

College for Financial Planning, Inc.; **APOLLO GROUP INC**

Colorscapes; **GEORGIA GULF CORPORATION**

ColorTyme, Inc.; **RENT-A-CENTER INC**

Columbia Paint & Coatings Co.; **SHERWIN WILLIAMS COMPANY (THE)**

Columbus Depot Equipment Company; **TOTAL SYSTEM SERVICES INC (TSYS)**

Columbus Productions; **TOTAL SYSTEM SERVICES INC (TSYS)**

Comcast Interactive Media; **COMCAST CORP**

Comcast Spectator; **COMCAST CORP**

Comedy Central; **VIACOM INC**

Commonwealth Edison Company; **EXELON CORPORATION**

Commonwealth Telephone Enterprises, Inc.; **FRONTIER COMMUNICATIONS CORPORATION**

CompBenefits Corporation; **HUMANA INC**

Comperio; **PRICEWATERHOUSECOOPERS**

CompuSafe; **BRINKS COMPANY (THE)**

Compuware Corp; **KEANE INC**

Condevor AB; **CIBER INC**

Congress Center (The); **LAS VEGAS SANDS CORP (THE VENETIAN)**

Connecticut Storage Fund; **PUBLIC STORAGE INC**

Conoco; **CONOCOPHILLIPS COMPANY**

Conor Medsystems, Inc.; **JOHNSON & JOHNSON**

Conrad Hotels and Resorts; **HILTON HOTELS CORP**

Conrail, Inc.; **NORFOLK SOUTHERN CORP**

Consolidated Edison Company of New York, Inc.; **CONSOLIDATED EDISON INC**

Consolidated Edison Development; **CONSOLIDATED EDISON INC**

Consolidated Edison Energy; **CONSOLIDATED EDISON INC**

Consolidated Edison Solutions; **CONSOLIDATED EDISON INC**

Consolidated Rail Corp.; **NORFOLK SOUTHERN CORP**

Constellation Energy Group; **BALTIMORE GAS AND ELECTRIC COMPANY**

Consumer Delivery Network; **EXEL TRANSPORTATION SERVICES INC (DHL EXEL)**

Contact Center Services; **SYKES ENTERPRISES INC**

Continuous Glucose Monitoring; **MEDTRONIC INC**

Convatec; **BRISTOL MYERS SQUIBB CO**

Converse Inc; **NIKE INC**

Cooper Cameron Corporation; **CAMERON INTERNATIONAL CORPORATION**

CooperSurgical, Inc.; **COOPER COMPANIES INC**

CooperVision, Inc.; **COOPER COMPANIES INC**

Coppertone; **SCHERING-PLOUGH CORP**

CopyCentre; **XEROX CORP**

CORA Health Services, Inc; **SELECT MEDICAL CORPORATION**

Cordis Corp; **JOHNSON & JOHNSON**

Cordovan; **TBC CORPORATION**

Core Payroll; **PAYCHEX INC**

Core Plan; **WEIGHT WATCHERS INTERNATIONAL INC**

Corian; **E I DU PONT DE NEMOURS & CO (DUPONT)**

Corliant, Inc.; **ACCENTURE LTD**

Corner Store; **VALERO ENERGY CORP**

Cornerstone Brands; **IAC/INTERACTIVECORP**

Cort Business Services Corporation; **BERKSHIRE HATHAWAY INC**

Cost Plus; **COST PLUS INC**

Cost Plus World Market; **COST PLUS INC**

Costa Cruises; **CARNIVAL CORPORATION**

Costco Wholesale Industries; **COSTCO WHOLESALE CORP**

CostTrack; **OWENS & MINOR INC**

Cotai Strip; **LAS VEGAS SANDS CORP (THE VENETIAN)**

Countrywide Financial Corp; **BANK OF AMERICA CORP**

Courtyard by Marriott; **LODGIAN INC**

Courtyard Residence Inn; **MARRIOTT INTERNATIONAL INC**

Cover Girl; **PROCTER & GAMBLE CO**

CoverageFirst; **ARTHUR J GALLAGHER & CO**

Cox Business Services; **COX COMMUNICATIONS INC**

Cox Cable; **COX COMMUNICATIONS INC**

Cox Digital Cable; **COX COMMUNICATIONS INC**

Cox Digital Telephone; **COX COMMUNICATIONS INC**

Cox Enterprises, Inc.; **COX COMMUNICATIONS INC**

Cox High Speed; **COX COMMUNICATIONS INC**

Cozaar; **MERCK & CO INC**

Crab House (The); **LANDRY'S RESTAURANTS INC**

Cracker Barrel Old Country Store; **CBRL GROUP INC**

Craftsman; **DANAHER CORP**

Creamland; **DEAN FOODS CO**

Creative Games International; **GTECH HOLDINGS CORP**

Creative Group (The); **ROBERT HALF INTERNATIONAL INC**

Credit Migration Solutions; **EXPERIAN AMERICAS**

CredStar; **FIRST ADVANTAGE CORPORATION**

Crescent Resources, LLC; **DUKE ENERGY CORP**

Crest; **PROCTER & GAMBLE CO**

Crestview Aerospace; **L-3 COMMUNICATIONS HOLDINGS INC**

CRI, Inc.; **MANPOWER INC**

Crisco; **JM SMUCKER CO**

Croissan'wich; **BURGER KING HOLDINGS INC**

Crowne Plaza; **LODGIAN INC**

Csi-The Remuneration Specialists; **HEWITT ASSOCIATES**

CSS Informatics; **PHARMACEUTICAL PRODUCT DEVELOPMENT INC**

CSX Corp; **CSX TRANSPORTATION INC**

INDEX OF SUBSIDIARIES, BRAND NAMES AND AFFILIATIONS, CONT.

CSX Corp; **NORFOLK SOUTHERN CORP**
CSX Hotels, Inc.; **CSX CORP**
CSX Intermodal, Inc.; **CSX CORP**
CSX Real Property, Inc.; **CSX CORP**
CSX Technology; **CSX CORP**
CSX Transportation, Inc.; **CSX CORP**
CTE; **AECOM TECHNOLOGY CORPORATION**
CTS Electronics Manufacturing Solutions; **CTS CORP**
Cub Condo; **BUILD-A-BEAR WORKSHOP INC**
CubCase; **BUILD-A-BEAR WORKSHOP INC**
Cubic Advanced Tactical Systems, LLC; **CUBIC CORP**
Cubic Applications, Inc.; **CUBIC CORP**
Cubic Defence New Zealand, Ltd.; **CUBIC CORP**
Cubic Defense Systems, Inc.; **CUBIC CORP**
Cubic Fiend Services, Ltd.; **CUBIC CORP**
Cubic Transportation Systems,Ltd.; **CUBIC CORP**
Cummins Power Generation; **CUMMINS INC**
Cunard Line; **CARNIVAL CORPORATION**
CuraScript, Inc.; **EXPRESS SCRIPTS INC**
Cusp; **NEIMAN MARCUS GROUP INC (THE)**
CVS Corp.; **CVS CAREMARK CORPORATION**
CVS/pharmacy; **CVS CAREMARK CORPORATION**
CyAn ADP Analyzer; **BECKMAN COULTER INC**
Dale Surgical Professional Supply, Inc.; **PATTERSON COMPANIES INC**
Dallas Semiconductor Corp; **MAXIM INTEGRATED PRODUCTS INC**
Damcos Holding A/S; **EMERSON ELECTRIC CO**
Dana Petroleum plc; **DEVON ENERGY CORPORATION**
Danaher Corp; **TEKTRONIX INC**
Dasani; **COCA COLA COMPANY (THE)**
Data ONTAP; **NETWORK APPLIANCE INC**
Data ONTAP; **NETWORK APPLIANCE INC**
Data Services; **FIRST ADVANTAGE CORPORATION**
DataFlux; **SAS INSTITUTE INC**
DaVita Clinical Research; **DAVITA INC**
DaVita Rx; **DAVITA INC**
Davol, Inc.; **CR BARD INC**
Days Inn; **WYNDHAM WORLDWIDE**
DAYTON; **WW GRAINGER INC**

DC; **QUIKSILVER INC**
DDB Worldwide; **OMNICOM GROUP INC**
dd's DISCOUNTS; **ROSS STORES INC**
De Beer; **VALSPAR CORPORATION (THE)**
Dealer Services; **FIRST ADVANTAGE CORPORATION**
Decision Power; **HEALTH NET INC**
Decus Insurance Brokers, Limited; **BROWN & BROWN INC**
Deerbrook; **ALLSTATE CORPORATION (THE)**
Defense Transformation; **SAIC INC**
Definity Health; **UNITEDHEALTH GROUP INC**
DEK Energy Company; **APACHE CORP**
Del Amo Storage Partners, Ltd.; **PUBLIC STORAGE INC**
Delaware Management Holdings, Inc.; **LINCOLN NATIONAL CORPORATION**
Deloitte & Touche LLP; **DELOITTE & TOUCHE USA LLP**
Deloitte Consulting; **DELOITTE & TOUCHE USA LLP**
Deloitte Financial Advisory Services; **DELOITTE & TOUCHE USA LLP**
Deloitte Tax; **DELOITTE & TOUCHE USA LLP**
Deloitte Touche Tohmatsu; **DELOITTE & TOUCHE USA LLP**
Deloitte Touche Tohmatsu; **DELOITTE CONSULTING LLP**
Delta Consolidated Industries; **DANAHER CORP**
Denny's Holdings, Inc.; **DENNY'S CORPORATION**
Denny's, Inc.; **DENNY'S CORPORATION**
Dent Demon; **ADESA INC**
Dental Benefits Providers; **UNITEDHEALTH GROUP INC**
Dentrix; **HENRY SCHEIN INC**
Department of Defense; **FLUOR CORP**
Department of Energy; **FLUOR CORP**
Department of Homeland Security; **FLUOR CORP**
Depend; **KIMBERLY-CLARK CORP**
Depuy Inc; **JOHNSON & JOHNSON**
Design Studio; **WILLIAMS SONOMA INC**
Detach; **STERIS CORP**
Detroit Edison Company (The); **DTE ENERGY COMPANY**
Deutsche Post; **EXEL TRANSPORTATION SERVICES INC (DHL EXEL)**
Deutsche Telekom AG; **T-MOBILE USA**
DeVry University; **DEVRY INC**
DeWALT; **BLACK & DECKER CORP**

DHL Worldwide Network; **EXEL TRANSPORTATION SERVICES INC (DHL EXEL)**
DHM Holding Company; **DOLE FOOD COMPANY INC**
Diabetes @ Home; **AMEDISYS INC**
Diabetes Healthways; **HEALTHWAYS INC**
DiaMed Holding AG; **BIO RAD LABORATORIES INC**
Diamond Offshore Drilling, Inc.; **LOEWS CORPORATION**
Diamond Shamrock; **VALERO ENERGY CORP**
Diamondoids; **CHEVRON CORPORATION**
Dianon Systems, Inc.; **LABORATORY CORP OF AMERICA HOLDINGS**
Diebold 450 ATM; **DIEBOLD INC**
Diebold Elections Systems, Inc.; **DIEBOLD INC**
Diebold International; **DIEBOLD INC**
Diebold North America; **DIEBOLD INC**
Digiplug S.A.S.; **ACCENTURE LTD**
Digital Insight Corp.; **INTUIT INC**
Digital Signal Controllers; **MICROCHIP TECHNOLOGY INC**
Dimensions International; **HONEYWELL INTERNATIONAL INC**
Dimetapp; **WYETH**
Direct-Q 3; **MILLIPORE CORP**
DIRECTV Latin America; **DIRECTV GROUP INC (THE)**
DIRECTV U.S.; **DIRECTV GROUP INC (THE)**
Discovery Verification Platform; **SYNOPSYS INC**
DISH Network Corp.; **ECHOSTAR CORP**
Disney Classics; **MATTEL INC**
Disney En Familia; **WALT DISNEY COMPANY (THE)**
Diversified Freight Logistics, Inc.; **BURLINGTON NORTHERN SANTA FE CORP**
DMJM Aviation; **AECOM TECHNOLOGY CORPORATION**
Dobson Communications Corp.; **AT&T INC**
DOCSIS 1.1; **BROADCOM CORP**
DocuColor; **XEROX CORP**
Documentum; **EMC CORP**
Dogwood Canyon; **BASS PRO SHOPS INC**
DolEx; **GLOBAL PAYMENTS INC**
Dollar Rent A Car, Inc.; **DOLLAR THRIFTY AUTOMOTIVE GROUP INC**
Dollar Thrifty Funding Corp.; **DOLLAR THRIFTY AUTOMOTIVE GROUP INC**
Domain; **MARY KAY INC**

INDEX OF SUBSIDIARIES, BRAND NAMES AND AFFILIATIONS, CONT.

DonJoy; **DJO INC**
Doritos; **PEPSICO INC**
DoubleClick; **GOOGLE INC**
Doublemint; **WM WRIGLEY JR COMPANY**
Douwe Egberts; **SARA LEE CORP**
Dow Jones & Co Inc; **NEWS CORP**
Dr. Scholl's; **SCHERING-PLOUGH CORP**
Dragon Development Corp.; **CACI INTERNATIONAL INC**
Draxxin; **PFIZER INC**
DreamWorks SKG; **VIACOM INC**
Dress Barn Woman; **DRESS BARN INC (THE)**
dsPIC; **MICROCHIP TECHNOLOGY INC**
DSX1/3; **ADC TELECOMMUNICATIONS INC**
DTE Biomass Energy; **DTE ENERGY COMPANY**
DTE Coal Services; **DTE ENERGY COMPANY**
DTE Energy Services; **DTE ENERGY COMPANY**
DTG Operations, Inc.; **DOLLAR THRIFTY AUTOMOTIVE GROUP INC**
Dual Core; **INTEL CORP**
Dual-Core Intel Itanium; **INTEL CORP**
Dual-Core Intel Xeon; **INTEL CORP**
Duane Arnold Energy Center; **FPL GROUP INC**
Duckworth Flavors; **CARGILL INC**
Duke Energy Field Services LLC; **CONOCOPHILLIPS COMPANY**
Duke Energy Generation Services; **DUKE ENERGY CORP**
Duke Energy International, LLC; **DUKE ENERGY CORP**
Duke Investments, LLC; **BRINKER INTERNATIONAL INC**
Dunn's; **CABELA'S INC**
Duron Inc; **SHERWIN WILLIAMS COMPANY (THE)**
Dustbuster; **BLACK & DECKER CORP**
Dutch Boy; **SHERWIN WILLIAMS COMPANY (THE)**
Dynastar; **QUIKSILVER INC**
E! Channel; **COMCAST CORP**
EA Casual Entertainment; **ELECTRONIC ARTS INC**
EA GAMES; **ELECTRONIC ARTS INC**
EA SPORTS; **ELECTRONIC ARTS INC**
EA-6B; **NORTHROP GRUMMAN CORP**
Eagle Family Foods Holdings, Inc.; **JM SMUCKER CO**
Easy Dental; **HENRY SCHEIN INC**
easyedge; **UNITED STATES CELLULAR CORP**
Easywell; **HALLIBURTON COMPANY**

EB Games; **GAMESTOP CORP**
eBay Express; **EBAY INC**
ebgames.com; **GAMESTOP CORP**
EchoStar Holding Corp.; **ECHOSTAR CORP**
Edge Wireless; **AT&T INC**
Edison Capital; **EDISON INTERNATIONAL**
Edison Mission Energy; **EDISON INTERNATIONAL**
Edwards and Kelcey; **JACOBS ENGINEERING GROUP INC**
EEPROM; **MICROCHIP TECHNOLOGY INC**
EG&G Division; **URS CORPORATION**
Eggo; **KELLOGG CO**
EGL Acquisition Corp.; **SELECT MEDICAL CORPORATION**
eKendleCollege; **KENDLE INTERNATIONAL INC**
Elan; **MANPOWER INC**
Electronics Japan, GK; **ARROW ELECTRONICS INC**
Electropura; **PEPSI BOTTLING GROUP INC**
Eletropaulo Metropolitana Electricidad; **AES CORPORATION (THE)**
Elfa; **CONTAINER STORE (THE)**
Elige; **MARY KAY INC**
Elite Protection Services; **ABM INDUSTRIES INC**
Elm Power Corp.; **PG&E CORPORATION**
Embassy Suits; **HILTON HOTELS CORP**
Embrace; **MARY KAY INC**
EMEND; **MERCK & CO INC**
Emerald Renewable Energy LLC; **CARGILL INC**
Emhart Teknologies; **BLACK & DECKER CORP**
Employer Services; **FIRST ADVANTAGE CORPORATION**
Enbrel; **AMGEN INC**
Encoda Systems Holdings, Inc.; **HARRIS CORPORATION**
Encom Holdings Pty Ltd.; **PITNEY BOWES INC**
Encompass; **ALLSTATE CORPORATION (THE)**
Encore Suites at Wynn Las Vegas; **WYNN RESORTS LIMITED**
Endius, Inc.; **ZIMMER HOLDINGS INC**
EndoArt S.A.; **ALLERGAN INC**
Energy Brands, Inc.; **COCA COLA COMPANY (THE)**
Energy Technology Company; **CHEVRON CORPORATION**
Enexus Energy Corporation; **ENTERGY CORP**
Enfamil; **BRISTOL MYERS SQUIBB CO**

Enlightened; **BAXTER INTERNATIONAL INC**
Enraf Holdings B.V.; **HONEYWELL INTERNATIONAL INC**
Ensure; **ABBOTT LABORATORIES**
Entergy Arkansas; **ENTERGY CORP**
Entergy Louisiana; **ENTERGY CORP**
Entergy Mississipi; **ENTERGY CORP**
Entergy New Orleans; **ENTERGY CORP**
Entergy Texas; **ENTERGY CORP**
Enterprise Car Sales; **ENTERPRISE RENT-A-CAR**
Enterprise Fleet Services; **ENTERPRISE RENT-A-CAR**
Enterprise Rent-a-Car; **ENTERPRISE RENT-A-CAR**
Enterprise Rent-a-Truck; **ENTERPRISE RENT-A-CAR**
Entrepreneur of the Year Award; **ERNST & YOUNG LLP**
Eon; **ST JUDE MEDICAL INC**
eONE Global, LP; **FIRST DATA CORP**
EP MedSystems, Inc.; **ST JUDE MEDICAL INC**
Epichem Group, Ltd.; **SIGMA-ALDRICH CORP**
EPOGEN; **AMGEN INC**
EPROM Memory; **MICROCHIP TECHNOLOGY INC**
Epsilon; **ALLIANCE DATA SYSTEMS CORPORATION**
Era Aviation Inc.; **SEACOR HOLDINGS INC**
EraMed LLC; **SEACOR HOLDINGS INC**
Ernst & Young International; **ERNST & YOUNG LLP**
Ernst & Young Online; **ERNST & YOUNG LLP**
E-Series; **JUNIPER NETWORKS INC**
E-site Marketing; **SABRE HOLDINGS CORP**
Esoterix, Inc.; **LABORATORY CORP OF AMERICA HOLDINGS**
ESPN Inc; **WALT DISNEY COMPANY (THE)**
Esprit Pharma Holdings; **ALLERGAN INC**
Ethicon Inc; **JOHNSON & JOHNSON**
Eurenov S.A.S.; **CATERPILLAR INC**
Europa Apotheek Venlo; **MEDCO HEALTH SOLUTIONS**
Europrint; **GTECH HOLDINGS CORP**
Ever; **AFLAC INC**
EverGreen; **SCOTTS MIRACLE GROW CO**
Everything About the Music; **HOT TOPIC INC**
Excalibur; **MGM MIRAGE**
Excede; **PFIZER INC**
Excedrin; **BRISTOL MYERS SQUIBB CO**

INDEX OF SUBSIDIARIES, BRAND NAMES AND AFFILIATIONS, CONT.

Excel Coal Ltd.; **PEABODY ENERGY CORP**
ExcellerateHRO; **TOWERS PERRIN**
ExecuStay; **MARRIOTT INTERNATIONAL INC**
Executive Choice; **BJ'S WHOLESALE CLUB INC**
Executive Risk Indemnity, Inc; **CHUBB CORPORATION (THE)**
Exel plc; **EXEL TRANSPORTATION SERVICES INC (DHL EXEL)**
Exelon Generation Company, LLC; **EXELON CORPORATION**
exp.o; **EXPEDITORS INTERNATIONAL OF WASHINGTON INC**
Experian Group; **EXPERIAN AMERICAS**
Experian Information Solutions, Inc.; **EXPERIAN AMERICAS**
Experimental & Applied Sciences Inc; **ABBOTT LABORATORIES**
EXPO Design Centers; **HOME DEPOT INC**
expresscopy.com; **INFOUSA INC**
Exxon Neftegas Limited; **EXXON MOBIL CORPORATION (EXXONMOBIL)**
ExxonMobil Chemica; **EXXON MOBIL CORPORATION (EXXONMOBIL)**
Ezeflow, Inc.; **SHAW GROUP INC (THE)**
F/A-18; **NORTHROP GRUMMAN CORP**
F-15 Eagle; **BOEING COMPANY (THE)**
F-35; **NORTHROP GRUMMAN CORP**
Faber Maunsell; **AECOM TECHNOLOGY CORPORATION**
Fabric.com; **AMAZON.COM INC**
Facconable; **NORDSTROM INC**
Fair, Isaac & Company, Inc.; **FAIR ISAAC CORPORATION**
Fairfield Inn; **MARRIOTT INTERNATIONAL INC**
Family Invest AB; **TWEEN BRANDS INC**
Fandango Inc; **COMCAST CORP**
Farm Fresh; **SUPERVALU INC**
Farrington American Express Travel Services Ltd.; **AMERICAN EXPRESS CO**
Fashion Bug; **CHARMING SHOPPES INC**
Fasson; **AVERY DENNISON CORP**
Federal Insurance Company; **CHUBB CORPORATION (THE)**
Federated Department Stores, Inc.; **MACY'S INC**
FedEx Custom Critical Inc; **FEDEX CORPORATION**
FedEx Express Corp; **FEDEX CORPORATION**

FedEx Freight Corp; **FEDEX CORPORATION**
FedEx Ground Package System Inc; **FEDEX CORPORATION**
FedEx Kinkos Office And Print Services Inc; **FEDEX CORPORATION**
FedEx Supply Chain Services Inc; **FEDEX CORPORATION**
FedEx Trade Networks Inc; **FEDEX CORPORATION**
Fentora; **CEPHALON INC**
Ferncliff TIH AS; **PRIDE INTERNATIONAL INC**
Ferrlecit; **WATSON PHARMACEUTICALS INC**
Fiber Guide Raceway; **ADC TELECOMMUNICATIONS INC**
FICO Score Simulator; **FAIR ISAAC CORPORATION**
Fifty-Four by Fossil; **FOSSIL INC**
Figi's; **CHARMING SHOPPES INC**
Filenet Corp; **INTERNATIONAL BUSINESS MACHINES CORP (IBM)**
Filet-O-Fish; **MCDONALD'S CORP**
Finish Line; **FINISH LINE INC (THE)**
Finn-Aqua; **STERIS CORP**
FinSecure LLC; **W R BERKLEY CORPORATION**
Finsoft; **GTECH HOLDINGS CORP**
Firestone Country Club; **CLUBCORP INC**
Firethorn Holdings, LLC; **QUALCOMM INC**
FireWire; **WESTERN DIGITAL CORP**
First Data Resources; **FIRST DATA CORP**
Fiserv Inc; **FIRST ADVANTAGE CORPORATION**
Fisher-Price; **MATTEL INC**
Fitigues; **CHICO'S FAS INC**
Fit-Rite Body Parts & Affilliates; **LKQ CORP**
Flash; **MICROCHIP TECHNOLOGY INC**
FLAVORx; **RITE AID CORPORATION**
FleetBoston; **BANK OF AMERICA CORP**
Fleming's Prime Steakhouse; **OSI RESTAURANT PARTNERS INC**
Flex Global View; **UNITED PARCEL SERVICE INC (UPS)**
Flex Plan; **WEIGHT WATCHERS INTERNATIONAL INC**
Flex Recubrimientos, Acabados Automotrices; **SHERWIN WILLIAMS COMPANY (THE)**
FlexRig3; **HELMERICH & PAYNE INC**
FlexRig4; **HELMERICH & PAYNE INC**
FlexRigs; **HELMERICH & PAYNE INC**
FlexVol; **NETWORK APPLIANCE INC**
Flight Options LLC; **RAYTHEON CO**

Flint Hills Resources; **KOCH INDUSTRIES INC**
Flip-Off; **WEST PHARMACEUTICAL SERVICES INC**
Florida Power & Light Company; **FPL GROUP INC**
Fluor Construction Company; **FLUOR CORP**
Focus Diagnostics, Inc.; **QUEST DIAGNOSTICS INC**
Focus Europe, S.r.l.; **GUESS? INC**
Food & Wine; **AMERICAN EXPRESS CO**
FootJoy; **FORTUNE BRANDS INC**
Foray; **OFFICE DEPOT INC**
Ford Motor Co.; **TELETECH HOLDINGS INC**
Forest Laboratories Europe; **FOREST LABORATORIES INC**
Forest Pharmaceuticals, Inc.; **FOREST LABORATORIES INC**
Forest Research Institute; **FOREST LABORATORIES INC**
Fosamax; **MERCK & CO INC**
Fossil; **FOSSIL INC**
Foster Wheeler Constructors; **FOSTER WHEELER LTD**
Foster Wheeler Energy, Ltd.; **FOSTER WHEELER LTD**
Foster Wheeler International Corp.; **FOSTER WHEELER LTD**
Foster Wheeler Power Machinery Co., Ltd.; **FOSTER WHEELER LTD**
Foster Wheeler Review; **FOSTER WHEELER LTD**
Four Points; **STARWOOD HOTELS & RESORTS WORLDWIDE INC**
Fox Broadcasting Company; **NEWS CORP**
Fox Entertainment Group Inc; **NEWS CORP**
Fox Filmed Entertainment; **FOX ENTERTAINMENT GROUP INC**
Fox Interactive Media; **FOX ENTERTAINMENT GROUP INC**
Fox Sports Net Inc; **NEWS CORP**
Fox Television Studios; **FOX ENTERTAINMENT GROUP INC**
FPL Energy Power Marking, Inc.; **FPL GROUP INC**
FPL Energy, LLC; **FPL GROUP INC**
FPL FiberNet, LLC; **FPL GROUP INC**
FPL Group Capitol; **FPL GROUP INC**
FRAM; **HONEYWELL INTERNATIONAL INC**
Franchised Electric & Gas Service; **DUKE ENERGY CORP**
Franciscan Health System; **CATHOLIC HEALTH INITIATIVES**
Franklin Group (The); **INVENTIV HEALTH INC**
Fred's; **FRED'S INC**

INDEX OF SUBSIDIARIES, BRAND NAMES AND AFFILIATIONS, CONT.

Fred's Pharmacies; **FRED'S INC**
Free People; **URBAN OUTFITTERS INC**
Freedom of the Seas; **ROYAL CARIBBEAN CRUISES**
Fresh 1 (The); **CH ROBINSON WORLDWIDE INC**
Fresh Apple Fries; **BURGER KING HOLDINGS INC**
Friends 2B Made; **BUILD-A-BEAR WORKSHOP INC**
Frito-Lay Inc; **PEPSICO INC**
Frontier Pages; **FRONTIER COMMUNICATIONS CORPORATION**
Frosty; **WENDYS INTERNATIONAL INC**
Fry's; **KROGER CO (THE)**
Fuji Xerox; **XEROX CORP**
Future Shop, Ltd.; **BEST BUY CO INC**
G.A. Pearson and Associates Insurance Brokers, Inc; **HILB ROGAL & HOBBS CO**
Galavision; **UNIVISION COMMUNICATIONS INC**
Galaxy Design Platform; **SYNOPSYS INC**
Gallagher Basset Services, Inc.; **ARTHUR J GALLAGHER & CO**
Gallagher Benefit Administrators; **ARTHUR J GALLAGHER & CO**
Gallagher RE; **ARTHUR J GALLAGHER & CO**
Galls; **ARAMARK CORPORATION**
Galpharm Healthcare, Ltd.; **PERRIGO CO**
Game Informer Magazine; **GAMESTOP CORP**
Games Media Limited; **SCIENTIFIC GAMES CORPORATION**
Games Media Ltd.; **SCIENTIFIC GAMES CORPORATION**
GameStop.com; **GAMESTOP CORP**
Garci Crespo; **PEPSI BOTTLING GROUP INC**
Gardasil; **MERCK & CO INC**
Gateway Energy and Coke Company; **SUNOCO INC**
Gatorade; **PEPSICO INC**
GE Aviation; **GENERAL ELECTRIC CO (GE)**
GE Commercial Finance; **GENERAL ELECTRIC CO (GE)**
GE Equipment Services; **GENERAL ELECTRIC CO (GE)**
GE Healthcare; **GENERAL ELECTRIC CO (GE)**
GE Industrial; **GENERAL ELECTRIC CO (GE)**
GE Infrastructure; **GENERAL ELECTRIC CO (GE)**
GE Money; **GENERAL ELECTRIC CO (GE)**

Geek Squad; **BEST BUY CO INC**
Geesink; **OSHKOSH CORPORATION**
GEICO Corporation; **BERKSHIRE HATHAWAY INC**
GemomeLab GeXP; **BECKMAN COULTER INC**
Gemzar; **ELI LILLY & COMPANY**
GeneOhm Sciences; **BECTON DICKINSON & CO**
General Dynamics Advanced Information Systems; **GENERAL DYNAMICS CORP**
General Dynamics C4 Systems; **GENERAL DYNAMICS CORP**
General Ledger Services; **PAYCHEX INC**
General Re Corporation; **BERKSHIRE HATHAWAY INC**
Genesco, Inc.; **FINISH LINE INC (THE)**
Genyx Medical, Inc.; **CR BARD INC**
GEO Care, Inc.; **GEO GROUP INC**
Georgia Power Company; **SOUTHERN COMPANY (THE)**
Georgia-Pacific Corp; **KOCH INDUSTRIES INC**
GEPetrol; **DEVON ENERGY CORPORATION**
Gestalt, LLC; **ACCENTURE LTD**
Get It Now; **RENT-A-CENTER INC**
getthere.com; **SABRE HOLDINGS CORP**
Gifts-To-Go; **COLDWATER CREEK INC**
Gillete; **PROCTER & GAMBLE CO**
Gilly Hicks; **ABERCROMBIE & FITCH CO**
Ginzton Technology Center; **VARIAN MEDICAL SYSTEMS INC**
Global Automotive Parts; **LKQ CORP**
Global Best Practices; **PRICEWATERHOUSECOOPERS**
Global Business Services; **PITNEY BOWES INC**
Global Hawk; **NORTHROP GRUMMAN CORP**
Global Imaging Systems, Inc.; **XEROX CORP**
Global Learning Center; **MANPOWER INC**
Global Mailstream Solutions; **PITNEY BOWES INC**
Global Payments Europe; **GLOBAL PAYMENTS INC**
Global Risk Services; **HEWITT ASSOCIATES**
Global Services; **INTERNATIONAL BUSINESS MACHINES CORP (IBM)**
Global Spectrum LP; **COMCAST CORP**
Global Valley Networks; **FRONTIER COMMUNICATIONS CORPORATION**
Global VATOnline; **PRICEWATERHOUSECOOPERS**

GlobalSantaFe Corp; **TRANSOCEAN INC**
Globelle Corp.; **TECH DATA CORP**
Gmarket Inc.; **YAHOO! INC**
Go-Go Taquitos; **7-ELEVEN INC**
Golden Nugget Hotels & Casinos; **LANDRY'S RESTAURANTS INC**
Golden Rule Insurance Company; **UNITEDHEALTH GROUP INC**
Goldston Engineering, Inc.; **CH2M HILL COMPANIES LTD**
Golf Channel (The); **COMCAST CORP**
Golf Galaxy; **DICK'S SPORTING GOODS INC**
Good Samaritan Health Systems; **CATHOLIC HEALTH INITIATIVES**
Goodby, Silverstein & Partners; **OMNICOM GROUP INC**
Goodhealth Worldwide; **AETNA INC**
Google; **GOOGLE INC**
Google AdSense; **GOOGLE INC**
Google AdWords; **GOOGLE INC**
Goowy Media, Inc.; **TIME WARNER INC**
GP Investments, Ltd.; **PRIDE INTERNATIONAL INC**
Grainger Caribe, Inc.; **WW GRAINGER INC**
Grainger China LLC; **WW GRAINGER INC**
Grainger Industrial Supply; **WW GRAINGER INC**
Grainger, S.A. de C.V.; **WW GRAINGER INC**
Grammaloy Holdings, L.P.; **NATIONAL OILWELL VARCO INC**
Grand Hyatt; **GLOBAL HYATT CORPORATION**
Grande Cuisine; **WILLIAMS SONOMA INC**
Grant Prideco Inc; **NATIONAL OILWELL VARCO INC**
Grant Thornton International; **GRANT THORNTON LLP**
Grant Thornton U.S.A.; **GRANT THORNTON LLP**
Grateful Harvest; **UNITED NATURAL FOODS INC**
Grayloc Products; **OCEANEERING INTERNATIONAL INC**
Greenbrier (The); **CSX CORP**
GroceryWorks; **SAFEWAY INC**
Group 1 Software, Inc.; **PITNEY BOWES INC**
Grove; **CAMERON INTERNATIONAL CORPORATION**
GS Capital Partners; **ARAMARK CORPORATION**
GSW Worldwide; **INVENTIV HEALTH INC**
Guard Libang; **SCIENTIFIC GAMES CORPORATION**

INDEX OF SUBSIDIARIES, BRAND NAMES AND AFFILIATIONS, CONT.

Guess? Jeans; **GUESS? INC**
Guidant; **BOSTON SCIENTIFIC CORP**
Gulf Power Company; **SOUTHERN COMPANY (THE)**
Gulfstream Aerospace; **GENERAL DYNAMICS CORP**
Guy Carpenter & Company, LLC; **MARSH & MCLENNAN COMPANIES INC**
GVN Services; **FRONTIER COMMUNICATIONS CORPORATION**
H.B. Fuller; **VALSPAR CORPORATION (THE)**
H.B. Maynard and Co., Inc.; **ACCENTURE LTD**
Haagen-Dazs; **GENERAL MILLS INC**
Hair Club for Men & Women; **REGIS CORPORATION**
Halogen; **NORDSTROM INC**
Hamilton Sundstrand; **UNITED TECHNOLOGIES CORPORATION**
Hampton Inn; **HILTON HOTELS CORP**
Hand Held Products, Inc.; **HONEYWELL INTERNATIONAL INC**
Happy Meal; **MCDONALD'S CORP**
Harborside Healthcare Corporation; **SUN HEALTHCARE GROUP**
Harmon Stores, Inc.; **BED BATH & BEYOND INC**
HarperCollins Publishers Inc; **NEWS CORP**
Harrah's; **HARRAH'S ENTERTAINMENT INC**
Harrah's Operating Company, Inc.; **HARRAH'S ENTERTAINMENT INC**
Hartford Fire Insurance Company; **HARTFORD FINANCIAL SERVICES GROUP INC (THE)**
Hartford International Management Services Company; **HARTFORD FINANCIAL SERVICES GROUP INC (THE)**
Hartford Investment Financial Services, LLC; **HARTFORD FINANCIAL SERVICES GROUP INC (THE)**
Hartford Life and Accident; **HARTFORD FINANCIAL SERVICES GROUP INC (THE)**
Hartford Life and Annuity; **HARTFORD FINANCIAL SERVICES GROUP INC (THE)**
Hartford Life Group Insurance Company; **HARTFORD FINANCIAL SERVICES GROUP INC (THE)**
Hartford Life Insurance Company; **HARTFORD FINANCIAL SERVICES GROUP INC (THE)**
Hartford Mutual Funds, Inc. (The); **HARTFORD FINANCIAL SERVICES GROUP INC (THE)**

Hartford Wolf Pack; **CABLEVISION SYSTEMS CORP**
Hat World Corporation; **GENESCO INC**
Hat Zone; **GENESCO INC**
Havok; **INTEL CORP**
Hawaiian Electric Company; **HAWAIIAN ELECTRIC INDUSTRIES INC**
Hawaiian Electric Light Company; **HAWAIIAN ELECTRIC INDUSTRIES INC**
Hawthorne Benefit Technologies, Inc.; **PAYCHEX INC**
HCR Manor Care; **MANOR CARE INC**
HDS Cosmetics Lab, Inc.; **PROCTER & GAMBLE CO**
Headwater LLC; **ANADARKO PETROLEUM CORPORATION**
HealthAmerica; **COVENTRY HEALTH CARE INC**
HealthAssurance; **COVENTRY HEALTH CARE INC**
HealthLink, Inc.; **WELLPOINT INC**
HealthSouth; **SELECT MEDICAL CORPORATION**
Healthy Choice; **CONAGRA FOODS INC**
Healthy Pet Corp.; **VCA ANTECH INC**
Heart @ Home; **AMEDISYS INC**
Heart of Florida Regional Medical Center; **HEALTH MANAGEMENT ASSOCIATES INC**
Heartland; **MANOR CARE INC**
H-E-B; **HE BUTT GROCERY COMPANY (HEB)**
H-E-B Insurance Agency; **HE BUTT GROCERY COMPANY (HEB)**
H-E-B Mobile; **HE BUTT GROCERY COMPANY (HEB)**
H-E-B plus!; **HE BUTT GROCERY COMPANY (HEB)**
HEI Diversified; **HAWAIIAN ELECTRIC INDUSTRIES INC**
Heil Beauty Supply; **ALBERTO-CULVER COMPANY**
Hennessy Industries; **DANAHER CORP**
HeptaCon; **HEWITT ASSOCIATES**
HEPTIMAX; **QUEST DIAGNOSTICS INC**
Herceptin; **GENENTECH INC**
Hershey Import Co.; **UNITED NATURAL FOODS INC**
Hershey's; **DEAN FOODS CO**
Herters; **CABELA'S INC**
Hertz Car Sales; **HERTZ GLOBAL HOLDINGS INC**
Hertz Equipment Rental Corp.; **HERTZ GLOBAL HOLDINGS INC**
Hertz Leasing; **HERTZ GLOBAL HOLDINGS INC**
Hertz Local Edition; **HERTZ GLOBAL HOLDINGS INC**

Hertz Rent A Car; **HERTZ GLOBAL HOLDINGS INC**
HFC Assessment Services; **HEALTH FITNESS CORP**
HFC Corporate Fitness Programs; **HEALTH FITNESS CORP**
HFC Fitness Programs; **HEALTH FITNESS CORP**
HFC Wellness Programs; **HEALTH FITNESS CORP**
Hhonors; **HILTON HOTELS CORP**
Hibbett Sports; **HIBBETT SPORTS INC**
Hibbett Team Sales, Inc.; **HIBBETT SPORTS INC**
HighMount Exploration & Production, LLC; **LOEWS CORPORATION**
HI-LITER; **AVERY DENNISON CORP**
Hill's Pet Nutrition; **COLGATE PALMOLIVE CO**
Hillshire Farm; **SARA LEE CORP**
Hilton Garden Vacations Company, LLC; **HILTON HOTELS CORP**
Hilton Group plc; **HILTON HOTELS CORP**
Hilton Group plc; **LODGIAN INC**
HIS; **IMS HEALTH INC**
HMSHost Corp.; **BRINKER INTERNATIONAL INC**
Höfer Vorsorge-Management; **MERCER INC**
Hold Everything; **WILLIAMS SONOMA INC**
Holiday Inn; **LODGIAN INC**
Holland America Line; **CARNIVAL CORPORATION**
Hollister Co.; **ABERCROMBIE & FITCH CO**
HollisterCo.com; **ABERCROMBIE & FITCH CO**
Home Way (The); **HOME DEPOT INC**
Homecraft; **PATTERSON COMPANIES INC**
HomeGoods; **TJX COMPANIES INC (THE)**
Homeland Security and Defense; **SAIC INC**
HomeSense; **TJX COMPANIES INC (THE)**
Homestead (The); **CLUBCORP INC**
Honeywell Aerospace Solutions; **HONEYWELL INTERNATIONAL INC**
Horchow; **NEIMAN MARCUS GROUP INC (THE)**
Horizon Health Corp.; **PSYCHIATRIC SOLUTIONS INC**
Horizon Organic; **DEAN FOODS CO**
Horseshoe; **HARRAH'S ENTERTAINMENT INC**
Hot Topic; **HOT TOPIC INC**
Hot Wheels; **MATTEL INC**
HotJobs.com, Ltd.; **YAHOO! INC**
HotTopic.com; **HOT TOPIC INC**

INDEX OF SUBSIDIARIES, BRAND NAMES AND AFFILIATIONS, CONT.

House of Kolor; **VALSPAR CORPORATION (THE)**
Hovensa; **HESS CORPORATION**
Howard Johnson; **WYNDHAM WORLDWIDE**
Howell Petroleum Corporation; **ANADARKO PETROLEUM CORPORATION**
HSN LP (Home Shopping Network); **IAC/INTERACTIVECORP**
Huarun Paints; **VALSPAR CORPORATION (THE)**
Huggies; **KIMBERLY-CLARK CORP**
Hughes Christensen; **BAKER HUGHES INC**
Humalog; **ELI LILLY & COMPANY**
Humana Dental; **HUMANA INC**
Humana Medicare; **HUMANA INC**
Humana Military Healthcare Services, Inc.; **HUMANA INC**
Humana Ventures; **HUMANA INC**
HumanaOne; **HUMANA INC**
Humira; **ABBOTT LABORATORIES**
Hunt's; **CONAGRA FOODS INC**
Hurley International, LLC; **NIKE INC**
HWC Energy Services, Inc.; **OIL STATES INTERNATIONAL INC**
Hyatt Gold Passport; **GLOBAL HYATT CORPORATION**
Hyatt Regency; **GLOBAL HYATT CORPORATION**
Hyatt Resorts; **GLOBAL HYATT CORPORATION**
Hyatt Summerfield Suites; **GLOBAL HYATT CORPORATION**
Hyatt Vacation Ownership, Inc.; **GLOBAL HYATT CORPORATION**
Hypak; **BECTON DICKINSON & CO**
Hypnion, Inc.; **ELI LILLY & COMPANY**
I. Arthur Yanoff & Co., Ltd.; **ARTHUR J GALLAGHER & CO**
IAC Search & Media; **IAC/INTERACTIVECORP**
IAP; **BUNGE LTD**
IBM Canada Ltd; **INTERNATIONAL BUSINESS MACHINES CORP (IBM)**
IBM Research; **INTERNATIONAL BUSINESS MACHINES CORP (IBM)**
ICG Communications Inc; **LEVEL 3 COMMUNICATIONS INC**
ICOMS; **CONVERGYS CORPORATION**
Icos Corporation; **ELI LILLY & COMPANY**
iDEN; **NII HOLDINGS INC**
Identeon; **SYNTEL INC**
Iditarod Systems, Inc.; **DELOITTE & TOUCHE USA LLP**
Ifokus Engineering AS; **OCEANEERING INTERNATIONAL INC**

iGATE Clinical Research International Private Ltd.; **IGATE CORPORATION**
iGATE Global Solutions; **IGATE CORPORATION**
iGATE Professional Services; **IGATE CORPORATION**
iGATE Shared Services; **IGATE CORPORATION**
iGATE Solutions; **IGATE CORPORATION**
IGN Entertainment; **NEWS CORP**
IGS; **IGATE CORPORATION**
IHOP Restaurant Training Program; **DINEEQUITY INC**
iLab; **BOSTON SCIENTIFIC CORP**
Ilypsa; **AMGEN INC**
IM Flash Technologies, LLC; **MICRON TECHNOLOGY INC**
Image Quest, Inc.; **XEROX CORP**
ImagineX; **COACH INC**
IMDb.com; **AMAZON.COM INC**
IMOnsite; **INGRAM MICRO INC**
InCircle; **NEIMAN MARCUS GROUP INC (THE)**
Indian Wells Country Club; **CLUBCORP INC**
Indiana Michigan Power; **AMERICAN ELECTRIC POWER COMPANY INC (AEP)**
Indianapolis Power & Light; **AES CORPORATION (THE)**
Industrial Automation; **EMERSON ELECTRIC CO**
Industrial Design and Construction; **CH2M HILL COMPANIES LTD**
Industrial Exchange; **DRESS BARN INC (THE)**
Industrial Transport; **EXEL TRANSPORTATION SERVICES INC (DHL EXEL)**
iNest Realty Inc; **IAC/INTERACTIVECORP**
Infinys; **CONVERGYS CORPORATION**
InfoBase; **ACXIOM CORP**
InfraStruXure; **AMERICAN POWER CONVERSION CORP**
INFUSE Bone Graft; **MEDTRONIC INC**
Ingenio; **AT&T INC**
Ingenix; **UNITEDHEALTH GROUP INC**
Ingram Micro Asia Pacific Pte. Ltd.; **INGRAM MICRO INC**
Ingram Micro Canada; **INGRAM MICRO INC**
Ingram Micro Channel Advisor; **INGRAM MICRO INC**
InGram Micro UK Ltd.; **INGRAM MICRO INC**
Inner Circle; **BJ'S WHOLESALE CLUB INC**

InnerLogix; **SCHLUMBERGER LIMITED**
Innogistics; **EXEL TRANSPORTATION SERVICES INC (DHL EXEL)**
Innoka; **GTECH HOLDINGS CORP**
InnoPharm, Ltd.; **PHARMACEUTICAL PRODUCT DEVELOPMENT INC**
Innova, S. de R.L. de C.V.; **DIRECTV GROUP INC (THE)**
Innovative Merchant Services; **INTUIT INC**
Innovative Paper Technologies; **3M COMPANY**
Insensys Oil & Gas, Ltd.; **SCHLUMBERGER LIMITED**
InsightIdentify; **ACXIOM CORP**
Inspur; **SCIENTIFIC GAMES CORPORATION**
Institute for Professional Development; **APOLLO GROUP INC**
Institute for Quality Management, Inc.; **CACI INTERNATIONAL INC**
Integra Group; **SMITH INTERNATIONAL INC**
Integrated Defense Systems; **BOEING COMPANY (THE)**
Integrated Group Benefits; **HILB ROGAL & HOBBS CO**
Integrated Investment Services; **JP MORGAN CHASE & CO INC**
Intel; **APPLE INC**
Intel Core 2 Quad; **INTEL CORP**
Intel Corp; **MICRON TECHNOLOGY INC**
IntelliCast; **WEST CORPORATION**
Intelligence; **SAIC INC**
Intensi-fi; **BROADCOM CORP**
InterCall, Inc.; **WEST CORPORATION**
InterContinental Hotels Group plc; **LODGIAN INC**
Interlott; **GTECH HOLDINGS CORP**
Intermix Media; **NEWS CORP**
International Business Machines Corp (IBM); **LEXMARK INTERNATIONAL INC**
International Business Machines Corp (IBM); **KEANE INC**
International Dairy Queen; **BERKSHIRE HATHAWAY INC**
International Delight; **DEAN FOODS CO**
International Direct Connect; **NII HOLDINGS INC**
International House of Pancakes; **DINEEQUITY INC**
International Logging, Inc.; **WEATHERFORD INTERNATIONAL LTD**
Internet Security Systems Inc; **INTERNATIONAL BUSINESS MACHINES CORP (IBM)**
InterQual; **MCKESSON CORPORATION**

INDEX OF SUBSIDIARIES, BRAND NAMES AND AFFILIATIONS, CONT.

Interstate Power and Light Company; **FPL GROUP INC**
Intrado, Inc.; **WEST CORPORATION**
Intuit Real Estate Solutions; **INTUIT INC**
inVentiv Clinical Services; **INVENTIV HEALTH INC**
inVentiv Commercial Services; **INVENTIV HEALTH INC**
inVentiv Communications; **INVENTIV HEALTH INC**
INVISTA; **KOCH INDUSTRIES INC**
Inwood Laboratories; **FOREST LABORATORIES INC**
IPALCO Enterprises, Inc.; **AES CORPORATION (THE)**
iPhone; **APPLE INC**
iPod; **APPLE INC**
IQ Guide Wire; **BOSTON SCIENTIFIC CORP**
Iridesse, Inc.; **TIFFANY & CO**
Irish Spring; **COLGATE PALMOLIVE CO**
iScript; **BIO RAD LABORATORIES INC**
IsoTherming Technology; **E I DU PONT DE NEMOURS & CO (DUPONT)**
I-Stat Corp; **ABBOTT LABORATORIES**
It's Your Life Wellsite; **HEALTH NET INC**
ITEDO Software LLC; **PARAMETRIC TECHNOLOGY CORP**
I-trax, Inc.; **WALGREEN CO**
It's a Girls World; **TWEEN BRANDS INC**
Ixempra; **BRISTOL MYERS SQUIBB CO**
J. Jill Group, Inc. (The); **TALBOTS INC (THE)**
J.C. Penney Corp., Inc.; **J C PENNEY COMPANY INC**
J.D. Edwards; **DELOITTE CONSULTING LLP**
J.P. Morgan Partners; **ARAMARK CORPORATION**
J.P. Morgan Securities; **JP MORGAN CHASE & CO INC**
JAC; **AVERY DENNISON CORP**
Jack in the Box; **JACK IN THE BOX INC**
Jack in the Box Foundation; **JACK IN THE BOX INC**
Jackfish; **DEVON ENERGY CORPORATION**
Jack's Ultimate Salads; **JACK IN THE BOX INC**
Jacobs; **KRAFT FOODS INC**
Jacobs Chuck Manufacturing Company; **DANAHER CORP**
Jacobs Vehicle Systems; **DANAHER CORP**
James Webb Space Telescope; **NORTHROP GRUMMAN CORP**

Jamilco; **COACH INC**
Japanese Practice; **KPMG LLP**
Java; **SUN MICROSYSTEMS INC**
JCPenney Custom Decorating; **J C PENNEY COMPANY INC**
JCPenney Optical Services; **J C PENNEY COMPANY INC**
JCPenney Portraits; **J C PENNEY COMPANY INC**
JCPenney Salon; **J C PENNEY COMPANY INC**
jcpenney.com; **J C PENNEY COMPANY INC**
Jefferson Pilot Variable Fund; **LINCOLN NATIONAL CORPORATION**
Jefferson Wells; **MANPOWER INC**
Jefferson-Pilot Corp.; **LINCOLN NATIONAL CORPORATION**
Jell-O; **KRAFT FOODS INC**
Jerr-Dan; **OSHKOSH CORPORATION**
Jersey Central Power & Light Co.; **FIRSTENERGY CORP**
JERZEES; **RUSSELL CORP**
JET; **CONOCOPHILLIPS COMPANY**
Jetway; **FMC TECHNOLOGIES INC**
Jewel-Osco; **SUPERVALU INC**
Jiangsu Five Star Appliance Co., Ltd.; **BEST BUY CO INC**
Jif; **JM SMUCKER CO**
Jimmy Dean; **SARA LEE CORP**
Jimmy'Z Surf Co., Inc.; **AEROPOSTALE INC**
JJWild, Inc.; **PEROT SYSTEMS CORP**
Jobcurry Systems Private Ltd.; **IGATE CORPORATION**
John Bean Technologies Corporation; **FMC TECHNOLOGIES INC**
John Deere; **DEERE & CO**
John Deere Agricultural Holdings, Inc.; **DEERE & CO**
John Deere Commercial Worksite Products, Inc.; **DEERE & CO**
John Deere Construction & Forestry Company; **DEERE & CO**
John Deere Construction Holdings, Inc.; **DEERE & CO**
John Deere Credit Company; **DEERE & CO**
John Deere Health Plan, Inc.; **DEERE & CO**
John Deere Lawn & Grounds Care Holdings, Inc.; **DEERE & CO**
John Middleton, Inc.; **ALTRIA GROUP INC**
Johnson Controls-Saft Advanced Power Solutions; **JOHNSON CONTROLS INC**
Johnston & Murphy; **GENESCO INC**
Journey; **MARY KAY INC**
Journeys; **GENESCO INC**
Journeys Kidz; **GENESCO INC**
JP Fruit Distributors Ltd.; **DOLE FOOD COMPANY INC**

JPMorgan Chase Vastera Inc; **JP MORGAN CHASE & CO INC**
JPMorgan Partners; **JP MORGAN CHASE & CO INC**
J-Series; **JUNIPER NETWORKS INC**
Juicy Fruit; **WM WRIGLEY JR COMPANY**
Jumbo Jack; **JACK IN THE BOX INC**
JUNOS; **JUNIPER NETWORKS INC**
Jupiter Telecommunication Co., Ltd. (J:Com); **LIBERTY GLOBAL INC**
Just4U; **ARAMARK CORPORATION**
Justice; **TWEEN BRANDS INC**
K&G; **MEN'S WEARHOUSE INC (THE)**
Kaiser Foundation Health Plan, Inc.; **KAISER PERMANENTE**
Kaiser Foundation Hospitals; **KAISER PERMANENTE**
Kaiser Permanente Healthcare Institute; **KAISER PERMANENTE**
Kangaroo Express; **PANTRY INC (THE)**
Katz Group of Companies (The); **CLEAR CHANNEL COMMUNICATIONS INC**
Katz Media; **CLEAR CHANNEL COMMUNICATIONS INC**
KD Innovation; **DJO INC**
Keebler; **KELLOGG CO**
Keller Graduate School of Management; **DEVRY INC**
Kellogg Snacks Division; **KELLOGG CO**
Kelly Office Services; **KELLY SERVICES INC**
Kelly Scientific Resources; **KELLY SERVICES INC**
KellyConnect; **KELLY SERVICES INC**
KellyDirect; **KELLY SERVICES INC**
Kendall; **CONOCOPHILLIPS COMPANY**
Kentucky Power; **AMERICAN ELECTRIC POWER COMPANY INC (AEP)**
Kerma; **QUIKSILVER INC**
Kerr-McGee Corporation; **ANADARKO PETROLEUM CORPORATION**
Ketchum; **OMNICOM GROUP INC**
Kevlar; **E I DU PONT DE NEMOURS & CO (DUPONT)**
Keystone Automotive Industries Inc; **LKQ CORP**
KFC; **YUM! BRANDS INC**
Kievoblenergo; **AES CORPORATION (THE)**
Kijiji; **EBAY INC**
Kimberly-Clark of South Africa; **KIMBERLY-CLARK CORP**
Kindred Healthcare, Inc.; **AMERISOURCEBERGEN CORP**
King Soopers; **KROGER CO (THE)**
Kiwi; **SARA LEE CORP**

INDEX OF SUBSIDIARIES, BRAND NAMES AND AFFILIATIONS, CONT.

KKR & Co LP (Kohlberg Kravis Roberts & Co); **DOLLAR GENERAL CORPORATION**
KKR & Co LP (Kohlberg Kravis Roberts & Co); **HCA INC**
Kleenex; **KIMBERLY-CLARK CORP**
KMG America Corporation; **HUMANA INC**
KnowItAll; **BIO RAD LABORATORIES INC**
Knurr AG; **EMERSON ELECTRIC CO**
Koch Chemical Technologies Group; **KOCH INDUSTRIES INC**
Koch Materials Company; **KOCH INDUSTRIES INC**
Koch Mineral Services; **KOCH INDUSTRIES INC**
Koch Pipeline Company; **KOCH INDUSTRIES INC**
Kohlberg Kravis Roberts & Co.; **FIRST DATA CORP**
Kohls.com; **KOHL'S CORP**
Komag Inc; **WESTERN DIGITAL CORP**
Kontos Kommentary; **ADESA INC**
KOS Pharmaceuticals Inc; **ABBOTT LABORATORIES**
Kotex; **KIMBERLY-CLARK CORP**
KP HealthConnect; **KAISER PERMANENTE**
KPMG International; **KPMG LLP**
KPMG TaxWatch Thought Leadership Series; **KPMG LLP**
K-Resin; **CHEVRON PHILLIPS CHEMICAL COMPANY LLC**
Kroll Inc; **MARSH & MCLENNAN COMPANIES INC**
KSL Capital LLC; **CLUBCORP INC**
Kuwait Oil Company; **FLUOR CORP**
Kwikset; **BLACK & DECKER CORP**
Kyphon, Inc.; **MEDTRONIC INC**
L.A. Dreyfus Company; **WM WRIGLEY JR COMPANY**
L-3 Communications Corporation; **L-3 COMMUNICATIONS HOLDINGS INC**
L-3 Communications Holdings Inc; **L-3 TITAN GROUP**
L-3 TITAN GROUP; **L-3 COMMUNICATIONS HOLDINGS INC**
La Electricidad de Caracas; **AES CORPORATION (THE)**
La Mer; **ESTEE LAUDER COMPANIES INC (THE)**
La Prairie; **RITZ-CARLTON HOTEL COMPANY LLC (THE)**
La Senza Corporation; **LIMITED BRANDS INC**
Lab Safety Supply, Inc.; **WW GRAINGER INC**
LabLink; **COVANCE INC**
LabOne; **QUEST DIAGNOSTICS INC**

Lady Speed Stick; **COLGATE PALMOLIVE CO**
Lake Norman Regional Medical Center; **HEALTH MANAGEMENT ASSOCIATES INC**
LAND O'LAKES; **DEAN FOODS CO**
Landmark; **HALLIBURTON COMPANY**
Landry's Seafood House; **LANDRY'S RESTAURANTS INC**
Lane Bryant; **CHARMING SHOPPES INC**
Lane Bryant Outlet; **CHARMING SHOPPES INC**
Lange; **QUIKSILVER INC**
LaSalle Bank Corp; **BANK OF AMERICA CORP**
Last Chance; **NORDSTROM INC**
Last-Call; **NEIMAN MARCUS GROUP INC (THE)**
LastMinute.com; **SABRE HOLDINGS CORP**
Latigent, LLC; **CISCO SYSTEMS INC**
LDK Solar Co; **FLUOR CORP**
Le Meridien; **STARWOOD HOTELS & RESORTS WORLDWIDE INC**
Lee Roy Selmon's; **OSI RESTAURANT PARTNERS INC**
Leisure Plus; **J C PENNEY COMPANY INC**
Leitch Technology Corporation; **HARRIS CORPORATION**
Lender Services; **FIRST ADVANTAGE CORPORATION**
LendingTree LLC; **IAC/INTERACTIVECORP**
Leonard Green & Partners; **CONTAINER STORE (THE)**
Leonard Green & Partners LP; **PETCO ANIMAL SUPPLIES INC**
Leumeta; **QUEST DIAGNOSTICS INC**
Lexapro; **FOREST LABORATORIES INC**
LGC Wireless; **ADC TELECOMMUNICATIONS INC**
Liberty Cablevision of Puerto Rico; **LIBERTY GLOBAL INC**
Liberty Electric PA, LLC; **RELIANT ENERGY INC**
Liberty Media Corp; **DIRECTV GROUP INC (THE)**
Liberty Mutual Insurance Co.; **SAFECO CORP**
Liberty of the Seas; **ROYAL CARIBBEAN CRUISES**
Liberty Reverse Mortgage, Inc.; **GENWORTH FINANCIAL INC**
Lids; **GENESCO INC**
Life Savers; **WM WRIGLEY JR COMPANY**
LifeScan Inc; **JOHNSON & JOHNSON**
LifeScan, Inc.; **MEDTRONIC INC**

LifeStent; **CR BARD INC**
Lightpath, Inc.; **CABLEVISION SYSTEMS CORP**
Limited (The); **INTIMATE BRANDS INC**
Limited Brands Inc; **TWEEN BRANDS INC**
Limited Brands, Inc.; **INTIMATE BRANDS INC**
Limited Too; **TWEEN BRANDS INC**
Limited, Inc. (The); **LIMITED BRANDS INC**
LiMo Foundation; **CELLCO PARTNERSHIP (VERIZON WIRELESS)**
Lincoln American Legacy Retirement; **LINCOLN NATIONAL CORPORATION**
Lincoln Director (The); **LINCOLN NATIONAL CORPORATION**
Lincoln Financial Media; **LINCOLN NATIONAL CORPORATION**
Lincoln UK; **LINCOLN NATIONAL CORPORATION**
Lincoln Variable Insurance Product; **LINCOLN NATIONAL CORPORATION**
Lingualcare; **3M COMPANY**
Lionville Systems, Inc.; **EMERSON ELECTRIC CO**
Lipitor; **PFIZER INC**
Lipton; **PEPSI BOTTLING GROUP INC**
Little Switzerland; **TIFFANY & CO**
LiveUpdate; **SYMANTEC CORP**
Livial; **SCHERING-PLOUGH CORP**
Loan-a-Tool; **AUTOZONE INC**
Lockwood Greene; **CH2M HILL COMPANIES LTD**
Loews Hotels Holding Corporation; **LOEWS CORPORATION**
Lone Star Medical Products, Inc.; **COOPER COMPANIES INC**
Long John Silver's; **YUM! BRANDS INC**
LongHorn Steakhouse; **DARDEN RESTAURANTS INC**
LopezGarcia Group, Inc.; **URS CORPORATION**
Lorillard Inc; **LOEWS CORPORATION**
Lottomatica S.p.A.; **GTECH HOLDINGS CORP**
Lovat, Inc.; **CATERPILLAR INC**
LSSi Data; **VOLT INFORMATION SCIENCES INC**
LUKOIL; **CONOCOPHILLIPS COMPANY**
Lumigan; **ALLERGAN INC**
Luminant; **SHELL OIL CO**
Luxor; **MGM MIRAGE**
Luxury Collection; **STARWOOD HOTELS & RESORTS WORLDWIDE INC**

INDEX OF SUBSIDIARIES, BRAND NAMES AND AFFILIATIONS, CONT.

LVL7 Systems, Inc.; **BROADCOM CORP**
Lynx S2S; **MILLIPORE CORP**
Lyovac; **STERIS CORP**
M&Ms; **MARS INC**
M.A.C; **ESTEE LAUDER COMPANIES INC (THE)**
M/DN Intermedullary Fixation; **ZIMMER HOLDINGS INC**
M1A1 Abrams Tank; **GENERAL DYNAMICS CORP**
Mac Acquisition LLC; **BRINKER INTERNATIONAL INC**
Mac OS X; **APPLE INC**
Macau Orient Golf; **HARRAH'S ENTERTAINMENT INC**
MacBook Pro; **APPLE INC**
Macromedia ColdFusion; **ADOBE SYSTEMS INC**
Macromedia Flash SDK; **ADOBE SYSTEMS INC**
MacTavish Furniture Industries; **AARON RENTS INC**
Macy's; **MACY'S INC**
Madden NFL; **ELECTRONIC ARTS INC**
Madison Dearborn Partners, LLC; **CDW CORPORATION**
Madison Square Garden; **CABLEVISION SYSTEMS CORP**
Maggiano's Little Italy; **BRINKER INTERNATIONAL INC**
Magnolia Audio Video; **BEST BUY CO INC**
Maison du Cafe; **SARA LEE CORP**
Major Market Services; **PAYCHEX INC**
Man Alive; **FINISH LINE INC (THE)**
Management Systens Designers, Inc.; **LOCKHEED MARTIN CORP**
Manah; **BUNGE LTD**
Mandalay Bay; **MGM MIRAGE**
ManorCare Health Services; **MANOR CARE INC**
Manpower Professional; **MANPOWER INC**
MapInfo Corp.; **PITNEY BOWES INC**
Marathon Petroleum Company LLC; **MARATHON OIL CORP**
Marciano; **GUESS? INC**
MarFlex; **CHEVRON PHILLIPS CHEMICAL COMPANY LLC**
Marie Callender's; **CONAGRA FOODS INC**
Marina Bay Sands; **LAS VEGAS SANDS CORP (THE VENETIAN)**
Marina Power Lighting; **EATON CORP**
Maritime Communications Services, Inc.; **HARRIS CORPORATION**
Mark; **AVON PRODUCTS INC**
Market Pantry; **TARGET CORPORATION**

Market Research Publications; **IMS HEALTH INC**
MarketZone; **INFOUSA INC**
Marks-A-Lot; **AVERY DENNISON CORP**
Marlex; **CHEVRON PHILLIPS CHEMICAL COMPANY LLC**
Marlex Energy Services Company; **NATIONAL OILWELL VARCO INC**
Marriott Hotels and Resorts; **MARRIOTT INTERNATIONAL INC**
Marriott International Inc; **RITZ-CARLTON HOTEL COMPANY LLC (THE)**
Marriott International Inc; **LODGIAN INC**
Marsh & McLennan Companies, Inc.; **MERCER INC**
Marsh & McLennan Risk Capital Holdings; **MARSH & MCLENNAN COMPANIES INC**
Marsh, Inc.; **MARSH & MCLENNAN COMPANIES INC**
Marshalls; **TJX COMPANIES INC (THE)**
MARTIN + OSA; **AMERICAN EAGLE OUTFITTERS INC**
MartinAndOsa.com; **AMERICAN EAGLE OUTFITTERS INC**
Martin-Senour; **SHERWIN WILLIAMS COMPANY (THE)**
MassLynx MS; **WATERS CORP**
MassTrak Immunosuppressant Kit; **WATERS CORP**
Mast Industries; **LIMITED BRANDS INC**
MasterBrand Cabinets, Inc.; **FORTUNE BRANDS INC**
MasterCuts; **REGIS CORPORATION**
Master-Pro; **O'REILLY AUTOMOTIVE INC**
Matador Cattle Company; **KOCH INDUSTRIES INC**
Matasys Building Management System; **JOHNSON CONTROLS INC**
Match.com; **IAC/INTERACTIVECORP**
Matchbox; **MATTEL INC**
Mathcad; **PARAMETRIC TECHNOLOGY CORP**
Mathsoft Engineering & Education, Inc.; **PARAMETRIC TECHNOLOGY CORP**
Maui Electric Company, Limited; **HAWAIIAN ELECTRIC INDUSTRIES INC**
Maurer Technology, Inc.; **NOBLE CORPORATION**
Maurice's; **DRESS BARN INC (THE)**
Maxamine; **ACCENTURE LTD**
MAXIM Systems, Inc.; **ACCENTURE LTD**
Maxon Corporation; **HONEYWELL INTERNATIONAL INC**

MAXTEK; **TEKTRONIX INC**
Maxwell House; **KRAFT FOODS INC**
May's Department Stores; **MACY'S INC**
MBNA Corp.; **BANK OF AMERICA CORP**
McAfee Anti-Virus; **MCAFEE INC**
McAfee Foundstone Professional Services; **MCAFEE INC**
McAfee Network Protection Solutions; **MCAFEE INC**
McAfee Spam Killer; **MCAFEE INC**
McAfee System Protection Solutions; **MCAFEE INC**
McKesson Canada; **MCKESSON CORPORATION**
McKesson Health Solutions; **MCKESSON CORPORATION**
McKesson Pharmacy Systems; **MCKESSON CORPORATION**
McKesson U.S. Pharmaceutical; **MCKESSON CORPORATION**
McKinsey & Co.; **MCKINSEY & COMPANY INC**
McKinsey Global Institute; **MCKINSEY & COMPANY INC**
McKinsey Quarterly (The); **MCKINSEY & COMPANY INC**
McLane Company; **PANTRY INC (THE)**
McNeilus; **OSHKOSH CORPORATION**
Meadowbrook Meat Company; **DENNY'S CORPORATION**
Meat Lover's Breakfast; **DENNY'S CORPORATION**
Medco Health Solutions; **HEALTHWAYS INC**
Medco Therapeutic Resource Centers; **MEDCO HEALTH SOLUTIONS**
MedFocus; **INVENTIV HEALTH INC**
Media Center; **WESTERN DIGITAL CORP**
MediaFLO USA, Inc.; **QUALCOMM INC**
Mediasenz; **ACCENTURE LTD**
Medical Management International, Inc.; **PETSMART INC**
Medicare Advantage; **HUMANA INC**
Medicare Part D Prescription Drug Program; **MEDCO HEALTH SOLUTIONS**
Medication Delivery; **BAXTER INTERNATIONAL INC**
Medimop Medical Projects, Ltd.; **WEST PHARMACEUTICAL SERVICES INC**
MedInitiatives; **IMS HEALTH INC**
Medmark Specialty Pharmacy; **WALGREEN CO**
MedStar PromptCare; **RITE AID CORPORATION**
Medtec; **OSHKOSH CORPORATION**
Medtronic ENT; **MEDTRONIC INC**
Medtronic Xomed; **MEDTRONIC INC**
Member's Mark; **SAM'S CLUB**

INDEX OF SUBSIDIARIES, BRAND NAMES AND AFFILIATIONS, CONT.

MEMCO Barge Line, Inc.; **AMERICAN ELECTRIC POWER COMPANY INC (AEP)**

Mendota Insurance Co; **TRAVELERS COMPANIES INC (THE)**

Mercer Global Investments; **MERCER INC**

Mercer HR; **MERCER INC**

Mercer HR Services; **MERCER INC**

Mercer Human Capital; **MERCER INC**

Mercer Inc; **MARSH & MCLENNAN COMPANIES INC**

Mercer Investment Consulting; **MERCER INC**

Mercer Retirement; **MERCER INC**

Mercer Specialty Consulting; **MARSH & MCLENNAN COMPANIES INC**

Merchant Solutions; **FIRST DATA CORP**

Merchants@; **AMAZON.COM INC**

Merck Institute for Science Education; **MERCK & CO INC**

Mercy Health Plans; **SISTERS OF MERCY HEALTH SYSTEMS**

Mercy Ministries of Laredo; **SISTERS OF MERCY HEALTH SYSTEMS**

Meritus University; **APOLLO GROUP INC**

Merona; **TARGET CORPORATION**

Merrill Lynch & Co Inc; **HCA INC**

Metamor Enterprise Solutions, LLC; **CIBER INC**

MetaSolv Software; **ORACLE CORP**

Metcalf & Eddy; **AECOM TECHNOLOGY CORPORATION**

MetLife Bank; **METLIFE INC**

Metri Medical, Inc.; **PATTERSON COMPANIES INC**

Metro Mechanical, Inc.; **JOHNSON CONTROLS INC**

Metropolitan Club; **CLUBCORP INC**

Metropolitan Edison Co.; **FIRSTENERGY CORP**

MGM Grand Las Vegas; **MGM MIRAGE**

MGM Grand Macau; **MGM MIRAGE**

M-I Drilling Fluids; **SCHLUMBERGER LIMITED**

M-I SWACO; **SMITH INTERNATIONAL INC**

Michigan Consolidated Gas (MichCon); **DTE ENERGY COMPANY**

Micro Logistics; **INGRAM MICRO INC**

MicroSafe, B.V.; **MILLIPORE CORP**

Microsoft Corp; **KEANE INC**

Microsoft Dynamics; **MICROSOFT CORP**

Microsroft Office; **MICROSOFT CORP**

Mid Atlantic Medical Services Inc; **UNITEDHEALTH GROUP INC**

MIDAS; **IMS HEALTH INC**

Midwest Energy Resources; **DTE ENERGY COMPANY**

MIHS Holdings, Inc.; **IMS HEALTH INC**

Milky Way; **MARS INC**

Millennium; **VARIAN MEDICAL SYSTEMS INC**

Miller Brewing Company; **ALTRIA GROUP INC**

MilliPROBE; **MILLIPORE CORP**

Minute Maid Company (The); **COCA COLA COMPANY (THE)**

MinuteClinic; **CVS CAREMARK CORPORATION**

Miracle-Gro; **SCOTTS MIRACLE GROW CO**

Mirage (The); **MGM MIRAGE**

Miramax Film Corp; **WALT DISNEY COMPANY (THE)**

Mirastar; **TESORO CORP**

Mirinda; **PEPSI BOTTLING GROUP INC**

Mission Hills Country Club; **CLUBCORP INC**

Mississippi Power Company; **SOUTHERN COMPANY (THE)**

Mitsukoshi Ltd.; **TIFFANY & CO**

Mix2Vial; **WEST PHARMACEUTICAL SERVICES INC**

Mixject; **WEST PHARMACEUTICAL SERVICES INC**

Mobile Power Pack; **AMERICAN POWER CONVERSION CORP**

Moen, Inc.; **FORTUNE BRANDS INC**

Molecular Medicine BioServices, Inc.; **SIGMA-ALDRICH CORP**

Monarch; **PAXAR CORP**

Monro Muffler Brake & Service; **MONRO MUFFLER BRAKE INC**

Monro Service Corporation; **MONRO MUFFLER BRAKE INC**

MONY Group; **AXA FINANCIAL INC**

MONY Life Insurance Company; **AXA FINANCIAL INC**

MONY Life Insurance Company of America; **AXA FINANCIAL INC**

Moores Clothing for Men; **MEN'S WEARHOUSE INC (THE)**

Morbid Makeup; **HOT TOPIC INC**

Morbid Metals; **HOT TOPIC INC**

Morbid Threads; **HOT TOPIC INC**

MorganMarkets; **JP MORGAN CHASE & CO INC**

MOSAID Technologies Incorporated; **SYNOPSYS INC**

Mossy Oak Apparel; **RUSSELL CORP**

Motiva Enterprises LLC; **SHELL OIL CO**

Motorola Inc; **NII HOLDINGS INC**

Motorola Q; **UNITED STATES CELLULAR CORP**

Mountain Dew; **PEPSI BOTTLING GROUP INC**

MountainView Software Corp.; **ARTHUR J GALLAGHER & CO**

Moving Comfort; **RUSSELL CORP**

Mr. Payroll Corp.; **CASH AMERICA INTERNATIONAL INC**

Mr. Tire; **MONRO MUFFLER BRAKE INC**

Mrs. Dash; **ALBERTO-CULVER COMPANY**

M-Series; **JUNIPER NETWORKS INC**

MSG Entertainment; **CABLEVISION SYSTEMS CORP**

MSN; **MICROSOFT CORP**

M-The Catalog for Men; **AVON PRODUCTS INC**

MTV Networks; **VIACOM INC**

MultiCare Express Clinics; **RITE AID CORPORATION**

Multifamily Services; **FIRST ADVANTAGE CORPORATION**

Multimax Incorporated; **HARRIS CORPORATION**

Multi-Mile; **TBC CORPORATION**

Multi-Platform Radar Technology Insertion Program; **NORTHROP GRUMMAN CORP**

Murco Petroleum, Ltd.; **MURPHY OIL CORPORATION**

Murphy Canada; **MURPHY OIL CORPORATION**

Murphy Oil Company, Ltd.; **MURPHY OIL CORPORATION**

Murphy Oil USA, Inc.; **MURPHY OIL CORPORATION**

Murphy USA; **MURPHY OIL CORPORATION**

MW; **FOSSIL INC**

MW Michele; **FOSSIL INC**

MW Tux; **MEN'S WEARHOUSE INC (THE)**

MX-Series; **JUNIPER NETWORKS INC**

My Contacts Backup; **UNITED STATES CELLULAR CORP**

myFICO; **FAIR ISAAC CORPORATION**

myfico.com; **FAIR ISAAC CORPORATION**

MyHealthways; **HEALTHWAYS INC**

MySpace; **NEWS CORP**

MySpace; **GOOGLE INC**

Nabisco Fruit Sancks; **KELLOGG CO**

Namenda; **FOREST LABORATORIES INC**

National Amusement, Inc.; **VIACOM INC**

National Car Rental; **ENTERPRISE RENT-A-CAR**

National Genetics Institute (The); **LABORATORY CORP OF AMERICA HOLDINGS**

National Geographic Channel; **FOX ENTERTAINMENT GROUP INC**

National Labor College; **KAISER PERMANENTE**

National Methanol Company; **DUKE ENERGY CORP**

INDEX OF SUBSIDIARIES, BRAND NAMES AND AFFILIATIONS, CONT.

National Processing; **BANK OF AMERICA CORP**
National Response Corp.; **SEACOR HOLDINGS INC**
National Tire & Battery; **TBC CORPORATION**
National-Oilwell, Inc.; **NATIONAL OILWELL VARCO INC**
Natura; **BRISTOL MYERS SQUIBB CO**
Natural Formula; **PERRIGO CO**
Natural Retail Group; **UNITED NATURAL FOODS INC**
Naturals; **AVON PRODUCTS INC**
Navini Networks, Inc.; **CISCO SYSTEMS INC**
NBC Universal; **GENERAL ELECTRIC CO (GE)**
NearStore; **NETWORK APPLIANCE INC**
Neca; **PERRIGO CO**
Neda by bebe; **BEBE STORES INC**
Neighborhood Market; **WAL-MART STORES INC**
Neiman Marcus Christmas Book; **NEIMAN MARCUS GROUP INC (THE)**
NeoPath Networks; **CISCO SYSTEMS INC**
Neste Jacobs Oy of Kilpilahti; **JACOBS ENGINEERING GROUP INC**
NetApp; **NETWORK APPLIANCE INC**
NetBeans IDE; **SUN MICROSYSTEMS INC**
NetCache; **NETWORK APPLIANCE INC**
NetEconomy, B.V.; **FISERV INC**
Netjets Inc; **BERKSHIRE HATHAWAY INC**
NetLink; **BROADCOM CORP**
NetOwl; **SRA INTERNATIONAL INC**
NetStore; **NETWORK APPLIANCE INC**
Network Power; **EMERSON ELECTRIC CO**
NetworkAIR; **AMERICAN POWER CONVERSION CORP**
Neulasta; **AMGEN INC**
NEUPOGEN; **AMGEN INC**
New Bakery Co., Inc. (The); **WENDYS INTERNATIONAL INC**
New Bridge Street Consultants; **HEWITT ASSOCIATES**
New Line Cinema; **TIME WARNER INC**
New York Knickerbockers; **CABLEVISION SYSTEMS CORP**
New York Rangers; **CABLEVISION SYSTEMS CORP**
Newport Bio Systems; **MILLIPORE CORP**
Newport Television, LLC; **CLEAR CHANNEL COMMUNICATIONS INC**
News Corp; **FOX ENTERTAINMENT GROUP INC**

NexGen; **ZIMMER HOLDINGS INC**
NexGen LPS-Flex Mobile Knee; **ZIMMER HOLDINGS INC**
Nextel Direct Connect; **NII HOLDINGS INC**
Nextel Online; **NII HOLDINGS INC**
Nextel Worldwide; **NII HOLDINGS INC**
Nexus Health Systems, Inc.; **SELECT MEDICAL CORPORATION**
Niceday; **OFFICE DEPOT INC**
Nickelodeon; **VIACOM INC**
Nike Bauer Hockey U.S.A., Inc; **NIKE INC**
Nike Bayer Hockey Corp.; **NIKE INC**
Nimbus Partners; **PHARMACEUTICAL PRODUCT DEVELOPMENT INC**
Nitco Paints; **SHERWIN WILLIAMS COMPANY (THE)**
Nobilon; **SCHERING-PLOUGH CORP**
Noble Amos Runner; **NOBLE CORPORATION**
Noble Category 5; **NOBLE CORPORATION**
Noble Downhole Technology; **NOBLE CORPORATION**
Noble Engineering & Development (NED); **NOBLE CORPORATION**
Norba; **OSHKOSH CORPORATION**
Nordstrom Bank; **NORDSTROM INC**
Nordstrom Rack; **NORDSTROM INC**
Norfolk Southern Railway Co.; **NORFOLK SOUTHERN CORP**
North American Components; **ARROW ELECTRONICS INC**
North American Financial Services; **FAIR ISAAC CORPORATION**
Northcountry; **COLDWATER CREEK INC**
Northwestern Flavors, LLC; **WM WRIGLEY JR COMPANY**
Norton; **SYMANTEC CORP**
Norton AntiVirus; **SYMANTEC CORP**
Norton Internet Security; **SYMANTEC CORP**
Norvasc; **PFIZER INC**
Nova Engineering; **L-3 COMMUNICATIONS HOLDINGS INC**
NQL Energy Services, Inc.; **NATIONAL OILWELL VARCO INC**
NuFlo Technologies, Inc.; **CAMERON INTERNATIONAL CORPORATION**
Nuflor; **SCHERING-PLOUGH CORP**
Nutri-Grain; **KELLOGG CO**
Nutropin; **GENENTECH INC**
Nuvigil; **CEPHALON INC**
NWC Research; **INFOUSA INC**
NXP Corporation; **TIFFANY & CO**
O'Brien's Group, Inc. (The); **SEACOR HOLDINGS INC**
Ocean Edge Resort & Golf Club (The); **CLUBCORP INC**

Oceaneering Intervention Engineering; **OCEANEERING INTERNATIONAL INC**
Oceaneering Multiflex; **OCEANEERING INTERNATIONAL INC**
Oceaneering Rotator; **OCEANEERING INTERNATIONAL INC**
Octalica, Inc.; **BROADCOM CORP**
Octal-PHY; **BROADCOM CORP**
OD Domestic; **OLD DOMINION FREIGHT LINE INC**
OD Expedited; **OLD DOMINION FREIGHT LINE INC**
OD Global; **OLD DOMINION FREIGHT LINE INC**
OD Technology; **OLD DOMINION FREIGHT LINE INC**
Odwalla; **COCA COLA COMPANY (THE)**
Office Tiger; **R R DONNELLEY & SONS CO**
OfficeCare; **DJO INC**
OfficeTeam; **ROBERT HALF INTERNATIONAL INC**
Offshore Angler; **BASS PRO SHOPS INC**
Ohio Edison Co.; **FIRSTENERGY CORP**
Olive Garden; **DARDEN RESTAURANTS INC**
Olive Garden Cafe; **DARDEN RESTAURANTS INC**
Oliver Wyman Group; **MARSH & MCLENNAN COMPANIES INC**
OM DIRECT; **OWENS & MINOR INC**
OMD Worldwide; **OMNICOM GROUP INC**
Omega; **FORTUNE BRANDS INC**
OmniCare; **COVENTRY HEALTH CARE INC**
Omnicare Clinical Research; **OMNICARE INC**
OmniReach FTTX Infrastructure Solutions; **ADC TELECOMMUNICATIONS INC**
Omnispark; **O'REILLY AUTOMOTIVE INC**
Omnium Worldwide, Inc.; **WEST CORPORATION**
On the Border Mexican Grill and Cantina; **BRINKER INTERNATIONAL INC**
On The Horizon; **GRANT THORNTON LLP**
Onan; **CUMMINS INC**
Onaro Inc; **NETWORK APPLIANCE INC**
Oncology Technology Network; **MCKESSON CORPORATION**
One Equity Partners; **JP MORGAN CHASE & CO INC**
ONEOK Partners, L.P.; **ONEOK INC**
OneSource Information Services Inc; **INFOUSA INC**
OneSpace; **PARAMETRIC TECHNOLOGY CORP**

INDEX OF SUBSIDIARIES, BRAND NAMES AND AFFILIATIONS, CONT.

OOO Burservice; **HALLIBURTON COMPANY**

OPEN: The Small Business Network; **AMERICAN EXPRESS CO**

Operations Management International; **CH2M HILL COMPANIES LTD**

Opinion Research Corp; **INFOUSA INC**

Opteva; **DIEBOLD INC**

Optima; **JOHNSON CONTROLS INC**

Optima MAX-MP; **BECKMAN COULTER INC**

Optimal Health; **MEDCO HEALTH SOLUTIONS**

Optimal Solutions, Inc.; **HARRIS CORPORATION**

Option Care, Inc.; **WALGREEN CO**

Optive; **ALLERGAN INC**

Oracle Corp; **DELOITTE CONSULTING LLP**

Oracle Human Capital Management; **DELOITTE CONSULTING LLP**

Orange and Rockland Utilities, Inc.; **CONSOLIDATED EDISON INC**

Oranje-Nassau Energie B.V.; **DEVON ENERGY CORPORATION**

O'Reilly Auto Parts; **O'REILLY AUTOMOTIVE INC**

Oreo; **KRAFT FOODS INC**

Organon Biosciences N.V.; **SCHERING-PLOUGH CORP**

Original Grand Slam; **DENNY'S CORPORATION**

Origins; **ESTEE LAUDER COMPANIES INC (THE)**

Orion; **LOCKHEED MARTIN CORP**

ORIONMagic; **SRA INTERNATIONAL INC**

Orkand Corp.; **HARRIS CORPORATION**

Orlandi Valuta; **WESTERN UNION COMPANY (THE)**

Ortho; **SCOTTS MIRACLE GROW CO**

Orthologic; **DJO INC**

Orthopedic Recovery @ Home; **AMEDISYS INC**

ORTHOsoft, Inc.; **ZIMMER HOLDINGS INC**

Orville Redenbacher's; **CONAGRA FOODS INC**

Oscar Mayer; **KRAFT FOODS INC**

Oshkosh; **OSHKOSH CORPORATION**

Oshkosh Truck Corporation; **OSHKOSH CORPORATION**

Osmocote; **SCOTTS MIRACLE GROW CO**

Otis Elevator Company; **UNITED TECHNOLOGIES CORPORATION**

Ouro Verde; **BUNGE LTD**

Outdoor World; **BASS PRO SHOPS INC**

OxyChem; **OCCIDENTAL PETROLEUM CORP**

OxyTec 900; **RESPIRONICS INC**

OxyTec Medical Corporation; **RESPIRONICS INC**

Oxytrol; **WATSON PHARMACEUTICALS INC**

Ozark Automotive Distributors, Inc.; **O'REILLY AUTOMOTIVE INC**

P&O Cruises; **CARNIVAL CORPORATION**

P&O Cruises Australia; **CARNIVAL CORPORATION**

P.A.L.S.; **PETCO ANIMAL SUPPLIES INC**

P.T. Kimberly-Lever Indonesia; **KIMBERLY-CLARK CORP**

Pacific Energy Conservation Services, Inc.; **HAWAIIAN ELECTRIC INDUSTRIES INC**

Pacific Gas and Electric Co.; **PG&E CORPORATION**

Pacific Indemnity Company; **CHUBB CORPORATION (THE)**

Pacific Sales; **BEST BUY CO INC**

Pacificare Health Systems Inc; **UNITEDHEALTH GROUP INC**

PacSun; **PACIFIC SUNWEAR OF CALIFORNIA INC**

PacSun Outlet; **PACIFIC SUNWEAR OF CALIFORNIA INC**

pacsun.com; **PACIFIC SUNWEAR OF CALIFORNIA INC**

PADCO; **AECOM TECHNOLOGY CORPORATION**

Pago Facil; **WESTERN UNION COMPANY (THE)**

Pain Management @ Home; **AMEDISYS INC**

Palazzo Resort Hotel Casino (The); **LAS VEGAS SANDS CORP (THE VENETIAN)**

Palmolive; **COLGATE PALMOLIVE CO**

Palo Alto Research Center; **XEROX CORP**

PanAmericana; **DIRECTV GROUP INC (THE)**

Pandac; **OWENS & MINOR INC**

Parallux; **IDEXX LABORATORIES INC**

Paramount Pictures Corp; **VIACOM INC**

PAREXEL APEX International; **PAREXEL INTERNATIONAL CORP**

PAREXEL Consulting & Medical Communications Svcs.; **PAREXEL INTERNATIONAL CORP**

PAREXEL International Synchron Private Limited; **PAREXEL INTERNATIONAL CORP**

Parsons Brinckerhoff Power, Inc.; **PARSONS BRINCKERHOFF INC**

Partners in Wound Care Program; **AMEDISYS INC**

Partnership Marketing Group; **ALLSTATE CORPORATION (THE)**

Passport Club; **CHICO'S FAS INC**

Pasta Pomodoro; **WENDYS INTERNATIONAL INC**

Patriot Air & Missile Defense System; **RAYTHEON CO**

Patterson Dental Co.; **PATTERSON COMPANIES INC**

Patterson Medical Holdings, Inc.; **PATTERSON COMPANIES INC**

Paxar Corp.; **AVERY DENNISON CORP**

Paychex FSA Debit Card; **PAYCHEX INC**

Paychex Online; **PAYCHEX INC**

Paychex Online Reports; **PAYCHEX INC**

PayPal; **EBAY INC**

PaySys International, Inc.; **FIRST DATA CORP**

PB Aviation, Inc.; **PARSONS BRINCKERHOFF INC**

PB Buildings, Inc.; **PARSONS BRINCKERHOFF INC**

PB Constructors, Inc.; **PARSONS BRINCKERHOFF INC**

PB Facilities, Inc.; **PARSONS BRINCKERHOFF INC**

PB Farradyne, Inc.; **PARSONS BRINCKERHOFF INC**

PB Research Library; **PARSONS BRINCKERHOFF INC**

PB Telecommunications, Inc.; **PARSONS BRINCKERHOFF INC**

PBteen; **WILLIAMS SONOMA INC**

PECO Energy Company; **EXELON CORPORATION**

Peking Union Lawke Biomedical Development, Ltd.; **PHARMACEUTICAL PRODUCT DEVELOPMENT INC**

Pemstar, Inc.; **BENCHMARK ELECTRONICS INC**

Pennsylvania Auto Dealers' Exchange; **ADESA INC**

Pennsylvania Electric Co.; **FIRSTENERGY CORP**

Pennsylvania Power Co.; **FIRSTENERGY CORP**

Pentium; **INTEL CORP**

Peoplefirst Rehabilitation; **KINDRED HEALTHCARE INC**

PeopleSoft; **DELOITTE CONSULTING LLP**

Pepsi; **PEPSICO INC**

PepsiAmericas Inc; **PEPSICO INC**

Pepsi-Cola; **PEPSI BOTTLING GROUP INC**

Percepta; **TELETECH HOLDINGS INC**

Perceptive Informatics, Inc.; **PAREXEL INTERNATIONAL CORP**

Perfect Fit; **MEN'S WEARHOUSE INC (THE)**

Permanente Medical Groups; **KAISER PERMANENTE**

INDEX OF SUBSIDIARIES, BRAND NAMES AND AFFILIATIONS, CONT.

Perrigo Israel Pharmaceuticals, Ltd.; **PERRIGO CO**
Perrigo New York, Inc.; **PERRIGO CO**
Perry-Judd's Holdings, Inc.; **R R DONNELLEY & SONS CO**
Per-Se Technologies Inc; **MCKESSON CORPORATION**
PersonalCare; **COVENTRY HEALTH CARE INC**
PersonicX; **ACXIOM CORP**
Petco Foundation (The); **PETCO ANIMAL SUPPLIES INC**
Peter Kiewit Sons', Inc. (PKS); **LEVEL 3 COMMUNICATIONS INC**
Peter Pan; **CONAGRA FOODS INC**
Petite Sophisticate Outlet; **CHARMING SHOPPES INC**
PetPerks; **PETSMART INC**
Petreco; **CAMERON INTERNATIONAL CORPORATION**
PetsHotels; **PETSMART INC**
PetSmart.com; **PETSMART INC**
petsmartbebettertogether.com; **PETSMART INC**
PG&E Strategic Capital, Inc.; **PG&E CORPORATION**
Phantom Works; **BOEING COMPANY (THE)**
PharmaCare Management Services; **CVS CAREMARK CORPORATION**
PharmaCare Pharmacy; **CVS CAREMARK CORPORATION**
Pharmaceutical Resource Solutions; **INVENTIV HEALTH INC**
Pharmaceutical World Review; **IMS HEALTH INC**
PharMerica Corp.; **KINDRED HEALTHCARE INC**
PharMerica Corporation; **AMERISOURCEBERGEN CORP**
Philadelphia; **KRAFT FOODS INC**
Philadelphia 76ers; **COMCAST CORP**
Philadelphia Flyers; **COMCAST CORP**
Philip Morris Capital Corp.; **ALTRIA GROUP INC**
Philip Morris International, Inc.; **ALTRIA GROUP INC**
Philip Morris U.S.A., Inc.; **ALTRIA GROUP INC**
Phillips 66; **CONOCOPHILLIPS COMPANY**
Phillips Casing & Tubing; **OIL STATES INTERNATIONAL INC**
Phoenix Marketing Group LLC; **EXPRESS SCRIPTS INC**
Phone Tools; **COX COMMUNICATIONS INC**
Physician Service Center; **MEDCO HEALTH SOLUTIONS**
PIC; **MICROCHIP TECHNOLOGY INC**
Pierce; **OSHKOSH CORPORATION**

Pigeon Cove; **WHOLE FOODS MARKET INC**
Pillsbury; **GENERAL MILLS INC**
Pillsbury; **JM SMUCKER CO**
PINK; **INTIMATE BRANDS INC**
Pintendre Autos Inc; **LKQ CORP**
Pioneer; **E I DU PONT DE NEMOURS & CO (DUPONT)**
Pitney Bowes Legal Solutions; **PITNEY BOWES INC**
Pixar Animation Studios Inc; **WALT DISNEY COMPANY (THE)**
Pizza Hut; **YUM! BRANDS INC**
PJM Interconnection, LLC; **BALTIMORE GAS AND ELECTRIC COMPANY**
PlantWeb Digital Plant Architecture; **EMERSON ELECTRIC CO**
Plavix; **BRISTOL MYERS SQUIBB CO**
Plus Membership Card; **SAM'S CLUB**
Poe & Brown, Inc.; **BROWN & BROWN INC**
Pogo.com; **ELECTRONIC ARTS INC**
Pollock NationaLease; **RYDER SYSTEM INC**
Polly Pocket!; **MATTEL INC**
Polo; **POLO RALPH LAUREN CORP**
Polo.com; **POLO RALPH LAUREN CORP**
PolyMedica Corporation; **MEDCO HEALTH SOLUTIONS**
Pop-Tarts; **KELLOGG CO**
Portal Software Inc; **ORACLE CORP**
PortalVision; **VARIAN MEDICAL SYSTEMS INC**
Porter Novelli; **OMNICOM GROUP INC**
Porter-Cable; **BLACK & DECKER CORP**
Pottery Barn; **WILLIAMS SONOMA INC**
Pottery Barn Kids; **WILLIAMS SONOMA INC**
Powell; **3M COMPANY**
Powerade; **COCA COLA COMPANY (THE)**
PowerChute; **AMERICAN POWER CONVERSION CORP**
PPD Development; **PHARMACEUTICAL PRODUCT DEVELOPMENT INC**
PPD Discovery; **PHARMACEUTICAL PRODUCT DEVELOPMENT INC**
PPD Medical Communications; **PHARMACEUTICAL PRODUCT DEVELOPMENT INC**
PPD Virtual; **PHARMACEUTICAL PRODUCT DEVELOPMENT INC**
Praair Surface Technologies, Inc.; **PRAXAIR INC**
Prakash Air Freight Pvt. Ltd.; **FEDEX CORPORATION**
Pratt & Whitney; **UNITED TECHNOLOGIES CORPORATION**

Praxair Distribution, Inc.; **PRAXAIR INC**
Precise ID; **EXPERIAN AMERICAS**
Precision Energy Services; **WEATHERFORD INTERNATIONAL LTD**
Precision International Contract Drilling; **WEATHERFORD INTERNATIONAL LTD**
Premarin; **WYETH**
Premier Health Partners; **CATHOLIC HEALTH INITIATIVES**
Premium Standard Firms Inc; **SMITHFIELD FOODS INC**
Preparation H; **WYETH**
Prescriptivees; **ESTEE LAUDER COMPANIES INC (THE)**
Prestone; **HONEYWELL INTERNATIONAL INC**
Price Pfister; **BLACK & DECKER CORP**
PricewaterhouseCoopers, LLP; **PRICEWATERHOUSECOOPERS**
Princess Cruises; **CARNIVAL CORPORATION**
Princeton Club; **DRESS BARN INC (THE)**
Principal Financial Services, Inc.; **PRINCIPAL FINANCIAL GROUP (THE)**
Principal International, Inc.; **PRINCIPAL FINANCIAL GROUP (THE)**
Principal Life Insurance Co.; **PRINCIPAL FINANCIAL GROUP (THE)**
Pringles; **PROCTER & GAMBLE CO**
Pro Line Printing, Inc.; **R R DONNELLEY & SONS CO**
Pro/ENGINEER; **PARAMETRIC TECHNOLOGY CORP**
ProCare; **DJO INC**
Process Dynamic; **E I DU PONT DE NEMOURS & CO (DUPONT)**
Process Management; **EMERSON ELECTRIC CO**
Procomp Industria Electronica S.A.; **DIEBOLD INC**
Proeton XPR36; **BIO RAD LABORATORIES INC**
Progress Rail Services, Inc.; **CATERPILLAR INC**
Progresso; **GENERAL MILLS INC**
Propecia; **MERCK & CO INC**
ProteomeLab; **BECKMAN COULTER INC**
Protiviti, Inc.; **ROBERT HALF INTERNATIONAL INC**
Provalliance; **REGIS CORPORATION**
Providence Equity Partners; **CLEAR CHANNEL COMMUNICATIONS INC**
Providence Equity Partners Inc.; **CDW CORPORATION**
Provigil; **CEPHALON INC**
Prozac; **ELI LILLY & COMPANY**

INDEX OF SUBSIDIARIES, BRAND NAMES AND AFFILIATIONS, CONT.

Prudential Bank; **PRUDENTIAL FINANCIAL INC**
Prudential Equity Group; **PRUDENTIAL FINANCIAL INC**
Prudential Insurance Company of America (The); **PRUDENTIAL FINANCIAL INC**
Prudential Real Estate Affiliates, Inc.; **PRUDENTIAL FINANCIAL INC**
Prudential Relocation; **PRUDENTIAL FINANCIAL INC**
Prudential Retirement Insurance and Annuity Co.; **PRUDENTIAL FINANCIAL INC**
PS Business Parks, Inc.; **PUBLIC STORAGE INC**
PS Partners, Ltd.; **PUBLIC STORAGE INC**
P-Serv; **KELLY SERVICES INC**
PSL Energy Services, Ltd.; **HALLIBURTON COMPANY**
PTI Group, Inc.; **OIL STATES INTERNATIONAL INC**
Public Service Co. of North Carolina, Inc.; **SCANA CORPORATION**
Public Service Company of Oklahoma; **AMERICAN ELECTRIC POWER COMPANY INC (AEP)**
Pullmantur; **ROYAL CARIBBEAN CRUISES**
Pull-Ups; **KIMBERLY-CLARK CORP**
Pulmozyme; **GENENTECH INC**
Pulsavac Plus Wound Debridement System; **ZIMMER HOLDINGS INC**
Pure Spring; **RITE AID CORPORATION**
Putnam LLC; **MARSH & MCLENNAN COMPANIES INC**
Pyxis; **CARDINAL HEALTH INC**
Q*VIEW; **COGNIZANT TECHNOLOGY SOLUTIONS CORP**
QAS; **EXPERIAN AMERICAS**
Qdoba Mexican Grill; **JACK IN THE BOX INC**
Qdoba Restaurant Corporation; **JACK IN THE BOX INC**
QFC; **KROGER CO (THE)**
Q-Prep Workstation; **BECKMAN COULTER INC**
QSS Group, Inc.; **PEROT SYSTEMS CORP**
Quaker Foods And Beverages; **PEPSICO INC**
Qualcomm Flarion Technologies, Inc.; **QUALCOMM INC**
Qualcomm Inc; **UNITED STATES CELLULAR CORP**
Qualcomm MEMS Technologies, Inc.; **QUALCOMM INC**
Quantum View; **UNITED PARCEL SERVICE INC (UPS)**
Quarter Pounder; **MCDONALD'S CORP**
Question Mark; **GUESS? INC**

Quick Stuff; **JACK IN THE BOX INC**
QuickBooks; **INTUIT INC**
QuickBooks Payroll; **INTUIT INC**
Quicken; **INTUIT INC**
Quicken.com; **INTUIT INC**
Quik Stop; **KROGER CO (THE)**
Quill Corp.; **STAPLES INC**
Quimica y Famarcia S.A. de C.V.; **PERRIGO CO**
Quota Monitor; **EXPEDITORS INTERNATIONAL OF WASHINGTON INC**
R E Austin Ltd.; **FIRST ADVANTAGE CORPORATION**
RABA Technologies, LLC; **SRA INTERNATIONAL INC**
Rachel's Organic; **DEAN FOODS CO**
RAD Data Communications; **MAXIM INTEGRATED PRODUCTS INC**
Radial Jaw; **BOSTON SCIENTIFIC CORP**
Rainbow Media Holdings LLC; **CABLEVISION SYSTEMS CORP**
Rainforest Cafe; **LANDRY'S RESTAURANTS INC**
Ralph Lauren; **POLO RALPH LAUREN CORP**
Ralph's; **KROGER CO (THE)**
Ramada; **WYNDHAM WORLDWIDE**
Ramcell; **CELLCO PARTNERSHIP (VERIZON WIRELESS)**
Rampage Clothing Co.; **CHARLOTTE RUSSE HOLDING**
Randall's Food Markets Inc; **SAFEWAY INC**
RapidArc; **VARIAN MEDICAL SYSTEMS INC**
Raptor; **WESTERN DIGITAL CORP**
Rational Software Corp; **INTERNATIONAL BUSINESS MACHINES CORP (IBM)**
RationalMed; **MEDCO HEALTH SOLUTIONS**
Raytheon Aircraft Company; **RAYTHEON CO**
Read-Rite Corp.; **WESTERN DIGITAL CORP**
RealEstate.com; **IAC/INTERACTIVECORP**
RealLife HR; **HEWITT ASSOCIATES**
Recycle America Alliance; **WASTE MANAGEMENT INC**
Red Lobster; **DARDEN RESTAURANTS INC**
RedHead; **BASS PRO SHOPS INC**
Reflexion Spiral X; **ST JUDE MEDICAL INC**
Refresh; **ALLERGAN INC**
Refuge; **CHARLOTTE RUSSE HOLDING**
Regentek; **DJO INC**
Regis Salons; **REGIS CORPORATION**

Rehab Therapy @ Home; **AMEDISYS INC**
Reinsurance Group of America, Inc.; **METLIFE INC**
Reliance; **STERIS CORP**
Reliant Energy Solutions East, LLC; **RELIANT ENERGY INC**
Reliant Resources, Inc.; **RELIANT ENERGY INC**
Relic; **FOSSIL INC**
Renaissance Hotels, Resorts and Suites; **MARRIOTT INTERNATIONAL INC**
Renal; **BAXTER INTERNATIONAL INC**
RenalSoft HD; **BAXTER INTERNATIONAL INC**
Renessen Feed & Processing; **CARGILL INC**
Renewable Hawaii, Inc.; **HAWAIIAN ELECTRIC INDUSTRIES INC**
Rent.com; **EBAY INC**
Rent-A-Centre; **RENT-A-CENTER INC**
Rental Car Finance Corp.; **DOLLAR THRIFTY AUTOMOTIVE GROUP INC**
Republic Services Inc; **WASTE MANAGEMENT INC**
Research Biotech; **SIGMA-ALDRICH CORP**
Research Essentials; **SIGMA-ALDRICH CORP**
Research Specialties; **SIGMA-ALDRICH CORP**
Residence Inn by Marriott; **LODGIAN INC**
Reslink; **SCHLUMBERGER LIMITED**
Resource Group, L.C. (The); **HILB ROGAL & HOBBS CO**
Respiratory Healthways; **HEALTHWAYS INC**
Restasis; **ALLERGAN INC**
Revolution/Stronghold; **PFIZER INC**
Reyataz; **BRISTOL MYERS SQUIBB CO**
RF Worx; **ADC TELECOMMUNICATIONS INC**
Rice Krispies; **KELLOGG CO**
RidemakerZ LLC; **BUILD-A-BEAR WORKSHOP INC**
Right Management; **MANPOWER INC**
Right Media, Inc.; **YAHOO! INC**
Rimadyl; **PFIZER INC**
Rintekno; **JACOBS ENGINEERING GROUP INC**
Rite Aid Health Solutions; **RITE AID CORPORATION**
Rituxan; **GENENTECH INC**
Ritz-Carlton (The); **MARRIOTT INTERNATIONAL INC**
Ritz-Carlton Club; **RITZ-CARLTON HOTEL COMPANY LLC (THE)**

INDEX OF SUBSIDIARIES, BRAND NAMES AND AFFILIATIONS, CONT.

River Oaks Health System; **HEALTH MANAGEMENT ASSOCIATES INC**
Rivneenergo; **AES CORPORATION (THE)**
RLM Systems, Ltd.; **LOCKHEED MARTIN CORP**
Road Runner; **VALERO ENERGY CORP**
RoadRailer; **NORFOLK SOUTHERN CORP**
Robert Half Finance & Accounting; **ROBERT HALF INTERNATIONAL INC**
Robert Half Legal; **ROBERT HALF INTERNATIONAL INC**
Robert Half Management Resources; **ROBERT HALF INTERNATIONAL INC**
Robert Half Technology; **ROBERT HALF INTERNATIONAL INC**
Robitussin; **WYETH**
Romano's Macaroni Grill; **BRINKER INTERNATIONAL INC**
Ronald McDonald House; **MCDONALD'S CORP**
Ronningen-Petter; **EATON CORP**
Roots & Fruits Cooperative Produce; **UNITED NATURAL FOODS INC**
Ross Dress for Less; **ROSS STORES INC**
Ross University; **DEVRY INC**
Rossignol; **QUIKSILVER INC**
Roto-Rooter Group, Inc.; **CHEMED CORPORATION**
Roxy; **QUIKSILVER INC**
Roxy Girl; **QUIKSILVER INC**
Royal Cargo Line; **BURLINGTON NORTHERN SANTA FE CORP**
Royal Caribbean International; **ROYAL CARIBBEAN CRUISES**
Royal Celebrity Tours; **ROYAL CARIBBEAN CRUISES**
Royal DuraPlank; **GEORGIA GULF CORPORATION**
Royal Dutch Shell (Shell Group); **SHELL OIL CO**
Royal Group, Inc.; **GEORGIA GULF CORPORATION**
Royal Philips Electronics NV; **RESPIRONICS INC**
Roy's; **OSI RESTAURANT PARTNERS INC**
RR Donnelley Global Document Solutions; **R R DONNELLEY & SONS CO**
Rubbish; **NORDSTROM INC**
RUEHL; **ABERCROMBIE & FITCH CO**
Rugby; **WATSON PHARMACEUTICALS INC**
Rugby; **POLO RALPH LAUREN CORP**
Rural Cellular Corp.; **CELLCO PARTNERSHIP (VERIZON WIRELESS)**

Russell Artwear; **RUSSELL CORP**
Russell Athletic; **RUSSELL CORP**
Russell Corp; **BERKSHIRE HATHAWAY INC**
Ryton; **CHEVRON PHILLIPS CHEMICAL COMPANY LLC**
Sabre Airline Solutions; **SABRE HOLDINGS CORP**
Sabre Travel Network; **SABRE HOLDINGS CORP**
Safari; **APPLE INC**
SAFC; **SIGMA-ALDRICH CORP**
SafeBoot Holding B.V.; **MCAFEE INC**
Safeway SELECT; **SAFEWAY INC**
Saint Alphonsus Express Care; **RITE AID CORPORATION**
Salesgenie.com; **INFOUSA INC**
Sally Beauty Company; **ALBERTO-CULVER COMPANY**
Saltgrass Steak House; **LANDRY'S RESTAURANTS INC**
Salud Con Health Net; **HEALTH NET INC**
Salute Fixation; **CR BARD INC**
Salve; **ALBERTO-CULVER COMPANY**
SAM Electronics GmbH; **L-3 COMMUNICATIONS HOLDINGS INC**
Sammons Preston Rolyan; **PATTERSON COMPANIES INC**
Sam's Café; **SAM'S CLUB**
SAM'S CLUB; **WAL-MART STORES INC**
San Diego Gas & Electric; **SEMPRA ENERGY**
Sanctura XR; **ALLERGAN INC**
Sandora, LLC; **PEPSICO INC**
Sands Expo and Convention Center (The); **LAS VEGAS SANDS CORP (THE VENETIAN)**
Sands Macao Casino (The); **LAS VEGAS SANDS CORP (THE VENETIAN)**
Sandwork Design; **SYNOPSYS INC**
SAP AG; **DELOITTE CONSULTING LLP**
SAS Enterprise BI Server; **SAS INSTITUTE INC**
SAS Enterprise Intelligence Platform; **SAS INSTITUTE INC**
SAS Promotion Optimization; **SAS INSTITUTE INC**
SAS Revenue Optimization; **SAS INSTITUTE INC**
SAS9; **SAS INSTITUTE INC**
Sat-Go; **DIRECTV GROUP INC (THE)**
Save-A-Lot; **SUPERVALU INC**
SBX; **DRESS BARN INC (THE)**
SCANA Communications, Inc.; **SCANA CORPORATION**
SCANA Energy Marketing, Inc.; **SCANA CORPORATION**
Scene7 Inc; **ADOBE SYSTEMS INC**

Scentinel; **CHEVRON PHILLIPS CHEMICAL COMPANY LLC**
SCF Marine Inc.; **SEACOR HOLDINGS INC**
Schaller Anderson, Inc.; **AETNA INC**
Schering-Plough Research Institute; **SCHERING-PLOUGH CORP**
Schlumberger Oilfield Services; **SCHLUMBERGER LIMITED**
Schneider Electric SA; **AMERICAN POWER CONVERSION CORP**
Scholar Ship (The); **ROYAL CARIBBEAN CRUISES**
Schreder-Hazemeyer; **EATON CORP**
Scicom Technologies Private Limited; **SAIC INC**
Science Advisory Board; **HEALTH FITNESS CORP**
Science Applications International Corporation; **SAIC INC**
Science Diet; **COLGATE PALMOLIVE CO**
Scientific Atlanta Inc; **CISCO SYSTEMS INC**
Scientific Games Racing LLC; **SCIENTIFIC GAMES CORPORATION**
Scios Inc; **JOHNSON & JOHNSON**
ScoreRight; **EXPERIAN AMERICAS**
Scorpio; **WESTERN DIGITAL CORP**
Scott; **KIMBERLY-CLARK CORP**
Scotts LawnService; **SCOTTS MIRACLE GROW CO**
SCS Technology; **BRINKS COMPANY (THE)**
sds business services GmbH; **AFFILIATED COMPUTER SERVICES INC**
SDX Service Deployment System; **JUNIPER NETWORKS INC**
Seabourn Cruise Line; **CARNIVAL CORPORATION**
SEACOR SMIT, Inc.; **SEACOR HOLDINGS INC**
Seasons 52; **DARDEN RESTAURANTS INC**
Secure Data Solutions; **BRINKS COMPANY (THE)**
Secure Mini-Storage; **PUBLIC STORAGE INC**
Securent, Inc.; **CISCO SYSTEMS INC**
Security DBS Drill Bits; **HALLIBURTON COMPANY**
Security Services of America; **ABM INDUSTRIES INC**
Seeds of Change; **MARS INC**
SEGCO; **SOUTHERN COMPANY (THE)**
Seidman Insurance Consultants, LLC; **BDO SEIDMAN LLP**
Seidman Private Advisors, LLC; **BDO SEIDMAN LLP**

INDEX OF SUBSIDIARIES, BRAND NAMES AND AFFILIATIONS, CONT.

Seidman Private Securities, LLC; **BDO SEIDMAN LLP**
Select Fish; **WHOLE FOODS MARKET INC**
Select Health Care Services; **RES CARE INC**
Select Nutrition Distributors, Inc.; **UNITED NATURAL FOODS INC**
Select Specialty Managers LLC; **W R BERKLEY CORPORATION**
Sempra Commodities; **SEMPRA ENERGY**
Sempra Financial; **SEMPRA ENERGY**
Sempra Generation; **SEMPRA ENERGY**
Sempra LNG; **SEMPRA ENERGY**
Sempra Pipeline & Storage; **SEMPRA ENERGY**
Sensient Dehydrated Flavors Company; **SENSIENT TECHNOLOGIES CORPORATION**
Sensient Flavors, Inc.; **SENSIENT TECHNOLOGIES CORPORATION**
Sensient Food Colors; **SENSIENT TECHNOLOGIES CORPORATION**
Sensient Imaging Technologies; **SENSIENT TECHNOLOGIES CORPORATION**
Sensient Pharmaceutical Technologies; **SENSIENT TECHNOLOGIES CORPORATION**
Senyuan International Holdings Limited; **EATON CORP**
Serologicals Corporation; **MILLIPORE CORP**
Serrana; **BUNGE LTD**
ServiceCare, Inc.; **SCANA CORPORATION**
Servicio Electronico De Pago S.A.; **WESTERN UNION COMPANY (THE)**
Sesame Street; **MATTEL INC**
Seven & I Holdings Co Ltd; **7-ELEVEN INC**
Shaw's Supermarkets; **SUPERVALU INC**
Sheba; **MARS INC**
Shell Chemicals Limited; **SHELL OIL CO**
Shell Exploration and Production; **SHELL OIL CO**
Shell Gas and Power; **SHELL OIL CO**
Shell Oil Products US; **SHELL OIL CO**
Sheraton; **STARWOOD HOTELS & RESORTS WORLDWIDE INC**
Shopping.com; **EBAY INC**
Shurgard Storage Centers, Inc.; **PUBLIC STORAGE INC**
Sierra Health Services0 Inc; **UNITEDHEALTH GROUP INC**
Sightline Technologies; **STRYKER CORP**
Sigma; **TBC CORPORATION**
Sikorsky; **UNITED TECHNOLOGIES CORPORATION**

Silcon UPS; **AMERICAN POWER CONVERSION CORP**
Silk; **DEAN FOODS CO**
Silver Lake Partners; **SABRE HOLDINGS CORP**
Silverhawk Security Specialists; **ABM INDUSTRIES INC**
SilverScript Insurance, Co.; **CVS CAREMARK CORPORATION**
Simcor; **ABBOTT LABORATORIES**
Similac; **ABBOTT LABORATORIES**
Simonton Holdings, Inc.; **FORTUNE BRANDS INC**
Sims (The); **ELECTRONIC ARTS INC**
Singulair; **MERCK & CO INC**
Sinograin; **BUNGE LTD**
SIR Warehouse Sports Store; **CABELA'S INC**
Sirna Therapeutics, Inc.; **MERCK & CO INC**
Sisters of Mercy-St. Louis Regional Community; **SISTERS OF MERCY HEALTH SYSTEMS**
Six Senses; **RITZ-CARLTON HOTEL COMPANY LLC (THE)**
Six Sigma; **BECHTEL GROUP INC**
Skunk Works; **LOCKHEED MARTIN CORP**
Sky Brasil Servicos Ltda.; **DIRECTV GROUP INC (THE)**
Skymark International, Inc.; **JOHNSON CONTROLS INC**
Skype; **EBAY INC**
Sleep Well Ventures; **RESPIRONICS INC**
Slim Jim; **CONAGRA FOODS INC**
Slurpee; **7-ELEVEN INC**
Smart Energy; **RELIANT ENERGY INC**
Smartphone; **UNITED STATES CELLULAR CORP**
SmartStyle; **REGIS CORPORATION**
Smart-UPS; **AMERICAN POWER CONVERSION CORP**
Smith & Hawken; **SCOTTS MIRACLE GROW CO**
Smith Borehole Enlargement; **SMITH INTERNATIONAL INC**
Smith International; **SCHLUMBERGER LIMITED**
Smith Services; **SMITH INTERNATIONAL INC**
Smith Technologies; **SMITH INTERNATIONAL INC**
Smithfield Beef Group; **SMITHFIELD FOODS INC**
Smith's; **KROGER CO (THE)**
Smith's Food & Drug Centers Inc; **KROGER CO (THE)**
Smuckers; **JM SMUCKER CO**
Sn@p; **EXPEDITORS INTERNATIONAL OF WASHINGTON INC**

SnakeLight; **BLACK & DECKER CORP**
SNAP; **IDEXX LABORATORIES INC**
SNC Technologies, Inc.; **GENERAL DYNAMICS CORP**
Snickers; **MARS INC**
Sobe; **PEPSI BOTTLING GROUP INC**
SoftMax, Inc.; **QUALCOMM INC**
Softsoap; **COLGATE PALMOLIVE CO**
Softswitch; **LEVEL 3 COMMUNICATIONS INC**
Software Inc; **INTERNATIONAL BUSINESS MACHINES CORP (IBM)**
Solar Turbines; **CATERPILLAR INC**
Solaris OS; **SUN MICROSYSTEMS INC**
Solid Phase Reversible Immobilization (SPRI); **BECKMAN COULTER INC**
Soltex; **CHEVRON PHILLIPS CHEMICAL COMPANY LLC**
Soma by Chico's; **CHICO'S FAS INC**
Sooner, Inc.; **OIL STATES INTERNATIONAL INC**
SOPIA Corporation; **ACCENTURE LTD**
Sound Technologies, Inc.; **VCA ANTECH INC**
South Carolina Electric & Gas Co.; **SCANA CORPORATION**
South Carolina Fuel Co., Inc.; **SCANA CORPORATION**
South Carolina Generating Co., Inc.; **SCANA CORPORATION**
Southern California Edison Company; **EDISON INTERNATIONAL**
Southern California Gas Company; **SEMPRA ENERGY**
Southern Health; **COVENTRY HEALTH CARE INC**
Southern Nuclear; **SOUTHERN COMPANY (THE)**
Southern Power; **SOUTHERN COMPANY (THE)**
SouthernLINC Wireless; **SOUTHERN COMPANY (THE)**
Southwestern Electric Power Company; **AMERICAN ELECTRIC POWER COMPANY INC (AEP)**
Spalding; **RUSSELL CORP**
Speakeasy, Inc.; **BEST BUY CO INC**
Specialized Health Products International, Inc; **CR BARD INC**
SpectraWatt, Inc.; **INTEL CORP**
SpectraWatt, Inc.; **INTEL CORP**
Spectrum Astro, Inc.; **GENERAL DYNAMICS CORP**
SPEEDAIRE; **WW GRAINGER INC**
Sperry Drilling Services; **HALLIBURTON COMPANY**
SpinaLogic; **DJO INC**
Spirit; **COLDWATER CREEK INC**
SPL World Group; **ORACLE CORP**
Sports & Co.; **HIBBETT SPORTS INC**
Sports Additions; **HIBBETT SPORTS INC**

INDEX OF SUBSIDIARIES, BRAND NAMES AND AFFILIATIONS, CONT.

Sports Illustrated; **TIME WARNER INC**
Sprint Nextel Corp; **EMBARQ CORP**
Sprint Nextel Corp; **NII HOLDINGS INC**
Sprite; **COCA COLA COMPANY (THE)**
SPUR; **MURPHY OIL CORPORATION**
SSG Precision Optronics, Inc.; **L-3 COMMUNICATIONS HOLDINGS INC**
SSL; **VERISIGN INC**
SSL VPN; **JUNIPER NETWORKS INC**
St. Ives Swiss Formula; **ALBERTO-CULVER COMPANY**
St. Paul Companies Inc; **TRAVELERS COMPANIES INC (THE)**
St. Regis; **STARWOOD HOTELS & RESORTS WORLDWIDE INC**
Stalla Review; **DEVRY INC**
Staples Business Advantage; **STAPLES INC**
Staples Business Delivery; **STAPLES INC**
Staples National Advantage; **STAPLES INC**
StarTek Connect; **STARTEK INC**
State Fair; **SARA LEE CORP**
Stellant, Inc.; **ORACLE CORP**
StepUp Commerce, Inc.; **INTUIT INC**
Steril S.p.A.; **FOSTER WHEELER LTD**
STERIS Isomedix Services; **STERIS CORP**
STERIS SYSTEM 1; **STERIS CORP**
Sterling Autobody Centers; **ALLSTATE CORPORATION (THE)**
Sterling Publishing Co., Inc.; **BARNES & NOBLE INC**
Stonefly; **INVENTIV HEALTH INC**
Stop N Go; **VALERO ENERGY CORP**
StorEdge; **SUN MICROSYSTEMS INC**
Stratagene Corp.; **AGILENT TECHNOLOGIES INC**
strategy+business; **BOOZ ALLEN HAMILTON**
Stroke Recovery @ Home; **AMEDISYS INC**
Stryker Biotech; **STRYKER CORP**
Stryker Endoscopy; **STRYKER CORP**
Stryker Instruments; **STRYKER CORP**
Stryker Medical; **STRYKER CORP**
Stryker Orthopaedics; **STRYKER CORP**
Stryker Osteosynthesis; **STRYKER CORP**
Stryker Spine; **STRYKER CORP**
Studio D; **BEST BUY CO INC**
Studio Y; **DRESS BARN INC (THE)**
Study Tracker; **COVANCE INC**
StumbleUpon; **EBAY INC**
Sun Fire; **SUN MICROSYSTEMS INC**
Sun Life Financial, Inc.; **GENWORTH FINANCIAL INC**
SunCoke Energy, Inc.; **SUNOCO INC**
SunCom Wireless Holdings, Inc.; **T-MOBILE USA**
Sundance Channel; **CABLEVISION SYSTEMS CORP**

SunDance Rehabilitation Corp.; **SUN HEALTHCARE GROUP**
Sunflower Market; **SUPERVALU INC**
Sunoco Chemicals; **SUNOCO INC**
Sunoco Logistic Partners L.P.; **SUNOCO INC**
Sunopsis; **ORACLE CORP**
SunPlus Home Health Services; **SUN HEALTHCARE GROUP**
Sunrise Assisted Living; **SUNRISE SENIOR LIVING**
SunSpectrum; **SUN MICROSYSTEMS INC**
Super 8; **WYNDHAM WORLDWIDE**
SuperCuts; **REGIS CORPORATION**
Superior; **SARA LEE CORP**
SuperPawn; **CASH AMERICA INTERNATIONAL INC**
SuperStart; **O'REILLY AUTOMOTIVE INC**
SuperTarget; **TARGET CORPORATION**
SureArrest; **AMERICAN POWER CONVERSION CORP**
SureWest Communications; **CELLCO PARTNERSHIP (VERIZON WIRELESS)**
SurgiTrack; **OWENS & MINOR INC**
Suttle Straus, Inc.; **TELEPHONE AND DATA SYSTEMS INC (TDS)**
Syan Holdings Limited; **AFFILIATED COMPUTER SERVICES INC**
SYGMA Network; **SYSCO CORP**
Symmetrix; **EMC CORP**
SymTech; **INGRAM MICRO INC**
Syncrude Canada, Ltd.; **MURPHY OIL CORPORATION**
Synflex; **EATON CORP**
Synovus Financial Corp.; **TOTAL SYSTEM SERVICES INC (TSYS)**
Synthetic American Fuel Enterprises I, LLC; **MARRIOTT INTERNATIONAL INC**
T.J. Maxx; **TJX COMPANIES INC (THE)**
T.K. Maxx; **TJX COMPANIES INC (THE)**
TA Instruments, Inc.; **WATERS CORP**
Taco Bell; **YUM! BRANDS INC**
Taiwan Green Point Enterprises Co., Ltd.; **JABIL CIRCUIT INC**
Taj Boston; **RITZ-CARLTON HOTEL COMPANY LLC (THE)**
Take Care Health Systems LLC; **WALGREEN CO**
Talbots Accessories & Shoes; **TALBOTS INC (THE)**
Talbots Mens; **TALBOTS INC (THE)**
Talbots Misses; **TALBOTS INC (THE)**
Talbots Outlet; **TALBOTS INC (THE)**
Talbots Petite; **TALBOTS INC (THE)**
Talbots Woman; **TALBOTS INC (THE)**

Talents Technology; **KELLY SERVICES INC**
Talty Insurance Agency, Inc.; **HILB ROGAL & HOBBS CO**
Tandem Labs., Inc.; **LABORATORY CORP OF AMERICA HOLDINGS**
Tarantella Inc; **SUN MICROSYSTEMS INC**
Target Card; **TARGET CORPORATION**
target.com; **TARGET CORPORATION**
Tax Governance Institute; **KPMG LLP**
Taxus; **BOSTON SCIENTIFIC CORP**
TBWA Worldwide; **OMNICOM GROUP INC**
T-Check Systems, Inc.; **CH ROBINSON WORLDWIDE INC**
TDS Metrocom; **TELEPHONE AND DATA SYSTEMS INC (TDS)**
TDS Telecom; **TELEPHONE AND DATA SYSTEMS INC (TDS)**
TeamSourcing; **SYNTEL INC**
Tech Data Germany AG; **TECH DATA CORP**
Technisys, Inc.; **FMC TECHNOLOGIES INC**
Teflon; **E I DU PONT DE NEMOURS & CO (DUPONT)**
Tekno S.A.; **VALSPAR CORPORATION (THE)**
Teknos Nova Coil TNC Oy; **VALSPAR CORPORATION (THE)**
TEKTRONIX; **TEKTRONIX INC**
Telcove Corp; **LEVEL 3 COMMUNICATIONS INC**
TeleCheck Services, Inc.; **FIRST DATA CORP**
Teledyne Brown Engineering; **TELEDYNE TECHNOLOGIES INCORPORATED**
Teledyne Cougar Inc; **TELEDYNE TECHNOLOGIES INCORPORATED**
Teledyne Energy Systems Inc; **TELEDYNE TECHNOLOGIES INCORPORATED**
Teledyne Isco Inc; **TELEDYNE TECHNOLOGIES INCORPORATED**
Teledyne Solutions Inc; **TELEDYNE TECHNOLOGIES INCORPORATED**
Teledyne Tekmar Co; **TELEDYNE TECHNOLOGIES INCORPORATED**
Teledyne Titan; **TELEDYNE TECHNOLOGIES INCORPORATED**
TeleFutura; **UNIVISION COMMUNICATIONS INC**
TeleHealth Services; **SYKES ENTERPRISES INC**
Telenet Group Holding NV; **LIBERTY GLOBAL INC**
Telephone and Data Systems Inc; **UNITED STATES CELLULAR CORP**
TELUS Corporation; **NII HOLDINGS INC**

INDEX OF SUBSIDIARIES, BRAND NAMES AND AFFILIATIONS, CONT.

Tempstaff Kelly; **KELLY SERVICES INC**

TerraTek, Inc.; **SCHLUMBERGER LIMITED**

TerraVici Drilling Solutions; **HELMERICH & PAYNE INC**

Tesoro Corp; **SHELL OIL CO**

Texaco; **CHEVRON CORPORATION**

Texaco Nederland B.V.; **CHEVRON CORPORATION**

Texas Pacific Group; **SABRE HOLDINGS CORP**

TextBooks.com; **BARNES & NOBLE COLLEGE BOOKSTORES**

THD Design Center; **HOME DEPOT INC**

The Capital Grille; **DARDEN RESTAURANTS INC**

The Capital Group; **JOHNSON CONTROLS INC**

The Carphone Warehouse; **BEST BUY CO INC**

The Global Draw Limited; **SCIENTIFIC GAMES CORPORATION**

The Tech Group; **WEST PHARMACEUTICAL SERVICES INC**

TheSimsOnStage.ea.com; **ELECTRONIC ARTS INC**

Think Adoption First; **PETCO ANIMAL SUPPLIES INC**

Think Green; **WASTE MANAGEMENT INC**

Thomas H Lee Partners LP; **CLEAR CHANNEL COMMUNICATIONS INC**

Thomas H. Lee Partners; **ARAMARK CORPORATION**

Thompson's; **SHERWIN WILLIAMS COMPANY (THE)**

Thrifty Canada, Ltd.; **DOLLAR THRIFTY AUTOMOTIVE GROUP INC**

Thrifty Car Sales, Inc.; **DOLLAR THRIFTY AUTOMOTIVE GROUP INC**

Thrifty Rent-A-Car System, Inc.; **DOLLAR THRIFTY AUTOMOTIVE GROUP INC**

Thrifty, Inc.; **DOLLAR THRIFTY AUTOMOTIVE GROUP INC**

TI Consulting; **DELOITTE & TOUCHE USA LLP**

Ticketmaster; **IAC/INTERACTIVECORP**

Tide; **PROCTER & GAMBLE CO**

Tiffany & Co. Japan, Inc.; **TIFFANY & CO**

Tiffany and Company; **TIFFANY & CO**

TigerWire; **ST JUDE MEDICAL INC**

Tilia Fe; **WATSON PHARMACEUTICALS INC**

Tillinghast; **TOWERS PERRIN**

Time Inc; **TIME WARNER INC**

Time Warner Cable Inc; **TIME WARNER INC**

TimeWise; **MARY KAY INC**

Tindall Technologies Inc; **TELEDYNE TECHNOLOGIES INCORPORATED**

Tire Kingdom, Inc.; **TBC CORPORATION**

Tivella, Inc.; **CISCO SYSTEMS INC**

TMBR/Sharp Drilling, Inc.; **PATTERSON-UTI ENERGY INC**

T-Mobile HotSpot; **T-MOBILE USA**

T-Mobile International AG; **T-MOBILE USA**

TNKase; **GENENTECH INC**

Toledo Edison Co. (The); **FIRSTENERGY CORP**

Tom's of Maine; **COLGATE PALMOLIVE CO**

Too, Inc.; **TWEEN BRANDS INC**

Torrid; **HOT TOPIC INC**

Torrid.com; **HOT TOPIC INC**

TOSS; **WASTE MANAGEMENT INC**

Total Distribution Services, Inc.; **CSX CORP**

Total Rewards; **HARRAH'S ENTERTAINMENT INC**

Total System Services de Mexico; **TOTAL SYSTEM SERVICES INC (TSYS)**

Towers Perrin Reinsurance; **TOWERS PERRIN**

TPG (Texas Pacific Group); **PETCO ANIMAL SUPPLIES INC**

TPG (Texas Pacific Group); **NEIMAN MARCUS GROUP INC (THE)**

TRACE; **EXPEDITORS INTERNATIONAL OF WASHINGTON INC**

Tracker Marine; **BASS PRO SHOPS INC**

TrackTek; **CHEVRON PHILLIPS CHEMICAL COMPANY LLC**

Trade Secret; **REGIS CORPORATION**

TradeFlow; **EXPEDITORS INTERNATIONAL OF WASHINGTON INC**

Transco; **WILLIAMS COMPANIES INC (THE)**

Transfer Express de Panama; **WESTERN UNION COMPANY (THE)**

TRANSFLO; **CSX CORP**

Transwheel Corporation; **LKQ CORP**

Travel+Leisure; **AMERICAN EXPRESS CO**

Travelocity.com LP; **SABRE HOLDINGS CORP**

Tread Quarters Discount Tire; **MONRO MUFFLER BRAKE INC**

Treanda for Injection; **CEPHALON INC**

Treasure Island; **MGM MIRAGE**

Trelstar Depot; **WATSON PHARMACEUTICALS INC**

Trendwest; **WYNDHAM WORLDWIDE**

Trenwith Group, LLC; **BDO SEIDMAN LLP**

TRESemme; **ALBERTO-CULVER COMPANY**

T-Rex Café; **LANDRY'S RESTAURANTS INC**

TRIAD; **FAIR ISAAC CORPORATION**

Trial Tracker; **COVANCE INC**

TrialBase; **KENDLE INTERNATIONAL INC**

TriaLine; **KENDLE INTERNATIONAL INC**

TrialView; **KENDLE INTERNATIONAL INC**

TrialWare; **KENDLE INTERNATIONAL INC**

TrialWeb; **KENDLE INTERNATIONAL INC**

Triangle Design; **GUESS? INC**

Tricone; **BAKER HUGHES INC**

Trinity Hospice, Inc.; **SUNRISE SENIOR LIVING**

TriPath Imaging; **BECTON DICKINSON & CO**

Triple Crown Services Co.; **NORFOLK SOUTHERN CORP**

TriPoint Global Communications, Inc.; **GENERAL DYNAMICS CORP**

Trisenox; **CEPHALON INC**

Triton Engineering Services; **NOBLE CORPORATION**

TriVascular; **BOSTON SCIENTIFIC CORP**

TRL Electronics; **L-3 COMMUNICATIONS HOLDINGS INC**

Tropicana Products Inc; **PEPSICO INC**

Truvia; **CARGILL INC**

T-Series; **JUNIPER NETWORKS INC**

TSYS Canada, Inc.; **TOTAL SYSTEM SERVICES INC (TSYS)**

TSYS Technology Center, Inc.; **TOTAL SYSTEM SERVICES INC (TSYS)**

TSYS Total Debt Management, Inc.; **TOTAL SYSTEM SERVICES INC (TSYS)**

Turf Builder; **SCOTTS MIRACLE GROW CO**

Turner Broadcasting System; **TIME WARNER INC**

Twentieth Century Fox Television; **FOX ENTERTAINMENT GROUP INC**

Twilight Wish Foundation; **SUN HEALTHCARE GROUP**

Twisted Frosty; **WENDYS INTERNATIONAL INC**

Twix; **MARS INC**

Tyvek; **E I DU PONT DE NEMOURS & CO (DUPONT)**

U.S. Franchise Systems, Inc.; **GLOBAL HYATT CORPORATION**

U.S. Trust; **BANK OF AMERICA CORP**

Ultima; **O'REILLY AUTOMOTIVE INC**

INDEX OF SUBSIDIARIES, BRAND NAMES AND AFFILIATIONS, CONT.

Ultraline Service Corp.; **HALLIBURTON COMPANY**
UltraSPARC; **SUN MICROSYSTEMS INC**
Uluwehiokama Biofuels Corp.; **HAWAIIAN ELECTRIC INDUSTRIES INC**
UMA; **AECOM TECHNOLOGY CORPORATION**
Uncle Ben's; **MARS INC**
Uncrustables; **JM SMUCKER CO**
Underground Station; **GENESCO INC**
Unicare; **WELLPOINT INC**
UniCel DxC 880i Sychrom Access Clinical System; **BECKMAN COULTER INC**
Union Pacific Railroad Company; **UNION PACIFIC CORP**
UnionPay Data Co., Ltd.; **TOTAL SYSTEM SERVICES INC (TSYS)**
Uniprise Incorporated; **UNITEDHEALTH GROUP INC**
United Bakers Group; **KELLOGG CO**
United Paramount Network (UPN); **VIACOM INC**
United Parcel Service Inc (UPS); **UPS SUPPLY CHAIN SOLUTIONS**
Universe Electron Corporation; **ARROW ELECTRONICS INC**
University of Phoenix Online; **APOLLO GROUP INC**
University of Phoenix, Inc. (The); **APOLLO GROUP INC**
Univision Online, Inc.; **UNIVISION COMMUNICATIONS INC**
Univision Radio, Inc.; **UNIVISION COMMUNICATIONS INC**
Univision Television Group; **UNIVISION COMMUNICATIONS INC**
UOP LLC; **HONEYWELL INTERNATIONAL INC**
UPC Broadband Division; **LIBERTY GLOBAL INC**
UPC Holding BV; **LIBERTY GLOBAL INC**
UPS Billing Analysis Tool; **UNITED PARCEL SERVICE INC (UPS)**
UPS Freight; **UNITED PARCEL SERVICE INC (UPS)**
UPS Hundredweight Services; **UNITED PARCEL SERVICE INC (UPS)**
UPS Next Day Air; **UNITED PARCEL SERVICE INC (UPS)**
UPS Supply Chain Solutions; **UNITED PARCEL SERVICE INC (UPS)**
UPS Trade Direct; **UPS SUPPLY CHAIN SOLUTIONS**
UPS WorldShip; **UNITED PARCEL SERVICE INC (UPS)**
Urban Outfitters; **URBAN OUTFITTERS INC**
URS Division; **URS CORPORATION**

US Cellular; **TELEPHONE AND DATA SYSTEMS INC (TDS)**
US Pathology Labs, Inc.; **LABORATORY CORP OF AMERICA HOLDINGS**
USAA Alliance Services; **USAA**
USAA Educational Foundation; **USAA**
USAA Investment Management Company; **USAA**
UTC Fire and Security; **UNITED TECHNOLOGIES CORPORATION**
UTC Power; **UNITED TECHNOLOGIES CORPORATION**
Vacutainer; **BECTON DICKINSON & CO**
Valero Refining & Marketing Company; **VALERO ENERGY CORP**
Valspar Refinish; **VALSPAR CORPORATION (THE)**
ValueMedics Research LLC; **IMS HEALTH INC**
Van Nuys Storage Partners, Ltd.; **PUBLIC STORAGE INC**
Vanderbilt Tires; **TBC CORPORATION**
VanDyke's; **CABELA'S INC**
Vanguard Car Rental USA Inc; **ENTERPRISE RENT-A-CAR**
Vanilla Frosty; **WENDYS INTERNATIONAL INC**
Varco International, Inc.; **NATIONAL OILWELL VARCO INC**
Varta; **JOHNSON CONTROLS INC**
VCA Animal Hospitals; **VCA ANTECH INC**
VECO; **CH2M HILL COMPANIES LTD**
Vector Products, Inc.; **BLACK & DECKER CORP**
Veikkaus Oy; **GTECH HOLDINGS CORP**
Velocity; **MARY KAY INC**
Velveeta; **KRAFT FOODS INC**
Venetian Macao Resort Hotel (The); **LAS VEGAS SANDS CORP (THE VENETIAN)**
Venetian Resort Hotel Casino (The); **LAS VEGAS SANDS CORP (THE VENETIAN)**
Venezia; **CHARMING SHOPPES INC**
Venture Tape; **3M COMPANY**
Verid; **EMC CORP**
VeriSign; **EBAY INC**
Verizon Business; **VERIZON COMMUNICATIONS**
Verizon Communications, Inc.; **CELLCO PARTNERSHIP (VERIZON WIRELESS)**
Verizon Telecom; **VERIZON COMMUNICATIONS**
Verizon Wireless; **CELLCO PARTNERSHIP (VERIZON WIRELESS)**

Verizon Wireless; **VERIZON COMMUNICATIONS**
VerSys; **ZIMMER HOLDINGS INC**
Vertex Aerospace LLC; **L-3 COMMUNICATIONS HOLDINGS INC**
VetLab; **IDEXX LABORATORIES INC**
Viagra; **PFIZER INC**
Viasys Healthcare, Inc.; **CARDINAL HEALTH INC**
Vi-Cell; **BECKMAN COULTER INC**
Victoria's Secret; **INTIMATE BRANDS INC**
Victoria's Secret; **LIMITED BRANDS INC**
Victoria's Secret Beauty; **LIMITED BRANDS INC**
Victoria's Secret Direct; **INTIMATE BRANDS INC**
VIDEOJET; **DANAHER CORP**
Vigilant Insurance Company; **CHUBB CORPORATION (THE)**
Vigo; **WESTERN UNION COMPANY (THE)**
Vista Equity Partners; **HEWITT ASSOCIATES**
Vitae; **MANPOWER INC**
Vitas Group; **CHEMED CORPORATION**
Vitas Healthcare Corp.; **CHEMED CORPORATION**
Vitesse Semiconductor Corp.; **MAXIM INTEGRATED PRODUCTS INC**
Vivitrol; **CEPHALON INC**
VMware Inc; **EMC CORP**
Vodafone Group PLC; **CELLCO PARTNERSHIP (VERIZON WIRELESS)**
Volt Europe; **VOLT INFORMATION SCIENCES INC**
Volt Human Resources; **VOLT INFORMATION SCIENCES INC**
Volt Services Group; **VOLT INFORMATION SCIENCES INC**
VoltDelta; **VOLT INFORMATION SCIENCES INC**
Volume Logic; **PLANTRONICS INC**
Von Hoffmann; **R R DONNELLEY & SONS CO**
Vons Companies Inc (The); **SAFEWAY INC**
Vontu, Inc.; **SYMANTEC CORP**
VTR Global Com S.A.; **LIBERTY GLOBAL INC**
Vysis Inc; **ABBOTT LABORATORIES**
W; **STARWOOD HOTELS & RESORTS WORLDWIDE INC**
W. & J. Dunlop, Ltd.; **HENRY SCHEIN INC**
Wachovia Securities, LLC; **PRUDENTIAL FINANCIAL INC**
Wade & Assoicates, Inc.; **CH2M HILL COMPANIES LTD**

INDEX OF SUBSIDIARIES, BRAND NAMES AND AFFILIATIONS, CONT.

Waldorf=Astoria Collection (The);
HILTON HOTELS CORP
Walgreen Advance Care, Inc.;
WALGREEN CO
Walgreen's Health Services; **WALGREEN CO**
Wallach Surgical Decives Inc; **COOPER COMPANIES INC**
Wal-Mart Stores, Inc.; **SAM'S CLUB**
Wal-Mart Supercenter; **WAL-MART STORES INC**
Walt Disney Parks & Resorts; **WALT DISNEY COMPANY (THE)**
Walt Disney Pictures; **WALT DISNEY COMPANY (THE)**
Walt Disney Studios (The); **WALT DISNEY COMPANY (THE)**
Walter Karl; **INFOUSA INC**
Warburg Pincus LLC; **NEIMAN MARCUS GROUP INC (THE)**
Warburg Pincus LLC; **ARAMARK CORPORATION**
Warner Bros Entertainment Inc; **TIME WARNER INC**
Washington Division; **URS CORPORATION**
Washington Group International; **URS CORPORATION**
Watco Companies; **NORFOLK SOUTHERN CORP**
Waters Division; **WATERS CORP**
Watson Laboratories; **WATSON PHARMACEUTICALS INC**
Watson Pharma; **WATSON PHARMACEUTICALS INC**
Watson Wyatt & Company Holdings; **WATSON WYATT WORLDWIDE INC**
Watson Wyatt Brans & Co.; **WATSON WYATT WORLDWIDE INC**
WD Raptor X; **WESTERN DIGITAL CORP**
Webex Communications Inc; **CISCO SYSTEMS INC**
Webster Management LP; **PATTERSON COMPANIES INC**
Weedol; **SCOTTS MIRACLE GROW CO**
Weight Watchers eTools; **WEIGHT WATCHERS INTERNATIONAL INC**
Weight Watchers Online; **WEIGHT WATCHERS INTERNATIONAL INC**
Well Director Rotary Steerable System; **NOBLE CORPORATION**
Wella; **PROCTER & GAMBLE CO**
WellDynamics; **HALLIBURTON COMPANY**
WellPath; **COVENTRY HEALTH CARE INC**
WellPoint Behavioral Health; **WELLPOINT INC**
WellPoint Dental Services; **WELLPOINT INC**

WellPoint Pharmacy Management; **WELLPOINT INC**
Welsh, Carson, Anderson & Stowe; **SELECT MEDICAL CORPORATION**
Wendy's; **WENDYS INTERNATIONAL INC**
West Analytical Services; **WEST PHARMACEUTICAL SERVICES INC**
West Asset Management; **WEST CORPORATION**
West Business Services Corp.; **WEST CORPORATION**
West Elm; **WILLIAMS SONOMA INC**
West Interactive Corp.; **WEST CORPORATION**
West Telemarketing Corp.; **WEST CORPORATION**
West Virginia Wireless; **CELLCO PARTNERSHIP (VERIZON WIRELESS)**
Western Auto; **ADVANCE AUTO PARTS INC**
Western Gas Resources; **ANADARKO PETROLEUM CORPORATION**
Western International University, Inc.; **APOLLO GROUP INC**
Western Oil Sands Inc; **MARATHON OIL CORP**
WesternGeco; **SCHLUMBERGER LIMITED**
Westin; **STARWOOD HOTELS & RESORTS WORLDWIDE INC**
Westinghouse; **SHAW GROUP INC (THE)**
Westport, Ltd.; **DRESS BARN INC (THE)**
Wexford Group International; **CACI INTERNATIONAL INC**
W-H Energy Services, Inc.; **SMITH INTERNATIONAL INC**
Wheatley; **CAMERON INTERNATIONAL CORPORATION**
Wheelbrator; **WASTE MANAGEMENT INC**
White Barn Candle Co.; **INTIMATE BRANDS INC**
White Barn Candle Company; **LIMITED BRANDS INC**
White Hen Pantry, Inc.; **7-ELEVEN INC**
White House/Black Market; **CHICO'S FAS INC**
White River Fly Shops; **BASS PRO SHOPS INC**
WhiteWave Foods Company; **DEAN FOODS CO**
Whole Health Management; **WALGREEN CO**
Whole Kitchen; **WHOLE FOODS MARKET INC**
Whole Pantry; **WHOLE FOODS MARKET INC**

Whopper; **BURGER KING HOLDINGS INC**
WHP Health Initiatives, Inc.; **WALGREEN CO**
Wild Oats Markets Inc; **WHOLE FOODS MARKET INC**
Wild Wings; **CABELA'S INC**
Williams Field Services Group, LLC; **WILLIAMS COMPANIES INC (THE)**
Williams Gas Pipeline Co., LLC; **WILLIAMS COMPANIES INC (THE)**
Williams NAtural Gas Liquids, Inc.; **WILLIAMS COMPANIES INC (THE)**
Williams Partners L.P.; **WILLIAMS COMPANIES INC (THE)**
Williams Power Co., Inc.; **WILLIAMS COMPANIES INC (THE)**
Williams Production Co., LLC; **WILLIAMS COMPANIES INC (THE)**
Williams Production RMT Co.; **WILLIAMS COMPANIES INC (THE)**
Williams-Sonoma Home; **WILLIAMS SONOMA INC**
Willis Group Holdings Ltd.; **HILB ROGAL & HOBBS CO**
Wilson; **SMITH INTERNATIONAL INC**
Wilson Welding & Medical Gases; **PRAXAIR INC**
Windlok; **GEORGIA GULF CORPORATION**
Windows; **MICROSOFT CORP**
Windows Live; **MICROSOFT CORP**
Windows Mobile; **UNITED STATES CELLULAR CORP**
Windows Vista; **MICROSOFT CORP**
Wingate Inns; **WYNDHAM WORLDWIDE**
Winners; **TJX COMPANIES INC (THE)**
WISDOM; **OWENS & MINOR INC**
Withoutabox; **AMAZON.COM INC**
Wizard; **CONVERGYS CORPORATION**
Woodhead; **MOLEX INC**
Woodstock Farms; **UNITED NATURAL FOODS INC**
Woody Car Design; **AEROPOSTALE INC**
Workforce Services Group; **RES CARE INC**
WorkingRx Holding Co.; **FISERV INC**
Worklife; **OFFICE DEPOT INC**
World Financial Capital Bank; **ALLIANCE DATA SYSTEMS CORPORATION**
World Financial Network National Bank; **ALLIANCE DATA SYSTEMS CORPORATION**
World Market; **COST PLUS INC**
World Market Stores; **COST PLUS INC**
World Ovens Bakery; **7-ELEVEN INC**
World's Foremost Bank; **CABELA'S INC**

INDEX OF SUBSIDIARIES, BRAND NAMES AND AFFILIATIONS, CONT.

Wound Care - A Therapy Approach;
AMEDISYS INC
Wrafton Laboratories, Ltd.; **PERRIGO CO**
Wrigley's Spearmint; **WM WRIGLEY JR COMPANY**
www.progressiveresponds.com;
PROGRESSIVE CORPORATION (THE)
Wyeth K.K.; **WYETH**
Wyndham Hotels; **WYNDHAM WORLDWIDE**
Wyndham Worldwide; **LODGIAN INC**
Wynn Diamond Suites at Wynn Macau;
WYNN RESORTS LIMITED
Wynn Las Vegas, LLC; **WYNN RESORTS LIMITED**
Wynn Resorts (Macau), S.A.; **WYNN RESORTS LIMITED**
Xbox 360; **MICROSOFT CORP**
Xcelicor, Inc.; **DELOITTE & TOUCHE USA LLP**
Xcelicor, Inc.; **DELOITTE CONSULTING LLP**
Xerox Canada Inc; **XEROX CORP**
Xhilaration; **TARGET CORPORATION**
XPRL;
PRICEWATERHOUSECOOPERS
Xserve; **APPLE INC**
Xspedius Communications LLC; **TW TELECOM INC**
Yahoo! Mail; **YAHOO! INC**
Yahoo! Messenger; **YAHOO! INC**
Yahoo! Shopping; **YAHOO! INC**
Yahoo.com; **YAHOO! INC**
Yak & Yeti; **LANDRY'S RESTAURANTS INC**
Yardbirds; **HOME DEPOT INC**
Yesmail.com Inc; **INFOUSA INC**
Yoplait; **GENERAL MILLS INC**
York International; **JOHNSON CONTROLS INC**
YouTube; **GOOGLE INC**
Yum! China; **YUM! BRANDS INC**
Yum! Restaurants International; **YUM! BRANDS INC**
Zandar Technologies; **HARRIS CORPORATION**
ZAO Begun; **GOOGLE INC**
ZEE Medical; **MCKESSON CORPORATION**
Zoasis.com; **VCA ANTECH INC**
Zodiac; **FOSSIL INC**
Zoloft; **PFIZER INC**
Zyprexa; **ELI LILLY & COMPANY**

INDEX BY COMPANIES FOR SPECIFIC TYPES OF JOB SEEKERS

Indexed by the following categories:

Information Systems	654
Liberal Arts	663
Management	673
Professionals	687
Sales/Marketing	703
Technical/Scientific	714

Information Systems

Consulting/Other:

ACCENTURE LTD
AFFILIATED COMPUTER SERVICES INC
AGILENT TECHNOLOGIES INC
APPLE INC
BDO SEIDMAN LLP
BECHTEL GROUP INC
BOEING COMPANY (THE)
BOOZ ALLEN HAMILTON
CACI INTERNATIONAL INC
CH2M HILL COMPANIES LTD
CIBER INC
CISCO SYSTEMS INC
COGNIZANT TECHNOLOGY SOLUTIONS CORP
COVANCE INC
DELOITTE & TOUCHE USA LLP
DELOITTE CONSULTING LLP
DIEBOLD INC
ERNST & YOUNG LLP
FLUOR CORP
FOSTER WHEELER LTD
GENERAL DYNAMICS CORP
GRANT THORNTON LLP
HARRIS CORPORATION
HEWITT ASSOCIATES
HONEYWELL INTERNATIONAL INC
IGATE CORPORATION
INTEL CORP
INTERNATIONAL BUSINESS MACHINES CORP (IBM)
JACOBS ENGINEERING GROUP INC
KEANE INC
KENDLE INTERNATIONAL INC

KPMG LLP
L-3 COMMUNICATIONS HOLDINGS INC
L-3 TITAN GROUP
LOCKHEED MARTIN CORP
MCKESSON CORPORATION
MCKINSEY & COMPANY INC
MERCER INC
MICROSOFT CORP
NORTHROP GRUMMAN CORP
ORACLE CORP
PAREXEL INTERNATIONAL CORP
PARSONS BRINCKERHOFF INC
PEROT SYSTEMS CORP
PHARMACEUTICAL PRODUCT DEVELOPMENT INC
PRICEWATERHOUSECOOPERS
RAYTHEON CO
SAIC INC
SAS INSTITUTE INC
SRA INTERNATIONAL INC
SUN MICROSYSTEMS INC
SUNGARD DATA SYSTEMS INC
SYNTEL INC
TOWERS PERRIN
UNITED TECHNOLOGIES CORPORATION
URS CORPORATION
WATSON WYATT WORLDWIDE INC

Hardware Development

3M COMPANY
ADC TELECOMMUNICATIONS INC
ADVANCED MICRO DEVICES INC (AMD)
AGILENT TECHNOLOGIES INC
AMERICAN POWER CONVERSION CORP
ANALOG DEVICES INC
APPLE INC
BAXTER INTERNATIONAL INC
BECKMAN COULTER INC
BECTON DICKINSON & CO
BENCHMARK ELECTRONICS INC
BIO RAD LABORATORIES INC
BOEING COMPANY (THE)
BROADCOM CORP
CACI INTERNATIONAL INC
CIBER INC
CISCO SYSTEMS INC
COGNIZANT TECHNOLOGY

SOLUTIONS CORP
CTS CORP
CUBIC CORP
CUMMINS INC
DIEBOLD INC
EATON CORP
EMC CORP
EMERSON ELECTRIC CO
FOSSIL INC
GENERAL DYNAMICS CORP
GENERAL ELECTRIC CO (GE)
GTECH HOLDINGS CORP
HARRIS CORPORATION
HONEYWELL INTERNATIONAL INC
IDEXX LABORATORIES INC
INTEL CORP
INTERNATIONAL BUSINESS MACHINES CORP (IBM)
JABIL CIRCUIT INC
JOHNSON CONTROLS INC
JUNIPER NETWORKS INC
KEANE INC
L-3 COMMUNICATIONS HOLDINGS INC
L-3 TITAN GROUP
LEXMARK INTERNATIONAL INC
LOCKHEED MARTIN CORP
MATTEL INC
MAXIM INTEGRATED PRODUCTS INC
MEDTRONIC INC
MICROCHIP TECHNOLOGY INC
MICRON TECHNOLOGY INC
MICROSOFT CORP
MILLIPORE CORP
MOLEX INC
NETWORK APPLIANCE INC
NORTHROP GRUMMAN CORP
PEROT SYSTEMS CORP
PITNEY BOWES INC
PLANTRONICS INC
PLEXUS CORP
QUALCOMM INC
RAYTHEON CO
SCIENTIFIC GAMES CORPORATION
SRA INTERNATIONAL INC
ST JUDE MEDICAL INC
SUN MICROSYSTEMS INC
SYNTEL INC
TEKTRONIX INC
TELEDYNE TECHNOLOGIES

INCORPORATED	AMGEN INC	BUCKLE INC (THE)
UNITED TECHNOLOGIES CORPORATION	ANADARKO PETROLEUM CORPORATION	BUILD-A-BEAR WORKSHOP INC
VARIAN MEDICAL SYSTEMS INC	ANALOG DEVICES INC	BUNGE LTD
WATERS CORP	ANNTAYLOR STORES CORP	BURGER KING HOLDINGS INC
WEST PHARMACEUTICAL SERVICES INC	APACHE CORP	BURLINGTON NORTHERN SANTA FE CORP
WESTERN DIGITAL CORP	APOLLO GROUP INC	CABELA'S INC
XEROX CORP	APPLE INC	CABLEVISION SYSTEMS CORP

Information Management

3M COMPANY	ARAMARK CORPORATION	CACI INTERNATIONAL INC
7-ELEVEN INC	ARCHER DANIELS MIDLAND CO	CAMERON INTERNATIONAL CORPORATION
AARON RENTS INC	ARROW ELECTRONICS INC	CAPITAL SENIOR LIVING CORP
ABBOTT LABORATORIES	ARTHUR J GALLAGHER & CO	CARDINAL HEALTH INC
ABERCROMBIE & FITCH CO	AT&T INC	CARGILL INC
ABM INDUSTRIES INC	AUTOMATIC DATA PROCESSING INC	CARMAX GROUP
ACADEMY SPORTS & OUTDOORS LTD	AUTOZONE INC	CARNIVAL CORPORATION
ACCENTURE LTD	AVERY DENNISON CORP	CASH AMERICA INTERNATIONAL INC
ACXIOM CORP	AVIS BUDGET GROUP INC	CATERPILLAR INC
ADC TELECOMMUNICATIONS INC	AVON PRODUCTS INC	CATERPILLAR LOGISTICS
ADESA INC	AXA FINANCIAL INC	CATHOLIC HEALTH INITIATIVES
ADOBE SYSTEMS INC	BAKER HUGHES INC	CBRL GROUP INC
ADVANCE AUTO PARTS INC	BALTIMORE GAS AND ELECTRIC COMPANY	CDW CORPORATION
ADVANCED MICRO DEVICES INC (AMD)	BANK OF AMERICA CORP	CELLCO PARTNERSHIP (VERIZON WIRELESS)
AECOM TECHNOLOGY CORPORATION	BARNES & NOBLE COLLEGE BOOKSTORES	CEPHALON INC
AEROPOSTALE INC	BARNES & NOBLE INC	CH ROBINSON WORLDWIDE INC
AES CORPORATION (THE)	BASS PRO SHOPS INC	CH2M HILL COMPANIES LTD
AETNA INC	BAXTER INTERNATIONAL INC	CHARLOTTE RUSSE HOLDING
AFFILIATED COMPUTER SERVICES INC	BDO SEIDMAN LLP	CHARMING SHOPPES INC
AFLAC INC	BEBE STORES INC	CHEMED CORPORATION
AGILENT TECHNOLOGIES INC	BECHTEL GROUP INC	CHESAPEAKE ENERGY CORP
AIR PRODUCTS & CHEMICALS INC	BECKMAN COULTER INC	CHEVRON CORPORATION
ALBERTO-CULVER COMPANY	BECTON DICKINSON & CO	CHEVRON PHILLIPS CHEMICAL COMPANY LLC
ALLERGAN INC	BED BATH & BEYOND INC	CHICO'S FAS INC
ALLIANCE DATA SYSTEMS CORPORATION	BENCHMARK ELECTRONICS INC	CHRISTOPHER & BANKS CORP
ALLSTATE CORPORATION (THE)	BERKSHIRE HATHAWAY INC	CHUBB CORPORATION (THE)
ALTRIA GROUP INC	BEST BUY CO INC	CIBER INC
AMAZON.COM INC	BIO RAD LABORATORIES INC	CINTAS CORP
AMEDISYS INC	BJ SERVICES COMPANY	CISCO SYSTEMS INC
AMERICAN EAGLE OUTFITTERS INC	BJ'S WHOLESALE CLUB INC	CLEAR CHANNEL COMMUNICATIONS INC
AMERICAN ELECTRIC POWER COMPANY INC (AEP)	BLACK & DECKER CORP	CLUBCORP INC
AMERICAN EXPRESS CO	BLOOMBERG LP	COACH INC
AMERICAN POWER CONVERSION CORP	BOEING COMPANY (THE)	COCA COLA COMPANY (THE)
	BOOZ ALLEN HAMILTON	COCA COLA ENTERPRISES INC
AMERISOURCEBERGEN CORP	BOSTON SCIENTIFIC CORP	COGNIZANT TECHNOLOGY SOLUTIONS CORP
	BRINKER INTERNATIONAL INC	COLDWATER CREEK INC
	BRINKS COMPANY (THE)	COLGATE PALMOLIVE CO
	BRISTOL MYERS SQUIBB CO	COMCAST CORP
	BROADCOM CORP	
	BROWN & BROWN INC	

CONAGRA FOODS INC	EMBARQ CORP	GUESS? INC
CONOCOPHILLIPS COMPANY	EMC CORP	HALLIBURTON COMPANY
CONSOL ENERGY INC	EMERITUS CORP	HARRAH'S ENTERTAINMENT INC
CONSOLIDATED EDISON INC	EMERSON ELECTRIC CO	HARRIS CORPORATION
CONTAINER STORE (THE)	ENTERGY CORP	HARTFORD FINANCIAL SERVICES GROUP INC (THE)
CONVERGYS CORPORATION	ENTERPRISE RENT-A-CAR	
COOPER COMPANIES INC	ERNST & YOUNG LLP	HAWAIIAN ELECTRIC INDUSTRIES INC
COST PLUS INC	ESTEE LAUDER COMPANIES INC (THE)	
COSTCO WHOLESALE CORP		HCA INC
COVANCE INC	EXEL TRANSPORTATION SERVICES INC (DHL EXEL)	HE BUTT GROCERY COMPANY (HEB)
COVENTRY HEALTH CARE INC	EXELON CORPORATION	HEALTH FITNESS CORP
COX COMMUNICATIONS INC	EXPEDITORS INTERNATIONAL OF WASHINGTON INC	HEALTH MANAGEMENT ASSOCIATES INC
CR BARD INC		
CSX CORP	EXPERIAN AMERICAS	HEALTH NET INC
CSX TRANSPORTATION INC	EXPRESS SCRIPTS INC	HEALTHWAYS INC
CTS CORP	EXXON MOBIL CORPORATION (EXXONMOBIL)	HELMERICH & PAYNE INC
CUBIC CORP		HENRY SCHEIN INC
CUMMINS INC	FAIR ISAAC CORPORATION	HERTZ GLOBAL HOLDINGS INC
CVS CAREMARK CORPORATION	FAMILY DOLLAR STORES INC	HESS CORPORATION
DANAHER CORP	FEDEX CORPORATION	HEWITT ASSOCIATES
DARDEN RESTAURANTS INC	FINISH LINE INC (THE)	HIBBETT SPORTS INC
DAVITA INC	FIRST ADVANTAGE CORPORATION	HILB ROGAL & HOBBS CO
DEAN FOODS CO	FIRST DATA CORP	HILTON HOTELS CORP
DEERE & CO	FIRSTENERGY CORP	HOME DEPOT INC
DELOITTE & TOUCHE USA LLP	FISERV INC	HONEYWELL INTERNATIONAL INC
DELOITTE CONSULTING LLP	FLUOR CORP	HOT TOPIC INC
DENNY'S CORPORATION	FMC TECHNOLOGIES INC	HUMANA INC
DEVON ENERGY CORPORATION	FOREST LABORATORIES INC	IAC/INTERACTIVECORP
DEVRY INC	FORTUNE BRANDS INC	ICT GROUP INC
DIAMOND OFFSHORE DRILLING INC	FOSSIL INC	IDEXX LABORATORIES INC
DICK'S SPORTING GOODS INC	FOSTER WHEELER LTD	IGATE CORPORATION
DIEBOLD INC	FOX ENTERTAINMENT GROUP INC	IMS HEALTH INC
DINEEQUITY INC	FPL GROUP INC	INFOUSA INC
DIRECTV GROUP INC (THE)	FRED'S INC	INGRAM MICRO INC
DJO INC	FRONTIER COMMUNICATIONS CORPORATION	INTEL CORP
DOLE FOOD COMPANY INC		INTERNATIONAL BUSINESS MACHINES CORP (IBM)
DOLLAR GENERAL CORPORATION	GAMESTOP CORP	
DOLLAR THRIFTY AUTOMOTIVE GROUP INC	GENENTECH INC	INTIMATE BRANDS INC
	GENERAL DYNAMICS CORP	INTUIT INC
DRESS BARN INC (THE)	GENERAL ELECTRIC CO (GE)	INVENTIV HEALTH INC
DTE ENERGY COMPANY	GENERAL MILLS INC	J C PENNEY COMPANY INC
DUKE ENERGY CORP	GENESCO INC	JABIL CIRCUIT INC
DYCOM INDUSTRIES INC	GENWORTH FINANCIAL INC	JACK IN THE BOX INC
E I DU PONT DE NEMOURS & CO (DUPONT)	GEO GROUP INC	JACOBS ENGINEERING GROUP INC
	GEORGIA GULF CORPORATION	JM SMUCKER CO
EATON CORP	GLOBAL HYATT CORPORATION	JOHNSON & JOHNSON
EBAY INC	GLOBAL PAYMENTS INC	JOHNSON CONTROLS INC
ECHOSTAR CORP	GOOGLE INC	JP MORGAN CHASE & CO INC
EDISON INTERNATIONAL	GRANT THORNTON LLP	JUNIPER NETWORKS INC
ELECTRONIC ARTS INC	GTECH HOLDINGS CORP	KAISER PERMANENTE
ELI LILLY & COMPANY		

KEANE INC	MERCER INC	PETCO ANIMAL SUPPLIES INC
KELLOGG CO	MERCK & CO INC	PETSMART INC
KELLY SERVICES INC	METLIFE INC	PFIZER INC
KENDLE INTERNATIONAL INC	MGM MIRAGE	PG&E CORPORATION
KIMBERLY-CLARK CORP	MICROCHIP TECHNOLOGY INC	PHARMACEUTICAL PRODUCT DEVELOPMENT INC
KINDRED HEALTHCARE INC	MICRON TECHNOLOGY INC	PITNEY BOWES INC
KOCH INDUSTRIES INC	MICROSOFT CORP	PLANTRONICS INC
KOHL'S CORP	MILLIPORE CORP	PLEXUS CORP
KPMG LLP	MOLEX INC	POLO RALPH LAUREN CORP
KRAFT FOODS INC	MONRO MUFFLER BRAKE INC	PRAXAIR INC
KROGER CO (THE)	MURPHY OIL CORPORATION	PRICEWATERHOUSECOOPERS
L-3 COMMUNICATIONS HOLDINGS INC	NATIONAL OILWELL VARCO INC	PRIDE INTERNATIONAL INC
L-3 TITAN GROUP	NEIMAN MARCUS GROUP INC (THE)	PRINCIPAL FINANCIAL GROUP (THE)
LABORATORY CORP OF AMERICA HOLDINGS	NETWORK APPLIANCE INC	PROCTER & GAMBLE CO
	NEWS CORP	PROGRESSIVE CORPORATION (THE)
LANDRY'S RESTAURANTS INC	NII HOLDINGS INC	
LAS VEGAS SANDS CORP (THE VENETIAN)	NIKE INC	PRUDENTIAL FINANCIAL INC
	NOBLE CORPORATION	PSYCHIATRIC SOLUTIONS INC
LEVEL 3 COMMUNICATIONS INC	NORDSTROM INC	PUBLIC STORAGE INC
LEXMARK INTERNATIONAL INC	NORFOLK SOUTHERN CORP	PUBLIX SUPER MARKETS INC
LIBERTY GLOBAL INC	NORTHROP GRUMMAN CORP	QUALCOMM INC
LIMITED BRANDS INC	OCCIDENTAL PETROLEUM CORP	QUEST DIAGNOSTICS INC
LINCARE HOLDINGS INC	OCEANEERING INTERNATIONAL INC	QUIKSILVER INC
LINCOLN NATIONAL CORPORATION		R R DONNELLEY & SONS CO
LKQ CORP	ODYSSEY HEALTHCARE INC	RAYTHEON CO
LOCKHEED MARTIN CORP	OFFICE DEPOT INC	REGIS CORPORATION
LODGIAN INC	OIL STATES INTERNATIONAL INC	RELIANT ENERGY INC
LOEWS CORPORATION	OLD DOMINION FREIGHT LINE INC	RENT-A-CENTER INC
LOWE'S COMPANIES INC	OMNICARE INC	RES CARE INC
MACY'S INC	OMNICOM GROUP INC	RESPIRONICS INC
MANOR CARE INC	ONEOK INC	RITE AID CORPORATION
MANPOWER INC	ORACLE CORP	RITZ-CARLTON HOTEL COMPANY LLC (THE)
MARATHON OIL CORP	O'REILLY AUTOMOTIVE INC	
MARRIOTT INTERNATIONAL INC	OSHKOSH CORPORATION	ROBERT HALF INTERNATIONAL INC
MARS INC	OSI RESTAURANT PARTNERS INC	ROSS STORES INC
MARSH & MCLENNAN COMPANIES INC	OWENS & MINOR INC	ROYAL CARIBBEAN CRUISES
	PACIFIC SUNWEAR OF CALIFORNIA INC	RUSSELL CORP
MARY KAY INC		RYDER SYSTEM INC
MASSEY ENERGY COMPANY	PANTRY INC (THE)	SABRE HOLDINGS CORP
MATTEL INC	PARAMETRIC TECHNOLOGY CORP	SAFECO CORP
MAXIM INTEGRATED PRODUCTS INC	PAREXEL INTERNATIONAL CORP	SAFEWAY INC
	PARSONS BRINCKERHOFF INC	SAIC INC
MCAFEE INC	PATTERSON COMPANIES INC	SAM'S CLUB
MCDONALD'S CORP	PATTERSON-UTI ENERGY INC	SARA LEE CORP
MCKESSON CORPORATION	PAXAR CORP	SAS INSTITUTE INC
MCKINSEY & COMPANY INC	PAYCHEX INC	SCANA CORPORATION
MEDCO HEALTH SOLUTIONS	PEABODY ENERGY CORP	SCHERING-PLOUGH CORP
MEDTRONIC INC	PEPSI BOTTLING GROUP INC	SCHLUMBERGER LIMITED
MEIJER INC	PEPSICO INC	SCIENTIFIC GAMES CORPORATION
MEN'S WEARHOUSE INC (THE)	PEROT SYSTEMS CORP	
	PERRIGO CO	

SCOTTS MIRACLE GROW CO

SEACOR HOLDINGS INC

SELECT MEDICAL CORPORATION

SEMPRA ENERGY

SENSIENT TECHNOLOGIES CORPORATION

SHAW GROUP INC (THE)

SHELL OIL CO

SHERWIN WILLIAMS COMPANY (THE)

SIGMA-ALDRICH CORP

SISTERS OF MERCY HEALTH SYSTEMS

SMITH INTERNATIONAL INC

SMITHFIELD FOODS INC

SOUTHERN COMPANY (THE)

SOUTHWEST AIRLINES CO

SRA INTERNATIONAL INC

ST JUDE MEDICAL INC

STAPLES INC

STARTEK INC

STARWOOD HOTELS & RESORTS WORLDWIDE INC

STERIS CORP

STRYKER CORP

SUN HEALTHCARE GROUP

SUN MICROSYSTEMS INC

SUNGARD DATA SYSTEMS INC

SUNOCO INC

SUNRISE SENIOR LIVING

SUPERVALU INC

SYKES ENTERPRISES INC

SYMANTEC CORP

SYNOPSYS INC

SYNTEL INC

SYSCO CORP

TALBOTS INC (THE)

TARGET CORPORATION

TBC CORPORATION

TECH DATA CORP

TEKTRONIX INC

TELEDYNE TECHNOLOGIES INCORPORATED

TELEPHONE AND DATA SYSTEMS INC (TDS)

TELETECH HOLDINGS INC

TESORO CORP

TIFFANY & CO

TIME WARNER INC

TJX COMPANIES INC (THE)

T-MOBILE USA

TOTAL SYSTEM SERVICES INC (TSYS)

TOWERS PERRIN

TRANSOCEAN INC

TRAVELERS COMPANIES INC (THE)

TW TELECOM INC

TWEEN BRANDS INC

TYSON FOODS INC

UNION PACIFIC CORP

UNITED NATURAL FOODS INC

UNITED PARCEL SERVICE INC (UPS)

UNITED STATES CELLULAR CORP

UNITED TECHNOLOGIES CORPORATION

UNITEDHEALTH GROUP INC

UNIVISION COMMUNICATIONS INC

UPS SUPPLY CHAIN SOLUTIONS

URBAN OUTFITTERS INC

URS CORPORATION

USAA

VALERO ENERGY CORP

VALSPAR CORPORATION (THE)

VARIAN MEDICAL SYSTEMS INC

VCA ANTECH INC

VERISIGN INC

VERIZON COMMUNICATIONS

VIACOM INC

VOLT INFORMATION SCIENCES INC

W R BERKLEY CORPORATION

WALGREEN CO

WAL-MART STORES INC

WALT DISNEY COMPANY (THE)

WASTE MANAGEMENT INC

WATERS CORP

WATSON PHARMACEUTICALS INC

WATSON WYATT WORLDWIDE INC

WEATHERFORD INTERNATIONAL LTD

WEIGHT WATCHERS INTERNATIONAL INC

WELLPOINT INC

WENDYS INTERNATIONAL INC

WEST CORPORATION

WEST PHARMACEUTICAL SERVICES INC

WESTERN DIGITAL CORP

WESTERN UNION COMPANY (THE)

WHOLE FOODS MARKET INC

WILLIAMS COMPANIES INC (THE)

WILLIAMS SONOMA INC

WM WRIGLEY JR COMPANY

WW GRAINGER INC

WYETH

WYNDHAM WORLDWIDE

WYNN RESORTS LIMITED

XEROX CORP

YAHOO! INC

YUM! BRANDS INC

ZIMMER HOLDINGS INC

Software Development

3M COMPANY

7-ELEVEN INC

AARON RENTS INC

ABBOTT LABORATORIES

ABERCROMBIE & FITCH CO

ACADEMY SPORTS & OUTDOORS LTD

ACCENTURE LTD

ACXIOM CORP

ADC TELECOMMUNICATIONS INC

ADOBE SYSTEMS INC

ADVANCE AUTO PARTS INC

ADVANCED MICRO DEVICES INC (AMD)

AECOM TECHNOLOGY CORPORATION

AEROPOSTALE INC

AES CORPORATION (THE)

AETNA INC

AFFILIATED COMPUTER SERVICES INC

AFLAC INC

AGILENT TECHNOLOGIES INC

AIR PRODUCTS & CHEMICALS INC

ALBERTO-CULVER COMPANY

ALLERGAN INC

ALLIANCE DATA SYSTEMS CORPORATION

ALLSTATE CORPORATION (THE)

ALTRIA GROUP INC

AMAZON.COM INC

AMERICAN EAGLE OUTFITTERS INC

AMERICAN ELECTRIC POWER COMPANY INC (AEP)

AMERICAN EXPRESS CO

AMERICAN POWER CONVERSION CORP

AMERISOURCEBERGEN CORP

AMGEN INC

ANADARKO PETROLEUM CORPORATION

ANALOG DEVICES INC	BURLINGTON NORTHERN SANTA FE CORP	COST PLUS INC
ANNTAYLOR STORES CORP		COSTCO WHOLESALE CORP
APACHE CORP	CABELA'S INC	COVANCE INC
APOLLO GROUP INC	CABLEVISION SYSTEMS CORP	COVENTRY HEALTH CARE INC
APPLE INC	CACI INTERNATIONAL INC	COX COMMUNICATIONS INC
ARAMARK CORPORATION	CAMERON INTERNATIONAL CORPORATION	CR BARD INC
ARCHER DANIELS MIDLAND CO		CSX CORP
ARROW ELECTRONICS INC	CARDINAL HEALTH INC	CSX TRANSPORTATION INC
ARTHUR J GALLAGHER & CO	CARGILL INC	CTS CORP
AT&T INC	CARMAX GROUP	CUBIC CORP
AUTOMATIC DATA PROCESSING INC	CARNIVAL CORPORATION	CUMMINS INC
	CASH AMERICA INTERNATIONAL INC	CVS CAREMARK CORPORATION
AUTOZONE INC	CATERPILLAR INC	DANAHER CORP
AVERY DENNISON CORP	CATERPILLAR LOGISTICS	DARDEN RESTAURANTS INC
AVIS BUDGET GROUP INC	CATHOLIC HEALTH INITIATIVES	DEERE & CO
AVON PRODUCTS INC	CBRL GROUP INC	DELOITTE & TOUCHE USA LLP
AXA FINANCIAL INC	CDW CORPORATION	DELOITTE CONSULTING LLP
BAKER HUGHES INC	CELLCO PARTNERSHIP (VERIZON WIRELESS)	DENNY'S CORPORATION
BALTIMORE GAS AND ELECTRIC COMPANY		DEVON ENERGY CORPORATION
	CEPHALON INC	DEVRY INC
BANK OF AMERICA CORP	CH ROBINSON WORLDWIDE INC	DIAMOND OFFSHORE DRILLING INC
BARNES & NOBLE COLLEGE BOOKSTORES	CH2M HILL COMPANIES LTD	DICK'S SPORTING GOODS INC
	CHARLOTTE RUSSE HOLDING	DIEBOLD INC
BARNES & NOBLE INC	CHARMING SHOPPES INC	DINEEQUITY INC
BASS PRO SHOPS INC	CHESAPEAKE ENERGY CORP	DIRECTV GROUP INC (THE)
BAXTER INTERNATIONAL INC	CHEVRON CORPORATION	DOLE FOOD COMPANY INC
BDO SEIDMAN LLP	CHEVRON PHILLIPS CHEMICAL COMPANY LLC	DOLLAR GENERAL CORPORATION
BEBE STORES INC		DOLLAR THRIFTY AUTOMOTIVE GROUP INC
BECHTEL GROUP INC	CHICO'S FAS INC	
BECKMAN COULTER INC	CHRISTOPHER & BANKS CORP	DRESS BARN INC (THE)
BECTON DICKINSON & CO	CHUBB CORPORATION (THE)	DTE ENERGY COMPANY
BED BATH & BEYOND INC	CIBER INC	DUKE ENERGY CORP
BENCHMARK ELECTRONICS INC	CINTAS CORP	E I DU PONT DE NEMOURS & CO (DUPONT)
BERKSHIRE HATHAWAY INC	CISCO SYSTEMS INC	
BEST BUY CO INC	CLEAR CHANNEL COMMUNICATIONS INC	EATON CORP
BIO RAD LABORATORIES INC		EBAY INC
BJ SERVICES COMPANY	CLUBCORP INC	ECHOSTAR CORP
BJ'S WHOLESALE CLUB INC	COACH INC	EDISON INTERNATIONAL
BLACK & DECKER CORP	COCA COLA COMPANY (THE)	ELECTRONIC ARTS INC
BLOOMBERG LP	COCA COLA ENTERPRISES INC	ELI LILLY & COMPANY
BOEING COMPANY (THE)	COGNIZANT TECHNOLOGY SOLUTIONS CORP	EMBARQ CORP
BOOZ ALLEN HAMILTON		EMC CORP
BOSTON SCIENTIFIC CORP	COLDWATER CREEK INC	EMERSON ELECTRIC CO
BRINKER INTERNATIONAL INC	COLGATE PALMOLIVE CO	ENTERGY CORP
BRINKS COMPANY (THE)	COMCAST CORP	ENTERPRISE RENT-A-CAR
BRISTOL MYERS SQUIBB CO	CONAGRA FOODS INC	ERNST & YOUNG LLP
BROADCOM CORP	CONOCOPHILLIPS COMPANY	ESTEE LAUDER COMPANIES INC (THE)
BROWN & BROWN INC	CONSOLIDATED EDISON INC	
BUCKLE INC (THE)	CONTAINER STORE (THE)	EXEL TRANSPORTATION SERVICES INC (DHL EXEL)
BUILD-A-BEAR WORKSHOP INC	CONVERGYS CORPORATION	
BURGER KING HOLDINGS INC	COOPER COMPANIES INC	EXELON CORPORATION

EXPEDITORS INTERNATIONAL OF WASHINGTON INC	HENRY SCHEIN INC	LEVEL 3 COMMUNICATIONS INC
EXPERIAN AMERICAS	HERTZ GLOBAL HOLDINGS INC	LEXMARK INTERNATIONAL INC
EXPRESS SCRIPTS INC	HESS CORPORATION	LIBERTY GLOBAL INC
EXXON MOBIL CORPORATION (EXXONMOBIL)	HEWITT ASSOCIATES	LIMITED BRANDS INC
FAIR ISAAC CORPORATION	HIBBETT SPORTS INC	LINCOLN NATIONAL CORPORATION
FAMILY DOLLAR STORES INC	HILB ROGAL & HOBBS CO	LOCKHEED MARTIN CORP
FEDEX CORPORATION	HILTON HOTELS CORP	LOEWS CORPORATION
FINISH LINE INC (THE)	HOME DEPOT INC	LOWE'S COMPANIES INC
FIRST ADVANTAGE CORPORATION	HONEYWELL INTERNATIONAL INC	MACY'S INC
FIRST DATA CORP	HOT TOPIC INC	MANPOWER INC
FIRSTENERGY CORP	HUMANA INC	MARATHON OIL CORP
FISERV INC	IAC/INTERACTIVECORP	MARRIOTT INTERNATIONAL INC
FLUOR CORP	ICT GROUP INC	MARS INC
FMC TECHNOLOGIES INC	IDEXX LABORATORIES INC	MARSH & MCLENNAN COMPANIES INC
FOREST LABORATORIES INC	IGATE CORPORATION	MARY KAY INC
FORTUNE BRANDS INC	IMS HEALTH INC	MATTEL INC
FOSSIL INC	INFOUSA INC	MAXIM INTEGRATED PRODUCTS INC
FOSTER WHEELER LTD	INGRAM MICRO INC	MCAFEE INC
FOX ENTERTAINMENT GROUP INC	INTEL CORP	MCDONALD'S CORP
FPL GROUP INC	INTERNATIONAL BUSINESS MACHINES CORP (IBM)	MCKESSON CORPORATION
FRED'S INC	INTIMATE BRANDS INC	MCKINSEY & COMPANY INC
FRONTIER COMMUNICATIONS CORPORATION	INTUIT INC	MEDCO HEALTH SOLUTIONS
GAMESTOP CORP	INVENTIV HEALTH INC	MEDTRONIC INC
GENENTECH INC	J C PENNEY COMPANY INC	MEIJER INC
GENERAL DYNAMICS CORP	JABIL CIRCUIT INC	MEN'S WEARHOUSE INC (THE)
GENERAL ELECTRIC CO (GE)	JACK IN THE BOX INC	MERCER INC
GENERAL MILLS INC	JACOBS ENGINEERING GROUP INC	MERCK & CO INC
GENESCO INC	JOHNSON & JOHNSON	METLIFE INC
GENWORTH FINANCIAL INC	JOHNSON CONTROLS INC	MGM MIRAGE
GEORGIA GULF CORPORATION	JP MORGAN CHASE & CO INC	MICROCHIP TECHNOLOGY INC
GLOBAL HYATT CORPORATION	JUNIPER NETWORKS INC	MICRON TECHNOLOGY INC
GLOBAL PAYMENTS INC	KAISER PERMANENTE	MICROSOFT CORP
GOOGLE INC	KEANE INC	MILLIPORE CORP
GRANT THORNTON LLP	KELLOGG CO	MOLEX INC
GTECH HOLDINGS CORP	KELLY SERVICES INC	MONRO MUFFLER BRAKE INC
GUESS? INC	KENDLE INTERNATIONAL INC	NATIONAL OILWELL VARCO INC
HALLIBURTON COMPANY	KIMBERLY-CLARK CORP	NEIMAN MARCUS GROUP INC (THE)
HARRAH'S ENTERTAINMENT INC	KOCH INDUSTRIES INC	NETWORK APPLIANCE INC
HARRIS CORPORATION	KOHL'S CORP	NEWS CORP
HARTFORD FINANCIAL SERVICES GROUP INC (THE)	KPMG LLP	NII HOLDINGS INC
HAWAIIAN ELECTRIC INDUSTRIES INC	KRAFT FOODS INC	NIKE INC
HE BUTT GROCERY COMPANY (HEB)	KROGER CO (THE)	NOBLE CORPORATION
HEALTH MANAGEMENT ASSOCIATES INC	L-3 COMMUNICATIONS HOLDINGS INC	NORDSTROM INC
HEALTH NET INC	L-3 TITAN GROUP	NORFOLK SOUTHERN CORP
HEALTHWAYS INC	LABORATORY CORP OF AMERICA HOLDINGS	NORTHROP GRUMMAN CORP
	LANDRY'S RESTAURANTS INC	OCCIDENTAL PETROLEUM CORP
	LAS VEGAS SANDS CORP (THE VENETIAN)	OCEANEERING INTERNATIONAL INC
		OFFICE DEPOT INC

OIL STATES INTERNATIONAL INC	RENT-A-CENTER INC	TBC CORPORATION
OLD DOMINION FREIGHT LINE INC	RESPIRONICS INC	TECH DATA CORP
OMNICARE INC	RITE AID CORPORATION	TEKTRONIX INC
OMNICOM GROUP INC	ROBERT HALF INTERNATIONAL INC	TELEDYNE TECHNOLOGIES INCORPORATED
ONEOK INC	ROSS STORES INC	TELEPHONE AND DATA SYSTEMS INC (TDS)
ORACLE CORP	ROYAL CARIBBEAN CRUISES	
O'REILLY AUTOMOTIVE INC	RUSSELL CORP	TELETECH HOLDINGS INC
OSHKOSH CORPORATION	RYDER SYSTEM INC	TESORO CORP
OSI RESTAURANT PARTNERS INC	SABRE HOLDINGS CORP	TIFFANY & CO
OWENS & MINOR INC	SAFECO CORP	TIME WARNER INC
PACIFIC SUNWEAR OF CALIFORNIA INC	SAFEWAY INC	TJX COMPANIES INC (THE)
PANTRY INC (THE)	SAIC INC	T-MOBILE USA
PARAMETRIC TECHNOLOGY CORP	SAM'S CLUB	TOTAL SYSTEM SERVICES INC (TSYS)
PAREXEL INTERNATIONAL CORP	SARA LEE CORP	TOWERS PERRIN
PARSONS BRINCKERHOFF INC	SAS INSTITUTE INC	TRAVELERS COMPANIES INC (THE)
PATTERSON COMPANIES INC	SCANA CORPORATION	TW TELECOM INC
PATTERSON-UTI ENERGY INC	SCHERING-PLOUGH CORP	TWEEN BRANDS INC
PAXAR CORP	SCHLUMBERGER LIMITED	UNION PACIFIC CORP
PAYCHEX INC	SCIENTIFIC GAMES CORPORATION	UNITED NATURAL FOODS INC
PEPSI BOTTLING GROUP INC	SEACOR HOLDINGS INC	UNITED PARCEL SERVICE INC (UPS)
PEPSICO INC	SEMPRA ENERGY	
PEROT SYSTEMS CORP	SENSIENT TECHNOLOGIES CORPORATION	UNITED STATES CELLULAR CORP
PERRIGO CO		UNITED TECHNOLOGIES CORPORATION
PETCO ANIMAL SUPPLIES INC	SHELL OIL CO	
PETSMART INC	SHERWIN WILLIAMS COMPANY (THE)	UNITEDHEALTH GROUP INC
PFIZER INC	SIGMA-ALDRICH CORP	UNIVISION COMMUNICATIONS INC
PG&E CORPORATION	SISTERS OF MERCY HEALTH SYSTEMS	UPS SUPPLY CHAIN SOLUTIONS
PHARMACEUTICAL PRODUCT DEVELOPMENT INC		URBAN OUTFITTERS INC
	SMITH INTERNATIONAL INC	URS CORPORATION
PITNEY BOWES INC	SOUTHERN COMPANY (THE)	USAA
PLANTRONICS INC	SOUTHWEST AIRLINES CO	VALERO ENERGY CORP
PLEXUS CORP	SRA INTERNATIONAL INC	VALSPAR CORPORATION (THE)
POLO RALPH LAUREN CORP	ST JUDE MEDICAL INC	VARIAN MEDICAL SYSTEMS INC
PRAXAIR INC	STAPLES INC	VCA ANTECH INC
PRICEWATERHOUSECOOPERS	STARTEK INC	VERISIGN INC
PRIDE INTERNATIONAL INC	STARWOOD HOTELS & RESORTS WORLDWIDE INC	VERIZON COMMUNICATIONS
PRINCIPAL FINANCIAL GROUP (THE)		VIACOM INC
	STERIS CORP	VOLT INFORMATION SCIENCES INC
PROCTER & GAMBLE CO	STRYKER CORP	W R BERKLEY CORPORATION
PROGRESSIVE CORPORATION (THE)	SUN MICROSYSTEMS INC	WALGREEN CO
	SUNGARD DATA SYSTEMS INC	WAL-MART STORES INC
PRUDENTIAL FINANCIAL INC	SUNOCO INC	WALT DISNEY COMPANY (THE)
PUBLIX SUPER MARKETS INC	SUPERVALU INC	WASTE MANAGEMENT INC
QUALCOMM INC	SYKES ENTERPRISES INC	WATERS CORP
QUEST DIAGNOSTICS INC	SYMANTEC CORP	WATSON PHARMACEUTICALS INC
QUIKSILVER INC	SYNOPSYS INC	WATSON WYATT WORLDWIDE INC
R R DONNELLEY & SONS CO	SYNTEL INC	WEATHERFORD INTERNATIONAL LTD
RAYTHEON CO	SYSCO CORP	
REGIS CORPORATION	TALBOTS INC (THE)	WEIGHT WATCHERS INTERNATIONAL INC
RELIANT ENERGY INC	TARGET CORPORATION	

WELLPOINT INC	BURLINGTON NORTHERN SANTA FE CORP	EXPERIAN AMERICAS
WENDYS INTERNATIONAL INC		EXXON MOBIL CORPORATION (EXXONMOBIL)
WEST CORPORATION	CABLEVISION SYSTEMS CORP	
WEST PHARMACEUTICAL SERVICES INC	CACI INTERNATIONAL INC	FEDEX CORPORATION
	CARDINAL HEALTH INC	FIRST ADVANTAGE CORPORATION
WESTERN DIGITAL CORP	CARGILL INC	FIRST DATA CORP
WESTERN UNION COMPANY (THE)	CATERPILLAR INC	FISERV INC
WHOLE FOODS MARKET INC	CATERPILLAR LOGISTICS	FLUOR CORP
WILLIAMS COMPANIES INC (THE)	CELLCO PARTNERSHIP (VERIZON WIRELESS)	FOSTER WHEELER LTD
WILLIAMS SONOMA INC		FRONTIER COMMUNICATIONS CORPORATION
WM WRIGLEY JR COMPANY	CEPHALON INC	
WW GRAINGER INC	CH ROBINSON WORLDWIDE INC	GENENTECH INC
WYETH	CH2M HILL COMPANIES LTD	GENERAL DYNAMICS CORP
WYNDHAM WORLDWIDE	CHEVRON CORPORATION	GENERAL ELECTRIC CO (GE)
WYNN RESORTS LIMITED	CIBER INC	GENERAL MILLS INC
XEROX CORP	CISCO SYSTEMS INC	GLOBAL HYATT CORPORATION
YAHOO! INC	CLEAR CHANNEL COMMUNICATIONS INC	GOOGLE INC
YUM! BRANDS INC		GRANT THORNTON LLP
ZIMMER HOLDINGS INC	COCA COLA COMPANY (THE)	HALLIBURTON COMPANY
	COGNIZANT TECHNOLOGY SOLUTIONS CORP	HARRAH'S ENTERTAINMENT INC
		HARRIS CORPORATION
Systems Integration	COLGATE PALMOLIVE CO	HEALTHWAYS INC
3M COMPANY	COMCAST CORP	HEWITT ASSOCIATES
ACCENTURE LTD	CONOCOPHILLIPS COMPANY	HILTON HOTELS CORP
ADC TELECOMMUNICATIONS INC	CONSOLIDATED EDISON INC	HONEYWELL INTERNATIONAL INC
ADOBE SYSTEMS INC	COVANCE INC	HUMANA INC
ADVANCED MICRO DEVICES INC (AMD)	COX COMMUNICATIONS INC	IGATE CORPORATION
	CSX CORP	INFOUSA INC
AECOM TECHNOLOGY CORPORATION	CSX TRANSPORTATION INC	INGRAM MICRO INC
	CTS CORP	INTEL CORP
AFFILIATED COMPUTER SERVICES INC	CUBIC CORP	INTERNATIONAL BUSINESS MACHINES CORP (IBM)
	CUMMINS INC	
AGILENT TECHNOLOGIES INC	DEERE & CO	INTUIT INC
AMERICAN ELECTRIC POWER COMPANY INC (AEP)	DELOITTE & TOUCHE USA LLP	INVENTIV HEALTH INC
	DELOITTE CONSULTING LLP	JABIL CIRCUIT INC
AMERICAN EXPRESS CO	DENNY'S CORPORATION	JACOBS ENGINEERING GROUP INC
AMERISOURCEBERGEN CORP	DIEBOLD INC	JOHNSON & JOHNSON
APPLE INC	DIRECTV GROUP INC (THE)	JOHNSON CONTROLS INC
ARCHER DANIELS MIDLAND CO	DUKE ENERGY CORP	JP MORGAN CHASE & CO INC
ARROW ELECTRONICS INC	EBAY INC	JUNIPER NETWORKS INC
AUTOMATIC DATA PROCESSING INC	EDISON INTERNATIONAL	KAISER PERMANENTE
	ELECTRONIC ARTS INC	KEANE INC
BANK OF AMERICA CORP	ELI LILLY & COMPANY	KELLOGG CO
BDO SEIDMAN LLP	EMBARQ CORP	KELLY SERVICES INC
BECHTEL GROUP INC	EMC CORP	KENDLE INTERNATIONAL INC
BERKSHIRE HATHAWAY INC	EMERSON ELECTRIC CO	KPMG LLP
BJ'S WHOLESALE CLUB INC	ERNST & YOUNG LLP	KRAFT FOODS INC
BLOOMBERG LP	EXEL TRANSPORTATION SERVICES INC (DHL EXEL)	L-3 COMMUNICATIONS HOLDINGS INC
BOEING COMPANY (THE)		
BOOZ ALLEN HAMILTON		
BROADCOM CORP	EXPEDITORS INTERNATIONAL OF WASHINGTON INC	L-3 TITAN GROUP
BURGER KING HOLDINGS INC		LAS VEGAS SANDS CORP (THE

VENETIAN)	SAM'S CLUB	YAHOO! INC
LEVEL 3 COMMUNICATIONS INC	SAS INSTITUTE INC	
LEXMARK INTERNATIONAL INC	SCHERING-PLOUGH CORP	**Liberal Arts**
LOCKHEED MARTIN CORP	SCHLUMBERGER LIMITED	
LODGIAN INC	SEACOR HOLDINGS INC	**Broadcasting**
MANPOWER INC	SHELL OIL CO	CABLEVISION SYSTEMS CORP
MARRIOTT INTERNATIONAL INC	SOUTHERN COMPANY (THE)	CLEAR CHANNEL COMMUNICATIONS INC
MARS INC	SOUTHWEST AIRLINES CO	COMCAST CORP
MCAFEE INC	SRA INTERNATIONAL INC	COX COMMUNICATIONS INC
MCDONALD'S CORP	STAPLES INC	DIRECTV GROUP INC (THE)
MCKESSON CORPORATION	STARWOOD HOTELS & RESORTS WORLDWIDE INC	ECHOSTAR CORP
MCKINSEY & COMPANY INC	SUN MICROSYSTEMS INC	FOX ENTERTAINMENT GROUP INC
MEDTRONIC INC	SUNGARD DATA SYSTEMS INC	IAC/INTERACTIVECORP
MERCER INC	SYKES ENTERPRISES INC	NEWS CORP
MERCK & CO INC	SYMANTEC CORP	QUALCOMM INC
MGM MIRAGE	SYNOPSYS INC	TIME WARNER INC
MICRON TECHNOLOGY INC	SYNTEL INC	UNIVISION COMMUNICATIONS INC
MICROSOFT CORP	SYSCO CORP	VIACOM INC
MILLIPORE CORP	TARGET CORPORATION	WAL-MART STORES INC
MOLEX INC	TECH DATA CORP	WALT DISNEY COMPANY (THE)
NETWORK APPLIANCE INC	TEKTRONIX INC	
NEWS CORP	TELEPHONE AND DATA SYSTEMS INC (TDS)	**General Writing**
NII HOLDINGS INC	TELETECH HOLDINGS INC	3M COMPANY
NORFOLK SOUTHERN CORP	TIME WARNER INC	7-ELEVEN INC
NORTHROP GRUMMAN CORP	TOTAL SYSTEM SERVICES INC (TSYS)	ABERCROMBIE & FITCH CO
OFFICE DEPOT INC	TW TELECOM INC	ABM INDUSTRIES INC
ORACLE CORP	UNION PACIFIC CORP	ACADEMY SPORTS & OUTDOORS LTD
PARAMETRIC TECHNOLOGY CORP	UNITED PARCEL SERVICE INC (UPS)	ACCENTURE LTD
PAREXEL INTERNATIONAL CORP	UNITED STATES CELLULAR CORP	ADOBE SYSTEMS INC
PARSONS BRINCKERHOFF INC	UNITED TECHNOLOGIES CORPORATION	ADVANCE AUTO PARTS INC
PAYCHEX INC	UNITEDHEALTH GROUP INC	AEROPOSTALE INC
PEPSICO INC	UPS SUPPLY CHAIN SOLUTIONS	AES CORPORATION (THE)
PEROT SYSTEMS CORP	URS CORPORATION	AETNA INC
PETSMART INC	USAA	AFFILIATED COMPUTER SERVICES INC
PFIZER INC	VARIAN MEDICAL SYSTEMS INC	AFLAC INC
PG&E CORPORATION	VERISIGN INC	AGILENT TECHNOLOGIES INC
PHARMACEUTICAL PRODUCT DEVELOPMENT INC	VERIZON COMMUNICATIONS	ALBERTO-CULVER COMPANY
PITNEY BOWES INC	VIACOM INC	ALLERGAN INC
PLEXUS CORP	VOLT INFORMATION SCIENCES INC	ALLIANCE DATA SYSTEMS CORPORATION
POLO RALPH LAUREN CORP	WAL-MART STORES INC	ALLSTATE CORPORATION (THE)
PRICEWATERHOUSECOOPERS	WALT DISNEY COMPANY (THE)	ALTRIA GROUP INC
PROCTER & GAMBLE CO	WATSON WYATT WORLDWIDE INC	AMAZON.COM INC
QUALCOMM INC	WELLPOINT INC	AMERICAN EAGLE OUTFITTERS INC
RAYTHEON CO	WYNDHAM WORLDWIDE	AMERICAN ELECTRIC POWER COMPANY INC (AEP)
RELIANT ENERGY INC	WYNN RESORTS LIMITED	AMERICAN EXPRESS CO
RITZ-CARLTON HOTEL COMPANY LLC (THE)	XEROX CORP	AMERICAN POWER CONVERSION
ROBERT HALF INTERNATIONAL INC		
SABRE HOLDINGS CORP		
SAIC INC		

CORP	CAPITAL SENIOR LIVING CORP	DENNY'S CORPORATION
AMERISOURCEBERGEN CORP	CARDINAL HEALTH INC	DEVRY INC
AMGEN INC	CARMAX GROUP	DICK'S SPORTING GOODS INC
ANADARKO PETROLEUM CORPORATION	CARNIVAL CORPORATION	DIEBOLD INC
ANNTAYLOR STORES CORP	CATERPILLAR INC	DINEEQUITY INC
APOLLO GROUP INC	CATERPILLAR LOGISTICS	DIRECTV GROUP INC (THE)
APPLE INC	CATHOLIC HEALTH INITIATIVES	DOLE FOOD COMPANY INC
ARAMARK CORPORATION	CDW CORPORATION	DOLLAR GENERAL CORPORATION
ARCHER DANIELS MIDLAND CO	CELLCO PARTNERSHIP (VERIZON WIRELESS)	DOLLAR THRIFTY AUTOMOTIVE GROUP INC
ARROW ELECTRONICS INC	CH2M HILL COMPANIES LTD	DRESS BARN INC (THE)
AT&T INC	CHARLOTTE RUSSE HOLDING	DTE ENERGY COMPANY
AUTOMATIC DATA PROCESSING INC	CHARMING SHOPPES INC	DUKE ENERGY CORP
AUTOZONE INC	CHEVRON CORPORATION	E I DU PONT DE NEMOURS & CO (DUPONT)
AVERY DENNISON CORP	CHICO'S FAS INC	EBAY INC
AVIS BUDGET GROUP INC	CHRISTOPHER & BANKS CORP	ECHOSTAR CORP
AVON PRODUCTS INC	CHUBB CORPORATION (THE)	EDISON INTERNATIONAL
AXA FINANCIAL INC	CIBER INC	ELECTRONIC ARTS INC
BAKER HUGHES INC	CINTAS CORP	ELI LILLY & COMPANY
BALTIMORE GAS AND ELECTRIC COMPANY	CISCO SYSTEMS INC	ENTERGY CORP
BANK OF AMERICA CORP	CLEAR CHANNEL COMMUNICATIONS INC	ENTERPRISE RENT-A-CAR
BARNES & NOBLE COLLEGE BOOKSTORES	CLUBCORP INC	ERNST & YOUNG LLP
BARNES & NOBLE INC	COACH INC	ESTEE LAUDER COMPANIES INC (THE)
BASS PRO SHOPS INC	COCA COLA COMPANY (THE)	EXELON CORPORATION
BAXTER INTERNATIONAL INC	COCA COLA ENTERPRISES INC	EXPERIAN AMERICAS
BDO SEIDMAN LLP	COGNIZANT TECHNOLOGY SOLUTIONS CORP	EXPRESS SCRIPTS INC
BEBE STORES INC	COLDWATER CREEK INC	EXXON MOBIL CORPORATION (EXXONMOBIL)
BECHTEL GROUP INC	COLGATE PALMOLIVE CO	FAIR ISAAC CORPORATION
BECKMAN COULTER INC	COMCAST CORP	FAMILY DOLLAR STORES INC
BECTON DICKINSON & CO	CONAGRA FOODS INC	FEDEX CORPORATION
BED BATH & BEYOND INC	CONOCOPHILLIPS COMPANY	FINISH LINE INC (THE)
BERKSHIRE HATHAWAY INC	CONSOLIDATED EDISON INC	FIRST ADVANTAGE CORPORATION
BEST BUY CO INC	CONTAINER STORE (THE)	FIRST DATA CORP
BIO RAD LABORATORIES INC	CONVERGYS CORPORATION	FIRSTENERGY CORP
BJ'S WHOLESALE CLUB INC	COST PLUS INC	FISERV INC
BLACK & DECKER CORP	COSTCO WHOLESALE CORP	FLUOR CORP
BLOOMBERG LP	COVENTRY HEALTH CARE INC	FOREST LABORATORIES INC
BOEING COMPANY (THE)	COX COMMUNICATIONS INC	FORTUNE BRANDS INC
BOOZ ALLEN HAMILTON	CR BARD INC	FOSSIL INC
BOSTON SCIENTIFIC CORP	CSX CORP	FOX ENTERTAINMENT GROUP INC
BRINKER INTERNATIONAL INC	CUMMINS INC	FPL GROUP INC
BRINKS COMPANY (THE)	CVS CAREMARK CORPORATION	FRED'S INC
BRISTOL MYERS SQUIBB CO	DANAHER CORP	FRONTIER COMMUNICATIONS CORPORATION
BUCKLE INC (THE)	DARDEN RESTAURANTS INC	GAMESTOP CORP
BUILD-A-BEAR WORKSHOP INC	DAVITA INC	GENENTECH INC
BURGER KING HOLDINGS INC	DEAN FOODS CO	GENERAL DYNAMICS CORP
CABELA'S INC	DEERE & CO	GENERAL DYNAMICS CORP
CABLEVISION SYSTEMS CORP	DELOITTE & TOUCHE USA LLP	GENERAL ELECTRIC CO (GE)
	DELOITTE CONSULTING LLP	

GENERAL MILLS INC	KEANE INC	NORTHROP GRUMMAN CORP
GENESCO INC	KELLOGG CO	OCCIDENTAL PETROLEUM CORP
GENWORTH FINANCIAL INC	KELLY SERVICES INC	OFFICE DEPOT INC
GLOBAL HYATT CORPORATION	KIMBERLY-CLARK CORP	OMNICARE INC
GLOBAL PAYMENTS INC	KOHL'S CORP	OMNICOM GROUP INC
GOOGLE INC	KPMG LLP	ORACLE CORP
GRANT THORNTON LLP	KRAFT FOODS INC	O'REILLY AUTOMOTIVE INC
GTECH HOLDINGS CORP	KROGER CO (THE)	OSHKOSH CORPORATION
GUESS? INC	LABORATORY CORP OF AMERICA HOLDINGS	OSI RESTAURANT PARTNERS INC
HALLIBURTON COMPANY		OWENS & MINOR INC
HARRAH'S ENTERTAINMENT INC	LANDRY'S RESTAURANTS INC	PACIFIC SUNWEAR OF CALIFORNIA INC
HARRIS CORPORATION	LAS VEGAS SANDS CORP (THE VENETIAN)	
HARTFORD FINANCIAL SERVICES GROUP INC (THE)		PANTRY INC (THE)
	LEXMARK INTERNATIONAL INC	PAREXEL INTERNATIONAL CORP
HAWAIIAN ELECTRIC INDUSTRIES INC	LIBERTY GLOBAL INC	PARSONS BRINCKERHOFF INC
	LIMITED BRANDS INC	PATTERSON COMPANIES INC
HCA INC	LINCOLN NATIONAL CORPORATION	PAXAR CORP
HE BUTT GROCERY COMPANY (HEB)	LOCKHEED MARTIN CORP	PAYCHEX INC
	LODGIAN INC	PEPSI BOTTLING GROUP INC
HEALTH FITNESS CORP	LOEWS CORPORATION	PEPSICO INC
HEALTH MANAGEMENT ASSOCIATES INC	LOWE'S COMPANIES INC	PEROT SYSTEMS CORP
HEALTH NET INC	MACY'S INC	PETCO ANIMAL SUPPLIES INC
HENRY SCHEIN INC	MANOR CARE INC	PETSMART INC
HERTZ GLOBAL HOLDINGS INC	MANPOWER INC	PFIZER INC
HEWITT ASSOCIATES	MARRIOTT INTERNATIONAL INC	PG&E CORPORATION
HIBBETT SPORTS INC	MARS INC	PITNEY BOWES INC
HILTON HOTELS CORP	MARSH & MCLENNAN COMPANIES INC	POLO RALPH LAUREN CORP
HOME DEPOT INC		PRICEWATERHOUSECOOPERS
HONEYWELL INTERNATIONAL INC	MARY KAY INC	PRINCIPAL FINANCIAL GROUP (THE)
HOT TOPIC INC	MATTEL INC	
HUMANA INC	MCAFEE INC	PROCTER & GAMBLE CO
IAC/INTERACTIVECORP	MCDONALD'S CORP	PROGRESSIVE CORPORATION (THE)
ICT GROUP INC	MCKESSON CORPORATION	
IMS HEALTH INC	MCKINSEY & COMPANY INC	PRUDENTIAL FINANCIAL INC
INFOUSA INC	MEDCO HEALTH SOLUTIONS	PUBLIX SUPER MARKETS INC
INGRAM MICRO INC	MEDTRONIC INC	QUIKSILVER INC
INTEL CORP	MEIJER INC	R R DONNELLEY & SONS CO
INTERNATIONAL BUSINESS MACHINES CORP (IBM)	MEN'S WEARHOUSE INC (THE)	RAYTHEON CO
	MERCER INC	REGIS CORPORATION
INTIMATE BRANDS INC	MERCK & CO INC	RELIANT ENERGY INC
INTUIT INC	METLIFE INC	RENT-A-CENTER INC
INVENTIV HEALTH INC	MGM MIRAGE	RITE AID CORPORATION
J C PENNEY COMPANY INC	MICROSOFT CORP	RITZ-CARLTON HOTEL COMPANY LLC (THE)
JACK IN THE BOX INC	MONRO MUFFLER BRAKE INC	
JM SMUCKER CO	NEIMAN MARCUS GROUP INC (THE)	ROBERT HALF INTERNATIONAL INC
JOHNSON & JOHNSON	NETWORK APPLIANCE INC	ROSS STORES INC
JOHNSON CONTROLS INC	NEWS CORP	ROYAL CARIBBEAN CRUISES
JP MORGAN CHASE & CO INC	NII HOLDINGS INC	RUSSELL CORP
JUNIPER NETWORKS INC	NIKE INC	SABRE HOLDINGS CORP
KAISER PERMANENTE	NORDSTROM INC	SAFECO CORP
	NORFOLK SOUTHERN CORP	SAFEWAY INC

SAIC INC	UNITED NATURAL FOODS INC	ACCENTURE LTD
SAM'S CLUB	UNITED PARCEL SERVICE INC (UPS)	ADC TELECOMMUNICATIONS INC
SARA LEE CORP		ADOBE SYSTEMS INC
SAS INSTITUTE INC	UNITED STATES CELLULAR CORP	ADVANCE AUTO PARTS INC
SCANA CORPORATION	UNITED TECHNOLOGIES CORPORATION	ADVANCED MICRO DEVICES INC (AMD)
SCHERING-PLOUGH CORP	UNITEDHEALTH GROUP INC	AECOM TECHNOLOGY CORPORATION
SCHLUMBERGER LIMITED	UNIVISION COMMUNICATIONS INC	
SCIENTIFIC GAMES CORPORATION	UPS SUPPLY CHAIN SOLUTIONS	AEROPOSTALE INC
SCOTTS MIRACLE GROW CO	URBAN OUTFITTERS INC	AETNA INC
SEACOR HOLDINGS INC	USAA	AFFILIATED COMPUTER SERVICES INC
SEMPRA ENERGY	VALERO ENERGY CORP	AFLAC INC
SHELL OIL CO	VALSPAR CORPORATION (THE)	AGILENT TECHNOLOGIES INC
SHERWIN WILLIAMS COMPANY (THE)	VARIAN MEDICAL SYSTEMS INC	ALBERTO-CULVER COMPANY
	VCA ANTECH INC	ALLERGAN INC
SISTERS OF MERCY HEALTH SYSTEMS	VERISIGN INC	ALLSTATE CORPORATION (THE)
SMITHFIELD FOODS INC	VERIZON COMMUNICATIONS	ALTRIA GROUP INC
SOUTHERN COMPANY (THE)	VIACOM INC	AMAZON.COM INC
SOUTHWEST AIRLINES CO	VOLT INFORMATION SCIENCES INC	AMERICAN EAGLE OUTFITTERS INC
SRA INTERNATIONAL INC	WALGREEN CO	AMERICAN ELECTRIC POWER COMPANY INC (AEP)
ST JUDE MEDICAL INC	WAL-MART STORES INC	
STAPLES INC	WALT DISNEY COMPANY (THE)	AMERICAN EXPRESS CO
STARTEK INC	WASTE MANAGEMENT INC	AMERICAN POWER CONVERSION CORP
STARWOOD HOTELS & RESORTS WORLDWIDE INC	WATSON PHARMACEUTICALS INC	
	WATSON WYATT WORLDWIDE INC	AMERISOURCEBERGEN CORP
STRYKER CORP	WEIGHT WATCHERS INTERNATIONAL INC	AMGEN INC
SUN HEALTHCARE GROUP		ANADARKO PETROLEUM CORPORATION
SUN MICROSYSTEMS INC	WELLPOINT INC	
SUNGARD DATA SYSTEMS INC	WENDYS INTERNATIONAL INC	ANNTAYLOR STORES CORP
SUNRISE SENIOR LIVING	WEST CORPORATION	APOLLO GROUP INC
SUPERVALU INC	WESTERN UNION COMPANY (THE)	APPLE INC
SYMANTEC CORP	WHOLE FOODS MARKET INC	ARAMARK CORPORATION
SYSCO CORP	WILLIAMS SONOMA INC	ARCHER DANIELS MIDLAND CO
TALBOTS INC (THE)	WM WRIGLEY JR COMPANY	ARROW ELECTRONICS INC
TARGET CORPORATION	WW GRAINGER INC	AT&T INC
TBC CORPORATION	WYETH	AUTOMATIC DATA PROCESSING INC
TECH DATA CORP	WYNDHAM WORLDWIDE	
TELEPHONE AND DATA SYSTEMS INC (TDS)	WYNN RESORTS LIMITED	AUTOZONE INC
	XEROX CORP	AVERY DENNISON CORP
TELETECH HOLDINGS INC	YAHOO! INC	AVIS BUDGET GROUP INC
TIFFANY & CO	YUM! BRANDS INC	AVON PRODUCTS INC
TIME WARNER INC	ZIMMER HOLDINGS INC	AXA FINANCIAL INC
TJX COMPANIES INC (THE)		BAKER HUGHES INC
T-MOBILE USA	**Graphic Arts**	BANK OF AMERICA CORP
TOTAL SYSTEM SERVICES INC (TSYS)	3M COMPANY	BARNES & NOBLE COLLEGE BOOKSTORES
	7-ELEVEN INC	
TOWERS PERRIN	AARON RENTS INC	BARNES & NOBLE INC
TRAVELERS COMPANIES INC (THE)	ABBOTT LABORATORIES	BASS PRO SHOPS INC
TW TELECOM INC	ABERCROMBIE & FITCH CO	BAXTER INTERNATIONAL INC
TWEEN BRANDS INC	ACADEMY SPORTS & OUTDOORS LTD	BDO SEIDMAN LLP
TYSON FOODS INC		BEBE STORES INC

BECHTEL GROUP INC	CONAGRA FOODS INC	FIRSTENERGY CORP
BECKMAN COULTER INC	CONOCOPHILLIPS COMPANY	FISERV INC
BECTON DICKINSON & CO	CONTAINER STORE (THE)	FLUOR CORP
BED BATH & BEYOND INC	COST PLUS INC	FMC TECHNOLOGIES INC
BERKSHIRE HATHAWAY INC	COSTCO WHOLESALE CORP	FOREST LABORATORIES INC
BEST BUY CO INC	COVANCE INC	FORTUNE BRANDS INC
BIO RAD LABORATORIES INC	COVENTRY HEALTH CARE INC	FOSSIL INC
BJ'S WHOLESALE CLUB INC	COX COMMUNICATIONS INC	FOSTER WHEELER LTD
BLACK & DECKER CORP	CR BARD INC	FOX ENTERTAINMENT GROUP INC
BLOOMBERG LP	CUBIC CORP	FPL GROUP INC
BOEING COMPANY (THE)	CUMMINS INC	FRED'S INC
BOOZ ALLEN HAMILTON	CVS CAREMARK CORPORATION	GAMESTOP CORP
BOSTON SCIENTIFIC CORP	DANAHER CORP	GENENTECH INC
BRINKER INTERNATIONAL INC	DARDEN RESTAURANTS INC	GENERAL DYNAMICS CORP
BRINKS COMPANY (THE)	DEAN FOODS CO	GENERAL ELECTRIC CO (GE)
BRISTOL MYERS SQUIBB CO	DEERE & CO	GENERAL MILLS INC
BUCKLE INC (THE)	DELOITTE & TOUCHE USA LLP	GENESCO INC
BUILD-A-BEAR WORKSHOP INC	DELOITTE CONSULTING LLP	GENWORTH FINANCIAL INC
BURGER KING HOLDINGS INC	DENNY'S CORPORATION	GLOBAL HYATT CORPORATION
CABELA'S INC	DEVRY INC	GOOGLE INC
CABLEVISION SYSTEMS CORP	DICK'S SPORTING GOODS INC	GRANT THORNTON LLP
CACI INTERNATIONAL INC	DIEBOLD INC	GTECH HOLDINGS CORP
CARDINAL HEALTH INC	DINEEQUITY INC	GUESS? INC
CARGILL INC	DIRECTV GROUP INC (THE)	HALLIBURTON COMPANY
CARMAX GROUP	DJO INC	HARRAH'S ENTERTAINMENT INC
CARNIVAL CORPORATION	DOLE FOOD COMPANY INC	HARRIS CORPORATION
CATERPILLAR INC	DOLLAR GENERAL CORPORATION	HARTFORD FINANCIAL SERVICES GROUP INC (THE)
CATHOLIC HEALTH INITIATIVES	DOLLAR THRIFTY AUTOMOTIVE GROUP INC	
CDW CORPORATION		HCA INC
CELLCO PARTNERSHIP (VERIZON WIRELESS)	DRESS BARN INC (THE)	HE BUTT GROCERY COMPANY (HEB)
	DYCOM INDUSTRIES INC	
CEPHALON INC	EATON CORP	HEALTH FITNESS CORP
CH2M HILL COMPANIES LTD	EBAY INC	HEALTH MANAGEMENT ASSOCIATES INC
CHARLOTTE RUSSE HOLDING	ECHOSTAR CORP	
CHARMING SHOPPES INC	EDISON INTERNATIONAL	HEALTH NET INC
CHEVRON CORPORATION	ELECTRONIC ARTS INC	HENRY SCHEIN INC
CHICO'S FAS INC	ELI LILLY & COMPANY	HERTZ GLOBAL HOLDINGS INC
CHRISTOPHER & BANKS CORP	EMC CORP	HEWITT ASSOCIATES
CHUBB CORPORATION (THE)	EMERSON ELECTRIC CO	HIBBETT SPORTS INC
CIBER INC	ENTERGY CORP	HILTON HOTELS CORP
CISCO SYSTEMS INC	ENTERPRISE RENT-A-CAR	HOME DEPOT INC
CLEAR CHANNEL COMMUNICATIONS INC	ERNST & YOUNG LLP	HONEYWELL INTERNATIONAL INC
	ESTEE LAUDER COMPANIES INC (THE)	HOT TOPIC INC
CLUBCORP INC		HUMANA INC
COACH INC	EXPERIAN AMERICAS	IAC/INTERACTIVECORP
COCA COLA COMPANY (THE)	EXXON MOBIL CORPORATION (EXXONMOBIL)	IGATE CORPORATION
COGNIZANT TECHNOLOGY SOLUTIONS CORP		IMS HEALTH INC
	FAMILY DOLLAR STORES INC	INFOUSA INC
COLDWATER CREEK INC	FEDEX CORPORATION	INGRAM MICRO INC
COLGATE PALMOLIVE CO	FINISH LINE INC (THE)	INTEL CORP
COMCAST CORP	FIRST DATA CORP	INTERNATIONAL BUSINESS

MACHINES CORP (IBM)	METLIFE INC	LLC (THE)
INTIMATE BRANDS INC	MGM MIRAGE	ROBERT HALF INTERNATIONAL INC
INTUIT INC	MICRON TECHNOLOGY INC	ROSS STORES INC
INVENTIV HEALTH INC	MICROSOFT CORP	ROYAL CARIBBEAN CRUISES
J C PENNEY COMPANY INC	MILLIPORE CORP	RUSSELL CORP
JACK IN THE BOX INC	MONRO MUFFLER BRAKE INC	SAFECO CORP
JACOBS ENGINEERING GROUP INC	NEIMAN MARCUS GROUP INC (THE)	SAFEWAY INC
JM SMUCKER CO	NEWS CORP	SAIC INC
JOHNSON & JOHNSON	NIKE INC	SAM'S CLUB
JOHNSON CONTROLS INC	NORDSTROM INC	SARA LEE CORP
JP MORGAN CHASE & CO INC	NORTHROP GRUMMAN CORP	SAS INSTITUTE INC
JUNIPER NETWORKS INC	OFFICE DEPOT INC	SCHERING-PLOUGH CORP
KAISER PERMANENTE	OMNICOM GROUP INC	SCHLUMBERGER LIMITED
KEANE INC	ORACLE CORP	SCIENTIFIC GAMES CORPORATION
KELLOGG CO	O'REILLY AUTOMOTIVE INC	SCOTTS MIRACLE GROW CO
KELLY SERVICES INC	OSHKOSH CORPORATION	SHAW GROUP INC (THE)
KIMBERLY-CLARK CORP	OSI RESTAURANT PARTNERS INC	SHELL OIL CO
KOHL'S CORP	OWENS & MINOR INC	SHERWIN WILLIAMS COMPANY (THE)
KPMG LLP	PACIFIC SUNWEAR OF CALIFORNIA INC	SISTERS OF MERCY HEALTH SYSTEMS
KRAFT FOODS INC	PANTRY INC (THE)	
KROGER CO (THE)	PARSONS BRINCKERHOFF INC	SMITHFIELD FOODS INC
L-3 TITAN GROUP	PATTERSON COMPANIES INC	SOUTHERN COMPANY (THE)
LABORATORY CORP OF AMERICA HOLDINGS	PAXAR CORP	SOUTHWEST AIRLINES CO
LANDRY'S RESTAURANTS INC	PEPSICO INC	ST JUDE MEDICAL INC
LAS VEGAS SANDS CORP (THE VENETIAN)	PEROT SYSTEMS CORP	STAPLES INC
	PETCO ANIMAL SUPPLIES INC	STARTEK INC
LEXMARK INTERNATIONAL INC	PETSMART INC	STARWOOD HOTELS & RESORTS WORLDWIDE INC
LIMITED BRANDS INC	PFIZER INC	
LINCOLN NATIONAL CORPORATION	PHARMACEUTICAL PRODUCT DEVELOPMENT INC	STERIS CORP
LOCKHEED MARTIN CORP		STRYKER CORP
LODGIAN INC	PITNEY BOWES INC	SUN MICROSYSTEMS INC
LOEWS CORPORATION	PLANTRONICS INC	SUNGARD DATA SYSTEMS INC
LOWE'S COMPANIES INC	POLO RALPH LAUREN CORP	SUPERVALU INC
MACY'S INC	PRICEWATERHOUSECOOPERS	SYMANTEC CORP
MANPOWER INC	PRINCIPAL FINANCIAL GROUP (THE)	SYNTEL INC
MARRIOTT INTERNATIONAL INC		SYSCO CORP
MARS INC	PROCTER & GAMBLE CO	TALBOTS INC (THE)
MARSH & MCLENNAN COMPANIES INC	PROGRESSIVE CORPORATION (THE)	TARGET CORPORATION
		TBC CORPORATION
MARY KAY INC	PRUDENTIAL FINANCIAL INC	TECH DATA CORP
MATTEL INC	PUBLIX SUPER MARKETS INC	TELEPHONE AND DATA SYSTEMS INC (TDS)
MCAFEE INC	QUEST DIAGNOSTICS INC	
MCDONALD'S CORP	QUIKSILVER INC	TIFFANY & CO
MCKESSON CORPORATION	R R DONNELLEY & SONS CO	TIME WARNER INC
MCKINSEY & COMPANY INC	RAYTHEON CO	TJX COMPANIES INC (THE)
MEDTRONIC INC	REGIS CORPORATION	T-MOBILE USA
MEIJER INC	RENT-A-CENTER INC	TOWERS PERRIN
MEN'S WEARHOUSE INC (THE)	RESPIRONICS INC	TRAVELERS COMPANIES INC (THE)
MERCER INC	RITE AID CORPORATION	TW TELECOM INC
MERCK & CO INC	RITZ-CARLTON HOTEL COMPANY	TWEEN BRANDS INC

	Music	BUILD-A-BEAR WORKSHOP INC
TYSON FOODS INC	ELECTRONIC ARTS INC	BURGER KING HOLDINGS INC
UNITED NATURAL FOODS INC	FOX ENTERTAINMENT GROUP INC	CABLEVISION SYSTEMS CORP
UNITED PARCEL SERVICE INC (UPS)	HARRAH'S ENTERTAINMENT INC	CAPITAL SENIOR LIVING CORP
UNITED STATES CELLULAR CORP	IAC/INTERACTIVECORP	CARNIVAL CORPORATION
UNITED TECHNOLOGIES CORPORATION	LAS VEGAS SANDS CORP (THE VENETIAN)	CATHOLIC HEALTH INITIATIVES
UNITEDHEALTH GROUP INC	MGM MIRAGE	CELLCO PARTNERSHIP (VERIZON WIRELESS)
UNIVISION COMMUNICATIONS INC	MICROSOFT CORP	CHARLOTTE RUSSE HOLDING
UPS SUPPLY CHAIN SOLUTIONS	NEWS CORP	CHARMING SHOPPES INC
URBAN OUTFITTERS INC	ROYAL CARIBBEAN CRUISES	CHICO'S FAS INC
URS CORPORATION	TIME WARNER INC	CHRISTOPHER & BANKS CORP
USAA	UNIVISION COMMUNICATIONS INC	CHUBB CORPORATION (THE)
VALSPAR CORPORATION (THE)	VIACOM INC	CLEAR CHANNEL COMMUNICATIONS INC
VARIAN MEDICAL SYSTEMS INC	WALT DISNEY COMPANY (THE)	COACH INC
VERISIGN INC	WYNN RESORTS LIMITED	COCA COLA COMPANY (THE)
VERIZON COMMUNICATIONS		COLDWATER CREEK INC
VIACOM INC		COLGATE PALMOLIVE CO
VOLT INFORMATION SCIENCES INC	Other	COMCAST CORP
WALGREEN CO	3M COMPANY	CONTAINER STORE (THE)
WAL-MART STORES INC	ABERCROMBIE & FITCH CO	COSTCO WHOLESALE CORP
WALT DISNEY COMPANY (THE)	ACCENTURE LTD	COX COMMUNICATIONS INC
WASTE MANAGEMENT INC	ADOBE SYSTEMS INC	DARDEN RESTAURANTS INC
WATERS CORP	AEROPOSTALE INC	DELOITTE & TOUCHE USA LLP
WATSON PHARMACEUTICALS INC	AETNA INC	DELOITTE CONSULTING LLP
WATSON WYATT WORLDWIDE INC	AFLAC INC	DENNY'S CORPORATION
WEIGHT WATCHERS INTERNATIONAL INC	ALBERTO-CULVER COMPANY	DEVRY INC
WELLPOINT INC	ALLSTATE CORPORATION (THE)	DIRECTV GROUP INC (THE)
WENDYS INTERNATIONAL INC	AMAZON.COM INC	DRESS BARN INC (THE)
WEST PHARMACEUTICAL SERVICES INC	AMERICAN EAGLE OUTFITTERS INC	EBAY INC
WESTERN DIGITAL CORP	AMERICAN EXPRESS CO	ELECTRONIC ARTS INC
WESTERN UNION COMPANY (THE)	ANNTAYLOR STORES CORP	ERNST & YOUNG LLP
WHOLE FOODS MARKET INC	APOLLO GROUP INC	ESTEE LAUDER COMPANIES INC (THE)
WILLIAMS SONOMA INC	APPLE INC	FINISH LINE INC (THE)
WM WRIGLEY JR COMPANY	AT&T INC	FOSSIL INC
WW GRAINGER INC	AVON PRODUCTS INC	FOX ENTERTAINMENT GROUP INC
WYETH	AXA FINANCIAL INC	FRED'S INC
WYNDHAM WORLDWIDE	BANK OF AMERICA CORP	GAMESTOP CORP
WYNN RESORTS LIMITED	BARNES & NOBLE COLLEGE BOOKSTORES	GENERAL ELECTRIC CO (GE)
XEROX CORP	BARNES & NOBLE INC	GENESCO INC
YAHOO! INC	BDO SEIDMAN LLP	GENWORTH FINANCIAL INC
YUM! BRANDS INC	BEBE STORES INC	GLOBAL HYATT CORPORATION
ZIMMER HOLDINGS INC	BERKSHIRE HATHAWAY INC	GOOGLE INC
	BJ'S WHOLESALE CLUB INC	GRANT THORNTON LLP
	BLACK & DECKER CORP	GUESS? INC
Music	BLOOMBERG LP	HARRAH'S ENTERTAINMENT INC
APPLE INC	BOEING COMPANY (THE)	HCA INC
CARNIVAL CORPORATION	BOOZ ALLEN HAMILTON	HE BUTT GROCERY COMPANY (HEB)
CLEAR CHANNEL COMMUNICATIONS INC	BRINKER INTERNATIONAL INC	
	BUCKLE INC (THE)	

HEALTH FITNESS CORP	INC	WENDYS INTERNATIONAL INC
HEALTH MANAGEMENT ASSOCIATES INC	PEPSICO INC	WILLIAMS SONOMA INC
HEWITT ASSOCIATES	PETSMART INC	WYNDHAM WORLDWIDE
HILTON HOTELS CORP	POLO RALPH LAUREN CORP	WYNN RESORTS LIMITED
HOME DEPOT INC	PRICEWATERHOUSECOOPERS	YAHOO! INC
HOT TOPIC INC	PRINCIPAL FINANCIAL GROUP (THE)	YUM! BRANDS INC
HUMANA INC	PROCTER & GAMBLE CO	
IAC/INTERACTIVECORP	PROGRESSIVE CORPORATION (THE)	**Technical Writing**
IMS HEALTH INC	PRUDENTIAL FINANCIAL INC	3M COMPANY
INTEL CORP	QUIKSILVER INC	ABBOTT LABORATORIES
INTERNATIONAL BUSINESS MACHINES CORP (IBM)	ROBERT HALF INTERNATIONAL INC	ACCENTURE LTD
INTIMATE BRANDS INC	ROSS STORES INC	ACXIOM CORP
INVENTIV HEALTH INC	ROYAL CARIBBEAN CRUISES	ADC TELECOMMUNICATIONS INC
J C PENNEY COMPANY INC	RUSSELL CORP	ADOBE SYSTEMS INC
JP MORGAN CHASE & CO INC	SAFECO CORP	ADVANCED MICRO DEVICES INC (AMD)
KAISER PERMANENTE	SAIC INC	AECOM TECHNOLOGY CORPORATION
KELLY SERVICES INC	SAM'S CLUB	AES CORPORATION (THE)
KIMBERLY-CLARK CORP	SISTERS OF MERCY HEALTH SYSTEMS	AETNA INC
KOHL'S CORP	SOUTHWEST AIRLINES CO	AFFILIATED COMPUTER SERVICES INC
KPMG LLP	STAPLES INC	AFLAC INC
LANDRY'S RESTAURANTS INC	STARWOOD HOTELS & RESORTS WORLDWIDE INC	AGILENT TECHNOLOGIES INC
LAS VEGAS SANDS CORP (THE VENETIAN)	SUN HEALTHCARE GROUP	AIR PRODUCTS & CHEMICALS INC
LIMITED BRANDS INC	SUN MICROSYSTEMS INC	ALLERGAN INC
LINCOLN NATIONAL CORPORATION	SUNRISE SENIOR LIVING	ALLSTATE CORPORATION (THE)
LOEWS CORPORATION	TALBOTS INC (THE)	AMAZON.COM INC
LOWE'S COMPANIES INC	TARGET CORPORATION	AMEDISYS INC
MACY'S INC	TIFFANY & CO	AMERICAN ELECTRIC POWER COMPANY INC (AEP)
MANOR CARE INC	TIME WARNER INC	AMERICAN POWER CONVERSION CORP
MANPOWER INC	TJX COMPANIES INC (THE)	AMERISOURCEBERGEN CORP
MARRIOTT INTERNATIONAL INC	T-MOBILE USA	AMGEN INC
MARSH & MCLENNAN COMPANIES INC	TOWERS PERRIN	ANADARKO PETROLEUM CORPORATION
MARY KAY INC	TRAVELERS COMPANIES INC (THE)	ANALOG DEVICES INC
MATTEL INC	TWEEN BRANDS INC	APACHE CORP
MCDONALD'S CORP	UNITEDHEALTH GROUP INC	APPLE INC
MCKINSEY & COMPANY INC	UNIVISION COMMUNICATIONS INC	ARAMARK CORPORATION
MEN'S WEARHOUSE INC (THE)	URBAN OUTFITTERS INC	ARCHER DANIELS MIDLAND CO
MERCER INC	USAA	ARROW ELECTRONICS INC
METLIFE INC	VERIZON COMMUNICATIONS	ARTHUR J GALLAGHER & CO
MGM MIRAGE	VIACOM INC	AT&T INC
MICROSOFT CORP	VOLT INFORMATION SCIENCES INC	AUTOMATIC DATA PROCESSING INC
NEIMAN MARCUS GROUP INC (THE)	WALGREEN CO	AVERY DENNISON CORP
NEWS CORP	WAL-MART STORES INC	BAKER HUGHES INC
NIKE INC	WALT DISNEY COMPANY (THE)	BALTIMORE GAS AND ELECTRIC COMPANY
NORDSTROM INC	WATSON WYATT WORLDWIDE INC	BAXTER INTERNATIONAL INC
OFFICE DEPOT INC	WEIGHT WATCHERS INTERNATIONAL INC	
OSI RESTAURANT PARTNERS INC	WELLPOINT INC	
PACIFIC SUNWEAR OF CALIFORNIA		

BDO SEIDMAN LLP	CONOCOPHILLIPS COMPANY	FAIR ISAAC CORPORATION
BECHTEL GROUP INC	CONSOL ENERGY INC	FEDEX CORPORATION
BECKMAN COULTER INC	CONSOLIDATED EDISON INC	FIRST ADVANTAGE CORPORATION
BECTON DICKINSON & CO	COOPER COMPANIES INC	FIRSTENERGY CORP
BENCHMARK ELECTRONICS INC	COVANCE INC	FLUOR CORP
BERKSHIRE HATHAWAY INC	COVENTRY HEALTH CARE INC	FMC TECHNOLOGIES INC
BIO RAD LABORATORIES INC	COX COMMUNICATIONS INC	FOREST LABORATORIES INC
BJ SERVICES COMPANY	CR BARD INC	FORTUNE BRANDS INC
BLACK & DECKER CORP	CSX CORP	FOSSIL INC
BLOOMBERG LP	CSX TRANSPORTATION INC	FOSTER WHEELER LTD
BOEING COMPANY (THE)	CTS CORP	FPL GROUP INC
BOOZ ALLEN HAMILTON	CUBIC CORP	FRONTIER COMMUNICATIONS CORPORATION
BOSTON SCIENTIFIC CORP	CUMMINS INC	GENENTECH INC
BRISTOL MYERS SQUIBB CO	DANAHER CORP	GENERAL DYNAMICS CORP
BROADCOM CORP	DAVITA INC	GENERAL ELECTRIC CO (GE)
BROWN & BROWN INC	DEERE & CO	GENWORTH FINANCIAL INC
BUNGE LTD	DELOITTE & TOUCHE USA LLP	GEORGIA GULF CORPORATION
BURLINGTON NORTHERN SANTA FE CORP	DELOITTE CONSULTING LLP	GOOGLE INC
CABLEVISION SYSTEMS CORP	DEVON ENERGY CORPORATION	GRANT THORNTON LLP
CACI INTERNATIONAL INC	DIAMOND OFFSHORE DRILLING INC	GTECH HOLDINGS CORP
CAMERON INTERNATIONAL CORPORATION	DIEBOLD INC	HALLIBURTON COMPANY
CAPITAL SENIOR LIVING CORP	DIRECTV GROUP INC (THE)	HARRIS CORPORATION
CARDINAL HEALTH INC	DJO INC	HARTFORD FINANCIAL SERVICES GROUP INC (THE)
CARGILL INC	DTE ENERGY COMPANY	HAWAIIAN ELECTRIC INDUSTRIES INC
CARNIVAL CORPORATION	DUKE ENERGY CORP	HCA INC
CATERPILLAR INC	DYCOM INDUSTRIES INC	HEALTH MANAGEMENT ASSOCIATES INC
CATERPILLAR LOGISTICS	E I DU PONT DE NEMOURS & CO (DUPONT)	HEALTH NET INC
CATHOLIC HEALTH INITIATIVES	EATON CORP	HEALTHWAYS INC
CDW CORPORATION	EBAY INC	HELMERICH & PAYNE INC
CELLCO PARTNERSHIP (VERIZON WIRELESS)	ECHOSTAR CORP	HENRY SCHEIN INC
CEPHALON INC	EDISON INTERNATIONAL	HESS CORPORATION
CH ROBINSON WORLDWIDE INC	ELECTRONIC ARTS INC	HEWITT ASSOCIATES
CH2M HILL COMPANIES LTD	ELI LILLY & COMPANY	HILB ROGAL & HOBBS CO
CHEMED CORPORATION	EMBARQ CORP	HONEYWELL INTERNATIONAL INC
CHESAPEAKE ENERGY CORP	EMC CORP	HUMANA INC
CHEVRON CORPORATION	EMERITUS CORP	IDEXX LABORATORIES INC
CHEVRON PHILLIPS CHEMICAL COMPANY LLC	EMERSON ELECTRIC CO	IGATE CORPORATION
CHUBB CORPORATION (THE)	ENTERGY CORP	IMS HEALTH INC
CIBER INC	ERNST & YOUNG LLP	INGRAM MICRO INC
CISCO SYSTEMS INC	ESTEE LAUDER COMPANIES INC (THE)	INTEL CORP
COCA COLA COMPANY (THE)	EXEL TRANSPORTATION SERVICES INC (DHL EXEL)	INTERNATIONAL BUSINESS MACHINES CORP (IBM)
COCA COLA ENTERPRISES INC	EXELON CORPORATION	INTUIT INC
COGNIZANT TECHNOLOGY SOLUTIONS CORP	EXPEDITORS INTERNATIONAL OF WASHINGTON INC	INVENTIV HEALTH INC
COLGATE PALMOLIVE CO	EXPERIAN AMERICAS	JABIL CIRCUIT INC
COMCAST CORP	EXPRESS SCRIPTS INC	JACOBS ENGINEERING GROUP INC
CONAGRA FOODS INC	EXXON MOBIL CORPORATION (EXXONMOBIL)	JOHNSON & JOHNSON

JOHNSON CONTROLS INC	OCEANEERING INTERNATIONAL INC	SCANA CORPORATION
JUNIPER NETWORKS INC	ODYSSEY HEALTHCARE INC	SCHERING-PLOUGH CORP
KAISER PERMANENTE	OIL STATES INTERNATIONAL INC	SCHLUMBERGER LIMITED
KEANE INC	OLD DOMINION FREIGHT LINE INC	SCIENTIFIC GAMES CORPORATION
KELLY SERVICES INC	OMNICARE INC	SCOTTS MIRACLE GROW CO
KENDLE INTERNATIONAL INC	ONEOK INC	SEACOR HOLDINGS INC
KINDRED HEALTHCARE INC	ORACLE CORP	SELECT MEDICAL CORPORATION
KOCH INDUSTRIES INC	OSHKOSH CORPORATION	SEMPRA ENERGY
KPMG LLP	OWENS & MINOR INC	SENSIENT TECHNOLOGIES CORPORATION
L-3 COMMUNICATIONS HOLDINGS INC	PARAMETRIC TECHNOLOGY CORP	SHAW GROUP INC (THE)
L-3 TITAN GROUP	PAREXEL INTERNATIONAL CORP	SHELL OIL CO
LABORATORY CORP OF AMERICA HOLDINGS	PARSONS BRINCKERHOFF INC	SHERWIN WILLIAMS COMPANY (THE)
LEVEL 3 COMMUNICATIONS INC	PATTERSON COMPANIES INC	SIGMA-ALDRICH CORP
LEXMARK INTERNATIONAL INC	PATTERSON-UTI ENERGY INC	SISTERS OF MERCY HEALTH SYSTEMS
LINCARE HOLDINGS INC	PAXAR CORP	SMITH INTERNATIONAL INC
LKQ CORP	PEABODY ENERGY CORP	SOUTHERN COMPANY (THE)
LOCKHEED MARTIN CORP	PEPSI BOTTLING GROUP INC	SOUTHWEST AIRLINES CO
LOEWS CORPORATION	PEPSICO INC	SRA INTERNATIONAL INC
MANOR CARE INC	PEROT SYSTEMS CORP	ST JUDE MEDICAL INC
MANPOWER INC	PERRIGO CO	STARTEK INC
MARATHON OIL CORP	PFIZER INC	STERIS CORP
MARSH & MCLENNAN COMPANIES INC	PG&E CORPORATION	STRYKER CORP
MASSEY ENERGY COMPANY	PHARMACEUTICAL PRODUCT DEVELOPMENT INC	SUN HEALTHCARE GROUP
MATTEL INC	PITNEY BOWES INC	SUN MICROSYSTEMS INC
MAXIM INTEGRATED PRODUCTS INC	PLANTRONICS INC	SUNGARD DATA SYSTEMS INC
MCAFEE INC	PLEXUS CORP	SUNOCO INC
MCKESSON CORPORATION	PRAXAIR INC	SUNRISE SENIOR LIVING
MCKINSEY & COMPANY INC	PRICEWATERHOUSECOOPERS	SYKES ENTERPRISES INC
MEDCO HEALTH SOLUTIONS	PRIDE INTERNATIONAL INC	SYMANTEC CORP
MEDTRONIC INC	PRINCIPAL FINANCIAL GROUP (THE)	SYNOPSYS INC
MERCER INC	PROCTER & GAMBLE CO	SYNTEL INC
MERCK & CO INC	PROGRESSIVE CORPORATION (THE)	TECH DATA CORP
METLIFE INC	PRUDENTIAL FINANCIAL INC	TEKTRONIX INC
MICROCHIP TECHNOLOGY INC	PSYCHIATRIC SOLUTIONS INC	TELEDYNE TECHNOLOGIES INCORPORATED
MICRON TECHNOLOGY INC	QUALCOMM INC	TELEPHONE AND DATA SYSTEMS INC (TDS)
MICROSOFT CORP	QUEST DIAGNOSTICS INC	TESORO CORP
MILLIPORE CORP	R R DONNELLEY & SONS CO	TIME WARNER INC
MOLEX INC	RAYTHEON CO	T-MOBILE USA
MONRO MUFFLER BRAKE INC	RELIANT ENERGY INC	TOWERS PERRIN
MURPHY OIL CORPORATION	RES CARE INC	TRANSOCEAN INC
NATIONAL OILWELL VARCO INC	RESPIRONICS INC	TRAVELERS COMPANIES INC (THE)
NETWORK APPLIANCE INC	ROBERT HALF INTERNATIONAL INC	TW TELECOM INC
NII HOLDINGS INC	ROYAL CARIBBEAN CRUISES	UNION PACIFIC CORP
NOBLE CORPORATION	SABRE HOLDINGS CORP	UNITED PARCEL SERVICE INC (UPS)
NORFOLK SOUTHERN CORP	SAFECO CORP	UNITED STATES CELLULAR CORP
NORTHROP GRUMMAN CORP	SAIC INC	
OCCIDENTAL PETROLEUM CORP	SAS INSTITUTE INC	

UNITED TECHNOLOGIES CORPORATION	CORPORATION	BAXTER INTERNATIONAL INC
UNITEDHEALTH GROUP INC	AEROPOSTALE INC	BDO SEIDMAN LLP
UPS SUPPLY CHAIN SOLUTIONS	AES CORPORATION (THE)	BEBE STORES INC
URS CORPORATION	AETNA INC	BECHTEL GROUP INC
USAA	AFFILIATED COMPUTER SERVICES INC	BECKMAN COULTER INC
VALERO ENERGY CORP	AFLAC INC	BECTON DICKINSON & CO
VALSPAR CORPORATION (THE)	AGILENT TECHNOLOGIES INC	BED BATH & BEYOND INC
VARIAN MEDICAL SYSTEMS INC	AIR PRODUCTS & CHEMICALS INC	BENCHMARK ELECTRONICS INC
VCA ANTECH INC	ALBERTO-CULVER COMPANY	BERKSHIRE HATHAWAY INC
VERISIGN INC	ALLERGAN INC	BEST BUY CO INC
VERIZON COMMUNICATIONS	ALLIANCE DATA SYSTEMS CORPORATION	BIO RAD LABORATORIES INC
VOLT INFORMATION SCIENCES INC	ALLSTATE CORPORATION (THE)	BJ SERVICES COMPANY
W R BERKLEY CORPORATION	ALTRIA GROUP INC	BJ'S WHOLESALE CLUB INC
WASTE MANAGEMENT INC	AMAZON.COM INC	BLACK & DECKER CORP
WATERS CORP	AMEDISYS INC	BLOOMBERG LP
WATSON PHARMACEUTICALS INC	AMERICAN EAGLE OUTFITTERS INC	BOEING COMPANY (THE)
WATSON WYATT WORLDWIDE INC	AMERICAN ELECTRIC POWER COMPANY INC (AEP)	BOOZ ALLEN HAMILTON
WEATHERFORD INTERNATIONAL LTD	AMERICAN EXPRESS CO	BOSTON SCIENTIFIC CORP
WELLPOINT INC	AMERICAN POWER CONVERSION CORP	BRINKER INTERNATIONAL INC
WEST PHARMACEUTICAL SERVICES INC	AMERISOURCEBERGEN CORP	BRINKS COMPANY (THE)
WESTERN DIGITAL CORP	AMGEN INC	BRISTOL MYERS SQUIBB CO
WILLIAMS COMPANIES INC (THE)	ANADARKO PETROLEUM CORPORATION	BROADCOM CORP
WW GRAINGER INC	ANALOG DEVICES INC	BROWN & BROWN INC
WYETH	ANNTAYLOR STORES CORP	BUCKLE INC (THE)
XEROX CORP	APACHE CORP	BUILD-A-BEAR WORKSHOP INC
YAHOO! INC	APOLLO GROUP INC	BUNGE LTD
ZIMMER HOLDINGS INC	APPLE INC	BURGER KING HOLDINGS INC
	ARAMARK CORPORATION	BURLINGTON NORTHERN SANTA FE CORP
	ARCHER DANIELS MIDLAND CO	CABELA'S INC
	ARROW ELECTRONICS INC	CABLEVISION SYSTEMS CORP
	ARTHUR J GALLAGHER & CO	CACI INTERNATIONAL INC
	AT&T INC	CAMERON INTERNATIONAL CORPORATION
	AUTOMATIC DATA PROCESSING INC	CAPITAL SENIOR LIVING CORP
	AUTOZONE INC	CARDINAL HEALTH INC
	AVERY DENNISON CORP	CARGILL INC
	AVIS BUDGET GROUP INC	CARMAX GROUP
	AVON PRODUCTS INC	CARNIVAL CORPORATION
	AXA FINANCIAL INC	CASH AMERICA INTERNATIONAL INC
	BAKER HUGHES INC	CATERPILLAR INC
	BALTIMORE GAS AND ELECTRIC COMPANY	CATERPILLAR LOGISTICS
	BANK OF AMERICA CORP	CATHOLIC HEALTH INITIATIVES
	BARNES & NOBLE COLLEGE BOOKSTORES	CBRL GROUP INC
	BARNES & NOBLE INC	CDW CORPORATION
	BASS PRO SHOPS INC	CELLCO PARTNERSHIP (VERIZON WIRELESS)
		CEPHALON INC
		CH ROBINSON WORLDWIDE INC
		CH2M HILL COMPANIES LTD

Management

Experienced Management
3M COMPANY
7-ELEVEN INC
AARON RENTS INC
ABBOTT LABORATORIES
ABERCROMBIE & FITCH CO
ABM INDUSTRIES INC
ACADEMY SPORTS & OUTDOORS LTD
ACCENTURE LTD
ACXIOM CORP
ADC TELECOMMUNICATIONS INC
ADESA INC
ADOBE SYSTEMS INC
ADVANCE AUTO PARTS INC
ADVANCED MICRO DEVICES INC (AMD)
AECOM TECHNOLOGY

CHARLOTTE RUSSE HOLDING	DEVON ENERGY CORPORATION	FMC TECHNOLOGIES INC
CHARMING SHOPPES INC	DEVRY INC	FOREST LABORATORIES INC
CHEMED CORPORATION	DIAMOND OFFSHORE DRILLING INC	FORTUNE BRANDS INC
CHESAPEAKE ENERGY CORP	DICK'S SPORTING GOODS INC	FOSSIL INC
CHEVRON CORPORATION	DIEBOLD INC	FOSTER WHEELER LTD
CHEVRON PHILLIPS CHEMICAL COMPANY LLC	DINEEQUITY INC	FOX ENTERTAINMENT GROUP INC
CHICO'S FAS INC	DIRECTV GROUP INC (THE)	FPL GROUP INC
CHRISTOPHER & BANKS CORP	DJO INC	FRED'S INC
CHUBB CORPORATION (THE)	DOLE FOOD COMPANY INC	FRONTIER COMMUNICATIONS CORPORATION
CIBER INC	DOLLAR GENERAL CORPORATION	GAMESTOP CORP
CINTAS CORP	DOLLAR THRIFTY AUTOMOTIVE GROUP INC	GENENTECH INC
CISCO SYSTEMS INC	DRESS BARN INC (THE)	GENERAL DYNAMICS CORP
CLEAR CHANNEL COMMUNICATIONS INC	DTE ENERGY COMPANY	GENERAL ELECTRIC CO (GE)
CLUBCORP INC	DUKE ENERGY CORP	GENERAL MILLS INC
COACH INC	DYCOM INDUSTRIES INC	GENESCO INC
COCA COLA COMPANY (THE)	E I DU PONT DE NEMOURS & CO (DUPONT)	GENWORTH FINANCIAL INC
COCA COLA ENTERPRISES INC	EATON CORP	GEO GROUP INC
COGNIZANT TECHNOLOGY SOLUTIONS CORP	EBAY INC	GEORGIA GULF CORPORATION
COLDWATER CREEK INC	ECHOSTAR CORP	GLOBAL HYATT CORPORATION
COLGATE PALMOLIVE CO	EDISON INTERNATIONAL	GLOBAL PAYMENTS INC
COMCAST CORP	ELECTRONIC ARTS INC	GOOGLE INC
CONAGRA FOODS INC	ELI LILLY & COMPANY	GRANT THORNTON LLP
CONOCOPHILLIPS COMPANY	EMBARQ CORP	GTECH HOLDINGS CORP
CONSOL ENERGY INC	EMC CORP	GUESS? INC
CONSOLIDATED EDISON INC	EMERITUS CORP	HALLIBURTON COMPANY
CONTAINER STORE (THE)	EMERSON ELECTRIC CO	HARRAH'S ENTERTAINMENT INC
CONVERGYS CORPORATION	ENTERGY CORP	HARRIS CORPORATION
COOPER COMPANIES INC	ENTERPRISE RENT-A-CAR	HARTFORD FINANCIAL SERVICES GROUP INC (THE)
COST PLUS INC	ERNST & YOUNG LLP	HAWAIIAN ELECTRIC INDUSTRIES INC
COSTCO WHOLESALE CORP	ESTEE LAUDER COMPANIES INC (THE)	HCA INC
COVANCE INC	EXEL TRANSPORTATION SERVICES INC (DHL EXEL)	HE BUTT GROCERY COMPANY (HEB)
COVENTRY HEALTH CARE INC	EXELON CORPORATION	HEALTH FITNESS CORP
COX COMMUNICATIONS INC	EXPEDITORS INTERNATIONAL OF WASHINGTON INC	HEALTH MANAGEMENT ASSOCIATES INC
CR BARD INC	EXPERIAN AMERICAS	HEALTH NET INC
CSX CORP	EXPRESS SCRIPTS INC	HEALTHWAYS INC
CSX TRANSPORTATION INC	EXXON MOBIL CORPORATION (EXXONMOBIL)	HELMERICH & PAYNE INC
CTS CORP	FAIR ISAAC CORPORATION	HENRY SCHEIN INC
CUBIC CORP	FAMILY DOLLAR STORES INC	HERTZ GLOBAL HOLDINGS INC
CUMMINS INC	FEDEX CORPORATION	HESS CORPORATION
CVS CAREMARK CORPORATION	FINISH LINE INC (THE)	HEWITT ASSOCIATES
DANAHER CORP	FIRST ADVANTAGE CORPORATION	HIBBETT SPORTS INC
DARDEN RESTAURANTS INC	FIRST DATA CORP	HILB ROGAL & HOBBS CO
DAVITA INC	FIRSTENERGY CORP	HILTON HOTELS CORP
DEAN FOODS CO	FISERV INC	HOME DEPOT INC
DEERE & CO	FLUOR CORP	HONEYWELL INTERNATIONAL INC
DELOITTE & TOUCHE USA LLP		HOT TOPIC INC
DELOITTE CONSULTING LLP		
DENNY'S CORPORATION		

HUMANA INC	LODGIAN INC	OLD DOMINION FREIGHT LINE INC
IAC/INTERACTIVECORP	LOEWS CORPORATION	OMNICARE INC
ICT GROUP INC	LOWE'S COMPANIES INC	OMNICOM GROUP INC
IDEXX LABORATORIES INC	MACY'S INC	ONEOK INC
IGATE CORPORATION	MANOR CARE INC	ORACLE CORP
IMS HEALTH INC	MANPOWER INC	O'REILLY AUTOMOTIVE INC
INFOUSA INC	MARATHON OIL CORP	OSHKOSH CORPORATION
INGRAM MICRO INC	MARRIOTT INTERNATIONAL INC	OSI RESTAURANT PARTNERS INC
INTEL CORP	MARS INC	OWENS & MINOR INC
INTERNATIONAL BUSINESS MACHINES CORP (IBM)	MARSH & MCLENNAN COMPANIES INC	PACIFIC SUNWEAR OF CALIFORNIA INC
INTIMATE BRANDS INC	MARY KAY INC	PANTRY INC (THE)
INTUIT INC	MASSEY ENERGY COMPANY	PARAMETRIC TECHNOLOGY CORP
INVENTIV HEALTH INC	MATTEL INC	PAREXEL INTERNATIONAL CORP
J C PENNEY COMPANY INC	MAXIM INTEGRATED PRODUCTS INC	PARSONS BRINCKERHOFF INC
JABIL CIRCUIT INC		PATTERSON COMPANIES INC
JACK IN THE BOX INC	MCAFEE INC	PATTERSON-UTI ENERGY INC
JACOBS ENGINEERING GROUP INC	MCDONALD'S CORP	PAXAR CORP
JM SMUCKER CO	MCKESSON CORPORATION	PAYCHEX INC
JOHNSON & JOHNSON	MCKINSEY & COMPANY INC	PEABODY ENERGY CORP
JOHNSON CONTROLS INC	MEDCO HEALTH SOLUTIONS	PEPSI BOTTLING GROUP INC
JP MORGAN CHASE & CO INC	MEDTRONIC INC	PEPSICO INC
JUNIPER NETWORKS INC	MEIJER INC	PEROT SYSTEMS CORP
KAISER PERMANENTE	MEN'S WEARHOUSE INC (THE)	PERRIGO CO
KEANE INC	MERCER INC	PETCO ANIMAL SUPPLIES INC
KELLOGG CO	MERCK & CO INC	PETSMART INC
KELLY SERVICES INC	METLIFE INC	PFIZER INC
KENDLE INTERNATIONAL INC	MGM MIRAGE	PG&E CORPORATION
KIMBERLY-CLARK CORP	MICROCHIP TECHNOLOGY INC	PHARMACEUTICAL PRODUCT DEVELOPMENT INC
KINDRED HEALTHCARE INC	MICRON TECHNOLOGY INC	
KOCH INDUSTRIES INC	MICROSOFT CORP	PITNEY BOWES INC
KOHL'S CORP	MILLIPORE CORP	PLANTRONICS INC
KPMG LLP	MOLEX INC	PLEXUS CORP
KRAFT FOODS INC	MONRO MUFFLER BRAKE INC	POLO RALPH LAUREN CORP
KROGER CO (THE)	MURPHY OIL CORPORATION	PRAXAIR INC
L-3 COMMUNICATIONS HOLDINGS INC	NATIONAL OILWELL VARCO INC	PRICEWATERHOUSECOOPERS
	NEIMAN MARCUS GROUP INC (THE)	PRIDE INTERNATIONAL INC
L-3 TITAN GROUP	NETWORK APPLIANCE INC	PRINCIPAL FINANCIAL GROUP (THE)
LABORATORY CORP OF AMERICA HOLDINGS	NEWS CORP	
	NII HOLDINGS INC	PROCTER & GAMBLE CO
LANDRY'S RESTAURANTS INC	NIKE INC	PROGRESSIVE CORPORATION (THE)
LAS VEGAS SANDS CORP (THE VENETIAN)	NOBLE CORPORATION	
	NORDSTROM INC	PRUDENTIAL FINANCIAL INC
LEVEL 3 COMMUNICATIONS INC	NORFOLK SOUTHERN CORP	PSYCHIATRIC SOLUTIONS INC
LEXMARK INTERNATIONAL INC	NORTHROP GRUMMAN CORP	PUBLIC STORAGE INC
LIBERTY GLOBAL INC	OCCIDENTAL PETROLEUM CORP	PUBLIX SUPER MARKETS INC
LIMITED BRANDS INC	OCEANEERING INTERNATIONAL INC	QUALCOMM INC
LINCARE HOLDINGS INC		QUEST DIAGNOSTICS INC
LINCOLN NATIONAL CORPORATION	ODYSSEY HEALTHCARE INC	QUIKSILVER INC
LKQ CORP	OFFICE DEPOT INC	R R DONNELLEY & SONS CO
LOCKHEED MARTIN CORP	OIL STATES INTERNATIONAL INC	RAYTHEON CO

REGIS CORPORATION	SUNGARD DATA SYSTEMS INC	VIACOM INC
RELIANT ENERGY INC	SUNOCO INC	VOLT INFORMATION SCIENCES INC
RENT-A-CENTER INC	SUNRISE SENIOR LIVING	W R BERKLEY CORPORATION
RES CARE INC	SUPERVALU INC	WALGREEN CO
RESPIRONICS INC	SYKES ENTERPRISES INC	WAL-MART STORES INC
RITE AID CORPORATION	SYMANTEC CORP	WALT DISNEY COMPANY (THE)
RITZ-CARLTON HOTEL COMPANY LLC (THE)	SYNOPSYS INC	WASTE MANAGEMENT INC
ROBERT HALF INTERNATIONAL INC	SYNTEL INC	WATERS CORP
ROSS STORES INC	SYSCO CORP	WATSON PHARMACEUTICALS INC
ROYAL CARIBBEAN CRUISES	TALBOTS INC (THE)	WATSON WYATT WORLDWIDE INC
RUSSELL CORP	TARGET CORPORATION	WEATHERFORD INTERNATIONAL LTD
RYDER SYSTEM INC	TBC CORPORATION	
SABRE HOLDINGS CORP	TECH DATA CORP	WEIGHT WATCHERS INTERNATIONAL INC
SAFECO CORP	TEKTRONIX INC	
SAFEWAY INC	TELEDYNE TECHNOLOGIES INCORPORATED	WELLPOINT INC
SAIC INC		WENDYS INTERNATIONAL INC
SAM'S CLUB	TELEPHONE AND DATA SYSTEMS INC (TDS)	WEST CORPORATION
SARA LEE CORP		WEST PHARMACEUTICAL SERVICES INC
SAS INSTITUTE INC	TELETECH HOLDINGS INC	
SCANA CORPORATION	TESORO CORP	WESTERN DIGITAL CORP
SCHERING-PLOUGH CORP	TIFFANY & CO	WESTERN UNION COMPANY (THE)
SCHLUMBERGER LIMITED	TIME WARNER INC	WHOLE FOODS MARKET INC
SCIENTIFIC GAMES CORPORATION	TJX COMPANIES INC (THE)	WILLIAMS COMPANIES INC (THE)
SCOTTS MIRACLE GROW CO	T-MOBILE USA	WILLIAMS SONOMA INC
SEACOR HOLDINGS INC	TOTAL SYSTEM SERVICES INC (TSYS)	WM WRIGLEY JR COMPANY
SELECT MEDICAL CORPORATION		WW GRAINGER INC
SEMPRA ENERGY	TOWERS PERRIN	WYETH
SENSIENT TECHNOLOGIES CORPORATION	TRANSOCEAN INC	WYNDHAM WORLDWIDE
	TRAVELERS COMPANIES INC (THE)	WYNN RESORTS LIMITED
SHAW GROUP INC (THE)	TW TELECOM INC	XEROX CORP
SHELL OIL CO	TWEEN BRANDS INC	YAHOO! INC
SHERWIN WILLIAMS COMPANY (THE)	TYSON FOODS INC	YUM! BRANDS INC
	UNION PACIFIC CORP	ZIMMER HOLDINGS INC
SIGMA-ALDRICH CORP	UNITED NATURAL FOODS INC	
SISTERS OF MERCY HEALTH SYSTEMS	UNITED PARCEL SERVICE INC (UPS)	**International Business**
		3M COMPANY
SMITH INTERNATIONAL INC	UNITED STATES CELLULAR CORP	7-ELEVEN INC
SMITHFIELD FOODS INC	UNITED TECHNOLOGIES CORPORATION	AARON RENTS INC
SOUTHERN COMPANY (THE)		ABBOTT LABORATORIES
SOUTHWEST AIRLINES CO	UNITEDHEALTH GROUP INC	ABERCROMBIE & FITCH CO
SRA INTERNATIONAL INC	UNIVISION COMMUNICATIONS INC	ABM INDUSTRIES INC
ST JUDE MEDICAL INC	UPS SUPPLY CHAIN SOLUTIONS	ACCENTURE LTD
STAPLES INC	URBAN OUTFITTERS INC	ACXIOM CORP
STARTEK INC	URS CORPORATION	ADC TELECOMMUNICATIONS INC
STARWOOD HOTELS & RESORTS WORLDWIDE INC	USAA	ADESA INC
	VALERO ENERGY CORP	ADOBE SYSTEMS INC
STERIS CORP	VALSPAR CORPORATION (THE)	ADVANCE AUTO PARTS INC
STRYKER CORP	VARIAN MEDICAL SYSTEMS INC	ADVANCED MICRO DEVICES INC (AMD)
SUN HEALTHCARE GROUP	VCA ANTECH INC	
SUN MICROSYSTEMS INC	VERISIGN INC	AECOM TECHNOLOGY CORPORATION
	VERIZON COMMUNICATIONS	

AEROPOSTALE INC	BED BATH & BEYOND INC	COCA COLA COMPANY (THE)
AES CORPORATION (THE)	BENCHMARK ELECTRONICS INC	COCA COLA ENTERPRISES INC
AFFILIATED COMPUTER SERVICES INC	BERKSHIRE HATHAWAY INC	COGNIZANT TECHNOLOGY SOLUTIONS CORP
AFLAC INC	BEST BUY CO INC	COLGATE PALMOLIVE CO
AGILENT TECHNOLOGIES INC	BIO RAD LABORATORIES INC	COMCAST CORP
AIR PRODUCTS & CHEMICALS INC	BJ SERVICES COMPANY	CONAGRA FOODS INC
ALBERTO-CULVER COMPANY	BLACK & DECKER CORP	CONOCOPHILLIPS COMPANY
ALLERGAN INC	BLOOMBERG LP	CONSOL ENERGY INC
ALLIANCE DATA SYSTEMS CORPORATION	BOEING COMPANY (THE)	CONSOLIDATED EDISON INC
ALLSTATE CORPORATION (THE)	BOOZ ALLEN HAMILTON	CONVERGYS CORPORATION
ALTRIA GROUP INC	BOSTON SCIENTIFIC CORP	COOPER COMPANIES INC
AMAZON.COM INC	BRINKER INTERNATIONAL INC	COSTCO WHOLESALE CORP
AMERICAN EAGLE OUTFITTERS INC	BRINKS COMPANY (THE)	COVANCE INC
AMERICAN ELECTRIC POWER COMPANY INC (AEP)	BRISTOL MYERS SQUIBB CO	COX COMMUNICATIONS INC
AMERICAN EXPRESS CO	BROADCOM CORP	CR BARD INC
AMERICAN POWER CONVERSION CORP	BROWN & BROWN INC	CSX CORP
AMERISOURCEBERGEN CORP	BUILD-A-BEAR WORKSHOP INC	CSX TRANSPORTATION INC
AMGEN INC	BUNGE LTD	CTS CORP
ANADARKO PETROLEUM CORPORATION	BURGER KING HOLDINGS INC	CUBIC CORP
ANALOG DEVICES INC	BURLINGTON NORTHERN SANTA FE CORP	CUMMINS INC
ANNTAYLOR STORES CORP	CABELA'S INC	DANAHER CORP
APACHE CORP	CACI INTERNATIONAL INC	DARDEN RESTAURANTS INC
APOLLO GROUP INC	CAMERON INTERNATIONAL CORPORATION	DEAN FOODS CO
APPLE INC	CARDINAL HEALTH INC	DEERE & CO
ARAMARK CORPORATION	CARGILL INC	DELOITTE & TOUCHE USA LLP
ARCHER DANIELS MIDLAND CO	CARNIVAL CORPORATION	DELOITTE CONSULTING LLP
ARROW ELECTRONICS INC	CASH AMERICA INTERNATIONAL INC	DENNY'S CORPORATION
ARTHUR J GALLAGHER & CO	CATERPILLAR INC	DEVON ENERGY CORPORATION
AT&T INC	CATERPILLAR LOGISTICS	DEVRY INC
AUTOMATIC DATA PROCESSING INC	CDW CORPORATION	DIAMOND OFFSHORE DRILLING INC
AUTOZONE INC	CEPHALON INC	DIEBOLD INC
AVERY DENNISON CORP	CH ROBINSON WORLDWIDE INC	DINEEQUITY INC
AVIS BUDGET GROUP INC	CH2M HILL COMPANIES LTD	DIRECTV GROUP INC (THE)
AVON PRODUCTS INC	CHARLOTTE RUSSE HOLDING	DJO INC
AXA FINANCIAL INC	CHARMING SHOPPES INC	DOLE FOOD COMPANY INC
BAKER HUGHES INC	CHEMED CORPORATION	DOLLAR THRIFTY AUTOMOTIVE GROUP INC
BANK OF AMERICA CORP	CHEVRON CORPORATION	DUKE ENERGY CORP
BARNES & NOBLE COLLEGE BOOKSTORES	CHEVRON PHILLIPS CHEMICAL COMPANY LLC	E I DU PONT DE NEMOURS & CO (DUPONT)
BASS PRO SHOPS INC	CHICO'S FAS INC	EATON CORP
BAXTER INTERNATIONAL INC	CHUBB CORPORATION (THE)	EBAY INC
BDO SEIDMAN LLP	CIBER INC	ECHOSTAR CORP
BEBE STORES INC	CINTAS CORP	EDISON INTERNATIONAL
BECHTEL GROUP INC	CISCO SYSTEMS INC	ELECTRONIC ARTS INC
BECKMAN COULTER INC	CLEAR CHANNEL COMMUNICATIONS INC	ELI LILLY & COMPANY
BECTON DICKINSON & CO	CLUBCORP INC	EMC CORP
	COACH INC	EMERITUS CORP
		EMERSON ELECTRIC CO
		ENTERGY CORP

ENTERPRISE RENT-A-CAR	HEWITT ASSOCIATES	LOWE'S COMPANIES INC
ERNST & YOUNG LLP	HILB ROGAL & HOBBS CO	MACY'S INC
ESTEE LAUDER COMPANIES INC (THE)	HILTON HOTELS CORP	MANOR CARE INC
EXEL TRANSPORTATION SERVICES INC (DHL EXEL)	HOME DEPOT INC	MANPOWER INC
	HONEYWELL INTERNATIONAL INC	MARATHON OIL CORP
EXPEDITORS INTERNATIONAL OF WASHINGTON INC	HOT TOPIC INC	MARRIOTT INTERNATIONAL INC
	HUMANA INC	MARS INC
EXPRESS SCRIPTS INC	IAC/INTERACTIVECORP	MARSH & MCLENNAN COMPANIES INC
EXXON MOBIL CORPORATION (EXXONMOBIL)	ICT GROUP INC	
	IDEXX LABORATORIES INC	MARY KAY INC
FAIR ISAAC CORPORATION	IGATE CORPORATION	MATTEL INC
FEDEX CORPORATION	IMS HEALTH INC	MAXIM INTEGRATED PRODUCTS INC
FIRST ADVANTAGE CORPORATION	INFOUSA INC	
FIRST DATA CORP	INGRAM MICRO INC	MCAFEE INC
FISERV INC	INTEL CORP	MCDONALD'S CORP
FLUOR CORP	INTERNATIONAL BUSINESS MACHINES CORP (IBM)	MCKESSON CORPORATION
FMC TECHNOLOGIES INC		MCKINSEY & COMPANY INC
FOREST LABORATORIES INC	INTIMATE BRANDS INC	MEDTRONIC INC
FORTUNE BRANDS INC	INTUIT INC	MEN'S WEARHOUSE INC (THE)
FOSSIL INC	INVENTIV HEALTH INC	MERCER INC
FOSTER WHEELER LTD	J C PENNEY COMPANY INC	MERCK & CO INC
FOX ENTERTAINMENT GROUP INC	JABIL CIRCUIT INC	METLIFE INC
GAMESTOP CORP	JACOBS ENGINEERING GROUP INC	MGM MIRAGE
GENENTECH INC	JM SMUCKER CO	MICROCHIP TECHNOLOGY INC
GENERAL DYNAMICS CORP	JOHNSON & JOHNSON	MICRON TECHNOLOGY INC
GENERAL ELECTRIC CO (GE)	JOHNSON CONTROLS INC	MICROSOFT CORP
GENERAL MILLS INC	JP MORGAN CHASE & CO INC	MILLIPORE CORP
GENESCO INC	JUNIPER NETWORKS INC	MOLEX INC
GENWORTH FINANCIAL INC	KEANE INC	MURPHY OIL CORPORATION
GEO GROUP INC	KELLOGG CO	NATIONAL OILWELL VARCO INC
GEORGIA GULF CORPORATION	KELLY SERVICES INC	NETWORK APPLIANCE INC
GLOBAL HYATT CORPORATION	KENDLE INTERNATIONAL INC	NEWS CORP
GLOBAL PAYMENTS INC	KIMBERLY-CLARK CORP	NII HOLDINGS INC
GOOGLE INC	KOCH INDUSTRIES INC	NIKE INC
GTECH HOLDINGS CORP	KPMG LLP	NOBLE CORPORATION
GUESS? INC	KRAFT FOODS INC	NORDSTROM INC
HALLIBURTON COMPANY	L-3 COMMUNICATIONS HOLDINGS INC	NORFOLK SOUTHERN CORP
HARRAH'S ENTERTAINMENT INC		NORTHROP GRUMMAN CORP
HARRIS CORPORATION	L-3 TITAN GROUP	OCCIDENTAL PETROLEUM CORP
HARTFORD FINANCIAL SERVICES GROUP INC (THE)	LABORATORY CORP OF AMERICA HOLDINGS	OCEANEERING INTERNATIONAL INC
HCA INC	LAS VEGAS SANDS CORP (THE VENETIAN)	
HE BUTT GROCERY COMPANY (HEB)		OFFICE DEPOT INC
	LEVEL 3 COMMUNICATIONS INC	OIL STATES INTERNATIONAL INC
HEALTH FITNESS CORP	LEXMARK INTERNATIONAL INC	OMNICARE INC
HEALTHWAYS INC	LIBERTY GLOBAL INC	OMNICOM GROUP INC
HELMERICH & PAYNE INC	LIMITED BRANDS INC	ORACLE CORP
HENRY SCHEIN INC	LINCOLN NATIONAL CORPORATION	OSHKOSH CORPORATION
HERTZ GLOBAL HOLDINGS INC	LOCKHEED MARTIN CORP	OSI RESTAURANT PARTNERS INC
HESS CORPORATION	LODGIAN INC	PACIFIC SUNWEAR OF CALIFORNIA INC
	LOEWS CORPORATION	PARAMETRIC TECHNOLOGY CORP

PAREXEL INTERNATIONAL CORP	SAS INSTITUTE INC	TRANSOCEAN INC
PARSONS BRINCKERHOFF INC	SCHERING-PLOUGH CORP	TRAVELERS COMPANIES INC (THE)
PATTERSON COMPANIES INC	SCHLUMBERGER LIMITED	TWEEN BRANDS INC
PATTERSON-UTI ENERGY INC	SCIENTIFIC GAMES CORPORATION	TYSON FOODS INC
PAXAR CORP	SCOTTS MIRACLE GROW CO	UNITED PARCEL SERVICE INC (UPS)
PAYCHEX INC	SEACOR HOLDINGS INC	UNITED TECHNOLOGIES CORPORATION
PEABODY ENERGY CORP	SELECT MEDICAL CORPORATION	
PEPSI BOTTLING GROUP INC	SEMPRA ENERGY	UNIVISION COMMUNICATIONS INC
PEPSICO INC	SENSIENT TECHNOLOGIES CORPORATION	UPS SUPPLY CHAIN SOLUTIONS
PEROT SYSTEMS CORP		URBAN OUTFITTERS INC
PERRIGO CO	SHAW GROUP INC (THE)	URS CORPORATION
PETSMART INC	SHELL OIL CO	USAA
PFIZER INC	SHERWIN WILLIAMS COMPANY (THE)	VALERO ENERGY CORP
PG&E CORPORATION		VALSPAR CORPORATION (THE)
PHARMACEUTICAL PRODUCT DEVELOPMENT INC	SIGMA-ALDRICH CORP	VARIAN MEDICAL SYSTEMS INC
	SISTERS OF MERCY HEALTH SYSTEMS	VERISIGN INC
PITNEY BOWES INC	SMITH INTERNATIONAL INC	VERIZON COMMUNICATIONS
PLANTRONICS INC	SMITHFIELD FOODS INC	VIACOM INC
PLEXUS CORP	ST JUDE MEDICAL INC	VOLT INFORMATION SCIENCES INC
POLO RALPH LAUREN CORP	STAPLES INC	W R BERKLEY CORPORATION
PRAXAIR INC	STARTEK INC	WALGREEN CO
PRICEWATERHOUSECOOPERS	STARWOOD HOTELS & RESORTS WORLDWIDE INC	WAL-MART STORES INC
PRIDE INTERNATIONAL INC		WALT DISNEY COMPANY (THE)
PRINCIPAL FINANCIAL GROUP (THE)	STERIS CORP	WATERS CORP
	STRYKER CORP	WATSON PHARMACEUTICALS INC
PROCTER & GAMBLE CO	SUN MICROSYSTEMS INC	WATSON WYATT WORLDWIDE INC
PROGRESSIVE CORPORATION (THE)	SUNGARD DATA SYSTEMS INC	WEATHERFORD INTERNATIONAL LTD
	SUNOCO INC	
PRUDENTIAL FINANCIAL INC	SUNRISE SENIOR LIVING	WEIGHT WATCHERS INTERNATIONAL INC
QUALCOMM INC	SYKES ENTERPRISES INC	
QUEST DIAGNOSTICS INC	SYMANTEC CORP	WENDYS INTERNATIONAL INC
QUIKSILVER INC	SYNOPSYS INC	WEST CORPORATION
R R DONNELLEY & SONS CO	SYNTEL INC	WEST PHARMACEUTICAL SERVICES INC
RAYTHEON CO	SYSCO CORP	
REGIS CORPORATION	TALBOTS INC (THE)	WESTERN DIGITAL CORP
RENT-A-CENTER INC	TARGET CORPORATION	WESTERN UNION COMPANY (THE)
RES CARE INC	TBC CORPORATION	WHOLE FOODS MARKET INC
RESPIRONICS INC	TECH DATA CORP	WILLIAMS COMPANIES INC (THE)
RITZ-CARLTON HOTEL COMPANY LLC (THE)	TEKTRONIX INC	WILLIAMS SONOMA INC
	TELEDYNE TECHNOLOGIES INCORPORATED	WM WRIGLEY JR COMPANY
ROBERT HALF INTERNATIONAL INC		WW GRAINGER INC
ROSS STORES INC	TELETECH HOLDINGS INC	WYETH
ROYAL CARIBBEAN CRUISES	TESORO CORP	WYNDHAM WORLDWIDE
RUSSELL CORP	TIFFANY & CO	WYNN RESORTS LIMITED
RYDER SYSTEM INC	TIME WARNER INC	XEROX CORP
SABRE HOLDINGS CORP	TJX COMPANIES INC (THE)	YAHOO! INC
SAFECO CORP	T-MOBILE USA	YUM! BRANDS INC
SAFEWAY INC	TOTAL SYSTEM SERVICES INC (TSYS)	ZIMMER HOLDINGS INC
SAIC INC		
SAM'S CLUB	TOWERS PERRIN	
SARA LEE CORP		

Management Trainees
3M COMPANY
7-ELEVEN INC
AARON RENTS INC
ABBOTT LABORATORIES
ABERCROMBIE & FITCH CO
ABM INDUSTRIES INC
ACADEMY SPORTS & OUTDOORS LTD
ACCENTURE LTD
ACXIOM CORP
ADC TELECOMMUNICATIONS INC
ADESA INC
ADOBE SYSTEMS INC
ADVANCE AUTO PARTS INC
ADVANCED MICRO DEVICES INC (AMD)
AECOM TECHNOLOGY CORPORATION
AEROPOSTALE INC
AES CORPORATION (THE)
AETNA INC
AFFILIATED COMPUTER SERVICES INC
AFLAC INC
AGILENT TECHNOLOGIES INC
AIR PRODUCTS & CHEMICALS INC
ALBERTO-CULVER COMPANY
ALLERGAN INC
ALLIANCE DATA SYSTEMS CORPORATION
ALLSTATE CORPORATION (THE)
ALTRIA GROUP INC
AMAZON.COM INC
AMEDISYS INC
AMERICAN EAGLE OUTFITTERS INC
AMERICAN ELECTRIC POWER COMPANY INC (AEP)
AMERICAN EXPRESS CO
AMERICAN POWER CONVERSION CORP
AMERISOURCEBERGEN CORP
AMGEN INC
ANADARKO PETROLEUM CORPORATION
ANALOG DEVICES INC
ANNTAYLOR STORES CORP
APACHE CORP
APOLLO GROUP INC
APPLE INC
ARAMARK CORPORATION
ARCHER DANIELS MIDLAND CO

ARROW ELECTRONICS INC
ARTHUR J GALLAGHER & CO
AT&T INC
AUTOMATIC DATA PROCESSING INC
AUTOZONE INC
AVERY DENNISON CORP
AVIS BUDGET GROUP INC
AVON PRODUCTS INC
AXA FINANCIAL INC
BAKER HUGHES INC
BALTIMORE GAS AND ELECTRIC COMPANY
BANK OF AMERICA CORP
BARNES & NOBLE COLLEGE BOOKSTORES
BARNES & NOBLE INC
BASS PRO SHOPS INC
BAXTER INTERNATIONAL INC
BDO SEIDMAN LLP
BEBE STORES INC
BECHTEL GROUP INC
BECKMAN COULTER INC
BECTON DICKINSON & CO
BED BATH & BEYOND INC
BENCHMARK ELECTRONICS INC
BERKSHIRE HATHAWAY INC
BEST BUY CO INC
BIO RAD LABORATORIES INC
BJ SERVICES COMPANY
BJ'S WHOLESALE CLUB INC
BLACK & DECKER CORP
BLOOMBERG LP
BOEING COMPANY (THE)
BOOZ ALLEN HAMILTON
BOSTON SCIENTIFIC CORP
BRINKER INTERNATIONAL INC
BRINKS COMPANY (THE)
BRISTOL MYERS SQUIBB CO
BROADCOM CORP
BROWN & BROWN INC
BUCKLE INC (THE)
BUILD-A-BEAR WORKSHOP INC
BUNGE LTD
BURGER KING HOLDINGS INC
BURLINGTON NORTHERN SANTA FE CORP
CABELA'S INC
CABLEVISION SYSTEMS CORP
CACI INTERNATIONAL INC
CAMERON INTERNATIONAL

CORPORATION
CAPITAL SENIOR LIVING CORP
CARDINAL HEALTH INC
CARGILL INC
CARMAX GROUP
CARNIVAL CORPORATION
CASH AMERICA INTERNATIONAL INC
CATERPILLAR INC
CATERPILLAR LOGISTICS
CATHOLIC HEALTH INITIATIVES
CBRL GROUP INC
CDW CORPORATION
CELLCO PARTNERSHIP (VERIZON WIRELESS)
CEPHALON INC
CH ROBINSON WORLDWIDE INC
CH2M HILL COMPANIES LTD
CHARLOTTE RUSSE HOLDING
CHARMING SHOPPES INC
CHEMED CORPORATION
CHESAPEAKE ENERGY CORP
CHEVRON CORPORATION
CHEVRON PHILLIPS CHEMICAL COMPANY LLC
CHICO'S FAS INC
CHRISTOPHER & BANKS CORP
CHUBB CORPORATION (THE)
CIBER INC
CINTAS CORP
CISCO SYSTEMS INC
CLEAR CHANNEL COMMUNICATIONS INC
CLUBCORP INC
COACH INC
COCA COLA COMPANY (THE)
COCA COLA ENTERPRISES INC
COGNIZANT TECHNOLOGY SOLUTIONS CORP
COLDWATER CREEK INC
COLGATE PALMOLIVE CO
COMCAST CORP
CONAGRA FOODS INC
CONOCOPHILLIPS COMPANY
CONSOL ENERGY INC
CONSOLIDATED EDISON INC
CONTAINER STORE (THE)
CONVERGYS CORPORATION
COOPER COMPANIES INC
COST PLUS INC
COSTCO WHOLESALE CORP

COVANCE INC	EXEL TRANSPORTATION SERVICES INC (DHL EXEL)	HE BUTT GROCERY COMPANY (HEB)
COVENTRY HEALTH CARE INC	EXELON CORPORATION	HEALTH FITNESS CORP
COX COMMUNICATIONS INC	EXPEDITORS INTERNATIONAL OF WASHINGTON INC	HEALTH MANAGEMENT ASSOCIATES INC
CR BARD INC	EXPERIAN AMERICAS	HEALTH NET INC
CSX CORP	EXPRESS SCRIPTS INC	HEALTHWAYS INC
CSX TRANSPORTATION INC	EXXON MOBIL CORPORATION (EXXONMOBIL)	HELMERICH & PAYNE INC
CTS CORP	FAIR ISAAC CORPORATION	HENRY SCHEIN INC
CUBIC CORP	FAMILY DOLLAR STORES INC	HERTZ GLOBAL HOLDINGS INC
CUMMINS INC	FEDEX CORPORATION	HESS CORPORATION
CVS CAREMARK CORPORATION	FINISH LINE INC (THE)	HEWITT ASSOCIATES
DANAHER CORP	FIRST ADVANTAGE CORPORATION	HIBBETT SPORTS INC
DARDEN RESTAURANTS INC	FIRST DATA CORP	HILB ROGAL & HOBBS CO
DAVITA INC	FIRSTENERGY CORP	HILTON HOTELS CORP
DEAN FOODS CO	FISERV INC	HOME DEPOT INC
DEERE & CO	FLUOR CORP	HONEYWELL INTERNATIONAL INC
DELOITTE & TOUCHE USA LLP	FMC TECHNOLOGIES INC	HOT TOPIC INC
DELOITTE CONSULTING LLP	FOREST LABORATORIES INC	HUMANA INC
DENNY'S CORPORATION	FORTUNE BRANDS INC	IAC/INTERACTIVECORP
DEVON ENERGY CORPORATION	FOSSIL INC	ICT GROUP INC
DEVRY INC	FOSTER WHEELER LTD	IDEXX LABORATORIES INC
DIAMOND OFFSHORE DRILLING INC	FOX ENTERTAINMENT GROUP INC	IGATE CORPORATION
DICK'S SPORTING GOODS INC	FPL GROUP INC	IMS HEALTH INC
DIEBOLD INC	FRED'S INC	INFOUSA INC
DINEEQUITY INC	FRONTIER COMMUNICATIONS CORPORATION	INGRAM MICRO INC
DIRECTV GROUP INC (THE)		INTEL CORP
DJO INC	GAMESTOP CORP	INTERNATIONAL BUSINESS MACHINES CORP (IBM)
DOLE FOOD COMPANY INC	GENENTECH INC	INTIMATE BRANDS INC
DOLLAR GENERAL CORPORATION	GENERAL DYNAMICS CORP	INTUIT INC
DOLLAR THRIFTY AUTOMOTIVE GROUP INC	GENERAL ELECTRIC CO (GE)	INVENTIV HEALTH INC
DRESS BARN INC (THE)	GENERAL MILLS INC	J C PENNEY COMPANY INC
DTE ENERGY COMPANY	GENESCO INC	JABIL CIRCUIT INC
DUKE ENERGY CORP	GENWORTH FINANCIAL INC	JACK IN THE BOX INC
DYCOM INDUSTRIES INC	GEO GROUP INC	JACOBS ENGINEERING GROUP INC
E I DU PONT DE NEMOURS & CO (DUPONT)	GEORGIA GULF CORPORATION	JM SMUCKER CO
EATON CORP	GLOBAL HYATT CORPORATION	JOHNSON & JOHNSON
EBAY INC	GLOBAL PAYMENTS INC	JOHNSON CONTROLS INC
ECHOSTAR CORP	GOOGLE INC	JP MORGAN CHASE & CO INC
EDISON INTERNATIONAL	GRANT THORNTON LLP	JUNIPER NETWORKS INC
ELECTRONIC ARTS INC	GTECH HOLDINGS CORP	KAISER PERMANENTE
ELI LILLY & COMPANY	GUESS? INC	KEANE INC
EMBARQ CORP	HALLIBURTON COMPANY	KELLOGG CO
EMC CORP	HARRAH'S ENTERTAINMENT INC	KELLY SERVICES INC
EMERITUS CORP	HARRIS CORPORATION	KENDLE INTERNATIONAL INC
EMERSON ELECTRIC CO	HARTFORD FINANCIAL SERVICES GROUP INC (THE)	KIMBERLY-CLARK CORP
ENTERGY CORP	HAWAIIAN ELECTRIC INDUSTRIES INC	KINDRED HEALTHCARE INC
ENTERPRISE RENT-A-CAR		KOCH INDUSTRIES INC
ERNST & YOUNG LLP	HCA INC	KOHL'S CORP
ESTEE LAUDER COMPANIES INC (THE)		KPMG LLP

KRAFT FOODS INC	MONRO MUFFLER BRAKE INC	POLO RALPH LAUREN CORP
KROGER CO (THE)	MURPHY OIL CORPORATION	PRAXAIR INC
L-3 COMMUNICATIONS HOLDINGS INC	NATIONAL OILWELL VARCO INC	PRICEWATERHOUSECOOPERS
L-3 TITAN GROUP	NEIMAN MARCUS GROUP INC (THE)	PRIDE INTERNATIONAL INC
LABORATORY CORP OF AMERICA HOLDINGS	NETWORK APPLIANCE INC	PRINCIPAL FINANCIAL GROUP (THE)
LANDRY'S RESTAURANTS INC	NEWS CORP	PROCTER & GAMBLE CO
LAS VEGAS SANDS CORP (THE VENETIAN)	NII HOLDINGS INC	PROGRESSIVE CORPORATION (THE)
LEVEL 3 COMMUNICATIONS INC	NIKE INC	PRUDENTIAL FINANCIAL INC
LEXMARK INTERNATIONAL INC	NOBLE CORPORATION	PSYCHIATRIC SOLUTIONS INC
LIBERTY GLOBAL INC	NORDSTROM INC	PUBLIC STORAGE INC
LIMITED BRANDS INC	NORFOLK SOUTHERN CORP	PUBLIX SUPER MARKETS INC
LINCARE HOLDINGS INC	NORTHROP GRUMMAN CORP	QUALCOMM INC
LINCOLN NATIONAL CORPORATION	OCCIDENTAL PETROLEUM CORP	QUEST DIAGNOSTICS INC
LKQ CORP	OCEANEERING INTERNATIONAL INC	QUIKSILVER INC
LOCKHEED MARTIN CORP	ODYSSEY HEALTHCARE INC	R R DONNELLEY & SONS CO
LODGIAN INC	OFFICE DEPOT INC	RAYTHEON CO
LOEWS CORPORATION	OIL STATES INTERNATIONAL INC	REGIS CORPORATION
LOWE'S COMPANIES INC	OLD DOMINION FREIGHT LINE INC	RELIANT ENERGY INC
MACY'S INC	OMNICARE INC	RENT-A-CENTER INC
MANOR CARE INC	OMNICOM GROUP INC	RES CARE INC
MANPOWER INC	ONEOK INC	RESPIRONICS INC
MARATHON OIL CORP	ORACLE CORP	RITE AID CORPORATION
MARRIOTT INTERNATIONAL INC	O'REILLY AUTOMOTIVE INC	RITZ-CARLTON HOTEL COMPANY LLC (THE)
MARS INC	OSHKOSH CORPORATION	ROBERT HALF INTERNATIONAL INC
MARSH & MCLENNAN COMPANIES INC	OSI RESTAURANT PARTNERS INC	ROSS STORES INC
MARY KAY INC	OWENS & MINOR INC	ROYAL CARIBBEAN CRUISES
MASSEY ENERGY COMPANY	PACIFIC SUNWEAR OF CALIFORNIA INC	RUSSELL CORP
MATTEL INC	PANTRY INC (THE)	RYDER SYSTEM INC
MAXIM INTEGRATED PRODUCTS INC	PARAMETRIC TECHNOLOGY CORP	SABRE HOLDINGS CORP
MCAFEE INC	PAREXEL INTERNATIONAL CORP	SAFECO CORP
MCDONALD'S CORP	PARSONS BRINCKERHOFF INC	SAFEWAY INC
MCKESSON CORPORATION	PATTERSON COMPANIES INC	SAIC INC
MCKINSEY & COMPANY INC	PATTERSON-UTI ENERGY INC	SAM'S CLUB
MEDCO HEALTH SOLUTIONS	PAXAR CORP	SARA LEE CORP
MEDTRONIC INC	PAYCHEX INC	SAS INSTITUTE INC
MEIJER INC	PEABODY ENERGY CORP	SCANA CORPORATION
MEN'S WEARHOUSE INC (THE)	PEPSI BOTTLING GROUP INC	SCHERING-PLOUGH CORP
MERCER INC	PEPSICO INC	SCHLUMBERGER LIMITED
MERCK & CO INC	PEROT SYSTEMS CORP	SCIENTIFIC GAMES CORPORATION
METLIFE INC	PERRIGO CO	SCOTTS MIRACLE GROW CO
MGM MIRAGE	PETCO ANIMAL SUPPLIES INC	SEACOR HOLDINGS INC
MICROCHIP TECHNOLOGY INC	PETSMART INC	SELECT MEDICAL CORPORATION
MICRON TECHNOLOGY INC	PFIZER INC	SEMPRA ENERGY
MICROSOFT CORP	PG&E CORPORATION	SENSIENT TECHNOLOGIES CORPORATION
MILLIPORE CORP	PHARMACEUTICAL PRODUCT DEVELOPMENT INC	SHAW GROUP INC (THE)
MOLEX INC	PITNEY BOWES INC	SHELL OIL CO
	PLANTRONICS INC	SHERWIN WILLIAMS COMPANY
	PLEXUS CORP	

SIGMA-ALDRICH CORP	UNITED PARCEL SERVICE INC (UPS)	**MBA Graduates**
SISTERS OF MERCY HEALTH SYSTEMS	UNITED STATES CELLULAR CORP	3M COMPANY
SMITH INTERNATIONAL INC	UNITED TECHNOLOGIES CORPORATION	7-ELEVEN INC
SMITHFIELD FOODS INC	UNITEDHEALTH GROUP INC	AARON RENTS INC
SOUTHERN COMPANY (THE)	UNIVISION COMMUNICATIONS INC	ABBOTT LABORATORIES
SOUTHWEST AIRLINES CO	UPS SUPPLY CHAIN SOLUTIONS	ABERCROMBIE & FITCH CO
SRA INTERNATIONAL INC	URBAN OUTFITTERS INC	ABM INDUSTRIES INC
ST JUDE MEDICAL INC	URS CORPORATION	ACADEMY SPORTS & OUTDOORS LTD
STAPLES INC	USAA	ACCENTURE LTD
STARTEK INC	VALERO ENERGY CORP	ACXIOM CORP
STARWOOD HOTELS & RESORTS WORLDWIDE INC	VALSPAR CORPORATION (THE)	ADC TELECOMMUNICATIONS INC
STERIS CORP	VARIAN MEDICAL SYSTEMS INC	ADESA INC
STRYKER CORP	VCA ANTECH INC	ADOBE SYSTEMS INC
SUN HEALTHCARE GROUP	VERISIGN INC	ADVANCE AUTO PARTS INC
SUN MICROSYSTEMS INC	VERIZON COMMUNICATIONS	ADVANCED MICRO DEVICES INC (AMD)
SUNGARD DATA SYSTEMS INC	VIACOM INC	AECOM TECHNOLOGY CORPORATION
SUNOCO INC	VOLT INFORMATION SCIENCES INC	AEROPOSTALE INC
SUNRISE SENIOR LIVING	W R BERKLEY CORPORATION	AES CORPORATION (THE)
SUPERVALU INC	WALGREEN CO	AETNA INC
SYKES ENTERPRISES INC	WAL-MART STORES INC	AFFILIATED COMPUTER SERVICES INC
SYMANTEC CORP	WALT DISNEY COMPANY (THE)	AFLAC INC
SYNOPSYS INC	WASTE MANAGEMENT INC	AGILENT TECHNOLOGIES INC
SYNTEL INC	WATERS CORP	AIR PRODUCTS & CHEMICALS INC
SYSCO CORP	WATSON PHARMACEUTICALS INC	ALBERTO-CULVER COMPANY
TALBOTS INC (THE)	WATSON WYATT WORLDWIDE INC	ALLERGAN INC
TARGET CORPORATION	WEATHERFORD INTERNATIONAL LTD	ALLIANCE DATA SYSTEMS CORPORATION
TBC CORPORATION	WEIGHT WATCHERS INTERNATIONAL INC	ALLSTATE CORPORATION (THE)
TECH DATA CORP	WELLPOINT INC	ALTRIA GROUP INC
TEKTRONIX INC	WENDYS INTERNATIONAL INC	AMAZON.COM INC
TELEDYNE TECHNOLOGIES INCORPORATED	WEST CORPORATION	AMEDISYS INC
TELEPHONE AND DATA SYSTEMS INC (TDS)	WEST PHARMACEUTICAL SERVICES INC	AMERICAN EAGLE OUTFITTERS INC
TELETECH HOLDINGS INC	WESTERN DIGITAL CORP	AMERICAN ELECTRIC POWER COMPANY INC (AEP)
TESORO CORP	WESTERN UNION COMPANY (THE)	AMERICAN EXPRESS CO
TIFFANY & CO	WHOLE FOODS MARKET INC	AMERICAN POWER CONVERSION CORP
TIME WARNER INC	WILLIAMS COMPANIES INC (THE)	AMERISOURCEBERGEN CORP
TJX COMPANIES INC (THE)	WILLIAMS SONOMA INC	AMGEN INC
T-MOBILE USA	WM WRIGLEY JR COMPANY	ANADARKO PETROLEUM CORPORATION
TOTAL SYSTEM SERVICES INC (TSYS)	WW GRAINGER INC	ANALOG DEVICES INC
TOWERS PERRIN	WYETH	ANNTAYLOR STORES CORP
TRANSOCEAN INC	WYNDHAM WORLDWIDE	APACHE CORP
TRAVELERS COMPANIES INC (THE)	WYNN RESORTS LIMITED	APOLLO GROUP INC
TW TELECOM INC	XEROX CORP	APPLE INC
TWEEN BRANDS INC	YAHOO! INC	ARAMARK CORPORATION
TYSON FOODS INC	YUM! BRANDS INC	ARCHER DANIELS MIDLAND CO
UNION PACIFIC CORP	ZIMMER HOLDINGS INC	
UNITED NATURAL FOODS INC		

ARROW ELECTRONICS INC	CORPORATION	COVANCE INC
ARTHUR J GALLAGHER & CO	CAPITAL SENIOR LIVING CORP	COVENTRY HEALTH CARE INC
AT&T INC	CARDINAL HEALTH INC	COX COMMUNICATIONS INC
AUTOMATIC DATA PROCESSING INC	CARGILL INC	CR BARD INC
AUTOZONE INC	CARMAX GROUP	CSX CORP
AVERY DENNISON CORP	CARNIVAL CORPORATION	CSX TRANSPORTATION INC
AVIS BUDGET GROUP INC	CASH AMERICA INTERNATIONAL INC	CTS CORP
AVON PRODUCTS INC	CATERPILLAR INC	CUBIC CORP
AXA FINANCIAL INC	CATERPILLAR LOGISTICS	CUMMINS INC
BAKER HUGHES INC	CATHOLIC HEALTH INITIATIVES	CVS CAREMARK CORPORATION
BALTIMORE GAS AND ELECTRIC COMPANY	CBRL GROUP INC	DANAHER CORP
BANK OF AMERICA CORP	CDW CORPORATION	DARDEN RESTAURANTS INC
BARNES & NOBLE COLLEGE BOOKSTORES	CELLCO PARTNERSHIP (VERIZON WIRELESS)	DAVITA INC
BARNES & NOBLE INC	CEPHALON INC	DEAN FOODS CO
BASS PRO SHOPS INC	CH ROBINSON WORLDWIDE INC	DEERE & CO
BAXTER INTERNATIONAL INC	CH2M HILL COMPANIES LTD	DELOITTE & TOUCHE USA LLP
BDO SEIDMAN LLP	CHARLOTTE RUSSE HOLDING	DELOITTE CONSULTING LLP
BEBE STORES INC	CHARMING SHOPPES INC	DENNY'S CORPORATION
BECHTEL GROUP INC	CHEMED CORPORATION	DEVON ENERGY CORPORATION
BECKMAN COULTER INC	CHESAPEAKE ENERGY CORP	DEVRY INC
BECTON DICKINSON & CO	CHEVRON CORPORATION	DIAMOND OFFSHORE DRILLING INC
BED BATH & BEYOND INC	CHEVRON PHILLIPS CHEMICAL COMPANY LLC	DICK'S SPORTING GOODS INC
BENCHMARK ELECTRONICS INC	CHICO'S FAS INC	DIEBOLD INC
BERKSHIRE HATHAWAY INC	CHRISTOPHER & BANKS CORP	DINEEQUITY INC
BEST BUY CO INC	CHUBB CORPORATION (THE)	DIRECTV GROUP INC (THE)
BIO RAD LABORATORIES INC	CIBER INC	DJO INC
BJ SERVICES COMPANY	CINTAS CORP	DOLE FOOD COMPANY INC
BJ'S WHOLESALE CLUB INC	CISCO SYSTEMS INC	DOLLAR GENERAL CORPORATION
BLACK & DECKER CORP	CLEAR CHANNEL COMMUNICATIONS INC	DOLLAR THRIFTY AUTOMOTIVE GROUP INC
BLOOMBERG LP	CLUBCORP INC	DRESS BARN INC (THE)
BOEING COMPANY (THE)	COACH INC	DTE ENERGY COMPANY
BOOZ ALLEN HAMILTON	COCA COLA COMPANY (THE)	DUKE ENERGY CORP
BOSTON SCIENTIFIC CORP	COCA COLA ENTERPRISES INC	DYCOM INDUSTRIES INC
BRINKER INTERNATIONAL INC	COGNIZANT TECHNOLOGY SOLUTIONS CORP	E I DU PONT DE NEMOURS & CO (DUPONT)
BRINKS COMPANY (THE)	COLDWATER CREEK INC	EATON CORP
BRISTOL MYERS SQUIBB CO	COLGATE PALMOLIVE CO	EBAY INC
BROADCOM CORP	COMCAST CORP	ECHOSTAR CORP
BROWN & BROWN INC	CONAGRA FOODS INC	EDISON INTERNATIONAL
BUCKLE INC (THE)	CONOCOPHILLIPS COMPANY	ELECTRONIC ARTS INC
BUILD-A-BEAR WORKSHOP INC	CONSOL ENERGY INC	ELI LILLY & COMPANY
BUNGE LTD	CONSOLIDATED EDISON INC	EMBARQ CORP
BURGER KING HOLDINGS INC	CONTAINER STORE (THE)	EMC CORP
BURLINGTON NORTHERN SANTA FE CORP	CONVERGYS CORPORATION	EMERITUS CORP
CABELA'S INC	COOPER COMPANIES INC	EMERSON ELECTRIC CO
CABLEVISION SYSTEMS CORP	COST PLUS INC	ENTERGY CORP
CACI INTERNATIONAL INC	COSTCO WHOLESALE CORP	ENTERPRISE RENT-A-CAR
CAMERON INTERNATIONAL		ERNST & YOUNG LLP
		ESTEE LAUDER COMPANIES INC (THE)

EXEL TRANSPORTATION SERVICES INC (DHL EXEL)	HE BUTT GROCERY COMPANY (HEB)	KRAFT FOODS INC
EXELON CORPORATION	HEALTH FITNESS CORP	KROGER CO (THE)
EXPEDITORS INTERNATIONAL OF WASHINGTON INC	HEALTH MANAGEMENT ASSOCIATES INC	L-3 COMMUNICATIONS HOLDINGS INC
EXPERIAN AMERICAS	HEALTH NET INC	L-3 TITAN GROUP
EXPRESS SCRIPTS INC	HEALTHWAYS INC	LABORATORY CORP OF AMERICA HOLDINGS
EXXON MOBIL CORPORATION (EXXONMOBIL)	HELMERICH & PAYNE INC	LANDRY'S RESTAURANTS INC
FAIR ISAAC CORPORATION	HENRY SCHEIN INC	LAS VEGAS SANDS CORP (THE VENETIAN)
FAMILY DOLLAR STORES INC	HERTZ GLOBAL HOLDINGS INC	LEVEL 3 COMMUNICATIONS INC
FEDEX CORPORATION	HESS CORPORATION	LEXMARK INTERNATIONAL INC
FINISH LINE INC (THE)	HEWITT ASSOCIATES	LIBERTY GLOBAL INC
FIRST ADVANTAGE CORPORATION	HIBBETT SPORTS INC	LIMITED BRANDS INC
FIRST DATA CORP	HILB ROGAL & HOBBS CO	LINCARE HOLDINGS INC
FIRSTENERGY CORP	HILTON HOTELS CORP	LINCOLN NATIONAL CORPORATION
FISERV INC	HOME DEPOT INC	LKQ CORP
FLUOR CORP	HONEYWELL INTERNATIONAL INC	LOCKHEED MARTIN CORP
FMC TECHNOLOGIES INC	HOT TOPIC INC	LODGIAN INC
FOREST LABORATORIES INC	HUMANA INC	LOEWS CORPORATION
FORTUNE BRANDS INC	IAC/INTERACTIVECORP	LOWE'S COMPANIES INC
FOSSIL INC	ICT GROUP INC	MACY'S INC
FOSTER WHEELER LTD	IDEXX LABORATORIES INC	MANOR CARE INC
FOX ENTERTAINMENT GROUP INC	IGATE CORPORATION	MANPOWER INC
FPL GROUP INC	IMS HEALTH INC	MARATHON OIL CORP
FRED'S INC	INFOUSA INC	MARRIOTT INTERNATIONAL INC
FRONTIER COMMUNICATIONS CORPORATION	INGRAM MICRO INC	MARS INC
GAMESTOP CORP	INTEL CORP	MARSH & MCLENNAN COMPANIES INC
GENENTECH INC	INTERNATIONAL BUSINESS MACHINES CORP (IBM)	MARY KAY INC
GENERAL DYNAMICS CORP	INTIMATE BRANDS INC	MASSEY ENERGY COMPANY
GENERAL ELECTRIC CO (GE)	INTUIT INC	MATTEL INC
GENERAL MILLS INC	INVENTIV HEALTH INC	MAXIM INTEGRATED PRODUCTS INC
GENESCO INC	J C PENNEY COMPANY INC	MCAFEE INC
GENWORTH FINANCIAL INC	JABIL CIRCUIT INC	MCDONALD'S CORP
GEO GROUP INC	JACK IN THE BOX INC	MCKESSON CORPORATION
GEORGIA GULF CORPORATION	JACOBS ENGINEERING GROUP INC	MCKINSEY & COMPANY INC
GLOBAL HYATT CORPORATION	JM SMUCKER CO	MEDCO HEALTH SOLUTIONS
GLOBAL PAYMENTS INC	JOHNSON & JOHNSON	MEDTRONIC INC
GOOGLE INC	JOHNSON CONTROLS INC	MEIJER INC
GRANT THORNTON LLP	JP MORGAN CHASE & CO INC	MEN'S WEARHOUSE INC (THE)
GTECH HOLDINGS CORP	JUNIPER NETWORKS INC	MERCER INC
GUESS? INC	KAISER PERMANENTE	MERCK & CO INC
HALLIBURTON COMPANY	KEANE INC	METLIFE INC
HARRAH'S ENTERTAINMENT INC	KELLOGG CO	MGM MIRAGE
HARRIS CORPORATION	KELLY SERVICES INC	MICROCHIP TECHNOLOGY INC
HARTFORD FINANCIAL SERVICES GROUP INC (THE)	KENDLE INTERNATIONAL INC	MICRON TECHNOLOGY INC
HAWAIIAN ELECTRIC INDUSTRIES INC	KIMBERLY-CLARK CORP	MICROSOFT CORP
	KINDRED HEALTHCARE INC	MILLIPORE CORP
HCA INC	KOCH INDUSTRIES INC	MOLEX INC
	KOHL'S CORP	
	KPMG LLP	

MONRO MUFFLER BRAKE INC	POLO RALPH LAUREN CORP	SIGMA-ALDRICH CORP
MURPHY OIL CORPORATION	PRAXAIR INC	SISTERS OF MERCY HEALTH SYSTEMS
NATIONAL OILWELL VARCO INC	PRICEWATERHOUSECOOPERS	SMITH INTERNATIONAL INC
NEIMAN MARCUS GROUP INC (THE)	PRIDE INTERNATIONAL INC	SMITHFIELD FOODS INC
NETWORK APPLIANCE INC	PRINCIPAL FINANCIAL GROUP (THE)	SOUTHERN COMPANY (THE)
NEWS CORP	PROCTER & GAMBLE CO	SOUTHWEST AIRLINES CO
NII HOLDINGS INC	PROGRESSIVE CORPORATION (THE)	SRA INTERNATIONAL INC
NIKE INC		ST JUDE MEDICAL INC
NOBLE CORPORATION	PRUDENTIAL FINANCIAL INC	STAPLES INC
NORDSTROM INC	PSYCHIATRIC SOLUTIONS INC	STARTEK INC
NORFOLK SOUTHERN CORP	PUBLIC STORAGE INC	STARWOOD HOTELS & RESORTS WORLDWIDE INC
NORTHROP GRUMMAN CORP	PUBLIX SUPER MARKETS INC	STERIS CORP
OCCIDENTAL PETROLEUM CORP	QUALCOMM INC	STRYKER CORP
OCEANEERING INTERNATIONAL INC	QUEST DIAGNOSTICS INC	SUN HEALTHCARE GROUP
ODYSSEY HEALTHCARE INC	QUIKSILVER INC	SUN MICROSYSTEMS INC
OFFICE DEPOT INC	R R DONNELLEY & SONS CO	SUNGARD DATA SYSTEMS INC
OIL STATES INTERNATIONAL INC	RAYTHEON CO	SUNOCO INC
OLD DOMINION FREIGHT LINE INC	REGIS CORPORATION	SUNRISE SENIOR LIVING
OMNICARE INC	RELIANT ENERGY INC	SUPERVALU INC
OMNICOM GROUP INC	RENT-A-CENTER INC	SYKES ENTERPRISES INC
ONEOK INC	RES CARE INC	SYMANTEC CORP
ORACLE CORP	RESPIRONICS INC	SYNOPSYS INC
O'REILLY AUTOMOTIVE INC	RITE AID CORPORATION	SYNTEL INC
OSHKOSH CORPORATION	RITZ-CARLTON HOTEL COMPANY LLC (THE)	SYSCO CORP
OSI RESTAURANT PARTNERS INC	ROBERT HALF INTERNATIONAL INC	TALBOTS INC (THE)
OWENS & MINOR INC	ROSS STORES INC	TARGET CORPORATION
PACIFIC SUNWEAR OF CALIFORNIA INC	ROYAL CARIBBEAN CRUISES	TBC CORPORATION
PANTRY INC (THE)	RUSSELL CORP	TECH DATA CORP
PARAMETRIC TECHNOLOGY CORP	RYDER SYSTEM INC	TEKTRONIX INC
PAREXEL INTERNATIONAL CORP	SABRE HOLDINGS CORP	TELEDYNE TECHNOLOGIES INCORPORATED
PARSONS BRINCKERHOFF INC	SAFECO CORP	TELEPHONE AND DATA SYSTEMS INC (TDS)
PATTERSON COMPANIES INC	SAFEWAY INC	
PATTERSON-UTI ENERGY INC	SAIC INC	TELETECH HOLDINGS INC
PAXAR CORP	SAM'S CLUB	TESORO CORP
PAYCHEX INC	SARA LEE CORP	TIFFANY & CO
PEABODY ENERGY CORP	SAS INSTITUTE INC	TIME WARNER INC
PEPSI BOTTLING GROUP INC	SCANA CORPORATION	TJX COMPANIES INC (THE)
PEPSICO INC	SCHERING-PLOUGH CORP	T-MOBILE USA
PEROT SYSTEMS CORP	SCHLUMBERGER LIMITED	TOTAL SYSTEM SERVICES INC (TSYS)
PERRIGO CO	SCIENTIFIC GAMES CORPORATION	
PETCO ANIMAL SUPPLIES INC	SCOTTS MIRACLE GROW CO	TOWERS PERRIN
PETSMART INC	SEACOR HOLDINGS INC	TRANSOCEAN INC
PFIZER INC	SELECT MEDICAL CORPORATION	TRAVELERS COMPANIES INC (THE)
PG&E CORPORATION	SEMPRA ENERGY	TW TELECOM INC
PHARMACEUTICAL PRODUCT DEVELOPMENT INC	SENSIENT TECHNOLOGIES CORPORATION	TWEEN BRANDS INC
		TYSON FOODS INC
PITNEY BOWES INC	SHAW GROUP INC (THE)	UNION PACIFIC CORP
PLANTRONICS INC	SHELL OIL CO	UNITED NATURAL FOODS INC
PLEXUS CORP	SHERWIN WILLIAMS COMPANY	

UNITED PARCEL SERVICE INC (UPS)	
UNITED STATES CELLULAR CORP	
UNITED TECHNOLOGIES CORPORATION	
UNITEDHEALTH GROUP INC	
UNIVISION COMMUNICATIONS INC	
UPS SUPPLY CHAIN SOLUTIONS	
URBAN OUTFITTERS INC	
URS CORPORATION	
USAA	
VALERO ENERGY CORP	
VALSPAR CORPORATION (THE)	
VARIAN MEDICAL SYSTEMS INC	
VCA ANTECH INC	
VERISIGN INC	
VERIZON COMMUNICATIONS	
VIACOM INC	
VOLT INFORMATION SCIENCES INC	
W R BERKLEY CORPORATION	
WALGREEN CO	
WAL-MART STORES INC	
WALT DISNEY COMPANY (THE)	
WASTE MANAGEMENT INC	
WATERS CORP	
WATSON PHARMACEUTICALS INC	
WATSON WYATT WORLDWIDE INC	
WEATHERFORD INTERNATIONAL LTD	
WEIGHT WATCHERS INTERNATIONAL INC	
WELLPOINT INC	
WENDYS INTERNATIONAL INC	
WEST CORPORATION	
WEST PHARMACEUTICAL SERVICES INC	
WESTERN DIGITAL CORP	
WESTERN UNION COMPANY (THE)	
WHOLE FOODS MARKET INC	
WILLIAMS COMPANIES INC (THE)	
WILLIAMS SONOMA INC	
WM WRIGLEY JR COMPANY	
WW GRAINGER INC	
WYETH	
WYNDHAM WORLDWIDE	
WYNN RESORTS LIMITED	
XEROX CORP	
YAHOO! INC	
YUM! BRANDS INC	
ZIMMER HOLDINGS INC	

Professionals

Consulting
ACCENTURE LTD
AFFILIATED COMPUTER SERVICES INC
BDO SEIDMAN LLP
BECHTEL GROUP INC
BOOZ ALLEN HAMILTON
CACI INTERNATIONAL INC
CH2M HILL COMPANIES LTD
CIBER INC
COGNIZANT TECHNOLOGY SOLUTIONS CORP
COVANCE INC
DELOITTE & TOUCHE USA LLP
DELOITTE CONSULTING LLP
ERNST & YOUNG LLP
EXEL TRANSPORTATION SERVICES INC (DHL EXEL)
FEDEX CORPORATION
FLUOR CORP
FOSTER WHEELER LTD
GRANT THORNTON LLP
HEWITT ASSOCIATES
ICT GROUP INC
IGATE CORPORATION
INTERNATIONAL BUSINESS MACHINES CORP (IBM)
INVENTIV HEALTH INC
JACOBS ENGINEERING GROUP INC
KEANE INC
KPMG LLP
L-3 TITAN GROUP
MARSH & MCLENNAN COMPANIES INC
MCKINSEY & COMPANY INC
MERCER INC
OMNICOM GROUP INC
PAREXEL INTERNATIONAL CORP
PARSONS BRINCKERHOFF INC
PEROT SYSTEMS CORP
PHARMACEUTICAL PRODUCT DEVELOPMENT INC
PRICEWATERHOUSECOOPERS
SAIC INC
SAS INSTITUTE INC
SRA INTERNATIONAL INC
SUN MICROSYSTEMS INC
SYNTEL INC
TOWERS PERRIN
UNITED PARCEL SERVICE INC

(UPS)	
UPS SUPPLY CHAIN SOLUTIONS	
URS CORPORATION	
WATSON WYATT WORLDWIDE INC	

Finance/Accounting
3M COMPANY
7-ELEVEN INC
AARON RENTS INC
ABBOTT LABORATORIES
ABERCROMBIE & FITCH CO
ABM INDUSTRIES INC
ACADEMY SPORTS & OUTDOORS LTD
ACCENTURE LTD
ACXIOM CORP
ADC TELECOMMUNICATIONS INC
ADESA INC
ADOBE SYSTEMS INC
ADVANCE AUTO PARTS INC
ADVANCED MICRO DEVICES INC (AMD)
AECOM TECHNOLOGY CORPORATION
AEROPOSTALE INC
AES CORPORATION (THE)
AETNA INC
AFFILIATED COMPUTER SERVICES INC
AFLAC INC
AGILENT TECHNOLOGIES INC
AIR PRODUCTS & CHEMICALS INC
ALBERTO-CULVER COMPANY
ALLERGAN INC
ALLIANCE DATA SYSTEMS CORPORATION
ALLSTATE CORPORATION (THE)
ALTRIA GROUP INC
AMAZON.COM INC
AMEDISYS INC
AMERICAN EAGLE OUTFITTERS INC
AMERICAN ELECTRIC POWER COMPANY INC (AEP)
AMERICAN EXPRESS CO
AMERICAN POWER CONVERSION CORP
AMERISOURCEBERGEN CORP
AMGEN INC
ANADARKO PETROLEUM CORPORATION
ANALOG DEVICES INC
ANNTAYLOR STORES CORP

APACHE CORP	FE CORP	CONTAINER STORE (THE)
APOLLO GROUP INC	CABELA'S INC	CONVERGYS CORPORATION
APPLE INC	CABLEVISION SYSTEMS CORP	COOPER COMPANIES INC
ARAMARK CORPORATION	CACI INTERNATIONAL INC	COST PLUS INC
ARCHER DANIELS MIDLAND CO	CAMERON INTERNATIONAL CORPORATION	COSTCO WHOLESALE CORP
ARROW ELECTRONICS INC		COVANCE INC
ARTHUR J GALLAGHER & CO	CAPITAL SENIOR LIVING CORP	COVENTRY HEALTH CARE INC
AT&T INC	CARDINAL HEALTH INC	COX COMMUNICATIONS INC
AUTOMATIC DATA PROCESSING INC	CARGILL INC	CR BARD INC
	CARMAX GROUP	CSX CORP
AUTOZONE INC	CARNIVAL CORPORATION	CSX TRANSPORTATION INC
AVERY DENNISON CORP	CASH AMERICA INTERNATIONAL INC	CTS CORP
AVIS BUDGET GROUP INC		CUBIC CORP
AVON PRODUCTS INC	CATERPILLAR INC	CUMMINS INC
AXA FINANCIAL INC	CATERPILLAR LOGISTICS	CVS CAREMARK CORPORATION
BAKER HUGHES INC	CATHOLIC HEALTH INITIATIVES	DANAHER CORP
BALTIMORE GAS AND ELECTRIC COMPANY	CBRL GROUP INC	DARDEN RESTAURANTS INC
	CDW CORPORATION	DAVITA INC
BANK OF AMERICA CORP	CELLCO PARTNERSHIP (VERIZON WIRELESS)	DEAN FOODS CO
BARNES & NOBLE COLLEGE BOOKSTORES		DEERE & CO
	CEPHALON INC	DELOITTE & TOUCHE USA LLP
BARNES & NOBLE INC	CH ROBINSON WORLDWIDE INC	DELOITTE CONSULTING LLP
BASS PRO SHOPS INC	CH2M HILL COMPANIES LTD	DENNY'S CORPORATION
BAXTER INTERNATIONAL INC	CHARLOTTE RUSSE HOLDING	DEVON ENERGY CORPORATION
BDO SEIDMAN LLP	CHARMING SHOPPES INC	DEVRY INC
BEBE STORES INC	CHEMED CORPORATION	DIAMOND OFFSHORE DRILLING INC
BECHTEL GROUP INC	CHESAPEAKE ENERGY CORP	DICK'S SPORTING GOODS INC
BECKMAN COULTER INC	CHEVRON CORPORATION	DIEBOLD INC
BECTON DICKINSON & CO	CHEVRON PHILLIPS CHEMICAL COMPANY LLC	DINEEQUITY INC
BED BATH & BEYOND INC		DIRECTV GROUP INC (THE)
BENCHMARK ELECTRONICS INC	CHICO'S FAS INC	DJO INC
BERKSHIRE HATHAWAY INC	CHRISTOPHER & BANKS CORP	DOLE FOOD COMPANY INC
BEST BUY CO INC	CHUBB CORPORATION (THE)	DOLLAR GENERAL CORPORATION
BIO RAD LABORATORIES INC	CIBER INC	DOLLAR THRIFTY AUTOMOTIVE GROUP INC
BJ SERVICES COMPANY	CINTAS CORP	
BJ'S WHOLESALE CLUB INC	CISCO SYSTEMS INC	DRESS BARN INC (THE)
BLACK & DECKER CORP	CLEAR CHANNEL COMMUNICATIONS INC	DTE ENERGY COMPANY
BLOOMBERG LP		DUKE ENERGY CORP
BOEING COMPANY (THE)	CLUBCORP INC	DYCOM INDUSTRIES INC
BOOZ ALLEN HAMILTON	COACH INC	E I DU PONT DE NEMOURS & CO (DUPONT)
BOSTON SCIENTIFIC CORP	COCA COLA COMPANY (THE)	
BRINKER INTERNATIONAL INC	COCA COLA ENTERPRISES INC	EATON CORP
BRINKS COMPANY (THE)	COGNIZANT TECHNOLOGY SOLUTIONS CORP	EBAY INC
BRISTOL MYERS SQUIBB CO		ECHOSTAR CORP
BROADCOM CORP	COLDWATER CREEK INC	EDISON INTERNATIONAL
BROWN & BROWN INC	COLGATE PALMOLIVE CO	ELECTRONIC ARTS INC
BUCKLE INC (THE)	COMCAST CORP	ELI LILLY & COMPANY
BUILD-A-BEAR WORKSHOP INC	CONAGRA FOODS INC	EMBARQ CORP
BUNGE LTD	CONOCOPHILLIPS COMPANY	EMC CORP
BURGER KING HOLDINGS INC	CONSOL ENERGY INC	EMERITUS CORP
BURLINGTON NORTHERN SANTA	CONSOLIDATED EDISON INC	EMERSON ELECTRIC CO

ENTERGY CORP	HARTFORD FINANCIAL SERVICES GROUP INC (THE)	KIMBERLY-CLARK CORP
ENTERPRISE RENT-A-CAR		KINDRED HEALTHCARE INC
ERNST & YOUNG LLP	HAWAIIAN ELECTRIC INDUSTRIES INC	KOCH INDUSTRIES INC
ESTEE LAUDER COMPANIES INC (THE)		KOHL'S CORP
	HCA INC	KPMG LLP
EXEL TRANSPORTATION SERVICES INC (DHL EXEL)	HE BUTT GROCERY COMPANY (HEB)	KRAFT FOODS INC
		KROGER CO (THE)
EXELON CORPORATION	HEALTH FITNESS CORP	L-3 COMMUNICATIONS HOLDINGS INC
EXPEDITORS INTERNATIONAL OF WASHINGTON INC	HEALTH MANAGEMENT ASSOCIATES INC	
		L-3 TITAN GROUP
EXPERIAN AMERICAS	HEALTH NET INC	LABORATORY CORP OF AMERICA HOLDINGS
EXPRESS SCRIPTS INC	HEALTHWAYS INC	
EXXON MOBIL CORPORATION (EXXONMOBIL)	HELMERICH & PAYNE INC	LANDRY'S RESTAURANTS INC
	HENRY SCHEIN INC	LAS VEGAS SANDS CORP (THE VENETIAN)
FAIR ISAAC CORPORATION	HERTZ GLOBAL HOLDINGS INC	
FAMILY DOLLAR STORES INC	HESS CORPORATION	LEVEL 3 COMMUNICATIONS INC
FEDEX CORPORATION	HEWITT ASSOCIATES	LEXMARK INTERNATIONAL INC
FINISH LINE INC (THE)	HIBBETT SPORTS INC	LIBERTY GLOBAL INC
FIRST ADVANTAGE CORPORATION	HILB ROGAL & HOBBS CO	LIMITED BRANDS INC
FIRST DATA CORP	HILTON HOTELS CORP	LINCARE HOLDINGS INC
FIRSTENERGY CORP	HOME DEPOT INC	LINCOLN NATIONAL CORPORATION
FISERV INC	HONEYWELL INTERNATIONAL INC	LKQ CORP
FLUOR CORP	HOT TOPIC INC	LOCKHEED MARTIN CORP
FMC TECHNOLOGIES INC	HUMANA INC	LODGIAN INC
FOREST LABORATORIES INC	IAC/INTERACTIVECORP	LOEWS CORPORATION
FORTUNE BRANDS INC	ICT GROUP INC	LOWE'S COMPANIES INC
FOSSIL INC	IDEXX LABORATORIES INC	MACY'S INC
FOSTER WHEELER LTD	IGATE CORPORATION	MANOR CARE INC
FOX ENTERTAINMENT GROUP INC	IMS HEALTH INC	MANPOWER INC
FPL GROUP INC	INFOUSA INC	MARATHON OIL CORP
FRED'S INC	INGRAM MICRO INC	MARRIOTT INTERNATIONAL INC
FRONTIER COMMUNICATIONS CORPORATION	INTEL CORP	MARS INC
	INTERNATIONAL BUSINESS MACHINES CORP (IBM)	MARSH & MCLENNAN COMPANIES INC
GAMESTOP CORP		
GENENTECH INC	INTIMATE BRANDS INC	MARY KAY INC
GENERAL DYNAMICS CORP	INTUIT INC	MASSEY ENERGY COMPANY
GENERAL ELECTRIC CO (GE)	INVENTIV HEALTH INC	MATTEL INC
GENERAL MILLS INC	J C PENNEY COMPANY INC	MAXIM INTEGRATED PRODUCTS INC
GENESCO INC	JABIL CIRCUIT INC	
GENWORTH FINANCIAL INC	JACK IN THE BOX INC	MCAFEE INC
GEO GROUP INC	JACOBS ENGINEERING GROUP INC	MCDONALD'S CORP
GEORGIA GULF CORPORATION	JM SMUCKER CO	MCKESSON CORPORATION
GLOBAL HYATT CORPORATION	JOHNSON & JOHNSON	MCKINSEY & COMPANY INC
GLOBAL PAYMENTS INC	JOHNSON CONTROLS INC	MEDCO HEALTH SOLUTIONS
GOOGLE INC	JP MORGAN CHASE & CO INC	MEDTRONIC INC
GRANT THORNTON LLP	JUNIPER NETWORKS INC	MEIJER INC
GTECH HOLDINGS CORP	KAISER PERMANENTE	MEN'S WEARHOUSE INC (THE)
GUESS? INC	KEANE INC	MERCER INC
HALLIBURTON COMPANY	KELLOGG CO	MERCK & CO INC
HARRAH'S ENTERTAINMENT INC	KELLY SERVICES INC	METLIFE INC
HARRIS CORPORATION	KENDLE INTERNATIONAL INC	MGM MIRAGE

MICROCHIP TECHNOLOGY INC	PHARMACEUTICAL PRODUCT DEVELOPMENT INC	SENSIENT TECHNOLOGIES CORPORATION
MICRON TECHNOLOGY INC	PITNEY BOWES INC	SHAW GROUP INC (THE)
MICROSOFT CORP	PLANTRONICS INC	SHELL OIL CO
MILLIPORE CORP	PLEXUS CORP	SHERWIN WILLIAMS COMPANY (THE)
MOLEX INC	POLO RALPH LAUREN CORP	SIGMA-ALDRICH CORP
MONRO MUFFLER BRAKE INC	PRAXAIR INC	SISTERS OF MERCY HEALTH SYSTEMS
MURPHY OIL CORPORATION	PRICEWATERHOUSECOOPERS	SMITH INTERNATIONAL INC
NATIONAL OILWELL VARCO INC	PRIDE INTERNATIONAL INC	SMITHFIELD FOODS INC
NEIMAN MARCUS GROUP INC (THE)	PRINCIPAL FINANCIAL GROUP (THE)	SOUTHERN COMPANY (THE)
NETWORK APPLIANCE INC	PROCTER & GAMBLE CO	SOUTHWEST AIRLINES CO
NEWS CORP	PROGRESSIVE CORPORATION (THE)	SRA INTERNATIONAL INC
NII HOLDINGS INC	PRUDENTIAL FINANCIAL INC	ST JUDE MEDICAL INC
NIKE INC	PSYCHIATRIC SOLUTIONS INC	STAPLES INC
NOBLE CORPORATION	PUBLIC STORAGE INC	STARTEK INC
NORDSTROM INC	PUBLIX SUPER MARKETS INC	STARWOOD HOTELS & RESORTS WORLDWIDE INC
NORFOLK SOUTHERN CORP	QUALCOMM INC	STERIS CORP
NORTHROP GRUMMAN CORP	QUEST DIAGNOSTICS INC	STRYKER CORP
OCCIDENTAL PETROLEUM CORP	QUIKSILVER INC	SUN HEALTHCARE GROUP
OCEANEERING INTERNATIONAL INC	R R DONNELLEY & SONS CO	SUN MICROSYSTEMS INC
ODYSSEY HEALTHCARE INC	RAYTHEON CO	SUNGARD DATA SYSTEMS INC
OFFICE DEPOT INC	REGIS CORPORATION	SUNOCO INC
OIL STATES INTERNATIONAL INC	RELIANT ENERGY INC	SUNRISE SENIOR LIVING
OLD DOMINION FREIGHT LINE INC	RENT-A-CENTER INC	SUPERVALU INC
OMNICARE INC	RES CARE INC	SYKES ENTERPRISES INC
OMNICOM GROUP INC	RESPIRONICS INC	SYMANTEC CORP
ONEOK INC	RITE AID CORPORATION	SYNOPSYS INC
ORACLE CORP	RITZ-CARLTON HOTEL COMPANY LLC (THE)	SYNTEL INC
O'REILLY AUTOMOTIVE INC	ROBERT HALF INTERNATIONAL INC	SYSCO CORP
OSHKOSH CORPORATION	ROSS STORES INC	TALBOTS INC (THE)
OSI RESTAURANT PARTNERS INC	ROYAL CARIBBEAN CRUISES	TARGET CORPORATION
OWENS & MINOR INC	RUSSELL CORP	TBC CORPORATION
PACIFIC SUNWEAR OF CALIFORNIA INC	RYDER SYSTEM INC	TECH DATA CORP
PANTRY INC (THE)	SABRE HOLDINGS CORP	TEKTRONIX INC
PARAMETRIC TECHNOLOGY CORP	SAFECO CORP	TELEDYNE TECHNOLOGIES INCORPORATED
PAREXEL INTERNATIONAL CORP	SAFEWAY INC	TELEPHONE AND DATA SYSTEMS INC (TDS)
PARSONS BRINCKERHOFF INC	SAIC INC	TELETECH HOLDINGS INC
PATTERSON COMPANIES INC	SAM'S CLUB	TESORO CORP
PATTERSON-UTI ENERGY INC	SARA LEE CORP	TIFFANY & CO
PAXAR CORP	SAS INSTITUTE INC	TIME WARNER INC
PAYCHEX INC	SCANA CORPORATION	TJX COMPANIES INC (THE)
PEABODY ENERGY CORP	SCHERING-PLOUGH CORP	T-MOBILE USA
PEPSI BOTTLING GROUP INC	SCHLUMBERGER LIMITED	TOTAL SYSTEM SERVICES INC (TSYS)
PEPSICO INC	SCIENTIFIC GAMES CORPORATION	TOWERS PERRIN
PEROT SYSTEMS CORP	SCOTTS MIRACLE GROW CO	TRANSOCEAN INC
PERRIGO CO	SEACOR HOLDINGS INC	SELECT MEDICAL CORPORATION
PETCO ANIMAL SUPPLIES INC	SELECT MEDICAL CORPORATION	TRAVELERS COMPANIES INC (THE)
PETSMART INC	SEMPRA ENERGY	
PFIZER INC		
PG&E CORPORATION		

TW TELECOM INC	XEROX CORP	JOHNSON & JOHNSON
TWEEN BRANDS INC	YAHOO! INC	KAISER PERMANENTE
TYSON FOODS INC	YUM! BRANDS INC	KENDLE INTERNATIONAL INC
UNION PACIFIC CORP	ZIMMER HOLDINGS INC	KINDRED HEALTHCARE INC
UNITED NATURAL FOODS INC		LABORATORY CORP OF AMERICA HOLDINGS
UNITED PARCEL SERVICE INC (UPS)	**Health Care**	
UNITED STATES CELLULAR CORP	3M COMPANY	LINCARE HOLDINGS INC
UNITED TECHNOLOGIES CORPORATION	ABBOTT LABORATORIES	LINCOLN NATIONAL CORPORATION
UNITEDHEALTH GROUP INC	AETNA INC	MANOR CARE INC
UNIVISION COMMUNICATIONS INC	AFLAC INC	MCKESSON CORPORATION
UPS SUPPLY CHAIN SOLUTIONS	ALLERGAN INC	MEDCO HEALTH SOLUTIONS
URBAN OUTFITTERS INC	AMEDISYS INC	MEDTRONIC INC
URS CORPORATION	AMERISOURCEBERGEN CORP	MERCK & CO INC
USAA	AMGEN INC	METLIFE INC
VALERO ENERGY CORP	AXA FINANCIAL INC	ODYSSEY HEALTHCARE INC
VALSPAR CORPORATION (THE)	BAXTER INTERNATIONAL INC	OMNICARE INC
VARIAN MEDICAL SYSTEMS INC	BECKMAN COULTER INC	OWENS & MINOR INC
VCA ANTECH INC	BECTON DICKINSON & CO	PAREXEL INTERNATIONAL CORP
VERISIGN INC	BIO RAD LABORATORIES INC	PATTERSON COMPANIES INC
VERIZON COMMUNICATIONS	BOSTON SCIENTIFIC CORP	PERRIGO CO
VIACOM INC	BRISTOL MYERS SQUIBB CO	PFIZER INC
VOLT INFORMATION SCIENCES INC	CAPITAL SENIOR LIVING CORP	PHARMACEUTICAL PRODUCT DEVELOPMENT INC
W R BERKLEY CORPORATION	CARDINAL HEALTH INC	
WALGREEN CO	CATHOLIC HEALTH INITIATIVES	PRINCIPAL FINANCIAL GROUP (THE)
WAL-MART STORES INC	CEPHALON INC	
WALT DISNEY COMPANY (THE)	CHEMED CORPORATION	PRUDENTIAL FINANCIAL INC
WASTE MANAGEMENT INC	COOPER COMPANIES INC	PSYCHIATRIC SOLUTIONS INC
WATERS CORP	COVANCE INC	QUEST DIAGNOSTICS INC
WATSON PHARMACEUTICALS INC	COVENTRY HEALTH CARE INC	RES CARE INC
WATSON WYATT WORLDWIDE INC	CR BARD INC	RESPIRONICS INC
WEATHERFORD INTERNATIONAL LTD	CVS CAREMARK CORPORATION	SCHERING-PLOUGH CORP
	DAVITA INC	SELECT MEDICAL CORPORATION
WEIGHT WATCHERS INTERNATIONAL INC	DJO INC	SISTERS OF MERCY HEALTH SYSTEMS
WELLPOINT INC	ELI LILLY & COMPANY	
WENDYS INTERNATIONAL INC	EXPRESS SCRIPTS INC	ST JUDE MEDICAL INC
WEST CORPORATION	FOREST LABORATORIES INC	STERIS CORP
WEST PHARMACEUTICAL SERVICES INC	GENENTECH INC	STRYKER CORP
	GENWORTH FINANCIAL INC	SUN HEALTHCARE GROUP
WESTERN DIGITAL CORP	HARTFORD FINANCIAL SERVICES GROUP INC (THE)	SUNRISE SENIOR LIVING
WESTERN UNION COMPANY (THE)		UNITEDHEALTH GROUP INC
WHOLE FOODS MARKET INC	HCA INC	VARIAN MEDICAL SYSTEMS INC
WILLIAMS COMPANIES INC (THE)	HEALTH MANAGEMENT ASSOCIATES INC	VCA ANTECH INC
WILLIAMS SONOMA INC		WALGREEN CO
WM WRIGLEY JR COMPANY	HEALTH NET INC	WATSON PHARMACEUTICALS INC
WW GRAINGER INC	HEALTHWAYS INC	WEIGHT WATCHERS INTERNATIONAL INC
WYETH	HENRY SCHEIN INC	
WYNDHAM WORLDWIDE	HUMANA INC	WELLPOINT INC
WYNN RESORTS LIMITED	IDEXX LABORATORIES INC	WEST PHARMACEUTICAL SERVICES INC
	IMS HEALTH INC	WYETH
	INVENTIV HEALTH INC	ZIMMER HOLDINGS INC

Human Resources/Other		
3M COMPANY	ARROW ELECTRONICS INC	CORPORATION
7-ELEVEN INC	ARTHUR J GALLAGHER & CO	CAPITAL SENIOR LIVING CORP
AARON RENTS INC	AT&T INC	CARDINAL HEALTH INC
ABBOTT LABORATORIES	AUTOMATIC DATA PROCESSING INC	CARGILL INC
ABERCROMBIE & FITCH CO		CARMAX GROUP
ABM INDUSTRIES INC	AUTOZONE INC	CARNIVAL CORPORATION
ACADEMY SPORTS & OUTDOORS LTD	AVERY DENNISON CORP	CASH AMERICA INTERNATIONAL INC
	AVIS BUDGET GROUP INC	
ACCENTURE LTD	AVON PRODUCTS INC	CATERPILLAR INC
ACXIOM CORP	AXA FINANCIAL INC	CATERPILLAR LOGISTICS
ADC TELECOMMUNICATIONS INC	BAKER HUGHES INC	CATHOLIC HEALTH INITIATIVES
ADESA INC	BALTIMORE GAS AND ELECTRIC COMPANY	CBRL GROUP INC
ADOBE SYSTEMS INC		CDW CORPORATION
ADVANCE AUTO PARTS INC	BANK OF AMERICA CORP	CELLCO PARTNERSHIP (VERIZON WIRELESS)
ADVANCED MICRO DEVICES INC (AMD)	BARNES & NOBLE COLLEGE BOOKSTORES	
		CEPHALON INC
AECOM TECHNOLOGY CORPORATION	BARNES & NOBLE INC	CH ROBINSON WORLDWIDE INC
	BASS PRO SHOPS INC	CH2M HILL COMPANIES LTD
AEROPOSTALE INC	BAXTER INTERNATIONAL INC	CHARLOTTE RUSSE HOLDING
AES CORPORATION (THE)	BDO SEIDMAN LLP	CHARMING SHOPPES INC
AETNA INC	BEBE STORES INC	CHEMED CORPORATION
AFFILIATED COMPUTER SERVICES INC	BECHTEL GROUP INC	CHESAPEAKE ENERGY CORP
	BECKMAN COULTER INC	CHEVRON CORPORATION
AFLAC INC	BECTON DICKINSON & CO	CHEVRON PHILLIPS CHEMICAL COMPANY LLC
AGILENT TECHNOLOGIES INC	BED BATH & BEYOND INC	
AIR PRODUCTS & CHEMICALS INC	BENCHMARK ELECTRONICS INC	CHICO'S FAS INC
ALBERTO-CULVER COMPANY	BERKSHIRE HATHAWAY INC	CHRISTOPHER & BANKS CORP
ALLERGAN INC	BEST BUY CO INC	CHUBB CORPORATION (THE)
ALLIANCE DATA SYSTEMS CORPORATION	BIO RAD LABORATORIES INC	CIBER INC
	BJ SERVICES COMPANY	CINTAS CORP
ALLSTATE CORPORATION (THE)	BJ'S WHOLESALE CLUB INC	CISCO SYSTEMS INC
ALTRIA GROUP INC	BLACK & DECKER CORP	CLEAR CHANNEL COMMUNICATIONS INC
AMAZON.COM INC	BLOOMBERG LP	
AMEDISYS INC	BOEING COMPANY (THE)	CLUBCORP INC
AMERICAN EAGLE OUTFITTERS INC	BOOZ ALLEN HAMILTON	COACH INC
	BOSTON SCIENTIFIC CORP	COCA COLA COMPANY (THE)
AMERICAN ELECTRIC POWER COMPANY INC (AEP)	BRINKER INTERNATIONAL INC	COCA COLA ENTERPRISES INC
	BRINKS COMPANY (THE)	COGNIZANT TECHNOLOGY SOLUTIONS CORP
AMERICAN EXPRESS CO	BRISTOL MYERS SQUIBB CO	
AMERICAN POWER CONVERSION CORP	BROADCOM CORP	COLDWATER CREEK INC
	BROWN & BROWN INC	COLGATE PALMOLIVE CO
AMERISOURCEBERGEN CORP	BUCKLE INC (THE)	COMCAST CORP
AMGEN INC	BUILD-A-BEAR WORKSHOP INC	CONAGRA FOODS INC
ANADARKO PETROLEUM CORPORATION	BUNGE LTD	CONOCOPHILLIPS COMPANY
	BURGER KING HOLDINGS INC	CONSOL ENERGY INC
ANALOG DEVICES INC	BURLINGTON NORTHERN SANTA FE CORP	CONSOLIDATED EDISON INC
ANNTAYLOR STORES CORP		CONTAINER STORE (THE)
APACHE CORP	CABELA'S INC	CONVERGYS CORPORATION
APOLLO GROUP INC	CABLEVISION SYSTEMS CORP	COOPER COMPANIES INC
APPLE INC	CACI INTERNATIONAL INC	COST PLUS INC
ARAMARK CORPORATION	CAMERON INTERNATIONAL	COSTCO WHOLESALE CORP
ARCHER DANIELS MIDLAND CO		

COVANCE INC	EXEL TRANSPORTATION SERVICES INC (DHL EXEL)	HE BUTT GROCERY COMPANY (HEB)
COVENTRY HEALTH CARE INC	EXELON CORPORATION	HEALTH FITNESS CORP
COX COMMUNICATIONS INC	EXPEDITORS INTERNATIONAL OF WASHINGTON INC	HEALTH MANAGEMENT ASSOCIATES INC
CR BARD INC	EXPERIAN AMERICAS	HEALTH NET INC
CSX CORP	EXPRESS SCRIPTS INC	HEALTHWAYS INC
CSX TRANSPORTATION INC	EXXON MOBIL CORPORATION (EXXONMOBIL)	HELMERICH & PAYNE INC
CTS CORP		HENRY SCHEIN INC
CUBIC CORP	FAIR ISAAC CORPORATION	HERTZ GLOBAL HOLDINGS INC
CUMMINS INC	FAMILY DOLLAR STORES INC	HESS CORPORATION
CVS CAREMARK CORPORATION	FEDEX CORPORATION	HEWITT ASSOCIATES
DANAHER CORP	FINISH LINE INC (THE)	HIBBETT SPORTS INC
DARDEN RESTAURANTS INC	FIRST ADVANTAGE CORPORATION	HILB ROGAL & HOBBS CO
DAVITA INC	FIRST DATA CORP	HILTON HOTELS CORP
DEAN FOODS CO	FIRSTENERGY CORP	HOME DEPOT INC
DEERE & CO	FISERV INC	HONEYWELL INTERNATIONAL INC
DELOITTE & TOUCHE USA LLP	FLUOR CORP	HOT TOPIC INC
DELOITTE CONSULTING LLP	FMC TECHNOLOGIES INC	HUMANA INC
DENNY'S CORPORATION	FOREST LABORATORIES INC	IAC/INTERACTIVECORP
DEVON ENERGY CORPORATION	FORTUNE BRANDS INC	ICT GROUP INC
DEVRY INC	FOSSIL INC	IDEXX LABORATORIES INC
DIAMOND OFFSHORE DRILLING INC	FOSTER WHEELER LTD	IGATE CORPORATION
DICK'S SPORTING GOODS INC	FOX ENTERTAINMENT GROUP INC	IMS HEALTH INC
DIEBOLD INC	FPL GROUP INC	INFOUSA INC
DINEEQUITY INC	FRED'S INC	INGRAM MICRO INC
DIRECTV GROUP INC (THE)	FRONTIER COMMUNICATIONS CORPORATION	INTEL CORP
DJO INC		INTERNATIONAL BUSINESS MACHINES CORP (IBM)
DOLE FOOD COMPANY INC	GAMESTOP CORP	
DOLLAR GENERAL CORPORATION	GENENTECH INC	INTIMATE BRANDS INC
DOLLAR THRIFTY AUTOMOTIVE GROUP INC	GENERAL DYNAMICS CORP	INTUIT INC
	GENERAL ELECTRIC CO (GE)	INVENTIV HEALTH INC
DRESS BARN INC (THE)	GENERAL MILLS INC	J C PENNEY COMPANY INC
DTE ENERGY COMPANY	GENESCO INC	JABIL CIRCUIT INC
DUKE ENERGY CORP	GENWORTH FINANCIAL INC	JACK IN THE BOX INC
DYCOM INDUSTRIES INC	GEO GROUP INC	JACOBS ENGINEERING GROUP INC
E I DU PONT DE NEMOURS & CO (DUPONT)	GEORGIA GULF CORPORATION	JM SMUCKER CO
	GLOBAL HYATT CORPORATION	JOHNSON & JOHNSON
EATON CORP	GLOBAL PAYMENTS INC	JOHNSON CONTROLS INC
EBAY INC	GOOGLE INC	JP MORGAN CHASE & CO INC
ECHOSTAR CORP	GRANT THORNTON LLP	JUNIPER NETWORKS INC
EDISON INTERNATIONAL	GTECH HOLDINGS CORP	KAISER PERMANENTE
ELECTRONIC ARTS INC	GUESS? INC	KEANE INC
ELI LILLY & COMPANY	HALLIBURTON COMPANY	KELLOGG CO
EMBARQ CORP	HARRAH'S ENTERTAINMENT INC	KELLY SERVICES INC
EMC CORP	HARRIS CORPORATION	KENDLE INTERNATIONAL INC
EMERITUS CORP	HARTFORD FINANCIAL SERVICES GROUP INC (THE)	KIMBERLY-CLARK CORP
EMERSON ELECTRIC CO		KINDRED HEALTHCARE INC
ENTERGY CORP	HAWAIIAN ELECTRIC INDUSTRIES INC	KOCH INDUSTRIES INC
ENTERPRISE RENT-A-CAR		KOHL'S CORP
ERNST & YOUNG LLP	HCA INC	KPMG LLP
ESTEE LAUDER COMPANIES INC (THE)		

KRAFT FOODS INC	MONRO MUFFLER BRAKE INC	POLO RALPH LAUREN CORP
KROGER CO (THE)	MURPHY OIL CORPORATION	PRAXAIR INC
L-3 COMMUNICATIONS HOLDINGS INC	NATIONAL OILWELL VARCO INC	PRICEWATERHOUSECOOPERS
L-3 TITAN GROUP	NEIMAN MARCUS GROUP INC (THE)	PRIDE INTERNATIONAL INC
LABORATORY CORP OF AMERICA HOLDINGS	NETWORK APPLIANCE INC	PRINCIPAL FINANCIAL GROUP (THE)
LANDRY'S RESTAURANTS INC	NEWS CORP	PROCTER & GAMBLE CO
LAS VEGAS SANDS CORP (THE VENETIAN)	NII HOLDINGS INC	PROGRESSIVE CORPORATION (THE)
LEVEL 3 COMMUNICATIONS INC	NIKE INC	PRUDENTIAL FINANCIAL INC
LEXMARK INTERNATIONAL INC	NOBLE CORPORATION	PSYCHIATRIC SOLUTIONS INC
LIBERTY GLOBAL INC	NORDSTROM INC	PUBLIC STORAGE INC
LIMITED BRANDS INC	NORFOLK SOUTHERN CORP	PUBLIX SUPER MARKETS INC
LINCARE HOLDINGS INC	NORTHROP GRUMMAN CORP	QUALCOMM INC
LINCOLN NATIONAL CORPORATION	OCCIDENTAL PETROLEUM CORP	QUEST DIAGNOSTICS INC
LKQ CORP	OCEANEERING INTERNATIONAL INC	QUIKSILVER INC
LOCKHEED MARTIN CORP	ODYSSEY HEALTHCARE INC	R R DONNELLEY & SONS CO
LODGIAN INC	OFFICE DEPOT INC	RAYTHEON CO
LOEWS CORPORATION	OIL STATES INTERNATIONAL INC	REGIS CORPORATION
LOWE'S COMPANIES INC	OLD DOMINION FREIGHT LINE INC	RELIANT ENERGY INC
MACY'S INC	OMNICARE INC	RENT-A-CENTER INC
MANOR CARE INC	OMNICOM GROUP INC	RES CARE INC
MANPOWER INC	ONEOK INC	RESPIRONICS INC
MARATHON OIL CORP	ORACLE CORP	RITE AID CORPORATION
MARRIOTT INTERNATIONAL INC	O'REILLY AUTOMOTIVE INC	RITZ-CARLTON HOTEL COMPANY LLC (THE)
MARS INC	OSHKOSH CORPORATION	ROBERT HALF INTERNATIONAL INC
MARSH & MCLENNAN COMPANIES INC	OSI RESTAURANT PARTNERS INC	ROSS STORES INC
MARY KAY INC	OWENS & MINOR INC	ROYAL CARIBBEAN CRUISES
MASSEY ENERGY COMPANY	PACIFIC SUNWEAR OF CALIFORNIA INC	RUSSELL CORP
MATTEL INC	PANTRY INC (THE)	RYDER SYSTEM INC
MAXIM INTEGRATED PRODUCTS INC	PARAMETRIC TECHNOLOGY CORP	SABRE HOLDINGS CORP
MCAFEE INC	PAREXEL INTERNATIONAL CORP	SAFECO CORP
MCDONALD'S CORP	PARSONS BRINCKERHOFF INC	SAFEWAY INC
MCKESSON CORPORATION	PATTERSON COMPANIES INC	SAIC INC
MCKINSEY & COMPANY INC	PATTERSON-UTI ENERGY INC	SAM'S CLUB
MEDCO HEALTH SOLUTIONS	PAXAR CORP	SARA LEE CORP
MEDTRONIC INC	PAYCHEX INC	SAS INSTITUTE INC
MEIJER INC	PEABODY ENERGY CORP	SCANA CORPORATION
MEN'S WEARHOUSE INC (THE)	PEPSI BOTTLING GROUP INC	SCHERING-PLOUGH CORP
MERCER INC	PEPSICO INC	SCHLUMBERGER LIMITED
MERCK & CO INC	PEROT SYSTEMS CORP	SCIENTIFIC GAMES CORPORATION
METLIFE INC	PERRIGO CO	SCOTTS MIRACLE GROW CO
MGM MIRAGE	PETCO ANIMAL SUPPLIES INC	SEACOR HOLDINGS INC
MICROCHIP TECHNOLOGY INC	PETSMART INC	SELECT MEDICAL CORPORATION
MICRON TECHNOLOGY INC	PFIZER INC	SEMPRA ENERGY
MICROSOFT CORP	PG&E CORPORATION	SENSIENT TECHNOLOGIES CORPORATION
MILLIPORE CORP	PHARMACEUTICAL PRODUCT DEVELOPMENT INC	SHAW GROUP INC (THE)
MOLEX INC	PITNEY BOWES INC	SHELL OIL CO
	PLANTRONICS INC	SHERWIN WILLIAMS COMPANY
	PLEXUS CORP	

Column 1	Column 2	Law
SIGMA-ALDRICH CORP	UNITED PARCEL SERVICE INC (UPS)	3M COMPANY
SISTERS OF MERCY HEALTH SYSTEMS	UNITED STATES CELLULAR CORP	7-ELEVEN INC
SMITH INTERNATIONAL INC	UNITED TECHNOLOGIES CORPORATION	AARON RENTS INC
SMITHFIELD FOODS INC	UNITEDHEALTH GROUP INC	ABBOTT LABORATORIES
SOUTHERN COMPANY (THE)	UNIVISION COMMUNICATIONS INC	ABERCROMBIE & FITCH CO
SOUTHWEST AIRLINES CO	UPS SUPPLY CHAIN SOLUTIONS	ABM INDUSTRIES INC
SRA INTERNATIONAL INC	URBAN OUTFITTERS INC	ACADEMY SPORTS & OUTDOORS LTD
ST JUDE MEDICAL INC	URS CORPORATION	ACCENTURE LTD
STAPLES INC	USAA	ACXIOM CORP
STARTEK INC	VALERO ENERGY CORP	ADC TELECOMMUNICATIONS INC
STARWOOD HOTELS & RESORTS WORLDWIDE INC	VALSPAR CORPORATION (THE)	ADESA INC
STERIS CORP	VARIAN MEDICAL SYSTEMS INC	ADOBE SYSTEMS INC
STRYKER CORP	VCA ANTECH INC	ADVANCE AUTO PARTS INC
SUN HEALTHCARE GROUP	VERISIGN INC	ADVANCED MICRO DEVICES INC (AMD)
SUN MICROSYSTEMS INC	VERIZON COMMUNICATIONS	AECOM TECHNOLOGY CORPORATION
SUNGARD DATA SYSTEMS INC	VIACOM INC	AEROPOSTALE INC
SUNOCO INC	VOLT INFORMATION SCIENCES INC	AES CORPORATION (THE)
SUNRISE SENIOR LIVING	W R BERKLEY CORPORATION	AETNA INC
SUPERVALU INC	WALGREEN CO	AFFILIATED COMPUTER SERVICES INC
SYKES ENTERPRISES INC	WAL-MART STORES INC	AFLAC INC
SYMANTEC CORP	WALT DISNEY COMPANY (THE)	AGILENT TECHNOLOGIES INC
SYNOPSYS INC	WASTE MANAGEMENT INC	AIR PRODUCTS & CHEMICALS INC
SYNTEL INC	WATERS CORP	ALBERTO-CULVER COMPANY
SYSCO CORP	WATSON PHARMACEUTICALS INC	ALLERGAN INC
TALBOTS INC (THE)	WATSON WYATT WORLDWIDE INC	ALLIANCE DATA SYSTEMS CORPORATION
TARGET CORPORATION	WEATHERFORD INTERNATIONAL LTD	ALLSTATE CORPORATION (THE)
TBC CORPORATION	WEIGHT WATCHERS INTERNATIONAL INC	ALTRIA GROUP INC
TECH DATA CORP	WELLPOINT INC	AMAZON.COM INC
TEKTRONIX INC	WENDYS INTERNATIONAL INC	AMEDISYS INC
TELEDYNE TECHNOLOGIES INCORPORATED	WEST CORPORATION	AMERICAN EAGLE OUTFITTERS INC
TELEPHONE AND DATA SYSTEMS INC (TDS)	WEST PHARMACEUTICAL SERVICES INC	AMERICAN ELECTRIC POWER COMPANY INC (AEP)
TELETECH HOLDINGS INC	WESTERN DIGITAL CORP	AMERICAN EXPRESS CO
TESORO CORP	WESTERN UNION COMPANY (THE)	AMERICAN POWER CONVERSION CORP
TIFFANY & CO	WHOLE FOODS MARKET INC	AMERISOURCEBERGEN CORP
TIME WARNER INC	WILLIAMS COMPANIES INC (THE)	AMGEN INC
TJX COMPANIES INC (THE)	WILLIAMS SONOMA INC	ANADARKO PETROLEUM CORPORATION
T-MOBILE USA	WM WRIGLEY JR COMPANY	ANALOG DEVICES INC
TOTAL SYSTEM SERVICES INC (TSYS)	WW GRAINGER INC	ANNTAYLOR STORES CORP
TOWERS PERRIN	WYETH	APACHE CORP
TRANSOCEAN INC	WYNDHAM WORLDWIDE	APOLLO GROUP INC
TRAVELERS COMPANIES INC (THE)	WYNN RESORTS LIMITED	APPLE INC
TW TELECOM INC	XEROX CORP	ARAMARK CORPORATION
TWEEN BRANDS INC	YAHOO! INC	ARCHER DANIELS MIDLAND CO
TYSON FOODS INC	YUM! BRANDS INC	
UNION PACIFIC CORP	ZIMMER HOLDINGS INC	
UNITED NATURAL FOODS INC		

ARROW ELECTRONICS INC	CORPORATION	COVANCE INC
ARTHUR J GALLAGHER & CO	CAPITAL SENIOR LIVING CORP	COVENTRY HEALTH CARE INC
AT&T INC	CARDINAL HEALTH INC	COX COMMUNICATIONS INC
AUTOMATIC DATA PROCESSING INC	CARGILL INC	CR BARD INC
AUTOZONE INC	CARMAX GROUP	CSX CORP
AVERY DENNISON CORP	CARNIVAL CORPORATION	CSX TRANSPORTATION INC
AVIS BUDGET GROUP INC	CASH AMERICA INTERNATIONAL INC	CTS CORP
AVON PRODUCTS INC	CATERPILLAR INC	CUBIC CORP
AXA FINANCIAL INC	CATERPILLAR LOGISTICS	CUMMINS INC
BAKER HUGHES INC	CATHOLIC HEALTH INITIATIVES	CVS CAREMARK CORPORATION
BALTIMORE GAS AND ELECTRIC COMPANY	CBRL GROUP INC	DANAHER CORP
BANK OF AMERICA CORP	CDW CORPORATION	DARDEN RESTAURANTS INC
BARNES & NOBLE COLLEGE BOOKSTORES	CELLCO PARTNERSHIP (VERIZON WIRELESS)	DAVITA INC
BARNES & NOBLE INC	CEPHALON INC	DEAN FOODS CO
BASS PRO SHOPS INC	CH ROBINSON WORLDWIDE INC	DEERE & CO
BAXTER INTERNATIONAL INC	CH2M HILL COMPANIES LTD	DELOITTE & TOUCHE USA LLP
BDO SEIDMAN LLP	CHARLOTTE RUSSE HOLDING	DELOITTE CONSULTING LLP
BEBE STORES INC	CHARMING SHOPPES INC	DENNY'S CORPORATION
BECHTEL GROUP INC	CHEMED CORPORATION	DEVON ENERGY CORPORATION
BECKMAN COULTER INC	CHESAPEAKE ENERGY CORP	DEVRY INC
BECTON DICKINSON & CO	CHEVRON CORPORATION	DIAMOND OFFSHORE DRILLING INC
BED BATH & BEYOND INC	CHEVRON PHILLIPS CHEMICAL COMPANY LLC	DICK'S SPORTING GOODS INC
BENCHMARK ELECTRONICS INC	CHICO'S FAS INC	DIEBOLD INC
BERKSHIRE HATHAWAY INC	CHRISTOPHER & BANKS CORP	DINEEQUITY INC
BEST BUY CO INC	CHUBB CORPORATION (THE)	DIRECTV GROUP INC (THE)
BIO RAD LABORATORIES INC	CIBER INC	DJO INC
BJ SERVICES COMPANY	CINTAS CORP	DOLE FOOD COMPANY INC
BJ'S WHOLESALE CLUB INC	CISCO SYSTEMS INC	DOLLAR GENERAL CORPORATION
BLACK & DECKER CORP	CLEAR CHANNEL COMMUNICATIONS INC	DOLLAR THRIFTY AUTOMOTIVE GROUP INC
BLOOMBERG LP	CLUBCORP INC	DRESS BARN INC (THE)
BOEING COMPANY (THE)	COACH INC	DTE ENERGY COMPANY
BOOZ ALLEN HAMILTON	COCA COLA COMPANY (THE)	DUKE ENERGY CORP
BOSTON SCIENTIFIC CORP	COCA COLA ENTERPRISES INC	DYCOM INDUSTRIES INC
BRINKER INTERNATIONAL INC	COGNIZANT TECHNOLOGY SOLUTIONS CORP	E I DU PONT DE NEMOURS & CO (DUPONT)
BRINKS COMPANY (THE)	COLDWATER CREEK INC	EATON CORP
BRISTOL MYERS SQUIBB CO	COLGATE PALMOLIVE CO	EBAY INC
BROADCOM CORP	COMCAST CORP	ECHOSTAR CORP
BROWN & BROWN INC	CONAGRA FOODS INC	EDISON INTERNATIONAL
BUCKLE INC (THE)	CONOCOPHILLIPS COMPANY	ELECTRONIC ARTS INC
BUILD-A-BEAR WORKSHOP INC	CONSOL ENERGY INC	ELI LILLY & COMPANY
BUNGE LTD	CONSOLIDATED EDISON INC	EMBARQ CORP
BURGER KING HOLDINGS INC	CONTAINER STORE (THE)	EMC CORP
BURLINGTON NORTHERN SANTA FE CORP	CONVERGYS CORPORATION	EMERITUS CORP
CABELA'S INC	COOPER COMPANIES INC	EMERSON ELECTRIC CO
CABLEVISION SYSTEMS CORP	COST PLUS INC	ENTERGY CORP
CACI INTERNATIONAL INC	COSTCO WHOLESALE CORP	ENTERPRISE RENT-A-CAR
CAMERON INTERNATIONAL		ERNST & YOUNG LLP
		ESTEE LAUDER COMPANIES INC (THE)

EXEL TRANSPORTATION SERVICES INC (DHL EXEL)	HE BUTT GROCERY COMPANY (HEB)	KRAFT FOODS INC
EXELON CORPORATION	HEALTH FITNESS CORP	KROGER CO (THE)
EXPEDITORS INTERNATIONAL OF WASHINGTON INC	HEALTH MANAGEMENT ASSOCIATES INC	L-3 COMMUNICATIONS HOLDINGS INC
EXPERIAN AMERICAS	HEALTH NET INC	L-3 TITAN GROUP
EXPRESS SCRIPTS INC	HEALTHWAYS INC	LABORATORY CORP OF AMERICA HOLDINGS
EXXON MOBIL CORPORATION (EXXONMOBIL)	HELMERICH & PAYNE INC	LANDRY'S RESTAURANTS INC
FAIR ISAAC CORPORATION	HENRY SCHEIN INC	LAS VEGAS SANDS CORP (THE VENETIAN)
FAMILY DOLLAR STORES INC	HERTZ GLOBAL HOLDINGS INC	LEVEL 3 COMMUNICATIONS INC
FEDEX CORPORATION	HESS CORPORATION	LEXMARK INTERNATIONAL INC
FINISH LINE INC (THE)	HEWITT ASSOCIATES	LIBERTY GLOBAL INC
FIRST ADVANTAGE CORPORATION	HIBBETT SPORTS INC	LIMITED BRANDS INC
FIRST DATA CORP	HILB ROGAL & HOBBS CO	LINCARE HOLDINGS INC
FIRSTENERGY CORP	HILTON HOTELS CORP	LINCOLN NATIONAL CORPORATION
FISERV INC	HOME DEPOT INC	LKQ CORP
FLUOR CORP	HONEYWELL INTERNATIONAL INC	LOCKHEED MARTIN CORP
FMC TECHNOLOGIES INC	HOT TOPIC INC	LODGIAN INC
FOREST LABORATORIES INC	HUMANA INC	LOEWS CORPORATION
FORTUNE BRANDS INC	IAC/INTERACTIVECORP	LOWE'S COMPANIES INC
FOSSIL INC	ICT GROUP INC	MACY'S INC
FOSTER WHEELER LTD	IDEXX LABORATORIES INC	MANOR CARE INC
FOX ENTERTAINMENT GROUP INC	IGATE CORPORATION	MANPOWER INC
FPL GROUP INC	IMS HEALTH INC	MARATHON OIL CORP
FRED'S INC	INFOUSA INC	MARRIOTT INTERNATIONAL INC
FRONTIER COMMUNICATIONS CORPORATION	INGRAM MICRO INC	MARS INC
GAMESTOP CORP	INTEL CORP	MARSH & MCLENNAN COMPANIES INC
GENENTECH INC	INTERNATIONAL BUSINESS MACHINES CORP (IBM)	MARY KAY INC
GENERAL DYNAMICS CORP	INTIMATE BRANDS INC	MASSEY ENERGY COMPANY
GENERAL ELECTRIC CO (GE)	INTUIT INC	MATTEL INC
GENERAL MILLS INC	INVENTIV HEALTH INC	MAXIM INTEGRATED PRODUCTS INC
GENESCO INC	J C PENNEY COMPANY INC	
GENWORTH FINANCIAL INC	JABIL CIRCUIT INC	MCAFEE INC
GEO GROUP INC	JACK IN THE BOX INC	MCDONALD'S CORP
GEORGIA GULF CORPORATION	JACOBS ENGINEERING GROUP INC	MCKESSON CORPORATION
GLOBAL HYATT CORPORATION	JM SMUCKER CO	MCKINSEY & COMPANY INC
GLOBAL PAYMENTS INC	JOHNSON & JOHNSON	MEDCO HEALTH SOLUTIONS
GOOGLE INC	JOHNSON CONTROLS INC	MEDTRONIC INC
GRANT THORNTON LLP	JP MORGAN CHASE & CO INC	MEIJER INC
GTECH HOLDINGS CORP	JUNIPER NETWORKS INC	MEN'S WEARHOUSE INC (THE)
GUESS? INC	KAISER PERMANENTE	MERCER INC
HALLIBURTON COMPANY	KEANE INC	MERCK & CO INC
HARRAH'S ENTERTAINMENT INC	KELLOGG CO	METLIFE INC
HARRIS CORPORATION	KELLY SERVICES INC	MGM MIRAGE
HARTFORD FINANCIAL SERVICES GROUP INC (THE)	KENDLE INTERNATIONAL INC	MICROCHIP TECHNOLOGY INC
	KIMBERLY-CLARK CORP	MICRON TECHNOLOGY INC
HAWAIIAN ELECTRIC INDUSTRIES INC	KINDRED HEALTHCARE INC	MICROSOFT CORP
	KOCH INDUSTRIES INC	MILLIPORE CORP
HCA INC	KOHL'S CORP	MOLEX INC
	KPMG LLP	

MONRO MUFFLER BRAKE INC	POLO RALPH LAUREN CORP	SIGMA-ALDRICH CORP
MURPHY OIL CORPORATION	PRAXAIR INC	SISTERS OF MERCY HEALTH SYSTEMS
NATIONAL OILWELL VARCO INC	PRICEWATERHOUSECOOPERS	SMITH INTERNATIONAL INC
NEIMAN MARCUS GROUP INC (THE)	PRIDE INTERNATIONAL INC	SMITHFIELD FOODS INC
NETWORK APPLIANCE INC	PRINCIPAL FINANCIAL GROUP (THE)	SOUTHERN COMPANY (THE)
NEWS CORP	PROCTER & GAMBLE CO	SOUTHWEST AIRLINES CO
NII HOLDINGS INC	PROGRESSIVE CORPORATION (THE)	SRA INTERNATIONAL INC
NIKE INC		ST JUDE MEDICAL INC
NOBLE CORPORATION	PRUDENTIAL FINANCIAL INC	STAPLES INC
NORDSTROM INC	PSYCHIATRIC SOLUTIONS INC	STARTEK INC
NORFOLK SOUTHERN CORP	PUBLIC STORAGE INC	STARWOOD HOTELS & RESORTS WORLDWIDE INC
NORTHROP GRUMMAN CORP	PUBLIX SUPER MARKETS INC	
OCCIDENTAL PETROLEUM CORP	QUALCOMM INC	STERIS CORP
OCEANEERING INTERNATIONAL INC	QUEST DIAGNOSTICS INC	STRYKER CORP
	QUIKSILVER INC	SUN HEALTHCARE GROUP
ODYSSEY HEALTHCARE INC	R R DONNELLEY & SONS CO	SUN MICROSYSTEMS INC
OFFICE DEPOT INC	RAYTHEON CO	SUNGARD DATA SYSTEMS INC
OIL STATES INTERNATIONAL INC	REGIS CORPORATION	SUNOCO INC
OLD DOMINION FREIGHT LINE INC	RELIANT ENERGY INC	SUNRISE SENIOR LIVING
OMNICARE INC	RENT-A-CENTER INC	SUPERVALU INC
OMNICOM GROUP INC	RES CARE INC	SYKES ENTERPRISES INC
ONEOK INC	RESPIRONICS INC	SYMANTEC CORP
ORACLE CORP	RITE AID CORPORATION	SYNOPSYS INC
O'REILLY AUTOMOTIVE INC	RITZ-CARLTON HOTEL COMPANY LLC (THE)	SYNTEL INC
OSHKOSH CORPORATION		SYSCO CORP
OSI RESTAURANT PARTNERS INC	ROBERT HALF INTERNATIONAL INC	TALBOTS INC (THE)
OWENS & MINOR INC	ROSS STORES INC	TARGET CORPORATION
PACIFIC SUNWEAR OF CALIFORNIA INC	ROYAL CARIBBEAN CRUISES	TBC CORPORATION
	RUSSELL CORP	TECH DATA CORP
PANTRY INC (THE)	RYDER SYSTEM INC	TEKTRONIX INC
PARAMETRIC TECHNOLOGY CORP	SABRE HOLDINGS CORP	TELEDYNE TECHNOLOGIES INCORPORATED
PAREXEL INTERNATIONAL CORP	SAFECO CORP	
PARSONS BRINCKERHOFF INC	SAFEWAY INC	TELEPHONE AND DATA SYSTEMS INC (TDS)
PATTERSON COMPANIES INC	SAIC INC	
PATTERSON-UTI ENERGY INC	SAM'S CLUB	TELETECH HOLDINGS INC
PAXAR CORP	SARA LEE CORP	TESORO CORP
PAYCHEX INC	SAS INSTITUTE INC	TIFFANY & CO
PEABODY ENERGY CORP	SCANA CORPORATION	TIME WARNER INC
PEPSI BOTTLING GROUP INC	SCHERING-PLOUGH CORP	TJX COMPANIES INC (THE)
PEPSICO INC	SCHLUMBERGER LIMITED	T-MOBILE USA
PEROT SYSTEMS CORP	SCIENTIFIC GAMES CORPORATION	TOTAL SYSTEM SERVICES INC (TSYS)
PERRIGO CO	SCOTTS MIRACLE GROW CO	
PETCO ANIMAL SUPPLIES INC	SEACOR HOLDINGS INC	TOWERS PERRIN
PETSMART INC	SELECT MEDICAL CORPORATION	TRANSOCEAN INC
PFIZER INC	SEMPRA ENERGY	TRAVELERS COMPANIES INC (THE)
PG&E CORPORATION	SENSIENT TECHNOLOGIES CORPORATION	TW TELECOM INC
PHARMACEUTICAL PRODUCT DEVELOPMENT INC		TWEEN BRANDS INC
	SHAW GROUP INC (THE)	TYSON FOODS INC
PITNEY BOWES INC	SHELL OIL CO	UNION PACIFIC CORP
PLANTRONICS INC	SHERWIN WILLIAMS COMPANY	UNITED NATURAL FOODS INC
PLEXUS CORP		

	Training	ARROW ELECTRONICS INC
UNITED PARCEL SERVICE INC (UPS)	3M COMPANY	ARTHUR J GALLAGHER & CO
UNITED STATES CELLULAR CORP	7-ELEVEN INC	AT&T INC
UNITED TECHNOLOGIES CORPORATION	AARON RENTS INC	AUTOMATIC DATA PROCESSING INC
UNITEDHEALTH GROUP INC	ABBOTT LABORATORIES	AUTOZONE INC
UNIVISION COMMUNICATIONS INC	ABERCROMBIE & FITCH CO	AVERY DENNISON CORP
UPS SUPPLY CHAIN SOLUTIONS	ABM INDUSTRIES INC	AVIS BUDGET GROUP INC
URBAN OUTFITTERS INC	ACADEMY SPORTS & OUTDOORS LTD	AVON PRODUCTS INC
URS CORPORATION	ACCENTURE LTD	AXA FINANCIAL INC
USAA	ACXIOM CORP	BAKER HUGHES INC
VALERO ENERGY CORP	ADC TELECOMMUNICATIONS INC	BALTIMORE GAS AND ELECTRIC COMPANY
VALSPAR CORPORATION (THE)	ADESA INC	BANK OF AMERICA CORP
VARIAN MEDICAL SYSTEMS INC	ADOBE SYSTEMS INC	BARNES & NOBLE COLLEGE BOOKSTORES
VCA ANTECH INC	ADVANCE AUTO PARTS INC	BARNES & NOBLE INC
VERISIGN INC	ADVANCED MICRO DEVICES INC (AMD)	BASS PRO SHOPS INC
VERIZON COMMUNICATIONS	AECOM TECHNOLOGY CORPORATION	BAXTER INTERNATIONAL INC
VIACOM INC	AEROPOSTALE INC	BDO SEIDMAN LLP
VOLT INFORMATION SCIENCES INC	AES CORPORATION (THE)	BEBE STORES INC
W R BERKLEY CORPORATION	AETNA INC	BECHTEL GROUP INC
WALGREEN CO	AFFILIATED COMPUTER SERVICES INC	BECKMAN COULTER INC
WAL-MART STORES INC	AFLAC INC	BECTON DICKINSON & CO
WALT DISNEY COMPANY (THE)	AGILENT TECHNOLOGIES INC	BED BATH & BEYOND INC
WASTE MANAGEMENT INC	AIR PRODUCTS & CHEMICALS INC	BENCHMARK ELECTRONICS INC
WATERS CORP	ALBERTO-CULVER COMPANY	BERKSHIRE HATHAWAY INC
WATSON PHARMACEUTICALS INC	ALLERGAN INC	BEST BUY CO INC
WATSON WYATT WORLDWIDE INC	ALLIANCE DATA SYSTEMS CORPORATION	BIO RAD LABORATORIES INC
WEATHERFORD INTERNATIONAL LTD	ALLSTATE CORPORATION (THE)	BJ SERVICES COMPANY
WEIGHT WATCHERS INTERNATIONAL INC	ALTRIA GROUP INC	BJ'S WHOLESALE CLUB INC
WELLPOINT INC	AMAZON.COM INC	BLACK & DECKER CORP
WENDYS INTERNATIONAL INC	AMEDISYS INC	BLOOMBERG LP
WEST CORPORATION	AMERICAN EAGLE OUTFITTERS INC	BOEING COMPANY (THE)
WEST PHARMACEUTICAL SERVICES INC	AMERICAN ELECTRIC POWER COMPANY INC (AEP)	BOOZ ALLEN HAMILTON
WESTERN DIGITAL CORP	AMERICAN EXPRESS CO	BOSTON SCIENTIFIC CORP
WESTERN UNION COMPANY (THE)	AMERICAN POWER CONVERSION CORP	BRINKER INTERNATIONAL INC
WHOLE FOODS MARKET INC	AMERISOURCEBERGEN CORP	BRINKS COMPANY (THE)
WILLIAMS COMPANIES INC (THE)	AMGEN INC	BRISTOL MYERS SQUIBB CO
WILLIAMS SONOMA INC	ANADARKO PETROLEUM CORPORATION	BROADCOM CORP
WM WRIGLEY JR COMPANY	ANALOG DEVICES INC	BROWN & BROWN INC
WW GRAINGER INC	ANNTAYLOR STORES CORP	BUCKLE INC (THE)
WYETH	APACHE CORP	BUILD-A-BEAR WORKSHOP INC
WYNDHAM WORLDWIDE	APOLLO GROUP INC	BUNGE LTD
WYNN RESORTS LIMITED	APPLE INC	BURGER KING HOLDINGS INC
XEROX CORP	ARAMARK CORPORATION	BURLINGTON NORTHERN SANTA FE CORP
YAHOO! INC	ARCHER DANIELS MIDLAND CO	CABELA'S INC
YUM! BRANDS INC		CABLEVISION SYSTEMS CORP
ZIMMER HOLDINGS INC		CACI INTERNATIONAL INC
		CAMERON INTERNATIONAL

Column 1	Column 2	Column 3
CORPORATION	COVANCE INC	EXEL TRANSPORTATION SERVICES INC (DHL EXEL)
CAPITAL SENIOR LIVING CORP	COVENTRY HEALTH CARE INC	EXELON CORPORATION
CARDINAL HEALTH INC	COX COMMUNICATIONS INC	EXPEDITORS INTERNATIONAL OF WASHINGTON INC
CARGILL INC	CR BARD INC	EXPERIAN AMERICAS
CARMAX GROUP	CSX CORP	EXPRESS SCRIPTS INC
CARNIVAL CORPORATION	CSX TRANSPORTATION INC	EXXON MOBIL CORPORATION (EXXONMOBIL)
CASH AMERICA INTERNATIONAL INC	CTS CORP	FAIR ISAAC CORPORATION
CATERPILLAR INC	CUBIC CORP	FAMILY DOLLAR STORES INC
CATERPILLAR LOGISTICS	CUMMINS INC	FEDEX CORPORATION
CATHOLIC HEALTH INITIATIVES	CVS CAREMARK CORPORATION	FINISH LINE INC (THE)
CBRL GROUP INC	DANAHER CORP	FIRST ADVANTAGE CORPORATION
CDW CORPORATION	DARDEN RESTAURANTS INC	FIRST DATA CORP
CELLCO PARTNERSHIP (VERIZON WIRELESS)	DAVITA INC	FIRSTENERGY CORP
CEPHALON INC	DEAN FOODS CO	FISERV INC
CH ROBINSON WORLDWIDE INC	DEERE & CO	FLUOR CORP
CH2M HILL COMPANIES LTD	DELOITTE & TOUCHE USA LLP	FMC TECHNOLOGIES INC
CHARLOTTE RUSSE HOLDING	DELOITTE CONSULTING LLP	FOREST LABORATORIES INC
CHARMING SHOPPES INC	DENNY'S CORPORATION	FORTUNE BRANDS INC
CHEMED CORPORATION	DEVON ENERGY CORPORATION	FOSSIL INC
CHESAPEAKE ENERGY CORP	DEVRY INC	FOSTER WHEELER LTD
CHEVRON CORPORATION	DIAMOND OFFSHORE DRILLING INC	FOX ENTERTAINMENT GROUP INC
CHEVRON PHILLIPS CHEMICAL COMPANY LLC	DICK'S SPORTING GOODS INC	FPL GROUP INC
CHICO'S FAS INC	DIEBOLD INC	FRED'S INC
CHRISTOPHER & BANKS CORP	DINEEQUITY INC	FRONTIER COMMUNICATIONS CORPORATION
CHUBB CORPORATION (THE)	DIRECTV GROUP INC (THE)	GAMESTOP CORP
CIBER INC	DJO INC	GENENTECH INC
CINTAS CORP	DOLE FOOD COMPANY INC	GENERAL DYNAMICS CORP
CISCO SYSTEMS INC	DOLLAR GENERAL CORPORATION	GENERAL ELECTRIC CO (GE)
CLEAR CHANNEL COMMUNICATIONS INC	DOLLAR THRIFTY AUTOMOTIVE GROUP INC	GENERAL MILLS INC
CLUBCORP INC	DRESS BARN INC (THE)	GENESCO INC
COACH INC	DTE ENERGY COMPANY	GENWORTH FINANCIAL INC
COCA COLA COMPANY (THE)	DUKE ENERGY CORP	GEO GROUP INC
COCA COLA ENTERPRISES INC	DYCOM INDUSTRIES INC	GEORGIA GULF CORPORATION
COGNIZANT TECHNOLOGY SOLUTIONS CORP	E I DU PONT DE NEMOURS & CO (DUPONT)	GLOBAL HYATT CORPORATION
COLDWATER CREEK INC	EATON CORP	GLOBAL PAYMENTS INC
COLGATE PALMOLIVE CO	EBAY INC	GOOGLE INC
COMCAST CORP	ECHOSTAR CORP	GRANT THORNTON LLP
CONAGRA FOODS INC	EDISON INTERNATIONAL	GTECH HOLDINGS CORP
CONOCOPHILLIPS COMPANY	ELECTRONIC ARTS INC	GUESS? INC
CONSOL ENERGY INC	ELI LILLY & COMPANY	HALLIBURTON COMPANY
CONSOLIDATED EDISON INC	EMBARQ CORP	HARRAH'S ENTERTAINMENT INC
CONTAINER STORE (THE)	EMC CORP	HARRIS CORPORATION
CONVERGYS CORPORATION	EMERITUS CORP	HARTFORD FINANCIAL SERVICES GROUP INC (THE)
COOPER COMPANIES INC	EMERSON ELECTRIC CO	HAWAIIAN ELECTRIC INDUSTRIES INC
COST PLUS INC	ENTERGY CORP	
COSTCO WHOLESALE CORP	ENTERPRISE RENT-A-CAR	HCA INC
	ERNST & YOUNG LLP	
	ESTEE LAUDER COMPANIES INC (THE)	

HE BUTT GROCERY COMPANY (HEB)	KRAFT FOODS INC	MONRO MUFFLER BRAKE INC
HEALTH FITNESS CORP	KROGER CO (THE)	MURPHY OIL CORPORATION
HEALTH MANAGEMENT ASSOCIATES INC	L-3 COMMUNICATIONS HOLDINGS INC	NATIONAL OILWELL VARCO INC
HEALTH NET INC	L-3 TITAN GROUP	NEIMAN MARCUS GROUP INC (THE)
HEALTHWAYS INC	LABORATORY CORP OF AMERICA HOLDINGS	NETWORK APPLIANCE INC
HELMERICH & PAYNE INC	LANDRY'S RESTAURANTS INC	NEWS CORP
HENRY SCHEIN INC	LAS VEGAS SANDS CORP (THE VENETIAN)	NII HOLDINGS INC
HERTZ GLOBAL HOLDINGS INC		NIKE INC
HESS CORPORATION	LEVEL 3 COMMUNICATIONS INC	NOBLE CORPORATION
HEWITT ASSOCIATES	LEXMARK INTERNATIONAL INC	NORDSTROM INC
HIBBETT SPORTS INC	LIBERTY GLOBAL INC	NORFOLK SOUTHERN CORP
HILB ROGAL & HOBBS CO	LIMITED BRANDS INC	NORTHROP GRUMMAN CORP
HILTON HOTELS CORP	LINCARE HOLDINGS INC	OCCIDENTAL PETROLEUM CORP
HOME DEPOT INC	LINCOLN NATIONAL CORPORATION	OCEANEERING INTERNATIONAL INC
HONEYWELL INTERNATIONAL INC	LKQ CORP	ODYSSEY HEALTHCARE INC
HOT TOPIC INC	LOCKHEED MARTIN CORP	OFFICE DEPOT INC
HUMANA INC	LODGIAN INC	OIL STATES INTERNATIONAL INC
IAC/INTERACTIVECORP	LOEWS CORPORATION	OLD DOMINION FREIGHT LINE INC
ICT GROUP INC	LOWE'S COMPANIES INC	OMNICARE INC
IDEXX LABORATORIES INC	MACY'S INC	OMNICOM GROUP INC
IGATE CORPORATION	MANOR CARE INC	ONEOK INC
IMS HEALTH INC	MANPOWER INC	ORACLE CORP
INFOUSA INC	MARATHON OIL CORP	O'REILLY AUTOMOTIVE INC
INGRAM MICRO INC	MARRIOTT INTERNATIONAL INC	OSHKOSH CORPORATION
INTEL CORP	MARS INC	OSI RESTAURANT PARTNERS INC
INTERNATIONAL BUSINESS MACHINES CORP (IBM)	MARSH & MCLENNAN COMPANIES INC	OWENS & MINOR INC
INTIMATE BRANDS INC	MARY KAY INC	PACIFIC SUNWEAR OF CALIFORNIA INC
INTUIT INC	MASSEY ENERGY COMPANY	PANTRY INC (THE)
INVENTIV HEALTH INC	MATTEL INC	PARAMETRIC TECHNOLOGY CORP
J C PENNEY COMPANY INC	MAXIM INTEGRATED PRODUCTS INC	PAREXEL INTERNATIONAL CORP
JABIL CIRCUIT INC		PARSONS BRINCKERHOFF INC
JACK IN THE BOX INC	MCAFEE INC	PATTERSON COMPANIES INC
JACOBS ENGINEERING GROUP INC	MCDONALD'S CORP	PATTERSON-UTI ENERGY INC
JM SMUCKER CO	MCKESSON CORPORATION	PAXAR CORP
JOHNSON & JOHNSON	MCKINSEY & COMPANY INC	PAYCHEX INC
JOHNSON CONTROLS INC	MEDCO HEALTH SOLUTIONS	PEABODY ENERGY CORP
JP MORGAN CHASE & CO INC	MEDTRONIC INC	PEPSI BOTTLING GROUP INC
JUNIPER NETWORKS INC	MEIJER INC	PEPSICO INC
KAISER PERMANENTE	MEN'S WEARHOUSE INC (THE)	PEROT SYSTEMS CORP
KEANE INC	MERCER INC	PERRIGO CO
KELLOGG CO	MERCK & CO INC	PETCO ANIMAL SUPPLIES INC
KELLY SERVICES INC	METLIFE INC	PETSMART INC
KENDLE INTERNATIONAL INC	MGM MIRAGE	PFIZER INC
KIMBERLY-CLARK CORP	MICROCHIP TECHNOLOGY INC	PG&E CORPORATION
KINDRED HEALTHCARE INC	MICRON TECHNOLOGY INC	PHARMACEUTICAL PRODUCT DEVELOPMENT INC
KOCH INDUSTRIES INC	MICROSOFT CORP	PITNEY BOWES INC
KOHL'S CORP	MILLIPORE CORP	PLANTRONICS INC
KPMG LLP	MOLEX INC	PLEXUS CORP

POLO RALPH LAUREN CORP	(THE)	UNITED NATURAL FOODS INC
PRAXAIR INC	SIGMA-ALDRICH CORP	UNITED PARCEL SERVICE INC (UPS)
PRICEWATERHOUSECOOPERS	SISTERS OF MERCY HEALTH SYSTEMS	UNITED STATES CELLULAR CORP
PRIDE INTERNATIONAL INC	SMITH INTERNATIONAL INC	UNITED TECHNOLOGIES CORPORATION
PRINCIPAL FINANCIAL GROUP (THE)	SMITHFIELD FOODS INC	UNITEDHEALTH GROUP INC
PROCTER & GAMBLE CO	SOUTHERN COMPANY (THE)	UNIVISION COMMUNICATIONS INC
PROGRESSIVE CORPORATION (THE)	SOUTHWEST AIRLINES CO	UPS SUPPLY CHAIN SOLUTIONS
PRUDENTIAL FINANCIAL INC	SRA INTERNATIONAL INC	URBAN OUTFITTERS INC
PSYCHIATRIC SOLUTIONS INC	ST JUDE MEDICAL INC	URS CORPORATION
PUBLIC STORAGE INC	STAPLES INC	USAA
PUBLIX SUPER MARKETS INC	STARTEK INC	VALERO ENERGY CORP
QUALCOMM INC	STARWOOD HOTELS & RESORTS WORLDWIDE INC	VALSPAR CORPORATION (THE)
QUEST DIAGNOSTICS INC	STERIS CORP	VARIAN MEDICAL SYSTEMS INC
QUIKSILVER INC	STRYKER CORP	VCA ANTECH INC
R R DONNELLEY & SONS CO	SUN HEALTHCARE GROUP	VERISIGN INC
RAYTHEON CO	SUN MICROSYSTEMS INC	VERIZON COMMUNICATIONS
REGIS CORPORATION	SUNGARD DATA SYSTEMS INC	VIACOM INC
RELIANT ENERGY INC	SUNOCO INC	VOLT INFORMATION SCIENCES INC
RENT-A-CENTER INC	SUNRISE SENIOR LIVING	W R BERKLEY CORPORATION
RES CARE INC	SUPERVALU INC	WALGREEN CO
RESPIRONICS INC	SYKES ENTERPRISES INC	WAL-MART STORES INC
RITE AID CORPORATION	SYMANTEC CORP	WALT DISNEY COMPANY (THE)
RITZ-CARLTON HOTEL COMPANY LLC (THE)	SYNOPSYS INC	WASTE MANAGEMENT INC
ROBERT HALF INTERNATIONAL INC	SYNTEL INC	WATERS CORP
ROSS STORES INC	SYSCO CORP	WATSON PHARMACEUTICALS INC
ROYAL CARIBBEAN CRUISES	TALBOTS INC (THE)	WATSON WYATT WORLDWIDE INC
RUSSELL CORP	TARGET CORPORATION	WEATHERFORD INTERNATIONAL LTD
RYDER SYSTEM INC	TBC CORPORATION	WEIGHT WATCHERS INTERNATIONAL INC
SABRE HOLDINGS CORP	TECH DATA CORP	
SAFECO CORP	TEKTRONIX INC	WELLPOINT INC
SAFEWAY INC	TELEDYNE TECHNOLOGIES INCORPORATED	WENDYS INTERNATIONAL INC
SAIC INC	TELEPHONE AND DATA SYSTEMS INC (TDS)	WEST CORPORATION
SAM'S CLUB		WEST PHARMACEUTICAL SERVICES INC
SARA LEE CORP	TELETECH HOLDINGS INC	
SAS INSTITUTE INC	TESORO CORP	WESTERN DIGITAL CORP
SCANA CORPORATION	TIFFANY & CO	WESTERN UNION COMPANY (THE)
SCHERING-PLOUGH CORP	TIME WARNER INC	WHOLE FOODS MARKET INC
SCHLUMBERGER LIMITED	TJX COMPANIES INC (THE)	WILLIAMS COMPANIES INC (THE)
SCIENTIFIC GAMES CORPORATION	T-MOBILE USA	WILLIAMS SONOMA INC
SCOTTS MIRACLE GROW CO	TOTAL SYSTEM SERVICES INC (TSYS)	WM WRIGLEY JR COMPANY
SEACOR HOLDINGS INC		WW GRAINGER INC
SELECT MEDICAL CORPORATION	TOWERS PERRIN	WYETH
SEMPRA ENERGY	TRANSOCEAN INC	WYNDHAM WORLDWIDE
SENSIENT TECHNOLOGIES CORPORATION	TRAVELERS COMPANIES INC (THE)	WYNN RESORTS LIMITED
	TW TELECOM INC	XEROX CORP
SHAW GROUP INC (THE)	TWEEN BRANDS INC	YAHOO! INC
SHELL OIL CO	TYSON FOODS INC	YUM! BRANDS INC
SHERWIN WILLIAMS COMPANY	UNION PACIFIC CORP	ZIMMER HOLDINGS INC

Sales/Marketing

Advertising Professionals
3M COMPANY
7-ELEVEN INC
AARON RENTS INC
ABBOTT LABORATORIES
ABERCROMBIE & FITCH CO
ACADEMY SPORTS & OUTDOORS LTD
ACCENTURE LTD
ADC TELECOMMUNICATIONS INC
ADOBE SYSTEMS INC
ADVANCE AUTO PARTS INC
ADVANCED MICRO DEVICES INC (AMD)
AEROPOSTALE INC
AES CORPORATION (THE)
AETNA INC
AFLAC INC
AGILENT TECHNOLOGIES INC
ALBERTO-CULVER COMPANY
ALLERGAN INC
ALLIANCE DATA SYSTEMS CORPORATION
ALLSTATE CORPORATION (THE)
ALTRIA GROUP INC
AMAZON.COM INC
AMERICAN EAGLE OUTFITTERS INC
AMERICAN ELECTRIC POWER COMPANY INC (AEP)
AMERICAN EXPRESS CO
AMERICAN POWER CONVERSION CORP
AMERISOURCEBERGEN CORP
ANALOG DEVICES INC
ANNTAYLOR STORES CORP
APOLLO GROUP INC
APPLE INC
ARAMARK CORPORATION
ARROW ELECTRONICS INC
ARTHUR J GALLAGHER & CO
AT&T INC
AUTOMATIC DATA PROCESSING INC
AUTOZONE INC
AVERY DENNISON CORP
AVIS BUDGET GROUP INC
AVON PRODUCTS INC
AXA FINANCIAL INC
BALTIMORE GAS AND ELECTRIC COMPANY

BANK OF AMERICA CORP
BARNES & NOBLE COLLEGE BOOKSTORES
BARNES & NOBLE INC
BASS PRO SHOPS INC
BAXTER INTERNATIONAL INC
BDO SEIDMAN LLP
BEBE STORES INC
BECKMAN COULTER INC
BECTON DICKINSON & CO
BED BATH & BEYOND INC
BENCHMARK ELECTRONICS INC
BERKSHIRE HATHAWAY INC
BEST BUY CO INC
BIO RAD LABORATORIES INC
BJ'S WHOLESALE CLUB INC
BLACK & DECKER CORP
BLOOMBERG LP
BOEING COMPANY (THE)
BOOZ ALLEN HAMILTON
BOSTON SCIENTIFIC CORP
BRINKER INTERNATIONAL INC
BRINKS COMPANY (THE)
BRISTOL MYERS SQUIBB CO
BROADCOM CORP
BROWN & BROWN INC
BUCKLE INC (THE)
BUILD-A-BEAR WORKSHOP INC
BURGER KING HOLDINGS INC
BURLINGTON NORTHERN SANTA FE CORP
CABELA'S INC
CABLEVISION SYSTEMS CORP
CARDINAL HEALTH INC
CARMAX GROUP
CARNIVAL CORPORATION
CASH AMERICA INTERNATIONAL INC
CATERPILLAR INC
CATERPILLAR LOGISTICS
CATHOLIC HEALTH INITIATIVES
CBRL GROUP INC
CDW CORPORATION
CELLCO PARTNERSHIP (VERIZON WIRELESS)
CH ROBINSON WORLDWIDE INC
CHARLOTTE RUSSE HOLDING
CHARMING SHOPPES INC
CHESAPEAKE ENERGY CORP
CHEVRON CORPORATION
CHICO'S FAS INC

CHRISTOPHER & BANKS CORP
CHUBB CORPORATION (THE)
CINTAS CORP
CISCO SYSTEMS INC
CLEAR CHANNEL COMMUNICATIONS INC
COACH INC
COCA COLA COMPANY (THE)
COCA COLA ENTERPRISES INC
COLDWATER CREEK INC
COLGATE PALMOLIVE CO
COMCAST CORP
CONAGRA FOODS INC
CONOCOPHILLIPS COMPANY
CONSOLIDATED EDISON INC
CONTAINER STORE (THE)
CONVERGYS CORPORATION
COOPER COMPANIES INC
COST PLUS INC
COSTCO WHOLESALE CORP
COVANCE INC
COVENTRY HEALTH CARE INC
COX COMMUNICATIONS INC
CR BARD INC
CSX CORP
CSX TRANSPORTATION INC
CUMMINS INC
CVS CAREMARK CORPORATION
DANAHER CORP
DARDEN RESTAURANTS INC
DEAN FOODS CO
DEERE & CO
DELOITTE & TOUCHE USA LLP
DELOITTE CONSULTING LLP
DENNY'S CORPORATION
DEVRY INC
DICK'S SPORTING GOODS INC
DIEBOLD INC
DINEEQUITY INC
DIRECTV GROUP INC (THE)
DJO INC
DOLE FOOD COMPANY INC
DOLLAR GENERAL CORPORATION
DOLLAR THRIFTY AUTOMOTIVE GROUP INC
DRESS BARN INC (THE)
DTE ENERGY COMPANY
DUKE ENERGY CORP
EATON CORP
EBAY INC
ECHOSTAR CORP

EDISON INTERNATIONAL	HCA INC	LODGIAN INC
ELECTRONIC ARTS INC	HE BUTT GROCERY COMPANY (HEB)	LOEWS CORPORATION
ELI LILLY & COMPANY		LOWE'S COMPANIES INC
EMBARQ CORP	HEALTH FITNESS CORP	MACY'S INC
EMC CORP	HEALTH NET INC	MANPOWER INC
EMERSON ELECTRIC CO	HENRY SCHEIN INC	MARRIOTT INTERNATIONAL INC
ENTERGY CORP	HERTZ GLOBAL HOLDINGS INC	MARS INC
ENTERPRISE RENT-A-CAR	HEWITT ASSOCIATES	MARSH & MCLENNAN COMPANIES INC
ERNST & YOUNG LLP	HIBBETT SPORTS INC	
ESTEE LAUDER COMPANIES INC (THE)	HILB ROGAL & HOBBS CO	MARY KAY INC
	HILTON HOTELS CORP	MATTEL INC
EXEL TRANSPORTATION SERVICES INC (DHL EXEL)	HOME DEPOT INC	MAXIM INTEGRATED PRODUCTS INC
	HONEYWELL INTERNATIONAL INC	
EXELON CORPORATION	HOT TOPIC INC	MCAFEE INC
EXPEDITORS INTERNATIONAL OF WASHINGTON INC	HUMANA INC	MCDONALD'S CORP
	IAC/INTERACTIVECORP	MCKESSON CORPORATION
EXPERIAN AMERICAS	IMS HEALTH INC	MCKINSEY & COMPANY INC
EXPRESS SCRIPTS INC	INFOUSA INC	MEDCO HEALTH SOLUTIONS
EXXON MOBIL CORPORATION (EXXONMOBIL)	INGRAM MICRO INC	MEDTRONIC INC
	INTEL CORP	MEIJER INC
FAMILY DOLLAR STORES INC	INTERNATIONAL BUSINESS MACHINES CORP (IBM)	MEN'S WEARHOUSE INC (THE)
FEDEX CORPORATION		MERCER INC
FINISH LINE INC (THE)	INTIMATE BRANDS INC	MERCK & CO INC
FIRST DATA CORP	INTUIT INC	METLIFE INC
FIRSTENERGY CORP	J C PENNEY COMPANY INC	MGM MIRAGE
FISERV INC	JABIL CIRCUIT INC	MICROCHIP TECHNOLOGY INC
FLUOR CORP	JACK IN THE BOX INC	MICRON TECHNOLOGY INC
FORTUNE BRANDS INC	JM SMUCKER CO	MICROSOFT CORP
FOSSIL INC	JOHNSON & JOHNSON	MILLIPORE CORP
FOX ENTERTAINMENT GROUP INC	JOHNSON CONTROLS INC	MOLEX INC
FPL GROUP INC	JP MORGAN CHASE & CO INC	MONRO MUFFLER BRAKE INC
FRED'S INC	JUNIPER NETWORKS INC	NEIMAN MARCUS GROUP INC (THE)
FRONTIER COMMUNICATIONS CORPORATION	KAISER PERMANENTE	NETWORK APPLIANCE INC
	KEANE INC	NEWS CORP
GAMESTOP CORP	KELLOGG CO	NII HOLDINGS INC
GENENTECH INC	KELLY SERVICES INC	NIKE INC
GENERAL DYNAMICS CORP	KIMBERLY-CLARK CORP	NORDSTROM INC
GENERAL ELECTRIC CO (GE)	KOHL'S CORP	NORFOLK SOUTHERN CORP
GENERAL MILLS INC	KPMG LLP	NORTHROP GRUMMAN CORP
GENESCO INC	KRAFT FOODS INC	OFFICE DEPOT INC
GENWORTH FINANCIAL INC	KROGER CO (THE)	OLD DOMINION FREIGHT LINE INC
GLOBAL HYATT CORPORATION	L-3 COMMUNICATIONS HOLDINGS INC	OMNICARE INC
GLOBAL PAYMENTS INC		OMNICOM GROUP INC
GOOGLE INC	LANDRY'S RESTAURANTS INC	ORACLE CORP
GRANT THORNTON LLP	LAS VEGAS SANDS CORP (THE VENETIAN)	O'REILLY AUTOMOTIVE INC
GUESS? INC		OSHKOSH CORPORATION
HARRAH'S ENTERTAINMENT INC	LEXMARK INTERNATIONAL INC	OSI RESTAURANT PARTNERS INC
HARRIS CORPORATION	LIBERTY GLOBAL INC	OWENS & MINOR INC
HARTFORD FINANCIAL SERVICES GROUP INC (THE)	LIMITED BRANDS INC	PACIFIC SUNWEAR OF CALIFORNIA INC
	LINCOLN NATIONAL CORPORATION	
HAWAIIAN ELECTRIC INDUSTRIES INC	LOCKHEED MARTIN CORP	PANTRY INC (THE)

PARAMETRIC TECHNOLOGY CORP	SISTERS OF MERCY HEALTH SYSTEMS	VARIAN MEDICAL SYSTEMS INC
PATTERSON COMPANIES INC	SMITHFIELD FOODS INC	VERISIGN INC
PAXAR CORP	SOUTHERN COMPANY (THE)	VERIZON COMMUNICATIONS
PAYCHEX INC	SOUTHWEST AIRLINES CO	VIACOM INC
PEPSI BOTTLING GROUP INC	SRA INTERNATIONAL INC	VOLT INFORMATION SCIENCES INC
PEPSICO INC	ST JUDE MEDICAL INC	W R BERKLEY CORPORATION
PEROT SYSTEMS CORP	STAPLES INC	WALGREEN CO
PETCO ANIMAL SUPPLIES INC	STARWOOD HOTELS & RESORTS WORLDWIDE INC	WAL-MART STORES INC
PETSMART INC		WALT DISNEY COMPANY (THE)
PFIZER INC	STERIS CORP	WASTE MANAGEMENT INC
PG&E CORPORATION	STRYKER CORP	WATERS CORP
PITNEY BOWES INC	SUN MICROSYSTEMS INC	WATSON WYATT WORLDWIDE INC
PLANTRONICS INC	SUNGARD DATA SYSTEMS INC	WEIGHT WATCHERS INTERNATIONAL INC
PLEXUS CORP	SUPERVALU INC	
POLO RALPH LAUREN CORP	SYMANTEC CORP	WELLPOINT INC
PRICEWATERHOUSECOOPERS	SYNOPSYS INC	WENDYS INTERNATIONAL INC
PRINCIPAL FINANCIAL GROUP (THE)	SYSCO CORP	WESTERN DIGITAL CORP
	TALBOTS INC (THE)	WESTERN UNION COMPANY (THE)
PROCTER & GAMBLE CO	TARGET CORPORATION	WHOLE FOODS MARKET INC
PROGRESSIVE CORPORATION (THE)	TBC CORPORATION	WILLIAMS SONOMA INC
	TECH DATA CORP	WM WRIGLEY JR COMPANY
PRUDENTIAL FINANCIAL INC	TEKTRONIX INC	WW GRAINGER INC
PUBLIX SUPER MARKETS INC	TELEDYNE TECHNOLOGIES INCORPORATED	WYETH
QUALCOMM INC		WYNDHAM WORLDWIDE
QUIKSILVER INC	TELEPHONE AND DATA SYSTEMS INC (TDS)	WYNN RESORTS LIMITED
RAYTHEON CO		XEROX CORP
REGIS CORPORATION	TELETECH HOLDINGS INC	YAHOO! INC
RELIANT ENERGY INC	TIFFANY & CO	YUM! BRANDS INC
RENT-A-CENTER INC	TIME WARNER INC	ZIMMER HOLDINGS INC
RESPIRONICS INC	TJX COMPANIES INC (THE)	
RITE AID CORPORATION	T-MOBILE USA	

RITZ-CARLTON HOTEL COMPANY LLC (THE)	TOTAL SYSTEM SERVICES INC (TSYS)	**Commercial/Industrial**
		3M COMPANY
ROBERT HALF INTERNATIONAL INC	TOWERS PERRIN	ABBOTT LABORATORIES
ROSS STORES INC	TRAVELERS COMPANIES INC (THE)	ABM INDUSTRIES INC
ROYAL CARIBBEAN CRUISES	TW TELECOM INC	ACCENTURE LTD
RUSSELL CORP	TWEEN BRANDS INC	ACXIOM CORP
RYDER SYSTEM INC	TYSON FOODS INC	ADC TELECOMMUNICATIONS INC
SAFECO CORP	UNION PACIFIC CORP	ADESA INC
SAFEWAY INC	UNITED PARCEL SERVICE INC (UPS)	ADOBE SYSTEMS INC
SAM'S CLUB		ADVANCE AUTO PARTS INC
SARA LEE CORP	UNITED STATES CELLULAR CORP	ADVANCED MICRO DEVICES INC (AMD)
SAS INSTITUTE INC	UNITED TECHNOLOGIES CORPORATION	
SCANA CORPORATION		AECOM TECHNOLOGY CORPORATION
SCHERING-PLOUGH CORP	UNITEDHEALTH GROUP INC	
SCIENTIFIC GAMES CORPORATION	UNIVISION COMMUNICATIONS INC	AES CORPORATION (THE)
SCOTTS MIRACLE GROW CO	UPS SUPPLY CHAIN SOLUTIONS	AETNA INC
SEMPRA ENERGY	URBAN OUTFITTERS INC	AFFILIATED COMPUTER SERVICES INC
SHELL OIL CO	USAA	
SHERWIN WILLIAMS COMPANY (THE)	VALERO ENERGY CORP	AFLAC INC
	VALSPAR CORPORATION (THE)	AGILENT TECHNOLOGIES INC
		AIR PRODUCTS & CHEMICALS INC

ALBERTO-CULVER COMPANY	BRISTOL MYERS SQUIBB CO	COX COMMUNICATIONS INC
ALLERGAN INC	BROADCOM CORP	CR BARD INC
ALLIANCE DATA SYSTEMS CORPORATION	BROWN & BROWN INC	CSX CORP
ALLSTATE CORPORATION (THE)	BUNGE LTD	CSX TRANSPORTATION INC
ALTRIA GROUP INC	BURLINGTON NORTHERN SANTA FE CORP	CTS CORP
AMEDISYS INC	CABLEVISION SYSTEMS CORP	CUBIC CORP
AMERICAN ELECTRIC POWER COMPANY INC (AEP)	CACI INTERNATIONAL INC	CUMMINS INC
AMERICAN EXPRESS CO	CAMERON INTERNATIONAL CORPORATION	DANAHER CORP
AMERICAN POWER CONVERSION CORP	CARDINAL HEALTH INC	DAVITA INC
AMERISOURCEBERGEN CORP	CARGILL INC	DEAN FOODS CO
AMGEN INC	CARMAX GROUP	DEERE & CO
ANADARKO PETROLEUM CORPORATION	CARNIVAL CORPORATION	DELOITTE & TOUCHE USA LLP
ANALOG DEVICES INC	CASH AMERICA INTERNATIONAL INC	DELOITTE CONSULTING LLP
APACHE CORP	CATERPILLAR INC	DEVON ENERGY CORPORATION
APPLE INC	CATERPILLAR LOGISTICS	DIAMOND OFFSHORE DRILLING INC
ARAMARK CORPORATION	CDW CORPORATION	DIEBOLD INC
ARCHER DANIELS MIDLAND CO	CELLCO PARTNERSHIP (VERIZON WIRELESS)	DJO INC
ARROW ELECTRONICS INC	CEPHALON INC	DOLE FOOD COMPANY INC
ARTHUR J GALLAGHER & CO	CH ROBINSON WORLDWIDE INC	DOLLAR THRIFTY AUTOMOTIVE GROUP INC
AT&T INC	CH2M HILL COMPANIES LTD	DTE ENERGY COMPANY
AUTOMATIC DATA PROCESSING INC	CHEMED CORPORATION	DUKE ENERGY CORP
AUTOZONE INC	CHESAPEAKE ENERGY CORP	DYCOM INDUSTRIES INC
AVERY DENNISON CORP	CHEVRON CORPORATION	E I DU PONT DE NEMOURS & CO (DUPONT)
AVIS BUDGET GROUP INC	CHEVRON PHILLIPS CHEMICAL COMPANY LLC	EATON CORP
AXA FINANCIAL INC	CHUBB CORPORATION (THE)	ECHOSTAR CORP
BAKER HUGHES INC	CIBER INC	EDISON INTERNATIONAL
BALTIMORE GAS AND ELECTRIC COMPANY	CINTAS CORP	ELECTRONIC ARTS INC
BANK OF AMERICA CORP	CISCO SYSTEMS INC	ELI LILLY & COMPANY
BAXTER INTERNATIONAL INC	CLEAR CHANNEL COMMUNICATIONS INC	EMBARQ CORP
BDO SEIDMAN LLP	CLUBCORP INC	EMC CORP
BECHTEL GROUP INC	COACH INC	EMERSON ELECTRIC CO
BECKMAN COULTER INC	COCA COLA COMPANY (THE)	ENTERGY CORP
BECTON DICKINSON & CO	COCA COLA ENTERPRISES INC	ENTERPRISE RENT-A-CAR
BED BATH & BEYOND INC	COGNIZANT TECHNOLOGY SOLUTIONS CORP	ERNST & YOUNG LLP
BENCHMARK ELECTRONICS INC	COLGATE PALMOLIVE CO	ESTEE LAUDER COMPANIES INC (THE)
BERKSHIRE HATHAWAY INC	COMCAST CORP	EXEL TRANSPORTATION SERVICES INC (DHL EXEL)
BEST BUY CO INC	CONAGRA FOODS INC	EXELON CORPORATION
BIO RAD LABORATORIES INC	CONOCOPHILLIPS COMPANY	EXPEDITORS INTERNATIONAL OF WASHINGTON INC
BJ SERVICES COMPANY	CONSOLIDATED EDISON INC	EXPERIAN AMERICAS
BLACK & DECKER CORP	CONTAINER STORE (THE)	EXPRESS SCRIPTS INC
BLOOMBERG LP	CONVERGYS CORPORATION	EXXON MOBIL CORPORATION (EXXONMOBIL)
BOEING COMPANY (THE)	COOPER COMPANIES INC	FAIR ISAAC CORPORATION
BOOZ ALLEN HAMILTON	COST PLUS INC	FEDEX CORPORATION
BOSTON SCIENTIFIC CORP	COVANCE INC	FIRST ADVANTAGE CORPORATION
BRINKS COMPANY (THE)	COVENTRY HEALTH CARE INC	FIRST DATA CORP

FIRSTENERGY CORP	INTEL CORP	MERCER INC
FISERV INC	INTERNATIONAL BUSINESS MACHINES CORP (IBM)	MERCK & CO INC
FLUOR CORP		METLIFE INC
FMC TECHNOLOGIES INC	INTUIT INC	MGM MIRAGE
FOREST LABORATORIES INC	INVENTIV HEALTH INC	MICROCHIP TECHNOLOGY INC
FORTUNE BRANDS INC	JABIL CIRCUIT INC	MICRON TECHNOLOGY INC
FOSSIL INC	JACOBS ENGINEERING GROUP INC	MICROSOFT CORP
FOSTER WHEELER LTD	JM SMUCKER CO	MILLIPORE CORP
FOX ENTERTAINMENT GROUP INC	JOHNSON & JOHNSON	MOLEX INC
FPL GROUP INC	JOHNSON CONTROLS INC	MURPHY OIL CORPORATION
FRONTIER COMMUNICATIONS CORPORATION	JP MORGAN CHASE & CO INC	NATIONAL OILWELL VARCO INC
	JUNIPER NETWORKS INC	NETWORK APPLIANCE INC
GENENTECH INC	KAISER PERMANENTE	NEWS CORP
GENERAL DYNAMICS CORP	KEANE INC	NII HOLDINGS INC
GENERAL ELECTRIC CO (GE)	KELLOGG CO	NIKE INC
GENERAL MILLS INC	KELLY SERVICES INC	NOBLE CORPORATION
GENESCO INC	KENDLE INTERNATIONAL INC	NORFOLK SOUTHERN CORP
GENWORTH FINANCIAL INC	KIMBERLY-CLARK CORP	NORTHROP GRUMMAN CORP
GEO GROUP INC	KOCH INDUSTRIES INC	OCCIDENTAL PETROLEUM CORP
GEORGIA GULF CORPORATION	KPMG LLP	OCEANEERING INTERNATIONAL INC
GLOBAL HYATT CORPORATION	KRAFT FOODS INC	
GLOBAL PAYMENTS INC	L-3 COMMUNICATIONS HOLDINGS INC	OFFICE DEPOT INC
GOOGLE INC		OIL STATES INTERNATIONAL INC
GRANT THORNTON LLP	L-3 TITAN GROUP	OLD DOMINION FREIGHT LINE INC
GTECH HOLDINGS CORP	LABORATORY CORP OF AMERICA HOLDINGS	OMNICOM GROUP INC
HALLIBURTON COMPANY		ONEOK INC
HARRAH'S ENTERTAINMENT INC	LAS VEGAS SANDS CORP (THE VENETIAN)	ORACLE CORP
HARRIS CORPORATION	LEVEL 3 COMMUNICATIONS INC	O'REILLY AUTOMOTIVE INC
HARTFORD FINANCIAL SERVICES GROUP INC (THE)	LEXMARK INTERNATIONAL INC	OSHKOSH CORPORATION
	LIBERTY GLOBAL INC	OWENS & MINOR INC
HAWAIIAN ELECTRIC INDUSTRIES INC	LINCARE HOLDINGS INC	PARAMETRIC TECHNOLOGY CORP
	LINCOLN NATIONAL CORPORATION	PAREXEL INTERNATIONAL CORP
HEALTH FITNESS CORP	LKQ CORP	PARSONS BRINCKERHOFF INC
HEALTH NET INC	LOCKHEED MARTIN CORP	PATTERSON COMPANIES INC
HEALTHWAYS INC	LOEWS CORPORATION	PATTERSON-UTI ENERGY INC
HELMERICH & PAYNE INC	LOWE'S COMPANIES INC	PAXAR CORP
HENRY SCHEIN INC	MANPOWER INC	PAYCHEX INC
HERTZ GLOBAL HOLDINGS INC	MARATHON OIL CORP	PEPSI BOTTLING GROUP INC
HESS CORPORATION	MARRIOTT INTERNATIONAL INC	PEPSICO INC
HEWITT ASSOCIATES	MARS INC	PEROT SYSTEMS CORP
HILB ROGAL & HOBBS CO	MARSH & MCLENNAN COMPANIES INC	PERRIGO CO
HILTON HOTELS CORP		PFIZER INC
HOME DEPOT INC	MATTEL INC	PG&E CORPORATION
HONEYWELL INTERNATIONAL INC	MAXIM INTEGRATED PRODUCTS INC	PHARMACEUTICAL PRODUCT DEVELOPMENT INC
HUMANA INC		
ICT GROUP INC	MCAFEE INC	PITNEY BOWES INC
IDEXX LABORATORIES INC	MCKESSON CORPORATION	PLANTRONICS INC
IGATE CORPORATION	MCKINSEY & COMPANY INC	PLEXUS CORP
IMS HEALTH INC	MEDCO HEALTH SOLUTIONS	POLO RALPH LAUREN CORP
INFOUSA INC	MEDTRONIC INC	PRAXAIR INC
INGRAM MICRO INC		PRICEWATERHOUSECOOPERS

PRIDE INTERNATIONAL INC	SYKES ENTERPRISES INC	WEST PHARMACEUTICAL SERVICES INC
PRINCIPAL FINANCIAL GROUP (THE)	SYMANTEC CORP	WESTERN DIGITAL CORP
PROCTER & GAMBLE CO	SYNOPSYS INC	WILLIAMS COMPANIES INC (THE)
PRUDENTIAL FINANCIAL INC	SYNTEL INC	WILLIAMS SONOMA INC
QUALCOMM INC	SYSCO CORP	WM WRIGLEY JR COMPANY
QUEST DIAGNOSTICS INC	TBC CORPORATION	WW GRAINGER INC
QUIKSILVER INC	TECH DATA CORP	WYETH
R R DONNELLEY & SONS CO	TEKTRONIX INC	WYNDHAM WORLDWIDE
RAYTHEON CO	TELEDYNE TECHNOLOGIES INCORPORATED	WYNN RESORTS LIMITED
RELIANT ENERGY INC	TELEPHONE AND DATA SYSTEMS INC (TDS)	XEROX CORP
RESPIRONICS INC		YAHOO! INC
RITZ-CARLTON HOTEL COMPANY LLC (THE)	TELETECH HOLDINGS INC	ZIMMER HOLDINGS INC
ROBERT HALF INTERNATIONAL INC	TESORO CORP	
ROYAL CARIBBEAN CRUISES	TIME WARNER INC	**Marketing Professionals**
RUSSELL CORP	T-MOBILE USA	3M COMPANY
RYDER SYSTEM INC	TOTAL SYSTEM SERVICES INC (TSYS)	7-ELEVEN INC
SABRE HOLDINGS CORP	TOWERS PERRIN	AARON RENTS INC
SAFECO CORP	TRANSOCEAN INC	ABBOTT LABORATORIES
SAIC INC	TRAVELERS COMPANIES INC (THE)	ABERCROMBIE & FITCH CO
SARA LEE CORP	TW TELECOM INC	ABM INDUSTRIES INC
SAS INSTITUTE INC	TYSON FOODS INC	ACADEMY SPORTS & OUTDOORS LTD
SCANA CORPORATION	UNION PACIFIC CORP	ACCENTURE LTD
SCHERING-PLOUGH CORP	UNITED NATURAL FOODS INC	ACXIOM CORP
SCHLUMBERGER LIMITED	UNITED PARCEL SERVICE INC (UPS)	ADC TELECOMMUNICATIONS INC
SCIENTIFIC GAMES CORPORATION	UNITED STATES CELLULAR CORP	ADOBE SYSTEMS INC
SCOTTS MIRACLE GROW CO	UNITED TECHNOLOGIES CORPORATION	ADVANCE AUTO PARTS INC
SEACOR HOLDINGS INC	UNITEDHEALTH GROUP INC	ADVANCED MICRO DEVICES INC (AMD)
SEMPRA ENERGY	UNIVISION COMMUNICATIONS INC	AECOM TECHNOLOGY CORPORATION
SENSIENT TECHNOLOGIES CORPORATION	UPS SUPPLY CHAIN SOLUTIONS	AEROPOSTALE INC
SHAW GROUP INC (THE)	URS CORPORATION	AES CORPORATION (THE)
SHELL OIL CO	VALERO ENERGY CORP	AETNA INC
SHERWIN WILLIAMS COMPANY (THE)	VALSPAR CORPORATION (THE)	AFFILIATED COMPUTER SERVICES INC
SIGMA-ALDRICH CORP	VARIAN MEDICAL SYSTEMS INC	AFLAC INC
SMITH INTERNATIONAL INC	VERISIGN INC	AGILENT TECHNOLOGIES INC
SMITHFIELD FOODS INC	VERIZON COMMUNICATIONS	AIR PRODUCTS & CHEMICALS INC
SOUTHERN COMPANY (THE)	VIACOM INC	ALBERTO-CULVER COMPANY
SRA INTERNATIONAL INC	VOLT INFORMATION SCIENCES INC	ALLERGAN INC
ST JUDE MEDICAL INC	W R BERKLEY CORPORATION	ALLIANCE DATA SYSTEMS CORPORATION
STAPLES INC	WALT DISNEY COMPANY (THE)	ALLSTATE CORPORATION (THE)
STARTEK INC	WASTE MANAGEMENT INC	ALTRIA GROUP INC
STARWOOD HOTELS & RESORTS WORLDWIDE INC	WATERS CORP	AMAZON.COM INC
STERIS CORP	WATSON PHARMACEUTICALS INC	AMEDISYS INC
STRYKER CORP	WATSON WYATT WORLDWIDE INC	AMERICAN EAGLE OUTFITTERS INC
SUN MICROSYSTEMS INC	WEATHERFORD INTERNATIONAL LTD	AMERICAN ELECTRIC POWER COMPANY INC (AEP)
SUNGARD DATA SYSTEMS INC	WELLPOINT INC	AMERICAN EXPRESS CO
SUNOCO INC	WEST CORPORATION	

AMERICAN POWER CONVERSION CORP	BRISTOL MYERS SQUIBB CO	COLGATE PALMOLIVE CO
AMERISOURCEBERGEN CORP	BROADCOM CORP	COMCAST CORP
AMGEN INC	BROWN & BROWN INC	CONAGRA FOODS INC
ANADARKO PETROLEUM CORPORATION	BUCKLE INC (THE)	CONOCOPHILLIPS COMPANY
ANALOG DEVICES INC	BUILD-A-BEAR WORKSHOP INC	CONSOLIDATED EDISON INC
ANNTAYLOR STORES CORP	BURGER KING HOLDINGS INC	CONTAINER STORE (THE)
APACHE CORP	BURLINGTON NORTHERN SANTA FE CORP	CONVERGYS CORPORATION
APOLLO GROUP INC	CABELA'S INC	COOPER COMPANIES INC
APPLE INC	CABLEVISION SYSTEMS CORP	COST PLUS INC
ARAMARK CORPORATION	CACI INTERNATIONAL INC	COSTCO WHOLESALE CORP
ARCHER DANIELS MIDLAND CO	CAMERON INTERNATIONAL CORPORATION	COVANCE INC
ARROW ELECTRONICS INC	CAPITAL SENIOR LIVING CORP	COVENTRY HEALTH CARE INC
ARTHUR J GALLAGHER & CO	CARDINAL HEALTH INC	COX COMMUNICATIONS INC
AT&T INC	CARGILL INC	CR BARD INC
AUTOMATIC DATA PROCESSING INC	CARMAX GROUP	CSX CORP
AUTOZONE INC	CARNIVAL CORPORATION	CSX TRANSPORTATION INC
AVERY DENNISON CORP	CASH AMERICA INTERNATIONAL INC	CTS CORP
AVIS BUDGET GROUP INC	CATERPILLAR INC	CUBIC CORP
AVON PRODUCTS INC	CATERPILLAR LOGISTICS	CUMMINS INC
AXA FINANCIAL INC	CATHOLIC HEALTH INITIATIVES	CVS CAREMARK CORPORATION
BAKER HUGHES INC	CBRL GROUP INC	DANAHER CORP
BALTIMORE GAS AND ELECTRIC COMPANY	CDW CORPORATION	DARDEN RESTAURANTS INC
BANK OF AMERICA CORP	CELLCO PARTNERSHIP (VERIZON WIRELESS)	DAVITA INC
BARNES & NOBLE COLLEGE BOOKSTORES	CEPHALON INC	DEAN FOODS CO
		DEERE & CO
BARNES & NOBLE INC	CH ROBINSON WORLDWIDE INC	DELOITTE & TOUCHE USA LLP
BASS PRO SHOPS INC	CH2M HILL COMPANIES LTD	DELOITTE CONSULTING LLP
BAXTER INTERNATIONAL INC	CHARLOTTE RUSSE HOLDING	DENNY'S CORPORATION
BDO SEIDMAN LLP	CHARMING SHOPPES INC	DEVON ENERGY CORPORATION
BEBE STORES INC	CHEMED CORPORATION	DEVRY INC
BECHTEL GROUP INC	CHESAPEAKE ENERGY CORP	DIAMOND OFFSHORE DRILLING INC
BECKMAN COULTER INC	CHEVRON CORPORATION	DICK'S SPORTING GOODS INC
BECTON DICKINSON & CO	CHEVRON PHILLIPS CHEMICAL COMPANY LLC	DIEBOLD INC
BED BATH & BEYOND INC		DINEEQUITY INC
BENCHMARK ELECTRONICS INC	CHICO'S FAS INC	DIRECTV GROUP INC (THE)
BERKSHIRE HATHAWAY INC	CHRISTOPHER & BANKS CORP	DJO INC
BEST BUY CO INC	CHUBB CORPORATION (THE)	DOLE FOOD COMPANY INC
BIO RAD LABORATORIES INC	CIBER INC	DOLLAR GENERAL CORPORATION
BJ SERVICES COMPANY	CINTAS CORP	DOLLAR THRIFTY AUTOMOTIVE GROUP INC
BJ'S WHOLESALE CLUB INC	CISCO SYSTEMS INC	DRESS BARN INC (THE)
BLACK & DECKER CORP	CLEAR CHANNEL COMMUNICATIONS INC	DTE ENERGY COMPANY
BLOOMBERG LP		DUKE ENERGY CORP
BOEING COMPANY (THE)	CLUBCORP INC	DYCOM INDUSTRIES INC
BOOZ ALLEN HAMILTON	COACH INC	E I DU PONT DE NEMOURS & CO (DUPONT)
BOSTON SCIENTIFIC CORP	COCA COLA COMPANY (THE)	
BRINKER INTERNATIONAL INC	COCA COLA ENTERPRISES INC	EATON CORP
BRINKS COMPANY (THE)	COGNIZANT TECHNOLOGY SOLUTIONS CORP	EBAY INC
		ECHOSTAR CORP
		EDISON INTERNATIONAL
	COLDWATER CREEK INC	ELECTRONIC ARTS INC

ELI LILLY & COMPANY	GUESS? INC	KELLOGG CO
EMBARQ CORP	HALLIBURTON COMPANY	KELLY SERVICES INC
EMC CORP	HARRAH'S ENTERTAINMENT INC	KENDLE INTERNATIONAL INC
EMERITUS CORP	HARRIS CORPORATION	KIMBERLY-CLARK CORP
EMERSON ELECTRIC CO	HARTFORD FINANCIAL SERVICES GROUP INC (THE)	KINDRED HEALTHCARE INC
ENTERGY CORP		KOCH INDUSTRIES INC
ENTERPRISE RENT-A-CAR	HAWAIIAN ELECTRIC INDUSTRIES INC	KOHL'S CORP
ERNST & YOUNG LLP		KPMG LLP
ESTEE LAUDER COMPANIES INC (THE)	HCA INC	KRAFT FOODS INC
	HE BUTT GROCERY COMPANY (HEB)	KROGER CO (THE)
EXEL TRANSPORTATION SERVICES INC (DHL EXEL)	HEALTH FITNESS CORP	L-3 COMMUNICATIONS HOLDINGS INC
EXELON CORPORATION	HEALTH MANAGEMENT ASSOCIATES INC	L-3 TITAN GROUP
EXPEDITORS INTERNATIONAL OF WASHINGTON INC	HEALTH NET INC	LABORATORY CORP OF AMERICA HOLDINGS
EXPERIAN AMERICAS	HEALTHWAYS INC	LANDRY'S RESTAURANTS INC
EXPRESS SCRIPTS INC	HENRY SCHEIN INC	LAS VEGAS SANDS CORP (THE VENETIAN)
EXXON MOBIL CORPORATION (EXXONMOBIL)	HERTZ GLOBAL HOLDINGS INC	
	HESS CORPORATION	LEVEL 3 COMMUNICATIONS INC
FAIR ISAAC CORPORATION	HEWITT ASSOCIATES	LEXMARK INTERNATIONAL INC
FAMILY DOLLAR STORES INC	HIBBETT SPORTS INC	LIBERTY GLOBAL INC
FEDEX CORPORATION	HILB ROGAL & HOBBS CO	LIMITED BRANDS INC
FINISH LINE INC (THE)	HILTON HOTELS CORP	LINCARE HOLDINGS INC
FIRST ADVANTAGE CORPORATION	HOME DEPOT INC	LINCOLN NATIONAL CORPORATION
FIRST DATA CORP	HONEYWELL INTERNATIONAL INC	LKQ CORP
FIRSTENERGY CORP	HOT TOPIC INC	LOCKHEED MARTIN CORP
FISERV INC	HUMANA INC	LODGIAN INC
FLUOR CORP	IAC/INTERACTIVECORP	LOEWS CORPORATION
FMC TECHNOLOGIES INC	ICT GROUP INC	LOWE'S COMPANIES INC
FOREST LABORATORIES INC	IDEXX LABORATORIES INC	MACY'S INC
FORTUNE BRANDS INC	IGATE CORPORATION	MANOR CARE INC
FOSSIL INC	IMS HEALTH INC	MANPOWER INC
FOSTER WHEELER LTD	INFOUSA INC	MARATHON OIL CORP
FOX ENTERTAINMENT GROUP INC	INGRAM MICRO INC	MARRIOTT INTERNATIONAL INC
FPL GROUP INC	INTEL CORP	MARS INC
FRED'S INC	INTERNATIONAL BUSINESS MACHINES CORP (IBM)	MARSH & MCLENNAN COMPANIES INC
FRONTIER COMMUNICATIONS CORPORATION	INTIMATE BRANDS INC	MARY KAY INC
GAMESTOP CORP	INTUIT INC	MATTEL INC
GENENTECH INC	INVENTIV HEALTH INC	MAXIM INTEGRATED PRODUCTS INC
GENERAL DYNAMICS CORP	J C PENNEY COMPANY INC	
GENERAL ELECTRIC CO (GE)	JABIL CIRCUIT INC	MCAFEE INC
GENERAL MILLS INC	JACK IN THE BOX INC	MCDONALD'S CORP
GENESCO INC	JACOBS ENGINEERING GROUP INC	MCKESSON CORPORATION
GENWORTH FINANCIAL INC	JM SMUCKER CO	MCKINSEY & COMPANY INC
GEORGIA GULF CORPORATION	JOHNSON & JOHNSON	MEDCO HEALTH SOLUTIONS
GLOBAL HYATT CORPORATION	JOHNSON CONTROLS INC	MEDTRONIC INC
GLOBAL PAYMENTS INC	JP MORGAN CHASE & CO INC	MEIJER INC
GOOGLE INC	JUNIPER NETWORKS INC	MEN'S WEARHOUSE INC (THE)
GRANT THORNTON LLP	KAISER PERMANENTE	MERCER INC
GTECH HOLDINGS CORP	KEANE INC	MERCK & CO INC

METLIFE INC	PHARMACEUTICAL PRODUCT DEVELOPMENT INC	SENSIENT TECHNOLOGIES CORPORATION
MGM MIRAGE	PITNEY BOWES INC	SHAW GROUP INC (THE)
MICROCHIP TECHNOLOGY INC	PLANTRONICS INC	SHELL OIL CO
MICRON TECHNOLOGY INC	PLEXUS CORP	SHERWIN WILLIAMS COMPANY (THE)
MICROSOFT CORP	POLO RALPH LAUREN CORP	SIGMA-ALDRICH CORP
MILLIPORE CORP	PRAXAIR INC	SISTERS OF MERCY HEALTH SYSTEMS
MOLEX INC	PRICEWATERHOUSECOOPERS	SMITH INTERNATIONAL INC
MONRO MUFFLER BRAKE INC	PRIDE INTERNATIONAL INC	SMITHFIELD FOODS INC
NATIONAL OILWELL VARCO INC	PRINCIPAL FINANCIAL GROUP (THE)	SOUTHERN COMPANY (THE)
NEIMAN MARCUS GROUP INC (THE)	PROCTER & GAMBLE CO	SOUTHWEST AIRLINES CO
NETWORK APPLIANCE INC	PROGRESSIVE CORPORATION (THE)	SRA INTERNATIONAL INC
NEWS CORP	PRUDENTIAL FINANCIAL INC	ST JUDE MEDICAL INC
NII HOLDINGS INC	PSYCHIATRIC SOLUTIONS INC	STAPLES INC
NIKE INC	PUBLIC STORAGE INC	STARTEK INC
NOBLE CORPORATION	PUBLIX SUPER MARKETS INC	STARWOOD HOTELS & RESORTS WORLDWIDE INC
NORDSTROM INC	QUALCOMM INC	STERIS CORP
NORFOLK SOUTHERN CORP	QUEST DIAGNOSTICS INC	STRYKER CORP
NORTHROP GRUMMAN CORP	QUIKSILVER INC	SUN HEALTHCARE GROUP
OCCIDENTAL PETROLEUM CORP	R R DONNELLEY & SONS CO	SUN MICROSYSTEMS INC
OCEANEERING INTERNATIONAL INC	RAYTHEON CO	SUNGARD DATA SYSTEMS INC
ODYSSEY HEALTHCARE INC	REGIS CORPORATION	SUNOCO INC
OFFICE DEPOT INC	RELIANT ENERGY INC	SUNRISE SENIOR LIVING
OIL STATES INTERNATIONAL INC	RENT-A-CENTER INC	SUPERVALU INC
OLD DOMINION FREIGHT LINE INC	RES CARE INC	SYKES ENTERPRISES INC
OMNICARE INC	RESPIRONICS INC	SYMANTEC CORP
OMNICOM GROUP INC	RITE AID CORPORATION	SYNOPSYS INC
ONEOK INC	RITZ-CARLTON HOTEL COMPANY LLC (THE)	SYNTEL INC
ORACLE CORP	ROBERT HALF INTERNATIONAL INC	SYSCO CORP
O'REILLY AUTOMOTIVE INC	ROSS STORES INC	TALBOTS INC (THE)
OSHKOSH CORPORATION	ROYAL CARIBBEAN CRUISES	TARGET CORPORATION
OSI RESTAURANT PARTNERS INC	RUSSELL CORP	TBC CORPORATION
OWENS & MINOR INC	RYDER SYSTEM INC	TECH DATA CORP
PACIFIC SUNWEAR OF CALIFORNIA INC	SABRE HOLDINGS CORP	TEKTRONIX INC
PANTRY INC (THE)	SAFECO CORP	TELEDYNE TECHNOLOGIES INCORPORATED
PARAMETRIC TECHNOLOGY CORP	SAFEWAY INC	TELEPHONE AND DATA SYSTEMS INC (TDS)
PAREXEL INTERNATIONAL CORP	SAIC INC	TELETECH HOLDINGS INC
PARSONS BRINCKERHOFF INC	SAM'S CLUB	TIFFANY & CO
PATTERSON COMPANIES INC	SARA LEE CORP	TIME WARNER INC
PATTERSON-UTI ENERGY INC	SAS INSTITUTE INC	TJX COMPANIES INC (THE)
PAXAR CORP	SCANA CORPORATION	T-MOBILE USA
PAYCHEX INC	SCHERING-PLOUGH CORP	TOTAL SYSTEM SERVICES INC (TSYS)
PEPSI BOTTLING GROUP INC	SCHLUMBERGER LIMITED	TOWERS PERRIN
PEPSICO INC	SCIENTIFIC GAMES CORPORATION	TRANSOCEAN INC
PEROT SYSTEMS CORP	SCOTTS MIRACLE GROW CO	TRAVELERS COMPANIES INC (THE)
PERRIGO CO	SEACOR HOLDINGS INC	TW TELECOM INC
PETCO ANIMAL SUPPLIES INC	SELECT MEDICAL CORPORATION	
PETSMART INC	SEMPRA ENERGY	
PFIZER INC		
PG&E CORPORATION		

TWEEN BRANDS INC	YAHOO! INC	DOLLAR THRIFTY AUTOMOTIVE GROUP INC
TYSON FOODS INC	YUM! BRANDS INC	DRESS BARN INC (THE)
UNION PACIFIC CORP	ZIMMER HOLDINGS INC	ENTERPRISE RENT-A-CAR
UNITED NATURAL FOODS INC		ESTEE LAUDER COMPANIES INC (THE)
UNITED PARCEL SERVICE INC (UPS)	**Retail Sales**	FAMILY DOLLAR STORES INC
UNITED STATES CELLULAR CORP	7-ELEVEN INC	FINISH LINE INC (THE)
UNITED TECHNOLOGIES CORPORATION	AARON RENTS INC	FOSSIL INC
UNITEDHEALTH GROUP INC	ABERCROMBIE & FITCH CO	FRED'S INC
UNIVISION COMMUNICATIONS INC	ACADEMY SPORTS & OUTDOORS LTD	GAMESTOP CORP
UPS SUPPLY CHAIN SOLUTIONS	ADVANCE AUTO PARTS INC	GENESCO INC
URBAN OUTFITTERS INC	AEROPOSTALE INC	GUESS? INC
URS CORPORATION	ALBERTO-CULVER COMPANY	HE BUTT GROCERY COMPANY (HEB)
USAA	AMAZON.COM INC	HERTZ GLOBAL HOLDINGS INC
VALERO ENERGY CORP	AMERICAN EAGLE OUTFITTERS INC	HIBBETT SPORTS INC
VALSPAR CORPORATION (THE)	ANNTAYLOR STORES CORP	HOME DEPOT INC
VARIAN MEDICAL SYSTEMS INC	APPLE INC	HOT TOPIC INC
VCA ANTECH INC	AT&T INC	INTIMATE BRANDS INC
VERISIGN INC	AUTOZONE INC	J C PENNEY COMPANY INC
VERIZON COMMUNICATIONS	AVIS BUDGET GROUP INC	KOHL'S CORP
VIACOM INC	AVON PRODUCTS INC	KROGER CO (THE)
VOLT INFORMATION SCIENCES INC	BARNES & NOBLE COLLEGE BOOKSTORES	LIMITED BRANDS INC
W R BERKLEY CORPORATION	BARNES & NOBLE INC	LOWE'S COMPANIES INC
WALGREEN CO	BASS PRO SHOPS INC	MACY'S INC
WAL-MART STORES INC	BEBE STORES INC	MARY KAY INC
WALT DISNEY COMPANY (THE)	BED BATH & BEYOND INC	MEIJER INC
WASTE MANAGEMENT INC	BERKSHIRE HATHAWAY INC	MEN'S WEARHOUSE INC (THE)
WATERS CORP	BEST BUY CO INC	NEIMAN MARCUS GROUP INC (THE)
WATSON PHARMACEUTICALS INC	BJ'S WHOLESALE CLUB INC	NIKE INC
WATSON WYATT WORLDWIDE INC	BUCKLE INC (THE)	NORDSTROM INC
WEATHERFORD INTERNATIONAL LTD	BUILD-A-BEAR WORKSHOP INC	OFFICE DEPOT INC
WEIGHT WATCHERS INTERNATIONAL INC	CABELA'S INC	O'REILLY AUTOMOTIVE INC
WELLPOINT INC	CARMAX GROUP	PACIFIC SUNWEAR OF CALIFORNIA INC
WENDYS INTERNATIONAL INC	CASH AMERICA INTERNATIONAL INC	PANTRY INC (THE)
WEST CORPORATION	CDW CORPORATION	PETCO ANIMAL SUPPLIES INC
WEST PHARMACEUTICAL SERVICES INC	CELLCO PARTNERSHIP (VERIZON WIRELESS)	PETSMART INC
WESTERN DIGITAL CORP	CHARLOTTE RUSSE HOLDING	POLO RALPH LAUREN CORP
WESTERN UNION COMPANY (THE)	CHARMING SHOPPES INC	PUBLIX SUPER MARKETS INC
WHOLE FOODS MARKET INC	CHICO'S FAS INC	QUIKSILVER INC
WILLIAMS COMPANIES INC (THE)	CHRISTOPHER & BANKS CORP	REGIS CORPORATION
WILLIAMS SONOMA INC	COACH INC	RENT-A-CENTER INC
WM WRIGLEY JR COMPANY	COLDWATER CREEK INC	RITE AID CORPORATION
WW GRAINGER INC	CONTAINER STORE (THE)	ROSS STORES INC
WYETH	COST PLUS INC	RYDER SYSTEM INC
WYNDHAM WORLDWIDE	COSTCO WHOLESALE CORP	SAFEWAY INC
WYNN RESORTS LIMITED	CVS CAREMARK CORPORATION	SAM'S CLUB
XEROX CORP	DICK'S SPORTING GOODS INC	SCOTTS MIRACLE GROW CO
	DOLLAR GENERAL CORPORATION	SHERWIN WILLIAMS COMPANY

(THE)	AUTOZONE INC	COX COMMUNICATIONS INC
STAPLES INC	AVERY DENNISON CORP	CVS CAREMARK CORPORATION
SUPERVALU INC	AVIS BUDGET GROUP INC	DANAHER CORP
TALBOTS INC (THE)	AVON PRODUCTS INC	DEAN FOODS CO
TARGET CORPORATION	AXA FINANCIAL INC	DICK'S SPORTING GOODS INC
TBC CORPORATION	BARNES & NOBLE COLLEGE BOOKSTORES	DIRECTV GROUP INC (THE)
TIFFANY & CO	BARNES & NOBLE INC	DOLE FOOD COMPANY INC
TJX COMPANIES INC (THE)	BASS PRO SHOPS INC	DOLLAR GENERAL CORPORATION
T-MOBILE USA	BAXTER INTERNATIONAL INC	DOLLAR THRIFTY AUTOMOTIVE GROUP INC
TWEEN BRANDS INC	BEBE STORES INC	DRESS BARN INC (THE)
UNITED STATES CELLULAR CORP	BED BATH & BEYOND INC	ECHOSTAR CORP
URBAN OUTFITTERS INC	BEST BUY CO INC	ELECTRONIC ARTS INC
VALERO ENERGY CORP	BJ'S WHOLESALE CLUB INC	ELI LILLY & COMPANY
VERIZON COMMUNICATIONS	BLACK & DECKER CORP	EMBARQ CORP
WALGREEN CO	BLOOMBERG LP	ENTERPRISE RENT-A-CAR
WAL-MART STORES INC	BRINKS COMPANY (THE)	ESTEE LAUDER COMPANIES INC (THE)
WHOLE FOODS MARKET INC	BRISTOL MYERS SQUIBB CO	EXPERIAN AMERICAS
WILLIAMS SONOMA INC	BUCKLE INC (THE)	EXXON MOBIL CORPORATION (EXXONMOBIL)
WW GRAINGER INC	BUILD-A-BEAR WORKSHOP INC	FAIR ISAAC CORPORATION
	CABELA'S INC	FAMILY DOLLAR STORES INC
Sales Trainees	CABLEVISION SYSTEMS CORP	FEDEX CORPORATION
3M COMPANY	CARDINAL HEALTH INC	FINISH LINE INC (THE)
7-ELEVEN INC	CARMAX GROUP	FIRST ADVANTAGE CORPORATION
AARON RENTS INC	CARNIVAL CORPORATION	FIRST DATA CORP
ABBOTT LABORATORIES	CASH AMERICA INTERNATIONAL INC	FORTUNE BRANDS INC
ABERCROMBIE & FITCH CO	CBRL GROUP INC	FOSSIL INC
ABM INDUSTRIES INC	CDW CORPORATION	FRED'S INC
ACADEMY SPORTS & OUTDOORS LTD	CELLCO PARTNERSHIP (VERIZON WIRELESS)	GAMESTOP CORP
ADESA INC	CHARLOTTE RUSSE HOLDING	GENENTECH INC
ADOBE SYSTEMS INC	CHARMING SHOPPES INC	GENERAL MILLS INC
ADVANCE AUTO PARTS INC	CHEMED CORPORATION	GENESCO INC
AEROPOSTALE INC	CHEVRON CORPORATION	GENWORTH FINANCIAL INC
AETNA INC	CHICO'S FAS INC	GLOBAL HYATT CORPORATION
AFLAC INC	CHRISTOPHER & BANKS CORP	GLOBAL PAYMENTS INC
ALBERTO-CULVER COMPANY	CHUBB CORPORATION (THE)	GUESS? INC
ALLSTATE CORPORATION (THE)	CINTAS CORP	HARRAH'S ENTERTAINMENT INC
ALTRIA GROUP INC	CLEAR CHANNEL COMMUNICATIONS INC	HARTFORD FINANCIAL SERVICES GROUP INC (THE)
AMAZON.COM INC	COACH INC	HE BUTT GROCERY COMPANY (HEB)
AMERICAN EAGLE OUTFITTERS INC	COCA COLA COMPANY (THE)	HEALTH FITNESS CORP
AMERICAN POWER CONVERSION CORP	COCA COLA ENTERPRISES INC	HENRY SCHEIN INC
AMERISOURCEBERGEN CORP	COLDWATER CREEK INC	HERTZ GLOBAL HOLDINGS INC
AMGEN INC	COLGATE PALMOLIVE CO	HIBBETT SPORTS INC
ANNTAYLOR STORES CORP	COMCAST CORP	HILTON HOTELS CORP
APPLE INC	CONOCOPHILLIPS COMPANY	HOME DEPOT INC
ARAMARK CORPORATION	CONTAINER STORE (THE)	HOT TOPIC INC
ARROW ELECTRONICS INC	COST PLUS INC	INFOUSA INC
AT&T INC	COSTCO WHOLESALE CORP	
AUTOMATIC DATA PROCESSING INC		

INGRAM MICRO INC	PRINCIPAL FINANCIAL GROUP (THE)	VALERO ENERGY CORP
INTERNATIONAL BUSINESS MACHINES CORP (IBM)	PROCTER & GAMBLE CO	VERIZON COMMUNICATIONS
INTIMATE BRANDS INC	PROGRESSIVE CORPORATION (THE)	VOLT INFORMATION SCIENCES INC
J C PENNEY COMPANY INC	PRUDENTIAL FINANCIAL INC	W R BERKLEY CORPORATION
JM SMUCKER CO	PUBLIX SUPER MARKETS INC	WALGREEN CO
JOHNSON & JOHNSON	QUIKSILVER INC	WAL-MART STORES INC
KELLOGG CO	R R DONNELLEY & SONS CO	WASTE MANAGEMENT INC
KELLY SERVICES INC	RENT-A-CENTER INC	WEIGHT WATCHERS INTERNATIONAL INC
KIMBERLY-CLARK CORP	RITE AID CORPORATION	WHOLE FOODS MARKET INC
KOHL'S CORP	RITZ-CARLTON HOTEL COMPANY LLC (THE)	WILLIAMS SONOMA INC
KRAFT FOODS INC	ROBERT HALF INTERNATIONAL INC	WM WRIGLEY JR COMPANY
KROGER CO (THE)	ROSS STORES INC	WW GRAINGER INC
LAS VEGAS SANDS CORP (THE VENETIAN)	ROYAL CARIBBEAN CRUISES	WYETH
LEXMARK INTERNATIONAL INC	RUSSELL CORP	WYNDHAM WORLDWIDE
LIMITED BRANDS INC	RYDER SYSTEM INC	WYNN RESORTS LIMITED
LINCOLN NATIONAL CORPORATION	SAFECO CORP	XEROX CORP
LOEWS CORPORATION	SAFEWAY INC	ZIMMER HOLDINGS INC
LOWE'S COMPANIES INC	SAM'S CLUB	

Technical/Scientific

MACY'S INC	SARA LEE CORP	
MANPOWER INC	SCHERING-PLOUGH CORP	**Engineers, Electrical**
MARRIOTT INTERNATIONAL INC	SCOTTS MIRACLE GROW CO	3M COMPANY
MARS INC	SHERWIN WILLIAMS COMPANY (THE)	ABBOTT LABORATORIES
MARY KAY INC		ACCENTURE LTD
MCKESSON CORPORATION	SMITHFIELD FOODS INC	ACXIOM CORP
MEDTRONIC INC	SOUTHWEST AIRLINES CO	ADC TELECOMMUNICATIONS INC
MEIJER INC	ST JUDE MEDICAL INC	ADOBE SYSTEMS INC
MEN'S WEARHOUSE INC (THE)	STAPLES INC	ADVANCED MICRO DEVICES INC (AMD)
MERCK & CO INC	STARWOOD HOTELS & RESORTS WORLDWIDE INC	AECOM TECHNOLOGY CORPORATION
METLIFE INC	SUPERVALU INC	AES CORPORATION (THE)
MGM MIRAGE	SYSCO CORP	AFFILIATED COMPUTER SERVICES INC
NEIMAN MARCUS GROUP INC (THE)	TALBOTS INC (THE)	AGILENT TECHNOLOGIES INC
NIKE INC	TARGET CORPORATION	AIR PRODUCTS & CHEMICALS INC
NORDSTROM INC	TBC CORPORATION	AMERICAN ELECTRIC POWER COMPANY INC (AEP)
OFFICE DEPOT INC	TECH DATA CORP	AMERICAN POWER CONVERSION CORP
OMNICARE INC	TELEPHONE AND DATA SYSTEMS INC (TDS)	AMGEN INC
O'REILLY AUTOMOTIVE INC	TIFFANY & CO	ANADARKO PETROLEUM CORPORATION
OWENS & MINOR INC	TJX COMPANIES INC (THE)	ANALOG DEVICES INC
PACIFIC SUNWEAR OF CALIFORNIA INC	T-MOBILE USA	APACHE CORP
PANTRY INC (THE)	TOTAL SYSTEM SERVICES INC (TSYS)	APPLE INC
PATTERSON COMPANIES INC	TRAVELERS COMPANIES INC (THE)	ARCHER DANIELS MIDLAND CO
PAYCHEX INC	TWEEN BRANDS INC	AT&T INC
PEPSI BOTTLING GROUP INC	TYSON FOODS INC	AUTOMATIC DATA PROCESSING INC
PEPSICO INC	UNITED NATURAL FOODS INC	
PETCO ANIMAL SUPPLIES INC	UNITED STATES CELLULAR CORP	BAKER HUGHES INC
PETSMART INC	URBAN OUTFITTERS INC	
PFIZER INC	USAA	
PITNEY BOWES INC		
POLO RALPH LAUREN CORP		

BALTIMORE GAS AND ELECTRIC COMPANY	DIRECTV GROUP INC (THE)	JOHNSON & JOHNSON
BAXTER INTERNATIONAL INC	DTE ENERGY COMPANY	JOHNSON CONTROLS INC
BECHTEL GROUP INC	DUKE ENERGY CORP	JUNIPER NETWORKS INC
BECKMAN COULTER INC	DYCOM INDUSTRIES INC	KEANE INC
BECTON DICKINSON & CO	E I DU PONT DE NEMOURS & CO (DUPONT)	KENDLE INTERNATIONAL INC
BENCHMARK ELECTRONICS INC		KOCH INDUSTRIES INC
BERKSHIRE HATHAWAY INC	EATON CORP	KRAFT FOODS INC
BIO RAD LABORATORIES INC	EBAY INC	L-3 COMMUNICATIONS HOLDINGS INC
BJ SERVICES COMPANY	ECHOSTAR CORP	
BLACK & DECKER CORP	EDISON INTERNATIONAL	L-3 TITAN GROUP
BLOOMBERG LP	ELECTRONIC ARTS INC	LEVEL 3 COMMUNICATIONS INC
BOEING COMPANY (THE)	ELI LILLY & COMPANY	LEXMARK INTERNATIONAL INC
BRISTOL MYERS SQUIBB CO	EMBARQ CORP	LIBERTY GLOBAL INC
BROADCOM CORP	EMC CORP	LOCKHEED MARTIN CORP
BURLINGTON NORTHERN SANTA FE CORP	EMERSON ELECTRIC CO	MARATHON OIL CORP
	ENTERGY CORP	MATTEL INC
CABLEVISION SYSTEMS CORP	EXELON CORPORATION	MAXIM INTEGRATED PRODUCTS INC
CACI INTERNATIONAL INC	EXXON MOBIL CORPORATION (EXXONMOBIL)	
CAMERON INTERNATIONAL CORPORATION		MCAFEE INC
	FEDEX CORPORATION	MEDTRONIC INC
CARGILL INC	FIRSTENERGY CORP	MERCK & CO INC
CATERPILLAR INC	FLUOR CORP	MICROCHIP TECHNOLOGY INC
CELLCO PARTNERSHIP (VERIZON WIRELESS)	FMC TECHNOLOGIES INC	MICRON TECHNOLOGY INC
	FOREST LABORATORIES INC	MICROSOFT CORP
CEPHALON INC	FOSSIL INC	MILLIPORE CORP
CH2M HILL COMPANIES LTD	FOSTER WHEELER LTD	MOLEX INC
CHESAPEAKE ENERGY CORP	FOX ENTERTAINMENT GROUP INC	MURPHY OIL CORPORATION
CHEVRON CORPORATION	FPL GROUP INC	NATIONAL OILWELL VARCO INC
CHEVRON PHILLIPS CHEMICAL COMPANY LLC	FRONTIER COMMUNICATIONS CORPORATION	NETWORK APPLIANCE INC
		NEWS CORP
CIBER INC	GENENTECH INC	NII HOLDINGS INC
CISCO SYSTEMS INC	GENERAL DYNAMICS CORP	NOBLE CORPORATION
CLEAR CHANNEL COMMUNICATIONS INC	GENERAL ELECTRIC CO (GE)	NORFOLK SOUTHERN CORP
	GOOGLE INC	NORTHROP GRUMMAN CORP
COGNIZANT TECHNOLOGY SOLUTIONS CORP	GTECH HOLDINGS CORP	OCCIDENTAL PETROLEUM CORP
	HALLIBURTON COMPANY	OCEANEERING INTERNATIONAL INC
COMCAST CORP	HARRIS CORPORATION	
CONAGRA FOODS INC	HAWAIIAN ELECTRIC INDUSTRIES INC	OIL STATES INTERNATIONAL INC
CONOCOPHILLIPS COMPANY		ONEOK INC
CONSOLIDATED EDISON INC	HELMERICH & PAYNE INC	ORACLE CORP
COX COMMUNICATIONS INC	HESS CORPORATION	OSHKOSH CORPORATION
CSX CORP	HONEYWELL INTERNATIONAL INC	PARAMETRIC TECHNOLOGY CORP
CSX TRANSPORTATION INC	IAC/INTERACTIVECORP	PAREXEL INTERNATIONAL CORP
CTS CORP	IDEXX LABORATORIES INC	PARSONS BRINCKERHOFF INC
CUBIC CORP	IGATE CORPORATION	PATTERSON-UTI ENERGY INC
CUMMINS INC	INTEL CORP	PEROT SYSTEMS CORP
DANAHER CORP	INTERNATIONAL BUSINESS MACHINES CORP (IBM)	PERRIGO CO
DEERE & CO		PFIZER INC
DEVON ENERGY CORPORATION	INTUIT INC	PG&E CORPORATION
DIAMOND OFFSHORE DRILLING INC	JABIL CIRCUIT INC	PHARMACEUTICAL PRODUCT DEVELOPMENT INC
DIEBOLD INC	JACOBS ENGINEERING GROUP INC	

PITNEY BOWES INC	VALERO ENERGY CORP	CARGILL INC
PLANTRONICS INC	VARIAN MEDICAL SYSTEMS INC	CARNIVAL CORPORATION
PLEXUS CORP	VERISIGN INC	CATERPILLAR INC
PRAXAIR INC	VERIZON COMMUNICATIONS	CELLCO PARTNERSHIP (VERIZON WIRELESS)
PRIDE INTERNATIONAL INC	VIACOM INC	CEPHALON INC
QUALCOMM INC	WALT DISNEY COMPANY (THE)	CH2M HILL COMPANIES LTD
RAYTHEON CO	WATERS CORP	CHESAPEAKE ENERGY CORP
RELIANT ENERGY INC	WATSON PHARMACEUTICALS INC	CHEVRON CORPORATION
RESPIRONICS INC	WEATHERFORD INTERNATIONAL LTD	CHEVRON PHILLIPS CHEMICAL COMPANY LLC
SABRE HOLDINGS CORP	WESTERN DIGITAL CORP	CLEAR CHANNEL COMMUNICATIONS INC
SAIC INC	WILLIAMS COMPANIES INC (THE)	
SAS INSTITUTE INC	WYETH	COLGATE PALMOLIVE CO
SCANA CORPORATION	XEROX CORP	COMCAST CORP
SCHERING-PLOUGH CORP	YAHOO! INC	CONAGRA FOODS INC
SCHLUMBERGER LIMITED		CONOCOPHILLIPS COMPANY
SCIENTIFIC GAMES CORPORATION		CONSOL ENERGY INC
SEACOR HOLDINGS INC	**Engineers, Other**	CONSOLIDATED EDISON INC
SEMPRA ENERGY	3M COMPANY	COOPER COMPANIES INC
SHAW GROUP INC (THE)	ABBOTT LABORATORIES	COX COMMUNICATIONS INC
SHELL OIL CO	AECOM TECHNOLOGY CORPORATION	CR BARD INC
SIGMA-ALDRICH CORP	AIR PRODUCTS & CHEMICALS INC	CSX CORP
SMITH INTERNATIONAL INC	ALLERGAN INC	CSX TRANSPORTATION INC
SOUTHERN COMPANY (THE)	AMERICAN ELECTRIC POWER COMPANY INC (AEP)	CUBIC CORP
SOUTHWEST AIRLINES CO	AMERICAN POWER CONVERSION CORP	CUMMINS INC
SRA INTERNATIONAL INC	AMGEN INC	DANAHER CORP
ST JUDE MEDICAL INC	ANADARKO PETROLEUM CORPORATION	DEAN FOODS CO
STERIS CORP	APACHE CORP	DEERE & CO
SUN MICROSYSTEMS INC	ARCHER DANIELS MIDLAND CO	DEVON ENERGY CORPORATION
SUNGARD DATA SYSTEMS INC	AT&T INC	DIAMOND OFFSHORE DRILLING INC
SUNOCO INC	BAKER HUGHES INC	DIRECTV GROUP INC (THE)
SYMANTEC CORP	BALTIMORE GAS AND ELECTRIC COMPANY	DJO INC
SYNOPSYS INC	BAXTER INTERNATIONAL INC	DTE ENERGY COMPANY
SYNTEL INC	BECHTEL GROUP INC	DUKE ENERGY CORP
TEKTRONIX INC	BECKMAN COULTER INC	DYCOM INDUSTRIES INC
TELEDYNE TECHNOLOGIES INCORPORATED	BECTON DICKINSON & CO	E I DU PONT DE NEMOURS & CO (DUPONT)
TELEPHONE AND DATA SYSTEMS INC (TDS)	BIO RAD LABORATORIES INC	EATON CORP
	BJ SERVICES COMPANY	ECHOSTAR CORP
TESORO CORP	BLACK & DECKER CORP	EDISON INTERNATIONAL
TIME WARNER INC	BOEING COMPANY (THE)	ELI LILLY & COMPANY
T-MOBILE USA	BOSTON SCIENTIFIC CORP	EMBARQ CORP
TRANSOCEAN INC	BRISTOL MYERS SQUIBB CO	ENTERGY CORP
TW TELECOM INC	BUNGE LTD	ESTEE LAUDER COMPANIES INC (THE)
UNION PACIFIC CORP	BURLINGTON NORTHERN SANTA FE CORP	
UNITED PARCEL SERVICE INC (UPS)	CABLEVISION SYSTEMS CORP	EXXON MOBIL CORPORATION (EXXONMOBIL)
UNITED STATES CELLULAR CORP	CAMERON INTERNATIONAL CORPORATION	FIRSTENERGY CORP
UNITED TECHNOLOGIES CORPORATION		FLUOR CORP
UNIVISION COMMUNICATIONS INC		FMC TECHNOLOGIES INC
URS CORPORATION		

FOREST LABORATORIES INC	OSHKOSH CORPORATION	VALSPAR CORPORATION (THE)
FORTUNE BRANDS INC	PARAMETRIC TECHNOLOGY CORP	VARIAN MEDICAL SYSTEMS INC
FOSTER WHEELER LTD	PARSONS BRINCKERHOFF INC	VERIZON COMMUNICATIONS
FOX ENTERTAINMENT GROUP INC	PATTERSON-UTI ENERGY INC	VIACOM INC
FPL GROUP INC	PEABODY ENERGY CORP	WALT DISNEY COMPANY (THE)
FRONTIER COMMUNICATIONS CORPORATION	PERRIGO CO	WASTE MANAGEMENT INC
GENENTECH INC	PFIZER INC	WATERS CORP
GENERAL DYNAMICS CORP	PG&E CORPORATION	WATSON PHARMACEUTICALS INC
GENERAL MILLS INC	PITNEY BOWES INC	WEATHERFORD INTERNATIONAL LTD
GEORGIA GULF CORPORATION	PRAXAIR INC	WEST PHARMACEUTICAL SERVICES INC
HALLIBURTON COMPANY	PRIDE INTERNATIONAL INC	WILLIAMS COMPANIES INC (THE)
HAWAIIAN ELECTRIC INDUSTRIES INC	PROCTER & GAMBLE CO	WYETH
HE BUTT GROCERY COMPANY (HEB)	RAYTHEON CO	XEROX CORP
HELMERICH & PAYNE INC	RELIANT ENERGY INC	ZIMMER HOLDINGS INC
HESS CORPORATION	RESPIRONICS INC	
HONEYWELL INTERNATIONAL INC	ROYAL CARIBBEAN CRUISES	**Health & Laboratory**
IDEXX LABORATORIES INC	SAIC INC	3M COMPANY
INTERNATIONAL BUSINESS MACHINES CORP (IBM)	SARA LEE CORP	ABBOTT LABORATORIES
JACOBS ENGINEERING GROUP INC	SCANA CORPORATION	AGILENT TECHNOLOGIES INC
JM SMUCKER CO	SCHERING-PLOUGH CORP	ALBERTO-CULVER COMPANY
JOHNSON & JOHNSON	SCHLUMBERGER LIMITED	ALLERGAN INC
JOHNSON CONTROLS INC	SCOTTS MIRACLE GROW CO	AMEDISYS INC
KELLOGG CO	SEACOR HOLDINGS INC	AMGEN INC
KENDLE INTERNATIONAL INC	SEMPRA ENERGY	BAXTER INTERNATIONAL INC
KOCH INDUSTRIES INC	SENSIENT TECHNOLOGIES CORPORATION	BECKMAN COULTER INC
KRAFT FOODS INC	SHAW GROUP INC (THE)	BECTON DICKINSON & CO
L-3 TITAN GROUP	SHELL OIL CO	BIO RAD LABORATORIES INC
LEVEL 3 COMMUNICATIONS INC	SIGMA-ALDRICH CORP	BOSTON SCIENTIFIC CORP
LIBERTY GLOBAL INC	SMITH INTERNATIONAL INC	BRISTOL MYERS SQUIBB CO
LKQ CORP	SOUTHERN COMPANY (THE)	CATHOLIC HEALTH INITIATIVES
LOCKHEED MARTIN CORP	SOUTHWEST AIRLINES CO	CEPHALON INC
MARATHON OIL CORP	ST JUDE MEDICAL INC	CHEMED CORPORATION
MASSEY ENERGY COMPANY	STERIS CORP	COLGATE PALMOLIVE CO
MEDTRONIC INC	STRYKER CORP	COOPER COMPANIES INC
MERCK & CO INC	SUNOCO INC	COVANCE INC
MURPHY OIL CORPORATION	TELEDYNE TECHNOLOGIES INCORPORATED	CR BARD INC
NATIONAL OILWELL VARCO INC	TELEPHONE AND DATA SYSTEMS INC (TDS)	DAVITA INC
NEWS CORP	TESORO CORP	DJO INC
NII HOLDINGS INC	TIME WARNER INC	E I DU PONT DE NEMOURS & CO (DUPONT)
NOBLE CORPORATION	T-MOBILE USA	ELI LILLY & COMPANY
NORFOLK SOUTHERN CORP	TRANSOCEAN INC	ESTEE LAUDER COMPANIES INC (THE)
NORTHROP GRUMMAN CORP	UNION PACIFIC CORP	FLUOR CORP
OCCIDENTAL PETROLEUM CORP	UNITED STATES CELLULAR CORP	FOREST LABORATORIES INC
OCEANEERING INTERNATIONAL INC	UNITED TECHNOLOGIES CORPORATION	GENENTECH INC
OIL STATES INTERNATIONAL INC	UNIVISION COMMUNICATIONS INC	HCA INC
ONEOK INC	URS CORPORATION	HEALTH MANAGEMENT ASSOCIATES INC
	VALERO ENERGY CORP	

HEALTHWAYS INC	BOOZ ALLEN HAMILTON	NORTHROP GRUMMAN CORP
IDEXX LABORATORIES INC	BRISTOL MYERS SQUIBB CO	ORACLE CORP
JOHNSON & JOHNSON	CEPHALON INC	PAREXEL INTERNATIONAL CORP
KAISER PERMANENTE	CHEVRON CORPORATION	PARSONS BRINCKERHOFF INC
KENDLE INTERNATIONAL INC	CHUBB CORPORATION (THE)	PERRIGO CO
LABORATORY CORP OF AMERICA HOLDINGS	CONOCOPHILLIPS COMPANY	PFIZER INC
LINCARE HOLDINGS INC	DELOITTE & TOUCHE USA LLP	PLANTRONICS INC
MEDTRONIC INC	DELOITTE CONSULTING LLP	PRICEWATERHOUSECOOPERS
MERCK & CO INC	DIEBOLD INC	PRINCIPAL FINANCIAL GROUP (THE)
MILLIPORE CORP	ELI LILLY & COMPANY	PROGRESSIVE CORPORATION (THE)
ODYSSEY HEALTHCARE INC	EMC CORP	PRUDENTIAL FINANCIAL INC
PAREXEL INTERNATIONAL CORP	EMERSON ELECTRIC CO	QUALCOMM INC
PERRIGO CO	ERNST & YOUNG LLP	RAYTHEON CO
PFIZER INC	EXPERIAN AMERICAS	SAS INSTITUTE INC
PHARMACEUTICAL PRODUCT DEVELOPMENT INC	EXXON MOBIL CORPORATION (EXXONMOBIL)	SCHERING-PLOUGH CORP
PROCTER & GAMBLE CO	FAIR ISAAC CORPORATION	SCHLUMBERGER LIMITED
QUEST DIAGNOSTICS INC	FEDEX CORPORATION	SHELL OIL CO
RESPIRONICS INC	FLUOR CORP	SUN MICROSYSTEMS INC
SCHERING-PLOUGH CORP	FOREST LABORATORIES INC	SYMANTEC CORP
SELECT MEDICAL CORPORATION	FOSTER WHEELER LTD	TELEDYNE TECHNOLOGIES INCORPORATED
SISTERS OF MERCY HEALTH SYSTEMS	GENENTECH INC	TRAVELERS COMPANIES INC (THE)
ST JUDE MEDICAL INC	GENERAL DYNAMICS CORP	UNITED PARCEL SERVICE INC (UPS)
STERIS CORP	GENERAL ELECTRIC CO (GE)	UNITED TECHNOLOGIES CORPORATION
STRYKER CORP	GENWORTH FINANCIAL INC	URS CORPORATION
VARIAN MEDICAL SYSTEMS INC	GTECH HOLDINGS CORP	USAA
WATERS CORP	HARRIS CORPORATION	VARIAN MEDICAL SYSTEMS INC
WATSON PHARMACEUTICALS INC	HARTFORD FINANCIAL SERVICES GROUP INC (THE)	W R BERKLEY CORPORATION
WEST PHARMACEUTICAL SERVICES INC	HONEYWELL INTERNATIONAL INC	WATSON PHARMACEUTICALS INC
WYETH	INTEL CORP	WESTERN DIGITAL CORP
ZIMMER HOLDINGS INC	INTERNATIONAL BUSINESS MACHINES CORP (IBM)	WYETH
	JOHNSON & JOHNSON	
Math & Other	JOHNSON CONTROLS INC	
ABBOTT LABORATORIES	JUNIPER NETWORKS INC	
ADVANCED MICRO DEVICES INC (AMD)	KENDLE INTERNATIONAL INC	**Petroleum/Chemicals**
AFLAC INC	KPMG LLP	ABBOTT LABORATORIES
AGILENT TECHNOLOGIES INC	L-3 COMMUNICATIONS HOLDINGS INC	AIR PRODUCTS & CHEMICALS INC
ALLERGAN INC	L-3 TITAN GROUP	ALLERGAN INC
ALLSTATE CORPORATION (THE)	LINCOLN NATIONAL CORPORATION	AMGEN INC
AMGEN INC	LOCKHEED MARTIN CORP	ANADARKO PETROLEUM CORPORATION
ANALOG DEVICES INC	LOEWS CORPORATION	APACHE CORP
APPLE INC	MARSH & MCLENNAN COMPANIES INC	BAKER HUGHES INC
AXA FINANCIAL INC	MCKINSEY & COMPANY INC	BALTIMORE GAS AND ELECTRIC COMPANY
BAKER HUGHES INC	MEDTRONIC INC	BECHTEL GROUP INC
BECHTEL GROUP INC	MERCK & CO INC	BJ SERVICES COMPANY
BERKSHIRE HATHAWAY INC	METLIFE INC	BRISTOL MYERS SQUIBB CO
BOEING COMPANY (THE)	MICROSOFT CORP	CEPHALON INC
		CHESAPEAKE ENERGY CORP

CHEVRON CORPORATION	PRIDE INTERNATIONAL INC	CARGILL INC
CHEVRON PHILLIPS CHEMICAL COMPANY LLC	PROCTER & GAMBLE CO	CEPHALON INC
COLGATE PALMOLIVE CO	RAYTHEON CO	CHEVRON CORPORATION
CONOCOPHILLIPS COMPANY	SCANA CORPORATION	CHEVRON PHILLIPS CHEMICAL COMPANY LLC
CONSOL ENERGY INC	SCHERING-PLOUGH CORP	CISCO SYSTEMS INC
CONSOLIDATED EDISON INC	SCHLUMBERGER LIMITED	COLGATE PALMOLIVE CO
DEVON ENERGY CORPORATION	SCOTTS MIRACLE GROW CO	CONOCOPHILLIPS COMPANY
DIAMOND OFFSHORE DRILLING INC	SEACOR HOLDINGS INC	COVANCE INC
DTE ENERGY COMPANY	SEMPRA ENERGY	CR BARD INC
DUKE ENERGY CORP	SENSIENT TECHNOLOGIES CORPORATION	CUBIC CORP
E I DU PONT DE NEMOURS & CO (DUPONT)	SHELL OIL CO	DAVITA INC
EDISON INTERNATIONAL	SHERWIN WILLIAMS COMPANY (THE)	DIEBOLD INC
ELI LILLY & COMPANY	SIGMA-ALDRICH CORP	E I DU PONT DE NEMOURS & CO (DUPONT)
ESTEE LAUDER COMPANIES INC (THE)	SMITH INTERNATIONAL INC	EATON CORP
EXELON CORPORATION	SOUTHERN COMPANY (THE)	ELI LILLY & COMPANY
EXXON MOBIL CORPORATION (EXXONMOBIL)	SUNOCO INC	EMC CORP
FIRSTENERGY CORP	TELEDYNE TECHNOLOGIES INCORPORATED	EMERSON ELECTRIC CO
FMC TECHNOLOGIES INC	TESORO CORP	ESTEE LAUDER COMPANIES INC (THE)
FOREST LABORATORIES INC	TRANSOCEAN INC	EXXON MOBIL CORPORATION (EXXONMOBIL)
FPL GROUP INC	VALERO ENERGY CORP	FMC TECHNOLOGIES INC
GENENTECH INC	VALSPAR CORPORATION (THE)	FOREST LABORATORIES INC
GEORGIA GULF CORPORATION	WATSON PHARMACEUTICALS INC	GENENTECH INC
HALLIBURTON COMPANY	WEATHERFORD INTERNATIONAL LTD	GENERAL DYNAMICS CORP
HELMERICH & PAYNE INC	WILLIAMS COMPANIES INC (THE)	GENERAL ELECTRIC CO (GE)
HESS CORPORATION	WYETH	GEORGIA GULF CORPORATION
JACOBS ENGINEERING GROUP INC		HALLIBURTON COMPANY
JOHNSON & JOHNSON		HARRIS CORPORATION
KENDLE INTERNATIONAL INC	**Scientists/Research**	HONEYWELL INTERNATIONAL INC
KOCH INDUSTRIES INC	3M COMPANY	IDEXX LABORATORIES INC
LINCARE HOLDINGS INC	ABBOTT LABORATORIES	INTEL CORP
MARATHON OIL CORP	ADC TELECOMMUNICATIONS INC	INTERNATIONAL BUSINESS MACHINES CORP (IBM)
MASSEY ENERGY COMPANY	ADVANCED MICRO DEVICES INC (AMD)	JOHNSON & JOHNSON
MERCK & CO INC	AGILENT TECHNOLOGIES INC	JOHNSON CONTROLS INC
MURPHY OIL CORPORATION	AIR PRODUCTS & CHEMICALS INC	JUNIPER NETWORKS INC
NATIONAL OILWELL VARCO INC	ALLERGAN INC	KENDLE INTERNATIONAL INC
NOBLE CORPORATION	AMGEN INC	L-3 TITAN GROUP
OCCIDENTAL PETROLEUM CORP	ANALOG DEVICES INC	LABORATORY CORP OF AMERICA HOLDINGS
OCEANEERING INTERNATIONAL INC	APPLE INC	LOCKHEED MARTIN CORP
OIL STATES INTERNATIONAL INC	ARCHER DANIELS MIDLAND CO	MAXIM INTEGRATED PRODUCTS INC
ONEOK INC	BAXTER INTERNATIONAL INC	MEDTRONIC INC
PATTERSON-UTI ENERGY INC	BECKMAN COULTER INC	MERCK & CO INC
PEABODY ENERGY CORP	BECTON DICKINSON & CO	MICROCHIP TECHNOLOGY INC
PERRIGO CO	BIO RAD LABORATORIES INC	MICRON TECHNOLOGY INC
PFIZER INC	BOEING COMPANY (THE)	MICROSOFT CORP
PG&E CORPORATION	BOSTON SCIENTIFIC CORP	MILLIPORE CORP
PRAXAIR INC	BRISTOL MYERS SQUIBB CO	
	BUNGE LTD	

NORTHROP GRUMMAN CORP
ORACLE CORP
PAREXEL INTERNATIONAL CORP
PEPSICO INC
PERRIGO CO
PFIZER INC
PHARMACEUTICAL PRODUCT DEVELOPMENT INC
PRAXAIR INC
PROCTER & GAMBLE CO
QUALCOMM INC
QUEST DIAGNOSTICS INC
RAYTHEON CO
RESPIRONICS INC
SAIC INC
SAS INSTITUTE INC
SCHERING-PLOUGH CORP
SCHLUMBERGER LIMITED
SENSIENT TECHNOLOGIES CORPORATION
SHELL OIL CO
SHERWIN WILLIAMS COMPANY (THE)
SIGMA-ALDRICH CORP
ST JUDE MEDICAL INC
STRYKER CORP
SUN MICROSYSTEMS INC
TEKTRONIX INC
TELEDYNE TECHNOLOGIES INCORPORATED
UNITED TECHNOLOGIES CORPORATION
VALSPAR CORPORATION (THE)
VARIAN MEDICAL SYSTEMS INC
WATERS CORP
WATSON PHARMACEUTICALS INC
WEST PHARMACEUTICAL SERVICES INC
WESTERN DIGITAL CORP
WYETH
XEROX CORP